VASCULAR SURGERY

VASCULAR SURGERY

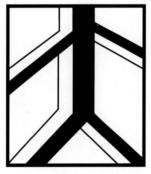

Fourth Edition

Robert B. Rutherford, M.D.

Professor of Surgery
University of Colorado Health Sciences Center
Denver, Colorado

Volume

II

W.B. SAUNDERS COMPANY
A Division of Harcourt Brace & Company
Philadelphia   London   Toronto   Montreal   Sydney   Tokyo

W.B. SAUNDERS COMPANY
A Division of
Harcourt Brace & Company

The Curtis Center
Independence Square West
Philadelphia, Pennsylvania 19106

Library of Congress Cataloging-in-Publication Data

Vascular surgery / [edited by] Robert B. Rutherford.—4th ed.

p. cm.

Includes bibliographical references.

ISBN 0–7216–3836–8 (set).—
ISBN 0–7216–3837–6 (v. 1).—ISBN 0–7216–3838–4 (v. 2)

1. Blood-vessels—Surgery.   I. Rutherford, Robert B.

[DNLM: 1. Vascular Surgery.   WG 170 V3311 1995]

RD598.5.V37   1995

617.4'13—dc20
DNLM/DLC   93–40051

VASCULAR SURGERY   ISBN Volume 1   0–7216–3837–6
                                            Volume 2   0–7216–3838–4
                                                 Set   0–7216–3836–8

Printed in the United States of America

Last digit is the print number: 9   8   7   6   5   4   3

CONTENTS

Arterial Aneurysms

Edited by William C. Krupski, M.D.

⌘

74

Overview

William C. Krupski, M.D.

• • •

Treatment of arterial aneurysms is a cornerstone of vascular surgery. It is ironic that no universally acknowledged definition of aneurysm exists, but most clinicians would accept a description of a permanent *localized* dilatation of an artery. The amount of dilatation required for an artery to be classified as aneurysmal is controversial. In general, enlargement to more than twice the size of the more proximal artery warrants the designation of aneurysm. Alternatively, Johnston and associates[1] have recommended defining aneurysms as a focal dilatation of arteries involving an increase in diameter of at least 50 per cent compared with the *expected normal* diameter. Unfortunately, with the exception of the abdominal aorta, which has been analyzed in large populations using measurements from computed tomography (CT) scans,[2] arterial size has not been rigorously studied. Thus, although there is general agreement that a 3-cm-wide abdominal aorta is aneurysmal, a precise size that characterizes a popliteal aneurysm, for example, is arbitrary. Further complicating this issue is the frequent coexistence of generally large arteries in patients with aneurysms, a condition known variously as arteriomegaly, arteriectasis, or dolichomegaly.

The chapters in this section discuss aneurysmal disease comprehensively. The purpose of this introductory chapter is to provide perspective and background with respect to the general process of aneurysm formation and treatment. In addition, the chapter introduces new information about pathophysiology, genetics, and techniques of repair of aneurysms.

HISTORICAL PERSPECTIVE

Arterial aneurysms have been recognized since ancient times. One of the earliest texts known, the Ebers Papyrus (2000 BC), contains a description of traumatic aneurysms of the peripheral arteries.[3] Galen (AD 131–200) defined an aneurysm as a localized pulsatile swelling that disappeared on pressure and wrote, "if an aneurysm be wounded, the blood is spouted out with so much violence that it can scarcely be arrested."[4] The first elective operation for treatment of an aneurysm was reported by Antyllus in the 2nd century AD. He recommended ligating the artery above and below the aneurysm and then incising the sac and evacuating its contents.[5] Antyllus also recognized the difference between true degenerative aneurysms and traumatic false aneurysms.

Antyllus' recommendations for aneurysm repair remained the basis of direct arterial operations for the next 1500 years, and few other operations have withstood the test of time so well. In the 7th century, details of operative repair of an arterial aneurysm were recounted by Aetius of Amida in his book *De Vasorum Dilatatione* ("On the Dilation of the Vessels"), now in the Vatican Library. Like Antyllus, Aetius noted that the pulsating swellings of arteries could arise spontaneously or follow trauma. He wrote:

An aneurysm located in the bend of the elbow is treated thus. First we carefully trace the artery leading to it, from armpit to elbow, along the inside of the upper arm. Then we make an incision on the inside of the arm, three or four finger-breadths below the armpit, where the artery is felt most easily. We gradually expose the bloodvessel and, when it can be lifted free with a hook, we tie it off with two firm ligatures and divide it between them. We fill the wound with incense and lint dressing, then apply a bandage. Next we open the aneurysm itself and no longer need fear bleeding. We remove the blood clots present, and seek the artery which brought the blood. Once found, it is lifted free with the hook, and tied as before. By again filling the wound with incense, we stimulate good suppuration.[6]

Modern surgeons will recognize the failure to obtain distal control in these instructions. Moreover, Aetius, like others of his times, believed Galen's teachings that no wound heals properly without the formation of pus, brought about by application of dried herbs (incense).

In medieval times brachial artery aneurysms were frequent complications of letting blood by puncture of the median cubital vein. Ambrose Paré (1510–1590), who contributed so much to the principles of proper wound care, applied his observations to aneurysm operations. He vividly described the death of a patient whose brachial artery aneurysm had been treated by application of a caustic, contrary to Paré's advice, resulting in a torrential fatal hemorrhage.[7] Paré's prestigious contemporary, Andreas Vesalius, wrote one of the first descriptions of an abdominal aortic aneurysm.[3]

In 1590, Peter Lowe (1550–1612), personal physician to King James VI in Scotland and founder of the medical and surgical faculty at Glasgow, reported that one of the highest-ranking officers in the Spanish Regiment presented with a peripheral arterial aneurysm. Whereas Lowe prescribed apothecary remedies against its growth, a second physician consulted a barber, who opened the swelling with a lance and "blood spewed out so violently that the Captain died some hours later."[6]

Almost a century later, Richard Wiseman (1625–1686), known as "the father of English surgery," described an aneurysm in the arm of a cooper from Maidenhead.[6] During operative exposure of the aneurysm it ruptured. Wiseman instructed an assistant to place his thumb over the hole. According to the detailed report, onlookers were eager to see the patient bleed to death. Instead, Wiseman inserted an instrument beneath the artery and ligated it, whereupon the assistant removed his finger and the bleeding subsided.

John Hunter (1728–1793) performed perhaps the most famous operation for an arterial aneurysm. Hunter had observed that the blood supply to the horns of deer changed under different conditions. A rich blood supply was present when the crest was full, but the blood vessels decreased in number and size when the horns shed. Hunter inferred that reserve vessels—now termed collaterals—might develop in humans if obstruction occurred in their arteries. In the autumn of 1785 a beer delivery man was admitted to St. George's Hospital with a pulsatile mass in the popliteal fossa, possibly secondary to repetitive trauma against the coachman's seat while driving on rough streets. He complained of leg pain on walking and rested frequently, presumably owing to arterial occlusion distal to the aneurysm. Standard treatment at that time entailed above-knee amputation, as strongly advocated by another renowned London surgeon, Percival Pott (1714–1788),[8] but Hunter's experiments with deer had suggested that collateral vessels must have formed around the obstruction or the leg would have developed gangrene. Thus, he incised above the knee at a location now known as Hunter's canal and tied four ligatures around the artery. Four sutures were used to avoid sawing through the vessel. After a bout of local infection, the patient survived and was discharged. Later, Hunter performed four similar operations and three were successful; the fourth patient died 26 days postoperatively.

Astley Paston Cooper (1768–1841) was John Hunter's most acclaimed disciple. In contrast to Hunter's irascible, sullen, and unsophisticated behavior, Cooper was handsome, charming, and well mannered. Although he is best remembered for his contributions to inguinal hernia repair and female breast anatomy, his most celebrated operation was performed for a leaking iliac artery aneurysm in 1817.[9] Before the operation he visited the autopsy room and practiced every detail of the procedure on a cadaver. His attempt to ligate the abdominal aorta seemed initially successful, but the patient died suddenly after 40 hours. Cooper also reported the first documented case of a spontaneous aortoenteric fistula due to aneurysmal disease and cautioned that patients who present with one aneurysm should be evaluated for the coexistence of others—advice that is equally applicable today.[9] The 18th century can be characterized as the era of arterial ligation for treatment of aneurysms with surgeons such as Anel, Brasdor, and Wardrop defending the merits of different sites of ligation in relation to the aneurysm. Interestingly, arterial ligation—accompanied by extra-anatomic bypass—was resurrected in the 1970s by the group at Albany, New York, for treatment of abdominal aortic aneurysms in high-risk patients. Unfortunately, many individuals so treated suffered outcomes similar to that of Cooper's patient.[10]

In 1804, Antonio Scarpa (1752–1832) wrote a definitive treatise on the forms and diagnosis of arterial aneurysms. About this time several ingenious treatments were introduced. Giovanni Monteggia (1762–1815) unwisely attempted to cure an aneurysm by injecting a sclerosant into it, which predictably failed because of rapid blood flow. Attempts to thrombose aneurysms by passing an electric current between needles stuck into the vessel were begun in 1832 and were still going on in the 1930s. Charles Hewitt Moore (1821–1870), at Middlesex Hospital in London, introduced obliteration of aneurysms by inserting steel wires in 1864, once using 26 yards of the material![6] One of the most prominent Americans known to have aneurysmal disease in the 19th century was Kit Carson, who died of a ruptured abdominal aortic aneurysm in rural Colorado in 1868.[11]

Albert Einstein also died of a ruptured abdominal aortic aneurysm.[12] Unlike Kit Carson, Einstein had been treated for his disorder by means of wrapping the aneurysm in cellophane, a technique introduced by Rea in 1948.[13] A better method of treatment of peripheral aneurysms had been developed in 1888 by the legendary New Orleans surgeon, Rudolph Matas (1860–1957). His technique of endoaneurysmorrhaphy involved clamping above and below the aneurysm, opening it, ligating branches from within, and buttressing the wall with imbricating sutures. By 1906 he had performed 22 obliterative operations and 7 restorative operations (preserving the arterial lumen) with no recurrences. Matas performed the first successful proximal ligation of an aortic aneurysm in 1923, some 106 years after Astley Cooper's innovative operation.[14] Matas' endoaneurysmorrhaphy presaged the current prevailing method of "internal" or intrasaccular reconstruction conceived by Oscar Creech and Michael DeBakey.[15]

Another notable achievement at the turn of the century is attributed to José Goyanes of Madrid.[16] In 1906 Goyanes excluded a popliteal aneurysm by proximal and distal ligation; in addition, he mobilized the adjacent popliteal vein and used it as an in situ interposition graft between the proximal femoral artery and the distal popliteal artery by means of end-to-end anastomoses. Unfortunately, this important contribution, which had a good outcome, remained largely ignored until many years later.

Modern techniques of aneurysm repair were made possible by Alexis Carrel (1873–1948), who demonstrated in animals that a segment of aorta could be replaced with a piece from another artery or vein and who successfully anastomosed blood vessels. Carrel won the Nobel Prize for this work in 1912. However, it was not until March 29, 1951, that his countryman Charles DuBost performed the first successful replacement of an aneurysm with a freeze-dried homograft.[17] He was inspired by a similar operation for an occluded abdominal aorta by Jacques Oudot in 1950.[18] The second and third aortic aneurysm repairs in which patients survived were both performed on October 25, 1952, one by Ormand Julian's group in Chicago and the other by Russel Brock and associates in London.[19, 20] DeBakey and Cooley in Houston soon reported survival of five of six patients operated on for replacement of abdominal aortic aneurysms.[21] In a series of 17 aortic aneurysm operations, Bahnson from Johns Hopkins described the first successful repair of a ruptured aortic aneurysm.[22] In 1953, Voorhees and colleagues introduced a major innovation by substituting Vinyon-N cloth for the unreliable homograft.[23] The modern era of aneurysm repair had truly begun.

The first successful repair of a thoracoabdominal aortic aneurysm was reported by Sam Etheredge in 1955.[24] E. Stanley Crawford became the authority on this formidable procedure beginning with his 1974 report delineating good results with 28 consecutive operations for thoracoabdominal aortic aneurysms.[25] Crawford's contributions to the repair of complex aortic aneurysms were extraordinary and have greatly reduced the risks of surgery.

In summary, throughout the late 1950s and early 1960s, aortic aneurysmectomy became a commonplace and safe surgical procedure throughout the world. The technical considerations of both emergent and elective repair have been firmly established. However, whereas the mortality of elective operations has progressively decreased, death rates after ruptured aortic aneurysms have remained dismally constant (see Chapter 76), emphasizing the importance of early detection and intervention when appropriate.

SCOPE OF THE PROBLEM

Repair of arterial aneurysms accounts for about 13 per cent of the vascular experience of residents in training and probably constitutes an even higher percentage of operations performed by vascular surgeons in practice.[26] The most common aneurysm occurs in the infrarenal abdominal aorta. In an epidemiologic study of mortality trends in the United States from 1951 to 1981, Lilienfield and associates found that the ratio of abdominal to thoracic aneurysms was 7:1 in men and 3:1 in women.[27] Likewise, the incidence of abdominal aneurysms among residents of Rochester, Minnesota, during the period from 1976 to 1980 was about seven times higher than the incidence of thoracic aneurysms.[28] Next in frequency are atherosclerotic aneurysms of the iliac (most often in association with aortic aneurysms), popliteal, femoral, and carotid arteries. Popliteal aneurysms account for 70 per cent of all peripheral aneurysms, whereas carotid aneurysms make up less than 4

per cent.[29, 30] The femoral artery is the most common site of anastomotic aneurysms (see Chapter 83) because bypass grafts commonly begin or end there. Moreover, it is now the most common location of infected aneurysms because of the prevalence of vascular reconstruction there and because it is the preferred entry site for radiologic procedures.

Because of its prevalence and proclivity to rupture and cause death, the abdominal aortic aneurysm is of paramount importance. The incidence of abdominal aortic aneurysms appears to be increasing. Two reports from the Mayo Clinic indicate a threefold increase in prevalence from 12.2 per 100,000 to 36.2 per 100,000 during the period 1951 through 1980.[28, 31] More aneurysms of all sizes were diagnosed from 1971 through 1980 than in the previous 2 decades, suggesting a real increase regardless of increased detection because of technologic advances.[32] The increasing median age of the population plays a role in the increasing incidence, as demonstrated in a European autopsy study in which men after the age of 55 years had a steadily increasing incidence of aortic aneurysms, reaching 5.9 per cent at the age of 90.[33] Women had an increased incidence of aneurysms after age 70 years, with a peak of 4.5 per cent at age 90. Mortality statistics also reflect a true increase in the prevalence of abdominal aortic aneurysms. Death rates in individuals under age 65 years have remained low since 1951, but rates have risen in older age groups, such that by 1984 a 20-fold and 11-fold increase in deaths from aortic aneurysms for men and women, respectively, has been observed in England and Wales.[34] The ratio of male-to-female death rates decreases from 11:1 in younger age groups to 3:1 in the oldest. Curiously, deaths most commonly occur in the winter months, like those from coronary artery disease.[35] It is also interesting that aneurysmal disease is increasing, whereas deaths from coronary heart disease, which shares the same risk factors, have decreased by 20 per cent in adults aged 30 to 74 years.[36]

The economic cost of ruptured aneurysms is staggering. One report estimated that $50 million and 2000 lives could have been saved if aneurysms had been repaired before they ruptured.[37] Another study, using cost reimbursement data for diagnosis-related groups (DRGs), showed that emergency operations for aneurysms resulted in a mean financial loss to the hospital of $24,655 per patient.[38]

PATHOGENESIS

The pathophysiology and causes of aneurysms are considered in detail in Chapters 13 and 75. For this overview it is enough to say that aneurysm formation depends on several factors that interact either to increase the expansile forces on the aortic wall or to decrease its ability to withstand them. In traumatic, anastomotic, and graft aneurysms, mural weakness and subsequent aneurysm formation can occur without unusual hemodynamic forces. In contrast, distinctive hemodynamic forces are of predominant significance in the development of the dilatations produced beyond the jet-stream effect of an arterial stenosis, the so-called poststenotic aneurysms. In a degenerative aneurysm, dilatation can begin in a previously normal artery because of hemodynamic factors and loss of integrity of the aortic wall, principally related to abnormalities in the two main components of the wall—collagen and elastin. Hypertension is a well-known risk factor for atherosclerotic aneurysms, and quantitative analysis shows a reduction in elastin content from about 35 per cent in the normal aorta to 8 per cent in the aneurysmal aorta.[39] Elastin has a half-life of about 70 years and cannot be synthesized by the adult aortic media. The structural properties of elastin and collagen are complementary. Elastin provides elastic recoil, whereas collagen adds strength at high loads. The more unusual causes of aneurysm, such as dissection and aneurysms associated with pregnancy are also related to fatigue of the vessel wall, usually in association with hypertension. The distinct causes of these different forms of aneurysmal disease have relevance to prevention, prediction of natural history, indications for operation, and modification of operative approach to avoid recurrence.

CLASSIFICATION SYSTEMS

Table 74–1 lists several strategies for the classification of arterial aneurysm. The classification systems have been designed to assist the clinician in establishing the correct diagnosis and planning treatment. In this regard, classifications based on shape, location, and structure have less value than methods based on etiology. In addition, the surgical literature most often conveys information with respect to etiology rather than other classification schemes. To be clinically relevant, a classification system of aneurysms, although principally organized according to etiology, should include categories whose features are unique and

Table 74–1.   Classification of Arterial Aneurysms

Shape	**Size**
Fusiform	Macroaneurysms
Saccular	Microaneurysms
Location	**Structure**
Central	True
Peripheral	False
Visceral	
Cerebral	

Etiology

Degenerative	**Inflammatory**
Nonspecific (atherosclerotic)	**Dissecting**
Fibrodysplasia	
Graft	**Aneurysms Associated With**
	Pregnancy
Congenital	
Idiopathic	**Inherited Abnormality of**
Tuberous sclerosis	**Connective Tissue**
Turner's syndrome	Marfan's syndrome
	Ehlers-Danlos syndrome
Infection	Cystic medial necrosis
Bacterial	Berry (cerebral)
Syphilitic	
Infection of false aneurysm	**Mechanical**
Fungal	Poststenotic
	Traumatic
Aneurysms Associated With	Anastomotic
Arteritis	Prosthetic
Systemic lupus erythematosus	
Takayasu's disease	
Giant cell arteritis	
Polyarteritis nodosa	
Behçet's disease	

sufficiently distinctive to warrant individual consideration. Clearly, no single scheme satisfies every clinical application. With this in mind, we have allocated the chapters in Section X to the following: infrarenal aortic aneurysms; ruptured aortic aneurysms; thoracoabdominal aortic aneurysms; peripheral vascular manifestations of acute aortic dissection; popliteal and femoral aneurysms; upper extremity aneurysms; splanchnic artery aneurysms; infected aneurysms; and anastomotic and traumatic aneurysms. Other aneurysms listed in this table are covered in detail in Chapter 13.

NOVEL DEVELOPMENTS

Genetic Factors. In 1977, Clifton was the first to note familial aggregation of abdominal aortic aneurysms, describing a family in which all three male siblings had undergone operation for a ruptured aneurysm.[40] During the 1980s, several studies have shown a familial clustering of abdominal aortic aneurysms, leading to sophisticated studies of the molecular genetics of arterial aneurysms.[41, 42] At least 18 per cent of patients with abdominal aortic aneurysms have a first-degree relative also affected.[43, 44] Genealogy studies have indicated that autosomal dominant, autosomal recessive, and sex-linked inheritance modes of transmission are plausible.[45] Most likely, degenerative arterial aneurysms are multi-factorial in etiology and genetically heterogeneous such that different genotypes produce the same phenotype. Genes involved in the synthesis and degradation of collagen and elastin are prime targets in this research. In Marfan's syndrome, which is associated with arterial dilations and dissections of the entire aorta, mutations in the fibrillin-1 gene (FBN1) on chromosome 15 have been implicated.[46] In patients with Ehlers-Danlos syndrome, who are at risk for sudden death from rupture of large arteries, defects in the type III collagen gene (COL3A1) have been described.[47]

There was some enthusiasm for implicating the COL3A1 gene as causative in familial degenerative aneurysm when a single U.S. family with a strong history of deaths from abdominal aortic aneurysms was identified, and analysis of their genomic DNA revealed a mutation in the COL3A1 gene, resulting in an amino acid substitution in the triple helical region of the molecule.[48] This occurred at a critical location that codes for amino acids that stabilize fibrillar collagen. However, the family was atypical in that all individuals were substantially younger than is routinely true for patients with abdominal aortic aneurysms, and the phenotype was not typical of atherosclerotic aneurysm. This mutation was not detected in any of 140 other patients with abdominal aortic aneurysm.[49] Nonetheless, variants of the COL3A1 gene may predispose to aneurysm in the presence of other components of the multi-factorial process.

Screening Programs and Management of Small Aortic Aneurysms. Screening the general population for abdominal aortic aneurysms is not cost-effective. From a theoretical screening model of a population of 100,000, it has been estimated that 1500 lives could be saved at a cost of $78,000 per life saved.[50] Most aneurysms detected by screening are small. Among 9777 subjects screened by ultrasound in 15 combined studies, relatively few aneurysms 6 cm in diameter or more were discovered in unselected populations (Table 74–2).[51–65] In contrast, selective screening may be cost-effective. For example, in 561 patients with peripheral vascular disease, nearly all of whom were cigarette smokers, aneurysms 3 cm or larger in diameter were found in 14 per cent.[61] Screening brothers of patients with aneurysms renders an incidence of aneurysms of 20 to 29 per cent.[56, 64] Thus, consideration should be given to screening those with a family history of aneurysm, patients between 55 and 80 years with peripheral vascular disease, and those with known extremity artery aneurysms, such as popliteal and femoral aneurysms.

Currently, screening programs (combined with trials to investigate the prognosis and optimal management of small asymptomatic abdominal aortic aneurysms) are being conducted in the United Kingdom, Canada, and the United States. Although follow-up regimens and precise size criteria differ slightly, the three studies are remarkably similar in design. In brief, aneurysms discovered by ultrasound screening are categorized by size. Patients with abdominal aortic aneurysms 3.0 to 3.9 cm in diameter are followed using serial abdominal ultrasonography. Patients with aneurysms measuring 4.0 to 5.5 cm in diameter are given a careful evaluation with respect to operative risk. If they are good candidates for operative repair, these patients are randomized to elective surgery or serial ultrasonography. Patients with aneurysms of 5.5 cm are offered elective repair unless they are unqualified for operation because of intercurrent illness (Fig. 74–1).

Endovascular Repair of Aortic Aneurysms. Palmaz in the United States, Parodi in Argentina, and Volodos and colleagues in the Ukraine have repaired abdominal aortic aneurysms by means of Dacron prostheses inserted through the common femoral artery.[66, 67] Experimental placement of these endovascular prostheses has been successful in animal models.[68] The basic principle of this technique involves a femoral artery exposure with intraluminal insertion of the graft (attached to a deployment device of various configurations). An expandable metal stent is used to anchor the proximal end of the Dacron graft in position in the infrarenal aorta. The distal end of the graft may or may not be stented because intravascular blood pressure may distend it and hold it in place. Recent computer-generated reconstructions of the abdominal aorta have suggested that a tube graft is not often possible, but bifurcated grafts can also be delivered.[69, 70] It is uncertain how durable such procedures

Table 74–2. Prevalence of Abdominal Aortic Aneurysms by Ultrasound Screening

Ref	First Author	Year	Location	No. Patients	Population	Number AAAs ≥ 3 cm (%)			
						Total	*3–4 cm*	*4–5 cm*	*5–6+ cm*
51	Thurmond	1988	Portland, USA	120	≥50-year-old men and women	27 (23)	21 (18)	6 (5)*	?
52	Collin	1988	Oxford, UK	426	65–74-year-old men	23 (5.4)	11 (2.6)	10 (2.3)	5 (2.5)
53	Lederle	1988	Minneapolis, USA	201	60–75-year-old men, veterans with HTN or CAD	18 (9)	8 (4)	5 (2.5)	5 (2.5)
54	Scott	1988	Chichester, UK	1312	60–80-year-old-men and women	76 (5.8)	—	—	—
55	Allardice	1988	London, UK	100	Men and women with PVD	10 (10)	—	—	—
56	Bengtsson	1989	Sweden	87	39–82-year-old siblings of AAA patients†	13 (15)	10 (12)	1 (1)	2 (2)
57	O'Kelly	1989	Stroud, UK	906	65–74-year-old men	71 (7.8)‡	—	14 (1.5)	—
58	Bengtsson	1989	Malmo, Sweden	183	34–74-year-old men and women with PVD	25 (14)	—	—	—
59	Berridge	1989	Nottingham, UK	104	Men and women with PVD	8 (7.7)¶	—	—	—
60	Akkersdijk	1991	Hague, Netherlands	1687	50–89-year-old men and women	82 (4.9)§	—	—	—
61	Galland	1991	Reading, UK	242	38–87-year-old men and women with PVD	34 (14)	17 (7)	10 (4)	7 (3)
62	Scott	1991	Chichester, UK	4122	65–80-year-old men and women	179 (4.3)	124 (3)	30 (0.7)	25 (0.6)
63	Webster	1992	Pittsburgh, USA	103	First-degree relatives of AAA patients	7 (7)**	—	—	—
64	Adamson	1992	London, UK	53	43–83-year-old siblings of AAA patients	6 (11)	—	—	—
65	Carty	1993	Saginaw, USA	131	40–93-year-old men and women with carotid disease	11 (8.4)	8 (6)	—	3 (2.4)

Abbreviations: *AAA, abdominal aortic aneurysm; HTN, hypertension; CAD, coronary artery disease; PVD, peripheral vascular disease.*
*> 4 cm.
†*29% in brothers, 6% in sisters.*
‡*AAA defined as ≥ 2.5 cm.*
¶*AAA defined as ≥ 3.5 cm or > 5 mm larger than adjacent vessel.*
§*11.4% in men > 60 years old.*
**Includes "focal bulge" as small as 1.9 cm; incidence increased to 25% in men >55 years old.*

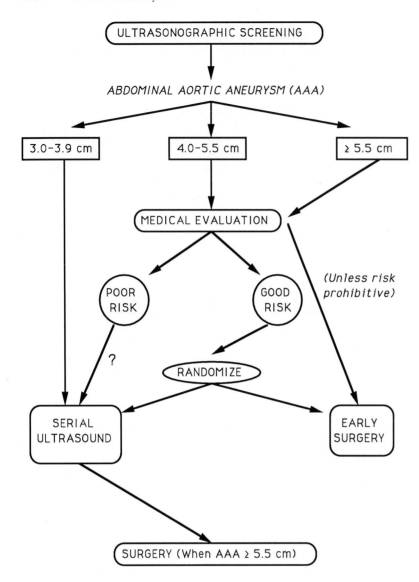

FIGURE 74–1. Ultrasound screening and management of small aneurysms: U.K., U.S., and Canada. The design of the three trials is outlined. Small differences exist between trials. For example, in the Canadian trial, the lower size limit is 4.5 cm. In all three, however, the upper size limit is 5.5 cm, thus allowing comparison of results. The U.S. Department of Veterans Affairs study (ADAM, for *Aneurysm Detection And Management*) will contribute the most screening information; after 1 year over 30,000 ultrasound screenings have been performed, and it is estimated that by the end of patient recruitment, 50,000 to 100,000 screenings will be available for review. Patients with aneurysms measuring 3.0 to 3.9 cm are followed by ultrasound surveillance every 6 months. Good-risk patients with aneurysms measuring 4.0 to 5.5 cm are randomized to either early elective operation or ultrasound surveillance every 6 months. Reasonable-risk patients are offered surgery when the aneurysm diameter exceeds 5.5 cm. The principal outcome is mortality in all three studies, but additional end-points will include quality of life, treatment costs, complication rates, and factors associated with aneurysm expansion.

will be and whether stents are the appropriate method for fixing the Dacron graft in the aneurysmal aorta. Currently, several clinical trials in humans are in the planning stages. This topic is covered in more detail in Chapter 75.

CLINICAL PRESENTATIONS AND MANAGEMENT

The clinical presentations of aneurysms depend on the type, size, location, and confounding factors in the patient (e.g., connective tissue disorders, hypertension, intravenous drug abuse). Some may present with rupture, others may embolize or thrombose, a few present with systemic sepsis, and still others remain completely asymptomatic. The relative frequency of these manifestations varies significantly from aneurysm to aneurysm. These matters are discussed in the following chapters. In addition, because renal and carotid artery aneurysms present special problems and are treated by methods similar to those used for other disorders of these vessels, they are discussed separately in Chapters 111 and 123.

The indications for surgical repair and a rational approach to management of each common type of aneurysm are discussed at length in the following chapters. In general, the operative approach is dictated by the natural or untreated course of the aneurysm, the ease of exposure and vascular control, the consequences of interrupting flow through the arterial segment, technical features of the repair, and—of great importance—the general status of the patient (see Chapters 2 and 22).

References

1. Johnston KW, Rutherford RB, Tilson MD, et al: Suggested standards for reporting on arterial aneurysms. J Vasc Surg 13:452, 1991.
2. Ouriel K, Green JRM, Donayre C, et al: An evaluation of new methods of expressing aortic aneurysm size; relationship to rupture. J Vasc Surg 15:12, 1992.
3. Osler W: Aneurysm of the abdominal aorta. Lancet 2:1089, 1905.
4. Erichsen JE: Observations on Aneurism. London, C & J Allard, 1844.
5. Osler W: Remarks on arterio-venous aneurysm. Lancet 2:949, 1915.
6. Haeger K: The Illustrated History of Surgery. New York, Bell Publishing, 1988.
7. Johnson T: The Workes of That Famous Chrurgeon Ambrose Paré. London, Coates & Dugard, 1649.

8. Pott P: Remarks of the Necessity and Propriety of the Operation of Amputation in Certain Cases. London, J Johnson, 1779.

9. Cooper AP: Lectures on the Principles and Practice of Surgery. 2nd ed. London, FC Westley, 1830.

10. Cho SI, Johnson WC, Bush HL, et al: Lethal complications associated with nonresective treatment of abdominal aortic aneurysms. Arch Surg 117:1214, 1982.

11. Abernathy CM, Baumgartner R, Butler HG, et al: The management of ruptured abdominal aortic aneurysms in rural Colorado: With a historical note on Kit Carson's death. JAMA 256:587, 1986.

12. Cohen JR, Graver LM: The ruptured abdominal aortic aneurysm of Albert Einstein. Surg Gynecol Obstet 170:455, 1990.

13. Rea CE: The surgical treatment of aneurysm of the abdominal aorta. Minn Med 31:153, 1948.

14. Matas R: Ligation of the abdominal aorta. Ann Surg 457:457, 1925.

15. Creech O Jr: Endoaneurysmorrhaphy and treatment of aortic aneurysm. Ann Surg 164:935, 1966.

16. Goyanes J: *In* Barker WF (ed): Clio Chirurgica: The Arteries, Part I. Austin, TX, Silvergirl, 1988.

17. DuBost C, Allary M, Deconomos N: Resection of an aneurysm of the abdominal aorta. Re-establishment of the continuity by a preserved human arterial graft, with a result after five months. Arch Surg 64:405, 1952.

18. Oudot J: La greffe vasculaire dans les thromboses du carrefour aortique. Press Med 59:234, 1951.

19. Julian OC, Grove WJ, Dye WS, et al: Direct surgery of atherosclerosis. Resection of abdominal aorta with homologous aortic graft replacement. Ann Surg 138:387, 1953.

20. Brock RC, Rob CG, Forty F: Reconstructive arterial surgery. Proc R Soc Med 46:115, 1953.

21. DeBakey ME, Cooley DA: Surgical treatment of aneurysm of abdominal aorta by resection of continuity with homograft. Surg Gynecol Obstet 97:257, 1953.

22. Bahnson HT: Considerations in the excision of aortic aneurysms. Ann Surg 97:257, 1953.

23. Voorhees A, Jaretzki A, Blakemore AH: The use of tubes constructed from Vinyon ''N'' cloth in bridging arterial defects. Am Surg 135:332, 1952.

24. Etheredge SN, Yee J, Smith JV, et al: Successful resection of a large aneurysm of the upper abdominal aorta and replacement with homograft. Surgery 38:1071, 1955.

25. Crawford ES: Thoraco-abdominal and abdominal aortic aneurysms involving renal, superior mesenteric and celiac arteries. Ann Surg 179:763, 1974.

26. Wheeler HB: Myth and reality in general surgery. Bull Am Coll Surg 78:21, 1993.

27. Lilienfield CE, Gunderson PD, Sprafka JM, Vargas C: Epidemiology of aortic aneurysms. 1. Mortality trends in the United States, 1951–1981. Arteriosclerosis 7:637, 1987.

28. Melton LJ, Bickerstaff LK, Hollier LH, et al: Changing incidence of abdominal aortic aneurysms: A population-based study. Am J Epidemiol 120:379, 1984.

29. Gaylis H: Popliteal arterial aneurysms. A review and analysis of fifty-five cases. S Afr Med J 48:75, 1974.

30. Welling RE, Taha JA, Goel T, et al: Extracranial carotid artery aneurysms. Surgery 93:319, 1983.

31. Bickerstaff LK, Hollier LH, Van Peenen HJ, et al: Abdominal aortic aneurysms: The changing natural history. J Vasc Surg 1:6, 1984.

32. Ernst CB: Abdominal aortic aneurysm. N Engl J Med 328:1167, 1993.

33. Bengtsson H, Bergqvist D, Sternby NH: Increasing prevalence of abdominal aortic aneurysm: A necropsy study. Eur J Surg 158:19, 1992.

34. Fowkes FGR, Macintyre CCA, Ruckley CV: Increasing incidence of aortic aneurysms in England and Wales. 298:33, 1989.

35. Castleden WM, Mercer JC: Abdominal aortic aneurysms in Western Australia: Descriptive epidemiology and patterns of rupture. Br J Surg 72:109, 1985.

36. Stern MP: The recent decline in ischemic heart disease mortality. Ann Intern Med 91:630, 1979.

37. Pasch AR, Ricotta JJ, May AG, et al: Abdominal aortic aneurysm: The case for elective resection. Circulation 70 (Suppl I):I–1, 1984.

38. Breckwoldt WL, Mackey WC, O'Donnell TF Jr: The economic implications of high-risk abdominal aortic aneurysms. J Vasc Surg 13:798, 1991.

39. Report of a meeting of physicians and scientists, University College London Medical School: Abdominal aortic aneurysm. Lancet 341:215, 1993.

40. Clifton MA: Familial abdominal aortic aneurysms. Br J Surg 64:765, 1977.

41. Tilson MD, Seashore MR: Fifty families with abdominal aortic aneurysms in two or more first-order relatives. Am J Surg 147:551, 1984.

42. Norrgard O, Angquist KA, Rais O: Familial occurrence of abdominal aortic aneurysms. Surgery 95:650, 1984.

43. Johansen K, Koepsell T: Familial tendency for abdominal aortic aneurysms. JAMA 256:1934, 1986.

44. Webster MW, St Jean PL, Steed DL, et al: Abdominal aortic aneurysm: Results of a family study. J Vasc Surg 13:366, 1991.

45. Tilson MD, Seashore MR: Human genetics of abdominal aortic aneurysm. Surg Gynecol Obstet 158:129, 1984.

46. Lee B, Godfrey M, Vitale E, et al: Linkage of Marfan syndrome and a phenotypically related disorder to two different fibrillin genes. Nature 352:330, 1991.

47. Kuivaniemi H, Tromp G, Prockop DJ: Mutations in collagen genes; causes of rare and some common diseases in humans. FASEB J 5:2025, 1991.

48. Kontusaari S, Tromp G, Kuivaniemi H, et al: A mutation in the gene for type III collagen (COL3A1) in a family with aortic aneurysms. J Clin Invest 86:1465, 1990.

49. Prockop DJ: Mutations in collagen genes as a cause of connective tissue diseases. N Engl J Med 326:540, 1992.

50. Quill DS, Colgan MP, Sumner DS: Ultrasonic screening for the detection of abdominal aortic aneurysms. Surg Clin North Am 69:713, 1989.

51. Thurmond AS, Semler HJ: Abdominal aortic aneurysm: Incidence in a population at risk. J Cardiovasc Surg 27:457, 1986.

52. Collin J, Araujo L, Walton J, Lindsell D: Oxford screening programme for abdominal aortic aneurysm in men aged 65–74 years. Lancet 2:613, 1988.

53. Lederle FA, Walker JM, Reinke DB: Selective screening for abdominal aortic aneurysms with physical examination and ultrasound. Arch Intern Med 148:1753, 1988.

54. Scott RAP, Ashton HA, Kay DN: Routine ultrasound screening in management of abdominal aortic aneurysm. Br Med J 296:1709, 1988.

55. Allardice JT, Allwright GJ, Wafula JMC, Wyatt AP: High prevalence of abdominal aortic aneurysm in men with peripheral vascular disease: Screening by ultrasonography. Br J Surg 75:240, 1988.

56. Bengtsson H, Norrgard O, Angquist KA, et al: Ultrasonic screening of the abdominal aorta among siblings of patients with abdominal aortic aneurysms. Br J Surg 76:589, 1989.

57. O'Kelly TJ, Heather BP: General practice-based population screening for abdominal aortic aneurysms: A pilot study. Br J Surg 76:479, 1989.

58. Bengtsson H, Ekberg O, Aspelin P, et al: Ultrasound screening of the abdominal aorta in patients with intermittent claudication. Eur J Vasc Surg 3:497, 1989.

59. Berridge DC, Griffith CDM, Amar SS, et al: Screening for clinically unsuspected abdominal aortic aneurysms in patients with peripheral vascular disease. Eur J Vasc Surg 3:421, 1989.

60. Akkersdijk GJM, Puylaert JBCM, de Vries AC: Abdominal aortic aneurysm as an incidental finding in abdominal ultrasonography. Br J Surg 78:1261, 1991.

61. Galland RB, Simmons MJ, Torrie EPH: Prevalence of abdominal aortic aneurysm in patients with occlusive peripheral vascular disease. Br J Surg 78:1259, 1991.

62. Scott RAP, Ashton HA, Kay DN: Abdominal aortic aneurysm in 4237 screened patients: Prevalence, development and management over 6 years. Br J Surg 78:1122, 1991.

63. Webster MW, Ferrell RE, St. Jean PL, et al: Ultrasound screening of first-degree relatives of patients with an abdominal aortic aneurysm. J Vasc Surg 13:9, 1991.

64. Adamson J, Powell JT, Greenhalgh RM: Selection for screening for familial aortic aneurysms. Br J Surg 79:897, 1992.

65. Carty GA, Nachtigal T, Magyar R, et al: Abdominal duplex ultrasound screening for occult aortic aneurysm during carotid arterial evaluation. J Vasc Surg 17:696, 1993.

66. Parodi JC, Palmaz JC, Barone HD: Transfemoral intraluminal graft implantation for abdominal aortic aneurysms. Ann Vasc Surg 5:491, 1991.

67. Volodos NL, Karpovich IP, Troyan VI, et al: Clinical experience of

the use of self-fixing synthetic prostheses for remote endoprostheses of the thoracic and the abdominal aorta and iliac arteries through the femoral artery as an intraoperative endoprosthesis for aorta reconstruction. Vasa (Suppl 33):93, 1991.

68. Laborde JC, Parodi JC, Clem MF, et al: Intraluminal bypass of abdominal aortic aneurysm: Feasibility study. Radiology 184:185, 1992.

69. Chuter T, Green JM, Ouriel K, et al: Infrarenal aortic aneurysm morphology: Implications for transfemoral repair. Presented at the International Society for Cardiovascular Surgery, Washington, DC, In press.

70. Lazarus HM: Endovascular grafting for the treatment of abdominal aortic aneurysms. Surg Clin North Am 72:959, 1992.

75

Infrarenal Aortic Aneurysms

Max B. Mitchell, M.D., Robert B. Rutherford, M.D., and William C. Krupski, M.D.

• • •

Since the first description of abdominal aortic aneurysm by the 16th century anatomist Vesalius,[120] the history of this disease has reflected the remarkable progress of vascular surgery. Prior to the development of modern surgical techniques, successful management was rare. Initial attempts at ligation of the aorta failed. In 1923, Matas performed the first successful aortic ligation in a patient with an abdominal aortic aneurysm.[129] Others attempted to induce thrombosis of aortic aneurysms by inserting intraluminal wires.[161] In 1948, Rea wrapped reactive cellophane around the neck and over the anterolateral surfaces of an aneurysm to induce a fibrotic reaction and thereby limit expansion.[163] In 1949, Nissen used this technique to treat the symptomatic aneurysm of Albert Einstein, who survived 6 years before succumbing to eventual rupture.[35] Durable and successful management of abdominal aortic aneurysms was finally achieved by resection and graft replacement, which was first performed in 1951. Although Dubost and coworkers published the first account of successful replacement of an abdominal aortic aneurysm,[57] a case subsequently reported by Schaffer and colleagues actually preceded that of Dubost.[172] The current standard procedure, endoaneurysmorrhaphy with intraluminal graft placement, was popularized by Creech and DeBakey and their colleagues.[44]

The infrarenal abdominal aorta is the most common site of arterial aneurysm. The term aneurysm refers to a permanent focal dilatation of a blood vessel with respect to the original or adjacent artery. Although used similarly, the term ectasia implies a lesser degree of vessel dilatation. Another associated term, arteriomegaly, refers to diffuse arterial enlargement and commonly occurs in conjunction with aneurysms of multiple vessels.[96] A uniform definition of abdominal aortic aneurysm is lacking, but most authors agree that a localized enlargement of the aorta greater than or equal to twice the normal diameter is aneurysmal.

Aneurysm size is an important factor in assessing the risk of rupture and the need for operative intervention.

When referring to the size of an aneurysm it is customary to use the maximal external transverse diameter of the aorta, regardless of how the measurement was obtained (i.e., ultrasound, computed tomography [CT], magnetic resonance imaging, or direct operative assessment). It is important to remember that enlargement of the aorta normally occurs with aging and also varies with gender.[182] CT measurement of the infrarenal aorta in adult men averages 2.3 cm, whereas the corresponding diameter in women is 1.9 cm.[145] These measurements are comparable to previous values determined by arteriography.[182] Normal adult aortic size in relation to gender and age is given in Table 75–1. Some practitioners have advocated relating the enlarged aorta to a more proximal unaffected portion of the aorta as a ratio, whereas others consider any aorta larger than an arbitrary size to be an aneurysm. Such recommendations have stemmed primarily from attempts to identify patients with small aneurysms that may be more prone to rupture than measurement of diameter alone would indicate.[187]

Macroscopically, most infrarenal aortic aneurysms are fusiform enlargements that begin below the origin of the renal arteries and extend into the aortic bifurcation. The aneurysmal aortic wall has atherosclerotic changes with marked thinning of the elastic media. Asymmetric weaken-

Table 75–1. Normal Size of the Infrarenal Aorta by Age and Sex*

| Sex | Age | | | | | Average |
	<40	40–49	50–59	60–69	≥70	
Male	2.1	2.2	2.3	2.3	2.4	2.3
Female	1.7	1.8	1.9	2.0	2.0	1.9

Data from Ouriel K, Green RM, Donayre C, et al: An evaluation of new methods of expressing aortic aneurysm size: Relationship to rupture. J Vasc Surg 15:12, 1992.

*Size in cm by computed tomography.

ing of the arterial wall may cause eccentric dilatation of the aorta, resulting in a spindle-shaped aneurysm. Large amounts of mural thrombus line the arterial lumen, narrowing it. The common iliac and hypogastric vessels are frequently involved; however, the external iliac arteries are less commonly affected. In approximately 5 per cent of cases, there is aneurysmal extension above the renal arteries. Operative management of the latter cases involves special technical considerations and is discussed separately in Chapter 77.

Diagnosed most commonly in the seventh decade of life, aneurysm of the abdominal aorta is primarily a disease of elderly males. Affected men outnumber women by approximately 4:1.[50, 184] Estimates of prevalence range from 2 to 5 per cent in men over the age of 60 years. The high morbidity and mortality consequent to aortic aneurysm attests to its clinical importance. Although potential complications include distal embolization, dissection, infection, adjacent organ obstruction, and thrombosis, it is the propensity for rupture and ensuing exsanguination that dominates clinical decision making in this disease. Abdominal aortic aneurysms account for at least 15,000 deaths per year in the United States. Furthermore, rupture of aortic aneurysm is the 10th leading cause of death in males over the age of 55.[207] The elderly constitute a rapidly growing segment of our population. This trend and the increasing use of newer diagnostic techniques, particularly ultrasound, are contributing to an increased rate of aneurysm detection. In a Rochester, MN, population-based study, Bickerstaff, Melton, and their associates documented a sevenfold increased prevalence of abdominal aortic aneurysms between 1951 and 1980.[21, 134] In part, aging of the population and enhanced diagnostic capabilities contributed to these findings; however, more aneurysms of all sizes were found between 1971 and 1980, suggesting a true increase in incidence. Similarly, Drott and colleagues reported that the annual incidence of rupture of abdominal aortic aneurysms in a defined Swedish population rose from 0.9/100,000 inhabitants in the 1950s to 6.9/100,000 in the 1980s.[56] Although deaths from rupture of abdominal aortic aneurysms have remained relatively constant in the United States (perhaps because of more elective aneurysm repairs),[122] such deaths have steadily increased in Great Britain.[69] Because of the frequency and catastrophic consequences of rupture, abdominal aortic aneurysms remain a central concern of vascular surgeons.

PATHOGENESIS OF AORTIC ANEURYSMS

Multiple factors are involved in the pathogenesis of aortic aneurysms. The predilection for aneurysm formation in the distal aorta suggests that mechanical and structural features may play a role. The architecture of the normal aorta changes progressively throughout its course. Aortic caliber decreases from its origin in the thorax to its bifurcation. This gradual tapering together with reflected pressure waves from the peripheral arterial tree increases mural tension in the infrarenal aorta. Furthermore, because fewer medial elastic lamellae are present in the distal aorta, elasticity is diminished, particularly just below the renal arte-

ries.[223] Finally, the nutrient vessels of the arterial wall, the vasa vasorum, are nearly absent in the infrarenal aorta.[215, 223] These normal anatomic features may predispose the infrarenal aorta to aneurysmal degeneration when it is exposed to unfavorable local or systemic factors.

Once vessel dilatation begins, regardless of the initiating factors, mural tension in the aneurysm increases dramatically, promoting further enlargement. Although somewhat of an oversimplification, the relationship between wall tension (T), vessel radius (r), and transmural pressure (p) generally conforms to the law of La Place, in which $T = pr$. At a given transmural pressure, wall tension is directly related to the radius. Thus, the law of La Place underscores the importance of aneurysm size as well as the influence of arterial hypertension in aneurysm rupture. In addition, wall strength is proportional to wall thickness. Thinning of the wall usually accompanies aneurysm formation, augmenting additional enlargement and eventual rupture. When mural tension exceeds the tensile strength of the vessel wall, rupture occurs.

Collectively, patients with abdominal aortic aneurysms have risk factors associated with occlusive vascular disease, particularly smoking and hypertension.[5] Because the aortic wall of most patients with aneurysms shows significant atherosclerosis, abdominal aortic aneurysms have customarily been classified as *atherosclerotic* aneurysms, and atherosclerosis was assumed to cause aneurysmal degeneration. This etiologic hypothesis was supported by the high incidence of concomitant atherosclerotic lesions of the cerebral and coronary vessels in patients with aneurysms.[29, 89, 201] Recently, however, controversy has erupted about the pathogenesis of abdominal aortic aneurysms.[166] Despite the frequency of coronary and carotid artery atherosclerotic occlusive disease in patients with aneurysms, concurrent occlusive disease in the aortoiliac distribution is uncommon. Furthermore, patients with infrarenal aneurysms are dissimilar to patients with aortic atherosclerotic occlusive disease. For example, Tilson and associates reported that 80 per cent of patients with aneurysms are men, whereas women account for more than half of those with aortic occlusive disease.[204] This study, like others,[31, 34] also found that patients with aortic occlusive disease were approximately 10 years younger at presentation than patients with aneurysms. There is now widespread belief that the presence of atherosclerosis in aneurysm patients is coincidental and does not indicate a cause and effect relationship. Therefore, atherosclerotic aneurysms are more appropriately described as *degenerative* or, alternatively, *nonspecific* aortic aneurysms. It is, however, quite possible that arterial occlusive disease and aneurysm of the aorta are simply different manifestations of atherosclerosis. Evidence for this was provided by Zarins and associates, who demonstrated that diseased arteries increase in external size in response to enlarging atherosclerotic plaques.[221] This phenomenon may explain in part why mean aortic diameters increase with age and has been interpreted as an adaptive response to preserve arterial flow. These authors have also presented experimental evidence suggesting that aneurysm formation may result from regression of atherosclerotic plaques.[219, 222] The reader is referred to Chapter 9 for a complete discussion of the pathogenesis of atherosclerosis.

A high incidence of aortic aneurysms in many members of several large families suggests that genetic factors are sometimes involved in the pathogenesis of this disorder.[103, 203] An abnormality on the long arm of chromosome 16 has been implicated in familial aneurysms.[159] Rare hereditary defects of collagen type III, a primary structural component of the arterial wall, are found in Ehlers-Danlos type IV syndrome, which is associated with aneurysms of many arteries.[190] Although variations in the genetic expression of minor collagen alleles have been reported,[158] no specific mutations of collagen have been identified in degenerative aortic aneurysms. Alterations in the metabolism of both collagen and the other primary structural arterial wall protein, elastin, are present in aneurysmal tissue relative to normal aorta.[36, 135, 213, 220] Resulting decreases in the tensile strength of the arterial wall may allow dilatation as well as longitudinal elongation, eventually resulting in aortic aneurysm formation. Changes in matrix structural protein content may reflect alterations in either degradation or synthesis of these constituents. Advances in molecular biology have provided evidence that altered gene expression may cause alterations in elastin and collagen contents in aortic aneurysms.[136] Elevated acute phase proteins in the serum of patients with degenerative aneurysms suggest that inflammatory processes play a role in aneurysm formation, even in patients who do not have the ''inflammatory'' aneurysm variant.[160] Similarly, chronic inflammatory cells present in the adventitia and media of aortic aneurysms suggest the presence of an immunologic response.[112] Cytokines elaborated by these cells may alter smooth muscle cell synthesis of matrix proteins that might contribute to the development of aneurysms.[151] Although these data promote understanding of aneurysm pathogenesis, they may reflect the results of the degenerative process rather than the causes. Clearly, the pathogenesis of aortic aneurysm remains incompletely understood. It is probable that the cause of aneurysmal degeneration is multi-factorial and that several distinct factors may be involved.[205]

Degenerative aneurysms account for more than 90 per cent of all infrarenal aortic aneurysms. Other causes include cystic medial necrosis, arteritis, trauma, genetic connective tissue disorders, and anastomotic disruption. The latter aneurysms account for approximately 5 per cent of all abdominal aortic aneurysms and are more precisely defined as pseudoaneurysms (see Chapter 37). The term *mycotic* aneurysm was coined by William Osler, when its definition did not imply fungal infection. A more precise term is *infected* aneurysm. Infected aneurysms result from localized infections of the arterial wall. A variety of pathologic mechanisms cause infected aneurysms. Most infected aneurysms develop from bacteremias originating at distant sites (e.g., endocarditis). Atheromatous ulcers of the arterial wall provide a nidus for inoculation of the arterial wall. Albeit rare, infected aneurysms are the most common type of aortic aneurysm in children.[186] Iatrogenic causes, in particular umbilical artery catheters, are responsible for most cases in this age group. *Luetic* aneurysms are a complication of tertiary syphilis, formerly a common cause of aortic aneurysms. Whereas the thoracic aorta is most frequently affected, syphilitic infrarenal aneurysms can also occur. Today, however, such aneurysms are extremely unusual in the United States. The different classifications of aneurysms are discussed in Chapters 13 and 74.

CLINICAL PRESENTATION

In clinical practice, approximately three fourths of all patients with abdominal aortic aneurysms are asymptomatic at the time of initial diagnosis.[21] This observation is partly explained by the fact that smaller aneurysms, which are more likely to be asymptomatic, constitute an increasing percentage of identified aneurysms. Reported operative series may underestimate the total percentage of asymptomatic aneurysms encountered because smaller aneurysms account for fewer operations. Aneurysms are commonly diagnosed during routine physical examination when an otherwise asymptomatic pulsatile epigastric mass is discovered. Patients themselves often find such masses and seek medical attention. Radiographic examinations performed for other reasons also commonly detect aneurysms. Not surprisingly, the widespread use of abdominal ultrasonography has increased detection of smaller asymptomatic aneurysms.[21] Ultrasound screening programs in high-risk populations will enhance this trend. Less commonly, aneurysms are discovered during laparotomy for other diseases or at postmortem examination following death from rupture or an unrelated disorder.

Vague abdominal pain is the most common complaint described by patients with symptoms from abdominal aortic aneurysms. Rapid expansion may cause more intense pain, probably from stretching of the overlying peritoneum. Pain is typically constant or ''throbbing'' and is located in the epigastrium. Not infrequently, the pain is described as penetrating through the epigastric region into the back. Rupture may be suspected, but the shock that normally accompanies rupture is absent if the aneurysm remains intact or the rupture remains temporarily contained. The potentially catastrophic result of misdiagnosis demands that aortic aneurysm be considered in any elderly patient with abdominal, back, or flank pain. Tenderness produced by direct palpation of the aneurysm suggests that symptoms are related to the aneurysm itself. Encroachment by an aneurysm on adjacent structures can produce a variety of symptoms. Vertebral body erosion is usually associated with large aneurysms, causing severe back pain; this symptom can occur even in the absence of any bony abnormality.[48] Gastrointestinal symptoms including early satiety, nausea, and weight loss may indicate intestinal compression. In advanced cases, complete gastrointestinal obstruction can occur, most commonly at the duodenum. Similarly, hydronephrosis from ureteral obstruction can result from both aortic and iliac aneurysms. Although ureteral involvement is common with inflammatory aneurysms, total obstruction of the ureters is surprisingly rare.[78] In contrast, ureteral obstruction is expected when aneurysms are associated with retroperitoneal fibrosis.[86] Ureteral obstruction also produces flank pain that may or may not radiate into the groin, along with bouts of pyelonephritis. Mural thrombus within the aneurysm can embolize and produce acute lower extremity ischemia. Thus, in the evaluation of lower extremity emboli, whenever a cardiac source of emboli cannot be found, aortic aneurysm should be considered. Thrombosis of an aneurysm with acute aortic occlusion can also occur, usually when aneurysms are accompanied by extensive aortoiliac occlusive disease. However, thrombosis is much more common in peripheral aneurysms.

Aneurysms often go undetected until sudden rupture prompts discovery because of dramatic symptoms and signs. Ruptured aneurysms account for between 10 and 30 per cent of operative vascular cases performed by general surgeons depending on the patient population and referral patterns, and up to two thirds of these are unrecognized prior to rupture.[76] Major vascular referral centers tend to attract more elective cases, whereas catastrophic aneurysm ruptures are more commonly encountered in city and county hospitals linked to emergency transport systems. If the aneurysm wall disrupts directly into the peritoneal cavity, death from rapid exsanguination usually occurs before the patient can reach a hospital. However, tamponade from surrounding structures or clot at the site of rupture may temporarily arrest massive hemorrhage, allowing survival long enough to obtain medical attention. Abdominal distention suggesting hemoperitoneum is often present, and if consciousness is maintained, patients usually complain of severe abdominal pain.[171] Nevertheless, patients with ruptured aneurysms often present in extremis, and despite rapid operative intervention, mortality is in excess of 50 per cent.[76, 84, 104]

Rupture of an aortic abdominal aneurysm most often occurs posteriorly into the retroperitoneum.[50] Survival is favored when a small initial leak is temporarily contained. In clinical practice, such cases are seen more frequently than ''free'' rupture because the slower onset of intractable hemorrhage allows for operative intervention. The triad of shock, pulsatile abdominal mass, and abdominal or back pain suggests contained rupture of an abdominal aortic aneurysm; however, shock may be absent or minimal depending on the magnitude of the initial blood loss. The pain of a ruptured aneurysm is usually severe, constant, and unaffected by position. Some patients report radiation of pain into the groins or posteriorly through the back in a ''boring'' fashion. Inability to palpate a pulsatile mass can lead to misdiagnosis,[128] and one should be aware that this finding is absent in up to 50 per cent of cases.[76] Operative intervention must be undertaken emergently because unconfined rupture into the peritoneal cavity can cause exsanguination at any moment. On occasion, concurrent myocardial ischemia causes angina pectoris after contained rupture. In such cases hypotension must not be mistakenly attributed to cardiogenic shock because death is inevitable without surgical intervention.

Rarely, a small perforation remains contained within the retroperitoneum, creating a chronic sealed rupture.[183] Patients with sealed ruptures usually experience back pain with the initiating event but can remain asymptomatic for variable periods of time. Because subsequent disruption is unpredictable, expeditious repair is indicated when this diagnosis is established.

Aneurysms may also present in unusual ways. A rare manifestation is *primary* aortoenteric fistula (see Chapter 38), which usually results from erosion of an aneurysm into the third portion of the duodenum.[164, 193] Affected patients develop abdominal pain or back pain accompanied by hematemesis or melena. Symptoms are insidious, and a so-called herald bleed often occurs prior to massive hemorrhage.[193] This premonitory bleeding is typically minor, occurs intermittently, and results from erosion of the duodenal mucosa. Subsequent rupture into the intestinal lumen produces catastrophic hemorrhage and death. Rarely, erosion of an aneurysm into the vena cava produces an aortocaval fistula (see Chapter 87).[140] In most cases, a loud, unremitting abdominal bruit is audible, and patients experience abdominal pain.[73] Regional venous hypertension may cause lower extremity cyanosis, edema, and hematuria. As with any large arteriovenous fistula, increased myocardial demand to compensate for reduced afterload commonly results in high output cardiac failure, evidenced by a ''water-hammer'' pulse and a widened pulse pressure. If aortocaval fistula remains uncorrected, intractable congestive heart failure and death result.

Because of the many special considerations involved in the management of ruptured abdominal aortic aneurysms, this entity is discussed in greater detail in Chapter 76.

NATURAL HISTORY AND RISK OF RUPTURE

The decision to operate on a patient with aortic aneurysm requires that the risk of death from the aneurysm exceed the risk of surgery. This assessment is complicated by the advanced age and the prevalence of significant concomitant disease in these patients, which increase both the likelihood of death due to causes other than aneurysm rupture and the risk of perioperative mortality (see Chapter 22). Knowledge of the natural history of abdominal aortic aneurysm is therefore essential to the management of this disease.

Early studies of aortic aneurysms, performed before safe techniques of repair were available, reported limited long-term survival in patients with aortic aneurysm, with rupture accounting for up to two thirds of all deaths.[63, 216] However, these early studies do not accurately reflect the true natural history of this disease for two reasons: (1) aneurysms of smaller size were less commonly identified, resulting in a disproportionate number of large aneurysms, and (2) symptomatic aneurysms were overrepresented. Thus, the expected survival rate in a modern population of patients with abdominal aortic aneurysm may be better than early studies suggested. In 1962, Schatz and colleagues reported a series consisting primarily of patients with asymptomatic aneurysms but still found that the 5-year survival of affected patients was only 36 per cent, less than half that of age-matched controls; one third of all deaths were due to rupture.[173] However, aneurysmectomy was developed during this period, and most of the patients in this study had been deemed unfit for surgery. Ideally, the true natural history should be defined by prospective analysis of a large population of patients with asymptomatic aneurysms of all sizes in which surgical intervention is not offered. However, following DeBakey and colleagues' report of a 58 per cent 5-year survival in a large series of patients undergoing operation (despite an operative mortality of 9 per cent),[52] ethical considerations have prevented initiation of a prospective study to delineate the true natural history of abdominal aortic aneurysms.

Although retrospective in design, the landmark study of Szilagyi and associates reported in 1966 validated aneurysm repair and provided data that continue to influence current surgical decision making.[198] This report was unique in that the long-term survival of a large number of patients, more than half of whom were *not* unfit for surgery, was compared with that of surgically treated patients with similar clinical characteristics. The authors demonstrated that the risk of rupture and the long-term survival of patients without operation were directly related to the size of the aneurysm. For patients with unrepaired small aneurysms (less than or equal to 6 cm in diameter), the 5-year survival was 47.8 per cent, compared with only 6 per cent for those with large (more than 6 cm) aneurysms. Twenty per cent of the 82 small aneurysms ruptured, whereas 43.3 per cent of the 141 larger aneurysms ruptured. In the 223 patients who did not undergo aneurysm repair, rupture accounted for 35 per cent of all deaths; coronary artery disease was the second leading cause, accounting for 17 per cent of deaths. Foster and associates confirmed these findings in a similar contemporaneous report of 75 patients with aneurysms that were not repaired.[68] Thirty-three per cent of all deaths were due to ruptured aneurysm, and 23 per cent were related to coronary artery disease. Furthermore, the rupture rate for aneurysms less than 6 cm in diameter was 16 per cent compared with 51 per cent for those larger than 6 cm. Because modern methods of early detection were not available in the 1960s, these studies were composed of a disproportionately high number of patients with large aneurysms compared with typical series of today. In addition, physical examination, which frequently overestimates aneurysm size, was used to estimate aneurysm size in many of these patients. Thus, a ruptured aneurysm that was recorded as 6 cm in diameter may have been found to be smaller if ultrasonography or computed tomography had been available. Despite these limitations, most authorities still agree with the general conclusions of the reports by Szilagyi and Foster and their associates. It is imprecise, however, to extrapolate the exact risk of rupture in relation to size using modern techniques of measurement. This caveat is particularly true for smaller aneurysms.

Results of studies in patients deemed unfit for aneurysm repair have an inherent bias toward death from other causes. Nevertheless, these series do provide useful information on natural history. In a rather significant contribution to the literature, Szilagyi and associates[196] followed 156 patients who had been rejected for aneurysm repair and examined the outcomes according to aneurysm size. Forty-three per cent of patients with aneurysms greater than 6 cm died from rupture, whereas 37 per cent died from myocardial infarction. In patients with aneurysms 6 cm or smaller, the two most common causes of death were the same but in reverse order. Myocardial infarction led to 36 per cent of all deaths, whereas rupture was responsible for 31 per cent. Bernstein and Chan more recently scrutinized 99 high-risk patients who had been initially diagnosed with aneurysms of less than 6 cm.[16] Forty-one eventually underwent operation owing to aneurysm expansion, development of symptoms, or rupture. At a mean follow-up of 2.4 years, there had been 34 deaths unrelated to aneurysm and only 4 deaths due to aneurysm rupture or surgery. Clearly, the number of deaths caused by aneurysms was reduced by operative intervention; however, more than one third of all deaths were due to cardiac disease. Two similar studies have also indicated that coronary disease is the most frequent cause of death in patients with small aneurysms, accounting for over 40 per cent of all deaths, whereas aneurysm-related mortality is 12 per cent or less.[46, 124] In studies subsequent to that of Szilagyi and associates,[196] operative intervention for symptoms or aneurysm expansion probably reduced the number of deaths due to aneurysm rupture. Thus, the true natural history of high-risk patients with smaller aneurysms is uncertain, but it is clear that coronary artery disease is still the major risk to life in these patients.

Autopsy studies also support the contention that risk of rupture rises dramatically with increasing size. In 1977, Darling and associates[50] reported that 10 per cent of all aneurysms less than or equal to 4 cm identified at autopsy had ruptured and caused death. In contrast, 46 per cent of all aneurysms between 7.1 and 10.1 cm had ruptured. For aneurysms ranging between 4.1 and 7.0 cm, one fourth had ruptured with no significant correlation with size. In a more recent examination of 297 patients with abdominal aortic aneurysms at autopsy, Sterpetti and colleagues[184] found a 5 per cent incidence of rupture for aneurysms 5.0 cm or less, 39 per cent for aneurysms measuring 5.1 to 6.9 cm, and 65 per cent for those above this size. In addition to confirming the correlation between size and rupture rate, these investigations are significant because they demonstrate that small aneurysms (i.e., less than 5.0 cm) can rupture. However, it is important to remember that a determination of aneurysm size at autopsy underestimates the actual size under physiologic arterial pressure. For this reason, and because patients dying of a ruptured aneurysm may be more likely to undergo autopsy, the incidence of rupture for small aneurysms may be overstated in these studies. Recently, population-based studies by Nevitt and coworkers[141] and Glimaker and associates[75] have reported a very low incidence of rupture of aneurysms with diameters of less than 5 cm. In contrast to autopsy studies, these reports probably underestimate the risk of rupture at this size. For example, in the former study, 24 per cent of patients with aneurysms of less than 5 cm were treated operatively, eliminating the possibility of rupture in this cohort.[98] In another series, however, only 6 per cent of 300 patients underwent elective operation, and only 2 per cent of the 4.0- to 4.9-cm aneurysms ruptured compared with 20 per cent of aneurysms 5.0 cm or larger.[81] It appears that small aneurysms can rupture but that this is a rare occurrence.

Some authors have contended that abdominal aortic aneurysms invariably continue to expand and eventually rupture unless death occurs from another cause.[50] Studies utilizing accurate noninvasive methods to follow aneurysm expansion serially indicate that this conclusion may not be valid. These studies have reported mean expansion rates ranging from 0.2 to 0.8 cm per year, for an average rate of expansion of about 0.4 cm per year.[17, 39, 45, 46, 75, 113, 124, 141, 187] Larger aneurysms generally expand more rapidly.[41, 123, 141] Some aneurysms may remain stable for long periods of time, exhibiting little or no enlargement, whereas others undergo progressive expansion. Still others remain stable and then undergo rapid expansion.[46] Although some authorities assert that hypertension and obstructive pulmonary disease are predictors of expansion and rupture,[45, 184] not all reports have confirmed this.[75, 113, 187] Architectural information provided by CT scans, such as an increased amount of luminal thrombus, may also be predictive of expansion rates.[113] The single factor that consistently correlates with aneurysm rupture is the size of the aneurysm. When confronted with an individual patient with a small aneurysm, one must recognize that aneurysm expansion and rupture are unpredictable.[45, 141, 187]

The available data, subject to the limitations mentioned previously, indicate that the 5-year rate of rupture of aneurysms 7.0 cm or larger exceeds 75 per cent.[50, 68, 196, 198] For aneurysms of 6 cm the 5-year rupture rate is approximately 35 per cent,[50, 68, 198] and for aneurysms between 5.0 and 5.9 cm it is approximately 25 per cent.[75, 141] Although the rate of rupture is substantially less for aneurysms smaller than 5.0 cm, small aneurysms can rupture.[45, 50, 124] There are insufficient data upon which to estimate accurately the risk of rupture of small aneurysms (less than 5 cm), primarily because most surgeons elect to operate on patients whose aneurysms reach the size of 5.0 cm or expand rapidly, provided that they are acceptable surgical risks.[27, 75, 141] Twenty to 45 per cent of patients in such ''natural history'' studies eventually underwent surgery; therefore, the true long-term risk of rupture of aneurysms less than 5.0 cm is uncertain. Large aneurysms, with their associated high risk of rupture, are clearly the dominant factor in the long-term survival of affected patients. In contrast, causes of death other than aneurysm are more important factors in determining the natural history of patients with small aneurysms.[118] In 1992 the Department of Veteran Affairs funded a multi-center randomized comparison of surgical versus observational treatment of aneurysms measuring 4.0 to 5.5 cm in diameter. The results of this study, which will be available in 2001, should provide important natural history data for small aneurysms.

The advanced age and associated diseases of patients with aneurysms occasionally necessitate unrelated operations in those patients whose aneurysms have not yet been repaired. It has been proposed that an unrelated operation may precipitate subsequent aneurysm rupture. This possibility was first suggested in a clinical report by Swanson and coworkers,[192] who hypothesized that activation of proteolytic enzymes by operation might provoke aneurysm weakening and rupture; however, no clinical or laboratory evidence was provided to support this hypothesis. Moreover, in 6 of the 10 patients reported, aneurysms had been exposed but not repaired by referring surgeons, thus potentially weakening the walls directly. The proposed association between unrelated surgery and subsequent aneurysm rupture is based largely on anecdotal reports and speculation. In a recent review of their experience and the related literature, Durham and associates reported a 2 per cent incidence of rupture after unrelated surgery in 45 patients with abdominal aortic aneurysms.[59] Thus, there is little support for a causative association between unrelated operations and subsequent rupture; however, the paucity of cases in this report and others does not exclude a possible relationship. Therefore, it seems prudent to follow such patients carefully.

RISK OF OPERATION

Survival after operative management of a ruptured aneurysm has not changed substantially in the past four decades. As noted in Chapter 76, the current average survival rate of 50 per cent also underestimates the mortality of rupture given that a large number of patients die before receiving treatment. In contrast, 30-day mortality rates in *electively* treated patients have improved greatly over the same period. This trend is true despite the fact that patients with comparatively more severe concurrent disease constitute a larger percentage of operatively treated patients than in the past. In a 25-year review, Crawford and associates[42] reported a drop in the elective mortality rate from 18 per cent between 1955 and 1966 to 1.4 per cent during the 1976 to 1980 period. As shown in Table 75–2, mortality

Table 75–2. Declining Mortality Associated With Elective Abdominal Aortic Aneurysm Repair

Author	Year	Early Era Mortality (dates)		Middle Era Mortality (dates)	Late Era Mortality (dates)
DeBakey and colleagues[52]	1964	9%	(1952–1964)	5% (1962–1964)	
Szilagyi and colleagues[198]	1966	21%	(1952–1955)	7.2% (1964–1965)	
Thompson and colleagues[201]	1975	17%	(1954–1961)	7.4% (1962–1967)	
Hicks and colleagues[92]	1975	13%	(1955–1965)		5.5% (1968–1974)
Volpetti and colleagues[209]	1976	16.5%	(1953–1957)		4.2% (1973–1975)
Young and colleagues[218]	1977	15.6%	(1958–1968)		0.8% (1971–1975)
Baird and colleagues[6]	1978	11.3%	(1955–1964)	9.8% (1965–1970)	6.3% (1968–1976)
Darling and Brewster[49]	1980	9.6%	(1953–1960)	4.7% (1961–1970)	1.2% (1971–1976)
Johnson and colleagues[105]	1980	15%	(1955–1960)		1.7% (1971–1979)
Whittemore and colleagues[214]	1981				0% (1972–1977)
Crawford and colleagues[42]	1981	18%	(1955–1960)	4.5% (1966–1975)	0.9% (1972–1979)
McCabe and colleagues[132]	1981				1.4% (1976–1980)
Diehl and colleagues[55]	1983				2.5% (1972–1979)
Hertzer and colleagues[88]	1984				5.1% (1974–1978)
Bernstein and colleagues[18]	1988				6.5% (1978–1981)
Johnston and Scobie[108]	1988				0.8% (1978–1985)
Branchereau and colleagues[24]	1990				4.5% (1986)
Clark and colleagues[34]	1990				2.5% (1980–1987)
Olsen and colleagues[144]	1991				2.0% (1981–1989)
					4.8% (1979–1988)

Table 75–3.   Operative Mortality for Urgent vs. Elective Abdominal Aortic Aneurysm Repair

Author	Year	Elective Mortality (No. Patients)	Urgent Mortality (No. Patients)
Baird and colleagues[6]	1978	1% (83)	17% (23)
Johnson and colleagues[105]	1980	0% (105)	18% (22)
Fielding and colleagues[65]	1981	8% (222)	19% (72)
McCabe and colleagues[132]	1981	2.5% (364)	14.3% (56)
Thomas and Stewart[200]	1988	8.3% (84)	13.3% (15)
Sullivan and colleagues[189]	1990	5.1% (117)	26% (19)
Olsen and colleagues[144]	1991	4.8% (287)	17.2% (151)

Note: *Numbers in parentheses represent the total number of patients in the respective category.*

rates for aneurysm repair ranging from approximately 13 to 15 per cent in the 1950s declined to about 6 per cent by the 1970s. Recent series commonly report elective mortality rates of between 2 to 5 per cent.[1, 108, 214] The death rate with operations for intact symptomatic aneurysms requiring urgent operation is much higher, averaging 18 per cent (Table 75–3).[6, 132, 189] The primary factor in the increased mortality for urgent operations is the lack of time available for careful evaluation and compensation for concurrent disease states.[189]

The improved outcome of elective aortic aneurysm surgery is the result of several factors. Abandonment of complete aneurysm resection in favor of endoaneurysmorrhaphy was largely responsible for the decrease in mortality observed in the 1960s.[42, 201] The development of improved prosthetic materials and other refinements in operative technique were also important.[201] Additionally, better anesthetic and postoperative management have contributed. For example, Whittemore and colleagues demonstrated that optimization of perioperative cardiac performance with the use of invasive monitoring, inotropic support, or afterload reduction when needed significantly enhanced survival.[214] Noninvasive diagnostic techniques have led to the earlier diagnosis and treatment of aneurysms. Lastly, improved preoperative detection and treatment of significant coronary disease and other concurrent diseases have increased the safety of aneurysm surgery.[18]

As with other major vascular procedures, the experience of the operating surgeon is an important factor in reducing perioperative morbidity and mortality,[1, 88] and the type of hospital does not appear to be crucial.[3] However, careful preoperative evaluation and adept postoperative management are as important as surgical skill in reducing morbidity and mortality. Patients with aneurysms are elderly, and concurrent diseases are common. Coronary artery disease, occurring in up to half of these patients, is the leading cause of perioperative mortality.[89, 169] Furthermore, coronary artery disease also causes most late deaths in patients who have undergone aneurysm surgery.[94, 156, 169] Minimizing the impact of coronary artery disease on surgical morbidity and mortality requires that special effort be directed toward preoperative detection, treatment when possible, and optimal perioperative cardiac support.[214]

The risk of elective aneurysm surgery is dependent on the physiologic status of the patient. Surgical risk is increased significantly by the presence of cardiac disease (recent myocardial infarction, abnormal electrocardiographic [ECG] findings, congestive heart failure), evidence of atherosclerotic disease elsewhere (claudication, absence of pulses, carotid bruits, symptoms of cerebral ischemia), hypertension, decreased renal function (24-hour creatinine clearance of less than 40 ml/min), emphysema or chronic obstructive pulmonary disease (forced expiratory volume in 1 second of less than 1 liter), and morbid obesity more than 50 kg or 100 per cent over ideal body weight). Table 75–4 lists criteria that place a patient at significantly increased risk for a major vascular procedure.[147]

Chronological age is not as important as physiologic age in determining the risk of surgery. O'Donnell and associates reported that 50 per cent of octogenarians with unrepaired aortic aneurysms died from rupture of their aneurysms.[143] This group and others[83, 168] have shown that aneurysm repair in octogenarians can be performed with low mortality. Therefore, chronologic age alone is not a reason for denying operative repair of aneurysms.

Other coexisting conditions are much more important than age in determining patient management. Local abdominal pathology substantially increases the risk of surgical complications. Multiple prior operations or prior abdominal abscesses may result in dense adhesions that make surgery more technically demanding. Retroperitoneal fibrosis, inflammatory bowel disease, prior irradiation, intestinal fistulae, and the presence of an enterostomy or ureterostomy

Table 75–4.   Criteria for Repair of Aortic Aneurysms

Age	>85 years
Cardiac	Class III–IV angina
	Resting LVEF <30%
	Recent CHF (<30 days)
	Recent MI
	Complex ventricular ectopy
	Large LV aneurysm
	Severe valvular disease
	Recurrent CHF or angina after CABG
	Severe CAD by angiography (not revascularized or unreconstructible)
Renal	Serum creatinine >3 mg/dl
Pulmonary	On oxygen at home
	Po₂ <50 mmHg
	FEV₁ <1 L
Hepatic	Biopsy-proven cirrhosis with ascites
Abdominal	Diffuse retroperitoneal fibrosis

LVEF, left ventricular ejection fraction; CHF, congestive heart failure; LV, left ventricular; CABG, coronary artery bypass grafting; MI, myocardial infarction; CAD, coronary artery disease; FEV₁, maximum forced expiratory volume in 1 second.

may complicate surgical approaches. Therefore, careful evaluation of each patient is of paramount importance in assessing the risk of surgery.

Operative repair of abdominal aortic aneurysms prolongs life in patients appropriately selected for surgical management, as suggested by Szilagyi and associates' early observations on the role of surgical treatment.[198] After patients were stratified according to the size of their aneurysms, 5-year survival after operation for aneurysms less than 6 cm in diameter was 66.7 per cent compared with 47.8 per cent for patients treated by observation alone. For aneurysms 6 cm or larger, the beneficial effect of surgery was even more dramatic, with a 5-year survival rate of 47.2 per cent after repair compared with only 6 per cent without operation. The most significant factor affecting the long-term survival in the surgical groups was perioperative mortality. The better 5-year survival for patients undergoing operation for aneurysms less than 6 cm compared with those with larger aneurysms (66.7 per cent versus 47.2 per cent) was primarily due to the 3 per cent perioperative mortality rate in the former group as opposed to 15 per cent in the latter. Although age- and sex-matched individuals without aneurysms have better survival than those undergoing operative repair, this difference can be explained by the prevalence of additional disorders in aneurysm patients. The effect of concurrent disease on late survival after surgery is demonstrated by Crawford and associates' observation that among patients having aneurysm repair, 84 per cent of those without coronary disease survived 5 years compared to 54 per cent of those with coronary artery disease.[42] In more recent studies the long-term survival reported for patients undergoing surgery more nearly approximates that of age-matched control populations, with 5-year survivals ranging from 63 to 84 per cent.[18, 42, 65, 144, 214] The steady reduction in elective surgical mortality is an important factor in the improved long-term survival of these patients. Finally, the overall assessment of surgical risk should also include the effect of long-term complications. Graft sepsis, anastomotic aneurysms, and other complications may account for as much as 2 per cent of all late postoperative deaths.[156, 169]

SELECTION OF PATIENTS FOR ANEURYSM SURGERY

Operative management of aortic aneurysm is indicated when the predicted risk of rupture exceeds the predicted risk of surgery. The necessity for careful individualized evaluation is obvious. Because death from ruptured or symptomatic aneurysm is predictable, *emergent* operation in the former case and *urgent* operation in the latter must be performed, regardless of the size of the aneurysm or the presence of concurrent disease. Exceptions to this policy include the patient with a very limited life expectancy or a severely limited quality of life in whom life-saving therapy of any nature would be withheld (e.g., a patient with advanced incurable cancer). The evaluation of a patient for elective operation must also include consideration of the patient's mental status because aneurysm repair would not enhance the life of a patient who is bedridden and has limited mental capacity.

Because aneurysm size is the best indicator of the risk of rupture, it is the dominant factor in selecting patients for *elective* aneurysm repair. Equally important is the estimation of operative mortality. Consequently, patients with aortic aneurysms are most appropriately managed by experienced surgeons with whom the risk of elective operative mortality is less than 5 per cent. Elective operative intervention is warranted for nearly all patients who have aneurysms with a maximal transverse diameter of 6 cm or larger because of the high incidence of rupture. Most authorities recommend a more selective management algorithm for patients with aneurysms ranging in size from 5 to 6 cm. In patients considered to be good surgical risks, the 20 to 25 per cent 5-year risk of rupture[75, 141] favors aneurysm repair. In contrast, high-risk patients should be observed by serial noninvasive imaging of the aneurysm at a minimum of 6-month intervals.[16, 187] Enlargement to 6 cm is an indication for operation in this population, because the risk of rupture at this size exceeds the risk of surgery in all but the sickest patients. Likewise, the onset of symptoms or other evidence of significant aneurysm expansion (0.5 cm enlargement or more in 6 months) should prompt operative therapy. In some patients the medical condition that places them at higher surgical risk can be treated so that subsequent aneurysm repair may be undertaken safely. This is particularly true for patients with coronary artery disease. Several groups have demonstrated that coronary revascularization in appropriately selected patients reduces the risk of subsequent aneurysm repair to the level of patients without coronary artery disease.[23, 77, 90]

The appropriate management of the patient with a small aneurysm (less than 5 cm) remains a subject of considerable controversy.[118] There is, however, general agreement that high-risk patients with aneurysms less than 5 cm in diameter should be observed. For good-risk patients some vascular surgeons recommend aneurysm repair when the diagnosis is made.[40, 42, 49, 98] Proponents of "immediate" operation argue that autopsy studies indicate that small aneurysms have a significant risk of rupture,[50] and that the low surgical mortality of modern surgical series justifies operative intervention. Furthermore, the operative risk of these patients is likely to increase with time, as is the probability of aneurysm enlargement.[98] Finally, the risk of surgery is increased in the symptomatic patient in whom urgent aneurysm repair is required,[132] suggesting that early intervention in all patients of reasonable surgical risk is appropriate.

In contrast, studies using noninvasive imaging to assess the progression of aneurysmal dilatation have revealed that expansion rates are quite variable and that factors other than initial size do not reliably correlate with expansion or rupture. Because a substantial number of patients with small aneurysms will die from causes unrelated to their aneurysms and because higher risk patients with medium size aneurysms (5 to 6 cm) have been successfully managed expectantly by careful observation,[16, 187] conservative management even for good-risk patients has been proposed.[27, 46, 124] Accordingly, low-risk patients with aneurysm diameters of less than 5 cm are generally observed at 6-month intervals by noninvasive imaging. Surgery is recommended when the aneurysm enlarges to a maximal transverse diameter of 5 cm, when "rapid" expansion is documented

(0.5 cm or more in 6 months),[27] or when symptoms of expansion are detected. For poor-risk patients the indications for surgery are similar except that the absolute size requirement is usually 6 cm. Proponents of ''selective'' management argue that autopsy studies overestimate the risk of rupture of small aneurysms. Indeed, as previously noted, recent population-based studies[75, 141] and other selective series[27, 101] suggest that aneurysm rupture at less than 5 cm is uncommon.

Table 75–5 summarizes the results of five prospective series of selective management of small abdominal aortic aneurysms.[16, 27, 46, 124, 187] Because most of these reports included large proportions of high-risk patients with higher mortality rates from other diseases, one could argue that aneurysm rupture rates may be falsely low and that the results cannot be directly extrapolated to the general population. However, these studies used a maximal aneurysm diameter of 6 cm as the threshold for operative repair in high-risk patients. Thus, lower rupture rates due to death from concurrent diseases may be offset by higher rupture rates for aneurysms between 5 and 6 cm compared with aneurysms less than 5 cm. Furthermore, the Kingston study,[27] consisting of 268 patients selected only on the basis of aneurysm size (less than 5 cm at initial diagnosis), yielded results similar to those of other series. Nearly 43 per cent of these patients underwent aneurysm repair after developing indications for operation during the mean follow-up time of 42 months. Only one rupture occurred; however, the aneurysm in this patient, in whom aneurysm repair was withheld because of severe Alzheimer's disease, had expanded to 7.5 cm at the time of rupture. From these analyses it can be concluded that after an average follow-up of 33 months, approximately 40 per cent of observed patients will meet the criteria for elective surgery. Two per cent will require either emergent or urgent surgery. The average annual rate of rupture for unoperated patients is 1 per cent. The average mortality rate of 5 per cent for elective operations and 60 per cent for urgent and emergent cases combined with the 1 per cent rate for unoperated rupture yields an overall aneurysm-related mortality of about 4 per cent. On average, 22 per cent of patients will die from unrelated causes leaving 28 per cent of patients

alive without operation. If followed to a final end-point, the latter patients would have one of three possible outcomes: elective operation, rupture, or death from unrelated disease. Assuming that enlargement and rupture rates in these series remain constant, a final aneurysm-related mortality rate of between 4 and 13 per cent can be projected.[118] When late complications of elective surgery are included, the overall aneurysm-related mortality rate of selective management appears to be similar to that of immediate surgery. Proponents of selective management therefore argue that the high cost of surgery and associated morbidity for the substantial number of patients in whom rupture would not occur without intervention outweighs any small survival advantage for the immediate approach.[101] Recently, other authors employing sophisticated computer modeling systems to evaluate numerous potential scenarios have concluded that early surgery is preferable to ''watchful waiting'' in the majority of low-risk patients with small aneurysms.[111, 138] However, important assumptions for which little hard data are available are required in any analysis of the management of small aortic aneurysms.

Fortunately, three separate trials, each designed to delineate the best approach to the management of small aortic aneurysms, are currently under way in Canada, the United Kingdom, and the United States. While awaiting the results of these randomized trials, we recommend the conservative approach to the management of small aortic aneurysms. However, it is important to individualize treatment. For psychological reasons some patients should be offered early intervention. Similarly, noncompliant patients who are unlikely to return for surveillance and those who live in remote areas should also be considered for early surgery. The age of the patient is also an important consideration. In the Kingston study 74 per cent of all patients under 70 years of age at the time of diagnosis eventually came to surgery, in contrast to only 27 per cent of those above this age. In addition, the likelihood of eventual development of operative indications increases the closer an aneurysm is to 5.0 cm at the initial diagnosis. Cronenwett and associates also demonstrated that younger age and larger aneurysm size each predicted eventual elective surgery.[46] Thus, for the experienced surgeon whose surgical mortality rate is low,

Table 75–5. Selective Management of Abdominal Aortic Aneurysms

	Bernstein and Chan[16]	Sterpetti and Colleagues[187]	Littooy and Colleagues[124]	Cronenwett and Colleagues[46]	Brown and Colleagues[27]
Number of patients	99	54	149	73	268
Mean follow-up (months)	29	24	35	37	42
AAA size criteria for surgery					
High-risk patients	≥6 cm	>6 cm	≥6 cm	≥6 cm	NA
Low-risk patients	NA	NA	≥5 cm	≥5 cm	≥5 cm
Total elective operations	41 (41%)	23 (43%)	58 (39%)	26 (36%)	114 (43%)
Mortality	2 (5%)	2 (9%)	2 (3%)	1 (4%)	2 (2%)
Urgent/emergent operations	3 (3%)	1 (2%)	5 (3%)	3 (4%)	0
Mortality	2 (67%)	1 (100%)	5 (100%)	1 (25%)	NA
Total operations for AAA	44 (44%)	24 (44%)	63 (42%)	29 (40%)	114 (43%)
Total ruptures unoperated	0	2	4	0	1
Total AAA-related mortality	4 (4%)	5 (9%)	11 (7%)	2 (3%)	3 (1%)
Non–AAA-related mortality	34 (34%)	14 (26%)	29 (19%)	26 (36%)	38 (14%)
Total patients alive unoperated	21 (21%)	14 (26%)	53 (36%)	18 (25%)	75 (28%)

AAA, Abdominal aortic aneurysm; NA, not applicable.

the decision to operate on a relatively young patient of good surgical risk who has an aneurysm of between 4 and 5 cm is reasonable in certain circumstances.[98]

In addition to size, symptoms, and evidence of rapid expansion, indications for aneurysm repair include the presence of chronic contained rupture, distal embolization, encroachment on adjacent viscera, aortoenteric hemorrhage, aortocaval fistula, aneurysms associated with severely symptomatic intra-abdominal occlusive disease, thrombosis, inflammatory aneurysms, saccular aneurysms, and aneurysms associated with a septic process.

DIAGNOSIS

Although the accuracy of physical examination varies widely, it remains essential in the diagnosis and evaluation of abdominal aortic aneurysms. Several considerations should be kept in mind when performing the physical examination. Aneurysms palpable in the obese patient are typically large. In very thin patients aneurysms are more easily detectable. However, because the lower lumbar vertebrae lie only a few inches from the abdominal wall of the thin patient, a prominent aortic pulsation can be mistaken for an aneurysm. One should also be aware that hyperdynamic patients (e.g., those with hypertension or hyperthyroidism) may have particularly prominent nonaneurysmal aortic pulsations. The bifurcation of the aorta lies at the level of the umbilicus; therefore, the pulsatile mass is located mostly at or above the umbilicus in the epigastrium. In some patients a tortuous aorta can easily be mistaken for an aneurysm. In such cases the aorta usually lies entirely to the left of the midline, whereas both expansile borders of an aneurysm are usually distinguishable, and the right border is commonly located to the right of the midline. Transmitted pulsations from tumors of the pancreas or other retroperitoneal structures can simulate aneurysms; however, the expansile nature of an aneurysm is absent. Aneurysm size can only be estimated by physical examination because even in the thin patient measurement is imprecise. The prevalence of concurrent atherosclerotic disease in these patients should prompt a careful search for its presence elsewhere. Auscultation of the abdomen should be performed because a bruit may indicate visceral or aortic occlusive disease or, more rarely, an aortocaval fistula. Finally, a careful peripheral vascular examination is essential. Femoral and popliteal aneurysms may be present, and carotid and lower extremity vascular insufficiency may also occur in this population.

Because the size of an abdominal aortic aneurysm is the most important predictor of the risk of rupture, newer noninvasive diagnostic imaging techniques capable of precise measurement now play an increasingly important role in operative decision making. *Ultrasonography* has become the preferred method for evaluating suspected abdominal aortic aneurysms. In experienced hands, its sensitivity and specificity for imaging and measuring aneurysms are excellent. This technology is now widely available, and examinations can be readily performed in most hospitals. Ultrasonography provides accuracy of size measurement to within 0.3 cm and allows imaging in both cross-sectional and longitudinal orientations, making it a useful initial test

in determining the need for further evaluation as well as operative management. One should be aware that imaging in the transverse plane, as with CT scanning, may result in oblique sectioning through the aorta, erroneously suggesting that an aneurysm is present. Improvements in ultrasonography continue to refine the resolution and increase the scope of anatomic detail detectable with this technology. However, ultrasonography currently has limited ability to show architectural details of aneurysms.[7] For example, the relationship of an aneurysm to the renal arteries is not reliably defined. Obesity and intestinal gas can obscure the abdominal aorta and commonly interfere with visualization of the iliac vessels. Most surgeons, therefore, use ultrasonography as an initial diagnostic tool to assist in determining appropriate patient management. If operative therapy is pursued, more detailed preoperative tests are performed. In patients who do not require immediate operation, ultrasonography is a convenient and cost-effective method of aneurysm surveillance.

Screening for Abdominal Aortic Aneurysm

The widespread use of ultrasonography for noninvasive visualization of intra-abdominal structures has resulted in increased detection of asymptomatic abdominal aortic aneurysms. Because undetected aortic aneurysms may be lethal and physical examination notoriously fails to make the diagnosis, several investigators have advocated the use of ultrasound to screen for aneurysms. Detection rates vary considerably and depend on the populations selected for screening.[162, 211] In populations chosen only on the basis of age and sex, aneurysms are detected in approximately 5 per cent of men between the ages of 65 and 79.[37, 38, 40, 176] Screening programs consistently indicate a lower prevalence of aneurysms in women.[13, 19, 211] Estimated costs for widespread ultrasonographic screening of the U.S. population (selected only by age 65 years or older) range between $108,000 and $360,000 per life saved.[162] When selection criteria focus on associated manifestations of atherosclerosis, the yield of detection is much higher, ranging from 5 to 9 per cent in individuals with coronary artery disease[119, 202] and from 9 to 16 per cent in those with occlusive peripheral vascular disease.[2, 13, 19, 32, 71] More than one fourth of men over the age of 55 who have a first-degree relative with an aortic aneurysm harbor occult aneurysms, whereas the corresponding incidence in women is about 6 per cent.[14, 211] Individuals over age 50 with a family history of aneurysm warrant screening. Patients with aortic aneurysms should also be advised to notify first-degree relatives of their increased risk. Patients over 65 with peripheral vascular disease in whom the aorta cannot be easily evaluated by physical examination should also be considered for screening. In addition, patients with peripheral aneurysms have a high incidence of aortic aneurysm, and abdominal ultrasonography screening should be performed in these patients as well.

Preoperative Studies

Plain abdominal radiographs and *excretory urography* are of limited use in the diagnosis of abdominal aortic aneurysms and are only rarely indicated. Occasionally, plain abdominal radiographs lead to incidental detection of aneurysms because the dilated aortic wall is identified by a fine rim of calcium (Fig. 75–1). In most cases, however, aneurysms have insufficient calcification to allow confident detection on plain radiographs. In addition, measurement of size is relatively imprecise even for heavily calcified aneurysms. Similarly, excretory urography has now been supplanted by CT scan, which more precisely delineates anatomic details such as the presence or absence of hydronephrosis.

Contrast-enhanced (*CT*) *scans* are the best study for the preoperative assessment of abdominal aortic aneurysms. Measurements are accurate to within 0.2 cm.[154] It must be remembered that CT scans may section through the aorta at an oblique angle, particularly when the aorta is tortuous, creating or magnifying an elliptical appearance of an aneurysm and suggesting a maximal diameter larger than that actually present.[145] The relationship of an aneurysm to surrounding structures is well delineated by CT. Preoperative identification of major venous and renal anomalies, which are accurately defined on CT, aids in determining the need for additional studies and enhances the safety of operation. Hydronephrosis as well as other unrelated pathologic conditions (e.g., unsuspected tumors) that may influence operative management can also be identified. CT provides an accurate image of the proximal and distal extent of most abdominal aortic aneurysms. Several investigators have shown that thin-section (2 mm), high-resolution CT correctly identifies the origin of aortic aneurysms in relation to the renal arteries in 94 to 99 per cent of cases.[79, 148, 206] Iliac

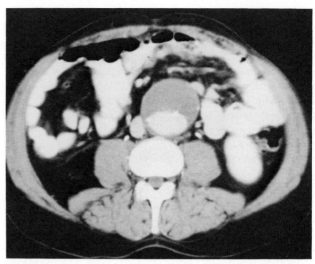

FIGURE 75–2.   Computed tomographic scan of the abdomen in a patient with a 6.3 cm aneurysm. Note the narrowed contrast-filled lumen surrounded by thick mural thrombus.

artery aneurysms are correctly identified in more than 85 per cent of cases.[80, 148, 206] Newer advances in three-dimensional and sagittal CT reconstructions also improve the definition of proximal and distal aneurysmal extension. Visualization of the aneurysm wall is excellent with CT. Mural thrombus is readily distinguished from the arterial lumen when contrast is used (Fig. 75–2). Although uncommon, CT may reveal an abnormal soft tissue collection with or without vertebral body erosion, indicating chronic contained rupture. CT is the diagnostic test of choice for suspected inflammatory aneurysms typified by thickened periaortic fibrous tissue that obliterates adjacent tissue planes.[47] In addition, retroperitoneal fibrosis is also evident on CT. Because most abdominal aortic aneurysms are straightforward, preoperative imaging alters the operation in roughly 10 per cent of cases. However, most surgeons believe that the information provided by CT scan justifies its routine use in the preoperative evaluation of abdominal aortic aneurysms.

Magnetic resonance imaging (MRI) accurately measures aneurysm size with a resolution of approximately 1 mm. In clinical studies MRI has compared favorably with other methods of evaluating aneurysms.[150] Like CT, surrounding anatomic relationships are well visualized. Images can be displayed in axial, coronal, or sagittal orientations, and the three-dimensional imaging of MRI is superior to that of CT reconstructions. Delineation of both proximal and distal aneurysm extension is excellent, as is the ability to determine the involvement of branching vessels. Details of the aortic wall including the presence of mural thrombus and inflammation can be detected with MRI. MRI is also a sensitive tool for detecting aortic dissections. A significant advantage of MRI is the excellent intravascular enhancement achieved without the need for contrast agents. MRI can quantitate and characterize blood flow patterns in aortic aneurysms.[130] Newer refinements in this technology can isolate and depict vascular anatomy. In fact, MRI angiography may eventually replace conventional angiography. Although the availability of this technology is increasing, MRI remains expensive. Other disadvantages include the

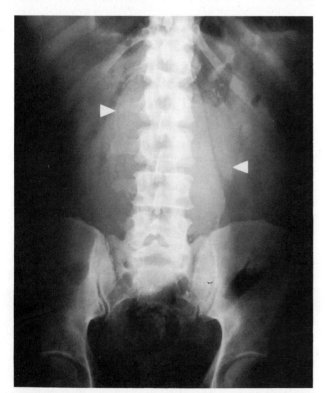

FIGURE 75–1.   Plain x-ray of the abdomen in a patient with an abdominal aortic aneurysm visible because of the calcified aneurysm wall *(arrows)*. Approximately 65 per cent of abdominal aortic aneurysms are visible on plain x-ray.

relatively slow time for image acquisition, the inability to scan patients with indwelling metallic devices (e.g., surgical clips, pacemakers) or patients requiring monitoring equipment, and the development of claustrophobia in patients during scanning. At present, although MRI is an excellent tool for the preoperative evaluation of aortic aneurysms, cost and availability favor CT in most patients. Further detailed discussion of these and other vascular imaging techniques is presented in Chapter 6.

Aortography is used routinely by some surgeons, whereas others obtain aortograms for aneurysms only in specific circumstances. Aortography does not accurately define aneurysm dimensions because of the presence of mural thrombus, which restricts contrast material to the more narrow central channel (Fig. 75–3). In some cases aortography may not even document the presence of an aneurysm, although subtle signs are usually present, such as the absence of lumbar vessels due to occluding mural thrombus. Because the proximal bulge of infrarenal aneurysms often curves back over and above the aneurysm neck, anteroposterior angiographic views may erroneously suggest involvement at or above the renal arteries, and lateral views should be obtained.

Absolute indications for aortography include (1) asso-

ciated renovascular hypertension, (2) unexplained impaired renal function, (3) symptoms of visceral angina, (4) unexplained abdominal or flank bruit, (5) evidence of significant iliofemoral occlusive disease, (6) suspicion of suprarenal involvement, (7) the presence of femoral or popliteal aneurysms, (8) evidence of horseshoe or pelvic kidney by other examination, because of the variability of arterial supply to the kidney in such cases, and (9) prior colectomy, which may alter the collateral circulation to the remaining colon, increasing the risk of intestinal ischemia.

In addition to imaging studies, patients under consideration for aneurysm repair should undergo other preoperative examinations appropriate for any major abdominal operation including electrocardiogram, chest radiographs, complete blood count, urinalysis, fasting blood sugar, blood urea nitrogen, and serum creatinine. Any prior medical conditions that might require special preoperative or postoperative care must be fully investigated. Systemic atherosclerosis is so common in patients with abdominal aortic aneurysms that this pathology requires special investigative effort (see Chapter 22). Carotid disease should be evaluated with duplex scanning when suspected. Lower extremity occlusive disease is detectable by history and physical examination, and its presence should prompt noninvasive vascular laboratory assessment with segmental limb pressures or segmental plethysmography. Because abdominal aortic aneurysms can interrupt the normal progressive amplification of systolic pressure as the aortic pulse is transmitted along the arterial tree, one should be aware that the characteristic elevated pressure in the upper thighs may not be present.[180] Significant occlusive arterial disease should be investigated with angiography because it may affect the type of arterial reconstruction required for aneurysm repair.

Evaluation and Management of Cardiac Disease

Coronary events are responsible for 50 to 60 per cent of all perioperative deaths associated with aortic aneurysm surgery, and the mortality associated with perioperative myocardial infarction may reach 70 per cent.[55] Coronary artery disease is also the leading cause of late mortality in patients undergoing aneurysm repair.[42, 87, 94, 165, 169] Thirty to 40 per cent of patients with aneurysms typically report either a history of past myocardial infarction or angina pectoris.[23, 77] Hertzer and associates performed routine coronary arteriography preoperatively in 246 patients with aneurysms and found an incidence of severe coronary artery disease of 36 per cent.[89] Of note, 17 per cent of the patients with severe coronary artery disease had no clinical evidence (i.e., on history or ECG) suggesting its presence. This study and others[23] suggest that the incidence of angiographically significant coronary disease in patients without clinical evidence of coronary disease is approximately one in five, underscoring the need for a careful preoperative search for cardiac disease.

Because myocardial infarction is the most frequent fatal complication of aneurysm repair, prophylactic myocardial revascularization in all patients with angiographically proven coronary disease has been advocated.[91, 133] Cor-

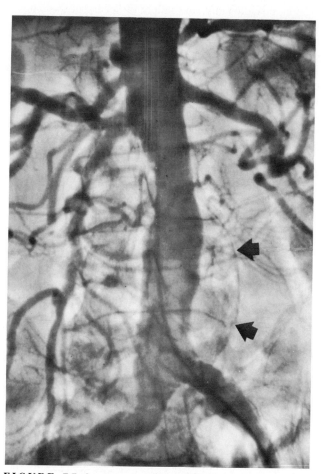

FIGURE 75–3. Digital subtraction aortography of an abdominal aortic aneurysm. Owing to the passage of contrast through a central channel lined by mural thrombus, aortography often gives a misleading impression of aneurysm size. *Arrows* mark the calcified aneurysm wall, indicating the true lateral extent of this aneurysm.

onary revascularization in this subset of patients clearly reduces the risk of perioperative myocardial infarction at subsequent aneurysm repair.[90] Furthermore, patients who survive both coronary revascularization and aneurysm repair have long-term survival rates approaching those of age-matched controls. However, routine coronary angiography for patients with abdominal aortic aneurysms is unwarranted because the incidence of perioperative coronary events in patients without clinical evidence of cardiac disease is less than 2 per cent.[23, 26, 77, 217] Coronary arteriography is expensive and carries risks. In addition, the substantial perioperative mortality for coronary bypass surgery, 5.7 per cent in the study of Hertzer and colleagues,[90] must be included in the overall risk assessment for this strategy. Other investigators employing selective evaluation of patients for coronary disease and coronary revascularization based on symptoms and noninvasive assessment have demonstrated excellent results.[77, 165, 169, 170] Finally, selective management of coronary artery disease in patients with abdominal aortic aneurysms appears to lead to long-term survival rates similar to those of prophylactic management protocols.[77, 94, 165] Noninvasive studies of cardiac disease, including stress ECG, stress thallium or dipyridamole-thallium imaging, or preoperative ambulatory ECG, aid in selecting patients at high risk for perioperative coronary events.[121] Coronary revascularization should be performed prior to aneurysm repair in patients in whom the severity of coronary disease would indicate surgical management on its own merits (i.e., left main coronary disease[199] or triple-vessel disease[208]). Table 75–6 illustrates the recommended algorithm for evaluating coronary artery disease in patients selected for aneurysm repair. This topic is discussed more thoroughly in Chapter 22.

MANAGEMENT OF ABDOMINAL AORTIC ANEURYSMS IN HIGH-RISK PATIENTS

The high risk of rupture for aneurysms exceeding 6 cm in size favors surgical management in most cases. However, patients with severe concurrent medical disease in whom aneurysm repair poses a significantly increased risk of perioperative mortality (see Table 75–4) are problematic. Currently, there are three possible alternatives for the management of these patients: (1) defer surgery indefinitely until symptoms develop or signs of aneurysm rupture be-

come evident; (2) perform aneurysm exclusion and bypass; or (3) undertake conventional aneurysm repair with intensive perioperative support. As noted previously, the high percentage of patients excluded from surgical management owing to advanced age who die of ruptured aneurysm indicates that age alone should not be a deterrent to surgery.[143] It is important to verify the severity of concurrent disease in presumed high-risk patients because fewer than half of these patients will eventually die from the condition for which they are excluded from surgical consideration.[67] Furthermore, 20 to 45 per cent of patients excluded from surgery for medical reasons experience aneurysm rupture.[50, 65, 101, 196] Therefore, nonoperative treatment of aortic aneurysms in high-risk patients does not afford optimal survival to these patients.

Prior to the development of current operative techniques, "nonresective" operations including aneurysm ligation, wrapping, and attempts at inducing aneurysm thrombosis yielded uniformly dismal results. Improvement in the results of extra-anatomic bypass has renewed interest in nonresective procedures combined with axillobifemoral bypass. In addition to extra-anatomic bypass, these procedures typically involve aneurysm exclusion by proximal and distal ligation[22] or distal ligation alone with or without transvascular induction of aneurysm thrombosis.[15, 110] Complications of these strategies include infection, visceral ischemia, coagulopathy, and failure of aneurysm thrombosis with continuing expansion, rupture, and death.[102, 175] The risk of subsequent rupture appears to be much higher after distal ligation alone compared with complete exclusion.[127] In the two largest series examining aneurysm exclusion and extra-anatomic bypass for high-risk patients, the overall aneurysm-related mortality rates were 10[110] and 18[100] per cent. Furthermore, the incidence of reoperation for complications of extra-anatomic bypass is considerable. For these reasons, aneurysm exclusion with extra-anatomic bypass offers no advantage over nonoperative therapy and is not advised. In contrast, Hollier and colleagues and Pairolero have reported an operative mortality of only 6 per cent in high-risk patients using conventional aneurysm repair with meticulous perioperative care.[95, 147] Long-term follow-up of these patients revealed that survival for high-risk patients undergoing conventional treatment paralleled that of non-high-risk patients for 30 months, suggesting a significant benefit for high-risk patients treated operatively. Thus, it appears that high-risk patients are best treated with conventional aneurysm repair when and where the resources for

Table 75–6. Schema of Cardiac Evaluation in Patients with Asymptomatic Abdominal Aortic Aneurysm

---

I. Asymptomatic cardiac status ⇒ AAA repair
II. Mild, stable cardiac symptoms ⇒ Noninvasive cardiac study:
    Study positive → Coronary angiography
    Study negative → AAA repair
III. Significant cardiac symptoms ⇒ Coronary angiography:
    Significant CAD → CABG, then staged AAA repair
    Insignificant CAD → AAA repair
IV. Very elderly, or LVEF <30%, or nonreconstructible CAD   } ⇒   AAA <6 cm → careful AAA surveillance
    AAA ≥ 6 cm → AAA repair with cardiac support

Key: *AAA, abdominal aortic aneurysm; LVEF, left ventricular ejection fraction; CAD, coronary artery disease; CABG, coronary artery bypass grafting.*

intensive intraoperative and postoperative support are available.

OPERATIVE TECHNIQUE

Transperitoneal Approach

The *transperitoneal* approach is the most widely used technique for the repair of infrarenal aortic aneurysms. (The operative details of the retroperitoneal approach, its advantages and disadvantages, and a comparison of the two techniques are discussed in the next section.) With the transperitoneal approach the patient is placed in the supine position, and the skin of the lower chest, entire abdomen, and both groins is prepared. Many surgeons also recommend preparing the legs to the ankles in case embolization occurs to the popliteal artery or its branches. Preoperative identification of the location of lower extremity pulses is helpful in assessing subsequent distal perfusion. The choice between a long midline incision and a wide transverse incision is a matter of personal preference. Factors such as the speed of incision and closure, the impact of postoperative pain, the extent of the aneurysm, the degree of obesity, and the coexistence of chronic pulmonary disease influence the choice of incision in individual patients. The operating surgeon may stand on either side of the table, but if the number of assistants is limited, the left side may allow better access to the aorta. If the surgeon stands on the patient's right side, mobilization and elevation of the right colon will improve exposure and freedom of movement, as will simply rolling the table toward the surgeon.

Preliminary exploration of the abdomen should always be performed in elective operations. The likelihood of a coexisting malignant tumor or other intra-abdominal pathologic condition is substantial in this age group, particularly in patients who present with abdominal symptoms that are not clearly due to the aneurysm.[188, 194] The surgical priorities in this situation are discussed later in this chapter. The extent of the aneurysm, especially its upper and lower limits, and the condition of the major adjacent arteries, particularly the renal and common iliac arteries, are determined by palpation. Extensive manipulation of the aneurysm should be avoided until proximal and distal control are established and all other preparations necessary for operative repair of the aneurysm are completed.

With the transverse colon retracted superiorly and the small bowel held to the right, a longitudinal incision is made in the peritoneum just to the left of the base of the small bowel mesentery to expose the aneurysm. This incision is then extended cephalad along the left margin of the distal duodenum to the inferior border of the pancreas and caudally over the right iliac artery. Care must be taken to identify and avoid the ureters. The parasympathetic nerves course anterior to the proximal left common iliac artery on their way to the pelvis.[212] In sexually potent males these nerves should be retracted with the peritoneum rather than incised. After the peritoneal incision is completed and the duodenum is mobilized, the small intestine is either packed into the right upper portion of the abdomen or eviscerated and retracted rightward after placing it in a plastic bag to reduce fluid loss. The newer self-retaining retraction de-

vices (e.g., Omnitract or Buchwalter) are extraordinarily helpful in maintaining exposure during the operation. After the ligament of Treitz is transected, the inferior mesenteric vein becomes apparent; it can be divided if necessary. The left renal vein lies more cephalad in a deeper plane. In order to obtain adequate exposure of larger aneurysms, it may be necessary to expose and retract this vein superiorly. Care must be taken not to injure its tributaries, particularly a descending lumbar vein, frequently encountered to the left of the aorta, which must be divided before the left renal vein is mobile enough to allow upward retraction. Occasionally, the left renal vein may be tightly stretched over the "neck" of the aneurysm. In such cases division medial to the adrenal and gonadal tributaries is usually well tolerated.[4] The safety of this maneuver should be tested beforehand by trial occlusion with a vascular clamp or Silastic loop. Elevation of distal venous pressure, which is usually obvious from the degree of distention and does not require measurement, dictates later reanastomosis. Fortunately, the high flow rate in this vessel usually preserves patency when reanastomosis is required.[195]

The upper part of the dissection is then pursued until control of the neck of the aneurysm is achieved. By first dissecting close to the anterior surface of the aortic segment immediately proximal to the aneurysm, and then staying in this "inside" plane as one proceeds laterally and posteriorly around the circumference of the aorta, control can usually be obtained quickly and easily. Once this plane has been established, the surgeon may safely insert a thumb and index finger, pinching them together posteriorly and using gentle upward traction to completely free the neck of the aneurysm. An opening behind the infrarenal aorta above the lumbar tributaries can usually be made sufficiently wide to admit a renal pedicle clamp so that an umbilical tape or a No. 14 rubber catheter can be drawn around the aorta. The advantage of the latter technique is that the lower jaw of a vascular clamp can later be placed in the catheter's flanged end and drawn into position for occlusion without catching or tearing adjacent structures. After exposure of an adequate segment of aorta above the aneurysm is obtained and before the aneurysm itself is dissected or otherwise manipulated, control of the iliac arteries is established in a similar fashion. When inflammatory reaction between the arteries and the underlying veins makes circumferential dissection of the iliac arteries hazardous, only the anterior two thirds of these vessels should be exposed. Later, care must be taken to avoid injury to the veins when applying vascular clamps. The quality of the renal, superior, and inferior mesenteric arteries should be assessed by palpation. If the inferior mesenteric artery is not already occluded, it may be controlled temporarily with a small vascular clamp or a double loop of Silastic tubing. The inferior mesenteric artery should never be ligated until the aneurysm is opened and backbleeding is assessed, particularly if the hypogastric arteries are diseased or if one may have to be sacrificed for technical reasons.

The available prosthetic grafts for aortic replacement include knitted Dacron, knitted Dacron impregnated with collagen or gelatin, woven Dacron, and polytetrafluoroethylene (PTFE). A detailed discussion of these and other graft choices is presented in Chapter 29. Because of its superior handling characteristics, knitted Dacron is the material most commonly chosen for elective aneurysm repair. The primary disadvantage of knitted Dacron is the requirement for preclotting, a process that can be time consuming and on occasion may still allow substantial blood loss. Impregnated knitted Dacron, PTFE, and woven Dacron grafts are nonporous, eliminating the need for preclotting; therefore, any of these grafts are preferable to knitted Dacron for ruptured aneurysms. Many surgeons also prefer nonporous grafts in elective cases. The advantages of one graft over the others have not been established by controlled trials. In a recent prospective randomized comparison of PTFE and Dacron, long-term patency was equivalent, but PTFE had a higher incidence of early graft failure and graft sepsis.[157] In contrast, in a smaller trial with shorter follow-up PTFE was found to be superior.[126] Thus, the optimal prosthesis for elective aortic replacement remains controversial.[155]

A graft of appropriate size is chosen according to the diameter of the proximal nonaneurysmal segment of the aorta. If knitted Dacron is selected, blood drawn from the aneurysm or the adjacent vena cava prior to systemic anticoagulation is used for preclotting. Heparin is given usually at an initial dose of 100 U/kg; sometimes, intraoperative activated clotting times (ACTs) are performed to ensure adequacy of anticoagulation. The distal vascular clamps are applied first (to prevent embolization from above) followed by the proximal clamp. The aneurysm is opened longitudinally along its anterior surface. The upper end of the incision is then incised horizontally in a T shape with the lateral extensions just below the neck of the aneurysm (Fig. 75–4). The posterior half of the aneurysm wall is not necessarily divided, although some surgeons prefer to transect the aorta completely. Intraluminal thrombotic material and atherosclerotic debris are extracted. The value of routine Gram's stain and culture of this material in predicting sub-

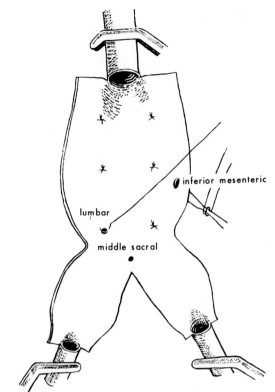

FIGURE 75–5. Method of internally controlling collateral flow into the aneurysm.

sequent graft sepsis is controversial;[28, 60, 131, 174] however, a recent review of routine cultures from 500 elective aneurysm repairs found that positive cultures did not predict subsequent graft sepsis.[64] Any signs of infectious aortitis demand intraoperative Gram's staining and culture.

After clearing the aneurysmal sac of its contents, an assistant controls bleeding from the lumbar arteries with pressure using a gauze pad moved progressively downward as the internal lumbar artery orifices are controlled individually with figure-of-eight suture ligatures (Fig. 75–5). Once collateral flow into the opened aneurysmal sac has been controlled in this manner, the upper anastomosis is begun (Fig. 75–6). From inside the aneurysm one can usually identify a distinct ring at its neck that is suitable for the upper anastomosis. Beginning at the posterior midline and using 000 polypropylene or Teflon-coated Dacron suture with double needles, deep bites are taken in an effort to include a double thickness of the posterior aortic wall for extra strength. The anterior half of the suture line is then completed with continuous deeply placed sutures because the diseased aorta does not hold sutures well. If the anterior wall is extremely friable, pledgets of Teflon or Dacron felt can be incorporated into the suture line. However, pledgets are rarely necessary if the curve of the needle is carefully observed as it penetrates the aortic wall and undue tension on the suture by the first assistant is avoided while "following" each new suture placement. This technique also provides better hemostasis and lessens the risk of suture line disruption as well as anastomotic aneurysm.

After completing the upper anastomosis, the distal graft is occluded with a vascular clamp, and the proximal aortic clamp is released briefly to check for suture line

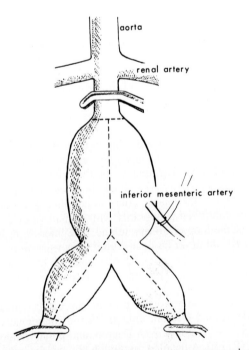

FIGURE 75–4. The incision in an aortic aneurysm using the "endoaneurysmal approach" in which the reconstruction is performed entirely intraluminally.

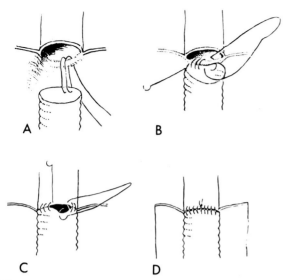

FIGURE 75–6. The upper anastomosis between a Dacron graft and the neck of the aneurysm, as described in the text.

bleeding. Particular attention should be paid to the posterior aspect of the suture line because it cannot be reached again once the distal anastomosis is undertaken. If the iliac arteries are not aneurysmal, only a segmental or tube graft is needed. A similar technique is used just above the bifurcation, suturing from within the lumen and encompassing both iliac artery orifices within the suture line. If iliac artery aneurysms exist, they are incised anteriorly so that the limbs of a bifurcated graft can be sutured into an oblique ellipse that includes the orifices of both the internal and external iliac arteries (Fig. 75–7). As previously emphasized, extension of the arteriotomy into the left iliac artery should be made only into the arterial wall while retracting the nerves laterally in sexually active men.[212] The iliac limbs of the graft should be placed beneath the ureters, if they are in the field, before these anastomoses are performed. Care should be taken to ensure distal patency with good backflow before completing each distal anastomosis; heparinized saline may be carefully flushed into the distal circulation.

As soon as the first iliac anastomosis is completed, flow into that extremity should be restored, releasing the clamps slowly to decrease "declamping" hypotension. Although declamping shock is rare if adequate intravenous fluid replacement has been administered (see later discussion), the sudden release of the aortic clamp, allowing blood flow into a dilated distal bed, and the concomitant venous return of vasoactive substances that have accumulated in the ischemic tissues may cause hypotension. Flow is released into the hypogastric arteries before the external iliac arteries if both of these arteries have been individually clamped, and warmed blood is infused rapidly when necessary to keep up with oozing through a knitted graft if this type is used. The authors have found that buffering and inotropic agents are only rarely necessary if an adequate circulating volume has been maintained and prefer to reclamp and restore further blood volume rather than resort to vasopressors. If the hypogastric artery has been isolated, releasing its clamp first has the additional advantage of

diverting any embolic debris into the hypogastric circulation rather than into the legs.

After restoration of flow into the iliac arteries, attention is turned to the inferior mesenteric artery and the circulation of the sigmoid colon. If the inferior mesenteric artery is already occluded, if it is small and not associated with palpable superior mesenteric artery occlusive disease, if it has good backflow on release of the controlling clamp, if the color and pulsations of the mesenteric arcade branches in the sigmoid colon are good, and if at least one hypogastric artery is patent, the inferior mesenteric artery can be ligated or occluded by a transfixing suture applied to its internal orifice. In questionable cases, Doppler signals[93] from the bowel or an adequate inferior artery "stump" pressure[62] may settle the question of bowel viability (see Chapter 99). In the rare circumstances when sigmoid colon perfusion appears marginal, particularly if the hypogastric arteries are diseased or excluded from the circulation, an elliptical cuff of the aortic wall around the inferior mesenteric artery orifice is excised and anastomosed to the left side of the graft (Fig. 75–8).

On occasion, embolization to the lower extremity can compromise distal perfusion. Prior to closure an assistant at the foot of the operating table can reach under the drapes and either palpate distal pulses or evaluate them with a Doppler probe. Alternatively, the feet can be placed in clear plastic bags during the draping procedure, allowing the surgeon to inspect the feet directly. A change in perfusion from preoperative status indicates the need for thromboembolectomy. Early discovery will decrease long-term morbidity from ischemia. In addition, lumbar sympathectomy should be considered in patients with multiple small emboli to digital arteries (see Chapter 59).

Finally, the remaining aneurysmal shell is trimmed and sutured around the graft to provide a natural tissue barrier over the prosthesis (Fig. 75–9) followed by closure of the

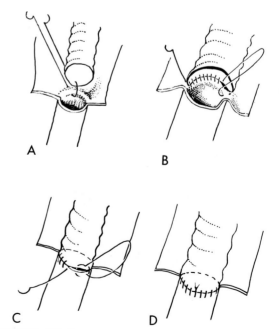

FIGURE 75–7. The lower or iliac anastomosis, which is also mostly performed from inside the arterial lumen.

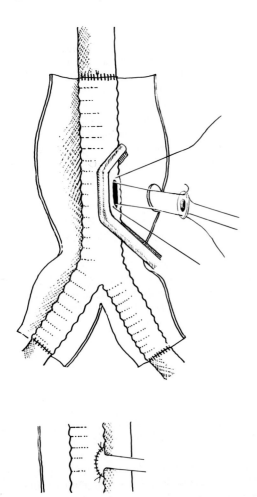

FIGURE 75–8. The technique of anastomosing the inferior mesenteric artery to the Dacron prosthesis. A similar approach may be used for reanastomosing aberrant or accessory renal arteries.

retroperitoneum. The aortic prosthesis and upper anastomosis must be isolated from the overlying duodenum during closure; if necessary, a pedicle of greater omentum can be interposed to achieve this purpose. The small bowel

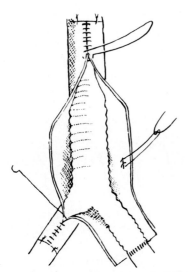

FIGURE 75–9. Closure of the aneurysm's shell around the Dacron prosthesis to reinforce and isolate it.

should be inspected carefully and replaced in its normal position. If retroperitoneal or graft hemorrhage is troublesome, reversal of heparin with protamine may be required. A diligent search for surgically correctable bleeding is mandatory, however.

Retroperitoneal Approach

Some surgeons routinely use the retroperitoneal approach for repairing infrarenal aortic aneurysms. Several retrospective series, mostly using historical transperitoneal controls, have suggested that this approach reduces postoperative pulmonary complications, paralytic ileus, and duration of hospital stay.[106, 117, 177] In contrast, Cambria and associates, in a recent prospective randomized trial, found that the only advantage of the retroperitoneal approach was a more rapid return of gastrointestinal function. Length of stay was not shortened in these patients.[30] Thus, there is little evidence to support the superiority of one approach over the other for routine aneurysm repairs.

There are advantages to each approach and certain situations in which one is clearly preferable to the other. The principal advantages of the transperitoneal approach are (1) opening and closing of the incision is faster and easier, (2) it allows exploration for intraperitoneal pathology, (3) it provides easier access to the right iliac artery, and (4) access to the right renal artery is superior. Access to the right iliac artery is limited in the retroperitoneal approach; therefore, if the right common iliac artery is aneurysmal, the transperitoneal approach is preferred. The authors also prefer the transperitoneal approach when associated right renal artery stenosis is encountered because access, particularly for distal disease, is limited with the retroperitoneal route. The advantages of the retroperitoneal approach are primarily evident in patients with less commonly encountered presentations of aortic aneurysms. Dense intraperitoneal adhesions from prior operations or peritonitis can be avoided with the retroperitoneal approach. Similarly, access to the aorta is improved in many patients with a colostomy or ileostomy. In patients with a left lower quadrant stoma, a right retroperitoneal approach can be used.[51] Most authors recommend the retroperitoneal approach for inflammatory aneurysms because adhesions between the aneurysm and the duodenum do not restrict access to the aorta by this route.[66, 137] Aortas embedded in retroperitoneal fibrosis are also more easily accessed through the flank. The presence of a horseshoe kidney is a relative indication for the retroperitoneal approach because it allows easier avoidance of the multiple and accessory renal arteries typical in this situation. Many surgeons prefer the retroperitoneal approach for juxtarenal aortic aneurysms. Finally, this approach is useful when replacing or removing an existing transperitoneally placed aortic prosthesis because of infection.

Proper patient positioning is essential in achieving optimal exposure with the retroperitoneal approach. For most infrarenal aneurysms an incision keyed on the 12th rib is adequate. If a need for higher exposure is anticipated (e.g., with juxtarenal or suprarenal aneurysms), the incision should be directed cephalad toward the 11th or 10th rib. Importantly, correct body positioning in the infrarenal and suprarenal exposures is different. In the more common former case, the patient's left shoulder is elevated to a 45- to 60-degree angle relative to the table while the pelvis is positioned as near horizontal as possible. The table should be flexed with the break positioned at the level of the lumbar spine midway between the iliac crest and the costal margin. An air-evacuating ''bean bag'' is helpful in maintaining the proper position and also allows the table to be rotated on its long axis to aid in optimal positioning. If the 10th or 11th rib exposures are used, the positioning differs in that the shoulders are positioned as near perpendicular to the table as possible, and following table flexion the trunk is twisted so that the angle between the pelvis and the table is about 30 degrees.

Beginning at the lateral border of the left rectus muscle midway between the symphysis and the umbilicus, the skin incision is carried superiorly and then curved laterally up to the tip of the 12th rib. If exposure of the right iliac artery is required, the incision can be extended inferolaterally into the right lower quadrant. For higher exposures the incision is curved upward to the left costal margin and posteriorly along the course of the selected rib, part of which is later resected. Using electrocautery the underlying muscles are divided, exposing the underlying peritoneum and, toward the leftward aspect of the incision, the anterior edge of the properitoneal fat layer. For most infrarenal exposures it is preferable to continue the dissection anteriorly over the left kidney and adrenal gland. After widely freeing up the peritoneal sac both inferiorly and superiorly, the retroperitoneal plane anterior to the kidney is entered by dissecting between the properitoneal fat and the peritoneum, achieving exposure of the infrarenal aorta with the kidney left in its native position. For juxtarenal aneurysms, for which more cephalad exposure is required, the kidney is mobilized by dissecting posterior to the properitoneal fat and Gerota's fascia. In this case, it is helpful to divide the left gonadal vein to avoid avulsion from the left renal vein. The ureter can be mobilized from the bifurcation of the common iliac artery to the ureteropelvic junction if necessary. Medial mobilization of the peritoneum exposes the inferior mesenteric artery, which, when ligated close to the aorta, permits access to the right side of the aorta and the confluence of the left renal vein and the inferior vena cava. Inferior and medial mobilization of the peritoneal sac provides exposure of the right iliac artery when necessary. After achieving adequate exposure, repair of the aneurysm is carried out according to the principles previously described. Once completed, the same considerations regarding assessment of lower extremity perfusion apply. One disadvantage of the retroperitoneal approach, however, is that bowel viability cannot be easily assessed without incising the peritoneum. Although most surgeons continue to favor the transperitoneal approach, the retroperitoneal approach is gaining in popularity. The advantages to each approach in the situations described make it advisable for the surgeon to become proficient with both alternatives.

Operative Management of the High-Risk Patient

As discussed previously, large abdominal aortic aneurysms in high-risk patients should generally be treated by conventional repair. Major concomitant risk factors that increase the morbidity of aneurysm repair include severe chronic obstructive pulmonary disease and severe cardiac disease. With meticulous perioperative care, even patients with pulmonary disease requiring home oxygen can undergo aneurysm repair with acceptable risk. Preoperative pulmonary preparation may include systemic antibiotics, bronchodilators, nebulizer or inhalational treatments, or postural drainage, depending on the specific underlying disorder. Direct transperitoneal repair can be performed safely in most cases; however, the retroperitoneal approach is preferred by surgeons who believe that it allows faster recovery of pulmonary function. Placement of an epidural catheter for administration of epidural analgesics is particularly beneficial because this provides pain relief without sedation and may improve pulmonary toilet.

Perioperative cardiac support in high-risk patients should start with determination of optimal myocardial performance curves using a Swan-Ganz catheter. Intraoperatively, serial observation of cardiac indices is used to direct appropriate volume replacement and the use of vasodilatory/or inotropic therapy. Recent improvements in transesophageal echocardiography that permit continuous evaluation of cardiac function may help to improve the maintenance of optimal myocardial performance in these patients.[72, 125] If afterload increases significantly, sodium nitroprusside is used to return peripheral vascular resistance to the optimal range. Volume replacement with crystalloid or blood should be given if cardiac output falls. Inotropic support, usually with low-dose dopamine, may be required if the cardiac output is low despite adequate intravascular volume. If the cardiac index cannot be maintained above 2 L/min/m^2 with these measures, insertion of an intra-aortic balloon counterpulsation device should be considered.[95, 97] After the proximal aortic anastomosis is completed, the intra-aortic balloon can be introduced percutaneously through the groin and advanced under direct vision or palpation through the iliac artery and passed through one limb of the graft. A tourniquet can then be placed on that limb, and the contralateral limb can be clamped. The proximal aortic clamp can then be removed, and the intra-aortic balloon can be positioned in the proximal descending thoracic aorta. Balloon counterpulsation is generally maintained at 1:1 counterpulsation for 24 to 48 hours until the patient is adequately stabilized. The patient can then be weaned off balloon assist over a 12-hour period and the balloon then removed. It is not necessary to administer heparin with balloon counterpulsation. Most cardiac dysfunction, even in high-risk patients, can be managed by careful monitoring using appropriate volume replacement and pharmacologic support. Optimizing oxygen delivery to patients with lower cardiac outputs requires maintaining the hematocrit above 30 per cent. In the series of high-risk patients reported by Hollier and colleagues, only 6 per cent of high-risk patients required intra-aortic balloon counterpulsation.[95]

Ruptured Abdominal Aortic Aneurysm

The surgical management of ruptured abdominal aortic aneurysm is discussed in detail in Chapter 76.

EARLY COMPLICATIONS OF AORTIC ANEURYSM SURGERY

Although the mortality associated with elective aortic aneurysm repair has declined to less than 5 per cent in recent series, major morbidity may occur. As noted earlier, myocardial infarction is the leading cause of both early and late mortality in patients undergoing aortic aneurysm surgery. Table 75–7 lists the incidences of complications reported in two recent large series of elective operations on abdominal aortic aneurysms.[55, 107] Several early complications specifically associated with aneurysm surgery warrant detailed discussion.

Intraoperative Hemorrhage

The use of endoaneurysmorrhaphy has markedly reduced the risk of intraoperative hemorrhage compared to that seen in the resection technique. Technological advances in autotransfusion have also reduced the need for blood transfusions during these operations. Major intraoperative hemorrhage usually increases cross-clamp times and contributes to coagulopathy. Not surprisingly, intraoperative blood loss correlates directly with postoperative morbidity and mortality.[55, 107] Major intraoperative hemorrhage during elective aneurysm repair is usually the result of technical misadventures. Intraoperative rupture of the aneurysm is rarely a problem when preliminary control of the proximal and distal vessels is obtained prior to dissection of the aneurysm itself. Persistent lumbar artery bleeding may occur if these vessels are not identified and suture-ligated promptly. Injuries to major veins are probably the most common cause of serious intraoperative hemorrhage. The left common iliac vein is most susceptible to injury where it courses beneath the right common iliac artery. This is particularly true when the iliac vessels are aneurysmal because the underlying venous structures may be adherent to the aneurysm. Venous injury is best avoided by minimiz-

ing attempts to free major venous structures from the aneurysm. It is often advisable to dissect only the anterior two thirds of the iliac arteries to apply occluding vascular clamps. Alternatively, Fogarty balloon catheters can be used to achieve intraluminal arterial control, thereby alleviating the need for dissection to isolate the arteries. Finally, the surgeon must be aware of and anticipate common venous anomalies to avoid their discovery through inadvertent injury. The major venous anomalies of particular importance in abdominal aortic aneurysm surgery are discussed in a subsequent section.

Aortic Declamping Shock

Hypotension after restoration of blood flow to the legs after extended aortic occlusion was once a significant cause of perioperative morbidity and mortality. With improved volume management and increased awareness of this phenomenon, prolonged declamping hypotension is now seen only rarely during elective aortic aneurysm repair. It remains much more of a problem with ruptured aortic aneurysms.

Three primary factors are thought to cause this complication. First, marked afterload reduction may result from sudden restoration of flow into a vasodilated distal circulation. Second, reduced myocardial performance may result from a sudden "washout" of potassium, acidic metabolites, and vasoactive humoral factors following reperfusion of distal ischemic tissues. Third, reduced preload due to increased venous capacitance or third-space volume loss in the distal tissues may contribute to depression of cardiac output. Careful intraoperative management can minimize declamping hypotension. The surgeon should notify the anesthesiologist well in advance of releasing the cross-clamp to administer volume. Distal perfusion should be restored gradually by slowly releasing flow into the lower extremities one at a time. Following completion of the first limb of a bifurcation graft, perfusion should be restored to the ipsilateral leg while the anastomosis of the opposite limb is completed.

Renal Failure

Renal failure after aneurysm repair formerly accounted for a 3 to 12 per cent operative mortality rate. This complication is now relatively uncommon following elective infrarenal aortic aneurysm surgery. Avoidance of intraoperative hypotension, improved volume resuscitation, and the shorter period of aortic occlusion required with the endoaneurysmal technique have contributed to improved outcome. Preoperative angiography can cause contrast-related renal toxicity when surgery is performed soon afterward. Consequently, it is wise to delay surgery for at least a day after angiography or CT scan and to hydrate patients adequately. Embolization of mural thrombus or atheromatous debris into the renal vessels can occur during mobilization of the proximal aorta. There is some evidence to support a beneficial effect of intravenous mannitol when mannitol is given prophylactically 15 to 30 minutes prior to aortic cross-clamping (12.5 to 25 gm).[139] Administration of intra-

Table 75–7. Perioperative Complications of Elective Abdominal Aortic Aneurysm Repair

Complication	Author	
	Diehl and Colleagues[155] *(n = 557)*	*Johnston*[107] *(n = 666)*
Mortality	5.1%	4.8%
Myocardial infarction	5.4%	5.2%
Congestive heart failure	2.9%	8.9%
Renal insufficiency	6.0%	5.4%
Dialysis required	NA*	0.6%
Pulmonary insufficiency	5.1%	8.4%
Ischemic colitis	1.1%	0.6%
Limb ischemia	NA	5.4%
Graft thrombosis	NA	0.9%
Wound infection	2.0%	2.0%
Graft infection	0.3%	0.2%
Stroke	0.9%	0.5%
Paraplegia	0	0.2%

NA, data not provided.

venous furosemide (20 to 40 mg) in addition to mannitol has been advocated, although its mechanism of action is less well understood. Tubular injury and disturbances in renal cortical blood flow distribution resulting from activation of the renin-angiotensin system have been implicated in postoperative renal failure.[139] It is sobering to realize that mortality in patients experiencing acute renal failure has not decreased despite the use of hemodialysis, which often serves only to prolong the time to death after this complication. Preoperative renal insufficiency is the only independent risk factor for postoperative acute renal failure;[139] therefore, maintenance of optimal hemodynamics is critical in these patients.

Gastrointestinal Complications

Some degree of bowel dysfunction occurs after any major abdominal procedure. However, the paralytic ileus that follows evisceration and dissection of the base of the mesentery for aneurysm repair often lasts much longer than that occurring after other procedures. Diarrhea may occur even when nasogastric drainage remains voluminous. Consequently, one must use caution in reinstituting oral feeding postoperatively. Dysmotility may be exacerbated by premature discontinuation of gastric decompression. Anorexia, periodic constipation, and diarrhea are commonly seen in the first few weeks following aneurysm surgery.

The most dreaded intestinal complication of aortic aneurysm surgery is "ischemic colitis," which usually involves the sigmoid colon and occurs in approximately 1 per cent of patients undergoing elective aneurysm repairs[11, 55, 107] (for detailed discussion see Chapter 99). Ischemic colitis is three to four times more common after emergent repair of ruptured aneurysm.[11] Although ligation of the inferior mesenteric artery can be a causative factor, interruption or significant occlusive disease of major collaterals, particularly in the superior mesenteric and hypogastric circulations, is usually present. The inferior mesenteric artery is often occluded as a consequence of the overlying mural thrombus within the aneurysms. Other contributing factors to ischemic colitis include postoperative colonic distention and reduced cardiac output. To avoid this complication one should preserve flow to at least one hypogastric artery[61] and avoid embolization into the hypogastric circulation. In addition, when backbleeding from a widely patent inferior mesenteric artery is minimal, reimplantation should be considered. When there is pulsatile backbleeding from the inferior mesenteric artery, it should be ligated from within the aneurysm as close to its origin as possible. Preoperative evidence of superior mesenteric artery occlusive disease may necessitate revascularization to avoid left colonic ischemia.

An excessive fluid requirement in the first 8 to 12 hours after abdominal aortic aneurysm repair may be the first indication of colonic ischemia. Subsequently, the appearance of bloody diarrhea, distention, signs of peritoneal irritation, unexplained fever, or leukocytosis should raise the suspicion of ischemic colitis. In this setting, colonoscopy is mandatory to establish the diagnosis of colonic ischemia and evaluate its extent. When present, mucosal changes are usually seen beginning 10 to 20 cm above the anal verge. In most cases, necrosis is limited to the mucosa; therefore, the management of this complication must be individualized. Bloody diarrhea *alone* is not an indication for laparotomy. If the necrosis is only mucosal and patchy, as is usually the case, spontaneous resolution is likely. Involvement of the muscular layers often leads to subsequent stricture that may require dilatation or resection at a later date. The development of strictures should be followed with serial barium enemas. The relatively benign course of many of these cases should not lead one to ignore persistent ileus, increasing abdominal tenderness, fever, leukocytosis, or signs of peritoneal irritation. In cases of full-thickness colonic necrosis, early operation is mandatory before massive contamination of the peritoneal cavity and the prosthesis occurs. Resection of the necrotic colon with a terminal descending colostomy, dependent pelvic drainage through the open rectal stump, and drainage of the iliac fossa through the flank are usually required because some degree of contamination is common. Primary anastomosis of the colon is not recommended.

Ureteral Injury

Ureteral injury is most common during emergency operation for a ruptured aneurysm. When this complication occurs during elective operations, the typical course of the ureter is usually distorted by the aneurysm or fibrosis and inflammation. In the latter case, a traction effect may draw the ureter much closer to the border of the aneurysm than normal, making this the most treacherous area for ureteral injury. The ureter is less likely to be injured in the location where one expects to encounter it while dissecting along the iliac arteries.

If injury occurs, it should be repaired immediately. A double-J stent should be inserted through the injury site to traverse the ureter from the renal pelvis to the urinary bladder. The ureter is then closed using 7–0 chromic sutures. Omentum can be mobilized on a vascular pedicle and wrapped around the site of injury. After copious irrigation, repair of the aneurysm can proceed. Early postoperative CT imaging is advised to detect possible urinoma formation. This is unlikely to occur if the stent is working properly, but if it does develop, percutaneous closed drainage can be instituted using CT or ultrasound guidance.

Embolization or Thrombosis of the Distal Arterial Tree

Acute arterial occlusion in one or both lower extremities can be a disastrous complication during aortic aneurysm repair. By carefully gaining both proximal and distal arterial control prior to manipulating the aneurysm itself, the likelihood of causing embolization of mural thrombus can be minimized. Avoidance of heparin anticoagulation during aneurysm repair, such as during emergency operations, can result in distal arterial thrombosis during the period of cross-clamping. In addition, thrombus formed above the proximal clamp can be flushed into the lower extremities when blood flow is restored. To minimize this possibility, flushing maneuvers should be performed prior to unclamping. Creation of an intimal flap from the arterial clamp that crushes the calcified plaque within the vessel is a common pitfall. If backbleeding is not present during flushing maneuvers, distal embolization or thrombosis may have occurred. Embolectomy or thrombectomy with a Fogarty balloon catheter should be attempted at this point but may be difficult because the iliac arteries are often tortuous (see Chapter 43).

Microembolization

Even when pedal pulses are palpable, microembolization can result in significant cutaneous necrosis. Sometimes termed "trash foot," microembolization can eventually result in persistent pain or skin loss, occasionally necessitating amputation. If recognized prior to closure of the abdomen, lumbar sympathectomy may be beneficial because it increases cutaneous circulation even in the area of ischemia (see Chapter 59). When microembolization is not discovered until after the patient has left the operating room, treatment should include the intravenous administration of 500 ml of low-molecular-weight dextran (Rheomacrodex-40 in 5 per cent dextrose in water) given over an 8- to 12-hour period. If extensive embolization causes tibial artery occlusion, thromboembolectomy should be performed.

Paraplegia

Paraplegia after thoracic aortic aneurysm repairs may occur in up to 16 per cent of cases.[191] This dreaded complication is rare after elective infrarenal aortic surgery, with reported incidences ranging from 0 to 0.9 per cent.[55, 82, 107, 153, 197] Spinal cord ischemia precipitates paraplegia. Important collateral vessels supporting flow to the anterior spinal artery, particularly the accessory spinal artery (the artery of Adamkewicz), arise from the descending thoracic or upper abdominal aorta. Occasionally, this critical collateral vessel or others may arise below the renal vessels as lumbar branches. Atherosclerotic disease of these vessels may contribute to ischemia of the spinal cord in conjunction with a low flow state and may lead to hypoperfusion or thrombosis. These factors are particularly important in the presence of a ruptured aneurysm with which paraplegia occurs up to 10 times more frequently than after elective operations.[197] Interestingly, paraplegia has been reported as the presenting symptom of infrarenal aortic aneurysm in several patients.[54, 109] This suggests that in some cases adequate blood supply to the lower spinal cord depends on collateral flow originating from the distal aorta, which may be occluded by aneurysmal thrombosis or mural thrombus. Recently, Picone and colleagues reported the occurrence of three cases of paraplegia following abdominal aortic aneurysm repair and four other cases after reconstruction for aortic occlusive disease.[153] Of these cases, five were associated with either the diminution or absence of *hypogastric artery perfusion*, underscoring the importance of these vessels. Fortunately, this complication is extremely unusual.

Infected Aortic Prosthesis

Infection of an aortic arterial prosthesis is one of the most dreadful complications of aortic aneurysm repair because the associated mortality rate varies from 25 to 50 per cent. The overall incidence of aortic graft infection following aneurysm repair ranges from 0.5 to 3 per cent,[55, 64, 107] with up to half of the cases occurring within 30 days. The incidence more than triples with ruptured aneurysms and is also increased when a groin incision is required. Because of the serious consequences, every effort must be made to avoid this complication. Prophylactic intravenous antibiotics are routinely given preoperatively and should be continued for the first 24 hours postoperatively. Intraoperative irrigation with an antibiotic-containing solution is usually performed. As previously noted, the predictive value of routine culture of intraluminal aneurysm contents is poor, and unless infection is strongly suspected at surgery, cultures are not recommended. To prevent the related complication of aortoenteric fistula, it is vital to separate the prosthesis from the overlying bowel. Reopposing the aneurysm wall and closing the parietal peritoneum is usually sufficient; however, in unusual cases a pedicle of omentum can be mobilized to provide complete coverage of the graft. The clinical presentation and management of aortoenteric fistulae are discussed in Chapter 38.

LATE COMPLICATIONS OF AORTIC ANEURYSM SURGERY

Late complications directly attributable to aortic aneurysm repair occur in approximately 10 per cent of patients.[94, 156] These complications primarily include anastomotic aneurysm (discussed in Chapter 37), aortoenteric fistula, and graft limb occlusion. As noted previously, graft infection may not become manifest until months or even years after implantation. Graft dilatation, reported mostly with knitted Dacron prostheses, can also occur.[53, 142] Usually graft dilatation is minimal; however, it may lead to graft disruption.[179]

Late occlusion of an aortoiliac Dacron prosthesis is less commonly associated with aneurysm repair than with bypass for aortic occlusive disease. Conversely, anastomotic aneurysms are a more common sequela of aneurysm repair. Plate and colleagues documented the occurrence of anastomotic aneurysms and late development of additional aneurysms (thoracic, thoracoabdominal, femoral) in 59 of 1017 patients (6 per cent) who were followed for 6 to 12 years after abdominal aneurysm repair.[156] Fourteen of these were anastomotic aneurysms. Patients with hypertension were three times more likely to develop additional aneurysms. In other series, the incidence of anastomotic aneurysms has ranged from 1 to 24 per cent.[53] Many of these complications remain asymptomatic until a sudden event such as rupture or embolization occurs. Consequently, careful follow-up with control of hypertension and periodic graft surveillance should be performed in all patients who undergo abdominal aortic aneurysm repair.

COMPLICATING PATHOLOGIC CONDITIONS

Horseshoe Kidney and Accessory Renal Arteries

Horseshoe kidney is uncommonly associated with aortic aneurysm. Although aortography reliably identifies horseshoe kidney, this study is not routinely obtained by all surgeons. Excretory urography is diagnostic in only half of cases. The predilection toward infection, stones, and hydronephrosis may have produced symptoms leading to previous diagnosis of this anomaly in many cases. Because ultrasonography and CT have become routine in the diagnostic evaluation of aortic aneurysms, unexpected discovery of horseshoe kidneys is unusual. Preoperative diagnosis mandates aortography to delineate the anomalous blood supply present in most cases.[181] Frequently, several renal arteries arise from the aneurysm or from the iliac arteries. In the event that horseshoe kidney is encountered unexpectedly, an intraoperative arteriogram may be helpful. A less desirable alternative is to open the aneurysm and gently probe the orifices within the aneurysm using palpation to determine the course of the vessels that supply the kidney.

Management of the multiple and anomalous renal arteries common with this condition is easier with the left retroperitoneal approach. However, with transperitoneal exposures the left colon and left portion of the horseshoe kidney can be mobilized and rotated medially, allowing opening of the aneurysm on its posterior aspect. In this way the graft can be placed, and the multiple accessory renal arteries can be implanted into the graft as one or more Carrel patches. It is almost never necessary to divide the isthmus or transverse portion of a horseshoe kidney. Preoperative recognition of horseshoe kidney also allows preparation for cold perfusion of the kidney during the period of interrupted blood flow.[99] Preoperative placement of ureteral stents may also be helpful in avoiding ureteral injury.

Inferior accessory renal arteries may be encountered independently or in association with horseshoe kidney. Rarely, accessory renal arteries may arise from the posterior aspect of the aorta, lending support to the argument of those who recommend routine preoperative aortography before undertaking aneurysm repair. The technique of preserving accessory renal arteries consists of excising them with a cuff of aorta and anastomosing this to the side of the graft, as described previously for the inferior mesenteric artery.

Associated Venous Anomalies

The complex embryologic development of major veins occasionally gives rise to anomalies that complicate aortic surgery. There are two significant variations of the inferior vena cava of which the surgeon should be aware.[8, 74] Duplication, or *double vena cava*, is present in 0.2 to 3.0 per cent of the population, and transposed or isolated *left-sided vena cava* has an incidence of 0.2 to 0.5 per cent. These variations can present technical problems that seriously complicate aortoiliac surgery. In addition to the large venous structures bordering the aorta on both sides, the surgeon should be aware that numerous retroaortic communications between the cavae may be present in a patient with double vena cava.[8] Injury to these communicating veins can produce severe hemorrhage. When left-sided vena cava occurs as an isolated condition without situs inversus, it presents technical problems because either the transposed inferior vena cava overlaps the infrarenal aorta obliquely, or the *right* renal vein crossing over the neck of the aneurysm is too short to retract. In addition, the overlapping positions of the iliac arteries and veins are reversed.[58] The proximal anastomosis may be done cephalad to the right renal vein; or if the vein has demonstrable adrenal or gonadal tributaries, it may be divided medially. If the vena cava does cross to the right near the upper part of the aneurysm, great care must be taken to avoid injuring it during maneuvers to isolate and cross-clamp the aneurysm neck.

Two anomalies of left renal venous drainage also present important technical considerations for abdominal aneurysm surgery. *Retroaortic left renal vein* is a rare anomaly, present in approximately 2 per cent of cases.[74] This may constitute the only venous drainage of the left kidney, or it may coexist with a normally positioned (anterior) left renal vein, a condition also known as *circumaortic venous ring*. The latter variation is more common and has a reported incidence of up to 6 per cent.[12, 25] Retroaortic left renal veins are well seen on CT scans[178] and should be suspected when the left renal vein is not readily visualized during routine dissection. Because of obvious exposure problems, injury to retroaortic renal veins can produce catastrophic hemorrhage requiring division of the infrarenal aorta. Circumaortic venous ring presents similar difficulties because the anterior component may be of normal size, leading to inadvertent injury of the unsuspected posterior component.[114]

Inflammatory Aneurysm

"Inflammatory" aortic aneurysms constitute approximately 5 per cent of all cases of infrarenal aortic aneurysms.[43, 78, 152, 210] Macroscopically, these aneurysms are obvious at operation because they are characterized by a translucent white appearance, marked thickness of the aortic wall, and a dense perianeurysmal fibrotic reaction in the retroperitoneum that incorporates adjacent structures. The latter feature involves the fourth part of the duodenum in over 90 per cent of cases. The inferior vena cava and left renal vein are adherent to the inflammatory aneurysmal mass in more than half the cases, and to the ureters in one quarter. Histopathologically, the media and adventitia show infiltration of inflammatory cells of variable intensity which is usually most prominent in the adventitia.

The etiology of inflammatory aneurysm remains unclear. However, because aneurysm repair usually is accompanied by resolution of the inflammation, the inflammatory process may be a response to the aneurysm rather than the aneurysm forming as a result of the inflammation. Mild chronic inflammation is often present in the walls of typical degenerative aneurysms.[112, 151, 167] Sterpetti and coworkers have suggested that inflammatory aneurysms may simply reflect an unusual accentuation of this reaction.[185] These authors postulate that aneurysm expansion may compress the lymphatic network along the anterolateral surface of the aorta, leading to stasis, edema, and secondary fibrosis. The observation that the posterior wall of the aorta, where the lymphatics are minimal or absent, is relatively uninvolved in the inflammatory process lends support to this hypothesis. Another possible cause is autoimmune disease. Less likely causes are infection and reaction to extravasated blood from chronic contained rupture.

Although inflammatory aneurysm may be a variant of degenerative aneurysm, it is a distinct clinical entity. In contrast to typical degenerative aneurysms, rupture of inflammatory aneurysms is less common. This fact may reflect a "protective" effect of the increased wall thickness and surrounding fibrosis. However, because more than two thirds of these patients present with clinical symptoms referable to their aneurysm,[152, 185] the lower rate of rupture may be due to increased detection and operative treatment. Abdominal pain or back pain is present in most patients with inflammatory aneurysms,[43, 78, 152] and many patients also present with weight loss. The erythrocyte sedimentation rate (ESR) is elevated in 75 per cent of cases, whereas only 30 per cent of patients with simple degenerative aneurysms have an elevated ESR. The triad of abdominal pain, weight loss, and elevated ESR in a patient with an aneurysm suggests the presence of an inflammatory aneurysm. However, this complete triad is present in only about 15 per cent of cases. Not surprisingly, symptoms from inflammatory aneurysms are often mistaken for acute rupture or dissection.

The preoperative diagnosis of inflammatory aneurysm is most readily made with CT, which typically reveals a four-layered appearance in the aneurysm that includes the innermost lumen, a mural thrombus, a thickened aortic wall, and a surrounding soft tissue density that enhances uniformly with contrast administration (Fig. 75–10).[47] MRI also accurately establishes the diagnosis. Ultrasonography, however, is less sensitive, and angiography is not useful. Excretory urography may suggest inflammatory aneurysm when the ureters are displaced or obstructed; however, this feature is present in fewer than half of all cases.

Treatment with steroids resolves the inflammatory response in some patients.[9, 85] Surgical therapy remains the only definitive treatment, however, because rupture following chronic steroid administration has been reported in several series.[78, 152] In general, steroids should be given only for treatment of associated urinary complications of perianeurysmal fibrosis. The effectiveness of this treatment is well established for idiopathic retroperitoneal fibrosis, a pathologically similar entity.

The perioperative mortality of inflammatory aneurysm repair in earlier series was higher than that for typical degenerative aneurysms, largely because adjacent adherent structures were injured. In addition, optimal preoperative preparation in patients with symptoms mimicking rupture often is not performed, contributing to increased mortality. Modifications of operative technique should include avoiding dissection of the duodenum, inferior vena cava, and left renal vein away from the aneurysm, which reduces operative mortality to levels nearing those achieved with routine aneurysm repair. Some surgeons advocate preoperative placement of stents to aid in identification of the ureters and the avoidance of injuries. Gaining infrarenal aortic control may prove difficult and hazardous. Suprarenal aortic control, obtained in the space between the left renal vein and the pancreas, requires care but is safer than attempting control below the renal arteries. Crawford and associates recommend supraceliac cross-clamping of the aorta, which minimizes the need for infrarenal dissection.[43] After the aorta is controlled, the aneurysm should be opened lateral to the duodenum without attempting to free the duodenum from the aneurysm. Ureterolysis should be performed only if there are symptoms or clear radiologic findings of obstruction. In recent years many authorities have adopted the retroperitoneal approach as the technique of choice when the diagnosis of inflammatory aneurysm has been established preoperatively.[66, 137] This technique avoids much of the perianeurysmal fibrotic reaction by approaching the aneurysm from its posterolateral aspect. Furthermore, the retroperitoneal approach offers easier access to the aorta both above and below the renal arteries. Nevertheless, because this entity is occasionally encountered unexpectedly, all surgeons who operate on aneurysms should be prepared to handle inflammatory aneurysms by the transperitoneal approach.

Incidental Procedures

Any procedure that could potentially contaminate the prosthesis, such as appendectomy or colotomy with polypectomy, should be avoided. Occasionally, a brief "clean" procedure that will be required eventually, such as ovarian cystectomy, can be performed. Vagotomy or any procedure that might compound the intestinal motility problems commonly associated with aneurysm repair should not be performed. Cholecystectomy can be performed concurrently,[146, 188] however, a substantial percentage of bile cultures from patients with asymptomatic cholelithiasis are positive. Thus, the potential for development of graft infection with its disastrous consequences argues against combined cholecystectomy in elective procedures.[70] When performed, any such additional procedure should be done after

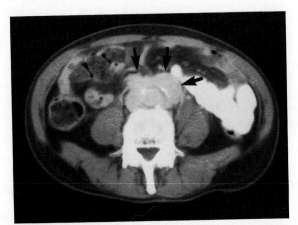

FIGURE 75–10. Computed tomographic scan of the abdomen of a patient with an inflammatory aneurysm. *Arrows* mark the thickened inflammatory tissue around the aorta.

the aneurysm is repaired and the retroperitoneal closure is complete, provided the patient's condition remains stable.

Associated Abdominal Malignancy

Occasionally a malignancy may be discovered unexpectedly during surgery for an aortic aneurysm. In a series of 803 aneurysm repairs, Szilagyi and colleagues reported that 4 per cent of patients harbored a concurrent intra-abdominal malignancy.[194] The most common malignancy encountered in conjunction with aortic aneurysm is carcinoma of the colon, which was present in 2 per cent of Szilagyi's patients. Concomitant malignancy is more likely to occur in the subset of aneurysm patients who present with abdominal pain. Therefore, because aneurysms are now more commonly discovered when they are small and asymptomatic, the prevalence of concurrent malignancy is probably lower than that reported in older studies.

Because malignancy and aneurysm each carry significant threat to life, their simultaneous presence can present a dilemma. Therefore, a careful assessment of each disorder is required. If widely metastatic disease is present and the associated life expectancy is short, aneurysm repair is precluded unless the aneurysm is very large, symptomatic, or ruptured. In general, each condition should be definitively treated at the initial operation according to its presentation. For example, rupture or acute occlusion would necessitate aneurysm repair, whereas hemorrhage, perforation, or obstruction by a tumor would dictate excision or intestinal bypass. In the absence of absolute indications, the aneurysm usually takes precedence because elective aneurysm repair can generally be accomplished with low mortality and minimal sequelae. The malignancy can then be resected at a second operation in 2 to 3 weeks. Conversely, if a malignancy such as colon carcinoma were resected initially, local septic complications may preclude aneurysm repair for weeks or months thereafter. The risk of graft infection for a subsequent elective or emergent repair may then be increased. Simultaneous resection of colon carcinoma and aneurysm repair should be avoided because of the risk of graft contamination. If a bowel resection is required at the initial operation and a septic complication occurs, subsequent aneurysm repair can usually be accomplished by the retroperitoneal approach, thereby avoiding a potentially hostile abdomen.

A retroperitoneal tumor such as a renal malignancy in close association with an aneurysm may present additional complicating factors. Operation for either condition may induce significant scar formation, making subsequent surgery for the other much more difficult. When the gastrointestinal tract is not involved, the risk of graft contamination is much lower with a concomitant operation. In the case of renal cell carcinoma, both conditions are usually known in advance, offering the opportunity to assess the relative threat to life of each condition. Simultaneous nephrectomy for renal malignancy and aneurysm repair should be considered in a patient who is in good general condition, has a large or symptomatic aneurysm, and has an opportunity for long-term survival.[10] Interestingly, despite the potential for contamination from the urinary tract, no reports of graft infection associated with simultaneous aneurysm repair and nephrectomy have been reported. However, the incidence of postoperative renal failure is reportedly increased; consequently, careful preoperative evaluation of renal function is necessary.[20]

As mentioned previously, the potentially increased risk of aneurysm rupture after a prior unrelated operation is based largely on anecdotal reports. Careful monitoring of an aneurysm is warranted, but this consideration should not play a decisive role in the selection of surgical priorities for aneurysm and concurrent disease.

FUTURE THERAPEUTIC OPTIONS FOR ABDOMINAL AORTIC ANEURYSM

Recently, the concept of "repairing" abdominal aortic aneurysms with an endoprosthesis introduced into the aorta through the femoral or external iliac arteries has quickly progressed to early clinical trials. At this writing, three different groups have developed delivery systems with actual or potential clinical applicability, and a number of other devices are in the design phase. After initial success in animals,[115] Parodi of Argentina and his group were the first investigators to apply this technique in humans using a device consisting of a compliant Dacron prosthesis attached to a Palmaz stent.[149] Introduced through an external iliac artery via a groin incision, the device is deployed in the neck of the aneurysm by balloon inflation, much as the Palmaz stent itself is expanded. After arterial inflow unfurls the graft, the distal end of the prosthesis is fixed at the bifurcation by a second stent. This approach has been applied in "close to 30 patients" at this writing. As yet, however, only anecdotal reports have been presented at professional meetings, and no objective data have been published.

In contrast to this straight graft, an endovascular bifurcated Dacron graft requiring a flexible 16- to 18-Fr introducer has been developed by Chuter and associates at the University of Rochester. It requires bilateral femoral artery exposure and has been successfully tested in canine experiments. Clinical trials are imminent.

A third endoprosthesis, the EVT endograft (Endovascular Technologies, Menlo Park, CA), has been developed. This device employs a spiked stent proximally and distally for better fixation. Lazarus initially tested this prosthesis in acute and chronic experiments in sheep.[116] Both straight and bifurcation models have been developed. These woven Dacron grafts are deployed by a sophisticated delivery system that requires a carrier measuring only 22 Fr. The EVT straight endograft is currently undergoing evaluation in a phase I clinical trial that is half completed at this writing. Subsequently, a prospective randomized multi-center phase II trial will compare the results of endoprosthesis repair with surgical repair for abdominal aortic aneurysms.

The need for a bifurcated prosthesis in addition to a straight graft was recently underscored in a report by Chuter and colleagues in which three-dimensional CT scanning was used to study aortic aneurysm dimensions and morphology in 22 patients.[33] Straight grafts appear feasible in only a minority of patients. For example, only 1 of 22 patients had a 2-cm distal aortic cuff. In contrast, a bifurcation graft was deemed feasible in 18 of 22 patients based on measurements of the proximal aortic neck and distal iliac cuffs. Equally important, roughly 1 in 3 aortic aneurysms were associated with iliac aneurysms, and 1 in 3 had severe posterior or lateral iliac angulation at the bifurcation. Additionally, 1 in 5 had very significant anterior or lateral proximal angulation at the neck, and 1 in 5 had more than a 5-mm difference between the diameters of the proximal neck and the distal aortic cuff. Wide application of endovascular grafts for aortic aneurysms faces the additional problems of (1) excluding important patent side branches (e.g., inferior mesenteric, aberrant renal or internal iliac arteries), (2) maneuvering through mural thrombus and avoiding embolism, (3) dealing with smaller than normal iliac arteries (9 to 10-mm diameter needed for passage), and (4) attaching the device securely to heavily calcified plaques at the proximal neck or distal cuff. Furthermore, the necessary manipulations may not be straightforward and will require considerable skill in endovascular techniques. Although these issues may initially limit this approach to carefully selected patients, the technology is likely to improve, considering the *potential* for cost savings (reduced intensive care unit and hospital stays), lower morbidity and mortality (particularly in high-risk patients), and decreased time to the return of normal activity compared with conventional repair. Assuming this technique proves safe and technically feasible, long-term studies will be necessary to ensure that no significant migration of the endoprosthesis occurs with time. A significant failure rate requiring subsequent surgery would negate the potential benefits of aortic endoprostheses. In the best scenario, low risk, durability, decreased morbidity, and reduced costs would ultimately demand wider application and extension to smaller aneurysms, for which one would otherwise not be able to justify surgical repair on the basis of a risk:benefit analysis. Future developments should prove interesting.

References

1. AbuRahma AF, Robinson PA, Boland JP, et al: Elective resection of 332 abdominal aortic aneurysms in a southern West Virginia community during a recent 5-year period. Surgery 109:244, 1991.
2. Allardice JT, Allwright GJ, Wafula JMC, et al: High prevalence of abdominal aortic aneurysm in men with peripheral vascular disease: Screening by ultrasound. Br J Surg 75:240, 1988.
3. Amundsen S, Skjaerven R, Trippestad A, et al: Abdominal aortic aneurysms. Is there an association between surgical volume, surgical experience, hospital type and operative mortality? Acta Chir Scand 156:323, 1990.
4. Andersen JC, Sjolin SU, Holstein P: Ligation of the renal vein during resection of abdominal aortic aneurysm. J Cardiovasc Surg (Torino) 27:454, 1986.
5. Auerbach O, Garfinkel L: Atherosclerosis and aneurysm of aorta in relation to smoking and age. Chest 78:805, 1980.
6. Baird RJ, Gurry JF, Kellam JF, et al: Abdominal aortic aneurysms: Recent experience with 210 patients. Can Med Assoc J 118:1229, 1978.
7. Bandyk DF: Preoperative imaging of aortic aneurysms. Surg Clin North Am 69:721, 1989.
8. Bartle EJ, Pearce WH, Sun JH, et al: Infrarenal venous anomalies and aortic surgery. J Vasc Surg 6:590, 1987.
9. Baskerville PA, Blakeney CG, Young AE, et al: The diagnosis and treatment of periaortic fibrosis ("inflammatory" aneurysms). Br J Surg 70:381, 1983.
10. Baskin LS, McClure RD, Rapp JH, et al: Simultaneous resection of renal cell carcinoma and abdominal aortic aneurysm. Ann Vasc Surg 5:363, 1991.
11. Bast TJ, van der Biezen JJ, Scherpenisse J, et al: Ischaemic disease of the colon and rectum after surgery for abdominal aortic aneurysm: A prospective study of the incidence and risk. Eur J Vasc Surg 4:253, 1990.
12. Beckman CF, Abrams HL: Circumaortic venous ring: Incidence and significance. Am J Radiol 132:561, 1979.
13. Bengtsson H, Ekberg O, Aspelin P, et al: Ultrasound screening of the abdominal aorta in patients with intermittent claudication. Eur J Vasc Surg 3:497, 1989.
14. Bengtsson H, Norrgard O, Angquist KA, et al: Ultrasonographic screening of the abdominal aorta among siblings with abdominal aortic aneurysms. Br J Surg 76:589, 1989.
15. Bergeur R, Schneider J, Wilner HI: Induced thrombosis of inoperable abdominal aortic aneurysm. Surgery 84:425, 1978.
16. Bernstein EF, Chan EL: Abdominal aortic aneurysms in high risk patients: Outcome of selective management based on size and expansion rate. Ann Surg 200:255, 1984.
17. Bernstein EF, Dilley RB, Goldberger LE, et al: Growth rates of small abdominal aortic aneurysms. Surgery 80:765, 1976.
18. Bernstein EF, Dilley RB, Randolph HF: The improving outlook for patients over seventy years of age with abdominal aortic aneurysms. Ann Surg 207:318, 1988.
19. Berridge DC, Griffith CPM, Amar SS, et al: Screening for clinically unsuspected abdominal aortic aneurysms in patients with peripheral vascular disease. Eur J Vasc Surg 3:421, 1989.
20. Bickerstaff LK, Hollier LH, Van Peenen HJ: Abdominal aortic aneurysm repair combined with a second surgical procedure: Morbidity and mortality. Surgery 95:487, 1984.
21. Bickerstaff LK, Hollier LH, Van Peenen HJ, et al: Abdominal aortic aneurysms: The changing natural history. J Vasc Surg 1:6, 1984.
22. Blaisdell FW, Hall AD, Thomas AN: Ligation treatment of abdominal aortic aneurysm. Am J Surg 109:560, 1965.
23. Blombery PA, Ferguson IA, Rosengarten DS, et al: The role of coronary artery disease in complications of abdominal aortic aneurysm surgery. Surgery 101:150, 1987.
24. Branchereau A, Nazet J, Colavolpe JC, et al: Combined morbidity and mortality of direct surgical treatment of abdominal aortic aneurysm. Ann Vasc Surg 4:10, 1990.
25. Brener BJ, Darling C, Frederick PL, et al: Major venous anomalies complicating abdominal aortic surgery. Arch Surg 108:160, 1974.
26. Brown OW, Hollier LH, Pairolero PC, et al: Abdominal aortic aneurysm and coronary artery disease. Arch Surg 116:1484, 1981.
27. Brown PM, Pattenden R, Gutelius JR: The selective management of small abdominal aortic aneurysms: The Kingston study. J Vasc Surg 15:21, 1992.
28. Buckels JAC, Fielding JWL, Black J, et al: Significance of positive cultures from aortic aneurysm contents. Br J Surg 72:440, 1985.
29. Cabellon S, Moncrief CL, Pierre DL, et al: Incidence of abdominal aortic aneurysm in patients with atheromatous arterial disease. Am J Surg 146:575, 1983.
30. Cambria RP, Brewster DC, Abbott WM, et al: Transperitoneal versus retroperitoneal approach for aortic reconstruction: A randomized prospective study. J Vasc Surg 11:314, 1990.
31. Cannon DJ, Read RC: Abdominal aortic aneurysm, Leriche's syndrome, inguinal herniation, and smoking. Arch Surg 119:387, 1984.
32. Carty GA, Nachtigal T, Magyar R, et al: Abdominal duplex ultrasound screening for occult aortic aneurysm during carotid arterial evaluation. J Vasc Surg 17:696, 1993.
33. Chuter T, Green RM, Ouriel K, et al: Infrarenal aortic aneurysm morphology: Implications for transfemoral repair. Presented at the International Society for Cardiovascular Surgery, Washington, D.C., June 7–8, 1993 (In press).
34. Clark ET, Gewertz BL, Bassiouny HS, et al: Current results of elective aortic reconstruction for aneurysmal and occlusive disease. J Cardiovasc Surg (Torino) 31:438, 1990.
35. Cohen JR, Graver LM: The ruptured abdominal aortic aneurysm of Albert Einstein. Surg Obstet Gynecol 170:455, 1990.
36. Cohen JR, Mandell C, Chang JB, et al: Elastin metabolism of the infrarenal aorta. J Vasc Surg 7:210, 1988.
37. Collin J, Araujo L, Lindsell D: Screening for abdominal aortic aneurysms. Lancet 2:736, 1987.
38. Collin J, Araujo L, Lindsell D: Oxford screening programme for abdominal aortic aneurysm in men aged 65 to 74 years. Lancet 2:613, 1988.

39. Collin J, Araujo L, Walton J: How fast do very small aneurysms grow? Eur J Vasc Surg 3:15, 1989.

40. Collin J, Araujo L, Walton J: A community detection program for abdominal aortic aneurysm. Angiology 41:53, 1990.

41. Collin J, Heather B, Walton J: Growth rates of subclinical abdominal aortic aneurysms—Implications for review and rescreening programmes. Eur J Vasc Surg 5:141, 1991.

42. Crawford ES, Saleh SA, Babb JW, et al: Infrarenal abdominal aortic aneurysm: Factors influencing survival after operation over a 25-year period. Ann Surg 193:699, 1981.

43. Crawford JL, Stowe CL, Safi HJ, et al: Inflammatory aneurysms of the aorta. J Vasc Surg 2:113, 1985.

44. Creech O Jr.: Endo-aneurysmorrhaphy and treatment of aortic aneurysm. Ann Surg 164:935, 1966.

45. Cronenwett JL, Murphy TE, Zelenock GB, et al: Actuarial analysis of variables associated with rupture of small abdominal aortic aneurysms. Surgery 98:472, 1985.

46. Cronenwett JL, Sargent SK, Wall MH, et al: Variables that affect the expansion rate and outcome of small abdominal aortic aneurysms. J Vasc Surg 11:260, 1990.

47. Cullenward MJ, Scanlan KA, Pozniak MA, et al: Inflammatory aortic aneurysm (periaortic fibrosis): Radiologic imaging. Radiology 159:75, 1986.

48. Darling RC: Ruptured arteriosclerotic abdominal aortic aneurysms. Am J Surg 119:397, 1970.

49. Darling RC, Brewster DC: Elective treatment of abdominal aortic aneurysm. World J Surg 4:661, 1980.

50. Darling RC, Messina CR, Brewster DC, et al: Autopsy study of unoperated abdominal aortic aneurysms. Circulation 56 (Suppl 2):II–161, 1977.

51. Davidson BR, Gardham R: Selective use of the right retroperitoneal approach to abdominal aortic aneurysm. Br J Surg 79:639, 1992.

52. DeBakey ME, Crawford ES, Cooley DA, et al: Aneurysm of abdominal aorta: Analysis of results of graft replacement therapy one to eleven years after operation. Ann Surg 160:622, 1964.

53. den Hoed PT, Veen HF: The late complications of aorto-ilio-femoral Dacron prostheses: Dilatation and anastomotic aneurysm formation. Eur J Vasc Surg 6:282, 1992.

54. Desai HB, Ralput AH, Uitti RJ: Recurrent spinal cord ischemia due to abdominal aortic aneurysm—a case report. Angiology 40:682, 1989.

55. Diehl JT, Cali RF, Hertzer NR, et al: Complications of abdominal aortic reconstruction: An analysis of perioperative risk factors in 557 patients. Ann Surg 197:49, 1983.

56. Drott C, Arfvidsson B, Ortenwall P, et al: Age-standardized incidence of ruptured aortic aneurysm in a defined Swedish population between 1952 and 1988: Mortality rate and operative results. Br J Surg 79:175, 1992.

57. Dubost C, Allary M, Oeconomos N: Resection of an aneurysm of the abdominal aorta: Reestablishment of the continuity by a preserved arterial graft, with result after five months. Arch Surg 64:405, 1952.

58. Dupont JR: Isolated left-sided vena cava and abdominal aortic aneurysm. Arch Surg 102:211, 1971.

59. Durham SJ, Steed DL, Moosa HH, et al: Probability of rupture of an abdominal aortic aneurysm after an unrelated operative procedure: A prospective study. J Vasc Surg 13:248, 1991.

60. Eriksson I, Forsberg O, Lundqvist B, et al: Significance of positive bacterial cultures from aortic aneurysms. Acta Chir Scand 149:33, 1983.

61. Ernst CB: Prevention of intestinal ischemia following abdominal aortic reconstruction. Surgery 93:102, 1983.

62. Ernst CB, Hagihara PF, Daugherty ME, et al: Inferior mesenteric artery stump pressure: A reliable index for safe IMA ligation during abdominal aneurysmectomy. Ann Surg 187:641, 1978.

63. Estes E: Abdominal aortic aneurysm: A study of one hundred and two cases. Circulation 2:258, 1950.

64. Farkas J, Fichelle J, Laurian C, et al: Long-term followup of positive cultures in 500 abdominal aortic aneurysms. Arch Surg 128:284, 1993.

65. Fielding JWL, Black J, Ashton F, et al: Diagnosis and management of 528 abdominal aortic aneurysms. Br Med J 283:355, 1981.

66. Fiorani P, Faraglia V, Speziale F, et al: Extraperitoneal approach for repair of inflammatory abdominal aortic aneurysm. J Vasc Surg 13:692, 1991.

67. Flannigan DP, Quinn T, Kraft RO: Selective management of high risk patients with an abdominal aortic aneurysm. Surg Gynecol Obstet 150:171, 1980.

68. Foster JH, Bolasny BL, Gobbel WG, et al: Comparative study of elective resection and expectant treatment of abdominal aortic aneurysm. Surg Gynecol Obstet 129:1, 1969.

69. Fowkes FGR, Macintyre CCA, Ruckley CV: Increasing incidence of aneurysms in England and Wales. Br Med J 298:33, 1989.

70. Fry RE, Fry WJ: Cholelithiasis and aortic reconstruction: The problem of simultaneous therapy. J Vasc Surg 4:345, 1986.

71. Galland RB, Simmons MJ, Torrie EP: Prevalence of abdominal aortic aneurysm in patients with occlusive peripheral vascular disease. Br J Surg 78:1259, 1991.

72. Gewertz BL, Kremser PC, Zarins CK, et al: Transesophageal echocardiographic monitoring of myocardial ischemia during vascular surgery. J Vasc Surg 5:607, 1987.

73. Gilling-Smith GL, Mansfield AO: Spontaneous abdominal arteriovenous fistulae: Report of eight cases and review of the literature. Br J Surg 78:421, 1991.

74. Giordano JM, Trout HH: Anomalies of the inferior vena cava. J Vasc Surg 3:924, 1986.

75. Glimaker H, Holmberg L, Elvin A, et al: Natural history of patients with abdominal aortic aneurysm. Eur J Vasc Surg 5:125, 1991.

76. Gloviczki P, Pairolero PC, Mucha P, et al: Ruptured abdominal aortic aneurysms: Repair should not be denied. J Vasc Surg 15:851, 1992.

77. Golden MA, Whittemore AD, Donaldson MC, et al: Selective evaluation and management of coronary artery disease in patients undergoing repair of abdominal aortic aneurysm. Ann Surg 212:415, 1990.

78. Goldstone J, Malone JM, Moore WS: Inflammatory aneurysms of the aorta. Surgery 83:425, 1978.

79. Gomes MN, Choyke PL: Improved identification of renal arteries in patients with aortic aneurysms by means of high resolution computed tomography. J Vasc Surg 6:262, 1987.

80. Gomes MN, Choyke PL: Preoperative evaluation of abdominal aortic aneurysms: Ultrasound or computed tomography? J Cardiovasc Surg 28:159, 1987.

81. Guirguis EM, Barber GG: The natural history of abdominal aortic aneurysms. Am J Surg 162:481, 1991.

82. Hands LJ, Collin J, Lamont P: Observed incidence of paraplegia after infrarenal aortic aneurysm repair. Br J Surg 78:999, 1991.

83. Harris KA, Ameli FM, Lally M, et al: Abdominal aortic aneurysm resection in patients more than 80 years old. Surg Gynecol Obstet 162:536, 1986.

84. Harris LM, Faggioli GL, Fiedler R, et al: Ruptured abdominal aortic aneurysms: Factors affecting mortality rates. J Vasc Surg 14:812, 1991.

85. Hedges AR, Bentley PG: Resection of inflammatory aneurysm after steroid therapy. Br J Surg 73:374, 1986.

86. Henry LG, Doust B, Korns ME, et al: Abdominal aortic aneurysms and retroperitoneal fibrosis. Arch Surg 113:1456, 1978.

87. Hertzer NR: Fatal myocardial infarction following abdominal aortic aneurysm resection. Ann Surg 192:667, 1980.

88. Hertzer NR, Avellone JC, Farrell CJ, et al: The risk of vascular surgery in a metropolitan community. J Vasc Surg 1:13, 1984.

89. Hertzer NR, Beven EG, Young JR, et al: Coronary artery disease in peripheral vascular patients. Ann Surg 199:223, 1984.

90. Hertzer NR, Young JR, Beven EG, et al: Late results of coronary bypass in patients with infrarenal aortic aneurysms. Ann Surg 205:360, 1987.

91. Hertzer NR, Young JR, Kramer RJ, et al: Routine coronary angiography prior to elective aortic reconstruction. Arch Surg 114:1336, 1979.

92. Hicks GL, Eastland MW, DeWeese JA, et al: Surgical improvement following aortic aneurysm resection. Ann Surg 181:863, 1975.

93. Hobson RW, Wright CB, Rich NP, et al: Assessment of colonic ischemia during aortic surgery by Doppler ultrasound. J Surg Res 20:231, 1976.

94. Hollier LH, Plate G, O'Brien PC, et al: Late survival after abdominal aortic aneurysm repair: Influence of coronary artery disease. J Vasc Surg 1:290, 1984.

95. Hollier LH, Reigel MM, Kazmier FJ, et al: Conventional repair of abdominal aortic aneurysm in the high-risk patient: A plea for abandonment of nonresective treatment. J Vasc Surg 3:712, 1986.

96. Hollier LH, Spittell JA, Gloviczki P, et al: Arteriomegaly: Classification and morbid implications of diffuse aneurysmal disease. Surgery 93:700, 1983.

97. Hollier LH, Spittell JA, Puga FJ: Intra-aortic balloon counterpulsation as adjunct to aneurysmectomy in high-risk patients. Mayo Clin Proc 56:565, 1981.

98. Hollier LH, Taylor LM, Oschner J: Recommended indications for operative treatment of abdominal aortic aneurysms. J Vasc Surg 15:1046, 1992.

99. Hollis HW, Rutherford RB: Abdominal aortic aneurysms associated with horseshoe or ectopic kidneys. Techniques of renal preservation. Semin Vasc Surg 1:148, 1988.

100. Inahara T, Geary GL, Mukherjee D, et al: The contrary position to the nonresective treatment for abdominal aortic aneurysm. J Vasc Surg 2:42, 1985.

101. Johannsen G, Nydahl S, Olofsson P, et al: Survival in patients with abdominal aortic aneurysms: Comparison between operative and nonoperative management. Eur J Vasc Surg 4:497, 1990.

102. Johansen K: Treatment options for aneurysm in high-risk patients. Surg Clin North Am 69:765, 1989.

103. Johansen K, Koepsell T: Familial tendency for abdominal aortic aneurysms. JAMA 256:1934, 1986.

104. Johansen KJ, Kohler TR, Nicholls SC, et al: Ruptured abdominal aortic aneurysm: The Harborview experience. J Vasc Surg 13:240, 1991.

105. Johnson G, McDevitt NB, Procter HJ, et al: Emergent or elective operation for symptomatic abdominal aortic aneurysm. Arch Surg 115:51, 1980.

106. Johnson JN, McLoughlin GA, Wahe PE, et al: Comparison of extraperitoneal and transperitoneal methods of aorto-iliac reconstruction. J Cardiovasc Surg 27:561, 1986.

107. Johnston KW: Multicenter prospective study of nonruptured abdominal aortic aneurysms. II. Variables predicting morbidity and mortality. J Vasc Surg 9:437, 1989.

108. Johnston KW, Scobie TK: Multicenter prospective study of nonruptured abdominal aortic aneurysms. I. Population and operative management. J Vasc Surg 7:69, 1988.

109. Joseph MG, Langsfeld MA, Lusby RJ: Infrarenal aortic aneurysm: Unusual cause of paraparesis. Aust NZ J Surg 59:743, 1989.

110. Karmody AM, Leather RP, Goldman M, et al: The current position of non-resective treatment for abdominal aortic aneurysm. Surgery 94:591, 1983.

111. Katz DA, Littenberg B, Cronenwett JL: Management of small abdominal aortic aneurysms: Early surgery vs watchful waiting. JAMA 268:2678, 1992.

112. Koch AE, Haines GK, Rizzo RJ, et al: Human abdominal aortic aneurysms immunophenotypic analysis suggesting an immune-mediated response. Am J Pathol 137:1199, 1990.

113. Krupski WC, Bass A, Thurston DW, et al: Utility of computed tomography for surveillance of small abdominal aortic aneurysms. Arch Surg 125:1345, 1990.

114. Kunkel JM, Weinstein ES: Preoperative detection of potential hazards in aortic surgery. Perspect Vasc Surg 2:1, 1989.

115. Laborde JC, Parodi JC, Clem MF, et al: Intraluminal bypass of abdominal aortic aneurysm: Feasibility study. Radiology 184:185, 1992.

116. Lazarus HM: Endovascular grafting for the treatment of abdominal aortic aneurysms. Surg Clin North Am 72:959, 1992.

117. Leather RP, Shah CM, Faufman JL, et al: Comparative analysis of retroperitoneal and transperitoneal aortic replacement for aneurysm. Surg Gynecol Obstet 168:387, 1989.

118. Lederle FA: Management of small abdominal aortic aneurysms. Ann Intern Med 113:731, 1990.

119. Lederle FA, Walker JM, Reinke DB: Selective screening for abdominal aortic aneurysms with physical examination and ultrasound. Arch Intern Med 148:1753, 1988.

120. Leonardo RA: History of Surgery. New York, Froben Press, 1943.

121. Lette J, Waters D, Lassonde J, et al: Multivariate clinical models and quantitative dipyridamole-thallium imaging to predict cardiac morbidity and death after vascular reconstruction. J Vasc Surg 14:160, 1991.

122. Lilienfield DE, Gunderson PD, Sprafka JM, et al: Epidemiology of aortic aneurysms: 1. Mortality trends in the United States. Arteriosclerosis 7:637, 1987.

123. Limet R, Sakalihassan N, Albert A: Determination of the expansion rate and incidence of rupture of abdominal aortic aneurysms. J Vasc Surg 14:540, 1991.

124. Littooy FN, Steffan G, Greisler HP, et al: Use of sequential B-mode ultrasonography to manage abdominal aortic aneurysms. Arch Surg 124:419, 1989.

125. London MJ, Tubau JJF, Wong MG, et al: The "natural history" of segmental wall motion abnormalities in patients undergoing noncardiac surgery. Anesthesiology 73:644, 1990.

126. Lord RSA, Nash PA, Raj PT, et al: Prospective randomized trial of polytetrafluoroethylene and Dacron aortic prosthesis. I. Perioperative results. Ann Vasc Surg 3:248, 1988.

127. Lynch K, Kohler T, Johansen K: Nonresective therapy for aortic aneurysm: Results of a survey. J Vasc Surg 4:469, 1986.

128. Marston WA, Ahlquist R, Johnson G, et al: Misdiagnosis of ruptured abdominal aortic aneurysm. J Vasc Surg 16:17, 1992.

129. Matas R: Ligation of the abdominal aorta: Report of the ultimate result, one year, five months and nine days after the ligation of the abdominal aorta for aneurysm of the bifurcation. Ann Surg 81:457, 1925.

130. Matsuoka H, Shigematsu Y, Ohtani T, et al: Analysis of bloodflow patterns in aortic aneurysm by cine magnetic resonance imaging—A review of case material. Angiology 43:181, 1992.

131. McAuley CE, Steed DL, Webster MW: Bacterial presence in aortic thrombus at elective aneurysm resection: Is it clinically significant? Am J Surg 147:322, 1984.

132. McCabe CJ, Coleman WS, Brewster DC: The advantage of early operation for abdominal aortic aneurysm. Arch Surg 116:1025, 1981.

133. McCollum CH, Garcia-Rinaldi R, Graham JM, et al: Myocardial revascularization prior to subsequent major surgery in patients with coronary artery disease. Surgery 81:302, 1978.

134. Melton LJ, Bickerstaff LK, Hollier LH, et al: Changing incidence of abdominal aortic aneurysms: A population-based study. Am J Epidemiol 120:379, 1984.

135. Menashi S, Campa JS, Greenhalgh RM, et al: Collagen in abdominal aortic aneurysm: Typing, content, and degradation. J Vasc Surg 6:578, 1987.

136. Mesh CL, Baxter BT, Pearce WH, et al: Collagen and elastin gene expression in aortic aneurysms. Surgery 112:256, 1992.

137. Metcalf RK, Rutherford RB: Inflammatory abdominal aortic aneurysm: An indication for the retroperitoneal approach. Surgery 109:555, 1991.

138. Michaels JA: The management of small abdominal aortic aneurysms: A computer simulation using Monte Carlo methods. Eur J Vasc Surg 6:551, 1992.

139. Miller DC, Meyers BD: Pathophysiology and prevention of acute renal failure associated with thoracoabdominal or abdominal aortic surgery. J Vasc Surg 5:518, 1987.

140. Nenhaus HP, Javid H: The distinct syndrome of spontaneous aortic-caval fistula. Am J Med 44:464, 1968.

141. Nevitt MP, Ballard DJ, Hallett JW: Prognosis of abdominal aortic aneurysms: A population based study. N Eng J Med 321:1009, 1989.

142. Nunn DB, Carter MM, Donohue MT, et al: Postoperative dilatation of knitted Dacron aortic bifurcation graft. J Vasc Surg 12:291, 1990.

143. O'Donnell TF, Darling C, Linton RR: Is 80 years too old for aneurysmectomy? Arch Surg 111:1250, 1976.

144. Olsen PS, Schroeder T, Agerskov K, et al: Surgery for abdominal aortic aneurysms: A survey of 656 patients. J Cardiovasc Surg 32:636, 1991.

145. Ouriel K, Green RM, Donayre C, et al: An evaluation of new methods of expressing aortic aneurysm size: Relationship to rupture. J Vasc Surg 15:12, 1992.

146. Ouriel K, Ricotta JJ, Adams JT, et al: Management of cholelithiasis in patients with abdominal aortic aneurysms. Ann Surg 198:717, 1983.

147. Pairolero PC: Repair of abdominal aortic aneurysm in high-risk patients. Surg Clin North Am 69:755, 1989.

148. Papanicolaou N, Wittenberg J, Ferrucci JT, et al: Preoperative evaluation of abdominal aortic aneurysms by computed tomography. Am J Radiol 146:711, 1986.

149. Parodi JC, Palmaz JC, Barone HD: Transfemoral intraluminal graft implantation for abdominal aortic aneurysms. Ann Vasc Surg 5:491, 1991.

150. Pavone P, Di Cesare E, Di Renzi P, et al: Abdominal aortic aneurysm evaluation: Comparison of US, CT, MRI, and angiography. Magn Reson Imaging 8:199, 1990.

151. Pearce WH, Sweis I, Yao JST, et al: Interleukin-1β and tumor necrosis factor-α release in normal and diseased human infrarenal aortas. J Vasc Surg 16:784, 1992.

152. Pennell RC, Hollier LH, Lie JT, et al: Inflammatory abdominal aortic aneurysms: A thirty-year review. J Vasc Surg 2:859, 1985.

153. Picone AL, Green RM, Ricotta JR, et al: Spinal cord ischemia following operations on the abdominal aorta. J Vasc Surg 3:94, 1986.

154. Pillari G, Chang JB, Zito J, et al: Computed tomography of abdominal aortic aneurysm. Arch Surg 123:727, 1988.

155. Piotrowski JJ, McCroskey BL, Rutherford RB: Selection of grafts currently available for repair of abdominal aortic aneurysms. Surg Clin North Am 69:827, 1989.

156. Plate G, Hollier LA, O'Brien PO, et al: Recurrent aneurysms and late vascular complications following repair of abdominal aortic aneurysms. Arch Surg 120:590, 1985.

157. Polterauer P, Prager M, Holzenbein T, et al: Dacron versus polytetrafluoroethylene for Y-aortic bifurcation grafts: A six-year prospective, randomized trial. Surgery 111:626, 1992.

158. Powell JT, Adamson J, MacSweeney STR, et al: Genetic variants of collagen III and abdominal aortic aneurysm. Eur J Vasc Surg 5:145, 1991.

159. Powell JT, Bashir A, Dawson S, et al: Genetic variation on chromosome 16 is associated with abdominal aortic aneurysm. Clin Sci 78:13, 1990.

160. Powell JT, Muller BR, Greenhalgh RM: Acute phase proteins in patients with abdominal aortic aneurysms. J Cardiovasc Surg 28:528, 1987.

161. Power DA: The palliative treatment of aneurysms by ''wiring'' with Colt's apparatus. Br J Surg 9:27, 1921.

162. Quill DS, Colgan MP, Sumner DL: Ultrasonic screening for the detection of abdominal aortic aneurysms. Surg Clin North Am 69:713, 1989.

163. Rea CE: The surgical treatment of aneurysm of the abdominal aorta. Minn Med 31:153, 1948.

164. Reckless JPD, McColl I, Taylor GW: Aorto-enteric fistula: An uncommon complication of abdominal aortic aneurysms. Br J Surg 59:458, 1972.

165. Reigel MM, Hollier LH, Kazmier FJ, et al: Late survival in abdominal aortic aneurysm patients: The role of selective myocardial revascularization on the basis of clinical symptoms. J Vasc Surg 5:222, 1987.

166. Reilly JM, Tilson MD: Incidence and etiology of aortic aneurysms. Surg Clin North Am 69:705, 1989.

167. Rizzo RJ, McCarthy WJ, Dixit SN, et al: Collagen types and matrix protein content in human abdominal aortic aneurysm. J Vasc Surg 10:365, 1989.

168. Robson AK, Currie IC, Poskitt KR, et al: Abdominal aortic aneurysm repair in the over eighties. Br J Surg 76:1018, 1989.

169. Roger VL, Ballard DJ, Hallett JW, et al: Influence of coronary artery disease on morbidity and mortality after abdominal aortic aneurysmectomy: A population-based study 1971–1987. J Am Coll Cardiol 14:1245, 1989.

170. Ruby ST, Whittemore AD, Couch NP, et al: Coronary artery disease in patients requiring abdominal aortic aneurysm repair. Selective use of a combined operation. Ann Surg 201:758, 1985.

171. Rutherford RB, McCroskey BL: Ruptured abdominal aortic aneurysms: Special considerations. Surg Clin North Am 69:859, 1989.

172. Schaffer PW, Hardin CW: The use of temporary and polythene shunts to permit occlusion, resection and frozen homologous artery graft replacement of vital vessel segments. Surgery 31:186, 1952.

173. Schatz IJ, Fairbairn JF, Jugens JL: Abdominal aortic aneurysms: A reappraisal. Circulation 26:200, 1962.

174. Schwartz JA, Powell TW, Burnham SJ, et al: Culture of abdominal aortic aneurysm contents. Arch Surg 122:777, 1988.

175. Schwartz RA, Nichols WK, Silver D: Is thrombosis of the infrarenal abdominal aortic aneurysm an acceptable alternative? J Vasc Surg 3:348, 1986.

176. Scott RA, Ashton HA, Kay DN: Abdominal aortic aneurysm in 4237 screened patients: Prevalence, development and management over 6 years. Br J Surg 78:1122, 1990.

177. Sicard GA, Freeman MB, VanderWoude JC, et al: Comparison between the transabdominal and retroperitoneal approach for reconstruction of the infrarenal abdominal aorta. J Vasc Surg 5:19, 1987.

178. Siegfried MS, Rochester D, Bernstein JR, et al: Diagnosis of inferior vena cava anomalies by computerized tomography. Comput Radiol 7:119, 1983.

179. Sladen JG, Gerein AN, Miyagishima RT: Late rupture of prosthetic aortic grafts. Am J Surg 153:453, 1987.

180. Spittell JA, Wallace RB: Aneurysms in peripheral vascular diseases. In Juergens JL, Spittell JA, Fairbairn JF (eds): Peripheral Vascular Diseases, 5th ed. Philadelphia, WB Saunders, 1980.

181. Starr DS, Foster WJ, Morris GC Jr: Resection of abdominal aortic aneurysm in the presence of horseshoe kidney. Surgery 89:387, 1981.

182. Steinberg CR, Morton A, Steinberg I: Measurement of the abdominal aorta after intravenous aortography in health and arteriosclerotic peripheral vascular disease. Am J Radiol 95:703, 1965.

183. Sterpetti AV, Blair EA, Schultz RD, et al: Sealed rupture of abdominal aortic aneurysms. J Vasc Surg 11:430, 1990.

184. Sterpetti AV, Cavallaro A, Cavallari N, et al: Factors influencing the rupture of abdominal aortic aneurysm. Surg Obstet Gynecol 173:175, 1991.

185. Sterpetti AV, Hunter WJ, Feldhaus RJ, et al: Inflammatory aneurysms of the abdominal aorta: Incidence, pathologic, and etiologic considerations. J Vasc Surg 9:643, 1989.

186. Sterpetti AV, Hunter WJ, Schultz RD: Congenital abdominal aortic aneurysms in the young: Case report and review of the literature. J Vasc Surg 7:763, 1988.

187. Sterpetti AV, Schultz RD, Feldhaus RJ, et al: Factors influencing enlargement rate of small abdominal aortic aneurysms. J Surg Res 43:211, 1987.

188. String ST: Cholelithiasis and aortic reconstruction. J Vasc Surg 1:664, 1984.

189. Sullivan CA, Rohrer MJ, Cutler BS: Clinical management of the symptomatic but unruptured abdominal aortic aneurysm. J Vasc Surg 11:799, 1990.

190. Superti-Furga A, Steinmann B, Ramirez F, et al: Molecular defects of type III procollagen in Ehlers-Danlos syndrome type IV. Hum Genet 82:104, 1989.

191. Svensson LG, Crawford ES, Hess KR, et al: Experience with 1509 patients undergoing thoraco-abdominal aortic operations. J Vasc Surg 17:357, 1993.

192. Swanson RJ, Littooy FN, Hunt TK, et al: Laparotomy as a precipitating factor in the rupture of intra-abdominal aneurysms. Arch Surg 115:299, 1980.

193. Sweeney MS, Gadacz TR: Primary aortoduodenal fistula: Manifestation, diagnosis, and treatment. Surgery 96:492, 1984.

194. Szilagyi DE, Elliott JP, Bergeur R: Coincidental malignancy and abdominal aortic aneurysm. Arch Surg 95:402, 1967.

195. Szilagyi DE, Elliott JP, Bergeur R: Temporary transection of the left renal vein: A technical aid in aortic surgery. Surgery 65:32, 1969.

196. Szilagyi DE, Elliott JP, Smith RF: Clinical fate of the patient with asymptomatic aortic aneurysm and unfit for surgical treatment. Arch Surg 104:600, 1972.

197. Szilagyi DE, Hageman JH, Smith RF, et al: Spinal cord damage in surgery of the abdominal aorta. Surgery 83:38, 1978.

198. Szilagyi DE, Smith RF, DeRusso FJ, et al: Contribution of abdominal aortic aneurysmectomy to prolongation of life. Ann Surg 164:678, 1966.

199. Taylor HA, Deumite NJ, Chaitman BR, et al: Asymptomatic left main coronary artery disease in the coronary artery surgery study (CASS) registery. Circulation 79:1171, 1989.

200. Thomas PRS, Stewart RD: Abdominal aortic aneurysm. Br J Surg 75:733, 1988.

201. Thompson JE, Hollier LH, Patman RD, et al: Surgical management of abdominal aortic aneurysms: Factors influencing mortality and morbidity—A 20-year experience. Ann Surg 181:654, 1975.

202. Thurmond AS, Semler HJ: Abdominal aortic aneurysm: Incidence in a population at risk. J Cardiovasc Surg 27:457, 1986.

203. Tilson DM, Seashore MR: Fifty families with abdominal aortic aneurysms in two or more first-order relatives. Am J Surg 147:551, 1984.

204. Tilson DM, Stansel HC: Differences in results for aneurysm vs. occlusive disease after bifurcation grafts. Results of 100 elective grafts. Arch Surg 107:1173, 1980.

205. Tilson MD: Status of research on abdominal aortic aneurysm disease. J Vasc Surg 9:367, 1989.

206. Todd GJ, Nowygrod R, Benvenisty A, et al: The accuracy of CT scanning in the diagnosis of abdominal and thoracoabdominal aortic aneurysms. J Vasc Surg 13:302, 1991.

207. United States Public Health Service: Vital Statistics of the United States, vol. II. Mortality, Part A. Department of Health and Human Service, Publ. No. (PHS) 87–1101. Washington DC, US Government Printing Office, 1987.

208. Varnauskas E, and European Coronary Artery Surgery Study Group: Twelve-year follow-up of survival in the randomized European coronary surgery study. N Engl J Med 391:332, 1988.

209. Volpetti G, Barker CF, Berkowitz H, et al: A twenty-two-year review of elective resection of abdominal aortic aneurysm. Surg Gynecol Obstet 142:321, 1976.

210. Walker DI, Bloor K, Williams G, et al: Inflammatory aneurysms of the abdominal aorta. Br J Surg 59:609, 1972.

211. Webster MW, Ferrell RE, St. Jean PI, et al: Ultrasound screening of first-degree relatives of patients with an abdominal aortic aneurysm. J Vasc Surg 13:9, 1991.

212. Weinstein MH, Machleder HI: Sexual function after aortoiliac surgery. Ann Surg 181:787, 1975.

213. White JV, Haas K, Phillips S, et al: Adventitial elastolysis is a primary event in aneurysm formation. J Vasc Surg 17:371, 1993.

214. Whittemore AD, Clowes AW, Hechtman HB, et al: Aortic aneurysm repair: Reduced operative mortality associated with maintenance of optimal cardiac performance. Ann Surg 192:414, 1980.

215. Wolinsky H, Glagov S: Nature of species differences in the medial distribution of aortic vasa vasorum in mammals. Circ Res 20:409, 1967.

216. Wright IS, Urdenata E, Wright B: Re-opening the case of the abdominal aortic aneurysm. Circulation 13:754, 1956.

217. Yeager RA, Weigel RM, Murphy ES, et al: Application of clinically valid risk factors to aortic aneurysm surgery. Arch Surg 121:278, 1986.

218. Young AE, Sandberg GW, Couch NP: The reduction of mortality of abdominal aortic aneurysm resection. Am J Surg 134:585, 1977.

219. Zarins CK, Glagov S, Vesselinovitch D, et al: Aneurysm formation in experimental atherosclerosis: Relationship to plaque formation. J Vasc Surg 12:246, 1990.

220. Zarins CK, Runyon-Hass A, Zatina MA, et al: Increased collagenase activity in early aneurysmal dilatation. J Vasc Surg 3:238, 1986.

221. Zarins CK, Weisenberg E, Kolettis G, et al: Differential enlargement of artery segments in response to enlarging atherosclerotic plaques. J Vasc Surg 7:386, 1988.

222. Zarins CK, Xu CP, Glagov S: Aneurysmal enlargement of the aorta during regression of experimental atherosclerosis. J Vasc Surg 15:90, 1992.

223. Zatina MA, Zarins CK, Gewertz BL, et al: Role of medial lamellar architecture in the pathogenesis of aortic aneurysms. J Vasc Surg 1:442, 1984.

76

Ruptured Abdominal Aortic Aneurysms

Peter Gloviczki, M.D.

• • •

Rupture is the most frequent and lethal complication of abdominal aortic aneurysms. Ruptured abdominal aortic aneurysm is the 15th leading cause of death in men in the United States[1] and is responsible for an annual death rate of 9.0 per 100,000 men and 2.8 per 100,000 women in Canada.[2] The incidence of ruptured abdominal aortic aneurysm has increased in the last three decades;[3] in England it caused death in 22 per 100,000 men aged 60 to 64 and 177 per 100,000 men aged 80 to 84.[4]

Without surgical treatment rupture invariably results in death. Unfortunately, the mortality following repair of ruptured abdominal aneurysms is also excessive. Except for two series from Houston (Lawrie and colleagues[5] in 1979 and Crawford[6] in 1991) that reported mortality rates of 15 and 23 per cent, respectively, death rates in multiple reports approached or exceeded 50 per cent.[7–40] When prehospital death was also accounted for, the mortality of ruptured aneurysm in one review was 94 per cent.[19] Even the most recent studies[34–40] failed to show any apparent improvement in death rate compared to those published in the 1960s[41–44] or to the initial surgical experience of Cooley and DeBakey in 1954, who reported three survivors among six patients undergoing repair of ruptured aneurysm using homograft.[45]

Differences in mortality rates from various centers can be attributed to different patient populations, variability in prehospital care and transport, delay in treatment, and dissimilar experience of surgeons. Mortality of ruptured aneurysm remains high, in marked contrast to the low mortality of elective repair. Despite all of our efforts, attempts to save the hypotensive patient with a ruptured abdominal aortic aneurysm still result in more failures than successes. The management of these patients continues to be one of the most challenging and formidable tasks that a vascular surgeon can undertake.

DIAGNOSIS

Rupture is frequently the first manifestation of an aortic aneurysm. Aneurysms are diagnosed in less than one third of patients before rupture.[40] The fundamental clinical triad of a ruptured abdominal aortic aneurysm is (1) abdominal or back pain of sudden onset, (2) hypotension, and (3) a pulsatile abdominal mass. Unfortunately, the complete triad is present in only about half of the patients. Sudden onset of abdominal pain is the most common symptom, and in the Mayo Clinic series it was noted in 82 per cent of patients (Table 76–1).[40] About half of the patients had back pain. The association of sudden abdominal discomfort with hypotension in any patient above 50 years of age, especially

Table 76–1. Clinical Presentation of 231 Patients With Ruptured Abdominal Aortic Aneurysm Treated at the Mayo Clinic (1980–1989)

Signs and Symptoms	No. of Patients	%
Abdominal pain	189	82
Hypotension	155	67
Back pain	131	57
Pulsatile mass	105	46
Cardiac arrest	56	24

From Gloviczki P, Pairolero PC, Mucha P Jr, et al: Ruptured abdominal aortic aneurysms: Repair should not be denied. J Vasc Surg 15:851, 1992.

those with other risk factors for atherosclerosis, strongly suggests a ruptured aneurysm. Patients with a perforated viscus may also present with shock and dramatic abdominal pain. However, signs of peritonitis with rigidity of the abdominal wall are striking features of perforation. In patients with acute mesenteric artery occlusion, pain is frequently out of proportion to the physical findings, and shock is late in appearance. Even if the initial diagnosis of a ruptured aneurysm is incorrect, it is important to note that most patients with abdominal pain and shock require urgent exploration. Myocardial infarction and pulmonary embolism must be included in the differential diagnosis. A normal electrocardiogram is helpful to exclude these disorders, but one should remember that hypovolemic shock causes decreased coronary artery perfusion resulting in myocardial ischemia.

The diagnosis of ruptured aneurysm is more difficult when hypotension is absent and the patient presents with abdominal pain alone. Irvin analyzed 1190 emergency hospitalizations of patients with abdominal pain in a general surgical unit.[46] In patients 60 years of age or older, ruptured abdominal aortic aneurysm caused symptoms in 3 per cent. The most frequent cause of abdominal pain was intestinal obstruction, followed by nonspecific abdominal pain, cholelithiasis, and colonic diverticular disease (Table 76–2). Retroperitoneal abdominal aortic aneurysmal rupture may result in compression and irritation of nerve roots, causing the pain to radiate along the sciatic nerve to the groin or

Table 76–2. Diagnoses for Abdominal Pain in 471 Emergency Admissions Into a General Surgery Unit (Age ≥ 60 Years)

Diagnosis	No. of Patients	%
Intestinal obstruction	132	28.0
Nonspecific abdominal pain	106	22.5
Cholelithiasis	42	8.9
Colonic diverticular disease	40	8.5
Abdominal malignancy	26	5.5
Acute appendicitis	20	4.2
Perforated peptic ulcer	20	4.2
Pancreatitis	18	3.8
Urologic	15	3.2
Ruptured aortic aneurysm	14	3.0
Mesenteric vascular occlusion	7	1.5
Medical (pneumonia, pulmonary embolism, myocardial infarction)	5	1.1
Miscellaneous	26	5.6

From Irvin TT: Abdominal pain: A surgical audit of 1190 emergency admissions. Br J Surg 76:1121, 1989. By permission of Butterworth-Heinemann Ltd.

scrotum. These unusual presentations of patients with ruptured aneurysm can lead to a mistaken initial diagnosis of lumbosacral radiculopathy,[47] incarcerated inguinal hernia,[48, 49] or ureteral colic.[50–53] The finding of microscopic hematuria does not exclude rupture of an abdominal aortic aneurysm.[51]

A pulsatile abdominal mass is a helpful clue to the diagnosis, but it is present in only half of patients with ruptured aneurysms.[40] In obese patients the aneurysm may not be palpable, whereas in others a large retroperitoneal hematoma or shock prevents detection of a pulsatile mass. Abdominal distention is a frequent finding, and in a hypotensive male patient over the age of 50 years it suggests ruptured abdominal aneurysm.[54] Distention is caused by retroperitoneal or intraperitoneal hematoma, by intraperitoneal bleeding, or by secondary ileus.

Lateral and distal extension of the retroperitoneal hematoma may result in ecchymoses and discoloration of the flank, groin, scrotum, or penis.[55] A massive retroperitoneal hematoma may cause obstruction of the left colon presenting as massive colonic dilatation proximal to the obstruction.[56] Proximal extension of the hematoma to the periduodenal tissue may mimic small intestinal obstruction. If the hematoma extends to the right upper abdomen, acute cholecystitis or biliary colic may be diagnosed mistakenly.[57] More proximal extension may irritate the diaphragm and cause hiccups, retching, or dry heaves.[58, 59] Rarely, the hematoma erodes the diaphragm, and the patient presents with massive hemothorax.[60]

The diagnosis of ruptured aortic aneurysm should be based on the clinical presentation. Diagnostic tests should be kept to a minimum. Injudicious delay incurred by performing unnecessary tests in hypotensive patients before taking them to the operating room is dangerous and further increases the already excessive mortality. If the clinical signs and symptoms are not sufficient to confirm the diagnosis of ruptured aneurysm, a few studies are permissible if they are performed simultaneously with the initial resuscitation of the patient.

Emergency B-mode ultrasound imaging is efficacious in confirming the presence of abdominal aortic aneurysms in patients with suspected rupture. In the Harborview experience, the aneurysm could be visualized in 95 per cent of patients.[36] It was obscured by gas or fat in the remainder. Shuman and colleagues also found emergency ultrasonography helpful in confirming the presence or absence of abdominal aortic aneurysm in 98 per cent of the patients studied.[61] Alternatively, although much less accurate, an anteroposterior or cross-table lateral roentgenogram may outline calcification in the wall of the aneurysm (Fig. 76–1). However, it confirms the diagnosis in only about 60 per cent of patients.[62] Neither ultrasound nor plain abdominal films are accurate, however, in determining the presence or absence of rupture. If the diagnosis is uncertain *and* the patient has been hemodynamically stable, computed tomography (CT) should be performed[63–67] (Fig. 76–2). However, this test should be undertaken with extreme caution and only after placement of large intravenous catheters. Vigilant supervision and monitoring during CT are mandatory, and preparations should be made to take the patient to the operating room immediately if necessary. Weinbaum and associates[67] reported that CT was 77 per cent sensitive for

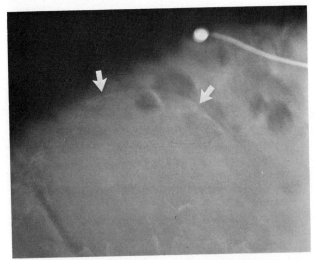

FIGURE 76–1. Emergency room cross-table lateral roentgenogram confirms the diagnosis of an abdominal aortic aneurysm. *Arrows* indicate calcification in the aneurysm wall.

demonstrating retroperitoneal blood; importantly, it was 100 per cent specific with an accuracy of 92 per cent. Transfemoral or translumbar aortography does *not* establish the diagnosis of ruptured abdominal aortic aneurysm, and we do not recommend it in this situation.

The importance of establishing a correct diagnosis early during resuscitation is emphasized by data from the Cleveland Vascular Society.[10] When the correct diagnosis was established initially, the mortality of ruptured abdominal aortic aneurysms was 35 per cent. However, the death rate increased to 75 per cent when rupture was not recognized initially, and a cardiopulmonary or cerebral cause was suspected.

RESUSCITATION

Resuscitation of hypotensive patients with ruptured aortic aneurysm should be initiated during rapid prehospital transport by a skilled team of paramedics. Infusion of crystalloid (lactated Ringer's) solution during transport is beneficial in patients with profound hypotension and may lower the incidence of perioperative renal failure.[36] After arrival in the emergency room, during the initial physical evaluation, large-bore catheters are placed in peripheral arm veins, and blood is sent for cross-matching and routine tests. Infusion of crystalloid solution is continued or, if not given previously, started immediately. The ideal amount of intravenous fluids infused in hypotensive patients in the preoperative period is controversial.[6, 68, 69] In general, intravenous fluids should be administered cautiously before placement of the aortic cross-clamp so that the patient's systolic blood pressure is elevated only to 80 to 100 mmHg. Additional increases in pressure and intravascular volume before placement of an aortic clamp may contribute to more blood loss through the ruptured aorta.

During the initial resuscitation an arterial line is also placed, and blood is obtained for arterial blood gas determination. A urinary catheter is placed to monitor urine

output. A chest roentgenogram and electrocardiogram are performed if time allows. The advisability of application of an antishock garment is controversial. If the likelihood of ruptured aneurysm is high, the patient is transferred immediately to the operating room, and no attempt is made to "stabilize" the patient in the emergency room. If the diagnosis is in question, emergency B-mode abdominal ultrasonography or, if this is not available, abdominal anteroposterior and cross-table lateral roentgenograms are obtained, as discussed previously. CT to establish the diagnosis should be performed *only in hemodynamically stable patients.* If CT confirms rupture, emergency aneurysm repair is required. However, if CT scan demonstrates an aneurysm with no evidence of rupture and no other abdominal pathology is suspected, the patient may undergo operative repair after a more thorough evaluation.

SURGICAL TECHNIQUE

The patient with a ruptured aneurysm should be transported from the emergency room to the operating room without delay. Immediate access to a constantly available operating room and operating team significantly reduces emergency room stay, which in the Harborview experience averaged only 12 minutes.[36] Anesthesia is not induced until the skin of the chest, abdomen, and groin is being prepared and sterile drapes are placed over the patient. If a pneumatic antishock garment has been applied, it is not removed in an unstable patient until after induction of anesthesia. The abdominal panel of the garment is decompressed first to facilitate preparation of the skin, and the leg compartments are deflated after anesthesia has been induced, or, in the severely hypotensive patient, after placement of the aortic clamp.

No time should be lost by attempting to place a Swan-Ganz catheter. If good peripheral venous access is not available, however, a Swan-Ganz introducer with a large bore

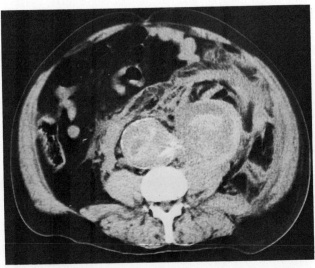

FIGURE 76–2. Computed tomography of a 70-year-old man confirms abdominal aortic aneurysm with rupture into the retroperitoneum.

and short shaft is useful for rapid infusion of intravenous fluid. It can be used subsequently for invasive monitoring. The Swan-Ganz catheter is inserted later during the course of the operation, when the aorta is cross-clamped and the patient is hemodynamically more stable.

Although selective use of a retroperitoneal exposure of ruptured aneurysms has been advocated recently,[33] most surgeons favor an expeditious midline incision from the xiphoid to the pubis for transperitoneal exposure of the abdominal aorta. The abdominal wall should be incised in layers to maintain a tamponading effect until the last moment before the peritoneal cavity is entered. Control of the proximal aorta should be obtained by the most experienced vascular surgeon.

The abdominal aorta can be isolated at the level of the diaphragm or at the infrarenal segment. Rapid control of the upper abdominal aorta below the diaphragm should be obtained if the patient is unstable, if there is free intraperitoneal bleeding, or if the retroperitoneal hematoma extends superiorly to the level of the left renal vein. Control is achieved by quickly incising the avascular portion of the gastrohepatic omentum, retracting the left lobe of the liver medially, and compressing the aorta manually against the spine[6] (Fig. 76–3). After control of the aorta is achieved, the patient is rapidly resuscitated with intravenous crystalloid solution, blood, fresh frozen plasma, and platelets. A low-dose intravenous infusion of dopamine may also be started. Intravenous antibiotics, usually a first-generation cephalosporin, should be given. Once replacement of adequate intravenous volume allows the surgeon to proceed, the crus of the diaphragm is incised longitudinally, and the muscle fibers are separated bluntly with finger dissection to gain access to both sides of the aorta.[70] A clamp is then temporarily applied to the aorta, replacing manual control (Fig. 76–4).

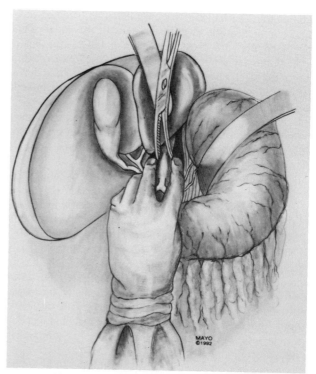

FIGURE 76–4. Cross-clamping of the supraceliac aorta is performed following blunt dissection of the crus of the diaphragm. (By permission of Mayo Foundation.)

Control of the infrarenal aorta is obtained in a manner similar to that used for elective repair of aneurysms. After laparotomy the small bowel and the right colon are retracted and eviscerated to the right. The retroperitoneum is incised between the duodenum and the inferior mesenteric vein, just distal to the left renal vein. The neck of the aneurysm is dissected bluntly distal to the renal arteries, and an aortic clamp is placed. The hematoma often pushes the overlying retroperitoneal structures anteriorly, facilitating this maneuver. "Blind" placement of an arterial clamp through a retroperitoneal hematoma that obscures the left renal vein should not be performed. As emphasized by Crawford,[6] this technique may cause inadvertent injury to the inferior vena cava, left renal, or lumbar veins, contributing to additional blood loss and possible exsanguination.

An alternative technique for controlling the proximal aorta is clamping the thoracic aorta through a left thoracotomy. A left anterolateral thoracotomy to control the descending thoracic aorta in patients with a ruptured infrarenal abdominal aortic aneurysm is seldom indicated. It can be useful, however, if intraperitoneal rupture is suspected in an unstable patient with previous upper abdominal surgery in whom excessive adhesions may prevent rapid access to the subdiaphragmatic aorta. Thoracoabdominal incision with control of the descending thoracic aorta is also required in patients with ruptured suprarenal or thoracoabdominal aortic aneurysms.

Another option in patients with presumed free abdominal aortic rupture is to control the aorta with an occlusive Fogarty balloon catheter introduced through direct cutdown into the brachial artery.[54] The 8 to 22 or 8 to 14 Fr aortic balloon catheter is advanced first into the descending tho-

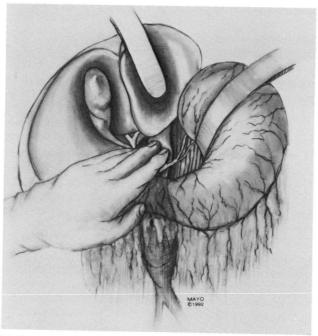

FIGURE 76–3. Technique of manual compression of the supraceliac abdominal aorta. (By permission of Mayo Foundation.)

racic aorta. The balloon is then inflated and floated down by aortic flow to the level of the neck of the aneurysm. If the blood pressure drops before an aortic clamp can be applied, the balloon is inflated. A large Foley balloon catheter or the same Fogarty catheter can also be inserted during the operation directly through the infrarenal aorta, immediately after opening the sac of the aneurysm (Fig. 76–5).[70]

After obtaining control of the proximal aorta, the aneurysm is incised, and thrombus from the aneurysm is carefully removed to avoid embolization. Bleeding from the iliac arteries is controlled by packs or balloon occlusion catheters. The iliac arteries are usually not clamped, to avoid injury to the iliac veins. Ernst suggests the use of iliac clamps; however, they should be placed without dissection or mobilization of the iliac arteries.[70] At this point, if bleeding from the proximal aorta is well controlled, 3000 to 5000 units of heparin can be administered intravenously. Alternatively, heparinized saline can be injected directly into the iliac arteries distally. Some surgeons, however, avoid the use of heparin altogether in patients with ruptured aneurysms.[71] Back-bleeding lumbar arteries are oversewn from within the aneurysm with heavy sutures, and bleeding from the inferior mesenteric artery is controlled temporarily with a vessel loop or a vascular clamp.

A low-porosity woven graft should be used to replace the abdominal aorta to minimize blood loss. Expanded polytetrafluoroethylene is also appropriate graft material. A knitted Dacron graft should be used only if the graft is coated with collagen, gelatin, or albumin. These ''zero-porosity'' fabrics are especially well suited to repair of ruptured aneurysms because, like expanded polytetrafluoroethylene grafts, they do not need preclotting. A straight infrarenal aortic graft should be used preferentially, but bifurcated graft may be needed because of either associated iliac artery aneurysm or iliac artery occlusive disease.

After the proximal anastomosis has been completed and the proximal aorta has been flushed, the aortic clamp is placed distally on the graft. If back-bleeding is not satisfactory, Fogarty balloon embolectomy catheters should be passed into the iliac arteries to remove thrombus or embolus and ensure distal patency. The distal anastomosis is then completed, and arterial inflow to both lower extremities is reestablished. The aortic clamp should be released slowly to avoid a sudden drop in arterial pressure and prevent ''declamping shock.''[54] As flow is restored to an ischemic, vasodilated distal arterial bed, the decreased peripheral vascular resistance produces decreased cardiac output. Perfusion to coronary, renal, and other important visceral beds is further decreased by return of flow to the lower extremities. To avoid ischemic insult to the myocardium during declamping, systolic blood pressure should not be allowed to drop more than 20 mmHg or below 100 mmHg.[54]

The retroperitoneal hematoma is *not* evacuated at the end of the procedure. At this point, the sigmoid colon, which is at high risk for ischemic injury,[72] is inspected. Unless there is unequivocal viability with a palpable pulse, pink color, and good peristalsis, we inject two ampules of fluorescein intravenously and observe the bowel under a Wood's lamp. If fluorescence is absent or if the pattern is patchy or perivascular, we reimplant the inferior mesenteric artery and ensure that there is pulsatile flow to at least one internal iliac artery. Additional methods of assessing colonic viability are discussed in Chapters 75 and 99. Reestablishment of pelvic flow is also important to prevent spinal cord injury, which occurs in 1 to 2 per cent of patients following aneurysm rupture.[73] Techniques used to decrease the incidence of injury to the spinal cord or lumbosacral plexus after aneurysm repair are detailed in Chapter 77.

A major cause of postoperative death after repair of ruptured aneurysms is persistent bleeding from the aorta, venous injuries, disseminated intravascular coagulation, or depletion of coagulation factors. Just as it is the surgeon's responsibility to minimize bleeding through proper surgical technique, an important task of the anesthesia team during surgery is to combat hypothermia and acidosis. Decreased core temperature plays an important role in the poor outcome for patients with massive blood loss. Hypothermia prolongs coagulation, interferes with normal platelet function, and contributes to disseminated intravascular coagulation.[74–76] Cold-induced injury to the vascular endothelium may result in release of large amounts of thromboplastin, a potent procoagulant.[77] The use of rapid autotransfusion of autologous blood has resulted in decreased requirements for banked blood and preservation of platelets.[78] In addition, the ability to warm the blood quickly with the autotransfu-

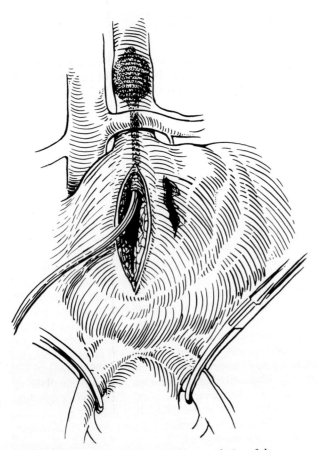

FIGURE 76–5. Intraluminal balloon occlusion of the suprarenal aorta. The catheter is placed during the operation after opening the sac of the ruptured aneurysm. (From Ernst CB: Emergency aortic reconstruction. *In* Bergan JJ, Yao JST [eds]: Techniques in Arterial Surgery. Philadelphia, WB Saunders, 1990, pp 42–55.)

sion device is useful for preventing and treating hypothermia. Prewarming of intravenous fluids and banked blood or blood products, the use of heated humidified air during ventilation, and additional maneuvers to increase core temperature should also be instituted. The use of a warming blanket, or the "bear hugger," covering the exposed extremities during the operation is recommended. At the end of the operation, the surgeon should irrigate the peritoneal cavity with warm saline. After reestablishment of circulation to the lower extremities, additional fresh frozen plasma and platelets should be given as necessary to correct coagulation abnormalities.

Before closure, an expeditious abdominal exploration is performed to exclude other abdominal pathology. Adequate circulation to both lower extremities should be confirmed before the patient is removed from the operating table. Thromboembolectomy, if needed, should be performed immediately, and the patient should not be transported to the intensive care unit with an ischemic extremity.

The management of rupture of an abdominal aortic aneurysm into the vena cava or iliac vein is discussed in detail in Chapter 87, and spontaneous rupture of an aneurysm into the duodenum is considered in Chapter 38.

POSTOPERATIVE COMPLICATIONS

Data from the Harborview experience delineate the number and severity of postoperative complications in patients undergoing repair of ruptured aneurysms. Despite expert postoperative care, 61 per cent of patients from that series admitted to the intensive care unit died, comprising 51 per cent of all deaths.[36] Prolonged mechanical ventilation was required in most patients. In the Mayo Clinic experience the median length of mechanical ventilation was 3 days, and the range was from 1 to 92 days.[40] Respiratory complications including atelectasis, pneumonia, interstitial pulmonary edema, and pleural effusions were the most frequent causes of postoperative morbidity (Table 76–3). In 30 per cent of patients with respiratory complications, a tracheostomy was required.

Acute renal failure is the second most frequent postoperative complication after repair of ruptured aneurysms.[40]

Table 76–3. Postoperative Complications in 174 Patients Following Repair of Ruptured Abdominal Aortic Aneurysm at the Mayo Clinic (1980–1989)

Complication	Patients		Mortality	
	No.	%	No.	%
Respiratory failure	83	48	28	34
Tracheostomy	25	14	11	44
Renal failure	50	29	38	76
Sepsis	42	24	19	45
Cardiac failure	41	24	27	66
Bleeding	29	17	25	86
Stroke	10	6	5	50
Ischemic colitis	9	5	6	67
Lower extremity ischemia	6	3	1	17
Paraplegia or paraparesis	4	2	2	50

From Gloviczki P, Pairolero PC, Mucha P Jr, et al: Ruptured abdominal aortic aneurysms: Repair should not be denied. J Vasc Surg 15:851, 1992.

Table 76–4. Main Cause of Postoperative Death in 57 Patients Following Repair of Ruptured Abdominal Aortic Aneurysm

Complication	Deaths (No.)	%
Bleeding	22	39
Multi-system failure	19	33
Cardiac failure	7	12
Respiratory failure	4	7
Renal failure	4	7
Sepsis	1	2

From Gloviczki P, Pairolero PC, Mucha P Jr, et al: Ruptured abdominal aortic aneurysms: Repair should not be denied. J Vasc Surg 15:851, 1992.

In the series of Wakefield and associates,[8] if dialysis was required mortality was 75 per cent. Perioperative hypotension, prolonged suprarenal cross-clamping, preexisting chronic renal failure or renal artery disease, and reperfusion of ischemic skeletal muscles following prolonged ischemia are potential causes of acute renal dysfunction. Increased intra-abdominal pressure in patients following repair of ruptured aneurysm is an important etiologic factor in renal and also in cardiopulmonary failure. Ischemia and reperfusion of the abdominal organs produce increased capillary and mucosal permeability, which results in the need for large amounts of intravenous fluids to maintain intravascular volume.[76] Rewarming from hypothermia also increases fluid requirements. Increased intra-abdominal pressure decreases effective tissue perfusion, results in further cellular swelling, and contributes to renal failure and mesenteric ischemia. Hemodynamic instability may occur owing to compression of the inferior vena cava, compromising venous return. Oxygenation and ventilation are also decreased in these patients. With marked abdominal distention, urine output is diminished despite high filling pressures and fails to respond to the usual pharmacologic treatments (low-dose dopamine, mannitol, loop diuretics). Elevated abdominal pressure is confirmed by elevated bladder pressures (e.g., more than 30 cmH$_2$O), as measured through the urinary catheter. Urgent decompressive laparotomy in these patients will result in dramatic improvement in urine output, oxygenation, and ventilation.[79] In such circumstances, the abdominal wall usually must be closed with the aid of a nonabsorbable prosthetic mesh.

Sepsis and cardiac failure also occur frequently after repair of ruptured aneurysms. Careful postoperative monitoring of intravascular volume and left ventricular performance is mandatory. Expert management is needed to compensate for the large fluid shifts, to maintain adequate oxygenation, to optimize cardiac output, to treat metabolic acidosis, and to administer appropriate antibiotics. Although postoperative bleeding occurred in only 17 per cent of the patients in the Mayo Clinic series, it was the most frequent cause of postoperative death[40] (Table 76–4). Multi-system organ failure, myocardial infarction, and congestive heart failure were other important causes of mortality.

Because ischemic colitis may also prove fatal, early postoperative diarrhea, bloody stool, sepsis, metabolic acidosis, and persistent coagulopathy demand immediate attention.[80] Flexible sigmoidoscopy should be performed when such signs appear in order to exclude colonic gangrene. Should transmural ischemic colitis develop, immediate reexploration with resection of the involved bowel is imperative. Eighteen per cent of the initial survivors at Harborview[36] manifested signs and symptoms of transmural colonic infarction, and ischemic colitis was the cause of death in 18 per cent of the patients who died in the intensive care unit. A recent review by Meissner and Johansen[81] suggested that maintenance of satisfactory perioperative cardiac output and avoidance of alpha-adrenergic vasopressor agents were the most critical elements in preventing colonic ischemia in patients with ruptured aneurysm. This problem is discussed in more detail in Chapter 99, and other generic complications are dealt with extensively in Section VI.

MORTALITY

In the Mayo Clinic series, the overall mortality in 231 patients admitted for ruptured abdominal aortic aneurysm was 49.4 per cent.[40] Seventeen deaths (7.4 per cent) occurred in the emergency room, 40 (17.3 per cent) in the operating room, 27 (11.7 per cent) during the first 48 postoperative hours, and 30 (13.0 per cent) later but during the same hospitalization. Thirty-day mortality was 45.9 per cent for all patients (106 of 231) and 41.6 per cent for patients who survived long enough to undergo repair (89 of 214). In the Harborview series, in which 96 per cent of patients had prehospital hypotension, 30-day mortality for all admissions was 70 per cent.[36] The early mortality of 1175 patients with ruptured abdominal aortic aneurysms reported in eight large series in the 1990s averaged 54 per cent[34-40] (Table 76–5).

The persistently high mortality rate following rupture can be attributed to several factors. Because of expert prehospital care and rapid transport, which includes helicopter service in many institutions, more patients reach the emergency room alive but in profound hypovolemic shock than at any time previously.[36] Many of these patients are of advanced age and have multiple cardiovascular risk factors. In other words, excellent prehospital emergency medical service programs with rapid transportation may save more lives but paradoxically increase the in-hospital mortality rate, whereas patients who can tolerate delays in referral and transportation selectively fare better, accounting for better institutional mortality rates with ruptured abdominal aortic aneurysms yet a (usually unrecognized) higher over-

Table 76–6. Association of Demographic Data and Clinical Variables With Hospital Mortality in 214 Patients Undergoing Repair for Ruptured Abdominal Aortic Aneurysm at the Mayo Clinic (1980–1989)

Variable	Univariate Analysis *p*-value	Multivariate Analysis *p*-value
APACHE II score	<.001	.0095
Hypotension	<.001	.0038
Hematocrit	<.001	.0075
Cardiac arrest	<.001	NS
Intraperitoneal rupture	.009	NS
Age	.010	NS
Transfusion needs	.037	NS
Gender	.038	NS
Chronic obstructive pulmonary disease	NS	.0140
Colon ischemia	NS	NS
Renal insufficiency*	NS	
Type of graft (straight, bifurcated)*	NS	
Coronary artery disease*	NS	
Diabetes mellitus*	NS	
Hypertension*	NS	

*Variables not included in multivariate analysis.
From Gloviczki P, Pairolero PC, Mucha P Jr, et al: Ruptured abdominal aortic aneurysms: Repair should not be denied. J Vasc Surg 15:851, 1992.

all mortality for the community or region. Thus, a simple comparison of mortality rates between institutions may be misleading.

The available experience from collated series indicates that patients with preoperative cardiac arrest or with profound hypotension on admission and immediately before the operation have the poorest likelihood of survival. In the Harborview experience, the highest mortality occurred in patients over 80 years of age, in women, and in those with preoperative hypotension and a low hematocrit on admission.[36] None of the 10 patients who had preoperative cardiac arrest survived. In the Mayo Clinic review the best preoperative predictors of death after ruptured aneurysm repair were a high APACHE II score, preoperative hypotension, a low admission hematocrit, and the presence of chronic obstructive pulmonary disease (Table 76–6).[40] Still, 38 per cent of patients with preoperative hypotension and 28 per cent of those with an admission hematocrit of less than 27 survived (Fig. 76–6). Forty-four per cent of patients 80 years old or older survived, as did 36 per cent of women. The mortality was highest (80 per cent) among those who underwent cardiopulmonary resuscitation for cardiac arrest.

The importance of surgical experience and technique with respect to outcome of operation for ruptured aneurysms is underscored by the excellent results of the personal series of E. Stanley Crawford. He reported a 90-day mortality rate of only 23 per cent in 87 patients who underwent repair of ruptured aortic aneurysms, with a mortality rate of 15 per cent in those 41 patients who underwent operation in the last decade.[6]

CONTRAINDICATIONS TO SURGICAL TREATMENT

Although the presence of certain preoperative risk factors predicts high mortality, patients may survive despite

Table 76–5. Mortality of Ruptured Abdominal Aortic Aneurysms (1990–1992)

First Author, Year	Total No. of Patients	Patients With Hypotension No.	Patients With Hypotension %	Mortality No.	Mortality %
Ouriel et al, 1990	243	97	51	133	55
Murphy et al, 1990	172	95	55	77	45
Johansen et al, 1991	186	178	96	130	70
Crawford, 1991	87	40	46	20	23
Cohen et al, 1991	70	43	39	47	67
Harris et al, 1991	113	34	30	72	64
AbuRahma et al, 1991	73	37	51	45	62
Gloviczki et al, 1992	231	155	67	106	46
Total	1175	679	58	630	54

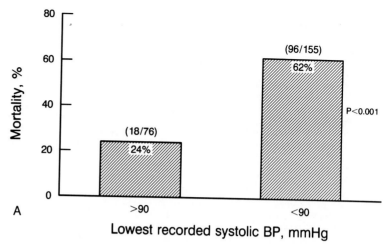

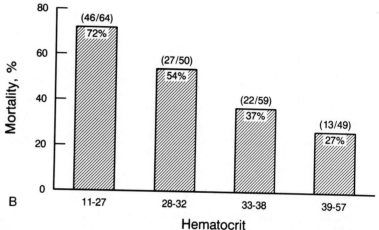

FIGURE 76-6. Mortality in patients admitted with ruptured abdominal aortic aneurysms. *A*, Association with hypotension. *B*, Association with admission hematocrit. (*B*, From Gloviczki P, Pairolero PC, Mucha P Jr, et al: Ruptured abdominal aortic aneurysms: Repair should not be denied. J Vasc Surg 15:851, 1992.)

preoperative shock, advanced age, and even cardiac arrest. Patients who arrive in moribund condition, unresponsive to prolonged cardiopulmonary resuscitation during transport, are usually not operative candidates. Similarly, operation is not performed in patients who are conscious, competent to make decisions, and refuse surgery. As suggested recently by the Joint Council of the Society for Vascular Surgery and the North American Chapter of the International Society of Cardiovascular Surgery, relative contraindications to surgical treatment include an unacceptable quality of life or short life expectancy, as in patients in the terminal phase of an underlying malignant disease or those with overwhelming medical problems.[82]

CONCLUSIONS

Rupture remains a lethal complication of abdominal aortic aneurysm. Timely referral, rapid transport, immediate resuscitation, early diagnosis, and prompt operative management with expeditious control of the proximal aorta offer the only hope for survival. Repair of the aneurysm, most frequently with a straight aortic graft, requires experience and technical skill. Attention to detail is needed to avoid intraoperative complications, such as continued bleeding from the aorta, diffuse hemorrhage from coagulopathy, injury to great veins, and compromise of the blood supply to the bowel, pelvis, or lower extremities. Proficient perioperative care is required to manage large fluid shifts, intravascular volume and bleeding abnormalities, metabolic acidosis, hypothermia, cardiac dysfunction, pulmonary edema, and renal failure. Regardless of skillful treatment, mortality from ruptured abdominal aortic aneurysms remains high. Screening of the high-risk population and timely *elective* repair of the aneurysm are the only practical means of significantly reducing death from this disease.

References

1. Vital Statistics of the United States, 1987. Washington, DC, US Government Printing Office, 1987.
2. Canadian Task Force on the Periodic Health Examination: Periodic health examination, 1991 update: Screening for abdominal aortic aneurysm. Can Med J 145:783, 1991.
3. Bickerstaff LK, Hollier LH, Van Peenen HJ, et al: Abdominal aortic aneurysms: The changing natural history. J Vasc Surg 1:6, 1984.
4. Collin J: Ruptured aortic aneurysm. Br J Surg 73:596, 1986.
5. Lawrie GM, Morris GC Jr, Crawford ES, et al: Improved results of operation for ruptured abdominal aortic aneurysm. Surgery 85:483, 1979.
6. Crawford ES: Ruptured abdominal aortic aneurysm [Editorial]. J Vasc Surg 13:348, 1991.
7. Lasonde J, Laurendeau F, Page P: Ruptured abdominal aortic aneurysm. Can J Surg 24:420, 1981.
8. Wakefield TW, Whitehouse WM, Wu SC, et al: Abdominal aortic aneurysm rupture: Statistical analysis of factors affecting outcome of surgical treatment. Surgery 91:586, 1982.

9. Scobie TK, Masters RG: Changing factors influencing abdominal aortic aneurysm repair. J Cardiovasc Surg 23:309, 1982.

10. Hoffman M, Avellone JC, Plecha FR, et al: Operation for ruptured abdominal aortic aneurysms: A community-wide experience. Surgery 91:597, 1982.

11. Makin GS: Some factors influencing hospital mortality in ruptured abdominal aortic aneurysms. J Cardiovasc Surg 24:646, 1983.

12. Hiatt JCG, Barker WF, Machleder HI, et al: Determinants of failure in the treatment of ruptured abdominal aortic aneurysm. Arch Surg 119:1264, 1984.

13. Fielding JWL, Black J, Ashton F, et al: Ruptured aortic aneurysms: Postoperative complications and their aetiology. Br J Surg 71:487, 1984.

14. Lawler M Jr: Aggressive treatment of ruptured abdominal aortic aneurysm in a community hospital. Surgery 95:38, 1984.

15. Crew JR, Bashour TT, Ellertson D, et al: Ruptured abdominal aortic aneurysms: Experience with 70 cases. Clin Cardiol 8:433, 1985.

16. Castleden WM, Mercer JC, and Members of the West Australia Vascular Service: Abdominal aortic aneurysms in Western Australia: Descriptive epidemiology and patterns of rupture. Br J Surg 72:109, 1985.

17. Donaldson MC, Rosenberg JM, Bucknam CA: Factors affecting survival after ruptured abdominal aortic aneurysm. J Vasc Surg 2:564, 1985.

18. Bodily KC, Buttorff JD: Ruptured abdominal aortic aneurysm. The Tacoma experience. Am J Surg 149:580, 1985.

19. Johansson G, Swedenborg J: Ruptured abdominal aortic aneurysms: A study of incidence and mortality. Br J Surg 73:101, 1986.

20. Meyer AA, Ahlquist RE Jr, Trunkey DD: Mortality from ruptured abdominal aortic aneurysms. A comparison of two series. Am J Surg 152:27, 1986.

21. Lambert ME, Baguley P, Charlesworth D: Ruptured abdominal aortic aneurysms. J Cardiovasc Surg 27:256, 1986.

22. Jenkins AML, Ruckley CV, Nolan B: Ruptured abdominal aortic aneurysm. Br J Surg 73:395, 1986.

23. Ingoldby CJH, Wajanto R, Mitchell JE: Impact of vascular surgery on community mortality from ruptured aortic aneurysms. Br J Surg 73:551, 1986.

24. Gangahar DM, Carveth SW, Reese HE, et al: Ruptured abdominal aortic aneurysm: Seven years experience in a community hospital. Nebr Med J 72:185, 1987.

25. Abernathy CM Jr, Baumgartner R, Butler HG, et al: Management of ruptured abdominal aortic aneurysms in rural Colorado (with a historical note on Kit Carson's death). JAMA 256:597, 1986.

26. Shackleton CR, Schechter MT, Bianco R, Hildebrand HD: Preoperative predictors of mortality risk in ruptured abdominal aortic aneurysm. J Vasc Surg 6:583, 1987.

27. Martin RS III, Edwards WH Jr, Jenkins JM, et al: Ruptured abdominal aortic aneurysm: A 25-year experience and analysis of recent cases. Am Surg 54:539, 1988.

28. Vohra R, Abdool-Carrim AT, Groome J, Pollock JG: Ruptured aortic aneurysms: Postoperative complications and their management. Ann Vasc Surg 2:114, 1988.

29. Thomas PRS, Stewart RD: Mortality of abdominal aortic aneurysm. Br J Surg 75:733, 1988.

30. Budd JS, Finch DR, Carter PG: A study of the mortality from ruptured abdominal aortic aneurysms in a district community. Eur J Vasc Surg 3:351, 1989.

31. Salo JA, Perhoniemi VJ, Lepantalo MJ, Mattila PS: Prognosis of patients over 75 years of age with a ruptured abdominal aortic aneurysm. World J Surg 13:484, 1989.

32. Slaney G: The management of ruptured abdominal aortic aneurysms. *In* Bergan JJ, Yao JST (eds): Aortic Surgery. Philadelphia, WB Saunders, 1989, pp 329–39.

33. Chang BB, Shah DM, Paty PS, et al: Can the retroperitoneal approach be used for ruptured abdominal aortic aneurysms? J Vasc Surg 11:326, 1990.

34. Ouriel K, Geary K, Green RM, et al: Factors determining survival after ruptured aortic aneurysm: The hospital, the surgeon, and the patient. J Vasc Surg 11:493, 1990.

35. Murphy JL, Barber GG, McPhail NV, Scobie TK: Factors affecting survival after rupture of abdominal aortic aneurysm: Effect of size on management and outcome. Can J Surg 33:201, 1990.

36. Johansen K, Kohler RT, Nicholls SC, et al: Ruptured abdominal aortic aneurysm: The Harborview experience. J Vasc Surg 13:240, 1991.

37. Cohen JR, Birnbaum E, Kassan M, Wise L: Experience in managing 70 patients with ruptured abdominal aortic aneurysms. NY State J Med 91:97, 1991.

38. Harris LM, Faggioli GL, Fiedler R, et al: Ruptured abdominal aortic aneurysms: Factors affecting mortality rates. J Vasc Surg 14:812, 1991.

39. AbuRahma AF, Woodruff BA, Lucente FC, et al: Factors affecting survival of patients with ruptured abdominal aortic aneurysm in a West Virginia community. Surg Gynecol Obstet 172:377, 1991.

40. Gloviczki P, Pairolero PC, Mucha P Jr, et al: Ruptured abdominal aortic aneurysms: Repair should not be denied. J Vasc Surg 15:851, 1992.

41. DeBakey ME, Crawford ES, Cooley DA et, et al: Aneurysm of the abdominal aorta: Analysis of results of graft replacement therapy one to eleven years after operation. Ann Surg 160:622, 1964.

42. Mannick JA, Brooks JW, Boshner LH, et al: Ruptured aneurysms of the abdominal aorta: A reappraisal. N Engl J Med 271:915, 1964.

43. Szilagyi DE, Smith RF, DeRusso FJ, et al: Contribution of aortic aneurysmectomy to prolongation of life. Ann Surg 164:678, 1966.

44. Stoney RJ, Wylie EJ: Surgical treatment of ruptured abdominal aortic aneurysm: Factors influencing outcome. West J Med 111:1, 1969.

45. Cooley DA, DeBakey ME: Ruptured aneurysms of abdominal aorta. Postgrad Med J 16:334, 1954.

46. Irvin TT: Abdominal pain: A surgical audit of 1190 emergency admissions. Br J Surg 76:1121, 1989.

47. Wilberger JE: Lumbosacral radiculopathy secondary to abdominal aortic aneurysm. Report of three cases. J Neurosurg 58:965, 1983.

48. Louras JC, Welch JP: Masking of ruptured abdominal aortic aneurysm by incarcerated inguinal hernia. Arch Surg 119:331, 1984.

49. Khaw H, Sottiurai VS, Craighead CC, et al: Ruptured abdominal aortic aneurysm presenting as symptomatic inguinal mass: Report of six cases. J Vasc Surg 4:384, 1986.

50. Moran CG, Edwards AT, Griffith GH: Ruptured abdominal aortic aneurysm presenting with ureteric colic [Letter to the editor]. Br Med J 294:1279, 1987.

51. O'Donnell D: Ruptured abdominal aortic aneurysm presenting with ureteric colic [Letter to the editor]. Br Med J 294:1689, 1987.

52. Stower MJ, Wyatt MG, Bristol JB: Ruptured abdominal aortic aneurysm presenting as ureteric colic [Letter to the editor]. Br Med J 295:670, 1987.

53. De Dombal FT, Telfer S: Ruptured abdominal aortic aneurysm presenting as ureteric colic [Letter to the editor]. Br Med J 295:1063, 1987.

54. Rutherford RB, McCroskey BL: Ruptured abdominal aortic aneurysms: Special considerations. Surg Clin North Am 69:859, 1989.

55. Ratzan R, Donaldson MC, Foster JH, et al: The blue scrotum sign of Bryant: A diagnostic clue to ruptured abdominal aortic aneurysm. J Emerg Med 5:323, 1987.

56. Politoske EJ: Ruptured abdominal aortic aneurysm presenting as an obstruction of the left colon. Am J Gastroenterol 85:745, 1990.

57. Chandler JJ: The Einstein sign: The clinical picture of acute cholecystitis caused by ruptured abdominal aortic aneurysm [Letter to the editor]. N Engl J Med 310:1538, 1984.

58. Finestone HM, Clifford JC: ''Dry heaves'': The sole presenting complaint in a case of ruptured abdominal aortic aneurysm. Can Med Assoc J 135:1154, 1986.

59. Page P, Page A: ''Dry heaves'' and ruptured abdominal aortic aneurysm. Can Med Assoc J 136:105, 1987.

60. Karam PG, Novick RJ, Glickman LT, et al: Right hemothorax: An unusual presentation of ruptured infrarenal abdominal aortic aneurysm. Can J Surg 29:133, 1986.

61. Shuman WP, Hastrup W Jr, Kohler TR, et al: Suspected leaking abdominal aortic aneurysm: Use of sonography in the emergency room. Radiology 168:117, 1988.

62. Darke SG, Eadie DDG: Abdominal aortic aneurysmectomy: A review of 60 consecutive cases contrasting elective and emergency surgery. J Cardiovasc Surg 14:484, 1973.

63. Rosen A, Korobkin M, Silverman PM, et al: CT diagnosis of ruptured abdominal aortic aneurysm. Am J Roentgenol 143:265, 1984.

64. Raptopoulos V, Cummings T, Smith EH: Computed tomography of life-threatening complications of abdominal aortic aneurysm. The disrupted aortic wall. Invest Radiol 22:372, 1987.

65. Gale ME, Johnson WC, Gerzof SG, et al: Problems in CT diagnosis of ruptured abdominal aortic aneurysms. J Comput Assist Tomogr 10:637, 1986.

66. Senapati A, Hurst PAE, Thomas ML, et al: Differentiation of ruptured aortic aneurysm from acute expansion by computerised tomography. J Cardiovasc Surg 27:719, 1986.
67. Weinbaum FI, Dubner S, Turner JW, et al: The accuracy of computed tomography in the diagnosis of retroperitoneal blood in the presence of abdominal aortic aneurysm. J Vasc Surg 6:11, 1987.
68. Friedman SG, Krishnasastry KV: Ruptured abdominal aortic aneurysm: An editorial. J Vasc Surg 15:456, 1992.
69. Bickel WH: Intravenous fluid administration and uncontrolled hemorrhage [Editorial]. J Trauma 29:409, 1989.
70. Ernst CB: Emergency aortic reconstruction. In Bergan JJ, Yao JST (eds): Techniques in Arterial Surgery. Philadelphia, WB Saunders, 1990, pp 42–55.
71. Mannick JA, Whittemore AD: Management of ruptured or symptomatic abdominal aortic aneurysms. Surg Clin North Am 68:377, 1988.
72. Bergman RT, Gloviczki P, Welch TJ, et al: The role of intravenous fluorescein in the detection of colon ischemia during aortic reconstruction. Ann Vasc Surg 6:74, 1992.
73. Gloviczki P, Cross SA, Stanson AW, et al: Ischemic injury to the spinal cord or lumbosacral plexus after aorto-iliac reconstruction. Am J Surg 162:131, 1991.
74. Kattlove HE, Alexander B: The effect of cold on platelets. I: Cold-induced platelet aggregation. Blood 38:39, 1971.
75. Hessell EA, Schner G, Dillard DH: Platelet kinetics during deep hypothermia. J Surg Res 28:23, 1980.
76. Patt A, McCroskey BL, Moore EE: Hypothermia-induced coagulopathies in trauma. Surg Clin North Am 68:775, 1988.
77. Mahajan SL, Myer TJ, Baldini MG: Disseminated intravascular coagulation during rewarming following hypothermia. JAMA 245:2517, 1981.
78. Bourchier RG, Gloviczki P, Larson MV, et al: The mechanisms and prevention of intravascular fluid loss after occlusion of the supraceliac aorta in dogs. J Vasc Surg 13:637, 1991.
79. Wakefield TW: Surgical treatment of ruptured infrarenal abdominal aortic aneurysm. In Ernst CB, Stanley JC (eds): Current Therapy in Vascular Surgery, 2nd ed. Philadelphia, B C Decker, 1991, pp 264–267.
80. Fietssam R Jr, Villalba M, Glover JL, et al: Intra-abdominal compartment syndrome as a complication of ruptured abdominal aortic aneurysm repair. Am Surg 55:396, 1989.
81. Meissner MH, Johansen KH: Colon infarction after ruptured abdominal aortic aneurysm. Arch Surg 127:979, 1992.
82. Hollier LH, Taylor LM, Ochsner J: Recommended indications for operative treatment of abdominal aortic aneurysms. Report of a subcommittee of the Joint Council of the Society for Vascular Surgery and the North American Chapter of the International Society for Cardiovascular Surgery. J Vasc Surg 15:1046, 1992.

77

Thoracoabdominal Aortic Aneurysm

Joseph S. Coselli, M.D.

• • •

Aneurysms that extend from the chest into the abdomen and those that involve the suprarenal segments of the abdominal aorta are traditionally classified as *thoracoabdominal*, either because both segments of the aorta are involved or because both body cavities are entered for the exposure necessary for operation. In either event, the disease is extensive, and the segment of abdominal aorta from which the visceral vessels arise is aneurysmal in the majority of cases. Effective treatment, as for similar lesions located elsewhere, is graft replacement, and its application requires extensive incisions for exposure, temporary aortic and visceral vessel occlusion, replacement of long segments of aorta, and restoration of circulation into branches of the involved aorta as well as the aorta itself. These unique features of the disease and the requirements for surgical treatment merit the special consideration that the author attempts to give them here on the basis of his experience and that of E. Stanley Crawford in the treatment of 1509 patients with aneurysms of this type[1–4, 10] (Tables 77–1 and 77–2).

Table 77–1. Early Results of Treatment of Thoracoabdominal Aortic Aneurysm, Nondissection

Extent of Aneurysm	No. of Patients	Survival	Paraplegia/Paraparesis*	Renal Failure*
I	292	276 (95%)	39 (13%)	19 (7%)
II	302	271 (90%)	93 (31%)	36 (12%)
III	312	280 (90%)	19 (6%)	30 (10%)
IV	327	309 (94%)	13 (4%)	29 (9%)
Total	1233	1136 (92%)	164 (13%)	114 (9%)

Both surviving and nonsurviving patients are included.

Table 77–2.   Early Results of Treatment of Thoracoabdominal Aortic Aneurysm, Dissection

Extent of Aneurysm	No. of Patients	Survival	Paraplegia/ Paraparesis*	Renal Failure*
I	86	76 (88%)	18 (21%)	8 (9%)
II	140	128 (91%)	46 (33%)	10 (7%)
III	31	29 (94%)	4 (13%)	4 (13%)
IV	19	17 (89%)	2 (11%)	0 (0%)
Total	276	250 (91%)	70 (25%)	22 (8%)

Both surviving and nonsurviving patients are included.

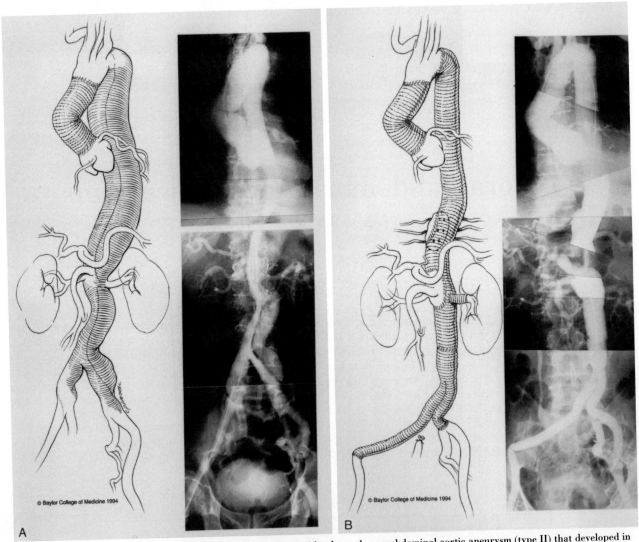

FIGURE 77–1.   *A*, Illustration and aortogram of a patient with a large thoracoabdominal aortic aneurysm (type II) that developed in the follow-up period after prior ascending aortic replacement for acute type I aortic dissection. *B*, Illustration and postoperative aortogram following resection and graft replacement of thoracoabdominal aortic dissection of aneurysm with reattachment of intercostal arteries, reattachment of the celiac axis and superior mesenteric and right renal arteries, Dacron bypass graft to distal left renal artery, and bifurcation graft replacement of distal abdominal aorta and both common iliac arteries. (*A* and *B*, © Baylor College of Medicine, 1987.)

NATURE OF THE DISEASE

The etiology of these aneurysms, in order of frequency, is medial degenerative disease (cystic medial necrosis, myxomatous or myxoid degeneration, senile aorta, Marfan's syndrome, and so on), aortic dissection, atherosclerosis, aortitis, infection, and trauma. Although they may differ from each other microscopically, macroscopically, chemically, or bacteriologically, all produce weakness and dilatation of the aortic wall, both of which are responsible for the complications presented by the disease. These complications are compression and erosion into adjacent structures such as nerves, lung, chest wall, esophagus, small bowel, colon, vena cava, ureter, and back. The most dreaded consequence is rupture, which may occur into the airway, the gut, or one of the body cavities.

Ninety-four patients were observed who did not have thoracoabdominal aortic replacement either because of their age, because of associated disease, because the aneurysm was not large enough to be replaced at the time it was first seen, or because treatment was staged, with a more proximal or distal operation performed first with the intent of performing thoracoabdominal aortic aneurysm replacement later. The 2-year survival rate of these patients was only 24 per cent, with half of the deaths due to aneurysm rupture, emphasizing the perilous nature of this disorder.[3]

Most causative conditions produce diffuse dilatation, and the aneurysms are fusiform in nature. The exception is infection, which produces saccular aneurysms, which characteristically occur in the aortic arch or in the abdominal aorta behind the origin of the visceral vessels. Usually only a part of the aortic circumference is affected, and this pattern of weakening results in a diverticular or saccular outpouching. Most saccular aneurysms, however, are of arteriosclerotic origin, and both infectious and degenerative types may be combined with fusiform aneurysms in patients with thoracoabdominal disease. Most thoracoabdominal dissections requiring prosthetic replacement are chronic and represent late diffuse dilatation of the outer wall or false lumen in DeBakey type I and type III dissections (see Chapter 78). In acute cases, operation is usually directed toward the origin of the dissection, either in the ascending aorta or just distal to the left subclavian artery; hence, many patients with such chronic thoracoabdominal aortic aneurysms will have had similar operations in the past, and the subsequent procedure or procedures will result in either replacement of the remaining descending thoracic and abdominal aorta or redo operations for complications of the previous ascending aorta and arch procedures and then complete replacement of the descending thoracic and abdominal aorta (Figs. 77–1 and 77–2). In still other cases in which the dissection arises in the ascending aorta and initial treatment is medical, the entire aorta may later require replacement (Fig. 77–3). Patients with Marfan's syndrome frequently have myxomatous degeneration of the ascending aorta producing annuloaortic ectasia and aortic insufficiency and associated dissection of either type I or type III. The former requires replacement of the valve and the ascending aorta, and the latter in the chronic stage may require replacement of all distal thoracic and abdominal aorta (Fig. 77–4).

Similarly, patients with major aortic ectasia ("mega aorta syndrome") may require graft replacement of the ascending aorta and aortic arch at one operation and varying segments distally (including the entire remaining aorta), usually at a second, staged operation. In fact, 40 per cent of the author's patients had other aortic segments replaced in addition to the thoracoabdominal aortic aneurysm. Thus, the true extent of aortic replacement was more extensive than that suggested by the classification discussed later.

EXTENT OF DISEASE

The extent to which both the aortic circumference and the aortic length are involved determines the type and extent of replacement. Thus, in the patient with a saccular aneurysm involving less than 50 per cent of the aortic circumference and located in the abdominal aorta behind the origin of the visceral vessels, treatment may be by excision and patch graft angioplasty. More extensive saccular aneurysms and those of a fusiform nature are treated with tube graft replacement. The length of the involved aortic segment in the latter cases is extremely variable but tends to assume four general patterns that determine the extent of operation, results of treatment, and nature and incidence of complications. In 378 patients (25 per cent) the aneurysm involved varying segments of the descending thoracic aorta and the upper abdominal aorta down to the celiac axis, permitting regular end-to-end anastomosis or anastomosis to the site of origin of the celiac axis anteriorly and to the renal arteries posteriorly, and requiring beveling of the graft to replace the posterior aneurysmal wall as a patch. To simplify discussion, these aneurysms are classified as *type I* (Fig. 77–5 and Table 77–3). Posterolateral thoracotomy incisions and separate diaphragm incisions enlarging the aortic hiatus that permitted retroperitoneal exposure were used in patients in whom abdominal extension was limited. Thoracoabdominal incisions were used in large or obese patients and in those with more extensive abdominal involvement.

Most of the descending thoracic and abdominal aortic segments were involved in 442 patients (29 per cent), and these aneurysms are classified as *type II* (Fig. 77–6; see also Figs. 77–3, 77–4, and 77–5).

Table 77–3. Classification of Thoracoabdominal Aneurysms

Extent	Description
Type I	Most of descending thoracic and upper abdominal aorta
Type II	Most of descending thoracic aorta and most or all of abdominal aorta
Type III	Distal descending thoracic aorta and most of the abdominal aorta
Type IV	Most or all of abdominal aorta including visceral vessel segment

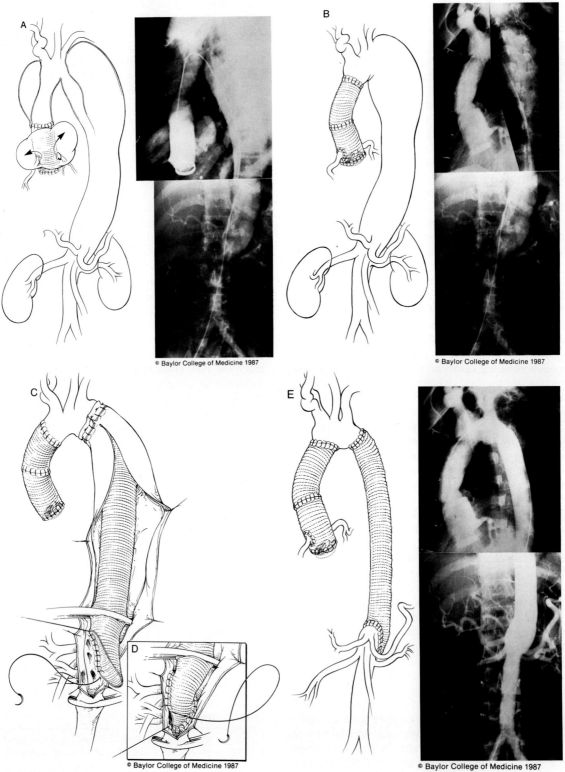

© Baylor College of Medicine 1987

© Baylor College of Medicine 1987

© Baylor College of Medicine 1987

© Baylor College of Medicine 1987

FIGURE 77–2. Type I chronic dissecting thoracoabdominal aortic aneurysm occurring after composite valve graft replacement of the aortic valve and ascending aorta, which became complicated by false aneurysm formation. *A*, Drawing and aortogram showing location and nature of aneurysms. *B*, Drawing and aortogram made after reconstruction of the ascending aorta and the complications of the first operation. *C* and *D*, Drawings showing technique of reconstruction for thoracoabdominal aortic aneurysm. *E*, Drawing and aortogram showing completed aortic reconstruction. (*A–E*, © Baylor College of Medicine, 1987.)

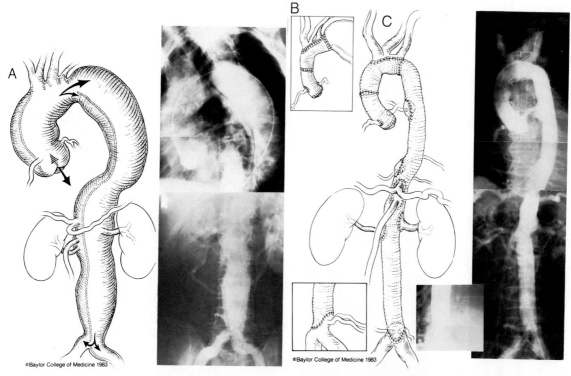

FIGURE 77–3. Illustrations of a patient with chronic dissection of the entire aorta associated with aortic valve insufficiency treated by total aortic replacement, including aortic valve (type II). *A*, Drawing and aortogram made before operation, showing extent of dissection. *B*, Drawing and aortogram after operative treatment consisting first of composite valve graft replacement of the aortic valve, ascending aorta, and transverse aortic arch at one operation, and then *C*, graft replacement of the entire descending thoracic and abdominal aorta at a later operation. (*A–C*, © Baylor College of Medicine, 1987.)

In 343 patients (23 per cent) the aneurysm, classified as *type III,* was located in the lower half of the descending thoracic aorta and varying segments of abdominal aorta, including that from which the visceral vessels arise (Fig. 77–7). The aneurysm in 346 patients (23 per cent) was located entirely in the abdominal aorta and involved its proximal segment, including the visceral vessel origins. These are classified as *type IV* (Figs. 77–8 and 77–9). Visceral vessel reconstruction or reattachment (or both) is required in types II, III, and IV. When technically feasible, the lower intercostal or upper lumbar arteries are reattached in patients with type I, II, or III lesions to avoid or reduce the incidence of spinal cord ischemia and neurologic disturbances of the lower extremities.

SYMPTOMS

Although thoracoabdominal aortic aneurysms may remain asymptomatic for varying periods of time, most ultimately produce a variety of symptoms before they rupture and cause death. Pain located in the chest, abdomen, flank, or back is the most common complaint and is due either to pressure on adjacent structures or to rupture. Compression of the trachea or bronchus may produce wheezing, cough, and pneumonitis distal to the area of obstruction. Erosion into the pulmonary parenchyma or airway may result in

hemoptysis. Similarly, compression or erosion of the esophagus may produce dysphagia or hematemesis. Erosion into the duodenum may cause intermittent or massive gastrointestinal bleeding. Compression of the liver or porta hepatis may produce jaundice. Traction of the vagus nerve at the aortic arch may cause recurrent laryngeal nerve paralysis, producing hoarseness. Vertebral body erosion may be present and cause back pain, and, in some of these patients, neurologic deficits may occur spontaneously from spinal cord compression. Thrombosis of spinal arteries with paraparesis or paraplegia has occurred and is seen most frequently in cases in which there is aortic dissection. Aortoinferior vena caval or iliac vein fistulae associated with heart failure have been observed. Secondary infection of the atheromatous debris and clot may occur, resulting in generalized sepsis. As with other aneurysms, distal embolization of clot or atheromatous debris or gradual obliteration and thrombosis of visceral and lower extremity branches are common.

DIAGNOSIS

Thoracic involvement of a palpable aortic aneurysm is rarely suspected on the basis of physical examination unless the abdominal component is so extensive that its cephalad projection is obscured to palpation by the costal margins of

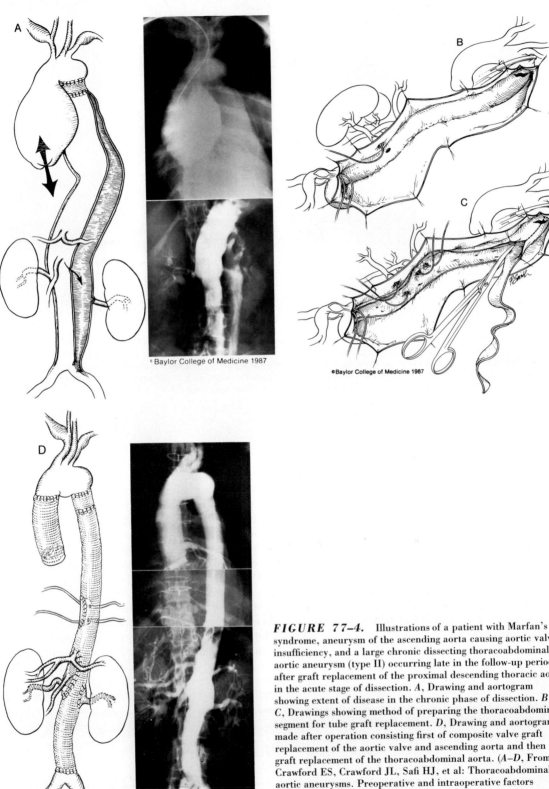

© Baylor College of Medicine 1987

©Baylor College of Medicine 1987

©Baylor College of Medicine 1987

FIGURE 77-4.   Illustrations of a patient with Marfan's syndrome, aneurysm of the ascending aorta causing aortic valve insufficiency, and a large chronic dissecting thoracoabdominal aortic aneurysm (type II) occurring late in the follow-up period after graft replacement of the proximal descending thoracic aorta in the acute stage of dissection. *A*, Drawing and aortogram showing extent of disease in the chronic phase of dissection. *B* and *C*, Drawings showing method of preparing the thoracoabdominal segment for tube graft replacement. *D*, Drawing and aortogram made after operation consisting first of composite valve graft replacement of the aortic valve and ascending aorta and then graft replacement of the thoracoabdominal aorta. (*A–D*, From Crawford ES, Crawford JL, Safi HJ, et al: Thoracoabdominal aortic aneurysms. Preoperative and intraoperative factors determining immediate and long-term results of operations in 605 patients. J Vasc Surg 3:389, 1986; © Baylor College of Medicine, 1987.)

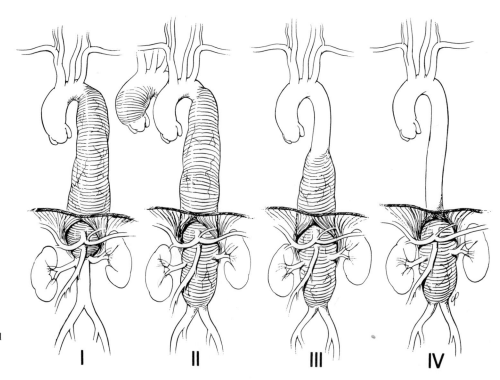

FIGURE 77–5.
Classification of thoracoabdominal aneurysms. (© Baylor College of Medicine, 1987.)

I   II   III   IV

the thoracic cage. In such cases, thoracoabdominal involvement should be strongly suspected. Plain chest roentgenograms may show widening of the descending thoracic aortic shadow emphasized by calcification that outlines the dilated aneurysmal wall. Similarly located calcification may also be seen in the upper abdomen in standard roentgenograms made in the anteroposterior and lateral position.

Precise diagnosis of aneurysm, including its location and extent, may be determined noninvasively either by magnetic resonance imaging (MRI) or by computed tomographic (CT) scanning. Ultrasonography may be helpful in identifying disease in the mid and lower abdomen but not in the upper abdomen and chest. Contrast aortography made with catheters and high-pressure injection in appropriate anteroposterior, oblique, and lateral views is used in patients selected for operation because this method of study best demonstrates the location and origins of the aortic branches. It also more clearly identifies the presence or absence of associated occlusive disease, which is present either in the visceral or iliac arteries in more than 20 per cent of cases. Separate small aneurysms involving these arteries may also be present in a small number of cases.

Special considerations are indicated in patients with compromised renal function and in those with a history of renal insufficiency occurring after prior exposure to contrast agents. To avoid recurrence of renal insufficiency or worsening of renal function, old (up to 3 months) arteriograms may be accepted provided that these studies are augmented by current non–contrast-enhanced CT scanning or MRI. Good quality CT scans may suffice in some instances. In any event, aortography is performed in a well-hydrated patient who is receiving intravenous fluids. It is our practice to increase the fluid intake of patients with borderline renal

function for several days before aortography and to give 25 gm of mannitol in 1000 ml of 5 per cent dextrose and Ringer's lactate solution immediately prior to the procedure. This usually reduces the blood urea nitrogen and creatinine levels before the procedure and may prevent increases afterward. Operation is delayed for 24 hours or longer to determine the effects of angiography on renal function and to permit diuresis of the contrast agent. If renal insufficiency occurs or increases, the operation is postponed until renal function becomes normal or stable.

ASSOCIATED DISEASE

Aneurysms involving other aortic segments had been present in 550 patients (36 per cent) and were present at the time of thoracoabdominal aneurysm repair in 128 patients (8.5 per cent)[11] (see Figs. 77–2, 77–3, and 77–4). Thus, ascending aortic or aortic arch aneurysmal disease was the most commonly associated condition, emphasizing the need for a study of the total aorta in patients with thoracoabdominal aneurysms. Cardiopulmonary disease and chronic renal disease are common accompaniments of thoracoabdominal aortic aneurysm owing to the nature of the underlying disease and the age of the patient population. Nevertheless, appropriate medical management permits operative therapy in over 90 per cent of these cases. Associated occlusive disease of the visceral and iliac arteries needing correction is present in 20 per cent of patients. Associated aneurysms of visceral vessels occur in a small number of cases. Other coexisting factors that complicated treatment in the author's cases included previous aortic operations, and unsuccessful attempts at repair in 10 per

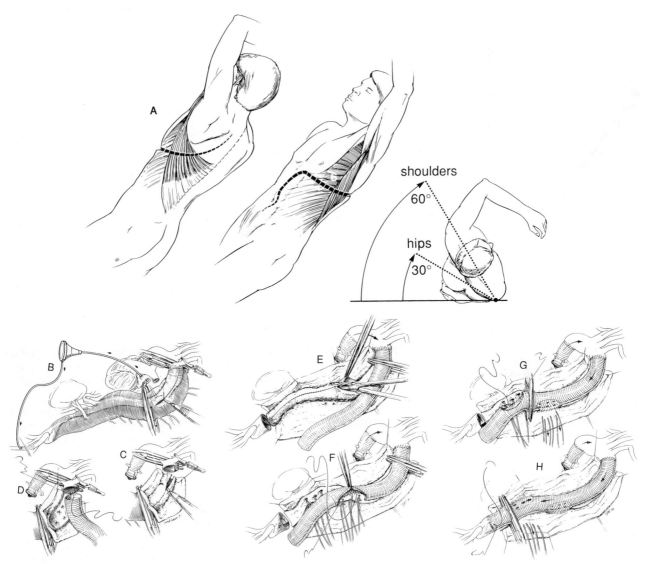

FIGURE 77–6. *A*, Location of proper incision for extensive thoracoabdominal aortic replacement and positioning of the body showing the relationship between the hip (placed at 30 degrees) and the shoulders (at 60 degrees) for maximal exposure as well as access to the left inguinal region. *B*, Drawing showing placement of bypass circuit from left atrium to left common femoral artery using Bio-Medicus pump. Proximal aortic clamping of the aorta is between the left common carotid and the left subclavian arteries. The left subclavian artery is occluded separately. A distal aortic clamp is placed to isolate the proximal aortic segment. *C*, The aorta is completely transected immediately distal to the left subclavian artery and separated from the esophagus. The false lumen, owing to its lateral position, is generally entered first. The aortic tissue separating the true and the false lumina is opened and completely excised. *D*, Proximal intercostal arteries are oversewn by direct suture. An end-to-end anastomosis is performed with running suture immediately distal to the left subclavian artery. *E*, The occluding clamp has been removed from the distal aortic arch and placed on the graft beyond the left subclavian artery. The left subclavian artery clamp has also been removed. Cardiofemoral bypass is discontinued following completion of the proximal anastomosis. The aneurysm is opened for its full length to the aortic bifurcation, and the remaining wall between the true and the false lumina throughout is completely excised. *F*, Back-bleeding from intercostal, visceral, and renal arteries is controlled with balloon catheters. Patent intercostal arteries in the region from T8 to T12 are reattached to an opening in the aortic graft. *G*, The cross clamp is sequentially moved further down on the aortic graft, restoring flow to reattached intercostal arteries while a separate opening in the graft is made for reattachment of the celiac axis and superior mesenteric and renal arteries. *H*, Following reattachment of the visceral and renal arteries, the cross clamp is again moved down on the graft to progressively restore flow. To complete the replacement, an end-to-end distal anastomosis is performed proximal to the aortic bifurcation.

Illustration continued on opposite page

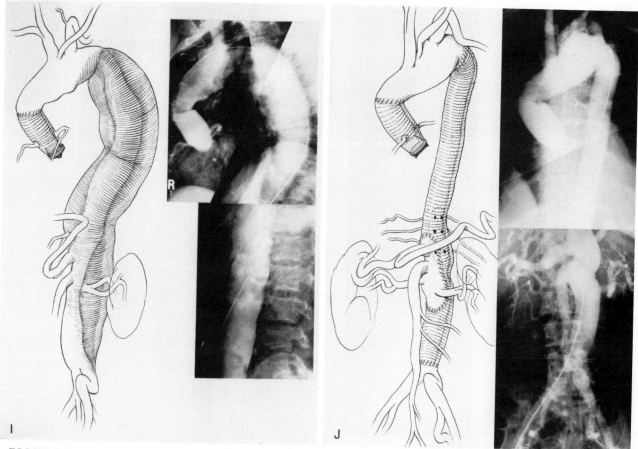

FIGURE 77–6 *Continued* *I*, Preoperative drawing and aortogram of patient with Marfan's syndrome and thoracoabdominal aortic aneurysm extending from the left subclavian artery to the aortic bifurcation, secondary to chronic dissection. This patient had previously undergone composite valve graft replacement of the aortic root. *J*, Postoperative drawing and aortogram following graft replacement of the thoracoabdominal aortic aneurysm with reattachment of multiple intercostal arteries, celiac axis, superior mesenteric artery, and both renal arteries.

cent of cases, rupture in 61 patients (4 per cent), aortoenteric fistulae in eight patients, and aortovenous fistulae in five patients. Concurrent gastrointestinal problems, including gallbladder disease, cancer, and peptic ulcer are not uncommon.

TREATMENT

Treatment of thoracoabdominal aortic aneurysms requires both aortic and visceral arterial reconstruction. Various procedures have been employed including (1) excision and graft replacement with direct reattachment of visceral vessels either to the graft or to a branch of the graft; (2) insertion of a permanent bypass, attachment of visceral vessels to branches of this graft, and then removal or imbrication of the aneurysm; (3) permanent bypass graft and reattachment of visceral vessels to branches of the graft, leaving the aneurysm in place with proximal inflow occluded; and (4) graft inclusion with direct visceral artery reattachment.[2–8] We prefer the last method because of the relative safety and simplicity with which it can be applied. This has been our choice during the past 25 years, and the technique is described in more detail later in this chapter.

Anesthetic Management

Improvements in anesthesia, physiologic monitoring, and blood component replacement have contributed to the success of treatment of thoracoabdominal aortic aneurysms. Because of advanced age and the prevalence of associated cardiac and occlusive disease in these patients, anesthesia is induced with agents that do not impair cardiac function, such as diazepam and fentanyl. Muscle relaxation is achieved with pancuronium bromide. A Carlens double-lumen endobronchial tube is inserted to allow selective ventilation of the right lung and deflation of the left lung. In addition to increasing exposure during the operation, this maneuver reduces trauma to the left lung and prevents excessive cardiac compression. Adequate intravenous access is essential to performance of the operation and should include insertion of a central venous catheter and four large peripheral catheters to allow rapid volume replacement. Bilateral radial arterial catheters allow continuous monitoring of upper extremity blood pressure during the frequent sampling for arterial blood gas and laboratory determinations. A Swan-Ganz catheter should be inserted via the subclavian or internal jugular vein in all patients to allow determination of right pulmonary artery and pulmonary capillary

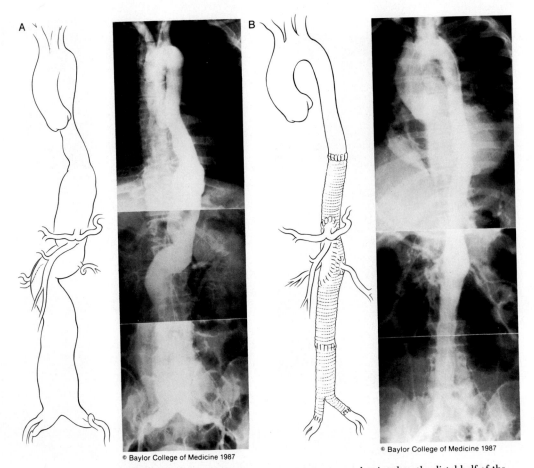

© Baylor College of Medicine 1987   © Baylor College of Medicine 1987

FIGURE 77–7.   Illustrations of a patient with degenerative aneurysm that involves the distal half of the descending thoracic aorta and the entire abdominal aorta (type III). *A*, Drawing and aortogram showing the location and extent of disease. *B*, Drawing and aortogram showing graft in place and functioning. (*A* and *B*, © Baylor College of Medicine, 1987.)

wedge pressures and cardiac output. Arterial blood gas and electrolyte measurements are performed every 30 minutes, and appropriate adjustments are made as indicated. Prophylactic antibiotics are begun 12 hours prior to surgery and are continued until the fifth postoperative day or until all catheters have been removed. Steroids are given at the onset of operation and Pentothal sodium at the time of aortic clamping, and blood sugar levels are controlled as recommended by others to protect the central nervous system.

Administration of crystalloid solutions is begun before the operation, and the first liter consists of lactated Ringer's solution with 5 per cent dextrose. Plain lactated Ringer's solution and blood elements are given during the remainder of the operation to maintain the central venous pressure between 7 and 10 cm/H_2O and the pulmonary capillary wedge pressure at normal or preanesthetic levels. Cardiac output is determined by thermodilution at the time of Swan-Ganz catheter insertion and as needed during the operation and postoperative recovery. At the time of induction of anesthesia, 25 gm of mannitol is given to promote vigorous diuresis. Proximal blood pressure, cardiac hemodynamics, and peripheral vascular resistance are maintained at optimal levels during the period of aortic cross-clamping by the administration of sodium nitroprusside solution in conjunc-

tion with replacement of fluid and blood losses. Nitroprusside administration is discontinued prior to the release of the aortic cross-clamp and restoration of flow through the graft. As the proximal aortic clamp is slowly released, blood components and crystalloid solutions are administered rapidly through peripheral venous lines so that declamping hypotension is avoided and normal cardiac hemodynamics are maintained. Sodium bicarbonate solution is routinely administered by continuous drip during the period of aortic cross-clamping to prevent acidosis.

Throughout the operation hemoglobin and coagulation parameters are carefully monitored, and adjustments are made by administering appropriate blood components. Fresh frozen plasma is given throughout the operation, and 10 to 16 units of platelet concentrate is administered at the time of aortic declamping. Problems related to coagulopathy induced by factor deficiency have been minimal when this approach is used. Requirements for banked blood for transfusion have been significantly reduced in recent years by the routine autotransfusion of washed red cells. Collection and transfusion of blood lost during resection of thoracoabdominal aneurysms is of immense importance because some large aneurysms may contain up to 2000 ml of blood. Salvage of this volume of blood contained within

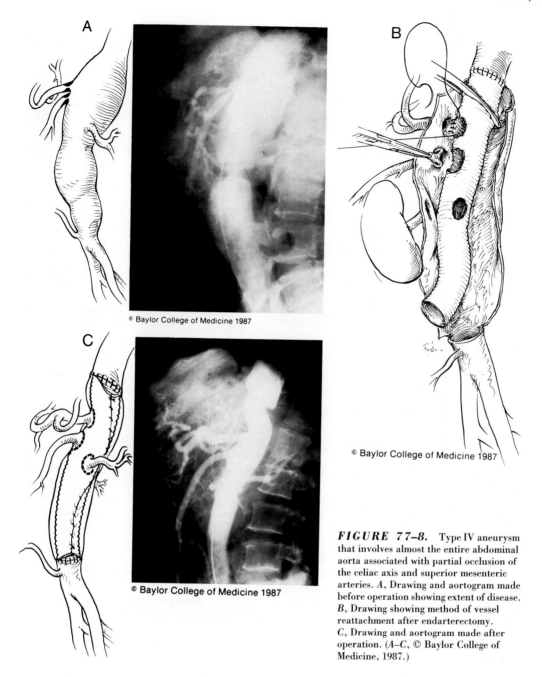

© Baylor College of Medicine 1987

© Baylor College of Medicine 1987

© Baylor College of Medicine 1987

FIGURE 77–8. Type IV aneurysm that involves almost the entire abdominal aorta associated with partial occlusion of the celiac axis and superior mesenteric arteries. *A,* Drawing and aortogram made before operation showing extent of disease. *B,* Drawing showing method of vessel reattachment after endarterectomy. *C,* Drawing and aortogram made after operation. (*A–C,* © Baylor College of Medicine, 1987.)

the aneurysm plus that lost during performance of the operation frequently makes it possible to save up to 45 units of packed, washed red cells per patient.

With the development of methods to monitor spinal cord function during operation using temporary pump bypass and somatosensory-evoked potentials, it was suggested that the incidence of paraplegia and renal insufficiency could be reduced using these techniques. This hypothesis was prospectively tested in a consecutive series of 198 patients.[9] The authors found the method completely unreliable in predicting postoperative spinal cord dysfunction and subsequent paraplegia. The incidence of both paraplegia and renal function disturbances was unchanged; consequently, this technique is not recommended.

Operation

The patient is positioned and maintained on the right side with the shoulders at 60 degrees and the hips at 30 degrees by utilizing a deflatable bean bag (see Fig. 77–6A). The entire left side of the chest and abdomen as well as the upper part of the groin in selected patients is prepared and draped in the usual sterile manner. Operative exposure is obtained through a thoracoabdominal incision in most patients. The level of the incision is determined by the proximal extent of the aneurysm in the thoracic aorta. Aortic lesions extending slightly above the diaphragm (type IV) are exposed through a low thoracic incision at about the level of the eighth or ninth rib, which is then extended

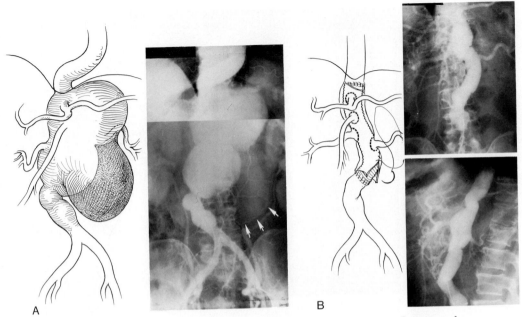

FIGURE 77–9. Huge aneurysm involving the upper abdominal aorta (type IV). *A,* Drawing and aortogram made before operation showing location and extent of disease. *B,* Drawing and aortogram made after operation showing graft in place and reattached visceral vessels. (*A* and *B,* From Crawford ES, Snyder DM, Cho CG, et al: Progress in treatment of thoracoabdominal and abdominal aortic aneurysms involving celiac, superior mesenteric, and renal arteries. Ann Surg 188:404, 1978.)

obliquely across the costal arch onto the abdomen and across to the level of the umbilicus. More extensive lesions extending into the mid or proximal descending thoracic aorta (types II and III) require exposure through a sixth intercostal space incision directed across the costal arch into the abdomen with extension to the pubis in the midline as needed. In some patients proximal exposure may require removal of the sixth rib. The incision across the costal arch is positioned lower than the standard anterior extent of a posterolateral thoracotomy to avoid sharp angulation and necrosis between the thoracic and abdominal components of the incision. Predominantly thoracic aortic aneurysms with thoracoabdominal extension through the diaphragm and to the level of the celiac artery (type I) may be approached completely through a thoracic incision, with provisions for detachment of the left vertebral diaphragmatic attachments and possible extension across the costal arch into the abdomen.

The thoracic portion of the thoracoabdominal aneurysm is exposed by gently retracting the collapsed lung medially. Adhesions between the aneurysm and left lung are left undisturbed to prevent inadvertent entry into the aneurysm and trauma to the lung. The vagus and recurrent laryngeal nerves are identified, and an adequate segment of the distal aortic arch or descending thoracic aorta is selected for placement of the aortic cross-clamp. Dividing the vagus nerve beyond the takeoff of the recurrent laryngeal nerve provides additional mobilization and reduces the likelihood of more proximal nerve injury. Minimal dissection is necessary to accomplish this without injury to the adjacent esophagus, pulmonary artery, or intercostal branches. The abdominal aorta is exposed through a left retroperitoneal approach following a radial division of the diaphragm from

the point of division of the costal arch to the aortic hiatus. With a retroperitoneal exposure, electrocautery is used to develop a relatively avascular tissue plane lateral to the left colon and posterior to the colon, left kidney, spleen, and pancreas. Maintaining the plane of dissection anterior to the left psoas muscle, the surgeon mobilizes and retracts the abdominal viscera medially, exposing the entire length of the posterolateral aspect of the abdominal aorta from the aortic bifurcation to the diaphragm. The abdominal aorta may be approached either intraperitoneally or extraperitoneally. The extraperitoneal approach is utilized in patients who have undergone multiple previous abdominal surgeries. The intraperitoneal approach allows thorough examination of the intra-abdominal organs both before and after aortic reconstruction. We have found no difference in fluid requirements, postoperative pulmonary status, and bleeding between these two approaches. The common iliac or femoral artery may be exposed in the groin if the iliac vessels are involved with occlusive disease or aneurysm.

With advance notice, the anesthesiologist begins infusion of nitroprusside to keep the proximal blood pressure and cardiac hemodynamics stable as the proximal aortic clamp is applied. In patients with severe peripheral vascular occlusive disease or distal arterial grafts, heparin is administered (1 mg/kg) prior to aortic clamping. Cardiofemoral bypass is used in patients with aortic dissection and extensive aneurysmal disease (types I and II) for distal organ perfusion and spinal cord protection during the time required for the proximal anastomosis. The proximal aorta is isolated between clamps (see Fig. 77–6). A woven Dacron tube of appropriate size (usually 20 to 26 mm in diameter) is selected for insertion. The proximal anastomosis to the uninvolved aorta is performed after complete aortic transection has been accomplished. Separation of the aorta from the esophagus prevents incorporation of the latter in the posterior portion of the suture line. The graft is clamped and the proximal aortic clamp temporarily released to assess hemostasis at the anastomosis. After completion of the proximal anastomosis, cardiofemoral bypass is discontinued and the distal extent of the aneurysm is opened in a longitudinal fashion in a posterolateral plane. The edges of the aneurysm wall are retracted with heavy stay sutures. Blood contained within the aneurysmal cavity and that lost by collateral circulation from the lumbar and intercostal vessels is collected in the autotransfusion unit. All atherosclerotic debris and clot is evacuated, and the origins of the celiac, superior mesenteric, and left and right renal arteries are identified. A No. 4 balloon occlusion catheter is gently inflated within the proximal portion of each vessel to prevent back-bleeding from the visceral vessels and distal embolization of debris at the time of aortic flushing. Selected intercostal or lumbar arteries or both are identified for reattachment to the graft, and the remaining vessels are suture ligated from within the aneurysm (see Figs. 77–1, 77–4, and 77–6). The selection of appropriate intercostal vessels for reattachment is based on the extent of the aneurysm, the potential risk of postoperative paraplegia, and the presence of suitable intercostal or lumbar vessels for reimplantation. Large intercostal branches in the region between T8 and L2 have the greatest potential as sources of accessory spinal arterial circulation and therefore are selected for reimplantation.

The graft is then placed under appropriate tension, and an oval opening is made opposite the pairs of intercostal vessels to be reattached. A circumferential anastomosis is performed between the graft and the orifice of these vessels with continuous over-and-over sutures, incorporating generous purchases of aortic wall (see Fig. 77–6F and G). The graft is placed under suitable tension, and similar appropriately sized openings are made in it for reattachment of the visceral and renal vessels. The number and size of openings may vary from one to four and depend upon the distance separating the vessel origins because of the aortic dilatation. The anastomoses are then performed in a similar manner, a circumferential running suture being used to attach the opening in the Dacron graft around the circumference of the visceral artery orifice to be reimplanted. Several variations in the degree of visceral artery origin separation may exist. In some patients, the celiac, superior mesenteric, and renal vessels may all be widely separated, requiring individual reattachment (see Fig. 77–9). In other instances, the visceral vessels are closely clustered and may be incorporated into one anastomosis or as an elliptical extension of the proximal or distal aortic anastomosis. Numerous variations of attachment are used, depending upon these variations in spacing of visceral artery origins and the proximity to normal uninvolved aorta (see Fig. 77–2). Occasionally, severe associated distal occlusive disease or wide separation of the vessel orifices on the aneurysm wall requires reattachment by separate bypass from the main Dacron graft by means of an 8-mm knitted Dacron tube extension.

Following completion of the visceral and renal artery reattachment, the patient's head is placed in a dependent position, and air and debris are flushed from the graft by temporarily releasing the proximal clamp. The graft is also vented by multiple needles as the patient's head is elevated. All balloon catheters are then deflated and removed as the aortic clamp is slowly removed. Flow is thus restored to the intercostal and visceral branches as the proximal aortic clamp is changed to an infrarenal position. The distal aortic reconstruction is then performed by either end-to-end anastomosis to uninvolved aorta or by attachment of a bifurcation graft with bypass to the iliac or femoral arteries (see Fig. 77–1). Flow is restored to the lower extremities, and a careful check for hemostasis at all suture lines is performed. The redundant aneurysm sac is not excised but is tightly sutured around the aortic reconstruction. This avoids additional and unnecessary dissection and bleeding as well as ensuring hemostasis and separation of the graft structures from adjacent organs. The abdominal visceral and renal vessels are then palpated for pulsations, and the viscera are returned to the abdomen in an orderly and anatomic fashion. The diaphragm is reapproximated, and an intercostal catheter is inserted for lung re-expansion and drainage. Finally, the wound is closed in layers.

Dissecting Aneurysms

Although dissection may be extensive and may involve the entire aorta, the segment of aortic circumference from which the intercostal and lumbar arteries arise may be spared. This fortuitous characteristic occurs in some patients and permits reconstruction that spares most of the spinal cord accessory circulation. Reconstruction is performed in such cases by replacing the dissected part of the aortic circumference with a corresponding portion of Dacron graft that is beveled to accommodate this part of the reconstruction (Fig. 77–10; see also Fig. 77–1). The orifices of the visceral vessels are usually spared or minimally involved in the dissection and are clustered close together. The septa of dissection are trimmed from the involved openings, and the origins of all four visceral arteries are attached to one opening made in the graft as shown in Figure 77–1. The infrarenal aortic and iliac arterial segments are reconstructed by using a bifurcation graft attached to the infrarenal segment of the upper tube graft inserted as described and illustrated in Figure 77–1.

This method of graft replacement of only the dissected segment of the aortic wall may be impossible and impractical owing to either quality of tissues or extreme volumes of back-bleeding through the intercostal vessels. Those cases are treated similarly to regular fusiform aneurysms of degenerative origin. The false lumen is first opened longitudinally, and then the inner wall of dissected true lumen is excised (see Fig. 77–4). The intercostal arteries necessary to reduce excessive bleeding are ligated, and those that are to be reattached are temporarily occluded by balloon catheters. Aortic reconstruction is then completed using a tubular graft to which the necessary arterial branches are reattached, as previously described (see Fig. 77–6). Following treatment for acute aortic dissection, we recommend continued surveillance of remaining aortic segments for dilatation of the false lumen. A CT or MRI scan is performed every 3 months for 1 year and, if the graft is stable in diameter, every year thereafter.

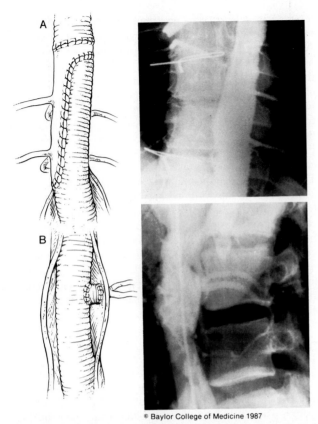

© Baylor College of Medicine 1987

FIGURE 77–10. Additional methods of reattaching intercostal or lumbar arteries. *A*, The beveled end of a tubular graft may be used to replace a short segment of dissected aortic circumference in order to spare several pairs of intercostal arteries. *B*, One end of a short segment of Dacron graft of appropriate diameter is first sutured around the origins of vessels to be reattached; the other end is attached to an oval opening made in the aortic graft. (*A* and *B*, © Baylor College of Medicine, 1987.)

Associated Vessel Disease

Associated occlusive lesions of the visceral arteries and iliac arteries are treated at the time of aneurysm operation. The former, when localized to the origin of the artery, are treated by endarterectomy performed from inside the aneurysm before reattachment to the graft (see Fig. 77–8). The cleavage plane between the diseased aortic intima and normal outer layers is entered around the vessel origin and continued distally into the involved part of the vessel beyond the atheromatous disease. Endarterectomy of at least one visceral artery was required in 82 patients (5 per cent) and endarterectomy of at least one renal artery was necessary in 190 patients (13 per cent). Bypass graft may be required in patients with more extensive involvement and in those with distal obstruction (see Fig. 77–4). The graft used to bypass the renal artery on the right extends from the iliac artery to the renal artery behind the viscera. The grafts used to bypass mesenteric, celiac axis, and left renal artery disease extend proximally either from graft or native aorta distally to the involved vessel. Iliac artery occlusive disease is treated with a bifurcated graft attached to the proximal end of the aortic graft. The limbs of the graft are then attached distally end-to-side to either the external iliac

or common femoral arteries, depending upon the extent of the disease.

RESULTS AND COMPLICATIONS

Of the 1509 patients submitted to operation by the authors, 1386 (92 per cent) were early (30-day) survivors. Preoperative variables predictive of early death were advanced age, the presence of pulmonary, cardiac, and renal disease, and rupture.[11] These variables were about equally present regardless of etiology, location, and extent of disease; consequently, the early survival rates were about equal for all groups of patients (see Tables 77–1 and 77–2). The long-term survival rate as determined by the Kaplan-Meier method in the 1509 patients submitted to operation and followed was 59 (± 3) per cent at 5 years and 32 (± 6) per cent at 10 years (Fig. 77–11). Risk factors predictive of late death (stepwise Cox regression model) were advanced age, rupture, renal dysfunction, extent of disease, and dissection. Long-term survival in patients with nondissecting aneurysms is compared with those with dissecting aneurysms in Figure 77–12. The 5-year survival rate of the former was about 6 per cent greater owing to the high frequency of rupture of another aneurysm in those with dissecting aneurysms.

The author has classified the complications of thoracoabdominal aneurysm repair as technical complications, blood volume disturbances, electrolyte imbalance, coagulation defects, neurologic complications, and disturbances in renal function. Awareness of these problems has allowed appropriate action in both prevention and treatment in some cases.

Technical Complications

Renal artery reconstruction may be difficult in patients with associated occlusive disease of the renal arteries and in some patients because of the position of origin of the left renal artery on the aortic wall. Unsuccessful reattachment in either instance is evidenced by lack of a palpable pulse in the renal artery on completion of reconstruction. This can be confirmed by intraoperative Doppler or duplex scanning. This complication is treated by insertion of an aorta–left renal artery bypass graft as previously described. Revision of the original attachment has not been successful and is not recommended. Postoperative occlusion of the right renal artery may not be evident because it is difficult to palpate with the standard exposure used for operation. Furthermore, occlusion of the left renal artery may be delayed. Bilateral renal artery occlusion is suspected when urine output during wound closure or the early postoperative period is poor. The time between intravenous administration of indigo carmine and the appearance of blue color in the urine closely correlates with the postoperative development of renal failure. Such findings dictate aortography; if occlusion is present, the patient is returned to the operating room for bilateral aortorenal bypass, as previously described.

The most serious technical problem occurring during operation is uncontrollable hemorrhage at the site of proxi-

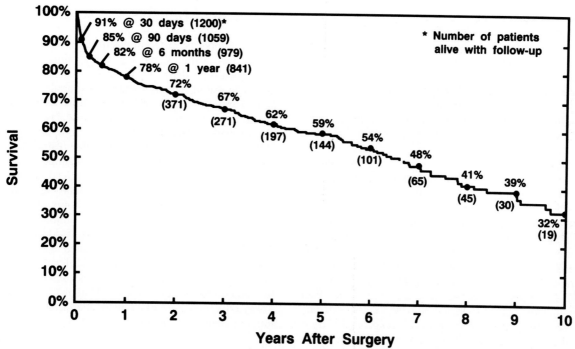

FIGURE 77–11. Long-term survival of entire population estimated by Kaplan-Meier method.

mal aortic clamping in the distal arch at or near the left subclavian artery in treatment of types I and II lesions. This complication may arise from transmural aortic injury during mobilization of the proximal aorta in patients with scarred cleavage planes resulting either from previous operation, inflammation, dissection, or rupture, or by the aortic clamp cutting the friable aorta during its application. This complication may be controlled by performing rapid, more proxi-

mal aortic exposure and then reapplying the clamps. This may not be possible; in fact, the aneurysm may be so large that the proximal structures cannot be exposed, or large contained ruptures may be entered even during chest entry. The left main pulmonary artery may also be accidentally entered in patients with scarred cleavage planes. Bleeding in the latter cases is controlled by finger pressure and closure of the common coverage of the pulmonary artery and

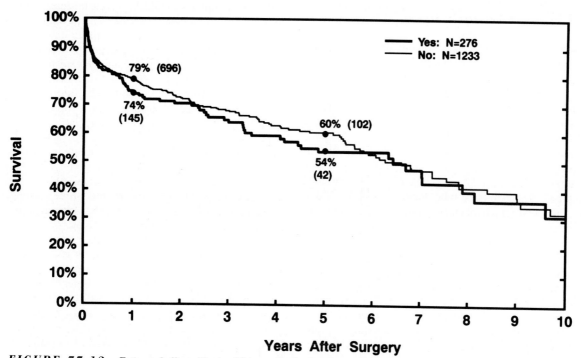

FIGURE 77–12. Estimated effects (Kaplan-Meier method) of etiology (nondissection vs. dissection) on long-term survival.

aorta. Proximal aortic exposure and graft anastomosis is performed in these cases without exposure and clamping by arresting circulation. This is accomplished by performing femoral artery–femoral vein cannulation and producing profound hypothermia (18°C, rectal) using partial cardio-pulmonary bypass. Crawford and colleagues have used this technique in 25 patients, with survival in 21.[10]

Balloon catheter rupture of intercostal, lumbar, mes-enteric, or renal artery may result from overdistention of the balloon. Moreover, this injury may be undetected dur-ing operation and may become evident only by signs of continued bleeding after operation. These injuries may be difficult to repair and emphasize the need for careful and gentle use of balloon occlusion catheters. Splenic tears are common regardless of gentle dissection and retraction dur-ing operation. Splenic salvage attempts after such injuries have proved unsafe. Capsular evulsion controlled by ''he-mostatic'' packing has resulted in early postoperative bleeding requiring reoperation and splenectomy. Suture re-pair of lacerations using various techniques has been associated with delayed sudden rupture and massive hemor-rhage, requiring reoperation several weeks later. Conse-quent to these experiences, the author recommends imme-diate splenectomy for treatment of splenic tears occurring during operation, since this procedure has not been associ-ated with either early or late complications.

Early reoperation for bleeding, in most cases resulting from technical complications, has been due to unsecured small bleeding vessels, suture holes at anastomoses, spon-taneous rearrangement of pleats in the end of the graft at the site of anastomosis, and wound disruption. The methods of preventing and treating these problems are obvious. Other causes of bleeding during and after operation are coagulopathies. Reoperation for bleeding in this series car-ried a mortality rate of 25 per cent.[11]

Blood Volume Disturbances

As discussed earlier, central venous pressure, pulmo-nary artery and pulmonary capillary wedge pressures, pe-ripheral arterial pressure, and urine output are monitored closely during and after operation. Normal values are main-tained primarily by intravenous fluid administration. Inade-quate blood volume, as reflected by low venous, pulmonary artery, and wedge pressures, may be due to inadequate replacement of large urine output, but wound and ''third-space'' losses are the usual cause in the presence of low urine output. Third-space loss may also be due to continued bleeding and excessive chest tube drainage; abdominal dis-tention and persistent hypotension despite blood replace-ment suggest ongoing hemorrhage. Regardless of cause, blood volume replacement and immediate reoperation to control bleeding are the indicated treatments. Prolonged volume deficits and associated renal hypoperfusion lead to renal ischemia and acute tubular necrosis. Vasopressors are contraindicated. When drugs are administered for hemody-namic support, we prefer dopamine and nitroprusside or nitroglycerin for the combined effects of elevating pressure and improving visceral perfusion by afterload reduction.

Electrolyte Imbalance

A number of different electrolyte imbalances may oc-cur in these patients, but the most common problem has been potassium depletion from diuresis soon after opera-tion. The use of mannitol and other diuretics together with administration of large volumes of fluid during the period of anuria associated with renal artery occlusion is responsi-ble for marked diuresis with hourly urine outputs of up to 250 to 1200 ml for 4 to 6 hours after restoration of renal inflow. Persistent diuresis of this magnitude may deplete intra- and extracellular potassium and lead to fatal cardiac dysrhythmias. Consequently, serum potassium is monitored *every 30 minutes* during and for 4 hours after operation, and normal values are maintained by administration of po-tassium solution. Potassium chloride is added at a rate of 20 mEq to each 1000 ml of lactated Ringer's solution administered postoperatively, and additional 10-mEq incre-ments are given via a central venous catheter as necessary to maintain blood potassium levels above 3.5 mEq/100 ml. To avoid aggravation of diuresis, the lactated Ringer's so-lution contains no glucose.

Coagulopathies

These patients are prone to disseminated intravascular coagulopathies before operation because of platelet and fi-brinogen consumption in the extensive aneurysms. This defect is aggravated during operation by loss of whole blood and its appropriate replacement with solutions lack-ing its normal clotting components, because the latter in itself produces a coagulopathy by diluting the patient's clot-ting substances. This, too, may be present before operation in the patient whose aneurysm has ruptured. The coagulant status of the patient should be determined prior to operation and every 30 to 40 minutes during operation; appropriate blood components should be given to correct any defects present and to prevent those that may develop. These com-ponents include fresh plasma, cryoprecipitate, and platelets. In the patient with normal preoperative coagulation, the author recommends giving 1 unit of fresh plasma per 2 units of red blood cells after the first transfusion of 3 con-secutive units of red blood cells. The frequency of plasma transfusions and the requirement for cryoprecipitate are de-pendent upon measurement of coagulation abnormalities. Heparin is not given intentionally, but activated clotting times (ACT) are determined at 30-minute intervals to detect heparin that may accompany blood given with the autoge-nous system of transfusion. Abnormal ACT is treated by administration of intravenous protamine sulfate. Fresh platelets (12 units) are routinely given when flow is restored to the distal aorta and lower extremities.

Unless the aforementioned precautions are taken, un-controllable diffuse bleeding will occur and persist until the coagulation defect is corrected. The wound should never be closed until coagulation is normal clinically and by labora-tory testing; otherwise, bleeding will continue in the post-operative period and reoperation will be required. Regard-less of the etiology of postoperative bleeding, this complication carries a high incidence of death and of such complications as paraplegia, renal failure, and sepsis. By following the principles mentioned previously for the treatment of these patients, good hemostasis has been achieved. Reoperation has been required in only 2 of the last 125 patients undergoing operation.

Neurologic Complications

The neurologic complications that are likely to occur in patients treated for thoracoabdominal aortic aneurysm disease may be of cerebral or spinal origin. Fortunately, cerebral complications resulting from either occlusive cerebrovascular lesions or air emboli from the long aortic grafts are rare. The former may be prevented by carotid endarterectomy and the latter by evacuation of air with the patient in the head-down position before restoration of flow through the graft as previously described. In this series of 1509 patients, known cerebrovascular occlusive disease was present in 230 patients (15 per cent). The postoperative complication of stroke occurred in 39 patients (3 per cent) and did not vary significantly with the extent of aortic replacement.

Postoperative development of paraplegia or paraparesis remains the most serious complication following surgery on these patients. The severity of the neurologic deficit has been variable, ranging from minimal weakness to flaccid paralysis with absent control of bladder and rectal sphincters. Patients who were able to move all joints against gravity were classified as having paraparesis. Those with less motion were considered paraplegic. In this series of 1509 patients, 234 (16 per cent) had paraplegia or paraparesis postoperatively. The cause of such neurologic deficits is multi-factorial and in general is related to the duration of spinal cord ischemia during aortic cross-clamping or to failure to reestablish the critical accessory arterial blood supply to the spinal cord. Up to one third of patients have had postoperative neurologic deficits delayed from 1 to 21 days following operation. The majority of these delayed complications were usually related to specific events such as myocardial infarction, respiratory failure, and other causes of hemodynamic instability.

Analysis of preoperative and operative variables significantly related to the development of postoperative neurologic paraplegia or paraparesis includes the following: extent of aorta replaced, aortic clamp time, presence of rupture, age, concurrent proximal aneurysmal disease, and history of preoperative renal dysfunction. Postoperative paraplegia or paraparesis was greatest in patients who required replacement of the entire descending thoracic and all of the abdominal aorta and occurred in 139 patients (31 per cent). In patients requiring replacement of the entire descending thoracic and upper abdominal aorta, paraplegia or paraparesis occurred in 57 patients (15 per cent). Deficits developed in 23 patients (7 per cent) requiring replacement of the lower descending thoracic and all of the abdominal aorta and in 15 patients (4 per cent) requiring replacement of the total abdominal aorta. In 1448 patients without rupture, 218 patients (15 per cent) developed postoperative neurologic deficits. Among the 61 patients with rupture of an aortic aneurysm 16 (26 per cent) developed deficits.

A reliable effective method of preventing paraplegia or paraparesis is not yet available. Theoretically, bypass from the left atrium to one of the common femoral arteries (atrial femoral bypass) using a centrifugal pump is capable of maintaining blood supply to the spinal cord via distal intercostal vessel arteries while the proximal anastomosis is being performed. Femorofemoral bypass with an oxygenator inserted could accomplish the same goal but has the distinct disadvantage of requiring heparinization.

Distal aortic perfusion was evaluated prospectively by Svensson and colleagues in 198 consecutive patients.[13] All patients survived operation and recovered from anesthesia and lived long enough for independent neurologic evaluation. In these 198 patients temporary distal aortic perfusion was combined with somatosensory evoked potential monitoring in an attempt to prevent the occurrence of neurologic complications after operation. In 99 patients adequate distal bypass with perfusion pressures of at least 60 mmHg was achieved. In 99 patients this goal could not be achieved for a variety of technical and anatomic reasons. Early and late neurologic complications were 8 per cent and 12 per cent, respectively, in the former group, and 7 per cent and 8 per cent, respectively, in the latter. No statistic difference in the incidence of neurologic complications was found between the two groups. The incidence of false-negative somatosensory-evoked potential response was 13 per cent, and the false-positive response rate was 67 per cent. Localization of critical spinal arteries for reattachment was not possible. Consequently, the author no longer uses somatosensory-evoked potential monitoring. However, distal arterial bypass using the atrial femoral technique without heparin is used in patients with friable aortas, particularly those with dissection or Marfan's syndrome, to allow gentle proximal clamping. Bypass has the additional advantage of reducing postclamping acidosis, and less pharmacologic intervention by anesthesia is needed to maintain a normal proximal pressure.

The influence of cerebrospinal fluid drainage on the incidence of neurologic deficit was evaluated by Crawford and associates in a prospective randomized series of patients with extensive aneurysmal disease of the thoracoabdominal aorta.[14] Of 98 patients evaluated, 46 patients had cerebrospinal fluid drainage and 52 patients did not (controls). Treatment included cerebrospinal fluid drainage along with graft replacement of the aneurysm, reattachment of intercostal and lumbar arteries, and temporary atrial femoral bypass during aortic occlusion. Cerebrospinal fluid drainage was *not* found to be beneficial in preventing paraplegia. In this study the only significant predictor of delayed neurologic deficit was the occurrence of postoperative hypotension.

Because permanent ligation of arteries supplying circulation to the spinal cord in operations for aortic aneurysm can lead to spinal cord infarct resulting in paraplegia, Svensson and Crawford reported a method of rapid intraoperative identification of specific arteries supplying the spinal cord using an intrathecal platinum electrode to detect a hydrogen solution injected into the aortic ostia.[13] The technique was used in both porcine experiments and in a pilot study of eight humans showing that the technique

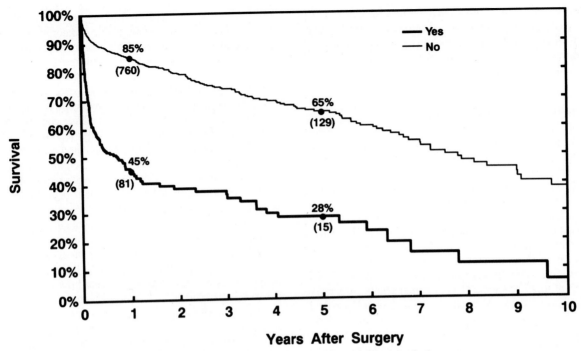

FIGURE 77–13. Effects of renal failure on long-term survival by Kaplan-Meier method.

could be satisfactorily utilized, but technical problems have yet to be resolved. If this technique is successful in larger numbers of patients, intraoperative identification of the arteries supplying the spinal cord may allow temporary perfusion and permanent reattachment, thus reducing the incidence of spinal cord ischemia and infarction after repair of thoracoabdominal aneurysms.

A variety of pharmacologic methods have been evaluated in an attempt to increase the tolerance of the spinal cord to ischemia. These have included the use of steroids, lidocaine, prostaglandin E_1, and thiopental. These and other methods may yet prove to be beneficial, either singly or in combination, but will require thorough evaluation in large numbers of patients.

The author has a contemporary experience in the treatment of 372 patients with thoracoabdominal aortic aneurysmal disease during the period from January 11, 1986, through March 1, 1994. There were 169 female patients and 203 male patients. The median age was 66 years. The distribution of aortic involvement from type I through type IV was 137, 96, 72, and 67, respectively. Ninety-five patients (25 per cent) were treated for acute or chronic dissection and 277 patients (75 per cent) had fusiform aneurysmal disease without dissection. For patients both with and without dissection, the 30-day survival rate was 95 per cent. Only 9 patients (2.4 per cent) were returned to the operating room for postoperative bleeding. Paraplegia or paraparesis in patients without dissection developed in 6.3 per cent of patients in type I; 19 per cent in type II; 3 per cent, type III; and 1.7 per cent, type IV; for an overall paraplegia and paraparesis rate of 7.2 per cent. In patients with dissection, the rate of paraplegia or paraparesis was 4.8 per cent for type I; 5.3 per cent for type II; and 0 per cent, types III and

IV; for an overall paraplegia and paraparesis rate of 4.2 per cent.

Disturbances in Renal Function

Renal failure is a common complication of thoracoabdominal aneurysm repair. In fact, it was second only to cardiac complications as a contributing cause of early death, and was third in late death (see Tables 77–1 and 77–2).[11] Renal function disturbances were related to a number of factors, including rupture, bleeding following operation, age, duration of renal artery occlusion, and the presence of renal insufficiency prior to operation. The latter was the most common contributing factor. Of the 1509 patients in the series, 210 (13 per cent) had chronic elevated blood creatinine levels (3 mg/dl or greater). Of these 210 patients, 105 (50 per cent) developed postoperative renal failure requiring hemodialysis following thoracoabdominal aneurysm repair. The effect on early and long-term survival is illustrated in Figure 77–13. In a retrospective review of 1525 patients who underwent replacement of the descending thoracic or thoracoabdominal aorta, the need for postoperative hemodialysis was not significantly altered by the use of cold perfusion of the kidneys with Ringer's lactate or with atrial femoral bypass.[12] Too few patients had renal ischemic times exceeding 45 minutes to analyze renal ischemic time as a separate variable. Consequently, the author continues to use cold perfusion for renal preservation in patients with preoperative renal dysfunction and in those requiring prolonged clamp times. Regardless of the renal function of the patient prior to operation, 65 per cent of those who required dialysis following operation died within 6 months of operation.

References

1. Crawford ES: Thoracoabdominal and abdominal aortic aneurysms involving renal, superior mesenteric, and celiac arteries. Ann Surg 179:763, 1974.
2. Crawford ES, Crawford JL, Safi HJ, et al: Thoracoabdominal aortic aneurysms: Preoperative and intraoperative factors determining immediate and long-term results of operations in 605 patients. J Vasc Surg 3:389, 1986.
3. Crawford ES, DeNatale RW: Thoracoabdominal aortic aneurysm: Observations regarding the natural course of the disease. J Vasc Surg 3:578, 1986.
4. Crawford ES, Snyder DM, Cho GC, et al: Progress in treatment of thoracoabdominal and abdominal aortic aneurysms involving celiac, superior mesenteric, and renal arteries. Ann Surg 188:404, 1978.
5. DeBakey ME, Creech O Jr, Morris GC Jr: Aneurysms of thoracoabdominal aorta involving the celiac, superior mesenteric, and renal arteries: Report of four cases treated by resection and homograft replacement. Ann Surg 144:459, 1956.
6. DeBakey ME, Crawford ES, Garrett HE, et al: Surgical considerations in the treatment of aneurysms of the thoracoabdominal aorta. Ann Surg 162:650, 1965.
7. Etheridge SN, Yee J, Smith JV, et al: Successful resection of a large aneurysm of the upper abdominal aorta and replacement with homograft. Surgery 38:1071, 1955.
8. Selle JG, Robicsek F, Daugherty HK, et al: Thoracoabdominal aortic aneurysms: A review and current status. Ann Surg 189:158, 1979.
9. Crawford ES, Mizrahi EM, Hess KR, et al: The impact of distal aortic perfusion and somatosensory evoked potential monitoring on prevention of paraplegia after thoracic cross-clamping. J Thorac Cardiovasc Surg 95:357, 1988.
10. Crawford ES, Coselli JS, Safi HJ: Partial cardiopulmonary bypass, hypothermic circulatory arrest, and posterolateral exposure for thoracic aortic aneurysm operation. J Thorac Cardiovasc Surg 94:824, 1987.
11. Svensson LG, Crawford ES, Hess KR, et al: Experience with 1509 patients undergoing thoracoabdominal aortic operations. J Vasc Surg 17:357, 1993.
12. Svensson LG, Coselli JS, Safi HJ, et al: Appraisal of adjuncts to prevent acute renal failure after surgery on the thoracic or thoracoabdominal aorta. J Vasc Surg 10(3):230, 1989.
13. Svensson LG, Patel V, Robinson MF, et al: Influence of preservation or perfusion of intraoperatively identified spinal cord blood supply on spinal motor evoked potentials and paraplegia after aortic surgery. J Vasc Surg 13(3):355, 1991.
14. Crawford ES, Svensson LG, Hess KR, et al: A prospective randomized study of cerebrospinal fluid drainage to prevent paraplegia after high-risk surgery on the thoracoabdominal aorta. J Vasc Surg 13(1):36, 1991.

78

Peripheral Vascular Manifestations of Acute Aortic Dissection

Philip J. Walker, M.D., M.B.B.S., F.R.A.C.S., George E. Sarris, M.D., and D. Craig Miller, M.D.

• • •

Acute aortic dissection, formerly and improperly called *dissecting aneurysm*, is the most common lethal catastrophe involving the aorta.[1-3] Although the incidence of dissection is at least twice that of ruptured abdominal aortic aneurysm,[4] the correct diagnosis is regrettably made far less regularly.[5,6] Despite significant advances in both diagnosis and treatment, acute aortic dissection remains one of the most formidable diseases faced by physicians today. Early diagnosis remains problematic, and mortality, although much improved, remains high, particularly for patients with complications such as aortic rupture or visceral or renal ischemia.[7-11] Delay in diagnosis is largely due to the perceived rarity of acute aortic dissection and variable presenting signs and symptoms, which can mimic those of a plethora of other, more common acute medical or surgical illnesses.[5,12] This explains its reputation as "the great clinical masquerader." During the first 48 hours, mortality for patients with undiagnosed, untreated acute type A aortic dissection (see later discussion) exceeds *1 per cent per hour*.[7,13-16] As a result, a soberingly large number of hospi-

talized patients die before the correct diagnosis is made and appropriate treatment can be instituted. Although clinical progress has been achieved since the 1950s, when a review of 735 cases revealed that the correct antemortem diagnosis had been made in only 11 per cent of patients,[17] a continuing need for improvement in recognition still exists, as shown by more contemporary studies from Vancouver (1982)[14] and the Massachusetts General Hospital (1984)[18] where more than 35 per cent and 11 per cent, respectively, of patients with acute type A dissections admitted to hospital died before a correct antemortem diagnosis could be established. Therefore, there is a compelling need to recognize the possibility of acute aortic dissection as early as possible so that appropriate diagnostic procedures can be undertaken and definitive therapy instituted without inordinate delay. Since occlusion of one or more aortic branches may herald acute aortic dissection in as many as 30 to 50 per cent of patients,[8,9,11,14,19-21] the vascular surgeon must maintain a high index of suspicion for this uncommon (but not rare) and highly lethal condition.

Optimal treatment is focused on control of the life-threatening thoracic aortic problem. Emergency surgical intervention (prosthetic graft replacement of the ascending aorta [using an "open" distal anastomosis during profound hypothermic circulatory arrest {PHCA}], aortic valve resuspension or replacement [if aortic insufficiency is present], and concomitant hemi-arch replacement in selected patients) is required for essentially all individuals with acute type A aortic dissections, but optimal management of those with acute type B dissections continues to be debated.[5, 6, 13, 14, 16, 18, 19, 22–42] In most centers, patients with acute type B dissections are treated medically.[6, 18, 22, 25, 27, 29] Surgical intervention (i.e., graft replacement of the descending thoracic aorta) is generally reserved for those with major complications, such as aortic rupture, ischemia of important distal end-organ systems, persistent or recurrent intractable pain, dissection progression, or uncontrollable hypertension.[22, 25, 27] At Stanford University[13] and Mt. Sinai (New York)[28] Medical Centers, carefully selected patients with *uncomplicated* acute type B aortic dissections are also offered early thoracic aortic repair. In most cases, this direct surgical approach to the thoracic aorta obviates the need for secondary aortic fenestration or other peripheral vascular revascularization procedures;[8, 14, 43] moreover, attempts at initial local peripheral revascularization (which all too often reflect an incorrect preoperative diagnosis) cause further delay, are usually unsuccessful if the central thoracic aortic problem remains untreated, and actually increase the patient's overall risk of dying. Alternative therapeutic approaches have been advocated, however, mainly in response to the high operative mortality for subgroups of patients with renal or mesenteric ischemia. It has been suggested that these patients be treated with primary aortic fenestration[41, 44] or local revascularization with or without interval thoracic aortic repair.[9] Some have proposed the use of intensive medical therapy alone.[9, 45, 46] More exciting is the advent of therapeutic percutaneous endovascular techniques (including balloon angioplasty, endovascular stenting, and septal fenestration) to alleviate these distal ischemic complications;[47, 48, 49, 108] if successful, endovascular intervention may well lead to future reevaluation of the clinical management algorithm.

INCIDENCE

It is not widely appreciated that acute aortic dissection is the most common catastrophic event involving the aorta; furthermore, its incidence may be increasing in the industrialized world. In a 1960s Danish study of 6480 autopsies, the incidence of aortic dissection was 5.2 per million population per year compared with 3.6 per million for ruptured abdominal aortic aneurysm and 1.2 per million for ruptured thoracic aortic aneurysm.[1] More recently, it has been estimated that the incidence of aortic dissection in the United States may be as high as 10 to 20 cases per million population per year,[2] or roughly 2000 to 4500 cases annually.[3] Importantly, these figures are undoubtedly underestimates because they do not include patients who die suddenly of aortic dissection but, in the absence of a postmortem examination, are presumed to have succumbed to a cardiac event. We tend to think that ruptured abdominal aortic aneurysms are more common, but this misperception has arisen only because it is diagnosed correctly more often than acute aortic dissection.

CLASSIFICATION SYSTEMS

It is important to understand and apply accurately the classification of aortic dissection to evaluate intelligently the results of diverse medical or surgical therapeutic strategies reported in the literature and to allow meaningful comparison of results between various institutions. Considerable confusion has arisen in the past in classifying aortic dissections. Numerous systems have been proposed, beginning with the nine categories suggested by DeBakey and colleagues in 1955.[50] The most widely used is the DeBakey type I, II, and III classification scheme initially introduced in 1965[51] and subsequently modified in 1982.[19] Despite the use of different terms, a consensus has been reached regarding the essential elements of a common functional classification system. The cardinal feature of all classification systems today is predicated upon the presence or absence of the involvement of the ascending aorta regardless of the location of the primary intimal tear and regardless of the distal extent of the dissection.[13] The Stanford classification approach as proposed by Daily and associates in 1970 has gained broad acceptance since the early 1980s.[52] If the ascending aorta is involved, the dissection is termed Stanford type A,[52] which corresponds to DeBakey type I,[19] University of Alabama "ascending,"[23] Massachusetts General Hospital "proximal,"[18] and Najafi "anterior" dissection.[32] DeBakey type I and II dissections both involve the ascending aorta; type I extends beyond the left subclavian artery, whereas type II does not. If the ascending aorta is *not* involved the dissection is called type B, type III, descending, distal, or posterior, respectively (Fig. 78–1). This functional classification system is pathophysiologically sound because involvement of the ascending aorta is the principal determinant of the expected biologic behavior of the dissection and predicts the most common complications and causes of death. It also simplifies diagnosis because it is easier to identify the presence of ascending aortic involvement than it is to determine the exact location of the primary intimal tear (or tears) or the full extent of distal propagation of the dissecting process. The site of the primary intimal tear and the distal extent of the dissection are less important prognostically.[53] Furthermore, the Stanford classification approach facilitates clinical decision making and surgical management. Patients with acute type A dissections should be treated by emergency operation in essentially all cases, whereas individuals with acute type B dissections can be treated either medically or with early surgical intervention. Patients with type A dissections require a median sternotomy and total cardiopulmonary bypass (CPB) and a brief period of PHCA, whereas those with type B dissections are approached through a left posterolateral thoracotomy, using partial CPB.

Two thirds of dissections involve the ascending aorta (Stanford type A),[1, 40, 54–56] and the primary intimal tear is usually located in the ascending aorta. Approximately one third of dissections are limited to the descending thoracic aorta (Stanford type B), with the intimal tear usually located

TYPE A   TYPE B

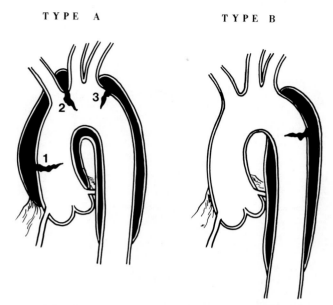

FIGURE 78-1. Schematic illustration of the Stanford classification system of aortic dissections: The ascending aorta is involved in patients with *type A* dissections, where the intimal tear can be located either in the ascending aorta (1), in the transverse aortic arch (2), or in the descending thoracic aorta (3). In *type B* dissections, the ascending aorta is not involved. Not shown here is the relatively rare but high-risk situation of a type B dissection due to antegrade propagation from an arch (2) tear. (From Miller DC, Stinson EB, Oyer PE, et al: Operative treatment of aortic dissections. J Thorac Cardiovasc Surg 78:365, 1979).

near the origin of the left subclavian artery. Although no patient in the Stanford 20-year (1963 to 1982) experience[7] had an abdominal aortic tear, it is estimated that 2 to 4 per cent of all aortic dissections may originate in the infradiaphragmatic aorta from which they may propagate distally or proximally.[54, 55, 57, 58] In approximately 10 per cent of patients, the intimal tear is located in the transverse arch, and the dissection extends to involve variable lengths of the ascending or descending thoracic aorta, or both. Rarely, a dissection can be limited to the transverse arch or to the abdominal aorta.[58] Aortic dissections detected within 14 days of the onset of pain or other presenting clinical symptoms are arbitrarily classified as acute; those diagnosed later than 2 weeks after onset are chronic.[12, 22, 27] DeBakey and colleagues used the term subacute to categorize dissections in the gray zone between 2 weeks and 2 months old.[19]

PATHOLOGY, PATHOPHYSIOLOGY, AND NATURAL HISTORY

The typical pathologic lesion found in patients with acute type B aortic dissection (who are usually older and frequently hypertensive) is smooth muscle degeneration within the aortic media; histopathologic investigation by Schlatmann and Becker has shown that this is not a novel pathologic entity but simply represents a normal manifestation of the aging process.[59] It is distinctly different from the elastic tissue degeneration seen in patients with type A dissections, who are usually younger and often have an inherited connective tissue abnormality in the elastic tissue

of the aortic media.[60] Type A dissections occur in patients with Marfan's or Ehlers-Danlos syndrome and those with annuloaortic ectasia. Two schools of thought exist concerning the initial event in dissection: Most believe that the initial event is tearing of the intima,[60–63] whereas the minority opinion postulates that intramural hemorrhage from the vasa vasorum weakens the aortic wall and causes secondary rupture of the intima.[56, 64–66] Type B aortic dissections can arise from rupture of an ulcerated atherosclerotic plaque in the arch or descending thoracic aorta, but this probably occurs infrequently.[5, 61]

Pathoanatomically, the aortic pathology is that of a false aneurysm because the aortic intima (true channel) actually is not aneurysmally dilated. The "aneurysmal" dilatation of the false lumen (which is usually the larger of the two channels) results in overall enlargement of the aorta beyond its normal dimensions. This usually is a diffuse, fairly uniform process extending along the entire length of the dissection. After a primary intimal tear occurs, propagation of the dissection depends on many factors, including the rate of rise of aortic systolic pressure (dP/dt), the magnitude of aortic diastolic recoil pressure, the mean aortic pressure, and the cohesive strength of the aortic wall.[59, 60, 62, 67–69]

Untreated acute aortic dissections are highly lethal.[1, 54–56] As nearly as one can discern from large autopsy reports, roughly one third of patients die within 24 hours, approximately one half by 48 hours, two thirds at 1 week, and 80 to 90 per cent by 1 month. Most patients with untreated acute type A dissection die from intrapericardial rupture with cardiac tamponade; other causes of death include free pleural rupture, aortic regurgitation with acute left ventricular failure, and compromise of cerebral or coronary blood flow. Most patients with untreated acute type B dissection die from free pleural rupture or occlusion of major aortic branches resulting in injury to vital organs.[27, 70] In our experience, limb ischemia and its complications do not significantly contribute to mortality,[7, 16] whereas occlusion of major abdominal tributaries resulting in renal or mesenteric infarction substantially increases the patient's risk.[7, 16]

Peripheral vascular complications arise when the dissecting process compromises blood flow to various branches. The usual mechanism is extrinsic compression of the true lumen by the false lumen or an intimal flap compromising the orifice of the branch artery,[7, 9, 14, 20, 56] as illustrated in Fig. 78–2. The false lumen ordinarily remains patent but rarely may thrombose. Depending on the circumferential extent of the dissection plane, some aortic tributaries may be spared and continue to be perfused from the true channel, while other branches at the same level may be perfused from the false lumen and subsequently become permanently dependent on false channel flow after "healing" of ostial flaps. The dissection often proceeds in a "spiral" fashion down the aorta. Fenestrations between the true and false lumina arise at points where tributaries are sheared off or as a result of spontaneous reentry into the true lumen. Compression by the false lumen may cause severe narrowing of the true aortic lumen,[43] which occasionally may result in subtotal aortic occlusion at the diaphragmatic hiatus;[10] distal perfusion in such circumstances is delivered through the aortic false lumen.

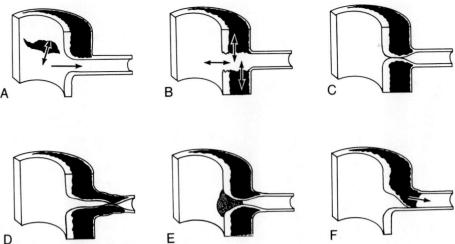

FIGURE 78–2. Examples of distal pathoanatomic complications of aortic dissections. Continued adequate perfusion of an aortic tributary is illustrated in panels *A*, *B*, and *F*; however, perfusion is via the true lumen in *A* and *B* and through the false channel in *F*. Obstruction of the aortic tributary due to extrinsic compression is shown in panels *C* and *D*, whereas compromise of the ostium of the true lumen with subsequent secondary thrombosis is shown in *E*. In *F*, reentry of the dissection into the branch vessel has created an intimal flap. This may become a permanent situation if the flap heals to the opposite wall of the vessel in the chronic phase, thus rendering this branch solely dependent on false channel perfusion. (*A–F*, From Miller DC: Surgical management of aortic dissections: Indications, perioperative management, and long-term results. *In* Doroghazi RM, Slater EE [eds]: Aortic Dissection, p 198. Copyright © 1983 by McGraw-Hill, Inc. Used by permission of McGraw-Hill Book Company.)

The pattern of branch artery involvement and the degree of compromise of perfusion determine the presenting symptoms and clinical signs, which may be extremely variable and often lead to a potentially fatal delay in diagnosis. The sudden, simultaneous occurrence of a variety of diverse acute clinical problems without a readily apparent unifying cause should prompt consideration of aortic dissection and hasten appropriate diagnostic studies. The relative frequency of involvement of aortic branches (in descending order) in a large autopsy series[56, 67] was the iliac arteries, followed by the innominate, left common carotid, left subclavian, coronary, renal, superior mesenteric, and celiac arteries (Fig. 78–3).

CLINICAL PRESENTATION

Patients with acute type A dissections are usually younger and include those with Marfan's syndrome and annuloaortic ectasia, whereas acute type B aortic dissection

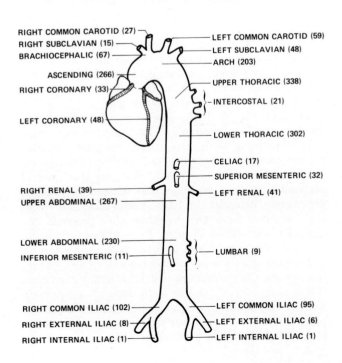

RIGHT COMMON CAROTID (27)
RIGHT SUBCLAVIAN (15)
BRACHIOCEPHALIC (67)
ASCENDING (266)
RIGHT CORONARY (33)
LEFT CORONARY (48)
RIGHT RENAL (39)
UPPER ABDOMINAL (267)
LOWER ABDOMINAL (230)
INFERIOR MESENTERIC (11)
RIGHT COMMON ILIAC (102)
RIGHT EXTERNAL ILIAC (8)
RIGHT INTERNAL ILIAC (1)

LEFT COMMON CAROTID (59)
LEFT SUBCLAVIAN (48)
ARCH (203)
UPPER THORACIC (338)
INTERCOSTAL (21)
LOWER THORACIC (302)
CELIAC (17)
SUPERIOR MESENTERIC (32)
LEFT RENAL (41)
LUMBAR (9)
LEFT COMMON ILIAC (95)
LEFT EXTERNAL ILIAC (6)
LEFT INTERNAL ILIAC (1)

FIGURE 78–3. Illustration of the frequency and distribution of dissection involvement of various segments of the aorta and its arterial branches in a series of 450 autopsies.[56, 67] In the authors' experience, the right coronary artery has been involved more frequently than the left main coronary. (From Hirst AE, Gore I: The etiology and pathology of aortic dissection. *In* Doroghazi RM, Slater EE [eds]: Aortic Dissection, p 193. Copyright © 1983 by McGraw-Hill, Inc. Used by permission of McGraw-Hill Book Company.)

is usually seen in middle-aged and elderly men; either type of dissection can occur in women (particularly young women during the third trimester of pregnancy or during labor and delivery) and also rarely in children.[5, 12] Older patients frequently have coexisting hypertension and generalized atherosclerosis[5, 18] as well as associated cardiac, pulmonary, renal, and cerebrovascular disease.

Most frequently, the hallmark of acute dissection is the hyperacute onset of severe, lancinating pain.[12, 13, 20, 69] The initial pain can be in any location but usually originates in the interscapular or anterior chest region. The pain, which characteristically is described as sharp or "tearing," is thought to be produced by stretching of the aortic adventitia by the dissecting hematoma. Persistence or migration of pain suggests continuing expansion or extension of the dissection. Occasionally, acute dissection can be painless; thus, vigilance is needed to recognize complications. Aside from the tearing back or chest pain due to the dissection per se, the large constellation of other symptoms and signs is largely related to which of the distal aortic tributaries has become involved by the dissecting hematoma and the extent of compromise of perfusion of various end-organs.

The patient appears subjectively to be in pain, "shocky," and poorly perfused peripherally, but elevated blood pressure is the rule. Blood pressure must be measured in both arms, and a complete examination of all peripheral pulses is imperative. Furthermore, the pulse check and neurologic examination should be repeated frequently because new deficits may appear with progression of the dissection. If the patient is hypotensive, aortic rupture should be suspected. Shock is usually due to intrapericardial rupture with tamponade, intrathoracic rupture with exsanguination, or a large myocardial infarction (MI). Symptoms of acute left ventricular failure can arise secondary to severe aortic valvular regurgitation or a MI due to compromised coronary blood flow. Unless the dissection is complicated by aortic branch vessel obstruction or occlusion, the remainder of the physical examination characteristically yields only nonspecific findings.

Approximately 25 per cent of patients, however, present with symptoms related to acute peripheral arterial occlusion or develop such symptoms early in the course of their illness. They may present with stroke, paraplegia, upper or lower extremity ischemia, or anuria or abdominal pain due to renal or mesenteric ischemia. Alternatively, loss of a peripheral pulse may be clinically asymptomatic. It

cannot be overemphasized that aortic dissection should always be considered in the differential diagnosis of acute limb ischemia, particularly when there is evidence of a generalized process affecting seemingly unrelated organ systems and no antecedent history of atherosclerotic peripheral vascular disease or cardiac symptoms that might suggest a source of thromboembolism. For example, in a patient presenting with chest pain, stroke, or acute abdominal pain in conjunction with a cold, pulseless leg, one should consider the possibility of aortic dissection and focus on the central life-threatening problem rather than attempting a local revascularization procedure or embolectomy. Indeed, many dissections have been correctly diagnosed only at the time of emergency femoral exploration when no thrombus or embolus is found in the femoral artery,[8] the so-called peak and shriek phenomenon (personal communication, Ronald J. Stoney, M.D.). Pulse loss may be evident at presentation or may evolve as the dissection progresses; therefore, frequent comprehensive pulse examinations are important. Most patients with this complication have a cold extremity and paresthesia with varying degrees of paresis; rarely, complete proximal aortic occlusion is present, and the patient presents with total ischemia of the lower half of the body.[10]

The frequency and distribution of various peripheral vascular manifestations of aortic dissection in several large series are shown in Table 78–1. In a recent review of the total Stanford experience by Fann and associates,[8] 31 per cent (85/272) of patients with all types of dissections sustained one or more peripheral vascular complications (38 per cent in the acute type A subgroup and 20 per cent of those in the acute type B subgroup [Fig. 78–4]), similar to other reported figures, which have been in the 30 to 50 per cent range.[9, 11, 14, 19–21] One hundred and twenty-eight patients (47 per cent) had an acute type A dissection, 70 (26 per cent) had a chronic type A, 40 (15 per cent) had an acute type B, and 34 (12 per cent), had a chronic type B dissection. Of the 85 patients with a vascular complication, 18 individuals (21 per cent) suffered two complications, 6 (7 per cent) had three, and 1 patient (0.4 per cent) had four separate vascular complications. Among the 168 patients sustaining an *acute dissection*, 7 patients (4 per cent) presented with acute carotid occlusion and stroke; 8 (5 per cent) had acute paraplegia secondary to spinal cord ischemia, 56 (33 per cent) sustained loss of one or more peripheral pulses, 18 (11 per cent) had impaired renal perfusion

Table 78–1. Peripheral Vascular Manifestations of Aortic Dissection

Series	Total	Type A	Type B	No. of Patients (All/Type A/Type B)			
				Stroke	*Paraplegia*	*Pulse Loss*	*Renal/ Visceral Ischemia*
Stanford[8]	272	198	74	7/7/0	9/8/1	66/55/11	38/23/15
Stanford[7, 16]	175	121	54	5/5/0	7/6/1	36/29/7	14/9/5
Vancouver[14]	141	89	53	—	6/0/6	50/32/18*	—
Baylor[19]†	527	195	332	21/8/13	10/4/6	36/18/18	35/7/28
Massachusetts General Hospital[20]	124	53	71	7/7/0	3/1/2	38/27/11	—

Includes carotid occlusions.

†DeBakey type I and II dissections considered together as type A.

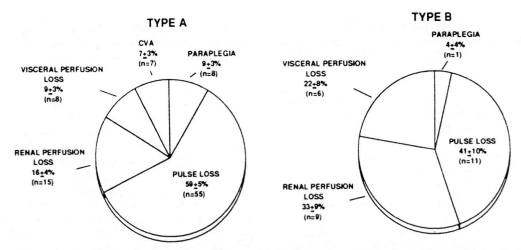

FIGURE 78–4. Distribution of peripheral vascular complications from among 168 patients in the Stanford experience segregated according to type of dissection (*A* or *B*); 85 patients sustained one or more complications. Note that these 85 patients had a total of 120 individual vascular complications. The number of patients (n) is indicated in each sector along with the associated mortality rate (± 70 per cent confidence limits) for those with this specific complication. (From Fann JI, Sarris GE, Mitchell RS, et al: Treatment of patients with aortic dissection presenting with peripheral vascular complications. Ann Surg 212:705, 1990.)

(demonstrated angiographically), and 10 patients (6 per cent) had compromised visceral perfusion by angiography. The incidence of these complications according to type and acuity of dissection together with the attendant operative mortality following definitive (intrathoracic) surgical treatment is summarized in Table 78–2. The distribution of specific sites of peripheral pulse loss in these patients is summarized in Table 78–3. Cambria and coworkers noted that the clinical course of peripheral limb ischemia is variable:[9] In this combined Yale-New Haven and Massachusetts General Hospital experience, one third of the group demonstrated either spontaneous resolution of peripheral pulse deficits or a fluctuating clinical picture.[9] This dynamic phenomenon can be explained by redirection of arterial flow into the true lumen through a spontaneous reentry tear, by changing pressure gradients between the two channels, or by fibrous contraction of the thrombus within the false lumen.

Neurologic findings can vary from minor sensory deficits in one leg or arm as a consequence of peripheral ischemic neuropathy to complete hemiplegia if arch involvement results in occlusion of a carotid artery, or paraplegia if the dissection compromises flow to the spinal cord by shearing off critical intercostal arteries, thereby interrupting flow in the radicularis magna artery.[5, 12, 13] Syncope or coma may also be acute manifestations of aortic dissection. Stroke or transient ischemic attack occurs relatively infrequently (usually in association with an acute type A dissection) and has an incidence ranging from 3 to 7 per cent.[8, 9, 19–21, 71, 72] The usual mechanism of stroke is an extracranial carotid obstruction,[9] although rarely the cause may be embolic with discharge of thrombus or atheroemboli into the aorta or at the site of a reentry tear in the innominate or carotid artery.[73] Paraplegia is a presenting symptom in approximately 2 to 6 per cent of cases[8, 9, 19, 71, 74] and is usually associated with extensive acute dissections; paraplegia may be the key diagnostic clue in instances of "painless" aortic dissection.[75]

The incidence of renal ischemia associated with acute aortic dissection varies from 3 to 60 per cent.[8, 9, 30, 41, 77–79] At Stanford, angiographically determined impaired renal perfusion occurred in 11 per cent of patients (18/168) with acute aortic dissection[8] compared with the 5 per cent rate of clinical renal ischemia or infarction reported by Cambria and coworkers.[9] This range probably reflects differences related to the method of detection (angiography versus pa-

Table 78–2. Peripheral Vascular Complications and Associated Operative Mortality Rates in a Series of 168 Patients With Acute Aortic Dissection

Vascular Complication	No. of Patients	OM Type A (n = 128)	No. of Patients Type B	OM (n = 40)
Stroke	7	1 (14 ± 14%)	0	—
Paraplegia	7	3 (43 ± 19%)	1	1 (100%)
Pulse loss	48	12 (25 ± 6%)	8	4 (50 ± 18%)
Renal ischemia	15	8 (53 ± 13%)	3	2 (67 ± 28%)
Visceral ischemia	8	4 (50 ± 18%)	2	1 (50 ± 37%)

Data from Fann JI, Sarris GE, Mitchell RS, et al: Treatment of patients with aortic dissection presenting with peripheral vascular complications. Ann Surg 212:705, 1990.

OM, Operative mortality rate (± 70 per cent confidence limits).

Table 78–3. Location of Peripheral Pulse Deficits in 56 of 168 Patients With Acute Aortic Dissection

	Type A (n = 128)	Type B (n = 40)
Right carotid	6	0
Left carotid	6	0
Right arm	25	0
Left arm	10	2
Right leg	21	4
Left leg	14	3
Total	82	9

Data from Fann JI, Sarris GE, Mitchell RS, et al: Treatment of patients with aortic dissection presenting with peripheral vascular complications. Ann Surg 212:705, 1990.

thology) rather than true population differences.[9] In contrast to a previous report that the left renal artery is more commonly involved in aortic dissection,[77] the right renal artery was more frequently involved in our experience.[8] Dissection or occlusion of the renal arteries resulting in ischemia or infarction of a kidney may be asymptomatic, that is, not detected until diagnostic imaging studies are performed. A history of flank pain and the presence of hematuria or oliguria should suggest a renovascular complication and prompt urgent angiography. Not infrequently, however, such symptoms are still misdiagnosed (e.g., ureteric colic). If the correct diagnosis is established promptly, urgent endovascular repair (balloon dilatation, renal artery stenting, or aortic septal fenestration) may be helpful in preserving renal function,[108] which is otherwise irreversibly lost within hours if the degree of renal arterial obstruction is complete.[80] Even if renal artery compromise is subtotal, renovascular hypertension that is difficult to control may develop subsequently.[81, 82]

Compromised mesenteric perfusion as a clinical entity is relatively uncommon, occurring in 5 per cent or less of cases,[8, 9, 19, 83] although autopsy investigation suggests that the dissection process involves the celiac or superior mesenteric arteries in more than 10 per cent of patients.[56] At Stanford, the incidence of angiographically demonstrated visceral arterial compromise was 6 per cent (8 of 128) in individuals with acute type A dissections and 5 per cent (2 of 40) for those with an acute type B dissection.[8] This complication portends a grave prognosis, with mortality rates as high as 88 per cent.[8–11] Mesenteric ischemia can be variable in its clinical presentation, ranging in severity from simple asymptomatic angiographic evidence of visceral hypoperfusion to frank gut infarction. Abdominal pain out of proportion to the physical findings should prompt consideration of visceral ischemia or infarction.[8, 9]

DEFINITIVE DIAGNOSIS AND INITIAL MANAGEMENT

All patients with suspected acute aortic dissection should immediately be given intensive medical antihypertensive and negative inotropic therapy.[6, 13] Intravenous (IV) beta blockade (propranolol, metoprolol, labetalol, or esmolol) is administered in small boluses (or as a continuous IV infusion) along with an IV infusion of sodium nitroprusside

while the appropriate diagnostic tests are being performed. Parenteral calcium channel antagonists that lower blood pressure and left ventricular dP/dt (e.g., verapamil) can also be used, especially in patients with bronchospastic lung disease. Because nitroprusside and angiotensin-converting enzyme inhibitors are arteriolar vasodilators, they theoretically increase arterial dP/dt; therefore, concomitant administration of a negative inotropic agent is essential. Although only rarely necessary today, an IV drip of trimethaphan camsylate can be added if satisfactory blood pressure control cannot be achieved. If surgical intervention is employed, antihypertensive and negative inotropic therapy is continued during anesthetic induction, intraoperatively, and postoperatively. Peak systolic, mean, and diastolic arterial pressures should be maintained at as low a level as possible consistent with adequate cerebral, cardiac, and renal perfusion (as determined from continuous monitoring of level of consciousness, electrocardiography, and urine output).

Definitive diagnostic procedures should be performed as expeditiously as possible to confirm or rule out the diagnosis of acute aortic dissection. Options include dynamic computed tomographic (CT) scanning, angiography, transesophageal echocardiography (TEE), and magnetic resonance imaging (MRI). Prior to the widespread availability of CT scanning, definitive diagnosis of aortic dissection was generally made by conventional (cut film) aortography or aortic cineangiography. Today, CT scanning has markedly facilitated the rapid and accurate diagnosis of acute aortic dissection in most hospitals, small or large. The sensitivity and specificity of CT scanning (with IV contrast) in making this diagnosis are relatively high (approximately 82 per cent and 99 per cent, respectively), but neither is absolute.[22, 25, 27, 53] A thrombosed false lumen can be confused with a laminated concentric thrombus within a fusiform atherosclerotic aneurysm or an ectatic aorta; also, because of the limited temporal sampling resolution, conventional CT scanning can miss a dissection flap if it is moving rapidly. High-speed cine CT scans and angiography can partially circumvent this problem but, again, are not 100 per cent sensitive or specific. In most cases, a CT scan with IV contrast can determine the type of dissection (type A or type B), which is of paramount importance in guiding further therapy. The extent of dissection, arch involvement, and the overall size of the aorta can also be assessed.

The recent advent of TEE employing Doppler color flow mapping has had a major positive impact on the diagnostic evaluation of patients in whom acute aortic dissection is suspected.[84–87] In Europe and Japan, TEE has been considered the initial diagnostic procedure of choice for many years, with most patients not requiring additional corroborative diagnostic studies. Erbel and colleagues reported sensitivity (98 per cent), specificity (99 per cent), and overall positive and negative predictive accuracy rates that exceed those of CT scanning and aortography using first-generation TEE equipment (single-plane transducer without color flow mapping).[84] Better results are expected after the introduction of biplane (or multi-plane) probes used in conjunction with color flow imaging.[86] This rapid, relatively noninvasive procedure can be performed at the bedside in the emergency room, intensive care unit, or operating room with minimal risk. Undesirable blood pressure elevation is a potential risk of TEE, and patient sedation is necessary. TEE is especially suitable for patients with aortic dissections because of the anatomic proximity of the descending thoracic aorta and the esophagus. In the past a TEE "blind spot" limited visualization of the distal ascending aorta and the proximal arch (owing to air in the trachea that interfered with ultrasonic transmission);[86] however, today this limitation has been resolved by the advent of multi-plane TEE probes. TEE with Doppler color flow mapping can demonstrate flow in both aortic channels, the flap separating the true and false lumina, and associated valvular or myocardial pathology.[84–87] Frequently, the primary intimal tear as well as secondary distal fenestrations between the two lumina can also be identified. The overall size of the dissected thoracic aorta (combined diameter of the true and false channels), extrinsic compression of the true lumen, and thrombus in the false channel can be determined, as well as the proximal extent of the dissection (which thereby defines the type [A or B] of the dissection). Definition of the abdominal aorta below the diaphragm is not possible;[88] therefore, a limitation of TEE in patients with acute aortic dissection is that the perfusion status of the renal and visceral arteries cannot be evaluated. In certain individuals, however, intragastric TEE can provide satisfactory images of the celiac axis or superior mesenteric artery.

Contrast biplane aortography, obtained using either cine or cut-film techniques, has long been considered the gold standard in the diagnosis of aortic dissection.[22, 25, 27, 53, 89] It is essential to determine whether the ascending or descending thoracic aorta is involved to guide surgical treatment focused on repair of the thoracic aorta. Angiography is associated with a low risk of morbidity and mortality, is invasive, is not infallible, and can be relatively time consuming.[53, 89] The sensitivity and specificity rates of angiography for the diagnosis of aortic dissection are approximately 81 per cent and 96 per cent, respectively. Because the most dangerous clinical diagnostic problem is one of a *false-negative* diagnosis, this relatively low sensitivity rate constitutes an important limitation of aortography. Compared with TEE and CT scanning, aortography provides more detailed information about the perfusion status of important branches (e.g., arch vessels, and the intercostal, renal, mesenteric, or iliac arteries) supplied by the dissected aorta. An aortic root injection can also detect coronary ostial involvement or severe coexisting proximal coronary artery disease. Dynamic blood flow in both the true and false lumina, perfusion of various aortic tributaries, motion of the dissection flap, and the site of the primary intimal tear can be characterized more precisely if the aortogram is recorded using high-speed (60-Hz) cine techniques.[90] Angiography can be followed immediately, if indicated, by therapeutic endovascular therapeutic procedures.[108]

Intravascular ultrasound (IVUS) has recently been described in the evaluation of patients with aortic dissection.[91–93] Usually one of the more conventional procedures (CT, TEE, or angiography) establishes the diagnosis, and IVUS is used to provide supplementary pathoanatomic information. For example, the location, extent, and condition of the septum separating the true and false aortic channels (i.e., intact or fenestrated) can be determined; IVUS can also demonstrate clearly which channel lumen is supplying

important aortic branches, such as the superior mesenteric, renal, or common iliac arteries. The miniature ultrasonic probe is inserted percutaneously into the femoral artery and advanced in retrograde fashion, providing visualization of the entire abdominal and thoracic aorta. We have also used IVUS to guide septal fenestration procedures and to monitor stent deployment in dissected renal and iliac arteries.

Currently, MRI scanning does not play a major diagnostic role in patients with acute dissection because these patients are critically ill; are connected to various monitoring devices, intravenous infusion pumps, or respirators; and cannot lie still for prolonged periods.[5, 22] Furthermore, the relatively long amount of time needed for the patient to remain in the magnet to obtain satisfactory gated MRI scans interferes with intensive patient monitoring. It is anticipated that newer scanners and more refined software will reduce the MRI capture time required; if so, MRI scanning (which is generally considered to have sensitivity and specificity rates approaching 98 per cent in the diagnosis of aortic dissection) may become clinically useful in acute cases. Today, MRI scans are most useful for serial follow-up of individuals with chronic dissections, including all postoperative patients and those treated medically. MRI scans can accurately demonstrate the intimal flap, both aortic channels, and the source of perfusion (true or false lumen) of major aortic tributaries (e.g., arch vessels, celiac axis, or superior mesenteric, renal, or iliac arteries). Unfortunately, in highly stenotic vessels (with more than 70 per cent stenosis), MRI can sometimes incorrectly indicate total occlusion. Spin-echo MRI images can differentiate between methemoglobin and oxyhemoglobin signals, which allows estimation of the age of the thrombus present within the false channel; this information can characterize the evolution of morphologic changes over time.

Having discussed the various diagnostic modalities available, it should be underscored that the best initial screening test is probably that which can be performed most rapidly and interpreted most accurately in any particular hospital; moreover, it is important to remember that no individual test is 100 per cent sensitive or specific.[53, 84, 85] Both false-positive and false-negative interpretations can occur. Therefore, if acute dissection is strongly suspected on clinical grounds and the initial diagnostic test is negative, additional imaging studies should be performed. Finally, it is advisable to transfer stable individuals with acute aortic dissections to tertiary medical centers where special expertise in surgery of the thoracic aorta for definitive acute medical therapy or surgical intervention is available because better survival rates have been reported by groups with more extensive experience.[13, 18, 25, 29, 39]

INDICATIONS FOR AND CHOICE OF OPERATION

The aim of therapy in patients with aortic dissection is to prevent death and irreversible end-organ damage. Attempts to control or treat any peripheral vascular complications of the dissection are meaningless if the most common causes of death from this condition are not dealt with directly and expeditiously.

All patients with acute type A aortic dissections should be considered for emergency definitive surgical repair of the thoracic aorta.[2, 7, 13–16, 18, 19, 26, 34, 52, 69, 94–99] This life-saving operation should precede (and usually obviates the need for) local revascularization for most peripheral vascular complications of the dissection. Exceptions to operative intervention on the thoracic aorta may include patients with a massive stroke[7, 13, 16] or those with other advanced systemic diseases (e.g., metastatic neoplasm) that preclude meaningful rehabilitation. Additionally, the rare patient in whom the false lumen has already thrombosed may (at least initially) be treated nonoperatively,[6, 7, 13, 18] but frequent serial imaging studies must be carried out because these patients are not immune to aortic rupture.

The primary goal of surgical treatment for patients with acute type A aortic dissection is to replace the ascending aorta to prevent rupture or proximal extension with resultant intrapericardial rupture and tamponade. Using a median sternotomy, the ascending aorta and proximal arch are replaced with a woven double-velour Dacron graft; an open distal aortic anastomosis employing PHCA is helpful, followed by antegrade reperfusion (achieved by inserting the arterial CPB cannula directly into the arch graft) and rewarming.[35, 109, 110] Aortic flow is redirected into the true lumen distally, which increases the likelihood of reperfusion of aortic branches previously jeopardized by extrinsic compression. Primary intimal tears located in the ascending aorta are resected; arch tears are resected by adding concomitant hemi-arch replacement, but only in selected patients.[40, 109, 110] If aortic regurgitation is present, it is corrected by means of valve resuspension and aortic root reconstruction in most cases.[35, 39, 112] In the Stanford experience, the native aortic valve was preserved in 84 per cent of cases of acute type A dissections; conversely, it should be replaced in patients with Marfan's or Ehlers-Danlos syndrome and those with gross annuloaortic ectasia using a composite valve graft with reimplantation of full-thickness Carrel coronary buttons (rather than the inclusion-wrap Bentall technique). Whether or not the primary intimal tear was capable of being resected had no statistically significant bearing on operative mortality, late reoperation, or late death rates in the 15-year Stanford experience,[7, 16] but the risks of operative death and late reoperation were higher if the tear was located in the transverse aortic arch.

In contrast, the optimal treatment method for patients with acute type B aortic dissections continues to be debated.[5–7, 13, 14, 16, 18, 19, 22–40, 56] This controversy pivots around the relatively good prognosis of these patients when treated medically compared with those with an acute type A dissection[6, 18] and the historically high operative mortality in patients with acute type B aortic dissection who are treated surgically (averaging 38 per cent in the 1960s and 1970s[34]). Patients with uncomplicated acute type B dissections are treated medically in most centers around the world,[6, 18, 22, 25, 27, 29] with surgical intervention generally reserved for those who sustain major complications, such as aortic rupture, severe distal ischemia, persistent or recurrent intractable pain, progression of the dissection, or uncontrollable hypertension.[22, 25, 27] Exceptions to this general policy[28, 35, 49] include carefully selected, young, good-risk patients with an uncomplicated acute type B aortic dissection (such as those with Marfan's syndrome or large [more than

5 cm] localized descending aortic false aneurysms[13, 18, 39]), who are offered early operation. This operation includes tubular graft replacement of a conservative segment of the descending thoracic aorta containing the most severe damage (with resection of the primary intimal tear, if possible) performed through a left thoracotomy and using partial (femorofemoral, pulmonary artery-femoral, or left atrial-femoral) CPB. Elderly, high-operative-risk patients with serious coexisting medical problems have a limited long-term prognosis and are best managed medically, if feasible. The therapeutic management policy of reserving operation for patients who fail to respond to medical treatment, however, has resulted in operative mortality rates as high as 75 to 100 per cent in these salvage circumstances;[7, 13, 26, 34] this is not surprising given the catastrophic clinical situation that sudden failure of medical therapy frequently represents. The indications for emergency operation in these dire circumstances (commonly aortic rupture or renal or mesenteric infarction) have been shown to be the statistically significant, independent determinants that portend an increased likelihood of operative death, together with older age.[7, 29] Nevertheless, emergency surgical intervention can be justified for these life-threatening complications if the patient's general condition and age justify aggressive attempts to prevent imminent death.

In an attempt to avoid this apparent therapeutic paradox, our policy at Stanford since 1977 has been to recommend early graft replacement of the descending thoracic aorta for carefully selected patients with uncomplicated acute type B dissections. The most severely traumatized segment of the descending thoracic aorta is resected to eliminate the most common cause of death, that is, aortic rupture. This policy is affirmed by the lower contemporary operative mortality risk;[7, 29, 35, 39] Svensson and colleagues' experience (when surgery was reserved for those with continued pain or other complications) showed that the operative survival rate plateaued at roughly 95 per cent after 1983 for patients with acute type B dissections undergoing thoracic aortic repair.[39] At Stanford, the operative mortality for patients with acute type B dissections improved from 45 per cent between 1963 and 1979[34] to 13 ± 12 per cent (± 70 per cent confidence limits) between 1977 and 1982.[7] In the combined Stanford-Duke database retrospective investigation, operative mortality for group III patients (those without a compelling indication for emergency operation or major coexisting medical problems) was approximately 10 per cent whether they were treated medically or surgically.[29] In this selected subset, the only statistically significant independent predictor of a high likelihood of early or late death was older age.[29] Other observations supporting our current policy of early operation for these selected patients include the high frequency (up to 84 per cent) of late deaths due to aortic rupture or other dissection-related complications in individuals treated medically, documented in a recent autopsy study,[38] and the fact that subsequent operation (possibly associated with an even higher operative risk compared with repair in the acute phase[13, 19, 100–102]) becomes necessary in many patients owing to progressive aneurysmal enlargement. Furthermore, early surgical replacement of the proximal descending aorta may possibly confer some degree of long-term protection, which reduces the chances of development of false aneurysms in other segments of the thoracic or thoracoabdominal aorta, of acute aortic redissection, or of other late ischemic complications involving compromise of blood flow to the kidneys, abdominal viscera, or lower extremities.

Our indications for operation for patients with chronic type A or type B dissections are more conservative. Surgical intervention is considered if symptoms referable to the dissection (e.g., congestive heart failure due to aortic valve insufficiency, pain, renovascular hypertension with or without renal dysfunction, mesenteric ischemia, and so on) or documented expansion of the chronic dissection occurs. Asymptomatic patients with large (5 to 6 cm in diameter or more) aortic dissections are also offered surgical intervention, but there is no compelling evidence favoring operation over continued expectant medical therapy (and imaging surveillance) for patients with small, asymptomatic, and nonexpanding chronic aortic dissections.[13] Serial CT or MRI scans are essential indefinitely in following these patients.[111]

MANAGEMENT OF PERIPHERAL VASCULAR COMPLICATIONS

Limb Ischemia. A variety of therapeutic approaches has been advocated for the management of aortic dissection complicated by ischemic peripheral vascular compromise, including initial surgical revascularization (aortic fenestration or local or extra-anatomic bypass[9, 10, 14, 41, 44, 82]) with interval thoracic aortic repair,[9] intensive medical therapy alone,[9, 45, 46] or, more recently, therapeutic endovascular therapy, including balloon dilatation, intravascular stenting, and fenestration procedures.[47, 48, 49, 108] Our policy at Stanford[8] (which is also corroborated by other investigators[39, 43]) has been to repair the central thoracic aortic defect initially. In most cases, this procedure has obviated the need for peripheral visceral or extremity revascularization. In the recently updated Stanford series,[8] local peripheral vascular procedures were *unnecessary* in 92 per cent of the 66 patients who presented with peripheral pulse loss following primary repair of the thoracic aorta. Only five patients (8 per cent) required a peripheral vascular procedure (two abdominal aortic fenestrations and three vascular reconstructions). Other authors[9, 41, 44–46, 105] recommend initial peripheral vascular reconstruction (including abdominal aortic fenestration) for patients with lower extremity ischemia, either adjunctively (in persons with acute type A dissections) or as an isolated surgical intervention (in individuals with acute type B dissections treated medically). Although these measures may successfully restore perfusion, the attendant mortality has been high.[9, 41] In Cambria and colleagues' experience, the early mortality was 70 per cent, and, as intuition would dictate, most deaths did not appear to be related to limb ischemia or its sequelae.[9] In Elefteriades and associates' report from Yale, restoration of distal perfusion was accomplished in all 12 (selected) patients treated by retroperitoneal infrarenal abdominal aortic fenestration.[41] Their rationale included the simplicity and effectiveness of this procedure, which avoided the risks of paraplegia and the need for partial CPB. Although no secondary revascularization procedures were necessary, the operative mortality (dating back to 1974) was 21 per cent.[41]

Notably, one patient died of rupture of an untreated ascending aortic dissection. We interpret these observations as indicating that a relatively high incidence of severe lower extremity and intra-abdominal ischemia can be expected if definitive surgical repair of the thoracic aortic dissection is not performed in a timely manner; moreover, once advanced ischemia or infarction of major intra-abdominal organs occurs, it is usually fatal. These suboptimal overall results may reflect only the serious complications associated with medical treatment of patients with acute aortic dissections rather than impugning the peripheral surgical procedures performed.

In summary, early surgical repair of the ascending or descending thoracic aorta in patients with acute aortic dissection is associated with fewer serious peripheral vascular complications in most patients and usually alleviates the cerebral or peripheral ischemic problem without the need to perform peripheral vascular reconstruction. Initial (local) peripheral revascularization is unnecessary and delays definitive thoracic aortic repair, often with fatal consequences. Local revascularization, however, does have a place in the high-risk patient with limb-threatening ischemia due to an acute type B dissection who is to be managed medically, although newer endovascular techniques may offer a more efficacious and lower risk alternative.[108]

Stroke. When stroke complicates an acute aortic dissection (usually type A), the Stanford policy has been to repair the thoracic aortic defect,[8, 103] whereas others defer operations until the neurologic status has resolved.[9] In our experience with seven patients (one of whom underwent concomitant carotid reconstruction), this approach has been associated with an operative survival rate of 86 per cent (6/7). In the overall Stanford analysis, stroke was not a significant independent predictor of operative death.[7, 16] Extension of stroke occurred in two patients, and stroke did indeed adversely influence late survival,[8, 16] because major irreversible neurologic deficits resulted in the death of two patients soon after discharge. Nonetheless, because a favorable outcome occurred in four patients (57 per cent), stroke complicating the presentation of aortic dissection probably should not constitute a strict contraindication to thoracic aortic repair.[8]

Paraplegia. Paraplegia, which occurred infrequently, did not alter this aggressive surgical policy at Stanford, although the operative mortality (50 per cent) was high; nonetheless, paraplegia per se was not a significant risk factor for operative or late death.[7, 16] In such cases it is clearly necessary that the patient, the patient's family, and the referring physician appreciate that the chances of postoperative neurologic recovery are highly unlikely;[9, 104] however, the probable irreversibility of the paraplegia in itself should not preclude operation to prevent other lethal complications. No intraoperative method of spinal cord protection offers complete immunity from the risk of paraplegia; using partial CPB for patients with type B dissections, the incidence of new paraplegia at Stanford was 3.5 per cent.[7] This potential postoperative complication must also be understood and accepted by all concerned parties preoperatively.

Renal Ischemia. The most appropriate management plan for patients presenting with acute aortic dissection complicated by impaired renal perfusion is problematic. Renal ischemia is a grave complication whether it occurs preoperatively or immediately postoperatively; in our experience, preoperative renal dysfunction and angiographic demonstration of impaired renal perfusion were significant independent predictors of operative death.[7] Immediate treatment is required to preserve renal function, control hypertension, or both.[9] Our policy has been to repair the thoracic aorta first, which restores compromised renal circulation;[106] however, the associated operative mortality has been relatively high (upward of 50 per cent).[8] Since postoperative angiographic evaluation was not available in most of the Stanford patients, the actual frequency of restoration of satisfactory renal or visceral perfusion following surgical repair of the thoracic aorta is not known. Nevertheless, close attention to the adequacy of renal or visceral blood flow immediately after thoracic aortic repair is imperative. Renal scans using a portable gamma camera or duplex ultrasound can be useful in the intensive care unit; if any doubt exists, early postoperative angiography is performed immediately.

Local renal revascularization in the acute phase of aortic dissection has been advocated by some authors;[9, 81] however, we do not agree that abdominal exploration and intestinal or renal revascularization should take priority over repair of the thoracic aorta, particularly for patients with acute type A dissections, in whom the unrepaired ascending aorta remains at risk of rupture.[9] In fact, initial local renal revascularization appears to have fairly disappointing results; as compiled by Cambria and colleagues, all four local revascularization procedures (two fenestrations and two direct grafts) failed to reverse the renal failure,[9] and renal artery compromise accompanied by functional renal deterioration was associated with a 50 per cent mortality.[9] Laas and coworkers, from Hannover, Germany, reported that two of three patients (67 per cent) with acute type B dissections complicated by abdominal aortic branch malperfusion died.[10] Each of these patients underwent fenestration, one transabdominally, one via a femoral arterial approach, and the third at the time of thoracic aortic replacement. In two other patients who initially underwent thoracic aortic graft replacement, malperfusion recurred 3 days and 4 weeks later and led to renal failure, necessitating abdominal aortic replacement and renal revascularization. These problems prompted this group to suggest that primary thoracoabdominal replacement may be the procedure of choice if the patient's clinical condition can tolerate such a extensive procedure.[10] In the Yale series,[41] despite the fact that the two patients with renal ischemia and uncontrolled hypertension both did well initially after operative infrarenal abdominal aortic fenestration, one of these patients died of multi-systemic failure.

Earlier renal revascularization is necessary to alter this dismal prognosis; endovascular restitution of adequate renal blood flow at the time of initial diagnostic angiography, either as definitive treatment or prior to thoracic aortic repair, may offer the best hope of improving the patient's prognosis.[108] This would optimize renal perfusion prior to the operative insult and minimize the overall renal ischemic time.[80] Additionally, the main surgical goal would remain focused on prompt repair of the central thoracic aortic problem. Such a policy of early identification and endovascular correction of renal artery compromise may prove to be preferable to the historical policy of intensive postoperative surveillance (e.g., renal nuclear scans, duplex sonography, angiography); unfortunately, these studies are usually undertaken at a time when the fate of the compromised kidney(s) may already have been irreversibly determined.

Visceral Ischemia. Mesenteric vascular compromise, which fortunately is uncommon, is a grave complication associated with mortality rates as high as 88 per cent.[8–11] The most optimal management strategy for visceral ischemia cannot be determined with certainty. At Stanford, we generally repair the thoracic aorta first and then, when indicated, perform supraceliac aortic fenestration or direct mesenteric revascularization (or bowel resection) as a secondary procedure.[8] This approach is associated with an operative mortality of 50 per cent among 10 patients with acute aortic dissection; however, if abdominal exploration is required the death rate rises to 80 per cent (4/5).[8] In very ill patients with visceral infarction or advanced ischemia, Cambria and colleagues attempted to restore visceral perfusion directly or to resect nonviable gut and reported an 88 per cent mortality (7/8).[9] Laas and coworkers had one successful case of direct SMA fenestration plus patch angioplasty.[10] In Elefteriades' series of operative abdominal aortic fenestrations, none of the 14 patients had mesenteric ischemia.[41] The rapidity of mesenteric reperfusion is vital because once small or large bowel infarction occurs, the mortality is excessively high regardless of surgical approach. Perhaps endovascular therapy employed earlier during initial diagnostic angiography might improve visceral perfusion more rapidly and, ideally, mitigate the devastating consequences of this complication.[108]

Newer Approaches. Very recently, endovascular catheter techniques aimed at treating peripheral ischemic complications of aortic dissection have been introduced.[47, 48, 49, 108] Percutaneous transluminal balloon angioplasty per se does not have much to offer except in cases of chronic dissection, in which the pathoanatomic consequences of the dissection have resulted in localized fibrous stenoses in major aortic tributaries. Intravascular stents placed using balloon angioplasty methods, however, can successfully revascularize important ischemic end-organs when the dissection flap or the false channel (patent or thrombosed) obstructs flow in the true lumen.[49] We have recently employed balloon angioplasty and stent placement in five patients for the management of ischemic complications of aortic dissection;[108] stents have been placed for iliac artery occlusion and renal artery stenosis. Intravascular ultrasound has been used to guide and monitor stent deployment. Today, these catheter-based techniques also permit interventional radiologists to fenestrate the aortic flap without resorting to operation.[47, 49] If fenestrations are absent or are small, and an important distal end-organ perfused exclusively by the false channel is not receiving adequate flow, balloon catheters can be threaded across small fenestrations in the flap and inflated. Alternatively, a fenestration can be created de novo in the flap if necessary.[47] This approach can also be employed when expansion of the false lumen extrinsically compromises antegrade flow in the adjacent aortic true channel; fenestration in this context "decompresses" the false lumen and provides a route that can increase blood flow in the distal true lumen. Complete evaluation (including contrast injections and filming in both aortic channels and assiduous measurement of arterial pressures in multiple locations within both lumens) precedes the decision to create or enlarge a fenestration. IVUS can provide additional pathoanatomic information to determine whether fenestration is warranted and to guide the procedure. Theoretically, there is some risk that balloon catheter (or surgical) fenestration may be complicated by intussusception of the flap downstream, which could result in catastrophic occlusion of either the distal aortic true or false lumen. Currently, clinical experience with these catheter-based procedures for patients with complicated aortic dissections is limited;[108] additional work is necessary before the full utility, safety, and limitations of the techniques can be fully determined. If additional clinical experience confirms that these endovascular approaches are safe and are durable long-term, a major therapeutic advance will have been accomplished for these particularly high-risk patients.

Impact of Peripheral Vascular Complications on Operative Mortality. The operative mortality for patients with acute aortic dissection has decreased markedly over the last decade, in large part due to earlier diagnosis and initiation of treatment.[7, 32, 107] Between 1977 and 1982, the operative risk in the Stanford series (Fig. 78–5) was 7 ± 5 per cent for patients with acute type A dissections and 13 ± 12 per cent for those with acute type B dissections.[7] In this study, multi-variate statistical analysis revealed that only earlier operative date, renal dysfunction, cardiac tamponade, and

(angiographic) renal or visceral ischemia or infarction were significant independent incremental risk factors portending a greater likelihood of operative death in the type A subgroup. For the type B subgroup, older age, aortic rupture, and renal or visceral ischemia were the predictors. When all patients were considered together, chronic pulmonary disease and site of tear (aortic arch > descending aorta > ascending aorta) emerged as additional incremental risk factors. Interestingly, several covariates did not attain statistic predictive significance, including stroke, paraplegia, peripheral pulse loss, type of dissection (A vs. B), acuity (acute vs. chronic), Marfan's syndrome, emergency operation, and whether or not the primary intimal tear was resected, the aortic valve was replaced, or concomitant coronary artery bypass grafting was performed.

In the recent Stanford report focusing on peripheral vascular complications,[8] the overall operative mortality was 25 ± 3 per cent (68 of 272 patients). The operative mortality rates were higher for subgroups of patients with compromised renal blood flow, compromised visceral blood flow, and those with paraplegia: 50 ± 11 per cent (11 of 22), 43 ± 14 per cent (6 of 14), and 44 ± 17 per cent (4 of 9), respectively. The mortality rates were lower for patients presenting with stroke (14 ± 14 per cent [1 of 7] patients) or peripheral pulse deficits (27 ± 6 per cent, [18/66], see Table 78–2). Multi-variate logistic analysis, however, revealed that only one of the five peripheral vascular complications—impaired renal perfusion—emerged as a significant independent predictor of operative death.[8] Renal dysfunction, hypertension, older age, tamponade, and earlier operative date were the other incremental risk factors.[8] Surprisingly, compromised visceral perfusion (despite the high associated operative mortality rate) per se did not

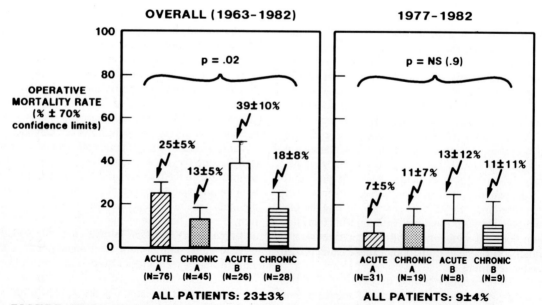

FIGURE 78–5. Operative mortality rates for patients with acute and chronic aortic dissections between 1963 and 1982 at Stanford. As shown in the *right panel*, early operative results improved in the more recent time frame (1977–1982), the current operative risk being 7 ± 5 per cent (±70 per cent confidence limits) for patients with acute type A dissections and 13 ± 12 per cent for those with acute type B dissections. Between 1963 and 1976, the overall mortality rate was 31 ± 5 per cent (34/108) compared with the more recent (1977–1982) overall risk of 9 ± 4 per cent. (From Miller DC, Mitchell RS, Oyer PE, et al: Circulation 70[Suppl I]:I–157, 1984. By permission of The American Heart Association, Inc.)

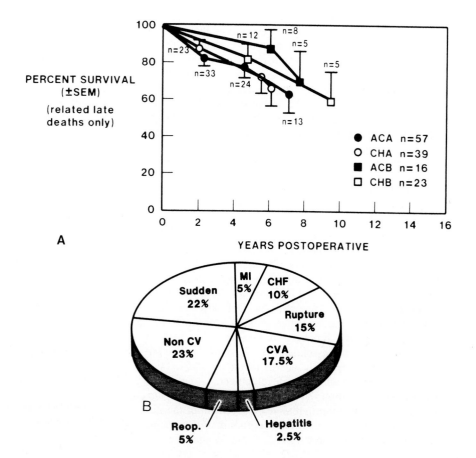

FIGURE 78–6. *A*, Actuarial survival curves for discharged patients with acute type A (ACA), acute type B (ACB), chronic type A (CHA), and chronic type B (CHB) aortic dissections after initial surgical repair of the thoracic aorta. These survival estimates apply only to late deaths that were definitely or possibly related to the aortic dissection or the previous surgical procedure. *B*, Cause of late deaths following surgical repair of the thoracic aorta. Rupture of another segment of the aorta (usually a false aneurysm) was responsible for 15 per cent of all late deaths; this figure was similar to that reported by Crawford's group,[39] but lower than the 29 per cent fraction in DeBakey and colleagues' long-term series.[19] (*A* and *B*, From Miller DC: Surgical emergencies of the thoracic aorta. *In* Bergan JJ, Yao JST [eds]: Vascular Surgical Emergencies. Orlando, FL, Grune & Stratton, 1987, p 331.)

emerge as a significant independent predictor of increased operative mortality risk in the multi-variate analysis; this may have been due to the small number of patients (beta or type II statistical error). Similarly, the low incidence of stroke and paraplegia may have prevented these factors from attaining statistical significance.

Long-Term Survival. The long-term survival for patients discharged from hospital in the earlier Stanford overall analysis[16] is illustrated in Figure 78–6. The 5-year actuarial survival estimate was 78 ± 6 per cent for patients with type A dissections and 88 ± 12 per cent in the type B dissection subgroup. Stroke, remote MI, renal dysfunc-

tion, and earlier operative era were the independent risk factors for late death. It should be emphasized that 15 per cent of late deaths were due to rupture of a contiguous or remote portion of the aorta (compared to 29 per cent of all late deaths in the 20-year long-term study from Baylor University).[19] This sobering figure should be amenable to future improvement if more careful patient follow-up is carried out.[13, 39, 111]

Late Reoperation. The incidence of late reoperation related to the dissection after thoracic aortic repair in the Stanford experience is shown in Figure 78–7; late reoperation was necessary in 13 ± 4 per cent of patients after 5

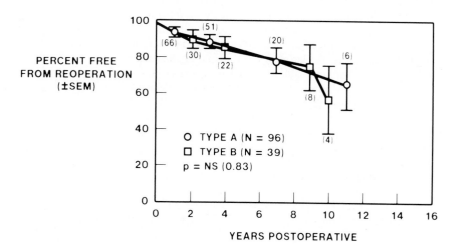

FIGURE 78–7. Actuarial incidence of freedom from reoperation (focusing solely on those surgical procedures related to the aorta or to complications of the dissection) after initial surgical repair of aortic dissections. Reoperations can be categorized into two distinct subgroups: Treatment Failures and Late Aortic Sequelae (see text). There was no statistically significant difference in reoperation rate between the two major types (A vs. B) of dissections. (From Haverich A, Miller DC, Scott WC, et al: Acute and chronic aortic dissections— Determinants of long-term outcome for operative survivors. Circulation 72[Suppl II]:II–26, 1985. By permission of The American Heart Association, Inc.)

years and 23 ± 6 per cent after 10 years. The independent incremental risk factors associated with a higher likelihood of late reoperation included younger age and site of tear (arch > descending aorta > ascending aorta), but resection of the tear and preservation versus replacement of the aortic valve had no real bearing on the probability of late death or reoperation.[16] Although some reoperations were related to the original repair (termed treatment failures—e.g., anastomotic disruption, false aneurysm formation, progressive aortic valvular insufficiency, failure of an inserted valve prosthesis), most were necessary to correct new problems arising in the remaining diseased aorta (called late aortic sequelae).[16, 111] These findings underscore the need for lifelong close medical supervision of all patients with aortic dissections, including serial CT or MRI scans to detect asymptomatic localized thoracic, thoracoabdominal, or abdominal aortic false aneurysms. Of note, such aneurysms developed in 45 per cent of patients with poor blood pressure control, but in only 17 per cent of those with well-controlled hypertension reported by DeBakey and colleagues.[19] Intensive medical management with antihypertensive and negative inotropic drugs (beta blockers or calcium antagonists) is essential, *even in normotensive patients*, to minimize the incidence of late acute redissection and progressive false aneurysm development.

Elective reoperation should be considered when symptoms occur or localized progressive enlargement of the dissected aorta is observed, or if the descending thoracic aorta or thoracoabdominal aorta exceed 6 cm in diameter (in asymptomatic patients). Diffuse, uniform enlargement of the aorta in the range of 4 to 4.5 cm (which usually consists mostly of the false lumen) is not necessarily an indication for reoperation in the absence of symptoms. In asymptomatic patients, the potential benefits of graft replacement need to be weighed against the risk of paraplegia (which pivots on the extent of aortic replacement and exceeds 30 per cent in patients undergoing extensive [Crawford type II] thoracoabdominal resection [see Chapter 77]),[39] the patient's general medical condition, and the operative risk.[35] Rarely, reoperation may be required for symptomatic aortic branch vessel compromise.

SUMMARY

The possibility of acute aortic dissection must be considered in the differential diagnosis of acute peripheral arterial ischemia, particularly when seemingly unrelated organ systems are involved simultaneously. It is important to be aware that aortic dissection is not rare and occurs twice as frequently as ruptured abdominal aortic aneurysm; however, the correct diagnosis is frequently missed or delayed. Furthermore, if not diagnosed and treated urgently, the mortality for patients with acute aortic dissection is inordinately high: on the order of *1 per cent per hour for the first 48 hours*. Appropriate management consists of administering antihypertensive and negative inotropic pharmacologic treatment while rapidly performing a definitive diagnostic procedure (TEE, CT scanning or aortography). Emergency surgical repair of the thoracic aorta is required for all patients with acute type A aortic dissections, as well as for those with acute type B dissections who sustain life-threatening complications. The optimal management of patients with *uncomplicated* acute type B aortic dissections remains controversial; we recommend early thoracic aortic repair in carefully selected patients. This policy may minimize the prohibitive operative mortality associated with emergency "salvage" operation when medical therapy fails suddenly. Initial or primary peripheral revascularization procedures have little or no role in the immediate treatment of individuals with acute aortic dissections because this delays diagnosis and definitive treatment, which can be potentially catastrophic. After the thoracic aorta is successfully repaired, preexisting compromise of the peripheral arterial circulation is usually restored spontaneously. Impaired renal or visceral perfusion, however, remains a vexing clinical problem and is associated with very high fatality rates. New endovascular techniques that can be performed at the time of initial diagnostic angiography are currently being investigated in an effort to ameliorate the impact of these devastating complications. All patients require lifelong administration of antihypertensive or negative inotropic drugs to reduce the risk of further aneurysmal degeneration or acute redissection. Rigorous surveillance with serial CT or MRI scanning to evaluate the entire thoracic and abdominal aorta for development of aneurysmal changes is mandatory on an indefinite basis.

Acknowledgment: *We thank Phoebe E. Taboada for her superb assistance in the preparation and assembly of this manuscript.*

References

1. Sorenson HR, Olsen H: Ruptured and dissecting aneurysms of the aorta. Incidence and prospects of surgery. Acta Chir Scand 128:644, 1964.
2. Pate JW, Richardson RL, Eastridge CE: Acute aortic dissections. Am Surgeon 42:395, 1976.
3. Bickerstaff LK, Pairolero PC, Hollier LH, et al: Thoracic aortic aneurysms: A population-based study. Surgery 92:1103, 1982.
4. Wheat MW Jr, Palmer RF: Dissecting aneurysms of the aorta. Curr Probl Surg 1:43, 1971.
5. Eagle KA, DeSanctis RW: Aortic dissection. Curr Probl Cardiol 14:225, 1989.
6. Wheat MW Jr: Intensive drug therapy. In Doroghazi RM, Slater EE (eds): Aortic Dissection. New York, McGraw-Hill, 1983, p 165.
7. Miller DC, Mitchell RS, Oyer PE, et al: Independent determinants of operative mortality for patients with aortic dissections. Circulation 70(Suppl I):I–153, 1984.
8. Fann JI, Sarris GE, Mitchell RS, et al: Treatment of patients with aortic dissection presenting with peripheral vascular complications. Ann Surg 212:705, 1990.
9. Cambria RP, Brewster DC, Gertler J, et al: Vascular complications associated with spontaneous aortic dissection. J Vasc Surg 7:199, 1988.
10. Laas J, Heinemann M, Schaefers H-J, et al: Management of thoracoabdominal malperfusion in aortic dissection. Circulation 84(Suppl III):III–20, 1991.
11. Pinet F, Froment JC, Guillot M, et al: Prognostic factors and indications for surgical treatment of acute aortic dissections: A report based on 191 observations. Cardiovasc Intervent Radiol 7:257, 1984.
12. Slater EE: Aortic dissection: Presentation and diagnosis. In Doroghazi RM, Slater EE (eds): Aortic Dissection. New York, McGraw-Hill, 1983, p 61.
13. Miller DC: Surgical management of aortic dissections: Indications, perioperative management, and long-term results. In Doroghazi RM, Slater EE (eds): Aortic Dissection. New York, McGraw-Hill, 1983, p 193.
14. Jamieson WRE, Munro AI, Miyagishima RT, et al: Aortic dissec-

tions: Early diagnosis and surgical management are the keys to survival. Can J Surg 25:145, 1982.

15. Miller DC: When to suspect aortic dissection: What treatment? Cardiovasc Med 9:811, 1984.

16. Haverich A, Miller DC, Scott WC, et al: Acute and chronic aortic dissections—Determinants of long-term outcome for operative survivors. Circulation 72(Suppl II):II–224, 1985.

17. Levinson DC, Edmeades DT, Griffith GC: Dissecting aneurysm of aorta: Its clinical, electrocardiographic, and laboratory features; Report of 58 autopsied cases. Circulation 1:360, 1950.

18. Doroghazi RM, Slater EE, DeSanctis RW, et al: Long-term survival of patients with treated aortic dissections. J Am Coll Cardiol 3:1026, 1984.

19. DeBakey ME, McCollum CH, Crawford ES, et al: Dissection and dissecting aneurysms of the aorta: Twenty-year follow-up of five hundred and twenty-seven patients treated surgically. Surgery 92:1118, 1982.

20. Slater EE, DeSanctis RW: The clinical recognition of dissecting aortic aneurysm. Am J Med 60:625, 1976.

21. Leonard JC, Hasleton PS: Dissecting aortic aneurysms: A clinicopathological study. I. Clinical and gross pathological findings. Q J Med 189:55, 1979.

22. Acute aortic dissection [Editorial]. Lancet 2:827, 1988.

23. Appelbaum A, Karp RB, Kirklin JW: Ascending vs. descending aortic dissections. Ann Surg 183:296, 1976.

24. Cipriano PR, Griepp RB: Acute retrograde dissection of the ascending thoracic aorta. Am J Cardiol 43:520, 1979.

25. Crawford ES: The diagnosis and management of aortic dissection. JAMA 264:2537, 1990.

26. Dalen JE, Alpert JS, Cohn LH, et al: Dissection of the thoracic aorta. Medical or surgical therapy? Am J Cardiol 34:803, 1974.

27. DeSanctis RW, Doroghazi RM, Austen WG, et al: Aortic dissection. N Engl J Med 317:1060, 1987.

28. Ergin MA, Lansman SL, Griepp RB: Acute dissections of the aorta. Cardiac Surgery: State of the Art Reviews 1:377, 1987.

29. Glower DD, Fann JI, Speier RH, et al: Comparison of medical and surgical therapy for uncomplicated descending aortic dissection. Circulation 82(Suppl IV):IV–39, 1990.

30. Glower DD, Speier RF, White WD, et al: Management and long-term outcome of aortic dissection. Ann Surg 214:31, 1991.

31. Jex RK, Schaff HV, Piehler JM, et al: Early and late results following repair of dissections of the descending thoracic aorta. J Vasc Surg 3:226, 1986.

32. Ming RL, Najafi H, Javid H, et al: Acute ascending aortic dissection: Surgical management. Circulation 64(Suppl II):II–231, 1981.

33. Miller DC: Acute dissection of the aorta—Continuing need for earlier diagnosis and treatment. Mod Concepts Cardiovasc Dis 54:51, 1985.

34. Miller DC, Stinson EB, Oyer PE, et al: Operative treatment of aortic dissections. J Thorac Cardiovasc Surg 78:365, 1979.

35. Miller DC: Surgical management of acute aortic dissection: New data. Semin Thorac Cardiovasc Surg 3:225, 1991.

36. Miller DC: Surgical treatment of aortic dissections. In Jamieson SW, Shumway NE (eds): Operative Surgery—Cardiac Surgery. London, Butterworths, 1986, p 526.

37. Reul GJ, Cooley DA, Hallman GL, et al: Dissecting aneurysm of the descending aorta. Improved surgical results in 91 patients. Arch Surg 110:632, 1975.

38. Roberts CS, Roberts WC: Aortic dissection with entrance tear in the descending thoracic aorta: Analysis of 40 necropsy patients. Ann Surg 213:356, 1991.

39. Svensson LG, Crawford ES, Hess KR, et al: Dissection of the aorta and dissecting aneurysms: Improving early and long-term surgical results. Circulation 82(Suppl IV):IV–24, 1990.

40. Yun KL, Glower DL, Miller DC, et al: Aortic dissection due to transverse arch tear: Is concomitant arch repair warranted? J Thorac Cardiovasc Surg 102:355, 1991.

41. Elefteriades JA, Hartleroad J, Gusberg RJ, et al: Long-term experience with descending aortic dissection: The complication-specific approach. Ann Thorac Surg 53:11, 1992.

42. Carpentier A, Deloche A, Fabiani JN, et al: New surgical approach to aortic dissection: Flow reversal and thromboexclusion. J Thorac Cardiovasc Surg 81:659, 1981.

43. Shumacker HB, Isch JH, Jolly WW: Stenotic and obstructive lesions in acute dissecting thoracic aortic aneurysms. Ann Surg 181:662, 1975.

44. Elefteriades JA, Hammond GL, Gusberg RJ, et al: Fenestration revisited: A safe and effective procedure for descending aortic dissection. Arch Surg 125:786, 1990.

45. Schoon IM, Holm J, Sudow G: Lower-extremity ischemia in aortic dissection. Scand J Thorac Cardiovasc Surg 19:93, 1985.

46. Shah PM, Clauss RH: Dissecting hematoma presents as acute lower limb ischemia: Diagnostic patient profile and management. J Cardiovasc Surg (Torino) 24:649, 1983.

47. Williams DM, Brothers TE, Messina LM: Relief of mesenteric ischemia in type III aortic dissection with percutaneous fenestration of the aortic septum. Radiology 174:450, 1990.

48. Shimshak TM, Giorgi LV, Hartzler GO: Successful percutaneous transluminal angioplasty of an obstructed abdominal aorta secondary to a chronic dissection. Am J Cardiol 61:486, 1988.

49. Miller DC: Acute dissection of the descending thoracic aorta. Chest Surg Clin North Am 2:347, 1992.

50. DeBakey ME, Cooley DA, Creech O Jr: Surgical considerations of dissecting aneurysm of the aorta. Ann Surg 142:586, 1955.

51. DeBakey ME, Henley SW, Cooley DA, et al: Surgical management of dissecting aneurysms of the aorta. J Thorac Cardiovasc Surg 49:130, 1965.

52. Daily PO, Trueblood HW, Stinson EB, et al: Management of acute aortic dissections. Ann Thor Surg 10:237, 1970.

53. Perez JE: Noninvasive diagnosis: Computed tomography and ultrasound. In Doroghazi RM, Slater EE (eds): Aortic Dissection. New York, McGraw-Hill, 1983, p 133.

54. Shennan T: Dissecting aneurysms. Medical Research Council, Special Report, Series No. 193. London: His Majesty's Stationary Office, 1934.

55. Gore I, Seiwert VJ: Dissecting aneurysm of the aorta. Pathological aspect and analysis of 85 fatal cases. Arch Pathol 53:121, 1952.

56. Hirst AE Jr, Johns VJ Jr, Kime SW Jr: Dissecting aneurysm of the aorta: A review of 505 cases. Medicine 37:217, 1958.

57. Graham D, Alexander JJ, Francheschi D, et al: The management of localized abdominal aortic dissections. J Vasc Surg 8:582, 1988.

58. Cambria RP, Morse S, August D, et al: Acute dissection originating in the abdominal aorta. J Vasc Surg 5:495, 1987.

59. Schlatmann TJM, Becker AE: Histologic changes in the normal aging aorta. Implications for dissecting aortic aneurysm. Am J Cardiol 39:13, 1977.

60. Schlatmann TJM, Becker AE: Pathogenesis of dissecting aneurysm of the aorta. Comparative histopathologic study of significance of medial changes. Am J Cardiol 39:21, 1977.

61. Larson EW, Edwards WD: Risk factors for aortic dissection: A necropsy study of 161 cases. Am J Cardiol 53:849, 1984.

62. Wheat MW Jr: Pathogenesis of aortic dissection. In Doroghazi RM, Slater EE (eds): Aortic Dissection. New York, McGraw-Hill, 1983, p 55.

63. Anagnostopoulos CE, Athanasuleas CL, Garrick TR: Acute Aortic Dissections. Baltimore, University Press, 1975.

64. Wilson SK, Hutchins GM: Aortic dissecting aneurysms: Causative factors in 204 subjects. Arch Pathol Lab Med 106:173, 1982.

65. Gore I, Hirst AE: Dissecting aneurysm of the aorta. Cardiovasc Clin 2:103, 1973.

66. Gore I: Pathogenesis of dissecting aneurysm of the aorta. Arch Pathol 53:142, 1952.

67. Hirst AE, Gore I: The etiology and pathology of aortic dissection. In Doroghazi RM, Slater EE (eds): Aortic Dissection. New York, McGraw-Hill, 1983, p 193.

68. Hirst AE, Gore I: Is cystic medial necrosis the cause of dissecting aortic aneurysm? Circulation 53:915, 1976.

69. Miller DC, Stinson EB: Acute and chronic aortic dissection. In Miller DC, Roon AJ (eds): Diagnosis and Management of Peripheral Vascular Disease. Menlo Park, CA, Addison-Wesley, 1982, p 179.

70. Lindsay J: Aortic dissection. Cardiovasc Clin 13:193, 1983.

71. Fradet G, Jamieson WRE, Janusz MT, et al: Aortic dissection: A six year experience with 117 patients. Am J Surg 155:697, 1988.

72. Walterbusch G, Oelert H, Borst HG: Restoration of cerebral blood flow by extraanatomic bypass in acute aortic dissection. Thorac Cardiovasc Surg 32:381, 1984.

73. Zirkle PK, Wheeler JR, Gregory RT, et al: Carotid involvement in aortic dissection diagnosed by duplex scanning. J Vasc Surg 1:700, 1984.

74. Scott RW, Sancetta SM: Dissecting aneurysm of aorta with hemorrhagic infarction of the spinal cord and complete paraplegia. Am Heart J 38:747, 1949.

75. Gerber O, Heyer EJ, Vieux U: Painless dissections of the aorta presenting as acute neurologic syndromes. Stroke 17:644, 1986.

76. Sutton MSJ, Oldershaw PJ, Miller GAH, et al: Dissection of the thoracic aorta: A comparison between medical and surgical treatment. J Cardiovasc Surg (Torino) 22:195, 1981.

77. Siegelman SS, Sprayregen S, Strasberg Z: Aortic dissection and the left renal artery. Radiology 95:73, 1970.

78. Burchell HB: Aortic dissection (dissecting hematoma; dissecting aneurysm of the aorta). Circulation 12:1068, 1955.

79. Stein HL, Steinberg I: Selective aortography, the definitive technique of diagnosis of dissecting aneurysm of the aorta. Am J Roentgenol 102:333, 1968.

80. Ouriel K, Andrus CH, Ricotta JJ, et al: Acute renal artery occlusion: When is revascularization justified? J Vasc Surg 5:348, 1987.

81. Bradbrook RA, Marshall AJ, Spreadbury PL: Hypertension with dissecting abdominal aortic aneurysm. Br Med J 4:23, 1974.

82. Noda Y, Fukiyama K, Omae T: Renin dependent hypertension by dissecting aortic aneurysm. Jpn Heart J 22:281, 1981.

83. Cogbill TH, Gundersen AE, Travelli R: Mesenteric vascular insufficiency and claudication following acute dissecting thoracic aortic aneurysm. J Vasc Surg 2:472, 1985.

84. Erbel R, Engbergbing R, Daniel W, et al: Echocardiography in the diagnosis of aortic dissection. Lancet 457, 1989.

85. Erbel R, Borner N, Brunier J, et al: Detection of aortic dissection by transesophageal echocardiography. Br Heart J 58:45, 1987.

86. Adachi H, Kyo S, Takamoto S, et al: Early diagnosis and surgical intervention of acute aortic dissection by transesophageal color flow mapping. Circulation 82(Suppl IV):IV–19, 1990.

87. Hashimoto S, Kumada T, Osakada G, et al: Assessment of transesophageal Doppler echography in dissecting aneurysm. J Am Coll Cardiol 14:1253, 1989.

88. Mohr-Kahaly S, Erbel R, Rennollet H, et al: Ambulatory follow-up of aortic dissection by transesophageal two-dimensional and color-coded Doppler echocardiography. Circulation 80:24, 1989.

89. Dinsmore RE, Willerson JT, Buckley MJ: Dissecting aneurysms of the aorta. Aortographic features affecting prognosis. Radiology 105:567, 1972.

90. Arciniegas JG, Soto B, Little WC, et al: Cineangiography in the diagnosis of aortic dissection. Am J Cardiol 47:890, 1981.

91. Pande A, Meier B, Fleisch M, et al: Intravascular ultrasound for diagnosis of aortic dissection. Am J Cardiol 67:662, 1991.

92. Weintraub AR, Schwartz SL, Pandian NG, et al: Evaluation of acute aortic dissection by intravascular ultrasound. N Engl J Med 323:1566, 1990.

93. Cavaye DM, French WJ, White RA, et al: Intravascular ultrasound imaging of an acute dissecting aortic aneurysm: A case report. J Vasc Surg 13:510, 1991.

94. Rubenson DS, Fowler RF, Miller DC, et al: Spontaneous dissection of the ascending aorta diagnosed by two-dimensional echocardiography. Chest 80:857, 1981.

95. Miller DC: Surgical emergencies of the thoracic aorta. *In* Bergan JJ, Yao JST (eds): Vascular Surgical Emergencies. Orlando, FL. Grune & Stratton, 1987, p 319.

96. Wolfe WG, Moran JF: The evolution of medical and surgical management of acute aortic dissection. Circulation 56:503, 1977.

97. Wheat MW Jr: Current status of medical therapy of acute dissecting aneurysms of the aorta. World J Surg 4:563, 1980.

98. Cachern JP, Vouhe RR, Loisance DY, et al: Surgical management of acute dissections involving the ascending aorta. J Thorac Cardiovasc Surg 82:576, 1981.

99. Miller DC, Stinson EB, Shumway NE: Realistic expections of surgical treatment of aortic dissection: The Stanford experience. World J Surg 4:571, 1980.

100. Carmutti VM, Dantur JR, Favaloro MR, et al: Deep hypothermia and circulatory arrest as an elective technique in the treatment of type B dissecting aneurysm of the aorta. J Cardiac Surg 4:206, 1989.

101. Crawford ES, Crawford JL, Stowe CL, et al: Total aortic replacement for chronic aortic dissection occurring in patients with and without Marfan's syndrome. Ann Surg 199:358, 1984.

102. Crawford ES, Coselli JS, Safi HJ: Partial cardiopulmonary bypass, hypothermic circulatory arrest, and posterolateral exposure for thoracic aneurysm operation. J Thorac Cardiovasc Surg 94:824, 1987.

103. Fann JI, Sarris GE, Miller DC, et al: Surgical management of acute aortic dissection complicated by stroke. Circulation 80(Suppl I):I–257, 1989.

104. Ross RT: Spinal cord infarction in disease and surgery of the aorta. Can J Neurol Sci 12:289, 1985.

105. White TJ III, Pinstein ML, Scott RL, et al: Aortic dissection manifested as leg ischemia. Am J Roentgenol 135:353, 1980.

106. Mulder DG, Kauffman JJ: Acute dissection of the thoracic aorta presenting as a renal artery occlusion. J Thorac Cardiovasc Surg 56:184, 1968.

107. Wolfe WG, Oldham HN, Rankin JS: Surgical treatment of acute ascending aortic dissection. Ann Surg 197:738, 1983.

108. Walker PJ, Dake MD, Mitchell RS, Miller DC: The use of endovascular techniques for the treatment of complications of aortic dissection. J Vasc Surg 18:1042, 1993.

109. Crawford ES, Kirklin JW, Naftel DC, et al: Surgery for acute dissection of ascending aorta: Should the arch be included? J Thorac Cardiovasc Surg 104:46, 1992.

110. Miller DC: Concomitant arch repair in acute type A aortic dissection. J Thorac Cardiovasc Surg 104:206, 1992.

111. Miller DC: Improved follow-up for patients with chronic dissections. Semin Thorac Cardiovasc Surg 3:270, 1991.

112. Fann JI, Glower DD, Miller DC, et al: Preservation of aortic valve in type A aortic dissection complicated by aortic valvular regurgitation. J Thorac Cardiovasc Surg 102:62, 1991.

Popliteal and Femoral Aneurysms

Kenneth Ouriel, M.D., and Cynthia K. Shortell, M.D.

• • •

Popliteal and femoral artery aneurysms constitute over 90 per cent of all peripheral arterial aneurysms.[9] True aneurysms are composed of all three layers of the vascular wall, may develop as a result of a degenerative process usually associated with atherosclerotic disease, and are frequently associated with arterial aneurysms in other sites. Popliteal aneurysms are almost exclusively of this variety. False aneurysms, consisting of encapsulated hematomas communicating with the vessel lumen, may occur after iatrogenic or traumatic injury or as a complication of vascular bypass graft procedures. Because of the increasing frequency of arteriographic studies and percutaneous vascular therapies performed through the femoral approach, false aneurysms have become the type of aneurysm most commonly encountered in the femoral artery.

Thrombosis, distal embolization, rupture, and compression of adjacent structures are the clinical manifestations generally produced by both true and false aneurysms, although the frequency with which they occur differs between the two types. Whereas patients with true aneurysms characteristically develop thrombosis and distal embolization, false aneurysms more often result in local pain and rupture. The natural history of untreated aneurysms of the popliteal and femoral arteries was best described in studies performed prior to the advent of modern reconstructive vascular techniques. Gifford and colleagues reported a series of 100 popliteal aneurysms in 1953; they observed an overall complication rate of 26 per cent in patients who were asymptomatic at the time of initial diagnosis.[12] No such early data exist for asymptomatic femoral aneurysms, but Graham and colleagues followed 105 patients with asymptomatic femoral aneurysms, documenting a complication rate of only 3 per cent during the period of follow-up observation.[13] These data suggest that asymptomatic popliteal and femoral aneurysms are associated with marked differences in morbidity; patients with popliteal aneurysms are prone to limb-threatening complications, whereas patients with femoral aneurysms only rarely develop significant symptoms.

POPLITEAL ANEURYSMS

The popliteal artery is the most frequent site of peripheral aneurysm formation, accounting for 84 per cent of all peripheral aneurysms in Dent and colleagues' series of 1488 patients with aneurysms of the aorta and its distal branches.[9] Atherosclerosis is the most common cause of popliteal aneurysms and is responsible for 84 to 100 per cent of lesions, depending on the series.[5, 11, 12, 31] The underlying mechanisms predisposing certain patients with atherosclerotic disease to popliteal aneurysm formation are not well understood.

The incidence of bilaterality in patients with popliteal aneurysms is high, ranging from 45 to 68 per cent.[29, 31] Similarly, the presence of aneurysmal disease elsewhere in the arterial tree is common. In his long-term follow-up of 147 patients with popliteal aneurysms, Vermillion and associates observed a 55 per cent incidence of associated aneurysms, with abdominal aortic aneurysms being the most common (40 per cent) followed by femoral aneurysms (34 per cent) and iliac aneurysms (25 per cent).[29] In addition, the authors reported that the incidence of extrapopliteal aneurysms was much higher in the group with bilateral popliteal aneurysms than in those with unilateral lesions, perhaps suggesting a generally more virulent degenerative process. Virtually all authors have observed that popliteal aneurysms occur almost exclusively in men,[12, 24, 31] with a median age of 60 to 65 years at the time of diagnosis.[8, 11]

Classification

Popliteal aneurysms can be divided into two types according to shape—fusiform and saccular. The majority of popliteal aneurysms are of the fusiform configuration. Fusiform aneurysms originate more proximally than saccular aneurysms and generally involve both the distal superficial femoral artery and the popliteal artery. They are small to moderate in diameter and are long in length. Fusiform aneurysms are densely atherosclerotic and may be associated with multiple focal stenoses along the length of the aneurysm, producing a scalloped appearance on arteriography (Fig. 79–1). Saccular aneurysms, by contrast, involve only the mid-popliteal artery, tend to be of a larger diameter and shorter length, and are associated with less atherosclerotic disease in the arterial segments proximal and distal to the dilatation (Fig. 79–2). The clinical implications of these two types of popliteal aneurysms have not yet been determined.

Clinical Manifestations

The proportion of patients with popliteal aneurysms who are symptomatic at the time of initial presentation has been reported to be between 52 and 86 per cent.[3, 8, 30, 31]

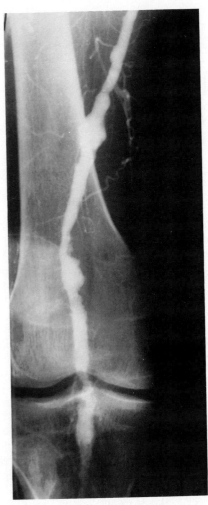

FIGURE 79–1. An arteriogram demonstrating the fusiform variety of popliteal aneurysm, with the aneurysmal process beginning in the superficial femoral artery and extending into the popliteal artery.

outflow from distal atheroembolization and retrograde thrombosis of the tibial arteries. The embolic process may proceed in a sequential fashion, progressing silently until the last tibial vessel is involved. Sudden onset of severe ischemia occurs at this time, frequently with irreversible compromise of the arterial supply to the foot.

Diagnosis

The most important element in the diagnosis of a popliteal aneurysm is a high index of suspicion in conjunction with a careful physical examination by an experienced observer. Popliteal aneurysms should be suspected in patients with other peripheral arterial aneurysms, particularly when a contralateral popliteal aneurysm exists and in patients with a family history of arterial aneurysms. Examination of the popliteal fossa in patients with *patent* popliteal aneurysms reveals a prominent popliteal pulse. The diagnosis may be suspected in patients with *thrombosed* popliteal aneurysms on the basis of a firm popliteal mass, a contralateral popliteal aneurysm, or a coexisting femoral or aortic aneurysm. Once the clinical diagnosis has been made, it can be confirmed by a number of noninvasive techniques. Ultrasound and computed tomography are useful in documenting the size and extent of the aneurysm and in detecting the presence of mural thrombus (see Fig. 79–3 on Color Plate IV). Ultrasound is the most appropriate modality with which to follow patients in whom operation is not performed. Arteriography is indicated for all patients in whom operation is anticipated because of the high incidence of distal disease due to thromboembolism as well as of inflow

Symptoms referable to popliteal aneurysms may be grouped according to their proximate cause: rupture, compression of adjacent structures, and ischemia (Table 79–1). Rupture of popliteal aneurysms is rare, occurring in only 4 (3 per cent) of 147 cases in the series of Vermillion and associates.[29] Compression of local venous and nervous structures may develop, particularly if the aneurysm is large and saccular. Venous obstruction was observed in 11 extremities (7 per cent), and nerve compression in 12 extremities (8 per cent). Ischemia is by far the most common presenting complication of popliteal aneurysms. The severity of ischemia ranges from mild claudication to rest pain and gangrene. Ischemia may occur as a result of distal embolism of thrombus or atheromatous debris to the tibial and pedal vessels, thrombosis of the aneurysm itself, or a combination of these two mechanisms. Thrombosis of the aneurysm may be due to the propagation of mural thrombus to the point where the lumen of the aneurysm is critically compromised. The ischemic symptoms are only moderately severe in this situation because the tibial arteries may remain patent through collateral circulation. Alternatively, aneurysm thrombosis may develop as a secondary event, preceded by a loss of

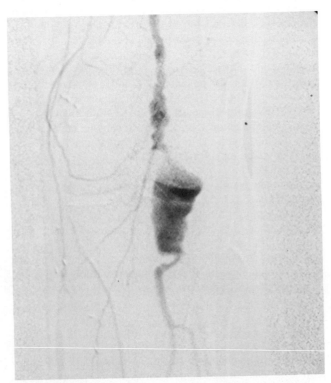

FIGURE 79–2. An arteriogram demonstrating the saccular variety of popliteal aneurysm, with the aneurysmal process limited to the popliteal artery.

Table 79–1. Presenting Symptoms of Popliteal Aneurysms

| Author | No. Aneurysms | No. Symptoms | Rupture | Local Compression | | Ischemia | |
				Nerve	*Vein*	*Claud*	*LTI*
Vermillion et al[29]	147	33%	3%	8%	7%	45%	37%
Dawson et al[8]	71	14%	5%	11%	0	46%	19%
Baird et al[5]	61	24%	0	4%	12%	43%	8%
Shortell et al[24]	51	29%	0	6%	2%	4%	22%

Claud, claudication; LTI, limb-threatening ischemia.

disease due to generalized atherosclerosis in this patient population. It is important to remember that arteriography may be misleading in the *diagnosis* of popliteal aneurysms owing to the presence of intraluminal thrombus.

In a subset of patients experiencing symptoms of acute lower limb ischemia due to occlusion of a popliteal aneurysm there is a significant delay in complete thrombosis of the unclotted blood in the aneurysm. This phenomenon may result from atheroembolic occlusion of the tibial artery outflow from the aneurysm, with persistence of a small amount of antegrade flow through the aneurysm to small collateral channels. These patients manifest a bounding popliteal pulse on physical examination, and delayed arteriographic images reveal extremely slow contrast entrance into a patent aneurysm. One should not be dissuaded from the diagnosis of a popliteal aneurysm as the cause of acute leg ischemia solely on the basis of a persistently palpable popliteal pulse.

Indications for Operation

The treatment of popliteal aneurysms remains somewhat controversial. In this regard, disagreement centers around the appropriate indications for operation; whereas some authors advocate operative repair for all popliteal aneurysms, others recommend reserving the operation for selected patients. Two criteria have been employed to select patients for operative repair; the presence of symptoms and the size of the aneurysm.

It is generally agreed that all patients with symptomatic popliteal artery aneurysms should undergo operative repair because the incidence of limb loss increases with the onset of symptomatic disease.[21, 24, 29, 31] Szilagyi and colleagues advocated repair of all symptomatic aneurysms regardless of size because limb loss was significantly more likely once complications referable to the aneurysm developed.[25] Other authors have advocated repair of all popliteal aneurysms regardless of size and symptoms, citing the low operative risk of repair and the high incidence of limb loss associated with the onset of complications.

It has been stated that smaller popliteal artery aneurysms are more prone to thrombosis than larger aneurysms; there is a mean diameter of only 2.5 cm in collected series of thrombosed popliteal aneurysms. Wychulis and associates observed a 31 per cent complication rate in patients managed conservatively, including three amputations in this group.[31] In contrast, no patients who were asymptomatic at the time of operative repair experienced limb loss, even if

the repaired artery subsequently occluded. In an operative series of 51 popliteal aneurysms, we found that limb loss and mortality occurred only in patients presenting with limb-threatening ischemia. No patients undergoing elective repair experienced limb loss, even in the presence of subsequent graft occlusion. We concluded that operative repair is indicated for all patients with popliteal aneurysms, given the negligible incidence of complications with elective repair contrasted with the significant morbidity and mortality associated with repair of complicated aneurysms (Fig. 79–4). In a series of 71 popliteal aneurysms, Dawson and colleagues reported that 74 per cent of all popliteal aneurysms managed nonoperatively developed complications within 5 years.[8] Szilagyi and colleagues, however, reported a low complication rate with nonoperative observation of asymptomatic popliteal aneurysms of less than 2 cm in diameter.[25] Similarly, Shellack and associates reported a low incidence of complications in a series of 95 popliteal aneurysms in which 26 small asymptomatic aneurysms were managed nonoperatively.[23] Only two (8 per cent) of these patients developed complications from their aneurysms.

The available data, subject to the limitations of inadequate natural history data (in the modern era) and absence of a randomized trial, indicate that asymptomatic popliteal aneurysms should be managed aggressively, with consideration of operative therapy when the aneurysm diameter reaches 2 cm. As a cautionary note, the availability of autogenous conduit material must be considered in deciding on the appropriateness of operation for an asymptomatic popliteal aneurysm. In general, the results of infragenicular prosthetic reconstructions are dismal, and the risks of graft failure and subsequent limb loss may outweigh the risks associated with expectant management of asymptomatic popliteal aneurysms.

OPERATIVE TECHNIQUE

The technique employed to bypass a popliteal aneurysm is dictated by a number of factors, including the configuration of the aneurysm, the vessels available for inflow and outflow, the elimination of an embolic source, and the prevention of continued enlargement of the aneurysm after operation.

Fusiform aneurysms of the popliteal artery usually begin in the superficial femoral artery. Elective therapy for fusiform aneurysms is directed at the prevention of embolic and thrombotic ischemic complications; resection of the

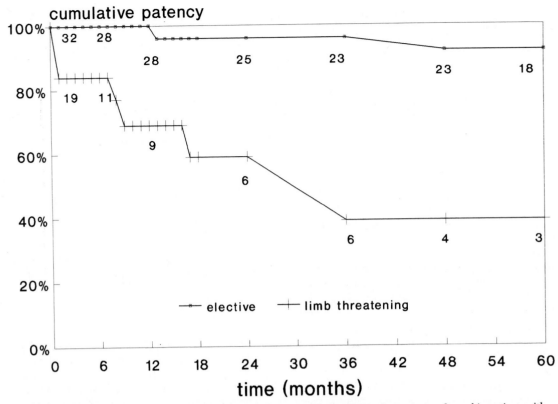

FIGURE 79–4. Life table analysis of the patency of lower extremity revascularization performed in patients with popliteal aneurysms; elective versus urgent (i.e., limb-threatening) procedures.

aneurysm is not necessary because the diameter is never great and symptoms of compression of surrounding structures or rupture are rare. The aims of operation are to bypass the aneurysmal process and to eliminate the risk of subsequent distal atheroembolization by excluding the potential embolic source. With the patient in the supine position, an autogenous vein bypass is constructed, originating from the common or superficial femoral artery proximal to the area of aneurysmal dilatation, terminating at the most distal popliteal artery where the vessel usually resumes a near normal diameter. Exclusion of the embolic source is accomplished with ligation of the native artery, either just beyond the proximal anastomosis or just proximal to the distal anastomosis (Fig. 79–5). We favor the former because it maximizes blood flow through the bypass graft (Fig. 79–5A).

Operative strategies for saccular popliteal aneurysms differ markedly from those of fusiform aneurysms, since the complications related to the compression of surrounding structures and thromboembolism must both be addressed. Proximal and distal aneurysm ligation does not eliminate the risk of subsequent aneurysm enlargement through collateral feeding vessels. Resection of the aneurysm and endoaneurysmorrhaphy are the two most effective means of preventing continued expansion.[24] Saccular popliteal aneurysms can be repaired using either a medial or posterior approach. Advantages of the medial approach include harvesting of the greater saphenous vein and exposure of the femoral vessels (if they are necessary for inflow) through

the same incision. However, excision of the aneurysm through the medial approach is arduous and may require division of the medial muscles and tendons of the knee. Using the posterior approach, resection of the aneurysm and endoaneurysmorrhaphy are easily accomplished, but proximal arterial exposure is difficult, and a separate incision is required to harvest the greater saphenous vein. Occasionally, the lesser saphenous vein may be of adequate caliber for use as a bypass graft, obviating the need for a second incision (Fig. 79–6).

There are two therapeutic choices for the acutely thrombosed popliteal aneurysm—operative revascularization and intra-arterial thrombolysis. If operative therapy is chosen, an inframalleolar bypass may be necessary because multiple atheroemboli may have rendered all three tibial arteries unusable. Recently, thrombolytic therapy has been utilized to reopen acutely occluded popliteal aneurysms. Thrombolysis of occluded popliteal aneurysms is problematic, however, because of the large amount of thrombus that may be present within the aneurysm cavity. Prolonged periods of thrombolytic infusion may be required for lysis, and the risk of secondary embolization with lysis is increased. Even if successful thrombolysis is achieved, distal nonlysable atheroemboli may prevent reperfusion of the foot. The poor results associated with any form of therapy for acutely thrombosed popliteal artery aneurysms reflect the severity of the problem and reemphasize the value of treating popliteal aneurysms at an early, asymptomatic stage (Table 79–2).

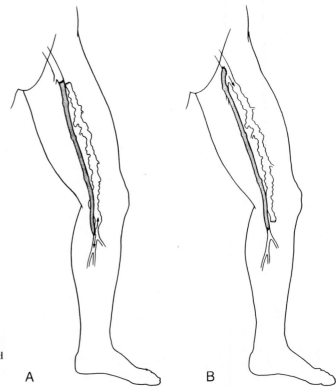

A

B

FIGURE 79–5. Technique of repair of a fusiform popliteal aneurysm. *A*, The aneurysm may be ligated proximally to maximize blood flow through the bypass graft. *B*, The aneurysm may be ligated distally, maintaining antegrade flow through the superficial femoral artery.

Table 79–2. Operative Results of Popliteal Aneurysm Repair

Author	No. Aneurysms	Cumulative Patency (10 yr)		Limb Salvage (10 yr)	
		Elective	*LTI*	*Elective*	*LTI*
Anton et al[3]	123	81%	48%	93%	79%
Dawson et al[8]	71	66%	60%	100%	60%
Shortell et al[24]	51	92%	39%	100%	84%

LTI, limb-threatening ischemia.

FIGURE 79–6. *A–C,* The posterior approach to resection of a saccular popliteal aneurysm, using an endoaneurysmorrhaphy technique and a vein bypass graft sewn from within the aneurysmal sac.

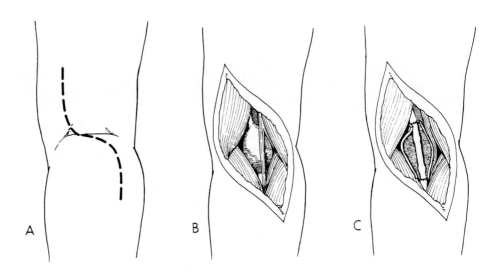

A

B

C

FEMORAL ARTERY ANEURYSMS

The femoral artery is the second most common site of peripheral aneurysm formation. The incidence of femoral artery aneurysms is rising, primarily because of an increase in the frequency of transfemoral arteriographic procedures and the associated sequelae of iatrogenic false aneurysm formation.[17] The complications of femoral artery aneurysms are identical to those of popliteal aneurysms and include embolism, thrombosis, and compression of surrounding structures. As with popliteal aneurysms, rupture is rare except for pseudoaneurysms. Atherosclerotic aneurysms are usually limited to the common femoral artery, with abrupt termination of the ectatic process at or immediately distal to the common femoral bifurcation. Diffuse aneurysmal change is common in the superficial femoral artery segment, and the process almost always continues to the popliteal level. We have grouped these superficial femoral aneurysms with the fusiform variety of popliteal aneurysms because of the similar scope of complications and treatment strategies. Unlike atherosclerotic femoral aneurysms, iatrogenic aneurysms frequently originate from the proximal profunda femoris or superficial femoral arteries because there appears to be an increased risk of false aneurysm formation when these vessels are inadvertently punctured.[16] Anastomotic aneurysms occur at the anastomotic site, usually over the common femoral artery. These aneurysms often extend proximal to the inguinal ligament, however, as the graft limb retracts into the retroperitoneum. Anastomotic aneurysms are discussed in detail in Chapter 83.

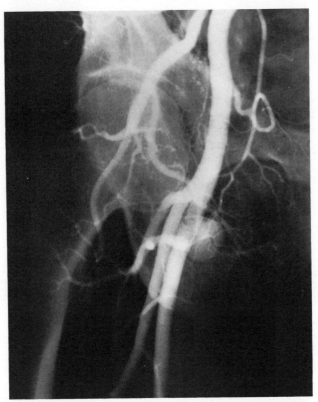

FIGURE 79–7. An arteriogram of an iatrogenic femoral false aneurysm that developed following coronary angioplasty through an inadvertent puncture of the superficial femoral artery. The lumen of the aneurysm was approximately 2.5 cm in diameter, whereas the external diameter of the sac was 4.0 cm in diameter, illustrating the exuberant pannus that forms on the aneurysm wall.

Classification

Femoral artery aneurysms may occur as a result of degenerative change, injury to the femoral vessels at the time of coronary or peripheral arteriographic procedures, or anastomotic disruption following bypass graft procedures. Infected aneurysms can occur at the femoral location and are observed most frequently in intravenous drug abusers. Amputation is necessary in up to one third of patients with infected femoral aneurysms, and the choice between ligation or reconstruction is controversial.[18, 20] Infected aneurysms are reviewed thoroughly in Chapter 82.

Degenerative (atherosclerotic) aneurysms are usually well localized to the common femoral artery; for unknown reasons aneurysmal change of the external iliac or profunda femoris artery is exceedingly rare.[27] Like their popliteal counterparts, atherosclerotic femoral aneurysms occur almost exclusively in men. Atherosclerotic femoral aneurysms are true aneurysms because the aneurysm wall contains all three layers of the normal arterial wall. The precise cause of atherosclerotic femoral aneurysms is unknown, but the observations that more than 50 per cent of femoral aneurysms are associated with aortic aneurysms, approximately 50 per cent are associated with popliteal aneurysms, and roughly 50 per cent are bilateral, suggest that a congenital or acquired defect in the structure of the arterial wall may be responsible (Table 79–3).[13, 26]

Iatrogenic pseudoaneurysms develop after percutaneous cannulation of the femoral vessels. An incidence of approximately one false aneurysm per 500 arteriograms has been reported.[22] These aneurysms consist of encapsulated outpouchings in communication with the arterial lumen through a relatively small defect (Fig. 79–7). The use of large-bore catheters increases the risk of femoral false aneurysm formation, as does the use of anticoagulant and throm-

Table 79–3. Associated Aneurysms in Patients With Femoral Aneurysms

Author	No. Patients	Aortic	Popliteal	Bilateral Femoral
Baird et al[4]	30	53%	17%	20%
Cutler and Darling[7]	45	51%	27%	40%
Graham et al[13]	100	85%	44%	72%
Tolstedt et al[28]	7	29%	29%	71%

bolytic agents, prolonged femoral cannulation, and unintentional cannulation of the profunda femoris or superficial femoral vessels.[16] The incidence of femoral false aneurysms is also increased in obese individuals in whom digital compression following removal of the arteriographic catheter is sometimes ineffective.

Anastomotic aneurysms of the femoral artery develop following infection of a bypass graft, fatigue of the graft or suture material, or disruption of the host arterial tissue (Fig. 79–8).[10] With improvements in the durability of vascular bypass graft and suture materials, host vessel wall deterioration has become the most frequent cause of anastomotic aneurysms.[2] Anastomotic aneurysms appear to occur more frequently following aortofemoral bypass procedures than infrainguinal procedures.[6] An infectious etiology is likely when the false aneurysm appears relatively soon after the primary revascularization procedure, and perioperative wound complications such as infection and lymph fistula predispose to the development of an anastomotic aneurysm. The most common offending organisms include *Staphylococcus aureus, Staphylococcus epidermidis,* and *Escherichia coli.*[26] By contrast, noninfectious femoral aneurysms characteristically appear long after the original procedure, developing in 2 to 3 per cent of aortofemoral anastomoses an average of 3 to 5 years after the primary revascularization procedure.[2, 10]

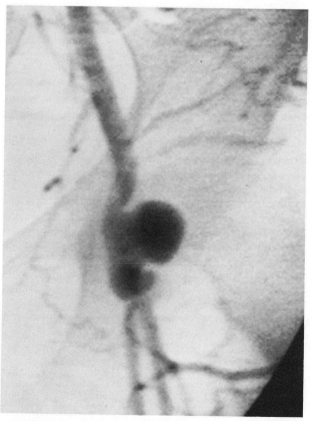

FIGURE 79–8. An arteriogram of an anastomotic femoral false aneurysm occurring several years after an aortobifemoral bypass with a woven Dacron prosthesis. The etiology of the process was degeneration of the host arterial tissue.

Clinical Manifestations

Patients with femoral artery aneurysms may present with symptoms of distal arterial ischemia, local compression of the femoral nerve or vein, and groin pain. Atherosclerotic aneurysms enlarge slowly over time, and the associated symptoms tend to be chronic, mild, and primarily related to the pressure associated with the gradual expansion of the mass. Encroachment on the femoral nerve is associated with nonspecific groin and anterior thigh pain, whereas femoral venous compression may produce unilateral leg edema secondary to venous hypertension. Arterial symptoms are common, with embolization to the small distal arterial branches of the leg. In this regard, atherosclerotic femoral aneurysms constitute one of the many causes of the "blue toe syndrome," whereby embolization of aneurysm thrombus or cholesterol debris lodges in the digital arteries, causing sudden onset of pain and discoloration of the affected toe. Occasionally, thrombosis of a femoral aneurysm produces acute limb ischemia that is frequently owing to the occlusion of arterial inflow to both the superficial femoral and profunda femoris vessels. Rupture of atherosclerotic femoral artery aneurysms is exceedingly uncommon, occurring in less than 5 per cent of patients.[13, 19]

Iatrogenic false aneurysms generally expand more rapidly than do femoral aneurysms of other causes. Symptoms may be acute, and early rupture of the aneurysm into the surrounding subcutaneous space is not infrequently observed. Iatrogenic aneurysms usually begin as large hematomas involving the subcutaneous space of the groin and anterior thigh. Pain is the most prominent symptom at this stage, and hemorrhage into the thigh, groin, and retroperitoneum can produce hypovolemic shock. A localized false aneurysm may become apparent with resolution of the acute hematoma, and physical examination may reveal a circumscribed pulsatile mass overlying the puncture site.

Anastomotic false aneurysms produce symptoms primarily related to discomfort resulting from compression of the femoral nerve and vein. These aneurysms may be classified into two varieties depending on whether the anastomosis is circumferentially disrupted or disrupted at a localized site along its length (Fig. 79–9). Complete circumferential disruption of an aortofemoral anastomosis results in retraction of the graft limb proximally, and the blood flow must traverse the aneurysm cavity to supply the leg. Localized disruption produces a situation analogous to that observed with iatrogenic false aneurysms, with an aneurysm cavity peripheral to the path of blood flow. The type of anastomotic false aneurysm has important clinical implications when spontaneous thrombosis occurs; thrombosis of circumferentially disrupted anastomoses results in devastating lower limb ischemia, whereas thrombosis of localized disruptions produces temporary or permanent resolution of the aneurysmal process without compromise of the arterial supply of the extremity.

Diagnosis

Femoral artery aneurysms are easily diagnosed on physical examination. The relatively superficial location of

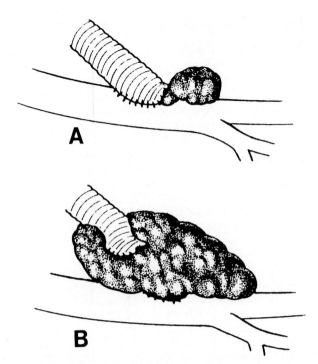

FIGURE 79–9.   Anastomotic femoral aneurysms may involve a segment of the anastomotic circumference or the complete circumference. *A,* Femoral anastomotic aneurysm developing as a result of dehiscence of the toe of the anastomosis. *B,* An anastomotic aneurysm with complete disruption of the anastomosis and retraction of the graft limb proximally.

the common femoral artery facilitates palpation of even mild degrees of dilatation. B-mode ultrasound is a rapid and inexpensive means of determining the size and extent of the aneurysm and provides an efficient means of screening for the presence of associated aneurysms in other locations. Arteriography is useful for precise localization of the femoral artery defect in iatrogenic false aneurysms and for defining the extent of coexisting occlusive disease. Arteriography is also important in delineating the anatomy of anastomotic false aneurysms, especially with respect to the degree of anastomotic disruption and the anatomic relationship between the site of the defect and the common femoral bifurcation. As with aneurysms at any location, the presence of intraluminal thrombus renders measurements of arteriographic diameter inaccurate.

Indications for Operation

Symptoms resulting from femoral artery aneurysms generally herald the development of the major limb-threatening and life-threatening complications of thromboembolism and rupture. Thus, all symptomatic femoral aneurysms should be repaired. By contrast, the appropriate treatment of asymptomatic femoral aneurysms is more controversial and can only be defined in the context of the natural history of the specific variety of aneurysm. The study of Graham and colleagues contained a subset of 105 femoral aneurysms that were initially followed conservatively.[13] The observation that only three of these aneurysms were the source of later limb-threatening complications justifies non-

operative management of small asymptomatic femoral aneurysms. With the exception of the 1961 study of Tolstedt and associates,[28] in which major amputation was required in five of seven initially asymptomatic femoral aneurysms, most series corroborate the findings of Graham and colleagues and recommend conservative management (Table 79–4).[1, 7, 14]

Iatrogenic false aneurysms occurring after arteriography have traditionally been treated by early operative intervention. Recently, Doppler ultrasonography has provided an objective method of following iatrogenic aneurysms. Several small series have documented spontaneous thrombosis and resolution of surprisingly large aneurysms, and the expectant management of asymptomatic iatrogenic aneurysms has not been associated with adverse clinical sequelae.[15, 17] The findings must be considered preliminary at present, however.

The natural history of femoral anastomotic false aneurysms is that of progressive enlargement with development of sudden limb-threatening complications in 20 per cent of patients.[6] Small anastomotic aneurysms less than 2 cm in diameter can be followed nonoperatively with a low frequency of complications.[10] Larger aneurysms are more prone to the complications of rupture and thrombosis, however, suggesting that operative intervention is indicated when the diameter of a femoral anastomotic aneurysm exceeds 2 cm (see Chapter 83).

Operative Technique

The operative strategies used in femoral aneurysm resection vary depending on the type of aneurysm. Isolated atherosclerotic femoral aneurysms are best approached through a standard groin incision. Proximal arterial control is achieved at the level of the inguinal ligament, although a separate retroperitoneal "transplant" incision may be appropriate to facilitate control of the external iliac artery with very large aneurysms. Control of the superficial femoral artery is achieved next, and gentle medial retraction of the superficial femoral and proximal common femoral arteries permit exposure and control of the profunda femoris artery. Balloon catheters have been utilized to control the outflow vessels from within the aneurysmal sac; however, early branching of the profunda femoris artery frequently renders balloon occlusion of backbleeding inadequate. Once the major inflow and outflow vessels have been controlled, the patient is given heparin, and vascular clamps are applied. The aneurysm may be resected, if small, taking care not to injure an adherent femoral vein. A Dacron or polytetrafluoroethylene graft approximating the normal arterial diame-

Table 79–4.   Follow-up of Asymptomatic Femoral Artery Aneurysms

Author	Aneurysms	Follow-up	Complications
Adiseshiah and Bailey[1]	19	48 months	0
Hands and Collin[14]	4	24 months	0
Graham et al[13]	105	28 months	3%
Tolsted et al[28]	7	—	71%

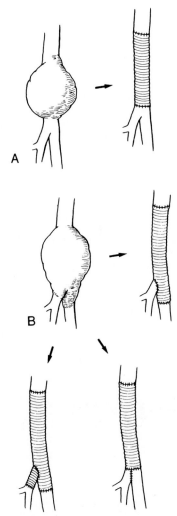

FIGURE 79–10. *A,* Resection and reconstruction of an aneurysm localized to the common femoral artery, using a Dacron interposition tube graft between the proximal and the distal portions of the common femoral artery. *B,* Resection of a femoral aneurysm that involves the most proximal portions of the deep and superficial femoral arteries. The profunda femoris artery may be reimplanted onto the body of the graft when the length of the aneurysmal profunda femoris artery is short, so that the nondilated portion of the vessel reaches to the graft. A separate limb of graft may be necessary to bridge the juncture between the main graft and the profunda femoris artery in some cases, or the orifices of the superficial femoral and profunda femoris vessels may be sewn together to form a common lumen. The distal anastomosis may then be constructed to this orifice.

ter (usually 8 mm) is placed using end-to-end anastomoses both proximally and distally. Saphenous vein may be used if it is of adequate caliber. If the aneurysm is large it may be left in place and the graft sewn from within the aneurysmal cavity in a manner similar to the technique employed for repair of aortic aneurysms. The aneurysmal sac is then reapproximated over the graft. Extension of the aneurysmal process to the proximal profunda femoris or superficial femoral vessels requires an innovative approach, including reanastomosis of the two vessels to one another to form a common lumen, reimplantation of the profunda femoris artery onto the side of the graft or the native superficial femoral artery, or utilization of a prosthetic graft side limb

between the main graft and the profunda femoris vessel (Fig. 79–10).

The repair of iatrogenic femoral aneurysms is usually less complex than the repair of other femoral aneurysms because the arterial defect is usually small and localized. It is safest to obtain control of the common, superficial, and deep femoral vessels prior to entering the false aneurysmal sac, although some surgeons prefer to open the aneurysm directly and to control bleeding digitally from the defect during suture placement. The femoral arterial hole is generally small, and one or two sutures are usually sufficient to achieve closure.

Anastomotic aneurysms represent a technical challenge for the surgeon. The reoperative situation renders dissection tedious, and the quality of the remaining femoral arterial wall may render construction of the new anastomosis technically demanding. Several caveats are important in the repair of anastomotic aneurysms. First, proximal and distal control is of critical importance because premature entry into the false aneurysmal sac may result in massive hemorrhage. Second, unless the aneurysm arose as a result of suture failure, one cannot hope merely to close a small defect in the original anastomotic line. The original site of anastomosis demonstrated its propensity for disruption, and a new, more distal site should be chosen. Finally, extension of the graft limb to a more distal location usually requires the interposition of a new graft segment to provide adequate length without imposing undue tension at the anastomosis.[10] This may necessitate separate anastomoses to the profunda femoris and superficial femoral arteries if an adequate sewing ring cannot be found at or proximal to the common femoral bifurcation.

References

1. Adiseshiah M, Bailey DA: Aneurysms of the femoral artery. Br J Surg 64:174, 1977.
2. Agrifoglio G, Costantini A, Lorenzi G, et al: Femoral noninfected anastomotic aneurysms. A report of 56 cases. J Cardiovasc Surg 31:453, 1990.
3. Anton GE, Hertzer NR, Beven EG, et al: Surgical management of popliteal aneurysms: Trends in presentation, treatment, and results from 1952–1984. J Vasc Surg 3:125, 1986.
4. Baird RJ, Gurry JF, Kellam J, et al: Arteriosclerotic femoral artery aneurysms. Can Med Assoc J 117:1306, 1977.
5. Baird RJ, Sivasankar R, Hayward R, et al: Popliteal aneurysms: A review and analysis of 61 cases. Surgery 59:911, 1966.
6. Clarke AM, Poskitt KR, Baird RN, et al: Anastomotic aneurysms of the femoral artery: Aetiology and treatment. Br J Surg 76:1014, 1989.
7. Cutler BS, Darling RC: Surgical management of arteriosclerotic femoral aneurysms. Arch Surg 74:764, 1973.
8. Dawson I, van Bockel JH, Brand R, et al: Popliteal artery aneurysms. Long-term follow-up of aneurysmal disease and results of surgical treatment. J Vasc Surg 13:398, 1991.
9. Dent TL, Lindenauer SM, Ernst CB, et al: Multiple arteriosclerotic arterial aneurysms. Arch Surg 105:338, 1972.
10. Ernst CB, Elliott JP Jr, Ryan CJ, et al: Recurrent femoral anastomotic aneurysms. A 30-year experience. Ann Surg 208:401, 1988.
11. Evans WE, Conley JE, Bernhard V: Popliteal aneurysms. Surgery 70:762, 1971.
12. Gifford RW Jr, Hines EA Jr, Janes JM: An analysis and follow-up study of one hundred popliteal aneurysms. Surgery 33:284, 1953.
13. Graham LM, Zelenock GB, Whitehouse WM Jr, et al: Clinical significance of arteriosclerotic femoral artery aneurysms. Arch Surg 115:502, 1980.
14. Hands LJ, Collin J: Infra-inguinal aneurysms: Outcome for patient and limb. Br J Surg 78:996, 1991.

15. Johns JP, Pupa LE Jr, Bailey SR: Spontaneous thrombosis of iatrogenic femoral artery pseudoaneurysms: Documentation with color Doppler and two-dimensional ultrasonography. J Vasc Surg 14:24, 1991.
16. Kim D, Orron DE, Skillman JJ, et al: Role of superficial femoral artery puncture in the development of pseudoaneurysm and arteriovenous fistula complicating percutaneous transfemoral cardiac catheterization. Cath Cardiovasc Diagn 25:91, 1992.
17. Oweida SW, Roubin GS, Smith RB, et al: Postcatheterization vascular complications associated with percutaneous transluminal coronary angioplasty. J Vasc Surg 12:310, 1990.
18. Padberg F Jr, Hobson R, Lee B, et al: Femoral pseudoaneurysm from drugs of abuse: Ligation or reconstruction? J Vasc Surg 15:642, 1992.
19. Pappas G, Janes JM, Bernatz PE, et al: Femoral aneurysms: Review of surgical management. JAMA 190:489, 1964.
20. Patel KR, Semel L, Clauss RH: Routine revascularization with resection of infection femoral pseudoaneurysms from substance abuse. J Vasc Surg 8:321, 1988.
21. Reilly MK, Abbott WM, Darling RC: Aggressive surgical management of popliteal aneurysms. Am J Surg 145:498, 1983.
22. Roberts SR, Main D, Pinkerton J: Surgical therapy of femoral artery pseudoaneurysm after angiography. Am J Surg 154:676, 1987.
23. Shellack J, Smith RB III, Perdue GD: Nonoperative management of selected popliteal aneurysms. Arch Surg 122:372, 1987.
24. Shortell CK, DeWeese JA, Ouriel K, et al: Popliteal artery aneurysms: A 25-year surgical experience. J Vasc Surg 14:771, 1991.
25. Szilagyi DE, Schwartz RL, Reddy DJ: Popliteal arterial aneurysms. Arch Surg 116:724, 1981.
26. Szilagyi DE, Smith RF, Elliott JP, et al: Infection in arterial reconstruction with synthetic grafts. Ann Surg 176:321, 1972.
27. Tait WF, Vohra RK, Carr HM, et al: True profunda femoris aneurysms: Are they more dangerous than other atherosclerotic aneurysms of the femoropopliteal segment? Ann Vasc Surg 5:92, 1991.
28. Tolstedt GE, Radke HM, Bell JW: Late sequela of arteriosclerotic femoral aneurysms. Angiology 12:601, 1961.
29. Vermillion BD, Dimmins SA, Pace WG, et al: A review of one hundred forty-seven popliteal aneurysms with long-term follow-up. Surgery 90:1009, 1981.
30. Whitehouse WM Jr, Wakefield TW, Graham LM, et al: Limb-threatening potential of arteriosclerotic popliteal artery aneurysms. Surgery 93:694, 1982.
31. Wychulis AR, Spittell JA Jr, Wallace RB: Popliteal aneurysms. Surgery 68:942, 1970.

80

Upper Extremity Aneurysms

G. Patrick Clagett, M.D.

· · ·

Upper extremity aneurysms are relatively rare in comparison with other peripheral arterial aneurysms.[18] However, their recognition and treatment are important because these aneurysms can cause major disability, lead to limb and digit loss, and, in the case of proximal aneurysms of the subclavian artery, result in death from rupture and exsanguination. In addition to rupture, proximal aneurysms are complicated by thromboembolism with ischemic upper extremity signs and symptoms (including gangrene), neuromuscular and sensory dysfunction from brachial plexus compression, and central neurologic deficits due to retrograde thromboembolism in the vertebral and right carotid circulations. In contrast, more distally located upper extremity aneurysms are almost exclusively manifested by thromboembolic complications of the hand and digits. Because of the relative rarity of upper extremity aneurysms, the natural history and the overall incidence of associated complications are unknown. However, in reviewing the reported cases in the literature, one is impressed by the serious morbidity encountered with the first manifestations of these aneurysms. Because of this, optimal surgical treatment should be carried out early, preferably before symptoms arise.

SUBCLAVIAN ARTERY ANEURYSM

Subclavian artery aneurysms arise from degenerative disease (e.g., atherosclerosis), thoracic outlet obstruction, or trauma. Aneurysms involving the proximal subclavian artery are usually caused by atherosclerosis,[39] and, less commonly, syphilis,[11] cystic medionecrosis,[65] invasion of the wall by contiguous tuberculous lymphadenitis,[35] and idiopathic congenital causes.[4, 19] In contrast, aneurysms of the distal subclavian artery, frequently with extension into the first portion of the axillary artery, are appropriately considered aneurysms of the subclavian-axillary arteries and are most commonly associated with a cervical rib or fibrous bands producing thoracic outlet syndrome.[63]

Aneurysms involving the proximal and mid-subclavian artery are most commonly atherosclerotic in etiology.[38] Thirty to 50 per cent of patients with atherosclerotic subclavian aneurysms have aortoiliac or other peripheral aneurysms.[59, 63] Therefore, patients presenting with subclavian aneurysms should be thoroughly evaluated for associated aneurysms.

Presenting symptoms of subclavian aneurysms include chest, neck, and shoulder pain from acute expansion or rupture; upper extremity acute and chronic ischemic symptoms from thromboembolism; upper extremity pain and neurologic dysfunction from brachial plexus compression; hoarseness from compression of the right recurrent laryngeal nerve; respiratory insufficiency from tracheal compression; transient ischemic attacks and stroke from retrograde thromboembolism in the vertebral and right carotid circulations; and, rarely, hemoptysis from erosion into the apex of the lung. Patients without symptoms may note the presence of a supraclavicular pulsatile mass. Most frequently, asymptomatic pulsatile masses in this area represent tortuous common carotid and subclavian arteries. These can usually be distinguished from true aneurysms by ultrasonography; however, on occasion arteriography is necessary (Fig. 80–1). In addition to a supraclavicular mass, physical signs may include a supraclavicular bruit; absent or diminished pulses in the upper extremity; normal pulses with signs of microembolization (blue finger syndrome); sensory and motor signs of brachial plexus compression; vocal cord paralysis; and Horner's syndrome due to compression of the stellate ganglion and other contributions to the cervical sympathetic chain at the base of the neck.[80]

Plain films of the chest may reveal a superior mediastinal mass that can be confused with a neoplasm. Ultrasonography or computed tomography will establish the diagnosis. Complete arch and upper extremity angiography is mandatory to delineate the extent of the aneurysm, to assess the sites of vascular occlusion in cases complicated by thromboembolism, and to note the competency of the contralateral vertebral circulation if the ipsilateral vertebral artery originates from an aneurysmal vessel. These points are crucial in planning appropriate surgical reconstruction.

The first attempted surgical correction of a proximal subclavian artery aneurysm was performed in 1818 by Valentine Mott of New York, who ligated the innominate artery.[11] The first successful treatment of a subclavian artery aneurysm was achieved in 1864 by Smyth of New Orleans, who ligated the right common carotid as well as the innominate artery.[11] Unfortunately, the aneurysm recurred and ruptured 10 years later. Halsted was the first to combine ligation successfully with resection of a subclavian artery aneurysm in 1892 at the Johns Hopkins Hospital.[33] In 1913, Matas reported 225 cases of treatment of aneurysms by endoaneurysmorrhaphy, and seven of these were subclavian aneurysms.[62]

Contemporary surgical repair of proximal and midsubclavian artery aneurysms involves resection and reestablishment of arterial continuity with an end-to-end anastomosis (for very small aneurysms) or, more commonly, an interposition arterial prosthesis. Although proximal and distal ligation of subclavian aneurysms has occasionally been successful in the past, ligation without reconstruction should generally not be performed because ischemic symptoms develop in 25 per cent of cases so treated.[63] For proximal right subclavian aneurysms, median sternotomy with extension into the supraclavicular fossa is usually necessary to gain adequate exposure for proximal control.[59] In cases of proximal left subclavian aneurysms, a left thoracotomy may be necessary. Extra-anatomic reconstruction combined with proximal and distal aneurysm ligation has also been described in unusual circumstances.[22] For aneurysms involving the mid and distal subclavian artery, a supraclavicular incision often gives adequate exposure and may be complemented by an infraclavicular incision for distal control. Division or resection of the mid-portion of the clavicle may be necessary to gain additional exposure,[38] and if so, the clavicle may be reconstructed at the completion of the operation. If the aneurysm involves the origin of the vertebral artery, reconstruction by reimplantation or other means is appropriate, particularly if the contralateral vertebral artery is hypoplastic or diseased.

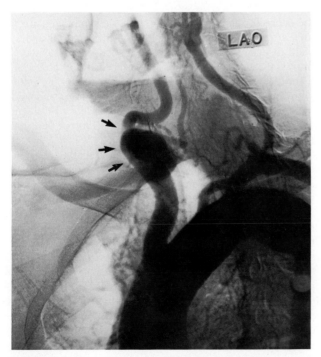

FIGURE 80–1. The confluence of elongated and tortuous innominate, subclavian, and common carotid arteries gives rise to a pulsatile mass in the right supraclavicular fossa and base of neck *(arrows)*. This common condition is harmless but is frequently confused on physical examination with a subclavian or common carotid aneurysm. Ultrasonography can usually differentiate between these; however, arteriography is sometimes required.

Subclavian-Axillary Artery Aneurysm: Post-Stenotic Dilatation From Cervical Rib

Although the first case of upper extremity ischemic complications associated with a cervical rib was reported by Hodgson in 1815,[40] it is not clear that the presence of an underlying subclavian-axillary artery aneurysm was recognized. Mayo, in 1813, described a subclavian aneurysm in association with thoracic outlet syndrome caused by exostosis of the first rib.[56] A cervical rib causing compression of the subclavian artery with resulting ischemia of the arm was reported in 1861 by Coote, who successfully performed the first decompressive operation by removing the cervical rib.[17] Halsted, in 1916, reported 27 cases of cervical rib in association with subclavian artery aneurysm and, based on experimental observation in dogs, hypothesized the rheologic mechanisms leading to post-stenotic dilatation and aneurysm formation.[34] The demonstration of thromboembolic complications emanating from cervical rib compression of the subclavian artery was made by Symonds in 1927, who reported two cases of contralateral hemiplegia from retrograde embolization in the carotid territory.[79] In 1934, Lewis and Pickering described the much more frequent occurrence of upper extremity thromboembolic complications.[47] The first case of arterial reconstruction for treatment of the thromboembolic complications from cervical rib was described by Schein and colleagues in 1956, who replaced the subclavian artery with a homograft.[70]

Aneurysms of the distal subclavian artery and proximal axillary artery are almost always associated with cervical ribs.[38, 73] Rarely, anomalous first ribs, nonunion of the clavicle, and other anatomic abnormalities of the thoracic outlet have been associated with subclavian-axillary aneurysms (see Chapter 70).[25, 45, 85] Although cervical ribs are estimated to occur in 0.6 per cent of the population,[2] most are asymptomatic, and arterial lesions are uncommon. In reviewing 716 patients with cervical ribs, Halsted found 27 cases (3.8 per cent) of associated subclavian aneurysms.[34] Six of these patients (0.8 per cent) suffered from gangrene of the fingers. Since cervical ribs are bilateral in 50 to 80 per cent of individuals with this anomaly,[2, 72] subclavian-axillary aneurysms in association with cervical ribs may also be bilateral.[75] Women may be more prone to develop arterial complications from cervical ribs (Fig. 80–2); in reviewing the literature, one is impressed with the overwhelming female predominance among reported cases. This may be because cervical ribs are more common in women.[2] The right-sided predominance of arterial complications is also evident, perhaps because more frequent muscular activity with the dominant upper extremity leads to earlier and more pronounced changes in the artery on that side.

Cervical ribs may compress the subclavian artery at the point where the vessel crosses the first rib (Fig. 80–3). This is most often the case with complete cervical ribs that join the first rib lateral to the subclavian artery.[45] In this region, the anterior end of the rib may unite with the first rib by a fibrous band, a diarthrodial joint, or a synostosis.[71] The resulting upward, medial, and anterior displacement of the subclavian artery against the tendinous portion of the scalenus anterior muscle causes stenosis of the vessel by extrinsic compression and angulation. Post-stenotic dilatation leads to aneurysmal changes, which begin in the distal subclavian artery and extend into the proximal axillary artery. Intraluminal thrombus, engendered by aneurysm formation and intimal damage, may become dislodged and embolize distally (Fig. 80–4). In some cases, the aneurysm may completely thrombose, and retrograde propagation may result in emboli in the vertebral circulation and, on the right side, in the common carotid artery (Fig. 80–5).[12, 26] Central neurologic sequelae can result from vertebral or carotid artery involvement.

Patients with subclavian-axillary aneurysms associated with cervical ribs may present with acute or chronic symptoms of upper extremity ischemia. On occasion, Raynaud's phenomenon may occur. If the cervical rib causes significant compression of the brachial plexus, neurologic symptoms typical of thoracic outlet obstruction predominate. On physical examination, the cervical rib may be palpated in

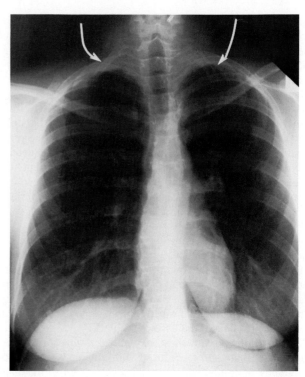

FIGURE 80–2. Bilateral, complete cervical ribs in a young female (arrows). Only the right cervical rib was associated with arterial dilatation and complications (complete thrombosis of the subclavian artery, as seen in the arteriogram of this patient shown in Figure 80–5).

the supraclavicular fossa along with the prominent subclavian artery pulsation that results from the anterior and upward displacement of this vessel. A loud, harsh subclavian bruit is usually present unless the artery is thrombosed, and a thrill is common. Patients with cervical ribs presenting with any ischemic symptoms need expeditious and complete upper extremity angiography. The urgency of diagnosis is mandated by the imminent threat of limb or digit loss, a point emphasized by most authors.[7, 10, 20, 42, 52, 54]

Surgical treatment of subclavian-axillary aneurysms associated with cervical ribs depends upon the size of the aneurysm, the symptomatic status of the patient, and the presence and extent of thromboembolic complications.[72] In asymptomatic individuals who are found to have a cervical rib with a prominent supraclavicular pulse and bruit, arteriography is recommended to assess the degree of post-stenotic dilatation of the subclavian artery (Fig. 80–6). Ultrasonography may also allow partial visualization of this portion of the subclavian artery and has been used to document dilatation.[45] If significant dilatation is present and the patient is an acceptable surgical risk, thoracic outlet decompression with cervical rib removal is indicated. In this early stage, relief of compression by removal of the rib may result in return to normal arterial caliber.[72]

Although it is unknown how many patients at this asymptomatic stage will go on to develop complications if untreated, the natural history of the disorder appears to be progressive with the eventual development of thromboembolic complications. Because the first manifestations may be limb or digit threatening, an aggressive approach is war-

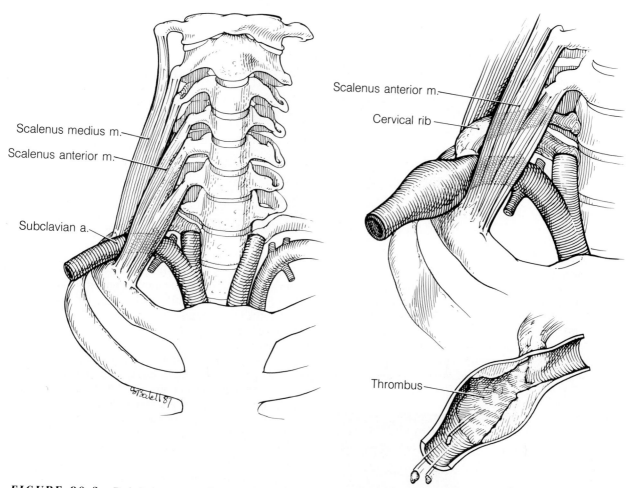

FIGURE 80–3. Pathologic anatomy of a cervical rib giving rise to subclavian-axillary aneurysm with mural thrombus and distal embolization.

FIGURE 80–4. There is embolic occlusion *(single arrow)* of the distal axillary and brachial arteries just proximal to the origin of the profunda brachial artery. The source of the embolus was an unimpressive-appearing subclavian-axillary aneurysm *(arrows)* associated with a cervical rib. The operative specimen of this resected artery is shown in Figure 80–7, which reveals the mural thrombus.

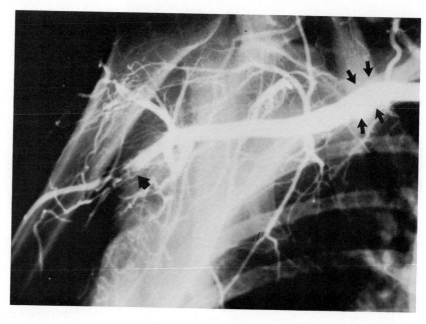

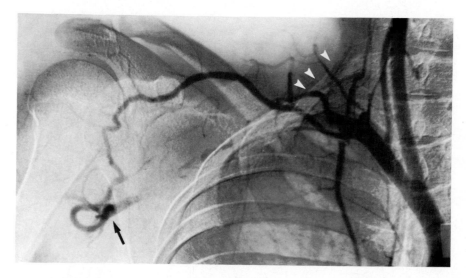

FIGURE 80–5. Arteriogram of the patient whose chest film is shown in Figure 80–2. There is complete occlusion of the subclavian artery with filling of the distal axillary artery *(arrow)* via the suprascapular branch of the subclavian artery to the circumflex scapular branch of the subscapular artery collateral pathway. The cervical rib is outlined by the *arrowheads*. Continued retrograde thrombosis of the subclavian artery would render the right vertebral and common carotid arteries susceptible to thromboembolism.

ranted. In asymptomatic individuals with more extensive aneurysmal change (greater than two times the normal vessel diameter), resection of the subclavian aneurysm in addition to cervical rib removal should be considered. Scher and associates observed that these aneurysms frequently contain thrombus, even in asymptomatic patients, and it is unlikely that regression to normal size will occur because of irreversible wall changes.[73] Operative inspection of the vessel to assess its size accurately and, in selected cases, its luminal aspect to look for mural irregularity and thrombus may be useful in determining the need for resection.[42, 45] Preoperatively, computed tomography (CT) or magnetic resonance imaging (MRI) may be useful to demonstrate intraluminal thrombus.

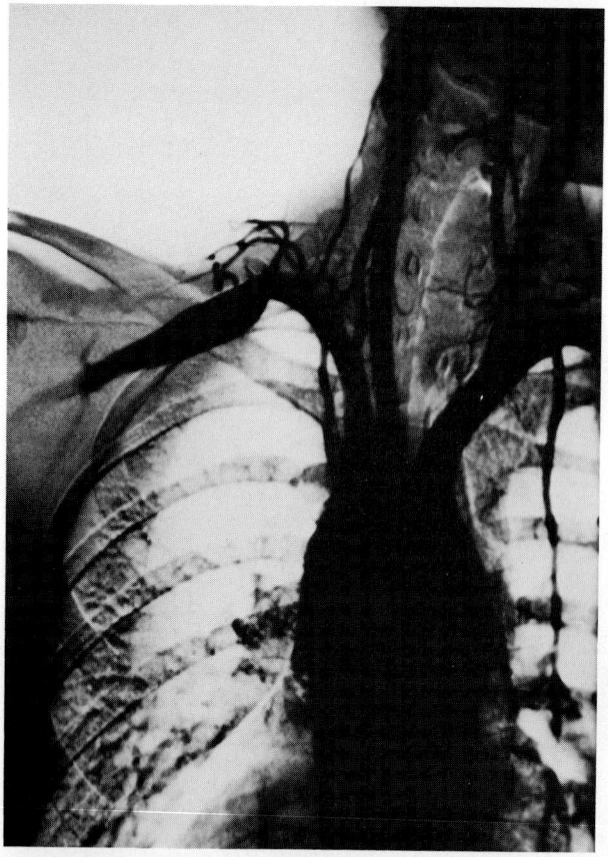

In patients with thromboembolic complications associated with a cervical rib, the distal subclavian artery should be resected regardless of the size of the aneurysm. The extent of intimal damage and thrombus present in the aneurysm is frequently underestimated by angiography (see Fig. 80–4); invariably, mural thrombus is found in the aneurysm, usually along the inferior wall (Fig. 80–7). In rare cases, vascular reconstruction can be accomplished by proximal and distal mobilization of the ends of the vessel and end-to-end anastomosis. However, most cases require a short interposition vein or prosthetic graft. To best accomplish this, supraclavicular and infraclavicular incisions are used to mobilize the distal subclavian and proximal axillary arteries, respectively.[73] Resection of the clavicle is unnecessary. The cervical rib is resected through the supraclavicular incision by standard techniques.[71] Key points in effectively relieving arterial compression include complete resection of bony, cartilaginous, and fibrous parts of the anterior portion of the cervical rib where it attaches or articulates with the first rib and complete resection of the scalenus anterior muscle at the scalene tubercle on the first rib. Resection of most of the posterior portion of the cervical rib should also be performed so that it is free of the brachial plexus, which is usually draped over the rib. Surprisingly, most patients with arterial complications of cervical ribs do not have neurologic symptoms of the thoracic outlet syndrome, and complete resection of the cervical rib along with arterial reconstruction is all that is required.[72] Although concomitant first rib resection has been advocated in the past by either the transaxillary or the supraclavicular approach,[45] this should rarely be necessary. Adequate decompression of the artery and the brachial plexus can almost always be accomplished by near-complete resection of the cervical rib and scalenus anterior muscle.

Balloon catheter thromboembolectomy is necessary to restore patency to recently occluded distal vessels critical

FIGURE 80–6. Large, asymptomatic subclavian-axillary aneurysm with a cervical rib in a young woman in whom a pulsatile right supraclavicular mass was found incidentally on physical examination. A harsh bruit and thrill were also present.

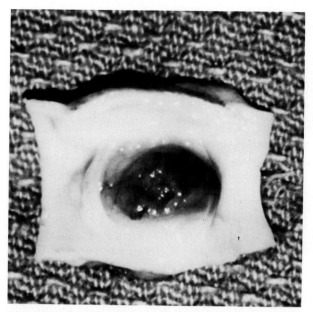

FIGURE 80–7. Mural thrombus within a minimally dilated segment of the subclavian artery distal to the cervical rib in a patient who presented with upper extremity rest pain and digital tip necrosis. The arteriogram of this patient is shown in Figure 80–4.

to limb viability. This may require separate exposure of the brachial and forearm arteries to effect complete thrombectomy. Unfortunately, many of these patients have suffered chronic repetitive embolic episodes, and the occluding thrombi may be partially organized and impossible to extract. In such cases, vein graft bypasses to arm and forearm arteries may be necessary to relieve critical ischemia and to promote healing of digital tip gangrene and ischemic ulcerations. Because of the inferior patency of prosthetic bypasses in this region, vein grafts are required for optimal results.[58] Adjunctive cervicodorsal sympathectomy has been advocated in the past, but most experts feel that this is unnecessary and that the emphasis should be placed on adequate arterial reconstruction.[45, 73] Sympathectomy might be considered in selected patients in whom vasospastic symptoms are prominent and complete restoration of pulsatile flow at the level of the hand is not possible.

Aneurysm of Aberrant Subclavian Artery: Kommerell's Diverticulum

An aberrant right subclavian artery arising from the proximal portion of the descending thoracic aorta is the most common congenital anomaly of the aortic arch.[6] Most patients with this anomaly are asymptomatic and the aberrant subclavian artery is of no clinical consequence. Rarely, the vessel compresses the esophagus against the posterior trachea and gives rise to difficulty in swallowing, a condition termed *dysphagia lusoria*.[81] Even more rarely, atherosclerotic aneurysmal change occurs in the anomalous vessel. This condition has been termed Kommerell's diverticulum after Kommerell, who in 1936 described a diverticulum of the aorta at the origin of the anomalous subclavian artery.[6] McCallen and Schaff first called attention to the

clinical significance of aneurysmal change in an anomalous right subclavian artery in a report in 1956,[57] and since then 32 cases have been reported.

Patients with aneurysm of an aberrant right subclavian artery may present with dysphagia from esophageal compression, dyspnea and coughing from tracheal compression, chest pain from expansion or rupture, or symptoms of right upper extremity ischemia due to thromboembolism. Death from rupture has been reported and appears to be unrelated to the size of the aneurysm.[6] Many reported cases were in asymptomatic patients whose aneurysm was found on chest radiography and interpreted as a superior mediastinal mass. Chest CT can diagnose this condition noninvasively, but angiography is necessary to plan surgical treatment. Approximately one fifth of reported patients with this anomaly have an associated abdominal aortic aneurysm.[6]

Because of the propensity of these aneurysms to cause symptoms and because of the possibility of lethal rupture, resection of the aneurysmal vessel with vascular reconstruction of the subclavian artery is recommended. This may be accomplished via a right or left posterolateral thoracotomy[6, 14] or median sternotomy.[6, 41] The subclavian artery is reconstructed by an interposition arterial prosthesis anastomosed proximally to the ascending arch of the aorta. Alternatively, a left posterolateral thoracotomy for proximal resection of the aneurysm coupled with a right supraclavicular incision for reconstruction of the subclavian artery by end-to-side anastomosis to the right common carotid artery has been described.[78] A staged approach with right carotid–subclavian bypass or transposition (end-subclavian to side-carotid) preceding left thoracotomy and aneurysm resection with oversewing of the origin from the aortic arch is attractive because the risk of cerebral and right upper extremity embolization is minimized.[86] Extra-anatomic reconstruction of the right subclavian artery has also been described.[23] Because it is necessary to resect the aneurysmal vessel near its origin from the aorta, the modified extrathoracic approach recently described for treatment of dysphagia lusoria would not be effective.[81]

AXILLARY ARTERY ANEURYSMS

With the exception of rare congenital causes,[4, 64] axillary aneurysms are caused by blunt or penetrating trauma (Fig. 80–8).[37] Crutch-induced blunt trauma producing aneurysmal dilatation of the axillary artery was first described by Rob in 1956[67] with subsequent cases reported by Brooks[13] and Abbott.[1] Pathologic examination of these aneurysms reveals markedly thickened walls and wrinkled, roughened intima. Instead of the typical intimal changes of atherosclerosis, there is severe fragmentation of medial elastic fibers and marked periadventitial fibrosis suggesting chronic trauma.[1] Thrombus, usually loosely adherent to the damaged intima, may become dislodged by further trauma from crutches and is the source of acute, chronic, or repetitive emboli. In many cases, the aneurysm thromboses completely when symptoms begin. The most common presenting complaints relate to upper extremity ischemia, and suspicion should be aroused when a patient who has been using crutches for a prolonged period presents with an absent brachial pulse.[1]

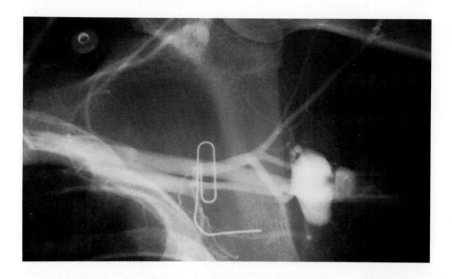

FIGURE 80–8.   False aneurysm of the axillary artery as a result of a stab injury.

False aneurysms of the axillary artery usually occur with penetrating trauma but may also occur with blunt trauma in the form of humeral fractures and anterior dislocation of the shoulder.[28, 51, 77] In the latter instance, the mechanism may be avulsion of the tethered thoracoacromial, subscapular, or circumflex humeral vessels at the time of dislocation. These aneurysms often present late as chronic false aneurysms because diagnosis is often delayed. This is especially true after blunt trauma, when lack of recognition is fostered by the difficulty of obtaining an adequate examination of the axillary artery because of the surrounding bone and muscles of the shoulder and the considerable pain and muscle spasm that prevent arm abduction to allow examination of the axilla.[28] Furthermore, because of the excellent collateral circulation in this area, distal perfusion may be adequate despite extensive axillary artery injury. However, these aneurysms can lead to serious and permanent neurologic disability because of hemorrhage into the axillary sheath and compression of the brachial plexus. Because of these considerations, arteriography should be obtained in all cases of significant penetrating trauma to the shoulder or arm, blunt trauma with abnormal pulse examination, and blunt trauma with normal pulse examination but brachial plexus palsy (the likelihood of concomitant vascular injury is great in these cases). Also, arteriography should be obtained in patients with blunt trauma to the shoulder or axilla with a normal neurovascular examination initially, but with signs of brachial plexus neuropathy on follow-up. The presence of an expanding chronic false aneurysm should be suspected in such cases.[28]

Surgical treatment of axillary aneurysms is straightforward and involves resection of the aneurysm and interposition vein graft. One must be careful to protect the brachial plexus and its major branches during dissection of the aneurysm. Prosthetic reconstruction of the axillary artery has been successful, but because of the superior patency of vein

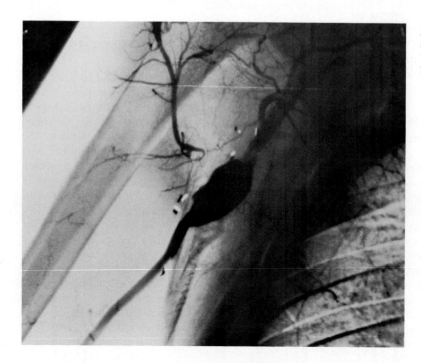

FIGURE 80–9.   Aneurysmal dilatation of an interposition brachial vein graft used to reconstruct the axillary artery at the time of penetrating trauma 4 years previously.

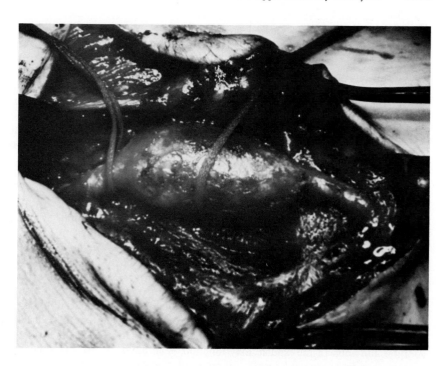

FIGURE 80–10. Operative dissection of the aneurysmal interposition brachial vein graft shown in Figure 80–9.

grafts in upper extremity reconstructions,[58] these are preferred. On occasion, an adjacent segment of the axillary or brachial vein has been used to reconstruct the artery (Fig. 80–9). However, this vein is extremely thin-walled and may itself become aneurysmal with time (Figs. 80–10 and 80–11). A segment of saphenous vein is the conduit of choice.

ULNAR ARTERY ANEURYSM: THE HYPOTHENAR HAMMER SYNDROME

Although rare, ulnar artery aneurysms are one of the most common causes of ischemia limited solely to the digits.[74] It is important to recognize this disorder because is-

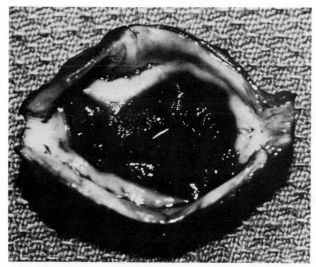

FIGURE 80–11. Mural thrombus lining the aneurysmal interposition brachial vein graft shown in Figures 80–9 and 80–10.

chemia arising from these aneurysms is frequently correctable and if untreated may lead to digital necrosis and severe disability. Diagnosis and treatment is all the more urgent when one considers that most individuals with the hypothenar hammer syndrome are middle-aged working men whose livelihood depends upon using their dominant hand, which is invariably involved. The first reported case occurred in a Roman coachman and was described by Guattani in 1772;[32] Middleton, in 1933, reported 16 cases,[60] Smith, in 1962, described 35 cases,[76] and Pineda and colleagues, in 1985, reviewed 53 cases.[66] All authors have identified trauma to the hand as the cause of this disorder and, in 1970, Conn and associates coined the term "hypothenar hammer syndrome."[16]

The syndrome develops in people who use the palms of their hands for pushing, pounding, or twisting. The practice of repeatedly striking with the dominant hand is common in many industries; the hypothenar hammer syndrome has been most often described in mechanics, automobile repairmen, lathe operators, pipe fitters, tire braiders, carpenters, and machinists. The disorder has also been described in individuals with hobbies (sculpting) and athletic pursuits (volleyball, skiing, and karate) that involve repetitive trauma to the hand.[3, 5, 8, 27, 29, 36, 49] The incidence is probably much higher than one would suspect from the number of patients reported in the literature (less than 150 cases). Little and Ferguson used noninvasive means to screen a population at risk.[48] Among 79 automobile repairmen who habitually used their hands as a hammer, 11 (14 per cent) showed some evidence of digital ischemia and were deemed to have the hypothenar hammer syndrome. Duration of employment was positively correlated with the syndrome, and there was no evidence of the syndrome in workers who did not use their hands as hammers. Many authors have stressed the importance of accuracy of diagnosis and its relationship to work activities because of insurance and workmen's compensation considerations.[16, 24, 48]

The pathophysiology is based on the unique vascular anatomy of the hand (Fig. 80–12).[76] The ulnar artery and nerve enter the hand by traversing Guyon's canal, bounded medially (ulnarly) by the pisiform bone, dorsally by the transverse carpal ligament, and superficially by the volar carpal ligament. Within this tunnel, the artery and the nerve each bifurcate into deep and superficial branches. The deep branch of the artery along with the motor branch of the ulnar nerve penetrate the hypothenar muscle mass where the artery becomes the deep palmar arch. The superficial division of the ulnar artery remains superficial to the hypothenar musculature and penetrates the palmar aponeurosis to form the superficial palmar arch, the main blood supply to the fingers via the common palmar digital arteries. Over this short distance of approximately 2 cm between the distal margin of Guyon's canal and the palmar aponeurosis, the artery lies just anterior to the hook of the hamate bone and is covered only by the slight palmaris brevis muscle, overlying skin, and subcutaneous tissue. With little protection above and the bony floor below, the artery is vulnerable to trauma. Fixation of the artery by the course of its deep branch allows little movement to escape blunt forces. In addition, the hook of the hamate may function as an anvil, accentuating the untoward results of repeated trauma. It should be noted that similar vulnerable conditions exist for a short segment of the superficial branch of the radial artery at the base of the thenar eminence, a much less frequent site of vessel trauma.[76] In an extensive study of arterial patterns of the hand, Coleman and Anson found that in 78 per cent of dissections, the superficial palmar arch was complete.[15] In approximately three quarters of these, the ulnar artery was the dominant component. In 22 per cent of dissections the arch was incomplete and there were diverse contributions to digital blood supply from the radial, ulnar, and, rarely, a persistent median artery. These anatomic variations are responsible for the diverse distribution of digital ischemic signs and symptoms in patients with the hypothenar hammer syndrome.

Trauma to the ulnar artery in this vulnerable area causes mural degeneration.[82] Damage to the intima alone results in thrombosis, whereas injury of the media leads to a true arterial aneurysm. Thrombosis of the ulnar artery or aneurysm is associated with downstream embolization. Pathologic studies of ulnar artery aneurysms have documented organizing thrombus adherent to the intimal surface and absence or severe fragmentation of the internal elastic lamina.[84] Fibrosis and focal intramural hemorrhage are also present, along with variable amounts of acute and chronic inflammation.[66] Although most authors have described true aneurysms with no loss in continuity of the arterial wall, some have reported false aneurysms of the ulnar artery, usually in association with penetrating trauma.[31, 69, 83]

Although the syndrome most often follows chronic, repetitive trauma, it may result from a single, acute episode.[66] The syndrome usually has a slow, insidious onset. At the time of injury, many patients report episodes of severe lacerating pain over the hypothenar eminence. Typically, dull aching pain and tenderness are present over the hypothenar area following these episodes, and ischemic symptoms develop weeks or months later. A variety of ischemic signs and symptoms may be present and often include pain, cold sensation, paresthesias, cyanosis, and mottling of the digits. The fourth and fifth fingers are most frequently symptomatic, but any digit or any combination of digits may be involved with the exception of the thumb, which is invariably spared because of its radial blood sup-

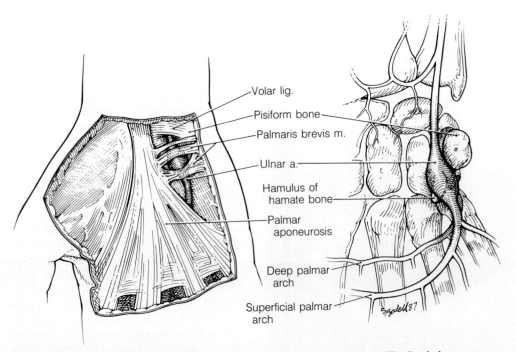

FIGURE 80–12. Pathologic anatomy of the hypothenar hammer syndrome. The distal ulnar artery is particularly vulnerable to external trauma in the 2-cm distance between its exit point from Guyon's canal (the roof of which is the volar carpal ligament) and the point where the artery dives under the tough palmar aponeurosis. In this short distance, the ulnar artery courses on top of the hook of the hamate bone and is covered incompletely by the thin palmaris brevis muscle and skin and subcutaneous tissue.

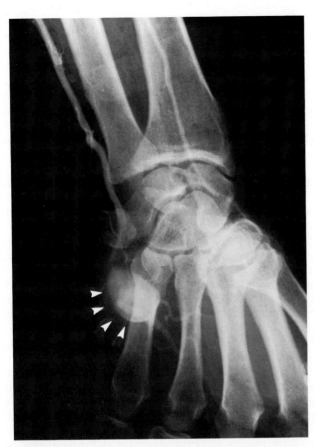

FIGURE 80–13. Large distal ulnar artery aneurysm *(arrowheads)* in a middle-aged man who frequently used his hand as a hammer in his work as an automobile repairman.

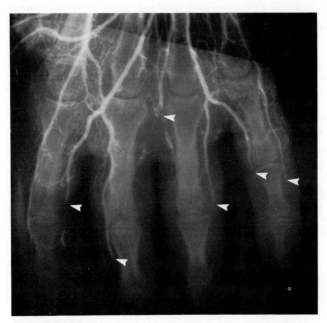

FIGURE 80–14. Delayed magnification views of the hand following papaverine injection, demonstrating multiple embolic occlusions *(arrowheads)* of the digital arteries in the patient whose initial arteriogram in Figure 80–15 showed only occlusion of the ulnar artery.

ply. Raynaud's phenomenon may be the chief presenting symptom and is distinguished from typical Raynaud's phenomenon in that it is unilateral, the thumb is not involved, and there is an absence of the classic triphasic color changes[66] because reactive hyperemia would not be expected to occur in the presence of fixed arterial obstruction.

On physical examination, in addition to the ischemic changes of the fingers, localized tenderness over the hypothenar eminence may be present with a pulsatile or nonpulsatile mass. A hypothenar callus may also be present. Atrophy and softening of the distal finger pads, ischemic fingertip ulcers, and subungual hemorrhages are sometimes evident. An abnormal Allen's test suggests occlusion or incomplete development of the superficial palmar arch or the distal ulnar artery and is present in the majority of patients with the hypothenar hammer syndrome.[66] Some patients may have an ulnar sensory deficit due to compression by the aneurysm of the superficial ulnar sensory branch.[43]

Noninvasive studies helpful in diagnosing the syndrome include digital plethysmography and Doppler flow studies. However, angiography is mandatory in patients suspected of having this disorder, and the angiographic features are virtually pathognomonic (Fig. 80–13).[9, 21, 50] These include irregularity, aneurysmal change, or occlusion

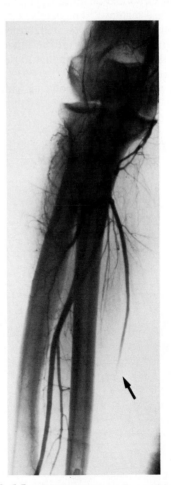

FIGURE 80–15. Initial arteriogram in a patient presenting with signs of small vessel embolism in the digits ("blue finger" syndrome). The arteriogram shows ulnar artery occlusion *(arrow).*

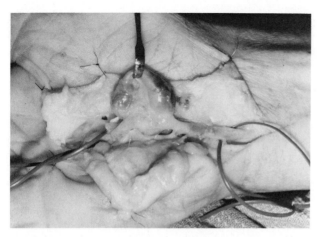

FIGURE 80–16. Operative exposure of an embolizing ulnar artery aneurysm in the right hand treated with resection and vein graft replacement.

of the ulnar artery segment overlying the hook of the hamate bone with occasional extension of these changes into the superficial palmar arch, embolic occlusion of the proper digital arteries in the distribution of the ulnar artery, and normal proximal and contralateral arteries (Fig. 80–14). Magnification views and pharmacoangiography are helpful in defining these features.[50] Frequently, distal ulnar artery occlusion is the only finding on initial arteriography (Fig. 80–15). Proximal angiography of the innominate, subclavian, and axillary arteries is important to rule out potential embolic sources.

Surgical therapy for the hypothenar hammer syndrome has included cervicodorsal sympathectomy, excision of the ulnar artery aneurysm with ligation of the ulnar artery, and aneurysmectomy with microsurgical reconstruction of the ulnar artery by reanastomosis or interposition vein graft (Fig. 80–16).[66] Although it is not clear which of these approaches is superior, most authors recommend microsurgical vascular reconstruction because it eliminates the thromboembolic source, removes the painful aneurysmal mass that may cause ulnar nerve compression, adds the vasodilatory benefits of a local periarterial sympathectomy, and improves digital perfusion.[30, 53, 55, 61, 74, 82] Resection of the aneurysm and placement of a vein interposition graft is the optimal treatment for either a patent ulnar aneurysm with clinical or radiographic evidence of distal embolization or a thrombosed ulnar aneurysm that has resulted in profound digital ischemia. Patients with minimal symptoms and no threat of digit loss after ulnar aneurysm thrombosis may not require revascularization.[87–89] Recently, adjunctive preoperative thrombolytic therapy has been reported with excellent results (Fig. 80–17).[44, 46] The principal benefit of thrombolytic therapy is the restoration of patency to digital arteries, thus reducing adverse sequelae and improving distal runoff, theoretically enhancing patency of the reconstruction. Because dextran 40 has been shown to improve patency of lower extremity complex reconstructions of small, distal arteries,[68] perioperative treatment with this agent is recommended. In patients in whom the ulnar artery and superficial palmar arch are chronically thrombosed and thrombolytic therapy is unsuccessful in restoring flow, medical therapy with calcium channel blockers may be helpful if vasospastic symptoms are prominent.[66] All patients with this disorder should be counseled to stop smoking and to avoid further hand trauma.

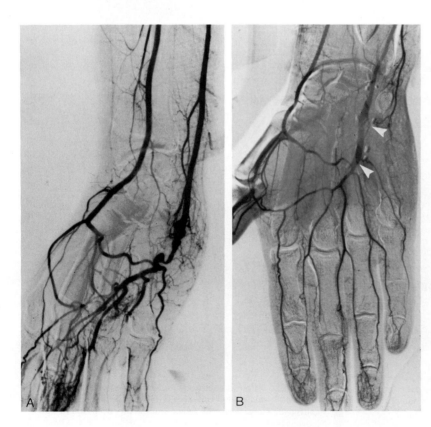

FIGURE 80–17. *A*, Urokinase was infused regionally for 24 hours in the patient whose initial arteriograms are shown in Figures 80–14 and 80–15. Near-complete lysis of thromboemboli restored patency to the distal ulnar artery, the superficial palmar arch, and some of the common digital arteries, in addition to demonstrating the underlying ulnar artery aneurysm. *B*, Repeat arteriogram in the same patient following microvascular resection of the ulnar artery aneurysm and reconstruction with an interposition vein graft *(arrowheads)* harvested from the forearm. Note restoration of complete circulation to the digits, all digital arteries being cleared of thrombus by the adjunctive preoperative use of regional urokinase infusion.

References

1. Abbott WM, Darling RC: Axillary artery aneurysms secondary to crutch trauma. Am J Surg 125:515, 1973.
2. Adson AW: Cervical ribs: symptoms, differential diagnosis and indications for section of the insertion of the scalenus anticus muscle. J Int Coll Surg 16:546, 1951.
3. Annetts DL, Graham AR: Traumatic aneurysm of the palmar arch: lemon squeezer's hand. Aust NZ J Surg 52:584, 1982.
4. Applebaum RE, Caniano DA, Sun C-C, et al: Synchronous left subclavian and axillary artery aneurysms associated with melorheostosis. Surgery 99:249, 1986.
5. Aulicino PL, Hutton PMJ, Du Puy TE: True palmar aneurysms—a case report and literature review. J Hand Surg 7:613, 1982.
6. Austin EH, Wolfe WG: Aneurysm of aberrant subclavian artery with a review of the literature. J Vasc Surg 2:571, 1985.
7. Banis JC, Rich N, Whelan TJ Jr: Ischemia of the upper extremity due to noncardiac emboli. Am J Surg 134:131, 1977.
8. Bayle E, Tran K, Benslamia H, et al: Ulnar artery aneurysm of the hand. Int Surg 68:215, 1983.
9. Benedict KT, Chang W, McCready FJ: The hypothenar hammer syndrome. Radiology 111:57, 1974.
10. Bertelsen S, Mathiesen RR, Ohlenschlaeger HH: Vascular complications of cervical rib. Scand J Thor Cardiovasc Surg 2:133, 1968.
11. Bjork VO: Aneurysm and occlusion of the right subclavian artery. Acta Chir Scand (Suppl) 356:103, 1965.
12. Blank RH, Connar RG: Arterial complications associated with thoracic outlet compression syndrome. Ann Thorac Surg 17:315, 1974.
13. Brooks A, Fowler B: Axillary artery thrombosis after prolonged use of crutches. J Bone Joint Surg 46-A:863, 1964.
14. Campbell CF: Repair of an aneurysm of an aberrant retroesophageal right subclavian artery arising from Kommerell's diverticulum. J Thorac Cardiovasc Surg 62:330, 1971.
15. Coleman SS, Anson BJ: Arterial patterns in the hand based upon a study of 650 specimens. Surg Gynecol Obstet 113:409, 1961.
16. Conn J Jr, Bergan JJ, Bell JL: Hypothenar hammer syndrome: posttraumatic digital ischemia. Surgery 68:1122, 1970.
17. Coote H: Pressure on the axillary vessels and nerve by an exostosis from a cervical rib. Interference with the circulation of the arm. Removal of the rib in exostosis. Recovery. Med Times Gaz 2:108, 1861.
18. Dent TL, Ernst CB: Multiple arteriosclerotic arterial aneurysms. Arch Surg 105:338, 1972.
19. Dobbins WO: Bilateral calcified subclavian arterial aneurysms in a young adult male. N Engl J Med 265:537, 1961.
20. Dorazio RA, Ezzet F: Arterial complications of the thoracic outlet syndrome. Am J Surg 138:246, 1979.
21. Dubois P, Stephen D: Angiographic findings in the hypothenar hammer syndrome. Aust Radiol 19:370, 1975.
22. Elefteriades JA, Kay HA, Stansel HC Jr, et al: Extraanatomical reconstruction for bilateral intrathoracic subclavian artery aneurysms. Ann Thorac Surg 35:188, 1983.
23. Esquivel CO, Miller GE Jr: Aneurysm of anomalous right subclavian artery. Contemp Surg 24:81, 1984.
24. Ettien JT, Allen JT, Vargas C: Hypothenar hammer syndrome. South Med J 74:491, 1981.
25. Fidler MW, Helal B, Barwegen GMH, et al: Subclavian artery aneurysm due to costoclavicular compression. J Hand Surg 9B:282, 1984.
26. Fields WS, Lemak NA, Ben-Menachem Y: Thoracic outlet syndrome: review and reference to stroke in a major league pitcher. AJR 146:809, 1986.
27. Foster DR, Cameron DC: Hypothenar hammer syndrome. Br J Radiol 54:995, 1981.
28. Gallen J, Wiss DA, Cantelmo N, et al: Traumatic pseudoaneurysm of the axillary artery: report of three cases and literature review. J Trauma 24:350, 1984.
29. Gaylis H, Kushlick AR: The hypothenar hammer syndrome. S Afr Med J 50:125, 1976.
30. Given KS, Puckett CL, Kleinert HE: Ulnar artery thrombosis. Plast Reconstr Surg 61:405, 1978.
31. Green DP: True and false traumatic aneurysms in the hand. J Bone Joint Surg 55-A:120, 1973.
32. Guattani C: De externis aneurysmaibus, manu chirurgica methodice perctrandis. Rome, 1771. Translated by Erischsen JE: London Sydenham Society 1844:268.
33. Halsted WS: Ligation of the first portion of the left subclavian artery and excision of a subclavio-axillary aneurysm. Johns Hopkins Hosp Bull 24:93, 1892.
34. Halsted WS: An experimental study of circumscribed dilation of an artery immediately distal to a partially occluding band, and its bearing on the dilation of the subclavian artery observed in certain cases of cervical rib. J Exp Med 24:271, 1916.
35. Hara M, Bransford RM: Aneurysm of the subclavian artery associated with contiguous pulmonary tuberculosis. J Thorac Cardiovasc Surg 46:256, 1963.
36. Ho PK, Dellon AL, Wilgis EFS: True aneurysms of the hand resulting from athletic injury. Report of two cases. Am J Sports Med 13:136, 1985.
37. Ho PK, Weiland AJ, McClinton MA, et al: Aneurysms of the upper extremity. J Hand Surg 12A:39, 1987.
38. Hobson RW II, Israel MR, Lynch TG: Axillosubclavian arterial aneurysms. *In* Bergen JJ, Yao JST (eds): Aneurysms—Diagnosis and Treatment. New York, Grune & Stratton, 1982, p 435.
39. Hobson RW II, Sarkaria J, O'Donnell JA, et al: Atherosclerotic aneurysms of the subclavian artery. Surgery 85:368, 1979.
40. Hodgson: Diseases of the Arteries and Veins. London, 1815, p 262.
41. Hunter JA, Dye WS, Najafi H, et al: Arteriosclerotic aneurysm of anomalous right subclavian artery. J Thorac Cardiovasc Surg 59:755, 1970.
42. Judy KL, Heymann RL: Vascular complications of thoracic outlet syndrome. Am J Surg 123:521, 1972.
43. Kalisman M, Laborde K, Wolff TW: Ulnar nerve compression secondary to ulnar artery false aneurysm at the Guyon's canal. J Hand Surg 7:137, 1982.
44. Kartchner MM, Wilcox WC: Thrombolysis of palmar and digital arterial thrombosis by intra-arterial thrombolysin. J Hand Surg 1:67, 1976.
45. Kieffer E: Arterial complications of thoracic outlet syndrome. In Bergan JJ, Yao JST (eds): Evaluation and Treatment of Upper and Lower Extremity Circulatory Disorders. Orlando, Grune & Stratton, 1984, p 249.
46. Lawhorne TW Jr, Sanders RA: Ulnar artery aneurysm complicated by distal embolization: management with regional thrombolysis and resection. J Vasc Surg 3:663, 1986.
47. Lewis T, Pickering GW: Observations upon maladies in which the blood supply to digits ceases intermittently or permanently, and upon bilateral gangrene of digits: Observations relevant to so-called "Raynaud's disease." Clin Sci 1:327, 1934.
48. Little JM, Ferguson DA: The incidence of the hypothenar hammer syndrome. Arch Surg 105:684, 1972.
49. Little JM, Grant AF: Hypothenar hammer syndrome. Med J Aust 1:49, 1972.
50. Maiman MH, Bookstein JJ, Bernstein EF: Digital ischemia: angiographic differentiation of embolism from primary arterial disease. AJR 137:1183, 1981.
51. Majeed L: Pulsatile haemarthrosis of the shoulder joint associated with false aneurysm of the axillary artery as a late complication of anterior dislocation of the shoulder. Injury 16:566, 1985.
52. Martin J, Gaspard DJ, Johnston PW, et al: Vascular manifestations of the thoracic outlet syndrome: A surgical urgency. Arch Surg 111:779, 1976.
53. Martin RD, Manktelow RT: Management of ulnar artery aneurysm in the hand: a case report. Can J Surg 25:97, 1982.
54. Mathes SJ, Salam AA: Subclavian artery aneurysm; sequela of thoracic outlet syndrome. Surgery 76:506, 1974.
55. May JW Jr, Grossman JAI, Costas B: Cyanotic painful index and long fingers associated with an asymptomatic ulnar artery aneurysm: case report. J Hand Surg 7:622, 1982.
56. Mayo H: Exostosis of the first rib with strong pulsations of the subclavian artery. Lon Med Phys J (NS) 11:40, 1831.
57. McCallen AM, Schaff B: Aneurysm of an anomalous right subclavian artery. Radiol 66:561, 1956.
58. McCarthy WJ, Flinn WR, Yao JST, et al: Result of bypass grafting for upper limb ischemia. J Vasc Surg 3:741, 1986.
59. McCollum CH, Da Gama AD, Noon GP, et al: Aneurysm of the subclavian artery. J Cardiovasc Surg 20:159, 1979.
60. Middleton DS: Occupational aneurysm of the palmar arteries. Br J Surg 21:215, 1933.
61. Millender LH, Nalebuff EA, Kasdon E: Aneurysms and thromboses of the ulnar artery in the hand. Arch Surg 105:686, 1972.
62. Muller GP: Subclavian aneurysm with report of a case. Ann Surg 101:568, 1935.

63. Pairolero PC, Walls JT, Payne WS, et al: Subclavian-axillary artery aneurysms. Surgery 90:757, 1981.

64. Perry SP, Massey CW: Bilateral aneurysms of the subclavian and axillary arteries. Radiology 61:53, 1953.

65. Persaud V: Subclavian artery aneurysm and idiopathic cystic medionecrosis. Brit Heart J 30:436, 1968.

66. Pineda CJ, Weisman MH, Bookstein JJ, et al: Hypothenar hammer syndrome. Form of reversible Raynaud's phenomenon. Am J Med 79:561, 1985.

67. Rob CG, Standeven A: Closed traumatic lesions of the axillary and brachial arteries. Lancet 1:597, 1956.

68. Rutherford RB, Jones DN, Bergentz S-E, et al: The efficacy of dextran 40 in preventing early postoperative thrombosis following difficult lower extremity bypass. J Vasc Surg 1:765, 1984.

69. Sanchez A, Archer S, Levine NS, et al: Traumatic aneurysm of a common digital artery—a case report. J Hand Surg 7:619, 1982.

70. Schein CJ, Haimovici H, Young H: Arterial thrombosis associated with cervical ribs. Surgical considerations. Surgery 40:428, 1956.

71. Schein CJ: A technic for cervical rib resection. Am J Surg 121:623, 1971.

72. Scher LA, Veith FJ, Haimovici H, et al: Staging of arterial complications of cervical rib: guidelines for surgical management. Surgery 95:644, 1984.

73. Scher LA, Veith FJ, Samson RH, et al: Vascular complications of thoracic outlet syndrome. Vasc Surg 3:565, 1986.

74. Silcott GR, Polich VL: Palmar arch arterial reconstruction for the salvage of ischemic fingers. Am J Surg 142:219, 1981.

75. Siu K, Ferguson I: Bilateral cervical rib and subclavian aneurysm. Aust NZ J Surg 42:245, 1973.

76. Smith JW: True aneurysms of traumatic origin in the palm. Am J Surg 104:7, 1962.

77. Stein E: Case report 374. Skeletal Radiol 15:391, 1986.

78. Stoney WS, Alford WC Jr, Burrus GR, et al: Aberrant right subclavian artery aneurysm. Ann Thorac Surg 19:460, 1975.

79. Symonds CP: Two cases of thrombosis of subclavian artery, with contralateral hemiplegia of sudden onset, probably embolic. Brain 50:259, 1927.

80. Temple LJ: Aneurysm of the first part of the left subclavian artery. A review of the literature and a case history. J Thorac Surg 19:412, 1950.

81. Valentine RJ, Carter DJ, Clagett GP: A modified extrathoracic approach to the treatment of dysphagia lusoria. J Vasc Surg 5:498, 1987.

82. Vayssairat M, Debure C, Cormier J-M, et al: Hypothenar hammer syndrome: seventeen cases with long-term follow-up. J Vasc Surg 5:838, 1987.

83. Walsh MJ, Conolly WB: False aneurysms due to trauma to the hand. Hand 14:177, 1982.

84. Von Kuster L, Abt AB: Traumatic aneurysms of the ulnar artery. Arch Pathol Lab Med 104:75, 1980.

85. Whelan TJ Jr: Management of vascular disease of the upper extremity. Surg Clin North Am 62:373, 1982.

86. Esposito RA, Khalil I, Galloway AC, et al: Surgical treatment for aneurysm of aberrant subclavian artery based on a case report and a review of the literature. J Thorac Cardiovasc Surg 95:888, 1988.

87. Mehlhoff TL, Wood MB: Ulnar artery thrombosis and the role of interposition vein grafting: patency with microsurgical technique. J Hand Surg 16A:274, 1991.

88. Nehler MR, Dalman RL, Harris EJ, et al: Upper extremity arterial bypass distal to the wrist. J Vasc Surg 16:633, 1992.

89. Rothkopf DM, Bryan DJ, Cuadros CL, et al: Surgical management of ulnar artery aneurysms. J Hand Surg 15A:891, 1990.

81

Splanchnic Artery Aneurysms

James C. Stanley, M.D., and Gerald B. Zelenock, M.D.

• • •

Aneurysms of splanchnic arteries represent an uncommon but important vascular disease. Nearly 22 per cent of all reported splanchnic artery aneurysms present as clinical emergencies, including 8.5 per cent that result in death.[78] The pathogenesis and natural history of these aneurysms have been reassessed, and in most instances redefined, within the past three decades.

More than 3000 splanchnic artery aneurysms have been documented in the literature. The increasing discovery of these lesions, particularly during arteriographic study, supports the contention that they are more common than previously claimed. Distribution of aneurysms among splanchnic arteries (Fig. 81–1) has varied little from that noted in earlier reviews.[15, 41, 83] Vessels affected, in descending order of involvement, include the splenic (60 per cent), hepatic (20 per cent), superior mesenteric (5.5 per cent), celiac (4 per cent), gastric and gastroepiploic (4 per cent), intestinal (jejunal, ileal, colic; 3 per cent), pancreaticoduodenal and pancreatic (2 per cent), gastroduodenal (1.5 per cent), and inferior mesenteric arteries (rare). Cumulative experience with some aneurysms is so meager that discussion of them is anecdotal. In other instances, evidence is sufficient to develop a rational basis for treatment. Specific biologic differences between individual aneurysms make it imperative to comment on them separately rather than collectively.

SPLENIC ARTERY ANEURYSMS

The most common abdominal visceral vessel affected by aneurysmal disease is the splenic artery. Aneurysms of this vessel make up 60 per cent of all splanchnic artery aneurysms. More than 1800 patients with splenic artery aneurysms have been described in previous publications, yet very few clinical series of more than 20 patients from a

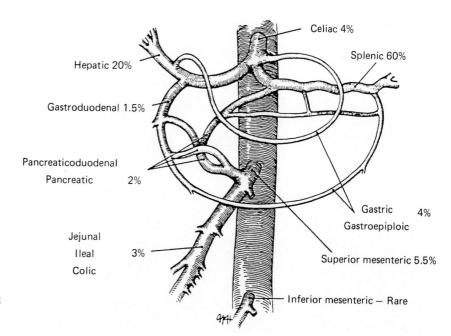

FIGURE 81–1. Relative incidence of aneurysms described in the literature affecting the visceral arteries of the splanchnic circulation.

single institution exist in the English literature.[57, 81, 85] The incidence of these lesions remains ill-defined,[44] ranging from 0.098 per cent among nearly 195,000 necropsies[56] to 10.4 per cent in a careful autopsy study of the splenic vessels in elderly patients.[7] Incidental demonstration of splenic aneurysms in 0.78 per cent of nearly 3600 abdominal arteriographic studies at the authors' institution may be a relatively accurate approximation of the actual frequency of these lesions in the general population.[81] Macroaneurysms of the splenic artery usually are saccular. These lesions occur most often at bifurcations of the distal vessel and are multiple in approximately 20 per cent of patients.

In sharp contrast to degenerative aneurysms in the abdominal aorta and lower extremity, splenic artery aneurysms exhibit an unusual sex predilection with a female-to-male ratio of 4 : 1. This fact and the propensity for aneurysm development in the splenic artery rather than in other splanchnic vessels has been attributed to acquired derangements of the vessel wall, including elastic fiber fragmentation, loss of smooth muscle, and internal elastic lamina disruption. Three distinct phenomena seemingly influence the evolution of these changes. First is the presence of systemic arterial fibrodysplasia. The recognized disruption of arterial wall architecture by medial dysplastic processes[82] is a logical forerunner of aneurysms, and in fact patients with medial fibrodysplasia exhibit splenic artery aneurysms with a frequency six times greater than that seen in the normal population.[81]

Portal hypertension with splenomegaly is a second disorder of alleged importance in the development of splenic artery aneurysmal disease.[8, 19, 52, 72, 81] Splenic artery aneurysms have been encountered in nearly 10 per cent of patients with portal hypertension and splenomegaly.[66, 79] In a recent survey, 30 per cent of 181 splenic artery aneurysms reported in Japan occurred in patients with portal hypertension and splenomegaly.[21] In these instances, aneurysms may be sequelae of the apparent hyperkinetic process that causes increased splenic artery diameters in portal hyperten-

sion.[52, 58] Whatever process underlies dilation of the artery, a similar process at vessel bifurcations would increase the likelihood of aneurysm formation. In this regard, aneurysm size in patients with portal hypertension has been directly correlated with splenic artery diameter.[66] These aneurysms are recognized often in patients undergoing orthotopic liver transplantation.[2]

The vascular effects of repeated pregnancy are a third factor relevant to evolution of splenic artery aneurysms.[15, 81, 85] Forty per cent of female patients described in a large series from our institution, with no obvious cause of their aneurysms, had completed six or more pregnancies.[81] The importance of pregnancy in the genesis of these lesions receives further support from the fact that 45 per cent of female patients with splenic artery aneurysms reported in the English-language literature from 1960 to 1970 in whom parity was stated were grand multi-paras.[83] Gestational alterations in the vessel wall due to hormonal and local hemodynamic events may have a causal relation to medial defects and aneurysmal formation. Such effects may be similar to those underlying the vascular complications of pregnancy associated with Marfan's syndrome. The predilection for aneurysms to occur in the splenic artery instead of in other similar-sized muscular vessels may reflect increased splenic arteriovenous shunting during pregnancy with excessive blood flow, or it may represent preexisting structural abnormalities inherent to this particular vessel.

Certain splenic artery aneurysms appear to have developed as a consequence of arteriosclerotic weakening of the vessel wall.[62] However, frequent localization of calcific arteriosclerotic changes to aneurysms, without involvement of the adjacent artery (Fig. 81–2), supports the contention that arteriosclerosis often is a secondary process rather than a primary etiologic event. Calcific arteriosclerotic changes in some but not all aneurysms where multiple lesions occur (Fig. 81–3) lend further credence to this hypothesis. Inflammatory processes adjacent to the splenic artery, particularly chronic pancreatitis with associated pseudocysts, are also

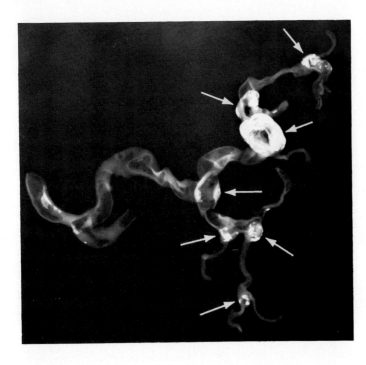

FIGURE 81-2. Splenic artery aneurysms (specimen roentgenogram). Marked calcific arteriosclerosis limited to splenic artery aneurysms occurring at vessel bifurcations *(arrows)*. Intervening arterial segments are unaffected by advanced arteriosclerotic changes.

known to cause aneurysms. In fact, peripancreatic pseudo-aneurysms occur in more than 10 per cent of patients with chronic pancreatitis, and many of these involve the splenic artery.[38] Similarly, penetrating and blunt trauma may precipitate aneurysmal development. Infected (mycotic) lesions, often associated with subacute bacterial endocarditis in intravenous drug addicts, are being encountered more frequently in contemporary times. Microaneurysms of intrasplenic vessels are usually a manifestation of a connective tissue disease such as periarteritis nodosa and are of less surgical importance than macroaneurysms due to other causes.

The presence of a splenic artery aneurysm may be suspected with radiographic demonstration of curvilinear, signet ring–like calcifications in the left upper quadrant (Fig. 81–4). Such findings have been reported in as many as 70 per cent of cases.[85] However, diagnoses of these aneurysms are most often the result of arteriographic studies in patients among whom there were no prior suspicions

of the lesion's presence (Fig. 81–5).[81] Clearly, arteriographic studies are needed to confirm the diagnosis of splenic artery aneurysm. Ultrasonography, computed axial tomography, and, more recently, magnetic resonance imaging[53] may prove useful in distinguishing certain aneurysms from other cystic and solid lesions in the vicinity of the splenic artery.

Splenic artery aneurysms usually are asymptomatic, although 17 and 20 per cent, respectively, of patients in two large series allegedly had symptoms referable to these lesions.[81, 85] Others have reported even higher incidences of symptomatic aneurysms. A common complaint among symptomatic patients is vague left upper quadrant or epigastric discomfort with occasional radiation to the left subscapular area. Acute expansion of splenic artery aneurysms intensifies these symptoms. Abdominal tenderness is an unlikely accompaniment of an intact aneurysm. Bruits ascribed to these lesions are more likely to arise from turbulent blood flow through the aorta and its branches than from

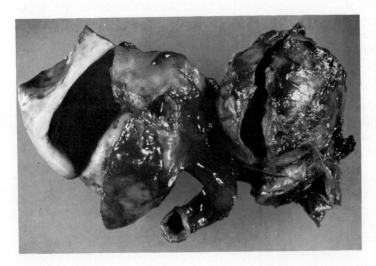

FIGURE 81-3. Splenic artery aneurysms. Multiple aneurysms involving a splenic artery with extensive arteriosclerosis and calcium deposition involving one aneurysm *(left)*, immediately adjacent to a thin nonatherosclerotic aneurysm *(right)*. Arteriosclerosis is considered a secondary event, not a primary factor in initiating splenic artery aneurysms.

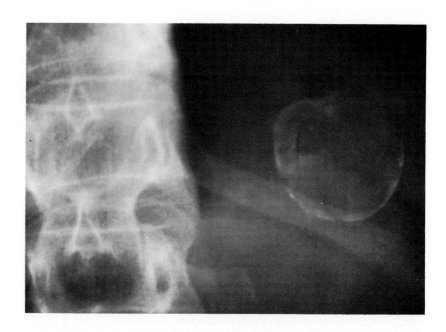

FIGURE 81-4. Splenic artery aneurysm. Curvilinear, signet ring–like calcifications in the left upper quadrant are characteristic of splenic artery aneurysms.

splenic aneurysmal disease. Most splenic artery aneurysms are less than 2 cm in diameter. Accordingly, pulsatile abdominal masses associated with these lesions are palpated infrequently.

Aneurysmal rupture and intraperitoneal hemorrhage account for the most dramatic clinical presentations of splenic artery aneurysms. In pregnant patients aneurysmal rupture often mimics common obstetric emergencies such as placental abruption, amniotic fluid embolization, or uterine rupture.[5, 47, 60] In nonpregnant patients, rupture often presents as an acute intra-abdominal catastrophe with associated cardiovascular collapse. In most cases bleeding initially occurs into the retrogastric area. Symptoms distant from the left upper quadrant and epigastrium may follow as blood escapes through the foramen of Winslow. Hemorrhage invariably proceeds to severe intraperitoneal bleeding

as lesser sac containment is lost. Such a "double rupture phenomenon" occurs in nearly 25 per cent of cases and often provides an opportunity for treatment before the onset of fatal hemorrhage. Occasionally, intermittent gastrointestinal bleeding may reflect a communication between the aneurysm and the intestinal tract. These latter lesions usually are products of an inflammatory process, and the communication most often occurs directly, as with penetrating gastric ulcers. In cases associated with pancreatitis, bleeding may occur through the pancreatic ducts.[34] Splenic arteriovenous fistulae are an even more uncommon complication of aneurysmal rupture, but when they do occur they are often associated with secondary portal hypertension.

Life-threatening rupture appears to affect fewer than 2 per cent of bland splenic artery aneurysms.[81] Factors contributing to rupture of previously asymptomatic splenic ar-

FIGURE 81-5. Splenic artery aneurysm. Arteriographic documentation of a pancreatitis-related aneurysm affecting the mid-splenic artery.

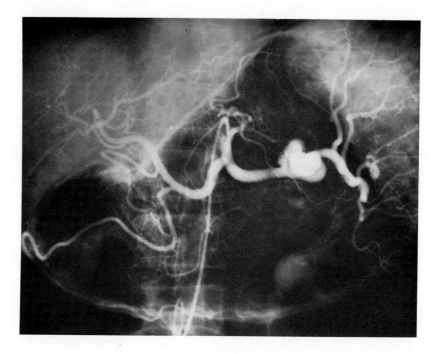

tery aneurysms remain poorly defined. There is no basis for the contention that rupture is less likely to occur in patients with calcified aneurysms, in normotensive as opposed to hypertensive patients, or in patients over 60 years of age. Aneurysms in patients who have received orthotopic liver transplants may be at greater risk of rupture than other bland aneurysms.[2, 10] The highest incidence of aneurysmal rupture occurs in young women during pregnancy. More than 95 per cent of aneurysms discovered during pregnancy have ruptured.[47, 81] Despite this fact, it is apparent that many splenic artery aneurysms develop during pregnancy, and the majority of these do not rupture during the pregnancy.

Indications for surgical therapy of splenic aneurysms have become better defined in recent years.[4, 81, 85] Symptomatic aneurysms warrant early surgical therapy. Operative intervention appears to be justified for splenic artery aneurysms encountered in pregnant patients or in females of childbearing age who subsequently may conceive. Maternal mortality of aneurysmal rupture during pregnancy is approximately 70 per cent, and fetal mortality exceeds 75 per cent.[5, 60, 81] Survival of both mother and child following rupture of a splenic artery aneurysm as of 1986 had been reported only eight times.[46, 71] In nonpregnant patients, operative mortality following surgical treatment for aneurysmal rupture is less than 25 per cent.[83] Although rupture has been reported to occur in 3.0 to 9.6 per cent of all patients with splenic artery aneurysms,[76, 81, 85] it is important to recall that disruption of bland lesions probably occurs in no more than 2 per cent of cases. Thus, elective operation for bland splenic artery aneurysms is appropriate only when the predicted surgical mortality rate is no greater than 0.5 per cent. This latter figure represents the product of the reported 2 per cent incidence of rupture and the 25 per cent mortality rate accompanying operative treatment. In certain patients in whom operative therapy entails a prohibitively high risk, transcatheter embolization of the aneurysm may be the preferred form of management.[50, 65]

Surgical techniques for treating splenic artery aneurysms have become standardized. Aneurysms of the proximal vessel may be treated by aneurysmectomy or simple ligation-exclusion without arterial reconstruction. In fact, restoration of splenic artery continuity when treating aneurysms of this vessel is rarely indicated. Proximal splenic artery aneurysms are easily exposed through the lesser sac after the gastrohepatic ligament has been incised. Entering and exiting vessels are ligated, and these lesions usually are excised if they are not embedded within pancreatic tissue. Certain mid-splenic artery aneurysms, especially those occurring as a result of pancreatic inflammatory disease, may not be removed so easily. Such false aneurysms, which often occur as a consequence of pancreatic pseudocyst erosion into the splenic artery, may be treated by arterial ligation from within the aneurysmal sac. Monofilament suture, such as polypropylene, is used to ligate vessels in this situation to lessen the risk of chronic infection that might occur in the presence of bacterial contamination of pseudocyst contents. Proximal splenic artery ligation or clamping, if easily accomplished, is recommended to lessen bleeding associated with opening of the false aneurysm. Internal or external drainage of these pseudocysts is often necessary following arterial ligation, and later extirpation of the diseased pancreas is frequently required. Distal pan-

createctomy including the affected artery is preferred when treating inflammatory false aneurysms involving the distal body and tail regions of the pancreas.

Surgical therapy of aneurysms within the hilus of the spleen in the past usually has entailed a conventional splenectomy. Given the importance of splenic preservation in maintaining host resistance, simple suture obliteration, aneurysmorrhaphy, or excision of distal aneurysms may become favored over traditional splenectomy. Mortality following surgical therapy for pancreatitis-related bleeding arterial aneurysms, most commonly affecting the splenic artery, approaches 30 per cent.[76] On the other hand, operative mortality following elective surgical treatment of bland noninflammatory splenic artery aneurysms, without concomitant vascular or gastrointestinal tract operations, has not been described among cases reported in the recent literature.[81, 83, 85]

HEPATIC ARTERY ANEURYSMS

Aneurysmal disease of the hepatic artery comprises 20 per cent of aneurysms affecting splanchnic vessels. Mycotic aneurysms, previously considered the most common type of hepatic artery aneurysm,[30] accounted for 16 per cent of lesions described in the literature from 1960 to 1970.[83] At present, they represent only 10 per cent of known hepatic artery aneurysms, occurring most often as a complication of illicit intravenous drug use. Atheromatous changes have been encountered in approximately 32 per cent of hepatic artery aneurysms. However, in most instances atherosclerosis is not considered an etiologic process but rather a secondary phenomenon. Medial degeneration, including alterations similar to those encountered in many splenic artery aneurysms, has been documented in approximately 24 per cent of these lesions. Medial defects appear to be acquired and are seemingly unrelated to congenital abnormalities. Specific events leading to development of aneurysms in this latter setting are unknown. True aneurysms or pseudoaneurysms developing as a consequence of trauma represent an additional 22 per cent of reported hepatic artery aneurysms, and the frequency of such lesions is increasing. Central hepatic rupture and deep parenchymal fractures subsequent to blunt abdominal injury or gunshot wounds are responsible for most traumatic aneurysms (Fig. 81–6). Periarteritis nodosa, cystic medial necrosis, and other more unusual arteriopathies have been associated with a very small number of these aneurysms. Lastly, periarterial inflammation, such as occurs with cholecystitis or pancreatitis, is a recognized but uncommon cause of hepatic artery aneurysms.

Hepatic artery aneurysms larger than 2 cm in diameter usually are saccular in character (Fig. 81–7). Smaller nontraumatic aneurysms tend to be fusiform. Eighty per cent of these lesions involve the extrahepatic vessels. Twenty per cent occur within the substance of the liver, with traumatic aneurysms dominating this latter group. A review of 163 aneurysms in which the specific site of the lesion could be ascertained revealed the following locations: common hepatic, 63 per cent; right hepatic, 28 per cent; left hepatic, 5 per cent; and both right and left hepatic arteries, 4 per cent.[83] Excluding multiple microaneurysms associated with

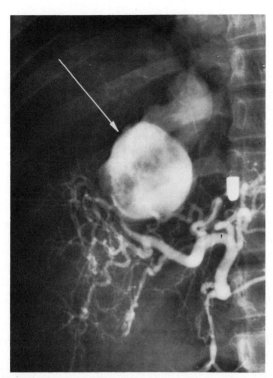

FIGURE 81–6. Traumatic hepatic artery aneurysm. Blunt abdominal injury and gunshot wounds cause most traumatic lesions. (From Whitehouse WM Jr, Graham LM, Stanley JC: Aneurysms of the celiac, hepatic, and splenic arteries. *In* Bergan JJ, Yao JST [eds]: Aneurysms, Diagnosis and Treatment. New York, Grune & Stratton, 1981, pp 405–415.)

connective tissue disorders, such as polyarteritis nodosa,[63] most hepatic artery aneurysms are solitary.

Men with hepatic artery aneurysms outnumber women 2:1. The majority of lesions, excluding traumatic aneurysms, occur in patients who have entered their sixth decade of life. Most aneurysms remain asymptomatic. Among symptomatic patients with intact aneurysms, the most com-

mon complaint is right upper quadrant or epigastric pain. Discomfort, although frequently vague, usually is persistent and is often attributed to cholecystitis. In most instances, pain is not related to meals. Expanding hepatic artery aneurysms usually cause severe upper abdominal discomfort, often with radiation to the back, similar to that accompanying pancreatitis. Exceedingly large aneurysms may compress the biliary tree and result in clinical manifestations similar to other forms of extrinsic extrahepatic bile duct obstruction. Pulsatile masses and abdominal bruits are uncommon findings in the presence of intact aneurysms.

Rupture of hepatic artery aneurysms occurs into the hepatobiliary tract and the peritoneal cavity with equal frequency. Rupture into bile ducts often is responsible for the characteristic findings of hematobilia.[18, 33, 39] In such a setting, patients may complain of intermittent abdominal pain similar to that of biliary colic. The majority exhibit massive gastrointestinal bleeding with periodic hematemesis. More than half of these patients become jaundiced when blood clots obstruct their biliary ducts. Most patients with hematobilia are febrile at some time during their illness. Symptoms of chronic anemia associated with insidious bleeding and melena are less common manifestations of aneurysmal communication with the biliary tree. Hematobilia occurs most often in the presence of traumatic intrahepatic pseudoaneurysms. Erosion of nontraumatic hepatic artery aneurysms into the stomach, duodenum, common bile duct, pancreatic duct, or portal vein is a recognized but relatively rare complication of these lesions. Intraperitoneal bleeding and exsanguinating hemorrhage, producing clinical signs of "abdominal apoplexy," frequently accompany extrahepatic aneurysmal rupture. In this regard, aneurysms associated with periarteritis nodosa that rupture into the intraperitoneal cavity are most likely to arise from the hepatic artery.[73] Unfortunately, many patients destined to develop such catastrophes do not exhibit prior symptoms.

The diagnosis of hepatic artery aneurysms in the past occurred most often at autopsy or at times of surgical exploration for major complications of these lesions. Vascular calcifications in the upper abdomen and displacement of

FIGURE 81–7. Hepatic artery aneurysms. Selective celiac arteriogram demonstrating a large saccular aneurysm at the bifurcation of the proper hepatic artery. Eighty per cent of hepatic artery aneurysms are extrahepatic.

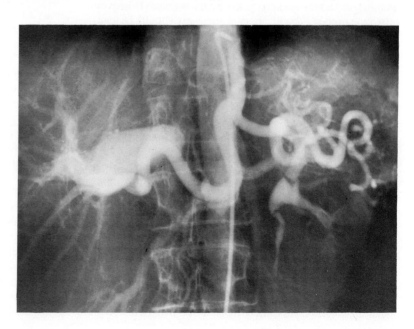

contiguous structures evident on barium studies or chole-cystography may suggest the presence of these aneurysms. More recently, arteriographic studies in patients with unknown causes of gastrointestinal hemorrhage and in those with major abdominal trauma have led to an increased recognition of hepatic artery aneurysms. Ultrasonography and computed axial tomography may be valuable in screening patients for suspected hepatic artery aneurysms and in maintaining noninvasive follow-up.[1]

Excision or obliteration of all hepatic artery aneurysms appears to be justified unless unusual risks preclude operation. Although not every aneurysm eventually ruptures, rupture occurred in 44 per cent of the lesions described in the literature from 1960 to 1970.[83] In recent isolated experiences high incidences of rupture have been reported,[70] but in general the overall rupture rate is probably less than 20 per cent. Mortality associated with rupture continues to be exceedingly high and certainly is not less than the 35 per cent previously reported.[12] An aggressive approach to managing these aneurysms seems appropriate.

Preoperative arteriographic delineation of the foregut and midgut arterial circulation is essential in planning optimal surgical therapy of these aneurysms.[90] Common hepatic artery aneurysms may often be treated by aneurysmectomy or aneurysmal exclusion without arterial reconstruction. Extensive foregut collateral circulation to the liver through the gastroduodenal and right gastric arteries frequently provides adequate hepatic blood flow despite common hepatic artery interruption. However, if blood flow to the liver appears compromised following a 5-minute trial of intraoperative hepatic artery occlusion, then aneurysmorrhaphy or formal hepatic revascularization should be pursued. Similarly, coexisting liver parenchymal disease makes ligation of the proximal hepatic artery less advisable and arterial reconstruction preferable.

Restoration of normal hepatic blood flow is most crucial in managing aneurysms involving the proper hepatic artery and its extrahepatic branches. Aneurysms of the hepatic artery are usually approached through an extended right subcostal or a vertical midline incision. Intact common hepatic artery aneurysms are easily isolated. However, proximal proper hepatic artery aneurysms should be cautiously dissected, especially near the gastroduodenal artery and its pancreaticoduodenal artery branch, which often cross over the common bile duct inferiorly. Similarly, distal proper hepatic or hepatic artery branch aneurysms must be carefully dissected to avoid bile duct injuries. Expeditious vascular control of entering and exiting vessels from within an aneurysm (after opening it) may be safer than dissecting the adjacent arteries when treating large or inflammatory aneurysms.

A number of therapeutic alternatives exist in repairing aneurysmal hepatic arteries. Aneurysmorrhaphy, with or without a vein patch closure, may be possible in managing select traumatic aneurysms. Fusiform and large saccular aneurysms that involve greater arterial circumferences are best treated by resection and arterial reconstriction. Use of autogenous saphenous vein, despite occasional failures,[69] is preferred over synthetic prostheses for these procedures. Anastomoses are best undertaken by spatulation of both the hepatic artery and vein graft to provide an ovoid anastomosis that will be less likely to be a site of stricture with

healing. Interposition grafts within the hepatic arterial circulation are often possible, and, when not, an aortohepatic bypass may be undertaken. An extended Kocher's maneuver with medial visceral rotation will allow exposure of the vena cava and aorta. A vein graft from the anterolateral aspect of the infrarenal aorta may then be carried behind the duodenum to the porta hepatis. After the aneurysmectomy has been performed, the spatulated vein is anastomosed in an end-to-end fashion to either the common or proper hepatic artery.

Resection of liver parenchyma for intrahepatic aneurysms that are unamenable to reconstruction is occasionally necessary. Control of bleeding intrahepatic aneurysms by means of simple ligation of the proximal vessel, despite the possibility of subsequent liver necrosis, may be preferable to undertaking a major liver resection in a critically ill patient. Similarly, percutaneous transcatheter balloon embolization with occlusion of hepatic artery aneurysms in high-risk cases may be an acceptable alternative to operative therapy.[4, 25, 40, 61]

SUPERIOR MESENTERIC ARTERY ANEURYSMS

The third most common splanchnic artery aneurysm, accounting for 5.5 per cent of these lesions, involves the main trunk of the superior mesenteric artery. These lesions, affecting the proximal 5 cm of this vessel, are most often infectious in etiology.[20] Mycotic aneurysms comprised 63 per cent of lesions reported nearly three decades ago[14] and 58 per cent of cases described more recently.[83] In this regard, the superior mesenteric artery harbors more infectious aneurysms than any other muscular artery. Nonhemolytic *Streptococcus*, related to left-sided bacterial endocarditis, has been the organism found most often in these lesions. A variety of other pathogens, especially staphylococcal organisms, have been described in aneurysms associated with noncardiac septicemia. Syphilitic aneurysms, frequently described in older reports, have not been observed in contemporary times. Dissecting aneurysms associated with medial defects are rare[13] but affect this vessel more than any other splanchnic artery (Fig. 81–8).[31] Arteriosclerosis, whether as a primary or secondary event, is evident in approximately 20 per cent of reported superior mesenteric artery aneurysms. Lastly, trauma is a rare cause of these aneurysms.

Intermittent upper abdominal discomfort that progresses to persistent and severe epigastric pain often accompanies symptomatic mycotic superior mesenteric artery aneurysms. In certain cases it may be difficult to distinguish symptomatology due to mesenteric ischemia from that due to aneurysmal expansion. Surprisingly, a tender pulsatile abdominal mass that is not rigidly fixed has been discovered in nearly half of these patients.

Females dominated earlier series of superior mesenteric artery aneurysms. More recent experience has not confirmed such a sex predilection, with men and women affected equally. Most reported mycotic aneurysms occur in patients under 50 years of age. Subacute bacterial endocarditis is usually present in these cases. Nonmycotic aneurysms of the superior mesenteric artery most often affect

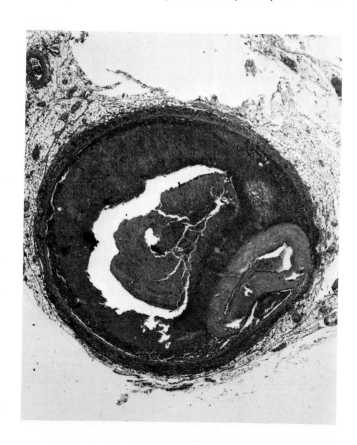

FIGURE 81–8. Superior mesenteric artery aneurysm. Microscopic cross-section of a dissecting aneurysm affecting the proximal superior mesenteric artery. (H&E.)

patients after the sixth decade of life. This older subgroup of patients often experiences prodromata of intestinal angina prior to aneurysm rupture.

Aneurysmal expansion with dissection, or propagation of intraluminal thrombus beyond the inferior pancreaticoduodenal and middle colic vessels effectively isolates the superior mesenteric artery from the collaterals of the celiac and inferior mesenteric artery circulations. In such circumstances, any compromise of blood flow through the superior mesenteric artery may cause intestinal angina. Because of the critical location of superior mesenteric artery aneurysms, the existence of numerous asymptomatic lesions is not as common as with many other splanchnic aneurysms. Antemortem diagnosis of uncomplicated superior mesenteric artery aneurysms is uncommon. In fact, recognition of asymptomatic solitary dissecting superior mesenteric artery aneurysms has not been reported.[13] Radiographic evidence of calcified mycotic aneurysms and abdominal angiograms made during studies for unrelated disease have been responsible for the majority of antemortem diagnoses.

Surgical treatment of most superior mesenteric artery aneurysms appears justified in light of the seemingly common occurrence of rupture or arterial occlusion. Nearly a third of reported superior mesenteric artery aneurysms have been successfully treated by operation.[48] This includes fewer than 20 mycotic aneurysms of this vessel.[20] Operative exposure for more distal lesions may be obtained by a transmesenteric route or for proximal lesions by a retroperitoneal approach after the lateral parietal tissues are incised and the left colon, pancreas, and spleen are reflected medially. Since the first successful surgical treatment of a supe-

rior mesenteric artery aneurysm was reported more than 35 years ago,[14] the most common procedures attempted have been ligation, in over a third of cases, and aneurysmorrhaphy. Ligation of the vessels entering and exiting these aneurysms without arterial reconstruction surprisingly has proved to be an acceptable, simple means of treatment.[24, 83] The existence of preformed collaterals involving the inferior pancreaticoduodenal and middle colic arteries increases the success of this approach. Temporary occlusion of the superior mesenteric artery with intraoperative assessment of bowel viability offers a means of identifying cases in which mesenteric revascularization is necessary.

Superior mesenteric artery aneurysmectomy may prove hazardous because of the close proximity of neighboring structures such as the superior mesenteric vein and pancreas. Endoaneurysmorrhaphy in selected patients with saccular aneurysms may be possible. Arterial reconstruction, using conventional interposition grafting or aortomesenteric bypass, to provide restoration of blood flow through the superior mesenteric artery after exclusion or excision of an aneurysm has been rarely accomplished.[48, 89, 94] Use of short synthetic prostheses, taking origin from the anterior aorta or intact proximal superior mesenteric artery and carried to normal vessel beyond the aneurysm, is acceptable in the absence of active aneurysmal infection or infarcted bowel. In the presence of infection or infarcted bowel, an autogenous saphenous vein is a more appropriate conduit for reconstruction. In such cases, long-term antibiotic therapy is also recommended. Contemporary surgical intervention for all types of superior mesenteric artery aneurysms carries a mortality of less than 15 per cent. Transcatheter occlusion of saccular aneurysms with discrete necks arising from the side of the superior mesenteric artery may occasionally be justified.[4]

CELIAC ARTERY ANEURYSMS

Aneurysms of the celiac artery are unusual lesions that account for 4 per cent of all splanchnic aneurysms. In 1985 only 108 celiac artery aneurysms had been described in the literature.[28] Arteriosclerosis and medial degeneration were the most common pathologic changes observed in these aneurysms. The former, noted in 27 per cent of patients, probably represents a secondary rather than a primary causative process. Preexisting reductions of elastic tissue and smooth muscle at major branchings appear to be a contributing factor in an additional 17 per cent of patients in whom developmental aneurysms were suspected. Traumatic aneurysms due to penetrating injuries are uncommon. Post-stenotic dilatation occasionally progresses to frank aneurysmal change and is an uncommon cause of these lesions. Mycotic celiac artery aneurysms are very rare,[91] and in recent times syphilitic and tuberculous lesions have not been encountered. Associated aortic aneurysms were noted in 18 per cent of patients with celiac artery aneurysms, and other splanchnic artery aneurysms affected 38 per cent of these patients.[28]

Most celiac artery aneurysms are asymptomatic. Although males outnumber females among all reported cases, there has been no sex predilection in patients reported during the past three decades. The average age of patients reported prior to 1950 was 40 years, in contrast to an average age of 52 years reported since then.[28]

Abdominal discomfort localized to the epigastrium accompanies more than 60 per cent of symptomatic celiac artery aneurysms. Intense discomfort, often with radiation to the back, as well as nausea and vomiting, has been attributed to aneurysmal expansion and may be confused with pancreatitis. Abdominal bruits are frequently heard in patients with celiac artery aneurysms. Nevertheless, such bruits are rarely attributable to the aneurysm. Celiac artery aneurysms are apparent as pulsatile abdominal masses in nearly 30 per cent of cases.[28] Symptomatology suggestive of intestinal angina is a rare accompaniment of celiac artery aneurysms and, when present, is usually due to significant coexisting arteriosclerotic occlusive disease affecting the superior mesenteric and inferior mesenteric arteries.

The most serious clinical complication of celiac artery aneurysmal disease is rupture. Although nearly 80 per cent of all previously reported lesions ruptured, clinical experience in the past 25 years has documented the risk of rupture as 13 per cent.[28] The contemporary incidence of rupture may be even lower. Aneurysmal disruption is most often associated with intraperitoneal hemorrhage, although communication with the gastrointestinal tract can occur.

Recognition of most celiac artery aneurysms encountered before 1950 occurred at the time of autopsy. Currently, unexpected discovery of aneurysms during angiography accounts for the diagnosis in nearly 65 per cent of cases (Fig. 81–9).[28] Calcification of aneurysmal walls, which affects 20 per cent of these lesions, and displacement of contiguous structures are occasional radiographic findings that suggest the diagnosis. Nearly 20 per cent of celiac artery aneurysms recognized before death were encountered at the authors' institution.[32, 83] Ultrasonography and computed axial tomography may be of diagnostic use in assessing certain lesions[32, 36] and should be useful in longitudinal follow-up of nonoperative cases.

Surgical treatment of celiac artery aneurysms is warranted except when operative risks contraindicate any abdominal operation.[28] Successful operations in more than 90 per cent of cases reported since the first successful surgical treatment nearly 30 years ago[74] support such a therapeutic approach.

Exposure of celiac artery aneurysms for symptomatic or large lesions is best obtained utilizing a thoracoabdom-

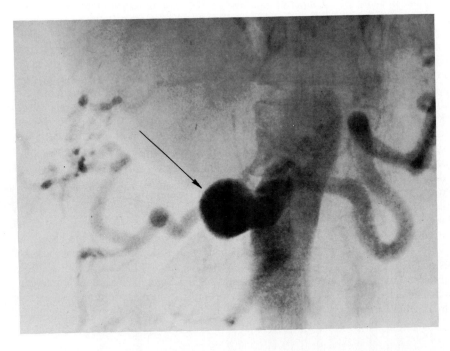

FIGURE 81–9. Celiac artery aneurysm *(arrow)*. Aortogram reveals saccular aneurysm that exhibited medial degenerative changes and secondary arteriosclerosis. (From Stanley JC, Whitehouse WM Jr: *In* Bergan JJ, Yao JST [eds]: Surgery of the Aorta and Its Body Branches. New York, Grune & Stratton, 1979, pp 497–519.)

inal approach with the incision extending from the mid-axillary line on the left, usually in the seventh intercostal space, across the costal margin into the abdomen. Small bland aneurysms, especially in patients in whom there is a broad angle at the costal margin, can often be treated by the abdominal route alone. In these instances, a transverse supraumbilical incision and subsequent medial visceral rotation of the left colon, spleen, and pancreas allow exposure of the aorta at the diaphagmatic hiatus. Transection of the left crus and median arcuate ligament of the diaphragm provides access to the origin of the celiac artery and adjacent aorta in this situation.

Aneurysmorrhaphy has been advocated in select cases, and although compromise of celiac artery blood flow is less likely with this form of therapy, it is favored only for discrete saccular aneurysms in which the integrity of the remaining arterial wall is considered normal. Aneurysmectomy with arterial reconstruction accounts for 50 per cent of reported operations.[28] Aneurysmectomy and primary reanastomosis of the celiac artery trunk are sometimes possible but should be undertaken only in the presence of a relatively normal and lengthy proximal celiac artery. When reanastomosis is not feasible, an aortoceliac bypass with a synthetic prosthesis or autogenous vein graft should be performed, originating from the supraceliac aorta.

Celiac axis ligation with interruption of antegrade blood flow through the common hepatic, left gastric, and splenic vessels has been undertaken in 35 per cent of reported operations.[28] Although celiac artery ligation rarely results in hepatic necrosis, it should be undertaken only when intraoperative findings suggest that liver blood flow will not be severely compromised.[26] Arterial ligation should not be performed in patients with known liver disease. Mortality for operative treatment of patients with ruptured celiac artery aneurysms is 40 per cent compared with only 5 per cent for those with nonruptured celiac artery aneurysms.[28]

GASTRIC AND GASTROEPIPLOIC ARTERY ANEURYSMS

Aneurysms of gastric and gastroepiploic arteries account for approximately 4 per cent of splanchnic aneurysms. These lesions appear to be acquired, although their exact cause often remains undefined.[87] Histologic evidence of arteriosclerosis in many aneurysms earlier led to a belief that this was an important etiologic factor.[55] It is more likely that medial degeneration of undetermined origin or degeneration resulting from periarterial inflammation precedes most arteriosclerotic changes. The latter are considered a secondary process. Most clinically important aneurysms involving vessels to the stomach are solitary. Aneurysms of gastric arteries are nearly ten times more common than those of gastroepiploic arteries. They are considered together because their natural history and management are similar.

Asymptomatic aneurysms of the gastric and gastroepiploic arteries are uncommon. Most reported aneurysms present as vascular emergencies, with rupture at the time of diagnosis occurring in more than 90 per cent of cases.

Nearly 70 per cent have been associated with serious gastrointestinal bleeding. A small number of patients describe antecedent dyspeptic epigastric discomfort, but the majority have no abdominal pain prior to aneurysmal rupture. Intestinal bleeding in these cases usually is manifest by acute massive hematemesis,[51] although a small number of patients experience chronic occult gastrointestinal bleeding. Rupture of gastric and gastroepiploic artery aneurysms causes life-threatening intraperitoneal bleeding in approximately 30 per cent of cases.[84] These aneurysms are second only to mesenteric branch aneurysms as a cause of abdominal apoplexy. As is the case with intestinal bleeding, most patients are asymptomatic prior to the occurrence of acute intraperitoneal aneurysmal disruption. The majority of cases affect individuals in their sixth and seventh decades of life. Males outnumber females approximately 3 : 1.

Antemortem diagnosis of gastric and gastroepiploic artery aneurysms most often occurs during urgent operation for gastrointestinal or intraperitoneal bleeding. Intraoperative search for gastric and gastroepiploic aneurysms entails careful palpation and transillumination of the entire stomach. Arteriographic studies for unexplained gastrointestinal bleeding result in occasional preoperative recognition of these lesions (Fig. 81–10). Mucosal alterations associated with these aneurysms are often minimal, and endoscopic recognition is difficult. Larger lesions may be mistaken for gastric ulcers or malignancies.

Treatment of gastric and gastroepiploic aneurysms is directed at controlling life-threatening hemorrhage. Early diagnosis and urgent operative intervention are necessary to improve survival. Approximately 70 per cent of patients reported to have these lesions succumb following aneurysm rupture.[83] Ligation of aneurysmal vessels, with or without excision of the aneurysm, is appropriate treatment for extraintestinal lesions and for those aneurysms associated with inflammatory processes adjacent to the stomach. Intramural aneurysms and those associated with bleeding into the gastrointestinal tract should be excised with portions of the involved gastric tissue.

JEJUNAL, ILEAL, AND COLIC ARTERY ANEURYSMS

Small intramural and intramesenteric aneurysms of jejunal, ileal, and colic arteries are uncommon,[37, 49, 59, 68] accounting for only 3 per cent of reported splanchnic aneurysms. With the exception of aneurysms associated with connective tissue disorders, 90 per cent of these lesions are solitary and range in size from a few millimeters to a centimeter in size. Occasionally, patients have two or three lesions, often in the same region of the intestinal circulation. The pathogenesis of these aneurysms is poorly understood. Most appear to be the result of congenital or acquired medial defects. Arteriosclerotic changes exist in approximately 20 per cent of these lesions.[49] As with other splanchnic aneurysms, arteriosclerosis most often is a secondary process. Multiple lesions may represent late sequelae of an endarteritis associated with an immunologic injury or septic emboli from subacute bacterial endocarditis.[86] Necrotizing vasculitides, such as periarteritis nodosa, are another rec-

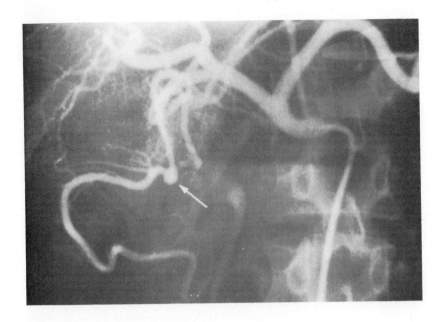

FIGURE 81–10. Gastroepiploic artery aneurysms. Selective celiac arteriogram. This saccular aneurysm (arrow) was responsible for massive gastrointestinal hemorrhage.

ognized cause of multiple mesenteric branch microaneurysms.[73]

There does not appear to be any sex predilection in the development of mesenteric branch aneurysms. The peak age of involvement is during the seventh decade of life. Intact aneurysms are rarely symptomatic. Most aneurysms are recognized at operation for complications of rupture into the mesentery, intestinal lumen, or peritoneal cavity. Rupture of aneurysms affecting the jejunal arteries is relatively rare.[16] Abdominal pain associated with aneurysmal rupture, the presence of a tender mass, or development of abdominal apoplexy with uncontained hemorrhage have been the initial manifestations of these lesions in 70 per cent of reported cases.[48] Mortality following rupture approaches 20 per cent.[83] Increasing contemporary recognition of intestinal artery aneurysms is the result of more frequent abdominal arteriographic studies for nonvascular

disease (Fig. 81–11),[42, 68] often during assessment of insidious gastrointestinal bleeding or massive rectal hemorrhage. Preoperative arteriographic localization of these small aneurysms is often essential for successful operative intervention.

Surgical therapy of mesenteric branch aneurysms necessitates arterial ligation, aneurysmectomy, and resection of ischemic small bowel or colon if the intestinal blood supply is compromised. An intraoperative search should always be undertaken for multiple aneurysms of the jejunal and ileal arteries. The risk of aneurysmal rupture remains undefined in the case of uncomplicated intestinal aneurysms. However, the seriousness of rupture and the limited risks of operative intervention support the contention that these lesions should be treated once their existence becomes known.

Aneurysms of the proximal inferior mesenteric artery

FIGURE 81–11. Ileal artery aneurysm. Mesenteric arteriogram documenting the presence of a saccular aneurysm (arrow) of a distal ileal artery.

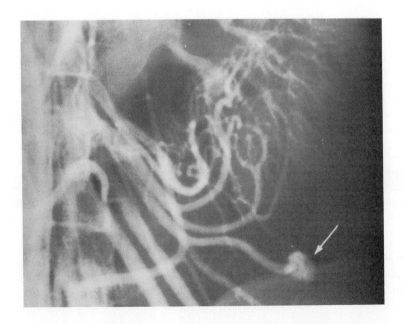

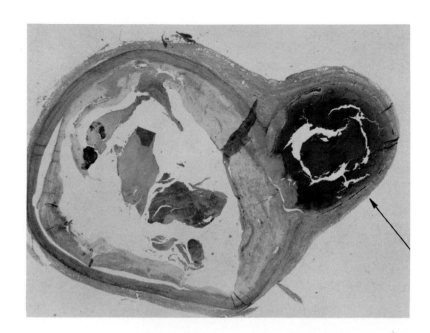

FIGURE 81–12. Inferior mesenteric artery aneurysm. Microscopic cross-section of aorta and a thrombus containing aneurysm *(arrow)* of the inferior mesenteric artery trunk. (H&E.)

or its branches are exceedingly rare (Fig. 81–12). As of 1985 only 13 of these lesions had been described in the literature.[27] Aneurysms of this vessel have diverse causes and varied clinical manifestations. Although their natural history remains ill defined, operative intervention seems justified in most instances.

GASTRODUODENAL, PANCREATICODUODENAL, AND PANCREATIC ARTERY ANEURYSMS

Periduodenal and peripancreatic aneurysmal disease of the communicating vessels between the celiac and superior mesenteric artery circulations is uncommon. Gastroduodenal artery aneurysms account for 1.5 per cent of all splanchnic artery aneurysms. These cases have all been reported since 1960. Aneurysms of pancreaticoduodenal and pancreatic vessels account for an additional 2 per cent of splanchnic artery aneurysms. The most common age of involvement is the sixth decade. Males are affected more often than females by nearly 4 : 1. This reflects the increased incidence of alcoholic pancreatitis in men and the fact that the majority of these lesions evolve as complications of acute or chronic pancreatitis.[17, 35, 80, 93] Periarterial inflammation, actual vascular necrosis, and erosion by expanding pancreatic pseudocysts all contribute to aneurysmal development in these cases.[22, 79] Noninflammatory pancreaticoduodenal artery aneurysms appear to have no sex predilection.[29] In some of these aneurysms increased blood flow, associated with celiac artery stenoses, may be an important etiologic factor.[67] Arteriosclerosis used to be considered the most common cause of these aneurysms,[83] but is now usually considered a secondary rather than a primary etiologic process.

Most patients with aneurysms involving the gastroduodenal, pancreaticoduodenal, or pancreatic arteries are symptomatic at the time of diagnosis. Epigastric pain, frequently with radiation to the back, is common. Silent inflammatory aneurysms are very uncommon. In some cases this discomfort is indistinguishable from that caused by underlying pancreatitis. This fact is particularly important because nearly 60 per cent of all gastroduodenal artery aneurysms and 30 per cent of all pancreaticoduodenal aneurysms are pancreatitis related.[17] Aneurysmal rupture is second only to abdominal pain as the most frequent manifestation of these lesions. Gastrointestinal hemorrhage affects nearly 75 per cent of these inflammatory aneurysms. Bleeding in these circumstances occurs most often into the stomach or duodenum and less often into the biliary or pancreatic ductal system.[23, 79] An occasional patient becomes jaundiced,[6] but a direct association with aneurysmal disease is not always easily documented. Rupture affects approximately 50 per cent of noninflammatory aneurysms, occurring into the intestinal tract and peritoneal cavity with equal frequency.

Arteriographic studies are essential in evaluating patients suspected of symptomatic gastroduodenal, pancreaticoduodenal, or pancreatic arterial aneurysms, especially those associated with pancreatitis (Figs. 81–13 and 81–14).[9, 17, 80] Endoscopic examinations, barium contrast studies, and ultrasonography may demonstrate coexisting gastroduodenal or pancreatic disease, but their usefulness in identifying aneurysms is limited. Computed axial tomography has greater usefulness as a means of evaluating these aneurysms (Fig. 81–15).[17]

Surgical intervention for aneurysms of the gastroduodenal or pancreaticoduodenal arteries is justified in all but the poorest-risk patients.[17, 29, 79, 88] Reported mortality following rupture of gastroduodenal artery aneurysms approaches 50 per cent. Mortality is somewhat less for ruptured pancreaticoduodenal artery aneurysms and is approximately 20 per cent for rupture of nonpancreatitis-related lesions.[29]

In general, pancreaticoduodenal and pancreatic artery aneurysms are more difficult to manage operatively than

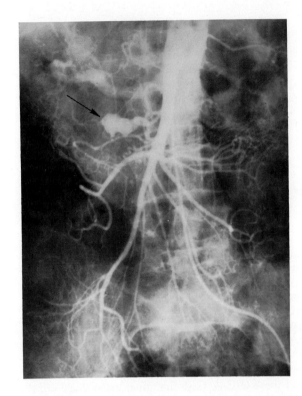

FIGURE 81–13.   Inferior pancreaticoduodenal artery aneurysm. Aortogram demonstrating false aneurysm *(arrow)* that evolved as a complication of pancreatitis. (From Stanley JC, Frey CF, Miller TA, et al: Major arterial hemorrhage. A complication of pancreatic pseudocysts and chronic pancreatitis. Arch Surg 111:435, 1976. Copyright 1976, American Medical Association.)

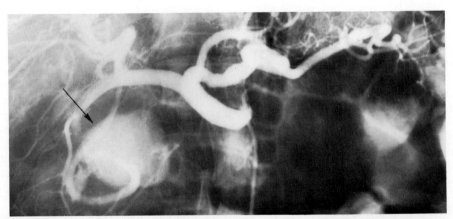

FIGURE 81–14.   Gastroduodenal artery aneurysm *(arrow)*. Selective celiac arteriogram. (From Eckhauser FE, Stanley JC, Zelenock GB, et al: Gastroduodenal and pancreaticoduodenal artery aneurysms: A complication of pancreatitis causing spontaneous gastrointestinal hemorrhage. Surgery 88:335, 1980.)

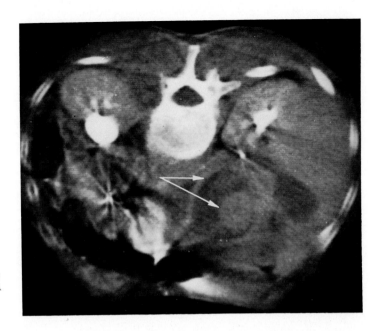

FIGURE 81–15. Gastroduodenal artery aneurysm. Computed axial tomography of a pancreatic pseudocyst *(short arrow)* containing an aneurysmal gastroduodenal artery *(long arrow)*. (From Eckhauser FE, Stanley JC, Zelenock GB, et al: Gastroduodenal and pancreaticoduodenal artery aneurysms: A complication of pancreatitis causing spontaneous gastrointestinal hemorrhage. Surgery 88:335, 1980.)

gastroduodenal artery aneurysms.[17, 92] The multiple vessels that communicate with these smaller aneurysms and the difficulty of identifying them within the substance of the pancreas limit the efficacy of aneurysmal exclusion by simple ligature alone. Intraoperative arteriography may prove useful in completing surgical therapy when lesions involve the proximal pancreas or other critical structures.[75] Suture ligature of entering and exiting vessels from within the aneurysmal sac rather than extra-aneurysmal dissection and arterial ligation is a more appropriate means of treating most gastroduodenal or pancreaticoduodenal artery aneurysms imbedded within the pancreas. When aneurysms are of a false type involving pancreatic pseudocysts, some manner of cyst decompression should be undertaken. The choice between external or internal drainage is usually determined on the basis of intraoperative findings. Major resections of pancreatic tissue, including pancreaticoduodenectomy, may be necessary eventually for successful treatment of selected patients with extensive aneurysmal involvement of the pancreatic arteries.[64]

Transcatheter embolization may be performed to ablate certain aneurysms.[50] Rebleeding and rupture may complicate this type of therapy.[45] Although embolization may prove a reasonable alternative to operation in some critically ill patients, it is perhaps better to view such a measure as a temporizing intervention before definitive surgical therapy is undertaken.

References

1. Athey PA, Sax SL, Lamki N, Cadavid G: Sonography in the diagnosis of hepatic artery aneurysms. AJR 147:725, 1986.
2. Ayalon A, Wiesner RH, Perkins JD, et al: Splenic artery aneurysms in liver transplant patients. Transplantation 45:386, 1988.
3. Babb RR: Aneurysm of the splenic artery. Arch Surg 111:924, 1976.
4. Baker JS, Tisnado J, Cho SR, Beachley MC: Splanchnic artery aneurysms and pseudoaneurysms: Transcatheter embolization. Radiology 163:135, 1987.
5. Barrett JM, Caldwell BH: Association of portal hypertension and ruptured splenic artery aneurysm in pregnancy. Obstet Gynecol 57:255, 1981.
6. Bassaly I, Schwartz IR, Pinchuck A, Lerner R: Aneurysm of the gastroduodenal artery presenting as common duct obstruction with jaundice. Am J Gastroenterol 59:435, 1973.
7. Bedford PD, Lodge B: Aneurysm of the splenic artery. Gut 1:321, 1960.
8. Boijsen E, Efsing HO: Aneurysm of the splenic artery. Acta Radiol [Diagn] (Stockh) 8:29, 1969.
9. Boijsen E, Gothlin J, Hallbook T, Sandblom P: Preoperative angiographic diagnosis of bleeding aneurysms of abdominal visceral arteries. Radiology 93:781, 1969.
10. Bronsther O, Merhav H, Van Thiel D, Starzl TE: Splenic artery aneurysms occurring in liver transplant recipients. Transplantation 52:4 723, 1991.
11. Buehler PK, Dailey TH, Lazarevic B: Spontaneous rupture of colic-artery aneurysms. Dis Colon Rectum 19:671, 1976.
12. Busuttil RW, Brin BJ: The diagnosis and management of visceral artery aneurysms. Surgery 88:619, 1980.
13. Cormier F, Ferry J, Artru B, et al: Dissecting aneurysms of the main trunk of the superior mesenteric artery. J Vasc Surg 15:424, 1992.
14. DeBakey ME, Cooley DA: Successful resection of mycotic aneurysm of superior mesenteric artery: Case report and review of the literature. Am Surg 19:202, 1953.
15. Deterling RA: Aneurysm of the visceral arteries. J Cardiovasc Surg 12:309, 1971.
16. Diettrich NA, Cacioppo JC, Ying DPW: Massive gastrointestinal hemorrhage caused by rupture of a jejunal branch artery aneurysm. J Vasc Surg 8:187, 1988.
17. Eckhauser FE, Stanley JC, Zelenock GB, et al: Gastroduodenal and pancreaticoduodenal artery aneurysms: A complication of pancreatitis causing spontaneous gastrointestinal hemorrhage. Surgery 88:335, 1980.
18. Erskine JM: Hepatic artery aneurysms. Vasc Surg 7:106, 1973.
19. Feist JH, Gajarej A: Extra and intrasplenic artery aneurysms in portal hypertension. Radiology 125:331, 1977.
20. Friedman SG, Pogo GJ, Moccio CG: Mycotic aneurysm of the superior mesenteric artery. J Vasc Surg 6:87, 1987.
21. Fukunaga Y, Usui N, Hirohashi K, et al: Clinical courses and treatment of splenic artery aneurysms—report of 3 cases and review of literature in Japan. Osaka City Med J 36(2):161, 1990.
22. Gadacz TR, Trunkey D, Kieffer RF: Visceral vessel erosion associated with pancreatitis. Case reports and a review of the literature. Arch Surg 113:1438, 1978.
23. Gangahar DM, Carveth SW, Reese HE, et al: True aneurysm of the pancreaticoduodenal artery: A case report and review of the literature. J Vasc Surg 2:741, 1985.
24. Geelkerken RH, van Bockel JH, de Roos WK, Hermans J: Surgical treatment of intestinal artery aneurysms. Eur J Vasc Surg 4:563, 1990.
25. Goldblatt M, Goldin AR, Shaff MI: Percutaneous embolization for

the management of hepatic artery aneurysms. Gastroenterology 73:1142, 1977.

26. Graham JM, McCollum CH, DeBakey ME: Aneurysms of the splanchnic arteries. Am J Surg 140:797, 1980.

27. Graham LM, Hay MR, Cho KJ, Stanley JC: Inferior mesenteric artery aneurysms. Surgery 97:158, 1985.

28. Graham LM, Stanley JC, Whitehouse WM Jr, et al: Celiac artery aneurysms: Historic (1745–1949) versus contemporary (1950–1984) differences in etiology and clinical importance. J Vasc Surg 5:757, 1985.

29. Granke K, Hollier LH, Bowen JC: Pancreaticoduodenal artery aneurysms: Changing patterns. South Med J 83:918, 1990.

30. Guida PM, Moore SW: Aneurysm of the hepatic artery. Report of five cases with a brief review of the previously reported cases. Surgery 60:299, 1966.

31. Guthrie W, Maclean H: Dissecting aneurysms of arteries other than the aorta. J Pathol 108:219, 1972.

32. Haimovici H, Sprayregen S, Eckstein P, Veith FJ: Celiac artery aneurysmectomy: Case report with review of the literature. Surgery 79:592, 1976.

33. Harlaftis NN, Akin JT: Hemobilia from ruptured hepatic artery aneurysm. Report of a case and review of the literature. Am J Surg 133:229, 1977.

34. Harper PC, Gamelli RL, Kaye MD: Recurrent hemorrhage into the pancreatic duct from a splenic artery aneurysm. Gastroenterology 87:417, 1984.

35. Harris RD, Anderson JE, Coel MN: Aneurysms of the small pancreatic arteries: A cause of upper abdominal pain and intestinal bleeding. Radiology 115:17, 1975.

36. Herzler GM, Silver TM, Graham LM, Stanley JC: Celiac artery aneurysm. J Clin Ultrasound 9:141, 1981.

37. Hoehn JG, Bartholomew LG, Osmundson PJ, Wallace RB: Aneurysms of the mesenteric artery. Am J Surg 115:832, 1968.

38. Hofer BO, Ryan JA Jr, Freeny PC: Surgical significance of vascular changes in chronic pancreatitis. Surg Gynecol Obstet 164:499, 1987.

39. Jeans PL: Hepatic artery aneurysms and biliary surgery: Two cases and a literature review. Aust NZ J Surg 58:889, 1988.

40. Jonsson K, Bjernstad A, Eriksson B: Treatment of a hepatic artery aneurysm by coil occlusion of the hepatic artery. Am J Roentgenol 134:1245, 1980.

41. Jorgensen BA: Visceral artery aneurysms. A review. Dan Med Bull 32:237, 1985.

42. Keehan MF, Kistner RL, Banis J: Angiography as an aid in extraenteric gastrointestinal bleeding due to visceral artery aneurysm. Ann Surg 187:357, 1978.

43. Kraft RO, Fry WJ: Aneurysms of the celiac artery. Surg Gynecol Obstet 117:563, 1963.

44. Kreel L: The recognition and incidence of splenic artery aneurysms. A historical review. Australas Radiol 16:126, 1972.

45. Lina JR, Jaques P, Mandell V: Aneurysm rupture secondary to transcatheter embolization. Am J Roentgenol 132:553, 1979.

46. Lowry SM, O'Dea TP, Gallagher DI, Mozenter R: Splenic artery aneurysm rupture: The seventh instance of maternal and fetal survival. Obstet Gynecol 67:291, 1986.

47. MacFarlane JR, Thorbjarnason B: Rupture of splenic artery aneurysm during pregnancy. Am J Obstet Gynecol 95:1025, 1966.

48. McNamara MF, Bakshi KR: Mesenteric artery aneurysms. In Bergan JJ, Yao JST (eds): Aneurysms. Diagnosis and Treatment. New York, Grune & Stratton, 1981, pp 285–403.

49. McNamara MF, Griska LB: Superior mesenteric artery branch aneurysms. Surgery 88:625, 1980.

50. Mandel SR, Jaques PF, Mauro MA, Sanofsky S: Nonoperative management of peripancreatic arterial aneurysms. A 10-year experience. Ann Surg 205:126, 1987.

51. Mandelbaum I, Kaiser GD, Lemple RE: Gastric intramural aneurysm as a cause for massive gastrointestinal hemorrhage. Ann Surg 155:199, 1962.

52. Manenti F, Williams R: Injection studies of the splenic vasculature in portal hypertension. Gut 7:175, 1966.

53. Martin KW, Morian JP, Lee JKT, Scharp DW: Demonstration of a splenic artery pseudoaneurysm by MR imaging. J Comput Assist Tomogr 9:190, 1985.

54. Michels NA: Collateral arterial pathways to the liver after ligation of the hepatic artery and removal of the celiac axis. Cancer 6:708, 1953.

55. Millard M: Fatal rupture of gastric aneurysm. Arch Pathol 59:363, 1955.

56. Moore SW, Guida PM, Schumacher HW: Splenic artery aneurysm. Bull Soc Int Chir 29:210, 1970.

57. Moore SW, Lewis RJ: Splenic artery aneurysm. Ann Surg 153:1033, 1961.

58. Nishida O, Moriyasu F, Nakamura T, et al: Hemodynamics of splenic artery aneurysm. Gastroenterology 90:1042, 1986.

59. Nordenstoft EL, Larsen EA: Rupture of a jejunal intramural aneurysm causing massive intestinal bleeding. Acta Chir Scand 133:256, 1967.

60. O'Grady JP, Day EJ, Toole AL, Paust JC: Splenic artery aneurysm rupture in pregnancy. A review and case report. Obstet Gynecol 50:627, 1977.

61. Okazaki M, Higashihara H, Ono H, et al: Percutaneous embolization of ruptured splanchnic artery pseudoaneurysms. Acta Radiol 32:349, 1991.

62. Owens JC, Coffey RJ: Aneurysm of the splenic artery including a report of six additional cases. Int Abstr Surg 97:313, 1953.

63. Parangi S, Oz MC, Blume RS, et al: Hepatobiliary complications of polyarteritis nodosa. Arch Surg 126:909, 1991.

64. Pitkaranta P, Haapiainen R, Kivisaari L, Schroder T: Diagnostic evaluation and aggressive surgical approach in bleeding pseudoaneurysms associated with pancreatic pseudocysts. Scand J Gastroenterol 26:58, 1991.

65. Probst P, Castaneda-Zuniga WR, Gomes AS, et al: Nonsurgical treatment of splenic-artery aneurysms. Radiology 128:619, 1978.

66. Puttini M, Aseni P, Brambilla G, Belli L: Splenic artery aneurysms in portal hypertension. J Cardiovasc Surg 23:490, 1982.

67. Quandalle P, Chambon JP, Marache P, et al: Pancreaticoduodenal artery aneurysms associated with celiac axis stenosis: Report of two cases and review of the literature. Ann Vasc Surg 4:540, 1990.

68. Reuter SR, Fry WJ, Bookstein JJ: Mesenteric artery branch aneurysms. Arch Surg 97:497, 1968.

69. Rutten APM, Sikkenk PJH: Aneurysm of the hepatic artery: Reconstruction with saphenous vein graft. Br J Surg 58:262, 1971.

70. Salo JA, Aarnio PT, Jarvinen AA, Kivilaakso EO: Aneurysms of the hepatic arteries. Am Surg 55:705, 1989.

71. Salo JA, Salmenkivi K, Tenhunen A, Kivilaakso EO: Rupture of splanchnic artery aneurysms. World J Surg 10:123, 1986.

72. Scheinin TM, Vanttinen E: Aneurysms of the splenic artery in portal hypertension. Ann Clin Res 1:165, 1969.

73. Sellke FM, Williams GB, Donovan DL, Clarke RE: Management of intra-abdominal aneurysms associated with periarteritis nodosa. J Vasc Surg 4:294, 1986.

74. Shumacker HB Jr, Siderys H: Excisional treatment of aneurysms of celiac artery. Ann Surg 148:885, 1958.

75. Spanos PK, Kloppedal EA, Murray CA: Aneurysms of the gastroduodenal and pancreaticoduodenal arteries. Am J Surg 127:345, 1974.

76. Spittell JA, Fairbairn JF, Kincaid OW, ReMine WH: Aneurysm of the splenic artery. JAMA 175:452, 1961.

77. Stabile BE, Wilson SE, Debas HT: Reduced mortality from bleeding pseudocysts and pseudoaneurysms caused by pancreatitis. Arch Surg 118:45, 1983.

78. Stanley JC: Abdominal visceral aneurysms. In Haimovici H (ed): Vascular Emergencies. New York, Appleton-Century-Crofts, 1981, pp 387–396.

79. Stanley JC, Eckhauser FE, Whitehouse WM Jr, Zelenock GB: Pancreatitis related splanchnic arterial microaneurysms and macroaneurysms. In Dent TL, Eckhauser FE, Vinik AI, Turcotte JG (eds): Pancreatic Disease. New York, Grune & Stratton, 1981, pp 325–341.

80. Stanley JC, Frey CF, Miller TA, et al: Major arterial hemorrhage. A complication of pancreatic pseudocysts and chronic pancreatitis. Arch Surg 111:435, 1976.

81. Stanley JC, Fry WJ: Pathogenesis and clinical significance of splenic artery aneurysms. Surgery 76:898, 1974.

82. Stanley JC, Gewertz BL, Bove EL, et al: Arterial fibrodysplasia. Histopathologic character and current etiologic concepts. Arch Surg 110:561, 1975.

83. Stanley JC, Thompson NW, Fry WJ: Splanchnic artery aneurysms. Arch Surg 101:689, 1970.

84. Thomford NR, Yurko JE, Smith EJ: Aneurysm of gastric arteries as a cause of intraperitoneal hemorrhage: Review of literature. Ann Surg 168:294, 1968.

85. Trastek VF, Pairolero PC, Joyce JW, et al: Splenic artery aneurysms. Surgery 91:694, 1982.
86. Trevisani MF, Ricci MA, Michaels RM, Meyer KK: Multiple mesenteric aneurysms complicating subacute bacterial endocarditis. Arch Surg 122:823, 1987.
87. Varekamp AP, Minder WH, VanNoort G, Wassenaar HA: Rupture of a submucosal gastric aneurysm, a rare cause of gastric hemorrhage. Neth J Surg 35:100, 1983.
88. Verta MJ Jr, Dean RH, Yao JST, et al: Pancreaticoduodenal artery aneurysms. Ann Surg 186:111, 1977.
89. Violago FC, Downs AR: Ruptured atherosclerotic aneurysm of the superior mesenteric artery with celiac axis occlusion. Ann Surg 174:207, 1971.
90. Weaver DH, Fleming RJ, Barnes WA: Aneurysm of the hepatic artery: The value of arteriography in surgical management. Surgery 64:891, 1968.
91. Werner K, Tarasoutchi F, Lunardi W, et al: Mycotic aneurysm of the celiac trunk and superior mesenteric artery in a case of infective endocarditis. J Cardiovasc Surg 32:380, 1991.
92. West JE, Bernhardt H, Bowers RF: Aneurysms of the pancreaticoduodenal artery. Am J Surg 115:835, 1968.
93. White AF, Baum S, Buranasiri S: Aneurysms secondary to pancreatitis. Am J Roentgenol 127:393, 1976.
94. Wright CB, Schoepfle J, Kurtock SB, et al: Gastrointestinal bleeding and mycotic superior mesenteric aneurysm. Surgery 92:40, 1982.

82

Infected Aneurysms

Daniel J. Reddy, M.D., and Calvin B. Ernst, M.D.

• • •

HISTORICAL BACKGROUND

Although aneurysmal disease was reported in Western literature in ancient times by Galen, 16 centuries passed until Ambroise Paré, writing in the mid-16th century, first noted the association between an aneurysm and infection. He described the fatal outcome and autopsy findings of a patient who suffered rupture of a syphilitic aneurysm of the descending thoracic aorta.[59]

In the last century, Rokitansky in Austria, Virkow and Koch in Germany, and Tufnell in Ireland predated Osler's landmark work with case reports associating endocarditis, septic emboli, arterial abscesses, and ruptured infected aneurysms of the superior mesenteric and popliteal arteries.[43, 73, 92, 94] Sir William Osler, in 1885, presented the first comprehensive discussion of an infected aneurysm, remarking on the "anatomical characters . . . , clinical features, and . . . etiological and pathological relations."[56] He used the term mycotic aneurysm to describe these infected aneurysms, which had developed as complications of bacterial endocarditis. Since there was no apparent association with fungal disease, Osler's choice of the term mycotic has been a source of discussion and confusion in the literature. Some have used the term mycotic aneurysm when referring to infected aneurysm regardless of pathogenesis.[1, 2, 7, 14, 16, 21, 32, 37, 55, 61, 63, 90, 96, 97] Fungal infection is *not* implied when using this designation. Strictly speaking, the term mycotic aneurysm should be used only when describing an infected aneurysm resulting from bacterial endocarditis complicated by septic arterial emboli or an infected aneurysm of the sinus of Valsalva resulting from contiguous spread from an infected aortic valve. Following Osler by 2 years, Eppinger provided evidence supporting the embolic etiology of a mycotic aneurysm when he documented identical strains of bacteria in both the peripheral embolus and the valvular vegetations of a patient with a mycotic aneurysm.[27]

At the turn of this century, Lewis and Schrager reviewed several cases of mycotic aneurysm occurring in young patients with endocarditis.[46] They commented on a case reported by Ruge involving a streptococcal coronary artery aneurysm in a 12-year-old boy with streptococcal osteomyelitis and advanced the hypothesis that not all infected aneurysms were "embolomycotic" in origin.

In 1923, Stengel and Wolferth described four patients and reviewed another 213 in whom a total of 382 bacterial aneurysms of intravascular origin had been found.[85] Multiple aneurysms were found in 49 patients. Although aortic, mesenteric, and intracranial mycotic aneurysms predominated, virtually every other named vessel in the arterial tree was also involved. Of greater significance in the evolving understanding of the pathogenesis of infected aneurysms was the finding that in 30 patients (14 per cent) there was no evidence of bacterial endocarditis, thereby demonstrating that infected aneurysms occur in connection with a variety of other septic conditions.

In 1937, Crane presented the clinical course and autopsy findings of a 35-year-old man with a primary multilocular infected aortic arch aneurysm in association with a hypoplastic aorta and infected superior mesenteric arterial aneurysm. He postulated that in arteries predisposed by disease, blood-borne bacteria could settle and produce infected aneurysms.[18] Six years later, this hypothesis—that bacteremia unassociated with endocarditis could cause an infected aneurysm—was confirmed by Revell.[72] Subsequent authors reported that atherosclerotic vessels were susceptible to bacterial infection, particularly by various Salmonella species.[10, 16, 22, 35, 36, 57, 61, 69, 83, 89, 91, 102] Such arterial infections are considered to be examples of microbial arteritis starting in nonaneurysmal arteries and producing infected aneurysms after the vessel wall has been destroyed by infection.

The classification of infected aneurysm was further refined by Sommerville's 1959 report of more than 20,000 Mayo Clinic autopsies as they related to atherosclerotic abdominal aortic aneurysms. In all, 178 aneurysms (0.8 per cent) were found. Of these, 172 were bland (97 per cent) and 6 were infected (3 per cent). Four of the six infected aneurysms had ruptured.[82] This report established the existence of a third type of arterial infection: namely, that which occurs in a preexisting atherosclerotic aneurysm. Bennett and Cherry in 1967, Mundth in 1969, and Jarrett in 1975 each reported series detailing the clinical course, bacteriology, treatment, and outcome for patients with this type of infected aneurysm.[9, 39, 54] With the advent of antibiotic therapy, the overall incidence of arterial infection declined, paralleling the successful treatment of bacterial endocarditis.[91]

In more recent years, however, the incidence of arterial infections and infected aneurysms has increased in response to the increasing prevalence of immune suppressed hosts,[35, 40, 44] invasive hemodynamic monitoring,[81] angiography,[5, 29] and drug addiction.[1, 42, 58, 62, 66] This change in pathogenesis has been noted by other authors who emphasize that a fourth type of infected aneurysm has emerged as a significant clinical entity: namely, post-traumatic infected false aneurysms.[100] The greatest number of such infected aneurysms have been associated with intravenous or intra-arterial drug injections.[42]

CLASSIFICATION

Based upon the foregoing historical review and the classifications suggested by others,[50, 100] this chapter considers four types of infected aneurysm: (1) mycotic aneurysms (i.e., from septic arterial emboli); (2) microbial arteritis with aneurysm; (3) infected preexisting aneurysms; and (4) post-traumatic infected false aneurysms. Excluded are aneurysms resulting from contiguous infection, spontaneous aortoenteric fistulae, and infections of synthetic vascular prostheses (Table 82–1).

MYCOTIC ANEURYSMS

Incidence

Mycotic aneurysms develop when septic emboli of cardiac origin lodge in the lumen or the vasa vasorum of peripheral arteries. This can occur in both normal and abnormal arteries.

In the preantibiotic era, approximately 90 per cent of all infected aneurysms were mycotic aneurysms.[46, 72, 85] They occurred in virtually every named artery intracranially, in the great vessels, the thoracoabdominal aorta, and the visceral, extremity, pulmonary, and coronary arteries. The century following Osler's initial description of this entity saw the discovery of antibiotic therapy, the advancement of microbiologic techniques allowing identification and treatment of specific bacterial infections, and the development of open heart surgery to permit replacement of the infected cardiac valve. These advances have sharply lowered the incidence of mycotic aneurysms occurring as embolic complications of infective endocarditis.[48]

In 1949, Cates and Christie reported the results of penicillin treatment of 442 patients with endocarditis.[15] One hundred and forty-five patients (35 per cent) suffered a major arterial embolization, and 20 (4.5 per cent) died after hemorrhage from a mycotic aneurysm, a marked improvement over previously quoted embolism rates of 80 per cent.[56] In a comprehensive review of infected aneurysms, Brown and associates found that endocarditis was implicated in the pathogenesis of only 16 per cent of all reported infected aneurysms and in only 10 per cent of cases since 1965.[12]

The relationship between bacterial endocarditis and peripheral arterial embolization has been reported from the Henry Ford Hospital.[24, 25, 47, 80] Hospital admissions for peripheral (extracranial) embolization during the period 1950 to 1964 were 23.1 per 100,000 and during the period 1960 to 1979 were 50.4 per 100,000. During this interval (1950 to 1979), 225 patients were admitted for 337 individual emboli.[48] Only two patients from this group developed a mycotic aneurysm from these emboli,[24] and both were treated between 1957 and 1961, giving a hospital incidence of mycotic aneurysm of 1 per 35,000 during that 5-year period. Since 1962, mycotic aneurysms occurring as an

Table 82–1. Clinical Characteristics of Infected Aneurysms

	Mycotic Aneurysm	Microbial Arteritis	Infection of Existing Aneurysm	Post-Traumatic Infected False Aneurysm
Etiology	Endocarditis	Bacteremia	Bacteremia	Narcotic addiction Trauma
Age (years)	30–50	>50	>50	<30
Incidence	Rare	Common	Unusual	Very common
Location	Aorta Visceral Intracranial Peripheral	Atherosclerotic Aortoiliac Intimal defects	Infrarenal Aorta	Femoral Carotid
Bacteriology	Gram-positive cocci	*Salmonella* Others	*Staphylococcus* Others	*Staphylococcus aureus* Polymicrobial
Mortality	25%	75%	90%	5%

From Wilson SE, Van Wagenen P, Passaro E Jr: Arterial infection. Curr Probl Surg 15:5, 1978. Reproduced with permission of Year Book Medical Publishers, Inc.

Table 82–2.   Frequency Distribution of Infected Aneurysms

Artery	Preantibiotic Era (1909–1943)			1968–1986	
Pulmonary	11	(3%)			
Coronary	8	(2%)			
Aorta	87	(25%)	Aorta	20	(12%)
Iliac	14	(4%)	Iliac	9	(5%)
Gluteal	2	(<1%)			
Upper extremity	35	(10%)	Upper extremity	10	(13%)
Subclavian (3)			Subclavian (3)		
Axillary (1)			Axillary (2)		
Brachial (8)			Brachial (3)		
Radial (1)			Radial (4)		
Ulnar (2)					
Lower extremity	40	(12%)	Lower extremity	69	(63%)
Femoral (10)			Femoral (69)		
Popliteal (2)					
Visceral	87	(25%)	Visceral	3	(2%)
Celiac (1)			Superior mesenteric (2)		
Hepatic (15)			Renal (1)		
Superior mesenteric (47)					
Splenic (18)					
Renal (5)					
Gastroepiploic (1)					
Extracranial cerebral vascular	3	(<1%)	Extracranial cerebral vascular	2	(1%)
Innominate (1)			Carotid (2)		
Carotid (1)					
Vertebral (1)					
Intracranial cerebral	50	(15%)	Intracranial cerebral	6	(4%)
Other	7	(2%)			
Totals	344	(100%)		168	(100%)

Compiled from various reports in references 1, 42, 46, 54, 66, 72, 85.

embolic complication of endocarditis have been encountered in only eight patients. Six of these eight aneurysms involved the intracranial arteries.[47]

During the period 1971 to 1983, Johansen and Devin reported that nine patients with infective endocarditis were treated for 14 episodes of mycotic embolization resulting in 17 individual emboli.[40] Six of these nine patients required cardiac valve replacement, but none developed a mycotic aneurysm. During the period 1972 to 1984, 91 patients underwent cardiac valve replacement for endocarditis, five of whom developed a mycotic cerebral aneurysm.[48] This decreasing incidence of mycotic aneurysms both in absolute terms and as a percentage of infected aneurysms has been noted by other authors.[1, 39, 46, 48, 82, 100]

Location

Even though mycotic aneurysms may occur in multiple sites in a given patient, certain anatomic locations predominate,[56] namely, the aorta and the intracranial, superior mesenteric, and femoral arteries (Table 82–2).[48, 85] The predilection of mycotic aneurysms for certain anatomic sites relates to their pathogenesis. For aneurysms of larger arteries, such as the aorta, infected emboli may lodge in the relatively large vasa vasorum, causing vessel wall ischemia and infection. As the media is destroyed by this process, an aneurysm forms. In smaller arteries, the infected macroscopic emboli may lodge in the vessel lumen or wall and initiate a similar pathologic process. Sites predisposed to

the formation of mycotic aneurysms are bifurcations, arteriovenous fistulae, and coarctations.[46, 70]

Bacteriology

Because mycotic aneurysms develop as a complication of endocarditis, the organisms isolated from arterial blood or cardiac valve vegetations of endocarditis cause mycotic aneurysms. In 1923, Stengel and Wolferth reported that the predominant organisms were nonhemolytic streptococci, pneumococci, and staphylocci.[85] In 1986, Magilligan and Quinn reported that the dominant infecting organisms in patients with no history of drug abuse (n = 55) with native valve endocarditis were *Streptococcus viridans* (22 per cent), *Staphylococcus aureus* (20 per cent), *Streptococcus faecalis* (14 per cent), and *Staphylococcus epidermidis* (11 per cent). Exotic bacteria such as *Eikenella corrodens* and *Propionibacterium acnes* and the fungus *Aspergillus* were also noted. In narcotic addicts (n = 36) the infecting organisms were *S. aureus* (36 per cent), *Pseudomonas* (16 per cent), polymicrobial species (15 per cent), *S. faecalis* (13 per cent), and *S. viridans* (11 per cent). Exotic organisms such as *Micrococcus, Corynebacterium,* and *Candida albicans* were also isolated.[48] The responsible organism in each of the six intracerebral mycotic aneurysms among these 91 patients was *S. faecalis* (3), *S. viridans* (1), *Pseudomonas* (1), and *C. albicans* (1).[48] Brown reported in 1984 that *S. aureus* and various streptococcal species accounted for 38 per cent of infected aneurysms of all types (Table 82–3).[12]

Table 82–3. Organisms Cultured From Infected Aneurysms: Collected Series From Review of English Language Literature

Organism	Prior to 1965	After 1965	Total
Salmonella species	14 (38%)	15 (10%)	29 (15%)
Staphylococcus aureus	7 (19%)	47 (30%)	54 (28%)
Streptococcus species	5 (14%)	15 (10%)	20 (10%)
Pseudomonas species	1	6	7
Staphylococcus epidermidis	1	5	6
Escherichia coli	—	4	4
Proteus species	2	1	3
Serratia species	—	3	3
Enterobacter species	—	3	3
Neisseria species	—	3	3
Clostridium species	—	2	2
Enterococcus group	—	2	2
Bacteroides species	—	2	2
Candida species	—	2	2
Klebsiella species	—	2	2
Bacteroides fragilis	—	1	1
Peptostreptococcus species	—	1	1
Corynebacterium species	—	1	1
Arizona hinshawii	—	1	1
Citrobacter freundii	—	1	1
Culture negative	7 (19%)	41 (25%)	48 (25%)
Total	37	158	195

From Brown SL, Busutill RW, Baker JD, et al: Bacteriologic and surgical determinants of survival in patients with mycotic aneurysms. J Vasc Surg 1:541, 1984.

MICROBIAL ARTERITIS WITH ANEURYSM

Incidence and Location

In the preantibiotic era, microbial arteritis with aneurysm occurred in approximately 14 per cent of patients.[85] In modern times, owing to the decline in rheumatic fever and bacterial endocarditis, microbial arteritis with aneurysm is becoming more prevalent than mycotic aneurysm.[12] This increase is due to the aging of the population and the corresponding increase in atherosclerosis, which is an important factor predisposing arteries to infection. The inci-

dence of infected aneurysms produced by microbial arteritis is estimated to be 0.06 to 0.65 per cent.[10, 69] Diseased intima, which, when normal, is highly resistant to infection, allows blood-borne bacteria to inoculate the arterial wall. Once infection is established, suppuration, localized perforation, and false aneurysm formation follow (Fig. 82–1). Supporting atherosclerosis as the principal predisposing factor in the pathogenesis of microbial arteritis is the fact that the aorta, the most frequent site of atherosclerosis, is also the most frequent location of these lesions (by a 3 to 1 margin over peripheral sites).[9, 16, 54, 55, 60, 63] In the authors' series, microbial arteritis accounted for 77 per cent of infected aortoiliac aneurysms (Table 82–4).[69] There has been

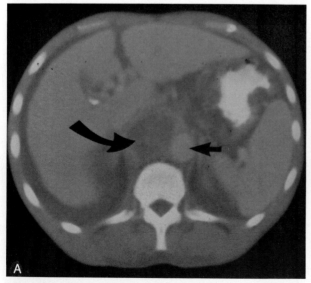
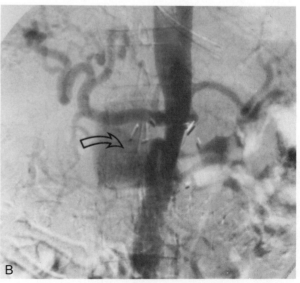

FIGURE 82–1. Diagnostic radiology studies of a patient with a *Staphylococcus aureus* microbial aortitis with aneurysm. *A,* contrast-enhanced computed tomogram demonstrates contained rupture of infected aneurysm *(curved arrow)* and the adjacent aorta *(straight arrow)*. *B,* Digital subtraction aortogram demonstrates saccular eccentric infected aneurysm of the infrarenal aorta *(arrow)*.

Table 82–4. Anatomic Location and Type of Infected Aneurysm

Type of Aneurysm	No. of Aneuryms*			Total No. (%) of Aneurysms
	SRAA	**IRAA**	**CIA**	
Microbial arteritis	3	5	2	10 (77)
Mycotic aneurysm	0	0	1	1 (7.7)
Infection in preexisting aneurysm	0	1	0	1 (7.7)
Adjacent soft-tissue infection	0	1	0	1 (7.7)
Total (%)	3 (23)	7 (54)	3 (23)	13 (100)

From Reddy DJ, Shepard AD, Evans JR, et al: Management of infected aorto-iliac aneurysms. Arch Surg 126:873–879, 1991. Copyright 1991, American Medical Association.

*SRAA, suprarenal abdominal aorta; IRAA, infrarenal abdominal aorta; CIA, common iliac artery.

speculation that patients with the acquired immunodeficiency syndrome may be susceptible to infectious aortitis. They could, therefore, represent a large cohort that will increase the incidence and alter the microbiology of this pathologic entity in the future.[22, 35]

Bacteriology

The predominant microorganisms associated with microbial arteritis leading to aneurysm are *Salmonella, Staphylococcus,* and *Escherichia coli.*[100] *Bacteroides fragilis* aneurysms of the suprarenal aorta have been reported recently, highlighting the necessity of culturing for anaerobes in these cases.[69, 86] The overall 25 per cent culture-negative rate may indicate a deficiency in obtaining anaerobic cultures (see Table 82–3).

The importance of *Salmonella* species in microbial arteritis, particularly microbial aortitis, has been highlighted in many series and confirmed in our own review at the Henry Ford Hospital.[69] The diseased aorta has a unique vulnerability to *Salmonella* (Fig. 82–2). The most virulent species are *S. choleraesuis* and *S. typhimurium,* which account for 62 per cent of the reported cases of *Salmonella* arteritis.[100]

INFECTION OF PREEXISTING ANEURYSMS

Incidence and Location

The incidence of infection in preexisting atherosclerotic aneurysms was estimated by Sommerville and associates to be 3.4 per cent.[82] Bennett and Cherry and Jarrett and colleagues each reported parallel findings noting the relative rarity of this lesion as well as its propensity for rupture.[9, 39]

The related entity of aortic aneurysms colonized by bacteria has been identified in two nearly simultaneous reports by Ernst and colleagues and Williams and Fisher.[28, 98] Patients undergoing abdominal aortic aneurysmectomy were studied prospectively with operative bacterial cultures taken from the aneurysm wall and contents and from bowel bag fluid. Overall, 15 per cent of cultures yielded positive results.[28] There was a higher incidence of positive cultures among patients with ruptured aneurysms (38 per cent) compared with those with asymptomatic (9 per cent) and symptomatic (13 per cent) aneurysms.[28] Even though the clinical significance of these findings is unknown, it appears that colonized aneurysms do not pose the same threat to patients as infected aneurysms.

The abdominal aorta is the predominant site reported for secondary infection of aneurysms. Lesions have been noted in other locations, and in earlier times, bacterial overgrowth in luetic aneurysms of the thoracic aorta was encountered.[100]

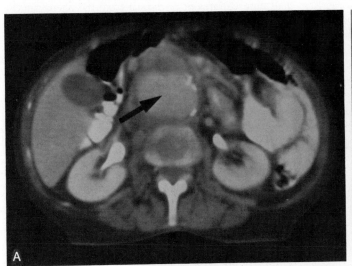
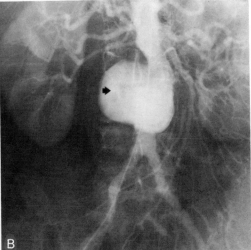

FIGURE 82–2. Diagnostic radiology studies of a patient with a *Salmonella* infection of a preexisting small atherosclerotic aneurysm. *A,* Contrast-enhanced computed tomogram demonstrates saccular aneurysm with calcification *(arrow). B,* Transfemoral aortogram demonstrates saccular atherosclerotic infrarenal aneurysm *(arrow).*

Table 82–5.   Etiology of Infected Aneurysms: Collected Series From a Published Review of English Literature

Etiology	Prior to 1965	After 1965	Total
Arterial trauma	4 (10%)	71 (51%)	75 (42%)
Endocarditis	15 (37%)	14 (10%)	29 (16%)
Local infection	3 (7%)	6 (4%)	9 (5%)
Bacteremia	—	9 (6%)	9 (5%)
Retroperitoneal abscess	2 (5%)	2 (1%)	4 (2%)
Gastrointestinal tract	1 (2%)	3 (2%)	4 (2%)
Oropharynx	—	3 (2%)	3 (2%)
Pneumonia	1 (2%)	—	1(<1%)
Carcinoma	—	1 (1%)	1(<1%)
Unknown	15 (36%)	30 (22%)	45 (25%)
Total	41	139	180

From Brown SL, Busutill RW, Baker JD, et al: Bacteriologic and surgical determinants of survival in patients with mycotic aneurysms. J Vasc Surg 1:541, 1984.

Bacteriology

Some authors have noted that the index of suspicion for infected abdominal aortic aneurysm is generally low, and as a consequence, these lesions may have been under-reported.[98] Jarrett and colleagues' series of infected preexisting abdominal aortic aneurysms showed a predominance of gram-positive organisms (59 per cent) over gram-negative organisms (35 per cent). The most prevalent organism was *Staphylococcus* (41 per cent). Though less common, gram-negative infections were more virulent than gram-positive infections from the standpoints of aneurysm rupture (84 per cent vs. 10 per cent) and patient mortality (84 per cent vs. 50 per cent).[39] In another study, colonized aneurysms yielded 81 per cent gram-positive and 19 per cent gram-negative organisms. The most prevalent organism was *S. epidermidis*, accounting for 53 per cent of positive cultures.[28]

POST-TRAUMATIC INFECTED FALSE ANEURYSMS

Incidence and Location

Post-traumatic infected false aneurysms have become the dominant type of infected aneurysm in recent decades (Table 82–5). The primary factor in this shifting emphasis in pathogenesis is drug addition. In the 25 years following Huebl and Read's initial report of two infected femoral artery false aneurysms in narcotic addicts,[38] there have been an additional 195 such cases reported (Table 82–6).

The femoral artery, used by narcotic addicts for repeated groin injections, is the most common site in which these lesions occur (Fig. 82–3). Other locations, such as the external iliac and carotid arteries have been reported (Fig. 82–4).[42, 45, 53]

Another factor contributing to the increasing incidence of these lesions is the proliferation of various invasive testing and monitoring procedures. In susceptible individuals, percutaneous arterial puncture may result in an iatrogenic post-traumatic infected false aneurysm.[5, 81]

Bacteriology

Since 1965, when the most prevalent form of infected aneurysm has been post-traumatic infected false aneurysm, the most likely infecting organism has been *S. aureus* (30 per cent).[12] In one report of infected femoral artery false aneurysms in drug addicts, 35 of 54 patients (65 per cent) had pure cultures of *S. aureus* from the aneurysm. Seventeen of these 35 staphylococcal cultures (48 per cent) were found to be methicillin resistant. An additional eight pa-

Table 82–6.   Summary of Reported Cases of Infected Femoral Artery False Aneurysms in Drug Addicts

Year of Report	First Author	No. of Cases
1966	Huebl[38]	2
1970	Fromm[32]	5
1974	Geelhoed[33]	1
1974	Anderson[1]	3
1977	Yellin[102]	2
1983	Feldman[31]	53
1983	Johnson[42]	38
1986	Reddy[66]	53
1988	Patel[62]	16
1992	Padberg[58]	23
Total		195

After Reddy DJ, Smith RF, Elliott JP, et al: Infected femoral artery false aneurysms in drug addicts: Evolution of selective vascular reconstruction. J Vasc Surg 3:718, 1986.

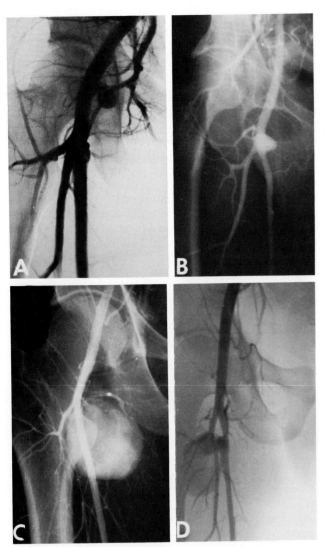

FIGURE 82–3. Arteriograms demonstrate the appearance of an infected femoral artery false aneurysm in each of four locations: *A*, common femoral artery; *B*, common femoral bifurcation; *C*, deep femoral artery; and *D*, superficial femoral artery. (*A–D*, From Reddy DJ, Smith RF, Elliott JP Jr, et al: Infected femoral artery false aneurysms in drug addicts: Evolution of selective vascular reconstruction. J Vasc Surg 3:718, 1986.)

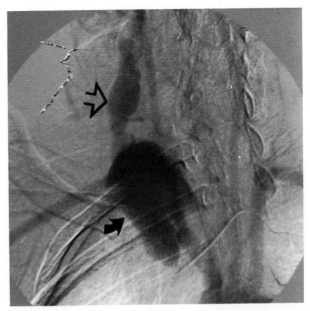

FIGURE 82–4. Digital subtraction angiogram of a patient with polymicrobial post-traumatic false aneurysm of the innominate artery caused by repeated cervical injections of narcotics *(closed arrow)*. There was an associated arteriovenous fistula to the internal jugular vein *(open arrow)* and a right recurrent laryngeal nerve paralysis.

tients (33 per cent) had mixed polymicrobial cultures including *S. aureus, E. coli, S. faecalis, Pseudomonas aeruginosa*, and various enterobacter organisms.[66] Johnson and coworkers, reporting on drug-related infected false aneurysms in a variety of anatomic locations, isolated *S. aureus* from a high percentage of blood (71 per cent) and wound (76 per cent) cultures.[42]

CLINICAL PRESENTATION

The clinical presentation of infected aneurysms depends upon the etiology and the anatomic site involved. Clinical characteristics of the different aneurysm types are summarized in Table 82–1.

Although infected aneurysms occur in all age groups, including neonates,[90] when there is no antecedent history of arterial injury, the typical patient is elderly and atherosclerotic.[8, 82] The principal signs and symptoms of an aneurysm and sepsis may be subtle (Table 82–7). Infection in a recognized abdominal aortic aneurysm may be very difficult to detect. Infected aortic aneurysms usually present with fever of unknown origin. Because of the insidious presentation of infected aneurysms, a high index of suspicion is needed whenever aneurysm patients have positive blood cultures, erosion of lumbar vertebrae, are women, have an uncalcified aneurysm, or have an aneurysm that first appeared after bacterial sepsis.[14, 16, 39, 95] As many as 40 per cent of infected abdominal aortic aneurysms may not be palpable and may go unrecognized until they rupture.[54, 93, 101] On the other hand, infected aneurysms of the femoral or carotid artery or other more easily examined peripheral locations are readily appreciated, and up to 90 per cent are palpable.[54] Infected femoral false aneurysms, for example, present with either a tender groin mass, indicating contained rupture; with some other manifestation of sepsis; or with bleeding in almost every patient.[58, 62, 66]

Table 82–7. Infected Aneurysms: Clinical Presentation

Clinical Marker	No. (%) of Patients
Abdominal pain	12 (92)
Fever	10 (77)
Leukocytosis*	9 (69)
Positive blood cultures	9 (69)
Palpable abdominal mass	6 (46)
Rupture	4 (31)

From Reddy DJ, Shepard AD, Evans JR, et al: Management of infected aorto-iliac aneurysms. Arch Surg 126:873–879, 1991. Copyright 1991, American Medical Association.

Leukocyte count >10.0 × 10⁹/L.

Fungal arterial infections are rare but characteristically occur in patients with chronic immune suppression[44] or diabetes mellitus[51] or after treatment for disseminated fungal disease.[52] The clinical presentation of these rare infections may be limited to fever or malaise or may be more apparent, with gangrene in an extremity following distal embolization.

Even though they can occur in virtually any artery and present with a variety of clinical signs and symptoms, infected aneurysms are alike in that they all lead to sepsis or hemorrhage. Consequently, whenever the surgeon suspects this diagnosis he or she must assume that the patient's life or limb is in jeopardy and proceed to confirmation of the diagnosis and urgent surgical therapy.

DIAGNOSIS

Laboratory Studies

In most patients, leukocytosis is a sensitive but nonspecific indicator of an infected aneurysm.[10, 39, 66, 69, 89] The sensitivity of this finding, however, may be limited by intercurrent antimicrobial therapy that has suppressed but not cured the infection.[52] A lack of specificity is also noted by reports indicating that sealed ruptures of bland, uninfected, atherosclerotic aneurysms may simulate sepsis and exhibit leukocytosis.[87] Likewise, an elevated erythrocyte sedimentation rate is often present but nonspecific. These limitations underscore the need for more specific and sensitive tests to confirm the presence of an infected aneurysm (see Table 82–7).

Positive blood cultures in a patient with an aneurysm are considered specific for an infected aneurysm until proved otherwise. However, positive cultures lack sensitivity. Anderson and colleagues found positive cultures in only 50 per cent of patients.[1] It follows that negative blood cultures alone are not sufficiently sensitive to rule out the diagnosis of an infected aneurysm.

When the diagnosis of an infected aneurysm is first entertained during operation, samples of the aneurysm wall and contents should be cultured for aerobic and anaerobic bacteria and fungi. Additional information may be gained by Gram's stains. However, these studies should not be considered sufficient to ensure that the aneurysm is not infected because neither negative blood cultures nor intraoperative Gram's stains are sufficiently sensitive to exclude the diagnosis of infected aneurysm.[12] Moreover, results of culture of the aneurysm wall and contents are not available during the operation and can only be used to direct postoperative antimicrobial therapy, and even final culture results may be misleading in patients treated with antibiotics. Some authors have advocated wider use of aneurysm content and wall cultures in routine operations for aortic aneurysm.[28, 39] In our experience with infected aortoiliac aneurysms, 69 per cent of patients had positive preoperative blood cultures, and 92 per cent had positive aneurysm wall cultures. Operative Gram's stains were positive in 50 per cent of those with ruptured infected aneurysms but in only 11 per cent of those with nonruptured but infected aneurysms.[69]

Radiologic Studies

Aortic aneurysms associated with vertebral body erosion or those devoid of calcification should raise the suspicion of an infected aneurysm. Plain films are not sufficiently sensitive to confirm the diagnosis, and additional studies are needed. Of value are computed tomography and either conventional or digital subtraction angiography. Although sonography of the abdominal aorta provides general information about aneurysm size and location, it is unreliable for diagnosing the presence or extent of arterial infection. When sonography has been used to evaluate infected femoral artery false aneurysms, it was found to be insensitive (Fig. 82–5).[66] In contrast, the utility of intravenous digital subtraction angiography in evaluating the femoral artery for infected aneurysm has been established.[79] It is of particular value in drug addicts and has been used to screen for similar lesions in the great vessels and the arteries of both the upper and lower extremities. Digital subtraction angiography is of comparable diagnostic accuracy and may be less expensive and more easily accomplished than conventional angiography.[79]

Arteriography, either digital subtraction or conventional, is indispensable in the evaluation of patients in whom an infected aneurysm is suspected. The angiographic criteria for infection in an aneurysm are (1) saccular aneurysm in an otherwise normal-appearing vessel; (2) multilobulated aneurysm; and (3) eccentric aneurysm with a relatively narrow neck (Figs. 82–1 to 82–6). However, an infected aneurysm may not exhibit any angiographic characteristics indicative of infection.[96]

Contrast-enhanced computed tomography is of value in determining etiology and assessing the presence or absence of aneurysm rupture (Figs. 82–1 and 82–2) but often fails to give specific information about the presence or absence of infection.[34] Magnetic resonance imaging may prove helpful in certain locations or in patients in whom radiography or contrast media are contraindicated.

Although some practitioners have found indium-111–labeled white blood cell scanning useful in diagnosing prosthetic graft infection, it has not been of demonstrated utility in confirming the diagnosis of infected aneurysm.[13]

MANAGEMENT

Preoperative Care

When an infected aneurysm is suspected but efforts to identify the specific organisms are unsuccessful, broad-spectrum antibiotic therapy should be initiated. Chloramphenicol or ampicillin should be included to cover *Salmonella*. Drug therapy is begun before operation and continued postoperatively and, in certain circumstances, for life.[16, 19] Treatment of narcotic addicts should include active and passive tetanus prophylaxis. Even though organism-specific antibiotic therapy is an essential element of successful surgical management of an infected aneurysm, patient survival depends on prompt diagnosis and operation.[39, 69] Rupture of infected aneurysms has been reported in patients undergoing antibiotic therapy while awaiting operation or in those who have completed anti-

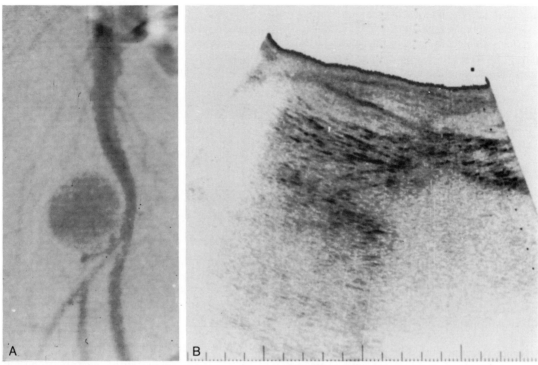

FIGURE 82–5.   Comparison of two diagnostic modalities in the same patient with an infected femoral false aneurysm. *A*, The digital subtraction angiogram confirms the diagnosis. *B*, The sonogram lacks diagnostic clarity and precision.

FIGURE 82–6.   Femoral arteriogram of patient with a post-traumatic infected false aneurysm of the common femoral artery demonstrates a lobulated aneurysm. *Inset*, Resected femoral artery specimen showing the injured and infected artery.

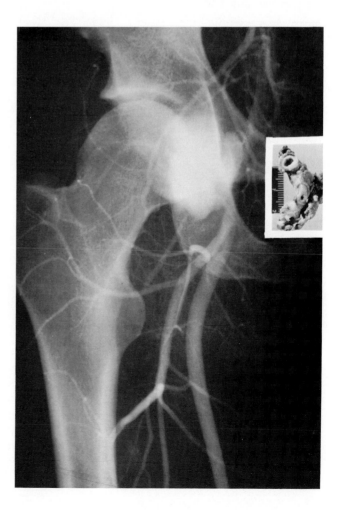

biotic therapy and are thought to have sterilized aneurysms.[15, 17, 82] Undue delay in operative intervention must be avoided. Reported spontaneous cures of infected aneurysms are exceptions.[40] In cases of a ruptured or symptomatic aneurysm, operation should be undertaken urgently.

Operation

General Principles. Six general principles apply in the operative management of infected aneurysms: (1) control of hemorrhage; (2) confirmation of the diagnosis, including tissue smears for Gram's stains and culture specimens for aerobic and anaerobic bacteria and fungi; (3) operative control of sepsis, including aneurysm resection and ligation of healthy artery followed by wide débridement of all surrounding infected tissue with antibiotic irrigation and placement of drains when needed; (4) thorough postoperative wound care, including dressing changes and necessary débridement; (5) continuation of antibiotics for a prolonged period after operation; (6) arterial reconstruction of vital arteries through uninfected tissue planes with selected use of interposition grafting through the bed of the resected aneurysm and use of autologous tissue for reconstruction.

The first five principles listed are established uncontroversial surgical tenets. Disagreement exists, however, about the selection of patients for arterial reconstruction and the timing and methods of reconstruction, particularly when the infected aneurysm involves the aorta, the femoral artery, or the carotid artery.*

---

*See references 2, 12, 16, 30, 31, 41, 42, 57, 58, 61, 66, 67, 68, 89 and 91.

Aorta. The classic approach to managing an infected aneurysm of the abdominal aorta parallels the treatment of infected aortic prostheses. The entire aneurysm is resected, the infected tissues are thoroughly débrided, drainage is established, and arterial reconstruction is carried out through uninfected planes by an axillobifemoral bypass.[25, 30, 39, 89] This conservative approach avoids the risks associated with the placement of a graft in the infected retroperitoneum, which is reported to be associated with an overall 23 per cent reoperation rate, which increases to 63 per cent when the infecting organism is gram negative.[30] Axillofemoral bypass, however, is a less durable reconstruction compared with successful interposition aortic grafting.[65, 69, 91] Moreover, some recent reports advocate ''in situ'' interposition aortic grafts as the principal mode of arterial reconstruction after resection of an infected aortic aneurysm.[12, 16, 41, 57, 91] The adjunctive use of antibiotic-releasing beads implanted in the perigraft tissue has been reported.[61] Others have speculated about the use of aortic homografts, but unfavorable previous experience with the late fate of homografts in noninfected sites argues against their use.[4, 88] It appears that this approach may be justified in favorable lesions with little or no gross sepsis, but it should be avoided when the retroperitoneum is grossly purulent. Even complex reconstruction of the suprarenal aorta may be accomplished with extra-anatomic techniques.[65] In infected aneurysms of the aortic arch, thoracic aorta and suprarenal abdominal aorta interposition grafting may be the only feasible approach.[2, 16]

Femoral Artery. Management options in the treatment of infected femoral artery aneurysms are arterial excision

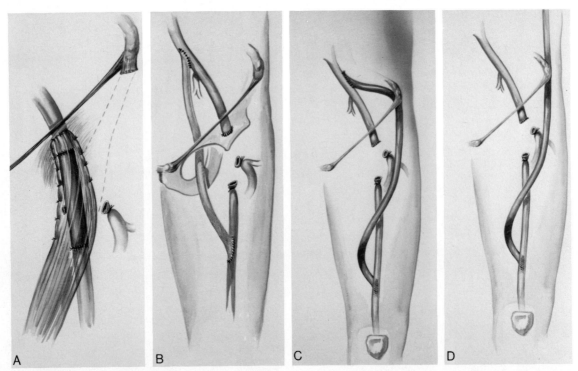

FIGURE 82–7. Methods of femoral artery reconstruction. *A*, Interposition vein autograft covered by rotated sartorius muscle; *B*, obturator bypass; *C*, lateral femoral bypass; *D*, axillodistal femoral bypass. (*A–D*, From Reddy DJ, Smith RF, Elliott JP Jr, et al: Infected femoral artery false aneurysms in drug addicts: Evolution of selective vascular reconstruction. J Vasc Surg 3:718, 1986.)

Table 82–8. Treatment Method and Results for Infected Femoral Artery False Aneurysms Resulting From Drug Addiction

	No.	Viable Limb	Graft Sepsis	Amputation
Common femoral artery				
Ligation-excision	14	14	—	0
Deep femoral artery				
Ligation-excision	11	11	—	0
Superficial femoral artery				
Ligation-excision	4	4	—	0
Common femoral bifurcation				
Ligation-excision	21	14	—	7 (33%)
Reconstruction with autogenous vein	6	6	1	0
Reconstruction with synthetic prosthesis	3	3	3 (100%)	0
Reconstruction by primary anastomosis	1	1	0	0
Totals	60	53	4	7 (12%)

From Reddy DJ, Smith RF, Elliott JP Jr, et al: Infected femoral artery false aneurysms in drug addicts: Evolution of selective vascular reconstruction. J Vasc Surg 3:718, 1986.

alone or arterial excision followed by arterial reconstruction. The various operative techniques for arterial reconstruction are illustrated in Figure 82–7.

If the cause of the infected aneurysm is other than drug injection, obturator bypass or interposition grafting appears to be the preferred method in most patients. Drug addicts are unsuitable candidates for arterial reconstruction with synthetic arterial prostheses because continued drug use carries a very high risk of graft infection (Table 82–8).[1, 58, 66] In this select group of patients, when reconstruction of the femoral artery is considered desirable, it is necessary to control groin sepsis and to use autogenous grafts. Surprisingly, greater saphenous vein from the mid-thigh usually is available even in patients with a long history of drug addiction (Fig. 82–8).[66]

Although selection criteria and methods of femoral arterial reconstruction in drug addicts are controversial, there is general agreement that most patients do not require reconstruction to avoid amputation.[31, 42, 58, 61, 66] Collateral circulation is usually sufficient to maintain limb viability even after the femoral artery bifurcation has been ligated (Fig. 82–9). In fact, amputation is almost always avoidable when femoral artery ligation-excision is limited to a single femoral artery segment—the common, superficial, or deep (Table 82–8) femoral artery. Patients at risk for amputation are those in whom the femoral artery bifurcation must be excised. Under these circumstances, autogenous vein interposition reconstruction may be considered when local wound conditions are favorable, although experience with this technique is limited.[66] The optimum management of these lesions is a matter of debate.[61, 62, 66, 67, 68] It is generally agreed that operative therapy is required, and prolonged use of antibiotics is inappropriate. Hyperbaric oxygen therapy may be of benefit.

Carotid Artery. Although ligation without arterial reconstruction is often safe when treating infected aneurysms of the innominate, common carotid, or upper extremity vessels, there is a major risk of stroke or death following ligation of the cervical internal carotid artery. Although it is unsettled, many authors favor ligation-excision without

reconstruction, preferring to avoid the potential disastrous consequences of postreconstruction graft sepsis and hemorrhage.[37, 45] Others favor primary reconstruction of the carotid artery with vein autograft[53, 76] or progressive clamp

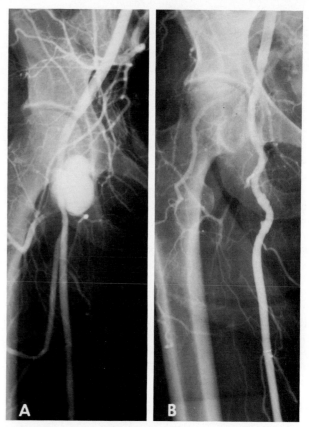

FIGURE 82–8. Angiographic sequence demonstrates preoperative appearance of infected false aneurysm of femoral bifurcation *(A)* and postoperative appearance of patent interposition vein graft after arterial reconstruction *(B)*. *(A and B, From Reddy DJ, Smith RF, Elliott JP Jr, et al: Infected femoral artery false aneurysms in drug addicts: Evolution of selective vascular reconstruction. J Vasc Surg 3:718, 1986.)*

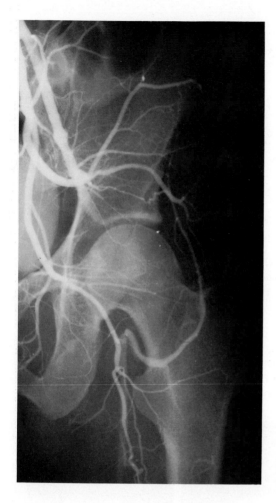

FIGURE 82-9. Arteriogram following ligation of femoral artery bifurcation demonstrates reconstitution of superficial femoral artery beyond the occlusion by numerous collaterals.

occlusion of the carotid while observing the awake patient for clinical signs of cerebral ischemia.[3]

Data to provide a rational basis for selection of patients for carotid artery ligation versus reconstruction have been reported by Ehrenfeld and his colleagues at the University of California at San Francisco. They found carotid ligation to be safe if carotid stump pressure exceeded 70 mmHg systolic. This was a selected group of patients who were anticoagulated and in whom systemic blood pressures were maintained at defined levels, which may not be a representative group.[23]

Visceral Arteries. Although visceral arterial aneurysms are uncommon, a high percentage are infected.[84] Treatment must be individualized and directed by angiography. When feasible, aneurysm ligation-excision is desirable, but arterial reconstruction with saphenous autografts may be required to preserve organ or bowel viability.[97]

Results

Successful surgical management of an infected aneurysm depends on the type of aneurysm, its location, and the microorganisms responsible, as well as the patient's general condition and clinical presentation. In general, results following treatment of infected aneurysms have steadily im-

proved because of prompt diagnosis, improved surgical techniques, and modern antimicrobial therapy. Bennett and Cherry reported in 1967 that infected aneurysms of the abdominal aorta were invariably fatal.[9] Since then, a number of successes have been reported, although management remains challenging (Table 82–9). Although recent reports have tended to emphasize the improved outlook for patient survival, the authors believe that infectious aneurysms of all types, particularly those that fail therapy, are underreported. To this end, Wilson estimated from a literature review that in treated patients mycotic aneurysm had a 25 per cent mortality rate, microbial arteritis with aneurysm had a 75 per cent mortality rate, infected preexisting aneurysms had a 75 per cent mortality rate, and post-traumatic infected false aneurysms had a 10 per cent mortality rate (see Table 82–1).[100]

Lower extremity amputation rates following treatment for infected femoral artery false aneurysms have ranged from 11 to 25 per cent.[1, 31, 42, 58, 61, 66] The above-knee amputation rate following ligation-excision of the femoral artery bifurcation in drug addicts approximates 33 per cent. When groin sepsis is not controlled, revascularization in an attempt to prevent amputation may pose an unnecessary and potentially lethal risk of graft sepsis and should be undertaken with caution. A certain number of amputations are unavoidable among patients with infected femoral false aneurysms.

Table 82–9.   Microbial Abdominal Aortitis With Aneurysm: 15-Year Survey 1978–1992

Author	Year	Number	% Surviving
Davis[21]	1978	3	100
Wilson[99]	1978	2	100
Mendelowitz[51]	1979	1	100
Scher[77]	1980	2	50
Bardin[6]	1981	2	50
McIntyre[49]	1982	1	100
Ewart[30]	1983	1	100
Johansen[41]	1983	4	100
Brown[12]	1984	3	66
Reddy[65]	1986	1	100
Suddleson[86]	1987	2	100
McNamara[50]	1987	4	25
Bitseff[10]	1987	5	60
Byard[14]	1988	1	0
Taylor[89]	1988	5	100
Yao[101]	1988	1	0
Oz[57]	1989	21	62
Atnip[2]	1989	1	100
Chan[16]	1989	13	92
Rutherford[75]	1989	1	100
Dupont[22]	1989	1	100
Trairatvorakul[91]	1990	7	57
Reddy[69]	1991	8	63
Cull[20]	1992	1	100
Gouny[35]	1992	3	100
Pasic[61]	1992	1	100
Van Damme[93]	1992	1	100
Totals*		96	74%

Totals excluding true mycotic, post-traumatic, iatrogenic, and drug-related aneurysms.

References

1. Anderson CB, Butcher HR Jr, et al: Mycotic aneurysms. Arch Surg 109:712, 1974.
2. Atnip RG: Mycotic aneurysms of the suprarenal abdominal aorta: Prolonged survival after in situ aortic and visceral reconstruction. J Vasc Surg 10:635, 1989.
3. Avellone JC, Ahmad MY: Cervical internal carotid aneurysm from syphilis. An alternative to resection. JAMA 241:238, 1979.
4. Bahnini A, Ruoyolo C, Koskas F, Kieffer E: In situ fresh allograft replacement of an infected aortic prosthetic graft: Eighteen months' follow-up. J Vasc Surg 14:98, 1991.
5. Baker WH, Moran JM, Dormer DB: Infected aortic aneurysm following arteriography. J Cardiovasc Surg 20:313, 1979.
6. Bardin JA, Collins GM, Devin JB, et al: Nonaneurysmal suppurative aortitis. Arch Surg 116:954, 1981.
7. Barker WF: Mycotic aneurysms. Ann Surg 139:84, 1954.
8. Bennett DE: Primary mycotic aneurysms of the aorta. Arch Surg 94:758, 1967.
9. Bennett DE, Cherry JK: Bacterial infection of aortic aneurysms: A clinicopathologic study. Am J Surg 113:321, 1967.
10. Bitseff EL, Edwards WA, Mulherin JL Jr, Kaiser AB: Infected abdominal aortic aneurysms. South Med J 80:309, 1987.
11. Blum L, Keefer E: Cryptogenic mycotic aneurysm. Ann Surg 155:398, 1962.
12. Brown SL, Busutill RW, Baker JD, et al: Bacteriologic and surgical determinants of survival in patients with mycotic aneurysms. J Vasc Surg 1:541, 1984.
13. Brunner MC, Mitchell RS, Baldwin JC, et al: Prosthetic graft infection: Limitations of indium white blood cell scanning. J Vasc Surg 3:42, 1986.
14. Byard RW, Leduc JR, Chambers J, Walley VM: The rapid evolution of a large mycotic aneurysm of the abdominal aorta. J Can Assoc Radiol 39:62, 1988.
15. Cates JE, Christie RV: Subacute bacterial endocarditis. Quart J Med 24:93, 1951.
16. Chan FY, Crawford ES, Coselli JS, et al: In situ prosthetic graft replacement for mycotic aneurysms of the aorta. Ann Thorac Surg 47:193, 1989.
17. Cooke PA, Ehrenfeld WK: Successful management of mycotic aortic aneurysm: Report of a case. Surgery 75:132, 1974.
18. Crane AR: Primary multiocular mycotic aneurysm of the aorta. Arch Pathol 24:634, 1937.
19. Crawford ES, Crawford JL (eds): Diseases of the Aorta Including an Atlas of Angiographic Pathology and Surgical Techniques. Baltimore, Williams & Wilkins, 1984.
20. Cull DL, Winter RP, Wheller JR, et al: Mycotic aneurysm of the suprarenal aorta. J Cardiovasc Surg 33:181, 1992.
21. Davies OG, Thorburn JD, Powell P: Cryptic mycotic abdominal aortic aneurysms. Am J Surg 136:96, 1978.
22. Dupont JR, Bonavita JA, DiGiovanni RJ, et al: Acquired immuno-deficiency syndrome and mycotic abdominal aortic aneurysms: A new challenge? Report of a case. J Vasc Surg 10:254, 1989.
23. Ehrenfeld WR, Stoney RJ, Wylie EJ: Relation of carotid stump pressure to safety of carotid arterial ligation. Surgery 93:299, 1983.
24. Elliott JP, Hageman JH, Szilagyi DE, et al: Arterial embolization: Problems of source, multiplicity, recurrence, and delayed treatment. Surgery 88:833, 1980.
25. Elliott JP, Smith RF, Szilagyi DE: Aortoenteric and paraprosthetic-enteric fistulas. Arch Surg 114:1041, 1974.
26. Elliott JP, Smith RF: Peripheral embolization. In Magilligan DJ, Quinn EL (eds): Endocarditis: Medical and Surgical Management, New York, Marcell Dekker, 1986, p 164.
27. Eppinger H: Pathogenesis (histogenesis und aetiologie) der anerysmen eimschliesslich des aneurysma equi verminosum. Arch Klin Chir 35:404, 1887.
28. Ernst CB, Campbell C Jr, Daugherty ME, et al: Incidence and significance of intra-operative bacterial cultures during abdominal aortic aneurysmectomy. Ann Surg 185:626, 1977.
29. Eshaghy B, Scanlon RJ, Amirparviz F, et al: Mycotic aneurysm of brachial artery: A complication of retrograde catheterization. JAMA 228:1574, 1974.
30. Ewart JM, Burke ML, Bunt TJ: Spontaneous abdominal aortic infections: Essentials of diagnosis and management. Am Surg 49:37, 1983.

31. Feldman AJ, Berguer R: Management of an infected aneurysm of the groin secondary to drug abuse. Surg Gynecol Obstet 157:519, 1983.

32. Fromm SH, Lucas CE: Obturator bypass for mycotic aneurysm of the drug addict. Arch Surg 100:82, 1970.

33. Geelhoed GW, Joseph WL: Surgical sequelae of drug abuse. Surg Gynecol Obstet 139:749, 1974.

34. Gomes MN, Schellinger D, Hufnagel CA: Abdominal aortic aneurysms: Diagnostic review and new techniques. Ann Thorac Surg 27:479, 1979.

35. Gouny P, Valverde A, Vincent D: Human immunodeficiency virus and infected aneurysm of the abdominal aorta: Report of three cases. Ann Vasc Surg 6:239, 1992.

36. Hankins JR, Yeager GH: Primary mycotic aneurysm. Surgery 40:747, 1956.

37. Howell HS, Barburao T, Graziano J: Mycotic cervical cartoid aneurysm. Surgery 81:357, 1977.

38. Huebl HC, Read RC: Aneurysmal abscess. Minn Med 49:11, 1966.

39. Jarrett F, Darling RC, Mundth ED, et al: Experience with infected aneurysms of the abdominal aorta. Arch Surg 10:1281, 1975.

40. Johansen K, Devin J: Spontaneous healing of mycotic aortic aneurysm. J Cardiovasc Surg 21:625, 1980.

41. Johansen K, Devin J: Mycotic aortic aneurysms: A reappraisal. Arch Surg 118:583, 1983.

42. Johnson JR, Ledgerwood AM, Lucas CE: Mycotic aneurysm: New concepts in surgery. Arch Surg 118:577, 1983.

43. Koch R: Ueber aneurysma der arteria mesenterica superior. In Inaug. Dural-Abhandlung. Erlangen, JJ. Barfus'schen Universitaets-Buch-druckerei, 1851.

44. Kyriakides GK, Simmons RL, Najarian JS: Mycotic aneurysms in transplant patients. Arch Surg 111:472, 1976.

45. Ledgerwood AM, Lucas CE: Mycotic aneurysm of the carotid artery. Arch Surg 109:496, 1974.

46. Lewis D, Schrager J: Embolomycotic aneurysms. JAMA 63:1808, 1909.

47. Magilligan DJ: Neurologic complications. In Magilligan DJ, Quinn EL (eds): Endocarditis: Medical and Surgical Management. New York, Marcel Dekker, 1986, p 187.

48. Magilligan DJ, Quinn EL: Active infective endocarditis. In Magilligan DJ Jr, Quinn EL (eds): Endocarditis: Medical and Surgical Management. New York, Marcel Dekker, 1986, p 207.

49. McIntyre KE, Malone JM, Richards E, et al: Mycotic aortic pseudoaneurysm with aortoenteric fistula caused by Arizona hinshawii. Surgery 91:173, 1982.

50. Mcnamara MF, Roberts AB, Bakshi KR: Gram-negative bacterial infection of aortic aneurysms. J Cardiovasc Surg 28:453, 1987.

51. Mendelowitz DS, Ramstedt R, Yao JST, et al: Abdominal aortic salmonellosis. Surgery 85:514, 1979.

52. Miller BM, Waterhouse G, Alford RH, et al: Histoplasma infection of abdominal aortic aneurysms. Ann Surg 197:57, 1983.

53. Monson RL, Alexander RH: Vein reconstruction of a mycotic internal carotid aneurysm. Ann Surg 191:47, 1980.

54. Mundth ED, Darling RC, Alvarado RH, et al: Surgical management of mycotic aneurysms and the complications of infection in vascular reconstructive surgery. Am J Surg 117:460, 1969.

55. Nabseth DC, Deterling RA: Surgical management of mycotic aneurysms. Surgery 50:347, 1961.

56. Osler W: The Gulstonian lectures on malignant endocarditis. Br Med J 1:467, 1885.

57. Oz MC, Brener BJ, Buda JA, et al: A ten-year experience with bacterial aortitis. J Vasc Surg 10:439, 1989.

58. Padberg F, Hobson R II, Lee B, et al: Femoral pseudoaneurysm from drugs of abuse: Ligation or reconstruction? J Vasc Surg 15:642, 1992.

59. Paré A: Of Aneurismas. In The apologie and treatise containing the voyages made into divers places with many of his writings upon surgery. The Classics of Surgery Library, Birmingham, Alabama, 1984.

60. Parkhurst GF, Decker JP: Bacterial aortitis and mycotic aneurysm of the aorta. Am J Pathol 31:821, 1955.

61. Pasic M, Segesser L, Turina M: Implantation of antibiotic-releasing carriers and in situ reconstruction for treatment of mycotic aneurysm. Arch Surg 127:745, 1992.

62. Patel KR, Semel L, Clauss RH: Routine revascularization with resec-tion of infected femoral pseudoaneurysms from substance abuse. J Vasc Surg: 8:321, 1988.

63. Patel S, Johnson KW: Classification and management of mycotic aneurysm. Surg Gynecol Obstet 144:691, 1977.

64. Perdue GD, Smith RB III: Surgical treatment of mycotic aneurysms. South Med J 60:848, 1967.

65. Reddy DJ, Lee RE, Oh HK: Suprarenal mycotic aortic aneurysm: Surgical management and follow up. J Vasc Surg 3:917, 1986.

66. Reddy DJ, Smith RF, Elliott JP Jr, et al: Infected femoral artery false aneurysms in drug addicts: Evolution of selective vascular reconstruction. J Vasc Surg 3:718, 1986.

67. Reddy DJ: Treatment of drug-related infected false aneurysms of the femoral artery—Is routine revascularization justified? J Vasc Surg 8:344, 1988.

68. Reddy DJ: Letter to editor. J Vasc Surg 10:358, 1989.

69. Reddy DJ, Shepard AD, Evans JR, et al: Management of infected aortoiliac aneurysms. Arch Surg 126:873, 1991.

70. Reid MR: Studies on abnormal arteriovenous communications, acquired and congenital. I. Report of a series of cases. Arch Surg 10:601, 1925.

71. Reister WH, Serrano A: Infrarenal mycotic pseudoaneurysm. J Thorac Cardiovasc Surg 71:633, 1975.

72. Revell STR: Primary mycotic aneurysms. Ann Intern Med 22:431, 1943.

73. Rokitansky CF: Handbuch der Pathologischen Anatomie, 2nd ed. 1844, p 55.

74. Rose HD, Stuart JL: Mycotic aneurysm of the thoracic aorta due to Aspergillus fumigatus. Chest 70:81, 1976.

75. Rutherford EJ, Eakins JW, Maxwell JG, et al: Abdominal aortic aneurysm infected with Campylobacter fetus subspecies fetus. J Vasc Surg 10:193, 1989.

76. Samson DS, Gewertz BL, Beyer CW Jr, et al: Saphenous vein interposition grafts in the microsurgical treatment of cerebral ischemia. Arch Surg 116:1578, 1981.

77. Scher A, Brener B, Goldendranz RJ, et al: Infected aneurysms of the abdominal aorta. Surgery 115:975, 1980.

78. Schumacker HB: Aneurysm development and degenerative changes in dilated artery proximal to arteriovenous fistula. Surg Gynecol Obstet 130:636, 1970.

79. Shetty PC, Krasicky GA, Sharma RP, et al: Mycotic aneurysms in intravenous drug abusers: The utility of intravenous digital subtraction angiography. Radiology 155:319, 1985.

80. Smith RF, Szilagyi DE, Colville JM: Surgical treatment of mycotic aneurysms. Arch Surg 85:663, 1967.

81. Soderstrom CA, Wasserman DJ, Ransom KJ, et al: Infected false femoral artery aneurysms secondary to monitoring catheters. J Cardiovasc Surg 24:63, 1983.

82. Sommerville RI, Allen EV, Edwards JE: Bland and infected arteriosclerotic abdominal aortic aneurysms. A clinicopathologic study. Medicine 38:207, 1959.

83. Sower ND, Whelan TJ: Suppurative arteritis due to Salmonella. Surgery 52:851, 1967.

84. Stanley JC, Thompson NW, Fry WJ: Splanchnic artery aneurysms. Arch Surg 101:689, 1970.

85. Stengel A, Wolferth CC: Mycotic (bacterial) aneurysms of intravascular origin. Arch Intern Med 31:527, 1923.

86. Suddleson EA, Katz SG, Kohl RD: Mycotic suprarenal aortic aneurysm. Ann Vasc Surg 1:426, 1987.

87. Szilagyi DE, Elliott JP, Smith RF: Ruptured abdominal aneurysms simulating sepsis. Arch Surg 91:263, 1965.

88. Szilgyi DE, Rodriquez FT, Smith RF, Elliott JP: Late fate of arterial allografts: Observations 6 to 15 years after implantation. Arch Surg 101:721, 1970.

89. Taylor LM Jr, Deitz DM, McConnell DB, Porter JM: Treatment of infected abdominal aneurysms by extraanatomic bypass, aneurysm excision, and drainage. Am J Surg 155:655, 1988.

90. Thompson TR, Tilleli J, Johnson DE, et al: Umbilical artery catheterization complicated by mycotic aortic aneurysm in neonates. Adv Pediatr 27:275, 1980.

91. Trairatvorakul P, Sriphojanart S, Sathapatayavongs B: Abdominal aortic aneurysms infected with salmonella: Problems of treatment. J Vasc Surg 12:16, 1990.

92. Tufnell J: On the influence of vegetation of the valves of the heart in the production of secondary arterial disease. Dublin Quart J Med 15:371, 1885.

93. Van Damme H, Belachew M, Damas P, et al: Mycotic aneurysm of the upper abdominal aorta ruptured into the stomach. Arch Surg 127:478, 1992.
94. Virkow R: Ueber die akute entzuendung der arterian. Virchows Arch Pathol 1:272, 1847.
95. Vogelzang RL, Sohaey R: Infected aortic aneurysms: CT appearance. J Comput Assist Tomogr 12(1):109, 1988.
96. Weintraub RA, Abrams HL: Mycotic aneurysm. Am J Roentgenol 102:354, 1968.
97. Werner K, Tarasoutchi F, Lunardi W, et al: Mycotic aneurysm of the celiac trunk and superior mesenteric artery in a case of infective endocarditis. J Cardiovasc Surg 32:380, 1991.
98. Williams RD, Fisher FW: Aneurysm contents as a source of graft infection. Arch Surg 112:415, 1977.
99. Wilson SE, Gordon E, Van Wagenen PB: Salmonella arteritis. Arch Surg 113:1163, 1978.
100. Wilson SE, Van Wagenen P, Passaro E Jr: Arterial infection. Curr Prob Surg 15:5, 1978.
101. Yao JST, McCarthy WJ: Contained rupture of a thoracoabdominal aneurysm. Contemp Surg 33:47, 1988.
102. Yellin AE: Ruptured mycotic aneurysm. Arch Surg 112:981, 1977.
103. Zak FG, Strauss L, Saphra I: Rupture of diseased large arteries in the course of enterobacterial (salmonella) infection. N Engl J Med 258:824, 1958.

83

Pseudoaneurysms

Elizabeth T. Clark, M.D., and Bruce L. Gewertz, M.D.

• • •

Pseudoaneurysms result from a variety of mechanisms including infection, trauma, and surgical procedures (Fig. 83–1). All have in common the disruption of arterial continuity with extravasation of blood into surrounding tissues. This ultimately results in the formation of a fibrous tissue capsule that progressively enlarges owing to unrelenting arterial pressure. This chapter focuses on the pathogenesis and natural history of pseudoaneurysms and considers the diverse clinical presentations, diagnostic modalities, and treatment options.

HISTORY

The first successful repair of a pseudoaneurysm was reported by Rudolph Matas in 1888.[1] He devised the technique of endoaneurysmorraphy for the repair of a traumatic aneurysm of the left brachial artery resulting from a gunshot wound sustained by the patient 2 months earlier. It was not until the early 1900s, following the introduction of Alexis Carrel's innovative techniques, that surgeons began

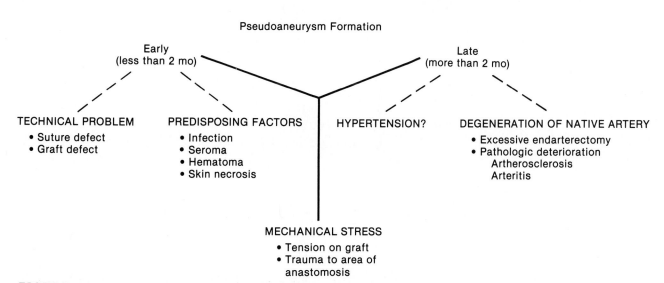

FIGURE 83–1. Depiction of the etiology and evolution of pseudoaneurysms. A disruption of arterial continuity usually precedes pseudoaneurysmal development, which is propagated by unrelenting arterial pressure.

treating arterial disease with regularity. Lexer in 1907 utilized an interposition vein graft for the repair of a large false aneurysm in the axilla.[2] Weglowski in Poland presented 51 cases of traumatic aneurysms repaired with "vein transplants" in 1925.[3]

ETIOLOGY

All causes of pseudoaneurysms involve a disruption of arterial continuity, whether due to arterial trauma, infection, vasculitis, or, most commonly, diverse complications of vascular surgery leading to anastomotic separation (Fig. 83–2). Pseudoaneurysms are also common following inter-

ventional diagnostic and therapeutic procedures that involve arterial puncture.

Iatrogenic Pseudoaneurysms

Most iatrogenic pseudoaneurysms occur as a result of arterial reconstructions. The incidence reflects the site of anastomosis and the use of prosthetic materials. The strength of an anastomosis and the union between the prosthetic graft and the artery depend primarily on the durability and integrity of the suture material. Regardless of the extent of soft tissue "incorporation" of prosthetic grafts, mesenchymal tissue ingrowth alone is inadequate to provide the

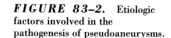

FIGURE 83–2. Etiologic factors involved in the pathogenesis of pseudoaneurysms.

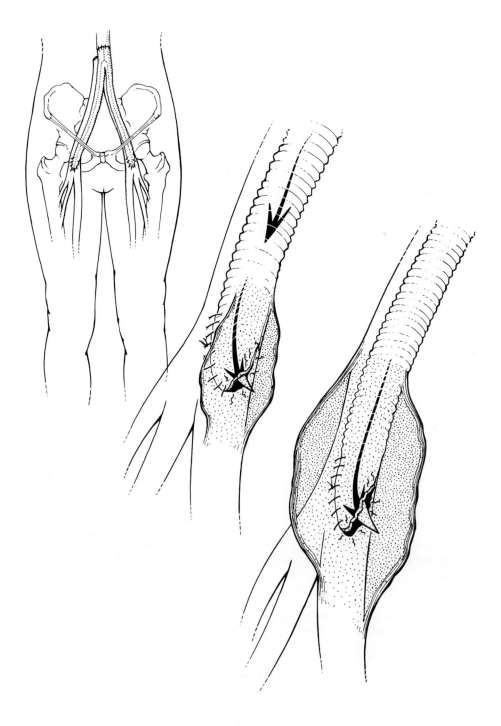

required strength.[4,5] Prior to 1967, when silk suture material was widely used, up to one fourth of all anastomoses between prosthetic grafts and femoral arteries resulted in pseudoaneurysm formation. There appears to a decline in the incidence of pseudoaneurysms in recent years owing to improvements in technique, suture materials, and graft materials. Nonetheless, graft-arterial disruption remains common even though few of these disruptions produce clinically important symptoms. In a study by Gooding and colleagues, 87 asymptomatic patients with functioning aortofemoral grafts were examined with ultrasonography, and 9 per cent were found to have developed pseudoaneurysms.[6]

Other factors implicated in anastomotic aneurysm formation include differences in compliance between native arteries and graft materials, shearing forces along anastomotic lines, vibratory fatigue, the position of the graft, and anticoagulation; all of these factors may allow blood to escape from the vessel via partial "dehiscence" of the suture line. Elongated end-to-side anastomoses may result in localized dilatation and increased tangential tension according to LaPlace's law ($T = P \times r$). Because most graft materials are less compliant than native arteries, there is preferential dilatation of the artery, which induces disruptive stress on the anastomosis.[7]

Loss of structural integrity results not only from suture material fatigue and prosthesis degeneration but also from degeneration of the host vessel independent of its relationship to prosthetic material. Fibrous degeneration of the media results in decreased elasticity, which inhibits arterial adaptability to diverse mechanical stresses. Stern has suggested that micro-occlusive disease of the vasa vasorum is involved in the pathogenesis of this fibrous degeneration.[8] Other causes of host vessel degeneration include the expected progression of atherosclerotic disease and local factors that may accelerate degeneration such as perigraft fluid collections, excessive endarterectomy, and extensive artery mobilization during the initial procedure.

Graft infections following bypass procedures undoubtedly play a role in the development of pseudoaneurysms. In surgically treated pseudoaneurysms with no clinical evidence of infection, as many as 60 per cent are found to be culture positive if meticulous bacteriologic techniques are employed. The most common organisms are *Staphylococcus epidermidis* or other coagulase-negative staphylococcal species.[9] Cytolysins from such bacteria cause disincorporation of the graft from host tissues and increase the propensity for pseudoaneurysm formation.

Angiography and thrombolytic therapy also may lead to pseudoaneurysm formation. Predictably, interventional procedures, such as percutaneous transluminal angioplasty, that require larger catheters and more aggressive manipulations are associated with a higher incidence of complications than simple diagnostic procedures. In one study by Messina and colleagues at the University of Michigan there was a 3.4 per cent incidence of complications in patients undergoing interventional therapeutic angiographic procedures; pseudoaneurysms accounted for 16 per cent of these complications.[10] Diagnostic studies were associated with a 0.7 per cent complication rate, 32 per cent of which were pseudoaneurysms.

Infectious Pseudoaneurysms

Infectious pseudoaneurysms result from septic emboli, contiguous infection, and intravenous drug abuse (IVDA)-related phenomena. The use of contaminated needles by addicts often leads to subacute bacterial endocarditis from which septic emboli lodge in atherosclerotic plaques or the vasa vasorum of larger vessels. Infarction or inflammation results in necrosis of the vessel wall and, ultimately, in aneurysm or pseudoaneurysm formation. Collagenases produced by bacteria may facilitate this process. Particularly worrisome are those pseudoaneurysms that occur in the abdominal aorta or mesenteric vessels because life-threatening complications may be the first indication of their existence.[11–14] An even more common mechanism is the direct deposit of infected materials into more superficial arteries during drug injections. These infected pseudoaneurysms occur most commonly in the groin, neck, and upper extremities.[15] Chapter 82 discusses this problem in detail.

Trauma

Both blunt and penetrating injuries may lead to pseudoaneurysm formation. Once formed, these traumatic pseudoaneurysms progressively expand or thrombose; in doing so, they may cause neural or venous compression, thrombosis of the native artery, or distal embolization. The popliteal artery and distal upper extremity arteries are particularly prone to blunt injury because of the muscular tethering of these vessels. In these regions, stretching and intimal disruption frequently accompany distracting skeletal injury. In contrast, the more superficial femoral and carotid vessels are more vulnerable to direct penetrating injury.

Vasculitis

Vasculitides have traditionally been associated with true aneurysm formation, but late sequelae such as medial destruction and vasa vasorum occlusion with transmural necrosis occasionally result in perforation and pseudoaneurysm formation. Because of intrinsic arterial wall fragility, anastomotic pseudoaneurysms and arterial puncture pseudoaneurysms are much more common in those vasculitides that involve the larger arteries. These include periarteritis nodosa, lupus erythematosus, thromboangiitis obliterans, giant cell arteritis, Behçet's disease, Kawasaki's syndrome, and the various rheumatoid arthritis syndromes.

DIAGNOSIS AND TREATMENT

Most pseudoaneurysms present with local symptoms such as pain, rapid expansion, or venous obstruction associated with a palpable mass. A palpable thrill or audible bruit may be detected. The most common site of presentation is the groin (Table 83–1). Combining data from a large number of clinical series yields an average age at presentation of 62 years, with a range of 20 to 86 years (Table 83–2). The average time interval from surgery to presentation

Table 83–1.   Incidence and Distribution of Pseudoaneurysms in Representative Studies

	Overall Incidence (%)	Aortic (%)	Iliac (%)	Femoral (%)	Popliteal (%)	Carotid (%)
Szilagyi and colleagues[16] 1957–1974	1.7	2.5	11.7	79.1	5.5	1.2
Nichols and colleagues[17] 1970–1979	2.6	7.0	7.0	83.7	0	—
Sedwitz and colleagues[18] 1965–1986	NA	14.8	14.8	75.3	9.9	—
Knox[19] 1970–1974	1.9	22.2	5.5	61.1	8.3	—
Millili and colleagues[20] 1960–1979	4.5	8.3	8.3	91.6	—	—
Richardson and McDowell[21] 1965–1975	NA	20.6	5.9	61.8	3.0	8.8
Sawyers and colleagues[22] 1956–1966	NA	—	—	90	10	—

NA, not applicable.

of an anastomotic aneurysm is 6.2 years with a range of 2.5 months to 19 years.[16–22] Earlier presentation is often correlated with infection or a second procedure performed upon the same anatomic area.

Diagnosis is aided by ultrasound or duplex imaging, computed tomography (CT), and angiography. Ultrasound is useful for defining the size and extent of the pseudoaneurysm as well as the presence of perigraft fluid collections. CT scanning is particularly helpful for evaluating the retroperitoneum. Color flow Doppler images are useful for detecting blood flow into the pseudoaneurysm cavities (Fig. 83–3). Coughlin and Paushter found sensitivity and specificity of 94 per cent and 97 per cent, respectively, using pulse wave Doppler imaging for the diagnosis of pseudoaneurysms.[23]

Angiography is also useful for evaluating the area of suspected pseudoaneurysm and other anastomotic sites and for planning the most appropriate surgical repair (Fig. 83–4). In a study of 51 patients with pseudoaneurysms, Yonkey and colleagues found that 60 per cent of patients had multiple pseudoaneurysms.[24]

Aortic pseudoaneurysms are notoriously difficult to diagnose, given their location and relative rarity. The paucity of symptoms associated with intra-abdominal pseudoaneurysms prior to catastrophic complications further compounds the problem. Patients may present with abdominal or back pain due to stretching of retroperitoneal structures;

an abdominal mass may be palpated. Acute thrombosis of aortic pseudoaneurysms occurs in as many as 25 per cent of patients. Renovascular hypertension and distal embolization may be evident. The most devasting and life-threatening complication is acute retroperitoneal or abdominal hemorrhage. Pseudoaneurysms of the abdominal aorta are rare (less than 2 per cent of all pseudoaneurysms) but occur most commonly in association with aortic aneurysm repairs; anastomotic aneurysms following aortobifemoral bypass for occlusive disease and traumatic pseudoaneurysms are less frequently seen.[25]

Iliac pseudoaneurysms are similarly difficult to diagnose and usually present when a complication such as thrombosis or distal embolization has occurred. They are most commonly associated with aortoiliac bypass procedures and occur less frequently as a sequela of trauma (Fig. 83–5). When they occur after pelvic trauma, iliac pseudoaneurysms may be associated with pelvic abscesses.[26] Operative repair of these pseudoaneurysms is challenging, especially in the presence of sepsis. Although some authors recommend primary repair with an interposition saphenous vein graft, even placement of autogenous tissue into the infected field may be unwise. If primary repair is impossible, iliac artery ligation and extra-anatomic bypass are recommended. Symptoms of iliac pseudoaneurysms result from encroachment on the ureters, bladder, sacral plexus, and iliac veins.

Femoral pseudoaneurysms are by far the most common type of pseudoaneurysm and account for more than three fourths of all clinically important pseudoaneurysms. The most common cause is disruption of a prosthetic arterial anastomosis. This occurs in 1.5 to 3.0 per cent of patients undergoing either aortofemoral or femoropopliteal bypass grafting.[27–30] If left untreated, femoral pseudoaneurysms may result in complications such as vessel thrombosis, distal embolization, or rupture. It is generally accepted that these sequelae are unusual if the pseudoaneurysm is less than 2 cm in diameter and is asymptomatic.[31] Since elective repairs of pseudoaneurysms have lower morbidity and mortality rates and higher long-term patency rates than emergent procedures, early diagnosis and treatment is the standard of care. In most instances, placement of an interposition conduit, composed of either prosthetic material or saphenous vein, is the preferred procedure (Fig. 83–6).

Table 83–2.   Age at Presentation and Interval From Original Operation to Time of Presentation in Representative Studies

	Age	Interval to Diagnosis
Nichols and colleagues[17] 1970–1979	42–85 yr	37 mo (16 day–16 yr)
Sedwitz and colleagues[18] 1965–1986	63 yr (20–86 yr)	5.2 yr (2 wk–12 yr)
Knox[19] 1970–1974	NA	29 mo
Millili and colleagues[20] 1960–1979	58 yr	3 mo–17 yr
Richardson and McDowell[21] 1965–1975	65 yr (43–80 yr)	5.4 yr (6 mo–14 yr)
Sawyers and colleagues[22] 1956–1966	51–85 yr	1–13 mo

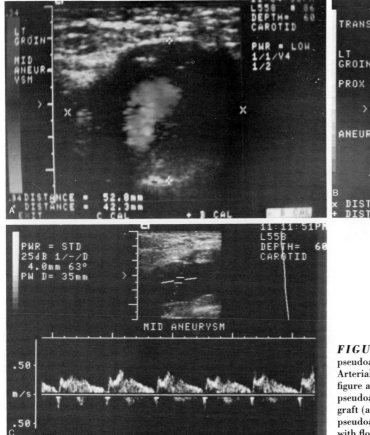

FIGURE 83–3. Duplex imaging of a left groin pseudoaneurysm in a patient with an aortobifemoral bypass. *A*, Arterial flow is demonstrated within the aneurysmal cavity. (This figure appears in color on Plate IV.) *B*, View of proximal pseudoaneurysm showing its relationship to the tubular prosthetic graft (at 12 o'clock). *C*, Velocity waveforms within the pseudoaneurysm cavity reflect turbulent flow (decreased flow velocity with flow reversal).

FIGURE 83–4. Angiogram showing a large left groin pseudoaneurysm with a smaller right groin pseudoaneurysm in a patient with an aortofemoral bypass graft.

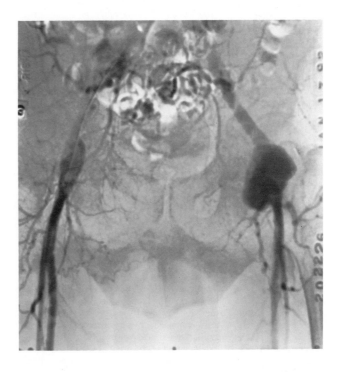

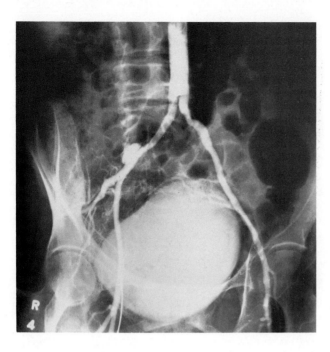

FIGURE 83–5. Illustration of a right iliac pseudoaneurysm in a patient who has had an infrarenal abdominal aortic aneurysm repair with a bifurcated graft to the common iliac arteries.

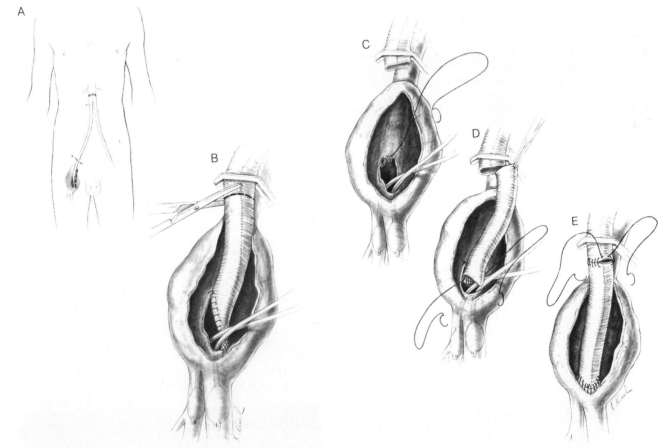

FIGURE 83–6. *A,* Most femoral pseudoaneurysms can be repaired through the previous groin incision. *B,* The pseudoaneurysm is exposed anteriorly, and control of the limb of the aortofemoral bypass is obtained above the aneurysm. After systemic heparinization, the graft is clamped, and the aneurysm is opened. The superficial and deep femoral branches are easily controlled from within the aneurysm with balloon catheters. The limb of the aortofemoral bypass is transected, the distal anastomosis is excised, and the distal graft segment is removed. *C,* The orifice of the native common femoral artery is oversewn from within the aneurysm. *D,* A new segment of prosthetic Dacron graft, with an appropriate diameter matching that of the original graft limb, is sutured to the orifices of the superficial femoral and deep femoral arteries. Large, deep bites are taken to ensure a full-thickness passage of each suture. *E,* After completion of the distal anastomosis, the balloon catheters are removed, and a clamp is placed on the Dacron graft for hemostasis. The new graft is then anastomosed end-to-end to the original Dacron graft: (*A–E,* From Zarins CK, Gewertz BL: Atlas of Vascular Surgery. Churchill Livingstone, New York, 1989.)

Such an approach results in less than a 4 per cent mortality and greater than 75 per cent 2-year patency rate according to most studies. Emergent procedures are associated with 24 to 47 per cent 2-year patency rate and a prohibitive mortality of 66 to 100 per cent.[32]

A study by Millili and colleagues examining the natural history of aortofemoral bypass for either arterial occlusive disease or aneurysmal disease found a 4.5 per cent incidence of pseudoaneurysm formation (4.0 per cent at the femoral anastamoses and 0.5 per cent at the level of the aorta).[20] In this study, 58 per cent of patients with pseudoaneurysmal disease had multiple aneurysms. Three types of repairs were performed. Resection of the pseudoaneurysm with reimplantation into the original arteriotomy resulted in a 40 per cent recurrence. Resection and prosthetic interposition grafting was associated with a 13 per cent recurrence. The best results were obtained with resection, oversewing of the arteriotomy, and distal bypass via a new arteriotomy; using this approach, no recurrences were noted.

The treatment of femoral pseudoaneurysms in the presence of infection is somewhat more involved. Reddy and associates reviewed 54 patients with IVDA-related femoral artery pseudoaneurysms who were treated operatively and noted an 11 per cent amputation rate and 0 per cent mortality.[33] The patients were divided into two groups: those with isolated common femoral arterial involvement and those with involvement of the common femoral artery and its bifurcation. In the former group there were no amputations if only the common or superficial femoral arteries were ligated or excluded. In the second group, some patients were treated with triple-vessel ligation and no reconstruction; there was a 21.4 per cent amputation rate, and claudication occurred in all patients postoperatively. In those whose arteries were reconstructed using prosthetic grafts, all grafts became infected and required removal. The subgroup of patients with saphenous vein grafts fared much better, experiencing lower rates of recurrent infection and acceptable long-term graft patency. Reddy and associates recommended aggressive débridement, saphenous vein graft reconstruction, and flap rotation of the sartorius muscle (first described by Barker in 1966).

Fromm and Lucas also noted a 30 per cent incidence of limb loss and a 25 per cent incidence of incapacitating arterial insufficiency following triple-vessel ligation in the treatment of infected femoral pseudoaneurysms.[34] They advocated initial exclusion of the area of pseudoaneurysm by ligation of the external iliac artery above the inguinal ligament and infra-inguinal ligation of the superficial femoral artery. This prevents bleeding from within the pseudoaneurysm and feeding of septic emboli to newly created suture lines. A bypass from the iliac artery to the popliteal artery via the obturator foramen is then performed, and the pseudoaneurysm is excised under local anesthesia at a later date.

Another less common cause of femoral pseudoaneurysm is femoral artery catheterization. The reported incidence of this complication ranges from 0.05 to 2.0 per cent of all femoral artery catheter procedures. The incidence may be increased with hypertension, anticoagulation, multiple punctures, the use of large-bore catheters and sheaths, and the cannulation of poorly compliant or calcific vessels. The clinical differentiation between hematoma and pseudoaneurysm is difficult, although the introduction of pulsed-wave Doppler and B-mode ultrasound has improved diagnostic accuracy.[35] Historically, confirmation of an acute pseudoaneurysm has prompted urgent repair. More recently, Kresowik and coworkers examined the natural history of such pseudoaneurysms.[36] They showed that restriction of physical activity alone resulted in a decrease in size of the groin mass and disappearance of flow in the pseudoaneurysmal cavity in all patients. Thus, thrombosis and resolution of most procedural-related pseudoaneurysms is the rule rather then the exception. Operative intervention is necessary if the pseudoaneurysm (1) is symptomatic, (2) is expanding, (3) is associated with an extremely large hematoma, or (4) persists for more than 6 weeks.[37]

Pseudoaneurysms of the *popliteal artery* are much less common than true aneurysms in this location (Fig. 83–7). Anastomotic popliteal aneurysms account for roughly 3 per cent of all pseudoaneurysms. In rare instances, blunt trauma

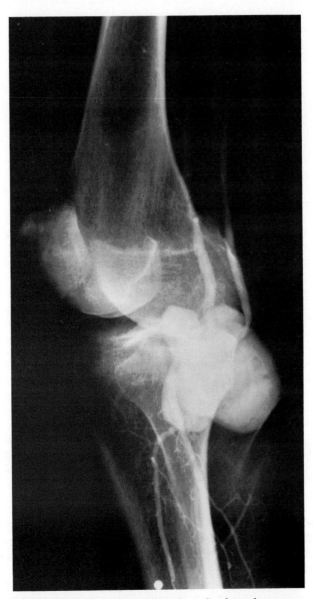

FIGURE 83–7. Example of a right popliteal pseudoaneurysm at the distal end of a femoropopliteal bypass. Disruption was caused by forceful knee extension during physical therapy.

may result in pseudoaneurysm formation in the popliteal area, given the degree of tethering of the vessel above and below the knee joint.[39] Percutaneous transluminal angioplasty (PTA) of the infrainguinal vessels is rarely associated with pseudoaneurysm development. In one series of 984 PTAs, only one pseudoaneurysm was noted.[40]

Distal peripheral arterial (e.g., radial) pseudoaneurysms occur most commonly as a result of catheter placement for continuous arterial pressure monitoring. These may be accurately assessed with duplex imaging as illustrated in Figure 83–8 on Color Plate IV. Treatment usually consists of excision of the pseudoaneurysm with ligation or interposition vein graft placement.

Carotid endarterectomy is rarely associated with pseudoaneurysm formation; the incidence in various studies ranges from 0.15 per cent to 0.6 per cent.[41, 42] Symptoms generally occur 4 to 6 months following operation and may include a painful pulsatile cervical mass, transient ischemic attacks secondary to emboli, and hoarseness due to recurrent laryngeal nerve compression.[43] Differential diagnosis includes chemodectoma of the carotid body, lymphadenopathy, and kinking of an endarterectomized carotid artery. These causes usually can be distinguished from pseudoaneurysmal or aneurysmal disease with duplex imaging. Prior to 1960, roughly half of all carotid pseudoaneurysms that occurred following endarterectomy were associated with prosthetic patching of the arteriotomy. This incidence may be more rationally attributed to the use of silk suture. Various reports from that era confirm an extremely high incidence of pseudoaneurysm formation (as great as 80 per cent) when silk suture material was utilized.[44]

Most patients with pseudoaneurysms following carotid endartectomy should undergo operative correction to eliminate the risk of embolization. Because ligation of this vessel is associated with at least a 20 per cent incidence of major stroke, interposition grafting is the preferred treatment. The dissection may be difficult owing to the presence of scar and problems with identification of important neural structures such as the vagus and hypoglossal nerves. Manipulation of the aneurysmal sac should be minimized; control of the common and internal and external carotid arteries should be obtained first.[38] When necessary, division of the posterior belly of the digastric muscle or mandibular subluxation facilitates exposure of the distal internal carotid artery. Once controlled, the aneurysmal sac is opened and a shunt placed if desired. Infection must be considered, and cultures of thrombus, prosthetic material, and degenerated arterial wall should be obtained.

If the pseudoaneurysm involves the carotid bifurcation, several options exist based on the size of the defect and the presence of infection. If the defect is small and there is no evidence of infection, primary closure may be possible. If the defect is large, patch angioplasty is indicated with either prosthetic material or saphenous vein. If the bifurcation has completely degenerated, a bypass graft from the more proximal common carotid artery to the internal carotid artery with a reversed saphenous vein graft is necessary (Fig. 83–9).

Recurrent carotid pseudoaneurysms are unusual and generally attributable to infection. They may be treated with either ligation or replacement of a prosthetic patch with autogenous vein. If ligation is necessary, the patient should

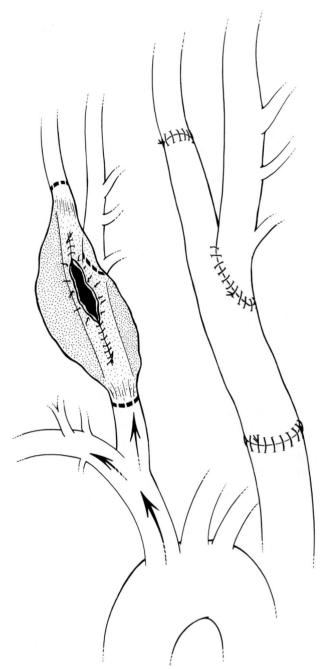

FIGURE 83–9. A reversed saphenous vein bypass graft from common carotid to internal carotid artery with inclusion of the origin of the external carotid artery.

be fully heparinized in the preoperative period; an extracranial-intracranial bypass may be performed if cerebral ischemia occurs.

Although primary mycotic carotid pseudoaneurysms are rare, they are associated with lethal complications. An aneurysmal abscess or pseudoaneurysm should be suspected in any drug-abusing patient with a painful neck mass and cellulitis. Angiography is indicated to define the extent of the pseudoaneurysm and assess the adequacy of collateral flow; duplex imaging may be a useful adjunct. Most lesions involve the common carotid rather than the internal carotid artery. Severe cellulitis should be treated with parenteral antibiotics for 7 to 14 days, at which time ligation of the involved artery and evacuation of infected hematoma is performed.[45, 46] Only rarely is bypass grafting feasible.

CONCLUSION

Pseudoaneurysms result from a variety of processes and occur most commonly following aortofemoral bypass. Avoidance of iatrogenic pseudoaneurysms requires meticulous surgical technique during the initial procedure. The use of permanent synthetic suture is mandatory. Minimal tension should be placed on anastomoses. Suture depth should be adequate to ensure full-thickness purchase on the arterial wall. An appropriately sized graft should be attached at an acute angle to minimize shear and hoop stress. Finally, one must minimize the occurrence of hematoma or lymphocele collections, which increase the risk of infection.

Diagnosis and treatment of pseudoaneurysms vary according to etiology and symptoms. In the absence of infection, interposition grafting with prosthetic material is widely accepted as the best form of treatment. When infection is obvious or suspected, autogenous vein is the best conduit. When pseudoaneurysms are identified early and treated appropriately, long-term results are excellent.

Acknowledgments: *The authors would like to acknowledge the expert secretarial assistance of Eileen Wayte and the artistic contributions of Kathy Hirsh in the preparation of this chapter.*

References

1. Matas R: Traumatic aneurysm of left brachial artery. Med News 53:462, 1888.
2. Lexer E: Die ideale Operation des Arteriellen und des arteriovenousen Aneurysm. Arch Klin Chir 83:459, 1907.
3. Haimovici H: Landmarks and present trends in vascular surgery. *In* Vascular Surgery: Principles and Techniques. Norwalk, CT, Appleton and Lange, 1989, pp 680–686.
4. Kottmeir CA, Wheat MW Jr: Strength of anastomoses in aortic prosthetic grafts. Am J Surg 31(2):128, 1965.
5. Edwards WS, Dalton D Jr, Quattlebaum R: Anastomoses between synthetic graft and artery. Arch Surg 92:123, 1966.
6. Gooding GA, Effency DJ, Goldstone J: The aortofemoral graft: Detection and identification of healing complications by ultrasonography. Surgery 89:94, 1981.
7. Brewster DC: Biologic behavior of grafts in arterial systems. *In* Haimovici H, Callow AD, DePalma RG, et al (eds): Vascular Surgery: Principles and Techniques. 3rd ed. Norwalk, CT, Appleton and Lange, 1989, pp 455–470.
8. Stern MS: Arteriosclerosis: Considerations as to etiology. South Med J 32:370, 1939.
9. Seabrook R, Schmitt DD, Bandyk DF, et al: Anastomotic femoral pseudoaneurysms: An investigation of occult infection as an etiologic factor. J Vasc Surg 11:629, 1990.
10. Messina LM, Brothers TE, Wakefield TW, et al: Clinical characteristics and surgical management of vascular complications in patients undergoing cardiac catheterization: Interventional versus diagnostic procedures. J Vasc Surg 13:593, 1991.
11. Potts RG, Alguire PC: Pseudoaneurysm of the abdominal aorta: A case report and review of the literature. Am J Med Sci 301(4):265, 1991.
12. Lavu J, Mattox KL, DeBakey ME: Mycotic aneurysm of the inferior mesenteric artery. Am J Surg 138:443, 1979.
13. Sterpetti AV, Feldhaus RJ, Schultz RD, Blair EA: Identification of abdominal aortic aneurysm patients with different clinical features and clinical outcomes. Am J Surg, 156:466, 1988.
14. Olsen WR, DeWeese MS, Fry WJ: False aneurysm of abdominal aorta. Arch Surg 92:123, 1966.
15. Ho KL, Rassekh ZS: Mycotic aneurysm of the right subclavian artery. Chest 74(1):116, 1978.
16. Szilagyi DE, Smith RF, Elliott JP, et al: Anastomotic aneurysms after vascular reconstruction: Problems of incidence, etiology and treatment. Surgery 78(6):800, 1975.
17. Nichols WK, Stanton M, Silver D, Keitzer WF: Anastomotic aneurysms following lower extremity revascularization. Surgery 88(3):366, 1980.
18. Sedwitz MM, Hye RJ, Stabile BE: The changing epidemiology of pseudoaneurysms: Therapeutic implications. Arch Surg 123:473, 1988.
19. Knox WG: Peripheral vascular and anastomotic aneurysms: A fifteen-year experience. Ann Surg 184(2):179, 1976.
20. Millili JJ, Lanes JS, Nemir P: A study of anastomotic aneurysms following aortofemoral prosthetic bypass. Ann Surg 192(1):69, 1980.
21. Richardson JV, McDowell HA: Anastomotic aneurysms following arterial grafting: A 10-year experience. Ann Surg 184(2):179, 1976.
22. Sawyers JL, Jacobs JK, Sutton JP: Peripheral anastomotic aneurysms: Development following arterial reconstruction with prosthetic grafts. Arch Surg 95:802, 1967.
23. Coughlin B, Paushter D: Peripheral pseudoaneurysms: Evaluation with duplex ultrasound. Radiology 108:339, 1988.
24. Yonkey JR, Clagett GP, Rich NM, et al: Anastomotic false aneurysms. Ann Surg 199:703, 1984.
25. Druny JK, Lieberman DP, Gilmour DG, Pollock JG: Operation for late complications of aortic grafts. Surg Gynecol Obstet 163:251, 1986.
26. Landrenau RJ, Snyder WH: Pelvic abscess or pseudoaneurysm: Diagnostic and therapeutic dilemma following iliac arterial trauma. Am J Surg 163:197, 1992.
27. Hollier LH, Batson RC, Cohn I Jr: Femoral anastomotic aneurysms. Ann Surg 191(6):715, 1979.
28. Gardner TJ, Brawley RK, Golt VL: Anastomotic false aneurysms. Surgery 72:474, 1972.
29. Sprah EM, Doran ML, Baird RJ: False aneurysms in the lower extremity. Surg Gynecol Obstet 144:562, 1967.
30. Moore WS, Hall AD: Late suture failure in the pathogenesis of anastomotic false aneurysms. Ann Surg 172(6):1064, 1970.
31. Ochsner J: Management of femoral pseudoaneurysms. Surg Clin North Am 62:431, 1982.
32. Dennis JW, Littooy FN, Greisler HP, Baker WH: Anastomotic pseudoaneurysms: A continuing late complication of vascular reconstructive procedures. Arch Surg 121:314, 1986.
33. Reddy DJ, Smith RF, Elliott JP, et al: Infected femoral artery false aneurysms in drug addicts: Evolution of selective vascular reconstruction. J Vasc Surg 3(5):718, 1986.
34. Fromm SH, Lucas CE: Obturator bypass for mycotic aneurysm in the drug addict. Arch Surg 100:82, 1970.
35. Johns JP, Pupa LE, Bailey SR: Spontaneous thrombosis of iatrogenic femoral artery pseudoaneurysms: Documentation with color Doppler and two dimensional ultrasonography. J Vasc Surg 14:24, 1991.
36. Kresowik TF, Khouny MD, Miller BV, et al: A prospective study of the incidence and natural history of femoral vascular complications after percutaneous transluminal coronary angioplasty. J Vasc Surg 13:328, 1991.
37. Rich NM, Hobson RW II, Fedde CW: Vascular trauma secondary to diagnostic and therapeutic procedures. Am J Surg 128:715, 1974.
38. Zarins CK, Gewertz BL: Atlas of Vascular Surgery. New York, Churchill Livingstone, 1989, pp 194–198.
39. Rosenbloom MS, Fellows BA: Chronic pseudoaneurysm of the popliteal artery after blunt trauma. J Vasc Surg 10:187, 1989.
40. Johnston KW, Raie M, Hogg-Johnston SA, et al: Five year results of a prospective study of percutaneous transluminal angioplasty. Ann Surg 206:403, 1987.
41. Hertzer NR: Postoperative management and complications following carotid endarterectomy. *In* Rutherford RB (ed): Vascular Surgery. 3rd ed. Philadelphia, WB Saunders, 1989, pp 1451–1471.
42. Thompson JE: Complications of carotid endarterectomy and their prevention. World J Surg 3:155, 1979.
43. Buscaglia LC, Moore WS, Hall AD: False aneurysm after carotid endarterectomy. JAMA 209:1529, 1969.
44. Branch OL Jr, Davis CH Jr: False aneurysm complicating carotid endarterectomy. Neurosurgery 19:421, 1986.
45. Maxwell TM, Olcott C IV, Blaisdell FW: Vascular complications of drug abuse. Arch Surg 100:82, 1970.
46. Ledgerwood AM, Lucas CE: Mycotic aneurysm of the carotid artery. Arch Surg 109:496, 1972.

Arteriovenous Communications and Congenital Vascular Malformations

Edited by Thomas S. Riles, M.D.

⌗

84

Overview

Thomas S. Riles, M.D.

• • •

The management of abnormal arteriovenous communications is one of the greatest challenges to the clinician. Unlike atherosclerotic vascular occlusive or aneurysmal disease, which tends to occur in recognized anatomic patterns, producing well-defined clinical syndromes, the etiology, distribution, and presentation of arteriovenous communications are far more varied. Their relative infrequency accounts for the fact that few physicians have encountered a sufficient number of patients with these disorders to qualify as experts in their management. Relatively few basic experimental studies have addressed the problem of congenital malformations of the arterial and venous systems and their associated communications. A notable exception is the classic work of Woolard,[11] discussed in Chapter 89. The physiology of shunting has been studied in more detail, with laboratory animal models having been used as far back as Vignolo.[9] The vast majority of information concerning human arteriovenous communications has come from two and a half centuries of observations by clinicians from all parts of the world, who carefully recorded the details of their patients' symptoms and physical findings. So many have shared in this heritage that it is impossible to mention but a few of the more recognizable names: William Hunter,[3] Rudolf Virchow,[10] Sir William Osler,[6] Rudolph Matas,[4] and Mont Reid.[7, 8] For an excellent review of the subject and an account of the hundreds of contributors to this field, the reader is referred to the works of Emile Holman[2] and Ernardo Malan.[5]

The subject of arteriovenous communications includes a vast array of conditions, most of which are abnormal but some of which are essential to normal development. It includes congenital anomalies, traumatic fistulae, erosions between an artery and a vein from infection or tumor, and even surgically created shunts. Arteriovenous communication, a very general term, refers to any connection between the arterial and the venous systems other than the pulmonary and systemic capillary beds. Communications can be multiple or single. A wide range of physiologic responses may result, depending on the location of the communication, the amount of blood per unit of time that passes from the artery to the vein, and the duration of the communication.

A discussion of arteriovenous communications is often hampered by an inadequate vocabulary and an unsatisfactory classification of the many varied conditions that share this common description. Unfortunately, there is no single system of classification suitable for all purposes. Many of the traditional systems, rich with descriptive terms and eponyms, have not been used in this section in order to avoid confusion with current terminology.

For the student and the diagnostician, a classification based on the etiology of the communication is quite helpful. Such a system is presented in Figure 84–1. Among the congenital lesions, those that are single communications are distinguished from those that have multiple channels. The latter usually result from the persistence of communications that normally exist at the earliest stages of development of arteriovenous systems. Although not truly arteriovenous communications, venous anomalies such as those found in the Klippel-Trenaunay syndrome are often included in this category because of their appearance and etiologic similarities. These are discussed further in Chapter 89. Although single fistulae may result from early developmental abnormalities, they may also be normal fetal communications

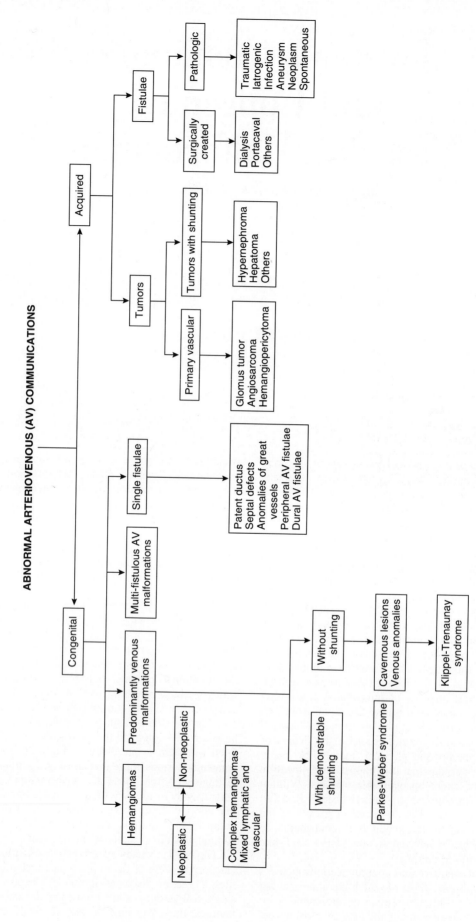

ABNORMAL ARTERIOVENOUS (AV) COMMUNICATIONS

FIGURE 84–1. Classification of abnormal arteriovenous communications.

that have failed to close at birth (patent ductus and septal defects).

Acquired communications are almost always single. One of the first descriptions of an acquired fistula involved a patient who developed a lesion from blood-letting, and medical procedures still account for the majority of traumatic fistulae. In addition to trauma, other etiologies such as infection, aneurysm (congenital and atherosclerotic), and neoplasm must be considered in evaluating acquired fistulae. Occasionally, spontaneous fistulae occur without an obvious underlying etiology.

A special category of therapeutic arteriovenous fistulae has evolved with modern surgery; it includes surgical fistulae for the correction of congenital defects of the heart and great vessels, access procedures for dialysis and chemotherapy, and fistulae created as an adjunct to other vascular operations, such as a femorotibial bypass or iliac vein thrombectomy. These are discussed in the following section on angioaccess.

The location, size, and physiologic effect of an abnormal arteriovenous communication are often more important than the etiology when planning a course of management. For example, the treatment of a spontaneous carotid–cavernous sinus fistula may be quite similar to that of a traumatic fistula of the kidney. To aid the clinician faced with the problems of management of these lesions, the chapters dealing with therapy have been organized into treatment-oriented groups. The arteriovenous fistulae are discussed in two chapters: one on the aorta and its major branches (Chapter 87) and the other dealing with the smaller vessels, in which both surgical and radiologic techniques have found a role (Chapter 88). The congenital vascular malformations are considered in Chapter 89.

A major advance that has occurred since the late 1970s is the development of percutaneous occlusion of arteriovenous communications. With the emergence of interventional radiology, new skills and new technology have developed. This has produced a renewed interest in the entire field of arteriovenous communications. Patients with malformations and fistulae that previously were considered untreatable have been skillfully managed by the use of embolic materials, balloons, glues, and other occlusive devices.[1] Appropriately, two interventional radiologists who have made significant contributions to the management of these difficult lesions are among the contributors to this edition of *Vascular Surgery.*

As experience grows, it is becoming clear that the best chance for cure of these complicated lesions is to coordinate the skills of many disciplines. In one memorable case, a patient with high-output cardiac failure and bleeding from a pelvic arteriovenous malformation, success was achieved only with the sustained efforts of the interventional radiologists, gynecologists, urologists, and vascular surgeons. Perhaps the greatest error in the handling of complicated arteriovenous communications is unnecessary ligation of the major feeding vessels as the initial step. This seldom works and hampers further therapy. In some cases, ligated vessels have had to be reconstructed so that embolization of the lesion could be performed. Cooperation among radiologists and surgical specialists is essential to avoid costly errors that could be disastrous for the patient or prevent successful therapy in the future.

In some cases, embolization followed by surgical resection has produced excellent cosmetic results. Otolaryngologists and plastic surgeons have been able to work closely with interventional radiologists and vascular surgeons to plan therapy for head and neck lesions or extremity malformations with minimal risk. Brain malformations or fistulae previously considered inoperable are now being successfully treated with catheter embolization or balloon occlusion. Clearly, this is the dawn of a new era in the management of arteriovenous communications.

In the following chapters, the many facets of this interesting and challenging aspect of vascular disease are explored. Few problems a vascular surgeon will encounter will be as complex with regard to anatomy, physiology, diagnosis, and therapy. The contributors to this edition of *Vascular Surgery* have provided an excellent review of the basic physiology as well as a guide to the management of abnormal arteriovenous communications.

References

1. Lasjaunias P, Berenstein A: Surgical Neuroangiography. Heidelberg, Springer Verlag, 1987, vol. II.
2. Holman E: Arteriovenous Aneurysm: Abnormal Communications Between the Arterial and Venous Circulations. New York, Macmillan, 1937.
3. Hunter W: The history of an aneurysm of the aorta, with some remarks on aneurysms in general. Med Observ Inq 1:323, 1757.
4. Matas R: On the systemic or cardiovascular effects of arteriovenous fistulae. Trans South Surg Assoc 36:623, 1923.
5. Malan E: Vascular Malformations (Angiodysplasias). Milan, Carlo Erba Foundation, 1974.
6. Osler W: Care of arteriovenous aneurysm of the axillary artery and vein of 14 years' duration. Ann Surg 17:37, 1893.
7. Reid MR: Studies on abnormal arteriovenous communications, acquired and congenital. I. Report of a series of cases. Arch Surg 10:601, 1925.
8. Reid MR, McGuire J: Arteriovenous aneurysms. Ann Surg 108:643, 1938.
9. Vignolo O: Un contributo sperimentale all'anatomia e fisiopathologia dell'aneurisma arterio-venoso. Policlinico [Chir] 9:197, 1902.
10. Virchow R: Pathologis des Tumeurs. Paris, Germer-Balliere, 1876.
11. Woolard HH: The development of the principal arterial system in the forelimb of the pig. Cont Embriol Carnegie Inst 14:139, 1922.

Hemodynamics and Pathophysiology of Arteriovenous Fistulae

David S. Sumner, M.D.

• • •

The "short circuit" between the high-pressure arterial system and the low-pressure venous system accounts for most of the symptoms and signs typical of an arteriovenous fistula. Electrical analogies are particularly apropos to the understanding of physiologic aberrations produced by arteriovenous fistulae. Let us suppose, for example, that a short circuit develops in the cord leading to a three-way floor lamp of a student intent on completing his or her evening studies (Fig. 85–1). Three problems may interfere with the completion of the work. First, the light may dim because the electrons have found a more direct route with less resistance back to the socket than that provided by the light bulb. Our enterprising student overcomes this difficulty by turning the switch to the high-intensity setting. However, just after the studies are again underway, all the lights go out. Too much current has burned out the fuse, which must be replaced. After the fuse has been replaced with one having a higher ampere rating, the student again begins work, only to be disturbed by the unmistakable odor of rubber burning. At last, the trouble is discovered: the local disruption of insulation, the overheated cord, and the threatened fire.

Likewise, patients with arteriovenous fistulae may experience three problems that parallel those of the electrical circuit. First, ischemia may develop in portions of the limb distal to the fistula. Even when peripheral vasodilatation is able to avert ischemia by compensating for the short circuit produced by the fistula, the demands on the heart may be excessive, resulting in cardiac failure. Finally, the blood vessels leading to and draining the fistula suffer degenerative changes. Thus, the pathophysiologic changes associated with arteriovenous fistula may be considered under the following three headings: *peripheral, central,* and *local* effects.

The magnitude and location of the leak determine the severity of the pathophysiologic changes. Whereas fistulae located centrally, near the heart, are more likely to produce cardiac failure, those located distally, in the extremities, are more likely to cause ischemia. Basically, the congenital and acquired forms of arteriovenous fistula are similar in principle from a hemodynamic point of view. However, the anatomy of the congenital fistula is far more complex. Instead of one major arteriovenous communication, there are usually many small, frequently innumerable, connections in parallel array. As a result, the central (cardiac) and the peripheral (ischemic) effects of congenital arteriovenous malformations are usually considerably less severe than those associated with acquired fistulae, and local effects

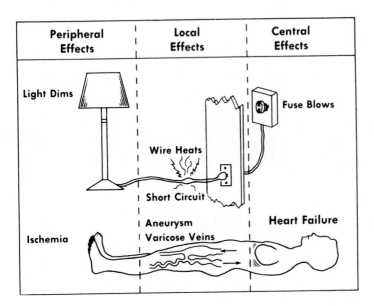

FIGURE 85–1. Like a short circuit in an electrical cord, arteriovenous fistulae produce peripheral, local, and central effects.

(e.g., venous hypertension, secondary varicosities, and limb hypertrophy) predominate. This is apparent from detailed discussions in Chapter 89. Because of these facts, it is much simpler to use the acquired form as a prototype for illustrating the hemodynamic features of arteriovenous fistulae.

In this chapter, the local, peripheral, and central effects of arteriovenous fistulae are described, as are how these effects dictate therapy and the design of fistulae for angioaccess. A brief discussion of naturally occurring arteriovenous communications is also included.

HEMODYNAMICS

Figure 85–2 illustrates the essential features of a typical side-to-side or H-type arteriovenous fistula. There is a *proximal* or *cardiad* artery and vein and a *distal* artery and vein. *Collateral arteries* connecting the proximal and distal arteries bypass the fistula. Similarly, *collateral venous channels* connect the distal vein with the proximal vein. A *peripheral vascular bed* that is supplied, at least in part, by the involved artery and drained by the involved vein lies distal to the fistula. Completing the circuit are the heart and the vessels that feed and drain the fistula.

Resistance of the Fistula

All the effects of an arteriovenous fistula (local, peripheral, and central) are inversely related to its hemodynamic resistance. As in all blood conduits, the greater the diameter of the fistula and the shorter its length, the less its resistance becomes. Side-to-side arteriovenous fistulae, such as those constructed between the radial artery and the cephalic vein or those that occur when an aortic aneurysm

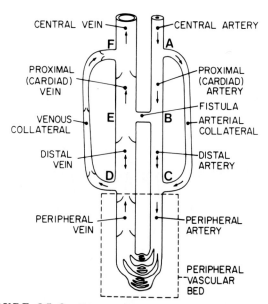

FIGURE 85–2. Diagram of a side-to-side arteriovenous fistula showing its relationship to collateral circulation and the peripheral vascular bed. (From Strandness DE Jr, Sumner DS: Arteriovenous fistulas. *In* Hemodynamics for Surgeons. New York, Grune & Stratton, 1975, pp 621–663.)

ruptures into the vena cava, have virtually no length. Although Poiseuille's law (see Eq. 3.15) suggests that a fistula with "zero" length should offer no resistance, some resistance is always present, owing to the inertial factors discussed in Chapter 3. Energy losses related to inertial factors, like those that are due to viscosity, are inversely proportional to the diameter of the opening. Consequently, small openings between contiguous arteries and veins may have a relatively high resistance despite their short length; however, beyond a certain critical diameter, the resistance becomes negligible in comparison with that of the other components of the fistulous circuit. When the transverse diameter of an elliptically shaped fistula approaches that of the proximal artery, extension of the longitudinal diameter will have little effect on blood flow through the parasitic circuit. Even though this may seem paradoxical in view of the lower resistance offered by the larger opening, the resistance of a fistula whose transverse diameter is near that of the proximal artery is so low that any further reduction in resistance will have essentially no effect on the total resistance of the entire circuit.[241]

On the other hand, the resistance of fistulous communications with a finite length—such as the H type illustrated in Figure 85–2 or those constructed for hemodialysis with a graft interposed between the artery and vein—is affected by both length and diameter. Both length and diameter influence viscous and inertial energy losses, and geometric factors, such as the compliance and curvature of the graft and the configuration of the proximal and distal anastomoses, affect inertial losses. As a result, H-type fistulae always have a greater resistance than side-to-side fistulae of equal diameter.

In an H-type fistula, most of the pressure is lost between between the donor artery and the arterial end of the graft and between the venous end of the graft and the recipient vein.[282] Fillinger and associates reported that 50 to 65 per cent of the pressure drop occurred at the arterial end of nontapered loop grafts, 25 to 30 per cent occurred at the venous end, and 11 to 18 per cent occurred along the grafts themselves.[265] When grafts were tapered with the larger diameter at the arterial end and the smaller diameter at the venous end, pressure drops at the arterial anastomosis were minimized, whereas those at the venous anastomosis were increased.[266] Reversing the taper changed these relationships in the opposite direction. The direction of the taper had little effect on the pressure drop within the grafts. Thus, flow disturbances at the junctions exact a greater toll in terms of fluid energy than viscous effects do in the main body of the graft, where the decline in pressure is gradual (see Chapter 3).

Experimentally, flow increases through an H-type fistula until its diameter exceeds twice that of the proximal artery.[156] Beyond this point, further increases in diameter may or may not have a discernible effect.

The combined resistance of fistulae in parallel equals the reciprocal of the sum of the reciprocals of their individual resistances (see Eq. 3.17). Therefore, the combined resistance must be less than the resistance of the fistula with the least resistance. Two parallel fistulae of equal size would have half the resistance of each fistula taken separately, but total blood flow through the two fistulae, although greatly increased, is seldom doubled.[154] Because of the increased flow, pressure at the proximal end of each fistula is reduced by opening the other; therefore, flow through each individual fistula is somewhat reduced. This explains why flow is more nearly doubled when the two fistulae are small than it is when they are large.

Local Effects

Blood Flow

Blood flow in the proximal artery is always increased (Fig. 85–3). The increase may be imperceptible when the fistula is small but will be multiplied manyfold when the fistula is large.[156] Although the size of the fistula is the main determinant of the magnitude of proximal artery blood flow, other factors, such as the resistance of the venous outflow, the arterial collaterals, and the peripheral vascular bed, also play a role.

Because the fistula markedly reduces the resistance "seen" by the proximal artery, diastolic flow is greatly increased. At times, diastolic flow may approach 80 to 90 per cent of the maximal flow rate during systole.[131, 211] This flow pattern is distinctly different from that observed in normal peripheral arteries. Under resting conditions, flow in normal arteries falls toward zero during diastole and often reverses for a brief period (see Fig. 85–3). Thus, the fistula not only increases the flow rate in the proximal artery but may also reduce its pulsatility.

Blood flow in the proximal vein not only is greatly increased but also becomes more pulsatile, with peak flow rates coinciding with arterial systole (Fig. 85–4). Because of the great compliance and low resistance of the proximal vein and its outflow channels, however, pulsations are rapidly damped out, usually within a few centimeters of the fistula. Pulsations are prominent only when the proximal vein is stenotic or occluded.

The direction of blood flow in the various components of the fistulous circuit is the key to understanding the essential hemodynamic features of this most interesting lesion

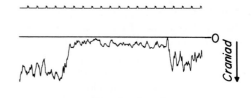

FISTULA OCCLUDED

FIGURE 85–4.   Blood flow in the cephalic vein proximal to a side-to-side radial artery–cephalic vein fistula. Because the Doppler probe was pointed craniad, flow in the normal direction is indicated by a downward deflection of the tracing. Note the large volume and pulsatile nature of the flow while the fistula is open and the low-volume, nonpulsatile flow with the fistula occluded.

(see Fig. 85–2). Flow in the proximal artery will always be directed toward the fistula, and flow in the proximal vein will always be directed centrally, toward the heart. Arterial collateral flow will always travel peripherally, bypassing the fistula, and venous collateral flow will always travel centrally, also bypassing the fistula. Blood in the distal artery and vein, however, may flow either toward or away from the fistula or may even be stagnant, depending on various anatomic and hemodynamic factors.

If the fistula is quite small, blood in the distal vein will continue to flow in the normal direction, past the fistula toward the heart (Fig. 85–5).[129, 211] This situation can occur only when the venous pressure at the nearest collateral junction exceeds that at the fistula site (see Fig. 85–2D and E). On the other hand, if the fistula is large, the pressure in the vein at the site of the fistula (see Fig. 85–2E) will exceed that farther distally in the vein (see Fig. 85–2D). This situation favors retrograde flow in the distal vein.[241] However, even in large acute fistulae, the presence of a single competent valve between the orifice of the fistula and the first venous collateral will prevent retrograde flow (Fig. 85–6A). Owing to increased pressure, the distal vein grad-

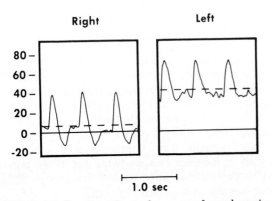

FIGURE 85–3.   Blood flow in the common femoral arteries of a 25-year-old man with an acute traumatic fistula between the left superficial femoral artery and vein. Mean velocity is indicated by the *broken line.* Calculated flow in the left common femoral artery (diameter, 9.0 mm) was 1680 ml/min, whereas that in the right common femoral artery (same diameter) was only 217 ml/min. Contrast the reversal of flow during diastole on the right (normal) side with the high diastolic flow on the left (fistulous) side. Note also that the pulse pressure is reduced on the side of the fistula.

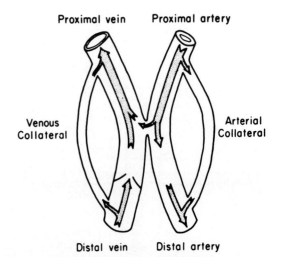

FIGURE 85–5.   Flow patterns in a small arteriovenous fistula. The direction of flow is normal in all parts of the circuit. (From Sumner DS: Arteriovenous fistula. *In* Strandness DE Jr [ed]: Collateral Circulation in Clinical Surgery. Philadelphia, WB Saunders, 1969, pp 27–90.)

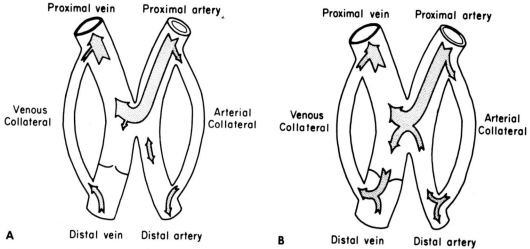

FIGURE 85-6. Flow patterns in large arteriovenous fistulae. *A*, Acute. *B*, Chronic. (*A* and *B*, From Sumner DS: Arteriovenous fistula. *In* Strandness DE Jr [ed]: Collateral Circulation in Clinical Surgery. Philadelphia, WB Saunders, 1969, pp 27–90.)

ually becomes more distended so that the valves no longer coapt properly. Therefore, in large chronic fistulae, blood will flow retrograde through incompetent valves down the distal vein until it is diverted into collateral venous channels (see Fig. 85–6*B*).[109, 136, 241] At some point, the excess pressure will be completely dissipated and retrograde flow will cease (see peripheral vein, Fig. 85–2).

The direction and quantity of blood flow in the distal artery depend on the relative magnitude of the pressure at the arterial end of the fistula and that at the site of collateral inflow (Fig. 85–2*B* and *C*).[241, 243] As shown in Figure 85–7, the fistula circuit can be compared to a Wheatstone bridge. In this model, the distal artery corresponds to the cross-arm of the bridge. The ratio of the resistance of the proximal artery to that of the fistula determines the pressure in the artery at the level of the fistula. Likewise, the ratio of the resistance of the collateral arteries to that of the distal vascular bed determines the pressure in the peripheral portion of the distal artery at the site of collateral inflow.

The following three possibilities exist for flow in the distal artery:

1. Flow in the normal peripheral direction will occur when the ratio of the fistula resistance to the proximal artery resistance exceeds that of the distal vascular bed to the arterial collaterals. This is most likely to occur in a small, high-resistance fistula, as shown in Figure 85–5, in which the arterial collaterals are not well developed and consequently have a high resistance.[109, 119, 129, 156, 165]

2. Flow in a retrograde direction will occur when the distal vascular bed resistance to the arterial collateral resistance ratio exceeds that of the fistula to the proximal artery. Typically, this occurs in large, chronic, low-resistance fistulae (see Fig. 85–6*B*) when the arterial collaterals are well developed.[6, 109, 119, 129, 152, 156, 165]

3. Stagnant flow exists only when the ratios are equal. This balance seldom occurs, but it can be seen in large acute fistulae before collaterals are well developed. In this case, blood may flow in the normal peripheral direction during systole but reverse during diastole (see Fig. 85–6*A*).[211]

Retrograde flow in the distal artery can deprive the peripheral vascular bed of nutrition and also increase the burden on the heart.

Pressure Levels

Blood pressure in the proximal artery is usually well maintained. Both systolic and diastolic pressures may be

FIGURE 85-7. A Wheatstone bridge model of an arteriovenous fistula. The distal artery corresponds to the crossarm of the bridge. (From Sumner DS: Arteriovenous fistula. *In* Strandness DE Jr [ed]: Collateral Circulation in Clinical Surgery. Philadelphia, WB Saunders, 1969, pp 27–90.)

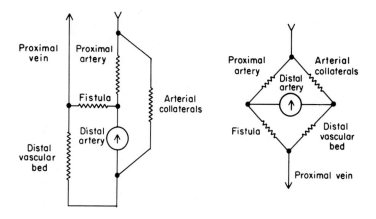

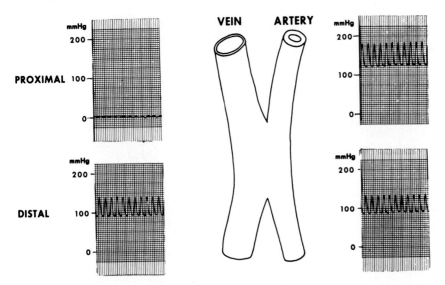

FIGURE 85–8. Blood pressures in the arteries and veins contributing to a large acute femoral arteriovenous fistula in a dog. Pressures were measured 1 cm away from the fistula. (From Sumner DS: Arteriovenous fistula. *In* Strandness DE Jr [ed]: Collateral Circulation in Clinical Surgery. Philadelphia, WB Saunders, 1969, pp 27–90.)

somewhat depressed, however, in the presence of a large acute fistula, owing to the energy losses associated with increased blood flow through a normal-sized artery.[133, 155, 178] When the proximal artery becomes dilated, as in a chronic fistula, pressures may even exceed those in comparable normal arteries at the same anatomic level.[128, 133]

In contrast, blood pressure in the distal artery is always reduced (Fig. 85–8). At any given distance from the fistula, both the mean and the pulse pressures will be lower than in the proximal artery.[23, 156, 211] When the fistula is small, pressure will gradually decrease from the proximal artery, past the fistula opening, to the distal artery (Fig. 85–9A). If the fistula is large, a pressure "sink" will exist at its opening. In other words, pressures will decrease from the proximal artery to the fistula but will rise again from the fistula to the distal artery (see Fig. 85–9B).[129] This reversal of the pressure gradient in the distal artery occurs in conjunction with reversal of blood flow and depends on the resistance relationships discussed earlier. In chronic fistulae, as collateral arteries increase in size, pressure in the distal artery tends to rise.[119, 212] This has the dual effect of encouraging

retrograde flow in the distal artery and of facilitating flow to the peripheral tissues.

Blood pressure in the proximal vein usually remains quite low despite the additional influx of blood from the fistula (cf. Figs. 85–8 and 85–9). One centimeter proximal to the fistula, the mean pressure ranges between 0 and 15 mmHg, and the pulse pressure seldom exceeds 5 mmHg.[129, 155, 211, 212] The low outflow resistance of the proximal vein, together with the remarkable compliance of the venous wall, accounts for the ability of the proximal vein to accommodate the increased flow rate with little change in pressure. If, however, the proximal vein is compressed or becomes obstructed, venous pressure will rise markedly, approaching that on the arterial side of the fistula.

The level of blood pressure in the distal vein depends on the size of the fistula and on the resistance offered to retrograde flow.[156] As mentioned previously, when the fistula is quite small, a normal pressure gradient will persist along the distal vein (see Fig. 85–9A). That is, there will be a slight but progressive fall in pressure from the periphery toward the fistula.[129, 211] However, when the fistula is large,

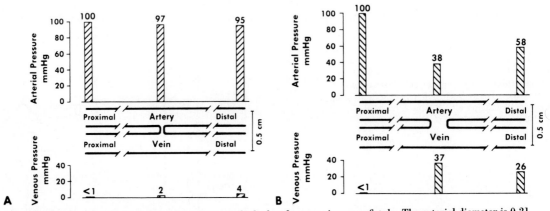

FIGURE 85–9. Theoretical blood pressures in the limbs of an arteriovenous fistula. The arterial diameter is 0.21 cm, and the venous diameter 0.24 cm. Proximal and distal pressures are measured 15 cm from the fistula. *A,* Small fistula, 0.02-cm diameter. *B,* Large fistula, 0.20-cm diameter. (*A* and *B,* Data from Strandness DE Jr, Sumner DS: Arteriovenous fistulas. *In* Hemodynamics for Surgeons. New York, Grune & Stratton, 1975, pp 621–663.)

venous pressure in the region of the fistula will be greatly increased (see Fig. 85–9B). This is especially true in acute fistulae when the venous valves are competent, prohibiting retrograde flow.[243] In such cases, the distal venous pressure may equal or even exceed that in the distal artery (see Fig. 85–8).[107, 108, 211, 256]

With the passage of time, resistance to retrograde flow diminishes as a result of the dilatation of the distal vein, the resulting incompetence of the venous valves, and the expansion of the venous collateral channels. Thus, blood pressure in distal venous segments tends to decrease as fistulae enter the chronic stage.[212]

Input Impedance

As one would predict, input impedance measured proximal to a large arteriovenous fistula is very low for the mean pressure-flow component (zero harmonic), reflecting the low outflow resistance (see Chapters 3 and 4).[281] The impedance curve remains flat across the spectrum of frequencies that correspond to higher harmonics, and the sine waves representing pressure and flow at each harmonic are roughly in phase. That pressure and flow are in phase is largely due to the absence of reflected waves from the low-resistance circuit. In contrast, the first harmonic of the input impedance in normal arteries is many orders of magnitude greater than that in arteries with distal arteriovenous fistulae, and phase angles for the higher harmonics are usually negative, indicating that the sine waves representing flow lead those representing pressure. Any impediment to the outflow of a fistula shifts the impedance curve toward that of normal arteries.

Turbulence

The bruit and thrill so characteristic of an arteriovenous fistula are the result of turbulent or disturbed flow patterns that cause vibrations in the walls of the associated blood vessels.[124, 157, 224] Several factors conspire to create these flow disturbances. Increased velocity of blood flow elevates the tube Reynolds number (see Eq. 3.12). Although the Reynolds number seldom reaches the critical value for turbulence in a smooth, straight pipe, it does reach that required for various geometric features to produce flow instability.[81, 181, 266] It is well known that bifurcations, bends, aneurysms, and sudden changes in the lumen of the blood vessel are responsible for flow disturbances.[8, 81, 181, 213, 232, 249] The circuit of an H-type fistula contains all these features. For example, the arterial flow stream either bifurcates at the entrance to the fistula—part flowing into the fistula and part into the distal artery—or, alternatively, is entirely diverted into the fistula, having been met head-on by a stream flowing proximally in the distal artery. The diameter of the lumen changes abruptly at the entrance to the fistula and again at its exit. This is particularly true if there is an intervening false aneurysm. As the flow stream emerges from the fistula, it may bifurcate into proximal and distal streams, swirl around in the distal vein, or join the proximally directed flow from the distal vein. Thus, there is little wonder that the flow pattern is markedly disturbed or that vibrations are set up in the walls of the contributing vascular channels.[265, 266]

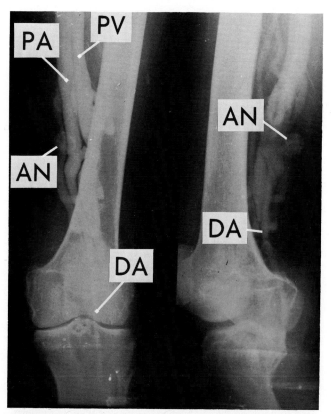

FIGURE 85–10. Chronic arteriovenous fistula of traumatic origin. Compare the dilatation of the proximal artery (PA) and vein (PV) with the normal dimensions of the distal artery (DA). Also, note the increased density of contrast medium in the proximal vessels, as compared with the faint visualization of the distal artery. Calcium occurs in the wall of the aneurysm. AN, associated aneurysm.

Anatomic Changes

With the exception of early traumatic fistulae, aortocaval fistulae that develop as a result of aneurysmal rupture, residual fistulae associated with in situ bypass grafting, and those created for hemodialysis, most fistulae that come to the attention of the surgeon are of the chronic variety. Even fistulae created for hemodialysis are usually allowed to "mature" for some time before use. Because of the increased arterial and venous blood flow, morphologic changes typically occur in the contributing vessels of chronic fistulae.

In general, the size of the opening between artery and vein increases with time; very few fistulae close spontaneously or become smaller.*

One of the most characteristic developments is the progressive elongation and distention of the proximal artery (Fig. 85–10).[33, 92, 111, 124, 133, 134, 194, 212] Indeed, many of these arteries become very tortuous and aneurysmal.[124, 163, 193, 207, 221] Although the arterial wall may initially become somewhat thickened, it eventually undergoes degenerative changes, with atrophy of smooth muscle, decrease in the quantity of elastic tissue, and formation of atheromatous plaques.† These changes may be irreversible if the fistula is allowed to persist for more than 1 or 2 years.[93, 163, 207]

*See references: increase with time, 117, 119; close or become smaller, 66, 121, 198, 220.
†See references: becomes thickened, 225; undergoes degenerative changes, 163, 193, 207, 221, 233.

Hemodynamic factors probably account for the changes observed in the proximal artery. It appears that the increased velocity of blood is in some way responsible.[134, 162, 252] Some investigators have suggested that the arterial endothelium senses the increased hydrodynamic drag produced by the interaction of the bloodstream on the interior surface of the artery. This, in turn, induces a reorganization of the structural elements of the arterial wall in an effort to reduce the effect of the wall shear stress.[146, 201] Other possibilities include the effect of vibration on the arterial wall.[134, 186, 224] The fact that the enlargement is most marked in the immediate vicinity of the fistula lends credence to this idea.[134] Vibration has been shown to play a role in post-stenotic dilatation, an anatomic change not dissimilar to aneurysm formation in the proximal artery.[115, 197]

Elongation and tortuosity of the proximal artery are also related to similar hemodynamic factors. The force that tends to stretch the artery along its long axis is directly proportional to the longitudinal pressure gradient, which is a function of the velocity of blood flow.[130, 153]

Similar changes are observed in the proximal vein, which also becomes dilated and tortuous (cf. Fig. 85–10).[92] Not only does the wall become irregularly thickened, owing to intimal proliferation and fibrosis, but also degenerative changes, such as atherosclerosis and aneurysms, may occur.* The internal elastic lamina tends to fragment and disappear. For these reasons, the term *arterialization,* often used to describe the changes in the venous wall, is inappropriate. Additional endothelial damage is produced in that

---

*See references: proliferation and fibrosis, 82, 233, 234; atherosclerosis and aneurysms, 235, 274.

portion of the vein wall immediately opposite the fistulous opening, presumably owing to the force of the jet of blood or to vibrations set up in the venous wall.[77, 224] Experiments with prosthetic graft fistulae in dogs suggest that thickening of the venous intima and media is correlated with turbulence at the distal anastomosis and kinetic energy transfer into the adjacent tissues.[265]

As mentioned in earlier portions of this chapter, with the passage of time, the distal vein dilates and elongates and its valves become incompetent. As venous collaterals develop, more and more of the fistula flow is carried distally by this vein, which suffers, albeit to a lesser degree, the same degenerative changes experienced by the proximal vein.[92, 109, 136]

The distal artery, in contrast to the proximal artery and the proximal and distal veins, tends to remain the same size, perhaps even shrinking a little (see Fig. 85–10).

About 60 per cent of traumatic fistulae will have an associated false aneurysm.[72] Calcium deposits, commonly found in the walls of these structures, can be seen in Figure 85–10.[82] As shown in Figure 85–11, the aneurysm may be a part of the fistulous tract itself, or it may be an outgrowth of either artery, vein, or both.[72, 166]

Collateral Development

Arteriovenous fistulae constitute the most powerful known stimuli to collateral development.[114, 141, 193] The extent of the collateral bed far exceeds that associated with an atherosclerotic occlusion of a comparable artery.

What factors are responsible for the remarkable growth? Two major theories have been proposed: that col-

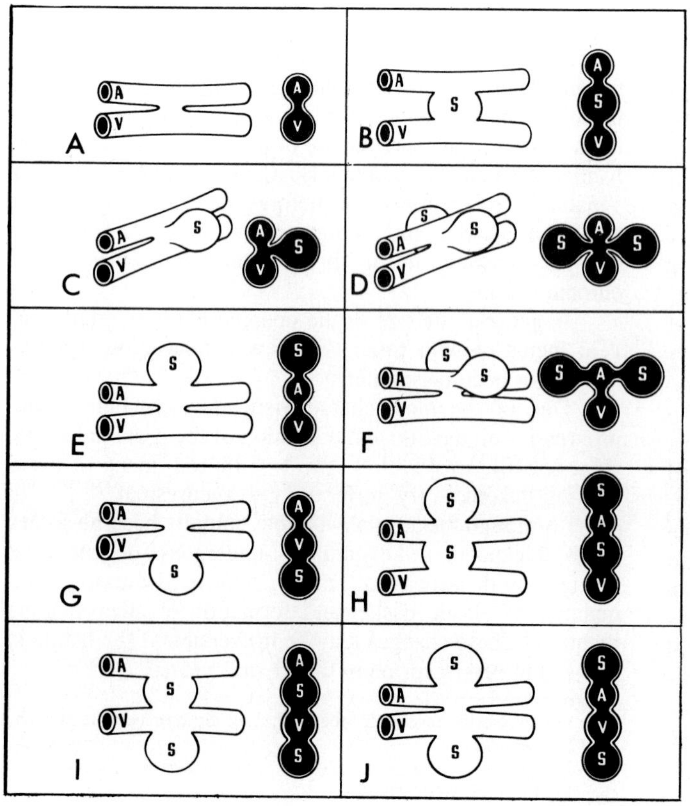

FIGURE 85–11. Relationship of aneurysmal sac to arteriovenous fistula. A, artery; V, vein; S, aneurysmal sac. (From Elkin DC, Shumacker HB Jr: Arterial aneurysms and arteriovenous fistulas: General considerations. *In* Elkin DC, DeBakey ME [eds]: Surgery in World War II: Vascular Surgery. Washington, DC, Office of the Surgeon General, Department of the Army, 1955, pp 149–180.)

lateral development is a function of an increased velocity of blood flow or of an increased pressure differential across the collateral bed.* The weight of the evidence appears to favor the first theory. For example, Holman[114] and Reid[193] observed that collateral formation after ligation of the femoral artery in dogs was less extensive than it was when a large femoral arteriovenous fistula had been created, despite the fact that the reduction in pressure in the artery distal to the obstruction or fistula was the same. An obvious difference between the two circuits is that flow through collaterals bypassing an arteriovenous fistula usually exceeds that through collaterals bypassing an occlusion. In the presence of a fistula, blood may flow retrograde in the distal artery toward the fistula; thus, the outflow resistance faced by the collateral channels is markedly reduced. In contrast, when the artery is obstructed, collaterals empty into the relatively high resistance offered by the peripheral vascular bed. As a result, *when there is reversed flow in the distal artery, collateral flow will always be higher in a limb containing a fistula than it will be in a limb with an arterial obstruction.*

In a series of elegant experiments, Holman demonstrated clearly the importance of retrograde flow in the distal artery.[114] He found that collateral development was markedly reduced when the fistula was constructed at the end of the proximal artery or when the distal artery was ligated just beyond the fistula. These preparations permitted no retrograde flow. When, however, the distal artery was ligated beyond a single branch, collateral development was extensive.

As mentioned earlier in this chapter, other investigators have shown convincingly that increased flow through a blood vessel stimulates the vessel to dilate, possibly as a result of increased shear stress on the endothelium (see Chapter 3).†

Several investigators have observed that the growth of venous collaterals may even exceed that of arterial collaterals.[61, 62, 109] As with arterial collaterals, the mechanism of development is probably related to increased velocity of blood flow. Lengthening and tortuosity are more pronounced in venous collaterals than in arterial collaterals. The superficial veins resemble primary varicose veins. Indeed, the presence of unilateral varicose veins should alert the clinician to the possible presence of an arteriovenous fistula.

Venous collaterals are required in large acute fistulae to transport blood around the distal venous segment, the valves of which are closed to prevent retrograde flow. As the fistula ages and the valves in the distal vein become incompetent, additional venous collaterals are recruited to handle the retrograde flow. Maximal venous collateral development is observed when the proximal vein is occluded, forcing all the fistula flow to travel retrograde in the distal vein.

Peripheral Circulation

Arteriovenous fistulae always constitute a threat to the blood supply of the peripheral tissues. Weak peripheral

---

*See references: velocity of blood flow, 67, 162, 201, 252; pressure differential, 114, 117, 141.

†See references: stimulates dilatation, 67, 134, 162, 252; as result of shear stress, 146, 201.

pulses, pallor, cyanosis, and edema are not uncommonly observed.[73, 124, 193] Plethysmographic pulses may be reduced in amplitude but usually retain a normal contour (Fig. 85–12).[31, 73, 242] Near the fistula, where arterial blood rapidly enters superficial and deep veins, the temperature of the skin, muscle, and bone is frequently elevated. However, distal to the fistula, these tissues tend to be cooler than normal.[61, 62, 73, 102, 108, 132, 136, 147, 193] Oxygen tension within the peripheral muscles and bones may be decreased.[132] Likewise, the venous blood draining these tissues may show a decreased oxygen saturation and an increased concentration of lactic acid, implying marginal perfusion.[132, 167] Some patients will describe pain and paresthesias of the digits distal to a fistula.[31, 69] Others may develop painful ulcerations or gangrene of the fingers or toes.[43, 50, 69, 195] A few patients will complain of intermittent claudication when the fistula is located proximally in the limb.[193]

Blood Flow and Blood Pressure

When the fistula is small, blood flowing in the normal peripheral direction within the distal artery will be joined by blood from the collaterals to supply the peripheral arteries and their recipient tissues (see Figs. 85–2 and 85–5). Even when the fistula is large and flow in the distal artery is retrograde, at one of the distal collateral junctions, flow must again turn toward the periphery to supply the tissues of the vascular bed (see Figs. 85–2 and 85–6). In other words, at some point toward the periphery, arterial flow always regains its normal peripheral orientation.[129, 241] For example, in patients with large radial artery–cephalic vein fistulae, flow in the digital artery, which is beyond any major collateral input, is peripherally directed even though flow in the distal radial artery is reversed (Fig. 85–13). In such cases, the point of division between retrograde and antegrade flow is in the superficial palmar arch.

When the fistula is small and the collateral arteries are large, there may be little or no decrease in peripheral blood flow because arteriolar dilatation will be sufficient to compensate for the leak. When the fistula is large, however, and the collaterals are poorly developed, arteriolar dilatation may not be adequate to maintain tissue nutrition. This is particularly likely to happen when there is a great deal of retrograde flow in the distal artery. In other cases, nutrition will not suffer, but there will be a relative reduction

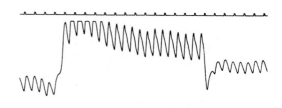

FISTULA OCCLUDED

FIGURE 85–12. Plethysmographic pulses from the tip of the index finger in a patient with a side-to-side radial artery–cephalic vein fistula. Note the marked increase in volume when the fistula is occluded. (From Strandness DE Jr, Sumner DS: Arteriovenous fistulas. *In* Hemodynamics for Surgeons. New York, Grune & Stratton, 1975, pp 621–663.)

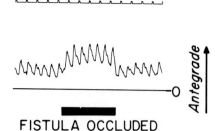

FISTULA OCCLUDED

FIGURE 85–13. Blood flow in the digital artery of the middle finger in a patient with a radial artery–cephalic vein fistula on the same side. Blood flows in the normal distal direction even though flow in the distal radial artery was reversed. Temporary occlusion of the fistula increases the velocity of blood flow. The Doppler probe was pointed craniad. (From Strandness DE Jr, Sumner DS: Arteriovenous fistulas. *In* Hemodynamics for Surgeons. New York, Grune & Stratton, 1975, pp 621–663.)

of blood flow in the distal portions of the involved extremity as compared with the uninvolved extremity.[31, 187, 200, 202, 241, 244, 258]

Although reduction in arteriolar resistance may permit blood flow to remain relatively normal, peripheral pressure will always be more or less reduced because of the obligatory energy losses associated with the fistula.* Of the patients with side-to-side radial artery–cephalic vein fistulae whom the author studied, 88 per cent had reduced digital artery pressures on the ipsilateral side. The average ratio of the pressure in the digital arteries to that in the brachial artery was 0.64 ± 0.24.[241, 244] As in the case of obstructive arterial disease, the drop in pressure is the most sensitive and reliable indicator of the hemodynamic severity of the lesion (see Chapters 3 and 5).[164]

Effect of Occluding the Fistula and Its Associated Vessels

Figure 85–14 illustrates the changes in finger blood pressure and blood flow produced by manual compression of a radial artery–cephalic vein fistula and the contributing vessels.[241, 244]

Peripheral pressure and flow are decreased when the proximal radial artery is occluded. This occurs no matter what the size of the fistula is. When the fistula is small, proximal artery compression eliminates the antegrade flow in the distal radial artery but permits blood to flow retrograde in the distal radial artery toward the fistula; in other words, flow in the distal radial artery reverses. When the fistula is large, proximal artery compression serves to increase the retrograde flow in the distal radial artery. Thus, proximal artery compression increases the "steal" of blood from the collateral channels bypassing the fistula and further deprives the peripheral tissues of nutritive flow.

Compression of the major collateral channel, the ulnar artery, also results in a marked decrease in digital artery pressure and flow. Although this maneuver may cause flow in the distal radial artery to switch from retrograde to antegrade when the fistula is large or to increase the antegrade

flow when the fistula is small, so much blood passes through the low-resistance fistula that peripheral perfusion is decreased. In fact, compression of the collateral arteries may produce a more severe deprivation of nutritive flow than does compression of the proximal artery.

Occlusion of any of the outflow channels of the fistula, such as the proximal or distal vein, increases the effective resistance of the fistula and increases the digital artery pressure and flow. However, a more striking increase in peripheral perfusion occurs when the radial artery distal to a large fistula is compressed. This is the result of eliminating retrograde flow through the distal artery, thereby permitting all the collateral flow to supply the distal tissues. If the fistula is of the small variety with antegrade flow in the distal artery, compression of the distal artery may decrease peripheral perfusion. The extent of the decrease would depend on the capacity of the collateral arteries.

Total occlusion of the fistula plus the proximal and distal arteries and veins may increase or decrease peripheral perfusion, depending on the size of the fistula and the functional capacity of the collateral vessels. If both the fistula and the collaterals are large, occlusion of the fistula and the four contributing vessels will increase the peripheral pressure and flow (see Fig. 85–14). On the other hand, if the fistula is small and the collaterals are poorly developed, this maneuver would result in decreased peripheral perfusion.

How these responses apply to the design of arteriovenous fistulae for hemodialysis and to therapy for congenital and acquired fistulae is discussed later in this chapter.

Systemic Effects

The introduction of an abnormal communication between the arterial and venous sides of the circulation produces a drop in *total peripheral resistance.* This is the essential pathophysiologic change responsible for all the systemic effects attributable to arteriovenous fistulae.

In order to discuss these effects, some definitions are necessary. *Total peripheral resistance* refers to the total resistance encountered by the left side of the heart. Its reciprocal equals the sum of the reciprocal of the *resistance of the fistula* plus the reciprocal of the *systemic resistance* offered by the peripheral vascular beds (see Eq. 3.17). *Systemic blood flow* is that part of the cardiac output that perfuses the peripheral tissues, and *fistula flow* is that part that passes exclusively through the parasitic circuit. Together, systemic blood flow and fistula flow equal the cardiac output.

If no circulatory adjustments were made, the reduction in total peripheral resistance accompanying an arteriovenous fistula would cause the arterial pressure to fall, the venous pressure to rise, and blood to be diverted from the peripheral tissues into the parasitic circuit. Arterial pressure could be maintained by increasing the systemic resistance, but this mechanism would further reduce flow to the peripheral tissues and would therefore be self-defeating. A more appropriate adjustment would be to augment the cardiac output by increasing heart rate and stroke volume. An increased cardiac output would maintain arterial pressure, reduce venous pressure, and supply enough blood to nour-

---

*See references: blood flow normal, 202; peripheral pressure reduced, 164, 241, 242.

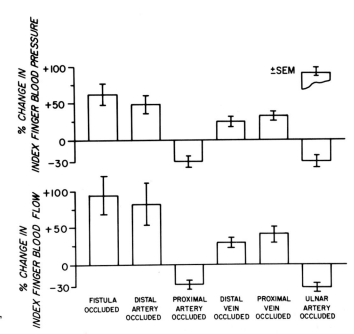

FIGURE 85–14.   Effect on peripheral blood flow and blood pressure of compressing various portions of the arteriovenous fistula circuit. Values represent the average percentage change in index finger blood pressure and blood flow. (From Strandness DE Jr, Sumner DS: Arteriovenous fistulas. *In* Hemodynamics for Surgeons. New York, Grune & Stratton, 1975, pp 621–663.)

ish the peripheral tissues. For the stroke volume to increase, venous return must become more efficient, the blood volume must increase, or both must occur.

All these mechanisms are called into play in patients with arteriovenous fistulae. Thus, heart rate, stroke volume, cardiac output, and blood volume are usually increased. In large fistulae in which compensatory mechanisms are inadequate, arterial blood pressure and systemic blood flow may be reduced, and the systemic resistance, the central venous pressure, and the left and right atrial pressure may be elevated.

Arterial and Left Ventricular Pressure

When an acute arteriovenous fistula is suddenly opened, there is a precipitous drop in arterial pressure as a result of the marked decrease in peripheral resistance (Fig. 85–15).[111, 177, 256] As the cardiac output increases and systemic resistance rises, the pressure rapidly returns toward baseline levels. Depending on the size of the fistula, however, the mean pressure often remains somewhat depressed.[177] In addition, the pulse pressure may increase because of a tendency for the diastolic pressure to be more depressed than the systolic, but this change is not consistently observed.* Closure of an acute fistula causes a sudden increase in arterial pressure to levels exceeding baseline values, as shown in Figure 85–15.[177] As the cardiac output and systemic resistance fall, the pressure rapidly returns to prefistula levels.[84, 177, 204, 256]

In most patients with chronic fistulae, the mean arterial pressure is maintained within normal limits but the diastolic pressure may be decreased, producing an increased pulse pressure (water-hammer pulse).[73, 161] The responses to compression or surgical closure of chronic fistulae are similar to those described for acute fistulae. Depending on the size

of the fistula, there may be no perceptible rise in pressure, or there may be an immediate increase, particularly in the diastolic pressure.*

Left ventricular systolic and end-diastolic pressures drop on opening of an acute arteriovenous fistula, but the end-diastolic pressure rapidly returns to near prefistula levels.[177] Closure of the fistula causes a momentary increase in systolic and end-diastolic pressures before they return to control values. In the presence of large chronic fistulae, left ventricular end-diastolic pressure gradually rises and may reach remarkably high levels in patients in whom cardiac failure is severe enough to cause death.[206]

Venous Pressure

Because the central venous pressure rises only a few millimeters of water (a fraction of a millimeter of mercury) when an arteriovenous fistula is opened, this change will not be detected unless careful serial measurements are made.[84, 96, 142, 177] Because the increased cardiac output serves to decompress the venous reservoir and because the compliant nature of the venous circulation easily absorbs the increased venous volume, central venous pressures ordinarily remain within normal limits.[142, 156, 194, 256]

Atrial, Right Ventricular, and Pulmonary Arterial Pressure

Opening an arteriovenous fistula causes a rise in right and left atrial pressure and in mean pulmonary arterial pressure (see Fig. 85–15).[96, 177, 178, 204, 268] The absolute magnitudes of these increases are small and are related to the quantity of blood flowing through the fistula.

The resistance of the pulmonary vascular bed tends to drop, paralleling the increase in fistula flow.[177] This has the

*See references: diastolic pressure depressed more than systolic, 177; not consistently, 211, 256.

*See references: no perceptible rise, 142, 226; immediate increase, 94, 110, 112, 113, 180, 182.

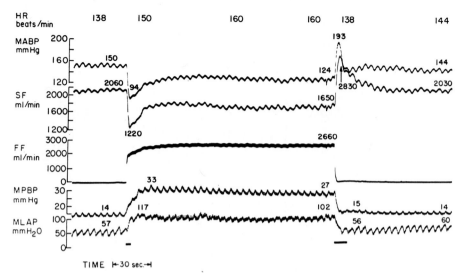

FIGURE 85–15. Effects of opening and closing a large acute arteriovenous fistula in an anesthetized dog. The fistula was opened at the *first bar* (base of graph) and closed at the *second bar*. HR, heart rate; MABP, mean systemic arterial blood pressure; SF, systemic blood flow; FF, fistula flow; MPBP, mean pulmonary arterial blood pressure; MLAP, mean left atrial blood pressure. (From Nakano J, DeSchryver C: Effects of arteriovenous fistula on systemic and pulmonary circulations. Am J Physiol 207:1319, 1964.)

effect of maintaining the same pressure drop across the pulmonary circuit. When flow through the fistula becomes very large, however, a minimal level of pulmonary resistance is reached. Increasing the flow beyond this level will cause a rise in the pressure gradient across the lung and an increase in mean pulmonary arterial pressure.[177]

Right ventricular systolic and end-diastolic pressures increase when an arteriovenous fistula is first opened, but the diastolic pressure rapidly returns to prefistula levels.[177] Closure of the fistula reverses this sequence.

Cardiac Output, Systemic Blood Flow, and Flow Through the Fistula

Cardiac output increases immediately after an acute arteriovenous fistula is opened, and peak flow is achieved within a few seconds. As a consequence of the rapid increase in fistula flow from zero to near maximal levels, there is an initial drop in blood flow through the systemic vascular beds, coinciding with the initial fall in mean arterial pressure. With the increase in cardiac output, systemic blood flow rises to stabilize at or somewhat below that existing before the introduction of the fistula into the circuit (see Fig. 85–15).[177, 178, 268]

Sudden closure of an acute arteriovenous fistula reverses the sequence. Fistula flow drops to zero, systemic blood flow is momentarily increased above prefistula levels, and cardiac output rapidly falls, as shown in Figure 85–15. The brief increase in systemic blood flow coincides with a temporary rise in systemic blood pressure and reflects the adjustment period during which excess cardiac output is forced to find egress through high-resistance peripheral vascular beds rather than through the low-resistance fistula.[84, 177]

When fistulae are small, the increase in cardiac output equals the blood flow through the fistula; consequently, there is no decrease in systemic blood flow. However, when fistulae are large and fistula flows exceed 27 to 40 per cent of the control (prefistula) cardiac output, the increase in cardiac output may not equal the fistula flow.[84, 158] Therefore, in such cases, blood is "stolen" from the peripheral vascular beds and systemic blood flow decreases. A fall in

the mean arterial pressure may be prevented by compensatory peripheral vasoconstriction until fistula flows exceed 60 per cent of the control cardiac output.[84, 177, 178, 256] Beyond this point, compensation is inadequate and systemic blood pressure falls. This situation develops clinically when an aortic aneurysm ruptures into the inferior vena cava, creating a massive arteriovenous fistula. Cardiac failure is rapid and death follows shortly unless the aneurysm is expeditiously removed and the fistula closed.[10, 12, 52, 56, 70, 199]

The percentage rise in systemic resistance always lags behind the percentage rise in fistula flow. Therefore, changes in systemic resistance are never able to compensate fully for the decrease in total peripheral resistance that follows the opening of an arteriovenous fistula. Were it not for the concomitant increase in cardiac output, blood pressure would fall to some extent in all cases.[178] Sympathoadrenal stimulation and increased levels of circulating catecholamines appear to be responsible for the increased systemic resistance.[177–179] As time passes and compensatory mechanisms are called into play, systemic resistance returns to normal levels.[268]

In most clinical cases, the increase in cardiac output is sufficient to prevent decreased blood flow to the systemic vascular beds. Depending on the size of the fistula, the cardiac output at rest may not be perceptibly elevated or it may be greatly increased.[14, 39, 76, 101, 142, 148, 176, 208, 214, 226, 231] Fistulae of moderate size do not appear to have an adverse effect on the increase in cardiac output induced by exercise.[64] Closure of a chronic arteriovenous fistula results in a decrease in cardiac output in 50 to 80 per cent of patients.[142, 182, 226, 261]

Heart Rate and Stroke Volume

There are two ways in which the cardiac output can be increased: an increase in heart rate and an increase in stroke volume. Both of these mechanisms are operational in the patient with an arteriovenous fistula, but an increase in stroke volume is the more significant of the two.[14, 79, 96, 177, 261]

Opening an acute arteriovenous fistula may produce a transient rise in pulse rate, but this response does not always occur. Closure of an acute fistula may cause the pulse rate to drop below control (prefistula) levels for a brief period before it returns to normal levels (see Fig. 85–15).[84, 96, 177, 178, 204, 256]

In patients with chronic arteriovenous fistulae, the heart rate is usually within normal limits. Slowing of the pulse rate with compression of the fistula or the proximal artery was first reported by Nicoladoni in 1875[183] and by Branham in 1890.[22] In the majority of patients, the decrease is more than 4 beats/min, averaging 3 ± 4 beats/min.[142, 182] This response appears to follow the temporary rise in systemic arterial pressure and is abolished by large doses of atropine, suggesting that it is initiated by the baroreceptors in the carotid sinus and aortic arch and that it is mediated through the vagus nerve.[110, 111, 161, 182] A more recent study has shown that tachycardia induced by opening an arteriovenous fistula may occur despite a controlled arterial pressure and that changes in heart rate do not necessarily depend on arterial baroreceptor reflexes.[95] The receptors mediating the cardioacceleratory reflexes may be in the heart or lung, and the vagus nerves appear to constitute the afferent and efferent pathways.

Although increasing the heart rate has little effect on cardiac output when venous return is normal, it does augment cardiac output in the presence of an arteriovenous fistula when venous return is elevated. This is especially true in the presence of increased catecholamine levels and heightened sympathetic activity, which accompany the opening of an arteriovenous fistula.[44]

Nevertheless, increased stroke volume alone accounts for 80 to 90 per cent of the rise in cardiac output associated with an acute or chronic arteriovenous fistula.[96, 177, 204, 268] The elevated stroke volume has been attributed to the Frank-Starling mechanism, which is initiated by a slight rise in atrial pressure.[96] It may also reflect an increase in myocardial contractility that develops in response to increased sympathetic adrenergic outflow and elevated levels of circulating catecholamines.[177-179]

Normally, the subendocardium exhibits greater oxygen extraction, coronary blood flow, and oxygen consumption than the subepicardium. These differences are not observed in the presence of a moderate-volume arteriovenous fistula, suggesting a relative decrease in subendocardial oxygen demand in response to an increase in volume work, especially at the apex of the left ventricle.[27]

Heart Size

Cardiac enlargement is frequently seen in patients with chronic arteriovenous fistulae. This well-known association has been recognized for more than 70 years.[192, 193, 238] The increase in heart size ranges from a small percentage in patients with small fistulae to nearly 80 per cent in those with large fistulae.[14]

A gradual enlargement of the heart begins immediately after the fistula is created and continues for several months.* When the fistula is large and uncompensated, the heart may initially decrease in size as a result of the displacement of blood into the capacious venous system.[112]

Closure of a chronic fistula may result in transient enlargement of the aorta and left ventricle, together with a

reduction in volume of the right atrium and pulmonary conus.[113] These effects are due to incomplete emptying of the left side of the heart and diminution of venous return to the heart. Permanent correction of a chronic fistula causes the heart to decrease steadily in size, frequently returning to normal dimensions within a few weeks.[137, 223, 261]

The increase in cardiac size may represent either dilatation or hypertrophy. Volume overload, like that which accompanies an arteriovenous fistula, causes both of these effects.[19, 63] Experimental studies suggest that the hearts of adult dogs respond primarily by dilatation, whereas the hearts of growing puppies tend to hypertrophy.[112] In rats with chronic aortocaval fistulae, an increase in heart weight of 86 per cent at 1 month has been shown to be due to hypertrophy of the individual myocytes rather than to hyperplasia.[272]

Blood Volume

Blood volume is often increased in the presence of a chronic arteriovenous fistula.[74, 113, 117, 148, 206, 214, 226, 260] In one series, the increase ranged from 200 to more than 1000 ml/m^2 of body surface.[260]

The excess blood is accommodated in all parts of the expanded fistulous circuit, including proximal arteries and veins, cardiac chambers, central veins, and collateral vessels.[117, 226] It aids peripheral perfusion by permitting the cardiac output to rise sufficiently to accommodate both the fistula and the systemic circulation, thus avoiding a steal.[84, 96] Indeed, transfusion may be necessary to preserve life in the presence of a large arteriovenous fistula.[51] It appears that the major factor limiting cardiac output in the presence of an acute fistula is an insufficient blood volume and not an inadequate cardiac reserve.[84] The organism tends to correct this volume deficit as the fistula becomes chronic.

Expansion of plasma volume, which accounts for most of the increase in blood volume,[53] is largely a result of sodium- and water-retaining mechanisms that are activated by the presence of a fistula.* This process appears to be triggered by a reduction in mean arterial pressure.[199] In response to the decreased perfusion pressure, renal blood flow and glomerular filtration rate decrease and reabsorption from the renal tubules increases. As a result, urine output falls, extracellular fluid accumulates, and blood volume expands.[268] In addition, decreased renal blood flow activates the renin-angiotensin-aldosterone system, which further increases renal sodium and fluid reabsorption.† Renal nerves evidently play an important role.[122] Once the proper volume elevation has been achieved, sodium and water excretion returns to normal.[54] In experimental animals with large arteriovenous fistulae, right atrial pressure rises in response to the elevated blood volume. The increase in right atrial pressure is accompanied by a marked increase in the level of circulating atrial natriuretic peptide.[268, 276] This substance augments glomerular filtration rate, inhibits sodium reabsorption in the medullary collecting duct, and opposes the antinatriuretic activity of the renin-angiotensin-

---

*See references: begins immediately, 161, 194; continues for months, 137.

*See references: expansion of plasma volume, 74; mechanisms activated by fistula, 106.

†See references; triggered by pressure changes, 250; mediated by renin-angiotensin-aldosterone system, 54, 255, 268, 276.

aldosterone system. Although it is attractive to postulate that atrial natriuretic peptide plays a role in achieving volume homeostasis in the presence of a chronic arteriovenous fistula, studies have cast doubt on this mechanism.[276]

In chronic cases, occlusion of the fistula results in increased sodium excretion.[75, 122] In addition to retention of sodium, protein stores are mobilized, thus maintaining the oncotic pressure of the plasma.[215] Without this mechanism, the intravascular volume could not expand.

Cardiac Failure

Cardiac failure rapidly develops when there is a massive leak of blood from the arterial to the venous side of the circulation.[199, 231] This is particularly true with large aorta–inferior vena cava fistulae, which are highly lethal.[10, 12, 51, 52, 70, 199, 206] On the other hand, failure may never occur or may be delayed for many years if the fistula is small.[65, 87] In experimental animals, a direct relationship between increased cardiac output and the development of heart failure has been demonstrated.[51] In humans, the situation is more complex, depending not only on the size of the fistula and the cardiac output but also on the presence of preexisting coronary or myocardial disease.[88] Children, with their generally healthy hearts, are able to sustain the increased circulatory load for prolonged periods without lapsing into cardiac failure.[26]

The continued expansion of the entire fistulous circuit that occurs with the passage of time results in a gradual increase in cardiac output and the delayed appearance of cardiac failure in some patients who initially were able to tolerate the fistula without evident physiologic strain.[118] Patients with congenital fistulae are less likely to have an elevated cardiac output and seldom develop heart failure.[15, 50, 148, 188, 247] Infants with massive congenital fistulae of the brain or liver are an exception to this rule. These large arteriovenous malformations may cause life-threatening cardiac failure, necessitating early operative intervention.[46, 91, 159, 259] Widely distributed arteriovenous malformations involving multiple organs are also known to cause greatly increased cardiac output and heart failure.[37] Treatment of these malformations is exceedingly difficult.

Edema formation in acute arteriovenous fistulae may be related to local elevation of venous pressure; however, when cardiac failure ensues, the full clinical picture of fluid retention appears, including peripheral edema, pulmonary edema, ascites, and weight gain.[5] Increased aldosterone secretion probably plays an important role at this stage.[54, 230, 255] Closure of chronic arteriovenous fistulae may result in massive diuresis.[134] Eiseman and Hughes reported that a patient lost 61 pounds (41.5 per cent of his body weight) in the first 12 days after repair of an aorta–vena cava fistula.[70]

Effect of Fistula Location

Arteriovenous fistulae involving vessels close to the heart have a more profound systemic effect than do those located in the periphery.[112, 116, 118] This is quite simply explained on the basis of the comparative resistance of the parasitic circuits. When the fistula lies between major central vessels (e.g., the aorta and the inferior vena cava), the proximal arteries and veins will have an extremely low resistance because of their wide diameter and short length, but when the fistula involves vessels in an extremity, the resistance of the circuit is much higher because of the smaller diameter of the vessels and the greater distance from the heart.[51, 73] Moreover, the diameter of the fistula itself can be much larger in central vessels than it can be in peripheral vessels, where its diameter is limited by the size of the involved artery and vein.

Fistulae of the pelvis and legs are said to exert a greater systemic effect than those of the head, neck, and arm.[223] This may be due to the hydrostatic effect of gravity, which tends to distend the involved vessels, thereby lowering their resistance.[85] There is, however, no good confirmatory evidence for this supposition.[158]

It is often stated that fistulae involving branches of the portal system have fewer systemic effects than would be expected from fistulae of similar size in other parts of the body. This may be related to the high outflow resistance offered by the hepatic sinusoids.[123, 174, 205, 239, 245] Nevertheless, some patients with fistulae between the superior mesenteric artery and vein do have significantly elevated cardiac outputs.[29, 227]

Outline of Systemic Effects

Opening an arteriovenous fistula produces an immediate reduction in total peripheral resistance. This causes the central arterial pressure to drop, the central venous pressure to rise, the systemic blood flow to decrease, and blood to be transferred from the arterial to the venous side of the circulation. A number of compensatory mechanisms are called into play to correct these physiologic aberrations.

The rise in central venous pressure distends the cardiac chambers, increasing the end-diastolic stretch of the myocardial fibers. The Frank-Starling mechanism, thus initiated, acts to increase stroke volume. Baroreceptor reflexes, responding to the fall in arterial pressure, cause the heart rate to rise, and myocardial contractility is strengthened through the effects of circulating catecholamines and sympathetic discharges on the cardiac muscle. Sympathoadrenal effects also stimulate systemic arteriolar constriction, which helps to maintain central arterial pressure but further decreases peripheral blood flow. Constriction of the central veins, on the other hand, facilitates venous return. Together these mechanisms cause the cardiac output and central aortic pressure to rise.

If compensation is adequate, as it usually is in most patients with good cardiac function, the cardiac output will increase sufficiently to permit central aortic pressure to approach normal prefistula values. Baroreceptor effects are thereby decreased, allowing the pulse rate to return to near-normal levels and the peripheral vascular constriction to be alleviated. Systemic blood flow returns to an adequate, although somewhat reduced, level. However, if the fistula is massive or if the myocardium is damaged, compensation will be incomplete. Cardiac output, although increased, will not be sufficient to maintain peripheral blood flow in the face of the great leak between the two sides of the circulation. Cardiac failure ensues, and early death may result.

Activation of the renin-angiotensin-aldosterone system causes retention of sodium and water. Together with mobilization of protein stores, this acts to increase the plasma volume. The resulting increase in blood volume allows the heart to enlarge and the remainder of the fistulous circuit to expand. This facilitates venous return, thereby improving the cardiac output. In the well-compensated system, systemic blood flow rises to prefistula levels and electrolyte metabolism returns to normal.

As time passes, the fistulous circuit often continues to expand as a result of the dilatation of the proximal arteries and veins, as well as of the fistula itself. In addition, both arterial and venous collaterals may continue to develop. The end-result is a further drop in total peripheral resistance and increased cardiac output. Sooner or later, depending on the presence or absence of coronary or myocardial disease, the cardiac reserve may be depleted, and cardiac failure occurs.

For more information, the reader is referred to a detailed study by Huang and colleagues of aortocaval fistulae in rats.[268] This study provides an excellent summary of the acute and chronic systemic effects of large arteriovenous fistulae and confirms the mechanisms outlined previously.

HEMODYNAMIC CONSIDERATIONS IN THE TREATMENT OF ARTERIOVENOUS FISTULAE

The indications for surgical therapy and the technical aspects of the various procedures are discussed in subsequent chapters. All modern operations are designed to eradicate the leak and, if possible, to restore the circulatory pattern to that which would normally exist in the absence of an arteriovenous fistula. Incomplete operations—in other words, those that merely decrease fistula flow—are avoided if at all possible.

Proximal Artery Ligation

Ligation of the artery leading to a fistula (the so-called Hunter operation) is a completely unsatisfactory and often dangerous procedure.[28] It has long been known that gangrene may result from this operation.[24]

Figure 85–16 shows the theoretical results of various operations in a model fistulous circuit in which the collateral artery resistance is no greater than that of the main arterial channel. In this illustration, proximal artery ligation would have little effect on the reduced peripheral blood flow and would further decrease peripheral blood pressure (see Fig. 85–16B). Although flow through the fistula would be reduced, it would still be appreciable. In many (perhaps most) cases, proximal arterial occlusion reduces both peripheral blood pressure and flow (cf. Fig. 85–14).

Thus, this operation not only decreases peripheral perfusion but also fails to eradicate flow through the fistula. When collateral channels are poorly developed, proximal arterial ligation can be expected to have devastating peripheral effects.[111] Because the fistula remains open, blood supplied by collateral arteries is further diverted into the distal artery, where it flows retrograde toward the fistula, thereby increasing the steal from the peripheral tissues.

It is probably safe to say that few surgeons today would knowingly treat an acquired arteriovenous fistula with proximal arterial ligation.[142] Unfortunately, physiologically similar procedures are sometimes performed inadvertently in the course of treating congenital arteriovenous fistulae. Most congenital fistulae are complex structures with many contributing arteries and veins and multiple arteriovenous communications, many of which are of microscopic size. Unless the fistula is very well localized, residual fistulae will be left behind following excisional therapy. With time, these residual fistulae and their communicating

FIGURE 85–16. Effects of proximal artery ligation (B), quadruple ligation and excision (C), and total reconstructive surgery (D) on flow through the fistula, peripheral arterial pressure, and peripheral blood flow. These theoretical results are based on a model with low-resistance arterial collaterals.

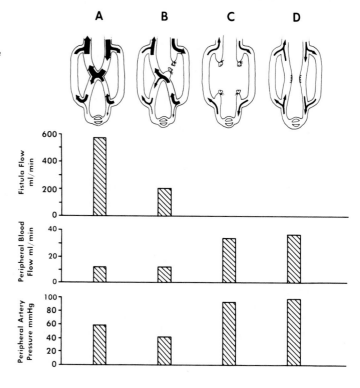

channels enlarge until the arteriovenous leak approaches that of the original lesion.[191] When any of the major arteries feeding the fistula are also responsible for supplying tissues peripheral to the lesion, their ligation jeopardizes tissue nutrition in the same way that ligation of the proximal artery does in cases of acquired fistula. Not only will the terminal tissues have to depend on collateral blood flow, but also retrograde flow through residual fistulous communication will create a steal, thus further reducing peripheral flow. For these reasons, a conservative, nonoperative approach is advocated for most congenital arteriovenous fistulae unless they are well localized and readily accessible.[207, 247, 248] When treatment is required because of skin ulceration, bleeding, excessive limb growth, or cardiac failure, embolic occlusion of the multiple arteriovenous communications is theoretically appealing.[37, 145, 184] This procedure should obliterate the leak while preserving the major arteries, veins, and collateral channels on which the peripheral tissues depend for their nutrition.

Quadruple Ligation and Excision

The advantages of ligating all communicating vessels together with total excision of the arteriovenous fistula were first recognized by Bramann over a century ago.[21] This operation remained the treatment most commonly employed before and even during World War II.[71]

Quadruple ligation is a physiologically sound procedure. By ligating the proximal artery and vein as well as the distal artery and vein and excising the fistula, the surgeon converts a complex hemodynamic circuit into one that is far more simple (see Fig. 85–16C). Because the distal artery and the fistula are eliminated, a steal can no longer occur. The afferent channels to the periphery consist of the collateral arteries, and the efferent channels are composed of the collateral veins. Thus, the success of quadruple ligation and excision depends on the resistance of the preexisting collateral vessels.

In order to ensure optimum collateral development, it was formerly customary to delay operation for several months after injury.[71] A number of tests were devised to help the surgeon recognize adequate collateral flow. In the Moschcowitz hyperemia test, blood flow to the involved limb was obstructed by a pneumatic cuff for 5 minutes. After the fistula had been occluded by external pressure, the cuff was suddenly deflated. As blood returned to the limb, a visible flush began proximally and extended distally. If the flush reached the end of the limb within 2 minutes, the collateral circulation was assumed to be satisfactory.[219]

The presence of pulsations in the distal artery after the proximal artery has been occluded (the Henle-Coenen phenomenon) is also good evidence that the collateral circulation is adequate. Perhaps a better method for estimating the functional capacity of the collaterals is to note whether the distal portion of the limb retains its normal color and warmth after the involved vessels have been occluded for 20 minutes.[222] Other, somewhat more objective tests that depend on measurement of pressure and flow have been devised. These are discussed in Chapter 86.

Figure 85–16C illustrates an optimal response to quad-ruple ligation and excision. In this model, flow through the fistula is totally eliminated and peripheral artery pressure and flow return to nearly normal levels. A similar response to compression of radial artery–cephalic vein fistulae is shown in Figure 85–14. In both of these examples, the collateral artery resistance is quite low. In many clinical situations, however, collaterals are not so well developed and the results may not be as good. Although few patients so treated will develop gangrene (none in Elkin's series), about 40 to 50 per cent will develop symptoms of arterial insufficiency—usually intermittent claudication.[13, 71, 82, 86, 90, 103, 121, 216] Clearly, the collateral arteries in these cases, although well developed, do not appear to be functionally superior to those that bypass chronic localized arterial obstructions in the lower limb.

Reconstructive Surgery

Despite the fact that Matas had advocated total reconstruction of arteriovenous fistulae as early as 1922, this approach was not widely adopted until after World War II.[168] During this war, a few innovative surgeons clearly demonstrated the superiority of reconstructive surgery over quadruple ligation and excision, and by the time of the Korean conflict, reconstructive surgery became the rule.* These developments were made possible by the availability of antibiotics, blood transfusions, improved vascular suture and instruments, autografts, and surgeons who were skilled in the disciplines required.

Obviously, successful elimination of the fistula and repair of the involved artery and vein return the circulation to normal (see Fig. 85–16D). Although some surgeons have adopted a cavalier approach to the vein, making no attempt at repair, more recent investigators have emphasized the importance of restoring venous continuity.[121, 196, 229] Ligation of the vein leads to varicose veins, chronic venous insufficiency, and sometimes gangrene.

Systemic Response

Elimination of the fistula, whether by reconstructive surgery or by quadruple ligation and excision, reverses the hemodynamic consequences of the leak from the arterial to the venous side of the circulation. Cardiac output falls to normal levels; blood pressure and pulse, if abnormal, return to prefistula values; and the heart, if enlarged, shrinks to normal size.[137, 176, 223, 226, 261] Blood volume decreases, and excess body fluid is eliminated.[70, 176, 226] In most cases, cardiac failure is rapidly cured.[88, 176, 231]

HEMODYNAMIC FACTORS IN THE DESIGN OF FISTULAE FOR VASCULAR ACCESS

The most important therapeutic application of arteriovenous fistulae is to provide a convenient access to the

---

*See references: demonstrated superiority, 86, 218; had become the rule, 135, 216, 229.

circulation in patients with chronic renal failure. Introduced in 1966 by Brescia and associates, this technique has rapidly supplanted the use of external shunts for long-term hemodialysis.[25] Chapter 90 discusses the technical aspects of these procedures.

Among the constraints placed on the design of fistulae to be used for hemodialysis are the following:

1. The fistula should transmit enough blood at sufficient pressure to permit a relatively high flow through the dialysis machine.

2. Fistula flow should not be excessively great, in order to avoid cardiac strain.

3. Circulation to the tissues peripheral to the fistula should not be jeopardized.

4. Congestion of the peripheral venous bed should be avoided.

5. Percutaneous access to the fistula output should be easily accomplished.

Diameter of the Fistula

Based on theoretical considerations, there would be no advantage to making a side-to-side anastomosis between the artery and vein any larger than the diameter of the proximal artery. Provided the fistula diameter is 60 to 80 per cent of the arterial diameter, its resistance is infinitesimally small in comparison with that of the artery.[241] Small fistulae, however, are difficult to construct, are prone to early occlusion as a result of fibrosis or thrombosis, and offer no advantages over large fistulae. Therefore, for practical purposes, most radial artery–cephalic vein fistulae are constructed with an anastomotic length of 6 to 10 mm— several times the diameter of the proximal artery.[32, 34, 69, 251, 253]

When the fistula itself is quite long, as in H-type arrangements constructed with prosthetic grafts or autogenous vein, the diameter of the fistula makes a difference.[152, 156] In order to minimize resistance, the fistula should be at least as large as the proximal artery and probably should have a diameter equal to that of the venous drainage. Aside from the question of flow, the graft must be large enough to avoid clotting and to facilitate percutaneous cannulation.

A common complication of polytetrafluoroethylene arteriovenous fistulae has been platelet deposition, intimal hyperplasia, and fibrosis in the runoff vein at the site of the anastomosis.[139] This occurs with both end-to-end and end-to-side anastomoses.[265] Progressive stenosis causes rising pressure in the venous dialysis line and eventual failure of the fistula.[282] Although the explanation for the fibrosis is unknown, it appears to be related to hemodynamic factors similar to those discussed earlier in this chapter (cf. Anatomic Changes). Animal experiments have shown that venous hyperplasia is decreased when tapered grafts are used and the larger end is anastomosed to the vein.[266] This configuration appears to minimize turbulence and kinetic energy transfer to the perivascular tissues.

Advantages and Disadvantages of Various Types of Fistulae

Radial Artery–Cephalic Vein

Radial artery–cephalic vein fistulae are well adapted to therapeutic use because they fulfill most of the requirements previously enumerated. Although these fistulae are capable of transmitting sufficient flow, they are situated far enough peripherally so that flow ordinarily is not excessive. Moreover, the ulnar artery provides an excellent collateral channel, fully capable of sustaining the circulation to the hand, thereby minimizing the risk of peripheral ischemia. Finally, the veins of the forearm are large, prominent, relatively straight, and easily punctured.

Several varieties of radial artery–cephalic vein anastomosis have been used. These include the classic side-to-side, the end of proximal artery–side of vein, the side of artery–end of proximal vein, and the end of proximal artery–end of vein. In addition, various H-type fistulae have been constructed. In these operations, autogenous vein or prosthetic grafts are used to link the artery with the vein.[2, 30, 40, 53, 69, 97, 143, 160, 170, 172, 253]

The hemodynamics described in the following paragraphs are illustrated by theoretical values listed in Table 85–1. These results were obtained by analogy with electrical circuit theory and are based on Kirchhoff's laws and

Table 85–1. Hemodynamic Properties of Various Radial Artery–Cephalic Vein Fistulae (Theoretical Values Based on a Standard Model System)

	Fistula Flow (ml/min)	Proximal Vein Flow (ml/min)	Arterial Blood Pressure in Hand (mmHg)	Venous Blood Pressure in Hand (mmHg)
No fistula	—	18	95	3
Side-to-side	571	434	58	26
End of proximal artery–side of vein (or distal artery ligated)	474	369	92	23
Side of artery–end of proximal vein (or distal vein ligated)	507	507	61	4
End-to-end proximal artery–proximal vein	435	435	91	6
Side-to-side (proximal vein occluded)	265	—	79	48
Side-to-side (proximal artery occluded)	194	152	41	9

From Strandness DE Jr, Sumner DS: Arteriovenous fistulas. In Hemodynamics for Surgeons. New York, Grune & Stratton, 1975, pp 621–663.

published values of flow and pressure in the various components of the fistula circuit. (Results of a similar analysis by van Gemert and Bruyninckx were consistent with clinical experience.[283])

Because blood can enter the anastomosis from both the proximal and the distal radial arteries and exit through both the proximal and the distal cephalic veins, the side-to-side fistula transmits more blood than other fistulae of similar size.[31, 34, 125] The high flow rate keeps the anastomosis open and facilitates hemodialysis. For these reasons, the side-to-side fistula is preferred by many surgeons.[32, 34, 40, 251] However, there are some problems associated with this arrangement.

Because the distal artery remains open, carrying blood in a retrograde fashion, the possibility of a steal exists.[23, 164] Indeed, the author's group found that the majority of such fistulae (88 per cent) were associated with decreased digital artery pressures.[241] In one series, hand claudication occurred in 42 per cent of the patients.[150] Fortunately, serious symptoms seldom develop unless there is concomitant obstructive disease of the digital arteries, the palmar arch, or the ulnar artery.[20, 31, 34, 40, 41, 69, 98, 172, 240, 253] Although ligation of the distal artery or construction of an end of artery–side of vein fistula will eliminate the possibility of a steal, fistula flow will be decreased somewhat.[20, 31, 241]

Another potential drawback of the side-to-side fistula is the relatively high pressure in the distal vein, as shown in Table 85–1. Usually, this is of little significance.[34] However, if the proximal vein becomes occluded, all the fistula flow will be diverted retrograde into the distal vein.[92] In such cases, the hand and fingers may become painful and swollen and may even develop ulcerations.[20, 60, 98, 173, 240] Moreover, blood flow in the distal vein, which seldom approaches that in the proximal vein, is rapidly dissipated into numerous venous collaterals. Thus, a vein capable of supplying enough blood for dialysis becomes difficult to find. When proximal vein thrombosis or narrowing occurs, the shunt must be reconstructed.[20, 60, 98] In rare instances in which the proximal vein remains patent, ligation of the distal vein has been curative.[60]

In an effort to avoid distal venous hypertension, many surgeons perform a side of artery–end of proximal vein anastomosis.[6, 36, 55, 60, 69, 97, 173, 185, 253] As indicated by the figures in Table 85–1, this procedure has much to recommend it. Fistula flow is high, and distal venous pressure is low. Because all the fistula output is diverted through the proximal vein, more flow is available for hemodialysis. Although the potential for a peripheral arterial steal exists, it is no worse than that associated with side-to-side fistulae.[6]

End-to-end fistulae have many theoretical advantages. Fistula flow and proximal vein flow are very good, distal venous pressure is low, and peripheral perfusion is maintained at near-normal levels. Because of these features, there has been some support for end-to-end fistulae.[9, 41, 60, 97, 175] Unfortunately, they have a tendency to thrombose in the early postoperative period.[253]

H grafts and other makeshift shunts are usually employed only when a radial artery–cephalic vein fistula cannot be fashioned or has failed.[251] In practice, up to two thirds of all fistulae are of this variety.[273, 280] Most interposition grafts are constructed of polytetrafluoroethylene,

have a straight or looped configuration, and connect the radial or brachial artery to the antecubital, cephalic, basilic, or axillary veins. The hemodynamics of these fistulae depend on the resistances of the fistula and the proximal and distal arterial and venous channels. In general, they fit one of the patterns already described.

Proximal Arteriovenous Fistulae

Because of their more proximal location, brachial fistulae have a higher blood flow than those toward the wrist.[5, 152] Although they function well, providing a good flow of blood through the fistula, they tend to shunt blood away from the peripheral tissues.[23, 32, 41, 241, 253] Many patients with these fistulae develop edema, skin ulcers, paresthesias, and pain.[98, 241, 253]

The major physiologic difference between the brachial artery and the radial artery locations is the quality of the collaterals that bypass the fistula. Although the brachial artery has several prominent collaterals, none compares with the ulnar artery. Therefore, in some cases, the peripheral tissues will have to be supplied, at least in part, by blood flowing past the fistula into the distal artery, where it continues in a normal centrifugal direction toward the hand. The total quantity of blood reaching the hand will depend on the magnitude of the leak through the fistula and the capacity of the collaterals. Even when the collaterals are moderately well developed, there may be significant distal flow deprivation. In this event, flow in the distal brachial artery may be reversed so that only a small portion of the collateral flow is available to nourish the hand and distal forearm. Nevertheless, the development of peripheral ischemia—and its severity—is less closely related to the magnitude of reversed flow than it is to the extent of peripheral arterial occlusive disease.[152] This is especially true in diabetics.[41] As time passes, the collateral arteries enlarge, the digital pressures tend to rise, and flow deprivation is usually alleviated.[23, 279]

When ischemic symptoms persist, reduction of fistula flow by plicating (or otherwise narrowing) the graft may be tried. Because the borderline between adequate reduction in flow and maintenance of graft patency is narrow, this approach often proves unsatisfactory. Monitoring digital pulses during the procedure has been advocated as a method of determining the point at which adequate reduction of the lumen has been achieved.[273, 278] When preservation of the hand requires fistula ligation, replacing the fistula with one using a branch of the axillary artery as the donor vessel has been advocated.[271] Because of the small size of the donor artery (3 mm in diameter), fistula flow is limited and a symptomatic steal no longer occurs. Another method of alleviating ischemia associated with brachial fistulae is to ligate the artery distal to the fistula (thus eliminating reversed flow in the distal artery).[279] This must be accompanied by the insertion of a bypass graft from a normal segment of the artery proximal to the fistula into the artery distal to the site of the ligature, thereby creating an additional low-resistance collateral to supply the peripheral tissues.

Serious steal phenomena have also been reported with femoral arteriovenous fistulae using bovine grafts, but they seem to occur infrequently.[11, 78] Even though blood flow through these fistulae is high, the arterial collaterals in the femoral area are good and the input through the iliofemoral system is less limited than it is in the brachial area. Resting ankle pressure may be reduced, but the ankle pressure response to exercise does not seem to be affected.[11]

Systemic Effects

Flow through upper extremity arteriovenous fistulae used for hemodialysis varies widely, ranging from 100 to 3000 ml/min, with an average level of about 200 to 400 ml/min.[4, 6, 69, 142, 195] Values as high as 3600 ml/min have been reported in the absence of cardiac failure.[4, 253]

High-output cardiac failure, although rare, does occur with fistulae in the arm.[1, 4, 34, 80, 88, 142, 171, 253] In these cases, fistula flows, measured intraoperatively, have ranged from 600 to 2900 ml/min. The decrease in cardiac output with fistula occlusion averages 2900 ml/min, although in one individual an 11 L/min decrease was reported.[4]

(Apparently, high-output congestive heart failure is much more common with lower extremity fistulae. According to one report, 59 per cent of patients with femoral arteriovenous bovine shunts developed heart failure within the 1st year.[79] Presumably, this is due to the high rate of flow through these "proximal" fistulae.)

Most cases of cardiac failure occurring in patients on hemodialysis can be attributed to anemia, hypertension, and excessive sodium and water retention. Even in the absence of these complications, patients with coronary arterial insufficiency or myocardial disease may not be able to sustain the increased circulatory load imposed by the fistula.[4, 253] Cardiac failure in these patients tends to be resistant to medical therapy. Reduction in fistula flow by surgical revision of the fistula or by narrowing of the involved vessels is necessary to correct the cardiac failure. If it is no longer needed—for example, after renal transplantation—the fistula can be eliminated. Results have usually been good with these procedures.[4, 71] There are, however, exceptions. In certain patients in whom left ventricular disease is primarily responsible for heart failure, occluding the fistula, which increases afterload, may have a detrimental effect on cardiac dynamics.[35, 254]

Several surgeons have reported success with banding procedures as a means of reducing fistula flow. In these operations, a 1-cm Teflon band is placed around the proximal artery or vein (or the fistula, when a graft is used) and tightened gradually until the desired flow rate is achieved.[3, 80] It is mandatory that flow be monitored with an electromagnetic flowmeter as the band is tightened because little reduction in flow will be achieved until the vessel has been narrowed to about 50 per cent of its original diameter, the so-called point of critical stenosis (see Chapter 3). Beyond this point, flow drops off rapidly (see Fig. 3–9). Flow should be fixed between 400 and 700 ml/min in upper extremity fistulae and between 300 and 900 ml/min in lower extremity fistulae.* In practice, this is often difficult to accomplish.

THERAPEUTIC USES OF ARTERIOVENOUS FISTULAE

In addition to their widespread use for vascular access, arteriovenous fistulae have been employed to enhance limb growth, to ensure the patency of vascular anastomoses, and to revascularize ischemic extremities.

Enhancement of Limb Growth

The presence of a congenital arteriovenous fistula or a traumatic fistula in a limb before epiphyseal closure appears to stimulate bone growth.[120] This same phenomenon has been demonstrated experimentally in puppies with iliac arteriovenous fistulae.[138] Because of these observations, surgeons have constructed superficial femoral arteriovenous fistulae in children in an effort to increase the length of legs shortened as a result of poliomyelitis or congenital absence of a hip joint. In about three quarters of these cases, there has been either no change or a relative increase in the length of the limb.[45, 105, 137] Unfortunately, a rare patient will develop a serious complication, such as edema, venous distention, stasis ulceration, hemorrhage, endarteritis, cystic degeneration of the femoral vein, or cardiac enlargement.[26, 105]

It is difficult to explain why an acquired arteriovenous fistula should stimulate bone growth. Ingebrigtsen and colleagues noted that the oxygen tension was decreased in the tibial metaphysis of canine limbs with femoral arteriovenous fistulae.[132] Rogers and Aust found that blood flow in bones distal to arteriovenous fistulae was reduced.[202] Moreover, Henrie and associates were unable to demonstrate increased rates of healing of femoral or fibular fractures in animals with iliac arteriovenous fistulae.[102] These observations are consistent with the dynamics of flow distal to acquired arteriovenous fistulae, as outlined previously in this chapter. Ordinarily, flow in the peripheral tissues ranges from normal to severely reduced, and blood pressure is inevitably decreased.

Other investigators, however, have reported experimental data suggesting increased perfusion of bony tissues distal to an arteriovenous fistula. These findings include elevated temperature on the surface and within the intramedullary portion of the bone; increased intramedullary pressure; and hypervascularity of the intramedullary small vessels and capillaries.* Apparently, vessels in the vicinity or within the bone contribute to the collateral pathways bypassing the fistula. Another explanation for increased bone growth involves the increased peripheral venous pressure that accompanies a proximally located fistula. Venous stasis has been shown to stimulate bone growth.[126]

The mechanism by which congenital fistulae accelerate bone growth is somewhat easier to comprehend. Typically these lesions are diffuse, and the arteriovenous communications often involve bone. Increased blood flow through these communications could stimulate bone growth as a result of the associated high oxygen tensions and elevated temperatures.

---

*See references: upper extremity, 3; lower extremity, 80.

*See references: elevated temperature, 147; increased intramedullary pressure and vascularity, 236.

Use in Reconstructive Vascular Surgery

Among the frequently reported causes of early failure of vascular operations is sluggish blood flow. Placing an arteriovenous fistula distal to the reconstructed segment will increase the rate of flow through the critical area, thereby decreasing the likelihood of thrombosis.

This method has been used successfully to maintain the patency of endarterectomies and bypass grafts in ischemic limbs with poor runoff.[16, 17, 127, 151] Initially, the use of an arteriovenous fistula for this purpose might seem counterproductive because all arteriovenous communications have a tendency to steal blood from the periphery. Indeed, the creation of a fistula between a distal artery (e.g., the posterior tibial artery in the lower leg) and an adjacent vein would be quite detrimental to the blood supply to the foot in the presence of severe obstructive disease in the inflow arteries. Diversion of blood away from the posterior tibial artery would further reduce the already low pressure perfusing the distal vascular bed. However, when all proximal obstructions have been bypassed by a graft of sufficiently large caliber to carry the augmented blood flow without a significant pressure drop, the pressure in the posterior tibial artery at the site of the anastomosis will be increased. Thus, patency of the graft is protected by the more rapidly flowing blood, and peripheral perfusion is improved by the increased pressure head. Placing the fistula at the site of the graft-artery anastomosis best fulfills the hemodynamic requirements outlined earlier.[264, 270] Although some surgeons have reported good clinical results when arteriovenous fistulae are constructed at some distance below the graft-artery anastomosis,[275, 277] there are theoretical arguments against this approach. If the intervening artery is widely patent, there is no problem; however, if this segment is or becomes stenotic, the increased blood flow supplying the fistula will cause an additional drop in blood pressure and consequently a reduction in the pressure head perfusing the distal tissues. In this situation, graft patency would be preserved and flow would be augmented in the intervening segment, but the tissues distal to the fistula would suffer.

Arteriovenous fistulae have also been used to increase blood flow through reconstructed venous segments.[68, 107, 144, 190] Here, the only consideration is to avoid a symptomatic peripheral steal by carefully adjusting the flow through the fistula.

By constructing an arteriovenous fistula in the forearm, surgeons have been able to convert cephalic veins, which were previously too narrow and thin-walled to serve as satisfactory bypass grafts, into conduits of adequate thickness and diameter.[104] These "arterialized" veins are suitable for distal tibial and peroneal reconstruction in the absence of a suitable saphenous vein.

Revascularization of Ischemic Extremities

Surgeons have long entertained the hope that arterialization of the venous system might be used to improve the circulation to ischemic extremities.[209] Most of these attempts have met with only limited success.[237] In an early review of the literature, only 3 of 42 patients who received arteriovenous fistulae for the treatment of threatened or existing gangrene of the extremity experienced any prolonged benefits from the procedure.[100] Szilagyi and associates, in 1951, reported nine consecutive failures of femoral arteriovenous fistulae used for treating occlusive arterial disease.[246] Nevertheless, sporadic reports of good results continue to appear in the literature.[42, 83, 269] Sheil described the use of the saphenous vein, in situ, to transport blood retrograde from a proximal arterial anastomosis at the femoral level to the dorsum of the foot.[217] He believed that this procedure avoided amputation in three of six limbs with severe ischemia.

Several groups have reported favorable results in experimental preparations with a Y-type arteriovenous fistula.[38, 89, 140, 169, 203, 257] Basically, a Y-type fistula consists of an end of proximal artery–side of vein anastomosis with the distal artery tied off. In most of these studies, enhanced limb survival associated with the construction of an arteriovenous fistula has been the major criterion for improved circulation. However, the paper by Gerard and colleagues does provide objective documentation of improved nutrition of previously ischemic tissues.[89] These investigators showed that the Y-type fistula increased intramuscular Po_2 in ischemic dog limbs from 5.3 mmHg to a nearly normal value of 45.5 mmHg; that the pH of the muscle surface increased from 7.06 to 7.40; that segmental blood pressures returned to normal; that toe pulse reappearance times decreased; and that toe plethysmograms approached normal volumes and configurations.

The following mechanisms have been postulated to explain the rationale for using this procedure: arteriovenous fistulae constitute a powerful stimulus for the development of collateral circulation, and retrograde arterial flow in the distal venous limb could nourish the peripheral tissues.

Based on current knowledge of the physiology of arteriovenous fistulae, it is difficult to understand how these changes would benefit the peripheral circulation. As Reid stated in 1925, "It would seem mere folly to expect any benefit from a fistula made between large vessels far removed from the part you are trying to help."[193] Although arteriovenous fistulae stimulate collateral development to a greater degree than simple occlusions do, *the increased size of the collaterals is due to their role in supplying retrograde flow to the distal artery rather than antegrade flow to the peripheral tissues.* Indeed, collateral development is markedly impaired when the artery is ligated just distal to the fistula, as it is in the Y-type anastomosis.[114] Therefore, there is little justification for believing that collaterals developed after such an anastomosis would significantly augment peripheral blood flow.[17] It is true that the Y-type fistula would have *fewer detrimental* effects than an H-type fistula because there would be no reversal of flow in the distal arterial limb and less steal from the peripheral tissues.

Although reversal of flow in the distal vein has been clearly demonstrated with Y- or H-type fistulae, it has never been shown that the blood flow in the capillary bed is reversed or even that this "arterialized" blood ever reaches the capillary bed. In fact, angiograms show that all of the blood containing enough contrast to be visible is transferred directly back to the heart by way of numerous venous collaterals. Some of the blood, however, could reach the venules and flow retrograde through the capillary bed and high-resistance terminal arterioles into the obstructed arteries of the ischemic extremity, which also would have a very high resistance. Once in these obstructed arteries, it could not flow retrograde into the major arteries but would have to be diverted back again to the venous system through terminal arterioles, capillaries, and venules. Clearly, the only way in which such a system could work is for the reversed venous flow to find its way into the terminal arterioles through low-resistance peripheral arteriovenous shunts and thence back through the capillaries proper into *another* nonarterialized vein.[269] Furthermore, most clinical and experimental observations have shown that high distal venous pressure is actually detrimental to the peripheral circulation.[17, 20, 60, 98, 173, 240] It is well known, for example, that large residual subcutaneous fistulae associated with in situ bypass grafting may cause localized edema, inflammation, and possibly even skin necrosis. If, indeed, arterialization of the venous system does improve tissue nutrition, the mechanism remains obscure. For these reasons, a healthy skepticism toward the use of arteriovenous fistulae for revascularization of ischemic limbs seems justified.[262]

ARTERIOVENOUS ANASTOMOSES

The preceding sections of this chapter deal with abnormal communications between arteries and veins. There are, however, normally occurring connections between arteries and veins, called arteriovenous anastomoses. Arteriovenous anastomoses are situated proximal to the capillary bed, have no connections with the capillaries, and shunt blood away from the capillaries. Most are short, thick-walled structures, but some are long and tortuous. The arteriovenous glomus is a complex form, consisting of multiple channels composed of epithelioid cells surrounded by a connective tissue sheath. All arteriovenous anastomoses are richly innervated by sympathetic nerve fibers. Because of their thick walls, it is unlikely that any exchange of nutrients or gases takes place between the anastomoses and the interstitial fluid. Unlike capillaries, which have a luminal diameter of about 7 μm and are composed of endothelial cells only, arteriovenous anastomoses commonly have an internal diameter of 20 to 40 μm (some exceed 100 μm) and have walls that are heavily invested with smooth muscle cells.

Arteriovenous anastomoses should be distinguished from thoroughfare or preferential channels, which have been described in some microvascular beds. Basically, these channels are enlarged capillaries that traverse a more direct route between arterioles and venules than true capillaries do. They have a few muscle fibers scattered in their walls, serve as the origin for most of the true capillaries, and probably function to regulate blood flow in the capillaries.

Although arteriovenous anastomoses have been found in most of the major vascular beds, those with diameters exceeding 20 μm are sparse or absent in the lung, liver, kidney, stomach, and intestine.[57] In muscles, they are confined to the intramuscular septa and tendons. They are most common in the nailbeds; are frequent in the volar or plantar surfaces of the fingers, toes, hands, and feet; and are virtually absent in the skin of the calf or forearm. They are also found in the skin of the nose and ears. In the canine hindlimb, removal of the paw and skin virtually eliminates arteriovenous shunting.

Although the volume of blood flowing through arteriovenous anastomoses can be estimated by measuring the "nutrient" or capillary blood flow with xenon-133 or sodium radioiodide (iodine-131) and then subtracting this value from the total organ blood flow measured with a plethysmograph or an electromagnetic flowmeter, a more direct estimation can be obtained by using radionuclide-labeled microspheres (see Chapter 86). Intra-arterially injected microspheres with a diameter of about 20 to 30 μm will be trapped in the peripheral capillaries but will pass unimpeded through arteriovenous anastomoses to the lungs, where they will be filtered out. If one knows the radioactivity of the injected microspheres and measures the radioactivity of the lungs, it is a relatively simple matter to calculate the fraction of blood that is diverted through arteriovenous shunts. Under normal circumstances, only 1 to 5 per cent of the total blood flow to the limb passes through these anastomoses.

Arteriovenous anastomoses are surgically important in that they may exert a detrimental effect on cellular nutrition in ischemic tissues, may divert blood away from the capillaries in septic areas, may contribute to the formation of varicose veins, and may provide a rational explanation for the conflicting opinions regarding the efficacy of sympathectomy. Moreover, when one attempts to estimate the physiologic significance of congenital or acquired arteriovenous fistulae, it is necessary to distinguish normal arteriovenous shunting from pathologic shunting (see Chapter 86).

Physiology

Arteriovenous anastomoses dilate in response to warmth and constrict in response to cold. They seem to serve a thermoregulatory function. Whereas local application of heat to the peripheral tissues has little effect on the degree of shunting, central body heating increases the fraction of blood shunted through arteriovenous anastomoses from a few per cent to about 25 per cent of the total blood flowing through the extremity.[263] Cooling, both central and peripheral, diminishes anastomotic flow almost to zero. It is postulated that the central nervous system senses the temperature of the arriving blood. When the temperature is elevated, sympathetic tone is relaxed and the arteriovenous anastomoses, which are innervated by sympathetic fibers, dilate. Because these structures are almost entirely confined to the skin and acral regions of the body, their dilatation acts to shunt blood from the deeper tissues into the superficial veins, where the excess heat can be radiated from the body. Closure of the anastomoses in response to cold conserves heat by reducing surface flow and by diverting blood into the deeper tissues.

Responses to various drugs indicate that the innervation of arteriovenous anastomoses is exclusively sympathetic and that the receptors are alpha-adrenergic. Administration of phenoxybenzamine and phentolamine, both alpha-receptor blockers, greatly increases shunting.[47, 59, 228] On the other hand, propranolol, a beta-blocker, and isoproterenol, a beta-stimulator, have no effect.[59, 228] Papaverine dilates both capillaries and arteriovenous anastomoses, but adenosine triphosphate only increases capillary flow and has no effect on shunt flow.[59] Anesthetic agents, both general and regional, augment arteriovenous shunting—an important consideration when one measures flow through arteriovenous fistulae in the anesthetized patient.

Short periods of ischemia (5 minutes) apparently have no effect on arteriovenous anastomoses.[47] Reactive hyperemia is therefore a manifestation of increased capillary blood flow. Long periods of ischemia (2 hours) likewise have no immediate effect on arteriovenous anastomoses, but 24 hours later shunting is greatly increased.[149] Thus, increased shunting is in part responsible for the delayed hyperemia that occurs when tourniquets are used to produce a bloodless field in certain operations.

Pathophysiology

Hypoxia greatly increases the flow of blood through arteriovenous anastomoses. Approximately one third of the blood flowing through an extremity may be shunted away from the capillary bed under the influence of hypoxia. Hypoventilation, which creates respiratory acidosis, hypercarbia, and mild hypoxia, has a similar effect. Both metabolic acidosis and pure hypercarbia increase flow through arteriovenous anastomoses, but the effect is less than that caused by hypoxia.[57]

Ischemic tissues are hypoxic, probably acidotic, and hypercarbic. Therefore, local ischemia—such as that occurring in conjunction with severe arterial disease—probably increases arteriovenous shunting. This in turn would have a further detrimental effect on tissue nutrition because blood diverted away from the capillaries would serve no metabolic function. The observations of Delaney provide some support for this concept. In two of seven severely ischemic human limbs, he found that 13 per cent and 25 per cent of the total limb blood flow, respectively, was being shunted.[57]

The effect of sepsis on flow through arteriovenous anastomoses remains controversial. It is known that oxygen utilization within septic tissues is not increased despite an increase in blood flow. Differences between the oxygen saturation of the arterial blood entering the affected region and that of the venous blood leaving the region are reduced. Using radionuclide-labeled microspheres, Cronenwett and Lindenauer demonstrated that 22 per cent of the blood entering the septic hindlimbs of dogs was being shunted through arteriovenous anastomoses.[48] On the other hand, Archie observed little change in the shunt fraction in dogs with septic, or endotoxin-induced, shock, except in areas of local inflammation.[7]

For many years, it has been suspected that arteriovenous anastomoses play a role in the genesis of varicose veins. Blalock reported increased oxygen tension in varicose veins,[18] and Haimovici and associates demonstrated numerous arteriovenous maculae in the soles of the feet of patients with varicose veins.[99] Using the operating microscope, Schalin visualized direct connections between arteries with a diameter of 100 μm and varicosities.[210] That arterial flow signals can be detected with Doppler flowmetry along the course of varicose veins lends some support to these observations,[267] but the possibility that these signals may represent hyperemic flow in inflamed tissues has not been excluded.

Increased flow through arteriovenous anastomoses occurs in patients with hypertrophic pulmonary osteopathy and cirrhosis but not in patients with Paget's disease.

Sympathectomy

Because arteriovenous anastomoses are controlled by the sympathetic nervous system, it is not surprising to find that surgical sympathectomy increases the fraction of shunt flow to 20 to 30 per cent of the total flow through the limb.[47, 49, 58] In ischemic canine hindlimbs, sympathectomy increases flow through arteriovenous anastomoses but has no effect on capillary perfusion, results in no increase in oxygen consumption, and causes no increase in tissue oxygen tension.[49, 189] All of the increased blood flow is confined to the skin and terminal regions of the extremities.[57, 58] There is no increase in blood flow through muscles, either at rest or during exercise. Therefore, these results question the rationale for using sympathectomy in the treatment of peripheral arterial disease (see Chapter 3). Any apparent relief of claudication must not be a function of increased muscle blood flow. Likewise, there is little evidence that the increased peripheral blood flow has any effect on tissue nutrition because most of the increased flow is diverted through arteriovenous anastomoses, where it serves no nutritive purpose.

References

1. Ahearn DJ, Maher JF: Heart failure as a complication of hemodialysis arteriovenous fistula. Ann Intern Med 77:201, 1972.
2. Alvarez JJP, Vargas-Rosendo R, Gutiérrez-Bosque R, et al: A new type of subcutaneous arteriovenous fistula for chronic hemodialysis in children. Surgery 67:355, 1970.
3. Anderson CB, Groce MA: Banding of arteriovenous dialysis fistulas to correct high-output cardiac failure. Surgery 78:552, 1975.
4. Anderson CB, Codd JR, Graff RA, et al: Cardiac failure and upper extremity arteriovenous dialysis fistulas. Case reports and a review of the literature. Arch Intern Med 136:292, 1976.
5. Anderson CB, Etheredge EE, Harter HR, et al: Blood flow measurements in arteriovenous dialysis fistulas. Surgery 81:459, 1977.
6. Anderson CB, Etheredge EE, Harter HR, et al: Local blood flow characteristics of arteriovenous fistulas in the forearm for dialysis. Surg Gynecol Obstet 144:531, 1977.
7. Archie JP Jr: Anatomic arterial-venous shunting in endotoxic and septic shock in dogs. Ann Surg 186:171, 1977.
8. Attinger EO, Sugawara H, Navarro A, et al: Pulsatile flow patterns in distensible tubes. Circ Res 18:447, 1966.
9. Baker CRF Jr: Complications and management of methods of dialysis access for renal failure. Am Surg 42:859, 1976.
10. Baker WH, Sharzer LA, Ehrenhaft JL: Aortocaval fistula as a complication of abdominal aortic aneurysms. Surgery 72:933, 1972.
11. Baur GM, Porter JM, Fletcher WS: Human umbilical cord vein allograft arteriovenous fistula for chemotherapy access. Am J Surg 138:238, 1979.
12. Beall AC Jr, Cooley DA, Morris GC Jr, et al: Perforation of arteriosclerotic aneurysms into inferior vena cava. Arch Surg 86:809, 1963.
13. Bigger IA: Treatment of traumatic aneurysms and arteriovenous fistulas. Arch Surg 49:170, 1944.
14. Binak K, Regan TJ, Christensen RC, et al: Arteriovenous fistula: Hemodynamic effects of occlusion and exercise. Am Heart J 60:495, 1960.

15. Björkholm M, Aschberg S: Hemodynamic influence of multiple congenital arteriovenous fistulas. Acta Med Scand 200:333, 1976.
16. Blaisdell FW, Lim RC Jr, Hall AD: Reconstruction of small arteries with an arteriovenous fistula, an experimental study. Arch Surg 92:206, 1966.
17. Blaisdell FW, Lim RC Jr, Hall AD, et al: Revascularization of severely ischemic extremities with an arteriovenous fistula. Am J Surg 122:166, 1966.
18. Blalock A: Oxygen content of blood in patients with varicose veins. Arch Surg 19:898, 1929.
19. Blundell PE, Tobin JR Jr, Swan HJC: Effect of right ventricular hypertrophy on infundibular pressure gradients in dogs. Am J Physiol 209:513, 1965.
20. Blutt KMH, Friedman EA, Kountz SL: Angioaccess. Curr Probl Surg 13(September):1, 1976.
21. Bramann F: Arterio-venous aneurism. Arch Klin Chir 33:1, 1886.
22. Branham HH: Aneurismal varix of the femoral artery and vein following a gunshot wound. Int J Surg 3:250, 1890.
23. Brener BJ, Brief DK, Alpert J, et al: The effect of vascular access procedures on digital haemodynamics. *In* Diethrich EB (ed): Noninvasive Cardiovascular Diagnosis. Current Concepts. Baltimore, University Park Press, 1978, pp 189–203.
24. Breschet G: Mémorie sur les aneurysmes. Mem Acad R Med Paris 3:101, 1833.
25. Brescia MJ, Cimino JE, Appel K, et al: Chronic hemodialysis using venipuncture and surgically created arteriovenous fistula. N Engl J Med 275:1089, 1966.
26. Breslau RC: Complications of arteriovenous fistula induced for augmentation of limb growth. Surgery 63:1012, 1968.
27. Briden KL, Weiss HR: Effect of moderate arterio-venous shunt on regional extraction, blood flow, and oxygen consumption in the dog heart. Cardiovasc Res 15:206, 1981.
28. Brooks B: The treatment of traumatic arteriovenous fistula. South Med J 23:100, 1930.
29. Brunner JH, Stanley RJ: Superior mesenteric arteriovenous fistula. JAMA 223:316, 1973.
30. Buselmeier TJ, Rattazzi LC, Kjellstrand CM, et al: A modified arteriovenous fistula applicable where there is thrombosis of standard Brescia-Cimino fistula vasculature. Surgery 74:551, 1973.
31. Bussell JA, Abbott JA, Lim RC: A radial steal syndrome with arteriovenous fistula for hemodialysis. Ann Intern Med 75:387, 1971.
32. Byrne JP, Stevens LE, Weaver DH, et al: Advantages of surgical arteriovenous fistulas for hemodialysis. Arch Surg 102:359, 1971.
33. Callander CL: Study of arterio-venous fistulae with analysis of 447 cases. Ann Surg 71:428, 1920.
34. Cerilli J, Limbert JG: Technique and results of the construction of arteriovenous fistulas for hemodialysis. Surg Gynecol Obstet 137:922, 1973.
35. Cerra FB, Shapiro RI, Anthone S, et al: Clinically significant arteriovenous fistulas: Physiologic response to acute occlusion. Surg Forum 28:208, 1977.
36. Cheek RC, Messina JJ, Acchiardo SR, et al: Arteriovenous fistulas for hemodialysis: Experience with 100 cases. Am Surg 42:386, 1976.
37. Coel MN, Alksne JF: Embolization to diminish high output failure secondary to systemic angiomatosis (Ullman's syndrome). Vasc Surg 12:336, 1978.
38. Cohen SE, Matolo NM, Wolfman EF Jr: Arteriovenous fistula for revascularization of the ischemic extremity. Vasc Surg 10:238, 1976.
39. Cohen SM, Edholm OG, Howarth S, et al: Cardiac output and peripheral blood flow in arteriovenous aneurysms. Clin Sci 7:35, 1948.
40. Cohn HE, Solit RW: Arteriovenous fistulas for chronic hemodialysis. Surg Clin North Am 53:673, 1973.
41. Corry RJ, Patel NP, West JC: Surgical management of complications of vascular access for hemodialysis. Surg Gynecol Obstet 151:49, 1980.
42. Courbier R, Jausseran JM, Reggi M: Le shunt saphéno-fémoral dans les ischémies sévères des membres inférieurs. J Chir (Paris) 105:441, 1973.
43. Coursley G, Ivins JC, Barker NW: Congenital arteriovenous fistulas in the extremities: An analysis of 69 cases. Angiology 7:201, 1956.
44. Cowley AW Jr, Guyton AC: Heart rate as a determinant of cardiac output in dogs with arteriovenous fistula. Am J Cardiol 28:321, 1971.
45. Cranley JJ: Arteriovenous fistulas. *In* Vascular Surgery. Peripheral Arterial Diseases. Hagerstown, MD, Harper and Row, 1972, vol. I, pp 171–185.

46. Crocker DW, Cleland RS: Infantile hemangioendothelioma of the liver: Report of three cases. Pediatrics 19:596, 1957.
47. Cronenwett JL, Lindenauer SM: Direct measurement of arteriovenous anastomotic blood flow after lumbar sympathectomy. Surgery 82:82, 1977.
48. Cronenwett JL, Lindenauer SM: Direct measurement of arteriovenous anastomotic blood flow in septic canine hind limb. Surgery 85:275, 1979.
49. Cronenwett JL, Lindenauer SM: Hemodynamic effects of sympathectomy in ischemic canine hind limbs. Surgery 87:417, 1980.
50. Cross FS, Glover DM, Simeone FA, et al: Congenital arteriovenous aneurysms. Ann Surg 148:649, 1958.
51. Crowe CP, Schenk WG Jr: Massive experimental arteriovenous fistulas. J Trauma 3:13, 1963.
52. Dardik H, Dardik I, Strom MG, et al: Intravenous rupture of arteriosclerotic aneurysms of the abdominal aorta. Surgery 80:647, 1976.
53. Dardik H, Ibrahim IM, Dardik I: Arteriovenous fistulas constructed with modified umbilical cord vein graft. Arch Surg 111:60, 1976.
54. Davis JO, Urquhart J, Higgins JT Jr, et al: Hypersecretion of aldosterone in dogs with a chronic aortic-caval fistula and high output heart failure. Circ Res 14:471, 1964.
55. Dawkins HG Jr, Vargish T, James PM Jr: Comparable hemodynamics of surgical arteriovenous fistulae in dogs. J Surg Res 18:169, 1975.
56. DeBakey ME, Cooley DA, Morris GC Jr, et al: Arteriovenous fistulae involving the abdominal aorta: Report of four cases with successful repair. Ann Surg 147:646, 1958.
57. Delaney JP: Control of arteriovenous anastomoses in the limb. *In* Rutherford RB (ed): Vascular Surgery. 1st ed. Philadelphia, WB Saunders, 1977, pp 785–791.
58. Delaney JP, Scarpino J: Limb arteriovenous shunting following sympathetic denervation. Surgery 73:202, 1973.
59. Delaney JP, Zanick DC, Scarpino JH: Control of arteriovenous shunting. Surg Forum 23:241, 1972.
60. Delpin EAS: Swelling of the hand after arteriovenous fistula for hemodialysis. Am J Surg 132:373, 1976.
61. Deterling RA Jr, Essex HE, Waugh JM: Arteriovenous fistula: Experimental study of influence of sympathetic nervous system on the development of collateral circulation. Surg Gynecol Obstet 84:629, 1947.
62. Deterling RA Jr, Essex HE, Waugh JM: Experimental studies of arteriovenous fistula with regard to the development of collateral circulation. Mayo Clin Proc 22:495, 1947.
63. Dodge HT, Kennedy JW, Petersen JL: Quantitative angiocardiographic methods in the evaluation of valvular heart disease. Prog Cardiovasc Dis 16:1, 1973.
64. Dongradi G, Rocha P, Baron B, et al: Hemodynamic effects of arteriovenous fistulae in chronic hemodialysis patients at rest and during exercise. Clin Nephrol 15:75, 1981.
65. Dorney ER: Peripheral A-V fistula of fifty-seven years' duration with refractory heart failure. Am Heart J 54:778, 1957.
66. Dry TJ, Horton BT: Traumatic arteriovenous fistula involving the right femoral artery and vein: Spontaneous closure. Arch Surg 33:248, 1936.
67. D'Silva J, Fouché RF: The effect of changes in flow on the caliber of the large arteries. J Physiol 150:23P, 1960.
68. Edwards WS: A-V fistula after venous reconstruction. Ann Surg 196:669, 1982.
69. Ehrenfeld WK, Grausz H, Wylie EJ: Subcutaneous arteriovenous fistulas for hemodialysis. Am J Surg 124:200, 1972.
70. Eiseman B, Hughes RH: Repair of an abdominal aortic vena caval fistula caused by rupture of an atherosclerotic aneurysm. Surgery 39:498, 1956.
71. Elkin DC: Operative treatment of aneurysm and arteriovenous fistula. South Med J 39:311, 1946.
72. Elkin DC, Shumacker HB Jr: Arterial aneurysms and arteriovenous fistulas: General considerations. *In* Elkin DC, DeBakey ME (eds): Surgery in World War II: Vascular Surgery. Washington, DC, Office of the Surgeon General, Department of the Army, 1955, pp 149–180.
73. Elkin DC, Warren JV: Arteriovenous fistulas: Their effect on the circulation. JAMA 134:1524, 1947.
74. Epstein FH, Ferguson TB: The effect of the formation of an arteriovenous fistula upon blood volume. J Clin Invest 34:434, 1955.
75. Epstein FH, Post RS, McDowell M: The effect of an arteriovenous

fistula on renal hemodynamics and electrolyte excretion. J Clin Invest 32:233, 1953.

76. Epstein FH, Shadle OW, Ferguson TB, et al: Cardiac output and intracardiac pressures in patients with arteriovenous fistulas. J Clin Invest 32:543, 1953.

77. Fallon JT, Stehbens WE: Venous endothelium of experimental arteriovenous fistulas in rabbits. Circ Res 31:546, 1972.

78. Fee HJ Jr, Golding AL: Lower extremity ischemia after femoral arteriovenous bovine shunts. Ann Surg 183:42, 1976.

79. Fee HJ Jr, Levisman JA, Dickmeyer JP, et al: Hemodynamic consequences of femoral arteriovenous bovine shunts. Ann Surg 184:103, 1976.

80. Fee HJ, Levisman J, Doud RB, et al: High-output congestive failure from femoral arteriovenous shunts for vascular access. Ann Surg 183:321, 1976.

81. Ferguson GG, Roach MR: Flow conditions at bifurcations as determined in glass models with reference to the focal distribution of vascular lesions. *In* Bergel DH (ed): Cardiovascular Fluid Dynamics. London, Academic Press, 1972, vol. 2, pp 141–156.

82. Foley PJ, Allen EV, Janes JM: Surgical treatment of acquired arteriovenous fistulas. Am J Surg 91:611, 1956.

83. Fontaine R, Kim M, Kieny R, et al: Résultats obtenus par 39 dérivations artério-veineuses pour oblitérations artérielles périphériques. J Chir (Paris) 83:321, 1962.

84. Frank CW, Wang H, Lammerant J, et al: An experimental study of the immediate hemodynamic adjustments to acute arteriovenous fistulae of various sizes. J Clin Invest 34:772, 1955.

85. Freeman LW, Shumacker HB Jr, Finneran JC, et al: Studies with arteriovenous fistulas. II. Influence of posture upon volume flow. Surgery 31:180, 1952.

86. Freeman NE: Arterial repair in the treatment of aneurysms and arteriovenous fistulae: A report of eighteen successful restorations. Ann Surg 124:888, 1946.

87. Frishman W, Epstein AM, Kulick S, et al: Heart failure 63 years after traumatic arteriovenous fistula. Am J Cardiol 34:733, 1974.

88. George CRP, May J, Schieb M, et al: Heart failure due to an arteriovenous fistula for hemodialysis. Med J Aust 1:696, 1973.

89. Gerard DF, Gausewitz SM, Dilley RB, et al: Acute physiologic effects of arteriovenous anastomosis and fistula in revascularizing the ischemic canine hind limb. Surgery 89:485, 1981.

90. Gerbode F, Holman E, Dickenson EH, et al: Arteriovenous fistulas and arterial aneurysms: The repair of major arteries injured in warfare, and the treatment of an arterial aneurysm with a vein graft inlay. Surgery 32:259, 1952.

91. Glass IH, Rowe RD, Duckworth JWA: Congenital arteriovenous fistula between the left internal mammary artery and the ductus venosus: Unusual cause of congestive heart failure in the newborn infant. Pediatrics 26:604, 1960.

92. Göthlin J, Lindstedt E: Angiographic features of Cimino-Brescia fistulas. AJR 125:582, 1975.

93. Graham JM, McCollum CH, Crawford ES, et al: Extensive arterial aneurysm formation proximal to ligated arteriovenous fistula. Ann Surg 191:200, 1980.

94. Gunderman W: Cited in Allen EV, Barker NW, Hines EA Jr: Peripheral Vascular Diseases. 3rd ed. Philadelphia, WB Saunders, 1962, p 476.

95. Gupta PD, Singh M: Neural mechanism underlying tachycardia induced by nonhypotensive a-v shunt. Am J Physiol 236:H35, 1979.

96. Guyton AC, Sagawa K: Compensations of cardiac output and other circulatory functions in areflex dogs with large A-V fistulas. Am J Physiol 200:1157, 1961.

97. Haimov M, Singer A, Schupak E: Access to blood vessels for hemodialysis: Experience with 87 patients on chronic hemodialysis. Surgery 69:884, 1971.

98. Haimov M, Baez A, Neff M, et al: Complications of arteriovenous fistulas for hemodialysis. Arch Surg 110:708, 1975.

99. Haimovici H, Steinman C, Caplan LH: Role of arteriovenous anastomoses in vascular disease of the lower extremity. Ann Surg 164:990, 1966.

100. Halstead AE, Vaugh RT: Arteriovenous anastomosis in the treatment of gangrene of the extremities. Surg Gynecol Obstet 14:1, 1912.

101. Harrison TR, Dock W, Holman E: Experimental studies in arteriovenous fistula: Cardiac output. Heart 11:337, 1924.

102. Henrie JN, Johnson EW Jr, Wakim KG, et al: The influence of experimental arteriovenous fistula on the healing of fractures and on

the blood flow distal to the fistula. Surg Gynecol Obstet 108:591, 1959.

103. Heringman EC, Rives JD, Davis HA: The repair of arteriovenous fistulas, evaluation of operative procedures, and analysis of fifty-three cases. JAMA 133:633, 1947.

104. Hertzer NR, Abud-Ortega AR: Cephalic vein arteriovenous fistula preceding lower-extremity arterial bypass. Vasc Diag Ther 2:57, 1981.

105. Hiertonn T: Arteriovenous fistula for discrepancy in length of lower extremities. Acta Orthop Scand 31:25, 1961.

106. Hilton JG, Kanter DM, Hays DR, et al: The effect of acute arteriovenous fistula on renal functions. J Clin Invest 34:732, 1955.

107. Hobson RW II, Wright CB: Peripheral side-to-side arteriovenous fistula. Hemodialysis and application in venous reconstruction. Am J Surg 126:411, 1973.

108. Hobson RW II, Croom RD III, Swan KG: Hemodynamics of the distal arteriovenous fistula in venous reconstruction. J Surg Res 14:483, 1973.

109. Hol R, Ingebrigtsen R: Experimental arteriovenous fistulae. Acta Radiol 55:337, 1961.

110. Holman E: Arteriovenous aneurysm: Clinical evidence correlating size of fistula with changes in the heart and proximal vessels. Ann Surg 80:801, 1924.

111. Holman E: Arteriovenous Aneurysm: Abnormal Communications Between the Arterial and Venous Circulations. New York, Macmillan, 1937.

112. Holman E: The anatomic and physiologic effects of an arteriovenous fistula. Surgery 8:362, 1940.

113. Holman E: Roentgenologic kymographic studies of the heart in the presence of an arteriovenous fistula and their interpretation. Ann Surg 124:920, 1946.

114. Holman E: Problems in the dynamics of blood flow. I. Conditions controlling collateral circulation in the presence of an arteriovenous fistula, following the ligation of an artery. Surgery 26:880, 1949.

115. Holman E: New Concepts in Surgery of the Vascular System. Springfield, IL, Charles C Thomas, 1955.

116. Holman E: Contributions to cardiovascular physiology gleaned from clinical and experimental observations of abnormal arteriovenous communications. J Cardiovasc Surg 3:48, 1962.

117. Holman E: The vicissitudes of an idea: The significance of total blood volume in the story of arteriovenous fistula. Rev Surg 20:153, 1963.

118. Holman E: Abnormal arteriovenous communications: Great variability of effects with particular reference to delayed development of cardiac failure. Circulation 32:1001, 1965.

119. Holman E, Taylor G: Problems in the dynamics of blood flow. II. Pressure relations at site of an arteriovenous fistula. Angiology 3:415, 1952.

120. Horton BT: Hemihypertrophy of extremities associated with congenital arteriovenous fistula. JAMA 98:373, 1932.

121. Hughes CW, Jahnke EJ Jr: The surgery of traumatic arteriovenous fistulas and aneurysms, a five-year followup study of 215 lesions. Ann Surg 148:790, 1958.

122. Humphreys MH, Al-Bander H, Eneas JF, et al: Factors determining electrolyte excretion and renin secretion after closure of an arteriovenous fistula in the dog. J Lab Clin Med 98:89, 1981.

123. Hunt TK, Leeds FH, Wanebo HJ, et al: Arteriovenous fistulas of major vessels in the abdomen. J Trauma 11:483, 1971.

124. Hunter W: Further observations upon a particular species of aneurysm. Med Observ Inq 2:390, 1764.

125. Hurwich BJ: Brachial arteriography of the surgically created radial arteriovenous fistula in patients undergoing chronic intermittent hemodialyses by venipuncture technique. AJR 104:394, 1968.

126. Hutchinson WJ, Bordeaux BD Jr: The influence of stasis on bone growth. Surg Gynecol Obstet 99:413, 1954.

127. Ibrahim IM, Sussman B, Dardik I, et al: Adjunctive arteriovenous fistula with tibial and peroneal reconstruction of limb salvage. Am J Surg 140:246, 1980.

128. Ingebrigtsen R, Husom O: Local blood pressure in congenital arteriovenous fistulae. Acta Med Scand 163:169, 1959.

129. Ingebrigtsen R, Wehn PS: Local blood pressure and direction of flow in experimental arteriovenous fistula. Acta Chir Scand 120:142, 1960.

130. Ingebrigtsen R, Fönstelien E, Solberg LA: Measurement of forces producing longitudinal stretching of the arterial wall, examined in

the artery proximal to an arteriovenous fistula. Acta Chir Scand 136:569, 1970.

131. Ingebrigtsen R, Krog J, Leraand S: Velocity and flow of blood in the femoral artery proximal to an experimental arteriovenous fistula. Acta Chir Scand 124:45, 1962.

132. Ingebrigtsen R, Krog J, Leraand S: Circulation distal to experimental arterio-venous fistulas of the extremities: A polarographic study. Acta Chir Scand 125:308, 1963.

133. Ingebrigtsen R, Johansen K, Müller O, et al: Blood pressure of the proximal artery in experimental arterio-venous fistulas of long standing. Acta Chir Scand 253(Suppl):134, 1960.

134. Ingebrigtsen R, Lie M, Hol R, et al: Dilatation of the iliofemoral artery following the opening of an experimental arteriovenous fistula in the dog. Scand J Clin Lab Invest 31:255, 1973.

135. Jahnke EJ Jr, Howard JM: Primary repair of major arterial injuries, a report of fifty-eight battle casualties. Arch Surg 66:646, 1953.

136. Jamison JP, Wallace WFM: The pattern of venous drainage of surgically created side-to-side arteriovenous fistulae in the human forearm. Clin Sci Mol Med 50:37, 1976.

137. Janes JM, Jennings WK Jr: Effect of induced arteriovenous fistula on leg length: 10-year observations. Mayo Clin Proc 36:1, 1961.

138. Janes JM, Musgrove JE: Effect of arteriovenous fistula on growth of bone: An experimental study. Surg Clin North Am 30:1191, 1950.

139. Jenkins A McL, Buist TAS, Glover SD: Medium-term follow-up of forty autogenous vein and forty polytetrafluoroethylene (Gore-Tex) grafts for vascular access. Surgery 88:667, 1980.

140. Johansen K, Bernstein EF: Revascularization of the ischemic canine hind limb by arteriovenous reversal. Ann Surg 190:243, 1979.

141. John HT, Warren R: The stimulus to collateral circulation. Surgery 49:14, 1961.

142. Johnson G Jr, Blythe WB: Hemodynamic effects of arteriovenous shunts used for hemodialysis. Ann Surg 171:715, 1970.

143. Johnson JM, Kenoyer MR, Johnson KE, et al: The modified bovine heterograft in vascular access for chronic hemodialysis. Ann Surg 183:62, 1976.

144. Johnson V, Eiseman B: Evaluation of arteriovenous shunt to maintain patency of venous autograft. Am J Surg 118:915, 1969.

145. Joyce PF, Sundaram M, Riaz MA, et al: Embolization of extensive peripheral angiodysplasias. Arch Surg 115:665, 1980.

146. Kamiya A, Togawa T: Adaptive regulation of wall shear stress to flow change in the canine carotid artery. Am J Physiol 239:H14, 1980.

147. Kelly PJ, Janes JM, Peterson LFA: The effect of arteriovenous fistulae on the vascular pattern of the femora of immature dogs, a microangiographic study. J Bone Joint Surg 41:1101, 1959.

148. Kennedy JA, Burwell CS: Measurement of the circulation in a patient with multiple arteriovenous communications. Am Heart J 28:133, 1944.

149. Kennedy TJ, Miller SH, Nellis SH, et al: Effects of transient ischemia on nutrient and arteriovenous shunting in canine hind limbs. Ann Surg 193:255, 1981.

150. Kinnaert P, Struyven J, Mathieu J, et al: Intermittent claudication of the hand after creation of an arteriovenous fistula in the forearm. Am J Surg 139:838, 1980.

151. Kusaba A, Inokuchi K, Furuyama M, et al: A new revascularization procedure for extensive arterial occlusions of lower extremity. A-V shunt procedure. J Cardiovasc Surg 23:99, 1982.

152. Kwun KB, Schanzer H, Finkler N, et al: Hemodynamic evaluation of angioaccess procedures for hemodialysis. Vasc Surg 13:170, 1979.

153. Lamport H, Baez S: Physical properties of small arterial vessels. Physiol Rev 42(Suppl 5):328, 1962.

154. Lavigne JE, Kerr JC, Swan KG: Hemodynamic effects of multiple arteriovenous fistulae in the canine hind limb. J Surg Res 20:571, 1976.

155. Lavigne JE, Brown CS, Fewel J, et al: Hemodynamics within a canine femoral arteriovenous fistula. Surgery 77:439, 1975.

156. Lavigne JE, Mesinna LM, Golding MR, et al: Fistula size and hemodynamic events within and about canine femoral arteriovenous fistulas. J Thorac Cardiovasc Surg 74:551, 1977.

157. Lees RS, Dewey CF Jr: Phonoangiography: A new noninvasive method for studying arterial disease. Proc Natl Acad Sci USA 67:935, 1970.

158. Leslie MB, Portin BA, Schenk WG: Cardiac output and posture studies in chronic experimental arteriovenous fistulas. Arch Surg 81:123, 1960.

159. Levine OR, Jameson AG, Nellkaus G, et al: Cardiac complications of cerebral arteriovenous fistula in infancy. Pediatrics 30:563, 1962.

160. Levowitz BS, Flores L, Dunn I, et al: Prosthetic arteriovenous fistula for vascular access in hemodialysis. Am J Surg 132:368, 1976.

161. Lewis T, Drury AN: Observations relating to arteriovenous aneurism. Heart 10:301, 1923.

162. Lie M, Sejersted OM, Kiil F: Local regulation of vascular cross-section during changes in femoral arterial blood flow in dogs. Circ Res 27:727, 1970.

163. Lindenauer SM, Thompson NW, Kraft RO, et al: Late complications of traumatic arteriovenous fistulas. Surg Gynecol Obstet 129:525, 1969.

164. Lindstedt E, Westling H: Effects of an antebrachial Cimino-Brescia arteriovenous fistula on the local circulation in the hand. Scand J Urol Nephrol 9:119, 1975.

165. Lough FC, Giordano JM, Hobson RW II: Regional hemodynamics of large and small femoral arteriovenous fistulas in dogs. Surgery 79:346, 1976.

166. Makins GH: The Bradshaw lecture on gunshot injuries of the arteries. Lancet 2:1743, 1913.

167. Marinescu V, Păuşescu E, Făgărăşanu D, et al: Metabolic factors in the cardiac insufficiency of arteriovenous fistula. Ann Surg 164:1027, 1966.

168. Matas R: Arteriovenous fistula of the femoral vessels (aneurysmal varix) on a level with the origin of the profunda. War injury of two years' duration. Dissection and mobilization of the femoral vessels with division and detachment of the anastomosis followed by separate lateral suture of the artery and vein, with perfect functional restoration of the circulation. Details of technic and commentaries. Surg Clin North Am 2:1165, 1922.

169. Matolo NM, Cohen SE, Wolfman EF Jr: Use of an arteriovenous fistula for treatment of the severely ischemic extremity: Experimental evaluation. Ann Surg 184:622, 1976.

170. May J, Tiller D, Johnson J, et al: Saphenous vein arteriovenous fistula in regular dialysis treatment. N Engl J Med 280:770, 1969.

171. McMillan R, Evans DB: Experience with three Brescia-Cimino shunts. Br Med J 3:781, 1968.

172. Merickel JH, Andersen RC, Knutson R, et al: Bovine carotid artery shunts in vascular access surgery. Complications in the chronic hemodialysis patient. Arch Surg 109:245, 1974.

173. Mindich B, Dunn I, Frumkin E, et al: Proximal venous thrombosis after side-to-side arteriovenous fistula. Arch Surg 108:227, 1974.

174. Mooney CS, Honaker AD, Griffen WO Jr: Influence of the liver on arteriovenous fistulas. Arch Surg 100:154, 1970.

175. Mozes M, Adar R, Eliahou HE, et al: Internal arteriovenous anastomoses for hemodialysis: Technical modifications and results of two years' experience. Vasc Surg 5:21, 1971.

176. Muenster JJ, Graettinger JS, Campbell JA: Correlation of clinical and hemodynamic findings in patients with systemic arteriovenous fistulas. Circulation 20:1079, 1959.

177. Nakano J: Effect of arteriovenous fistula on the cardiovascular dynamics. Jpn Heart J 12:392, 1971.

178. Nakano J, DeSchryver C: Effects of arteriovenous fistula on systemic and pulmonary circulations. Am J Physiol 207:1319, 1964.

179. Nakano J, Zekert H, Griege CW, et al: Effect of ventricular tachycardia and arteriovenous fistula on catecholamine blood level. Am J Physiol 200:413, 1961.

180. Nanu I, Alexandrescu-Dersca C, Lazeanu E: Les troubles cardiaques consécutifs. Aux anévrismes artério-veineux. Arch Mal Coeur 15:829, 1922.

181. Newman DL, Gosling RG, King DH, et al: Turbulence in bifurcation grafts. J Surg Res 13:63, 1972.

182. Nickerson JL, Elkin DC, Warren JV: The effect of temporary occlusion of arteriovenous fistulas on heart rate, stroke volume, and cardiac output. J Clin Invest 30:215, 1951.

183. Nicoladoni C: Phlebarteriectasie der rechten oberen Extremität. Arch Klin Chir 18:252, 1875.

184. Olcott C, Newton TH, Stoney RJ, et al: Intra-arterial embolization in the management of arteriovenous malformations. Surgery 79:3, 1976.

185. Paruk S, Koenig M, Levitt S, et al: Arteriovenous fistulas for hemodialysis in 100 consecutive patients. Am J Surg 131:552, 1976.

186. Pasch TH, Bauer RD, Von der Emde J: Hemodynamic effects of an experimental chronic arteriovenous fistula. Res Exp Med 161:110, 1973.

187. Pauporte J, Lowenstein JM, Richards V, et al: Blood turnover rates distal to an arteriovenous fistula. Surgery 43:828, 1958.

188. Pemberton J de J, Saint JH: Congenital arteriovenous communications. Surg Gynecol Obstet 46:470, 1928.

189. Perry MO, Horton J: Muscle and subcutaneous oxygen tension. Measurements by mass spectrometry after sympathectomy. Arch Surg 113:176, 1978.

190. Rabinowitz R, Goldfarb D: Surgical treatment of axillosubclavian venous thrombosis: A case report. Surgery 70:703, 1971.

191. Ravitch MM, Gaertner RA: Congenital arteriovenous fistula in the neck: 48-year follow-up of a patient operated upon by Dr. Halsted in 1911. Bull Johns Hopkins Hosp 107:31, 1960.

192. Reid MR: The effect of arteriovenous fistula upon the heart and blood-vessels: An experimental and clinical study. Bull Johns Hopkins Hosp 31:43, 1920.

193. Reid MR: Abnormal arteriovenous communications, acquired and congenital. III. The effects of abnormal arteriovenous communications on the heart, blood vessels, and other structures. Arch Surg 11:25, 1925.

194. Reid MR, McGuire J: Arteriovenous aneurysms. Ann Surg 108:643, 1938.

195. Reilly DT, Wood RFM, Bell PRF: Arteriovenous fistulas for dialysis: Blood flow, viscosity, and long-term patency. World J Surg 6:628, 1982.

196. Rich NM, Hughes CW, Baugh JH: Management of venous injuries. Ann Surg 171:724, 1970.

197. Roach MR: An experimental study of the production and time course of post-stenotic dilatation in the femoral and carotid arteries of adult dogs. Circ Res 13:537, 1963.

198. Rob C, Eastcott HHG: Five unusual arteriovenous fistulae. Br J Surg 42:68, 1954.

199. Robertson MG: Spontaneous rupture of an abdominal aortic aneurysm into the inferior vena cava. Am J Med 42:1011, 1967.

200. Robertson RL, Dennis EW, Elkin DC: Collateral circulation in the presence of experimental arteriovenous fistula, determination by direct measurement of extremity blood flow. Surgery 27:1, 1950.

201. Rodbard S, Ikeda K, Montes M: An analysis of mechanisms of post stenotic dilatation. Angiology 18:348, 1967.

202. Rogers W, Aust JB: The effect of arteriovenous fistula on tissue blood flow in the canine limb. Vasc Surg 8:238, 1974.

203. Root HD, Cruz AB Jr: Effects of an arteriovenous fistula on the devascularized limb. JAMA 191:645, 1965.

204. Rowe GG, Castillo CA, Afonso S, et al: The systemic and coronary hemodynamic effects of arteriovenous fistulas. Am Heart J 64:44, 1962.

205. Ryan KG, Lorber SH: Traumatic fistula between hepatic artery and portal vein. Report of a case. N Engl J Med 279:1215, 1968.

206. Sabiston DC Jr, Theilen EO, Gregg DE: Physiologic studies in experimental high output cardiac failure produced by aortic-caval fistula. Surg Forum 6:233, 1955.

207. Sako Y, Varco RL: Arteriovenous fistula: Results of management of congenital and acquired forms, blood flow measurements, and observations on proximal arterial degeneration. Surgery 67:40, 1970.

208. Samet P, Berstein WH, Jacobs W, et al: Indicator-dilution curves in systemic arteriovenous fistulas. Am J Cardiol 13:176, 1964.

209. San Martin y Satrustegui A: Anastomose arterioveineuse pour remedier à obliteration des artères des membres. Bull Med 16:451, 1902.

210. Schalin L: Arteriovenous communications in varicose veins localized by thermography and identified by operative microscopy. Acta Chir Scand 147:409, 1981.

211. Schenk WG Jr, Bahn RA, Cordell AR, et al: The regional hemodynamics of experimental acute arteriovenous fistulas. Surg Gynecol Obstet 105:733, 1957.

212. Schenk WG Jr, Martin JW, Leslie MB, et al: The regional hemodynamics of chronic experimental arteriovenous fistulas. Surg Gynecol Obstet 110:44, 1960.

213. Scherer PW: Flow in axisymmetrical glass model aneurysms. J Biomech 6:695, 1973.

214. Schreiner GE, Freinkel N, Athens JW, et al: Cardiac output, central volume and dye injection curves in traumatic arteriovenous fistulas in man. Circulation 7:718, 1953.

215. Schreiner GE, Freinkel N, Athens JW, et al: Dynamics of T-1824 distribution in patients with traumatic arteriovenous fistulas. Circ Res 1:548, 1953.

216. Seeley SF, Hughes CW, Cook FN, et al: Traumatic arteriovenous fistulas and aneurysms in war wounded: A study of 101 cases. Am J Surg 83:471, 1952.

217. Sheil AGR: Treatment of critical ischemia of the lower limb by venous arterialization: An interim report. Br J Surg 64:197, 1977.

218. Shumacker HB Jr: The problem of maintaining the continuity of the artery in the surgery of aneurysms and arteriovenous fistulae: Notes on the development and clinical application of methods of arterial suture. Ann Surg 127:207, 1948.

219. Shumacker HB Jr: Test for and means of improving the collateral circulation in cases of aneurysm and arteriovenous fistula of the extremities. Angiology 5:167, 1954.

220. Shumacker HB Jr: Arterial aneurysms and arteriovenous fistulas: Spontaneous cures. In Elkin DC, DeBakey ME (eds): Surgery in World War II: Vascular Surgery. Washington, DC, Office of the Surgeon General, Department of the Army, 1955, pp 361–374.

221. Shumacker HB Jr: Aneurysm development and degenerative changes in dilated artery proximal to arteriovenous fistula. Surg Gynecol Obstet 130:636, 1970.

222. Shumacker HB Jr, Carter KL: Tests for collateral circulation in the extremities. Arch Surg 53:359, 1946.

223. Shumacker HB Jr, Stahl NMD: A study of the cardiac frontal area in patients with arteriovenous fistulas. Surgery 26:928, 1949.

224. Simkins TE, Stehbens WE: Vibrations recorded from the adventitial surface of experimental aneurysms and arteriovenous fistulas. Vasc Surg 8:153, 1974.

225. Solberg LA, Harkness RD, Ingebrigtsen R: Hypertrophy of the median coat of the artery in experimental arteriovenous fistula. Acta Chir Scand 136:575, 1970.

226. Solti F, Soltész L, Bodor E: Hemodynamic changes of systemic and limb circulation in extremital arteriovenous fistula. Angiologica 9:69, 1972.

227. Spellman MW, Mandal A, Freeman HP, et al: Successful repair of an arteriovenous fistula between the superior mesenteric vessels secondary to a gunshot wound. Ann Surg 165:458, 1967.

228. Spence RJ, Rhodes BA, Wagner HN Jr: Regulation of arteriovenous anastomotic and capillary blood flow in the dog leg. Am J Physiol 222:326, 1972.

229. Spencer FC, Grewe RV: Management of arterial injuries in battle casualties. Ann Surg 141:304, 1955.

230. Spielman WS, Davis JO, Gotshall RW: Hypersecretion of renin in dogs with a chronic aortic-caval fistula and high-output heart failure. Proc Soc Exp Biol Med 143:479, 1973.

231. Spurny OM, Pierce JA: Cardiac output in systemic arteriovenous fistulas complicated by heart failure. Am Heart J 61:21, 1961.

232. Stehbens WE: Turbulence of blood flow in the vascular system of man. In Copley AL, Stainsby G (eds): Flow Properties of Blood. London, Pergamon Press, 1960, pp 137–140.

233. Stehbens WE: Blood vessel changes in chronic experimental arteriovenous fistulas. Surg Gynecol Obstet 127:327, 1968.

234. Stehbens WE: The ultrastructure of the anastomosed vein of experimental arteriovenous fistulae in sheep. Am J Pathol 76:377, 1974.

235. Stehbens WE, Karmody AM: Venous atherosclerosis associated with arteriovenous fistulas for hemodialysis. Arch Surg 110:176, 1975.

236. Stein AH, Morgan HC, Porras R: The effect of an arteriovenous fistula on intramedullary bone pressure. Surg Gynecol Obstet 109:287, 1959.

237. Stetton D: The futility of arteriovenous anastomosis in the treatment of impending gangrene of the lower extremity. Surg Gynecol Obstet 20:381, 1915.

238. Stewart FT: Arteriovenous aneurysm treated by angiorrhaphy. Ann Surg 57:574, 1913.

239. Stone HH, Jordan WD, Acker JJ, et al: Portal arteriovenous fistulas: Review and case report. Am J Surg 109:191, 1965.

240. Storey BG, George CRP, Stewart JH, et al: Embolic and ischemic complications after anastomosis of radial artery to cephalic vein. Surgery 66:325, 1969.

241. Strandness DE Jr, Sumner DS: Arteriovenous fistulas. In Hemodynamics for Surgeons. New York, Grune & Stratton, 1975, pp 621–663.

242. Strandness DE Jr, Gibbons GE, Bell JW: Mercury strain gauge plethysmography: Evaluation of patients with acquired arteriovenous fistula. Arch Surg 85:215, 1962.

243. Sumner DS: Arteriovenous fistula. In Strandness DE Jr (ed): Collat-

eral Circulation in Clinical Surgery. Philadelphia, WB Saunders, 1969, pp 27–90.

244. Sumner DS, Wilcox MW, Strandness DE Jr: Physiological studies of arteriovenous fistulas constructed for hemodialysis. Unpublished data.

245. Sumner RG, Kistler PC, Barry WF Jr, et al: Recognition and surgical repair of superior mesenteric arteriovenous fistula. Circulation 27:943, 1963.

246. Szilagyi DE, Jay GE, Munnel ED: Femoral arteriovenous anastomosis in the treatment of occlusive arterial disease. Arch Surg 63:435, 1951.

247. Szilagyi DE, Elliott JP, DeRusso FJ, et al: Peripheral congenital arteriovenous fistulas. Surgery 57:61, 1965.

248. Szilagyi DE, Smith RF, Elliott JP, et al: Congenital arteriovenous anomalies of the limbs. Arch Surg 111:423, 1976.

249. Szilagyi DE, Whitcomb JG, Schenker W, et al: The laws of fluid flow and arterial grafting. Surgery 47:55, 1960.

250. Taylor RR, Covell JW, Ross J Jr: Left ventricular function in experimental aorto-caval fistula with circulatory congestion and fluid retention. J Clin Invest 47:1333, 1968.

251. Tellis VA, Veith FJ, Soberman RJ, et al: Internal arteriovenous fistula for hemodialysis. Surg Gynecol Obstet 132:866, 1971.

252. Thoma R: Untersuchungen über die Histogenese und Histomechanik des Gefasssystems. Stuttgart, Enke, 1893.

253. Thompson BW, Barbour G, Bissett J: Internal arteriovenous fistula for hemodialysis. Am J Surg 124:785, 1972.

254. Timmis AD, McGonigle RJS, Weston MJ, et al: The influence of hemodialysis fistulas on circulating dynamics and left ventricular function. Int J Artif Organs 5:101, 1982.

255. Urquhart J, Davis JO, Higgins JT: Simulation of spontaneous secondary hyperaldosteronism by intravenous infusion of angiotensin II in dogs with an arteriovenous fistula. J Clin Invest 43:1355, 1964.

256. Van Loo A, Heringman EC: Circulatory changes in the dog produced by acute arteriovenous fistula. Am J Physiol 158:103, 1949.

257. Vetto RM, Belzer FO: Use of an arterio-bone fistula in advanced ischemia. Surg Forum 16:131, 1965.

258. Wakim KG, Janes JM: Influence of arteriovenous fistula on the distal circulation in the involved extremity. Arch Phys Med 39:413, 1958.

259. Walker WJ, Mullins CE, Knovick GC: Cyanosis, cardiomegaly, and weak pulses: A manifestation of massive congenital systemic arteriovenous fistula. Circulation 24:777, 1964.

260. Warren JV, Elkins DC, Nickerson JL: The blood volume in patients with arteriovenous fistulas. J Clin Invest 30:220, 1951.

261. Warren JV, Nickerson JL, Elkins DC: The cardiac output in patients with arteriovenous fistulas. J Clin Invest 30:210, 1951.

262. Warren R: Can the venous system be made to act in situ for the arterial system? Arch Surg 112:1238, 1977.

263. Zanick DC, Delaney JP: Temperature influences on arteriovenous anastomoses. Proc Soc Exp Biol Med 144:616, 1973.

264. Dardik H, Berry SM, Dardik A, et al: Infrapopliteal prosthetic graft patency by use of the distal adjunctive arteriovenous fistula. J Vasc Surg 13:685, 1991.

265. Fillinger MF, Kerns DB, Bruch D, et al: Does the end-to-end venous anastomosis offer a functional advantage over the end-to-side venous anastomosis in high-output arteriovenous grafts? J Vasc Surg 12:676, 1990.

266. Fillinger MF, Reinitz ER, Schwartz RA, et al: Graft geometry and venous intimal-medial hyperplasia in arteriovenous loop grafts. J Vasc Surg 11:556, 1990.

267. Haimovici H: Arteriovenous shunting in varicose veins. Its diagnosis by Doppler ultrasound flow detector. J Vasc Surg 2:684, 1985.

268. Huang M, Hester RL, Guyton AC: Hemodynamic changes in rats after opening an arteriovenous fistula. Am J Physiol 262:H846, 1992.

269. Inoue G, Tamura Y: The use of an afferent arteriovenous fistula in digit replantation surgery: A report of two cases. Br J Plast Surg 44:230, 1991.

270. Jacobs MJHM, Gregoric ID, Reul GJ: Prosthetic graft placement and creation of a distal arteriovenous fistula for secondary vascular reconstruction in patients with severe limb ischemia. J Vasc Surg 15:612, 1992.

271. Jendrisak MD, Anderson CB: Vascular access in patients with arterial insufficiency. Construction of proximal bridge fistulae based on inflow from axillary branch arteries. Ann Surg 212:187, 1990.

272. Liu Z, Hilbelink DR, Crokett WB, Gerdes AM: Regional changes in hemodynamics and cardiac myocyte size in rats with aortocaval fistulas. 1. Developing and established hypertrophy. Circ Res 69:52, 1991.

273. Odland MD, Kelly PH, Ney AL, et al: Management of dialysis-associated steal syndrome complicating upper extremity arteriovenous fistulas: Use of intraoperative digital photoplethysmography. Surgery 110:664, 1991.

274. Patel KR, Chan FA, Batista RJ, Clauss RH: True venous aneurysms and arterial "steal" secondary to arteriovenous fistulae dialysis. J Cardiovasc Surg 33:185, 1992.

275. Paty PSK, Shah DM, Saifi J, et al: Remote distal arteriovenous fistula to improve infrapopliteal bypass patency. J Vasc Surg 11:171, 1990.

276. Reiser IW, Chou S-Y, Porush JG: Failure of atrial natriuretic peptide to induce natriuresis in aortocaval fistula dogs. Kidney Int 42:867, 1992.

277. Ricco JB, Gauthier JB, Richer J-P, et al: Remote arteriovenous fistula with infrapopliteal polytetrafluoroethylene bypass for critical ischemia. Ann Vasc Surg 5:525, 1991.

278. Rivers SP, Scher LA, Veith FJ: Correction of steal syndrome secondary to hemodialysis access fistulas: A simplified quantitative technique. Surgery 112:593, 1992.

279. Schanzer H, Schwartz M, Harrington E, Haimov M: Treatment of ischemia due to "steal" by arteriovenous fistula with distal artery ligation and revascularization. J Vasc Surg 7:770, 1988.

280. Schuman ES, Gross GF, Hayes JF, et al: Long-term patency of polytetrafluoroethylene graft fistulas. Am J Surg 155:644, 1988.

281. Schwartz LB, Purut CM, O'Donohoe MK, et al: Quantitation of vascular outflow by measurement of impedance. J Vasc Surg 14:353, 1991.

282. Sullivan KL, Besarab A, Dorrell S, Moritz MJ: The relationship between dialysis graft pressure and stenosis. Invest Radiol 27:352, 1992.

283. van Gemert MJC, Bruyninckx CMA: Simulated hemodynamic comparison of arteriovenous fistulas. J Vasc Surg 6:39, 1987.

86

Diagnostic Evaluation of Arteriovenous Fistulae

Robert B. Rutherford, M.D., and David S. Sumner, M.D.

• • •

The clinical features that play a role in the diagnosis of acquired and congenital arteriovenous fistulae are discussed in Chapters 88 and 89 and need not be repeated here. This chapter reviews a variety of methods that may assist the clinician in making the diagnosis, in evaluating the hemodynamic effects of the lesion, and in planning a therapeutic approach. Some have broad applications; others are useful only in certain settings.

PRESSURE MEASUREMENTS AND COMPRESSION TESTING

As pointed out in Chapter 85, the mean arterial blood pressure distal to an arteriovenous fistula is always reduced to some degree. This is the result of blood being shunted away from the peripheral vascular bed into the low-resistance pathway offered by the arteriovenous communication.[54] The reduction in pressure is particularly severe when the fistula is large and the arterial collaterals are small. Even when collaterals are well developed, reversal of flow in the distal artery further decreases peripheral arterial pressure because much of the collateral flow is diverted back into the fistulous circuit and never reaches the periphery. On the other hand, when the fistula is small and the collaterals are large, there may be little or no perceptible effect on the peripheral pressure. Thus, the magnitude of the pressure drop across a fistula can provide the surgeon with an objec-

tive assessment of its hemodynamic consequences (Fig. 86–1).[4, 11, 29, 46, 54, 55]

Although arterial pressures can be measured most accurately with a transducer, this technique requires percutaneous puncture of the vessel, a rather sophisticated apparatus, and some technical skill. Noninvasive methods of measuring systolic blood pressure are usually sufficiently accurate and are painless, rapid, and much less cumbersome. A pneumatic cuff is placed around the part at the required site and inflated to above systolic pressure. As the cuff is deflated, the point at which blood flow returns distal to the cuff is noted on an aneroid or mercury manometer. Return of flow can be detected with a Doppler flowmeter, a mercury-in-Silastic strain-gauge, a photoplethysmograph, or a pulse volume recorder. These methods are described in more detail in Chapter 5. In the upper extremity, pressure measurements can be made at the upper arm, forearm, wrist, or finger levels; in the lower extremity, pressure measurements can be made at the thigh, calf, ankle, foot, or toe.

Of course, a low peripheral pressure does not necessarily imply the presence of an arteriovenous fistula because low pressures in limbs or digits are far more frequently due to obstructive arterial disease. If, however, compression of a pulsatile mass, the artery distal to a suspicious lesion, or a large proximal or distal vein causes the peripheral pressure to *rise*, the diagnosis of an arteriovenous fistula is established (see Fig. 85–14). No other lesion of the arterial

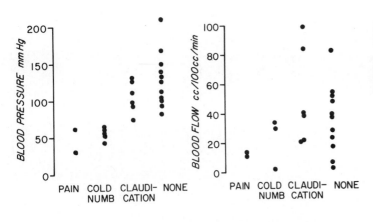

FIGURE 86–1. Relationship between symptoms and hemodynamic measurements in the index fingers of patients with side-to-side radial artery–cephalic vein fistulae. Blood pressure was measured at the proximal phalanx, and blood flow was measured in the distal phalanx. Note that pressure measurements correlate well with the patient's symptoms, whereas flow measurements do not.

or venous tree behaves in this fashion. Compression of these vessels in aneurysmal disease, in obstructive arterial disease, or in venous disorders either will cause no change in the pressure or, as is usually the case, will cause the pressure to *fall*.

On the other hand, a drop in peripheral blood pressure with compression of a suspicious lesion does not rule out the possibility that it is a fistula. In most cases, it is impossible to exert pressure on a localized fistula without also narrowing the lumen of the associated artery. Therefore, when the peripheral tissues continue to depend on antegrade flow in the artery distal to the arteriovenous communication, compression of the fistula—by interfering with this flow—will cause a fall in peripheral blood pressure (see Fig. 85–5). This is especially likely to happen when the fistula is small or the collateral arteries are poor.

It must also be pointed out that finding a normal peripheral pressure does not rule out the presence of a congenital arteriovenous fistula. In fact, the *systolic* pressure may even be elevated in comparison with that of the opposite limb at the same level.[47] This apparent paradox occurs when the pressure cuff has been placed over the site of the fistula or its afferent tributaries. Because the arteries supplying the fistula are dilated, having a reduced resistance to blood flow, there is less pressure drop than would normally be expected at the same anatomic level. This same phenomenon has been noted in the proximal artery leading to an acquired fistula. In addition, the pressure may normally be elevated if it is measured *proximal* to the fistula and only *systolic* pressure is measured. Even though mean pressure is reduced in the arterial tree as one approaches an arteriovenous fistula, the pressure swings between systolic and diastolic (i.e., the pulse pressure) may be increased so that systolic pressure may in fact be elevated proximal to a fistula.

By noting the effect on peripheral blood pressure produced by compression of the various vessels that make up the fistulous circuit, the clinical investigator can gain a clear idea of their contribution to fistula flow.[11, 54] If compression of the distal or proximal veins produces little or no change in peripheral pressure, it is probable that only a small amount of the total fistula flow is exiting through that particular vein. If, however, there is a distinct rise in pressure at the periphery, it is safe to assume that the vein constitutes an important outflow channel for the fistula. If compression of the distal artery causes a rise in peripheral pressure, it is likely that there is retrograde flow in this vessel; however, if compression causes a drop in peripheral pressure, the distal artery flow is almost certainly antegrade.

Compression of the proximal artery will always cause some decrease in peripheral pressure. When flow in the distal artery is derived in its entirety from the proximal artery, cessation of proximal arterial flow will cause a decrease in peripheral perfusion. Antegrade flow in the distal artery will come to a halt and may even be replaced by retrograde flow. When flow in the distal artery is already in a retrograde direction, compression of the proximal artery will result in an increase in this retrograde flow, thus further aggravating the peripheral steal.

Compression of collateral arteries will give some idea of the extent to which they contribute to the nutrition of the peripheral tissues.[11, 54] Obviously, if cessation of flow in

these vessels causes a marked fall in peripheral pressure, it can be assumed that they play a vital role in supplying blood to the distal portions of the extremity.

Collateral arteries may also be evaluated by noting the effect of compressing the fistula and the immediately associated vessels on peripheral pressure.[4, 11, 54, 55] If the pressure rises or does not change significantly with occlusion of the fistula plus the proximal and distal arteries and veins, the limb would certainly tolerate quadruple ligation and excision. On the other hand, if the peripheral pressure falls markedly, excisional surgery would be hazardous, and some sort of arterial reconstruction must be performed to ensure the viability of the limb.

Pressure measurements are also useful in assessing the physiologic results of surgical therapy. Successful reconstruction should return peripheral pressures to normal levels.[29, 55] Pressures should improve (or at least not fall) after quadruple ligation and excision, provided that the collateral input is adequate. Finally, the efficacy of ligating individual component vessels of a surgically created arteriovenous fistula to decrease a steal or restrict retrograde venous flow can be evaluated by pressure measurement. The latter is extremely important in dealing with a symptomatic distal steal associated with an angioaccess arteriovenous fistula (see Chapter 90).

Invasive pressure measurements are useful during surgery to determine the magnitude of the steal.[10] Swan-Ganz catheterization provides valuable hemodynamic data that not only facilitate the diagnosis of massive fistulae, such as those that develop between the aorta and the inferior vena cava or renal veins, but also aid in their perioperative management.[27, 33]

PLETHYSMOGRAPHY

Examination of plethysmographic pulses in the arms, legs, fingers, or toes may be helpful in making the diagnosis of arteriovenous fistula and in assessing its hemodynamic significance. Air-filled cuffs (the pulse volume recorder), photoplethysmographs, or mercury-in-Silastic strain-gauges (Chapter 5) can be used.

Although the pulse contour may be normal (or nearly so) in a limb distal to an arteriovenous fistula, its volume is frequently reduced, particularly in the presence of a steal (Fig. 86–2).[4, 8, 11, 46, 54, 55] As in the case of peripheral pressure

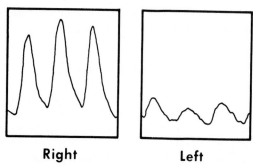

Right   **Left**

FIGURE 86–2. Plethysmographic pulses from the second toes of a patient with an acute fistula between the left superficial femoral artery and vein.

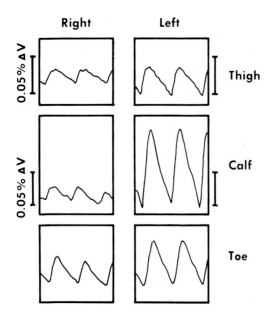

Right   **Left**

Thigh

Calf

Toe

FIGURE 86–3. Plethysmographic pulses obtained with a mercury-in-Silastic strain-gauge at thigh, calf, and toe levels in a 4-year-old girl with a congenital arteriovenous fistula of the left pelvic region. The pulses measured: right thigh, 0.02 per cent ΔV; left thigh, 0.04 per cent ΔV; right calf, 0.03 per cent ΔV; and left calf, 0.11 per cent ΔV. Increased pulses on the left side suggest the presence of further arteriovenous malformations at multiple levels in the leg.

measurements, the reduction in pulse volume depends on the size of the fistula and the adequacy of the collateral arteries. Successful reconstruction will return the pulse volume and contour to normal.[8, 55] Although the volume of the pulse may increase after quadruple ligation and excision, the pulse will usually have an "obstructive" contour (see Fig. 5–11).

When the pulse-sensing device is placed over the fistula or just proximal to it, the pulse volume may actually be increased.[46, 47] This is commonly seen in limbs with congenital arteriovenous malformations, the increased pulsation being almost diagnostic (Fig. 86–3).

If compression of a lesion suspected of being an arteriovenous fistula—or the distal artery or venous drainage—causes an immediate increase in pulse volume, the diagnosis of arteriovenous fistula is virtually assured (see Fig. 85–12). Although it is true that a similar reaction might be observed in other situations involving an arterial steal (e.g., in the donor limb when a cross-pubic femorofemoral graft is compressed), it will not occur in other spontaneous or traumatic lesions.

VOLUME FLOW MEASUREMENTS

It might seem that volume flow measurements would be a valuable approach in the diagnostic assessment of arteriovenous fistulae; however, depending on the technique used and the location of the fistula, they may be either difficult to perform or not accurate and reproducible.

Measurement of blood flow with venous occlusion plethysmography may be used to estimate the quantity of

blood flowing through a limb harboring an arteriovenous fistula.[24, 57] Unfortunately, the accuracy of this technique is compromised when the occluding cuff is proximal to the fistula because the venous pressure rises almost immediately to equal cuff pressure. This causes the limb volume to increase so rapidly that a good slope is difficult to obtain. Nevertheless, venous occlusion plethysmography can be used to measure flow distal to the fistula with a fair degree of accuracy.[4, 54]

With the use of the Doppler principle, volume measurements can be made in individual vessels (unlike with venous occlusion plethysmography, which measures total flow to a limb segment). This requires the measurement of mean velocity, the angle of the ultrasound beam, and the cross-sectional area. This can be done using a duplex scanner, but its absolute accuracy is not very good, so it is used to measure *relative changes* in volume flow. However, even here reproducibility limits its value (e.g., ± 20 per cent or more). The highly turbulent flows *near the fistula* make it difficult to obtain accurate velocity measurements, and the angle of the sound beam, although constant to the vessel wall, is different for different red blood cells because the flow is not laminar. One alternative is to monitor flow upstream over a major inflow artery in the affected and contralateral unaffected limbs. The difference should estimate fistula flow. These studies, however, are somewhat cumbersome and time consuming. This and problems with accuracy have prevented this approach from playing a major diagnostic role in evaluating arteriovenous fistulae until now, but continuing technologic advances can be expected to change this, particularly when cross-sectional areas can be integrated using one mode and mean velocity integrated from all the velocity signals obtained by another.

Furthermore, the results of these flow measurements are seldom as revealing as those obtained much more easily by means of pressure measurements (see Fig. 86–1). Peripheral blood flow (particularly in the digits) is extremely variable, depending heavily on environmental conditions and sympathetic tone. Moreover, peripheral blood flow usually remains adequate despite the presence of a significant steal, owing to the tendency of the arterioles to dilate in order to compensate for the reduction in perfusion pressure. Only when the steal is quite marked or the collaterals are quite poor will the peripheral blood flow fall into the ischemic range (see Fig. 86–1).

Increases in peripheral blood flow with compression of the fistula, distal artery, or proximal and distal veins are ordinarily seen when a steal is present, and they coincide with increases in plethysmographic pulsations and distal blood pressure (see Fig. 85–14).

DOPPLER VELOCITY DETECTION

For many if not most clinical purposes, a qualitative estimate of flow velocity and pulse contour obtained with a directional Doppler velocity detector with analog tracings or "waveforms" provides sufficient information for clinical decision making. Finding a high-velocity flow pattern in an artery leading to a suspicious lesion is good evidence that the lesion is an arteriovenous fistula (Fig. 86–4; cf. Fig.

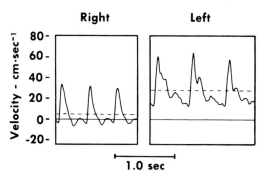

FIGURE 86–4. Blood flow in the common femoral arteries of a 4-year-old girl with a left iliofemoral arteriovenous fistula. The Doppler probe was held at a 45-degree angle to the underlying vessel. The right common femoral artery measured 0.45 cm in diameter, and the left measured 0.55 cm (see Fig. 86–10). Mean flow velocity *(dashed line)* was 5 cm/sec on the right and 28 cm/sec on the left. Total flow was estimated to be 48 ml/min on the right and 397 ml/min on the left. Contrast the reversal of flow on the right during diastole with the high velocity of flow throughout diastole on the left.

85–3).[4, 47, 52, 54] Although increased flow velocities are encountered when a part is inflamed, this problem is usually evident on clinical examination. Hyperdynamic flow associated with conditions such as beriberi or thyrotoxicosis is generalized and therefore should cause no confusion. Other causes of hyperemia isolated to an individual vessel or limb (e.g., exercise or reactive hyperemia following a period of ischemia) are transient, lasting only a few minutes. Externally applied heat, local infection (e.g., cellulitis or abscess), or sympathetic blockade can also increase flow.

The character of the audible flow signal is helpful. Flow in an artery feeding an arteriovenous fistula will be pulsatile but will lack the three sounds typical of the normal arterial signal (see Chapter 5). In the *normal* signal, the first sound coincides with the rapid forward surge of blood during systole; the second sound reflects a period of reversed flow during early diastole; and the third sound represents a second diastolic forward flow phase of much reduced volume. In the presence of an arteriovenous fistula, the proximal arterial signal will be louder than normal, higher pitched, and more continuous. These changes are due to an elevation of diastolic flow and to the absence of any reversed flow component, as shown in Figures 85–3 and 86–4.

The signal heard over veins draining a fistula will be increased in volume and may be pulsatile if the probe is near the fistula (see Fig. 85–4).[4, 52, 54] These findings are often helpful in diagnosing and localizing arteriovenous fistulae in patients with unilateral varicose veins (Fig. 86–5).[56]

All these audible Doppler signals have characteristic equivalents when seen on analog tracings obtained using a zero-crossing or some other frequency-to-voltage converter. This feature is not on the simpler bedside Doppler units but is a standard feature of the Doppler instruments used in most vascular diagnostic laboratories. The characteristic arterial pattern, shown in Figure 86–4, consists of an elimination of end-systolic reversal and a marked increase in diastolic velocity, which "elevates" the entire tracing above the zero-velocity baseline. The degree of elevation in

end-diastolic velocity correlates directly with the flow increase caused by the arteriovenous fistula.[46, 47]

By using these characteristic arterial and venous flow signals as a guide, one can detect and localize congenital or traumatic arteriovenous communications that otherwise might escape detection.[9, 41, 56] Care must be taken to compare the signal from one limb with that from the other at the same anatomic location. Also, one must appreciate the fact that similar signals can be heard in hyperemic tissues. For example, pulsatile flow is often detected in the inflamed skin associated with superficial thrombophlebitis, lymphangitis, bacterial infection, or thermal or mechanical trauma.

The Doppler probe may also be used during operation to help locate the fistula (or fistulae) and to assess the completeness of the surgery.[8, 16, 29, 32, 39, 52] Following successful operation, the arterial and venous flow signals should regain their normal character.

The direction of blood flow in the various arteries and veins contributing to the fistulous circuit can be determined with a direction-sensing Doppler velocity detector.[4, 54] For example, recognition of reversed flow in the distal artery unequivocally establishes the diagnosis of a steal (Fig. 86–

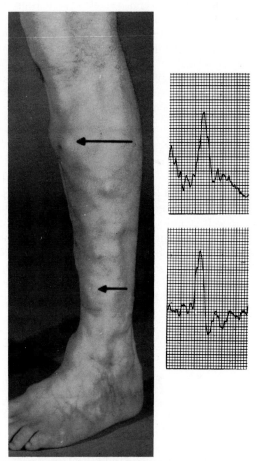

FIGURE 86–5. Tender unilateral varicose veins in a 33-year-old man who had sustained an injury to the lower part of the leg several years previously. Pulsatile venous flow was heard over two subcutaneous venous "lakes" *(arrows)*. Arteriovenous fistulae were found at these two sites. (From Strandness DE Jr, Schultz RD, Sumner DS, Rushmer RF: Ultrasonic flow detection: A useful technic in the evaluation of peripheral vascular disease. Am J Surg 113:311, 1967. Reprinted by permission.)

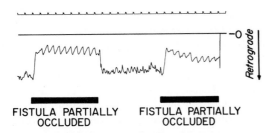

FIGURE 86–6.   Velocity of blood flow in the radial artery distal to a side-to-side radial artery–cephalic vein fistula. Note that flow is reversed and the partial compression of the fistula decreases the volume of retrograde flow. The Doppler probe was pointed craniad. (From Strandness DE Jr, Sumner DS: Arteriovenous fistula. *In* Hemodynamics for Surgeons. New York, Grune & Stratton, 1975, pp 621–663.)

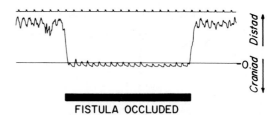

FIGURE 86–8.   Blood flow in the cephalic vein distal to a side-to-side radial artery–cephalic vein fistula. Note the great volume of reversed, highly pulsatile flow when the fistula is open. When the fistula is compressed, flow decreases markedly and regains its normal cephalad orientation. The Doppler probe was pointed craniad. (From Strandness DE Jr, Sumner DS: Arteriovenous fistula. *In* Hemodynamics for Surgeons. New York, Grune & Stratton, 1975, pp 621–663.)

6). The contribution of the collateral arteries to flow through the fistula can also be estimated by noting the decrease in flow through these arteries when the fistula is compressed (Fig. 86–7). The direction of blood flow and its course back to the heart can be mapped out in the distal vein (Fig. 86–8). Examinations such as these may be helpful in recognizing the cause of venous hypertension in the hand of the patient with a radial artery–cephalic vein fistula.

The Doppler signal in arteries far distal to an arteriovenous fistula may be reduced in volume if there is a significant flow steal.[4, 29, 52, 54] When the collateral arteries are good, compression of the fistula will increase the flow in these peripheral arteries (see Fig. 85–13). Examples of many of these applications are presented later.

DUPLEX SCANNING

The duplex scanner has simplified many of the Doppler methods described previously, and in turn, color-coding of velocity signals has simplified the use of the duplex scanner as well as provided colored images that are diagnostic in themselves. Its application in obtaining volume flow measurements has already been described, as have the characteristic velocity changes detected by the Doppler probe. Duplex scanning simply allows the Doppler beam to be more precisely localized at a point in the vessel visual-

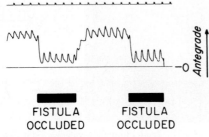

FIGURE 86–7.   Velocity of blood flow in the ulnar artery of a patient with a side-to-side radial artery–cephalic vein fistula. Note the large volume of antegrade flow and the marked reduction in flow that occurs when the fistula is occluded. The excess flow was finding its way back through the fistula via the distal radial artery. The Doppler probe was pointed craniad. (From Strandness DE Jr, Sumner DS: Arteriovenous fistula. *In* Hemodynamics for Surgeons. New York, Grune & Stratton, 1975, pp 621–663.)

ized on the B-mode image. In addition, the duplex scan will probably obtain its signal by a range-gated pulsed Doppler focused on a small area of insonation rather than the entire vessel when interrogated by a continuous-wave instrument. Furthermore, the display on the duplex scan will be adapted for spectral analysis rather than using simple analog velocity tracings. Nevertheless, the same basic information can be obtained, using the same interpretive principles discussed for the Doppler velocity detector.

However, the images obtained with color duplex scanning provide an entirely new diagnostic dimension (see Chapter 6). Traumatic arteriovenous fistulae, particularly the iatrogenic variety produced by the percutaneous introduction of catheters via the femoral vessels, are readily seen as multi-colored, orange to white "flashes" between the red and blue artery and vein. The nearby tissues transmitting the thrill will appear to "light up" with each cardiac cycle because of a motion artifact. Congenital arteriovenous fistulae are more complex, but their high-flow patterns are readily recognized and the nature and extent of the more localized lesions can be well characterized. Having performed this initial evaluation, duplex scanning can then be used to follow up and evaluate the results of interventional therapy, whether embolotherapy or surgical resection. Channels thrombosed by embolotherapy or sclerotherapy will "lose color" (i.e., their velocity signal) and will be incompressible when pressure is applied by the duplex scanner head. This approach is ideal for superficial, localized congenital vascular malformations, whereas magnetic resonance imaging is better for follow-up of deeper, more extensive lesions.

TEMPERATURE MEASUREMENTS

Direct measurement of skin temperature with a thermistor or detection of "hot spots" with a thermograph may help locate the site of arteriovenous fistulae (Table 86–1). Temperatures are usually elevated over the fistula and over the veins that drain it.[1, 20] Because retrograde flow in distal veins is common, the area of increased skin temperature may extend for considerable distances down the limb away from the fistula.[61] Similarly, temperatures will be elevated proximal to the fistula as a result of the presence of arterial blood that has been diverted into the proximal vein. In

Table 86–1. Temperature Measurements at Various Sites Along the Legs

	Temperature (°C)*	
Site	**Right**	**Left**
Thigh	31.6	32.4
Knee	31.1	35.8
Calf	30.6	33.0
Foot	31.0	31.9

Room temperature was 26°C.

contrast, temperatures in the distal part of a limb containing a proximal arteriovenous fistula will often be decreased.[18] This is especially likely when there is a significant flow steal.

Because of the diffuse nature of the temperature elevation, this technique cannot be relied on for precise identification of fistula location, and with the advancement of other noninvasive technologies, the use of thermography has greatly diminished.

VENOUS OXYGEN TENSION

The oxygen saturation of the venous blood draining a limb containing an arteriovenous fistula will always be more or less elevated in comparison with that of the opposite normal limb.[1, 60] This finding may be of significant help in making the diagnosis of congenital arteriovenous fistula, particularly in obscure cases. Because the concentration of oxygen in the venous blood bears a direct relationship to the quantity of blood leaked from the arterial to the venous side of the circulation, this test aids in assessing the hemodynamic significance of the fistula. However, it is much less helpful in congenital vascular malformations, in which lesions are more diffuse and single sampling sites less representative. Furthermore, these lesions are usually associated with varicose veins, and even simple varicose veins are known to contain blood with a higher oxygen saturation. Nevertheless, the widespread introduction of transcutaneous techniques (e.g., pulse oximetry) may restore the practical value of this approach in certain settings.

CARDIAC OUTPUT

Cardiac output can be measured by the direct oxygen-Fick method, indicator dilution methods, thermodilution, ballistocardiography, echocardiography, or other techniques. Using an ultrasound beam aimed at the aortic root from the suprasternal notch, cardiac output (minus coronary flow) can be readily monitored. Although many patients with arteriovenous fistulae will have little or no perceptible increase in cardiac output, in others the cardiac output may be quite high. By noting the magnitude of the decrease in cardiac output with fistula compression, the clinician can estimate the quantity of blood flowing through the fistula.[3, 6, 25, 37, 44, 50, 59] In addition, the efficacy of surgical therapy can be assessed by measuring the decrease in cardiac output.[14, 19, 35, 62]

From a diagnostic point of view, finding an exceptionally high cardiac output should alert the physician to the possible existence of an arteriovenous fistula.[33] When indicator dilution methods are employed, early recirculation of dye in the systemic arterial tree and early appearance in right-sided heart samples are typical patterns observed in the presence of arteriovenous fistulae.[49] Manual compression of the fistula corrects these abnormalities temporarily.

RADIONUCLIDE ASSESSMENT

Radionuclide-labeled microspheres can be used to diagnose and quantitate arteriovenous shunting. The rationale is quite simple: microspheres too large to pass through capillaries are introduced into an artery; those passing through arteriovenous communications are trapped in the lung; and the fraction of microspheres reaching the lung is determined. If the microspheres have been well mixed with the arterial inflow, the fraction of the total quantity injected that reaches the lung is proportional to the fraction of blood flow to the extremity that passes through the arteriovenous shunt. Although naturally occurring arteriovenous shunts are present in normal human extremities, less than 3.2 per cent of the total blood flow (and usually much less) is diverted through these communications.[43] When the fraction of microspheres reaching the lung exceeds this value, abnormal shunting is present.

The method described by Rhodes and Rutherford and their colleagues is as follows: With the patient lying supine, the lungs are monitored by means of a gamma camera or a rectilinear scintillation scanner maintained in a fixed position over a limited pulmonary field.[43, 45, 46] The patient is instructed not to move during the period of study. The agent used consists of a suspension of 35-μ human albumin microspheres labeled with technetium-99m (similar to that commonly used in lung scans). In order to obtain a background counting rate for unbound technetium-99m, a sample of the suspending solution is initially injected through a cannula inserted into the major inflow artery of the extremity being studied. This is followed by one or more intraarterial injections of the suspended microspheres, each of which has a volume of about 1.0 ml and an activity of 2 to 4 mCi.

After each injection, counting is continued for 3 to 5 minutes in order to reach a plateau. Finally, a dose of microspheres is administered through a superficial vein in another extremity. Because 100 per cent of the intravenously injected microspheres will reach and be trapped by the lung, the counts obtained after the venous injection represent the baseline situation of no shunting. To ensure similar counting efficiencies, the suspension injected into the vein contains one fourth to one third of the activity of that injected into the artery, approximately 0.5 to 1.0 mCi. The relative radioactivity of the microsphere suspensions is measured by scintillation counting of the syringes before and after the microspheres have been administered. It is important that no microspheres be lost by extravasation.

The formula used to estimate the percentage of arteriovenous shunting is as follows:

$$\% \text{ shunt} = \frac{(Pa - Bg)}{(Pv - Pa)} \cdot \frac{(Iv_i - Iv_r)}{(Ia_i - Ia_r)} \cdot (100)$$

where Bg is background pulmonary counts per unit time, Pa is pulmonary counts per unit time after arterial injection, Pv is pulmonary counts per unit time after venous injection, Iv_i is counts per unit time of venous syringe before injection, Iv_r is residual counts per unit time of venous syringe after injection, Ia_i is counts per unit time of arterial syringe before injection, and Ia_r is residual counts per unit time of arterial syringe after injection.[43]

For example, if the pulmonary radioactivity following the arterial injection (Pa − Bg) was half that measured following the venous injection (Pv − Pa) and the ratio of the activity of the venous injectate (Iv_i − Iv_r) to that of the arterial injectate (Ia_i − Ia_r) was one fourth, the estimated shunt volume would be 12.5 per cent of the total flow to the extremity, or

$$(\tfrac{1}{2})\,(\tfrac{1}{4})\,(100) = 12.5\%$$

Although the study is minimally invasive, it is relatively simple to perform, causes little discomfort, and carries a negligible risk. It can be undertaken as a separate procedure, in conjunction with arteriography, or during operation. When measurements are made during operation, it is necessary to obtain baseline estimations of arteriovenous shunting because anesthesia, both general and regional, increases shunting through naturally occurring arteriovenous communications. Moreover, the percentage of blood shunted through such communications can reach 40 per cent in the limbs of patients with sympathetic denervation, cirrhosis, or hypertrophic pulmonary osteopathy.[45] The examiner must be aware of these potential pitfalls and make the proper allowances when the test results are interpreted.

Radionuclide-labeled microspheres are most useful for studying patients with suspected congenital arteriovenous fistulae.[45–47] As a diagnostic modality, the test can be performed before arteriography in patients with ''hemangiomas,'' limb overgrowth, or atypical varicose veins, as well as in those with obvious congenital vascular malformations in whom the presence and degree of arteriovenous shunting are in doubt. Arteriography occasionally may fail to demonstrate the fistula or fistulae, either because they are too small or because the flow is too rapid. Early venous filling may be the only clue to their existence. In such cases, injection of microspheres in conjunction with arteriography can be used to establish the diagnosis. In diffuse or extensive congenital vascular malformations, it may be difficult to distinguish clinically between the so-called microfistulous lesions, in which the arteriovenous communications cannot be visualized angiographically, and predominantly venous malformations. The labeled microsphere study solves this dilemma.

Because shunt flow can be quantified, the results have prognostic value.[45–47] One can estimate the hemodynamic significance of the lesion and the likelihood that it will cause heart failure, limb overgrowth, distal arterial insufficiency, ulceration, or skin changes. With this knowledge, the surgeon is better equipped to determine the need for operative intervention. By applying occlusive pneumatic tourniquets to different levels of the limb and repeating the microsphere injections, one can locate multiple fistulae and compare their hemodynamic significance. However, with the ubiquity of magnetic resonance imaging (discussed later), this particular application is of less value. Arteriovenous fistulae persisting after previous excisional operations or embolotherapy may be detected and quantified by this approach.

During operation, after all overt lesions have been excised, the injections can be repeated to determine whether residual communications have been overlooked. Follow-up studies may be used to evaluate the results of therapeutic procedures such as ablative surgery or embolotherapy. Finally, serial measurements will indicate whether the fistula is following a stable or progressive course and whether previously dormant arteriovenous communications have begun to open up or grow.

COMPUTED TOMOGRAPHY AND MAGNETIC RESONANCE IMAGING

Angiographic studies tend to underestimate the full anatomic extent of vascular malformations. Computed tomography (CT) will usually demonstrate the location and extent of the lesion and even the involvement of specific muscle groups and bone.[7, 42, 63] Deep intramuscular lesions give a mottled appearance, and with the bolus administration of contrast, there is enhancement that depends on the rate of arteriovenous shunting in, and the degree of cellularity of, the lesion. Offsetting these desirable features are the need for contrast, the lack of an optimum protocol for its administration, and the practical limitation of having to use multiple transverse images to reconstruct the anatomy of the lesion.

Magnetic resonance imaging (MRI) possesses a number of distinct advantages over CT in evaluating congenital vascular malformations (CVMs). There is no need for contrast, the anatomic extent is more clearly demonstrated, longitudinal as well as transverse sections may be obtained, and the flow patterns in the CVM can be characterized. As a result, *MRI has become the pivotal diagnostic study in the evaluation of most CVMs.* The MRI signal intensity depends on the proton density, the magnetic relaxation times (T_1 and T_2), and the bulk proton flux (the last-named reflecting blood flow). If an image is obtained after the pulsed protons (in rapidly moving blood) have left the field, a (black) flow void appears on T_2-weighted scans, identifying high-flow vascular spaces and their feeding arteries and draining veins. In contrast, a predominantly venous malformation with its slow flow would appear white. Another MRI technique, even-echo rephasing, identifies vessels in which there is slow laminar flow. Hemorrhage into soft tissues can be seen and roughly aged. Cellularity can be appreciated because stromal tissues ''relax'' at different rates. Thus, cellularity produces a higher-intensity signal than blood-filled spaces.[34] Magnetic resonance angiography, which uses the time-of-flight principle, is being applied to the study of both acquired and congenital arteriovenous fistulae. It holds the promise of three-dimensional reconstruction, but as of this writing, it is not clear how much valuable *new* information it adds over that of earlier MRI techniques. Clinical examples of the value of MRI in the setting of CVMs are illustrated in Figures 86–9 to 86–11.

Because of favorable experiences with MRI in evaluating patients with CVMs,[38] one of the authors now uses a

Text continued on page 1203

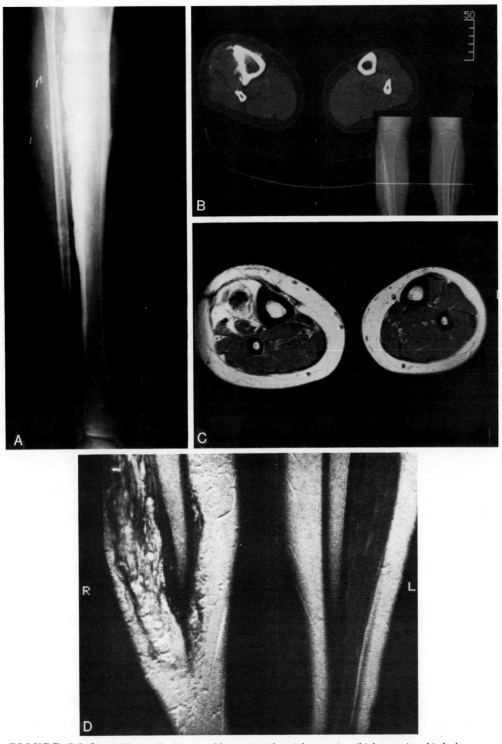

FIGURE 86–9. *A,* X-ray of a 29-year-old woman with a right anterior tibial mass since birth shows speckled calcifications, metal clips from multiple previous operations, and tibial cortical irregularities. An arteriogram (not shown) revealed "hypervascularity and one area of early venous filling." *B,* Computed tomographic scan also suggests bone involvement. *C,* Transverse magnetic resonance imaging (MRI) view shows lesion filling the anterior tibial compartment, but the margins of the tibia are clean. *D,* Longitudinal MRI view also demonstrates the lack of fast-flow voids. Total excision of the lesion was performed without difficulty or significant blood loss. Histologic study revealed a "highly cellular and fibrotic cavernous (venous) malformation." (*A–D,* From Pearce WH, Rutherford RB, Whitehill TA, Davis K: Nuclear magnetic resonance imaging: Its diagnostic value in patients with congenital vascular malformations of the limbs. J Vasc Surg 8:64, 1988.)

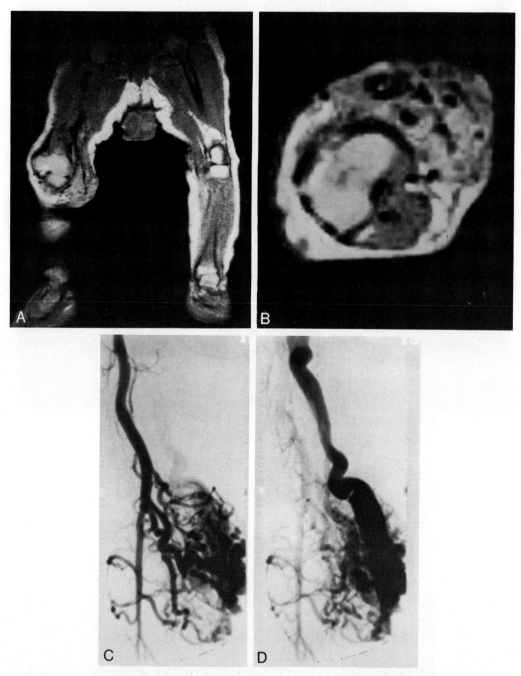

FIGURE 86–10.   A 4-day-old infant presented with a medial lower thigh mass with palpable thrill. *A*, Longitudinal MRI view shows the mass with a large, high-flow draining vein. *B*, Transverse MRI view shows multiple fast-flow voids with involvement of muscle and bone. *C*, After several months, this arteriogram was obtained because of the onset of high-output heart failure. *D*, Later-phase view shows the same large draining vein seen on MRI. Therapeutic embolization was carried out, resulting in transient disseminated intravascular coagulation but with a diminution of the mass and control of heart failure. (*A–D*, From Pearce WH, Rutherford RB, Whitehill TA, Davis K: Nuclear magnetic resonance imaging: Its diagnostic value in patients with congenital vascular malformations of the limbs. J Vasc Surg 8:64, 1988.)

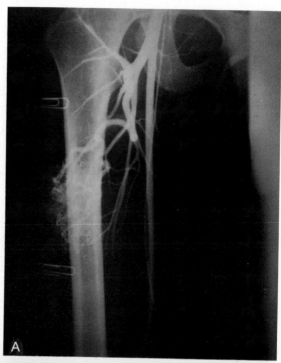

FIGURE 86–11. A 24-year-old man had been aware of a painless soft mass on his upper anterolateral thigh for many years. *A,* An arteriogram was obtained, which showed a localized arteriovenous malformation fed by the profunda femoris artery. The patient was referred for operation. *B,* Sagittal MRI view shows high-flow voids and large draining veins. *C,* Transverse MRI shows not only the high-flow voids but also diffuse involvement of the anterior thigh muscles. Operation was withheld in this asymptomatic man because excision would have produced an immediate neuromuscular disability. There was no distal steal or cardiac embarrassment.

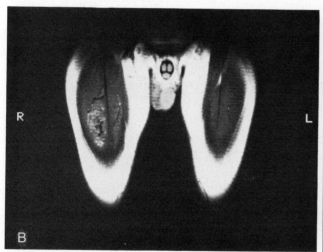

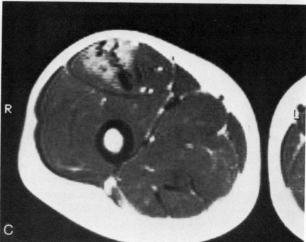

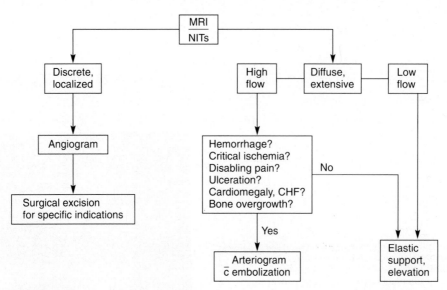

FIGURE 86–12. Algorithm showing how the use of noninvasive tests (NITs), including MRI, can help guide the management of peripheral congenital vascular malformations (CVMs). The treatment options and indications are over-simplified here (see Chapter 89). CHF, congestive heart failure.

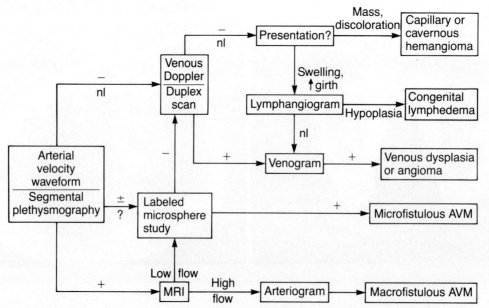

FIGURE 86–13. Algorithm of the diagnostic approach for categorizing peripheral CVMs. In most cases, lymphoscintigraphy would be used before or instead of lymphangiography, and in each instance angiography would be withheld if there were no indications for therapeutic intervention because it is not needed just to confirm the diagnosis. MRI would be used in its place. AVM, arteriovenous malformation.

combination of MRI and the noninvasive tests described earlier in the initial diagnostic approach in children with CVMs, avoiding angiography unless and until therapeutic intervention is indicated. An algorithm of this approach appears in Figure 86–12. Finally, one can *selectively* combine the different studies described earlier in a logical manner to arrive at a definitive categorical diagnosis of CVM. This approach, shown algorithmically in Figure 86–13, allows CVMs to be separated into macrofistulous and microfistulous arteriovenous malformations, venous dysplasias, lymphatic abnormalities, and capillary-cavernous hemangiomas.

ANGIOGRAPHY

With the advent of MRI, angiography is no longer necessary to diagnose CVMs or even to manage most of the low-flow lesions. This is particularly important in children, in whom angiography requires general anesthesia. Fortunately, noninvasive tests allow parents to be given an accurate diagnosis and prognosis and will at least guide initial therapy. Furthermore, duplex scanning can diagnose most iatrogenic arteriovenous fistulae and serve as the instrument for compression therapy. However, angiography is necessary with most other acquired (e.g., traumatic) arteriovenous fistulae with "intent to treat" CVMs, in which one may proceed with embolotherapy at the same time. These techniques are well described in Chapters 88 and 89 (see also Chapter 20).[12, 22, 51] Cineangiography or serial films (two or three per second) made with a rapid changer are necessary in order to visualize the fistula and to time the appearance of the radiopaque medium in the venous channels.[5]

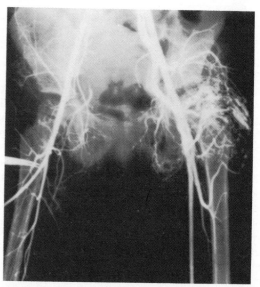

FIGURE 86–15. Arteriogram showing a large arteriovenous malformation in a 4-year-old girl. Branches of the hypogastric and profunda femoris arteries are involved. Note the pronounced enlargement of the hypogastric, external iliac, common femoral, and profunda femoris arteries.

Acquired Arteriovenous Fistulae

The actual communication between artery and vein may be apparent in radiographs of acquired fistulae; otherwise, the site of the fistula is indicated by the point of initial venous opacification (Fig. 86–14). Not uncommonly, aneurysms will be noted in the vicinity of the fistula (see Fig. 85–10). Flow in the proximal artery and proximal vein is usually quite rapid. When the fistula is large, flow in the distal artery will be sluggish or absent altogether, and there may be retrograde opacification of the distal vein. As a rule, the proximal artery will be dilated, sometimes to aneurysmal dimensions, and it may be tortuous if the fistula is chronic. Similarly, the proximal vein is dilated, especially adjacent to the fistula. Valvular incompetence may be demonstrated for a variable distance when the distal vein is distended.

On the other hand, if the fistula is small, opacification of the peripheral arteries may not be delayed appreciably and the appearance of dye in the communicating veins will be relatively slow.

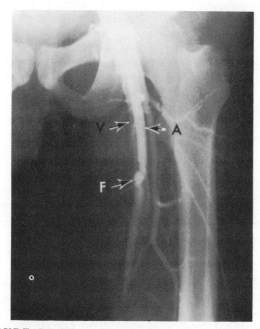

FIGURE 86–14. Acute traumatic arteriovenous fistula (F) between the left superficial femoral artery (A) and vein (V). Note the large, well-developed profunda femoris artery.

Congenital Arteriovenous Fistulae

The radiographic appearance of congenital arteriovenous fistulae is much more complicated (Fig. 86–15).[36, 58] Indirect signs of an abnormal arteriovenous communication (i.e., increased flow in the afferent arteries, decreased flow in the peripheral arteries, and rapid venous filling) are nearly always present. The fistula or, more commonly, the multiple fistulae may not be visible, however, because they may be quite small and often are of microscopic size. This occurred in close to 30 per cent in one large series.[58] Furthermore, the array of overlying arteries and veins adds to the complexity. Numerous arteries may feed and numerous veins may drain a single arteriovenous malformation. For this reason, selective angiography of the afferent artery, by reducing the number of opacified vessels, may be helpful in delineating the extent of the fistula.

Sometimes, localized dilated contrast-filled spaces will indicate the site of the fistula with some precision. On other occasions, small fistulae will be revealed as faint, diffuse opacifications between major arterial and venous channels. Other clues include abnormal vessels arising from the parent artery, horizontal branches connecting parallel vessels, and venous retia.[36]

Because the radiopaque medium tends to seek out the fistulae that are most proximal and those that carry the greatest volume of flow, smaller and more distally located communications may escape detection.[15] This is particularly unfortunate in cases of congenital arteriovenous malformations because of the tendency for multiple sites to be involved. MRI has overcome this problem.

Phlebography

Phlebography may be helpful in some cases of CVMs.[58] Lindenauer found that deep veins in the popliteal and superficial femoral regions were absent in a number of limbs with the Klippel-Trenaunay syndrome ("hemangioma," varicose veins, and unilateral increase in leg size).[30] Characteristically, arteriographic findings are normal in this condition; no arteriovenous fistulae are evident.

Phlebography, as commonly used to identify deep venous thrombosis, will often underestimate venous malformations because of grape-like clusters of venous "angiomas" that lie outside the mainstream of venous flow. Selective catheterization, direct percutaneous puncture, or passive filling under inflow occlusion (much as used for Bier block) may be necessary for proper visualization. Again, MRI is best for diagnosis; phlebography is needed only to guide therapy (e.g., sclerotherapy with absolute alcohol or sodium tetradecyl sulfate [Sotradecol]).

ARTERIOVENOUS FISTULAE FOR HEMODIALYSIS: DIAGNOSTIC CONSIDERATIONS

Although the topic of arteriovenous fistulae for hemodialysis access is covered in detail in the next section (see Chapter 90), most of the diagnostic studies are covered in this chapter. To avoid repetition and burdening of the chapter on clinical management with extensive coverage of diagnosis, the application of the previously described studies in this particular setting is described here.

Preoperative Studies

For primary access procedures, or the initial procedure in a new limb, normal arteries and adequate veins may be presumed from palpating bounding peripheral pulses and seeing adequate veins distended by tourniquet application. If this is not the case, the arterial tree may be studied noninvasively by segmental pressure measurements and plethysmography,[46, 47] and the adequacy of superficial veins can be determined by Duplex scanning.[28, 48] On the basis of these findings, and particularly in complicated or reoperative cases, arteriography and phlebography may still be required. Patients with long-standing azotemia and diabetes often have significant distal arterial occlusive disease, which may be occult. Patients with debilitating diseases require frequent admissions, during which intravenous infusions may have produced obliterative phlebitis of the superficial arm veins. Those with previous dialysis through proximal sites in the neck or groin may have occult thrombosis there, which may greatly complicate attempts to create an arteriovenous fistula distally in the same extremity.[40, 53]

Postoperative Studies

Palpation of a prominent thrill over the outflow vein after creation of an arteriovenous fistula or a shunt may suffice when present, but Doppler interrogation offers more objective evidence of adequate fistula flow in the perioperative period. Actual flow rates may be estimated as described earlier (see Volume Flow Measurements), but reproducible measurements require exacting technique and serial study in uncomplicated cases to detect a failing fistula cannot be justified. Flow rates observed during dialysis offer a more practical clue. However, other late complications, usually producing persistent symptoms such as extremity pain or swelling, deserve investigation, and they are described and illustrated.

Late complications of radial artery–cephalic vein fistulae are relatively rare; however, some patients will complain of ischemic symptoms in the hand or fingers, and others may suffer from the effects of elevated peripheral venous pressure.[13, 17, 26] In addition, a few patients have markedly increased cardiac output, and some of these may develop cardiac failure.

Pressure, flow, and plethysmographic measurements of the digital circulation will often elucidate the cause of any discomfort experienced by the patient, ruling in or out the presence of ischemia (see Fig. 86–1). Selective compression of the vessels contributing to the fistulous circuit usually permits identification of the problem area: there may be reversed flow in the distal radial artery, retrograde flow in the distal cephalic vein, or an obstructed proximal cephalic vein (Fig. 85–14).[54] Directional Doppler ultrasonic studies are valuable supplements to the foregoing information in that they can be used to define the direction of flow in the various vessels (see Figs. 85–4, 85–13, 86–6, 86–7, and 86–8). Findings elicited by these techniques will often enable the surgeon to correct the problem. Moreover, after surgical correction, the extent of the resulting benefits can be assessed objectively.

When the problem is one of inadequate supply of blood to the dialysis machine, noninvasive studies may be helpful. Obstruction to the proximal vein (perhaps related to repeated venipunctures) and excessive diversion of flow into the distal vein are easily recognized. If there is little or no reduction in digital blood pressure or if compression of the fistula produces no rise in pressure, it is likely that the

Table 86–2. Case 1: Radial Steal—Effect of Ligating Distal Radial Artery on Blood Pressure in Index Finger Ipsilateral to Radial Artery–Cephalic Vein Fistula

	Before Ligation of Distal Radial Artery (mmHg)	After Ligation of Distal Radial Artery (mmHg)
Brachial pressure	100	100
Index finger pressure		
Fistula open	32	80
Fistula occluded	68	92
Distal artery occluded	60	—
Ulnar artery occluded	0	0

problem is poor fistula flow. (If compression of the fistula causes the digital pressure to fall, the collateral arteries—usually the ulnar artery and its branches—are inadequate.) Stenoses of the fistula or afferent artery are among the causes of inadequate fistula flow. Sometimes the site of obstruction can be located with the Doppler flowmeter.[5] Confirmation by arteriography may be necessary.[2, 21]

Cardiac output studies are useful in patients experiencing heart failure. The change in cardiac output with compression of the fistula gives an estimate of fistula flow.[3, 25] Such information is important when one attempts to discover the cause of cardiac failure in patients undergoing hemodialysis, because cardiac failure frequently results from causes other than high output. Again, the success or failure of any surgical procedure designed to correct the excess fistula flow can be assayed by cardiac output measurements in the postoperative period.[3]

Case 1. A 29-year-old man with a side-to-side radial artery–cephalic vein fistula complained of pain in the thumb and index finger. This pain was especially severe during dialysis. Although his brachial systolic pressure was 100 mmHg, his index finger pressure was only 32 mmHg (Table 86–2). When the fistula was compressed, the index finger pressure rose to 68 mmHg. Compression of the radial artery distal to the fistula caused the index finger pressure to rise to 60 mmHg. Directional Doppler studies revealed reversal of flow in the distal radial artery. Compression of the ulnar artery caused the index finger pressure to drop to 0. Doppler flow signals in the ulnar artery decreased markedly with compression of the fistula.

These data were interpreted as showing a steal of blood from the finger by the fistula, with retrograde flow through the distal radial artery. In addition, they indicated that the ulnar artery was the sole supplier of blood to the finger and that much of the ulnar flow was being siphoned off to feed the fistulous circuit. On the basis of this information, the distal radial artery was ligated. Postoperatively, the index finger pressure rose to 80 mmHg even though the arm pressure remained

at 100 mmHg. Although compression of the fistula continued to cause a rise in pressure (to 92 mmHg), the percentage change was reduced compared with that obtained preoperatively, implying that the steal had been reduced appreciably (see Table 86–2). The patient's symptoms were distinctly improved: he no longer had pain while off dialysis, and pain during dialysis appeared only after about 5 hours.

Comment. Although this patient's symptoms were typical of a radial steal, confirmation of the role of the distal radial artery by pressure measurement in the index finger and by Doppler flow studies was helpful in establishing the diagnosis. Additionally, the low pressure in the index finger with the fistula open provided objective proof that the fistula was severely restricting blood flow to the hand.

The efficacy of distal artery ligation was shown by the rise of the index finger pressure out of the ischemic range and by the fact that compression of the fistula had a lesser effect on distal blood pressure.

Case 2. Three and a half years after a side-to-side radial artery–cephalic vein fistula had been constructed in the left wrist of a 40-year-old man, he began to experience increasing swelling and pain in his hand. Index finger pressures were lower than arm pressures, indicating a significant steal that could be corrected by manual compression of the fistula and partially corrected by compression of the distal radial artery (Table 86–3). However, the level of the digital artery pressure was well above the ischemic range. Although manual compression of the proximal vein had little effect on digital pressure, compression of the distended distal vein returned digital pressures to near-normal levels, as shown in Table 86–3, implying that the distal vein constituted the major outflow tract of the fistula. This was confirmed by directional Doppler studies.

Relief of his symptoms was obtained by ligation of the distal vein followed by a carpal tunnel release.[23, 31] Flow to the dialysis machine, obtained from the proximal veins, was improved. Postoperatively, arterial blood pressure in the index finger was essentially unchanged, but manual compression of

Table 86–3. Case 2: Distal Venous Hypertension—Effect of Ligating Distal Vein on Blood Pressure in Index Finger Ipsilateral to Radial Artery–Cephalic Vein Fistula

	Before Ligation of Distal Vein (mmHg)	After Ligation of Distal Vein (mmHg)
Brachial pressure	156	160
Index finger pressure		
Fistula open	100	110
Fistula occluded	160	186
Distal artery occluded	140	178
Proximal vein occluded	110	140
Distal vein occluded	152	110

the proximal vein raised the pressure in the finger appreciably, indicating that this vein was now the major outflow tract of the fistula. Compression of distal veins no longer had an effect.

Comment. Measurements of digital pressure in this patient revealed that his hand pain was not of ischemic origin. They also demonstrated that the distal vein was carrying most of the venous outflow, thus creating painful venous hypertension in the hand and causing congestion within the carpal tunnel. Correction of these defects produced circulatory dynamics that were more favorable to dialysis and relieved the pain in the hand.

References

1. Allen EV, Barker NW, Hines EA Jr: Arteriovenous fistulas. *In* Peripheral Vascular Diseases. 3rd ed. Philadelphia, WB Saunders, 1965, pp 475–494.
2. Anderson CB, Gilula LA, Harter HR, et al: Venous angiography and the surgical management of subcutaneous hemodialysis fistulas. Ann Surg 187:194, 1978.
3. Anderson CB, Codd JR, Graff RA, et al: Cardiac failure and upper extremity arteriovenous dialysis fistulas. Arch Intern Med 136:292, 1976.
4. Barnes RW: Noninvasive assessment of arteriovenous fistula. Angiology 29:691, 1978.
5. Bell D, Cockshott WP: Angiography of traumatic arteriovenous fistulae. Clin Radiol 16:241, 1965.
6. Bergrem H, Flatmark A, Simonsen S: Dialysis fistulas and cardiac failure. Acta Med Scand 204:191, 1978.
7. Bernardino ME, Jing BS, Thomas JL, et al: The extremity soft-tissue lesion: A comparative study of ultrasound, computed tomography, and xeroradiography. Radiology 189:53, 1981.
8. Bingham HG, Lichti E: Use of ultrasound transducer (Doppler) to localize peripheral arteriovenous fistulae. Plast Reconstr Surg 46:151, 1970.
9. Bingham HG, Lichti EL: The Doppler as an aid in predicting the behavior of congenital cutaneous hemangioma. Plast Reconstr Surg 47:580, 1971.
10. Boley SJ, Sammartano R, Brandt LJ, et al: Vascular ectasias of the colon. Surg Gynecol Obstet 149:353, 1979.
11. Brener BJ, Brief DK, Alpert J, et al: The effect of vascular access procedures on digital hemodynamics. *In* Diethrich EB (ed): Noninvasive Cardiovascular Diagnosis: Current Concepts. Baltimore, University Park Press, 1978, pp 189–203.
12. Bron KM: Femoral arteriography. *In* Abrams HL (ed): Angiography. 2nd ed. Boston, Little, Brown, 1971, vol. II, pp 1221–1249.
13. Bussell JA, Abbott JA, Lim RC: A radial steal syndrome with arteriovenous fistula for hemodialysis. Ann Intern Med 75:387, 1971.
14. Cantelmo NL, Alpert JS, Cutler BS, et al: Arteriovenous fistula masquerading as valvular heart disease. JAMA 245:1936, 1981.
15. Coleman CC: Diagnosis and treatment of congenital arteriovenous fistulas of the head and neck. Am J Surg 126:557, 1973.
16. Cooperman M, Martin EW Jr, Evans WE, et al: Use of Doppler ultrasound in intraoperative localization of intestinal arteriovenous malformation. Ann Surg 190:24, 1979.
17. Delpin EAS: Swelling of the hand after arteriovenous fistula for hemodialysis. Am J Surg 132:373, 1976.
18. Elkin DC, Warren JV: Arteriovenous fistulas: Their effect on the circulation. JAMA 134:1524, 1947.
19. Fee HJ, Levisman J, Doud RB, et al: High-output congestive failure from femoral arteriovenous shunts for vascular access. Ann Surg 183:321, 1976.
20. Galera GR, Martinez CA: Thermography in the management of carotid-cavernous fistulas. J Neurosurg 43:352, 1975.
21. Göthlin J, Lindstedt E: Angiographic features of Cimino-Brescia fistulas. Am J Roentgenol Radium Ther Nucl Med 125:582, 1975.
22. Hewitt RL, Smith AD, Drapanas T: Acute traumatic arteriovenous fistulas. J Trauma 13:901, 1973.
23. Holtmann B, Anderson CB: Carpal tunnel syndrome following vascular shunts for hemodialysis. Arch Surg 112:65, 1977.
24. Hurwich BJ: Plethysmographic forearm blood flow studies in mainte-

nance patients with radial arteriovenous fistulae. Nephron 6:673, 1969.
25. Johnson G Jr, Blythe WB: Hemodynamic effects of arteriovenous shunts used for hemodialysis. Ann Surg 171:715, 1970.
26. Kinnaert P, Struyven J, Mathieu J, et al: Intermittent claudication of the hand after creation of an arteriovenous fistula in the forearm. Am J Surg 139:838, 1980.
27. Kwaan JHM, McCart PM, Jones SA, et al: Aortocaval fistula detection using a Swan-Ganz catheter. Surg Gynecol Obstet 144:919, 1977.
28. Leather RP, Kupinski AM: Preoperative evaluation of the saphenous vein as a suitable graft. Semin Vasc Surg 1:51, 1988.
29. Lichti EL, Erickson TG: Traumatic arteriovenous fistula: Clinical evaluation and intraoperative monitoring with the Doppler ultrasonic flowmeter. Am J Surg 127:333, 1974.
30. Lindenauer SM: The Klippel-Trenaunay syndrome: Varicosity, hypertrophy, and hemangioma with no arteriovenous fistula. Ann Surg 162:303, 1965.
31. Mancusi-Ungaro A, Corres JJ, DiSpaltro F: Median carpal tunnel syndrome following a vascular shunt procedure in the forearm. Plast Reconstr Surg 57:96, 1976.
32. Matjasko MJ, Williams JP, Fontanilla M: Intraoperative use of Doppler to detect successful obliteration of carotid-cavernous fistulas. J Neurosurg 43:634, 1975.
33. Merrill WH, Ernst C: Aorta–left renal vein fistula: Hemodynamic monitoring and timing of operation. Surgery 89:678, 1981.
34. Mills CM, Brant-Zawadzki M, Crooks LE: Nuclear magnetic resonance: Principles of blood flow imaging. AJR 142:165, 1984.
35. Muenster JJ, Graettinger JS, Campbell JA: Correlation of clinical and hemodynamic findings in patients with systemic arteriovenous fistulas. Circulation 20:1079, 1959.
36. Murphy TO, Margulis AR: Roentgenographic manifestations of congenital peripheral arteriovenous communications. Radiology 67:26, 1956.
37. Nickerson JL, Elkin DC, Warren JV: The effect of temporary occlusion of arteriovenous fistulas on heart rate, stroke volume, and cardiac output. J Clin Invest 30:215, 1951.
38. Pearce WH, Rutherford RB, Whitehill TA, Davis K: Nuclear magnetic resonance imaging: Its diagnostic value in patients with congenital vascular malformations of the limbs. J Vasc Surg 8:64, 1988.
39. Pinkerton JE Jr: Intraoperative Doppler localization of intestinal arteriovenous malformation. Surgery 85:472, 1979.
40. Piotrowski JJ, Rutherford RB: Proximal vein thrombosis secondary to hemodialysis catheterization complicated by arteriovenous fistula. J Vasc Surg 5:876, 1987.
41. Pisko-Dubienski ZA, Baird RJ, Bayliss CE, et al: Identification and successful treatment of congenital microfistulas with the aid of directional Doppler. Surgery 78:564, 1975.
42. Rauch RF, Silverman PM, Korobkin M, et al: Computed tomography of benign angiomatous lesions of the extremities. J Comput Assist Tomogr 8:1143, 1984.
43. Rhodes BA, Rutherford RB, Lopez-Majano V, et al: Arteriovenous shunt measurement in extremities. J Nucl Med 13:357, 1972.
44. Riley SM, Blackstone EH, Sterling WA, et al: Echocardiographic assessment of cardiac performance in patients with arteriovenous fistulas. Surg Gynecol Obstet 146:203, 1978.
45. Rutherford RB: Clinical applications of a method of quantitating arteriovenous shunting in extremities. *In* Vascular Surgery. 1st ed. Philadelphia, WB Saunders, 1977, pp 781–783.
46. Rutherford RB: Noninvasive testing in the diagnosis and assessment of arteriovenous fistula. *In* Bernstein EF (ed): Noninvasive Diagnostic Techniques in Vascular Disease. St. Louis, CV Mosby, 1982, pp 430–442.
47. Rutherford RB, Fleming PW, McLeod FD: Vascular diagnostic methods for evaluating patients with arteriovenous fistulas. *In* Diethrich EB (ed): Noninvasive Cardiovascular Diagnosis: Current Concepts. Baltimore, University Park Press, 1978, pp 189–203.
48. Salles-Cunha SX, Andros G, Harris RW, et al: Preoperative noninvasive assessment of arm veins to be used as bypass grafts in the lower extremities. J Vasc Surg 3:813, 1986.
49. Samet P, Berstein WH, Jacobs W, et al: Indicator-dilution curves in systemic arteriovenous fistulas. Am J Cardiol 13:176, 1964.
50. Solti F, Soltész L, Bodor E: Hemodynamic changes of systemic and limb circulation in extremital arteriovenous fistula. Angiologica 9:69, 1972.
51. Steinberg I, Tillotson PM, Halpern M: Roentgenography of systemic (congenital and traumatic) arteriovenous fistulas. AJR 89:343, 1963.

52. Stella A, Pedrini LD, Curti T: Use of ultrasound technique in diagnosis and therapy of congenital arteriovenous fistulas. Vasc Surg 15:77, 1981.
53. Stone WJ, Wall MN, Powers TA: Massive upper extremity edema with arteriovenous fistula for hemodialysis: A complication of previous pacemaker insertion. Nephron 31:184, 1982.
54. Strandness DE Jr, Sumner DS: Arteriovenous fistula. *In* Hemodynamics for Surgeons. New York, Grune & Stratton, 1975, pp 621–663.
55. Strandness DE Jr, Gibbons GE, Bell JW: Mercury strain gauge plethysmography—Evaluation of patients with acquired arteriovenous fistula. Arch Surg 85:215, 1962.
56. Strandness DE Jr, Schultz RD, Sumner DS, Rushmer RF: Ultrasonic flow detection: A useful technic in the evaluation of peripheral vascular disease. Am J Surg 113:311, 1967.
57. Sumner DS: Mercury strain-gauge plethysmography. *In* Bernstein EF (ed): Noninvasive Diagnostic Techniques in Vascular Disease. St. Louis, CV Mosby, 1982, pp 117–135.
58. Szilagyi DE, Smith RF, Elliott JP, et al: Congenital arteriovenous anomalies of the limbs. Arch Surg 111:423, 1976.
59. Timmis AD, McGonigle RJS, Weston MJ, et al: The influence of hemodialysis fistulas on circulatory dynamics and left ventricular function. Int J Artif Organs 5:101, 1982.
60. Veal JR, McCord WM: Congenital abnormal arteriovenous anastomoses of the extremities with special reference to diagnosis by arteriography and by the oxygen saturation test. Arch Surg 33:848, 1936.
61. Wallace WFM, Jamison JP: Effect of a surgically created side-to-side arteriovenous fistula on heat elimination from the human hand and forearm: Evidence for a critical role of venous resistance in determining fistular flow. Clin Sci Mol Med 55:349, 1978.
62. Warren JV, Nickerson JL, Elkins DC: The cardiac output in patients with arteriovenous fistulas. J Clin Invest 30:210, 1951.
63. Wilson JS, Korobkin M, Genant HK, et al: Computed tomography of musculoskeletal disorders. AJR 131:55, 1978.

87

Arteriovenous Fistulae of the Aorta and Its Major Branches

William H. Baker, M.D.

• • •

Arteriovenous fistulae of the aorta and its major branches present an unparalleled challenge in patient care. Because of their central location, blood flow through these fistulae may be massive; the associated complications are usually dramatic, resulting in severe refractory congestive heart failure, massive venous hypertension, or extensive hemorrhage during an ill-fated surgical repair.

The average vascular surgeon does not have extensive experience with this disorder owing to its relative rarity. For this reason, it behooves the surgeon to become well acquainted with the problem in order to avoid morbid complications and thus ensure optimal patient care.

ETIOLOGY

Arteriovenous fistulae of the aorta and its major branches are classified as congenital or acquired. The congenital types are briefly considered here; they are discussed more extensively in Chapter 89.

Any disease that spontaneously weakens the wall of the aorta or one of its major branches might logically lead to the formation of an arteriovenous fistula. Rare causes are erosion of false aneurysms secondary to sepsis and specific aortitis. There has been one report of a mesenchymal tumor between the aorta and inferior vena cava leading to aorta–vena cava fistula, but arteriovenous fistulae secondary to tumors are most often reported with hypernephromas.[3, 5]

Rupture of an atherosclerotic aneurysm is a relatively common cause of acquired fistulae.

Trauma is the major cause of arteriovenous fistulae. Relatively low velocity trauma from a knife or small-caliber missile, for example, leads to fistula formation, whereas higher-velocity wounds made by large-caliber missiles tend to disrupt the major vessels, leading to more immediate exsanguination.

The surgeon may unwittingly be another source of trauma. If, during lumbar disc operations, the rongeur penetrates the anterior longitudinal ligament, the immobile major vessels may be injured. The aorta and inferior vena cava are injured opposite the L4–L5 disc space, whereas the iliac vessels are injured opposite the L5–S1 space. Lumbar arteries and veins can be injured at any level. The popularity of microdiscectomy seems to have decreased the incidence of this complication. Closure of the mesentery following gastrectomy and small bowel resections has damaged adjacent arteries and veins and led to arterioportal venous fistulae. Mass ligations of major arteries and veins, such as the renal and splenic pedicle, have produced fistulae. Finally, needle biopsy of the kidney has led to renal arteriovenous fistulae.

DIAGNOSIS

The diagnosis of a major arteriovenous fistula is not usually difficult for the wary physician but may escape the casual examiner. The patient will often complain of a noise or a thrill over the fistula. There may be a pulsating mass due to a false aneurysm. If there is a large flow of blood through the fistula, congestive heart failure may be evident. There may be symptoms related to the "stealing" of blood from a variety of end-organs, producing renal ischemia and hypertension, visceral ischemia and abdominal angina, cerebrovascular insufficiency, and intermittent claudication.

The classic signs of increased pulse pressure, a bruit over the fistula, pulsating veins, venous hypertension and edema, and diminished distal pulses may or may not be present. In addition, renal function may be impaired, either because of reduced arterial flow through the kidney or because of venous hypertension leading to lower glomerular filtration rates.

Many of these arteriovenous fistulae have an associated false aneurysm or are secondary to aneurysm rupture. These aneurysms notoriously are partially filled with thrombus. The thrombus may partially, completely, or intermittently cover the fistula, and symptoms may be intermittently present or totally absent.[1] The surgeon may be misled until the clot is removed in the operating room and the surgical field is flooded with venous blood.

The precise site of any arteriovenous fistula is best located by arteriography, although both computed tomography[11] and ultrasound[9] have diagnosed this condition. Frequent films must be taken because of the increased velocity of flow through the fistula. In a patient who is bleeding actively from either trauma or ruptured aneurysm, there will be insufficient time to obtain arteriograms; therefore, the diagnosis must, of necessity, be made in the operating room. In elective cases, arteriography will not only inform the surgeon of the exact arterial site (suprarenal as opposed to infrarenal aorta) but often yield information concerning venous drainage (left renal vein as opposed to the inferior vena cava) (Fig. 87–1).

PRINCIPLES OF THERAPY

Preoperative recognition of an arteriovenous fistula of the aorta or its major branches is of paramount importance. It is an absolute necessity that the surgeon spend the extra time needed to examine the patient completely. Is there a to-and-fro bruit over the aneurysm? Does the patient with penetrating abdominal trauma have distended leg veins? If the diagnosis is delayed until the patient is going into congestive heart failure from overtransfusion or until the thrill of the fistula is first felt through an inadequate or misplaced incision, the patient ultimately will suffer.

The fluid dynamics in patients with arteriovenous fistulae were reviewed previously. Patients with acute fistulae may have associated blood loss and be hypovolemic despite the presence of pulsating veins. Those with chronic fistulae are usually hypervolemic. In general, they do not need volume-for-volume blood replacement; thus, the surgeon should beware of overtransfusion in the patient who will become overloaded when the fistula is closed.

The central venous pressure is abnormally elevated in the patient with a central arteriovenous fistula, and this measurement cannot be used to guide fluid administration. A Swan-Ganz catheter, however, facilitates fluid manage-

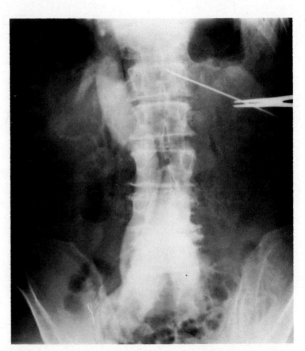

FIGURE 87–1. A translumbar aortogram reveals that this abdominal aortic aneurysm has eroded into the distal inferior vena cava. (From Baker WH, Sharzer LA, Ehrenhaft JL: Aortocaval fistula as a complication of abdominal aortic aneurysms. Surgery 72:933, 1972.)

ment and allows the surgical team to measure the pulmonary wedge pressure and cardiac output and thus assess the function of the left ventricle. Transesophageal echography should also be helpful in assessing cardiac performance. Although these principles are well known to the modern surgical team, when hypotension and hemorrhage occur during the hurried repair of these fistulae, fluid administration is both difficult and critical.

Whenever surgery is to be undertaken, enough blood must be available in case of hemorrhagic catastrophes. Acute fistulae are easily entered. Chronic fistulae have thinned large arteries and bulging veins and are encased in a fibrotic or inflammatory mass. The dissection may be extremely difficult and bloody. Autotransfusion is an ideal way to replace large amounts of blood lost by hemorrhage in a clean surgical field and has been used successfully in patients with aorta–vena cava fistulae.[4] Total circulatory arrest has also been successfully used in patients with large central arteriovenous fistulae.[6]

The goals of surgical therapy for a major arteriovenous fistula are to close the fistula, thereby restoring normal hemodynamics, and to reestablish or maintain vascular continuity. There is little place in modern surgery for quadruple ligation of a major fistula involving the aorta or its major branches.

Before the patient is brought to the operating room, some care must be taken in planning the incision. It is always best to prepare an extensive area so that an adequate incision can be made to control major bleeding. For example, if the wound is at the base of the neck, the thorax is always prepared so that a thoracotomy or sternotomy can be performed for control of the major vessels as they come off the aortic arch. For treating high abdominal fistulae, the thorax is prepared so that the descending thoracic aorta can be controlled if major bleeding is encountered.

It is imperative that the surgeon obtain proximal and distal control of the artery involved. If arterial control is obtained at some distance from the fistula, the uncontrolled branches should then be individually isolated.

Occlusion of the aorta from the level of the aortic arch to the level of the renal arteries may cause significant hypertension. This can usually be tolerated by a young, vigorous heart, but the increased afterload may cause cardiac failure with diminished cardiac output and hypoperfusion. In this situation, the pressure and peripheral resistance should be pharmacologically controlled until the afterload caused by the occluding clamp is removed. At the time of clamp removal, the administration of antihypertensive drugs must be carefully stopped lest profound hypotension ensue.

Ideally, proximal and distal venous control should be obtained, but often this is most difficult. The veins are distended from the increased pressure and the increased volume of blood. Blood under arterial pressure gushes forth from every little venous tributary that ordinarily retracts and bleeds but a few drops. If indeed venous control is obtained, it is facilitated by intermittent clamping of the proximal and distal artery. This maneuver diminishes the flow through the fistula, reduces the venous hypertension, and thereby makes dissection easier. Transvenous balloon tamponade has been successfully used.[7]

When venous control is obtained, the surgeon must have careful communication with the anesthesiologists. Control of the inferior vena cava may seriously diminish the venous return to the heart, and this may cause dire cardiac effects in an already hypovolemic patient. Many times the patient can tolerate this hemodynamic insult for only a few seconds, and intermittent flow through the vena cava may be necessary to maintain acceptable hemodynamics.

More often, the vein is not encircled, but proximal and distal arterial control is obtained and the artery is opened. The fistula can be controlled by a finger or thumb placed over the communication. Compression with sponge sticks caudad and cephalad to the fistula will diminish blood flow through the vein (Fig. 87–2). This maneuver ordinarily takes but a few seconds and only temporarily disturbs the patient's venous return. If the surgeon is careful in sewing under his or her finger, blood loss can be kept at a minimum.

After the vein is repaired, the preferred method for restoring arterial continuity is with a graft. Ordinarily, a Dacron graft is used to bridge the deficit. If the surgical field is contaminated by concomitant injury to the adjacent viscera or by a wounding missile, however, the care becomes much more complicated. These patients should be managed like those with arterial infections. That is, the area of sepsis should be débrided, the artery should be closed proximally and distally, and arterial continuity should be restored extra-anatomically. After the abdomen is closed, a subcutaneous bypass can be performed in a clean surgical field to maintain viability of the extremities.

An alternative plan is to place a prosthetic graft into the potentially contaminated field. The operative area is completely débrided and irrigated with saline or antibiotic

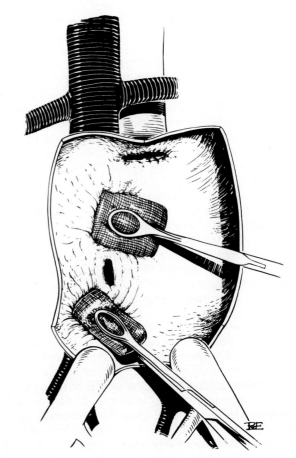

FIGURE 87–2. Sponge stick control of the inferior vena cava as seen through the open aortic aneurysm. (From Baker WH, Sharzer LA, Ehrenhaft JL: Aortocaval fistula as a complication of abdominal aortic aneurysms. Surgery 72:933, 1972.)

solution. After the prosthetic graft is sutured into place, it is isolated from the contaminated peritoneal cavity, using an omental pedicle if necessary.

These patients should be given massive doses of antibiotics, and they must be followed up continuously for many months to ensure that graft infection, false aneurysm formation, and exsanguination will not result.

FISTULAE AT SPECIFIC SITES

Base of the Neck

It is rare to find an arteriovenous fistula involving the thoracic aorta and superior vena cava or involving the great vessels as they come off the thoracic arch. Thoracic aortic aneurysms tend to dissect rather than form saccular aneurysms that erode into adjacent veins. Wounds of this area are, by and large, operated on immediately, before a fistula has had a chance to develop. Direct puncture of the carotid and vertebral arteries for arteriography is an uncommon cause of fistulae.

Subclavian artery and vein fistulae present with the symptoms that are discussed in Chapter 88 and with local symptoms of a palpable mass and thrill. They may be secondary to trauma (penetrating or blunt, causing fractures of the thoracic outlet) or congenital. Associated brachial plexus symptoms may be present, depending on the size of the aneurysm or the extent of the trauma.

A fistula between the carotid artery and the internal jugular vein may divert enough blood from the carotid system to create symptoms of cerebrovascular insufficiency. In addition, thrombus from the false aneurysm may embolize cephalad to the eye or brain. The patient usually complains of a mass in the neck, which represents the false aneurysm. In addition, a thrill or bruit is present over the fistula.

If the fistula is low in the base of the neck, the surgeon should electively gain proximal control by thoracotomy or median sternotomy. The left common carotid artery and the innominate artery can be controlled through a full or limited median sternotomy (trapdoor incision), but the left subclavian artery is best controlled through a left anterior thoracotomy because of its posterior position on the arch. In most patients, the artery is opened, the fistula is closed from the arterial side, and the divided artery is repaired with an end-to-end anastomosis. If too much artery is resected to allow reanastomosis without undue tension, an interposition graft of vein or Dacron can be used with good results.

When the carotid circulation is interrupted during repair of a fistula involving the great vessels of the neck, an indwelling shunt may be used to ensure adequate cerebral circulation. The use of these shunts is a debatable topic. Ordinarily, at the base of the neck there is enough collateral circulation so that a shunt is unnecessary most, if not all, of the time.

There is little place for nonoperative therapy in the management of acquired arteriovenous fistulae at the base of the neck. Their natural history is that they will continue to grow, and the patient will have either rupture of the false aneurysm or symptoms of cerebrovascular insufficiency. The risk of repair is related to cerebral complications and blood loss. Because these risks can be kept to a minimum, surgical repair is the treatment of choice.

Aorta and Vena Cava

Aorta–vena cava fistulae are most commonly due to rupture of aortic abdominal aneurysms of atherosclerotic origin. In a series of six such patients from the University of Iowa, classic symptoms (abdominal bruit, widened pulse pressure, venous hypertension, edema, arterial insufficiency, and congestive heart failure) were present in three, and a proper preoperative diagnosis was made in one.[1] Proximal and distal control of the aortic aneurysm was obtained in the usual manner. Venous control was not attempted, but the aneurysm was opened and the fistula controlled with compression, as mentioned earlier. The fistula was closed and the aneurysm replaced with a graft. In a subsequent series from Boston of perhaps less urgent cases, 75 per cent were correctly diagnosed preoperatively and the mortality rate was reduced from 50 to 10 per cent.[2]

Special care should be taken to manipulate the aortic aneurysm as little as possible before closure of the fistula. These aneurysms are notoriously filled with thrombus, and if this clot becomes dislodged, it will embolize through the

fistula and return via the inferior vena cava to the right side of the heart and the pulmonary artery (Fig. 87–3). This complication can be avoided by careful surgical technique.

Traumatic fistulae between the aorta and the inferior vena cava are less common. Direct trauma usually causes massive blood loss, and most patients do not make it to the operating room.

The formation of arteriovenous fistulae between the aorta and the vena cava or the iliac vein following total discectomies is fortunately uncommon. Half of these patients will not have extreme blood loss noted during their operation. Many will have unexplained hypotension during the discectomy. However, the blood loss is into the retroperitoneum and may not present to the operating surgeon posteriorly through the disc space. The treatment of these fistulae is surgical because they will continue to grow. They are located relatively caudad in the abdominal aorta, and thus exposure is usually not difficult. It is safer to close the fistula through the artery because dissection at the confluence of the iliac veins and the inferior vena cava can be extremely hazardous in the presence of arterialized venous pressure.

Aorta and Renal Vein

Aortic abdominal aneurysms can rupture anteriorly into the left renal vein as it crosses in its normal position over the aorta, but they most often rupture into a retroaortic left renal vein. They should be treated as other aorta–inferior vena cava fistulae. The vein is closed from within the

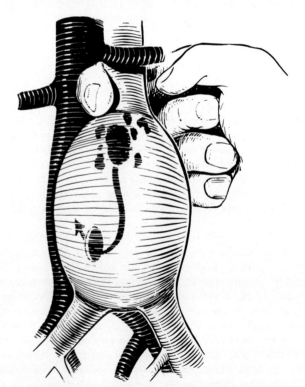

FIGURE 87–3.   Dissection of the clot-containing aneurysm must be delicate lest the thrombus become dislodged, enter the inferior vena cava, and embolize to the pulmonary artery. (From Baker WH, Sharzer LA, Ehrenhaft JL: Aortocaval fistula as a complication of abdominal aortic aneurysms. Surgery 72:933, 1972.)

artery, and a graft is used to replace the aortic abdominal aneurysm. Sacrifice of the vein is possible without sequelae if the adrenal or gonadal vein is left intact to provide collateral venous circulation.

Renal Artery and Vein

Renal arteriovenous fistulae are covered separately in Chapter 111. Suffice it to say that most are secondary to mass ligation of the renal hilum during nephrectomy.[10] Traumatic fistulae are caused by knife and missile wounds. The renal biopsy needle is a cause of intrarenal arteriovenous fistulization. Hypernephromas commonly grow caudad through the renal veins. Such a tumor has been reported to grow into the renal artery, producing a major arteriovenous fistula.[8] The indication for repair is usually the presence of a fistula. Rarely will a fistula be small and fail to enlarge. Hypertension, if present, is usually poorly controlled until the fistula is repaired or the kidney is removed.

Portal Vein and Systemic Artery

Systemic artery–portal vein fistulae are extremely rare.[12] They may follow surgical procedures, sepsis that erodes adjacent arteries and veins, rupture of aneurysms, and trauma. Splenic arteriovenous fistulae occur when splenic artery aneurysms rupture into the splenic vein. Congenital fistulae are reported to be most common between the hepatic artery and the portal vein and are associated with hemangiomas and telangiectasia.

These fistulae characteristically do not cause symptoms of congestive heart failure, presumably because of the buffer of the hepatic venous circulation. Portal venous hypertension is produced, however, and esophageal, gastric, or small bowel varices may lead to gastrointestinal hemorrhage, ascites, or both.

The treatment of these fistulae depends on the vessels involved. Splenic fistulae may be excised by splenectomy. Peripheral mesenteric fistulae may be simply excised, but more centrally located fistulae should be excised, the arterial flow restored to maintain bowel viability, and the portal venous flow restored to correct the portal hypertension and to avoid venous infarction of the bowel. Peripheral hepatic aneurysms and fistulae may be treated by percutaneous embolization.

References

1. Baker WH, Sharzer LA, Ehrenhaft JL: Aortocaval fistula as a complication of abdominal aortic aneurysms. Surgery 72:933, 1972.
2. Brewster DC, Cambria RP, Moncure AC, et al: Aortocaval and iliac arteriovenous fistulas: Recognition and treatment. J Vasc Surg 13:253, 1991.
3. Crawford ES, Turrell DJ, Alexander JK: Aorto-inferior vena caval fistula of neoplastic origin. Circulation 27:414, 1963.
4. Doty DB, Wright CB, Lamberth WC, et al: Aortocaval fistula associated with aneurysm of the abdominal aorta: Current management using autotransfusion techniques. Surgery 84:250, 1978.
5. Gomes MMR, Bernatz PE: Arteriovenous fistulas: A review and ten-year experience. Mayo Clin Proc 45:81, 1970.
6. Griffin LH Jr, Fishback ME, Galloway RF, et al: Traumatic aortorenal vein fistula: Repair using total circulatory arrest. Surgery 81:480, 1977.
7. Ingoldby CJ, Case WG, Primrose JN: Aortocaval fistulas and the use of transvenous balloon tamponade. Ann R Coll Surg Engl 72(5):335, 1990.
8. Jantet GH, Foot EC, Kenyon JR: Rupture of an intrarenal arteriovenous fistula secondary to carcinoma. A case report. Br J Surg 49:404, 1962.
9. Mansour MA, Russ PD, Jubber SW, Pearce WH: Aorto left renal vein fistula: Diagnosis by duplex sonography. AJR 152(5):1107, 1989.
10. Matos A, Moreira A, Mendonca M: Renal arteriovenous fistula after nephrectomy. Ann Vasc Surg 6:378, 1992.
11. Sheward SE, Spencer RR, Hinton RT, et al: Computed tomography of primary aorto caval fistula. Comput Med Imaging Graph 16(2):121, 1992.
12. Strodel WE, Eckhauser FE, Lemmer JH, et al: Presentation and perioperative management of arterioportal fistulas. Arch Surg 127:563, 1987.

88

Peripheral Arteriovenous Fistulae

Thomas S. Riles, M.D., Robert J. Rosen, M.D., and Alejandro Berenstein, M.D.

• • •

PATHOGENESIS

The etiology of an arteriovenous fistula, which is simply defined as an abnormal single communication between the arterial and venous systems, may be quite varied. Acquired fistulae most often result from trauma. Penetrating injuries from knives, bullets, needles, and catheters injure adjacent arteries and veins, opening communications between the two vascular systems. Blunt trauma that causes fracture or joint disarticulation may lead to the development of an arteriovenous fistula as well. Carotid-cavernous fistulae from facial trauma and hypogastric artery fistulae from pelvic injuries are examples. Arteriovenous fistulae may also result from neoplasm, infection, and atherosclerotic aneurysms, although this occurs quite rarely.

Congenital arteriovenous fistulae are usually associated with malformations of the great vessels or result from failure of the fetal arteriovenous communications of the atrial septum and patent ductus to close. Congenital fistulae may also be found in the peripheral circulation. First cousins of the multi-fistulous congenital arteriovenous malformations discussed in Chapter 89, congenital fistulae also result from the failure of the embryonic vascular network to differentiate into separate arterial and venous systems with an intervening capillary network. Although the existence of congenital arteriovenous fistulae has long been noted and has occasionally been observed on routine angiography, these fistulae are seldom of clinical significance. The diagnosis of congenital arteriovenous fistula is usually made by the exclusion of other, more common etiologies.

Arteriovenous fistulae created for therapeutic purposes such as dialysis or for the maintenance of arterial bypasses and venous repairs are discussed in a separate section devoted to this topic (see Section XII).

In some instances, the distance between the artery and the vein may be quite short, with the fistula consisting of no more than the walls of the adjacent vessels. In other cases, a fibrotic channel may separate the artery and vein. False aneurysms are frequently found in association with fistulae, particularly with those that result from trauma (Fig. 88–1). Of the 195 patients with traumatic arteriovenous fistulae examined by Elkin and Shumacker, 60 per cent had an associated false aneurysm.[10] Although the majority of the aneurysms were interposed between the artery and vein, the remainder were at various locations, separate from or on the venous side of the fistula (see Fig. 85–11).

PHYSIOLOGY AND CLINICAL MANIFESTATIONS

The physiology of arteriovenous fistulae is extensively reviewed in Chapter 85. In brief, a peripheral arteriovenous fistula may lead to local changes in the region of the abnormal communication, to central changes due to the stress on the entire cardiovascular system, or to both local and central changes. The extent of the clinical manifestations is related to the size of the fistula, the duration of the fistula, and the precise location of the fistula. For example, a small-caliber

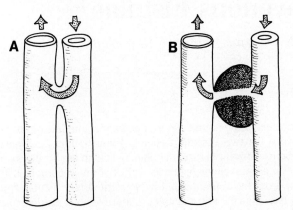

FIGURE 88–1. *A*, Arteriovenous fistula between two adjacent vessels. *B*, Arteriovenous fistula with an intervening false aneurysm.

fistula of recent onset in an extremity may be appreciated only by the presence of an audible bruit or a palpable thrill. A chronic fistula in the same location may create venous hypertension and valvular incompetence. Fistulae of long duration are typically associated with dilatation and elongation of the feeding artery.[19] The venous system proximal to the fistula similarly dilates. Venous hypertension, incompetence, and hypertrophy commonly lead to distal swelling. A large fistula, acute or chronic, in the same area may result in extensive shunting (''steal'') of peripheral blood flow, loss of pulse, and ischemia to the distal tissues.

In addition to the local changes, the heart and the remainder of the vascular system may be profoundly affected. The major determinant of the systemic response is the size of the shunt, which is measured in terms of the percentage of cardiac output that passes through the fistula. Other factors include the duration of the shunt and other medical conditions such as coronary artery disease, valvular incompetence, and myocardial dysfunction. Lesser shunts over a longer period may lead to ventricular dilatation, myocardial hypertrophy, and congestive heart failure. Massive shunts may quickly lead to hypotension, heart failure, and death.

DIAGNOSIS

Although many imaginative studies have been described for the diagnosis of arteriovenous fistulae, most fistulae are easily detected by a careful history and physical examination. In trauma patients, an arteriovenous fistula should be considered with any penetrating injury. A stethoscope placed over the site of injury may detect the continuous murmur characteristic of an arteriovenous fistula. If surgery is not immediately indicated in patients with deep wounds, arteriography should be performed to rule out an arteriovenous fistula, as well as other arterial pathology.

In the case of a chronic arteriovenous fistula, a history of penetrating injury is usually obtained. The patient usually presents with a complaint of a pulsatile mass, a buzzing sound, or a vibrating sensation. Swelling may also be present. It is rare that the diagnosis has not been made before symptoms of ischemia and heart failure develop.

Examination of the patient reveals a site of recent injury or a scar from an old injury over the course of an artery. A to-and-fro (''machinery'') murmur is usually best heard directly over the fistula and is often associated with a thrill. It is to be distinguished from the loud systolic and separate, faint diastolic murmur of the false aneurysm, and from the systolic murmur of arterial stenosis. The temperature of the skin overlying the arteriovenous fistula may be elevated, whereas distally, the skin temperature is often decreased. Veins, especially peripheral to the fistula, are distended and at times tortuous and varicose. In the long-standing fistula, chronic venous hypertension may cause dermatitis and ulceration similar to that seen in the postphlebitic state. The tachycardia observed in some patients may decrease when the artery leading to the fistula or the fistula itself is occluded (Branham's sign).[5] Studies to document the increase in cardiac output and blood volume that accompanies some fistulae, although of physiologic interest, rarely help in making the diagnosis or in treating these patients. The use of a Doppler probe and other noninvasive methods for diagnosing this condition are described in Chapter 86.

Angiography should be performed in most cases of suspected arteriovenous fistula to confirm the diagnosis and clarify the anatomic location of the abnormal vascular communication. Demonstration of the actual site of communication may be quite difficult because of the very high flow and dilatation of the venous system. The diagnostic study should be as selective as possible. Rapid contrast injection and very rapid imaging are often essential for visualizing the communication. Even more taxing are chronic arteriovenous fistulae in patients who have had unsuccessful previous surgical or radiologic attempts at closure. After arterial ligation or embolization, complex patterns of collateral inflow obscure the view of the fistula. The use of balloon catheters to retard or arrest flow may greatly aid in localization of the lesion.[2] False aneurysms and secondary changes, such as dilatation and tortuosity of the feeding artery and reversal of venous flow distal to the fistula, may also be seen with angiography. Identification of these related changes may be important in planning therapy.

TREATMENT: A HISTORICAL PERSPECTIVE

The history of the treatment of arteriovenous fistulae is a fascinating tale of clinical frustration, scientific observation, and surgical ingenuity. Hunter's vivid description of an arteriovenous fistula, presented in 1762, was apparently the first to be recorded.[16] With the frequent use of bloodletting in the mid-1800s, surgeons had the opportunity to deal with numerous fistulae involving the brachial artery and vein. The debate over whether to do nothing, to ligate the proximal and distal arteries, or to use the "ancient method" of opening the sac and tying off the feeding vessels continued into the 1900s.[23]

In 1833, Breschet recognized that proximal artery ligation of an arteriovenous fistula was ill-advised because the development of collateral circulation allowed the abnormal communication to persist (Fig. 88–2B).[6] Dupuytren, in 1854, continued to recommend proximal arterial ligation.[9] In 1843, Norris, while attempting proximal and distal arterial ligation, had numerous complications that "were such as would prevent my ever again having recourse to it" and recommended the "old operation of laying open the sac and securing the vessel above and below the wounded point."[23]

In 1897, Murphy closed a small hole in the vein of an arteriovenous fistula and then performed the first end-to-end anastomosis of the artery (see Fig. 88–2C).[22] Despite this, Matas, in 1902, after extensive review of arteriovenous fistulae involving the subclavian vessels, concluded that "the old rule of non-intervention is still in order and should be followed."[20] He added, however, that when the lesion is not well tolerated, it is justifiable to operate with a view to extirpating the lesion.

After 1902, when Carrel demonstrated the ability to create a vascular anastomosis, extirpation of the arteriovenous fistula with end-to-end anastomosis gradually became

the treatment of choice for the fistula of short duration.[7] By 1922, Matas believed that "quadruple ligation with resection of both vessels has become an almost obsolete practice"[21] (see Fig. 88–2D).

It is interesting to note that in a report by Elkin and Shumacker of 585 arteriovenous fistulae treated during World War II, 526 of the 585 were treated by quadruple ligation and excision.[10] Despite this, extirpation of the lesion with maintenance or restoration of the continuity of the artery was considered to be the ideal treatment.[10, 12]

Foley and associates, in 1956, noted that "post-operative arterial insufficiency" developed in 50 per cent of all patients at the Mayo Clinic who had interruption of arterial continuity of the lower extremity for treatment of arteriovenous communications.[11] As a result of this observation, they made a plea for early surgical treatment of traumatic arteriovenous fistulae with an attempt to reestablish arterial and venous continuity. This advice was echoed by Beall and associates in 1963.[1] Spencer and Grewe[27] and Hughes and Jahnke[15] urged simultaneous venous repair to prevent swelling of the distal extremity. Reports from Vietnam in 1966 and 1969 noted that arteriovenous fistulae were infrequently encountered when the policy of early repair of arterial injuries was maintained.[14, 26]

Thus, the repair of arteriovenous fistulae has evolved from simple arterial ligation through extirpation of the fistula to the currently recommended treatment of reconstructive surgery. Added to this now is the possibility of closure of fistulae with percutaneous catheters (see Fig. 88–2I to K).[25] With the techniques currently available, there should be few chronic traumatic arteriovenous fistulae in the practice of vascular surgery.

CURRENT THERAPY

Except in very rare instances, the goal of treatment should be complete closure of an arteriovenous fistula, regardless of the etiology.

Proximal arterial ligation has repeatedly been shown to fail and should be avoided at all costs. In addition to the persistence of the fistula, the patient's condition usually worsens immediately because of ischemia of the distal tissues. Percutaneous closure with detachable balloons, a treatment that may ultimately be the procedure of choice, is virtually impossible once proximal arterial ligation has been performed.

After the location of the fistula is determined by angiography, a decision must be made as to how it may best be managed. The alternatives include various surgical options, as well as a selection of catheter occlusion techniques that have come about with modern interventional radiology. The choice of technique is largely determined by the size, the accessibility, and the etiology of the fistula. Other factors include the relative risk of either the percutaneous or the surgical approach. It is essential that the interventional radiologist and the surgeon review together the various possibilities and develop a unified plan with alternatives and contingencies. With very complex communications, both must be alert for the unexpected.

As previously mentioned, the majority of peripheral arteriovenous fistulae are the result of trauma.[13, 24] If the fistula arises from a branch artery or a nonessential artery,

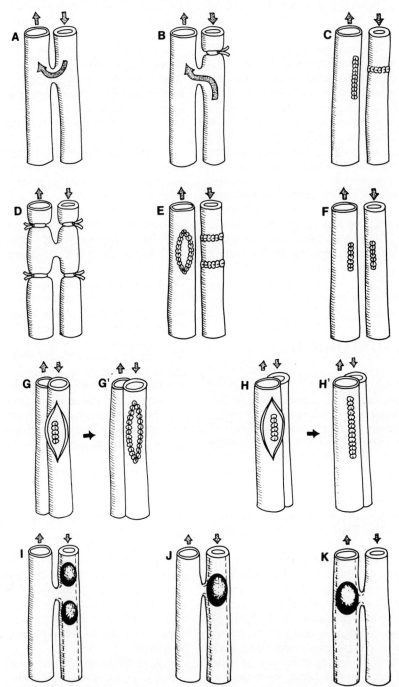

FIGURE 88–2. Methods of surgical and percutaneous treatment of arteriovenous fistulae. *A*, Arteriovenous fistula. *B*, Proximal ligation fails to control the fistula because of collateral circulation to the distal artery. *C*, Resection of the fistula with end-to-end reanastomosis of the artery and primary vessel closure. *D*, Quadruple ligation without reconstruction, which is reserved for small fistulae. *E*, Resection of the fistula with an interposition graft to reconstruct the artery and patch angioplasty repair of the vein. *F*, Simple division of the fistula and primary closure of the artery and the vein. *G*, Closure of the fistula through an arteriotomy, with patch closure of the arteriotomy (*G¹*). *H*, Closure of the fistula through a venotomy, with primary closure of the venotomy (*H¹*). *I* and *J*, Closure of the fistula by percutaneous placement of detachable balloons, which is an acceptable method for small fistulae with adequate collateral circulation around the site of communication. *K*, Closure of the fistula by percutaneous placement of a balloon on the venous site of the fistula.

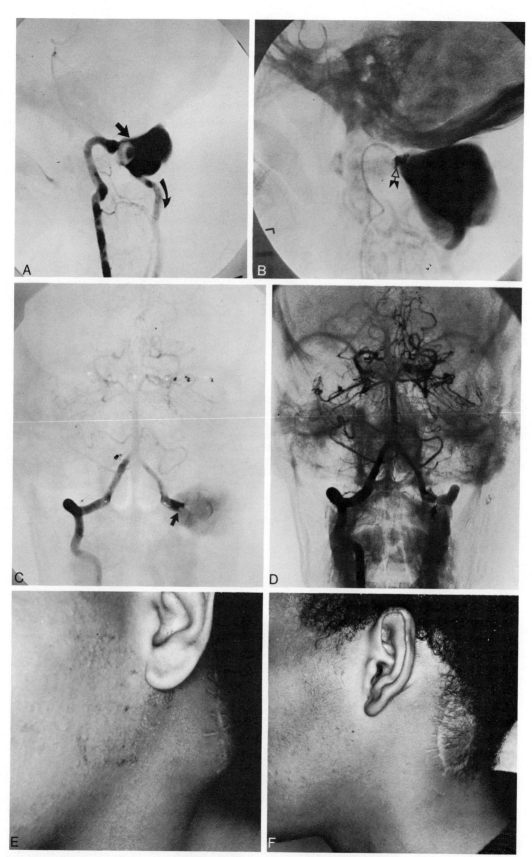

FIGURE 88-3. Traumatic fistula of the left vertebral artery at the base of the skull following a penetrating injury. *A,* Lateral subtraction angiogram of the left vertebral artery demonstrates an aneurysmally dilated venous structure *(straight arrow)* with filling of the paravertebral venous drainage *(curved arrow). B,* Lateral view of the superselective catheterization of the fistula *(arrow)* as it enters into the aneurysmally dilated venous sac. *C,* Right (contralateral) vertebral injection demonstrates the upper extent of the laceration in the vertebral artery *(arrow).* *D,* Right vertebral angiogram for control after balloon trapping of the left-sided fistula. Note the retrograde flow into the left vertebral artery up to the balloon site without filling of the fistula *(arrow). E,* Clinical appearance before treatment. Note the aneurysmal dilatation producing a pulsatile mass. *F,* Three weeks after treatment.

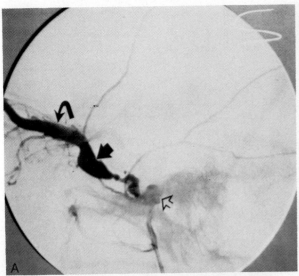

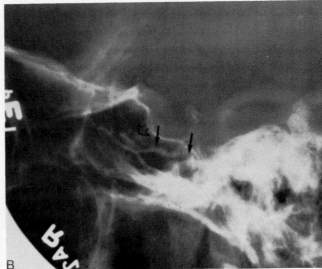

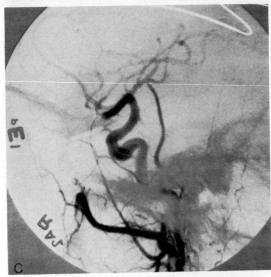

FIGURE 88-4. Fistula of the middle meningeal artery. *A,* Lateral subtraction angiogram of the superselective catheterization of the middle meningeal artery at the level of the foramen spinosum. This fills a fistula of the cavernous sinus *(open arrow)* draining into the common ophthalmic *(broad arrow)* and superior division *(curved arrow)* of the ophthalmic venous system. *B,* Lateral skull roentgenogram after embolization demonstrates the radiopaque isobutyl 2-cyanoacrylate in the cavernous sinus *(arrows)* up to the common ophthalmic vein *(open arrow). C,* Lateral subtraction angiogram of the common carotid artery after embolization. Note the preservation of all normal branches and occlusion of the fistula.

FIGURE 88-5. *A,* Arteriovenous fistula of the dorsalis pedis artery secondary to a surgically placed screw for fracture. *B,* Subtraction angiogram of the same patient after successful closure of the fistula with a liquid embolic agent placed by a percutaneous catheter.

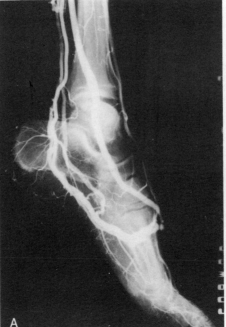

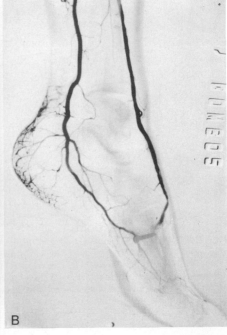

simple obliteration of the fistula without concern for the maintenance of arterial continuity may be the treatment of choice. Obliteration of the fistula may be accomplished by surgical ligation of the artery above and below the fistula. The addition of venous ligation (quadruple ligation) is of historical importance but is seldom necessary as long as the arterial component is properly performed. Failure to obliterate the artery exactly at the site of the fistula may lead to a recurrence as collateral blood flow finds its way to the fistula.

The same result may be obtained by percutaneous placement of detachable balloons or liquid embolic agents at the site of the fistula.[2–4, 25] Vessels amenable to this occlusion-obliteration technique include branches of the profunda or hypogastric artery; tibial or peroneal arteries; and subclavian, vertebral, and small branch arteries (Figs. 88–3 to 88–5). Rapid polymerizing agents, such as the cyanoacrylate tissue adhesives, are most suitable for very small vessels. These agents will polymerize in 1 to 2 seconds after contact with blood, hardening to form an occlusive cast of the artery almost instantaneously. Some type of flow control, such as an occlusive balloon catheter, may be used to prevent loss of the embolic agent into the venous circulation.[8] Whether the fistula is closed by surgery or by a percutaneous technique, it is important to be sure that the remaining collateral circulation is sufficient to maintain the distal tissues.

When major vessels are involved, sacrifice of the artery is not an option. In these cases, direct surgical repair is most often the treatment of choice. In addition to arteriography, preoperative measures include the prophylactic administration of antibiotics. At the time of surgery, catheters for monitoring central venous pressure and blood replacement are placed. Preparation should be made for harvesting saphenous vein if vascular reconstruction is anticipated.

It is generally advised that the dissection begin with the artery proximal and distal to the fistula to allow for clamping if early bleeding is encountered. With chronic fistulae, it may be necessary to dissect the proximal and distal vein as well. With recent fistulae of small caliber, such as those from catheters and needles, this may not be necessary. Heparin may be given if prolonged vascular occlusion is expected.

Once the vessels have been controlled and clamped, the repair may be as simple as separating the artery and vein and suture ligating the holes in the respective vessels. An alternative is to incise the artery opposite the fistula, repair the hole by suture ligation of the back wall of the artery, and then close the front wall by direct suture or patch angioplasty. Alternatively, the fistula may be approached through the vein. Care must be taken to avoid air emboli during these procedures.[17] More extensive injuries may require end-to-end reanastomosis of the artery, patching, or replacing segments of the artery and/or vein with interposition grafts. Saphenous vein is the preferred conduit for reconstruction. Completion angiography should be performed if any question remains about the arterial repair. The authors generally advise repair for all major veins the size of the popliteal vein or larger. Tibial-sized veins may simply be ligated. Venous repairs have a high rate of thrombosis. Heparin therapy or dextran therapy has been advised by some clinicians to try to minimize this problem. These issues are discussed in detail in the section on venous surgery (see also Chapter 17).

Finally, some arteriovenous fistulae occur in areas that are surgically inaccessible. An example of this is the carotid-cavernous fistula. In these cases, it is obviously preferable to maintain carotid artery continuity while closing the fistula. The technique that has evolved for the management of this problem is the percutaneous placement of balloons through the fistula and their detachment on the venous side of the communication (Fig. 88–6).[18, 20] This maneuver has provided excellent results, allowing the preservation of the carotid artery while closing the fistula.

The management of fistulae between large vessels, such as the aortocaval fistula, is discussed in Chapter 87.

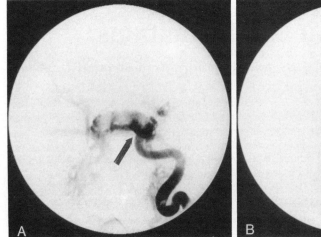 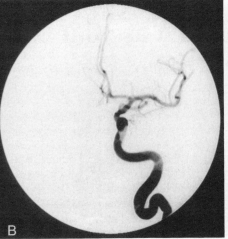 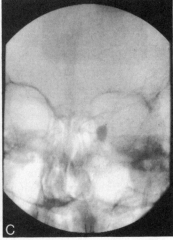

FIGURE 88–6. *A,* Lateral subtraction angiogram of the left internal carotid artery demonstrating a carotid-cavernous fistula *(arrow)* in a patient presenting with chemosis, proptosis, exophthalmos, and a bruit over the orbit. *B,* Angiogram of the same patient after placement of a balloon through the fistula into the cavernous sinus, successfully closing the fistula without losing continuity of the internal carotid artery. *C,* Radiograph of the same patient showing the balloon in the cavernous sinus. The balloon is filled with a radiopaque fluid.

Acknowledgment: The authors wish to acknowledge the earlier contributions to this text by Dr. George Johnston, Jr., particularly the historical section, which was borrowed almost verbatim from his writings in the third edition of Vascular Surgery.

References

1. Beall AC, Harrington DB, Crawford ES, et al: Surgical management of traumatic arteriovenous aneurysms. Am J Surg 106:610, 1963.
2. Berenstein A, Kricheff II: Balloon catheters for the investigation of carotid cavernous fistulas. Radiology 132(3):762, 1979.
3. Berenstein A, Scott J, Choi IS, Persky M: Percutaneous embolization of arteriovenous fistulas of the external carotid artery. AJNR 7:937, 1986.
4. Berenstein A, Kricheff II: Catheter and material selection for transarterial embolization. Technical considerations. II. Materials. Radiology 132(3):631, 1979.
5. Branham HH: Aneurysmal varix of the femoral artery and vein following a gunshot wound. Int J Surg 3:250, 1890.
6. Breschet G: Memoire sur les aneurysmes. Mem Acad R Med (Paris) 3:101, 1833.
7. Carrel A: La technique operatoire des anatomoses vasculaires et la transplantation des visceres. Lyon Med 98:859, 1902.
8. Debrun G, Lacour P, Caron JP, et al: Inflatable and released balloon techniques. Experimental in dog, application in men. Neuroradiology 9:267, 1975.
9. Dupuytren G: False aneurysm of the brachial artery and varicose aneurysm. *In* Lesions of the Vascular System, Diseases of the Rectum, and Other Surgical Complaints. Part I, Section IV. London, Sydenham Society, 1854.
10. Elkin DC, Shumacker HB Jr: Arterial aneurysms and arteriovenous fistula. *In* Elkin DC, DeBakey ME (eds): Surgery in World War II. Vascular Surgery. Washington, DC, Office of the Surgeon General, Department of the Army, 1955.
11. Foley PJ, Allen EV, Janes JM: Surgical treatment of acquired arteriovenous fistulas. Am J Surg 91:611, 1956.
12. Freeman NE, Shumacker HB Jr: Arterial aneurysms and arteriovenous fistulas. Maintenance of arterial continuity. *In* Elkin DC, DeBakey ME (eds): Surgery in World War II. Vascular Surgery. Washington, DC, Office of the Surgeon General, Department of the Army, 1955.
13. Glaser RL, McKellar D, Sher KS: Arteriovenous fistulas after cardiac catheterization. Arch Surg 124:1313, 1989.
14. Heaton LD, Hughes CW, Rosegay H, et al: Military surgical practice of the United States Army in Viet Nam. Curr Probl Surg, November, p 1, 1966.
15. Hughes CW, Jahnke EJ Jr: Surgery of traumatic arteriovenous fistulas and aneurysms. A five-year follow-up study of 215 lesions. Ann Surg 148:790, 1958.
16. Hunter W: Further observations upon a particular species of aneurysm. Med Observ Inquiries 2:390, 1762.
17. Johnson G Jr, Dart CH, Peters RM, et al: The importance of venous circulation in arteriovenous fistula. Surg Gynecol Obstet 123:995, 1966.
18. Lasjaunias P, Berenstein A: Surgical Neuroangiography. Heidelberg, Springer-Verlag, 1987, vol. II, p 175.
19. Lindenauer SM, Thompson NW, Kraft RO, et al: Late complications of traumatic arteriovenous fistulas. Surg Gynecol Obstet 129:525, 1969.
20. Matas R: Traumatic arteriovenous aneurysms of the subclavian vessels, with an analytical study of fifteen reported cases, including one operated upon. JAMA 38:103, 1902.
21. Matas R: Arteriovenous fistula of the femoral vessels (aneurysmal varix) on a level with the origin of the profunda. War injury of two years' duration. Dissection and mobilization of the femoral vessels with division and detachment of the anastomosis followed by separate lateral suture of the artery and vein, with perfect functional restoration of the circulation. Details of technic and commentaries. Surg Clin North Am 2:1165, 1922.
22. Murphy JB: Resection of arteries and veins injured in continuity, end to end suture. Med Rec 1073, 1897.
23. Norris GW: Varicose aneurysm at the bend of the arm; ligature of the artery above and below the sac; secondary hemorrhages with a return of the aneurysmal thrill on the tenth day; care. Am J Med Sci 5:27, 1843.
24. Oweida SW, Roubin GS, Smith RB III, et al: Postcatheterization vascular complications associated with percutaneous transluminal coronary angioplasty. J Vasc Surg 12:310, 1990.
25. Peters FLM, Kromhout JG, Reekers JA, et al: Treatment of solitary arteriovenous fistulas. Surgery 109:220, 1991.
26. Rich NM, Baugh JH, Hughes CW: Popliteal artery injuries in Vietnam. Am J Surg 118:531, 1969.
27. Spencer FC, Grewe RB: Management of arterial injuries in battle casualties. Ann Surg 141:304, 1955.

89

Congenital Vascular Malformations

Robert J. Rosen, M.D., Thomas S. Riles, M.D., and Alejandro Berenstein, M.D.

• • •

Although vascular malformations have been recognized as a clinical entity for more than 100 years, they continue to be a source of confusion in terms of diagnosis, classification, and treatment. It is impossible to categorize precisely every lesion encountered clinically; however, "arteriovenous lesions" can be divided into four major types: (1) true arteriovenous malformations, which are congenital anomalies; (2) predominantly venous lesions, including dysplasias and cavernous hemangiomas; (3) infantile hemangiomas, which are benign neoplasms; and (4) arteriovenous fistulae, which are usually acquired lesions and are discussed elsewhere in this section.

CONGENITAL ARTERIOVENOUS MALFORMATIONS

General Considerations

Arteriovenous malformations (AVMs) are congenital anomalies resulting from faulty development of arterial, capillary, venous, or lymphatic structures or any combination thereof. These lesions are thought to be present from birth and do not represent neoplasms.

The early work of Woollard on the embryology of the vascular system provides some insight into the developmental origin of these lesions (Fig. 89-1).[1] The vascular system in the embryo initially consists of interlacing blood spaces in the primitive mesenchyme. Subsequent differentiation involves the development of a primitive capillary network (stage 1), which is followed by a "retiform stage" in which the primitive capillaries coalesce into large plexiform structures (stage 2). The capillary endothelial cell contains all of the genetic material to create this capillary network. Through a process that is not understood, blood begins to flow through the retiform plexus from an "arterial" to a "venous" side. In the maturation phase (stage 3), the primitive elements are replaced by mature vascular stems, with the remodeling apparently being influenced by blood flow. The factors that appear to be most important in this remodeling process were first described by Thoma in 1893 and are commonly referred to as Thoma's laws:[2]

1. The caliber of blood vessels is determined by the velocity of blood flow.

2. Vessel length is determined by the pull on vessel walls from surrounding organs and tissues.

3. Vessel thickness is determined by the blood pressure within it.

4. New capillaries will form in response to increased terminal blood pressure in the region, whereas capillary size is reduced in the presence of decreased pressure.

Congenital vascular malformations are presumed to represent a focal persistence of primitive vascular elements. Depending on the stage at which this failure occurs, the abnormal communication may range from just above capillary level to large vessel (macrofistulous) communications.

Although AVMs generally occur as isolated anomalies in otherwise healthy individuals, associated abnormalities in regional skeletal structures may occur. Some of these seem to be coexistent congenital anomalies, whereas others occur in response to abnormal local blood flow (e.g., overgrowth, undergrowth, and focal gigantism). The observed association between AVMs and regional autonomic dysfunction (e.g., hyperhidrosis), as well as the common presence of café-au-lait spots, also suggests connections between abnormal vascular and neural tissue development. Finally, there is evidence that some vascular malformations, particularly the venous and lymphatic types, may develop in response to acquired vascular obstructions occurring in utero.

Vascular malformations differ from true hemangiomas

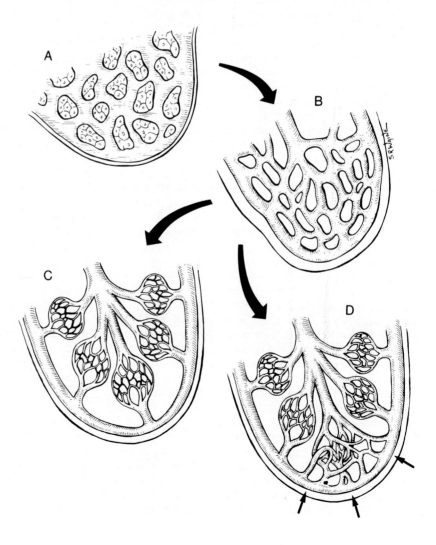

FIGURE 89-1. Stages of embryonic vascular development. *A*, Interlacing blood spaces in the primitive mesenchyme differentiate into a primitive capillary network (stage 1). *B*, Primitive capillaries coalesce into large plexiform structures (stage 2). *C*, Disappearance of primitive elements and the appearance of mature vascular stems and capillary beds (stage 3). *D*, Focal failure of the developmental sequence with the persistence of primitive vascular structures, resulting in an arteriovenous malformation (AVM).

in that they are not neoplasms. The work of Folkman,[3] Mulliken and associates,[4] and Mulliken and Glowacki[5] has shown that there is no endothelial proliferation and no cellular stroma in these lesions and that they do not show growth in tissue culture. These lesions do not exhibit the sequence of rapid proliferation followed by spontaneous involution that is characteristic of hemangiomas encountered in infancy and childhood.

In summary, congenital AVMs, like other congenital anomalies, remain incompletely understood in terms of pathogenesis. From a clinical standpoint, patients can be assured that (1) they are malformations, not neoplasms; (2) they are generally isolated anomalies; (3) they are rarely genetically transmitted; and (4) they are often stable lesions requiring no specific treatment.

Clinical Aspects

The clinical behavior of vascular malformations is quite variable. They can remain "dormant" for years, and many undoubtedly go undetected throughout life. There is no apparent sexual predominance, as there is with infantile hemangiomas.[5] Gradual enlargement of the malformation occurs in proportion to the growth of the individual. Detection may result from observation of a skin discoloration, palpation of a mass, recognition of secondary effects of the lesion on adjacent normal structures, or evaluation of complications of the malformation, such as hemorrhage, venous ulceration, or ischemia of regional tissues due to the "steal" effect. Some lesions appear to be activated by factors such as trauma or hormonal stimulation as in menarche or pregnancy. Although a history of trauma is sometimes elicited in patients with AVMs, the relationship is unclear. In the vast majority of cases, the lesion represents a traumatic arteriovenous fistula or the trauma has called attention to a preexisting congenital lesion. It appears that true congenital AVMs occasionally can be "activated" by trauma through the creation of new arteriovenous communications or the disturbance of a previously stable pattern of collateral circulation.[8] It should be emphasized that rapid expansion or apparent invasion of adjacent structures seems to be due to the enlargement of vascular channels and the recruitment of collaterals rather than to any pathologically observable proliferation of cellular elements.[5]

Vascular malformations can occur anywhere in the body, although certain anatomic sites, such as the pelvis, the extremities, and the intracranial circulation, seem to be more commonly affected. The vast majority of AVMs are isolated lesions or are at least confined to one anatomic region. Multiple lesions may be encountered in some congenital syndromes, such as Rendu-Osler-Weber syndrome. Even extensive malformations may be clinically silent if they are located in deep structures and do not cause any functional impairment. These lesions seldom cause pain and rarely bleed spontaneously, although the authors have encountered patients who presented with hemoptysis, gastrointestinal bleeding, and hematuria. Measured cardiac output may be increased, but clinically significant cardiovascular effects are uncommon, in contrast to the situation with acquired arteriovenous fistulae. The relative rarity of high-output failure is not well understood because the degree of

angiographically observed shunting in some lesions is striking. Some authors have postulated that the multiple tortuous vessels that comprise these lesions may allow peripheral resistance to be maintained despite a large total cross-sectional area of arteriovenous communication.[6] Clinically significant high-output states associated with AVMs tend to occur in two settings: lesions in infancy and extremely large (usually pelvic or intra-abdominal) lesions in adults. A lesion that is relatively asymptomatic or even silent clinically may thus require treatment because of its generalized cardiovascular effects.

AVMs that are in locations accessible to physical examination may or may not show associated pigment changes in the overlying skin. When a mass is palpable, it is usually firm, spongy, and noncompressible, except in the case of purely venous lesions. Prominent pulsations and a thrill are characteristic findings, and auscultation usually reveals a continuous or oscillating bruit. Enlarged draining veins are characteristic, and these veins may or may not be pulsatile. Over time, the increased flow and pressure in the draining veins often result in varicosities, which can be extremely troublesome. Superficial phlebitis, manifested by localized pain and tenderness and inflammatory changes in the overlying skin, may complicate the situation; thrombosed veins may also be palpable.

Extremity lesions presenting in childhood may be associated with overgrowth of bones and soft tissue, which can be extreme and disfiguring. Leg length discrepancies may not be apparent until late childhood, when limping or scoliosis is observed. Often, the limb is not only longer but larger overall; recording serial measurements may be helpful in determining the rate of growth and the need for intervention, in which timing may be critical. Pulses in the involved extremity are commonly increased in strength, and prominent draining veins may also be present. Ischemic ulcerations or areas of tissue breakdown with bleeding are sometimes seen in association with extremity lesions. This problem can be intractable and is due to both arterial ischemia (by a proximal steal through the AVM) and venous hypertension. The ulcerations and other skin changes seen in association with AVMs are strikingly similar to the chronic ulcerations seen with long-standing venous disease of the legs. The pathologic steps that occur in response to an abnormal arteriovenous communication were outlined in 1936 by Holman (Fig. 89–2).[7]

As stated, the pelvis is one of the more common anastomic sites of vascular malformations. These lesions may be asymptomatic and discovered incidentally, but they may also produce pelvic pain, pain referred to the leg, sexual dysfunction, pressure effects on pelvic organs, high-output failure, and occasionally hemorrhage. In female patients, these malformations tend to be complex, with multiple feeding arteries. Although the primary supply is generally from one or both hypogastric arteries, secondary supply is often noted from the inferior mesenteric artery, middle sacral artery, lumbar arteries, common femoral branches, and deep femoral branches. Because of their complex supply, these lesions are extremely difficult to eradicate completely, and recurrences are common. Patients must be aware of this, and symptoms must be severe enough to warrant initial intervention.

In the male patient, the authors have encountered a

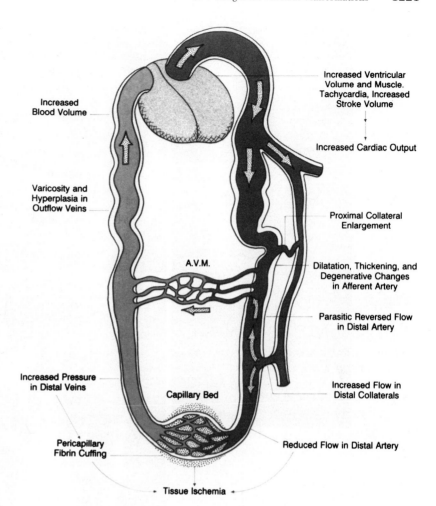

FIGURE 89–2. Pathologic steps that occur in response to an abnormal arteriovenous communication as first described by Holman (1936). (From Young AE: Arteriovenous malformations. *In* Mulliken JB, Young AE [eds]: Vascular Birthmarks, Hemangiomas and Malformations. Philadelphia, WB Saunders, 1988, p 234.)

distinctive pattern of malformation characterized by supply from only one hypogastric artery with massively dilated draining veins. The venous component of the lesion is usually the cause of symptoms, which are related to pressure on surrounding structures. Presenting complaints have commonly included pelvic pain (particularly after sexual activity), urinary outlet obstruction, and rectal pain. These lesions tend to respond to embolization much more favorably because of their simpler blood supply. In contrast to the "female type" of AVM, many of these lesions can be completely eradicated with a much lower incidence of recurrence.

Laboratory and Radiologic Findings

Routine laboratory studies in these patients are usually unrevealing. Plain radiographs generally show no abnormality but may demonstrate bone and soft tissue hypertrophy, with differences in limb length in extremity lesions presenting in childhood. Regional bone demineralization or, more rarely, bone destruction may be seen in high-flow lesions in adults. Phleboliths may be seen in lesions with a cavernous venous component.

Both computed tomography and magnetic resonance imaging are extremely helpful in delineating the true extent of these lesions.[9–11] The lesion itself and the involvement of

adjacent structures (including muscle and bone) are well demonstrated in most cases (Fig. 89–3). Magnetic resonance imaging distinguishes between high- and low-flow components. Often, these studies show the lesion to be much more extensive than expected on the basis of clinical or even angiographic findings (see Chapter 86).

Although noninvasive vascular studies have not had a major role in the diagnosis and management of congenital AVMs, abnormal findings may be encountered.[12] The feeding vessels to the malformation may show extremely high velocity flow, which is easily detected with a Doppler probe in the extremity or a duplex scan in the abdominal cavity. Decreased arterial pressures and flattened pulse volume recordings may be encountered in affected extremities. These findings may mimic those seen in arterial occlusive disease, when in fact the abnormality is due to the shunting of blood into the venous system, away from the distal tissues. Depending on the degree of shunting, the venous Doppler findings may also be altered proximal to the malformation, showing high flow and often pulsatile flow. These findings and others are described in Chapter 86.

Other types of examinations have been described that can document, semi-quantitatively, the presence of arteriovenous shunting. One technique involves measurement of increased oxygen saturation in venous blood draining a site of suspected arteriovenous shunting, and another consists of injecting radionuclide-labeled microspheres of a known

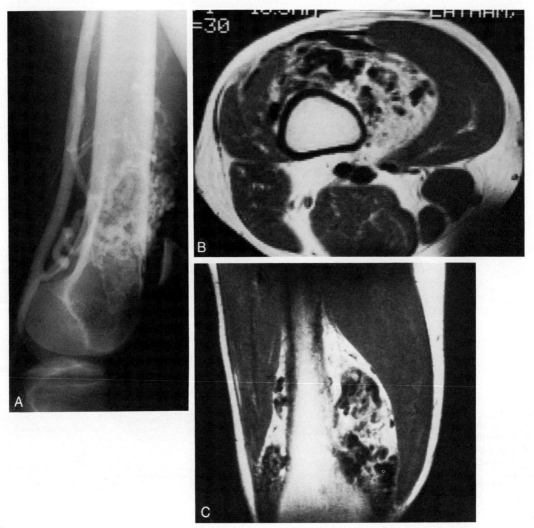

FIGURE 89–3.   AVM of the distal thigh in a 36-year-old man. *A,* Lateral view of a femoral arteriogram shows a typical AVM supplied by branches of the superficial femoral and popliteal arteries. *B* and *C,* Axial and coronal magnetic resonance images of the same AVM demonstrate the relationship of the malformation to bone and muscular structures.

size into arteries suspected of feeding an arteriovenous communication.[13] The microspheres are significantly larger than the diameter of red blood cells and would be trapped in a normal capillary bed, but they can pass through an area of abnormal arteriovenous communication. Lung scanning is performed to detect and quantify the percentage of trapped versus shunted microspheres, thus providing a quantitative estimation of the presence and degree of shunting. This is described in more detail in Chapter 86.

Any lesion of significant size that is symptomatic enough to warrant therapeutic intervention should undergo angiographic evaluation. Angiography will confirm the presence of a vascular lesion and generally (although not always) allow its differentiation from a vascular tumor. The study will demonstrate the flow characteristics of the lesion, as well as delineate feeding arteries and draining veins and their relationship to the normal circulation of the region.

Selective angiographic studies should be performed, rather than simple flush studies. A characteristic finding is marked hypertrophy and tortuosity of the feeding arteries,

which may enlarge to several times their normal diameter. The nidus, or center, of the lesion is quite variable in appearance, ranging from large tortuous channels to innumerable small vessels appearing as an intense blush. In either case, arteriovenous shunting may be rapid and massive, with almost immediate opacification of the draining veins (Fig. 89–4). In Szilagyi and coworkers' series of 82 cases, which included all types of congenital arteriovenous anomalies, 60 per cent of cases were reported to demonstrate arteriovenous communications angiographically, whereas 28 per cent were considered normal.[14] The latter group undoubtedly reflected the inclusion of predominantly venous lesions, which often show no angiographic abnormalities. In some of these cases, persistent venous staining can be demonstrated using large volumes of contrast and prolonged filming.

Extensive collateral arteries are often demonstrated, particularly when there has been previous surgical ligation or embolization (Fig. 89–5). Although collateral vessels tend to have a characteristic corkscrew appearance and do not show shunting, it may be impossible to distinguish reliably between extensive collaterals and areas of vascular malformation.

Treatment

Congenital vascular malformations present an extremely difficult therapeutic challenge. Asymptomatic or mildly symptomatic lesions do not require treatment once the nature of the mass has been confirmed. Szilagyi and associates reported no worsening of symptoms in 20 of 23 patients in whom only conservative measures were applied.[6]

Absolute indications for treatment include hemorrhage, secondary ischemic complications, and congestive heart failure from arteriovenous shunting. Relative indications include pain (often from nonhealing ulcers), functional impairment, and cosmetic deformity, including limb asymmetry associated with extremity lesions.

Hemorrhage is uncommon but may occur when the lesion is in an area subject to trauma or when there is a potential communication between the lesion and a viscus, such as the gastrointestinal tract or urinary bladder. Bleeding from a high-flow AVM may be profuse and is notoriously difficult to control surgically. In this setting, emergency ligation of feeding vessels or surgical packing when there is a closed space may be effective, if only temporarily.

Transcatheter embolization is a valuable treatment modality in this setting because control can often be obtained non-surgically and there is less likelihood of making subsequent therapy more difficult, as can occur after proximal ligation.

Ischemic complications result from the stealing of flow from normal structures. They can be manifested by pain and ulceration in extremity lesions and by neurologic symptoms when the lesion involves the central nervous system. These ischemic complications can often be significantly reduced by decreasing the magnitude of arteriovenous shunting, even if the lesion cannot be eradicated completely. Pain and ulceration may also be related to chronic venous hypertension. In this situation, the usual measures employed for chronic venous lesions (i.e., local wound care, elastic compression, elevation, and removal of specific symptomatic veins) can be used in addition to efforts to treat the underlying problem.

If treatment is required, careful planning is mandatory. A team approach is often required, involving the appropriate specialists to achieve the optimum result. The patient must be made aware of the complex nature of the problem and of the considerable uncertainties involved in treatment. Although these lesions are not neoplastic, their clinical behavior can, in some cases, be as devastating as that of any malignancy.

Patients who have symptomatic lesions judged to be resectable by careful preoperative evaluation should probably undergo surgery because complete removal provides

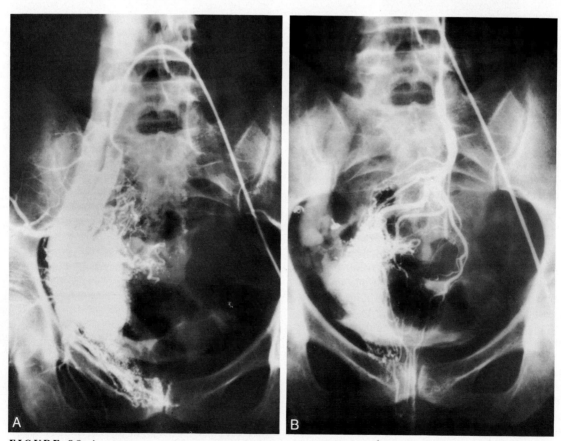

FIGURE 89–4. A 38-year-old woman with a large AVM of the right pelvis. *A*, Selective injection into the right hypogastric artery shows intense blush of the malformation, with rapid shunting into the iliac vein. *B*, Medial portion of the malformation is also supplied by branches of the inferior mesenteric artery.

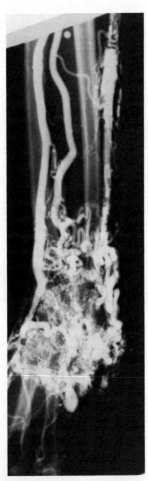

FIGURE 89–5.   Arteriogram of a 48-year-old man with AVMs of the forearm and hand. The patient underwent numerous surgical ligations and amputations. Many of the abnormal vessels demonstrated on this study are extensive collaterals that developed in response to the ligations, rather than actual areas of malformation.

the best chance for cure. This is most suitable for superficial lesions of the trunk, scalp, face, and extremities. The goal of surgery should be complete resection of the lesion. Ligation of feeding arteries is only temporarily effective, and the rapid recruitment of collateral channels makes further treatment, especially embolization, difficult or impossible (Fig. 89–6). "Surgical skeletonization" of complex lesions can be performed in some cases. This option, which consists of meticulous dissection and ligation of all branches feeding the lesion, often appears more feasible preoperatively than in the operating room. Resection of large lesions may be associated with significant blood loss. In anticipation of this possibility, provisions should be made for large-volume blood replacement. Intraoperative hypotension, autotransfusion, and proximal tourniquets have been successfully employed.[15, 16] Complete circulatory arrest, extracorporeal bypass, or both have occasionally been required. Preoperative embolization can facilitate surgical resection and reduce operative blood loss (Fig. 89–7). In such cases, embolization should be performed as near to the time of surgery as feasible in order to prevent recurrence or enlargement of collateral vessels.

Transcatheter embolization now plays a significant role in the treatment of many vascular malformations.[17–21] Advances in instrumentation and imaging that have been made since the early 1980s now routinely permit superselective catheterization to be performed with a high degree of control and safety. Numerous embolic materials have been developed, ranging from simple Gelfoam pledgets to complex systems employing microcatheters and detachable balloons.[20] Temporary occluding materials, such as Gelfoam or autologous clot, are unsuitable when embolization is being performed for long-term or definitive therapy because recanalization and recurrence are virtually guaranteed.

Permanent embolic materials include stainless steel coils, detachable balloons, polyvinyl alcohol particles (Ivalon), liquid silicone, and acrylic tissue adhesives. Some of these materials, such as coils and balloons, occlude large-caliber vessels and are equivalent to a surgical ligation. Such macrovascular occluding devices should not, in general, be used in these cases. Proximal occlusion, whether performed surgically or with embolization, may produce an impressive result initially, but recurrence can nearly always be anticipated. Recurrences after proximal ligation or embolization are extremely difficult to treat because of the recruitment of multiple new sources of blood supply to the lesion (Fig. 89–8). The authors have encountered patients in whom mildly symptomatic lesions became severely symptomatic or even life threatening because of hemorrhage or ischemia following proximal occlusion.

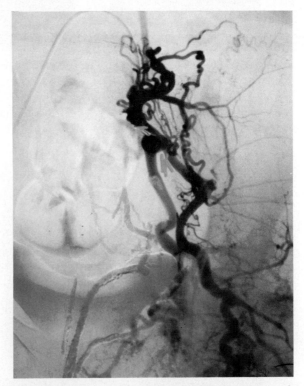

FIGURE 89–6.   A 32-year-old woman with an extensive pelvic AVM. Selective injection into the stump of the left hypogastric artery, which was ligated 3 years previously, demonstrates extensive collateral vessels bypassing the ligation and supplying the malformation. Proximal ligation nearly always results in recurrence.

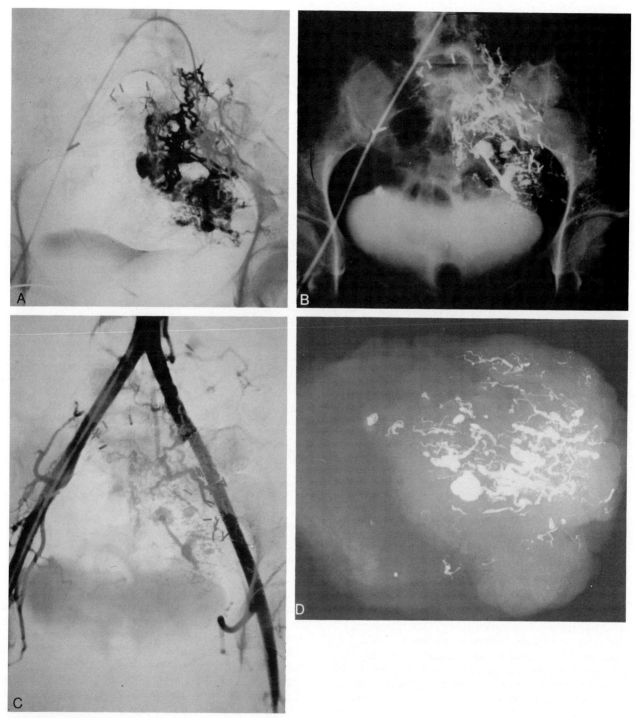

FIGURE 89–7.   A 24-year-old woman who underwent attempted resection of an extensive posterior pelvic AVM that was terminated because of extensive blood loss. *A,* Selective injection into the stump of one of the previously ligated feeders demonstrates extensive malformation. *B,* Cyanoacrylate cast of the lesion obtained using transcatheter embolization. *C,* Flush study following embolization demonstrates no filling of the malformation. *D,* Nidus of the AVM was removed en bloc with minimal blood loss following embolization. Note the radiopaque embolic material in the specimen radiograph.

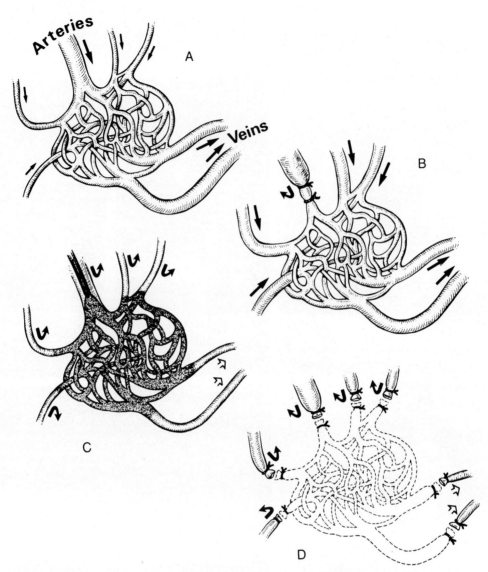

FIGURE 89–8.   Schematic representation of AVM. *A*, Typical AVM has multiple feeding arteries.
B, Proximal ligation of the major feeder results in hypertrophy of the secondary feeders and the
recruitment of new collateral vessels. *C* and *D*, Nidus of the lesion must be obliterated if lasting results
are to be achieved. This can be done by using transcatheter embolization to form a cast of the nidus
(C), by complete surgical excision *(D)*, or by using a combination of these approaches.

Transcatheter obliteration of the center of the lesion
with deeply penetrating particulate or liquid permanent embolic agents is a feasible alternative to surgery, offering the
advantages of decreased hospitalization and recovery time,
decreased morbidity, and decreased cost (Fig. 89–9). The
two agents that have provided the best results in the authors' experience are polyvinyl alcohol foam (Ivalon) particles, which are available in graded sizes from 50 to 1000
μ in diameter, and cyanoacrylate, a rapidly polymerizing
liquid tissue adhesive.

Embolization procedures for treating vascular malformations must be as carefully planned as any surgical approach to the problem. A detailed selective angiographic
examination must be performed initially to determine which
vessels supply the lesion, likely sources of collateral resup-
ply, and the routes of venous drainage. The embolization is
then performed as a separate procedure, usually under gen-

eral anesthesia. Anesthesia is commonly used because of
the length of time required for many of these complex
procedures and because of the discomfort involved in numerous selective injections of radiographic contrast material. The feeding vessels are identified, superselectively
catheterized, and embolized, with the goal of penetration
and obliteration of the lesion. Newer coaxial microcatheter
systems allow catheterization of remarkably small branches,
which aids in reaching the nidus of the lesion. Complex
lesions may require multiple staged embolization procedures because of limitations in anesthetic time and in the
volume of contrast material that can be safely administered.

Liquid agents, such as the cyanoacrylate adhesives,
can be used to form an actual cast of the nidus (see Fig.
89–8). If this can be achieved, there is much less likelihood
of collateral recruitment and recurrence of the lesion. Particulate agents, such as polyvinyl alcohol particles, can pen-

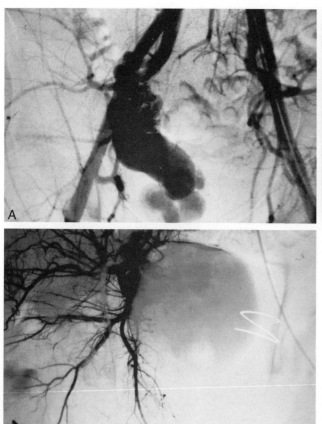

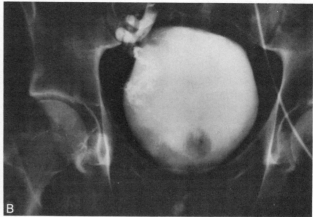

FIGURE 89–9. A 21-year-old man who presented with rectal bleeding and a pulsatile mass on rectal examination. *A,* Flush pelvic angiogram demonstrates an AVM supplied by branches of the right hypogastric artery with shunting into massively dilated pelvic veins. *B,* Radiopaque cast of the lesion after selective embolization. *C,* Postembolization angiogram shows no filling of the lesion. An angiogram obtained 5 years after embolization demonstrated no evidence of recurrence. Male pelvic AVMs appear to be simpler lesions than those found in females, with fewer feeding vessels and a better response to therapy.

etrate distally, but they incompletely occlude vessels and eventually tend to be incorporated into vessel walls. Studies performed months or years later may demonstrate what appears to be reabsorption of this "permanent" embolic material, with recurrence of the malformation. Although absolute alcohol has been injected directly into venous lesions with good results, it should be used with great caution intra-arterially because of its extreme tissue toxicity, which may result in skin or mucosal sloughing or permanent nerve damage. Nevertheless, some authors have reported good results with the intra-arterial use of ethanol for the treatment of AVMs.[22] Extremely fine particulate agents, such as Gelfoam powder, can occlude at the capillary level and produce similar complications.

Potential complications of any embolization procedure include tissue necrosis, inadvertent embolization of normal tissues, and passage of embolic materials through arteriovenous communications, resulting in pulmonary embolization. In the authors' series of 120 congenital vascular malformations outside the central nervous system treated by transcatheter embolization over a 12-year period, the overall incidence of complications was 6 per cent. Three patients had major complications, including temporary hemiparesis in two patients with thoracic lesions and intractable hematuria in a patient with an extensive pelvic malformation. In three patients, embolization of embolic materials to the lungs was documented radiographically. None of these patients demonstrated any clinical sequelae or any change in pulmonary function study results. No deaths occurred in this series.

Some of the agents currently employed have not been in clinical use long enough to completely rule out adverse long-term effects. The risks and potential benefits must be carefully weighed by the clinician and presented to the patient before any course of therapy is embarked on.

Because many therapeutic interventions produce an early response, only to be followed by recurrence, the efficacy of any given form of treatment must be judged on the basis of long-term results. For the 120 patients the authors have treated to date, adequate follow-up data are available on 108. Of these patients, 25 per cent were asymptomatic and had no radiologic evidence of residual or recurrent malformation at least 3 years after treatment. Thirty per cent were asymptomatic but showed evidence of residual or recurrent malformation clinically or on computed tomographic, magnetic resonance imaging, or angiographic studies. Another 21 per cent had significant improvement but were still symptomatic. Twenty per cent had little or no change in symptoms, and 4 per cent were more symptomatic or had different but more severe symptoms related to a complication of the procedure. Thus, it is apparent that although a significant number of patients (76 per cent in this series) can be helped, these malformations remain extremely difficult to treat and only a minority can be completely eradicated. Although it is impossible to compare results of different series directly for such a disparate group of patients, the results of embolization therapy compare favorably with those reported by Szilagyi in 18 patients treated surgically.[6] In this series, 55 per cent had improvement, 11 per cent remained the same, and 33 per cent were worse following treatment. It must be noted that the length of follow-up is significantly greater in Szilagyi's series than in the authors', a factor that may strongly influence results with a condition so prone to recurrence. Treatment must obviously be individualized, and in many cases a combination of embolization followed by surgery may provide the best long-term result.

VENOUS MALFORMATIONS

Clinical Aspects

Venous malformations represent a specific type of lesion composed of large venous spaces under low pressure, with no clinical or angiographic evidence of significant arteriovenous shunting. They may occur anywhere in the body. When close to the skin surface, they have a distinct bluish discoloration, and the overlying skin may be thinned, even to the extent that ulceration and spontaneous bleeding occur. Cavernous lesions can often be emptied by manual compression or elevation and show slow refilling when pressure is released or the lesion is placed in a dependent position.

Venous lesions are often asymptomatic, but they may be disfiguring if they are large or in an exposed area. Pain may occur with venous distention, after activity, or when the lesion is in a dependent position. Localized pain and tenderness can also result from focal areas of thrombosis within a lesion, with findings similar to those of a superficial phlebitis on physical examination.

Klippel-Trenaunay syndrome is a specific complex of congenital abnormalities affecting one or more limbs. It consists of venous anomalies, cutaneous hemangiomas (port wine stains), lymphatic abnormalities, and hypertrophy of bones and soft tissue (Fig. 89–10).[23] The venous abnormalities consist of extensive varicosities, absence or maldevelopment of the deep veins, and venous hypertension. Similar findings of venous engorgement and limb hypertrophy, as well as cutaneous pigmentation, may accompany AVMs or congenital fistulae, but demonstrable shunting is consistently absent when angiography is performed on patients with this syndrome. Some authors have postulated that congenital obstructions in the deep venous system are responsible for the findings,[24] whereas others attribute the abnormalities to microscopic arteriovenous fistulae that cannot be seen angiographically.[25] This can be documented in some cases by injecting radionuclide-labeled microspheres (see Chapter 86). When these fistulous communications are demonstrable angiographically, the condition is termed Parkes-Weber syndrome.[26] The syndrome most likely represents a mesodermal defect primarily affecting angiogenesis, with secondary changes in the bones and soft tissues.[27]

Radiologic Findings

Plain films often demonstrate phleboliths (bead-like calcifications), which are pathognomonic for venous lesions (Fig. 89–11A). These lesions are often more extensive than they appear on clinical examination, with irregular extensions into deep tissues and infiltration of muscle planes. For

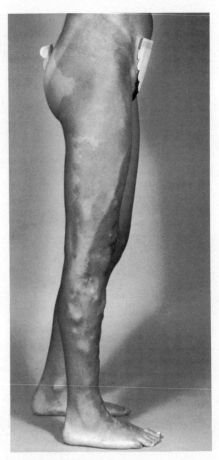

FIGURE 89–10. A 22-year-old woman with typical findings of Klippel-Trenaunay syndrome, including cutaneous hemangioma, mild limb hypertrophy, and extensive varicosities.

this reason, evaluation of their true extent often requires computed tomographic or magnetic resonance imaging studies.

Arteriography is generally unrevealing, demonstrating normal-caliber arteries and no evidence of significant shunting (see Fig. 89–11B). If high-volume injections of contrast media are performed, small "puddles" may be seen on late-phase films, representing stasis within venous spaces. This contrast staining may persist for several minutes.

A more effective method of studying these lesions is direct puncture angiography (Fig. 89–12), which is performed by entering the lesion directly with a small-caliber sheathed needle.[28] The actual skin entry is made through adjacent normal skin, with the lesion entered subcutaneously to avoid bleeding. Slow contrast injection under fluoroscopic control will show filling of irregular venous spaces, with the eventual opacification of draining veins in most cases. Because these lesions may be compartmentalized, more than one injection may be required to study the entire lesion. A small amount of a collagen suspension (Avitene) is injected through the sheath as it is withdrawn to seal the tract and prevent bleeding.

Treatment

Localized symptomatic lesions may be treated by excision, although as mentioned previously, they may be

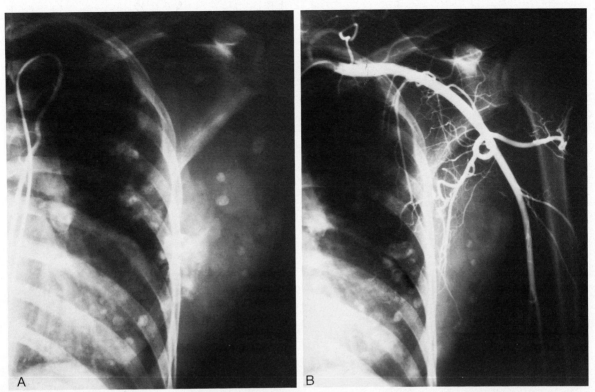

FIGURE 89-11. A 33-year-old man with an extensive venous malformation over the left chest wall. *A*, Numerous phleboliths in soft tissues are seen. These are characteristic calcifications found in venous lesions. *B*, Subclavian arteriogram shows essentially normal arterial branches with no evidence of arteriovenous shunting.

more extensive than is evident clinically. Considerable cosmetic deformity may also result from the excision.

Embolization of arterial branches supplying the lesion has been attempted, but results have been disappointing, as might be anticipated from the fact that the lesion does not contain significant arteriovenous communications. Direct puncture, as described earlier, followed by sclerosis using absolute ethanol, has been much more effective, with marked shrinkage of the lesion in many cases (see Fig. 89–12).[29]

The treatment of Klippel-Trenaunay syndrome is controversial, but most authors advocate conservative management with support stockings, epiphysiodesis in the case of marked leg length discrepancy, and vein stripping only for specific veins causing discomfort.[30] Contrast venography should be performed to evaluate the adequacy of the deep veins before any vein-stripping procedure. Extensive venous stripping often results in marked worsening of symptoms.[30] Servelle reported good clinical results after operations to repair sites of venous obstruction, which he postulates to be the primary cause of the entire syndrome.[24] The syndrome generally follows a benign but troublesome course in the majority of patients.

INFANTILE HEMANGIOMAS

General Considerations

Hemangiomas encountered in infancy and childhood, commonly called strawberry birthmarks, are vascular neo-

plasms, as opposed to congenital malformations.[5] These lesions show a 5:1 female predominance and are present at birth in 30 per cent of cases, with the remaining 70 per cent appearing in the first few months of life. Typically, they undergo a period of rapid growth in the first 6 months of life, pathologically demonstrating marked proliferation of endothelial cells. The proliferative phase is generally followed by spontaneous gradual involution, beginning at about 1 year and continuing to complete resolution by age 7 in 95 per cent of patients. The distinction between the pathology and clinical behavior of this lesion and those of true congenital vascular malformations has been emphasized in the classification of Mulliken and Glowacki (Table 89–1).[5]

Clinical Aspects and Treatment

True hemangiomas, as defined previously, appear as red or reddish-blue, flat or slightly raised lesions involving any part of the body. During the proliferative phase, endothelial proliferation is manifested clinically by rapid growth that can be not only disfiguring but also life threatening in extreme cases, owing to involvement of respiratory structures, congestive heart failure, or consumption coagulopathy (Fig. 89–13). The latter complications are particularly common in diffuse hepatic hemangiomas encountered in infancy.[31, 32]

Because spontaneous resolution occurs in the majority of cases, conservative management should be the rule. Treatment is reserved for lesions producing functional im-

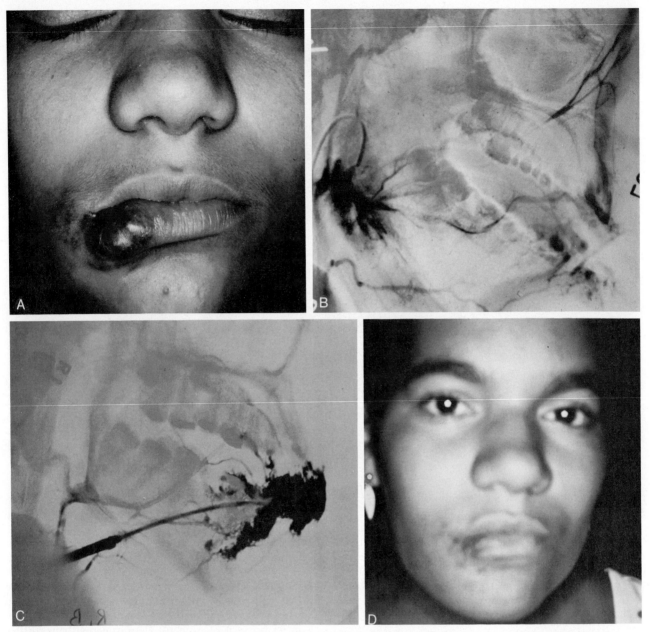

FIGURE 89–12. A 19-year-old woman with a venous malformation of the lower lip. *A*, Lesions are characteristically bluish, nonpulsatile, and soft and can be emptied by manual compression. *B*, Selective facial arteriogram shows normal-caliber arteries and minimal staining in venous spaces. *C*, Direct puncture angiogram clearly shows the extent of the lesion. Note the opacification of the small draining veins. *D*, Marked regression of the lesion following direct injections of alcohol over a 6-month period.

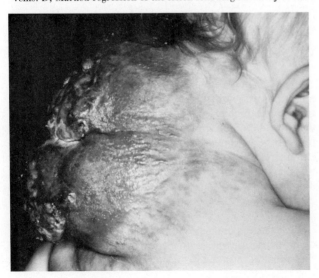

FIGURE 89–13. A 6-month-old infant with a large hemangioma in the proliferative stage.

89 / Congenital Vascular Malformations **1231**

Table 89–1. Distinguishing Features of Hemangiomas and Arteriovenous Malformations

Hemangioma	Arteriovenous Malformation
Neoplasm	Congenital anomaly
30% present at birth; remainder present in first 3 mo	90% present at birth, although many not manifest
Proliferative phase: 1st year	Female:male ratio of 1:1
Female:male ratio of 5:1	No cellular proliferation
Endothelial proliferation	No growth in tissue culture
Growth in tissue culture	No mast cells
Cellular stroma	No spontaneous involution—grow with individual
Increased mast cells	May or may not require treatment
Spontaneous involution in 95% by age 7	
No treatment required in vast majority	

Data from Mulliken JB, Glowacki J: Hemangiomas and vascular malformations in infants and children: A classification based on endothelial characteristics. Plast Reconstr Surg 69:412, 1982.

pairment or life-threatening complications. Even in these cases, the therapeutic options are extremely limited. Corticosteroid therapy and radiation therapy have been used, but neither is consistently effective.[33, 34] Transcatheter embolization has been used successfully in some patients to speed the onset of involution.[29, 35]

In all but localized lesions, surgical resection is difficult and potentially disfiguring. Surgery should be reserved for lesions producing life-threatening complications or for disfiguring lesions that fail to involute.

SUMMARY

Congenital vascular malformations include a wide range of lesions, most of which can be traced to a focal failure in the vascular development of the embryo. They must be distinguished from true hemangiomas and acquired arteriovenous fistulae.

True hemangiomas are benign neoplasms occurring in infancy. They characteristically undergo a proliferative phase followed by spontaneous involution during early childhood, so that treatment is rarely required. Acquired arteriovenous fistulae usually result from trauma and in most cases consist of simple shunts associated with high flow. They respond well to closure of the fistula, which is often necessary because of complications such as hemorrhage, high-output failure, or ischemia of regional tissues.

Congenital AVMs are complex lesions with multiple feeding arteries and draining veins that range clinically from asymptomatic to life threatening. Treatment is extremely difficult and is not indicated for asymptomatic lesions. Proximal ligation of feeding vessels, whether performed surgically or with embolization, has been shown to be ineffective at best and potentially deleterious. When treatment is indicated, it should be directed at eradicating the nidus of the lesion by surgical resection, transcatheter embolization, or a combination of the two.

Purely venous malformations, often referred to as cavernous hemangiomas, are composed of large venous spaces with slow flow. The true anatomic extent is often greater than would be expected by clinical examination. Treatment options include surgical resection and, more recently, direct injection of sclerosing agents.

References

1. Woollard HH: The development of the principal arterial stems in the forelimb of the pig. Cont Embryol 14:139, 1922.
2. Malan E: Vascular Malformations (Angiodysplasias). Milan, Carlo Erba Foundation, 1974, p 20.
3. Folkman J: Toward a new understanding of vascular proliferative disease in children. Pediatrics 74:850, 1984.
4. Mulliken JB, Zetter BR, Folkman J: In vitro characteristics of endothelium from hemangiomas and vascular malformations. Surgery 92:348, 1982.
5. Mulliken JB, Glowacki J: Hemangiomas and vascular malformations in infants and children: A classification based on endothelial characteristics. Plast Reconstr Surg 69:412, 1982.
6. Szilagyi DE, Elliott JP, DeRusso FJ, et al: Peripheral congenital arteriovenous fistulas. Surgery 57:61, 1965.
7. Holman E: Abnormal Arteriovenous Communications. 2nd ed. Springfield, IL, Charles C Thomas, 1968.
8. Lawton RC, Tidrick RT, Brintnall ES: A clinico-pathological study of multiple congenital arteriovenous fistulae of the lower extremities. Angiology 8:161, 1957.
9. Cohen JM, Weinreb JC, Redman HC: Arteriovenous malformations of the extremities: MR imaging. Radiology 158:475, 1986.
10. Rauch RF, Silverman PM, Korobkin M, et al: Computed tomography of benign angiomatous lesions of the extremities. J Comput Assist Tomogr 8(6):1143, 1984.
11. Amparo EG, Higgins CB, Hricak H: Primary diagnosis of abdominal arteriovenous fistulae by MR imaging. J Comput Assist Tomogr 8(6):1140, 1984.
12. Rutherford RB: Noninvasive testing in the diagnosis and assessment of arteriovenous fistula. *In* Berenstein EF (ed): Noninvasive Diagnostic Techniques in Vascular Disease. St. Louis, CV Mosby, 1985, pp 666–679.
13. Rhodes BA, Rutherford RB, Lopez-Majano V, et al: Arteriovenous shunt measurements in extremities. J Nucl Med 13:357, 1972.
14. Szilagyi DE, Smith RF, Elliott JP, et al: Congenital arteriovenous anomalies of the limbs. Arch Surg 111:423, 1976.
15. Trout HH, McAllister HA, Giordano JM, et al: Vascular malformations. Surgery 97:36, 1985.
16. Natali J, Jue-Denis P, Kieffer E, et al: Arteriovenous fistulae of the internal iliac vessels. J Cardiovasc Surg 25:165, 1984.
17. Kaufman SL, Kumar AAJ, Roland JA, et al: Transcatheter embolization in the management of congenital arteriovenous malformations. Radiology 137:21, 1980.
18. Palmaz JC, Newton TH, Reuter SR, et al: Particulate intraarterial embolization in pelvic arteriovenous malformations. Am J Roentgenol 137:117, 1981.
19. Gomes AS, Mali WP, Oppenheim WL: Embolization therapy in the management of congenital arteriovenous malformations. Radiology 144:41, 1982.
20. Berenstein A, Kricheff II: Catheter and material selection for transarterial embolization. II. Materials. Radiology 132:631, 1979.
21. Rosen RJ: Embolization in the treatment of arteriovenous malformations. *In* Goldberg HI, Higgins CB, Ring EJ (eds): Contemporary Imaging. San Francisco, University of California Press, 1985, p 153.
22. Yakes WF, Luethke JM, Merland JJ, et al: Ethanol embolization of arteriovenous fistulas; A primary model of therapy. J Vasc Interv Radiol 1:89, 1990.
23. Klippel M, Trenaunay P: Du naevus variqueux osteohypertrophique. Arch Gen Med (Paris) 3:611, 1900.
24. Servelle M: Klippel and Trenaunay's syndrome: 768 operated cases. Ann Surg 201:365, 1985.
25. Cotton LT, Sykes BJ: The treatment of diffuse congenital arteriovenous fistulae of the leg. Proc R Soc Med 62:245, 1969.
26. Parkes WF: Haemangiectatic hypertrophy of limbs: Congenital varicose veins. Br J Child Dis 15:31, 1918.
27. Baskerville PA, Ackroyd JS, Browse NL: The etiology of the Klippel-Trenaunay syndrome. Ann Surg 202:624, 1985.

28. Boxt LM, Levin DC, Fellows KE: Direct puncture angiography in congenital venous malformations. Am J Roentgenol 140:135, 1983.

29. Lasjaunias P, Berenstein A: Surgical Neuroangiography. Heidelberg, Springer-Verlag, 1987, vol. 2.

30. Lindenauer SM: Congenital arteriovenous fistula and the Klippel-Trenaunay syndrome. Ann Surg 174:248, 1971.

31. Crocker DW, Cleland RS: Infantile hemangioendothelioma of the liver. Pediatrics 19:596, 1957.

32. Stanley P, Gates GF, Eto RS, et al: Hepatic cavernous hemangiomas and hemangioendotheliomas in infancy. Am J Roentgenol 129:317, 1977.

33. Jackson C, Greene H, O'Neill J, et al: Hepatic hemangioendothelioma: Angiographic appearances and apparent prednisone responsiveness. Am J Dis Child 131:74, 1977.

34. Rotan M, John M, Stowe S, et al: Radiation treatment of pediatric hepatic hemangiomatosis and coexisting cardiac failure. N Engl J Med 302:852, 1980.

35. Stanley P, Grinnell VS, Stanton RE, et al: Therapeutic embolization of infantile hepatic hemangioma with polyvinyl alcohol. Am J Roentgenol 141:1047, 1983.

Angioaccess

Edited by Anthony J. Comerota, M.D.

90

Vascular Access for Hemodialysis

Timothy P. Connall, M.D., and Samuel E. Wilson, M.D.

• • •

Hemodialysis access surgery has seen enormous growth and innovation since the first practical dialysis machine was designed and implemented by Kolff in 1944.[1] At that time and for several years thereafter, vascular access for hemodialysis was achieved by surgical cutdown and placement of metal, glass, or plastic cannulas into an artery and vein. After each dialysis treatment, or at best after a few sessions, the cannulas were removed and the vessels ligated. This limited approach to circulatory access confined hemodialysis to the treatment of acute renal failure. In 1960 Quinton and colleagues designed the Teflon external arteriovenous shunt for long-term access.[2] With this shunt, the era of hemodialysis for chronic renal failure began. Six years later another breakthrough occurred when Brescia and coworkers introduced the radiocephalic fistula.[3] Indeed, the subcutaneous fistula, whether the autogenous radiocephalic type or the many prosthetic bridge fistulae that soon followed, remains the primary means of permanent hemodialysis access today.

As our ability to access the circulation has developed and dialysis techniques have improved, so have the numbers of patients requiring dialysis grown. The 1991 report of the United States Renal Data System indicates that approximately 200,000 Americans are currently being treated for end-stage renal disease (ESRD).[4] The yearly incidence of those treated nearly doubled during the last decade, and now the number of new cases of ESRD per year is over 41,000.[4] Diabetes and hypertension account for about 60 per cent of new cases (Table 90–1). Sixty per cent of ESRD patients are treated by hemodialysis, 25 per cent have a functioning renal transplant, and 9 per cent are treated with peritoneal dialysis (Fig. 90–1). Renal transplantation is the preferred treatment for many patients, but owing primarily to limited donor organ availability, there has been only modest growth in the number of transplants from 1986 to 1990 (Fig. 90–2).[4–6] Thus, the majority of patients continue to require hemodialysis as their primary renal replacement therapy. In addition to these patients, many patients without ESRD also require two-way circulatory access for the treatment of acute renal failure and for the implementation of continuous arteriovenous hemofiltration and plasmapheresis.

CENTRAL VENOUS CANNULATION

Percutaneous major vessel cannulation has largely replaced the Scribner shunt for dialysis access in the many patients in whom short-term access is needed. Venous cannulation is indicated for patients with acute renal failure requiring temporary dialysis or for those in emergency situations such as poisonings. Most patients with chronic renal failure also require percutaneous access at the initiation of dialysis; as a temporary method while waiting for maturation of a permanent hemodialysis fistula or while waiting for transplantation or peritoneal dialysis; or during complications of their primary renal replacement therapy. Further, for some patients with ESRD, percutaneous cannulation must serve as a means of long-term dialysis access because of exhausted fistula sites (Table 90–2).

Table 90–1. Etiologies of End-Stage Renal Disease

Primary Disease	Incidence (%)
Diabetes	33.1
Hypertension	28.5
Glomerulonephritis	14.9
Interstitial nephritis	3.7
Cystic kidney diseases	3.6
Obstructive nephropathy	2.5
Collagen vascular diseases	2.3
Malignancies	1.4
Other/unknown	10.0

United States Renal Data System: 1991 Annual Report. Am J Kidney Dis 18 (Suppl 2):9, 1991.

Prevalence by Modality

Per Cent of Patients Alive on December 31st by Treatment Modality. All Patients by Year, 1981-1989

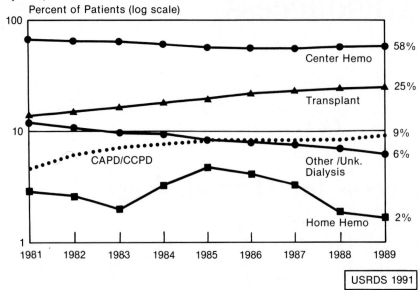

FIGURE 90-1.   Percent distribution of end-stage renal disease (ESRD) patients by treatment modality and year, 1981–1989. Logarithmic scale is used to show more detail for smaller modalities. Medicare patients only. (From United States Renal Data System: 1991 Annual Report. Am J Kidney Dis 18[Suppl 2]: 9, 1991.)

The double-lumen subclavian hemodialysis catheter introduced by Uldall and colleagues in 1980 has been subsequently refined and is now the preferred method for percutaneous access.[7] Dialysis catheters may have a side-by-side or coaxial configuration. The PermCath catheter has proximal "arterial" ports for drawing blood into the dialysis machine and distal "venous" ports for return flow, thus creating a circuit that allows conventional continuous flow hemodialysis (Fig. 90–3). With this system mean flow rates of approximately 225 ml/min and mean recirculation rates of 6.5 per cent are typically achieved.[8, 9] The catheter may be placed solely percutaneously or, if it is needed for more

than several days, a tunneled, indwelling catheter with a Dacron cuff may be placed. Indwelling catheters function on average 3 months and have been reported to continue functioning for up to 28 months.[8, 9]

The method of catheter insertion is similar to the placement of other central venous catheters. (See Chapter 92 for a complete discussion of the placement of venous catheters.) The traditional subclavian approach has the drawback of causing subclavian vein stenosis (reported to be as high as 50 per cent), which can result in venous obstruction and upper extremity edema.[10–14] Placement in the internal jugular vein has a lower incidence of associated

Transplants

Kidney Transplants by Donor Type and Patients Awaiting a Transplant, 1982–1990

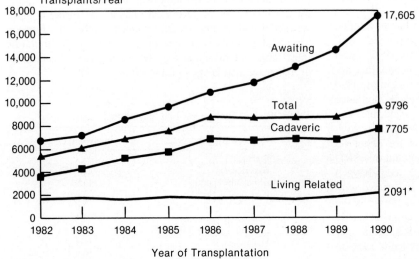

*Includes 90 living unrelated transplants.

FIGURE 90-2.   Counts of kidney transplants performed by donor type and counts of patients awaiting cadaver transplants by year, 1982–1990. Includes Medicare and non-Medicare patients. Patients awaiting transplants may be overstated owing to multiple listing. (From United States Renal Data System: 1991 Annual Report. Am J Kidney Dis 18[Suppl 2]:9, 1991.)

Table 90–2.   Indications for Percutaneous Dialysis Access

Acute renal failure
   Temporary dialysis
   Treatment of fluid overload
Emergency dialysis
   Drug overdose
   Poisoning
ESRD hemodialysis patient
   During maturation of arteriovenous fistula or graft
   Failed access
   Access revision required
   Long-term access if arteriovenous fistula sites are exhausted
Peritoneal dialysis patient
   Access during abdominal surgery
   Peritonitis
Transplant patient
   Awaiting transplant
   Recent nonfunctional transplant
   Failed transplant
Others
   Continuous arteriovenous hemofiltration
   Plasmapheresis

stenosis and is the preferred cannulation site by some surgeons, but positioning is more awkward for the patient.[10, 12] The catheter may be placed by surgical cutdown of the external or internal jugular veins or by percutaneous cannulation of the internal jugular or subclavian veins using the Seldinger technique. Ideally, under fluoroscopy, the catheter tip is positioned in the largest portion of the superior vena cava—that is, at the second intercostal space, and the proximal arterial port is positioned in the center of the superior vena cava (see Fig. 90–3). This orientation minimizes the possibility of obstruction of the arterial port by suction against the caval wall during dialysis.[9] Flow

through each lumen is tested with a syringe, and the lumina are injected with 1.5 ml of saline containing 5000 units of heparin.

Approximately 15 per cent of catheters require removal because of thrombotic or infectious complications.[8, 9] Thrombosis of the catheter lumen is the most common complication, but it can be treated successfully with urokinase or streptokinase infusion and results in catheter removal in only 3 per cent of cases.[8, 9] Likewise, subclavian vein thrombosis ipsilateral to the catheter occurs frequently, and associated catheter malfunction usually resolves with thrombolytic infusion.[8] Exit site infections present with erythema and often purulent discharge around the catheter. These infections are often treated with local care and parenteral antibiotics, leaving the catheter in place.[8, 15] Catheter-associated bacteremia, which occurs in 10 per cent of catheters, may also be treated with the catheter left in place, but a much lower success rate should be expected.[8, 9, 15] In a report by Moss and colleagues, bacteremia resolved in only 25 per cent of patients with parenteral antibiotics alone, and bacteremia never resolved in diabetic patients without catheter removal.[8] Technical complications such as pneumothorax, hemothorax, hemomediastinum, subclavian vein or superior vena cava perforation, air embolism, right atrial thrombus, and exit site hematomas account for less than 3 per cent of catheter-related complications.[8, 9, 14] Although these complications are rare, one should keep in mind that they can easily be fatal. Vanholder and associates' review of the complications of single-lumen central venous hemodialysis catheters found that of six catheter-associated fatalities, four were due to technical complications. The other two deaths were caused by bacteremia.[16]

Other methods of achieving major vessel dialysis access include single-lumen subclavian or jugular vein can-

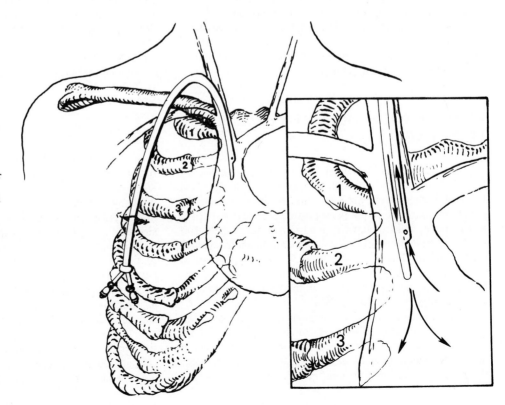

FIGURE 90–3.   The PermCath double-lumen hemodialysis catheter is inserted through the internal jugular vein. The catheter is externalized over the anterolateral chest, with an approximately 3-cm distance between the skin exit and the Dacron cuff. The inset depicts the catheter tip positioned at the second intercostal space with the proximal arterial port oriented away from the wall of the superior vena cava. Arrows denote bidirectional blood flow. (Adapted from Bour ES, Weaver AS, Yang HC, et al: Experience with the double-lumen Silastic catheter for hemoaccess. Surg Gynecol Obstet 171:33, 1990. By permission of Surgery, Gynecology and Obstetrics.)

nulation and femoral cannulation. Single-lumen subclavian vein cannulation was described by Erben and colleagues in 1969.[17] This technique requires the use of single-needle dialysis and has largely been supplanted by the double-lumen catheter. Shaldon and associates introduced femoral vein and artery cannulation in 1961 as a primary access modality for patients with chronic renal failure.[18] Later, femoral vein–vein cannulation was used. This technique requires frequent recannulation of the femoral vessels. Except for femoral artery and vein cannulation for continuous arteriovenous hemofiltration (CAVH), there are few indications for this technique today. The associated complications include the relatively high incidence of infection attendant to the groin location, bleeding, and limited mobility. Further, as with any form of femoral cannulation, this technique causes potential harm to the femoral and iliac vessels. With any of these access procedures, the surgeon should be cognizant that in the renal patient an effort should be made to preserve the integrity of the femoral and iliac vessels to facilitate potential kidney transplantation.

THE EXTERNAL ARTERIOVENOUS SHUNT

With the popularization of central venous cannulation, the external arteriovenous shunt is now seldom used. This shunt requires operation for its placement, necessitates ligation of the distal artery and vein upon its construction, and has relatively high rates of infection and failure. The Scribner arteriovenous shunt consists of curved Teflon tips for vessel cannulation, two Silastic extension tubes, and a Teflon connector for placement between the arterial and venous Silastic tubes. The shunt is typically constructed by isolation and cannulation of the radial artery and cephalic vein in the distal forearm. The resulting external shunt is then easily accessed by clamping the venous and arterial Silastic limbs, removing the Teflon connector, and attaching the dialysis machine tubing.

AUTOGENOUS ARTERIOVENOUS FISTULAE

The radiocephalic autogenous fistula, introduced by Brescia, Cimino, and colleagues in 1966, remains the best form of hemodialysis access.[3] This fistula is technically simple to construct, requires no prosthetic material, is easy to cannulate, and has superior long-term patency rates and fewer associated complications compared to the polytetrafluoroethylene (PTFE) bridge fistula.[19] The Brescia-Cimino fistula also allows preservation of proximal sites for potential secondary access procedures in the form of fistula revision or bridge fistula construction.

Judicious site selection is crucial for the construction of a successful fistula. Two frequent causes of early fistula failure are poor arterial flow secondary to arterial narrowing and calcification (usually seen in diabetic patients) and thrombosis of the forearm veins, commonly due to repeated venipunctures. To minimize these potential pitfalls a thorough examination of the arterial and venous systems of the proposed, preferably nondominant, extremity should be carried out preoperatively (Figs. 90–4 and 90–5). The Allen test is performed to determine the adequacy of ulnar blood supply to the hand, and the radial pulse is palpated. The venous network is evaluated by placing a tourniquet on the upper arm. Patency of the cephalic vein is confirmed by gentle percussion of the vein at the wrist and observation of a transmitted wave to the antecubital fossa. If the clinical examination is equivocal or poor, diagnostic studies such as sequential pressures, plethysmography, duplex scanning, and angiography may be performed.

The surgeon should be aware that subclavian vein cannulation for dialysis access leads to a high incidence (up to 50 per cent has been reported) of occult subclavian vein stenosis.[10–13, 20–22] In the presence of increased flow caused by creation of an arteriovenous shunt, the stenosis can be flow limiting and can lead to venous hypertension. To avoid this complication, before placing a permanent vascular access fistula or graft, the subclavian vein should be evaluated radiographically in patients with a history of a dialysis catheter in the ipsilateral subclavian vein.

The fistula may be constructed using local infiltration, upper extremity nerve block, or general anesthesia. Microsurgical instruments and loupes are used, and the surgeons should be seated. An oblique or longitudinal incision is made over the radial artery, just proximal to the wrist. A 5-cm length of cephalic vein is dissected free, and its tributaries are ligated. A comparable length of the radial artery is also isolated and prepared. Effective mobilization of the vein to allow easy juxtaposition of the vein to the artery is critical to prevent angulation and rotation at the anastomosis and to minimize associated fistula failure. The anastomosis may be constructed side-to-side, end-to-end, arterial end to vein side, or vein end to arterial side (Fig. 90–6). In configurations in which the arterial end is anastomosed, the possibility of arterial steal is eliminated; however, these configurations also have the lowest fistula flow. When the venous end is used, the risk of distal venous hypertension is minimized. The side-to-side fistula is the easiest to construct and has the highest flow, though the risk of associated venous hypertension is higher. The end of vein to side of radial artery is our first choice (Fig. 90–7). A fistula opening of approximately 1 cm is fashioned, and an anastomosis is made using 6–0 polypropylene suture. Before completing the anastomosis, patency is checked by passing a coronary artery dilator. On completion, a thrill should be felt over the fistula and for a moderate distance proximally. A transmitted pulse but not a thrill may indicate an outflow obstruction or clotted fistula. Approximately 3 weeks should be allowed before accessing the fistula to allow for resolution of edema, wound healing, dilation of the vein, and development of a hypertrophied muscular vein wall. If venipuncture is performed before arterialization of the vein has occurred, complications such as bleeding, hematoma, and false aneurysm are more likely to occur.

If the vessels of the distal arm are inadequate, other sites are available as secondary configurations. The basilic vein in the mid-forearm may be transposed and anastomosed end-to-side to the radial artery; the basilic vein may

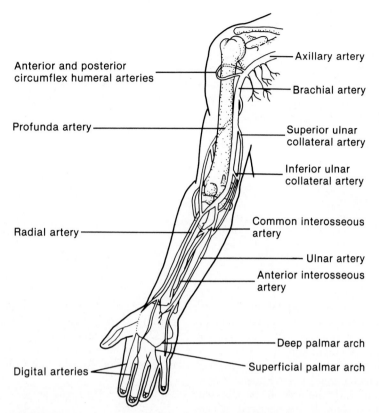

FIGURE 90–4.   Arterial anatomy of the upper extremity. (Reprinted with permission from Snell RS: Clinical Anatomy for Medical Students. 2nd ed. Boston, Little, Brown and Company, 1981, p 389.)

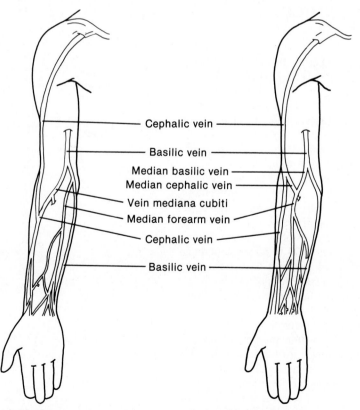

FIGURE 90–5.   Venous anatomy of the upper extremity. (From Hollinshead WH: Anatomy for Surgeons. 3rd ed. Philadelphia, Harper & Row, 1982, vol. 3, p 254.)

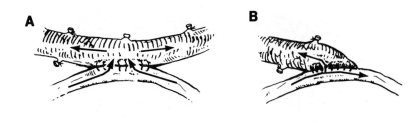

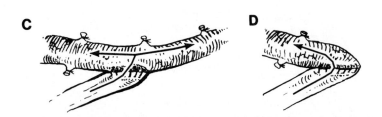

FIGURE 90-6.   Types of arteriovenous anastomoses. *A*, Side-to-side artery to vein. *B*, End of vein to side of artery. *C*, End of artery to side of vein. *D*, End of artery to end of vein. (From Fernando ON: Arteriovenous fistulas by direct anastomosis. *In* Wilson SE [ed]: Vascular Access Surgery. 2nd ed. Chicago, Year Book Medical, 1988, p 204.)

be anastomosed to the ulnar artery; and the cephalic or basilic veins may be anastomosed to the brachial artery in the antecubital fossa or upper arm. As with any vascular construction, the possibility of compromise to distal perfusion of one of these proximal fistulae (especially with use of the ulnar artery if the radial artery is inadequate or if a previous radiocephalic fistula has failed) should be assessed carefully. Should a Scribner shunt be encountered, it can easily be converted to an end-to-end arteriovenous fistula.

ARTERIOVENOUS BRIDGE FISTULAE

Even though the Brescia-Cimino fistula is the first choice for primary dialysis access, many patients require placement of an arteriovenous bridge fistula due either to a failed Brescia-Cimino fistula or to distal circulation not amenable to its construction. Early bridge fistulae were constructed with autogenous vein as the conduit. Since then, several biologic and prosthetic arterial substitutes have been used. Several studies have found that PTFE is superior to autogenous saphenous vein and bovine carotid artery heterografts with regard to patency, complication rates, and ease of revision (Fig. 90–8).[23–26] Human umbilical vein homografts have reported patency rates at 1 year of 57 per cent and 63 per cent and at 2 years of 47 per cent.[27] For PTFE fistulae 1-year patency rates of 71 to 80 per cent and 2-year patency rates of 60 to 70 per cent have been reported.[19, 28, 29] Because of its availability, ease of handling and repair, and comparatively low failure and complication rates, PTFE is widely accepted as the conduit of choice.

Although most imaginable anatomic configurations have been employed for bridge fistula placement, upper extremity configurations are preferred. Arm sites are chosen over thigh sites because of a lower incidence of infection and ischemia.[30] Also, complications such as infection, aneurysm, and ischemia are managed in the arm with less risk of limb loss, whereas the same complications involving the larger superficial femoral or common femoral arteries may be limb or life threatening. These considerations outweigh

the increased patency rates found with thigh grafts.[31] According to the proximity of the arterial and venous anastomoses, the subcutaneously placed conduit may be positioned in either a straight or looped fashion. In the experience of Rizzuti and colleagues, patency rates for

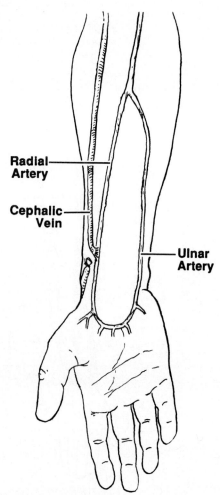

FIGURE 90-7.   The radiocephalic end-to-side arteriovenous fistula.

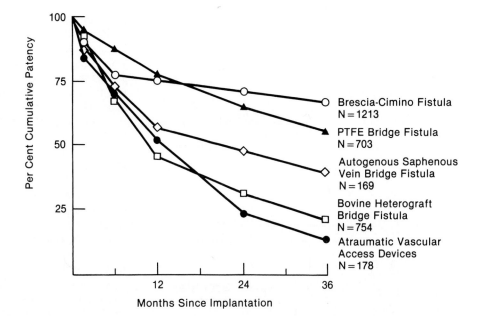

FIGURE 90–8. Meta-analysis of cumulative patency over 3 years of various vascular access devices. (From Wilson SE: Complications of vascular access procedures. *In* Wilson SE [ed]: Vascular Access Surgery. 2nd ed. Chicago, Year Book Medical, 1988, p 293.)

looped forearm grafts are 10 to 20 per cent higher compared to those for straight forearm grafts.[29] Looped grafts, however, require a counter incision for their construction, are somewhat more difficult to position accurately, and may require a secondary graft opening to pass a thrombectomy catheter for declotting.

Our first choice is the straight forearm graft from the distal radial artery to the cephalic or brachial vein in the antecubital fossa (Fig. 90–9A). This site makes use of a peripheral artery, thus minimizing serious ischemic

changes. The area is easy to prepare antiseptically and has a low infection rate. Local infiltration anesthesia can be used, and the ulnar and brachial arteries are preserved for potential proximal procedures. As described for the construction of the Brescia-Cimino fistula, physical examination of the proposed extremity is performed to evaluate the fullness of the radial pulse, the collateral ulnar blood supply to the palmar arches, and the adequacy of the antecubital veins. Diagnostic studies of the arm may be required. If the ipsilateral subclavian vein has been used for percutaneous

FIGURE 90–9. Two common upper extremity bridge fistula configurations. *A*, Distal radial artery to brachial vein. *B*, Brachial artery to cephalic vein forearm loop graft. PTFE, polytetrafluorotetraethylene.

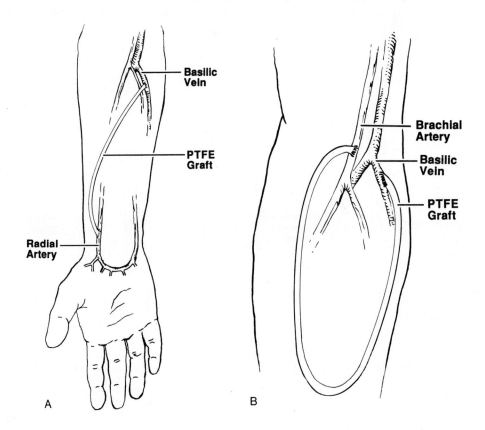

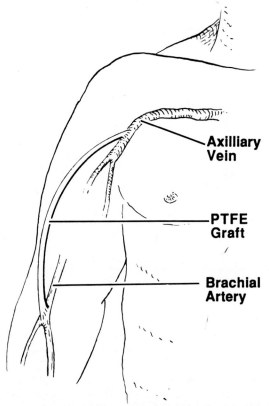

FIGURE 90–10. The brachial artery to axilliary vein bridge fistula.

diameter graft is used. The graft is anastomosed end-to-side to the radial artery, tunneled along the lateral aspect of the forearm, and then anastomosed end-to-side to the largest vein in the antecubital fossa. Other upper extremity fistulae are the brachial artery to cephalic vein forearm loop fistula and the brachial artery to axillary vein straight upper arm fistula (Figs. 90–9B and 90–10).

When upper extremity sites are unsuitable or are exhausted, the thigh may be used. Patency rates for thigh grafts are superior to those in the upper extremity because of higher fistula flow due to the larger vessels.[29, 32] Preoperative evaluation should include measurement of the ankle-brachial pressure index (ABI). If the ABI is less than 0.75 or if the patient has claudication, the risk of ischemia to the leg by means of a steal phenomenon requires further evaluation, possibly including arteriography. Our preferred configuration in the thigh is the superficial femoral artery to the saphenous vein (Fig. 90–11A). An 8-mm graft is anastomosed end-to-side to the superficial femoral artery in any location distal to the profunda femoris origin and proximal to the abductor canal. This placement is chosen so that if occlusion of the superficial femoral artery occurs, adequate collateral channels derived from the profunda may provide filling of the popliteal segment. The graft is tunneled over the lateral aspect of the thigh and anastomosed to the proximal saphenous vein. The graft may be anastomosed to the common femoral or superficial femoral veins as well. A common femoral artery to saphenous vein loop graft may also be placed (Fig. 90–11B). The risk of ischemia from arterial insufficiency, potential complications at the arterial suture line, and associated risks of limb loss make this configuration less desirable.

As peripheral sites are spent, more proximal configurations may be required. These include the axillary artery to the contralateral axillary vein, the subclavian artery to

dialysis access, ultrasonography or radiographic evaluation of potential subclavian stenosis should be performed.[10–13, 20–22] Immediately before surgery intravenous antibiotics are given.[30] A 6-mm diameter graft or a 4- to 7-mm increasing

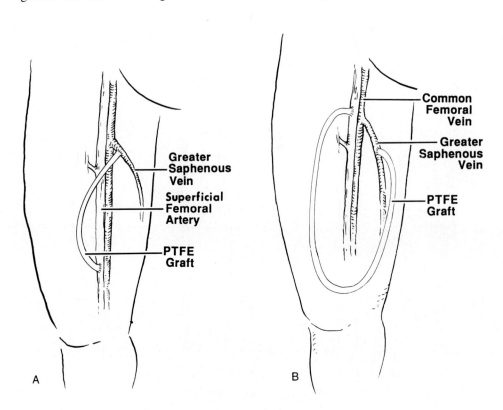

FIGURE 90–11. *A,* Superficial femoral artery to saphenous vein bridge fistula. *B,* Common femoral artery to saphenous vein loop bridge fistula.

the contralateral subclavian vein, and the brachial artery to the ipsilateral internal jugular vein.

To avoid early thrombosis care must be taken not to compress the graft with bandages. We prefer to allow 2 weeks for the graft to be incorporated in the subcutaneous tissue prior to use; however, if other sites are not available, we use the site as early as 24 hours after construction.[33] Early use carries an increased risk of perigraft hematoma and infection.[34]

COMPLICATIONS OF SURGICALLY CONSTRUCTED FISTULAE

Thrombosis

Thrombosis is the most common complication of Brescia-Cimino or bridge fistulae.[31, 35–37] Early thrombosis (thromboses occurring within 3 months of graft placement) is greater for Brescia-Cimino compared with PTFE fistulae, but long-term patency of autogenous fistulae is superior.[19, 26] Early thrombosis is typically caused by technical flaws of fistula construction, such as an inadequately sized anastomosis, twisting or kinking of the fistula or graft, or low flow secondary to compression or hypotension.[19, 26, 38] Late thrombosis of bridge fistulae is most often due to stenosis at the venous anastomosis caused by intimal hyperplasia resulting from high pressure and turbulent blood flow, and possibly to compliance mismatch at the graft-vein interface.[19, 26, 37] Late thrombosis of Brescia-Cimino fistulae is typically due to fibrosis and stenosis caused by repeated needle punctures. Arterial stenosis is the cause in 7 to 19 per cent of thrombosed grafts.[37, 39]

The thrombosed graft is first assessed by palpation and auscultation. When a strong pulse is felt at the arterial limb, thrombectomy is directed to the venous side. Radiographic evaluation may be done with Doppler ultrasound or angiography. Simple balloon thrombectomy may be effective in some patients who have early Brescia-Cimino or bridge fistula thromboses.[19, 39] If thrombectomy fails or if late thrombosis causes occlusion of the autogenous fistula, it may be necessary to proceed with construction of a bridge fistula. Thrombosed bridge fistulae may be revised by construction of a PTFE extension graft to bypass the venous runoff stenosis, revision of the venous limb with a new venous anastomosis at a proximal site, or venous endarterectomy and patch venoplasty.[19, 37, 39–42]

Thrombolytic therapy and percutaneous transluminal angioplasty (PTA) are alternative approaches. For early fistula thrombosis due to technical error these modalities have a limited role; however, recanalization rates for late thromboses treated with urokinase infusion range from 58 to 90 per cent.[37] Once recanalization is achieved, dilation of hemodynamically significant stenoses can be performed with PTA. Glanz and colleagues, in their experience with dilation of stenotic lesions in autogenous and prosthetic fistulae, report an initial success rate of 82 per cent and 1-year patency rates of 45 per cent.[42] As with surgical repair, percutaneous treatment of thromboses and stenoses typically needs to be repeated many times during the life of a fistula.[37, 41, 42] Though superior patency rates for thrombolysis and PTA are not established, the percutaneous techniques have the significant advantage of sparing proximal venous sites for fistula construction in the future. Some surgeons recommend PTA of stenoses in locations that are difficult to access surgically such as the axillary or subclavian veins.[36, 37, 42]

Indicators of poor fistula performance during dialysis, such as high recirculation rates and high venous dialysis pressures, are frequently indicative of venous stenosis. In a study by Schwab and colleagues the specificity of a venous dialysis pressure greater than 150 mmHg for detection of venous stenosis on angiography was 93 per cent, and its sensitivity was 86 per cent. This group went on to perform PTA or surgery on stenoses of greater than 50 per cent. This treatment strategy resulted in a decrease in the incidence of thrombosis and fistula replacement, per patient year on hemodialysis, of more than threefold compared with data prior to the use of these methods.[36]

Infection

Physiologic and technical factors unique to the dialysis patient account for the approximately 10 per cent acute and delayed infection rate found with PTFE grafts. Chronic renal failure patients have altered humoral and cellular immune responses, including impaired granulocyte adherence, phagocytosis, and bacteriocidal activity.[43] The skin, nose, and throat of 60 to 70 per cent of dialysis patients are colonized with *Staphylococcus aureus,* whereas carriage rates of only 10 to 14 per cent are found in control populations.[43] Natural barriers to infection of the subcutaneous tissue and blood are violated with each cannulation of the graft for dialysis, and prosthetic grafts lack the endogenous structures and functions required to resist infection.

Dialysis graft infections range from localized cellulitis to abscess formation and bacteremia. A tailored approach to management can lead to salvage of a number of infected grafts.[39, 44–46] Antibiotic therapy should be instituted in all patients with infected fistulae. Because the majority of infections are caused by *S. aureus* (followed by *S. epidermidis*), the authors use vancomycin until culture and sensitivity results can be used as a guide to more specific therapy. Localized graft infection not involving a suture line may be treated with incision, drainage, and packing with betadine-soaked gauze.[44] Alternatively, Raju has described incision and drainage and isolation of the infected segment by ligating the graft on each side of the abscess.[39] Graft continuity is then restored by constructing a PTFE bypass graft through a new subcutaneous tunnel, either immediately or after 1 to 2 weeks. In soft tissue infections resulting in chronically exposed grafts, McKenna and Leadbetter have reported fistula salvage with the use of flexor carpi ulnaris and flexor digitorum superficialis muscle flaps for graft coverage.[46]

If these approaches fail, if the entire graft is involved, or if systemic infection is too severe to delay definitive treatment, then the entire graft should be excised without delay. Before a new bridge fistula is placed a full course of antimicrobial therapy should be completed and all signs of infection should be resolved.

To minimize bacterial seeding during operation perioperative antibiotics (with activity against *Staphylococcus*) should be given, and thigh graft sites should be avoided.[30] If the patient has a history of methicillin-resistant *S. aureus* infection, vancomycin should be used for prophylaxis. To minimize subsequent seeding, scrupulous aseptic technique must be practiced by dialysis nurses and technicians in cannulating the fistula during each dialysis session.

Venous Hypertension

The high pressures achieved with venous arterialization can cause retrograde venous flow and resultant venous hypertension. Symptoms include edema, pain, discoloration, and at times venous stasis ulceration. Venography should be performed to assess potential venous stenosis at the graft site due to technical error, thrombosis, or intimal hyperplasia. If there is no stenosis requiring repair, venous hypertension can often be corrected by ligation of the arterialized venous tributary just distal to the graft anastomosis.[47]

For patients with edema throughout the upper extremity central vein stenosis should be suspected as the cause. As discussed previously, this is especially true given the wide use of subclavian vein catheters for temporary access and the attendant high thrombosis rate.[11–13] Venography reveals the causative lesion (Fig. 90–12). Resolution of venous hypertension has been achieved by local bypass to the

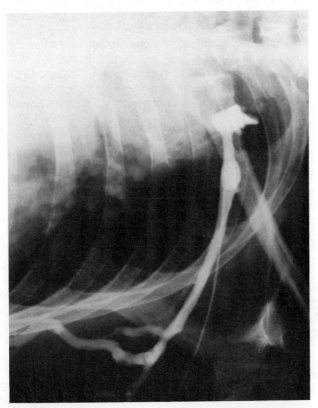

FIGURE 90–12. Venogram demonstrating complete obstruction of the left subclavian vein near its junction with the left internal jugular vein.

internal jugular vein.[20, 22] Angioplasty has also been successful in a small series of patients.[21] Many central thromboses are subclinical before fistula construction increases venous flow and pressure, and the clinical symptoms and edema quickly resolve with ligation of the arteriovenous connection.[48]

Arterial Insufficiency

Symptomatic ischemia distal to autogenous or prosthetic fistulae is reported to occur in 3 to 7 per cent of patients.[31, 49, 50] This complication can be quite debilitating and potentially limb threatening, particularly in the lower extremity.[31] Patients with arterial insufficiency or steal typically present with, pain, coldness, numbness, and, occasionally motor dysfunction of the fingers and hand. Also, ischemia may affect the median nerve, causing symptoms that mimic the carpal tunnel syndrome. Ischemia is the result of excessive shunting of arterial blood through the low-pressure fistula, reversal of flow in the artery distal to the anastomosis, and inadequate arterial collateral flow.[51] Arterial steal in a radiocephalic fistula occurs when blood from the superficial and deep palmar arches is diverted from the tissues of the hand to the hemodialysis fistula through retrograde flow in the radial artery and the ulnar collateral flow is insufficient. The diagnosis is confirmed by measuring digital and forearm blood pressures with plethysmography or Doppler techniques.[50, 51] Measurable augmentation of flow and improvement of symptoms should occur with compression of the fistula or graft.[50]

Correction of ischemia depends on reducing or eliminating shunted blood flow through the fistula. Some surgeons achieve this in the Brescia-Cimino fistula by converting the side-to-side anastomosis to an effective end-to-side anastomosis (thus eliminating reversal of flow) by ligating the radial artery just distal to the fistula. In many cases of arterial insufficiency, ligation of the artery may increase the ischemia, and in some fistula configurations, especially those using the femoral and brachial arteries, artery ligation should not be done. Attempts to salvage fistulae without ligating the artery have been made by banding the prosthesis with PTFE and narrowing the anastomosis with sutures to reduce blood flow.[50] These techniques, however, have limited utility and are not widely practiced owing to the surgeon's inability to restrict blood flow precisely.[51] In many cases, arterial insufficiency can be corrected only by removing the fistula and performing lateral arteriorrhaphy to restore antegrade arterial inflow. If a more conventional configuration is not available, construction of a bridge fistula using branches of the axillary artery, such as the subscapular and thoracodorsal arteries, has been reported without recurrence of ischemia.[51]

Neuropathy

Peripheral neuropathy has long been recognized in up to 25 per cent of hemodialysis patients.[52] Peripheral nerve entrapment (carpal tunnel syndrome) is a distinct pathologic entity that affects approximately 10 per cent of dialysis patients.[52, 53] Peripheral nerve entrapment presents with paresthesias and pain in the median or ulnar nerve distribution in the hand and fingers; these symptoms are often exacerbated during dialysis sessions.[52, 53] Thenar atrophy and motor dysfunction occur in approximately 25 per cent of patients.[52] The process is nearly always associated with either an existing dialysis fistula or a history of a long-standing fistula in the affected extremity. Reflecting the possible systemic nature of the pathologic process, many patients present with bilateral complaints, even though in some, dialysis access has been confined to one extremity.[52] In contrast to the diffuse distribution observed with peripheral neuropathy, the diagnosis of carpal tunnel syndrome is made by the clinical picture of an isolated, anatomically distributed neurologic deficit; it is confirmed by electromyography and nerve conduction studies.[52, 53]

The etiology of nerve entrapment in dialysis patients is unknown. Some patients also have peripheral neuropathy, and 11 of 46 patients reported by Gilbert and associates had radial artery steal.[52] Venous hypertension, expanded extracellular fluid volume, flexor synovitis, and deposition of amyloid have all been implicated as putative causes.[52, 53] Release of the compressed nerve by release of the transverse carpal ligament, neurolysis, and epineurotomy typically produce relief of the symptoms.[52] Intraoperative findings are typically thickening of the transverse carpal ligament, compression and narrowing of the median nerve with or without perineural edema, and fibrotic changes of the epineurium.[52]

Congestive Heart Failure

An arteriovenous fistula results in decreased peripheral resistance, and if mean arterial pressure is to remain normal, an increase in cardiac output must occur. If flow through a fistula is great, high-output heart failure may result.[54] Cardiac failure in patients with surgically constructed fistulae has occurred, but case reports (which mostly involve the Brescia-Cimino fistula) are relatively few.[54–56] It is estimated that cardiac failure occurs when at least 20 to 50 per cent of the cardiac output is shunted through a fistula.[56] In a review of Brescia-Cimino arteriovenous fistulae resulting in congestive heart failure, fistula flow ranged from 0.6 to 2.9 L/min and averaged 1.5 L/min.[56] In bridge fistulae, especially those in the upper extremity, resting flow rates range from 200 to 400 ml/min, and therefore they run little risk of producing a hemodynamically detrimental shunt. Several reviews of hemodialysis fistulae and associated complications have reported no instances of cardiac failure.[31, 34, 35, 39, 47] Many dialysis patients have risk factors, including hypertension, anemia, fluid retention, and coronary artery disease that are more likely causes of congestive heart failure. In those in whom the fistula is implicated, the Nicoladoni-Branham sign—that is, slowing of the pulse rate upon temporary occlusion of the fistula—may be elicited.[54] Cardiac output and flow studies are performed to confirm the diagnosis. Symptoms typically resolve with surgical correction of the high-flow fistula either by narrowing the fistula with a 1-cm strip of 4-mm PTFE, suture

narrowing, or revising the anastomosis, or by fistula ligation.[54, 56]

ANEURYSMS

Pseudoaneurysms of PTFE fistulae are reported to occur in 2 to 10 per cent of grafts.[28, 29, 31, 49] Pseudoaneurysm formation is most commonly due to needle punctures. Today's PTFE grafts are generally not susceptible to true aneurysm formation. Autogenous fistulae may also form pseudoaneurysms but at a lower rate than PTFE grafts.[31] Local excision and interposition of a small segment of graft or, occasionally, local suture repair of the graft defect corrects most pseudoaneurysms.

References

1. Kolff WJ, Berk HTJ, terWelle M, et al: The artificial kidney: A dialyzer with a great area. Acta Med Scand 117:121, 1944.
2. Quinton WE, Dillard DH, Scribner BH: Cannulation of blood vessels for prolonged hemodialysis. Trans Am Soc Artif Intern Organs 6:104, 1960.
3. Brescia M, Cimino J, Appel K, et al: Chronic hemodialysis using venipuncture and a surgically created arteriovenous fistula. N Engl J Med 275:1089, 1966.
4. United States Renal Data System: 1991 Annual data report. Am J Kidney Dis 18 (Suppl 2):9, 1991.
5. Suranyi MG: Current status of renal transplantation. West J Med 152:687, 1990.
6. Evans RW, Orians CE, Ascher NL: The potential supply of organ donors. JAMA 267:239, 1992.
7. Uldall PR, Woods F, Merchant N, et al: A double-lumen subclavian cannula for temporary hemodialysis access. Trans Am Soc Artif Intern Organs 26:93, 1980.
8. Moss AH, Vasilakis BS, Holley JL, et al: Use of a silicone dual-lumen catheter with a Dacron cuff as a long-term vascular access for hemodialysis patients. Am J Kidney Dis 16:211, 1990.
9. Bour ES, Weaver AS, Yang HC, et al: Experience with the double lumen Silastic catheter for hemoaccess. Surg Gynecol Obstet 171:33, 1990.
10. Schillinger F, Schillinger D, Montagnac R, et al: Post catheterisation vein stenosis in haemodialysis: Comparative angiographic study of 50 subclavian and 50 internal jugular accesses. Nephrol Dial Transplant 6:722, 1991.
11. Surratt RS, Picus D, Hicks ME, et al: The importance of preoperative evaluation of the subclavian vein in dialysis access planning. AJR 156:623, 1991.
12. Cimochowski GE, Worley E, Rutherford RE, et al: Superiority of the internal jugular over the subclavian access for temporary dialysis. Nephron 54:154, 1990.
13. Clark DD, Albina JE, Chazan JA: Subclavian vein stenosis and thrombosis: A potential serious complication in chronic hemodialysis patients. Am J Kidney Dis 15:265, 1990.
14. Fincher ME, Caruana RJ, Humphries A, et al: Right atrial thrombus formation following central venous dialysis catheter placement. Am Surg 54:652, 1988.
15. Dryden S, Samson A, Ludlam HA, et al: Infective complications associated with the use of the Quinton "Permcath" for long-term central vascular access in haemodialysis. J Hosp Infect 19:257, 1991.
16. Vanholder R, Hoenich N, Ringoir S: Morbity and mortality of central venous catheter hemodialysis: A review of 10 years' experience. Nephron 47:274, 1987.
17. Erben J, Kvansnicka J, Bastecky J, et al: Experience with routine use of subclavian vein cannulation in hemodialysis. Proc Eur Dial Transplant Assoc 6:59, 1969.
18. Shaldon S, Chiandussi L, Higgs B: Hemodialysis by percutaneous catheterization of the femoral artery and vein with regional heparinisation. Lancet 2:857, 1961.

19. Kherlakian GM, Roedersheimer LR, Arbaugh JJ, et al: Comparison of autogenous fistula versus expanded polytetrafluoroethylene graft fistula for angioaccess in hemodialysis. Am J Surg 152:238, 1986.

20. Fulks KD, Hyde GL: Jugular-axillary vein bypass for salvage of arteriovenous access. J Vasc Surg 9:169, 1989.

21. Schwab SJ, Quarles LD, Middleton JP, et al: Hemodialysis-associated subclavian vein stenosis. Kidney Int 33:1156, 1988.

22. Campistol JM, Abad C, Torras A, et al: Salvage of upper arm access graft in the presence of symptomatic subclavian vein thrombosis. Nephron 51:551, 1989.

23. Lilly L, Nighiem D, Mendez-Picon G, et al: Comparison between bovine heterograft and expanded PTFE grafts for dialysis access. Am Surg 46:694, 1980.

24. Haimov M, Burrows L, Schanzer H, et al: Experience with arterial substitutes in the construction of vascular access for hemodialysis. J Cardiovasc Surg 21:149, 1980.

25. Butler IHG, Baker JLD, Johnson JM: Vascular access for chronic hemodialysis: Polytetrafluoroethylene (PTFE) versus bovine heterograft. Am J Surg 134:791, 1977.

26. Wilson SE: Complications of vascular access procedures. *In* Wilson SE (ed): Vascular Access Surgery. 2nd ed. Chicago, Year Book, 1988, p 285.

27. Andersen RC, Ney Al, Madden MC, et al: Biologic conduits for vascular access: Saphenous veins, umbilical veins, bovine carotid arteries. *In* Sommer BG, Henry ML (eds): Vascular Access for Hemodialysis. Chicago, Pluribus Press, 1989, p 65.

28. Palder SB, Kirkman RL, Whittemore AD, et al: Vascular access for hemodialysis. Ann Surg 202:235, 1985.

29. Rizzuti RP, Hale JC, Burkart TE: Extended patency of expanded polytetrafluoroethylene grafts for vascular access using optimal configuration and revisions. Surg Gynecol Obstet 166:23, 1988.

30. Bennion RS, Hiatt JR, Williams RA, et al: A randomized, prospective study of preoperative antimicrobial prophylaxis for vascular access surgery. J Cardiovasc Surg 26:270, 1985.

31. Zibari GB, Rohr MS, Landreneau MD, et al: Complications from permanent hemodialysis vascular access. Surgery 104:681, 1988.

32. Owens ML, Stabile BE, Gahr MD, et al: Vascular grafts for hemodialysis: An evaluation of site and materials. Dial Transplant 8:521, 1979.

33. Jaffers G, Angstadt JD, Bowman JS III: Early cannulation of plasma TFE and Gore-Tex grafts for hemodialysis: A prospective randomized study. Am J Nephrol 11:369, 1991.

34. Connolly JE, Brownell DA, Levine EF, et al: Complications of renal dialysis access procedures. Arch Surg 119:1325, 1984.

35. Hill SL, Donato AT: Complications of dialysis access: A six-year study. Am J Surg 162:265, 1991.

36. Schwab SJ, Raymond JR, Saeed M, et al: Prevention of hemodialysis fistula thrombosis. Early detection of venous stenoses. Kidney Int 36:707, 1989.

37. Kumpe DA, Cohen MA: Angioplasty/thrombolytic treatment of failing and failed hemodialysis access sites: Comparison with surgical treatment. Prog Cardiovasc Dis 34:263, 1992.

38. Ryan JJ, Dennis MJS: Radiocephalic fistula in vascular access. Br J Surg 77:1321, 1990.

39. Raju S: PTFE grafts for hemodialysis access. Ann Surg 206:666, 1987.

40. Schulak JA, Lukens ML, Mayes JT: Salvage of thrombosed forearm polytetrafluoroethylene vascular access grafts by reversal of flow direction and venous bypass grafting. Am J Surg 161:485, 1991.

41. Bell DD, Rosental JJ: Arteriovenous graft life in chronic hemodialysis. A need for prolongation. Arch Surg 123:1169, 1988.

42. Glanz S, Gordon DH, Butt KMH, et al: The role of percutaneous angioplasty in the management of chronic hemodialysis fistulas. Ann Surg 206:777, 1987.

43. Buckels JAC: Management of infection in hemodialysis. *In* Wilson SE (ed): Vascular Access Surgery. 2nd ed. Chicago, Year Book, 1988, p 305.

44. Bhat DJ, Tellis VA, Kohlberg WI, et al: Management of sepsis involving expanded polytetrafluoroethylene grafts for hemodialysis access. Surgery 87:445, 1980.

45. McMullen K, Hayes D, Hussey JL, et al: Salvage of hemodialysis access in infected arteriovenous fistulas. Arch Surg 126:1303, 1991.

46. McKenna PJ, Leadbetter MG: Salvage of chronically exposed Gore-Tex vascular access grafts in the hemodialysis patient. Plast Reconstr Surg 82:1046, 1988.

47. Corry RJ, Patel NP, West JC: Surgical management of complications of vascular access for hemodialysis. Surg Gynecol Obstet 151:49, 1980.

48. McCready RA, Hyde GL, Schwartz RW, et al: Massive upper extremity edema following vascular access surgery. Ann Vasc Surg 2:75, 1988.

49. Munda R, First RF, Alexander JW, et al: Polytetrafluoroethylene graft survival in hemodialysis. JAMA 249:219, 1983.

50. Mattson WJ: Recognition and treatment of vascular steal secondary to hemodialysis prostheses. Am J Surg 154:198, 1987.

51. Jendrisak MD, Anderson CB: Vascular access in patients with arterial insufficiency. Construction of proximal bridge fistulae based on inflow from axillary branch arteries. Ann Surg 212:187, 1990.

52. Gilbert MS, Robinson A, Baez A, et al: Carpal tunnel syndrome in patients who are receiving long-term renal hemodialysis. J Bone Joint Surg [Am] 70:1145, 1988.

53. Semer NB, Goldberg NH, Cuono CB: Upper extremity entrapment neuropathy and tourniquet use in patients undergoing hemodialysis. J Hand Surg [Am] 14:897, 1989.

54. Ahearn DJ, Maher JF: Heart failure as a complication of hemodialysis arteriovenous fistula. Ann Intern Med 77:201, 1972.

55. von Bibra H, Castro L, Autenrieth G, et al: The effects of arteriovenous shunts on cardiac function in renal dialysis patients—an echocardiographic evaluation. Clin Nephrol 77:201, 1978.

56. Anderson CB, Codd JR, Graff RA, et al: Cardiac failure and upper extremity arteriovenous dialysis fistulas. Arch Intern Med 136:292, 1976.

91

Peritoneal Dialysis

Julie A. Freischlag, M.D.

• • •

The history of peritoneal dialysis dates back to 1923 when Ganter first performed peritoneal dialysis in rabbits and guinea pigs that had undergone ureteral ligation.[1] In this uremic model, peritoneal fluid exchanges lasting 2 to 4 hours were analyzed. He then treated a patient who had obstructive uropathy in a similar manner. In 1938 Rhoads used intermittent peritoneal dialysis to treat two nephrotic patients with some success.[2] Attention was then directed toward the problem of maintenance peritoneal dialysis with the observation that dialysis would need to be performed frequently in a sterile setting. Other patient problems such as dietary restrictions and nutritional supplementation were also recognized as essential for patient survival. It was not until the 1960s that peritoneal dialysis became a viable option for use in many patients.[3] By that time, catheters had been developed that could be managed over a long-term period and dialysate mixtures had become commercially available. Automated machines also were available for home use, which made peritoneal dialysis an acceptable option for patients.[4]

In 1965 Weston and Roberts reported on the use of a catheter for acute peritoneal dialysis.[5] Palmer and associates were the first to describe the concept of an indwelling peritoneal catheter in 1964 and performed intermittent peritoneal dialysis for the first time.[6] Unfortunately, inadequate dialysis due to this technique resulted, and the procedure was complicated by peritonitis. In 1968 Tenckhoff and Schecter devised and utilized a silicone catheter with two Dacron cuffs in patients who would need chronic peritoneal dialysis.[7] This catheter in a modified form is still the one most frequently used.[8-11] In 1976 Popovich and Moncrief and their associates first reported on a portable equilibrium method of peritoneal dialysis that has evolved to the present continuous ambulatory peritoneal dialysis technique used by many patients today.[12, 13] According to the National Institutes of Health (NIH) Registry Report, approximately 35,000 patients throughout the world are on peritoneal dialysis.[14] Of these, approximately 16,000, which includes 17 per cent of the patients in the United States who are on dialysis, use peritoneal dialysis as opposed to hemodialysis. The cost of peritoneal dialysis is less than that of hemodialysis and can be done at home by most patients.[15]

The peritoneum acts as a biologic membrane that is available for exchange of solutes and fluid volume.[16-18] The capillary endothelium and the endothelial basement membrane, interstitium, and mesothelium act as the surface membranes that provide the surfaces for this exchange.

Smaller molecules such as urea equilibrate in 4 hours or less, and larger ones take up to twice that amount of time.[19] Protein losses occur with peritoneal dialysis and average 6 to 12 gm/day depending on the size of the patient and the frequency of the exchanges.[20, 21] Amino acids are also lost at a rate of 2.0 to 3.5 gm/day.[22-24] Serum levels of vitamins C, B_1, B_6, and folic acid are decreased in patients on peritoneal dialysis.[25, 26] Glucose absorption from the dialysate is substantial in these patients and approaches 100 to 200 gm/day, which can lead to obesity, impaired glucose tolerance, and hypertriglyceridemia if the patient's diet is not monitored closely.[27-30]

Glucose acts as an osmotic agent that facilitates the removal of fluid through the peritoneal cavity. The pH of the dialysate needs to be acidic to prevent caramelization of the glucose.[31] The low pH of the solutions can lead to pain when the solution is instilled into the peritoneal cavity. There is also evidence that the low pH can inhibit the function of the peritoneal white blood cells and lead to peritonitis.[32] Other substances have been utilized as osmotic agents in the dialysate fluids that may prove to be better than glucose. These include amino acids,[33, 34] glycerol,[35] xylitol,[36, 37] sorbitol,[38, 39] mannitol,[40] fructose,[41, 42] dextran,[43, 44] and other glucose polymers.[45] Amino acids may be as effective as glucose in their osmotic action and may also provide better nutrition for these patients. Glycerol has a higher pH than glucose and delivers a lower caloric load to the patient; however, its osmotic action is not as good.

Intermittent peritoneal dialysis (IPD) can be used effectively in patients needing acute care but is not adequate for chronic use because malnutrition, acidosis, anemia, and poor control of the state of the patient's hydration are seen beyond the first year.[46, 47] IPD is usually offered only to patients with some residual renal function or to those who refuse other methods of peritoneal dialysis for whatever reason. IPD uses 2 to 3 liters of dialysate with peritoneal cavity dwell times of 20 to 30 minutes between drainage of the peritoneal cavity. Ten-hour sessions every other night or three sessions per week are usually performed. IPD can be done manually or by means of an automated reverse osmosis delivery system.

Continuous ambulatory peritoneal dialysis (CAPD) is a low-flow rate continuous dialysis technique that utilizes 2 liters of dialysate with peritoneal cavity dwell times of 4 to 8 hours before drainage of the peritoneal cavity.[48-56] The cycle is continuous throughout all 24 hours of the day. Continuous cycling peritoneal dialysis (CCPD) is similar to

CAPD except that most of the cycles occur at night, and there is only one diurnal cycle with a prolonged dwell time during the day using 1500 to 2000 ml of dialysate.[57, 58] CCPD patients have been shown to develop fewer peritoneal infections than CAPD patients because they need to disconnect less frequently for exchanges.

Nocturnal peritoneal dialysis (NPD) is another method whereby the cycles occur primarily during the night with 20- to 60-minute cycles continuing over 8 to 10 hours. High dialysate flows are required to maintain such exchange rates, and this type of peritoneal dialysis is best for patients with high peritoneal transfer rates and for those who cannot tolerate large peritoneal volumes due to pain or discomfort from the increased abdominal pressure.[59] Therefore, patients with abdominal leaks, hernias, bladder prolapse, low back pain, and restrictive lung disease may benefit from this form of peritoneal dialysis. Clearances of urea and creatinine are lower with NPD, and the procedure is more expensive because of the need for higher flows from the exchanger.

Tidal peritoneal dialysis (TPD) is a recently devised experimental method of peritoneal dialysis that keeps a larger reservoir of fluid in the peritoneal cavity at all times and exchanges smaller volumes.[60–62] The rationale for this type of peritoneal dialysis is that the dialysate is kept in contact with the peritoneal cavity at all times. TPD requires a special automated cycler that is modified by volume rather than by time. No real benefit from this type of peritoneal dialysis has yet been shown.

No matter which form of peritoneal dialysis is chosen, its success is determined by patient education and motivation. Training sessions are required prior to institution of peritoneal dialysis at home. Between 5 and 15 sessions may be required to reduce the threat of contamination and other technical problems.[63] Peritoneal dialysis patients can successfully undergo renal transplantation in the future without increased risk of peritonitis and graft failure.[64]

INDICATIONS

Acute Peritoneal Dialysis

Acute peritoneal dialysis is an easy procedure to perform, especially in children.[65–68] Indications include all those variables that dictate the need for acute dialysis—hyperkalemia, fluid overload, metabolic acidosis, electrolyte disorders, and congestive heart failure due to fluid overload.[69–72] Patients who have a contraindication to heparinization, which is required for hemodialysis, are ideal candidates for acute peritoneal dialysis because heparinization is not necessary. Also, patients with poor venous access can undergo acute dialysis with peritoneal dialysis. If the patient's cardiovascular status is borderline, peritoneal dialysis can be performed with fewer hemodynamic consequences than hemodialysis.[73]

Drug intoxication can also be treated with acute peritoneal dialysis. Usually hemodialysis is utilized for drug intoxication; however, if it is unavailable or is contraindicated, peritoneal dialysis can be used instead.[74, 75] The pH of the peritoneal dialysate can be altered to enhance anion diffusion. The addition of albumin can bind with the drug and prevent its absorption. Intraperitoneal administration of other reagents can facilitate their absorption through the peritoneal cavity.[76–78]

Other indications for acute peritoneal dialysis include profound hypothermia,[79–81] hypoglycemia from chronic use of oral hypoglycemic agents, poisoning, congenital lactic acidosis,[82, 83] maple sugar urine disease, urea cycle defects, severe hyperuricemia associated with gouty nephropathy,[84–86] hepatic coma, and psoriasis.[87] Intraperitoneal deferoxamine has been used to chelate aluminum.[88, 89] Acute pancreatitis can be treated with acute peritoneal dialysis,[90, 91] but the results for this indication are not very encouraging according to reviews of controlled clinical trials. The reason for these poor results is that the dialysate can irrigate only the intraperitoneal space; it cannot reach the retroperitoneal area where most of the damaging enzymes and debris from the necrotizing pancreas are located.

Chronic Peritoneal Dialysis

Indications for chronic peritoneal dialysis include end-stage renal disease in those patients who are capable and competent to manage the catheter and its machine or who have a family member who can do so for them. Children are ideal candidates for chronic peritoneal dialysis.[92–95] Children weighing less than 10 kg have very small arteries and veins, which makes creation of a hemodialysis fistula technically difficult. Patients with diabetes and congestive heart failure also do well with peritoneal dialysis.[96–98] Because heparin is not used for chronic peritoneal dialysis, patients with a contraindication to heparinization (i.e., retinal or vitreous hemorrhages) are also good candidates for peritoneal dialysis.

CONTRAINDICATIONS

Contraindications are similar for patients on either acute or chronic peritoneal dialysis. Major contraindications include recent abdominal surgery; inflammatory bowel disease; presence of a colostomy, ileostomy, or ileal conduit; extensive peritoneal fibrosis; or immunosuppression. Patients with a significant neurologic deficit, psychosis, or poor intellect or those who are not motivated should not be considered candidates for chronic peritoneal dialysis. Patients who are blind or who have crippling arthritis of the hands cannot be candidates for chronic peritoneal dialysis unless there is a family member who can help them with the procedure. Minor contraindications include severe chronic obstructive pulmonary disease, diverticulosis, polycystic kidney disease, hyperlipidemia, obesity, lumbar back disease, and protein malnutrition. Patients who need acute peritoneal dialysis immediately after surgery also may not be candidates owing to the presence of surgical drains and wounds. Previous abdominal surgery may lead to the formation of adhesions, which prevent performance of adequate dialysis. Diaphragmatic, abdominal, or inguinal hernias may become more symptomatic during peritoneal dialysis and therefore may need repair prior to peritoneal dialysis.[99–101] Severe gastroesophageal reflux can prevent the use of peritoneal dialysis in some patients.

TYPES OF PERITONEAL CATHETERS

One of the first peritoneal dialysis catheters used was a latex rubber catheter designed by Boen and colleagues in 1961.[102] Weston and Roberts devised a nylon catheter for peritoneal dialysis in 1965.[5] This acute peritoneal dialysis catheter demonstrated outflow problems in 8 to 69 per cent of patients in all series evaluated. Gutch first introduced silicone as the material of choice for use in peritoneal dialysis catheters due to its biocompatibility.[103, 104] The most frequently used peritoneal access device is the Tenckhoff catheter.[7, 8] It is a soft, nonreactive Silastic tube with multiple sideholes along the distal peritoneal portion of the tube as well as a hole in the end of the catheter. It has been shown experimentally that it is more difficult to drain the peritoneal cavity than to to fill it; therefore, during outflow the majority of the dialysate returns via the sideholes and not through the tip of the catheter. Catheters with only an endhole have a higher incidence of outflow drainage malfunction.

The Tenckhoff catheter has two Dacron cuffs that help to fix the catheter in place. The inner cuff prevents leakage around the catheter from the peritoneal cavity. Initially, the Dacron cuff initiates an inflammatory reaction around itself with formation of a fibrin clot followed by infiltration of granulocytes and fibroblasts with giant cells. Simple squamous epithelium grows around the inner cuff over time to seal the peritoneal cavity. The outer cuff is placed in the subcutaneous space where fibrous tissue ingrowth occurs, preventing bacterial growth from the skin from contaminating the catheter. Stratified squamous epithelium grows around the skin exit site as well and also helps to seal the catheter.[105] Single-cuff catheters have a lower 1-year survival rate and a higher infection rate than do the double-cuff catheters.[106] Curled-tip catheters have no clear advantage over straight-tip catheters.

Newer types of catheters have been invented but have not been shown to have a particular advantage over the Tenckhoff catheter. Twardowski and coworkers have described a Swan-Neck catheter, which is similar to the Tenckhoff catheter except that the subcutaneous portion of the catheter is formed with a sharp arc as in the neck of a swan.[107, 108] The subcutaneous tunnel is made at such an angle, and the catheter retains that shape. It was thought that such a configuration might prevent tunnel infections; however, no such improvement has yet been documented. A polytetrafluoroethylene catheter has been tried but had an increased number of tunnel infections compared with the Tenckhoff catheter. A polyurethane catheter (Corpak catheter) designed by Thermedics has an inner catheter diameter that is 1.5 times that of the Tenckhoff catheter.[109] Good tissue ingrowth has been shown with the polyurethane catheter. Polyurethrane may possess more strength than the Silastic catheter and may remain patent longer and be more resistant to infection. Silicone catheters become impregnated with a protein biofilm that inhibits the white blood cell function of engulfing bacteria that migrate along the catheter.[110] This process may lead to more catheter infections and is not seen in polyurethrane catheters.

The Goldberg catheter has a saline fluid-filled balloon, which was devised to keep the catheter in position in the lower abdomen.[111] It has shown no real advantage in preventing catheter migration, however. The Toronto Western Hospital has promoted the use of a catheter that has two silicone discs perpendicular to the catheter tube that were devised to hold the catheter in place.[112] A 10 per cent outflow failure due to obstruction from either bowel or omentum has been shown despite the presence of these silicone discs. Another new type of catheter is the Lifecath catheter, which has an intraperitoneal silicone disc placed just under the abdominal wall in the peritoneal cavity.[113] This catheter shows a 6 per cent outflow failure rate owing to obstruction because the omentum can still attach itself to the disc even though it has a large peripheral port. The half-life of this catheter may be a bit longer than that of the Tenckhoff catheter because it is associated with less migration and infection; however, increased leakage has been reported.[114]

PERITONEAL CATHETER PLACEMENT

Acute peritoneal dialysis catheters can be placed percutaneously, a method that is more efficient and less expensive. Most physicians choose to place the catheter at McBurney's point or on the left side of the abdomen just opposite McBurney's point. A Foley catheter should be placed prior to insertion of the dialysis catheter if the patient still makes urine. An enema can be used prior to placement of the catheter to decompress the colon. Antibiotics should be given prior to insertion as well as for prophylaxis. Xylocaine is infiltrated in the skin, and intravenous sedation can be used for patient comfort. A stylet or guidewire is used to advance the catheter into the peritoneal cavity.[115]

Chronic peritoneal dialysis catheters should be inserted in the operating room for maximal patient comfort and sterility. Local, regional, or general anesthesia can be utilized depending on the patient. General anesthesia is preferred in children because relaxation of the abdominal musculature facilitates placement of the catheter. Chronic peritoneal catheters may be inserted with a closed technique using a trocar. The preferred method, however, is an open operative technique, which allows direct vision for positioning the catheter and viewing the contents of the peritoneal cavity. Preoperatively, the patient fasts from midnight the night before, and an enema is given. Systemic antibiotic prophylaxis with a broad-spectrum antimicrobial agent is also given. A cephalosporin or vancomycin is suitable for such prophylaxis because these drugs have antistaphylococcal coverage.

Many types of incisions have been used for insertion of peritoneal dialysis catheters including the paramedian, midline below the umbilicus, and transverse incision in either lower quadrant. The method preferred by the author is a small longitudinal incision placed below the umbilicus, which allows excellent exposure. This incision is carried down through the anterior rectus fascia, and the muscle is then split bluntly to expose the peritoneum. The peritoneum is grasped between clamps and lifted, and a scalpel is used to incise it, allowing access to the peritoneal cavity. Care must be taken if there are adhesions to the parietal peritoneum from previous procedures. Some surgeons recommend omentectomy to prevent later envelopment of the catheter by the omentum, which would lead to catheter occlusion. This is not routinely done by the author.

The catheter is introduced through the peritoneal opening and directed toward the pelvis because this is the most dependent area of the peritoneal cavity in both the upright and supine positions. A guidewire placed through the lumen of the catheter may help facilitate placement of the catheter. A nonabsorbable suture is placed on the internal aspect of the anterior abdominal wall and tied loosely around the catheter to secure it in place in the pelvis. A pursestring suture is placed to secure the edges of the peritoneal opening to the first Dacron cuff. This ensures a watertight closure so that peritoneal dialysis can be started early in the postoperative period. This suture is reinforced with a second pursestring suture that incorporates the transversalis fascia around the cuff to further strengthen the seal. A nonabsorbable suture such as prolene is used.

The catheter exit site is chosen preoperatively and is positioned below the belt line for patient comfort. The catheter should be positioned through the rectus muscle to prevent migration later. A small stab incision is made in the skin, and either a long clamp or a tunneling device is used to create a tunnel in the subcutaneous plane that is brought out medially through the midline incision.[116] The catheter is advanced through the tunnel and is positioned so that the second Dacron cuff lies at least 2 cm from the skin exit opening in the subcutaneous space. No suture is placed at the exit site because that can create an inflammatory reaction and may lead to infection. Irrigation of the catheter with heparinized saline documents patency of the catheter at the time of the operation, flushes out any debris or blood clots, and ensures that there is no leakage from around the first cuff. The fluid instilled should drain out of the abdominal cavity spontaneously with gravity only.

The rectus fascia is closed using interrupted 2–0 or 0 nonabsorbable sutures, and the skin is closed using 3–0 nylon sutures or skin staples. The catheter is connected to a bag of dialysate in the operating room, and peritoneal dialysis is begun with a small volume. The fluid should flow freely, and there should be no demonstrable leaks. A sterile gauze dressing is placed over the midline wound, and a clear, semi-permeable dressing such as Opsite is placed over the catheter exit site. If peritoneal dialysis does not need to be started for a period of time, daily flushes of the catheter should be performed in a sterile manner to maintain patency of the catheter. If peritoneal dialysis needs to begin immediately, small volumes should be exchanged at frequent intervals with the patient in a supine and inactive position to prevent leakage from the wounds. The patient should not lift anything weighing more than 30 pounds for 2 weeks so that proper healing can take place.

Another method of placement of the peritoneal dialysis catheter that has been used by some surgeons involves the use of peritoneoscopy.[117, 118] This procedure permits documentation of good peritoneal catheter placement using the closed trocar technique. By placing a scope through a separate stab incision, exact placement of the catheter can be ensured. The first cuff can be placed at the level of the peritoneum using this technique. The only disadvantage is that the inner cuff cannot be sutured securely in place to prevent leakage of fluid and later migration. However, only a small stab incision needs to be made instead of a larger incision as in the open technique, and this may be a key factor in preventing those complications.

COMPLICATIONS OF PERITONEAL DIALYSIS

Interestingly, there has been no change in the incidence of early and late complications following Tenckhoff catheter placement since 1977. During the first months following Tenckhoff catheter placement, the major complication is that of outflow failure, which in reported series occurs in 1 to 20 per cent of cases.[119] Rarely, early catheter infections occur. During the first month, outflow failure is due to malposition of the catheter if it develops during the first few days postoperatively and is due to obstruction of the catheter sideholes by the omentum if it occurs in the first few weeks after placement. If there are inflow problems as well, there may be a kink or clot in the catheter. Inflow pain may also indicate poor positioning of the catheter. If a change in dialysate composition to increase pH by adding sodium bicarbonate does not relieve the pain experienced when the infusion of dialysate is begun, one must suspect that the catheter is pushing against some portion of the abdominal cavity and its contents, thus causing discomfort. This usually occurs when the catheter becomes dislodged and shifts into a poor position, most commonly under the diaphragm. Using radiographic dye to delineate the problem can be helpful, but in most cases, especially if the obstruction occurs early in the postoperative period, the catheter must be repositioned surgically.

Outflow failure is also the leading cause of catheter failure after 1 month. The incidence ranges from 5 to 20 per cent. If the catheter itself is obstructed, streptokinase or urokinase can be instilled into the catheter to dissolve the fibrin clot.[120, 121] If successful, heparin should be used in the dialysate for the next few days to ensure patency of the catheter.[122] Peritoneoscopy can be helpful to document whether outflow failure is due to bowel or omentum obstructing the catheter's sideholes. During peritoneoscopy, therapeutic manipulation of the abdominal contents may release the obstruction of the catheter. In most cases, however, reexploration is required to alleviate the obstruction. Repositioning under fluoroscopy can be attempted but is not usually successful unless the catheter was recently placed.

Intraperitoneal bleeding can occur immediately following placement of the catheter. The most common sites from which the blood originates are small visceral or abdominal wall vessels. If the hematocrit of the effluent is less than 2 per cent or if the red blood cell count is less than $60,000/cm^3$, the bleeding is insignificant and can be watched expectantly with good results. Heparin (1000 U/2 L dialysate) should be added while the effluent remains bloody to prevent clotting of the catheter.[123] If bleeding is noted more than 1 month after placement of the peritoneal dialysis catheter, one must suspect other causes of such bleeding. These include inflammation, which may lead to peritonitis; perforation of a viscus; or IgA glomerulonephritis, which often occurs in association with upper respiratory tract infections. Bleeding may also be seen in female patients secondary to endometriosis or at the time of a normal menstrual period.[124, 125] Diagnostic evaluation should be performed to determine the cause of late bleeding associated with peritoneal dialysis catheters.[126]

Leakage of dialysate from around the catheter exit site or from the midline wound can occur immediately after the operation.[127] Leakage may be manifested by edema in the abdominal wall, legs, or scrotum.[128] Leakage usually occurs because the volume of dialysate is too large. By decreasing the amount of dialysate and increasing the number of exchanges, the leak can be allowed to seal itself without reoperation. Only if the inner Dacron cuff has been extruded from its original position will the pericatheter leak not seal with conservative management.

Pericatheter hernias may occur during the course of peritoneal dialysis.[129–131] These occur more frequently in older patients, multiparous women, and patients who experienced leakage from the abdominal wound immediately postoperatively. Most of these pericatheter hernias need to be repaired surgically. Other preexisting hernias may become enlarged during peritoneal dialysis because of the increased intra-abdominal pressure and volume.[132] These include inguinal hernias (especially if there is a patent processus vaginalis), umbilical hernias, and surgical incisional hernias. Acute hydrothorax on either the left or right side can occur early in the course of peritoneal dialysis if the pleuroperitoneal communication is still patent.[133, 134] In children, an asymptomatic Bochdalek or Morgagni hernia may also be revealed after peritoneal dialysis has begun.

Other symptoms that might be experienced owing to the increased intra-abdominal pressure of peritoneal dialysis include delayed gastric emptying, which may lead to gastroesophageal reflux.[135] Patients with impaired pulmonary function may worsen when the peritoneal cavity is filled with dialysate fluid.[136] Cardiac output and stroke volume in patients on peritoneal dialysis are decreased owing to the decreased preload that results from compression of the inferior vena cava. In patients with marginal cardiac status, this could pose a problem. Decreasing the volume of dialysate can help to lessen the patient's symptoms.

Metabolic complications can occur in patients on peritoneal dialysis. These include dehydration, which can be treated by decreasing the osmolarity of the dialysate, and overhydration which can be treated by decreasing the dwell time and increasing the dialysate glucose concentration. Severe hyperglycemia and a hyperosmolar state can occur in peritoneal dialysis patients who are diabetic.[28, 137] Protein malnutrition can occur owing to the daily obligatory losses of protein and amino acids through the dialysis process.[18, 20] Malnutrition can be treated with diet supplements, but if it is refractory to that treatment, peritoneal dialysis may have to be terminated. The increased caloric load resulting from glucose absorption can result in obesity, uncontrolled hyperglycemia, or hypertriglyceridemia in some patients.[30] Changing to an osmotic agent other than glucose may help, but often peritoneal dialysis must be stopped. Important vitamins that are depleted can be replenished through dietary supplements.[25, 26] Renal osteodystrophy may be seen in

those patients on peritoneal dialysis.[138, 139] Both osteitis fibrosis and osteomalacia are seen. Other metabolic alterations such as hyponatremia, hypernatremia, hypokalemia, and hyperkalemia can be avoided with appropriate changes in dialysate mixtures.[140]

The disequilibrium syndrome has also been described in patients on peritoneal dialysis and is characterized by headaches, nausea, vomiting, hypertension, seizures, and, rarely, coma, which is associated with cerebral edema.[141] This syndrome is thought to develop when a rapid osmotic gradient is created between the brain and the extracellular compartment owing to delay in the removal of urea across the blood–brain barrier. Treatment of this syndrome is symptomatic; the syndrome can be avoided by decreasing the osmolality of the dialysate.

Visceral perforation may be seen early and late in the course of patients on peritoneal dialysis.[142, 143] The catheter may penetrate the hollow viscera, solid organs, and the pelvic wall as well as the retroperitoneal space.[144] Visceral perforation can be detected by the presence of feculent effluent from the catheter, diarrhea following dialysate infusion, high volumes of urine following dialysate infusion, bloody effluent from the catheter, retention of dialysate after infusion, or the presence of a polymicrobial peritonitis with a predominance of enteric organisms in culture. Visceral perforation needs to be addressed surgically, and most often the catheter must be removed to allow the peritonitis to clear.[145]

Peritonitis

Infectious complications of the catheter are frequent and lead to catheter failure in 5 to 20 per cent of catheters placed.[146, 147] Data collected from the NIH National Registry documented 4.6 episodes of infection per year per patient in 1978 and 1.7 episodes in 1982.[14] The 12-month period risk rate of infection in peritoneal dialysis patients is 65 per cent.[148] The most common catheter infections include exit site infections, deep cuff infections, and unresolving peritonitis.[149, 150] It is estimated that one third of hospitalizations of patients on peritoneal dialysis are due to peritonitis.[129] The reason why most patients stop using peritoneal dialysis is frequent recurrent peritonitis, which occurs in 25 to 60 per cent of cases.[151, 152] It is also estimated that 15 per cent of deaths of patients on continuous ambulatory peritoneal dialysis are due to peritonitis.[137] These infections are common because the catheter itself provides a direct route for contamination of the peritoneal cavity. The infused dialysate dilutes the concentrations of opsonins (IgG and C_3) and peritoneal macrophages, which are needed to fight intra-abdominal infections.[153] The fluid within the abdominal cavity impairs the ability to localize infection by the omentum. Phagocytic and bactericidal white blood cell activity is also diminished by the hypertonicity and acidic nature of the dialysate.[154, 155]

Peritonitis most commonly is manifested by the presence of a cloudy effluent accompanied by abdominal discomfort.[156] The white blood cell count of the effluent increases to over 100 white blood cells/cm³.[157] Monocytes are normally the predominant cell, accounting for 70 per cent of white blood cells. With peritonitis, the majority of white blood cells (more than of 50 per cent) retrieved from the peritoneal cavity are neutrophils.[158] Some patients experience nausea and vomiting (27 per cent), rebound tenderness (40 per cent), fever (27 per cent), and peripheral leukocytosis (23 per cent).[148]

The pathogen often can be cultured from the catheter fluid, which directs appropriate antibiotic therapy.[116] The pathogens most commonly responsible for catheter-related peritonitis are coagulase-negative *Staphylococcus* (55 to 80 per cent) and *S. aureus* (17 to 30 per cent).[160, 161] Fungus can also cause peritonitis in these patients.[162–166] These contaminants originate from the patient's own skin flora, nasal flora, catheter exit site colonization, and sometimes from transmural contamination from the bowel. As mentioned previously, a perforated viscus can present with signs and symptoms of peritonitis. Cultures obtained from patients with a perforated viscus reveal a polymicrobial flora with a predominance of enteric organisms rather than staphylococcal organisms.

Peritonitis due to one predominant organism and not associated with a perforated viscus can be treated initially with antimicrobial therapy, which can be instilled through the peritoneal catheter itself.[167] Eradication of the organisms, as proved by culture and resolution of the patient's symptoms, should be apparent in 3 to 5 days. Organisms that produce slime, which is an amorphous glycocalyx that can adhere to plastic surfaces, may make eradication of these substances more difficult.[168] The slime protects the bacteria from opsonization owing to the fluid environment and prevents white blood cells from engulfing the bacteria. Organisms that produce slime include coagulase-negative *Staphylococcus, S. aureus, Candida albicans,* and *Pseudomonas aeruginosa.*[169]

The majority of patients with peritonitis can be treated initially at home. Hospitalization is reserved for those patients with gram-negative infections, anaerobic infections, *Pseudomonas* infections, fungal infections, or toxic symptoms. Antimicrobial therapy should be selected to treat the offending organism cultured from the peritoneal cavity.[170] Initially, antibiotic coverage should be a cephalosporin plus an aminoglycoside or vancomycin. If the peritonitis does not resolve, the catheter may need to be removed. If recurrent episodes of peritonitis occur, the catheter may have to be removed because the catheter itself may be harboring the organisms causing the peritonitis.

Catheter tunnel infections may lead to peritonitis, or they can exist as localized infections confined to the catheter alone. It is estimated that patients on peritoneal dialysis experience one tunnel infection episode for every 16 patient months on peritoneal dialysis.[147] An increased number of tunnel infections are associated with inadequate surgical technique, poor catheter maintenance, exit site skin irritation from tape and dressings, and undue tension placed on the catheter causing protrusion of the outer Dacron cuff. If the exit site and the tract are erythematous but not purulent, the tunnel infection can be treated with local measures such as cleansing with hydrogen peroxide or Betadine.[171, 172] Topical antibiotic ointment as well as systemic antibiotics can be used. If there is frank purulence, however, it is very difficult to eradicate the tunnel infection. Removal of the outer Dacron cuff has been advocated by some to help cure the tunnel infection, but that is rarely successful.[173–175]

After placement of the Tenckhoff catheter, the peritoneum becomes thickened in some patients, leading to a loss of ultrafiltration capacity.[176] Inclusion collections of silicone and aluminum have been found within the peritoneal membrane as well.[177] Peripheral eosinophilia may be seen in the first few days after catheter placement, and in some patients eosinophilic peritonitis can occur.[178–180] The pathophysiology of the eosinophilic peritonitis is unknown but has been linked to exposure of the peritoneal cavity to the talc found in surgical gloves, air exposure alone, peritoneal administration of antibiotics, or perhaps an allergic response to the silicone or aluminum polymers that are deposited in the peritoneum over time.[181, 182] No treatment is needed for eosinophilic peritonitis.

Peritoneal membrane dysfunction may occur and is characterized by increased peritoneal permeability, which results in rapid absorption of the dialysate. This alters the osmotic gradient that is needed for adequate dialysis. The transport of solutes remains the same, but transfer of water does not occur. This phenomenon may result from the use of acetate in the dialysate solutions.[183] Treatment includes the use of shorter dwell times with higher flow rates and elimination of long diurnal dwell times.

Peritoneal sclerosis can occur and can lead to abandonment of peritoneal dialysis in these patients because of the inability to achieve adequate dialysis.[184–189] A thickened peritoneal scar develops and envelops the intra-abdominal organs. The surface area available for dialysis is thus decreased.[190] The cause is unknown but may be related to repeated bouts of peritonitis, acetate, hyperosmolar dialysate solutions, or particulate matter in the dialysate.[191, 192] The process can be fatal if bowel obstruction and strangulation occurs. No treatment is known to aid in preventing this complication or improving this condition.

SUMMARY

Peritoneal dialysis is a viable option for many patients who need dialysis. Children especially are excellent candidates for peritoneal dialysis. Despite the frequency of the complications previously described, overall 60 to 90 per cent of catheters placed are still functioning after 1 year. Patient survival is similar to that of patients on hemodialysis with 3-year survival rates of 60 per cent. Of those who survive 3 years, 60 per cent are still being maintained on peritoneal dialysis therapy. Infectious complications, such as recurrent bouts of peritonitis, lead to abandonment of peritoneal dialysis in the majority of patients.

References

1. Ganter G: Ueber die Beseitigung giftiger Stoffe aus dem Blute durch Dialyse. Munch Med Wochschr 70-II:1478, 1923.
2. Rhoads JE: Peritoneal lavage in the treatment of renal insufficiency. Am J Med Sci 192:642, 1938.
3. Oreopoulos DG, Robson M, Faller B, et al: CAPD: A new era in the treatment of chronic renal failure. Clin Nephrol 11:125, 1979.
4. Gutman RA: Automatic peritoneal dialysis for home use. Q J Med 47:261, 1978.
5. Weston RE, Roberts M: Clinical use of stylet-catheter for peritoneal dialysis. Arch Intern Med 115:659, 1965.
6. Palmer RA, Quinton W, Gray JE: Prolonged peritoneal dialysis for chronic renal failure. Lancet 1:700, 1964.

7. Tenckhoff H, Schecter H: A bacteriologically safe peritoneal access device. Trans Am Soc Artif Intern Organs 14:181, 1968.

8. Tenckhoff H, Shilipetar G, Boen ST: One year's experience with home peritoneal dialysis. Trans Am Soc Artif Intern Organs 11:11, 1965.

9. Striker GE, Tenckhoff H: A transcutaneous prosthesis for prolonged access to the peritoneal cavity. Surgery 69:70, 1971.

10. Tenckhoff H: Catheter implantation. Dial Transplant 1:18–20, 1972.

11. Bullmaster JR, Miller SF, Finley RK, et al: Surgical aspects of the Tenckhoff peritoneal dialysis catheter. A seven-year experience. Am J Surg 149:339, 1985.

12. Popovich RP, Moncrief JW, Decherd JF, et al: The definition of a portable-wearable equilibrium peritoneal technique. Abstr Am Soc Artif Intern Organs 5:64, 1976.

13. Moncrief JW, Sorrels PAJ, Druger VG, et al: Development of training programs for continuous ambulatory peritoneal dialysis—Historical review. *In* M Legrain (ed): Continuous Ambulatory Peritoneal Dialysis. Amsterdam, Excerpta Medica, 1980, pp 149–151.

14. Steinberg SM, Cutler SJ, Novak JW, et al: Report of the national CAPD registry of the National Institutes of Health. Washington, DC, NIH, 1986.

15. Roxe DM, del Greco F, Krumlovsky F, et al: A comparison of maintenance hemodialysis to maintenance peritoneal dialysis in the maintenance of end-stage renal disease. Trans Am Soc Artif Intern Organs 25:81, 1979.

16. Clark AJ: Absorption from the peritoneal cavity. J Pharmacol 16:415, 1921.

17. Putnam TJ: The living peritoneum as a dialyzing membrane. Am J Physiol 63:548, 1922.

18. Gjessing J: Absorption of amino acids and fat from the peritoneum. Opuscula Medica 13:251, 1968.

19. Nolph KD, Twardowski ZJ, Popovich RV, Rubin J: Equilibration of peritoneal dialysis solutions during long dwell exchanges. J Lab Clin Med 93:246, 1979.

20. Rubin J, Nolph KD, Arfania D, et al: Protein losses in continuous ambulatory peritoneal dialysis. Nephron 28:218, 1981.

21. Blumenkrantz MJ, Gahl GM, Kopple JD, et al: Protein losses during peritoneal dialysis. Kidney Int 19:593, 1981.

22. Dombros N, Oren A, Marliss EB, et al: Plasma amino acid profiles and amino acid losses in patients undergoing CAPD. Perit Dial Bull 2:27, 1982.

23. Giordano C, De Santo NG, Capodicasa G, et al: Amino acid losses during CAPD. Clin Nephrol 14:230, 1980.

24. Kopple JD, Blumenkrantz MJ, Jones MR, et al: Plasma amino acid levels and amino acid losses during continuous ambulatory peritoneal dialysis. Am J Clin Nutr 36:395, 1982.

25. Blumberg A, Hanck A, Sander G: Vitamin nutrition in patients on continuous ambulatory peritoneal dialysis. Clin Nephrol 20:244, 1983.

26. Henderson IS, Leung ACT, Shenkin A: Vitamin status in continuous ambulatory peritoneal dialysis. Perit Dial Bull 4:143, 1984.

27. Robson MD, Levi J, Rosenfeld JB: Hyperglycaemia and hyperosmolarity in peritoneal dialysis: Its prevention by the use of fructose. Proc Eur Dial Transplant Assoc 6:300, 1969.

28. Grodstein GP, Blumenkrantz MJ, Kopple JD, et al: Glucose absorption during continuous ambulatory peritoneal dialysis. Kidney Int 19:564, 1981.

29. Alvestrand A, Ahlberg M, Furst P, Bergstrom J: Clinical results of long-term treatment with a low protein diet and a new amino acid preparation in patients with chronic uremia. Clin Nephrol 19:67, 1982.

30. Shen FH, Sherrard DJ, Scollard D, et al: Thirst, relative hypernatremia, and excessive weight gain in maintenance peritoneal dialysis. Trans Am Soc Artif Intern Organs 24:142, 1978.

31. Nolph KD, Rubin J, Wiegman DL, et al: Peritoneal clearances with three types of commercially available peritoneal dialysis solutions: Effects of pH adjustment and intraperitoneal nitroprusside. Nephron 24:35, 1979.

32. Vas SI, Suwe A, Weatherhead J: Natural defense mechanisms of the peritoneum. The effect of peritoneal dialysis fluid on polymorphonuclear cells. *In* Atkins RC, Thomson NM, Farrell PC (eds): Peritoneal Dialysis. Edinburgh, Churchill Livingstone, 1981, pp 41–51.

33. Williams PF, Marliss E, Anderson GH, et al: Amino acid absorption following intraperitoneal administration in CAPD patients. Perit Dial Bull 2:124, 1982.

34. Gjessing J: Addition of amino acids to peritoneal dialysis fluid. Lancet 2:812, 1968.

35. Matthys E, Dolkart R, Lameire N: Extended use of glycerol-containing dialysate in diabetic CAPD patients. Perit Dial Bull 7:10, 1987.

36. Buoncristiani U, Carobi C, Cozzari M, et al: Xylitol as osmotic agent in CAPD: A reappraisal. Perit Dial Bull 7:S11, 1987.

37. Bazzato G, Coli U, Landini S, et al: Xylitol and low doses of insulin: New perspectives for diabetic uremic patients on CAPD. Perit Dial Bull 2:161, 1982.

38. Yutuc W, Ward G, Shilipetar G, Tenckhoff H: Substitution of sorbitol for dextrose in peritoneal irrigation fluid: A preliminary report. Trans Am Soc Artif Intern Organs 13:168, 1967.

39. Mailloux L, Allerhand J: Comparison of glucose and sorbitol peritoneal dialysis. Abstr Am Soc Nephrol p 52, 1970.

40. Olmstead WH: The metabolism of mannitol and sorbitol. Diabetes 2:132, 1953.

41. Raja RM, Kramer MS, Manchanda R, et al: Peritoneal dialysis with fructose dialysate. Ann Intern Med 79:511, 1973.

42. Robson M, Rosenfeld JB: Fructose for dialysis. Ann Intern Med 75:975, 1971.

43. Gjessing J: The use of dextran as a dialyzing fluid in peritoneal dialysis. Acta Med Scand 185:237, 1969.

44. Jirka J, Kotkova E: Peritoneal dialysis in iso-oncotic dextran solution in anesthetized dogs. Intraperitoneal fluid volume and protein concentration in the irrigation fluid. Proc Eur Dial Transplant Assoc 4:141, 1967.

45. Twardowski ZJ, Nolph KD, McGary TJ, Moore HL: Polyanions and glucose as osmotic agents in simulated peritoneal dialysis. Artif Organs 7:420, 1983.

46. Ahmad S, Gallagher N, Shen F: Intermittent peritoneal dialysis: Status reassessed. Trans Am Soc Artif Intern Organs 25:86, 1979.

47. Diaz-Buxo JA, Walker PJ, Chandler JT, et al: Experience with intermittent peritoneal dialysis and continuous cyclic peritoneal dialysis. Am J Kidney Dis 4:242, 1984.

48. Popovich RP, Moncrief JW, Nolph KD, et al: Continuous ambulatory peritoneal dialysis. Ann Intern Med 88:449, 1978.

49. Oreopoulos DG, Robson M, Izatt S, et al: A simple and safe technique for continuous ambulatory peritoneal dialysis. Trans Am Soc Artif Intern Organs 24:484, 1978.

50. Nolph KD, Sorkin M, Rubin J, et al: Continuous ambulatory peritoneal dialysis: Three-year experience at one center. Ann Intern Med 92:609, 1980.

51. Diaz-Buxo JA, Walker PJ, Farmer CD, et al: Continuous cyclic peritoneal dialysis—a preliminary report. Artif Organs 5:157, 1981.

52. Twardowski Z, Ksiazek A, Majdan M, et al: Kinetics of continuous ambulatory peritoneal dialysis (CAPD) with four exchanges per day. Clin Nephrol 15:119, 1981.

53. Oren A, Wu G, Anderson GH, et al: Effective use of amino acid dialysate over four weeks in CAPD patients. Perit Dial Bull 3:66, 1983.

54. Nolph KD, Ryan L, Moore H, et al: Factors affecting ultrafiltration in continuous ambulatory peritoneal dialysis. First report of an international cooperative study. Perit Dial Bull 4:14, 1984.

55. Nolph KD, Cutler SJ, Steinberg SM, Novak JW: Continuous ambulatory peritoneal dialysis in the United States: A three-year study. Kidney Int 28:198, 1985.

56. Nolph KD: Continuous ambulatory peritoneal dialysis (CAPD) 1987: A therapy in evolution. Contemp Dial Nephrol 8:26, 1987.

57. Diaz-Buxo JA, Farmer CD, Walker PJ, et al: Continuous cyclic peritoneal dialysis: A preliminary report. Artif Organs 5:157, 1981.

58. Diaz-Buxo JA, Farmer CD, Chandler JT, et al: Continuous cycling peritoneal dialysis (CCPD)—"wet" is better than "dry." Perit Dial Bull 7:S22, 1987.

59. Twardowski ZJ, Nolph KD, Khanna R, et al: Choice of peritoneal dialysis regimen based on peritoneal transfer rates. Perit Dial Bull 7:S79, 1987.

60. Frock J, Twardowski Z, Nolph K, et al: Tidal peritoneal dialysis [Abstract]. Kidney Int 31:250, 1987.

61. Twardowski ZJ, Nolph KD, Khanna R, et al: Eight hour tidal peritoneal dialysis matches 24-hour CAPD and surpasses 8 hour nightly intermittent peritoneal dialysis clearances. Perit Dial Bull 7:S79, 1987.

62. Twardowski ZJ, Prowant BF, Nolph KD, et al: High volume, low frequency continuous ambulatory peritoneal dialysis. Kidney Int 23:64, 1983.

63. Clayton S, Quinton C, Oreopoulos D: Training technique for continuous ambulatory peritoneal dialysis. Perit Dial Bull 1:S23, 1981.

64. Cardella CJ, Izatt SJ: What should one do with the peritoneal dialysis catheter in a patient receiving a transplant? Perit Dial Bull 2:90, 1982.

65. Posen GA, Luiscello J: Continuous equilibration peritoneal dialysis in the treatment of acute renal failure. Perit Dial Bull 1:6, 1980.

66. Firmat J, Zucchini A: Peritoneal dialysis in acute renal failure. Contrib Nephrol 17:33, 1979.

67. Segar WE, Gibson RK, Rhamy R: Peritoneal dialysis in infants and small children. Pediatrics 27:603, 1961.

68. Chan JCM, Campbell RA: Peritoneal dialysis in children, a survey of its indications and applications. Clin Pediatr 12:131, 1973.

69. Raja RM, Krasnoff SO, Moros JG, et al: Repeated peritoneal dialysis in treatment of heart failure. JAMA 213:2268, 1970.

70. Shapira J, Lang R, Jutrin I, et al: Peritoneal dialysis in refractory congestive heart failure, Part I: Intermittent peritoneal dialysis. Perit Dial Bull 3:130, 1983.

71. Chopra MP, Gulati RB, Portal RW, Aber CP: Peritoneal dialysis for pulmonary edema after acute myocardial infarction. Br Med J 3:77, 1970.

72. Mailloux LU, Swartz CD, Onesti GO, et al: Peritoneal dialysis for refractory congestive heart failure. JAMA 199:873, 1967.

73. Rubin J, Ball R: Continuous ambulatory peritoneal dialysis as treatment of severe congestive heart failure in the face of chronic renal failure. Arch Intern Med 146:1533, 1986.

74. Winchester JF, Gelfand MC, Knepshield JH, Schreiner GE: Dialysis and hemoperfusion of poisons and drugs—Update. Trans Am Soc Artif Intern Organs 23:762, 1977.

75. Maher JF: Principles of dialysis and dialysis of drugs. Am J Med 62:475, 1977.

76. Di Paolo N, Capotondo L, De Mia M, et al: Phosphatidylcholine: Physiological modulator of peritoneal transport. Perit Dial Bull 7:S23, 1987.

77. Dombros N, Balaskas E, Savidis N, et al: Phosphatidylcholine increases ultrafiltration in CAPD patients. Perit Dial Bull 7:S24, 1987.

78. Miller FN, Wiegman DL, Joshua JG, et al: Effects of vasodilators and peritoneal dialysis solution on the microcirculation of the rate cecum. Proc Soc Exp Biol Med 161:605, 1979.

79. Reuler JB, Parker RA: Peritoneal dialysis in the management of hypothermia. JAMA 240:2289, 1978.

80. Zawada ET Jr: Treatment of profound hypothermia with peritoneal dialysis. Dial Transplant 9:255, 1980.

81. O'Connor J: The treatment of profound hypothermia with peritoneal dialysis. Perit Dial Bull 2:171, 1982.

82. Sheppard JM, Lawrence JR, Oon RCS, et al: Lactic acidosis: Recovery associated with the use of peritoneal dialysate. Aust NZ J Med 4:389, 1972.

83. Hayat JC: The treatment of lactic acidosis in the diabetic patient by peritoneal dialysis using sodium acetate. A report of two cases. Diabetologia 10:485, 1974.

84. Knochel JP, Mason AD: Effect of alkalinization on peritoneal diffusion of uric acid. Am J Physiol 210:1160, 1966.

85. Maher JF, Rath CE, Schreiner GE: Hyperuricemia complicating leukemia. Treatment with allopurinol and dialysis. Arch Intern Med 123:198, 1969.

86. Molitoris BA, Alfrey PS, Miller NL, et al: Efficacy of intramuscular and intraperitoneal deferoxamine for aluminum chelation. Kidney Int 31:986, 1987.

87. Twardowski ZJ, Nolph KD, Rubin J, Anderson PC: Peritoneal dialysis for psoriasis, an uncontrolled study. Ann Intern Med 88:349, 1978.

88. Sorkin MI, Nolph KD, Anderson HO, et al: Aluminum mass transfer during continuous ambulatory peritoneal dialysis. Perit Dial Bull 1:91, 1981.

89. Bertholf RL, Roman JM, Brown S, et al: Aluminum hydroxide induced osteomalacia, encephalopathy and hyperaluminemia in CAPD treatment with desferrioxamine. Perit Dial Bull 4:30, 1984.

90. Wall AJ: Peritoneal dialysis in the treatment of severe acute pancreatitis. Med J Aust 52:281, 1965.

91. Glenn LD, Nolph KD: Treatment of pancreatitis with peritoneal dialysis. Perit Dial Bull 2:63, 1982.

92. Stefanidis C, Balfe JW, Arbus GS, et al: Renal transplantation in children treated with continuous ambulatory peritoneal dialysis. Perit Dial Bull 1:5, 1983.

93. Diaz-Buxo JA: CCPD is even better than CAPD. Kidney Int 28:S26, 1985.

94. Fine RN, Salusky IB: CAPD/CCPD in children: Four years' experience. Kidney Int 30:S7, 1986.

95. Leichter HE, Salusky IB, Fine RN: Renal transplantation in patients on CAPD and CCPD—special focus in pediatrics. Perspect Perit Dial 4:12, 1986.

96. White N, Snowden SA, Parsons U, et al: The management of terminal renal failure in diabetic patients by regular dialysis therapy. Nephron 11:261, 1973.

97. Blumenkrantz MJ, Shapiro DJ, Mimura N, et al: Maintenance peritoneal dialysis as an alternative in the patient with diabetes mellitus and end-stage uremia. Kidney Int 6:S108, 1974.

98. Amair P, Khanna R, Leibel B, et al: Continuous ambulatory peritoneal dialysis in diabetics with end-stage renal disease. N Engl J Med 306:625, 1982.

99. Digenis GE, Khanna R, Mathews R, et al: Abdominal hernias in patients undergoing CAPD. Perit Dial Bull 2:115, 1982.

100. Rubin J, Raju S, Teal N, et al: Abdominal hernia in patients undergoing continuous ambulatory peritoneal dialysis. Arch Intern Med 142:1453, 1982.

101. Rocco MV, Stone WJ: Abdominal hernias in chronic peritoneal dialysis patients: A review. Perit Dial Bull 5:171, 1985.

102. Boen ST, Mulinari AS, Dillard DH, et al: Periodic peritoneal dialysis in the treatment of chronic uremia. Trans Am Soc Artif Intern Organs 8:256, 1962.

103. Gutch CF: Peritoneal dialysis. Trans Am Soc Artif Intern Organs 10:406, 1964.

104. Gutch CF, Stevens SC: Silastic catheter for peritoneal dialysis. Trans Am Soc Artif Intern Organs 12:106, 1966.

105. Diaz-Buxo JA, Chandler JT, Farmer CD, et al: Long-term observations of peritoneal clearances in patients undergoing peritoneal dialysis. ASAIO J 5:21, 1983.

106. Diaz-Buxo JA, Geissinger WT: Single cuff versus double cuff Tenckhoff catheter. Perit Dial Bull 4:S100, 1984.

107. Twardowski ZJ, Nolph KD, Khanna R, et al: The need for a "swan neck" permanently bent, arcuate peritoneal dialysis catheter. Perit Dial Bull 5:219, 1985.

108. Twardowski ZJ, Khanna R, Nolph KD, et al: Preliminary experience with the swan neck peritoneal dialysis catheters. Trans Am Soc Artif Intern Organs 32:64, 1986.

109. Oreopoulos DG, Zellerman G, Izatt S, Gotloib L: Catheters and connectors for chronic peritoneal dialysis: Present and future. In Atkins RC, Thomson NM, Farrel PC (eds): Peritoneal Dialysis. New York, Churchill Livingstone, 1981, pp 313–319.

110. Keane WF, Peterson PK: Host defense mechanisms of the peritoneal cavity and continuous ambulatory peritoneal dialysis. Perit Dial Bull 4:122, 1984.

111. Goldberg EM, Hill W: A new peritoneal access prosthesis. Proc Clin Dial Transplant Forum pp 122–123, 1973.

112. Khanna R, Izatt S, Burke D, et al: Experience with the Toronto Western Hospital permanent peritoneal catheter. Perit Dial Bull 4:95, 1984.

113. Thornhill JA, Dhein CR, Johnson H, Ash SR: Drainage characteristics of the column disc catheter: A new chronic peritoneal access catheter. Proc Clin Dial Transplant Forum pp 119–125, 1980.

114. Ash SR, Slingeneyer A, Schardin KE: Further clinical experience with the Lifecath peritoneal implant. Perspect Perit Dial 1(2):9, 1983.

115. Olcott C, Feldman CA, Coplon NS, et al: Continuous ambulatory peritoneal dialysis: Technique of catheter insertion and management of associated surgical complications. Am J Surg 146:98, 1983.

116. Oreopoulous DG, Baird-Helfrich G, Khanna R, et al: Peritoneal catheters and exit-site practices: Current recommendations. Perit Dial Bull 7(3):130, 1987.

117. Ash SR, Wolf GC, Bloch R: Placement of the Tenckhoff peritoneal dialysis catheter under peritoneoscopic visualization. Dial Transplant 10:383, 1981.

118. Ash SR, Handt AE, Bloch R: Peritoneoscopic placement of the Tenckhoff catheter: Further clinical experience. Perit Dial Bull 3:8, 1983.

119. Khanna R, Wu G, Vas S, Oreopoulos DG: Mortality and morbidity on continuous ambulatory peritoneal dialysis. ASAIO J 6:197, 1983.

120. Palacios M, Schley W, Dougherty J: Use of streptokinase to clear peritoneal catheters. Dial Transplant 11:172, 1982.

121. Wiegmann TB, Stuewe B, Duncan KA, et al: Effective use of strep-

tokinase for peritoneal catheter failure. Am J Kidney Dis 6:119, 1985.

122. Thayssen P, Pindborg T: Peritoneal dialysis and heparin. Scand J Urol Nephrol 12:73, 1978.

123. Furman KL, Gomperts ED, Hockle J: Activity of intraperitoneal heparin during peritoneal dialysis. Clin Nephrol 9:15, 1978.

124. Blumenkrantz MJ, Gallagher N, Bashore RA, Tenckhoff H: Retrograde menstruation in women undergoing chronic peritoneal dialysis. Obstet Gynecol 57:667, 1981.

125. Coronel F, Marenjo P, Torrente J, Pratts D: The risk of retrograde menstruation in CAPD patients. Perit Dial Bull 4:190, 1984.

126. Twardowski ZJ, Tully RJ, Nichols WK, Sunderrajan S: Computerized tomography CT in the diagnosis of subcutaneous leak sites during continuous ambulatory peritoneal dialysis. Perit Dial Bull 4:163, 1984.

127. Nolph KD, Cutler SJ, Steinberg SM, et al: Factors associated with morbidity and mortality among patients on CAPD. Trans Am Soc Artif Intern Organs 33:57, 1987.

128. Orfei R, Seybold K, Blumberg A: Genital edema in patients undergoing continuous ambulatory peritoneal dialysis. Perit Dial Bull 4:251, 1984.

129. Chan MK, Baillod RA, Tanner A, et al: Abdominal hernias in patients receiving continuous ambulatory peritoneal dialysis. Br Med J 283:826, 1981.

130. Digenis GE, Khanna R, Oreopoulos DG: Abdominal hernias in patients undergoing continuous ambulatory peritoneal dialysis. Perit Dial Bull 2:115, 1982.

131. Jorkasky D, Goldfarf S: Abdominal wall hernia complicating chronic ambulatory peritoneal dialysis. Am J Nephrol 2:323, 1982.

132. Wetherington GM, Leapman SB, Robison RJ, Filo RS: Abdominal wall and inguinal hernias in continuous ambulatory peritoneal dialysis patients. Am J Surg 150:357, 1985.

133. Singh S, Vaidya P, Dale A, et al: Massive hydrothorax complicating continuous ambulatory peritoneal dialysis. Nephron 34:168, 1983.

134. Grefberg N, Danielson BG, Benson L, et al: Right-sided hydrothorax complicating peritoneal dialysis. Nephron 34:130, 1983.

135. Brown-Cartwright D, Smith HJ, Feldman M: Delayed gastric emptying: A common problem in patients on continuous ambulatory peritoneal dialysis. Perit Dial Bull 7:S10, 1987.

136. Berlyne GM, Lee HA, Ralston AJ, Woodlock JA: Pulmonary complications of peritoneal dialysis. Lancet 2:75, 1966.

137. Rottembourg J, Gahl GM, Poignet JL, et al: Severe abdominal complications in patients undergoing continuous ambulatory peritoneal dialysis. Proc Eur Dial Transplant Assoc 20:236, 1983.

138. Buccianti G, Bianchi ML, Valenti G: Progress of renal osteodystrophy during continuous ambulatory peritoneal dialysis. Clin Nephrol 22:279, 1984.

139. Delmez JA, Fallon MD, Bergfeld MA, et al: Continuous ambulatory peritoneal dialysis and bone. Kidney Int 30:379, 1986.

140. Gault MH, Fergusson EL, Sidhu JS, Corbin RP: Fluid and electrolyte complications of peritoneal dialysis. Choice of dialysis solutions. Ann Intern Med 75:253, 1971.

141. Port F, Johnson WJ, Klass DW: Prevention of dialysis disequilibrium syndrome by use of high sodium concentration in the dialysate. Kidney Int 3:327, 1973.

142. Watson LC, Thompson JC: Erosion of the colon by a long-dwelling peritoneal dialysis catheter. JAMA 243:2156, 1980.

143. Rubin J, Oreopoulos DG, Lio TT, et al: Management of peritonitis and bowel perforation during chronic peritoneal dialysis. Nephron 16:220, 1976.

144. Coward RA, Gokal R, Wise M, et al: Peritonitis associated with vaginal leakage of dialysis fluid in continuous ambulatory peritoneal dialysis. Br Med J 284:1529, 1982.

145. Vas SI: Indications for removal of the peritoneal catheter. Perit Dial Bull 1:149, 1981.

146. Steigbigel RT, Cross AS: Infections associated with hemodialysis and chronic peritoneal dialysis. *In* Remington JS, Swarts MN (eds): Current Clinical Topics in Infectious Diseases. New York, McGraw-Hill, 1987, pp 124–145.

147. Montgomerie JZ, Kalmanson GM, Guze LB: Renal failure and infection. Medicine 47:1, 1968.

148. Gokal R, Ramos JM, Francis DMA, et al: Peritonitis in continuous ambulatory peritoneal dialysis. Lancet 2:1388, 1982.

149. Prowant B, Nolph K, Ryan L, et al: Peritonitis in continuous ambulatory peritoneal dialysis. Analysis of an 8 year experience. Nephron 43:105, 1986.

150. Rubin J, Rogers WA, Taylor HM, et al: Peritonitis during continuous ambulatory peritoneal dialysis. Ann Intern Med 92:7, 1980.

151. Wu G: A review of peritonitis episodes that caused interruption of continuous ambulatory peritoneal dialysis. Perit Dial Bull 3(Suppl):S11, 1983.

152. Piraino B, Bernardini J, Sorkin M: The influence of peritoneal catheter exit-site infections on peritonitis, tunnel infections and catheter loss in patients on CAPD. Am J Kidney Dis 8:436, 1986.

153. Keane WF, Comty CM, Verbrugh HA, et al: Opsonic deficiency of peritoneal dialysis effluent in continuous ambulatory peritoneal dialysis. Kidney Int 25:539, 1984.

154. Verbrugh HA, Keane WF, Hoidal JR, et al: Peritoneal macrophage and opsonins: Antibacterial defense in patients on chronic peritoneal dialysis. J Infec Dis 147:1018, 1983.

155. Peresecenschi G, Blum M, Aviram A, Spirer ZH: Impaired neutrophil response to acute bacterial infection in dialyzed patients. Arch Intern Med 141:1301, 1982.

156. Prowant BF, Nolph KD: Clinical criteria for diagnosis of peritonitis. *In* Atkins RC, Thomson NM, Farrel PC (eds): Peritoneal Dialysis. Edinburgh, Churchill Livingstone, 1981, pp 257–263.

157. Males BM, Walshe JJ, Amsterdam D: Laboratory indices of clinical peritonitis, total leukocyte count, microscopy and microbiological culture of peritoneal dialysis effluent. J Clin Microbiol 25:2367, 1987.

158. Williams P, Pantalony D, Vas ST, et al: The value of dialysate cell count in the diagnosis of peritonitis in patients on continuous ambulatory peritoneal dialysis. Perit Dial Bull 1:59, 1981.

159. Keane WF, Everett ED, Fine RN, et al: CAPD related peritonitis management and antibiotic therapy recommendations. Perit Dial Bull 7:55, 1987.

160. Eisenberg ES, Ambalu M, Szylagi G, et al: Colonization of skin and development of peritonitis due to coagulase-negative staphylococci in patients under-going peritoneal dialysis. J Infect Dis 156:478, 1987.

161. Walshe JJ, West TE, West MR, Gunnerson NJ: Carriage of staphylococci among CAPD patients and the significance of adherence and exopolysaccharide production. X Int Cong Nephrol, London, 1987, p 203.

162. Rault R: Candida peritonitis complicating peritoneal dialysis: A report of five cases and review of the literature. Am J Kidney Dis 2:544, 1983.

163. Johnson RJ, Ramsey PJ, Gallagher N, et al: Fungal peritonitis in patients on peritoneal dialysis: Incidence, clinical features and prognosis. Am J Nephrol 5:169, 1985.

164. Rubin J: Management of fungal peritonitis. Perspect Perit Dial 4:10, 1986.

165. Khanna R, McNeely DJ, Oreopoulos DG, et al: Treating fungal infections: Fungal peritonitis in CAPD. Br Med J 280:1147, 1980.

166. Kerr CM, Perfect JR, Craven PC, et al: Fungal peritonitis in patients on continuous ambulatory peritoneal dialysis. Ann Intern Med 99:334, 1983.

167. Digenis GE, Khanna R, Pierratos A, et al: Morbidity and mortality after treatment of peritonitis with prolonged exchanges and intraperitoneal antibiotics. Perit Dial Bull 2:45, 1982.

168. Reed WP, Light PD, Newman KA: Biofilm on Tenckhoff catheters: A possible source for peritonitis. Proceedings of Third International Symposium on Peritoneal Dialysis, Washington, DC, June, 1984, p 176.

169. Kilmos HJ, Anderson KEH: Peritonitis with *Pseudomonas aeruginosa* in hospitalized patients treated with peritoneal dialysis. Scand J Infect Dis 11:207, 1979.

170. Williams P, Khanna R, Vas SI, et al: The treatment of peritonitis in patients on CAPD: To lavage or not. Perit Dial Bull 1:12, 1980.

171. Nichols WK, Nolph KD: A technique for managing exit site and cuff infection in Tenckhoff catheters. Perit Dial Bull Suppl 3, p S4, 1983.

172. Andreoli SP, West KW, Grosfeld JL, Bengstein JM: A technique to eradicate tunnel infection without peritoneal dialysis catheter removal. Perit Dial Bull 4:156, 1984.

173. Poirier VL, Daly BDT, Dasse KA, et al: Elimination of tunnel infection. *In* Maher JF, Winchester JF (eds): Frontiers in Peritoneal Dialysis. New York, Field, Rich and Associates, 1986, pp 210–217.

174. Helfrich GB, Winchester JF: Shaving of external cuff of peritoneal catheter. Perit Dial Bull 2:183, 1982.

175. Piraino B, Bernardini J, Peitzman A, Sorkin M: Failure of peritoneal catheter cuff shaving to eradicate infection. Perit Dial Bull 7(3):179, 1987.

176. Faller B, Marichal JF: Loss of ultrafiltration in continuous ambulatory peritoneal dialysis: A role for acetate. Perit Dial Bull 4:10, 1984.

177. Taber T, Hageman T, York S, Miller R: Removal of aluminum with intraperitoneal deferoxamine. Perit Dial Bull 6:213, 1986.

178. Gokal R, Ramos JM, Ward MK, et al: Eosinophilic peritonitis in continuous ambulatory peritoneal dialysis. Clin Nephrol 15:328, 1981.

179. Nolph KD, Sorkin MI, Prowant BF, et al: Asymptomatic eosinophilic peritonitis in continuous ambulatory peritoneal dialysis. Dial Transpl 11:309, 1982.

180. Digenis GE, Khanna R, Pantalony D: Eosinophilia after implantation of the peritoneal catheter. Perit Dial Bull 2:98, 1982.

181. Daugirdas JT, Leehey DJ, Popli S, et al: Induction of peritoneal fluid eosinophilia by intraperitoneal air in patients on continuous ambulatory peritoneal dialysis. N Engl J Med 313:1481, 1985.

182. Daugirdas JT, Leehey DJ, Popli S, et al: Induction of peritoneal fluid eosinophilia and/or monocytosis by intraperitoneal air injection. Am J Nephrol 7:116, 1987.

183. Katirtzoglou A, Digenis GE, Kontensis P, et al: Is peritoneal ultrafiltration influenced by acetate of lactate buffers? *In* Maher JF, Winchester JF (eds): Frontiers in Peritoneal Dialysis. New York, Field, Rich and Associates, 1986, pp 270–273.

184. Gandhi VC, Ing TS, Jablokow JT, et al: Thickened peritoneal membrane in maintenance peritoneal dialysis patients. Kidney Int 14:675, 1978.

185. Gandhi VC, Humayun HM, Ing TS, et al: Sclerotic thickening of the peritoneal membrane in maintenance peritoneal dialysis patients. Arch Intern Med 140:1201, 1980.

186. Slingeneyer A, Faller B, Beraud JT: Progressive sclerosing peritonitis: Late and severe complication of maintenance peritoneal dialysis. Trans Am Soc Artif Intern Organs 29:633, 1983.

187. Bradley JA, McWhinnie DL, Hamilton DNH, et al: Sclerosing obstructive peritonitis after continuous ambulatory peritoneal dialysis. Lancet 2:113, 1983.

188. Ing TS, Daugirdas JT, Gandhi VC: Peritoneal sclerosis in peritoneal dialysis patients. Am J Nephrol 4:173, 1984.

189. Novello AC, Port FK: Sclerosing encapsulating peritonitis. Int J Artif Organs 9:393, 1986.

190. Verger C, Brunschvicg O, Le Charpentier Y, et al: Structural and ultrastructural peritoneal membrane changes and permeability alterations during CAPD. Proc Eur Dial Transpl Assoc 18:199, 1981.

191. Nielsen LH, Nolph KD, Khanna R, Moore H: Sclerosing peritonitis on CAPD; The acetate-lactate controversy. Am J Nephrol 17:82A, 1984.

192. Junor BJR, Briggs JD, Forwell MA, et al: Sclerosing peritonitis: Role of chlorhexidine alcohol. Perit Dial Bull 5:101, 1985.

92

Long-Term Venous Access

Gail T. Tominaga, M.D., and John A. Butler, M.D.

• • •

Long-term venous access is assuming increasing importance in surgical and medical practice as a method of infusion of total parenteral nutrition, multi-agent chemotherapy, antibiotics, and blood products as well as for hemodialysis.

Peripheral access with needles or polyethylene catheters is the most commonly used method of short-term administration of isosmolar solutions or noncaustic medications. Peripheral venous access in chronically ill and debilitated patients has several limitations including venous sclerosis, thrombosis, infection, infiltration, and extravasation. The incidence of these problems increases with the administration of hyperosmolar or vesicant solutions. To avoid these problems, alternative means of vascular access have been employed.

Arteriovenous fistulae have been utilized in the past as a more reliable means of access in nonuremic patients.[1] Reported infection rates were favorably low at 0 to 3 per cent. However, due to the high rate of failure related to thrombosis in nonuremic patients, this method has not gained widespread use.[2–3] Bridge fistulae have been described using conduits between superficial veins and arte-

ries when use of direct arteriovenous fistulae is not feasible.[4] The preferred conduit material is autogenous saphenous vein, although polytetrafluoroethylene, Teflon, umbilical vein, and bovine carotid artery have also been used.[4–6] The benefit of reduced infection rates is countered by the increased thrombogenicity compared with use of direct fistulae.

Central venous access has become the preferred method of circulatory access for long-term use. A large central vein allows high flow and liberal administration of hyperosmolar solutions not tolerated by the smaller peripheral veins. Various types of long-term central venous catheters have been developed, including the Broviac and Hickman type catheters and totally implantable subcutaneous ports (implantable central venous access devices [ICVADs]).

DEVELOPMENT OF LONG-TERM VENOUS ACCESS

The first intravenous infusion was performed using a cannula made from a quill by Sir Christopher Wren in

1657. Following experimental work with dogs, Robert Boyle transfused animal blood into humans in 1663. The first successful human transfusion was performed by Richard Lower in 1667.[7] At that time interest in the circulation was modest, and progress was slow.

In 1929, Forssmann, a German urologist, introduced a catheter from a peripheral vein into his right atrium and confirmed the catheter position by radiograph.[8] The importance of this technique was not recognized until after World War II.

Percutaneous subclavian venipuncture was first described in 1951 by Aubaniac, a French military surgeon, for the resuscitation of patients.[9] The first percutaneous placement of a subclavian vein catheter was reported in 1956.[10] As the use of this procedure increased, complications such as thrombosis, phlebitis, and sepsis became more frequent. With progress in industrial technology, materials that combined greater pliancy with reduced thrombogenicity became available, and complication rates decreased.

A new technique for catheter insertion was described by Seldinger in 1953. Direct venipuncture was performed with a guidewire introduced through the needle. After removal of the needle, the catheter was introduced over the guidewire.[11] This technique gained widespread acceptance in vascular access surgery. With the advent of softer catheters, however, this technique has been modified by the use of a peel-away introducer sheath.

In 1968 Dudrick and colleagues reported the use of percutaneous infraclavicular subclavian catheterization for the administration of hypertonic parenteral nutrition solutions.[12] This led to the development of a long-term indwelling right atrial Silastic catheter by Broviac and associates in 1973 for total parenteral nutrition at home.[13] These catheters were inserted directly by a cutdown technique into the cephalic or internal jugular vein. The catheter was then tunneled subcutaneously with the external end of the catheter exiting the skin on the lower anterior chest wall. Advantages included decreased thrombogenicity and a reduced infection rate that was thought to be secondary to the bacterial barrier provided by the subcutaneous tunnel and fibrous adhesions to the Dacron cuff.

In 1979 Hickman and colleagues modified the Broviac catheter by increasing the size of the catheter to facilitate care of patients undergoing bone marrow transplantation.[14] The larger-bore catheter had a greater internal diameter and a thicker wall, which increased durability.

To avoid the external component of the Broviac and Hickman catheters, a totally implantable device consisting of a small-volume subcutaneous injection port and a Silastic catheter was developed in 1982.[15]

CATHETER TYPES

Temporary central venous polyethylene catheters were popularized in the hospital setting in the 1970s. Long-term success with central venous catheters of Teflon, polyethylene, and polyvinyl chloride has been limited by unacceptable rates of sepsis and thrombosis. Advances in catheter technology have made available silicone rubber catheters. Advantages of the silicone catheter include greater flexibility, decreased thrombogenicity.[16–18] and decreased incidence

of sepsis compared to polyethylene catheters. Silicone catheters are more expensive but have a longer life expectancy than polyethylene catheters.

In 1973, Broviac and associates introduced a silicone rubber right atrial catheter (with an internal/external diameter of 1.0/2.2 mm) for prolonged parenteral alimentation. Hickman and colleagues modified the Broviac catheter, making it both larger (internal/external diameter of 1.6/3.2 mm) and suitable for blood sampling and infusion of drugs, intravenous solutions, and blood products. The Broviac and Hickman catheters are 90 cm long, radiopaque, and have a Dacron cuff 30 cm from the Luer-Lok at the external end. These catheters come with one, two, or three lumina and one or two Dacron cuffs placed on the extravascular segment. The catheter is inserted into a central vein and then tunneled subcutaneously with the Dacron cuff placed distant from the venipuncture site. This Dacron cuff was designed to prevent infection by promoting tissue fibroblastic ingrowth and forming an anatomic barrier to organisms ascending along the outer aspect of the catheter.[19] Subsequent studies,[20–21] however, have shown that tunneling catheters does not decrease catheter sepsis and that the origin of most catheter sepsis is bacteria migrating intraluminally from the infected hub.[21–22]

The Broviac and Hickman catheters require daily heparin flushes to avoid thrombosis. The Groshong catheter requires only weekly saline flushes when not in use. It is a thin-walled Silastic catheter (internal/external diameter 1.5/2.5 mm) with a pressure-sensitive "three-way" valve.[23] The proposed advantage is the Groshong valve, which reduces the risk of air embolism and blood reflux and eliminates the need for catheter clamping and heparin flushes. It is available with one or two lumina and in percutaneous or cutdown kits.

ICVADs were developed in an attempt to further reduce complications associated with central venous access.[15] These devices consist of a Silastic catheter attached to a port with a self-sealing silicone septum. ICVADs are available with one or two ports. The port is implanted subcutaneously and is accessed by a specially designed Huber needle. This needle has a deflected point and an opening on the side wall to avoid taking a core of silicone from the diaphragm during each puncture. The integrity of the septum is maintained for 1500 to 2000 cannulations. A 90-degree Huber needle is used for continuous infusion. Because they are totally implanted, ICVADs eliminate the need for daily catheter care. Blood sampling can be performed but requires flushing with heparinized saline after sampling. When not in use, the system requires flushing every 4 weeks. Catheter obstruction by thrombosis is rare when an adequate protocol for care of the catheter is maintained. The major disadvantage is that it requires repeated puncture of the port each time it is accessed. Because of this there is the risk of extravasation if the port chamber is not entered.

CATHETER PLACEMENT

Two techniques of catheter insertion have been described: (1) the cutdown method using the cephalic, internal, or external jugular vein as described by Heimbach and

Ivey,[24] and (2) the percutaneous method using a wire and peel-away introducer described by Cohen and Wood.[25] The latter technique can substantially reduce operating time at the expense of the potential complications of pneumothorax, hemothorax, vascular trauma, thoracic duct injuries, and bleeding.

The choice of cutdown versus percutaneous catheter placement should be made on an individual basis according to the patient's body habitus, venous anatomy, and coagulation status. The cutdown method may be preferred in obese patients and in patients with thrombocytopenia or coagulopathy.

Often venous access in the upper torso is precluded by anatomic constraints such as burns of the upper body, cervicothoracic trauma, planned radiation therapy to the mediastinum, bilateral radical neck dissection, infected median sternotomy incisions, and venous thrombosis. In these circumstances, cannulation of the inferior vena cava (IVC) can be successfully performed.[26–27] Access is obtained by saphenous vein cutdown with a subcutaneous tunnel to the abdominal wall. The catheter tip is placed below the renal veins. Infection rates have been comparable to those reported with catheters placed in the superior vena cava (SVC); however, there appears to be an increased risk of iliofemoral thrombosis. Williard and colleagues[27] reported on 31 catheters placed infra-umbilically in 26 patients and found a statistically significant difference in central venous thrombosis compared with catheters placed in the SVC (13 per cent vs. 1.5 per cent, respectively). It is not clear whether these patients would benefit from low-level anticoagulation.

Successful translumbar insertion of an IVC Hickman catheter has been reported in two patients with thrombosis of the upper great vessels.[28] In addition, the gonadal vessels can be cannulated through a retroperitoneal approach in patients with thrombosis of both the SVC and bilateral iliofemoral veins.[29]

Patients who have had central lines placed previously often have clinically silent venous thrombosis. To avoid this problem, these patients can be evaluated preoperatively with Doppler ultrasonic imaging of vascular structures.[30]

Traditionally, placement of long-term central venous access catheters has been done by surgeons in the operating room; however, there have been recent reports of catheter placement performed by interventional radiologists in the radiology suite. Morris and colleagues[31] reported successful placement of 102 infusion ports in the interventional radiology suite. They noted major complications in 13.6 per cent (0.88/1000 access days), catheter-related infection in 5 per cent (0.31/1000 access days), and refractory thrombosis rates of 4 per cent (0.25/1000 access days). These results are comparable to those of surgically placed ports.

INDICATIONS FOR USE

Since the work of Dudrick and Ruberg,[32] total parenteral nutrition (TPN) has become an important therapeutic technique in the management of seriously injured or ill patients. TPN must be given through a central vein owing to the high osmolarity of the solutions.

Cancer patients undergoing chemotherapy often require multiple courses of intravenous drugs. Intravenous catheters and needles rapidly cause sclerosis and thrombosis of available peripheral veins and have an unacceptable rate of local infection and thrombophlebitis. As venous cannulation becomes increasingly more difficult, the risk of extravasation with possible tissue necrosis is increased. Hence, most cancer patients requiring chemotherapy need placement of a long-term venous access device. In addition, cancer patients may need venous access to allow for intravenous hydration, antiemetics, analgesics, and blood sampling.

Patients requiring chronic intravenous medications may benefit from long-term venous access. This group includes patients with bleeding disorders such as hemophilia[33] and Christmas disease,[34] who often require repeated transfusion of coagulation factors. Other patients with chronic anemias such as sickle-cell disease need frequent blood transfusions.[35]

CHOICE OF DEVICE

Broviac and Hickman catheters are similar, the main difference being size. The Hickman catheter with its larger internal diameter is more durable. Complication rates are similar. Pasquale and colleagues[36] compared 55 Groshong with 53 Hickman catheters placed in cancer patients. There was an overall complication rate of 71 per cent for Groshong catheters and a rate of 42 per cent for Hickman catheters, but no significant difference in septic complications and thrombus formation. The main difference was that Groshong catheters had a higher incidence of malfunction (29.1 per cent vs. 9.4 per cent, respectively).

The choice of catheter or subcutaneous port/ICVAD can be difficult; however, there are certain situations when one is preferred over another. If the vascular access device is to be used for a short period of time (i.e., less than 3 months) a catheter should be used because it is easier to insert and remove. For vesicant drug administration the catheter might be preferred, to lessen the chance of extravasation injury. If the patient requires chemotherapy and hyperalimentation, a multi-lumen catheter or a double-port ICVAD can be used. Catheters are often preferred in children because cannulation of the port may be problematic. The disadvantage of the catheter is that it requires daily maintenance and is cosmetically less appealing. In addition, dislodgment is more common with catheters than with ICVADs.

Subcutaneous ports have the advantage of requiring less maintenance and are ideal for intermittent long-term therapy. ICVADs appear to have increased longevity,[37] lower complication rates,[37–39] and improved cosmetic appearance. The disadvantages are that they are more difficult to insert and remove, require trained personnel and a special needle to achieve access, and require repeated puncture through the skin.

There is some controversy about whether ports or catheters are better for infusion of hyperalimentation. Many argue that the hyperalimentation fluid in the infusion port may increase the risk of infection. Because most patients on TPN require daily catheter use for prolonged periods of time, multiple punctures of the skin and port would be required if an ICVAD were used for this purpose. This could result in skin breakdown. In addition, the risk of extravasation of hyperosmolar TPN fluid is increased in ports compared with catheters. In contrast, Pomp and colleagues[40] demonstrated the safe use of ICVADs for cyclic TPN administration in 15 patients. They found a 13 per cent infection rate with ports compared with an 11 to 42 per cent infection rate with Hickman catheters previously reported in the literature.

It is difficult to determine the superiority of subcutaneous ports over catheters or vice versa. The device chosen should be tailored to the needs of the patient weighing the advantages and disadvantages of each.

COMPLICATIONS

One of the ongoing problems with venous access devices is the risk of infection and sepsis. Because the infectious focus is usually found at the level of the hub, there should be strict rules concerning its use. It has been clearly shown that when TPN solutions are used, the same line must not be used for taking blood samples or for any other purpose.[41] Manipulation of the needle and the hub should be kept to a minimum, and strict protocols for dressing and tubing changes should be followed.[42]

Infection is the most common long-term complication of permanent access devices, with rates reported as high as 30 per cent. It is difficult to compare data on the incidence of infection because of differences in the definition of catheter sepsis as well as differences in patient populations and manner of reporting (e.g., incidence per patient, incidence per catheter days). Press and colleagues[43] reported on 129 Hickman catheters placed in 102 patients with acute non-lymphocytic leukemia and found an infection rate of 0.14/100 catheter days. They found that most exit site infections could be cured with antibiotics alone (84.6 per cent) without catheter removal, even in the presence of bacteremia. However, they recommend catheter removal if there is no clinical improvement after 48 hours of antibiotic therapy. Raff[44] reported a series in which up to 90 per cent of "catheter sepsis" was successfully treated without catheter removal.

Infections and septic complications appear to be lower with the totally implantable system than with externalized devices. Harvey and coworkers[45] reported an infection rate of 0.04/100 port days with the use of subcutaneous ports. Although infection rates with these devices appear to be lower than with catheters, it should be noted that if infection occurs in a subcutaneous port, removal is necessary in approximately 85 per cent of patients. Skin breakdown or frank pus aspirated from the port pocket requires removal of the access device.

Maki and colleagues[46] demonstrated reduced infection rates with temporary central venous catheters that have attachable subcutaneous cuffs. The Vitacuff is a cuff of collagen impregnated with bactericidal silver ion. The cuff is placed around the catheter and into the subcutaneous tunnel near the exit site. There is immediate bactericidal activity with the silver ion, and subsequent tissue ingrowth occurs into the collagen, forming a physical barrier. Permanent central venous catheters such as the Broviac and Hickman catheters are available with Vitacuffs. Additional benefits with permanent catheters have not been established. The rationale for their use is bactericidal action prior to fixation of the Dacron cuff.

The incidence of catheter or port occlusion varies from 9 to 24 per cent, and usually it can be cleared by instillation of urokinase using a small-volume syringe. Catheter thrombogenicity and pliancy are directly related, and only polyurethane and silicone elastomers are sufficiently pliant to ensure a very low incidence of thrombotic complications.[18] To decrease the incidence of catheter thrombosis Broviac and Hickman catheters should be flushed with heparinized saline once a day. Silastic catheters with Groshong valves need to be flushed with normal saline weekly. Subcutaneous ports or ICVADs require heparin flushing after blood sampling or once every 4 weeks if not in use. When catheter occlusion occurs, thrombolytic agents such as urokinase can be placed in the catheter. Bern and colleagues[47] reported a lower thrombosis rate in subcutaneous ports in which low-dose warfarin prophylaxis was used.

Many catheter complications are related to the experience of the clinician inserting the catheter. Bernard and Stahl[48] reported a complication rate of 8 per cent for 101 catheterizations performed by inexperienced physicians (less than 50 catheterizations each) compared with no complications for 90 catheterizations performed by experienced physicians (more than 50 catheterizations each). Such complications included pneumothorax, hemothorax, bleeding, thoracic duct injury, cardiac arrhythmias, air embolism, malposition of the catheter, transection of the catheter, and arteriovenous fistula formation. Other complications include spontaneous catheter migration,[49] catheter compression by the clavicle and first rib,[50–51] and extravasation.[52] Rare complications such as endocardial abscess[53] and superior vena cava syndrome[54–55] have been reported.

Death due to central venous catheterization is unusual. Borja[56] reviewed 61 reports of subclavian vein catheterization and found 15 fatalities. The reported deaths were due to air embolism in five, pneumothorax in three, hemothorax in two, and cardiac perforation, innominate vein perforation, and catheter sepsis in one each. The complicating cause of death was not given for two deaths caused by subclavian catheterization.

FUTURE TRENDS

Peripherally inserted central venous silicone elastomer catheters were first reported in 1975 by Horshal.[57] He reported on the placement of 36 catheters and noted a 17 per cent phlebitis rate. Bottino and associates[58] reported a 23 per cent incidence of phlebitis and a 1 per cent incidence of catheter-related sepsis in 87 catheters placed in 81 hospitalized cancer patients. This compares favorably with peripherally inserted central polyvinyl catheters, which have a 40 per cent rate of phlebitis at 6 days when used for hyperalimentation.[16] With the advent of Broviac and Hickman catheters as well as totally implantable devices, these peripherally inserted central venous silicone catheters (PIC lines) declined in popularity.

There has been a recent resurgence in the popularity of the PIC catheter. A modification of this device is the peripheral implantable port (Port-A-Cath P.A.S. Port, Pharmacia Deltec Inc., St Paul, MN). The peripheral access system (P.A.S.) port is smaller than other systems (5.6 gm in weight, 26.7 mm in length, 16.5 mm wide, 7.4 mm high, 6.6 mm septum diameter) and is designed for a peripheral location in the arm. These devices have been used for administration of chemotherapy, antibiotics, antivirals, antifungals, and blood products. A Cath-finder Tracking System has been developed to aid in catheter placement.[59] Winters and coworkers[60] reported the use of the P.A.S. port in 14 patients. There were 19 complications in 14 patients (3.9/1000 catheter days), with an infection rate of 3 per cent (0.2/1000 catheter days), port pocket cellulitis in 3 per cent (0.2/1000 catheter days), phlebitis in 12.5 per cent (0.8/1000 catheter days), and thrombosis in 6.2 per cent (0.4/1000 catheter days). Although these authors report that PIC ports are less expensive and are comparable to standard subcutaneous ports, the experience reported in the literature is limited.

Newer modes of access are being investigated. These include a port device placed in the bone marrow known as the Osteoport (LifeQuest Medical Inc., San Antonio, TX). In addition, the search continues for improved materials for catheters that are potentially less thrombogenic and are resistant to fibrin sleeves.

SUMMARY

The development of permanent central venous catheters and ICVADs has improved the care of chronically ill patients. It has made administration of long-term intravenous regimens clinically possible with relatively low complication rates.

References

1. Ries CA, Klock JC, Perkins HA, et al: Arteriovenous fistulas for vascular access in patients with hematologic disorders. N Engl J Med 295:342, 1976.
2. Engels LGJ, Skotnicki SH, Buskens FGM, et al: Home parenteral nutrition via arteriovenous fistulae. 7:412, 1983.
3. Wobbes T, Slooff MJH, Sleijfer DT, et al: Five years' experience in access surgery for polychemotherapy. Cancer 52:978; 1983.
4. Raaf JH: Vascular access grafts for chemotherapy: Use in forty patients at M.D. Anderson Hospital. Ann Surg 190:614, 1979.
5. Dardik H, Ibrahim M, Baier R: Human umbilical cord—a new source for vascular prosthesis. JAMA 236:2859, 1976.
6. Chinitz JL, Yokoyama T, Bower R, et al: Self sealing prosthesis for arteriovenous fistula in man. Trans Am Soc Artif Intern Organs 18:452, 1972.
7. Gordon HE: Historical development of vascular access procedures. In Wilson SE (ed): Vascular Access Surgery. 2nd ed. Chicago, Year Book, 1988, p 1.
8. Forssmann W: Die Sondierung des rechten Herzens. Klin Wochenschr 8:2085, 1929.
9. Aubaniac R: L'injection intraveineuse sous-claviculaire: Advantages et technique. Presse Med 60:1456, 1952.
10. Kerri-Szantu M: The subclavian vein, a constant and convenient intravenous injection site. Arch Surg 72:179, 1956.
11. Seldinger SI: Catheter replacement of the needle in percutaneous arteriography. Acta Radiol (Stockh) 39:368, 1953.
12. Dudrick JJ, Wilmore DW, Vars HM, et al: Long-term total parenteral nutrition with growth, development, and positive nitrogen balance. Surgery 64:134, 1968.
13. Broviac JW, Cole JJ, Scribner BH: A silicone rubber atrial catheter for prolonged parenteral alimentation. Surg Gynecol Obstet 136:602, 1973.
14. Hickman RO, Buckner CD, Clift RA, et al: A modified right atrial catheter for access to the venous system in marrow transplant recipients. Surg Gynecol Obstet 148:871, 1979.
15. Niederhuber JE, Ensminger W, Gyves JW, et al: Totally implanted venous and arterial access system to replace external catheters in cancer treatment. Surgery 92:706, 1982.
16. MacDonald AS, Master SKP, Moffitt EA: A comparative study of peripherally inserted silicone catheters for parenteral nutrition. Can Anaesth Soc J 24:263, 1977.
17. Welch GW, McKeel DW, Jr, Silverstein P, et al: The role of catheter composition in the development of thrombophlebitis. Surg Gynecol Obstet 138:421, 1974.
18. Stenqvist O, Curelaru I, Linder LE, et al: Stiffness of central venous catheters. Acta Anaesthesiol Scand 27:153, 1983.
19. Wagman LD, Kirkemo A, Johnston MR: Venous access: a prospective, randomized study of the Hickman catheter. Surgery 95:303, 1983.
20. Garden OJ, Sim AJW: A comparison of tunnelled and untunnelled subclavian catheters: a prospective study of complications during parenteral feeding. Clin Nutr 2:51, 1983.
21. Sitges-Serra A, Liñares J: Tunnels do not protect against venous-catheter–related sepsis. Lancet 1:459, 1984.
22. Sitges-Serra A, Liñares J, Garau J: Catheter sepsis: The clue is the hub. Surgery 97:355, 1985.
23. Malviya VK, Deppe G, Gove N, et al: Vascular access in gynecologic cancer using the Groshong right atrial catheter. Gynecol Oncol 33(3):313, 1989.
24. Heimbach DM, Ivey TD: Technique for placement of a permanent home hyperalimentation catheter. Surg Gynecol Obstet 143:634, 1976.
25. Cohen AM, Wood WC: Simplified technique for placement of long term central venous silicone catheters. Surg Gynecol Obstet 154:721, 1982.
26. Curtas S, Bonaventura M, Meguid MM: Cannulation of inferior vena cava for long term central venous access. Surg Gynecol Obstet 168:121, 1989.
27. Williard W, Coit D, Lucas A, et al: Long-term vascular access via the inferior vena cava. J Surg Oncol 46:162, 1991.
28. Denny DF, Dorfman GS, Greenwood LH, et al: Translumbar inferior vena cava Hickman catheter replacement for total parenteral nutrition. AJR 148:621, 1987.
29. Coit DG, Turnbull ADM: Long-term central vascular access through the gonadal vein. Surg Gynecol Obstet 175:362, 1992.
30. Jaques PF, Mauro MA, Keefe B: Ultrasound guidance for vascular access. Technical note. J Vasc Interv Radiol 3(2):427, 1992.
31. Morris SL, Jaques PF, Mauro MA: Radiology-assisted placement of implantable subcutaneous infusion ports for long-term venous access. Radiology 184:149, 1992.
32. Dudrick SJ, Ruberg RL: Principles and practice of parenteral nutrition. Gastroenterology 61:901, 1971.
33. Sussman L, Lozman H: Arteriovenous fistula for self-treatment of hemophilia. JAMA 230:437, 1974.
34. Yates AJ, Harvie A, Lowe G, et al: Mandril-Grown graft for vascular access in Christmas disease. Br Med J 2:1108, 1976.
35. Greenberg HL, Berk SH: Creation of an arteriovenous fistula for transfusion. N Engl J Med 285:787, 1971.
36. Pasquale MD, Campbell JM, Magnant CM: Groshong versus Hickman catheters. Surg Gynecol Obstet 174(5):408, 1992.
37. Stanislav GV, Fitzgibbons RJ, Bailey RT, et al: Reliability of implantable central venous access device in patients with cancer. Arch Surg 122:1280, 1987.
38. Shaw JHF, Douglas R, Wilson T: Clinical performance of Hickman and Portacath atrial catheters. Aust NZJ Surg 58:657, 1988.
39. Ross MN, Haase GM, Poole MA, et al: Comparison of totally implanted reservoirs with external catheters as venous access devices in pediatric oncologic patients. Surg Gynecol Obstet 167:141, 1988.
40. Pomp A, Caldwell MD, Albina JE: Subcutaneous infusion ports for administration of parenteral nutrition at home. Surg Gynecol Obstet 169:329, 1989.
41. Ryan JA Jr, Abel RM, Abbott WM, et al: Catheter complications in total parenteral nutrition. N Engl J Med 290:757, 1974.
42. Johnson A, Oppenheim BA: Vascular catheter-related sepsis: Diagnosis and prevention. J Hosp Infect 20(2):67, 1992.

43. Press OW, Ramsey PG, Larson EB, et al: Hickman catheter infections in patients with malignancies. Medicine 63:189, 1984.

44. Raff JH: Results from use of 826 vascular access devices in cancer patients. Cancer 55:1312, 1985.

45. Harvey WH, Pick TE, Reed K, et al: A prospective evaluation of the Port-a-cath implantable venous access system in chronically ill adults and children. Surg Gynecol Obstet 169:495, 1989.

46. Maki DG, Cobb L, Garman JK: An attachable silver-impregnated cuff for prevention of infection with central venous catheters: A prospective randomized muticenter trial. Am J Med 85:307, 1988.

47. Bern MM, Lokich JJ, Wallach SR, et al: Very low doses of warfarin can prevent thrombosis in central venous catheters. Ann Intern Med 112:423, 1990.

48. Bernard RW, Stahl WM: Subclavian vein catheterizations: A prospective study. I. Noninfectious complications. Ann Surg 173:184, 1971.

49. Rasuli P, Hammond DI, Peterkin IR: Spontaneous intrajugular migration of long-term central venous access catheters. Radiology 182:822, 1992.

50. Hinke DH, Zandt-Stastny DA, Goodman LR, et al: Pinch-off syndrome: a complication of implantable subclavian venous access devices. Radiology 177:353, 1990.

51. Aitken DR, Minton JP: The "pinch-off sign": a warning of impending problems with permanent subclavian catheters. Am J Surg 148:633, 1984.

52. Gemlo BT, Rayner AA, Swanson RJ, et al: Extravasation—a serious complication of the split-sheath introducer technique for venous access. Arch Surg 123:490, 1988.

53. George RL, Cornel G: Subendocardial abscess as a complication of prolonged central venous access for parenteral nutrition. Can J Surg 35(1):91, 1992.

54. Matthews JA, Blake HA, Hall DJ: Iatrogenic superior vena cava syndrome treated with streptokinase. Gynecol Oncol 26:119, 1987.

55. Smith NL, Ravo B, Soroff HS, et al: Successful fibrinolytic therapy for superior vena cava thrombosis secondary to long-term total parenteral nutrition. JPEN 9(1):55, 1985.

56. Borja AR: Current status of infraclavicular subclavian vein catheterization: Review of the English literature. Ann Thorac Surg 13:615, 1972.

57. Horshal VL: Total intravenous nutrition with peripherally inserted silicone elastomer central venous catheters. Arch Surg 110:644, 1975.

58. Bottino J, McCredie KB, Groschel DH, et al: Long-term intravenous therapy with peripherally inserted silicone elastomer central venous catheters in patients with malignant diseases. Cancer 43:1937, 1979.

59. Pearl JM, Goldstein L, Ciresi KF: Improved methods in long term venous access using the P.A.S. port. Surg Gynecol Obstet 173:313, 1991.

60. Winters V, Peters B, Coila S, et al: A trial with a new peripheral implanted vascular access device. Oncol Nurs Forum 17(6):891, 1990.

93

Iatrogenic Complications of Arterial and Venous Catheterizations

John W. Hallett, Jr., M.D., F.A.C.S.

• • •

Since the late 1970s, arterial and venous catheterizations have become increasingly common in hospitalized patients.[1] Critically ill patients seldom escape without an arterial line and a pulmonary artery catheter. Hundreds of thousands of subclavian vein lines are placed each year for fluid resuscitation, parenteral nutrition, chemotherapy, hemodialysis, and cardiac pacemakers. A more aggressive approach to cardiac and vascular disease has resulted in the exponential growth of coronary and peripheral angiograms, thrombolytic therapy, various types of angioplasty, and intravascular stents. Cardiac balloon pumps have also been placed percutaneously as well as surgically. The introducing sheaths for these interventions leave vascular puncture sites as large as small-caliber gunshot wounds (7 to 12 Fr). It should not be surprising that the number of iatrogenic complications of arterial and venous access has reached almost epidemic proportions.

Iatrogenic arterial and venous injuries currently represent the most common type of vascular trauma in most hospitals (Fig. 93–1).[1-4] Iatrogenic injuries exceed all vascular trauma from gunshot and knife wounds. Because they can occur in any major hospital, every surgeon must be prepared to manage them.

It must be emphasized that an iatrogenic vascular injury is *not* minor but major trauma. These injuries frequently require surgical repair with its attendant risks of anesthesia, blood transfusion, and wound complications. Hospital stay and costs are generally doubled for patients with injuries. Some patients have long-term limb dysfunction after the vascular injury. Such complications can include local neuralgias, claudication, and limb loss. Four key concepts underlie a successful approach to iatrogenic vascular injuries.[1-4]

1. Dedication to Prevention. Most of these injuries are due to errors in technique and consequently are avoidable. Certain patient characteristics (e.g., aberrant anatomy, underlying vascular disease, obesity) and therapeutic adjuncts (e.g., multiple anticoagulants) set the stage for a complica-

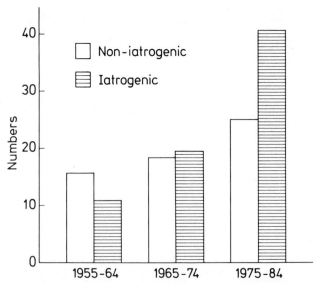

FIGURE 93–1. Increasing incidence of iatrogenic *(lined bar)* compared with noniatrogenic *(white bar)* vascular injuries in Sweden (1955–1984) (From Bergqvist D, Helfer M, Jensen N, Tägil M: Trends in civilian vascular trauma during 30 years. A Swedish perspective. Acta Chir Scand 153:417, 1987.)

tion. Prevention, however, ultimately depends on the technical expertise of the physician.

2. Early Recognition. Most iatrogenic injuries are symptomatic or are evident by physical examination within minutes or hours of catheter placement or removal. Nonetheless, delayed recognition remains a problem. Clearly, early recognition can minimize serious hemorrhage and ischemia. Nurses and house staff must be trained to recognize such injuries and to initiate prompt therapy.

3. Prompt Management. The operative words here are prompt, precise, and gentle. Bleeding at arterial or venous puncture sites can often be stopped promptly by precise finger compression for 20 to 30 minutes. Likewise, operative repair must emphasize gentle handling of tissues because local hematomas can predispose to tissue necrosis and infection. Adjacent nerves (e.g., the median nerve at the brachial artery and the femoral nerve in the groin) must be carefully avoided during dissection and wound closure.

4. Late Surveillance for Sequelae. Catheter complications such as pseudoaneurysm and arteriovenous fistulae may not become manifest or be recognized until weeks, months, or even years after the catheterization. Consequently, it is important to check catheter sites at subsequent office visits or whenever patients direct complaints to previous catheter sites.

INCIDENCE

The risk of catheter-related vascular complications depends upon vessel location and type of catheterization (Fig. 93–2) and treatment employed.[1–11]

Arterial. The lowest complication rates occur with the transfemoral approach (1 to 2 per cent) and increase with translumbar (2 to 3 per cent) and transaxillary (3 to 4 per cent) cannulation.[1, 5] Routine diagnostic arteriograms have the lowest risk of complication at any site (1 to 2 per cent), whereas interventions such as thrombolytic therapy, balloon angioplasty, atherectomy, stenting, and valvuloplasty dramatically increase complication rates (5 to 10 per cent). Traditional transbrachial arterial catheterization, whether percutaneous or cutdown, carries about a 1.5 per cent risk of occlusion necessitating surgical repair. In the operating room or intensive care unit, radial artery catheters seldom cause serious complications, although asymptomatic arterial thrombosis is common (33 per cent).[1] Severe finger ischemia with gangrene occurs in less than 0.5 per cent of patients and usually occurs in critically ill patients with low cardiac output who are taking vasopressors. These figures probably underestimate the actual complication rates because some patients are asymptomatic or the complication is never recognized during hospitalization.

Venous. Subclavian vein thrombosis complicates approximately 10 to 20 per cent of prolonged catheterizations for parenteral nutrition, hemodialysis, or cardiac pacemakers. The next most common complication of central venous cannulation is intravascular embolization of a guidewire or piece of a catheter (1 per cent). Serious arterial injury from subclavian venous access is rare and is known only from case reports of arterial laceration with hemopneumothorax, pseudoaneurysms, and arteriovenous fistulae. In contrast, internal jugular venous thrombosis after catheterization is uncommon, although inadvertent carotid artery puncture with serious hemorrhage, pseudoaneurysm, or chronic arteriovenous fistula is well recognized, especially in cardiac transplant patients undergoing serial transjugular endocardial biopsies. In addition, common use of pulmonary artery catheters has added the rare but serious complication of catheter-induced pulmonary artery perforation with intrabronchial hemorrhage.

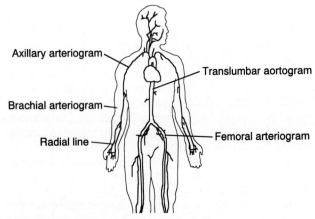

FIGURE 93–2. Most common sites of arterial cannulation complicated by iatrogenic trauma.

TYPES OF INJURIES

The types of vascular injury have changed during the past 25 years. Previously, arterial thrombosis was the most common complication following angiography.[7] Currently, expanding hematomas and pseudoaneurysms predominate.[11, 18] This change is due primarily to large catheter sheaths, thrombolytic agents and anticoagulants, and longer duration of catheter use. The most common complication of central venous cannulation is venous thrombosis. The frequency of this problem has risen considerably with so many therapeutic interventions through the subclavian vein. The subsequent discussion emphasizes prevention, recognition, and management of iatrogenic vascular complications.

FEMORAL ARTERY CATHETERIZATION

Certain measures effectively reduce femoral artery catheter–related complications (Fig. 93–3). Precatheterization evaluation of limb perfusion is important because chronic aortoiliac or femoropopliteal atherosclerosis is common in many of these patients. Consequently, the quality of pulses should be documented, and if they are found to be diminished, ankle-brachial pressure indices should be measured. If aortoiliac occlusive disease is evident, alternative arterial access should be considered. If aortofemoral or femoropopliteal grafts are present, their puncture should be avoided whenever possible. If they must be punctured, prophylactic intravenous antibiotics (e.g., cefazolin 1 gm) should be given before the catheter is inserted.

Catheter complications can be minimized by using correct anatomic landmarks to locate and cannulate the common femoral artery.[12] The common femoral artery begins at the inguinal ligament, which spans a line between the anterior superior iliac spine and the pubic tubercule. The groin fat crease is inferior to the inguinal ligament and is sometimes mistaken for it. Puncture at the fat crease often results in puncture of the superficial femoral or deep femoral artery, both of which are more difficult to compress adequately after catheter removal (Fig. 93–4). Some angiographers use fluoroscopy to identify the head of the femur, which is generally deep to the common femoral artery. Despite the proper use of these landmarks, improper catheter angulation can place the puncture site above the inguinal ligament, in the external iliac artery, where compression after catheter removal can also be difficult.

Anticoagulation should be reduced or stopped before the catheter is removed. Current protocols following thrombolysis, angioplasty, and vascular stenting call for contin-

FIGURE 93–3. Types of iatrogenic vascular injuries associated with femoral catheterization. (By permission of Mayo Foundation.)

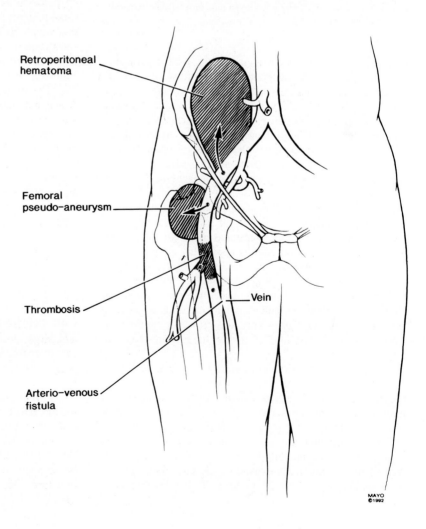

Retroperitoneal hematoma

Femoral pseudo-aneurysm

Thrombosis

Arterio–venous fistula

Vein

MAYO ©1992

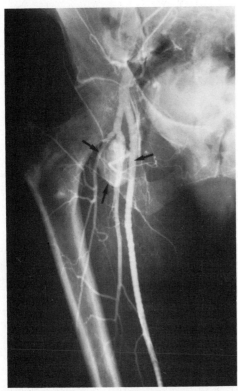

FIGURE 93-4. Acute pseudoaneurysm of the profunda femoris artery *(arrows)* after a low groin puncture for transfemoral coronary angiography.

ued anticoagulation, which increases the risk of groin hematomas and pseudoaneurysms. These drugs can usually be reduced or temporarily halted until the catheters are out and hemostasis is achieved. Holding or reducing these drugs for 1 to 2 hours before catheter removal and for 1 to 2 hours afterward is helpful and seldom leads to thrombosis of any treated coronary or peripheral artery. Immobilization for 6 to 8 hours after catheter removal is also reasonable, especially when thrombolytic and anticoagulant drugs are being used.

The key to avoiding hematomas and pseudoaneurysms is adequate point compression by the fingers over the puncture site for at least 20 to 30 minutes after catheter extraction. Ideally, this compression is applied by a knowledgeable individual. Massive compressive bandages, sandbags, and compressive C clamps do not provide point pressure and therefore are not a reliable substitute for point finger compression. Bandages and sandbags can hide expanding hematomas, and C clamps can cause pressure necrosis of the skin if improperly applied for too long (more than 4 to 6 hours).

Despite compression, *expanding hematomas* and *pseudoaneurysms* can occur. They generally start within 12 hours, either immediately or as patients begin to move the limb. Consequently, a nurse, physician assistant, or physician should monitor the puncture site during this vulnerable period. In particular, any complaints of groin or lower limb pain, coolness, or numbness must be immediately evaluated. If the hematoma is expanding, point pressure should be reapplied for 20 to 30 minutes. If the hematoma is

pulsatile and a pseudoaneurysm is suspected, emergent color flow Doppler ultrasound should be done. If a pseudoaneurysm is confirmed, ultrasound-guided compression can be effectively applied to an increasing number of patients[13] (see Fig. 93-5 on Color Plate V).

Since its introduction by Fellmeth and colleagues in 1991, ultrasound-guided compression of acute pseudoaneurysms has become the initial treatment of choice.[14, 15, 17] A large recent series from the Cleveland Clinic achieved closure of pseudoaneurysms in over 90 per cent of 100 cases.[16] Mean compression time was 30 minutes using 10-minute compression intervals. Intravenous sedation and analgesics may be necessary because this procedure can be quite uncomfortable. Bed rest overnight with a compression bandage is advisable. The compression site must be rechecked prior to discharge because about 20 per cent of pseudoaneurysms recur and require additional compression. Outcome does not appear to be affected by the size, duration, site of injury, or size of the arterial sheath of the pseudoaneurysm. Continued anticoagulation, however, reduces the success rate from 98 per cent to 86 per cent. Contraindications to ultrasound-guided compression include local infection, skin ischemia, and severe local pain, which exist in approximately 15 to 20 per cent of patients. Another 10 per cent of patients experience spontaneous thrombosis between the time of identification and compression.

Consequently, a surgeon must still repair about 20 to 30 per cent of femoral catheter injuries.[17–24] Although in some patients repairs can be performed under local anesthesia, about 50 to 60 per cent of patients require general anesthesia. Hemorrhage resulting in anemia and requiring blood transfusion occurs in 40 to 50 per cent, and approximately 15 per cent experience hemorrhagic shock.

The surgical approach to a pseudoaneurysm should be direct and gentle. A longitudinal groin incision over the femoral pulse is best. Instead of entering the hematoma, dissection should be carried directly to the inguinal ligament, where the femoral artery or distal external iliac artery can be exposed and controlled. Further dissection should be minimized because hematoma may obscure the femoral nerve branches and the deep and superficial femoral arteries. If *femoral artery thrombosis* has occurred or arterial repair with a graft or patch angioplasty appears necessary, a low dose of intravenous heparin (2000 to 3000 units) should be considered. After the femoral artery is clamped at the inguinal ligament, the hematoma can be incised and evacuated. The puncture site can be identified and controlled with finger pressure. A simple suture suffices in most cases. Large hematoma cavities should be drained with a closed suction catheter. Vigorous use of retractors and large closing sutures should be avoided because they can overstretch or entrap fibers of the femoral cutaneous nerve, resulting in a painful femoral neuralgia[18] (Fig. 93-6).

Ongoing uncontrolled hemorrhage after catheter removal affects about 10 to 15 per cent of patients with catheter injuries and rapidly progresses to shock. Fluid resuscitation with Ringer's lactate should be started while blood is typed and cross-matched. Anticoagulants should be stopped. If the bleeding is originating from the groin puncture site, direct pressure for 20 to 30 minutes may

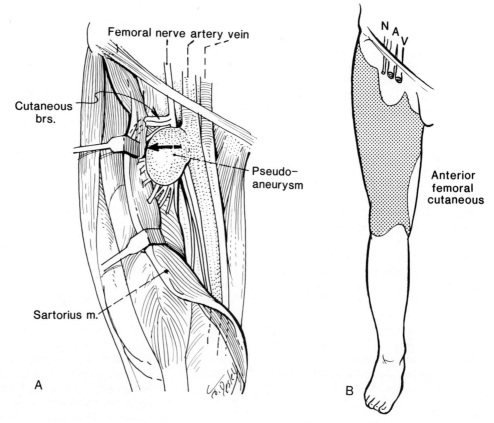

FIGURE 93–6. Mechanism (*A*) and cutaneous distribution (*B*) of femoral cutaneous neuralgia syndrome after catheter-induced pseudoaneurysm. Compression, stretching, or suture entrapment may disturb cutaneous branches (brs.) of the femoral nerve. (*A* and *B*, From Hallett JW, Wolk SW, Cherry KJ, et al: The femoral neuralgia syndrome after arterial catheter trauma. J Vasc Surg 11:702, 1990.)

suffice. If local compression fails after 30 to 40 minutes, the patient needs operative exposure and closure.

If the patient slips into shock and no groin bleeding or hematoma is evident, an inadvertent puncture of the external iliac artery with a hidden *retroperitoneal hemorrhage* must be suspected. When the patient is stable, an abdominal CT scan should be considered to ascertain the diagnosis. For patients who cannot be quickly stabilized, an immediate operation is indicated through an extended groin incision that takes down the inguinal ligament for access to the distal external iliac artery or a lower abdominal retroperitoneal (transplant-type) incision. Occasionally, a guidewire perforates the common iliac artery or aorta, but the retroperitoneal hemorrhage usually tamponades, and surgical exploration and repair are rarely necessary.

An *arteriovenous fistula* (Fig. 93–7) usually occurs after a low groin puncture and involves the deep or superficial femoral arteries and their adjacent veins. Such fistulae are usually asymptomatic. They are recognized by a palpable thrill or a continuous machinery murmur. Sometimes they are incidentally diagnosed by ultrasound evaluation of an associated pseudoaneurysm. Some fistulae close spontaneously, and others can be closed with compression. Large chronic or symptomatic arteriovenous fistulae require surgical repair, but small asymptomatic fistulae are probably more common than we recognize and can be left alone in many patients.

Arterial dissection usually occurs in patients with underlying aortoiliac atherosclerosis and tortuous pelvic arteries. Dissections are often recognized by the angiographer using fluoroscopy for guidewire and catheter advancement. Most dissections stabilize after catheter withdrawal. If sudden iliac occlusion occurs, resulting in severe limb ischemia, a femorofemoral crossover graft can be the simplest solution. More extensive aortofemoral grafting is seldom necessary.

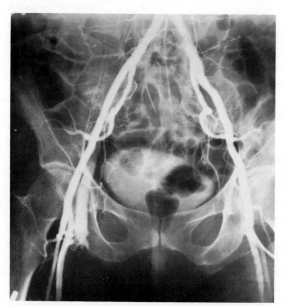

FIGURE 93–7. Arteriovenous fistula between the superficial femoral artery and vein after transfemoral coronary angiography.

TRANSLUMBAR AORTOGRAPHY

Translumbar aortic puncture was once a common approach for aortograms, but in the majority of patients it has been replaced by transfemoral or transaxillary cannulation.

The most common complication of translumbar aortography is *retroperitoneal hemorrhage*. Extravasation of angiographic contrast during the aortogram is one indication that a through-and-through aortic puncture has occurred and may be leaking. If several hundred milliliters of blood extravasate, the patient may become hypotensive and may complain of back pain. Generally, these hematomas are self-limiting. Fluid resuscitation can quickly stabilize blood pressure, and the diagnosis can be made by an abdominal CT scan. Bed rest and observation are sufficient therapy for most patients, and surgical exploration is rarely required.

An occasional complication of translumbar aortography is contrast injection into the aortic wall or plaque with *dissection*. A gentle test injection of contrast through the angiographic needle before the power injection usually shows the beginning of a subintimal dissection and prevents a catastrophic arterial occlusion. Aspiration of the contrast and repositioning of the needle prevent serious damage. Intraplaque contrast injection with acute infrarenal aortic occlusion occurs occasionally. If ischemia is severe, emergent aortic grafting is necessary.

BRACHIAL ARTERY CATHETERIZATION

Mason Sones of the Cleveland Clinic introduced transbrachial cardiac angiography more than three decades ago.[23] It continues to be a common approach for diagnostic arteriograms.[22-24] From its inception, brachial artery catheterization has been complicated by local arterial thrombosis. Because of the rich collateral network around the elbow, occlusion may initially cause few or no ischemic symptoms.

Brachial artery thrombosis after catheterization occurs in about 1 to 12 per cent of patients as reported in large series.[1] Routine Doppler ultrasound examination demonstrates acute brachial artery occlusion in 17 per cent of patients, but two thirds have no symptoms.[1] Despite the absence of initial symptoms, up to 75 per cent of patients eventually experience forearm claudication or hand coolness and discomfort after exercise or cold exposure.[1] This is a substantial disability for those who do manual labor, housework, or handwriting or who work in cold environments. Consequently, most experts recommend immediate brachial artery repair when acute thrombosis is recognized, especially if it is associated with exercise-induced forearm claudication 1 hour after catheter removal.[24]

Local thrombectomy and brachial artery repair can be easily performed under local anesthesia. In a consecutive series of 532 (1.5 per cent) brachial artery repairs after 34,291 transbrachial cardiac catheterizations at the Cleveland Clinic, 97 per cent of patients were discharged with a normal radial pulse.[23] Delay of operative repair of more than 1 day increased the risk of rethrombosis to 12 per cent compared to 2 per cent in those treated within 24 hours. Although some practitioners argue against repair of asymptomatic brachial artery occlusions, this viewpoint is difficult to defend in light of the late limb disability and the ease of most brachial artery repairs.

In addition to brachial artery thrombosis, other complications include arteriovenous fistula, pseudoaneurysm, and median nerve injury. An arteriovenous fistula can be closed more easily under sterile tourniquet occlusion of the upper arm. This approach is also useful for repair of pseudoaneurysms. The tourniquet offers constant hemostasis and allows minimal dissection, avoiding neurovascular injury. If a patient demonstrates median nerve weakness after brachial artery repair, the wound should be reexplored to be certain that sutures have not entrapped the median nerve.

TRANSAXILLARY ARTERIAL CATHETERS

The transaxillary approach is associated with the highest risk of neurologic complications following arteriography. Although the incidence is relatively low (2 to 4 per cent), it is several times greater than that seen with either the transfemoral or transaortic approach. The most common problem is axillary sheath hematoma with motor deficit followed by local arterial thrombosis, pseudoaneurysm, and an occasional central neurologic deficit related to thromboembolism from the ipsilateral vertebral artery or from the aortic arch.

Two factors can minimize brachial plexus damage: (1) meticulous attention to initial axillary puncture, and (2) urgent exploration of the axillary sheath and artery when a neurologic deficit occurs and persists after 1 hour. Patients with a neurologic problem related to axillary sheath hematoma usually complain of hand paresthesias or numbness, which can progress to hand weakness within hours. A small amount of blood in a tense axillary sheath (compartment syndrome) can cause a neurologic deficit. A large hematoma is not necessary, so one should not hesitate to explore the axillary sheath whenever a neurologic deficit is detected and persists for more than 1 hour. *Early exploration* is essential to prevent a chronic neurologic deficit.

INTRA-AORTIC BALLOON PUMPS

Counterpulsation with an intra-aortic balloon pump for circulatory support was developed in the early 1960s and was introduced clinically by Kantrowitz and colleagues in 1967.[25] Passage through the femoral artery has been the most common approach. Because the balloon pumps are large (10.5 to 12 Fr), femoral artery injury or obstruction with distal ischemia are significant risks. Overall, complication rates average 10 per cent with reports as high as 25 to 35 per cent.[26-28] Patients at greatest risk are those with underlying peripheral vascular disease or aneurysms as well as women with small arteries. Complications approach 60 per cent of patients with chronic arterial occlusive disease or aortoiliac aneurysms.

Arterial complications associated with intra-aortic balloon pumps occur in three categories: (1) *thrombosis* of the femoral artery at the insertion site or in the iliac artery through which the catheter was passed, (2) *peripheral emboli,* more commonly seen in patients with aneurysms lined with atheroma and clot, and (3) a *technical mishap* such as arterial perforation or laceration of the aortoiliac segments, catheter-associated groin infection, or bleeding around the catheter site. Currently, it is still debatable whether complications differ significantly between balloon pumps passed by surgical cutdown versus those passed percutaneously.

The management of arterial ischemia associated with a balloon pump depends both on the severity of the ischemia and on the continued need for the balloon pump. If distal pulses are reduced but the patient is asymptomatic and pedal Doppler flow is present, the limb can often be managed by observation alone. When ischemia threatens limb viability, however, several options exist. First, cardiac output must be optimized. Second, the balloon pump should be removed and moved to the contralateral groin, if feasible. Proximal and distal Fogarty thromboembolectomy and local arterial repair usually salvage the affected limb unless severe microemboli to the toes and foot have occurred. Third, a femorofemoral crossover graft below the balloon pump can be limb saving and allows continuation of balloon support[26] (Fig. 93–8). A review of 1454 patients with intra-aortic balloons revealed that 5 per cent had severe ischemia requiring a femorofemoral graft. However, only 36 per cent of such critically ill patients survived.[27] In

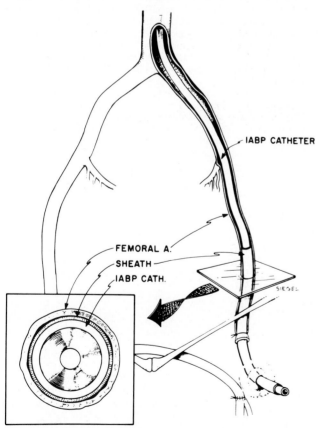

FIGURE 93–8. Femorofemoral crossover graft with intra-aortic balloon pump (IABP) in place (From Friedell ML, Alpert J, Parsonnet V, et al: Femorofemoral grafts for lower limb ischemia caused by intra-aortic balloon pump. J Vasc Surg 5:180, 1987.)

addition, 18 per cent of survivors had irreversible ischemia before grafting that ended in amputation, persistent paresthesias, or foot drop. Another 7 per cent developed graft infection. These data indicate that the need for a femorofemoral crossover graft during intra-aortic balloon support is a bad prognostic sign not only for the limb but also for life.

RADIAL ARTERY CATHETERS

Complications rarely occur after routine radial artery lines are placed.[1] Before radial artery recannulation, one should check for symptoms or signs of chronic hand ischemia. An Allen test is a minimal screening examination. If the hand became ischemic after catheter insertion, the cannula should be removed. If severe ischemia persists, one should consider radial artery exploration, thromboembolectomy, and repair under local anesthesia and magnification. Sometimes hand ischemia in critically ill patients is due to low cardiac output and high-dose vasopressors. Optimizing cardiac function and discontinuing vasopressors are obviously essential steps in preserving hand function.

SUBCLAVIAN VEIN CATHETERS

Subclavian vein catheterization is one of the most common vascular access procedures. Although subclavian vein thrombosis is a relatively common complication of long-term catheters, acute injury of the adjacent subclavian artery is rare. Occasionally the artery is punctured, but immediate removal of the needle and local pressure usually solve the problem. Sudden hemodynamic collapse of the patient should quickly raise suspicion of a pneumothorax. If the chest x-ray shows fluid in the chest, a *hemopneumothorax* may also be present. If insertion of a chest tube is followed by continuing hemorrhage, an emergent thoracotomy with vessel repair may be necessary. An arteriovenous fistula between the subclavian artery and vein is rare.

JUGULAR VEIN CATHETERS

Cannulation of the internal jugular vein is associated with several potential vascular problems: carotid artery puncture with hemorrhage, pseudoaneurysm, or arteriovenous fistula; thyrocervical trunk pseudoaneurysm; hemopneumothorax; and vertebral arteriovenous fistula.[29] If the carotid artery is punctured, simple removal of the needle and local point pressure for 20 to 30 minutes seals most puncture sites. Occasionally ongoing hemorrhage or an expanding pseudoaneurysm requires an operation. A chronic thyrocervical trunk pseudoaneurysm or a vertebral arteriovenous fistula is less common and requires clear arteriographic delineation before operative repair.

PULMONARY ARTERY CATHETERS

The most life-threatening risk of the Swan-Ganz pulmonary artery catheter is perforation of the pulmonary artery with *massive hemoptysis.* Fortunately, this life-threatening catastrophe is very uncommon, occurring in about 1 in 1000 pulmonary artery catheter placements.[1] This complication is due primarily to one of three causes: (1) eccentric balloon configuration, propelling the balloon through the vessel wall, (2) excessive balloon pressure (i.e., 250 mmHg or higher), and (3) tip perforation of the vasculature.[1] Whenever hemoptysis (more than 15 to 30 ml) occurs after pulmonary artery catheter insertion, a pulmonary artery perforation should be suspected. The diagnosis can be made by a "wedge angiogram" demonstrating contrast extravasation. A double-lumen endotracheal tube should be placed immediately to facilitate ventilation and prevent aspiration of the noninvolved lung. Emergency pneumonectomy or lobectomy may be life saving.

References

1. Bergentz SE, Bergquist D: Iatrogenic Vascular Injuries. Berlin, Springer-Verlag, 1989.
2. Adar R, Bass A, Walden R: Iatrogenic complications in surgery: Five years' experience in general and vascular surgery in a university hospital. Ann Surg 196:725, 1982.
3. Lazarides MK, Arvanitis DP, Liatas AC, et al: Iatrogenic and noniatrogenic arterial trauma: A comparative study. Eur J Surg 157:17, 1991.
4. Mills JL, Wiedeman JE, Robison JG, et al: Minimizing mortality and morbidity from iatrogenic arterial injuries: The need for early recognition and prompt repair. J Vasc Surg 4:22, 1986.
5. Hessel SJ, Adams DF, Abrams HL: Complications of angiography. Radiology 138:273, 1981.
6. Mortensen JD: Clinical sequelae from arterial needle puncture, cannulation, and incision. Circulation 35:1118, 1967.
7. Kottke BA, Fairbairn JF, Davis GD: Complications of aortography. Circulation 30:843, 1964.
8. Haut G, Amplatz K: Complication rates of transfemoral and transaortic catheterization. Surgery 63:594, 1968.
9. Rich NM, Hobson RW, Fedde CW: Vascular trauma secondary to diagnostic and therapeutic procedures. Am J Surg 128:715, 1974.
10. Youkey JR, Clagett GP, Rich NM, et al: Vascular trauma secondary to diagnostic and therapeutic procedures: 1974 through 1982. Am J Surg 146:788, 1983.
11. Skillman JJ, Kim D, Baim DS: Vascular complications of percutaneous femoral cardiac interventions. Arch Surg 123:1207, 1988.
12. Kim D, Orron DE, Skillman JJ, et al: Role of superficial femoral artery puncture in the development of pseudoaneurysm and arteriovenous fistula complicating percutaneous transfemoral cardiac catheterization. Cathet Cardiovasc Diagn 25:91, 1992.
13. Johns JP, Pupa LE, Bailey SR: Spontaneous thrombosis of iatrogenic femoral artery pseudoaneurysms: Documentation with color Doppler and two-dimensional ultrasonography. J Vasc Surg 14:24, 1991.
14. Fellmeth BD, Roberts AC, Bookstein JJ, et al: Postangiographic femoral artery injuries: Nonsurgical repair with US-guided compression. Radiology 178:671, 1991.
15. Dorfman GS, Cronan JJ: Postcatheterization femoral artery injuries: Is there a role for nonsurgical treatment? Radiology 178:629, 1991.
16. Cox GS, Young JR, Gray BR, et al: Ultrasound guided compression repair of traumatic pseudoaneurysms: Results of treatment in 100 cases. J Vasc Surg (In press).
17. Rivers SP, Lee ES, Lyon RT, et al: Successful conservative management of iatrogenic femoral arterial trauma. Ann Vasc Surg 6:45, 1992.
18. Hallett JW, Wolk SW, Cherry KJ, et al: The femoral neuralgia syndrome after arterial catheter trauma. J Vasc Surg 11:702, 1990.
19. Oweida SW, Roubin GS, Smith RB, et al: Postcatheterization vascular complications associated with percutaneous transluminal coronary angioplasty. J Vasc Surg 12:310, 1990.
20. Kresowik TF, Khoury MD, Miller BV, et al: A prospective study of the incidence and natural history of femoral vascular complications after percutaneous transluminal coronary angioplasty. J Vasc Surg 13:328, 1991.
21. McCann RL, Schwartz LB, Pieper KS: Vascular complications of cardiac catheterization. J Vasc Surg 14:375, 1991.
22. Campion BC, Frye RL, Pluth JR, et al: Arterial complications of retrograde brachial arterial catheterization. Mayo Clin Proc 46:589, 1971.
23. Kline RM, Hertzer NR, Beven EG, et al: Surgical treatment of brachial artery injuries after cardiac catheterization. J Vasc Surg 12:20, 1990.
24. Walton J, Greenhalgh RM: Brachial artery damage following cardiac catheterization: When to re-explore. Eur J Vasc Surg 4:219, 1990.
25. Iverson LIG, Herfindahl G, Ecker RR, et al: Vascular complications of intraaortic balloon counterpulsation. Am J Surg 154:99, 1987.
26. Perler BA, McCabe CJ, Abbott WM, et al: Vascular complications of intra-aortic balloon counterpulsation. Arch Surg 118:957, 1983.
27. Friedell ML, Alpert J, Parsonnet V, et al: Femorofemoral grafts for lower limb ischemia caused by intra-aortic balloon pump. J Vasc Surg 5:180, 1987.
28. Kvilekval KH, Mason RA, Newton GB, et al: Complications of percutaneous intra-aortic balloon pump use in patients with peripheral vascular disease. Arch Surg 126:621, 1991.
29. Jobes DR, Schwartz AJ, Greenhow DE, et al: Safer jugular vein cannulation: Recognition of arterial puncture and preferential use of the external jugular route. Anesthesiology 59:353, 1983.

The Management of Visceral Ischemic Syndromes

Edited by Lloyd M. Taylor, Jr., M.D.

94

Diagnosis of Intestinal Ischemia

Gregory L. Moneta, M.D., and Raymond W. Lee, M.D.

• • •

The clinical importance of vascular pain in the abdomen lies in the fact that it may be the precursor of fatal mesenteric vascular occlusion.

J. E. Dunphy[1]

There is surely no greater wisdom than well to time the beginning and onsets of things.

Bacon, Essay on "Delay"[2]

The quotations by Dunphey and Bacon summarize the two most important points in any discussion of intestinal ischemia. First, missed or delayed diagnosis of intestinal ischemia may result in fatal intestinal infarction. Second, even with improved understanding of the pathophysiology of intestinal ischemia and new diagnostic methods, intestinal arterial insufficiency remains primarily a clinical diagnosis dependent on proper performance and interpretation of the history and physical examination.

This section of *Vascular Surgery* focuses on gut ischemia. The emphasis in this chapter is on the diagnosis of the surgically important etiologies of chronic, acute occlusive, and acute nonocclusive intestinal ischemia caused by arterial insufficiency. The diagnosis of intestinal ischemia caused by venous thrombosis is considered in Chapter 97. The treatment of intestinal ischemia is considered in later chapters.

CHRONIC INTESTINAL ISCHEMIA

Differential Diagnosis

Chronic intestinal ischemia results from occlusion or severe stenosis of the major visceral arteries. In the vast majority of cases, this is caused by atherosclerosis involving the proximal (ostial) portion of these arteries. A number of other conditions may also result in chronic intestinal ischemia. These conditions, which may affect large or small arteries, are listed in Table 94–1.[3–15] The remainder of this segment is devoted to the discussion of chronic intestinal ischemia caused by large artery obstruction, because it is these conditions that may be treated by vascular surgical procedures.

Failure to achieve normal postprandial hyperemic intestinal arterial flow is the basic pathophysiologic mechanism of chronic intestinal ischemia. It is therefore necessary to consider briefly selected aspects of intestinal anatomy and physiology relevant to chronic intestinal ischemia before available diagnostic methods are discussed.

Table 94–1. Conditions Associated With Mesenteric Ischemia[3–15]

Visceral artery atherosclerosis	Systemic lupus erythematosus
Neurofibromatosis	Polyarteritis nodosa
Visceral artery dissection	Cogan's syndrome
Fibromuscular hyperplasia	Coarctation repair
Buerger's disease	Ergot poisoning
Radiation injury	Cocaine abuse
Rheumatoid arthritis	

Visceral Atherosclerosis and Collateral Circulation

Symptomatic intestinal ischemia is rare, but atherosclerotic stenosis or occlusion of the intestinal arteries is frequently observed. Six to 10 per cent of unselected autopsy specimens demonstrate 50 per cent or greater stenosis of at least one of the three main intestinal arterial trunks.[16] The prevalence of atherosclerosis in visceral arteries increases with age and is higher in patients with other forms of symptomatic peripheral artery atherosclerosis. In one study, 27 per cent of patients undergoing aortography before peripheral vascular surgery were found to have an asymptomatic stenosis of 50 per cent or more of either the celiac or the superior mesenteric artery.[17] These observations illustrate the ability of the visceral arterial circulation to collateralize efficiently under most circumstances.

The importance of the intestinal collateral circulation has been recognized for more than 100 years. In 1868, the autopsy of a 65-year-old woman revealed complete occlusion of the superior mesenteric artery and the celiac artery. The patient had, however, died of causes unrelated to the intestinal circulation. The bowel, which appeared normal, derived its arterial supply from a hypertrophied superior hemorrhoidal artery.[18]

A number of collateral pathways provide intestinal arterial supply when either the celiac artery or the superior mesenteric artery is significantly stenosed or occluded.[19] When only one of these arteries is narrowed and the other vessel remains patent, the pancreaticoduodenal arteries are the most important collaterals. With stenosis or occlusion of the superior mesenteric artery, flow proceeds from the hepatic artery to the gastroduodenal artery and into the superior mesenteric artery distribution via the superior and inferior pancreaticoduodenal arteries. Narrowing of the celiac artery in the face of a patent superior mesenteric artery leads to flow along the same pathway but in the opposite direction (Fig. 94–1).

If both the superior mesenteric artery and the celiac artery are severely diseased, the inferior mesenteric artery serves as the collateral blood supply to the small intestine and the organs of the upper abdomen. Blood proceeds from the inferior mesenteric artery through the arch of Riolan (basically an ascending branch of the left colic artery) to marginal anastomotic arteries and then to the middle colic and pancreaticoduodenal arteries to supply areas normally perfused via the celiac artery or the superior mesenteric artery (Fig. 94–2). The colon can be supplied by flow in the opposite direction when the inferior mesenteric artery is occluded and the superior mesenteric artery remains patent. The internal iliac arteries may also serve as a collateral source of intestinal circulation by inferior mesenteric artery branches contiguous with a patent inferior mesenteric artery and marginal and pancreaticoduodenal arteries. However, when the inferior mesenteric artery is occluded, the principal source of collateral circulation to the left colon is the superior mesenteric artery rather than the internal iliac arteries.[20]

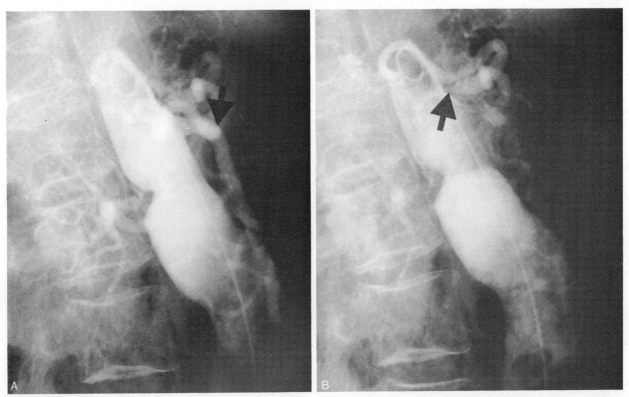

FIGURE 94–1. *A,* In this aortogram from a patient with a juxtarenal aortic aneurysm, the superior mesenteric artery *(arrow)* fills before the celiac artery, suggesting a high-grade celiac artery stenosis. *B,* In a later film from the same injection, the celiac artery lesion is well seen *(arrow)* and there is little contrast remaining in the superior mesenteric artery, indicating celiac artery filling via superior mesenteric artery collaterals.

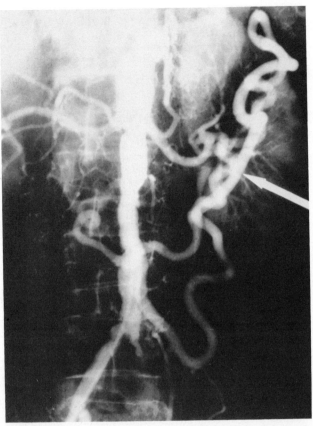

FIGURE 94-2. Angiogram from an asymptomatic patient with proximal occlusion of the celiac and superior mesenteric arteries. The arterial supply to the fore- and mid-gut is via a large collateral vessel of the inferior mesenteric artery, the arch of Riolan *(arrow)*.

Undoubtedly, the ability of the visceral circulation to tolerate atherosclerotic occlusions and stenoses of its major arterial trunks reflects the slow progression of the atherosclerotic process, which allows time for the gradual enlargement of potential collateral circulation pathways. For the rare patients who develop clinically evident intestinal ischemia, symptoms are not usually present until at least two of the three major splanchnic arteries are highly stenosed or occluded.[21, 22] However, significant symptoms of chronic intestinal ischemia can occasionally result from atherosclerotic occlusion of a single vessel, usually the superior mesenteric artery. This situation can occur especially in patients who have undergone previous abdominal surgery that has interrupted important collaterals. In contrast, isolated narrowing or occlusion of the celiac artery or the inferior mesenteric artery is virtually always well tolerated.

Postprandial Intestinal Hyperemia

An appreciation of the dynamic metabolic requirements of the gut is important in understanding the pathophysiology of chronic intestinal ischemia. Intestinal arterial blood flow increases markedly after a meal.[23] Postprandial hyperemia varies in duration and magnitude depending on the size and nutrient composition of the meal as well as on the species studied.[24, 25] Although small changes in intestinal

blood flow may occur in anticipation of feeding, the presence of food in the stomach and intestine is required to achieve the greatest magnitude of increase in intestinal blood flow over baseline. The large majority of this hyperemic flow is distributed to the small intestine and pancreas, with little or no increase in stomach or colonic arterial flow.[26] Total hepatic flow increases, but this is secondary to an increase in portal venous flow. Hepatic artery flow does not change.[27, 28] In humans, intestinal hyperemia is maximal 30 to 90 minutes after food reaches the intestine. The duration of the hyperemic response is 4 to 6 hours.[25]

The mechanism of postprandial intestinal hyperemia is complex and incompletely understood. Humoral, metabolic, and possibly neural factors all appear to participate in its production.[29, 30] Gastrin, secretin, and especially cholecystokinin all clearly mediate postprandial intestinal hyperemia to some extent. Other intestinal hormones, such as neurotensin, glucagon, vasoactive intestinal peptide, substance P, and somatostatin, have also been observed to influence intestinal blood flow when given in pharmacologic doses.[29, 31, 32] Because the various gastrointestinal hormones probably act in a paracrine fashion, these substances may also be of physiologic importance, even though large peripheral doses are required to demonstrate an effect on intestinal arterial blood flow experimentally.

Duplex ultrasound has provided a means of studying human visceral arterial blood flow regulation in vivo. Duplex-derived superior mesenteric artery waveforms from a fasting subject are usually triphasic, reflecting high vascular resistance of the fasting intestinal circulation.[25, 31, 33, 34] After feeding, the superior mesenteric artery waveform demonstrates a large increase in end-diastolic velocity, indicating a decrease in intestinal vascular resistance. Systolic velocities also increase significantly.[25, 31, 33] As in animal studies, the intestinal blood flow response depends on the composition of the test meal. Maximal blood flow response is seen following a mixed-nutrient meal when compared with meals of pure protein, fat, or carbohydrate of equal caloric content, osmolality, and volume[25] (Fig. 94–3).

Fasting celiac artery velocity waveforms reflect the relatively low but constant vascular resistance of the splenic and hepatic arterial circulations. Celiac artery waveforms therefore demonstrate higher levels of diastolic flow than superior mesenteric artery waveforms.[35]

Mesenteric Ischemic Pain

Mesenteric ischemic pain simplistically represents an imbalance between oxygen supply and demand. The pain associated with eating in patients with chronic intestinal ischemia is analogous to that of angina pectoris. It is known that the active absorption of nutrients and the increased motor activity of the postprandial bowel require increased intestinal oxygen consumption.[36] The metabolic demands of nutrient absorption and intestinal motility in the setting of significant arterial obstruction may lead to the production of one or many anaerobic metabolic by-products, and these may be the source of postprandial pain in patients with chronic intestinal ischemia.

An alternative hypothesis for the abdominal pain of chronic intestinal ischemia has been suggested. It is postu-

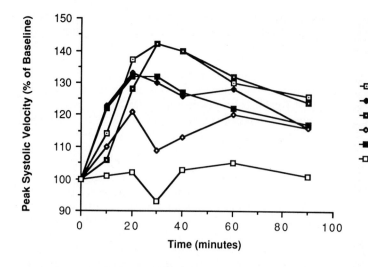

FIGURE 94–3. Increases in superior mesenteric artery duplex-derived peak systolic velocities following equal-caloric test meals of varying compositions, with mannitol and water controls for osmolality and volume. (From Moneta GL, Taylor DC, Helton WS, et al: Duplex ultrasound measurement of postprandial intestinal blood flow: Effect of meal composition. Gastroenterology 95:1294, 1988.)

lated that in the presence of superior mesenteric artery obstruction, increased blood flow in the distal small intestinal branches is achieved at the expense of flow to the stomach (gastric steal). Decreased gastric blood flow then results in increased gastric acid production, transient peptic ulceration, and abdominal pain.[37] The theory is supported by endoscopic observations of superficial gastric ulcerations in some patients with chronic intestinal ischemia. However, patients with chronic intestinal ischemia have usually been initially treated with H_2 blocking agents or other antiulcer medications, without symptom improvement. It has been noted, however, that patients with chronic intestinal ischemia who have successful revascularization do have a significant increase in gastric mucosal pH compared with preoperative values.[38]

Although intestinal infarction is frequently marked by acidosis, leukocytosis, and hyperamylasemia, these are not markers of the reversible ischemic abdominal pain encountered in patients with chronic intestinal ischemia. Currently, abdominal pain in patients with acute or chronic intestinal ischemia without intestinal infarction has not been attributed to any specific metabolite. As a result, no serum or intraluminal marker is currently available to aid definitively in the diagnosis of intestinal ischemia.

Symptoms and Signs

The usual patient with chronic intestinal ischemia is female (female : male ratio of 3 : 1), is between 40 and 70 years of age (mean age, 59), and has undergone an extensive evaluation for long-standing abdominal pain.[39] In one series, patients with chronic intestinal ischemia were symptomatic for an average of 18 months before diagnosis.[40]

The pain of chronic intestinal ischemia is mid-abdominal or epigastric and may be described as colicky or as a dull, deep, intense ache occasionally radiating to the back. It begins 15 to 30 minutes after eating, lasts 1 to 3 hours (often less), is not associated with signs of peritonitis, and usually varies in intensity with the size of the meal ingested.

Early in the course of chronic intestinal ischemia, patients may consume some meals without pain. Partially

because of this, as well as because of the rarity of chronic intestinal ischemia, many physicians mistake the pain of chronic intestinal ischemia for that associated with abdominal malignancy. An ulcer diathesis or cholelithiasis may also be suspected. As the disease progresses, patients gradually come to associate eating with abdominal pain and begin to limit their meals. This so-called food fear and the resultant weight loss are invariably present in well-established cases of chronic intestinal ischemia. Weight loss is often so great that an advanced and incurable malignancy is diagnosed. Although frequently suspected, malabsorption is not a consistent feature of chronic intestinal ischemia; the weight loss in patients with chronic intestinal ischemia has been shown to result entirely from decreased nutritional intake.[41]

On occasion, severely symptomatic patients with chronic intestinal ischemia complain of constant mild, generalized abdominal discomfort not associated with eating that ultimately disappears with intestinal revascularization. Physical examination reveals no signs of peritonitis or intestinal infarction. Although this may represent critical resting ischemia or a preintestinal infarction state, this has not been proved.

Other than a history of recurring postprandial abdominal pain and weight loss, there are no other symptoms or signs reliably associated with chronic intestinal ischemia. Physical examination and history most often reveal atherosclerotic involvement of other organ systems, but occasional patients with chronic intestinal ischemia do not have widespread detectable atherosclerosis. Most patients with chronic intestinal ischemia have abdominal bruits, but this finding is so nonspecific that it is not useful. No pattern of bowel evacuation is constant. Diarrhea, constipation, and normal bowel habits have all been described in patients with well-documented chronic intestinal ischemia.

Diagnostic Tests

Diagnostic tests in patients with suspected chronic intestinal ischemia have included tests of intestinal absorptive and excretory function, arteriography, and most recently, duplex scanning to evaluate visceral artery stenosis noninvasively.

Tests of Intestinal Absorption and Excretion

Tests of intestinal function have not been found useful for diagnosing possible chronic intestinal ischemia. A number have been evaluated. The results are inconsistent and correlate so poorly with the presence of arterial lesions that these tests are not recommended in the evaluation of possible chronic intestinal ischemia.[42] The most widely publicized test was the measurement of urinary D-xylose levels after orally administered D-xylose. Urine is collected from the patient for 5 hours after an oral dose of 25 gm of D-xylose. Malabsorption is present if less than 5 gm of D-xylose can be recovered from the urine over 5 hours.[43] A modification of this test involved oral administration of 5 gm of D-xylose, with subsequent hourly determination of blood levels corrected for body surface area.[44] When results are positive, the D-xylose test indicates malabsorption, but unfortunately not chronic intestinal ischemia.

Arteriography

Arteriography is the primary diagnostic procedure in patients with suspected chronic intestinal ischemia (Fig. 94–4). Lateral and anteroposterior views of the aorta are

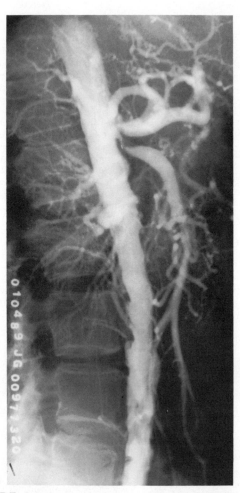

FIGURE 94–4. Lateral aortogram demonstrating high-grade stenoses of the celiac and superior mesenteric arteries. Symptoms of postprandial abdominal pain were relieved with splanchnic artery bypass. (From Moneta GL: Diagnosis of chronic intestinal ischemia. Semin Vasc Surg 3:176, 1990.)

required to evaluate fully the severity of visceral stenosis and the extent of collateral development. A transfemoral Seldinger technique suffices in most cases. Iliofemoral occlusive disease occasionally necessitates a transaxillary or translumbar approach. Sixty to 100 ml of contrast is required for appropriate lateral and anteroposterior views of the abdominal aorta. Because visceral arterial lesions are usually ostial, selective catheterization of the main intestinal arteries is neither necessary nor advisable. Most surgeons prefer full-sized cut films, but intra-arterial digital subtraction techniques are usually adequate for lateral views and require less contrast. Arteriography also demonstrates coexisting lesions of the aorta and of the renal and iliac arteries to aid in planning revascularization.

Some investigators believe that arteriographically demonstrated visceral artery collaterals indicate hemodynamic significance of visceral artery lesions.[45] However, the presence or absence of demonstrable collaterals is not useful in ascribing abdominal symptoms to mesenteric ischemia. Poor collateralization may indicate that the visceral artery lesion is either hemodynamically insignificant or poorly compensated. A technically inadequate study secondary to poor timing of the contrast injection or injection at sites distal to collateral origins may also be an explanation for poor angiographic demonstration of collateral vessels. Extensive collateralization found in association with visceral artery stenosis may reflect either an adequate collateral blood supply to the intestine or a vigorous but insufficient attempt at collateralization. Like peripheral and renal arteriography, visceral arteriography should be regarded as a means of demonstrating lesions that are compatible with arterial insufficiency, not as a means of ascribing symptoms to specific lesions (Fig. 94–5).

Duplex Ultrasound

Duplex ultrasound has been advocated as a possible method of identifying high-grade visceral arterial lesions in patients with possible chronic intestinal ischemia[46–48] (Fig. 94–6). Some investigators have speculated that the availability of a noninvasive method of screening patients for possible visceral artery stenosis would lead to earlier diagnosis of chronic intestinal ischemia in selected patients. Given the small numbers of patients with recognized chronic intestinal ischemia, the number of patients with chronic intestinal ischemia thus far studied with duplex ultrasound is small. Investigators have therefore focused on developing criteria for duplex detection of high-grade celiac and superior mesenteric artery stenosis.

The first duplex ultrasound criteria for splanchnic artery stenosis were proposed in 1991.[48] Investigators at the Oregon Health Sciences University retrospectively reviewed 34 lateral aortograms and correlated them with splanchnic artery duplex scans. On the basis of these data, a superior mesenteric artery peak systolic velocity of greater than 275 cm/sec and a celiac artery peak systolic velocity of greater than 200 cm/sec appeared to be good predictors of 70 per cent superior mesenteric artery and 70 per cent celiac artery stenosis, respectively. These retrospectively derived criteria were subsequently evaluated in a blinded, prospective study of 100 patients undergoing visceral artery duplex scanning and lateral aortography.[49] The

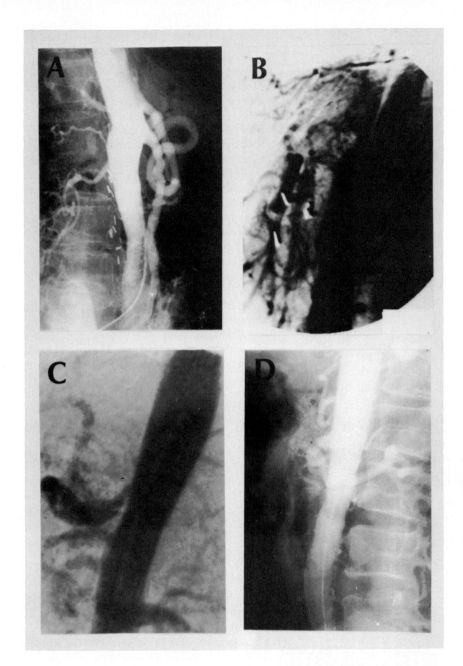

FIGURE 94-5. Lateral aortograms demonstrating the often poor correlation between visceral artery stenoses and symptoms of chronic intestinal ischemia. *A,* Patient with normal celiac and superior mesenteric arteries despite symptoms of weight loss and postprandial abdominal pain. *B* and *C,* Despite both celiac artery and superior mesenteric artery occlusion in *B* and superior mesenteric artery occlusion with high-grade celiac artery stenosis in *C,* both patients were asymptomatic. *D,* Patient with severe chronic mesenteric ischemia relieved by visceral artery bypass. (*A–D,* From Moneta GL: Diagnosis of chronic intestinal ischemia. Semin Vasc Surg 3:176, 1990.)

FIGURE 94-6. B-mode ultrasound image of the abdominal aorta (Ao). The celiac (Cel) and superior mesenteric (SMA) arteries are shown.

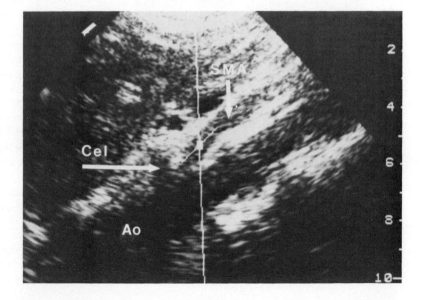

results of this study showed that a fasting superior mesenteric artery peak systolic velocity of greater than 275 cm/sec or no flow signal predicted more than 70 per cent angiographic stenosis with a sensitivity of 92 per cent, a specificity of 96 per cent, a positive predictive value of 80 per cent, and a negative predictive value of 99 per cent. For the ability of a fasting celiac artery peak systolic velocity of greater than 200 cm/sec to predict 70 per cent celiac artery angiographic stenosis, the results were 87, 80, 63, and 94 per cent, respectively (Fig. 94–7). Other investigators have proposed end-diastolic velocity criteria for detecting superior mesenteric artery stenosis. On the basis of retrospective data, it has been suggested that a superior mesenteric artery end-diastolic velocity of greater than 45 cm/sec is predictive of 50 per cent angiographic superior mesenteric artery stenosis.[50] Such end-diastolic velocity criteria have not, however, been evaluated in a prospective fashion. It also

appears that reversal of the normal flow direction in the hepatic and splenic arteries provides an important indirect clue to the presence of a high-grade stenosis or occlusion of the celiac axis.[51]

Although duplex ultrasound of the visceral vessels is potentially useful in screening patients with possible chronic intestinal ischemia for intestinal artery stenosis, a number of practical concerns have thus far limited its widespread application. The examination is technically demanding, with respiratory motion, depth of the vessels, and intra-abdominal gas all combining to make insonation of the visceral arteries difficult. Indeed, even with careful patient preparation (overnight fast, morning examinations, and pre-examination oral simethicone), the vessels cannot always be satisfactorily visualized. It is also critically important to perform the examination with the Doppler angle as near as possible to 60 degrees, and this is difficult. Doppler angles

FIGURE 94–7. *A,* The Doppler sample volume is positioned in the proximal portion of the superior mesenteric artery in this patient with persistent postprandial abdominal pain following repair of a thoracic aortic dissection. The greater than 300 cm/sec peak systolic velocity indicates a more than 70 per cent diameter reducing superior mesenteric artery stenosis. *B* and *C,* Anteroposterior and lateral aortograms confirm the presence of splanchnic artery stenosis. Not demonstrated is the patient's 8-cm infrarenal aortic aneurysm. Postprandial abdominal pain was relieved following aneurysm repair coupled with superior mesenteric artery bypass.

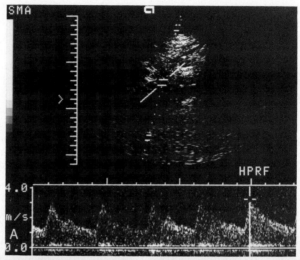

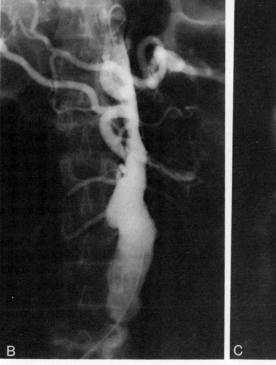

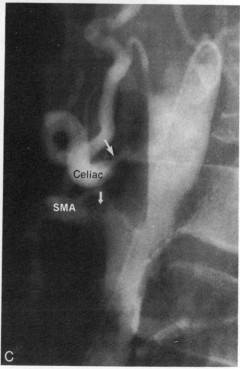

of more than 70 degrees result in falsely elevated peak systolic velocities and therefore contribute to false-positive results.[52]

As is true with arteriography, ascribing a patient's symptoms to visceral artery stenoses detected by duplex ultrasound is not advisable. Intestinal blood flow studies using indocyanine green have suggested that total intestinal blood flow does not increase following a test meal in patients with abdominal angina.[53] Because it is known that superior mesenteric artery peak systolic velocity and end-diastolic velocity normally increase after feeding[25, 33] (see Fig. 94–3), it has been suggested that failure to detect increased superior mesenteric artery flow velocities post-prandially might be a marker for chronic intestinal ischemia. This, however, has *not* been proved and fails to consider that there may be increased postprandial flow to the intestine via collaterals without significant increases in proximal superior mesenteric artery flow. Duplex scanning has detected increased postprandial flow within hypertrophied inferior mesenteric arteries after a test meal in patients with both superior mesenteric artery and celiac artery occlusion.[54] Therefore, although visceral artery duplex scanning clearly can be used to demonstrate mesenteric postprandial blood flow changes, it currently cannot be used to distinguish physiologically appropriate from inadequate blood flow responses. No true ''stress test'' of the intestinal circulation with definite end-points currently exists.

CELIAC AXIS COMPRESSION SYNDROME

External compression of the celiac artery by the median arcuate ligament of the diaphragm has been reported to result in a variant of chronic intestinal ischemia.[55, 56] Diaphragmatic compression of the celiac axis is frequently reversible and varies with respiration. During inspiration the aorta and the celiac axis move downward with the abdominal viscera, whereas in expiration the vessels move upward to result in maximal external compression (Fig. 94–8). Reversible celiac axis compression can be demonstrated with both angiography and duplex scanning in many asymptomatic individuals.[57] Indeed, autopsy studies have indicated that the median arcuate ligament significantly compresses the celiac axis in up to one third of persons.[58] Patients described as having symptomatic celiac axis compression have manifested poorly defined symptoms and signs. These include cramping epigastric pain that changes with body position, nausea, vomiting, and diarrhea. Many patients treated surgically have had a known psychiatric disorder or a history of substance abuse or have undergone previous abdominal surgery. In only one third of patients was the abdominal pain clearly postprandial. Weight loss was often not present.[59]

Postprandial studies of the celiac artery using duplex ultrasound demonstrate little if any increase in celiac artery blood flow following a test meal.[25] This finding is inconsistent with the concept of isolated celiac artery occlusive disease or external compression of the celiac artery producing postprandial abdominal pain solely on the basis of impaired celiac artery blood flow. Some investigators have argued that angiographically demonstrated celiac artery compression is simply a marker of abnormal celiac ganglion splanchnic nerve fiber entrapment. In this theory, pain relief with decompression of the celiac artery results not from improvement in postprandial flow but from destruction of the splanchnic nerves during the surgical exposure of the artery.[60]

Given the nonspecific nature of this syndrome and the inconsistent surgical results reported with celiac artery decompression, Reilly and colleagues evaluated the experience at the University of California, San Francisco.[61] They subsequently developed a group of positive and negative criteria believed to predict good relief of symptoms with celiac axis decompression. These criteria, which have not been prospectively evaluated, include female gender, postprandial pain, age of 40 to 60 years, weight loss of greater than 20 pounds, absence of a psychiatric or drug abuse history, and arteriographic findings of celiac artery compression with post-stenotic dilatation or collateral flow.

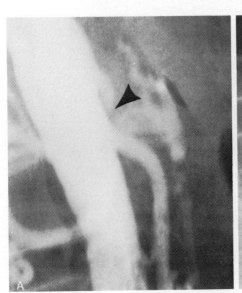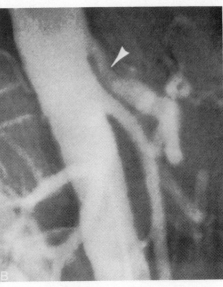

FIGURE 94–8. Lateral aortograms showing extrinsic compression of the celiac artery *(arrowhead)* in expiration *(A)* and compression relief with deep inspiration *(B)*.

Symptomatic external compression of the visceral vessels is possible. A well-documented case by Lawson and Ochsner of concurrent celiac artery and superior mesenteric artery compression serves as a likely example.[62] However, it is obvious isolated symptomatic celiac artery compression has at best an uncertain pathophysiology. The diagnosis remains one of exclusion and should be made only with very careful deliberation. Only a single case, with unclear benefit, has come to operation at the authors' institution in the last 20 years.

ACUTE OCCLUSIVE INTESTINAL ISCHEMIA

Acute intestinal ischemia is defined as a sudden, symptomatic reduction in intestinal blood flow of sufficient magnitude to potentially result in intestinal infarction. In this section the term *acute intestinal ischemia* means abrupt occlusion of the proximal portion of a major splanchnic arterial trunk. The diagnosis of nonocclusive acute intestinal ischemia is discussed in the following section.

Acute intestinal ischemia is usually caused by embolism of organized thrombi to the superior mesenteric artery or from its thrombotic occlusion. Acute intestinal ischemia has, however, been reported to occur from thrombotic emboli to the celiac trunk,[63] from tumor emboli,[64] and from iatrogenically induced cholesterol emboli. Superior mesenteric artery thrombosis usually occurs as an end-result of proximal superior mesenteric artery atherosclerotic stenosis; therefore, in many cases it can be regarded as a complication of untreated chronic intestinal ischemia.

The mortality rate for all cases of occlusive acute intestinal ischemia exceeds 70 per cent in most series.[65, 66] Occlusive acute intestinal ischemia secondary to superior mesenteric artery embolism has a more favorable prognosis than that resulting from superior mesenteric artery thrombosis. Survival following acute intestinal ischemia resulting from superior mesenteric artery thrombosis is, in fact, quite uncommon. The more favorable prognosis with embolism results from the fact that emboli characteristically lodge distally in the superior mesenteric artery (beyond the origin of the middle colic artery), thus allowing partial perfusion of the proximal intestine via middle colic and jejunal artery branches. Thrombotic occlusion of the superior mesenteric artery occurs proximal to the middle colic artery and therefore virtually totally interrupts mid-gut arterial perfusion in patients with poorly developed celiac artery or inferior mesenteric artery collaterals.

Clinical Presentation

Approximately two thirds of patients with acute intestinal ischemia are women. The median age is 70 years. Abdominal pain is present in all cases of acute intestinal ischemia. The nature, location, and duration of the pain may vary. The usual presentation is of a sudden onset of steady abdominal pain referred to the anterior abdomen that is of sufficient severity that the patient, if capable, seeks immediate medical attention. Presentation may, however, be delayed for up to several days, and the pain may be felt most severely in the epigastrium or suprapubic areas. Interestingly, the duration of symptoms does not appear to correlate with the reversibility of intestinal injury.[65]

Physical examination usually reveals at least some degree of abdominal distention. Vomiting is present in more than half the patients, and diarrhea in about one third. Bowel sounds may or may not be present, and when they are present, their quality is too nonspecific to be of any significant diagnostic value. Signs of peritoneal irritation are frequently striking by their absence; this is a well-known feature of acute intestinal ischemia referred to as "pain out of proportion to physical findings." Occult gastric or rectal blood is found in 25 per cent of patients.[65]

Laboratory Evaluation

Routine laboratory evaluation is not helpful. Most patients have a moderate to marked leukocytosis, but about 10 per cent have a normal white blood cell count (less than 10,000/mm^3). Serum amylase levels are mildly but not strikingly elevated in about 50 per cent of patients.[65–67] Plain abdominal x-ray studies usually reveal only distended loops of bowel.

A number of serum markers have been evaluated as potentially useful diagnostic aids early in the course of acute intestinal ischemia. These include familiar seromuscular enzymes such as lactic dehydrogenase, creatine phosphokinase, and alkaline phosphatase, as well as hexosaminidase.[68–71] Their low specificity and failure to identify acute intestinal ischemia before intestinal infarction have limited their clinical utility. Because the intestinal mucosa is most sensitive to ischemia and the intestine can survive with ischemia-induced mucosal sloughing, enzymes such as diamine oxidase, which is present primarily in intestinal mucosa, have also been evaluated as suitable early serum markers in patients with acute intestinal ischemia.[72] Unfortunately, intestinal mucosa enzymes offer no advantage in detecting acute intestinal ischemia over the seromuscular enzymes noted earlier. As is the case with chronic intestinal ischemia, thus far no reliable serum marker for acute intestinal ischemia has been found.

Arteriography

The proper use of arteriography in the diagnosis of acute intestinal ischemia is controversial. Preoperative arteriography requires time and can result in unnecessary delay before laparotomy. Advocates suggest liberal use of arteriography in patients with abdominal pain and possible acute intestinal ischemia may actually result in a more rapid diagnosis of acute intestinal ischemia by identifying patients with acute abdominal pain who have visceral artery occlusions.[73] In addition, arteriography may help avoid operation in some patients without peritoneal signs. This is because intestinal ischemia from nonocclusive causes (discussed later) and occasionally from both proximal and distal superior mesenteric artery embolism has been treated successfully with systemic anticoagulation or the selective infusion of vasodilating agents into the superior mesenteric artery.[74, 75] At the time of laparotomy, knowledge of the extent and distribution of atherosclerosis, emboli, or both, in the abdominal vasculature aids in the performance of optimal revascularization at the time of the initial operation.

No randomized trial of patients with acute intestinal ischemia managed with and without preoperative arteriography exists, nor is one ever likely to be performed. The decision to employ arteriography in patients with possible acute intestinal ischemia before emergency laparotomy is best made on a case-by-case basis. Patients whose clinical history suggests embolic or thrombotic superior mesenteric artery occlusion rather than nonocclusive intestinal ischemia and who truly present acutely so that there is a real possibility of saving threatened but not infarcted intestine are probably best managed by prompt operation by a surgeon capable of rapidly correcting either embolic or thrombotic occlusion of the superior mesenteric artery. Patients who have a more delayed presentation or who are likely to have nonocclusive mesenteric ischemia (discussed later) should be considered for angiography before laparotomy. In such cases, the potential advantages of the added information provided by angiography probably outweigh the risk of further intestinal infarction resulting from the time required to perform angiography.

Ultrasound

Duplex ultrasound is a theoretically attractive and more rapid alternative to angiography in patients with abdominal pain and possible acute intestinal ischemia. The technical limitations on duplex scanning imposed by abdominal distention and excessive intraluminal gas, however, make it less useful in patients with possible acute intestinal ischemia than in those examined for possible chronic intestinal ischemia.

NONOCCLUSIVE MESENTERIC ISCHEMIA

Acute intestinal ischemia may occur without actual occlusion of the mesenteric vessels, a condition termed nonocclusive mesenteric ischemia. Infarction of the intestine in the absence of arterial or venous occlusion has been documented in the American medical literature since 1943.[76] The cause of this condition has been shown to be severe and prolonged intestinal arterial spasm to the point that infarction occurs. Although a hypoperfusion state is present in most patients with nonocclusive mesenteric ischemia, some have nonocclusive mesenteric ischemia from visceral vasoconstriction alone, as is the case with cocaine or ergot intoxication.[14, 15]

The largest percentage of patients with nonocclusive mesenteric ischemia have severe cardiac failure.[77-79] The precise circumstances surrounding the cardiac decompensation are not as important as the associated hypoperfusion itself. Nonocclusive mesenteric ischemia is clearly associated with acute exacerbation of chronic congestive heart failure and acute congestive heart failure following myocardial infarction. Many cases have appeared in cardiac surgery patients whose postoperative course was marked by prolonged vasopressor dependency.[80-82] Nonocclusive mesenteric ischemia has also been reported as a complication of gastroenteritis, pneumonia, hemoconcentration, and spinal shock.[78, 83]

Many patients with nonocclusive mesenteric ischemia have received long-term treatment with digitalis preparations.[79] In animal experiments, baseline intestinal arterial resistance is not altered by digitalis. However, arterial resistance in animals treated with digitalis does increase in response to intestinal venous hypertension when compared with that in nondigitalized controls.[84] Thus, digitalized patients with increases in portal pressure, such as occur with worsening heart failure, may be more susceptible to the development of nonocclusive mesenteric ischemia as a result of arterial mesenteric vasoconstriction. The availability and preferential use of medications other than digitalis for the treatment of congestive failure may in part explain the anecdotal impression that many clinicians have of a decreasing incidence of nonocclusive mesenteric ischemia.

No findings on physical examination or laboratory evaluation can confirm the diagnosis of nonocclusive mesenteric ischemia. With the exception of the presence of a preexisting shock state induced by severe cardiac or multisystem organ failure, the signs and symptoms of nonocclusive mesenteric ischemia are similar to those encountered in patients with the occlusive forms of acute mesenteric ischemia discussed previously. The diagnosis is often delayed because patients afflicted with this disease are generally quite ill, making history and physical examination more difficult. Nonocclusive mesenteric ischemia should therefore be considered in severely ill patients who demonstrate further deterioration accompanied by any new signs or symptoms referable to the abdomen.

Arteriography is required to confirm the diagnosis of nonocclusive mesenteric ischemia. The diagnosis depends on the demonstration of patent mesenteric arterial trunks with tapering spastic narrowing of the visceral artery branches. Arteriography may also be used for therapy in many patients with nonocclusive mesenteric ischemia.[74] It should be liberally employed in seriously ill patients with a clinical picture suggestive of acute intestinal ischemia.

References

1. Dunphy JE: Abdominal pain of vascular origin. Am J Med 192:109, 1936.
2. Cope Z: The Early Diagnosis of the Acute Abdomen. 14th ed. London, Oxford University Press, 1972.
3. Snyder MS, Mahoney EB, Rob CG: Symptomatic celiac artery stenosis due to constriction by the neurofibrous tissue of the celiac ganglion. Surgery 61:372, 1967.
4. Krupski WC, Effency DJ, Ehrenfeld WK: Spontaneous dissection of the superior mesenteric artery. J Vasc Surg 2:731, 1985.
5. Ripley HR, Levin SR: Abdominal angina associated with fibromuscular hyperplasia of the celiac and superior mesenteric arteries. Angiology 17:297, 1966.
6. Wylie EJ, Binkley FM, Palubinskas AJ: Extrarenal fibromuscular hyperplasia. Am J Surg 112:149, 1966.
7. Wolf EA, Sumner DS, Strandness DE Jr: Disease of the mesenteric circulation in patients with thromboangiitis obliterans. Vasc Surg 6:218, 1972.
8. Deucker H, Hison-Holmdahl K, Lunderquist A, et al: Mesenteric

angiography in patients with radiation injury of the bowel after pelvis irradiation. AJR 114:476, 1972.

9. Williams LF Jr: Vascular insufficiency of the intestines. Gastroenterology 61:757, 1971.

10. McCauley RL, Johnston MR, Fanci AS: Surgical aspects of systemic necrotizing vasculitis. Surgery 97:104, 1985.

11. LaRaja RD: Cogan syndrome associated with mesenteric vascular insufficiency. Arch Surg 111:1028, 1976.

12. Sealy WC: Indications for surgical treatment of coarctation of the aorta. Surg Gynecol Obstet 97:301, 1953.

13. Mays ET, Sergeant CK: Postcoarctectomy syndrome. Arch Surg 91:58, 1965.

14. Green FL, Ariyan S, Stausel HC Jr: Mesenteric and peripheral vascular ischemia secondary to ergotism. Surgery 81:176, 1977.

15. Nalbaudiau H, Sheth N, Dietrich R, et al: Intestinal ischemia caused by cocaine ingestion: Report of two cases. Surgery 97:374, 1985.

16. Croft RJ, Menon GP, Marston A: Does intestinal angina exist? A critical study of obstructed visceral arteries. Br J Surg 68:316, 1981.

17. Valentine RJ, Martin JD, Myers SI, et al: Asymptomatic celiac and superior mesenteric artery stenoses are more prevalent among patients with unsuspected renal artery stenoses. J Vasc Surg 14:195, 1991.

18. Chiene J: Complete obliteration of the celiac and mesenteric arteries. J Anat Physiol 3:65, 1869.

19. Olofsson PA, Connelly DP, Stoney RJ: Surgery of the celiac and mesenteric arteries. In Haimovici H (ed): Vascular Surgery—Principles and Techniques. Norwalk, CT, Appleton & Lange, 1989, p 750.

20. Iliopoulos JI, Pierce GE, Hermreck AS, et al: Hemodynamics of the inferior mesenteric arterial circulation. J Vasc Surg 11:120, 1990.

21. Mikkelsen WP, Berne CJ: Intestinal angina. Its surgical significance. Am J Surg 94:262, 1957.

22. Hansen HJB: Abdominal angina. Acta Chir Scand 142:319, 1976.

23. Fara JW: Postprandial mesenteric hyperemia. In Shephard AP, Granger DN (eds): Physiology of the Intestinal Circulation. New York, Raven Press, 1984, p 99.

24. Siregar H, Chou CC: Relative contribution of fat, protein, carbohydrate and ethanol to intestinal hyperemia. Am J Physiol 242:G27, 1982.

25. Moneta GL, Taylor DC, Helton WS, et al: Duplex ultrasound measurement of postprandial intestinal blood flow: Effect of meal composition. Gastroenterology 95:1294, 1988.

26. Bond JH, Prentiss RA, Levitt MD: The effects of feeding on blood flow to the stomach, small bowel, and colon of the conscious dog. J Lab Clin Med 93:594, 1979.

27. Dobson A, Barnes RJ, Comeline RS: Changes in the sources of hepatic portal blood flow with feeding in the sheep. Physiologist 24:15, 1981.

28. Gallavan RH, Chou CC, Kvietys PR, et al: Regional blood flow during digestion in the conscious dog. Am J Physiol 238:H220, 1980.

29. Chou CC, Mangino MJ, Sawmiller DR: Gastrointestinal hormones and intestinal blood flow. In Shephard AP, Granger DN (eds): Physiology of the Intestinal Circulation. New York, Raven Press, 1984, p 121.

30. Greenway CV: Neural control and autoregulatory escape. In Shephard AP, Granger DN (eds): Physiology of the Intestinal Circulation. New York, Raven Press, 1984, p 61.

31. Lilly MP, Harwood TRS, Flinn WR, et al: Duplex ultrasound measurement of changes in mesenteric flow velocity with pharmacologic and physiologic alteration of intestinal blood flow in man. J Vasc Surg 9:18, 1989.

32. Mulholland MW, Sarpa MS, Delvalle J, et al: Splanchnic and cerebral vasodilatory effects of calcitonin gene related peptide I in humans. Ann Surg 214:440, 1991.

33. Jager K, Bollinger A, Valli C, et al: Measurement of mesenteric blood flow by duplex scanning. J Vasc Surg 3:462, 1986.

34. Quamar MI, Read AE, Skidmore R, et al: Transcutaneous Doppler ultrasound measurement of superior mesenteric artery blood flow in man. Gut 27:100, 1986.

35. Quamar MI, Read AE, Skidmore R, et al: Transcutaneous Doppler ultrasound measurement of coeliac axis blood flow in man. Br J Surg 72:391, 1985.

36. Chou CC: Relationship between intestinal blood flow and motility. Ann Rev Physiol 44:29, 1982.

37. Poole JW, Sammartano RJ, Boley SJ: Hemodynamic basis of pain of chronic mesenteric ischemia. Am J Surg 153:171, 1987.

38. Fiddian-Green RG, Stanley JC, Nostrant T, et al: Chronic gastric

ischemia: A cause of abdominal pain or bleeding identified from the presence of gastric mucosal acidosis. J Cardiovasc Surg 30:852, 1989.

39. Olofsson PA, Connelly DP, Stoney RJ: Surgery of the celiac and mesenteric arteries. In Haimovici H (ed): Vascular Surgery—Principles and Techniques. Norwalk, CT, Appleton & Lange, 1989, p 750.

40. Schneider PA, Ehrenfeld WK, Cunningham CG, et al: Recurrent chronic visceral ischemia. J Vasc Surg (In press).

41. Marston A, Clarke JMF, Garcia J, et al: Intestinal function and intestinal blood supply. Gut 26:656, 1985.

42. Marston A: Chronic intestinal ischemia. In Vascular Disease of the Gastrointestinal Tract: Pathophysiology, Recognition and Management. Baltimore, Williams & Wilkins, 1986, p 116.

43. Farmer RG: Tests for intestinal absorption. In Brown CH (ed): Diagnostic Procedures in Gastroenterology. St. Louis, CV Mosby, 1967, p 143.

44. Haeney MR, Culank LS, Montgomery RD, et al: Evaluation of xylose absorption as measured in blood and urine: A one hour blood xylose screening test in malabsorption. Gastroenterology 75:393, 1978.

45. Pollak AA, Beckmann CF: Angiographic diagnosis of visceral vascular disease. In Persson AV, Skudder PA Jr (eds): Visceral Vascular Surgery. New York, Marcel Dekker, 1987, p 17.

46. Nicholls SC, Kohler TR, Martin RL, et al: Use of hemodynamic parameters in the diagnosis of mesenteric insufficiency. J Vasc Surg 3:507, 1986.

47. Taylor DC, Moneta GL: Duplex ultrasound scanning of the renal and mesenteric circulations. Semin Vasc Surg 1:23, 1988.

48. Moneta GL, Yeager RA, Dalman R, et al: Duplex ultrasound criteria for diagnosis of splanchnic artery stenosis or occlusion. J Vasc Surg 14:511, 1991.

49. Lee RW, Moneta GL, Yeager RA, et al: Mesenteric artery duplex scanning: A blinded, prospective study. J Vasc Surg 17:79, 1993.

50. Bowersox JC, Zwalak RM, Walsh DB, et al: Duplex ultrasonography in the diagnosis of celiac and mesenteric artery occlusive disease. J Vasc Surg 14:780, 1991.

51. LaBombard FE, Musson A, Bowersox JC, et al: Hepatic artery duplex as an adjunct in the evaluation of chronic mesenteric ischemia. J Vasc Tech 16:7, 1992.

52. Rizzo RJ, Sandager G, Astleford P, et al: Mesenteric flow velocities as a function of angle of insonation. J Vasc Surg 11:688, 1990.

53. Hansen HJB, Engell HC, Ring-Larsen H: Splanchnic blood flow in patients with abdominal angina before and after arterial reconstruction: A proposal for a diagnostic test. Ann Surg 186:216, 1977.

54. Moneta GL, Cummings C, Castor J, et al: Duplex ultrasound demonstration of postprandial mesenteric hyperemia in splanchnic circulation collateral vessels. J Vasc Tech 15:37, 1991.

55. Curl JH, Thompson NW, Stanley JC: Medial arcuate ligament compression of the celiac and superior mesenteric arteries. Ann Surg 173:314, 1981.

56. Dunbar JD, Molnar W, Beman FF, et al: Compression of the celiac trunk and abdominal angina. Preliminary report of 15 cases. AJR 95:731, 1965.

57. Taylor DC, Moneta GL, Cramer MM, et al: Extrinsic compression of the celiac artery by the median arcuate ligament of the diaphragm: Diagnosis by duplex ultrasound. J Vasc Tech 11:236, 1987.

58. Linder HH, Kemprud E: A clinicoanatomical study of the arcuate ligament of the diaphragm. Arch Surg 103:600, 1971.

59. Taylor LM, Porter JM: Nonatherosclerotic diseases of the visceral vasculature. In Persson AV, Skudder PA Jr (eds): Visceral Vascular Surgery. New York, Marcel Dekker, 1987, p 101.

60. Carey JP, Stemmer EA, Connolly JE: Median arcuate ligament syndrome. Arch Surg 99:441, 1969.

61. Reilly LM, Ammar AD, Stoney RJ, et al: Late results following operative repair for celiac artery compression syndrome. J Vasc Surg 2:79, 1985.

62. Lawson JD, Ochsner JL: Median arcuate ligament syndrome with severe two-vessel involvement. Arch Surg 119:226, 1984.

63. Fratesi SJ, Barber GG: Celiac artery embolism: Case report. Can J Surg 24:512, 1981.

64. Low DE, Frenkel VJ, Manley PN, et al: Embolic mesenteric infarction: A unique initial manifestation of renal cell carcinoma. Surgery 106:925, 1989.

65. Ottinger LW: The surgical management of acute occlusion of the superior mesenteric artery. Ann Surg 188:72L, 1978.

66. Buchardt Hansen HJ, Oigaard A: Embolization to the superior mesenteric artery. Acta Chir Scand 142:451, 1976.

67. Wittenberg J, Athanasoulis CA, Shapiro JH: A radiological approach to the patient with acute, extensive bowel ischemia. Radiology 106:13, 1973.

68. Graeber GM, Cafferty PJ, Wolf RE: An analysis of creatinine phosphokinase in the mucosa and muscularis of the gastrointestinal tract. J Surg Res 37:376, 1984.

69. Graeber GM, Wolf RE, Harmon JW: Serum creatinine kinase and alkaline phosphatase in experimental small bowel infarction. J Surg Res 37:25, 1984.

70. Marks WH, Salvino C, Newell K, et al: Circulating concentrations of porcine ileal peptide but not hexosaminidase are elevated following one hour of mesenteric ischemia. J Surg Res 45:134, 1988.

71. Jamiesen WG, Lozon A, Durand D, et al: Changes in serum phosphate levels associated with intestinal infarction and necrosis. Surg Gynecol Obstet 140:19, 1975.

72. Thompson JS, Bragg LE, West WW: Serum enzyme levels during intestinal ischemia. Ann Surg 211:369, 1990.

73. Boley SJ, Feinstein FR, Sammartano R, et al: New concepts in the management of emboli of the superior mesenteric artery. Surg Gynecol Obstet 153:561, 1981.

74. Boley SJ, Sprayregan S, Siegelman SS: Initial results from an aggressive roentgenological and surgical approach to acute mesenteric ischemia. Surgery 82:848, 1977.

75. Kaufman SL, Harrington DP, Siegelman SS: Superior mesenteric artery embolization: An angiographic emergency. Radiology 124:625, 1977.

76. Thorek M: Surgical Errors and Safeguards. 4th ed. Philadelphia, JB Lippincott, 1943, p 478.

77. Aldrete JS, Hansy SY, Laws HL, et al: Intestinal infarction complicating low cardiac output states. Surg Gynecol Obstet 144:371, 1977.

78. Williams LF, Anastasia LF, Hasiotis CA: Nonocclusive mesenteric infarction. Am J Surg 114:376, 1967.

79. Britt LG, Cheek RC: Nonocclusive mesenteric vascular disease: Clinical and experimental observations. Ann Surg 169:704, 1969.

80. Moneta GL, Misbach GA, Ivey TD: Hypoperfusion as a possible factor in the development of gastrointestinal complications after cardiac surgery. Am J Surg 149:648, 1985.

81. Rosemurgy AS, McAllister E, Karl RC: The acute surgical abdomen after cardiac surgery involving extracorporeal circulation. Ann Surg 207:323, 1988.

82. Allen KB, Salam AA, Lumsden AB: Acute mesenteric ischemia following cardiopulmonary bypass. J Vasc Surg 16:391, 1992.

83. Landreueau RJ, Fry WJ: The right colon as a target organ of nonocclusive mesenteric ischemia. Arch Surg 125:591, 1990.

84. Kim EH, Gewertz BL: Chronic digitalis administration alters mesenteric vascular reactivity. J Vasc Surg 5:382, 1987.

95

Treatment of Acute Intestinal Ischemia Caused by Arterial Occlusions

Lloyd M. Taylor, Jr., M.D., and John M. Porter, M.D.

• • •

The clinical course of acute intestinal ischemia sufficiently severe to produce intestinal infarction is familiar to most surgeons. An elderly person complaining of severe abdominal pain is admitted to the hospital. Initially, there is a lack of accompanying physical findings, leading to an orderly diagnostic work-up. Within a few hours, the patient develops tachycardia, hypotension, acidosis, and marked abdominal tenderness, leading to emergency laparotomy. Extensive necrosis of the intestine is discovered. Despite treatment, the outcome is nearly always fatal. For the few patients who survive after extensive intestinal resection, a lifetime need for parenteral nutrition is nearly inescapable.

Although considerable advances have been made in the overall diagnosis and treatment of intestinal ischemia in the past several decades, as outlined in the other chapters of this section, the same cannot be said for the results of treatment of acute intestinal ischemia caused by arterial obstructions. Even the briefest literature review reveals prohibitive mortality rates, little changed from those of historical reports and averaging 75 to 80 per cent, as shown in Table 95–1.[1–8] The reason for this grim prognosis is found in the time course of the clinical signs of the disease. The

pain of intestinal ischemia is initially unaccompanied by physical signs, leading to an almost inevitable delay in diagnosis. By the time physical signs are prominent and the diagnosis of surgical abdominal disease becomes obvious, the pathology is typically so advanced that survival is doubtful. For the few patients fortunate enough to encounter an appropriately suspicious surgeon early, major abdominal arterial surgery in the emergency setting is required,

Table 95–1. Mortality Associated With Treatment of Acute Intestinal Ischemia From Arterial Obstructions

Study	No. of Patients	Mortality (%)
Ottinger and Austen, 1967[1]	51	43 (84)
Slater and Elliott, 1972[2]	4	4 (100)
Singh et al, 1975[3]	30	24 (81)
Smith and Patterson, 1976[4]	23	21 (91)
Kairaluoma et al, 1977[5]	44	31 (70)
Hertzer et al, 1978[6]	10	7 (70)
Sachs et al, 1982[7]	30	23 (77)
Levy et al, 1990[8]	45	20 (44)

often with the resection of various but significant lengths of bowel.

These considerations suggest that the mortality rate for patients with acute intestinal ischemia will probably always remain high. Nevertheless, there is potential for salvage with patients seen sufficiently early in the course of the disease and with those in whom the extent of the intestinal ischemia is limited. An approach to the management of such patients is the basis for this chapter. Systematic management of patients with acute intestinal ischemia caused by arterial obstructions requires the physician to confirm the diagnosis, determine the etiology and location of the arterial obstruction, and perform appropriate treatment. The acute nature of the disease process means that for the majority of patients, each of these steps will be conducted during the course of an operation.

CONFIRMATION OF THE DIAGNOSIS OF ACUTE INTESTINAL ISCHEMIA

The diagnosis of intestinal ischemia is discussed in detail in Chapter 94. With regard to acute intestinal ischemia, the factor most essential to correct diagnosis is a *high index of suspicion* on the part of the examining physician. The foundation of this suspicion is recognition of the pattern of presentation of acute intestinal ischemia. The clinical presentations of acute intestinal ischemia caused by venous disease and that resulting from nonocclusive causes are discussed in Chapters 96 and 97. Acute intestinal ischemia caused by arterial obstructions most often results from thrombosis or embolism of the superior mesenteric artery, each of which is briefly described. In a few patients with chronic occlusion or stenosis of the superior mesenteric artery, acute intestinal ischemia may result from occlusion of collaterals.

Large Artery Thrombosis

An unknown number of patients with severe stenosis of the superior mesenteric artery develop thrombosis of this vessel with resulting acute intestinal ischemia. The majority of these patients are elderly and female, have evidence of symptomatic vascular disease at other sites, and have often had previous vascular surgery. About one half have a history of chronic abdominal pain and weight loss suggestive of chronic visceral ischemia.[1-8] The occurrence of acute severe abdominal pain out of proportion to physical findings in such a patient is strongly suggestive of acute intestinal ischemia.

Intestinal Artery Embolism

In the past, most arterial emboli were cardiac in origin. About 5 per cent of cardiac emboli lodge within visceral vessels.[9] The likelihood of cardiac embolism to intestinal arteries should be considered when patients with known cardiac disease (e.g., atrial arrhythmias, cardiomyopathy,

acute myocardial infarction, and rheumatic valvular disease) experience the sudden onset of severe abdominal pain. The proportion of arterial emboli arising from the heart is decreasing in association with more widespread anticoagulant treatment of heart disease, especially atrial fibrillation, and the decrease in the prevalence of rheumatic heart disease. Proximal arterial sites have become an increasingly important source of emboli. Arterioarterial emboli can arise from ulcerated atherosclerotic plaques or from arterial aneurysms. A particularly important source of arterioarterial embolism has become diagnostic or interventional arteriographic catheter manipulation. The mechanism of embolism appears to be dislodgment of atherothrombotic material during the manipulation of guidewires and catheters within the arterial lumen. The clinical occurrence of severe abdominal pain after cardiac catheterization or other diagnostic or interventional proximal aortic arteriographic procedures should lead to an immediate consideration of intestinal ischemia resulting from intestinal artery embolism.

The Decision to Perform Arteriography

Although the diagnosis of acute intestinal ischemia caused by arterial obstructions is facilitated by arteriography, the treatment of intestinal ischemia is a true surgical emergency, and performing visceral arteriography typically requires several hours, hours that may be crucial to the successful treatment of a critically ill patient. The authors obtain arteriograms for patients suspected of having intestinal ischemia based on the presence of *pain alone* in the typical clinical setting. In these patients, a diagnosis is necessary because pain alone is usually not an indication for surgery. For patients with typical pain and physical findings such as rebound tenderness or abdominal rigidity clearly indicating the need for operation, arteriography is contraindicated. A typical arteriogram obtained from a patient with acute intestinal ischemia caused by superior mesenteric artery thrombosis is seen in Figure 95–1. Because the arteriosclerotic stenosis causing the thrombosis is almost always located at or near the origin of the artery, the entire superior mesenteric artery fails to visualize. An arteriogram from a patient with superior mesenteric artery embolism is seen in Figure 95–2. The vessel is occluded beyond the origin of several proximal branches, there is a sharp cutoff of a normal-appearing artery, and thrombus is visible at the site of the occlusion, all of which are angiographic signs of embolism.

INTERVENTIONAL ARTERIOGRAPHIC TREATMENT OF ACUTE INTESTINAL ISCHEMIA

Acute intestinal ischemia from arterial obstruction is usually caused by localized arterial thrombus or by localized atherosclerotic stenosis. It thus appears reasonable to consider the potential roles of thrombolytic treatment, bal-

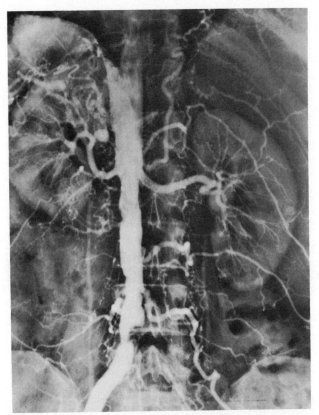

FIGURE 95-1. Aortogram from a patient with acute intestinal ischemia caused by superior mesenteric artery thrombosis. Note the complete absence of filling of any intestinal arteries, as well as evidence of severe arterial disease in the aorta and the iliac arteries.

loon angioplasty, or both as definitive treatments. This may be especially true in patients undergoing arteriography in whom the arterial occlusion causing acute intestinal ischemia has just been visualized. To date, to the authors' knowledge, the successful use of interventional arteriographic treatment of acute intestinal ischemia has not been reported. The obvious reason is that the extent and degree of intestinal ischemia cannot be predicted from the physical examination or from any known laboratory or diagnostic test short of laparotomy. Although thrombolytic or catheter interventional therapy may restore arterial vascular supply to ischemic intestine, most patients with acute intestinal ischemia have at least some intestine that is frankly necrotic at the time of diagnosis. If resection of this portion of intestine is delayed until the need for the procedure becomes obvious after initial attempts at nonoperative therapy, the outcome is predictably fatal. The only hope for survival for patients with acute intestinal ischemia lies in immediate revascularization of intestine that has the potential to recover and resection of the remainder. To date, this objective has been achieved only through operation.

OPERATIVE TREATMENT OF ACUTE INTESTINAL ISCHEMIA

Findings at Operation

At laparotomy, the etiology and appropriate treatment of intestinal ischemia are determined by the appearance of

the intestines and the status of the circulation in the superior mesenteric artery. Acutely ischemic bowel that is not yet necrotic may be deceptively normal in appearance. The physical appearance of ischemic intestine includes loss of normal sheen, dull-gray discoloration (which may be especially difficult to detect if global), and lack of peristalsis. These subjective signs may be overlooked. Objective signs of intestinal ischemia include absence of palpable pulse in the proximal superior mesenteric artery, lack of visible pulsations in mesenteric arcade vessels, and absence of pulsatile flow detected by Doppler examination of these vessels and of the intestine itself. Fluid is present within the abdomen in advanced cases, and it may be foul smelling even in the absence of intestinal perforation.

The distribution of the ischemic intestine provides important information about the cause of ischemia (Fig. 95–3).[10] In superior mesenteric artery thrombosis, the small intestine is usually ischemic throughout its length, with sparing of only the stomach and duodenum and the distal portion of the colon. In embolic occlusions of the superior mesenteric artery, the proximal jejunum frequently remains normal, reflecting the propensity of cardiac emboli to lodge beyond the first few branches of the superior mesenteric artery. Arterioarterial embolism may produce a patchy distribution of ischemia, with multiple areas of involvement and skipped sections of normal-appearing intestine.

The plan for operative treatment is based on these findings. Regardless of the etiology of ischemia, the goals of therapy are assurance of normal pulsatile flow to the superior mesenteric artery, restoration of adequate arterial inflow to ischemic but viable intestine, and resection of nonviable intestine. These steps in treatment are discussed in the following sections.

Revascularization of Acutely Ischemic Intestine

In patients with advanced intestinal ischemia, bowel necrosis may be widespread and obvious. The systemic

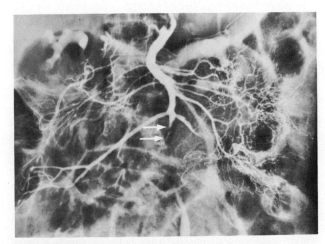

FIGURE 95-2. Selective arteriogram of the superior mesenteric artery in a patient with embolism. Note the patent proximal branches, the sharp cutoff at the site of the occlusion, and the visible thrombus *(arrows)* at the site of the occlusion.

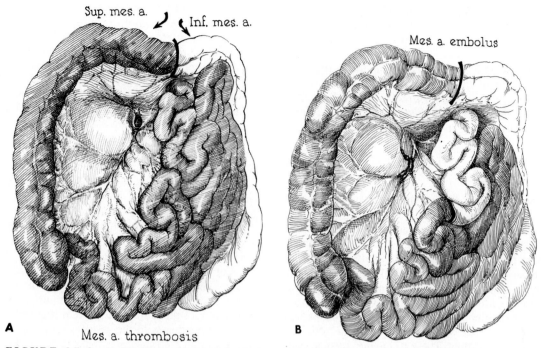

FIGURE 95–3. *A,* Distribution of intestinal ischemia with superior mesenteric artery thrombosis. The entire small bowel and the proximal colon are ischemic. *B,* Distribution of intestinal ischemia with superior mesenteric artery embolism. The proximal jejunum is spared. (*A* and *B,* From Bergan JJ: Recognition and treatment of intestinal ischemia. Surg Clin North Am 47:109, 1967.)

effects of such a lesion are catastrophic and rapidly fatal. This means that most patients undergoing surgery for intestinal ischemia are in an earlier stage of the evolution of necrosis and at least a portion of the bowel is of questionable viability. This has important implications for treatment. It is not possible to predict accurately the potential for revascularization to restore viability to ischemic-appearing intestine. This means that except in the most advanced cases, *revascularization should precede resection.* Restoration of pulsatile flow to the superior mesenteric artery may produce a remarkable change in bowel that appeared hopelessly ischemic at first inspection. One of two techniques is used: mesenteric artery embolectomy or intestinal artery bypass. The choice of technique depends on the cause of the ischemia.

Superior Mesenteric Artery Embolectomy

For embolectomy, the superior mesenteric artery is exposed from within the abdomen, at the base of the junction of the small bowel and transverse colon mesenteries, just as it emerges from beneath the inferior border of the pancreas. At this point, the artery has several major branches, each of which should be carefully exposed and isolated. The authors prefer to open the artery with a longitudinal incision because its size in most persons prevents adequate visualization of the lumen through a transverse incision. Proximal embolectomy is performed with a balloon catheter (size 3 or 4 Fr). Failure to establish copious pulsatile inflow from the aorta should lead to a diagnosis of mesenteric artery thrombosis and the performance of a bypass procedure as described in the next section. Distal em-

bolectomy of the superior mesenteric artery and its branches is difficult because of the size of the vessels, their fragility, and their multiplicity. The authors believe it is best performed with a size 2 Fr balloon catheter, and the technique must be quite gentle in comparison to that used in the less fragile arteries of the extremities. Once all possible thrombus has been removed, the arteriotomy is closed with a patch of autogenous vein. If adequate pulsatile inflow cannot be restored, the arteriotomy becomes the site of anastomosis for a bypass graft.

Superior Mesenteric Artery Bypass

For patients with mesenteric artery thrombosis seen early in whom the entire intestine appears salvageable by revascularization, the technique of superior mesenteric artery bypass using a prosthetic graft described in Chapter 98 is used to restore arterial flow. In some patients, this degree of intestinal ischemia will be accompanied by the presence of a foul smell within the abdomen in the absence of intestinal perforation or of obvious intestinal necrosis. This finding is not a contraindication to performing a prosthetic bypass.

In the majority of patients with acute intestinal ischemia from mesenteric artery thrombosis, at least some of the intestine is obviously necrotic, requiring resection, and in some patients perforation will have occurred. For these patients, the authors believe that prosthetic bypass is contraindicated. In this situation, they prefer to perform a bypass to the superior mesenteric artery using the proximal greater saphenous vein in reversed fashion, with the graft configuration exactly as described for prosthetic bypass in

Chapter 98. The authors' first choice is retrograde bypass from the infrarenal aorta. If this vessel is severely diseased, antegrade bypass from the supraceliac aorta is performed with saphenous vein.

For patients with arterioarterial embolism, the very small particle size of the embolic material means that a number of emboli lodge in peripheral arteries. Embolectomy is usually not possible, and bypass beyond the point of embolic obstruction is also not possible. For these patients, resection of nonviable intestine is the only practical operative therapy.

Determination of Intestinal Viability

Once revascularization has been completed, the need for intestinal resection must be determined. In early cases, restoration of pulsatile flow may be the only therapy necessary. In most, however, the bowel will contain obviously necrotic areas, obviously viable areas, and areas of questionable viability. Multiple techniques have been proposed to aid in differentiating bowel that will remain viable and recover from bowel that will become frankly necrotic despite the restoration of flow. These techniques include clinical judgment based on inspection and palpation, the use of Doppler ultrasound, the administration of intravenous fluorescein, infrared photoplethysmography, surface oximetry, and laser Doppler velocimetry.

Clinical inspection of viable intestine reveals visible pulsations in the mesenteric arcade vessels, bleeding from cut surfaces, a normal color, and peristaltic motions. None of these criteria is absolute, all are inherently subjective, and none is easily quantitated. Despite this, clinical inspection by experienced surgeons enables viable bowel to be distinguished from nonviable bowel in a large majority of cases. In the prospective study reported on by Bulkley and associates, this method had a sensitivity of 82 per cent and a specificity of 91 per cent.[11]

The use of a sterilized, continuous-wave Doppler ultrasound flow detector (9 to 10 MHz) for determining intestinal viability was first reported in a canine model by Wright and Hobson.[12] With this method, pulsatile Doppler signals are sought on the intestinal surface. Segments with absent signals are deemed nonviable. Successful clinical use of this method has been reported in humans.[13, 14] This method has the distinct advantage of using instrumentation that is available sterile in most vascular surgery operating rooms.

With the fluorescein fluorescence method, 10 to 15 ml/kg of fluorescein is injected intravenously, and the intestine is inspected using Wood's lamp. A complete absence of fluorescence is diagnostic of nonviability, whereas rapid, confluent, bright fluorescence is diagnostic of viability. There is a large area between these two extremes, however, and interpretation of the pattern and intensity of fluorescence is inherently subjective. Carter and coworkers described the use of a quantitative method of fluorescein testing using a perfusion fluorometer.[15] In their experimental setting, the quantitative method had a sensitivity and specificity of 100 per cent for detecting nonviable segments of intestine, compared with a sensitivity of 11 per cent and a specificity of 100 per cent for qualitative visual inspection.

The requirement for special equipment and the possibility of serious allergic reactions resulting from the injection of this medication into patients who are already critically ill are significant drawbacks to the clinical use of this method.

Locke and colleagues used surface oximetry and demonstrated in a canine model that abnormal Po_2 values from intestine with various degrees of ischemia were predictive of failure of anastomotic healing.[16] The feasibility of this method for detecting nonviable segments of bowel using simpler equipment (the pulse oximeter) was demonstrated in dogs by Ferrara and associates[17] and by DeNobile and coworkers.[18]

Infrared photoplethysmography uses a small probe to detect changes in tissue blood volume resulting from changes in reflected infrared light. Sensitivity and specificity for this method comparable to those achieved with Doppler ultrasound and with the fluorescein method were demonstrated by Pearce and colleagues.[19]

Yet another method with experimental success in detecting ischemic intestinal segments was demonstrated by Oohata and coworkers.[20] These authors used laser Doppler velocimetry of the surface of the intestine and showed excellent correlation with the results of hydrogen gas clearance testing in the same intestinal segments. The hydrogen gas method, an extremely accurate method of quantifying blood flow in the intestine, is not applicable in the clinical setting.

To date, only one study has evaluated various methods of determining intestinal viability in prospective, controlled fashion.[11] Bulkley and associates compared clinical judgment, Doppler ultrasound, and fluorescein injection in 78 intestinal segments of 28 consecutive patients with intestinal ischemia. The results of this study are seen in Table 95–2. Interestingly, standard clinical judgment proved to be very reliable, at least as reliable as the other two methods. Although these authors found perfect reliability for the fluorescein method, this has not been duplicated by other investigators.

Whitehill and colleagues provided some explanation for why the various techniques for determining bowel viability are less than perfect.[21] These authors evaluated Doppler ultrasound, photoplethysmography, and fluorescein injection and discovered that each was capable of detecting intestinal blood flow at levels below the minimum required for viability. This means that each method has the potential for false-negative testing—the most dangerous incorrect result for patients.

Given the vagaries of these methods and the documented high reliability of clinical judgment, the authors of

Table 95–2.   Diagnostic Ability of Reported Techniques for Determining the Viability of Acutely Ischemic Intestine

Technique	Sensitivity (%)	Specificity (%)	Accuracy (%)
Clinical judgment	82	91	89
Fluorescein injection (qualitative)	100	100	100
Doppler ultrasound	63	88	84

Adapted from Bulkley GB, Zuidema GD, Hamilton SR, et al: Intraoperative determination of small intestinal viability following ischemic injury. Ann Surg 193:628, 1981.

this chapter rely on a combination of clinical judgment and Doppler ultrasound to determine intestinal viability. This choice is based on the lack of documented superiority of any method and on the ready availability of sterile Doppler probes in the authors' operating room. In deciding which bowel to resect, the choices are clearly influenced by the length of the obviously viable segment remaining. If this segment is large and is clearly adequate for life (more than 6 feet of small intestine), the resection of remaining bowel should be quite liberal, with removal of any questionably viable segments. If the length of obviously viable bowel is quite limited, however, the resection of questionably viable segments should be deferred to a "second-look" operation. Resection of multiple segments of necrotic bowel separated by skipped areas of normal viability is appropriate if the overall remaining bowel is limited, even if this means that multiple anastomoses will be required.

The authors' preference for treatment of the remaining bowel is to perform anastomoses to restore bowel continuity. The reasons for this preference are that segments of intestine used for stomas are rarely functional in an absorptive capacity, additional bowel is invariably lost during reanastomosis, and the stoma segment is more ischemic than adjacent bowel by virtue of detachment from the mesentery, compression by the body wall, and so on.

Second-Look Surgery

Because it is usually advisable to avoid resection of questionably viable bowel at the time of the initial operation, second-look operations are frequently performed after revascularization for acute intestinal ischemia. The decision to perform such surgery must be made at the time of the original operation, and the second procedure must be performed as planned *regardless of the condition of the patient.* The desperate condition of patients with severe acute intestinal ischemia may deceptively and dramatically improve after resection of the majority of ischemic bowel. Despite this, a small segment of remaining necrotic bowel will ultimately prove just as fatal as the original large segment if it is not detected and treated. At the second-look operation, performed 18 to 36 hours after the first, any remaining nonviable bowel is resected, the integrity of vascular repairs is ensured, and the anastomoses are checked. In some cases, especially when precarious anastomoses are made in revascularized intestine, the authors have used a "third-look" procedure 4 to 6 days after the first procedure, the intent of which is to detect and treat any anastomotic leaks before the occurrence of peritonitis and sepsis.

PERIOPERATIVE CARE OF PATIENTS WITH ACUTE INTESTINAL ISCHEMIA

Acute intestinal ischemia is a life-threatening condition that most frequently affects elderly patients with serious underlying medical conditions. The only hope such patients have for survival lies in the skilled performance of early surgery to revascularize ischemic intestine and resect nonviable segments. Both the ischemic intestine and the surgical treatment required contribute to major hemodynamic instability and dysfunction of multiple organ systems. The most intensive care possible, including full hemodynamic monitoring, is required for maximal safety.

If patients recover from the acute illness and surgery, prolonged parenteral nutrition is an integral part of postoperative management. There is frequently severe ischemic damage to the remaining viable intestine, and motility and absorptive function may be compromised, requiring a prolonged recovery period that may extend for months. In the authors' experience, most patients do not require lifelong parenteral nutrition if the remaining small bowel is at least a few feet in length and has been revascularized.

SUMMARY

This chapter emphasizes that acute intestinal ischemia caused by arterial obstructions is associated with a very high patient mortality rate because severe symptoms occur only when disease is advanced and because the patient population affected is often elderly, with preexisting multisystem disease. Early diagnosis based on a high index of suspicion is the key to achieving survival in some patients seen early in the course of the disease. The differences between arterial thrombosis and arterial embolism are described, as each has a different treatment, and the steps in operative therapy are described in some detail, with an emphasis on revascularization of intestine, resection of necrotic bowel, and second-look surgery to determine the viability of questionable segments. The importance of intensive perioperative care using hemodynamic monitoring and parenteral nutrition is also emphasized. With the use of these principles, it should be possible to achieve survival in some patients with acute intestinal ischemia who are seen sufficiently early in the course of disease that some viable small bowel remains.

References

1. Ottinger L, Austen WG: A study of 136 patients with mesenteric infarction. Surg Gynecol Obstet 124:1251, 1967.
2. Slater H, Elliott PW: Primary mesenteric infarction. Am J Surg 123:309, 1972.
3. Singh RP, Shah RC, Lee ST: Acute mesenteric vascular occlusion: A review of thirty-two patients. Surgery 78:613, 1975.
4. Smith JS Jr, Patterson LT: Acute mesenteric infarction. Am Surg 42:562, 1976.
5. Kairaluoma MI, Karkola P, Heikkinen E, et al: Mesenteric infarction. Am J Surg 133:188, 1977.
6. Hertzer NR, Beven EG, Humphries AW: Acute intestinal ischemia. Am Surg 44:744, 1978.
7. Sachs SM, Morton JH, Schwartz SI: Acute mesenteric ischemia. Surgery 92:646, 1982.
8. Levy PJ, Krausz MM, Manny J: Acute mesenteric ischemia: Improved results—A retrospective analysis of ninety-two patients. Surgery 107:372, 1990.
9. Elliott JP Jr, Hageman JH, Szilagyi E, et al: Arterial embolization: Problems of source, multiplicity, recurrence, and delayed treatment. Surgery 88:833, 1980.
10. Bergan JJ: Recognition and treatment of intestinal ischemia. Surg Clin North Am 47:109, 1967.
11. Bulkley GB, Zuidema GD, Hamilton SR, et al: Intraoperative determination of small intestinal viability following ischemic injury. Ann Surg 193:628, 1981.
12. Wright CB, Hobson RW: Prediction of intestinal viability using Doppler ultrasound technique. Am J Surg 129:642, 1975.

13. O'Donnell JA, Hobson RW: Operative confirmation of Doppler ultrasound evaluation of intestinal ischemia. Surgery 87:109, 1980.
14. Cooperman M, Paca WG, Martin EW, et al: Determination of viability of ischemic intestine by Doppler ultrasound. Surgery 83:705, 1978.
15. Carter MS, Fantini GA, Sammartano RJ, et al: Qualitative and quantitative fluorescein fluorescence in determining intestinal viability. Am J Surg 147:117, 1984.
16. Locke R, Hauser CJ, Shoemaker WC: The use of surface oximetry to assess bowel viability. Arch Surg 119:1252, 1984.
17. Ferrara J, Dyess D, Lasecki M, et al: Surface oximetry: A new method to evaluate intestinal perfusion. Am Surg 54:10, 1988.
18. DeNobile J, Guzzetta P, Patterson K: Pulse oximetry as a means of assessing bowel viability. J Surg Res 48:21, 1990.
19. Pearce WH, Jones DN, Warren GH, et al: The use of infrared photoplethysmography in identifying early intestinal ischemia. Arch Surg 122:108, 1987.
20. Oohata Y, Mibu R, Hotokezaka M, et al: Comparison of blood flow assessment between laser Doppler velocimetry and the hydrogen gas clearance method in ischemic intestine in dogs. Am J Surg 160:511, 1990.
21. Whitehill TA, Pearce WH, Rosales C, et al: Detection thresholds of nonocclusive intestinal hypoperfusion by Doppler ultrasound, photoplethysmography, and fluorescein. J Vasc Surg 8:28, 1988.

96

Nonocclusive Mesenteric Ischemia

Steven P. Rivers, M.D., and Frank J. Veith, M.D.

• • •

Although embolic or thrombotic obstruction of the arterial or venous circulation is the usual source of acute mesenteric vascular insufficiency, intestinal ischemia also occurs in the absence of mechanical vascular obstruction. The most frequent clinical setting producing nonocclusive mesenteric ischemia is severe systemic illness with circulatory insufficiency and end-organ shock.[1, 2] In this setting, the cause of the ischemia that occurs has been demonstrated to be severe and prolonged visceral arterial vasospasm, frequently resulting in intestinal necrosis. Severe intestinal arterial vasospasm also occurs in response to drug intoxication, as with cocaine and ergot derivatives, and after repair of aortic coarctations. Each of these conditions is described in this chapter.

The true prevalence of nonocclusive mesenteric ischemia is unknown because mesenteric ischemia without infarction undoubtedly occurs and resolves in some patients in whom the diagnosis is never confirmed. At the authors' institution, a policy of liberal use of angiography for all suspected cases of intestinal ischemia has produced a large number of arteriograms for review. On the basis of this experience, it is estimated that nonocclusive mesenteric ischemia is currently responsible for 20 per cent of all cases of splanchnic vascular insufficiency (Fig. 96–1). This incidence is lower than that previously reported by others,[3] when nonocclusive mesenteric ischemia was responsible for approximately 50 per cent of mesenteric infarctions. In the authors' opinion, this declining incidence has resulted directly from improved treatment of critically ill patients in the intensive care setting. Specifically, the widespread use of invasive hemodynamic monitoring and a shift in emphasis from the use of peripheral vasoconstrictors to the use of peripheral vasodilatation for the treatment of refractory congestive heart failure and cardiogenic shock are probably responsible for much of the decline in the prevalence of nonocclusive mesenteric ischemia.

PATHOPHYSIOLOGY

Mesenteric vasoconstriction occurs normally in response to both normovolemic and hypovolemic shock states and may persist for several hours after the reversal of all other manifestations of shock.[4] Intestinal mucosal permeability increases in direct proportion to the duration and severity of the vascular insult, although greater permeability is found with total occlusion than with a low but persistent flow of blood.[5] In the normal setting, the increasing local ischemia resulting from this vasoconstriction eventually leads to vasodilatation and restoration of adequate blood flow before the occurrence of necrosis. The specific reasons this sequence does not occur in some cases of shock have been difficult to ascertain. Angiographically demonstrated hypoperfusion from vasospasm does not always result in mucosal damage and has in fact been shown to correlate poorly with histologic evidence of ischemia in a dog model.[6] It has been suggested that autoregulatory vasodilatation, which usually results from local ischemia, requires a normal perfusion pressure,[7] a circumstance not usually present in the standard clinical setting for nonocclusive mesenteric ischemia. This may explain the failure of normal autoregulation to permit reperfusion before the occurrence of intestinal necrosis in the shock setting. In patients with cocaine or ergot poisoning, the mechanism of persistent vasospasm due to the persistence of extrinsic vasoconstrictor overriding local autoregulatory control seems clear. Whether the mechanism is centrally mediated decreased perfusion, as occurs with shock; locally induced vasospasm,

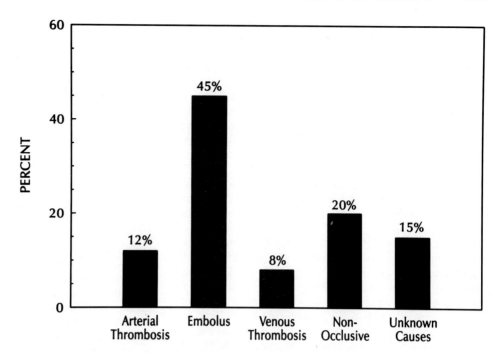

FIGURE 96-1. Etiology of mesenteric ischemia, 1980 to 1990. (From Rivers S: Acute nonocclusive mesenteric ischemia. Semin Vasc Surg 3:172, 1990.)

as occurs with drug intoxication; or a combination of the two, as occurs when shock is treated with vasoconstrictors, it is clear that vasoconstriction is the source of the ischemia sufficient to produce intestinal necrosis in patients with nonocclusive mesenteric ischemia.

Interestingly, the renin-angiotensin axis appears to be an important mediator of vasospasm in nonocclusive mesenteric ischemia. Experimentally, bilateral nephrectomy or the administration of angiotensin-converting enzyme inhibitors before the onset of shock will alleviate the ischemic response in the visceral circulation. Surprisingly, blockade of the alpha-adrenergic system before an episode of hypoperfusion does not seem to alter the incidence or severity of nonocclusive mesenteric ischemia.[8, 9]

The etiology of mesenteric ischemia may be multifactorial in some patients in whom no single lesion would be sufficient to cause symptoms. For example, patients with intestinal distention, previously asymptomatic proximal mesenteric artery stenoses, or both may develop intestinal ischemia and necrosis when a systemic low-flow state is superimposed.[10, 11]

PRESENTATION

Nonocclusive mesenteric ischemia appears in clinical settings in which severe, often multi-systemic illnesses result in low-flow states and visceral vasoconstriction. Congestive heart failure, with or without other manifestations of cardiogenic shock, is by far the most frequent isolated etiology. Sepsis, dehydration, and renal or hepatic disease may occasionally be sufficiently severe to produce the necessary low-flow state and splanchnic vasospasm, but nonocclusive mesenteric ischemia is rarely seen in the absence of significant, clinically apparent cardiac dysfunction, vasoconstrictor drug administration (including self-administration), or both.

The signs and symptoms of nonocclusive mesenteric ischemia are similar to those of other forms of acute intestinal ischemia. Abdominal pain is the most common symptom, noted in at least 75 per cent of patients. However, pain may be undetected or unreported in the critically ill patient. For this reason, a high index of suspicion is required for the diagnosis of nonocclusive mesenteric ischemia when isolated findings such as abdominal distention, gastrointestinal bleeding, fever, or leukocytosis occur in the appropriate clinical setting. Mild cases of nonocclusive mesenteric ischemia that are never clearly diagnosed probably occur frequently. These cases present as localized or intermittent abdominal pain secondary to fluctuating local perfusion, and they resolve spontaneously as the overall condition improves. The presentation of severe cases with impending or actual intestinal necrosis is indistinguishable from the presentations of the other types of acute mesenteric ischemia discussed in Chapters 95, 97, and 98.

Postcoarctectomy Syndrome

Nonocclusive mesenteric ischemia has been reported in as many as 4 per cent of patients after repair of an aortic coarctation.[12] The syndrome is thought to be related to the paradoxical postoperative hypertension seen in many patients, with the sudden increase in pressure below the coarctation causing a necrotizing vasculitis of the mesenteric vessels.[13] Angiographic studies demonstrate mesenteric arterial spasm, which rapidly reverses in response to local intra-arterial papaverine infusion or treatment of hypertension with systemic vasodilating agents.[13] The problem occurs more frequently in the youngest patients[12, 14] and is one reason surgery is usually postponed whenever possible until the child reaches 3 to 5 years of age.

Drug-Induced Mesenteric Ischemia

Digoxin and vasopressor agents used to treat patients with multi–organ system failure have also been implicated in the development of nonocclusive mesenteric ischemia. In therapeutic doses, these medications do not usually cause significant intestinal ischemia. However, their vasoconstrictive effect on the splanchnic circulation undoubtedly contributes to the development of mesenteric ischemia in patients already suffering from a low-flow situation. The shift away from the use of these medications and the corresponding decrease in the incidence of nonocclusive mesenteric ischemia provide strong evidence of the contributory role of these medications.

Otherwise healthy patients may rarely develop nonocclusive mesenteric ischemia from ergot poisoning or cocaine abuse,[15, 16] and in this setting, abdominal pain and intestinal ischemia may be the presenting symptoms of these drug intoxications. The vasoactive properties of the various ergot alkaloids differ in intensity. Ergonovine has only a slight vasoconstrictive effect, dihydroergotamine has a much more active one, and ergotamine tartrate has the most severely vasoconstrictive effect.[17] The diagnosis of ergot-induced mesenteric ischemia is not difficult because ergotism today is almost entirely the result of the medicinal use of ergot alkaloids for migraine headaches. Cocaine poisoning may be somewhat more difficult to establish if the history of ingestion is withheld.

DIAGNOSIS

Certain confirmation of the diagnosis of nonocclusive mesenteric ischemia would require actual observation of ischemic bowel in the absence of any organic vascular occlusion. In practice, the angiographic demonstration of intestinal arterial vasospasm in symptomatic patients at risk is acceptable for diagnosis. The radiologic signs of splanchnic arterial vasoconstriction include narrowed origins of major branches of the superior mesenteric artery; beading, tapering, or segmental narrowing of intestinal branches; spasm of intestinal arcades; and reduced or absent filling of intramural vessels.[18] The arteriographic findings are similar for any etiology of nonocclusive mesenteric ischemia; they are relatively specific only for the complication of mesenteric insufficiency.

In symptomatic patients at risk for nonocclusive mesenteric ischemia, plain abdominal radiographs are obtained first to rule out other causes of abdominal pain. Aortography and selective mesenteric arteriography may then be performed. On completion of the study, the catheter can be secured in place with the tip in the orifice of the superior mesenteric artery for subsequent papaverine infusion. This technique is useful even for patients requiring surgery for thrombotic or embolic occlusions because postoperative vasospasm may still occur.

A critical issue in patients with suspected intestinal ischemia and possible infarction is the requisite delay in operative intervention imposed by angiography. In the authors' opinion, the decision to perform arteriography or to proceed directly to surgery should be individualized. Patients with mild or intermittent abdominal pain thought to be ischemic in nature might not require angiography at all. Prompt correction of the low-flow state and bowel decompression may resolve the problem and eliminate the need for invasive studies. At the other end of the clinical spectrum, patients with peritoneal signs and a high probability of intestinal infarction can ill afford a significant delay in laparotomy. Even in the most well prepared centers, the transport of an intensive care unit patient with infusion pumps, monitors, and respirators and the need for selective and biplane angiography will be time consuming and risk further intestinal necrosis or acidosis.

Nevertheless, arteriography is clearly a useful diagnostic tool and should be considered whenever feasible. Of the first 50 patients with suspected acute mesenteric ischemia examined angiographically at the authors' institution, the diagnosis was confirmed in 35 patients (70 per cent), 15 of whom had nonocclusive mesenteric ischemia. Of the 15 patients with other causes of abdominal pain, arteriography facilitated the correct diagnosis in 8.[19] Furthermore, some patients with early signs of peritoneal irritation will show improvement after the institution of intra-arterial papaverine therapy and will be able to avoid laparotomy. Only patients with physical findings that mandate urgent exploration should forego this critical study. After thrombectomy, resection of gangrenous bowel, or both, adjunctive vasodilator therapy can be initiated intraoperatively or postoperatively.

Several interesting new diagnostic approaches developed to address the risks and limitations of angiography are currently being evaluated. These include duplex scanning,[20, 21] phosphorus magnetic resonance imaging,[22] radiolabeled leukocyte scintigraphy,[23] and intraperitoneal xenon injection.[24] At present, none is sufficiently developed to replace angiography. The more direct approach of diagnostic laparoscopy has also been proposed for patients for whom arteriography is unsuitable.[25] However, this approach detects only grossly ischemic bowel and has no therapeutic ability. Furthermore, the attendant increase in intraperitoneal pressure risks a further decrease in mesenteric blood flow.[26]

TREATMENT

In contrast to the reversal of intestinal ischemia caused by mesenteric arterial occlusions, the reversal of nonocclusive mesenteric ischemia essentially depends on nonoperative methods of increasing mesenteric blood flow. Measures such as pulmonary artery catheterization to optimize fluid therapy and improve cardiac output, the reduction or elimination of digitalis or vasopressor agents, and the management of cardiogenic shock with vasodilators have all contributed to both prevention and treatment of nonocclusive mesenteric ischemia. In particular, agents such as captopril are valuable because of the sensitivity of the mesenteric vasculature to the renin-angiotensin axis.

Treatment of the underlying disease process is also critical for patients with a noncardiac source of nonocclusive mesenteric ischemia. Patients with postcoarctectomy syndrome should respond to prompt and adequate control of postoperative hypertension. Although the treatment of

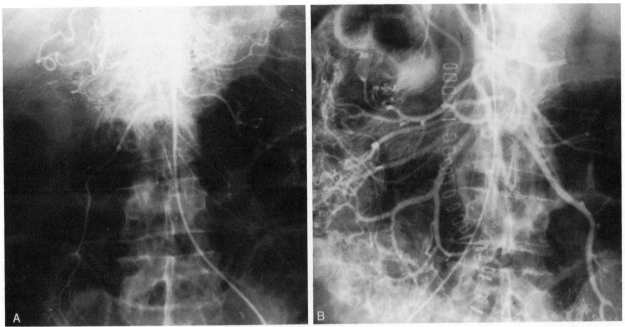

FIGURE 96–2. *A,* Nonocclusive mesenteric ischemia diagnosed arteriographically. There is diffuse spasm of the intestinal arcades with poor filling of intramural vessels. *B,* Relief of spasm and filling of distal vessels are observed after several hours of intra-arterial papaverine infusion. A laparotomy was performed for early peritoneal irritation, but no resection was required after the initiation of vasodilator therapy. (*A* and *B,* From Rivers S: Acute nonocclusive mesenteric ischemia. Semin Vasc Surg 3:172, 1990.)

cocaine and ergot poisoning is not significantly different from that of the usual nonocclusive mesenteric ischemia in patients with multi–organ system failure, the response of patients with ergotism to vasodilators or sympatholytic drugs is noteworthy because experimental attempts to displace ergotamine from alpha-receptors have not been successful. In this setting, the adjunctive use of anticoagulants has been recommended.[17]

Direct superior mesenteric artery infusion of vasodilators has been recommended for the optimal management of nonocclusive mesenteric ischemia. Although the effectiveness of this therapy has been difficult to confirm experimentally and clinically, papaverine is unequivocally able to reverse mesenteric artery vasoconstriction, even in low-flow states.[18] The relative contribution of intra-arterial infusion to ultimate patient outcome is hard to assess because treatment of the underlying shock state occurs simultaneously. The most impressive clinical data come from the observation of affected patients with severe abdominal pain and vasospasm whose symptoms and angiographic abnormalities resolve within hours of intra-arterial papaverine infusion (Fig. 96–2). Direct mesenteric drug administration should clearly be regarded as complementary to, rather than competitive with, systemic correction of hypoperfusion.

The authors' protocol for papaverine administration involves a constant infusion of 30 to 60 mg/hr directly into the superior mesenteric artery as soon as the diagnostic study is completed. The infusion is continued for at least 24 hours, after which arteriography is repeated. Obviously, patient physical findings are also closely monitored throughout the treatment period. Additional 24-hour treatment intervals are determined by the clinical and radiologic reassessment. However, most favorable responses will oc-

cur within the first 24 hours. As an adjunct to laparotomy for mesenteric thrombosis or bowel resection, the infusion may be continued during and after surgery to maximize the perfusion of ischemic but viable segments of intestine. Although other medications such as nitroglycerine, tolazoline, and prostaglandin E_1 would logically be expected to produce similar results, most of the clinical experience has been obtained with papaverine.

A new approach to the treatment of intestinal ischemia uses intraluminal instillation of oxygenated perfluorocarbons.[27, 28] Although the concept is intriguing, its clinical application has not yet been established.

The role of surgical treatment in nonocclusive mesenteric ischemia is limited to identification and resection of nonviable segments of bowel. Initial resection should be limited to clearly gangrenous segments because vasodilator therapy and treatment of the underlying disease may improve areas of uncertain viability.

The survival of patients with an established diagnosis of nonocclusive mesenteric ischemia has been reported to be as low as 0 to 29 per cent, with or without papaverine infusion.[29–31] The results in the authors' institution have been somewhat better, probably because of an aggressive posture regarding early angiography of high-risk patients. The cause of death in most cases is irreversible shock or advanced intestinal necrosis at the time of diagnosis. The high mortality rate is a reflection of the seriousness of the underlying diseases and of the failure to recognize nonocclusive mesenteric ischemia in its earlier, treatable phase. Beneficial measures such as intra-arterial papaverine infusion directed toward specific end-organ damage remain entirely appropriate and are probably effective, despite the generally high mortality.

Acknowledgment: *This chapter was supported in part by the Manning Foundation, the Anna S. Brown Trust, and the New York Institute for Vascular Studies.*

References

1. Wilson R, Qualheim RD: A form of acute hemorrhagic enterocolitis affecting chronically ill individuals. A description of twenty cases. Gastroenterology 27:431, 1954.
2. Ende N: Infarction of the bowel in cardiac failure. N Engl J Med 258:879, 1958.
3. Ottinger LW, Austen WG: A study of 136 patients with mesenteric infarction. Surg Gynecol Obstet 124:251, 1967.
4. Boley SJ, Regan JA, Tunick PA, et al: Persistent vasoconstriction—A major factor in nonocclusive intestinal ischemic injury. Curr Top Surg Res 3:435, 1971.
5. Parks DA, Grogaard B, Granger DN: Comparison of partial and complete arterial occlusion models for studying intestinal ischemia. Surgery 92:896, 1982.
6. Bookstein JJ, Goldberger L, Niwayama G, et al: Angiographic aspects of experimental nonocclusive intestinal ischemic injury. Am J Roentgenol 128:923, 1971.
7. Mellander S, Johansson B: Control of resistance, exchange, and capacitance functions in the peripheral circulation. Pharmacol Rev 20:117, 1968.
8. Bailey RW, Bulkley GB, Hamilton SR, et al: Protection of the small intestine from nonocclusive mesenteric ischemic injury due to cardiogenic shock. Am J Surg 153:108, 1987.
9. Bailey RW, Hamilton SR, Morris JB, et al: Pathogenesis of nonocclusive ischemic colitis. Am Surg 203:590, 1986.
10. Boley SJ, Agarwal GP, Warren AR, et al: Pathophysiologic effects of bowel distension on intestinal blood flow. Am J Surg 117:228, 1969.
11. Russ JE, Haid SP, Yao JST, et al: Surgical treatment of nonocclusive mesenteric infarction. Am J Surg 134:38, 1977.
12. Cheatham JE Jr, Williams GR, Thompson WM, et al: Coarctation: A review of 80 children and adolescents. Am J Surg 138:889, 1979.
13. Kawauchi M, Tada Y, Asano K, et al: Angiographic demonstration of mesenteric arterial changes in postcoartectomy syndrome. Surgery 98:602, 1985.
14. Behl PR, Sante P, Blesovsky A: Isolated coarctation of the aorta: Surgical treatment and late results. Eighteen years' experience. J Cardiovasc Surg 29:509, 1988.
15. Greene FL, Ariyan S, Stansel HC Jr: Mesenteric and peripheral vascular ischemia secondary to ergotism. Surgery 81:176, 1977.
16. Nalbandian H, Sheth N, Dietrich R, et al: Intestinal ischemia caused by cocaine ingestion: Report of two cases. Surgery 97:374, 1985.
17. Merhoff GC, Porter JM: Ergot intoxication: Historical review and description of unusual clinical manifestations. Ann Surg 180:773, 1974.
18. Siegelman SS, Sprayregan S, Boley SJ: Angiographic diagnosis of mesenteric arterial vasoconstriction. Diagn Radiol 112:533, 1974.
19. Boley SJ, Sprayregan S, Siegelman SS, et al: Initial results from an aggressive roentgenological and surgical approach to acute mesenteric ischemia. Surgery 82:848, 1977.
20. Jager K, Bollinger A, Valli C, et al: Measurement of mesenteric blood flow by duplex scanning. J Vasc Surg 3:462, 1986.
21. Lilly MP, Harward TRS, Flinn WR, et al: Duplex ultrasound measurement of changes in mesenteric flow velocity with pharmacologic and physiologic alteration of intestinal blood flow in man. J Vasc Surg 9:18, 1989.
22. Blum H, Barlow C, Chance B, et al: Acute intestinal ischemia studies by phosphorus nuclear magnetic resonance spectroscopy. Ann Surg 204:83, 1986.
23. Bardfeld PA, Boley SJ, Sammartano RJ, et al: Scintigraphic diagnosis of ischemic intestine with technetium 99m sulfur colloid labelled leukocytes. Radiology 124:439, 1977.
24. Gharagozloo F, Bulkley GB, Zuidema GD, et al: The use of intraperitoneal xenon for early diagnosis of acute mesenteric ischemia. Surgery 95:404, 1984.
25. Serreyn RF, Schoofs PR, Baetens PR, et al: Laparoscopic diagnosis of mesenteric venous thrombosis. Endoscopy 18:249, 1986.
26. Kleinhaus S, Sammartano RJ, Boley SJ: Variations in blood flow during laparoscopy. Physiologist 19:255, 1976.
27. Ricci JL, Sloviter HA, Ziegler MM: Intestinal ischemia: Reduction of mortality utilizing intraluminal perfluorochemical. Am J Surg 149:84, 1985.
28. Oldham KT, Guice KS, Gore D, et al: Treatment of intestinal ischemia with oxygenated intraluminal perfluorocarbons. Am J Surg 153:291, 1987.
29. Sachs SM, Morton JH, Schwartz SI: Acute mesenteric ischemia. Surgery 92:646, 1982.
30. Hildebrand HD, Zierler RE: Mesenteric vascular disease. Am J Surg 139:188, 1980.
31. Bergan JJ, McCarthy WJ, Flinn WR, et al: Nontraumatic mesenteric vascular emergencies. J Vasc Surg 5:903, 1987.

97

Intestinal Ischemia Caused by Venous Thrombosis

Andris Kazmers, M.D., M.S.P.H.

• • •

Thrombotic occlusions of the mesenteric veins infrequently cause intestinal ischemia.[1-15] As with all forms of acute intestinal ischemia, the reported mortality associated with this rare clinical problem is substantial. In 1935, Warren and Eberhard reported a mortality rate of 34 per cent after intestinal resection for venous thrombosis.[1] Despite the subsequent development of anticoagulants and potent antibiotics, in addition to many improvements in clinical care, currently reported mortality rates are comparable.[2, 9, 10] Warren and Eberhard also reported that intestinal infarction *inevitably* resulted from intestinal ischemia due to venous thrombosis. Only 5 per cent of their patients with intestinal ischemia from venous thrombosis left the hospital alive if they did not undergo surgery.[1] The current understanding of mesenteric venous thrombosis indicates that some patients are less severely affected and do not necessarily develop gut infarction; thus, selective nonoperative management is possible. In this chapter, the present understanding of the epidemiology, pathophysiology, diagnosis, and management of intestinal ischemia caused by venous thrombosis is discussed.

EPIDEMIOLOGY

Warren and Eberhard reported that mesenteric venous thrombosis was present in 0.003 per cent of the general hospital population and in 0.05 per cent of autopsy cases.[1] A more recent report indicated that gut infarction from splanchnic venous occlusion comprised 0.006 per cent of hospital admissions and less than 0.2 per cent of autopsy cases.[12] Only 372 patients with mesenteric venous thrombosis had been reported by 1984.[2] Acute intestinal ischemia of any cause is a rare clinical problem, and these figures confirm that mesenteric venous thrombosis is responsible for only a small percentage of cases of acute intestinal ischemia. One study reported that 0.38 per cent of laparotomies performed for "acute abdomen" revealed mesenteric infarction, and only 17 per cent of these infarctions were due to venous thrombosis.[14] By inference, intestinal infarction from venous thrombosis will be encountered in less than 1 in 1000 laparotomies for acute abdomen.

Prior understanding of the natural history and incidence of intestinal ischemia from venous thrombosis was biased toward more severe cases because most were diagnosed at laparotomy or autopsy.[1, 16, 17] Duplex ultrasound, computed tomography (CT), and magnetic resonance imaging (MRI), as well as the aggressive use of arteriography for the evaluation of patients with possible acute intestinal ischemia, have all facilitated preoperative or antemortem diagnosis.[18–49] Although portomesenteric venous thrombosis appears to be increasing in incidence, this is probably due to improved diagnostic capability rather than a true increase in disease frequency.

Acute intestinal ischemia from venous thrombosis occurs at any age and in either sex. Clinical characteristics associated with increased probability of this problem are few. Correct clinical diagnosis is therefore rare.[17] For practical purposes, the diagnosis is usually made at laparotomy, at autopsy, or incidentally from diagnostic imaging studies. A history of portomesenteric or lower extremity venous thrombosis in someone with abdominal pain, however, warrants inclusion of intestinal ischemia from venous thrombosis in the differential diagnosis. In one series, the majority of patients with this disorder had a history of venous thrombosis.[9]

ETIOLOGY

Mesenteric venous occlusions have been categorized as primary or secondary (Table 97–1). Primary occlusions have no known underlying cause, whereas secondary thromboses are associated with other disorders producing at

Table 97–1.   Etiology of Mesenteric Venous Thrombosis

Primary (idiopathic, agnogenic, spontaneous)	Mechanical venous occlusion
Secondary	Malignancy
Trauma	Portal hypertension
Operative trauma	Volvulus
Postsplenectomy	Intussusception
Blunt abdominal injury	Strangulated obstruction
Penetrating abdominal injury	Infection
Endoscopic sclerotherapy	Septic pylephlebitis
Hematologic diseases	Appendicitis
Protein C deficiency	Diverticulitis
Antithrombin III deficiency	Intra-abdominal abscess
Protein S deficiency	Peritonitis
Abnormal plasminogen	Generalized sepsis
Oral contraceptives	Other causes
Thrombocytosis	Congestive heart failure
Sickle cell disease	Renal failure
Pregnancy	Renal transplantation
Polycythemia vera	Decompression sickness

From Kispert JF, Kazmers A: Acute intestinal ischemia caused by mesenteric venous thrombosis. Semin Vasc Surg 3:158, 1990.

least one element of Virchow's triad.[50–87] These disorders may promote portal venous stasis (i.e., liver cirrhosis), splanchnic venous injury (i.e., following splenectomy), or hypercoagulability. Hypercoagulable states associated with splanchnic venous thrombosis have included protein C or S deficiency, antithrombin III deficiency, the presence of anticardiolipin antibody, and certain malignancies.[57, 58, 61, 64, 76–80, 82–85] Obviously, some venous occlusions currently regarded as primary may be due to yet undefined coagulation abnormalities.

Secondary portomesenteric thrombosis may be associated with intra-abdominal infection or inflammation. Infection is the most common cause in children.[60] In some cases, the mesenteric venous thrombus itself becomes infected, a condition known as pylephlebitis.

In patients with intra-abdominal malignancy, secondary intestinal venous thrombosis can result from direct invasion or obstruction of venous trunks or from hypercoagulability.[60] Splenectomy patients have a recognized increased incidence of portomesenteric venous thrombosis due to a combination of factors, including trauma to the splenic vein, stasis in the splenic vein stump, reduced portomesenteric venous flow, and perhaps postsplenectomy thrombocytosis. The role of thrombocytosis, if any, requires further assessment. When splenectomy is performed for hematologic disease, the underlying disorder may contribute to the venous thrombosis. This is particularly true after splenectomy in those with myeloid metaplasia.[50]

Secondary mesenteric venous thrombosis has been reported in women using oral contraceptives and in men receiving estrogen therapy for prostate cancer.[2, 86] One report suggested that mortality due to splanchnic venous thrombosis related to oral contraceptive use may be lower than that with other secondary causes.[2]

Portomesenteric venous thrombosis also occurs in patients with cirrhosis and portal hypertension.[55, 58, 81] In this setting, splanchnic venous thrombosis may occur spontaneously or may follow sclerotherapy for esophageal varices or selective transhepatic portal angiography.[52, 63, 71, 72] The etiology of splanchnic venous thrombosis after sclerotherapy is postulated to be the entry of sclerosing agent into the portomesenteric venous circulation.[71]

CLINICAL PRESENTATION

Mesenteric venous thrombosis may present with various manifestations, ranging from an asymptomatic state to a catastrophic illness.[1–6, 8, 9, 11, 30, 69, 74, 87] Prolonged abdominal discomfort is common. Symptoms tend to develop less rapidly than with acute arterial insufficiency of the intestines. Abdominal pain is typically generalized. Rebound tenderness is present only with transmural bowel infarction. Pain out of proportion to physical findings, although a rare presenting symptom, suggests the presence of acute intestinal ischemia, which may be caused by venous thrombosis.

Abdominal distention is frequently present and may be disproportionate to the expected degree of tympany on physical examination. This is because the distention is due to bowel wall edema, as well as to intraluminal sequestration of fluid and blood. Bloody peritoneal fluid is present in advanced cases and has adverse prognostic significance.[25] Occult gastrointestinal bleeding is frequently associated with mesenteric venous thrombosis. Significant gastrointestinal hemorrhage is usually caused by variceal hemorrhage.[60, 81, 88, 89]

PATHOPHYSIOLOGY

Acute portomesenteric venous occlusions abruptly increase portal venous pressure, promoting the formation of varices. Thus, variceal hemorrhage may be the presenting sign of splanchnic venous thrombosis.[60, 81] Portal vein thrombosis is commonly associated with portal hypertension, varices, and splenomegaly, with or without hypersplenism. Ascites may appear or, if already present, may worsen abruptly. Such portal vein occlusions may result in intestinal ischemia by blockage of superior mesenteric venous outflow or by direct extension of thrombus into the superior mesenteric vein. Isolated splenic vein thrombosis, usually associated with pancreatic disease, may result in upper gastrointestinal bleeding from isolated gastric varices, a condition called sinistral portal hypertension.[53, 66] When such venous thromboses are confined to the splenic vein, intestinal ischemia does not occur.

Thrombosis involving the superior mesenteric vein results in intestinal ischemia confined to the small intestine.[1–5, 8] Colon infarction has been reported but is unusual after superior mesenteric vein thrombosis. The clinical manifestations occurring in any one patient depend on the location and, importantly, on the rapidity of venous occlusion.[16] Thus, splanchnic venous thrombosis presents with a spectrum of severity ranging from ascites, variceal hemorrhage, and intestinal ischemia to asymptomatic occlusion of the portal or superior mesenteric veins.[30, 74, 90] Occlusion of the inferior mesenteric vein is nearly always asymptomatic.

The most rapid occlusion of portomesenteric veins occurs with surgical ligation. Acute ligation of the inferior mesenteric vein is well tolerated. Acute ligation of the portal or superior mesenteric veins is less well tolerated.[59, 62, 91–95] Portal vein ligation may be appropriate in managing irreparable portal vein injuries. Similarly, acute ligation of the superior mesenteric vein has been advocated for unstable patients with severe superior mesenteric vein injuries. Some patients, however, do not tolerate portal or superior mesenteric vein ligation.[93] It is not currently possible to predict the consequences of ligation of these major splanchnic venous trunks for a given patient. Therefore, most authorities recommend repair of injuries to the portal and superior mesenteric veins when possible, reserving ligation for severely unstable patients with truly massive injuries.

Advances in understanding the pathophysiology of portomesenteric venous thrombosis have resulted from the availability of CT, abdominal duplex scanning, and MRI, which facilitate preoperative or antemortem diagnosis. Because in the past most cases were diagnosed at operation or autopsy, a biased understanding of the natural history of mesenteric venous occlusions was responsible for the opinion that nonoperative management is associated with poor outcome. Currently, cases of mesenteric venous thrombosis are occasionally diagnosed by CT before they become clinically evident. Autopsy series suggest that roughly 50 per cent (range, 45 to 61 per cent) of patients dying with portomesenteric venous thrombosis do not have bowel infarction.[16, 90]

Extensive acute mesenteric venous obstruction results in massive intestinal fluid sequestration with resultant hypovolemia and hemoconcentration.[96–103] Intestinal arteriolar vasoconstriction results from elevations in portal venous pressure.[98, 99, 104] Experimental studies suggest that arterial spasm and intestinal blood flow reduction persist after removal of such venous obstructions.[98, 99] In addition, reduction of intestinal perfusion may follow in a fashion similar to that found in phlegmasia cerulea dolens.[54] In both situations, massive obstruction of venous outflow impairs arterial inflow. Hemorrhagic intestinal infarction results.[101, 102]

Other adverse physiologic consequences follow intestinal ischemia. Ischemia impairs the ability of the gastrointestinal tract to protect itself from its own luminal contents, and intestinal autodigestion may ensue.[105, 106] Loss of intestinal wall integrity is associated with the release of vasoactive agents from intestinal cells, as well as the loss of boundary function for intestinal organisms.[106] This loss of boundary function is thought to be associated with the development of multiple organ failure.[107]

The presenting symptoms and signs of acute mesenteric venous thrombosis outlined previously, including bowel ischemia, may occur in any combination. Those with secondary mesenteric venous thrombosis also exhibit signs and symptoms of their underlying disorder, further confusing the clinical picture. Mesenteric venous thrombosis may mimic commonly encountered disorders such as appendicitis, gastroenteritis, and bowel obstruction. Unlike acute superior mesenteric artery embolism, which has a characteristic clinical presentation, intestinal ischemia from portomesenteric venous thrombosis usually presents in an indistinct fashion. Although earlier recognition might allow diagnosis before venous congestion progresses to transmural bowel infarction, the correct preoperative diagnosis is made in only a small fraction of patients.

DIAGNOSIS

Laboratory tests or plain abdominal x-ray findings cannot identify intestinal ischemia caused by mesenteric venous thrombosis. Hemoconcentration and leukocytosis are expected but nonspecific findings. Other blood studies, including serum phosphorus levels, are not diagnostic. Abdominal x-ray findings are nonspecific and may include small bowel dilatation, small bowel wall thickening (Fig. 97–1), air in the portal venous system, and free intra-abdominal air. Barium contrast gastrointestinal studies may reveal thumbprinting or a peculiar type of small intestinal narrowing.[19] Once performed, such contrast studies interfere with angiographic evaluation. The latter consideration, together with the low yield of barium contrast studies, limits their utility.

When the differential diagnosis suggests that mesenteric venous thrombosis is possible or likely, abdominal duplex scanning, CT with contrast, angiography, or a combination, may be used to confirm the diagnosis. As equipment and operator skills have improved, duplex scanning has played a greater role in the diagnosis and follow-up of patients with mesenteric vascular disease, both venous and arterial. Duplex scanning for portomesenteric venous thrombosis is less sensitive than CT, particularly for assessment of the superior mesenteric and splenic veins. Thrombus in the portal and hepatic veins is difficult to distinguish from surrounding liver tissue by ultrasound. An inability to image the portal vein should raise suspicion for portal venous thrombosis when failure of insonation is not due to overlying bowel gas or hepatic parenchymal abnormalities. The presence of worm-like vascular channels in the area of the portal vein suggests cavernomatous transformation from prior portal venous thrombosis. Intraluminal thrombus and cavernomatous transformation are the most frequent ultrasound findings in portal venous thrombosis (Fig. 97–2). Other findings suggestive of splanchnic venous thrombosis include enlargement of splanchnic veins, intravenous echogenic thrombus, abnormal or absent flow within veins, and lack of either compressibility or respiratory variation in vein size. Ultrasound and other diagnostic techniques cannot reliably differentiate clot from tumor thrombus in the

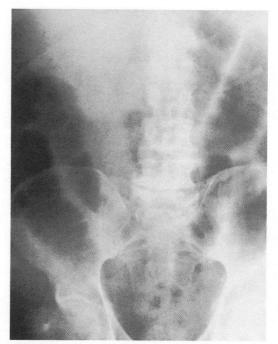

FIGURE 97–1. Plain abdominal x-ray study of a patient with mesenteric venous thrombosis. Positive findings, which are nonspecific, include small bowel dilatation, small bowel wall thickening, and absence of colonic gas. (From Kispert JF, Kazmers A: Acute intestinal ischemia caused by mesenteric venous thrombosis. Semin Vasc Surg 3:163, 1990.)

portal vein. The portal vein is ordinarily less than 13 mm in diameter in adults without portal hypertension.[42] The size of thrombosed portal veins ranges from 15 to 26 mm. Massive venous enlargement has been mistaken for a pancreatic pseudocyst.[33]

The typical CT appearance of superior mesenteric venous thrombosis is enlargement of the thrombosed vein with a central area of low attenuation, associated with clot within the lumen, that is surrounded by a well-defined contrast-enhanced venous wall (Fig. 97–3).[25] Some investigators suggest the venous wall enhancement is due to contrast

FIGURE 97–2. Sonogram demonstrating portal vein thrombosis. The occlusive thrombus (clot, *arrow*) is echogenic. There was Doppler flow signal in the portal vein (PV). IVC, inferior vena cava.

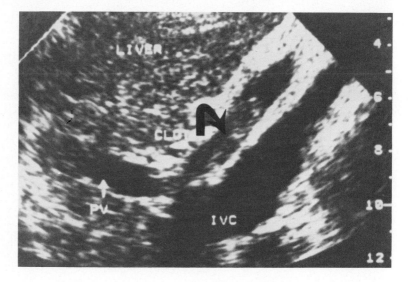

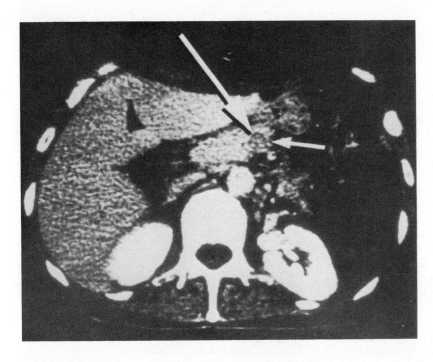

FIGURE 97–3. Abdominal computed tomographic (CT) scan with contrast from a patient with superior mesenteric vein thrombosis treated nonoperatively. The *arrows* point to a dense (contrast-enhanced) superior mesenteric vein wall with central lucency. There is no intra-abdominal fluid or other sign of intestinal infarction. (From Kispert JF, Kazmers A: Acute intestinal ischemia caused by mesenteric venous thrombosis. Semin Vasc Surg 3:159, 1990.)

in the vasa vasorum and not to contrast flowing around thrombus, whereas others believe it is related to the visual contrast between low-density thrombus and the superior mesenteric vein wall. Such vein wall enhancement is not always present. CT may define the presence of an underlying intra-abdominal problem that has caused secondary portomesenteric venous thrombosis. In portomesenteric venous thrombosis, multi-vein occlusion is more frequent than appreciated. The CT triad of hypodensity in the superior mesenteric vein, thickening of the intestinal wall and valvulae conniventes in the small intestine, and a significant amount of peritoneal fluid suggests intestinal infarction (Fig. 97–

4).[25] The presence of peritoneal fluid suggests greater severity of intestinal ischemia from venous occlusion. Clavien and colleagues found that all of their patients with irreversible bowel ischemia had a "significant amount of hemorrhagic ascites."[25] They suggested that the absence of peritoneal fluid was a reassuring finding. Absence of ascites supports the decision to treat a patient with mesenteric venous thrombosis nonoperatively. Clavien and colleagues suggested that the development of ascites in such patients was an indication for surgery. Other important CT findings may include the abnormal presence of gas in the intestinal wall, venous system, or peritoneal cavity. Pneumatosis in-

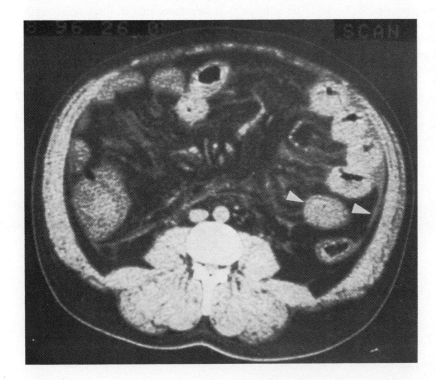

FIGURE 97–4. Abdominal CT scan from a patient with intestinal infarction caused by mesenteric venous thrombosis. There is marked bowel wall edema with obliteration of the bowel lumen *(medial white arrow)*, and free intra-abdominal fluid *(lateral white arrow)* is seen as well. (From Kispert JF, Kazmers A: Acute intestinal ischemia caused by mesenteric venous thrombosis. Semin Vasc Surg 3:161, 1990.)

testinalis is more easily detected by CT than by plain film radiography. Portal or mesenteric venous gas strongly suggests the presence of bowel infarction.

Multiple angiographic techniques have been reported in the diagnosis of mesenteric venous thrombosis. These include splenoportography (percutaneous needle insertion into the spleen with contrast injection, outlining the mesenteric veins), transhepatic portography (percutaneous needle insertion into the hepatic parenchyma, with identification and catheterization of the portal system and subsequent contrast injection), and arterial portography (catheterization of the superior mesenteric artery with contrast injection and venous phase filming). In addition to providing diagnostic information, angiographic techniques have the potential for therapy, such as directed thrombolytic infusions and balloon dilatation.

Splenoportography is not recommended for diagnosing mesenteric venous thrombosis because of its potential complications, its inability to reliably outline the superior mesenteric vein, and the availability of other diagnostic modalities. This technique is currently of historic interest only. Transhepatic portography has been used to embolize bleeding esophageal varices and could also be used for diagnosis. One complication associated with this technique, however, is portal vein thrombosis. On the other hand, at least one group has reported successful transhepatic, transvenous selective clot lysis for the management of portomesenteric venous thrombosis.[108] This unique approach may prove useful in selected patients.

Arterial portography remains the favored method for confirming the presence of portal or superior mesenteric venous thrombosis when other tests such as CT, MRI, and abdominal duplex scanning are unavailable or their results are equivocal. Angiography may reveal intraluminal thrombus, nonvisualization of the venous outflow, or venous occlusion (Figs. 97–5 and 97–6). Experimental and clinical reports suggest that superior mesenteric arterial spasm, prolongation of the arterial phase, and other subtle findings also result from superior mesenteric venous occlusion (Fig. 97–7).[22, 23, 46] Angiography and CT with contrast can serve as complementary studies in difficult cases.

MRI may also confirm the diagnosis. Diagnostic MRI criteria for portomesenteric venous thrombosis are being developed.[26, 32] Early work suggests that MRI will be a very sensitive test for detection of splanchnic venous thrombosis. MRI may even be able to differentiate clot from tumor thrombus. The role of MRI for the evaluation of portomesenteric thrombosis requires further definition.

Diagnostic testing for suspected mesenteric venous thrombosis should begin with the least invasive test (i.e., duplex scanning). Abdominal duplex scanning is operator dependent, may be unavailable at all hours or in all hospitals, and is difficult to perform with abdominal tenderness or gaseous distention. For these reasons, negative duplex scanning results should not be regarded as diagnostic, and scanning should be followed by confirmatory tests. CT's greater sensitivity for the detection of splanchnic venous thrombosis and its ability to detect bowel wall thickening and other associated findings render it superior to duplex ultrasound for the work-up of those with possible splanchnic venous thrombosis. CT is currently preferable to MRI because of its greater availability and familiarity.

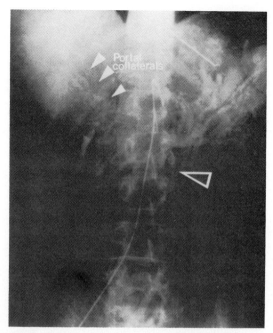

FIGURE 97–5. Venous phase of a superior mesenteric arteriogram demonstrates thrombosis with cavernous transformation of the portal vein *(white arrows)*. The *dark arrow* points to a patent inferior mesenteric vein. (From Kispert JF, Kazmers A: Acute intestinal ischemia caused by mesenteric venous thrombosis. Semin Vasc Surg 3:159, 1990.)

Ancillary tests that may be used in patients with mesenteric venous thrombosis include paracentesis, laparoscopy, and gastrointestinal endoscopy. Abdominal paracentesis may provide indirect evidence (bloody ascites) and laparoscopy may provide direct evidence of intestinal ischemia from portomesenteric venous thrombosis.[109] In venous gut infarction, the mid–small intestine is usually involved, thus eluding colonoscopy and upper gastrointestinal tract endoscopy.[110] Although upper endoscopy may not provide important diagnostic information in the absence of upper gastrointestinal tract bleeding, it is reasonable to assess the development of gastroesophageal varices, particularly in patients receiving long-term anticoagulant therapy for mesenteric venous thromboses. Endoscopy is clearly indicated for the evaluation of gastrointestinal bleeding to determine whether the source is varices.

INTRAOPERATIVE ASSESSMENT

Because of the rarity of mesenteric venous thrombosis, most cases are diagnosed only at laparotomy or autopsy. When the diagnosis of visceral infarction is made at laparotomy, particularly in patients who have not undergone preoperative arteriography or CT, systematic evaluation is required to determine the etiology. Cyanotic intestinal discoloration and pronounced edema of the mesentery and the intestine are characteristic of mesenteric venous thrombosis. Serosanguineous fluid is also consistent with, but not specific for, venous infarction. The pattern of infarction also suggests the etiology. Infarction from mesenteric venous thrombosis commonly involves the mid–small intestine.

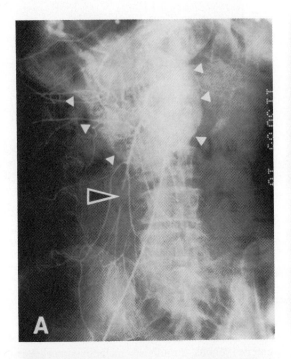

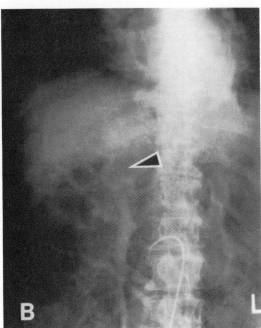

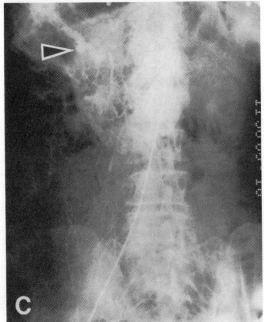

FIGURE 97–6.   Superior mesenteric arteriogram in a patient with portal vein occlusion from thrombus. *A,* Arterial phase shows segmental occlusion of a minor gastroduodenal artery branch *(black arrow)* and marked venous congestion in the upper intestine *(white arrows). B,* Venous phase shows a patent superior mesenteric vein but an occluded portal vein *(black arrow). C,* Later venous phase demonstrates portal vein collaterals, one of which is dominant *(black arrow).* (A–C, From Kispert JF, Kazmers A: Acute intestinal ischemia caused by mesenteric venous thrombosis. Semin Vasc Surg 3:160, 1990.)

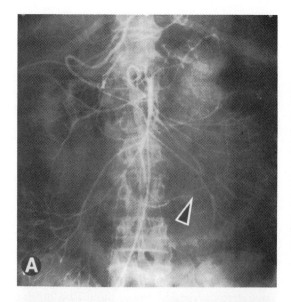

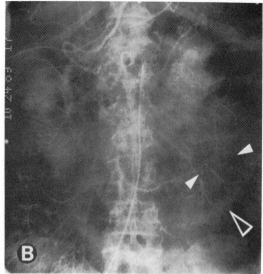

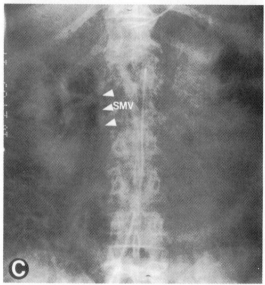

FIGURE 97–7. Superior mesenteric arteriogram from a patient with mesenteric venous thrombosis and resulting intestinal infarction. *A,* Arterial phase shows peripheral occlusion and spasm of arcade vessels *(black arrow). B,* Later arterial phase shows persistent opacification of jejunal vessels *(white arrows)* and intensified opacification of a markedly thickened bowel wall *(black arrow). C,* Venous phase shows patency of the superior mesenteric vein (SMV) with intraluminal thrombus *(white arrows).* The portal vein is occluded, and there is persistent opacification of the bowel wall. *(A–C,* From Kispert JF, Kazmers A: Acute intestinal ischemia caused by mesenteric venous thrombosis. Semin Vasc Surg 3:162, 1990.)

With venous occlusion, the extent of intestinal infarction may be massive but is usually segmental, and the colon is usually not affected. Duodenal or colon involvement suggests that infarction is not venous in origin. The presence of mesenteric arteriolar pulsations and palpable superior mesenteric artery pulsations also confirms that intestinal infarction is due to mesenteric venous thrombosis. Extrusion of venous thrombi from the divided edge of the mesentery is characteristic of venous thrombosis. Some investigators have employed intraoperative venography to confirm the diagnosis and evaluate the extent of portomesenteric venous thrombosis.[111] Angioscopy has also been used to assess portomesenteric thrombosis.[112] In most cases, neither of these techniques is necessary because the diagnosis is obvious from the gross findings described.

TREATMENT

Patients with acute intestinal ischemia due to mesenteric venous thrombosis require vigorous blood volume re-

expansion. Broad-spectrum antibiotics with anaerobic coverage are recommended for those with intestinal infarction. The utility of mesenteric vasodilators has not been established for mesenteric venous thrombosis. Anticoagulation is absolutely mandatory to limit the thrombotic process and prevent recurrence. If not begun preoperatively, anticoagulation should begin intraoperatively. On the basis of experimental studies, either heparin or low-molecular-weight dextran can be used, but heparin is preferable.[2, 6, 100, 103] Recurrent thrombosis can be expected in almost one third (29 per cent) of those with mesenteric venous thrombosis.[113, 114] Anticoagulation reduces recurrence and overall mortality. Naitove and Weissman reported that no deaths occurred in patients with primary mesenteric venous thrombosis who received anticoagulation postoperatively, whereas 50 per cent of those who did not receive postoperative anticoagulation died.[6] A literature review of mesenteric venous thrombosis reported that of 173 patients undergoing bowel resection for mesenteric venous thrombosis, 38 (22 per cent) had recurrent thrombosis.[2] Of those treated surgically, recurrence was significantly lower in the heparin-treated group than in untreated patients. Only 14 per cent of those treated with heparin had recurrence, whereas 26 per cent of those not treated with heparin had recurrence, a statistically significant difference.[2] Of patients with recurrence, 22 per cent (2 of 9) of those treated with anticoagulants died, whereas 59 per cent (17 of 29) of those not treated with heparin died.[2]

Heparin should be continued until anticoagulation with warfarin can be accomplished. The required duration of anticoagulation therapy is unknown because insufficient information about the natural history is available. Some authors have suggested that most recurrent thromboses occur within 6 weeks of prior portomesenteric thrombosis.[6] A short course of anticoagulation would protect the majority of patients from such recurrence. For those with coagulation disorders, anticoagulation should be continued indefinitely. All patients with thrombosis of the portomesenteric venous circulation without obvious cause should have their coagulation systems assessed. A list of currently available tests is provided in Table 97–2. When the results of these coagulation studies are normal, the patient should be considered to have primary venous occlusion. Patients with primary mesenteric venous thrombosis and those with identified disorders of coagulation should be anticoagulated indefinitely. This recommendation is based on the supposition that those with primary thrombosis may harbor yet undefined coagulation disorders. Management of secondary splanchnic venous occlusion must take into consideration the underlying disorder. For example, in patients with splanchnic venous injury, discontinuation of anticoagulation can be considered. Anticoagulation in the presence of cirrhosis, portal hypertension, and gastrointestinal varices is problematic. Although it seems that anticoagulation may increase the risk of variceal hemorrhage, it will reduce the incidence of recurrent splanchnic venous thrombosis and has reduced mortality; it is therefore recommended.

Lytic therapy with urokinase or streptokinase has no well-defined role in mesenteric venous thrombosis.[108, 115, 116] In an animal model of temporary mesenteric venous obstruction, streptokinase improved survival in subjects with temporary but not permanent venous obstruction.[116] The risk of hemorrhage from fibrinolytic agents in someone with an acute abdominal process that may evolve into hemorrhagic gut infarction makes the use of these agents less appealing. Despite this reservation, fibrinolytic agents have had experimental and anecdotal clinical success in the splanchnic venous circulation. One report described successful lysis of superior mesenteric venous thrombosis using recombinant tissue-type plasminogen activator.[115] The presence of gastroesophageal varices did not serve as a contraindication to lytic therapy in another case report, and bleeding did not ensue.[108] Interestingly, the varices disappeared after clot lysis. The role of lytic agents in the management of splanchnic venous thrombosis will need further clarification.

In the majority of patients, the diagnosis of intestinal venous thrombosis is made during laparotomy. If the diagnosis is made before surgery on the basis of the diagnostic studies listed earlier, the indications for operation include physical findings of peritonitis, hemodynamic instability, and CT findings indicating a strong possibility of intestinal infarction (intra-abdominal fluid or air, or intramural or intraportal air). For those undergoing surgery, infarcted intestine should be resected with wide margins. The thrombotic process may involve the mesentery of viable intestine adjacent to the infarcted intestine. Intestinal reanastomosis is permissible in stable patients with focal infarction confined to the small intestine when the remaining gut looks normal. Exteriorizing the intestine after resection is appropriate when conditions are not optimal for primary anastomosis. If the infarction is extensive, limited resection of necrotic bowel should be performed initially. Recurrent infarction from repeated venous thrombosis involves the area adjacent to the anastomosis in 60 per cent of patients. Anticoagulation reduces the likelihood of such recurrences.[113]

In mesenteric venous occlusion, recurrent thrombosis tends to occur later in the postoperative period than is usual with arterial occlusions.[102, 117] Second-look procedures are not mandatory after segmental venous infarction has been widely resected in stable patients who are anticoagulated with heparin. Intraoperative assessment of gut viability may be difficult because the accuracy of Doppler and fluorescein techniques is not established in intestinal ischemia from venous thrombosis.[118–120] Experimentally, the use of fluorescein appears more accurate than clinical or Doppler assessment of intestinal viability in venous infarction.[120] These considerations should lead to the use of second-look procedures when the viability of unresected intestine is in question or when massive intestinal resection would otherwise be required. Second-look operations may also be useful for the rare patient who undergoes portomesenteric venous thrombectomy.

Anecdotal reports suggest that portomesenteric venous thrombectomy may be useful, particularly when the alternative is massive intestinal resection.[70, 97, 111, 121–125] Removal of all thrombus from the smaller veins is not likely, and continued patency of the main venous trunks after thrombectomy has not been shown to be responsible for clinical improvement. Nevertheless, portomesenteric venous thrombectomy has successfully reestablished venous patency in some transplanted livers, as well as in some with acute intestinal ischemia from venous thrombosis.[70, 97, 111, 121–128] Portomesenteric venous thrombectomy therefore has a role in managing selected patients with portomesenteric venous thromboses.

Surgeons may not be familiar with the operative approach that has been used for portomesenteric venous thrombectomy (Fig. 97–8). Inahara isolated the superior mesenteric vein, performed linear venotomy, and removed the small clots from the peripheral veins by milking the bowel and mesentery (Fig. 97–9).[121] A Fogarty catheter can be used to retrieve more centrally located thrombus in the proximal superior mesenteric and portal veins. A variety of surgical approaches to the splanchnic venous system can be envisioned, but the one successfully used by Inahara is

Table 97–2. Coagulation Tests Performed in Patients With Mesenteric Venous Thrombosis

Prothrombin time	Antithrombin III
Partial thromboplastin time	Anticardiolipin antibody
Platelet count	Lupus anticoagulant
Protein C	Platelet aggregation studies
Protein S	

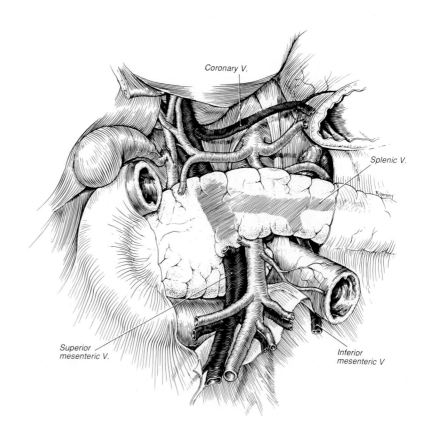

Coronary V.

Splenic V.

Superior mesenteric V.

Inferior mesenteric V

FIGURE 97–8. Exposure of the superior mesenteric vein in the base of the small bowel mesentery below the inferior border of the pancreas and to the right of the superior mesenteric artery.

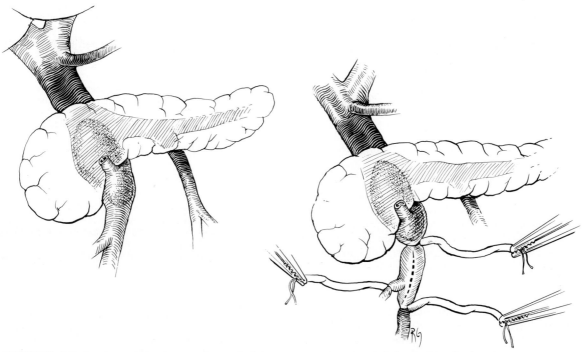

FIGURE 97–9. Method of isolation and control of the superior mesenteric vein before incision for thrombectomy *(dotted line).*

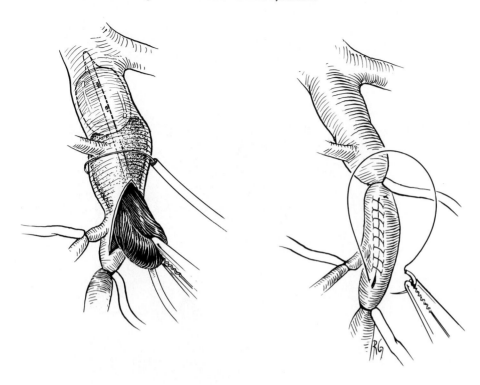

FIGURE 97–10. Use of the Fogarty balloon catheter for thrombectomy via a superior mesenteric venotomy, followed by closure of the venotomy.

comparable to that used by others (Fig. 97–10).[111, 121] The approach to the superior mesenteric vein is similar to that for superior mesenteric artery embolectomy. The vein is to the right of the artery and is much more fragile. Both linear and transverse venotomies in the superior mesenteric vein have been used successfully.

SUMMARY

Improved ability to make the preoperative or antemortem diagnosis of portomesenteric venous thrombosis by CT, duplex scanning, or MRI has resulted in the realization that this disorder does not invariably proceed to intestinal infarction or death without operative intervention. Nonoperative management with anticoagulation is appropriate for patients in whom intestinal ischemia from venous thrombosis has not progressed to transmural infarction. The continued absence of peritoneal fluid on CT, the absence of peritoneal signs, and the absence of sepsis are favorable findings that permit continued nonoperative management. The presence of any of these findings is an indication for laparotomy. As an adjunct to surgical therapy, anticoagulation has been proved to reduce the incidence and mortality from recurrent thrombosis. It has also been shown to reduce overall mortality for patients who have had intestinal infarction from venous thrombosis. Lytic therapy and thrombectomy have historically been of minimal importance in the management of splanchnic venous thrombosis, perhaps unjustifiably. Both techniques have been associated with anecdotal success. With the improved ability to diagnose and follow up patients with portomesenteric venous thrombosis and intestinal ischemia, it is likely that further improvements will be added to what has been until now the mainstay of therapy: resection of infarcted intestine.

References

1. Warren S, Eberhard TP: Mesenteric venous thrombosis. Surg Gynecol Obstet 61:102, 1935.
2. Abdu RA, Zakhour BJ, Dallis DJ: Mesenteric venous thrombosis 1911 to 1984. Surgery 101:383, 1987.
3. Grendell JH, Ockner RH: Mesenteric venous thrombosis. Gastroenterology 82:358, 1982.
4. Harward RS, Green D, Bergan JJ, et al: Mesenteric venous thrombosis. J Vasc Surg 9:328, 1989.
5. Mathews JE, White RR: Primary mesenteric venous occlusive disease. Am J Surg 122:579, 1971.
6. Naitove A, Weissman RE: Primary mesenteric venous thrombosis. Ann Surg 161:516, 1965.
7. Adar R, Walden R: Mesenteric venous thrombosis [Letter to the editors]. J Vasc Surg 15:257, 1992.
8. Kazmers A: Mesenteric venous occlusion. *In* Stanley JC, Ernst C (eds): Current Therapy in Vascular Surgery. Philadelphia, BC Decker, 1987, pp 320–323.
9. Clavien PA, Durig M, Harder F: Venous mesenteric infarction, a particular entity. Br J Surg 75:252, 1988.
10. Clavien PA, Muller C, Harder F: Treatment of mesenteric infarction. Br J Surg 74:500, 1987.
11. Montany PF, Finley RK: Mesenteric venous thrombosis. Am Surg 54:161, 1988.
12. Ottinger LW, Austen WG: A study of 136 patients with mesenteric infarction. Surg Gynecol Obstet 124:251, 1967.
13. Picardi E, Peoples JB: Mesenteric venous thrombosis: Ten year record review and evaluation of difficulties with the ICD coding system. S D J Med 44:33, 1991.
14. Rius X, Escalante JF, Jover J, Puig La Calle J: Mesenteric infarction. World J Surg 3:489, 1979.
15. Umpleby HC: Thrombosis of the superior mesenteric vein. Br J Surg 74:694, 1987.
16. Johnson CC, Baggenstoss AH: Mesenteric venous occlusion. Study of 99 cases of occlusion of veins. Mayo Clin Proc 24:628, 1949.
17. Donaldson JK, Stout BF: Mesenteric thrombosis: Arterial and venous types as separate clinical entities; A clinical and experimental study. Am J Surg 29:208, 1935.
18. Tomchik FS, Wittenberg J, Ottinger LW: The roentgenographic spectrum of bowel infarction. Radiology 96:249, 1970.
19. Clemett AR, Chung J: The radiologic diagnosis of spontaneous mesenteric venous thrombosis. Am J Gastroenterol 63:209, 1975.

20. Bolondi L, Mazziotti A, Arienti V, et al: Ultrasonographic study of portal venous system in portal hypertension and after portosystemic shunt operations. Surgery 95:261, 1984.

21. Miller VE, Berland LL: Pulsed Doppler duplex sonography and CT scan of portal venous thrombosis. AJR 145:73, 1985.

22. Friedenberg MJ, Polk HC, McAlister WH, et al: Superior mesenteric arteriography in experimental mesenteric venous thrombosis. Radiology 85:38, 1965.

23. Siegelman SS, Sprayregen S, Boley SJ: Angiographic diagnosis of mesenteric arterial vasoconstriction. Radiology 112:533, 1974.

24. Rosen A, Korobkin M, Silverman PM, et al: Mesenteric vein thrombosis: CT identification. AJR 143:83, 1984.

25. Clavien PA, Huber O, Mirescu D, Rohner A: Contrast enhanced CT scan as a diagnostic procedure in mesenteric ischaemia due to mesenteric venous thrombosis. Br J Surg 76:93, 1989.

26. Williams DM, Eckhauser FE, Aisen A, et al: Assessment of portosystemic shunt patency and function with magnetic resonance imaging. Surgery 102:602, 1987.

27. Johansen K, Paun M: Duplex ultrasonography of the portal vein. Surg Clin North Am 70:181, 1990.

28. Alpern MB, Glazer GM, Francis IR: Ischemic or infarcted bowel: CT findings. Radiology 166:149, 1988.

29. Federle MP, Chun G, Jeffrey RB, Rayor R: Computed tomographic findings in bowel infarction. AJR 142:91, 1984.

30. Harch JM, Radin RD, Yellin AE, Donovan AJ: Pylethrombosis: Serendipitous radiologic diagnosis. Arch Surg 122:1116, 1987.

31. Kane RA, Katz SG: The spectrum of sonographic findings in portal hypertension: A subject review and new observations. Radiology 142:453, 1982.

32. Levy HM, Newhouse JH: MR imaging of portal vein thrombosis. AJR 151:283, 1988.

33. Martin K, Balfe DM, Lee JKT: Computed tomography of portal vein thrombosis: Unusual appearances and pitfalls in diagnosis. J Comput Assist Tomogr 13:811, 1989.

34. Mori H, Hayashi K, Uetani M, et al: High-attenuation recent thrombus of the portal vein: CT demonstration and clinical significance. Radiology 163:353, 1987.

35. Nordback I, Sisto T: Ultrasonography and computed tomography in the diagnosis of portomesenteric vein thrombosis. Int Surg 76:179, 1991.

36. Schwerk WB: Portal vein thrombosis: Real-time sonographic demonstration and follow-up. Gastrointest Radiol 11:312, 1986.

37. Tessler FN, Gehring BJ, Gomes AS, et al: Diagnosis of portal vein thrombosis: Value of color Doppler imaging. AJR 157:293, 1991.

38. Tey H, Sprayregen S, Ahmed A, Chan KF: Mesenteric vein thrombosis. Angiography in two cases. AJR 136:809, 1981.

39. Vogelzang RL, Gore RM, Anschuetz SL, Blei AT: Thrombosis of the splanchnic veins: CT diagnosis. AJR 150:93, 1988.

40. Vujic I, Rogers CI, LeVeen HH: Computed tomographic detection of portal vein thrombosis. Radiology 135:697, 1980.

41. Webb L, Berger LA, Sherlock S: Grey-scale ultrasonography of portal vein. Lancet 2:675, 1977.

42. Weinreb J, Kumari S, Phillips G, Pochaczevsky R: Portal vein measurements by real-time sonography. AJR 139:497, 1982.

43. Zerhouni EA, Barth KH, Siegelman SS: Demonstration of venous thrombosis by computed tomography. AJR 134:753, 1980.

44. Ivatury RR, Nallathambi M, Rohman M, et al: Portal vein injuries: Noninvasive follow-up of venorrhaphy. Ann Surg 206:733, 1987.

45. Al Karawi MA, Quaiz M, Clark D, et al: Mesenteric vein thrombosis, noninvasive diagnosis and follow-up (US + MRI), and noninvasive therapy by streptokinase and anticoagulants. Hepatogastroenterology 37:507, 1990.

46. Subramanyam BR, Balthazar J, Lefleur RS, et al: Portal venous thrombosis: Correlative analysis of sonography, CT, and angiography. Am J Gastroenterol 79:773, 1984.

47. Verbanck JJ, Rutgeerts LJ, Haerens MH: Partial splenoportal and superior mesenteric venous thrombosis. Gastroenterology 86:949, 1984.

48. Matos C, Van-Gansbeke D, Zalcman M, et al: Mesenteric vein thrombosis: Early CT and US diagnosis and conservative management. Gastrointest Radiol 11:322, 1986.

49. Hricak H, Amparo E, Fisher MR, et al: Abdominal venous system: Assessment using MR. Radiology 156:415, 1985.

50. Broe RJ, Conley CL, Cameron JL: Thrombosis of the portal vein following splenectomy for myeloid metaplasia. Surg Gynecol Obstet 152:488, 1981.

51. Witte CL, Brewer ML, Witte MH, et al: Protean manifestations of pylethrombosis. Ann Surg 202:191, 1985.

52. Ashida H, Kotoura Y, Nishioka A, et al: Portal and mesenteric venous thrombosis as a complication of endoscopic sclerotherapy. Am J Gastroenterol 84:306, 1989.

53. Keith RG, Mustard RA, Saibil EA: Gastric variceal bleeding due to occlusion of splenic vein in pancreatic disease. Can J Surg 25:301, 1982.

54. Mergenthaler FW, Harris MN: Superior mesenteric vein thrombosis complicating pancreaticoduodenectomy: Successful treatment by thrombectomy. Ann Surg 167:106, 1968.

55. Belli L, Romani F, Sansalone CV, et al: Portal thrombosis in cirrhotics. Ann Surg 203:286, 1986.

56. Belli L, Romani F, Riolo F, et al: Thrombosis of portal vein in absence of hepatic disease. Surg Gynecol Obstet 169:46, 1989.

57. Bemelman WA, Butzelaar RMJM, Khargi K, Keeman JN: Mesenteric venous thrombosis caused by deficiency of physiologic anticoagulants: Report of a case. Neth J Surg 42I:16, 1990.

58. Brown KM, Kaplan MM, Donowitz M: Extrahepatic portal venous thrombosis: Frequent recognition of associated diseases. J Clin Gastroenterol 7(2):153, 1985.

59. Cohen D, Johansen K, Cottingham K, et al: Trauma to major visceral veins: An underemphasized cause of accident mortality. J Trauma 20:928, 1980.

60. Cohen J, Edelman RR, Chopra S: Portal vein thrombosis: A review. Am J Med 92:173, 1992.

61. Collins GJ, Zuck TF, Zajtchuk R, Heymann RL: Hypercoagulability in mesenteric venous occlusion. Am J Surg 132:389, 1976.

62. Courcy PA, Brotman S, Oster-Granite ML, et al: Superior mesenteric artery and vein injuries from blunt abdominal trauma. J Trauma 24(9):843, 1984.

63. Deboever G, Elegeert I, Defloor E: Portal and mesenteric venous thrombosis after endoscopic injection sclerotherapy. Am J Gastroenterol 84:1336, 1989.

64. De Clerck LS, Michielsen PP, Ramael MR, et al: Portal and pulmonary vessel thrombosis associated with systemic lupus erythematosus and anticardiolipin antibodies. J Rheumatol 18:1919, 1991.

65. Engelhardt TC, Kerstein MD: Pregnancy and mesenteric venous thrombosis. South Med J 82:1441, 1989.

66. Evans G, Yellin AE, Weaver FA, Stain SC: Sinistral (left-sided) portal hypertension. Am Surg 56:758, 1990.

67. Hansen HJ, Christoffersen JK: Occlusive mesenteric infarction. Acta Chir Scand 472:103, 1976.

68. Hickman A, Wilson SK, Stein M, et al: Portal and superior mesenteric venous thrombosis following splenectomy. J Tenn Med Assoc 84:329, 1991.

69. Ikeda N, Umetsu K, Suzuki T, et al: Sudden unexpected death from a superior mesenteric venous thrombosis after a gastrectomy. Jpn J Legal Med 43:328, 1989.

70. Jaffe V, Lygidakis NJ, Blumgart LH: Acute portal vein thrombosis after right hepatic lobectomy: Successful treatment by thrombectomy. Br J Surg 69:211, 1982.

71. Korula J, Yellin A, Kanel GC, Nichols P: Portal vein thrombosis complicating endoscopic variceal sclerotherapy. Dig Dis Sci 36:1164, 1991.

72. Leach SD, Meier GH, Gusberg RJ: Endoscopic sclerotherapy: A risk factor for splanchnic venous thrombosis. J Vasc Surg 10:9, 1989.

73. Mattox KL, Guinn GA: Mesenteric infarction. Am J Surg 126:332, 1973.

74. Barro L, Vicente M, et al: Trombosis venosa mesenterica: Un nuevo caso de evolucion favorable con tratamiento conservador. Rev Esp Enferm Ap Dig 75:720, 1989.

75. Britton BJ, Royle G: Mesenteric venous thrombosis. Br J Surg 69:118, 1982.

76. Olson JF, Steuber CP, Hawkins E, Mahoney DH: Functional deficiency of protein C associated with mesenteric venous thrombosis and splenic infarction. Am J Pediatr Hematol Oncol 13:168, 1991.

77. Orozco H, Guraieb E, Takahashi T, et al: Deficiency of protein C in patients with portal vein thrombosis. Hepatology 8:1110, 1988.

78. Berry FB, Bougas JA: Agnogenic venous mesenteric thrombosis. Ann Surg 132:450, 1950.

79. Valla D, Casadevall N, Huisse MG, et al: Etiology of portal vein thrombosis in adults. Gastroenterology 94:1063, 1988.

80. Valla D, Denninger MH, Delvigne JM, et al: Portal vein thrombosis with ruptured oesophageal varices as presenting manifestation of hereditary protein C deficiency. Gut 29:856, 1988.

81. Webb L, Sherlock S: The aetiology, presentation and natural history of extra-hepatic portal venous obstruction. Q J Med 192:627, 1979.

82. Yates P, Cumber PM, Sanderson S, Harrison MS: Mesenteric venous thrombosis due to protein C deficiency. Clin Lab Haematol 13:137, 1991.

83. Maung R, Kelly JK, Schneider MP, et al: Mesenteric venous thrombosis due to antithrombin III deficiency. Arch Pathol Lab Med 112:37, 1988.

84. Green D, Ganger DR, Blei AT: Protein C deficiency in splanchnic venous thrombosis. Am J Med 82:1171, 1987.

85. Broekmans AW, van Rooyen W, Westerveld BD, et al: Mesenteric vein thrombosis as presenting manifestation of hereditary protein S deficiency. Gastroenterology 92:240, 1987.

86. Sahdev P, Wolff M, Widmann WD: Mesenteric venous thrombosis associated with estrogen therapy for treatment of prostatic carcinoma. J Urol 134:563, 1985.

87. Witte CL, Brewer ML, Witte MH, et al: Protean manifestations of pylethrombosis. Ann Surg 202:191, 1985.

88. Soper NJ, Rikkers LF, Miller FJ: Gastrointestinal hemorrhage associated with chronic mesenteric venous occlusion. Gastroenterology 88:1964, 1985.

89. Miyaki CT, Park YS, Gopalswamy N: Upper gastrointestinal bleeding in acute mesenteric thrombosis. J Clin Gastroenterol 10(1):84, 1988.

90. Laufman H, Scheinberg S: Arterial and venous mesenteric occlusion. Am J Surg 58:84, 1942.

91. Mattox KL: Abdominal venous injuries. Surgery 91:497, 1982.

92. Donahue TK, Strauch GO: Ligation as definitive management of injury to the superior mesenteric vein. J Trauma 28:541, 1988.

93. Patterson RB, Fowl RJ, Braunstein PW, et al: Ligation as definitive management of injury to the superior mesenteric vein. [Letter to the editors]. J Trauma 25:1684, 1988.

94. Sheldon GF, Lim RC, Yee ES, Petersen SR: Management of injuries to the porta hepatis. Ann Surg 202:539, 1985.

95. Sirinek KR, Levine BA: Traumatic injury to the proximal superior mesenteric vessels. Surgery 98:831, 1985.

96. Kispert JF, Kazmers A: Acute intestinal ischemia caused by mesenteric venous thrombosis. Semin Vasc Surg 3:157, 1990.

97. Polk H: Experimental mesenteric venous occlusion. Ann Surg 163:432, 1966.

98. Turner MD, Neely WA, Barnett WO: The effects of temporary arterial, venous, and arteriovenous occlusion upon intestinal blood flow. Surg Gynecol Obstet 108:347, 1959.

99. Laufman H, Method H: Role of vascular spasm in recovery of strangulated intestine: Experimental study. Surg Gynecol Obstet 85:675, 1943.

100. Nelson LE, Kremen AJ: Experimental occlusion of the superior mesenteric vessels with special reference to the role of intravascular thrombosis and its prevention by heparin. Surgery 28:819, 1950.

101. Khanna SD: An experimental study of mesenteric occlusion. J Pathol Bacteriol 77:575, 1959.

102. Khodadadi J, Rozencwajg J, Nacash N, et al: Mesenteric vein thrombosis. Arch Surg 115:315, 1980.

103. Lepley D, Mani CJ, Ellison EH: Superior mesenteric venous occlusion: A study using low molecular weight dextran to prevent infarction. J Surg Res 2:403, 1962.

104. Granger DN, Richardson PDI, Kvietys PR, Mortillaro NA: Intestinal blood flow. Gastroenterology 78:837, 1980.

105. Montgomery A, Borgstrom A, Haglund U: Pancreatic proteases and intestinal mucosal injury after ischemia and reperfusion in the pig. Gastroenterology 102:216, 1992.

106. Kazmers A, Zwolak R, Appleman HD, et al: Pharmacologic interventions in acute mesenteric ischemia: Improved survival with intravenous glucagon, methylprednisolone, and prostacyclin. J Vasc Surg 1:472, 1984.

107. Zhi-Young S, Yuan-Lin D, Xiao-Hong W: Bacterial translocation and multiple system organ failure in bowel ischemia and reperfusion. J Trauma 32:148, 1992.

108. Bilbao JI, Rodriguez-Cabello J, Longo J, et al: Portal thrombosis: Percutaneous transhepatic treatment with urokinase—A case report. Gastrointest Radiol 14:326, 1989.

109. Serreyn RF, Schoofs PR, Baetens PR, et al: Laparoscopic diagnosis of mesenteric venous thrombosis. Endoscopy 18:249, 1986.

110. Jabbari M, Cherry R, Goresky CA: The endoscopic diagnosis of mesenteric venous thrombosis. Gastrointest Endosc 31:405, 1985.

111. Bergentz SE, Ericsson B, Hedner U, et al: Thrombosis in the superior mesenteric and portal veins: Report of a case treated with thrombectomy. Surgery 76:286, 1974.

112. Yamashita Y, Kimitsuki H, Hiraki M, et al: Direct observation of the portal vein interior by intra-operative angioscopy in the dog and man. J Gastroenterol Hepatol 5:234, 1990.

113. Jona J, Cummins GM, Head HB, et al: Recurrent primary mesenteric venous thrombosis. JAMA 227:1033, 1974.

114. Dada FB, Balan AD, Newark D: Recurrent primary mesenteric venous thrombosis. South Med J 80:1329, 1987.

115. Robin P, Gruel Y, Lang M, et al: Complete thrombolysis of mesenteric vein occlusion with recombinant tissue-type plasminogen activator. Lancet 1(2):1391, 1988.

116. Picardi E, Rundell WK, Peoples JB: Effects of streptokinase on experimental mesenteric venous thrombosis in a feline model. Curr Surg 46:378, 1989.

117. Levy PJ, Krausz MM, Manny J: The role of second-look procedure in improving survival time for patients with mesenteric venous thrombosis. Surg Gynecol Obstet 170:287, 1990.

118. Bulkley GB, Zuidema GD, Hamilton SR, et al: Intraoperative determination of small intestinal viability following ischemic injury: A prospective controlled trial of two adjuvant methods (Doppler and fluorescein) compared with standard clinical judgement. Ann Surg 193:628, 1981.

119. Cooperman M, Martin EW, Carey LC: Determination of intestinal viability by Doppler ultrasonography in venous infarction. Ann Surg 191:57, 1980.

120. Gorey TF: Prediction of intestinal recovery after ischaemic injury due to arterial, venous and mixed arterial and venous occlusions. J R Soc Med 73:631, 1980.

121. Inahara T: Acute superior mesenteric venous thrombosis treatment by thrombectomy. Ann Surg 174:956, 1971.

122. Fontaine R, Pietri J, Masson JC, et al: Two recent cases of intestinomesenteric infarct of venous origin: The place of thrombectomy in the treatment. J Chir 97:145, 1969.

123. Ghaly M, Frawley JE: Superior mesenteric vein thrombosis. Aust N Z J Surg 56:277, 1986.

124. Harrison TA: Portal phlebothrombosis: The role of thrombectomy. Ann R Coll Surg Engl 60:320, 1978.

125. Marty A, Krampf K, Lauber A: Beitrag zur Klinik und Therapie der isolierten Mesenterialvenenthrombose. Helv Chir Acta 55:25, 1988.

126. Langnas AN, Marujo WC, Stratta RJ, et al: A selective approach to preexisting portal vein thrombosis in patients undergoing liver transplantation. Am J Surg 163:132, 1992.

127. Shaked A, Busuttil RW: Liver transplantation in patients with portal vein thrombosis and central portacaval shunts. Ann Surg 214:696, 1991.

128. Neuhas P, Bechstein WO, Blumhardt G, Steffen R: Management of portal venous thrombosis in hepatic transplant recipients. Surg Gynecol Obstet 171:251, 1990.

98

Treatment of Chronic Visceral Ischemia

Lloyd M. Taylor, Jr., M.D., and John M. Porter, M.D.

· · ·

Vascular surgeons become accustomed to diagnosing and treating disorders of the circulation caused by atherosclerosis, the most frequently encountered pathologic process in our aging population. This means that most atherosclerotic syndromes are encountered in large numbers, and individual surgeons quickly accumulate large personal case experiences. Similarly, the literature contains many articles describing the natural history and clinical outcome of patient series composed of hundreds or even thousands of individuals. Chronic intestinal ischemia, in contrast, is quite rare. All authorities agree that the clinical syndrome produced by inadequate blood supply to the intestines is encountered infrequently. Even major institutions with the accumulated experience of many thousands of arterial reconstructions rarely report an entire institutional experience exceeding 100 cases of chronic intestinal ischemia.[1-6] It is clear that few surgeons will accumulate sufficient case material to develop principles of treatment based on personal experience.

Unfortunately, the available literature describing chronic intestinal ischemia is vague at best. There are no large-scale natural history studies and no randomized or controlled clinical trials. Published anecdotal clinical reports do not present consistent recommendations for operative treatment, and in many reports technical details of operative procedures are simply not described. Others describe technically demanding procedures requiring extensive dissections in areas not frequently approached by most vascular surgeons.[7, 8] For all these reasons, there is no consensus regarding the treatment of chronic visceral ischemia.

This chapter summarizes available information on chronic visceral ischemia. The topics addressed include the natural history, indications for treatment, and treatment options, among them nonoperative therapy, balloon angioplasty, and surgical revascularization. The operations discussed are arterial bypass, both antegrade and retrograde and using vein or prosthetic grafts, and visceral artery endarterectomy. The recommendations for treatment in this chapter are based on the patient experience accumulated by the vascular surgery service at Oregon Health Sciences University. This service was founded by the senior author (JMP) in 1971, allowing some conclusions to be drawn from the long-term follow-up of patients treated with standardized methods.

NATURAL HISTORY OF CHRONIC INTESTINAL ISCHEMIA

Interestingly, the existence of a clinical syndrome in which chronic episodic abdominal pain results from the obstruction of intestinal arteries was postulated before it was clinically recognized. Conner speculated in 1933 that some patients with fatal intestinal infarction might have suffered earlier from misdiagnosed abdominal pain.[9] This speculation was confirmed by the important study conducted by Dunphy.[10] He reviewed the case records of 12 patients who died of intestinal infarction at the Peter Bent Brigham Hospital and found that 7 (58 per cent) had well-documented histories of "chronic recurrent abdominal pain preceding the fatal attack by weeks, months, or years."

After Dunphy's report, it was generally accepted that patients with "intestinal angina" existed and that, untreated, at least some of these patients progressed to fatal intestinal infarction.[11, 12] The possibility that surgical treatment might relieve the symptoms and prevent these deaths was proposed by Mikkelsen in 1957.[13] He described the typical orificial atherosclerotic lesions of the celiac and superior mesenteric artery that led to mesenteric thrombosis. Mikkelsen also noted that most frequently the distal arteries were spared in the atherosclerotic process and that this feature made surgical reconstruction before intestinal infarction feasible. In the next year, Shaw and Maynard performed the first reported arterial reconstructive surgery for the treatment of chronic intestinal ischemia.[14] Since then, many papers have documented successful surgical relief of the symptoms of chronic intestinal ischemia, including abdominal pain, food fear, and weight loss.[1-8]

Important questions about the natural history of chronic intestinal ischemia include the following: (1) How frequently do the typical arterial lesions occur? (2) How often are symptoms associated with the lesions? and (3) How often do symptomatic or asymptomatic individuals with intestinal arterial obstructions develop intestinal infarction? Although there is considerable information suggesting that atherosclerotic obstruction of the intestinal arteries is quite frequent, there is little information on the implications of these lesions in asymptomatic patients.

Significant atherosclerotic obstruction of the visceral arteries is present in 6 to 10 per cent of unselected autopsy cases.[15] In the more selected population undergoing abdominal aortography, significant stenosis of the celiac artery, the superior mesenteric artery, or both is present in 14 to 24 per cent.[16] An aortogram showing superior mesenteric artery occlusion in an asymptomatic patient is seen in Figure 98–1. Despite the frequency of visceral artery stenosis, symptomatic chronic intestinal ischemia is rare because of the excellent collateral circulatory network supplying the intestine. It is widely believed that intestinal collaterals are so extensive that at least two of the three intestinal vessels (the celiac, superior mesenteric, and inferior mesenteric arteries) must be stenotic or occluded for symptoms to occur.[13, 17] Although this aphorism serves to illustrate the principle, it is not true. Cases of bona fide symptomatic chronic intestinal ischemia to the point of infarction caused by single-vessel disease have occurred in the authors' experience and in the reported experience of others.[18] Single-vessel obstructions producing symptoms are almost always limited to the superior mesenteric artery. Isolated occlusions of the celiac artery or the inferior mesenteric artery appear to be well tolerated.

At present, no studies have allowed determination of the proportion of patients with asymptomatic intestinal arterial occlusions who subsequently become symptomatic with intestinal angina or develop catastrophic bowel infarction. Without such knowledge, it is impossible to make informed recommendations about the treatment of asymptomatic individuals with arteriographic findings such as those seen in Figure 98–1. This unanswered question represents a serious gap in the knowledge of the natural history of arterial occlusive disease. The frequency with which such lesions are seen on arteriography, combined with the rarity of symptomatic intestinal ischemia, suggests that progression to symptomatic visceral ischemia must be unusual.

Some information suggests caution with regard to the prognosis for at least one select subgroup of individuals with asymptomatic mesenteric arterial obstructions. This subset includes patients with superior mesenteric artery occlusion or high-grade stenosis who must undergo abdominal vascular surgery for other indications, such as aortoiliac or renal artery occlusive disease. Shaw and Maynard reported on a patient who developed acute intestinal ischemia after aortic surgery for lower extremity ischemia.[14] Connolly and Stemmer later reported on a series of patients who developed severe intestinal ischemia following aortic surgery.[19] Preoperatively, the patients had had no symptoms of intestinal ischemia. Connolly and Stemmer attributed this to a "steal" syndrome, although it appears more likely that the ischemia resulted from the disruption of vital retroperitoneal collaterals coincident with the aortic surgery. These reports, however, clearly indicate that individuals with asymptomatic superior mesenteric artery obstruction are at risk for postoperative intestinal ischemia when they undergo aortic surgery.

The natural history of symptomatic chronic intestinal ischemia appears to be well documented. Patients suffer intermittent abdominal pain and progressive weight loss resulting from voluntary food avoidance. The usual outcome following what may be a prolonged period of symptoms, ranging from months to years, is death from inanition or from intestinal infarction. Interestingly, there are presently insufficient data from which to predict the anticipated duration of illness, the likelihood of remission, and the frequency of the development of infarction.

NONOPERATIVE TREATMENT OF CHRONIC INTESTINAL ISCHEMIA

Because the symptoms of chronic visceral ischemia occur with food ingestion, it is logical that cessation of oral intake will eliminate the pain. This is indeed the case, and most patients voluntarily or involuntarily limit food intake, which inevitably results in the profound weight loss characteristic of chronic intestinal ischemia. It is possible to offset this by the administration of parenteral nutrition and to achieve both reversal of weight loss and relief of symptoms. This treatment is impractical as a solution to chronic visceral ischemia but may be of value in preparation for more definitive treatment.

Patients with chronic visceral ischemia are inevitably severely malnourished as a result of simple starvation. The increased operative risk associated with malnutrition in elderly atherosclerotic patients is well documented.[20] It is not known whether this risk can be reduced by a period of preoperative nutritional supplementation.[21] Despite this, it is the authors' practice to treat patients who have chronic visceral ischemia with cessation of oral intake and total parenteral nutrition for 7 to 10 days before elective revascularization is performed. The authors have not recognized an adverse outcome associated with this practice, and the benefits of reestablishing a positive nitrogen balance seem intuitively attractive. Obviously, such treatment is inappropriate for patients with signs of acute visceral ischemia.

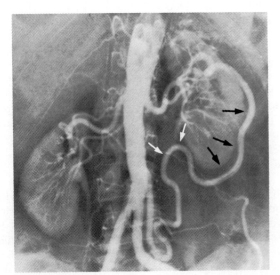

FIGURE 98–1.   Aortogram of a patient with superior mesenteric and celiac artery occlusions. A meandering mesenteric artery collateral is prominent *(arrows)*. The patient had no symptoms of intestinal ischemia. (From Taylor LM Jr, Porter JM: Treatment of chronic intestinal ischemia. Semin Vasc Surg 3:187, 1990.)

BALLOON ANGIOPLASTY TREATMENT OF CHRONIC INTESTINAL ISCHEMIA

Surgical reconstruction of obstructed intestinal arteries necessitates performing a major operative procedure on an elderly patient, who usually has both multi-system disease and profound recent weight loss. Minimally invasive percutaneous treatment is obviously an attractive alternative. Balloon angioplasty of the superior mesenteric artery was first reported by Furrer and coworkers in 1980.[22] Since this initial report appeared, many others have described the technical feasibility and the anecdotal results of visceral angioplasty.[23–28]

As described by Mikkelsen,[13] a frequent feature of atherosclerotic lesions producing intestinal artery obstruction is their location at the origin of the artery from the aorta. These "orificial" lesions are in fact composed mostly of aortic plaque, a portion of which extends into the visceral vessel. This location of plaque is the feature that makes visceral stenoses quite amenable to surgical repair but relatively unattractive for balloon angioplasty. As has been thoroughly documented in the renal circulation,[26] dilatation of orificial lesions has a low success rate. A similar lack of success with dilatation of visceral orificial lesions has also been described.[29]

For patients in whom balloon angioplasty has been successful, early recurrence of stenosis has been frequent in the visceral arteries. Tegtmeyer and Selby summarized the results of several reported series.[30] Of the procedures described, follow-up information was available on 35 patients. These patients were selected for their suitability for angioplasty, which means that most patients with typical orificial lesions were not selected for treatment. For example, the series of Odurny and associates, the largest of those reviewed, included only 1 patient (of a total of 10) with an orificial lesion.[24] Angioplasty was initially successful, as judged by angiographic appearance and relief of symptoms in 28 patients (80 per cent). The mean follow-up period was 28 months. During this interval, 8 patients (29 per cent of those with successful procedures) required surgery or repeated dilatation for recurrence of symptoms. More importantly, 7 of the 18 patients with follow-up intervals of greater than 12 months experienced a recurrence (39 per cent). Thus, the overall success rate of the procedure for patients with at least 12 months of follow-up was only 48 per cent (61 per cent of 80 per cent). Arteriograms of a patient with superior mesenteric artery stenosis before and after successful balloon angioplasty are shown in Figure 98–2. This patient experienced initial relief of symptoms associated with the angiographic improvement demonstrated in the figure. The symptoms and the stenosis recurred after 3 months, at which time the patient had successful surgical repair.

The use of expandable endovascular stents has been proposed to improve the results of dilatation of aortic orificial lesions involving the renal arteries. A preliminary trial has reported initial success in some patients.[31] A similar use of stents has also been proposed for intestinal arterial ostial stenoses. To date, the results of such procedures have not been reported.

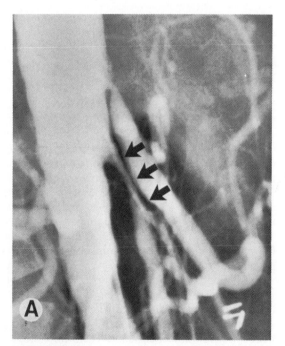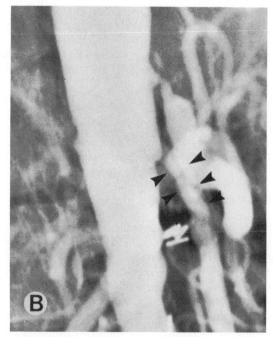

FIGURE 98–2. *A,* Lateral aortogram of a patient with intestinal ischemia and stenosis of the celiac and superior mesenteric arteries. Note that the superior mesenteric stenosis is distal to the aortic orifice *(arrows).* *B,* After balloon angioplasty, the lumen is considerably larger *(arrows).* The patient became asymptomatic for 3 months, when the symptoms and stenosis recurred. She was treated with bypass surgery. (*A* and *B,* From Taylor LM Jr, Porter JM: Treatment of chronic intestinal ischemia. Semin Vasc Surg 3:189, 1990.)

At present, the low likelihood of success for balloon angioplasty and the high reported recurrence rate influence the authors not to recommend this modality as initial therapy for patients with typical lesions. There are obviously exceptions. Rare lesions such as those caused by fibromuscular disease[23] or isolated short-segment atherosclerotic lesions beyond the first 1 to 2 cm of the superior mesenteric artery may be quite amenable to percutaneous interventional therapy. It is unlikely that this treatment will be of benefit to the large majority of symptomatic patients with typical lesions.

SURGICAL TREATMENT OF CHRONIC INTESTINAL ISCHEMIA

Indications for Surgery

As discussed previously, a few patients with chronic visceral ischemia may be adequately treated with balloon angioplasty. Except for these individuals, patients with symptomatic chronic visceral ischemia should be treated by operation. In the majority of cases, such patients will have been subjected to extensive diagnostic evaluation before surgical referral. Occasionally, however, vascular surgeons encounter patients with abdominal pain in whom only angiography showing typical lesions has been performed. It is wise to remember that chronic visceral ischemia is rare, and other conditions producing abdominal pain and weight loss occur much more frequently, especially visceral malignancy. In view of this relationship, it seems prudent to perform at least a gastrointestinal examination with endoscopy or radiology and abdominal CT before visceral revascularization.

At present, no information justifies visceral revascularization for asymptomatic lesions, with the important exception of patients with asymptomatic stenoses or occlusions of the superior mesenteric artery who must undergo other indicated aortic or renal artery operations. The occurrence of acute intestinal ischemia following such procedures is sufficiently well documented[14, 19] that the authors routinely perform superior mesenteric artery grafting at the time of the aortic surgery. Asymptomatic obstructions of the celiac artery do not require surgery.

Operative Techniques

A wide variety of operative techniques to revascularize obstructed superior mesenteric and celiac arteries have been reported, which serves as an ongoing source of confusion to surgeons with little experience in this field. Given the rarity of the clinical syndrome, a majority of surgeons are included in this category. Even a brief perusal of the literature yields techniques ranging from visceral artery reimplantation to endarterectomy to bypass. Bypass grafting has been performed with vein or prosthetics, and originating from almost any imaginable abdominal vessel.[1–8, 14, 32–46] A partial list of described techniques of visceral revascularization is given in Table 98–1. Interestingly, some authoritative reports on visceral revascularization have failed to describe operative technique beyond enumerating the visceral

Table 98–1. Techniques of Intestinal Arterial Revascularization

SMA or celiac reimplantation
Retrograde endarterectomy ("blind")
Direct vision endarterectomy
Transaortic endarterectomy
Antegrade infrarenal aorta–SMA vein graft
Retrograde infrarenal aorta–SMA or celiac artery vein graft, or both
Retrograde infrarenal aorta–SMA or celiac artery prosthetic graft, or both
Antegrade supraceliac aorta–SMA or celiac artery prosthetic graft, or both

SMA, superior mesenteric artery.

vessels revascularized, further compounding the difficulty of analyzing the suitability of different operations.[39–46]

Although it is tempting to conclude that the lack of technical detail in many reports, combined with the wide variety of described procedures, means that operative technique is not critical, this is clearly not the case. Meticulous operative technique is the foundation of successful vascular surgery. Many of the operations described for visceral revascularization have been performed in only small numbers, and little long-term follow-up information is available. Three basic operations have been widely described for the treatment of visceral ischemia, and each of these is discussed. They include endarterectomy, vein bypass grafting, and prosthetic bypass grafting.

Visceral Endarterectomy

As has been the history of most operations for atherosclerotic occlusive disease, the initial reports of surgery for visceral ischemia described the use of endarterectomy. Endarterectomy of the superior mesenteric artery can be accomplished in a blind retrograde fashion through a distal arteriotomy in the superior mesenteric artery,[14] although this approach is primarily of historical interest only. A more reliable approach is surgery performed under direct vision with control of the suprarenal aorta and incision across the origin of the superior mesenteric artery.[40] A third technique of visceral endarterectomy, termed transaortic endarterectomy[7] by its developers at the University of California at San Francisco, involves a posterolateral approach to the aorta and a "trapdoor" aortic incision, with subsequent visceral-origin endarterectomy through the opened aorta. This approach allows for simultaneous endarterectomy of the renal arteries and of the suprarenal aorta in selected patients.

Although significant numbers of patients have undergone visceral arterial endarterectomy, particularly transaortic endarterectomy, with excellent published results, most surgeons choose to use various forms of arterial bypass to treat chronic intestinal ischemia. There are multiple reasons for this decision. Surgical exposure of the proximal visceral vessels and the portion of the aorta from which they arise is infrequently performed by most surgeons and requires extensive dissection. The risks of suprarenal aortic clamping and direct operation on the origins of the visceral vessels include renal and lower extremity embolization, renal ischemia, and paraplegia, as well as a significantly increased risk of cardiac complications. Given the lack of familiarity with the required dissection on the part of most surgeons, as well as the significant inherent risks of the procedure, the choice of bypass by most surgeons is easily understood.

Infrarenal Aorta–Visceral Artery Vein Bypass

If not severely diseased, the infrarenal aorta may serve as the origin for visceral bypass grafts. If it is diseased, replacement with a prosthesis may be indicated, and this may obviously serve as a site for mesenteric graft origin. A technique shown as standard for these bypasses in many reference works consists of placement of a very short saphenous vein from the cephalad portion of the anterior wall of the infrarenal aorta to the superior mesenteric artery just below the inferior border of the pancreas.[47] Although this graft configuration is diagrammatically simple, there are several problems with it. When the patient is in the recumbent position, the proximal superior mesenteric artery is directly anterior to the aorta. The mass of the mesentery and the intestines normally rests on the retroperitoneum containing the aorta. Saphenous vein grafts from the infrarenal aorta to the superior mesenteric artery must be at right angles to both vessels, if they are short. If the graft is lengthened, in an effort to avoid acute angulation, the origin must be more distal, and the anastomoses remain acutely angulated. Thus, short grafts are particularly prone to kinking, and longer grafts do little to reduce this tendency (Fig. 98–3). Besides being subject to kinking and compression, saphenous vein grafts of average size will rarely carry more than 500 ml of blood per minute at physiologic pressures. Electromagnetic and noninvasive flow measurements indicate normal superior mesenteric artery flow in excess of 750 ml/min.[48]

Given these considerations, it is not surprising that several authors have found saphenous vein grafts generally

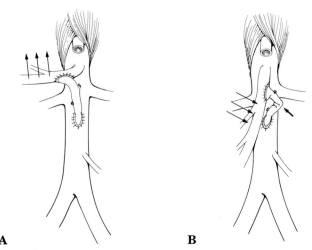

A   **B**

FIGURE 98–3. Potential for kinking that occurs with the use of short saphenous vein grafts from the infrarenal aorta to the superior mesenteric artery.

unsatisfactory for use as visceral bypass grafts.[2, 7, 49] The authors of this chapter prefer prosthetic grafts, usually 6- to 7-mm double-velour Dacron. An exception is made in cases in which perforation or necrosis of bowel has occurred and intestinal resection is required. In these cases, surgical judgment suggests avoiding prosthetics. The saphenous vein grafts are placed using the configuration described in the next section.

Current Approach to Visceral Revascularization

The procedure chosen for visceral revascularization for individual patients is based on the extent and location of aortic disease and on the need for other vascular procedures, such as infrarenal aortic grafting. The authors' clear first choice for the origin of a visceral artery bypass graft is the infrarenal aorta. There are several reasons for this choice. The exposure is familiar. The risks associated with dissection and clamping are less than those with the suprarenal or supraceliac aorta, and the procedure can be readily combined with other intra-abdominal procedures.

Avoiding the problems of kinking associated with saphenous vein grafts requires careful attention to graft configuration. The authors' preference for the origin of the graft is from the distal infrarenal aorta or from the junction of the aorta and the right common iliac artery. Crimped woven Dacron bifurcation grafts (12 × 7 mm) are used if both the superior mesenteric and the celiac arteries are to be revascularized. For superior mesenteric revascularization alone, a single limb is cut from a bifurcation graft in the manner described by Wylie and colleagues[50] to create a "flange" for sewing and to prevent constriction of the proximal anastomosis. The ligament of Treitz is dissected. The graft to the superior mesenteric artery is then passed as illustrated in Figure 98–4: first cephalad, then turning anteriorly and inferiorly a full 180 degrees to terminate in an antegrade anastomosis to the anterior wall of the superior mesenteric artery just beyond the inferior border of the pancreas. Exclusion of the graft from the peritoneal cavity and contact with the intestine is performed by closing the posterior parietal peritoneum, the ligament of Treitz, and the mesenteric peritoneum. When a celiac artery limb is included, the course is retropancreatic, with anastomosis to the hepatic or (rarely) the splenic artery. Obviously, an infrarenal aortic graft serves equally well as the origin for this configuration.

Infrarenal aorta–visceral artery grafting serves the majority of patients requiring operation. Occasionally, patients have contraindications to the use of the infrarenal aorta. These include severe atherosclerotic disease of the infrarenal aorta for which concomitant aortic grafting is not indicated. An example is shown in Figure 98–5. Another relative contraindication to the use of the infrarenal aorta is previous surgery in this area, with resultant scarring and hazardous redissection. In these cases, bypass grafts from the supraceliac aorta to the visceral arteries are an excellent alternative. Some surgeons have advocated the use of the supraceliac aortic graft origin as the procedure of choice for visceral artery bypass, based on a perception of improved

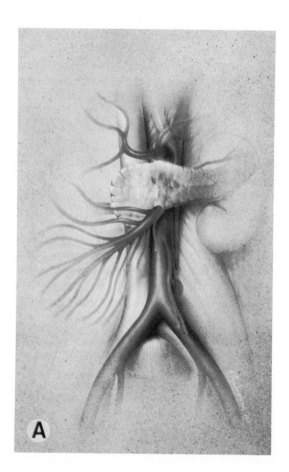

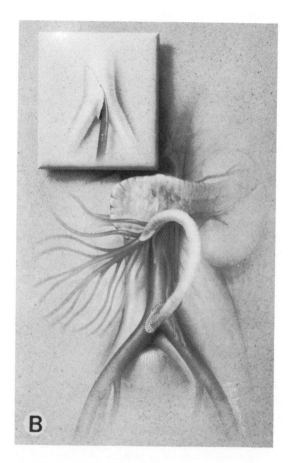

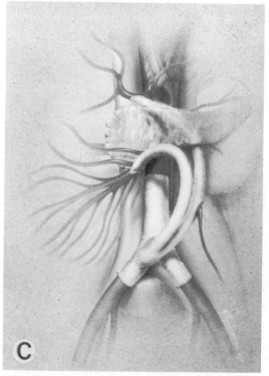

FIGURE 98–4.   *A*, Exposure of the infrarenal aorta and the superior mesenteric and celiac arteries. *B*, Method of infrarenal aorta–superior mesenteric artery bypass. *Inset*, Method of forming the graft origin. *C*, Method of infrarenal aortic graft placement with bypass to the superior mesenteric and hepatic arteries. Note the reimplantation of the inferior mesenteric artery. (*A–C*, From Taylor LM Jr, Porter JM: Treatment of chronic intestinal ischemia. Semin Vasc Surg 3:193, 1990.)

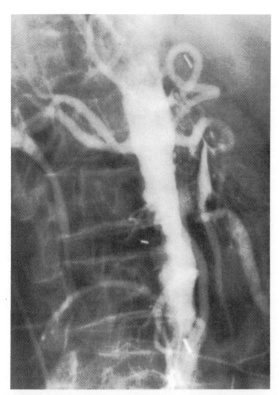

FIGURE 98–5. Severe disease of the infrarenal aorta in a patient with intestinal ischemia without symptoms of lower extremity ischemia. The supraceliac aorta was used for the visceral bypass origin. (From Taylor LM Jr, Porter JM: Treatment of chronic intestinal ischemia. Semin Vasc Surg 3:194, 1990.)

results with this procedure.[5, 8, 51] Such a conclusion is not justified by these reports. All based their conclusions of improved results on comparisons with historical control patients treated by other methods. Obviously, much has changed over time, not just operative methods. In particular, the results of prosthetic supraceliac aorta–visceral artery bypass grafting have been compared with those achieved with vein grafts or with prosthetic grafts from the infrarenal aorta that had a disadvantageous graft configuration, which is hardly an appropriate comparison.

The authors reserve the use of the supraceliac graft origin for special indications because of the added potential risks associated with supraceliac surgery, which include proximal aortic clamping and possible renal, hepatic, and lower extremity embolization or prolonged ischemia. These are obviously relative risks. Visceral bypass grafts can be anastomosed to most supraceliac aortas with partial-occlusion clamping. Hepatic, intestinal, and renal ischemia is usually well tolerated, in part because well-formed collaterals already exist. To minimize the risks associated with supraceliac aortic surgery, the procedure should be reserved for patients in whom this arterial segment is *angiographically normal*. Severely diseased supraceliac aortas are not suitable for partial-occlusion clamping or for use as visceral artery bypass origins.[52] An example of such an aorta is seen in Figure 98–6.

Supraceliac aorta–visceral artery bypass is performed through a mid-line abdominal incision, with the use of a

self-retaining retractor. The gastrohepatic ligament is incised; this is followed by incision of the diaphragmatic crus and exposure of the anterior surface of the aorta (Fig. 98–7). Woven Dacron bifurcation grafts or single limbs cut from a bifurcation graft are used (12 × 7 mm or 10 × 6 mm). After completion of the proximal anastomosis, celiac revascularization is accomplished by end-to-side anastomosis to the common hepatic artery. Grafts to the superior mesenteric artery are normally tunneled behind the pancreas and anastomosed to the anterior wall of the superior mesenteric artery in end-to-side fashion. In some patients, the retropancreatic space is narrow, and great care is necessary with the tunneling. Some surgeons advocate prepancreatic tunneling to avoid possible compression.[53]

Currently, the surgical literature favors revascularization of multiple visceral vessels over single-vessel repairs.[51, 54] There are no controlled or randomized studies to support this widely held opinion. Authors advocating this position have invariably performed more multiple-vessel operations in their more recent experience, leaving comparison to historical controls as the basis for this recommendation. The results obtained by the authors of this chapter, which are described in the following sections, do not justify this opinion. The critical vessel in chronic intestinal ischemia is the superior mesenteric artery, and adequate revascularization of this vessel will provide durable relief of symptoms in most patients. At present, the authors reserve multiple-vessel revascularization for patients in whom the superior mesenteric artery is diffusely diseased and there is a question about the durability of bypass to this vessel or for patients in whom previous surgery (especially gastrectomy or colectomy) has disrupted the normal collateral connections between the superior mesenteric and celiac beds.

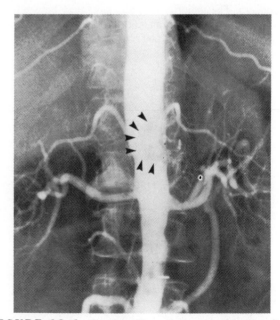

FIGURE 98–6. Extensive plaque *(arrows)* in the supraceliac aorta, making it unsuitable for safe clamping or for use as the origin of visceral bypass grafts. (From Taylor LM Jr, Porter JM: Treatment of chronic intestinal ischemia. Semin Vasc Surg 3:194, 1990.)

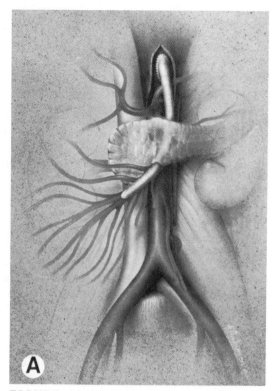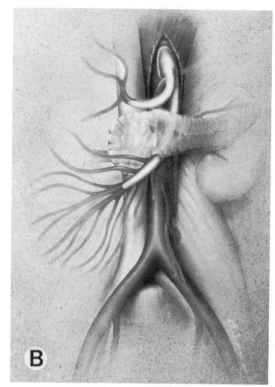

FIGURE 98–7. *A*, Supraceliac aorta–superior mesenteric artery bypass. The graft origin is best cut from a bifurcation graft, as illustrated in Figure 98–4*B*. *B*, Supraceliac aorta–superior mesenteric and hepatic bypass. (*A* and *B*, From Taylor LM Jr, Porter JM: Treatment of chronic intestinal ischemia. Semin Vasc Surg 3:195, 1990.)

Assurance of Technical Success

Electromagnetic flow measurement is helpful to ensure unobstructed intestinal revascularization. Flow below 400 ml/min in either celiac or superior mesenteric grafts is cause for concern. The majority of grafts have flow between 500 and 800 ml/min. Occasional grafts have flow exceeding 1000 ml/min. It is important that flow measurements be performed after all packs and retractors have been removed and after the viscera have returned to their normal position of repose. This approach should minimize technical failures from graft kinking.

In contrast to the situation with most other vascular repairs, continuous postoperative monitoring of the patency of visceral revascularizations is impossible, and early postoperative duplex scanning is difficult or impossible. Be-

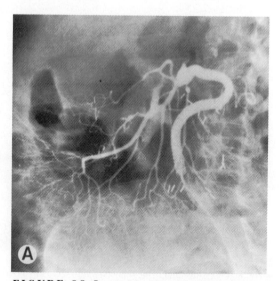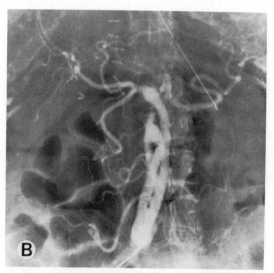

FIGURE 98–8. *A*, Selective postoperative arteriogram of an infrarenal aorta–superior mesenteric artery bypass. *B*, Postoperative arteriogram of an infrarenal aorta–superior mesenteric and hepatic bypass. (*A* and *B*, From Taylor LM Jr, Porter JM: Treatment of chronic intestinal ischemia. Semin Vasc Surg 3:196, 1990.)

cause most patients with chronic visceral ischemia have symptoms only with eating, it is quite possible for postoperative occlusion of bypass grafts to go unrecognized. Because of the normal incisional pain, fluid shifts, leukocytosis, and temperature elevation characteristic of the postoperative state, diagnosis of acute graft occlusion is difficult or impossible in the early postoperative period. When symptoms do occur with resumption of oral intake, reoperation may be difficult because of postoperative inflammatory scarring. Because of this, the authors routinely obtain arteriograms 5 to 7 days postoperatively to confirm visceral revascularization patency. Examples of these arteriograms are seen in Figures 98–8 and 98–9. If graft occlusion is discovered, reoperation and restoration of patency are mandatory.

Postoperative Care

Patients with chronic visceral ischemia often have significant ischemic bowel injury, which requires time for recovery. In addition, the preoperative symptom of ''food fear'' is in part a learned behavior that does not resolve rapidly postoperatively. Prolonged periods of inability to achieve adequate oral nutrition are frequent following visceral revascularization. For this reason, total parenteral nutrition is continued postoperatively.

Some patients with severe preoperative ischemia develop a ''revascularization syndrome'' consisting of abdominal pain, tachycardia, leukocytosis, and intestinal edema. Gewertz and Zarins described postoperative abdominal pain caused by intestinal vasospasm after revascularization.[55] Any deviation from a totally normal postoperative course should suggest the need for arteriography, re-exploration, or both. Problems are usually readily corrected if discovered early. Delayed diagnosis of graft occlusion or intestinal necrosis is invariably fatal. Even in the face of a totally normal postoperative course, angiography before hospital discharge is mandatory in the authors' opinion.

RESULTS OF REVASCULARIZATION FOR CHRONIC INTESTINAL ISCHEMIA

Table 98–2 lists the reported results of several large series of operations for the treatment of chronic intestinal ischemia. These results represent the outcome of revascularization with multiple operative methods, including bypass by antegrade and retrograde techniques and endarter-

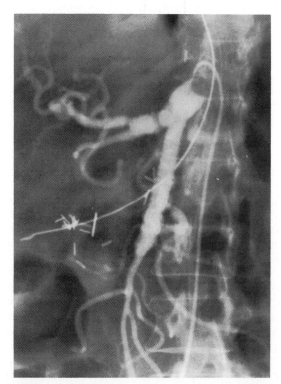

FIGURE 98–9. Selective postoperative arteriogram of a supraceliac aorta–superior mesenteric and hepatic bypass. (From Taylor LM Jr, Porter JM: Treatment of chronic intestinal ischemia. Semin Vasc Surg 3:197, 1990.)

ectomy. The reported results are quite similar to those achieved by the vascular surgery service at Oregon Health Sciences University.

From 1972 to 1993, 58 patients with chronic visceral ischemia were operated on by the vascular surgery service at Oregon Health Sciences University. The mean age of the patients was 61 years (range, 13 to 87 years), and the majority were female (66 per cent). Interestingly, no patients had diabetes. Most had had previous vascular surgery at some other site (64 per cent). These details are given in Table 98–3.

Of the 58 patients, 13 (22 per cent) had symptoms of acute visceral ischemia at the time of their operations, in addition to the clear history of chronic symptoms. Nine patients (15 per cent) had no symptoms of visceral ischemia. Their superior mesenteric artery occlusions were repaired at the time of indicated aortic or renal artery surgery. Twenty-six operations (45 per cent) included aortic grafting, renal artery grafting, or both.

Table 98–2.   Results of Revascularization for Chronic Intestinal Ischemia

Study	No. of Patients	Operative Mortality (%)	Female (%)	Follow-Up (yr)	Late Success (%)
McAfee et al, 1992[51]	58	10	79	5*	90
Cunningham et al, 1991[54]	74	12	82	5*	85
Rheudasil et al, 1988[56]	41	5	51	3.5	84
Current series	58	7	66	4.5	96

*Life table follow-up.

Table 98–3.   Chronic Intestinal Ischemia: Patient Data

Number	58
Age	61 yr (mean); 13–87 yr (range)
Sex	66% female
Diabetes	0
Previous vascular surgery	64%

All 58 patients had occlusion or severe stenosis of the superior mesenteric artery, emphasizing the central role of this vessel in chronic intestinal ischemia. Stenosis or occlusion of the celiac artery was present in 45 patients (78 per cent), and stenosis or occlusion of the inferior mesenteric artery was present in 35 patients (60 per cent). Only 5 patients had occlusions of the superior mesenteric artery without stenosis or occlusion of at least one other vessel. These angiographic results are summarized in Table 98–4.

All patients were treated with arterial bypass grafting procedures, 47 (81 per cent) of which were retrograde, from the infrarenal aorta, and 11 (19 per cent) of which were antegrade, from the supraceliac aorta. Grafting to the superior mesenteric artery was performed in all cases. The celiac artery was revascularized in 29 (50 per cent), and the inferior mesenteric artery was revascularized in 9 (16 per cent). Renal artery revascularization was performed simultaneously in 5 patients in this group. The operations performed are listed in Table 98–5.

Four patients (7 per cent) died postoperatively. All deaths occurred in patients with acute intestinal ischemia; three were from myocardial infarction, and one was from extensive intestinal infarction, which in retrospect was irreversible. There were no operative deaths in patients with chronic symptoms only and no operative deaths in patients without symptoms.

Postoperative complications included one hemorrhage requiring reoperation, one stroke, and three graft limb thromboses. All three thromboses were asymptomatic, were discovered by routine postoperative arteriography, and were corrected by reoperation. There were no episodes of postoperative bowel necrosis.

The follow-up for these patients ranged from 6 months to 13 years (mean follow-up, 4.5 years). Late complications include one graft infection occurring 3 years postoperatively in a patient whose initial operation was complicated by gangrenous cholecystitis, the complications of which were fatal. There were two late graft occlusions, both occurring in retrograde grafts to the superior mesenteric artery. One graft occlusion occurred 10 years postoperatively and resulted in fatal intestinal infarction. The second occurred 11 years postoperatively and resulted in recurrent intestinal ischemia. This patient was successfully revascularized with an antegrade graft.

Table 98–4.   Chronic Intestinal Ischemia:
Angiographic Findings

SMA stenosis or occlusion	100%
Celiac stenosis or occlusion	78%
IMA stenosis or occlusion	60%
Single-vessel stenosis or occlusion (all SMA)	9%

SMA, superior mesenteric artery; IMA, inferior mesenteric artery.

Table 98–5.   Chronic Intestinal Ischemia: Operations Performed

Operation	No. of Patients (%)
Retrograde bypass	47 (81)
Antegrade bypass	11 (19)
Graft to SMA	58 (100)
Graft to celiac artery	29 (50)
Graft to IMA	9 (16)
Simultaneous aortic graft, renal graft, or both	26 (45)

SMA, superior mesenteric artery; IMA, inferior mesenteric artery.

OVERVIEW AND CONCLUSIONS

Chronic intestinal ischemia is a rare symptomatic manifestation of atherosclerosis, and there are important gaps in our knowledge of the natural history of this condition. When it does occur, the results given in Table 98–2 and those described from the authors' service demonstrate that when properly diagnosed, chronic intestinal ischemia is amenable to surgical treatment by standard techniques, with predictably good immediate and long-term results. Although some unusual intestinal arterial lesions are amenable to treatment by balloon angioplasty, the anatomic nature of the most frequently encountered stenoses and occlusions means that for the foreseeable future, most patients will require surgery. The authors' clear preference for surgical technique involves prosthetic bypass from the infrarenal aorta to the superior mesenteric artery, with antegrade bypass and multiple-vessel revascularization reserved for special indications. The authors believe that aggressive postoperative care and angiographic confirmation of technical success are important for optimal results.

References

1. Crawford ES, Morris GC Jr, Myhre HO, Roehm JOF Jr: Celiac axis, superior mesenteric artery, and inferior mesenteric artery occlusion: Surgical considerations. Surgery 82:856, 1977.
2. Zelenock GB, Graham LM, Whitehouse WM, et al: Splanchnic arteriosclerotic disease and intestinal angina. Arch Surg 115:497, 1980.
3. MacFarlane SD, Beebe HG: Progress in chronic mesenteric arterial ischemia. J Cardiovasc Surg 30:178, 1989.
4. Baur GM, Millay DJ, Taylor LM Jr, Porter JM: Treatment of chronic visceral ischemia. Am J Surg 148:138, 1984.
5. Rapp JH, Reilly LM, Qvarfordt PG, et al: Durability of endarterectomy and antegrade grafts in the treatment of chronic visceral ischemia. J Vasc Surg 3:799, 1986.
6. Hollier LH, Bernatz PE, Pairolero PC, et al: Surgical management of chronic intestinal ischemia: A reappraisal. Surgery 90:940, 1981.
7. Stoney RJ, Ehrenfeld WK, Wylie EJ: Revascularization methods in chronic visceral ischemia. Ann Surg 186:468, 1977.
8. Beebe HG, MacFarlane S, Raker EJ: Supraceliac aortomesenteric bypass for intestinal ischemia. J Vasc Surg 5:749, 1987.
9. Conner LA: A discussion of the role of arterial thrombosis in the visceral diseases of middle life, based upon analogies drawn from coronary thrombosis. Am J Med Sci 185:13, 1933.
10. Dunphy JE: Abdominal pain of vascular origin. Am J Med Sci 192:109, 1936.
11. Benjamin D: Mesenteric thrombosis. Am J Surg 76:338, 1948.
12. McClenahan JE, Fisher B: Mesenteric thrombosis. Surgery 23:778, 1948.
13. Mikkelsen WP: Intestinal angina: Its surgical significance. Am J Surg 94:262, 1957.
14. Shaw RS, Maynard EP III: Acute and chronic thrombosis of the mesenteric arteries associated with malabsorption: A report of two cases successfully treated by thromboendarterectomy. N Engl J Med 258:874, 1958.

15. Croft RJ, Menon GP, Marston A: Does intestinal angina exist? A critical study of obstructed visceral arteries. Br J Surg 68:316, 1981.
16. Moneta GL, Lee RW, Yeager RA, et al: Mesenteric duplex scanning: A blinded prospective study. J Vasc Surg 17:79, 1993.
17. Hansen HJB: Abdominal angina. Acta Chir Scand 142:319, 1976.
18. Bergan JJ, Yao JST: Chronic intestinal ischemia. In Rutherford RB (ed): Vascular Surgery. 3rd ed. Philadelphia, WB Saunders, 1989, pp 1097–1103.
19. Connolly JE, Stemmer EA: Intestinal gangrene as the result of mesenteric arterial steal. Am J Surg 126:197, 1973.
20. Christou NV, Meakins JL: Neutrophil function in anergic surgical patients: Neutrophil adherence and chemotaxis. Ann Surg 190:557, 1979.
21. Fischer JE: Metabolism in surgical patients. In Sabiston DC Jr (ed): Textbook of Surgery. 14th ed. Philadelphia, WB Saunders, 1991, pp 103–140.
22. Furrer J, Gruntzig A, Kugelmeier J, Goebel N: Treatment of abdominal angina with percutaneous dilation of an arteria mesenterica superior stenosis. Cardiovasc Intervent Radiol 3:43, 1980.
23. Golden DA, Ring EJ, McLean GK, Freiman DB: Percutaneous angioplasty in the treatment of abdominal angina. AJR 139:247, 1982.
24. Odurny A, Sniderman KW, Colapinto RF: Intestinal angina: Percutaneous transluminal angioplasty of the celiac and superior mesenteric arteries. Radiology 167:59, 1988.
25. Birch SJ, Colapinto RF: Transluminal dilatation in the management of mesenteric angina: A report of two cases. J Can Assoc Radiol 33:46, 1982.
26. Roberts L, Wertman DA, Mills SR, et al: Transluminal angioplasty of the superior mesenteric artery: An alternative to surgical revascularization. AJR 141:1039, 1983.
27. Wilms G, Baert AL: Transluminal angioplasty of superior mesenteric artery and celiac trunk. Ann Radiol 29:535, 1986.
28. Levy PJ, Haskell L, Gordon RL: Percutaneous transluminal angioplasty of splanchnic arteries: An alternative method to elective revascularization in chronic visceral ischaemia. Eur J Radiol 7:239, 1987.
29. Cicuto KP, McLean GK, Oleaga JA, et al: Renal artery stenosis: Anatomic classification for percutaneous transluminal angioplasty. AJR 137:599, 1981.
30. Tegtmeyer CJ, Selby JB: Balloon angioplasty of the visceral arteries (renal and mesenteric circulation): Indications, results, and complications. In Moore WS, Ahn SS (eds): Endovascular Surgery. Philadelphia, WB Saunders, 1989, pp 223–257.
31. Rees CR, Palmaz JC, Becker GJ, et al: Palmaz stent in atherosclerotic stenoses involving the ostia of the renal arteries: Preliminary report of a multicenter study. Radiology 181:507, 1991.
32. Bergan JJ, Dean RH, Conn J Jr, Yao JST: Revascularization in treatment of mesenteric infarction. Ann Surg 182:430, 1975.
33. Nunn DB: Chronic intestinal angina: A report of two patients treated successfully by operation. Ann Surg 175:523, 1972.
34. Eidemiller LR, Nelson JC, Porter JM: Surgical treatment of chronic visceral ischemia. Am J Surg 138:264, 1979.
35. Jaxheimer EC, Jewell ER, Persson AV: Chronic intestinal ischemia. Surg Clin North Am 64:123, 1985.
36. Hollier LH: Revascularization of the visceral artery using the pantaloon vein graft. Surg Gynecol Obstet 155:415, 1982.
37. Daily PO, Fogarty TJ: Simplified revascularization of the celiac and superior mesenteric arteries. Am J Surg 131:762, 1976.
38. Rogers DM, Thompson JE, Garrett WV, et al: Mesenteric vascular problems. Ann Surg 195:554, 1982.
39. Rob C: Stenosis and thrombosis of the celiac and superior mesenteric arteries. Am J Surg 114:363, 1967.
40. Hansen HJB: Abdominal angina: Results of arterial reconstruction in 12 patients. Acta Chir Scand 142:319, 1976.
41. McCollum CH, Graham JM, DeBakey ME: Chronic mesenteric arterial insufficiency: Results of revascularization in 33 cases. South Med J 69:1266, 1976.
42. MacFarlane SD, Beebe HG: Progress in chronic mesenteric ischemia. J Cardiovasc Surg 30:178, 1989.
43. Reul GJ Jr, Wukasch DC, Sandiford FM, et al: Surgical treatment of abdominal angina: Review of 25 patients. Surgery 75:682, 1974.
44. Pokrovsky AV, Kasantchjan PO: Surgical treatment of chronic occlusive disease of the enteric branches of the abdominal aorta. Ann Surg 191:51, 1980.
45. Hollier LH, Bernatz PE, Pairolero PC, et al: Surgical management of chronic intestinal ischemia: A reappraisal. Surgery 90:940, 1981.
46. Stanton PE Jr, Hollier PA, Seidel TW, et al: Chronic intestinal ischemia: Diagnosis and therapy. J Vasc Surg 4:338, 1986.
47. Bergan JJ, Yao JST: Chronic intestinal ischemia. In Rutherford RB (ed): Vascular Surgery. 3rd ed. Philadelphia, WB Saunders, 1989, pp 1097–1103.
48. Moneta GL, Taylor DC, Helton WS, et al: Duplex ultrasound measurement of postprandial intestinal blood flow: Effect of meal composition. Gastroenterology 95:1294, 1988.
49. Hertzer NR, Humphries AW: Chronic intestinal ischemia. Surg Gynecol Obstet 145:321, 1977.
50. Wylie EJ, Stoney RJ, Ehrenfeld WK: Visceral atherosclerosis. In Manual of Vascular Surgery. New York, Springer-Verlag, 1980, p 211.
51. McAfee MK, Cherry KJ Jr, Naessens JM, et al: Influence of complete revascularization on chronic mesenteric ischemia. Am J Surg 164:220, 1992.
52. Taylor LM Jr, Porter JM: Supraceliac aortic bypass. In Bergan JJ, Yao JST (eds): Aortic Surgery. Orlando, FL, Grune & Stratton, 1988, pp 195–210.
53. Cooley DA, Wukasch DC: Techniques in Vascular Surgery. Philadelphia, WB Saunders, 1979, p 120.
54. Cunningham CG, Reilly LM, Rapp JH, et al: Chronic visceral ischemia. Ann Surg 214:276, 1991.
55. Gewertz BL, Zarins CK: Postoperative vasospasm after antegrade mesenteric revascularization: A report of three cases. J Vasc Surg 14:382, 1991.
56. Rheudasil JM, Stewart MT, Schellack JV, et al: Surgical treatment of chronic mesenteric arterial insufficiency. J Vasc Surg 8:495, 1988.

99

Colon Ischemia Following Aortic Reconstruction

Calvin B. Ernst, M.D.

· · ·

Refinements in operative technique, improved preoperative and postoperative care, and sophisticated perioperative monitoring methods have contributed to a progressive reduction in mortality and morbidity for abdominal aortic reconstruction. This steady decline since the late 1950s to an operative death rate of about 2 per cent for aortic aneurysmectomy has been gratifying.[13, 54, 55] Achievement of better results and reduction of operative deaths and morbidity to the ideal minimum of zero depend not only on prevention but also on recognition and appropriate treatment of morbid and potentially lethal events following operation. Intestinal ischemia, particularly colonic, is such a complication. Identification of patients at risk should aid in its prevention. Furthermore, prediction may preclude its occurrence by identifying which patients require reconstruction of the inferior or the superior mesenteric artery during aortic reconstruction.

The overall mortality rate for colon ischemia approximates 50 per cent, and it approaches 90 per cent with transmural involvement.[5, 16, 28, 35, 42, 49, 51, 56, 64] Conservative estimates of the number of aortic reconstructions for aneurysmal disease performed in 1985 in the United States placed the number at 33,000. Added to this were about 30,000 aortic reconstructions for occlusive disease, for a total of 63,000 aortic reconstructive procedures performed annually.[18] If the accepted incidence of 2 per cent for ischemic colitis developing after aortic reconstruction is assumed, with an attendant mortality rate of 50 per cent, it is clear that colon ischemia contributes significantly to the total operative deaths for aortic reconstruction. Preventing this complication should therefore improve results of aortic reconstruction and thereby help realize the ideal operative death rate of zero.

CLASSIFICATION AND INCIDENCE

Colon ischemia may follow abdominal aortic reconstruction for aneurysmal or occlusive disease.[6, 16, 23, 28, 37, 42, 56, 60] Reports of clinically manifest cases following aneurysmectomy predominate. Almost all reports describe arterial ischemia. Venous ischemia is so rare after aortic reconstruction that for practical purposes it may be ignored.

Depending on the severity of ischemia and the thickness of bowel wall involved, three forms of ischemic colitis have been recognized: mucosal ischemia, which is transient and mild; mucosal and muscularis involvement, which may result in healing with fibrosis and stricture; and transmural ischemia, which results in gangrene and perforation (Table 99–1). More than 60 per cent of reported cases describe transmural ischemia.

The most commonly encountered type of intestinal ischemia following aortic reconstruction involves the sigmoid colon after aneurysmectomy with inferior mesenteric artery ligation.[3–6, 20, 23, 28, 35, 41, 42, 45, 46, 51, 56, 60]

The incidence of ischemic colitis following aortic reconstruction varies from 0.2 to 10 per cent.[3–5, 16, 23, 27, 28, 37, 42, 46, 47, 51, 56, 60] Several authors have suggested that the actual incidence may be greater than the commonly accepted 2 per cent because most reports in the literature are retrospective studies of clinically manifest cases. In such reports, ischemic colitis is three to four times as common following aneurysmectomy as it is following reconstruction for occlusive disease.[28] In a prospective study of abdominal aortic reconstructive procedures for both aneurysmal and occlusive disease, the overall incidence of ischemic colitis, iden-

Table 99–1. Classification and Clinical Course

Type	Pathologic Findings	Clinical Findings	Clinical Outcome
I	Mucosal ischemia, submucosal edema or hemorrhage; mucosal slough ulceration may follow	Diarrhea with or without blood; presence or absence of fever; onset usually in 24–48 hr	Reversible; no sequelae; near-zero mortality
II	As above, with penetration of muscularis	Symptoms vary between type I and type II	Reversible; residual ischemic stricture possible
III	Transmural bowel involvement	Profound physiologic changes; sepsis, acidosis, cardiovascular collapse; may develop feculent peritonitis or late fecal fistula	Irreversible; mortality = $70 \pm 10\%$

From Tollefson DFJ, Ernst CB: Colon ischemia following aortic reconstruction. Ann Vasc Surg 5:485–489, 1991. Reprinted by permission of Blackwell Scientific Publications, Inc.

tified by routine postoperative colonoscopy, was 6 per cent.[16] Ischemic changes were noted in 4.3 per cent of patients who underwent reconstruction for occlusive disease and in 7.4 per cent of those who underwent aneurysmectomy. When aneurysmectomy for ruptured aneurysm was included, the overall incidence of ischemic colitis approached 12 per cent. Among patients studied after reconstruction for ruptured aneurysm, the incidence of ischemic colitis was 60 per cent.[23] Other authors have confirmed a high incidence of ischemic colitis following aneurysm rupture.[1, 30]

ANATOMY AND PATHOPHYSIOLOGY

The inferior mesenteric artery and its branches are connecting links between the superior mesenteric artery and hypogastric artery circulations. Among these three circuits, the inferior mesenteric artery provides the chief blood supply to the left colon. After arising at a 30-degree angle from the left anterolateral aspect of the aorta, the inferior mesenteric branches into the left colic artery, three to four sigmoid vessels, and the superior rectal artery. Inferior mesenteric branching occurs 3 to 4 cm from its aortic origin.

The marginal artery of Drummond, originally described by von Haller in 1786, is an important connecting link between the superior and inferior mesenteric arteries. At the splenic flexure, the left colic branch of the superior mesenteric and the left colic artery from the inferior mesenteric anastomose to provide marginal artery of Drummond continuity. This is Griffiths' point.[22] Griffiths noted a critical area in the region of the splenic flexure where functional anastomoses may be marginal or lacking in 5 per cent of individuals. In addition, noting the absence of the middle colic artery in 20 per cent of individuals, he emphasized the importance of both the right colic branch from the superior mesenteric artery and the hypogastric arteries in ligation of the inferior mesenteric artery in such patients.

The meandering mesenteric artery is a large, continuous communicating link between the left branch of the middle colic and the left colic arteries (Fig. 99–1). The meandering mesenteric artery has also been termed the central anastomotic artery of the colon, the marginal artery, the mesomesenteric artery, the middle-left colic collateral, the artery of Drummond, the arc of Riolan, and the arch of Treves. Such a profusion of names has caused confusion about colonic collateral circulation in general and the meandering mesenteric artery in particular. The preferred term for this vital collateral channel between the superior and inferior mesenteric arterial circuits is the *meandering mesenteric artery*.[40] This vessel is *potentially* present in about two thirds of normal individuals. It has been identified on routine preoperative aortography in 35 and 27 per cent of patients with aortoiliac occlusive disease and aneurysmal disease, respectively.[16]

The hypogastric arteries through the middle and inferior rectal branches provide a communication between the systemic and visceral circulations to the left colon by way of the superior rectal branch of the inferior mesenteric artery.

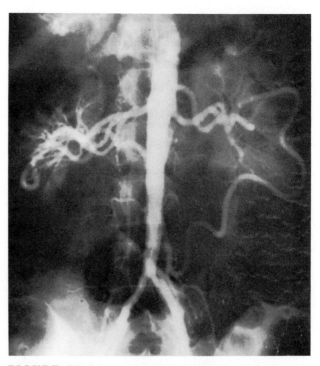

FIGURE 99–1. Aortographic documentation of a large meandering mesenteric artery.

The superior mesenteric artery provides blood to the small bowel and the right half of the colon. If the small bowel derives a significant amount of its blood supply from the inferior mesenteric by way of the meandering mesenteric artery because of complete or partial superior mesenteric artery occlusion, interruption of the meandering mesenteric artery during aortic reconstruction may eventuate in mid-gut gangrene.[4, 12, 21, 28, 50, 58]

Data have suggested, however, that after acute occlusion of the inferior mesenteric artery, branches of the superior mesenteric artery provide the major collateral blood flow to the inferior mesenteric artery circulation and collateral contributions from the hypogastric arteries are insignificant.[61] However, hypogastric collateral blood flow cannot be completely ignored, particularly among patients with celiac and superior mesenteric artery stenoses, in whom gut circulation depends on meandering mesenteric artery blood flow contributed by the hypogastric vessels.

Precise knowledge of anatomic pathways of collateral circulation to the bowel assumes importance when the vascular surgeon undertakes aortic reconstruction. Preservation of as many collateral circuits and restoration of flow to as many vital arterial branches as possible are imperative to prevent ischemic colitis.

Many factors affect the development of colon ischemia after aortic reconstruction. Among them are caliber of the vessel occluded, duration and degree of ischemia, rapidity of onset of the ischemic process, adequacy and efficiency of collateral circulation, state of the general circulation, metabolic requirements of the affected bowel, presence of bacteria within the bowel lumen, and associated conditions such as colonic distention.[7] Although ligation of the inferior mesenteric artery is the main factor in the development of

Table 99–2. Predisposing Factors for the Development of Ischemic Colitis Following Aortic Reconstruction

Improper IMA ligation
Loss of IMA-hypogastric blood flow
Ruptured aneurysm
Perioperative hypotension and hypoperfusion
Manipulative trauma
Inadequate collateral development and recruitment
IMA to SMA flow in the meandering mesenteric artery

IMA, inferior mesenteric artery; SMA, superior mesenteric artery.

ischemic colitis in most reports, other causes are also cited. Identifiable predisposing factors include improper ligation of the inferior mesenteric artery, failure to restore inferior mesenteric or hypogastric artery blood flow, ruptured aneurysm with mesenteric compression by hematoma, manipulative trauma to the colon by retractors, persistent hypotension and hypoperfusion, congenitally inadequate collateral communications between mesenteric circulations, and damage of vital existing collateral vessels, such as the meandering mesenteric artery (Table 99–2).

Ischemia and reperfusion result in the release of toxic metabolites of molecular oxygen, superoxide and hydroxyl free radicals.[59] Xanthine oxidase is a source of the superoxide radical. Superoxide species are very toxic to the intracellular matrix and cell membranes.

The abundance in intestinal mucosa of xanthine dehydrogenase, which is rapidly converted to xanthine oxidase during ischemia, provides a potential mechanism for free radical generation and subsequent cellular destruction with loss of integrity of the mucosal barrier. Loss of the mucosal barrier results in translocation of bacteria into the systemic circulation. The ensuing systemic sepsis and endotoxemia may exacerbate or eventuate in multiple organ system failure, the adult respiratory distress syndrome, hepatic failure, and renal failure.

The precise clinical application of inhibitors of the conversion of xanthine dehydrogenase to xanthine oxidase, such as superoxide dismutase, catalase, allopurinol, soybean trypsin inhibitor, mannitol, and dimethyl sulfoxide, to prevent or treat colonic ischemia has not yet been delineated.

CLINICAL MANIFESTATIONS AND DIAGNOSIS

Awareness of the potential development of ischemic colitis following aortic reconstruction should alert the surgeon to early diagnosis. Knowledge of the predisposing factors cited earlier enhances this awareness. The reported overall 50 per cent mortality rate from this complication suggests that delay in diagnosis may preclude effective therapy.[28] A high index of suspicion for patients at greatest risk for developing ischemic colitis is mandatory to reduce deaths and morbidity.

Depending on the degree of bowel ischemia, clinical manifestations vary from the subclinical form to bowel gangrene with perforation, peritonitis, and death (see Table 99–1). Undoubtedly, among many patients, minor degrees of ischemia go unrecognized and the patients recover.[5, 16, 42, 46]

Some minor and all major episodes of ischemia produce symptoms.

Clinical manifestations of colonic ischemia may be masked or complicated by the systemic responses and altered abdominal findings that normally follow major operations. The most common symptom is diarrhea, either brown liquid or bloody.[3, 5, 28, 31, 35, 46, 49, 51, 56] Although its onset may occur as long as 14 days after operation, diarrhea usually begins within 24 to 48 hours of operation in 75 per cent of patients. Bloody diarrhea has been reported to be more ominous than nonbloody diarrhea.[5] However, some investigators have noted no correlation between extent of ischemic injury, prognosis, and presence of bloody diarrhea.[42] Any diarrhea, bloody or not, should prompt immediate endoscopic evaluation.

Other symptoms include extraordinary postoperative pain, particularly in the left side of the abdomen. Progressive abdominal distention not relieved by intestinal decompression and accompanied by signs of peritoneal irritation points to bowel perforation. Signs and symptoms of sepsis, such as unexplained leukocytosis of 20,000 to 30,000 cells/mm³, severe or refractory acidosis, progressive oliguria, and elevated temperature, should cause the surgeon to consider colon ischemia. Unexplained metabolic acidosis, unusual requirements for crystalloid and colloid solutions, and development of hypotension in the absence of sepsis or hypovolemia are not specific for, but should suggest, bowel infarction. Severe thrombocytopenia (fewer than 90,000 platelets/mm³) has been suggested as a marker of bowel necrosis and should arouse suspicion of ischemic colitis in symptomatic patients.[31]

Biochemical markers such as serum phosphorus, urea, uric acid, lactic dehydrogenase, creatine, phosphokinase, alkaline phosphatase, aspartate aminotransferase, alanine aminotransferase, hexosaminidase, and vasoactive intestinal polypeptide have not proved to be specific for documentation of ischemic colitis. Nevertheless, with normal liver and renal function, marked elevations in any of these should alert the clinician to possible colonic ischemia.

Endoscopy, employing the fiberoptic colonoscope, is the most reliable diagnostic modality available.[17, 23] Repeated studies over several days are required to document resolution or progression of the ischemic process. Passage of the colonoscope up to 40 cm is usually sufficient to detect ischemic colitis. Ischemia in other segments of the colon without left colon involvement is rare.[23] If colonic ischemia is identified, colonoscopy must be terminated. Passage of the instrument beyond the involved bowel segment should be avoided lest perforation occur.

Flexible colonoscopy may be performed at the bedside and does not require transport to a specialized area. Early changes include circumferential petechial hemorrhages and edema. Finding pseudomembranes, erosions, and ulcers documents advanced stages of ischemia. A yellowish-green, necrotic, noncontractile surface defines gangrene.

Barium contrast studies, although helpful in documenting late sequelae of ischemic colitis, are usually not required for diagnosis in the immediate postoperative period. Hazards of barium enema include those involved in moving a critically ill patient from the intensive care unit to the radiology suite and possible perforation with barium peritonitis.

Frequent re-examination of the abdomen; repeated colonoscopy; and monitoring of blood gases, urine output, fluid requirements, and vital signs are required when ischemic colitis has been identified. Progression of the ischemic process, documented by deteriorating clinical signs and worsening of symptoms, requires prompt operation. Increasing abdominal tenderness, fever, leukocytosis, thrombocytopenia, and worsening diarrhea that may progress from nonbloody to bloody indicate progression. Colonoscopy under these circumstances must be performed cautiously.

Progressive clinical deterioration associated with advancing colonic ischemia, such as that described earlier, requires reoperation. Ischemia of the colon requires resection of all compromised bowel. Preoperative colonoscopy may be helpful to determine the extent of resection necessary. Primary anastomosis following resection is contraindicated. Colostomy with Hartmann's pouch or distal mucous fistula construction is necessary. During bowel resection, isolation of the retroperitoneum and the recently placed aortic prosthesis is necessary to prevent graft contamination. Rectal necrosis requires removal of the rectum and perineal drainage, but wide excision of the rectal segment as employed for treatment of rectal cancer is not necessary. Removal of the necrotic muscular and mucosal elements is all that is required to achieve pelvic débridement. Under these circumstances, every effort must be made to avoid exposing the aortic prosthesis. During reperitonealization of the pelvic floor, the area of the prosthesis must be isolated from the open perineum. An omental graft sutured into the pelvis may be required to achieve this objective.

Improvement, evidenced by subsidence of symptoms (e.g., lessening of diarrhea), stabilization of or improvement in laboratory parameters, and resolution of the ischemic process documented by repeated colonoscopy, permits nonoperative treatment. Under such circumstances, bowel rest must be maintained by nasogastric tube decompression. Broad-spectrum bacteriocidal antibiotics are administered intravenously.

Reversible lesions should improve within 7 to 10 days.[7, 17] Continued bleeding and diarrhea beyond 2 weeks strongly suggest walled-off colonic perforation requiring operation.

A minimally symptomatic or asymptomatic patient with a colonic stricture does not require surgery. Such strictures usually occur 6 to 10 weeks after the acute process. Some of these may respond to dilatation, but many symptomatic strictures require bowel resection.

PREVENTION

Although both awareness that patients are at risk for developing ischemic colitis and early diagnosis allow effective therapy, prevention of this catastrophe is eminently more successful in minimizing mortality and morbidity than is therapy for clinically manifest disease. Prediction of the development of ischemic colitis may prevent this complication altogether by identifying patients who require reconstruction of the inferior mesenteric artery. Prediction, however, may prove challenging because of the many diverse predisposing factors (see Table 99–2). Thorough preoperative assessment, including aortography, and attention to operative technical details greatly assist in avoiding the development of ischemic bowel complications after aortic reconstruction.

Aortography

Preoperative aortography has proved useful in identifying patients at risk for developing ischemic bowel disorders.[2, 6, 8, 16, 17, 28, 48] This is particularly true when the history and physical examination findings suggest intestinal angina. Under such circumstances, documentation of precarious visceral circulation dependent on the inferior mesenteric artery requires aortography.[12, 21] Aortographic documentation of a meandering mesenteric artery signals concomitant superior or inferior mesenteric artery arteriosclerosis, as shown in Figure 99–1.[12, 16, 21] Inferior mesenteric artery opacification from the superior mesenteric by the meandering mesenteric artery is predictive of minimal risk of ischemic colitis developing after aortic reconstruction, provided this important collateral vessel is preserved. Documentation of reversal of blood flow in the meandering mesenteric artery from the inferior to the superior mesenteric artery demands lateral filming following a second contrast medium injection to document occlusion or stenosis of the superior mesenteric artery. Under such conditions, prophylactic revascularization of the superior mesenteric or reconstruction of the inferior mesenteric during aortic reconstruction is required to prevent catastrophic small bowel ischemia.[12, 28]

Arteriographic identification of the presence or absence of hypogastric artery patency is helpful in planning aortic reconstruction so that pelvic blood flow may be preserved or restored. When the inferior mesenteric artery is ligated, the hypogastric arteries assume an important role in collateral circulation to the rectum.

Operative Technical Details

Strict attention to operative technical details is probably more influential in avoiding the development of ischemic colitis than are preoperative or postoperative factors. Common to almost all instances of ischemic colitis following aneurysmectomy is ligation of the inferior mesenteric artery. Improper ligation interrupts communications between the ascending left colic artery and the descending sigmoid branches. To preserve these branches, the inferior mesenteric artery must be dissected and ligated at its origin, or its orifice must be sutured closed from within after the aneurysm has been opened.

Gentleness during dissection of the aorta minimizes dispersion of embolic debris and prevents "trash colon." Manipulative trauma from overly vigorous retraction or packing may occlude mesenteric collateral channels, particularly in the left colon mesentery and mesosigmoid. Avoidance of such manipulation or opening and evacuating the mesentery in managing a ruptured aneurysm with its associated mesocolic hematoma may prove critical in preserving tenuous collateral blood flow.

Operative or postoperative hypotension and hypoperfusion must be prevented by proper administration of blood and fluids. In critically ill patients, analysis of central venous pressure and pulmonary wedge pressure data is essential to balance fluid therapy properly. Colonic circulation reliant on collateral blood flow following ligation of the inferior mesenteric artery may be more susceptible to hypotension and hypoperfusion than if the artery were intact. That intact collateral circuits maintain inferior mesenteric artery blood pressure near preligation levels has been documented.[17] Using inferior mesenteric artery stump blood pressure measurements as an index of the adequacy of inferior mesenteric artery collateral blood flow, the author's group found that 54 per cent of patients had greater inferior mesenteric artery stump pressures recorded following aneurysmectomy. However, if postoperative hypotension occurs, collateral perfusion may be jeopardized, with the resultant development of ischemic colitis. Preservation of vital pelvic collateral circulation by the restoration of pulsatile flow to one or both hypogastric arteries is required to minimize the development of ischemic colitis or proctitis.[3, 17, 32, 36, 51, 52] Adequate perfusion of at least one hypogastric artery may be accomplished in more than 90 per cent of cases. If hypogastric blood flow cannot be restored without resorting to complex reconstructive techniques, inferior mesenteric stump pressure measurements may document that hypogastric reconstruction may not be required, as is discussed later.

Clinical prediction of the viability of bowel, in particular the colon, is notoriously unreliable. Predictive criteria of viability using color, arterial pulsations, and peristalsis have proved unsatisfactory in distinguishing viable from nonviable bowel.[7, 10, 29, 38, 42, 46] Several techniques for predicting gut viability have been described, including radioisotope scanning, surface temperature determinations, electromyographic findings, and dye injection and detection techniques.[9, 10, 29, 38, 44, 53, 57] Such studies require specially designed equipment and may be time consuming, cumbersome, and complex.

As they pertain to colonic viability, two techniques for determining when the inferior mesenteric artery may be safely ligated and when reconstruction is required have merit.[17, 25, 26] One technique employs Doppler ultrasound to document arterial blood flow in the inferior mesenteric artery, in the large bowel mesentery, and on the serosal surface of the colon before and after occlusion of the artery (Fig. 99–2).[25, 26, 33] The other uses measurement of inferior mesenteric stump blood pressure (Fig. 99–3).[17] Two other described techniques, neither of which has undergone adequate clinical trials, have appeal.[19, 43] One employs indirect measurements of intramural pH by a silicone tonometer to measure PCO_2 changes in the lumen of the colon. Intramural pH measurements of less than 6.86 suggest colon ischemia.[19] The other employs a photoplethysmographic method using a sterile pulse oximeter probe to detect arterial pulsatility and transcolonic oxygen saturation. Unmeasurable transcolonic oxygen saturations and loss of pulsatility suggest colon ischemia.[43]

Hobson and colleagues, employing the Doppler technique, concluded that the presence of arterial flow sounds along the left colon confirmed adequacy of collateral flow, whereas the absence of Doppler sounds during inferior mes-

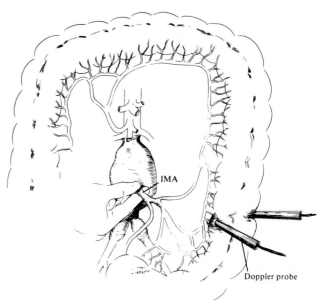

FIGURE 99–2. Application of a Doppler probe to the antimesenteric and mesenteric borders of the left colon during digital compression of the inferior mesenteric artery (IMA) documents the presence or absence of collateral blood flow. (From Bernhard VM, Towne JB: Complications in Vascular Surgery. New York, Grune & Stratton, 1980, p 398.)

enteric artery occlusion suggested potential colon ischemia.[26] Whether or not reconstruction of the artery is necessary when Doppler signals are lost, however, cannot be determined from this study because control data were not presented. Furthermore, routine postoperative colonoscopy

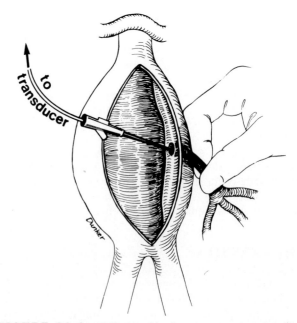

FIGURE 99–3. IMA stump blood pressure measurement. The cannula is threaded into the IMA orifice through the opened aneurysm sac. The cannula is secured into the arterial lumen by compression of the IMA and adjacent mesentery between the thumb and forefinger. (From Ernst CB: Prevention of intestinal ischemia following abdominal aortic reconstruction. Surgery 93:102, 1983. Reprinted by permission.)

to detect colon ischemia was not employed. The Doppler technique may be used for both occlusive and aneurysmal disease.

Inferior mesenteric artery stump pressure measurements are obtained by cannulating the divided distal artery with an 18-gauge Teflon catheter. Alternatively, and consistent with the author's preference, the catheter may be threaded into the arterial orifice from inside the open aneurysmal sac (see Fig. 99–3).[15] When mean stump blood pressures measure greater than 40 mmHg, the inferior mesenteric artery may be safely ligated, even when hypogastric pulsatile flow cannot be detected.[15, 17] Mean pressures of less than 40 mmHg forewarn of the possible development of ischemic colitis. It must be emphasized that reliance on stump pressure measurements assumes that systemic blood pressure and regional perfusion are maintained in the postoperative period at levels at least as high as when the operative measurements were determined. To impugn the usefulness of inferior mesenteric artery stump pressure measurements when postoperative bleeding and hypotension occur as a result of technical misadventures is not appropriate.[34] Even the best predictive test is not infallible under such circumstances.

At this time, controlled data are insufficient to endorse any of these techniques as foolproof predictors of the development of ischemic colitis or the need for inferior mesenteric artery reconstruction. Continued experience with them, however, may provide these data.[15] Measurement of inferior mesenteric artery stump blood pressure may offer advantages over hearing Doppler flow signals because audible flow may be present even though perfusion pressure is less than the critical closing pressure of the nutrient bed, namely 40 mmHg. A false sense of security may accompany hearing Doppler flow signals if perfusion pressure is less than 40 mmHg. Complete cessation of flow, however, appears to be a discriminating end-point with Doppler evaluation.

It must be recognized that the stump blood pressure technique may not be applicable in the management of occlusive disease because here the inferior mesenteric artery orifice is not available for cannulation, as it is when aneurysmal disease is being treated. Under these circumstances, Doppler evaluation is suggested.

Indirect intramural pH monitoring has appeal because it may be applicable to both occlusive and aneurysmal disease, but more importantly, it may serve as a continuing postoperative monitor of bowel viability.

Table 99–3 summarizes methods of operative assessment of colon viability.

Routine rather than selective reconstruction of all patent inferior mesenteric arteries may be justified, but only if the rate of complications after routine reconstruction is acceptably low. In a multi-center study, inferior mesenteric artery reconstruction was associated with an increased frequency of postoperative bleeding.[62] However, two reports in which 75 inferior mesenteric arteries were reconstructed provide support for routine inferior mesenteric artery reconstruction.[63, 65] Nevertheless, it could not be proved that routine inferior mesenteric artery reconstruction was superior to selective ligation, particularly when the safety of ligation was documented by objective evaluation of the adequacy of colonic collateral circulation with the use of the tests previously described.

INFERIOR MESENTERIC ARTERY RECONSTRUCTION

When to reconstruct the inferior mesenteric artery cannot be conclusively determined from reports in the literature. Some surgeons use objective data,[17, 26] whereas others rely on clinical intuitive methods.[3, 21, 24, 28, 39, 42] Nonetheless, the following techniques have proved effective: reimplantation of the inferior mesenteric origin as a button from the aorta into the prosthesis; the Carrel patch technique; and anastomosis of a portion of the aneurysmal sac including the orifice of the artery into the prosthesis (the inclusion technique, popularized by Crawford) (Figs. 99–4 and 99–5).[11, 14] Alternative methods include reimplantation of the inferior mesenteric artery without an aortic button and interposition grafting of prosthetic material or autogenous tissue from the aortic graft to the artery.

Table 99–3. Operative Assessment of Colon Viability

Test	Advantages	Disadvantages
Inspection	Easy	Inaccurate
Second look	Accurate	Second operation
Doppler ultrasound	Easy; inexpensive; 80% accurate	Limited bowel area sampled (2 cm²); one-time measurement during operation only
IMA stump pressure	Easy; inexpensive; highly accurate	One-time measurement during operation only; IMA must be cannulated
Colonic intramural pH	Able to monitor colonic blood flow operatively and postoperatively	Requires preoperative catheter placement in colon through rectum
Photoplethysmography with transcolonic oxygen saturation	Relatively easy; moderately accurate	Limited bowel area sampled; one-time measurement during operation only

From Tollefson DFJ, Ernst CB: Colon ischemia following aortic reconstruction. Ann Vasc Surg 5:485–489, 1991. Reprinted by permission of Blackwell Scientific Publications, Inc.
IMA, inferior mesenteric artery.

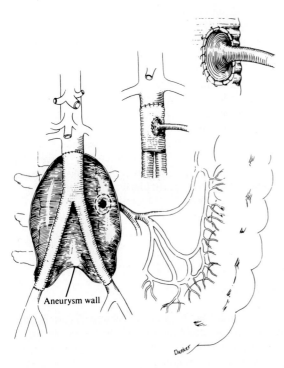

Aneurysm wall

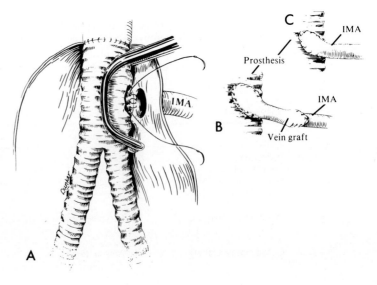

FIGURE 99–4.   Carrel patch technique for reconstruction of the IMA. Excision of a button of aneurysm wall surrounding the artery's orifice facilitates repair. (From Bernhard VM, Towne JB: Complications in Vascular Surgery. New York, Grune & Stratton, 1980, p 402.)

FIGURE 99–5.   Reconstruction of the IMA. *A*, Anastomosis of the rim of the aneurysmal sac including the arterial orifice to the prosthesis (suture of hole-to-hole technique). *B*, Reconstruction with autogenous saphenous vein graft. *C*, Implantation of the large artery into the prosthesis. A button of prosthesis must be excised to ensure a patulous anastomosis.

Table 99–4.   Risk Prediction for Bowel Ischemia Following Aortic Reconstruction

Greatest risk
Symptoms of visceral ischemia
Aortic aneurysm (ruptured)
Patent IMA
No operative Doppler flow
IMA stump pressure <40 mmHg
Critical intramural pH decrease
Loss of photoplethysmographic pulsatility and transcolonic oxygen saturation
IMA to SMA flow in the meandering mesenteric artery

IMA, inferior mesenteric artery; SMA, superior mesenteric artery.

SUMMARY

The prevention of ischemic colitis following aortic reconstruction is preferable to its successful management. Avoidance of this complication hinges on identification of the high-risk patient; precise, gentle, meticulous operative technique; knowledge of bowel blood supply; and methods of preventing damage to the blood supply or preserving it by inferior mesenteric artery reconstruction. Patients at greatest risk for developing ischemic colitis after aortic reconstruction include those with ruptured aneurysms, those with a patent inferior mesenteric artery, those whose post–aortic reconstruction mean inferior mesenteric stump pressures are below 40 mmHg, those whose Doppler arterial flow signals cease following division or occlusion of the inferior mesenteric artery, and those in whom a meandering mesenteric artery is not recognized and is damaged (Table 99–4).

Diagnosis of ischemic colitis depends on early recognition of vague and variable symptoms and on prompt fiberoptic colonoscopy. Aggressive management, at times employing colon resection, provides the only chance for successful outcome once the process has been established.

References

1. Bandyk DF, Florence MG, Johansen KH: Colon ischemia accompanying ruptured abdominal aortic aneurysm. J Surg Res 30:297, 1981.
2. Baur GM, Porter JM, Eidemiller LR, et al: The role of arteriography in abdominal aortic aneurysm. Am J Surg 136:184, 1978.
3. Bernatz PE: Necrosis of the colon following resection for abdominal aortic aneurysms. Arch Surg 81:373, 1960.
4. Bernstein WC, Bernstein EF: Ischemic ulcerative colitis following inferior mesenteric arterial ligation. Dis Colon Rectum 6:54, 1963.
5. Bicks RO, Bale GF, Howard H, et al: Acute and delayed colon ischemia after aorta aneurysm surgery. Arch Intern Med 122:249, 1968.
6. Birnbaum W, Rudy L, Wylie EJ: Colonic and rectal ischemia following abdominal aneurysmectomy. Dis Colon Rectum 7:293, 1964.
7. Boley SJ, Brandt LJ, Veith FJ: Ischemic disorders of the intestines. Curr Probl Surg 15:1, 1978.
8. Brewster DC, Retana A, Waltman AC, et al: Angiography in the management of aneurysms of the abdominal aorta. N Engl J Med 292:822, 1975.
9. Bulkley GB, Zuidema GD, Hamilton SR, et al: Intraoperative determination of small intestinal viability following ischemic injury: A prospective, controlled trial of two adjuvant methods (Doppler and fluorescein) compared with standard clinical judgement. Ann Surg 193:628, 1981.
10. Bussemaker JB, Lindeman J: Comparison of methods to determine viability of small intestine. Ann Surg 176:97, 1972.
11. Carrel A: Technique and remote results of vascular anastomoses. Surg Gynecol Obstet 14:246, 1912.
12. Connolly JE, Kwaan JHM: Prophylactic revascularization of the gut. Ann Surg 190:514, 1979.
13. Crawford ES, Saleh SA, Babb JW III, et al: Infrarenal abdominal aortic aneurysm: Factors influencing survival after operation performed over a 25-year period. Ann Surg 193:699, 1981.
14. Crawford ES, Snyder DM, Cho GC, et al: Progress in treatment of thoracoabdominal and abdominal aortic aneurysms involving celiac, superior mesenteric, and renal arteries. Ann Surg 188:404, 1978.
15. Ernst CB: Prevention of intestinal ischemia following abdominal aortic reconstruction. Surgery 93:102, 1983.
16. Ernst CB, Hagihara PF, Daugherty ME, et al: Ischemic colitis incidence following abdominal aortic reconstruction: A prospective study. Surgery 80:417, 1976.
17. Ernst CB, Hagihara PF, Daugherty ME, Griffen WO Jr: Inferior mesenteric artery stump pressure: A reliable index for safe IMA ligation during abdominal aortic aneurysmectomy. Ann Surg 187:641, 1978.
18. Ernst CB, Rutkow IM, Cleveland RJ, et al: Vascular surgery in the United States. J Vasc Surg 6:611, 1987.
19. Fiddian-Green RG, Amelin PM, Herrimann JB, et al: Prediction of the development of sigmoid ischemia on the day of aortic operations. Arch Surg 121:654, 1986.
20. Gibson WE III, Pearce CW, Creech O Jr: Infarction of the left hemicolon due to primary vascular occlusion. Dis Colon Rectum 12:323, 1969.
21. Gonzalez LL, Jaffe MS: Mesenteric arterial insufficiency following abdominal aortic resection. Arch Surg 93:10, 1966.
22. Griffiths JD: Surgical anatomy of the blood supply of the distal colon. Ann R Coll Surg Engl 19:241, 1956.
23. Hagihara PF, Ernst CB, Griffen WO Jr: Incidence of ischemic colitis following abdominal aortic reconstruction. Surg Gynecol Obstet 149:571, 1979.
24. Hardy JD: Preservation of accessory arterial supply in abdominal aneurysm resection. Surg Gynecol Obstet 123:1317, 1966.
25. Hobson RW II, Wright CB, O'Donnell JA, et al: Determination of intestinal viability by Doppler ultrasound. Arch Surg 114:165, 1979.
26. Hobson RW II, Wright CB, Rich NM, et al: Assessment of colonic ischemia during aortic surgery by Doppler ultrasound. J Surg Res 20:231, 1976.
27. Javid H, Julian OC, Dye WS, et al: Complications of abdominal aortic grafts. Arch Surg 85:142, 1962.
28. Johnson WC, Nabseth DC: Visceral infarction following aortic surgery. Ann Surg 180:312, 1974.
29. Katz S, Wahab A, Murray W, et al: New parameters of viability in ischemic bowel disease. Am J Surg 127:136, 1974.
30. Kim MW, Hundahl SA, Dang CR, et al: Ischemic colitis after aortic aneurysmectomy. Am J Surg 141:392, 1983.
31. Lannerstad O, Bergentz SE, Bergqvist D, et al: Ischemic intestinal complications after aortic surgery. Acta Chir Scand 151:599, 1985.
32. Launer DP, Miscall BG, Beil AR Jr: Colorectal infarction following resection of abdominal aortic aneurysms. Dis Colon Rectum 21:613, 1978.
33. Lee BY, Trainor FS, Kavner D, et al: Intraoperative assessment of intestinal viability with Doppler ultrasound. Surg Gynecol Obstet 149:671, 1979.
34. Lie M, Normann E, Ovrum E: Necrosis of distal colon after abdominal aneurysmectomy despite high retrograde pressure in inferior mesenteric artery. Ann Chir Gynaecol 71:347, 1982.
35. McBurney RP, Howard H, Bicks RO, et al: Ischemia and gangrene of the colon following abdominal aortic resection. Am Surg 36:205, 1970.
36. McKain J, Shumacker HB Jr: Ischemia of the left colon associated with abdominal aortic aneurysms and their treatment. Arch Surg 76:355, 1958.
37. Miller RE, Knox WG: Colon ischemia following infrarenal aorta surgery: Report of four cases. Ann Surg 163:639, 1966.
38. Moosa AR, Skinner DB, Stark V, et al: Assessment of bowel viability using ⁹⁹ᵐtechnetium-tagged albumin microspheres. J Surg Res 16:466, 1974.
39. Morris GC Jr: In discussion of Ernst CB, Hagihara PF, Daugherty ME, Griffen WO Jr: Inferior mesenteric artery stump pressure: A reliable index for safe IMA ligation during abdominal aortic aneurysmectomy. Ann Surg 187:641, 1978.
40. Moskowitz M, Zimmerman H, Felson B: The meandering mesenteric artery of the colon. Am J Roentgenol 92:1088, 1964.

41. Movius HJ II: Resection of abdominal arteriosclerotic aneurysm. Am J Surg 90:298, 1955.

42. Ottinger LW, Darling RC, Nathan MJ, Linton RR: Left colon ischemia complicating aortoiliac reconstruction. Arch Surg 105:841, 1972.

43. Ouriel K, Fiore WM, Geary JE: Detection of occult colonic ischemia during aortic procedures: Use of an intraoperative photoplethysmographic technique. J Vasc Surg 7:5, 1988.

44. Papachristou D, Fortner JG: Prediction of intestinal viability by intraarterial dye injection: A simple test. Am J Surg 132:572, 1976.

45. Papadopoulos CD, Mancini HW, Marino AWM Jr: Ischemic necrosis of the colon following aortic aneurysmectomy. J Cardiovasc Surg 15:494, 1974.

46. Perdue GD, Lowry K: Arterial insufficiency to the colon following resection of abdominal aortic aneurysms. Surg Gynecol Obstet 115:39, 1962.

47. Rob C, Snyder M: Chronic intestinal ischemia: A complication of surgery of the abdominal aorta. Surgery 60:1141, 1966.

48. Robicsek F: In discussion of Ottinger LW, Darling RC, Nathan MJ, Linton RR: Left colon ischemia complicating aortoiliac reconstruction. Arch Surg 105:841, 1972.

49. Schroeder T, Christoffersen JK, Andersen J, et al: Ischemic colitis complicating reconstruction of the abdominal aorta. Surg Gynecol Obstet 160:299, 1985.

50. Shaw RS, Green TH: Massive mesenteric infarction following inferior mesenteric artery ligation in resection of the colon for carcinoma. N Engl J Med 248:890, 1953.

51. Smith RF, Szilagyi DE: Ischemia of the colon as a complication in the surgery of the abdominal aorta. Arch Surg 80:806, 1960.

52. Steward JA, Rankin FW: Blood supply of large intestine: Its surgical considerations. Arch Surg 26:843, 1933.

53. Stolar CJH, Randolph JG: Evaluation of ischemic bowel viability with a fluorescent technique. J Pediatr Surg 13:221, 1978.

54. Volpetti G, Barker CF, Berkowitz HD, et al: A twenty-two year review of elective resection of abdominal aortic aneurysms. Surg Gynecol Obstet 142:321, 1976.

55. Whittemore AD, Clowes AW, Hechtman HB, et al: Aortic aneurysm repair: Reduced operative mortality associated with maintenance of optimal cardiac performance. Ann Surg 192:414, 1980.

56. Young JR, Humphries AW, deWolfe VG, et al: Complications of aortic surgery. Part II: Intestinal ischemia. Arch Surg 86:65, 1963.

57. Zarins CK, Skinner DB, Rhodes HA, et al: Predictions of the viability of revascularized intestine with radioactive microspheres. Surg Gynecol Obstet 138:578, 1974.

58. Zimberg YH, Sullivan JM: Midgut gangrene after resection of an infrarenal aortic aneurysm. Am J Surg 107:785, 1964.

59. Bulkley GB: Pathophysiology of free-radical mediated reperfusion injury. J Vasc Surg 5:512, 1987.

60. Farkas JC, Calvo-Verjat N, Laurain C, et al: Acute colorectal ischemia after aortic surgery: Pathophysiology and prognostic criteria. Ann Vasc Surg 6:11, 1992.

61. Iliopoulos JI, Pierce GE, Hermreck AS: Hemodynamics of the inferior mesenteric arterial circulation. J Vasc Surg 11:120, 1990.

62. Johnson KW, Scobie TK: Multicenter prospective study of nonruptured abdominal aortic aneurysms. I. Population and operative management. J Vasc Surg 7:69, 1988.

63. Seeger JM, Coe DA, Kaelin LD, et al: Routine reimplantation of patent inferior mesenteric arteries limits colon infarction after aortic reconstruction. J Vasc Surg 15:635, 1992.

64. Tollefson DFJ, Ernst CB: Colon ischemia following aortic reconstruction. Ann Vasc Surg 5:485, 1991.

65. Zelenock GB, Strodel WE, Knoll JA, et al: A prospective study of clinically and endoscopically documented colonic ischemia in 100 patients undergoing aortic reconstructive surgery with aggressive colonic and direct pelvic revascularization, compared with historic controls. Surgery 106:771, 1989.

The Management of Portal Hypertension

Edited by Kaj H. Johansen, M.D., Ph.D.

100

Overview

Kaj H. Johansen, M.D., Ph.D.

• • •

Portal hypertension—elevated pressure in the portal vein or its tributary branches—is a ubiquitous condition with diverse manifestations. Whether arising as a consequence of alcoholic cirrhosis—most common in industrialized Western countries—or as a result of various postviral, parasitic, or toxic states—as seen in the developing world— the medical and surgical implications of portal hypertension are costly, morbid, and frequently lethal. In this chapter the epidemiology and natural history, pathologic anatomy and physiology, and clinical presentation of the various manifestations of this condition are discussed, and a diagnostic and therapeutic algorithm, to be used as early as possible in the evaluation of such patients, is proposed. In Chapter 101, emergency management of patients with portal hypertension is discussed, including how to resuscitate, stabilize, and diagnose such patients. Endoscopic techniques for controlling both acute and chronic variceal hemorrhage are reviewed in Chapter 102. Chapter 103 critically analyzes various nonoperative interventional techniques for management of the complications of portal hypertension. Finally, Chapter 104 discusses various operative techniques for treating bleeding esophageal varices, including the proper role of liver transplantation.

The magnitude and severity of the problem of portal hypertension and the fact that, depending upon an individual patient's status, appropriate management may vary from pharmacologic to endoscopic to radiographic to operative means, have resulted in a voluminous and sometimes contradictory literature. The interested reader is referred to several recent reviews of this topic for different perspectives and more detailed discussion.[1–5]

ANATOMY AND PATHOPHYSIOLOGY

In a healthy adult the portal vein conducts 1000 to 1500 ml of blood per minute from the splanchnic viscera to the hepatic sinusoids.[2] Despite this high flow and the density of the liver parenchyma, resistance to flow within the liver is normally very low, as manifested by a pressure differential between the portal vein and the suprahepatic vena cava (the portacaval pressure gradient) that rarely exceeds 5 to 7 mmHg. In the normal physiologic setting portal collateral flow is negligible.

However, obstruction to portal venous flow before (presinusoidal, extrahepatic or intrahepatic), within (perisinusoidal), or beyond (postsinusoidal) the liver results in increased resistance to flow and a rise in portal venous pressure as well as a rise in portal collateral flow. Portal hypertension is present when the corrected portal pressure (the portacaval pressure gradient) exceeds 15 mmHg, or when absolute portal venous pressure exceeds 25 mmHg. Pressures as high as 50 mmHg may be measured.

Collateral routes for the hypertensive portal vein are numerous (Fig. 100–1). Many, such as those in the retroperitoneum and around the left renal vein, are clinically silent. Others are of physiologic importance or interest, either as diagnostic markers for the underlying condition (dilated abdominal wall veins, or caput medusae) or as potential sites of major bleeding (esophagogastric, rectal, or stomal varices; portal hypertensive gastropathy).

In portal hypertension portal venous flow falls precip-

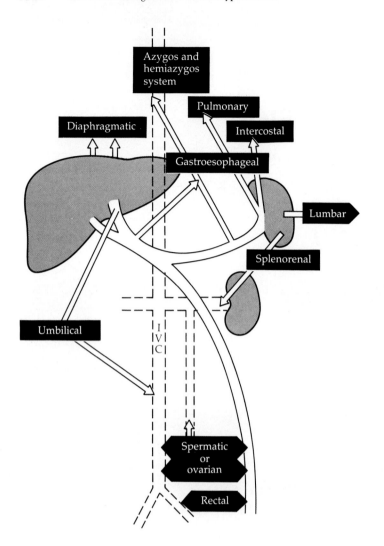

FIGURE 100-1. Multiple collateral pathways develop in response to the development of portal hypertension. Most important clinically from the perspective of variceal hemorrhage are pathways from the portal vein to the azygos or hemiazygos system via the gastroesophageal variceal plexus, and those communicating with hemorrhoidal tributaries of the hypogastric venous circuit. (From Sherlock S: The portal venous system and portal hypertension. *In* Diseases of the Liver and Biliary System. 8th ed. Oxford, Blackwell Scientific Publications, 1989, p 166.)

itously in parallel with a rise in portal collateral flow. Depending upon the nature and severity of the obstruction, portal venous flow may stagnate or even reverse; in other words, resistance to flow in the portal vein may exceed that within the portal collateral bed, and portal vein flow reverses as it is converted into a venous outflow tract for the liver. As portal venous flow diminishes, compensatory increases occur in hepatic arterial flow (which in normal circumstances provides only 25 per cent of total hepatic blood flow). In fact, the capacity to increase hepatic arterial flow may be an independent determinant of hepatic survival when portal venous perfusion of the liver is lost,[6] as for example when spontaneous reversal of flow occurs in the portal vein or following portal vein thrombosis or "total" portasystemic shunt.

The chronic liver dysfunction that coexists with most of the manifestations of portal hypertension must constantly be considered in the evaluation and management of this condition. The majority of such patients display various disorders of hepatocellular function—clotting abnormalities, volume overload, jaundice, portal systemic encephalopathy, hypoprothrombinemia, malnutrition—at one time or another. The Child-Pugh classification (see later discussion) is a clinical scoring system that takes into account many of these issues. Certain other implications of these

patients' disease states must be confronted as well; for example, pancreatitis or acute alcohol withdrawal in patients with Laennec's cirrhosis, hepatitis seropositivity, and a sharply increased risk of hepatoma in patients with postviral cirrhosis.

Extrahepatic manifestations of severe liver dysfunction are manifold. The first sign of clinically relevant portal hypertension is splenomegaly,[2] and the hematologic manifestations of hypersplenism, especially thrombocytopenia and leukopenia, are commonplace. For incompletely understood reasons, advanced liver disease is associated with a hyperdynamic circulatory state, including elevated cardiac outputs and diminished peripheral resistance. The clinical picture may initially be confused with sepsis; however, the latter is characterized by a high pulmonary vascular resistance, whereas hepatic failure is accompanied by low resistance in both the systemic and pulmonary circuits. In fact, the same opening of precapillary arteriovenous communications that leads to "spider" angiomata and palmar erythema in patients with advanced liver disease can also be found in the pulmonary circulation; hypoxemia due to a physiologic shunt is frequently observed in cirrhotic subjects.[7]

A poorly characterized but stereotypic neuropsychiatric disorder, portal systemic encephalopathy, is frequently observed in advanced cirrhosis. Both portasystemic shunting (either spontaneous or resulting from a shunt procedure) and hepatocellular dysfunction must be present for hepatic encephalopathy to be manifest. The pathogenesis probably relates to excessive systemic levels of ammonia and other products of bacterial peptide metabolism in the gut,[8] a conclusion derived in part from the observation that encephalopathy can be improved by oral antibiotics, colon resection or bypass, cathartics, liver transplantation, or portasystemic shunt occlusion.

Ascites is a common presentation in patients with portal hypertension and is found almost universally in those with decompensated or terminal liver failure. The pathogenesis of ascites is still incompletely understood but is based primarily on the superimposition of a disordered Starling equilibrium (an increased hepatic sinusoidal hydrostatic pressure and a diminished serum oncotic pressure) on hepatic lymphatic (space of Disse) obstruction, thereby producing excessive extracellular fluid. Secondary hyperaldosteronism resulting from the diseased liver's inability to metabolize endogenous steroids further complicates normal removal of ascites. Other fluid and electrolyte disturbances in cirrhotic patients may include, besides sodium excess, an extreme total body potassium deficit and a resulting metabolic alkalosis.

Renal dysfunction frequently accompanies decompensated liver failure. The hepatorenal syndrome is characterized by oliguria and rising serum creatinine values in the absence of evidence of prerenal or renal parenchymal disease; hepatic dysfunction is advanced, and urine sodium levels are less than 10 mEq/L.[9] Redistribution of regional blood flow within the kidney, with extreme renal cortical vasoconstriction, is characteristic.[10] Recent observations suggest that elevated serum endothelin levels may play a pathogenetic role. The mortality rate of *established* hepatorenal failure exceeds 90 per cent; the only effective therapy is liver transplantation, successful performance of which can result in a return of normal renal function.

EPIDEMIOLOGY, RISK FACTORS, AND NATURAL HISTORY

Although portal hypertension and its complications may arise from diverse disease states (Table 100–1), cirrhosis due to alcoholic liver disease predominates in Western societies. In the United States alcoholic liver disease accounts for about 90 per cent of patients with portal hypertension. Worldwide, the leading causes of portal hypertension are the consequence of past infectious states, either postnecrotic (hepatitis B virus) or secondary to schistosomal involvement of the liver.[11] Other less common but clinically important causes of portal hypertension—congenital, toxic, inflammatory, or vascular—are enumerated in Table 100–1. Because of its predominance in industrialized Western countries, cirrhosis arising from alcoholic liver disease will be the focus of much of the subsequent discussion.

Conservative estimates suggest that as many as 30 million adults—10 per cent of the North American population—manifest signs and symptoms of chronic alcohol-

Table 100–1. Causes of Portal Hypertension

Presinusoidal
  Extrahepatic
    Portal vein thrombosis
    Splenic vein occlusion
    Increased splenic blood flow (e.g., myelofibrosis)
  Intrahepatic
    Schistosomiasis
    Congenital hepatic fibrosis
    Portal zone infiltrations (reticulosis, sarcoidosis)
    Primary portal hypertension (Indian childhood cirrhosis)
Sinusoidal
  Cirrhosis
  Sinusoidal occlusion (vitamin A toxicity, Gaucher's disease, myeloid metaplasia)
  Alcoholic hepatitis
Postsinusoidal
  Hepatic vein occlusion (vascular occlusion due to malignancy, Budd-Chiari syndrome)
  Veno-occlusive disease
  Alcoholic central hyaline necrosis
Other Causes Not Defined by Pre, Intra-, or Postsinusoidal Terminology
  Hematologic disorders (lymphoma, leukemia, myeloproliferative disorders)
  Hemodynamic causes (increased splanchnic blood flow [e.g., splenic arteriovenous or hepatic arterioportal fistula])
  Hepatic parenchymal abnormalities (partial nodular transformation, regenerative hyperplasia)
  Idiopathic (portal phlebosclerosis, Banti's syndrome)

ism.[12] Accordingly, although only 10 per cent of alcoholics develop hepatic cirrhosis, and of that group only 30 per cent develop signs and symptoms of portal hypertension, alcoholic liver disease is clearly a major public health problem. Hepatic cirrhosis ranks ninth among all causes of death in the United States.[13] In many developing countries variceal hemorrhage is one of the major nontraumatic causes of death in adults. Bleeding from varices is the leading cause of death from gastrointestinal hemorrhage worldwide and is a major cause of disability and death in persons between the ages of 35 and 59, when employment and family-rearing are particularly important. The human, public health, and societal costs of this condition are substantial.

The natural history of cirrhosis and portal hypertension relates primarily to the persistence and severity of the underlying hepatic dysfunction. For example, abstinence from alcohol can frequently result in stabilization of the scarring-regenerating process that characterizes Laennec's cirrhosis. Bleeding from esophageal varices most commonly occurs in cirrhotics who continue to consume alcohol, whereas hemorrhage is unusual in patients with alcoholic cirrhosis who have been abstinent from alcohol for more than 1 year. For patients with postnecrotic cirrhosis, the hepatic inflammation and fibrosis resulting from the underlying process often "burns out," thus explaining these patients' somewhat better long-term prognosis compared to those with alcoholic cirrhosis. On the other hand, viral hepatitis may persist as a chronic relapsing infection; such patients also have a substantial risk of developing hepatocellular carcinoma.[14]

Without any management, the outcome of hepatic cirrhosis is poor. Classic older studies must be consulted to demonstrate the natural history of the condition because medical or surgical intervention is the contemporary norm in most such patients. The famous Boston Interhospital Liver Group studies demonstrated that cirrhotics who developed ascites had only a 10 per cent survival rate at 1 year.[15] Development of jaundice was even more ominous; such patients had a median survival of 4 months. Orloff and associates demonstrated, prior to the liver transplantation era, that patients displaying the clinical tetrad of jaundice, ascites, encephalopathy, and severe muscle wasting had a mortality rate approaching 100 per cent at one year, optimal medical and surgical therapy notwithstanding.[16] In schistosomal disease of the liver, because hepatocellular function is relatively better preserved than in patients with cirrhosis, mortality is less; nevertheless, the development of gastrointestinal hemorrhage is commonplace.

The stereotypic nature of advanced liver disease allows semi-objective quantitation of hepatocellular dysfunction. The scoring systems of Child[17] and Pugh and colleagues,[18] originally established to predict outcome following (respectively) emergency portacaval shunt and esophageal transection for the treatment of bleeding esophageal varices, can also be used to classify such patients in numerous other therapeutic and prognostic settings (Table 100–2). Child's system includes assessment of ascites, encephalopathy, muscle wasting, and levels of serum albumin and bilirubin. Pugh's scale deletes muscle wasting and adds prothrombin time. A certain degree of controversy attends the use of these classifications;[19] nevertheless, they are simple and reproducible and remain remarkably useful in predicting ultimate outcome in cirrhotic patients.

Because the complications of portal hypertension—variceal hemorrhage, ascites, hypersplenism, and portal systemic encephalopathy—always occur in patients with advanced liver dysfunction (and, not infrequently, other major medical conditions), hospitalization and even intensive care unit admission are usually required in these patients. The likelihood of various complications and prolonged hospitalization is high as well. The mortality risk associated with hospitalization for a first episode of bleeding from esophageal varices approaches 50 per cent.[1] The condition is extraordinarily costly in a fiscal sense as well: In 1980 hospitalization in the United States for the management of bleeding esophageal varices resulted in average hospital charges of $50,000.[20]

The optimal solution to the excessive mortality and other societal costs incurred by patients with cirrhosis and portal hypertension ultimately revolves around prevention. Unfortunately, alcoholism (and abuse of other substances) appears to be an almost unavoidable aspect of the human condition; prohibition, taxation, education, and other attempts at mitigation have shown only minimal success. Alcohol treatment programs are notoriously unsuccessful; a critical review of such regimens suggests that their effect is brief, their costs substantial, and recidivism common.[21] Other maneuvers directed against hepatitis, such as widespread hepatitis B vaccination,[22] screening of community blood supplies, or even more controversial public health measures such as needle-sharing programs for intravenous drug abusers, may have some useful prophylactic impact. Attempts have been made to develop an antischistosomal vaccine.[23]

Table 100–2.   Child-Pugh Classification

Child Classification	Class		
	A	B	C
Bilirubin (mg/dl)	<2.0	2.0–3.0	>3.0
Albumin (mg/dl)	>3.5	3.0–3.5	<3.0
Ascites	None	Reversible	Refractory
Encephalopathy	None	Minimal	Spontaneous
Nutrition (muscle mass)	Normal	Fair	Poor

Pugh Classification	Points Scored for Increasing Abnormality		
	1	2	3
Encephalopathy (grade)	Normal	1 or 2	3 or 4
Albumin (mg/dl)	>3.5	2.8–3.5	<2.8
Bilirubin (mg/dl)	1.0–2.0	2.0–3.0	>3.0
Ascites	Absent	Slight	Significant
Prothrombin time (seconds prolonged)	1–4	4–6	>6
Grade A		5 or 6	
Grade B		7, 8, or 9	
Grade C		10–15	

From Child CG: Surgery and portal hypertension. In Dunphy JE (ed): The Liver and Portal Hypertension. Philadelphia, WB Saunders, 1964; and Pugh RNH, Murray-Lyon IM, Dawson JL, Williams R: Transsection of the esophagus for bleeding esophageal varices. Br J Surg 60:646, 1973, by permission of Butterworth Heinemann, Ltd, Oxford, publisher.

CLINICAL APPROACH TO THE PATIENT WITH PORTAL HYPERTENSION

Subsequent chapters demonstrate that many different therapies—pharmacologic, endoscopic, interventional radiologic, and operative—may be considered for the patient manifesting the complications of portal hypertension. Which approach is pursued depends upon the patient's clinical and physical status, the underlying cause of the hepatic dysfunction being treated, and, to some degree, the availability of various therapies. Whether such a patient should be cared for in a major medical center or can be effectively managed in the community setting is unclear. On the presumption that a patient with bleeding esophageal varices or intractable ascites is being managed in a setting where all contemporary modes of therapy are possible, optimal management can be attained by answering the following questions.

1. *Is the patient a liver transplantation candidate?* As noted in Chapter 104, this question generally implies the presence of end-stage *nonalcoholic* liver disease in a patient under the age of 60 who manifests no other significant medical comorbidity. The portal vein should be patent, and scarring from prior right upper quadrant operations should be minimal or absent. It is much more difficult to achieve successful transplantation in patients with portal or diffuse splanchnic venous thrombosis or those with prior right upper quadrant operations, especially portasystemic shunts.[24] A patient with variceal hemorrhage who is considered a transplant candidate should be managed medically (intravenous vasoconstrictor therapy, balloon tamponade, beta blockers), endoscopically (variceal sclerotherapy or banding), or by angiographic shunt (transjugular intrahepatic portasystemic shunt, or TIPS); if operative portal decompression is required, it should be done as a splenorenal

or mesocaval shunt, thereby avoiding dissection and subsequent adhesions in the right upper quadrant and the hepatic hilum.

Patients with cirrhosis and portal hypertension whose liver function is relatively well preserved (Child-Pugh class A or B) should be considered for alternative nontransplant therapies, as should those who are actively consuming alcohol, have advanced cardiopulmonary or other serious medical comorbidity, are elderly, or are seropositive for hepatitis B. Most patients with variceal hemorrhage or other complications of portal hypertension fit into one of these categories. However, patients with variceal hemorrhage are acceptable candidates for liver transplantation.[25]

2. *Is the patient compliant and responsible? Does he or she live nearby?* Some patients, for example, many of those who are actively drinking alcohol, are noncompliant; their ability to maintain the long-term follow-up required by various palliative treatments for portal hypertension is limited. Similarly, for some patients definitive treatment removes anxiety about future recurrent variceal hemorrhage. Still others living at great distances from the medical center are at grave risk if drug or endoscopic therapy should fail.[26] In such circumstances, *definitive* therapy—operative shunt or liver transplantation—may be preferable. Conversely, compliant patients living near the medical center, especially those with nonalcoholic liver disease, may do well with *palliative* therapies such as chronic endoscopic variceal bandings or sclerotherapy, beta-blocker administration, or TIPS.

3. *Are there anatomic, physiologic, or other clinical abnormalities that might affect certain therapies?* Operative or angiographic portacaval shunt cannot be performed in the presence of portal vein thrombosis. The presence of a diminutive splenic vein or one that is anatomically distant from the renal vein is a contraindication to distal splenorenal shunt, as is the presence of significant ascites or hepatofugal portal vein flow.[27] Preoperative encephalopathy of significant degree often becomes worse following an otherwise successful portasystemic shunt, either by operative or angiographic means. Endoscopic sclerotherapy is dangerous in the presence of significant esophageal ulceration secondary to prior sclerotherapy. Beta-blocker therapy intended to reduce portal hypertension pharmacologically is contraindicated in the presence of asthma or congestive heart failure. General anesthetics and operations are poorly tolerated by patients with decompensated cirrhosis.

SUMMARY

Portal hypertension, usually arising from various forms of advanced chronic liver disease, is a complicated and lethal condition wherein gastrointestinal hemorrhage, sometimes torrential in nature, occurs against a backdrop of chronic hepatocellular dysfunction and (not infrequently) other medical comorbidities. Other related problems may include hypersplenism, ascites, and portal systemic encephalopathy. Therapy for the complications of portal hypertension depends upon the nature and extent of the underlying liver disease as well as on other clinical factors such as the availability of various treatment modalities, patient compliance, and proximity to a major medical center. Subsequent chapters detail the selection of the appropriate diagnostic and therapeutic approach for the patient with portal hypertension.

References

1. Burroughs AK: The management of bleeding due to portal hypertension. Part 1. The management of acute bleeding episodes. Q J Med 67:447, 1988. Part 2. Prevention of variceal bleeding and prevention of the first bleeding episode in patients with portal hypertension. Q J Med 68:507, 1988.
2. Sherlock S: The portal venous system and portal hypertension. *In* Diseases of the Liver and Biliary System. 8th ed. Oxford, Blackwell Scientific Publications, 1989, pp 151–207.
3. Terblanche J, Burroughs AK, Hobbs KEF: Controversies in the management of bleeding varices. N Engl J Med 21:89, 1989.
4. Henderson JM, Millikan WJ (eds): W. Dean Warren Memorial Issue. Am J Surg 160:138, 1990.
5. Johansen K, Helton WS: Portal hypertension and bleeding esophagogastric varices. Ann Vasc Surg 6:553, 1992.
6. Burchell AR, Moreno AH, Panke WF, Nealon TF: Hepatic artery flow improvement after portacaval shunt: A single hemodynamic clinical correlate. Ann Surg 192:9, 1976.
7. Yao EH, Kong BC, Hsue GL, et al: Pulmonary function changes in cirrhosis of the liver. Am J Gastroenterol 82:352, 1987.
8. Zieve L: Pathogenesis of hepatic encephalopathy. Metab Brain Dis 2:147, 1987.
9. Schelling JR, Linas S: Hepatorenal syndrome. Semin Nephrol 10:565, 1990.
10. Bosch J: Splanchnic vasodilatation and renal vasoconstriction: A key to the hepatorenal syndrome? Hepatology 12:1445, 1990.
11. Raia S, Mies S, Alfieri F: Portal hypertension in mansonic schistosomiasis. World Surg 15:176, 1991.
12. Vaillant EE: The Natural History of Alcoholism. Cambridge, Harvard University Press, 1983.
13. Vital Statistics of the United States. Washington, D.C., U.S. Government Printing Office, 1993.
14. Simonetti RG, Camma C, Fiorello F, et al: Hepatocellular carcinoma: A worldwide problem and the major risk factors. Dig Dis Sci 36:962, 1991.
15. Garceau AJ and the Boston Interhospital Liver Group: The natural history of cirrhosis. I. Survival with esophageal varices. N Engl J Med 268:469, 1962; II. The influence of alcohol and prior hepatitis on pathology and prognosis. N Engl J Med 271:1173, 1964.
16. Orloff MJ, Chandler JG, Charters AC, et al: Comparison of end-to-side and side-to-side portacaval shunt in dogs and humans with cirrhosis and portal hypertension. Am J Surg 128:195, 1974.
17. Child CG: Surgery and portal hypertension. *In* Dunphy JE (ed): The Liver and Portal Hypertension. Philadelphia, WB Saunders, 1964.
18. Pugh RNH, Murray-Lyon IM, Dawson JL, Williams R: Transsection of the esophagus for bleeding esophageal varices. Br J Surg 60:646, 1973.
19. Conn HO: A peek at the Child-Turcotte classification. Hepatology 1:673, 1981.
20. O'Donnell TF, Gembarowicz RM, Callow AD, et al: The economic impact of acute variceal bleeding: Cost-effectiveness implications for medical and surgical therapy. Surgery 88:643, 1980.
21. Smart R, Gray C: Multiple predictors of dropout from alcoholism treatment. Arch Gen Psychiatry 35:363, 1978.
22. Margolis HS, Alter MJ, Hadler SC: Hepatitis B: Evolving epidemiology and implications for control. Semin Liver Dis 11:84, 1991.
23. Bergquist R: Prospects of vaccination against schistosomiasis. Scand J Infect Dis 76:60, 1990.
24. Brems JJ, Hiatt JR, Klein AS, et al: Effect of prior portasystemic shunt on subsequent liver transplantation. Ann Surg 209:51, 1989.
25. Iwatsuki S, Starzl TE, Todo S, et al: Liver transplantation in the treatment of bleeding esophageal varices. Surgery 104:697, 1988.
26. Rikkers LF, Burnett DA, Valentine GD, et al: Shunt surgery versus endoscopic sclerotherapy for long-term treatment of variceal bleeding. Early results of a randomized trial. Ann Surg 206:261, 1987.
27. Zeppa R: The distal splenorenal shunt. *In* Orloff MJ, Stipa S, Ziparo V (eds): Medical and Surgical Problems of Portal Hypertension. New York, Academic Press, 1980, pp 153–158.

Diagnosis and Emergency Management of Variceal Hemorrhage

John Terblanche, Ch.M., F.C.S.(S.A.), F.R.C.S.(Eng.), F.A.C.S.(Hon.), F.A.C.P.(Hon.)
• • •

Controlled and uncontrolled studies have indicated a rate of death during the first bleeding episode from esophageal varices in cirrhotic patients that varies from 30 to 80 per cent. It has been stated that, "As with a volcano it is difficult to know when a varix will erupt."[7] When a varix does erupt, it often does so without warning, with massive bleeding that constitutes a terrifying experience for the patient's relatives and friends. For the patient, it often heralds the commencement of a series of disastrous events that eventually culminate in death. Management of variceal hemorrhage presents one of the most exacting challenges in clinical medicine. The lethality of the event depends on the underlying liver disease, the degree of hepatic decompensation, and the efficacy of treatment. Comparison of data from the 1930s, the 1950s, and the 1970s revealed that standard conventional therapy had reduced neither the early nor the delayed death rate.[10]

The broad aims of therapy must be to stop bleeding, improve survival, and render the patient as fit as possible for any subsequent treatment required to prevent recurrent bleeding. Although few will qualify, all patients must be evaluated as potential liver transplant recipients. Emphasis should be placed on simple but effective measures designed to give the patient the best chance of surviving the early stages of this disorder. Extensive surgical measures during the emergency phase, when the patient is at greatest risk, are contraindicated if lesser surgical procedures will suffice. This is particularly true if a liver transplant is being considered. Because most deaths occur early after a variceal bleed, Graham and Smith have stressed that "any substantial improvement in long-term survival must improve survival for the early period."[10] Thus, effective emergency management is vital.

In this discussion, only adults, particularly those with underlying cirrhosis, are considered. The principles of treatment in children with life-threatening variceal hemorrhage are much the same, although children with portal vein thrombosis are usually easier to manage.

Patients whose variceal bleeding stops soon after admission to the hospital pose fewer problems. It is those who continue to bleed that constitute the difficult group to manage and that also have a significant mortality rate.

The importance of bleeding gastric varices is uncertain. In the Cape Town experience, they appear to have been rare. Even if they were underdiagnosed and had been a cause of bleeding, control was usually achieved by the management policy detailed in this chapter. Attention has also been focused on bleeding from the gastric mucosa in portal hypertension as a result of portal hypertensive congestive gastropathy.[24, 29, 32, 40]

The management schedule that has proved successful in the author's hands is described.[16, 48, 52] Alternative forms of treatment are presented in an attempt to place them in perspective. Many of the older procedures are not discussed because they are of historical interest only.

CLINICAL PRESENTATION

When a patient with previously diagnosed portal hypertension presents with massive upper gastrointestinal hemorrhage, the diagnosis of bleeding esophageal varices will be suspected by the attending doctor. This diagnosis must be confirmed endoscopically prior to initiating complex therapy because a third to a half of the patients may be bleeding from another lesion.[16, 26, 47, 48, 52] In patients without known portal hypertension who present with massive upper gastrointestinal bleeding, the physician must bear portal hypertension in mind because of the need for specialized therapy. An adequate history, together with a thorough physical examination looking for signs of either cirrhosis or portal hypertension, is essential. The diagnosis is simple in patients with gross evidence of liver dysfunction. Patients with milder liver dysfunction should be evaluated for subtle signs such as splenomegaly, mild ascites or encephalopathy, and spider angiomata. In the author's institution, all patients admitted with upper gastrointestinal hemorrhage undergo routine diagnostic endoscopy following initial resuscitation. A number of patients with unsuspected variceal bleeding have been diagnosed by this method.

Can patients with bleeding esophageal varices be managed adequately in a community hospital or should they be referred to a specialist center with expertise in the management of portal hypertension? The author believes that these patients must be referred to an institution with a special interest in hepatology. Not only is therapy complex and specialized, but if improved survival is to be achieved, the early management phase is the most important.[10] The author's group advises the primary physician to consult the specialist center by telephone to ensure that a rational decision is made regarding transport, particularly for patients who are a long distance from the specialist center. Depending on the expertise available in the community hospital, pharmacologic therapy may be instituted and, in patients with severe bleeding, an initial diagnostic endoscopic procedure followed by correct insertion of a balloon tube is sometimes required prior to transporting the patient by road or air. Protection of the airway is vital, and the patient should be accompanied by an experienced nurse, medical technician, or physician.

DIAGNOSTIC INVESTIGATIONS

When major variceal hemorrhage is suspected, all early efforts should be directed toward resuscitation, diagnosis, and arrest of the hemorrhage. Routine diagnostic investigations must be kept to a minimum. The exceptions are coagulation studies and emergency diagnostic fiberoptic endoscopy.

After resuscitation has begun, blood samples should be sent for emergency hematologic evaluations, including a platelet count and prothrombin level. A simple coagulation profile should be obtained if possible. Except for serum electrolyte and acid-base measurements, the remaining biochemical, immunologic, and liver function tests should be performed later as routine rather than emergency procedures and the results evaluated as a baseline for subsequent management.

INITIAL MANAGEMENT

Immediate hospitalization is mandatory, preferably in an intensive care unit in an institution with a special interest in hepatology. If the patient is in shock or continues to hemorrhage, one or more large-bore intravenous lines are inserted, and crystalloid infusion is commenced immediately. While awaiting results of a blood cross-match, one should establish a central venous line and catheterize the bladder. Fresh blood or blood components are administered as soon as they are available. The subsequent management policy should be decided by immediate consultation with the relevant senior internal medicine and surgical staff. Junior or inexperienced physicians should not proceed on their own. Further emergency measures, particularly endoscopy, are required to confirm the diagnosis and stop bleeding.

PHARMACOLOGIC CONTROL

The role of emergency pharmacologic control of variceal bleeding has focused on agents that lower portal pressure. These include vasopressin, glypressin, and somatostatin. Various sympatholytic or serotonin-active agents are, for the moment, of speculative interest. The role and efficacy of pharmacologic therapy for acute variceal bleeding remains controversial.

Vasopressin was the first drug used and remains the most widely employed agent. Its precise mechanism of action is not fully understood but is thought to be mainly that of lowering portal pressure. There is even dispute about whether it is effective in the presence of the hemodynamic alterations that occur in acute variceal hemorrhage. One

study suggests that it is less effective than in patients in a stable state,[55] whereas another shows that it remains effective in this setting.[34] The author uses a continuous intravenous infusion of vasopressin at the rate of 0.4 U/min combined with sublingual nitroglycerin (1 tablet every half hour for up to 6 hours). The latter reputedly potentiates the action of vasopressin while reducing the side effects.[50, 52] Unless contraindicated, vasopressin plus nitroglycerin therapy is commenced when variceal bleeding is suspected in the hope that it may have controlled active variceal bleeding by the time emergency diagnostic endoscopy is performed.

Although controlled trials suggest that glypressin is more effective than vasopressin,[9, 56] the design of the trials has been criticized and the agent is expensive. Its advantage is that it is effective when administered as 6-hourly intravenous bolus doses rather than by the more complex continuous intravenous route required for vasopressin. Some groups use a single bolus dose prior to transporting a patient with suspected variceal bleeding.

Somatostatin has been shown to be highly effective and is probably the best of the candidate drugs for acute variceal bleeding.[5] Analogues such as octreotide may be preferable and have been shown to be simple to use with few side effects.[25] Somatostatin has also been shown to be highly effective in controlling bleeding from esophageal ulcers resulting as a complication of injection sclerotherapy.[14]

Metoclopramide, which increases lower esophageal sphincter pressure, has been shown to decrease transmural variceal pressure significantly in cirrhotic patients without exerting an effect on portal hemodynamics.[20, 46] It has also been shown to be effective in controlling acute variceal hemorrhage.[12]

There is a high rebleeding rate after vasopressin therapy is discontinued. Therefore, further emergency management, particularly sclerotherapy, has been recommended for most patients. The same principle probably applies following the use of the newer pharmacologic agents for emergency management.

EMERGENCY DIAGNOSIS OF THE SOURCE OF BLEEDING

Not all patients with suspected cirrhosis have esophageal varices. In fact, in one third or more of cirrhotic patients with varices, other lesions may be the cause of bleeding.[16, 26, 47, 48, 52] Such lesions include portal hypertensive gastropathy, erosive gastritis, peptic ulceration, and Mallory-Weiss tears, all of which require completely different management. Thus, a definitive diagnosis of bleeding from varices is required prior to initiating therapy.

Emergency Endoscopy

Emergency endoscopy is mandatory in all patients with suspected variceal bleeding. The author's group currently performs emergency endoscopy as soon as the patient is stable, usually within 4 hours of admission and after volume resuscitation and commencement of intravenous vasopressin therapy. The only exception is the rare patient with life-threatening uncontrolled hemorrhage, for whom balloon tamponade should be instituted immediately and other procedures, including endoscopy, should be performed subsequently.

Although there are problems with emergency endoscopy, the patient cannot be managed rationally unless the source of bleeding is diagnosed. A confident diagnosis can be made only if a bleeding varix is seen or a lesion other than a varix is noted to be bleeding. With massive upper gastrointestinal hemorrhage, one's vision is often obscured and the diagnosis of bleeding varices is less secure. Thus, the procedure must be undertaken by an experienced endoscopist.

After the patients without varices have been differentiated and excluded, patients with varices can be classified into three groups: those whose variceal bleeding is active; those whose variceal bleeding has stopped (no other lesion noted; with or without a blood clot on a varix); and those who have varices but are bleeding from another lesion.[16, 26, 48] Approximately one third of patients fall into each of the three groups.[16, 26, 47, 48]

Patients with varices who are bleeding from another lesion are treated appropriately. Patients with either active variceal bleeding or variceal bleeding that has stopped should be treated by immediate emergency sclerotherapy at the time of the first diagnostic endoscopy whenever possible. In a controlled trial, immediate sclerotherapy was shown to be both safe and effective even in the presence of major hemorrhage and proved superior to pharmacologic management with combined vasopressin and nitroglycerin.[57]

Other Emergency Investigations

Unlike endoscopy, angiography has not proved accurate in diagnosing the source of bleeding, and is no longer used as an emergency procedure in suspected esophageal variceal bleeding. Emergency barium studies are contraindicated because they do not provide useful information and may obscure subsequent endoscopic or angiographic studies.

BALLOON TUBE TAMPONADE

Despite views expressed to the contrary, balloon tube tamponade is not hazardous when properly used.[16, 26, 48, 50] Failures are usually due to faulty technique in the hands of inexperienced junior staff. If the balloon is correctly placed and the patient is appropriately managed, this method temporarily stops acute variceal bleeding in virtually all cases.[16, 48] Because of its potential dangers, balloon tamponade should only be used in patients in whom initial or subsequent sclerotherapy fails. Further bleeding after insertion of the tube invariably indicates either that the tube is incorrectly placed or that the patient is bleeding from another source. The tube should immediately be repositioned

by an expert; if bleeding continues, repeat endoscopy usually reveals another source of bleeding.

Although a balloon tube controls bleeding temporarily in most patients, the rebleed rate after removal of the tube is high (60 per cent in the Cape Town trial).[16, 26, 47, 48] Therefore, further definitive emergency management is required after removal of the tube.

Balloon Tube Tamponade Technique

Meticulous attention to detail is required for successful use.[33, 52] The four-lumen tube with a gastric and an esophageal balloon is recommended. In stuporous, comatose, or uncooperative patients the airway should be protected by an endotracheal tube to prevent aspiration.

A new tube is always used. The inflated gastric and esophageal balloons are tested under water to confirm a complete air seal. After inducing adequate topical pharyngeal anesthesia, the deflated lubricated tube is passed through the mouth, protected by a biteguard. The nose should not be used because of the risk of pressure necrosis of the nasal cartilage. The initial passage of the tube is assisted by the operator's left index finger in the patient's mouth that guides the tip of the tube over the posterior tongue and through the cricopharyngeus and prevents coiling of the tube in the pharynx. A McGill forceps and laryngoscope can be used to assist in negotiating the cricopharynx. It is important to insert the balloon tube almost "to the hilt" to ensure that it is placed well within the stomach. Air is instilled via the aspirating lumen using a 50-ml syringe, and the position of the tube in the stomach is checked by auscultation over the epigastrium. The gastric balloon is inflated with 200 ml of air using 50-ml increments. If the patient shows any signs of discomfort, the tube may be sited in the lower esophagus; inflation should be stopped immediately and the position of the tube rechecked. Once the gastric balloon is fully inflated, the tube is pulled back until the balloon engages at the esophagogastric junction and abuts the cardia of the stomach. A football helmet is applied, with the tube taped securely to the face mask; alternatively, a split tennis ball is firmly secured to the tube at the patient's mouth to maintain firm traction against the biteguard. This ensures constant compression on the cardia by the gastric balloon (Fig. 101–1). It is necessary to inflate the esophageal balloon only if bleeding continues after traction on the gastric balloon. When used, the esophageal balloon is inflated to 40 mmHg using a three-way stopcock and a blood pressure gauge. The gastric lumen is used for suction and to instill medications (e.g., lactulose), and the esophageal lumen is kept on constant suction in order to clear the esophagus of secretions above the esophageal balloon, thereby preventing aspiration.

The patient should be aggressively resuscitated in an intensive care unit. The balloons should not be left inflated for more than 6 to 12 hours, in order to avoid troublesome mucosal slough, which may ulcerate and bleed. Thereafter, sclerotherapy or a definitive procedure should be undertaken.

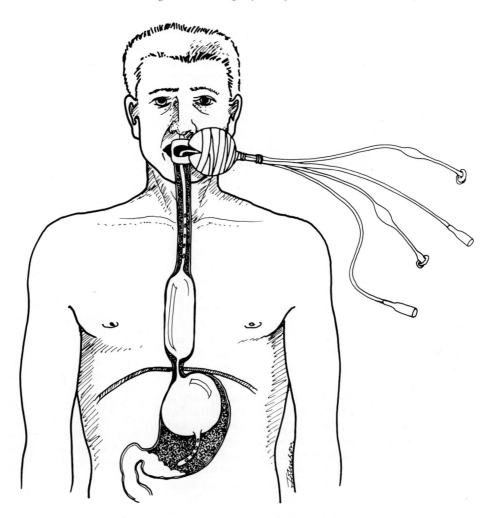

FIGURE 101–1. The four-lumen balloon tube has a gastric and an esophageal balloon and two separate lumina for suction of the stomach and upper esophagus. Traction is maintained with a split tennis ball strapped firmly to the tube at the patient's mouth.

SUBSEQUENT EMERGENCY MANAGEMENT

Both immediate sclerotherapy and balloon tube tamponade are effective in providing temporary acute variceal bleeding control in most patients. The role of pharmacologic therapy is less clearly defined. The early rebleeding rate after balloon tamponade or pharmacologic therapy is high. Thus, patients controlled by these measures require further emergency treatment.

In the author's view, all patients, including those who have had successful immediate sclerotherapy, should proceed to further elective treatment within that hospital admission to prevent subsequent variceal bleeding. Those patients being considered for a liver transplant should proceed to injection sclerotherapy.

Further emergency treatment options are endoscopic injection sclerotherapy, endoscopic variceal ligation, a portasystemic shunt, or an esophageal transection procedure. Each is considered separately. The more major surgical options are usually reserved for patients in whom sclerotherapy has failed.

Endoscopic Injection Sclerotherapy

Sclerotherapy is currently the accepted definitive treatment for acute variceal bleeding in the majority of major

centers. This therapy is supported by controlled trial data.[1, 21, 30] Sclerotherapy should be performed at the time of the first emergency endoscopy[57] whenever possible or within 6 to 12 hours of insertion of a balloon tube when this is required. The surgical alternatives of shunting or esophageal transection should be reserved for patients in whom sclerotherapy has failed.[4, 50, 53, 54] Using sclerotherapy, control of acute variceal bleeding is achieved in 90 to 95 per cent of patients. A single injection treatment suffices in 70 per cent of subjects;[50, 52–54] some 30 per cent of patients rebleed and require further injection treatments. Sclerotherapy fails in 5 to 10 per cent of patients, in whom the subsequent risk of death is high. For this reason, the failures of sclerotherapy should be identified as early as possible. Failure has been defined as a further variceal bleed occurring after two emergency injection treatments during a single hospital admission.[3, 4] In patients defined as having failed sclerotherapy the variceal hemorrhage should be recontrolled by balloon tube tamponade, and the patient should be further resuscitated and submitted urgently to some other form of therapy, usually one of the surgical options or a transjugular intrahepatic portasystemic shunt (TIPS). Unless failure is recognized, the mortality is prohibitive, particularly in poor-risk Child's class C patients.[3, 4, 53] There is still debate about whether, under certain circumstances, a surgical shunt or a transection operation may have a place as a primary procedure in some subsets of patients.[4, 53] The potential role of newer modalities of therapy is discussed below.

Although many other procedures used in the management of acute variceal bleeding are standardized, sclerotherapy techniques are far from standardized. Injection techniques, sclerosant solutions, levels of technical skill, frequency of injection treatments, and underlying disease entities vary widely in reviews of this topic. This variation is frequently lost sight of in assessing controlled trials in which a specific form of treatment is compared with one of several possible techniques of sclerotherapy. It is therefore not surprising that these trials have produced conflicting data.

Sclerosants can be injected intravariceally with the aim of thrombosing the varices (Fig. 101–2A) or in a paravariceal fashion with the aim of compressing the varices initially by edema and subsequently producing fibrous thickening of the overlying mucosa (Fig. 101–2C). Although it was once believed that the intravariceal technique using a fiberoptic endoscope could be enhanced by using an oversheath with a slot, this method is infrequently used today (Fig. 101–2B). A new concept of sclerotherapy has been proposed by Kitano and colleagues[18] whereby ethanolamine oleate 5 per cent is injected into the varices on the first one or two occasions until the varices are thrombosed. These authors subsequently inject the same agent paravariceally at repeat sessions until a circumferential superficial ulcer has been formed over the thrombosed varices. This is followed by healing with new mucosa and complete variceal eradication. Their results have been remarkably good, but their data require confirmation. The most widely used technique today for acute control of variceal bleeding is a combination of intra- and paravariceal injections (Fig. 101–2D).

Our group has continued to use ethanolamine oleate 5 per cent,[16, 50] which has been shown to be superior to other sclerosants in several controlled trials.[50] The earlier North American groups used sodium morrhuate 5 per cent and, more recently, have shifted to sodium tetradecyl sulfate 1 per cent or various combination solutions. The most widely used solution for an entirely paravariceal technique has been polidocanol 0.5 per cent or 1 per cent concentration.[30, 31]

When injection sclerotherapy is used for the control of acute variceal bleeding, repeat sclerotherapy is usually continued at intervals as part of the long-term management until the varices are eradicated. Because early eradication is important, most techniques today incorporate weekly endoscopy and sclerotherapy treatments unless these are precluded by local ulceration.

Endoscopic Variceal Ligation

Endoscopic variceal ligation or variceal banding, as devised by Stiegmann and Goff and their colleagues,[43] is described in Chapter 102 and is used both in the treatment of acute variceal bleeding and in long-term management. It has even been suggested that a combination of endoscopic variceal ligation and simultaneous low-volume injection sclerotherapy might eradicate varices more rapidly.[35] Banding has also been used for patients with failed injection sclerotherapy.[38] In a recent controlled randomized trial comparing sclerotherapy with banding,[43] the latter was shown to be superior with respect to complications, survival, recurrent hemorrhage, and the number of treatments required to eradicate varices. Although the preliminary data from other controlled trials look encouraging, this controlled trial must be confirmed by other groups before this new technique is widely adopted. It should be noted that the sclerosant chosen, sodium tetradecyl sulfate 1 per cent, administered by multiple 2-ml injections, is not necessarily the best injection sclerotherapy technique. Banding needs to be compared with other sclerotherapy techniques. A survival difference was shown only in the better-risk Child's A and B category patients and was not noted in the limited number of Child's C patients included in the study.[43] Because these poor-risk patients pose the major challenge in most Western series, further studies of banding in Child's C patients are required. Banding is an exciting new technique that, after further evaluation, may either supplement or replace injection sclerotherapy.

Emergency Portasystemic Shunts

Although an emergency operative portacaval shunt procedure will effectively stop acute variceal bleeding, few authorities advocate its routine use because of the high operative mortality rate associated with it, particularly for poor-risk cirrhotic patients in the hands of the average surgeon. The widespread use and apparent success of sclero-

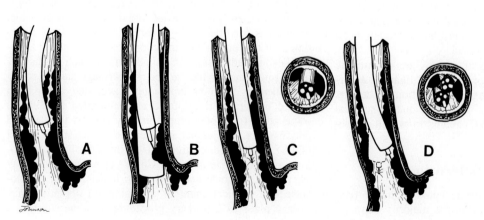

FIGURE 101–2. Injection sclerotherapy with the fiberoptic esophagoscope. *A,* Freehand intravariceal injection. *B,* Intravariceal injection using an oversheath with slot. *C,* Submucosal (paravariceal) injection technique. *D,* Combined submucosal and intravascular injection sclerotherapy (Cape Town technique).

therapy have caused it to become the first line of treatment. The author has subscribed to the view that the availability of alternative lesser procedures, which can at least temporarily stop acute variceal hemorrhage, makes the use of emergency surgical portosystemic shunts difficult to justify.

The recent introduction of the invasive radiologic technique of angiographic portal decompression (TIPS) (Fig. 101–3) has stimulated interest in this form of shunting for acute variceal bleeding (see Chapter 103).[36, 37, 58] TIPS appears to be valuable as a "bridge" to liver transplantation,[37] but its durability remains to be proved, as the transhepatic channel may progressively stenose and ultimately close.

Surgical Portasystemic Shunts

The available shunts that have been used for emergency portasystemic shunting are depicted in Figure 101–4. Although all of these shunts have been used in the long-term management of patients with portal hypertension, only the end-to-side portacaval and side-to-side portacaval shunts (Fig. 101–4*A* and *B*) and the narrow diameter portacaval interposition H-graft (Fig. 101–4*D*) or mesocaval shunt[39] (Fig. 101–4*C*) are used today for managing acute variceal bleeding. For long-term management the distal splenorenal shunt is most commonly used (Fig. 101–4*F*); this is occasionally used also in emergency situations in good-risk patients who do not have continued active variceal bleeding.

The role of emergency portacaval shunting has not yet been clearly defined. It remains one of the two main surgical options for sclerotherapy failures. Shunting may be-

come a routine procedure in some subsets of patients in the future, but the indications for such usage remain to be determined.[53] It is apparent that sclerotherapy in acute situations, which fails to control variceal bleeding in 5 to 10 per cent of patients, has been overused in the past and that other procedures should be introduced earlier for sclerotherapy failures.[3, 4, 50, 52, 53] Our group currently prefers the narrow diameter PTFE portacaval shunt as the emergency shunt of choice,[39] a standard portacaval shunt being the alternative. We use shunting for patients in whom sclerotherapy has failed and in whom a staple gun esophageal transection[15, 41] is technically not possible. Orloff and associates have been the main proponents of emergency shunting;[27] their work is supported by other recent studies.[6, 8, 42, 59] Orloff and colleagues' updated data have demonstrated remarkable results with a high survival and low encephalopathy rate in Child's class C patients. The discussion published with their paper introduces a note of caution, however.[59]

Emergency Devascularization and Transection Operations

A variety of esophagogastric devascularization[11, 17, 23, 44] or esophageal transection[4, 13, 15, 28, 41, 45] procedures has been advocated. The high mortality rate associated with these procedures, especially in poor-risk alcoholic cirrhotic patients, raises the question whether the widespread use of such operations is justified. Other problems are that varices recur in time, with a variable but high rebleed rate, and that these major operations cannot be repeated without undue

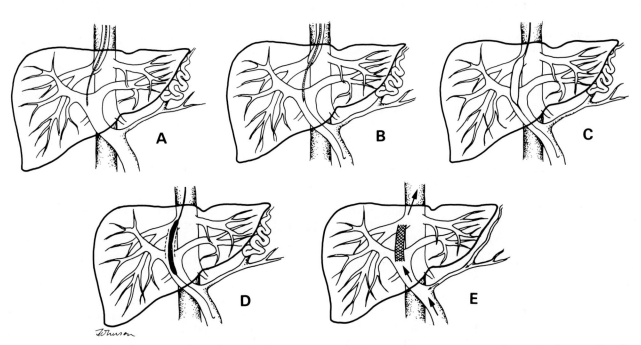

FIGURE 101–3. Transjugular intrahepatic portasystemic shunting (TIPS). *A*, A catheter is passed via the transjugular route into the hepatic vein, and a robust needle is passed through the liver substance into the portal vein. *B*, A guidewire is passed into the portal vein. *C*, The tract is dilated with an angioplasty balloon. *D*, An expandable metal stent is inserted through the tract. *E*, The stent is expanded, and the guidewire and catheter are withdrawn.

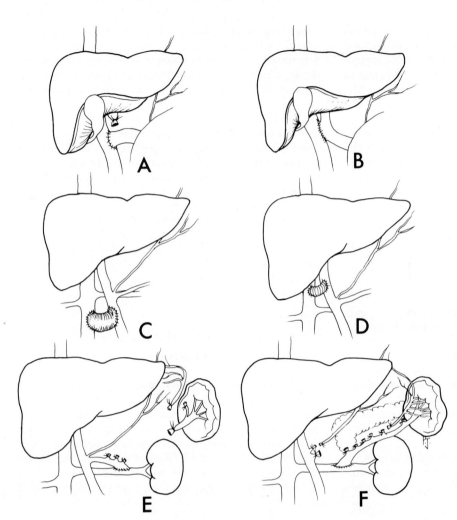

FIGURE 101–4. Portasystemic shunts used for the treatment of variceal bleeding. *A*, End-to-side portacaval shunt. *B*, Side-to-side portacaval shunt. *C*, Mesocaval interpositional H-graft. *D*, Portacaval interpositional H-graft. *E*, Central splenorenal shunt. *F*, Selective distal splenorenal shunt (Warren shunt). (*A–F*, From Terblanche J, Burroughs AK, Hobbs KEF: Controversies in the management of bleeding esophageal varices. Reprinted with permission from The New England Journal of Medicine 320:1393, 1989.)

risk to the patient.[23] Finally, bleeding from gastric varices, or from portal hypertensive gastropathy, cannot be controlled predictably by such operations.

A randomized controlled clinical trial compared sclerotherapy with staple transection for the emergency control of bleeding from esophageal varices.[4] The authors concluded that staple transection of the esophagus is as safe as sclerotherapy and more effective than a single sclerotherapy procedure. Nevertheless, they recommended sclerotherapy as the primary treatment with staple transection for the failures of sclerotherapy as defined earlier. This is the author's current policy, simple staple gun transection being the favored procedure in Cape Town for the failures of sclerotherapy.

A major concern has been the use of the staple gun for transection in patients who have had initial injection sclerotherapy. Prior sclerotherapy has not proved to be a problem in practice after one or two initial injection attempts, but the procedure can be substantially more difficult in patients who have undergone chronic sclerotherapy and subsequently have experienced a failure of control of an acute bleed by sclerotherapy.

Staple transection of the esophagus has not been compared with operative or angiographic portal decompression in patients with variceal hemorrhage. Devascularization procedures may be advantageous in certain settings because they should not complicate a planned future liver transplant.

Other Forms of Emergency Therapy

Percutaneous transhepatic embolization of the coronary and short gastric veins, approached via the portal vein, has been abandoned because of problems, particularly a high rebleed rate and portal vein thrombosis.[2] Other modifications of this procedure have been described but have not gained widespread acceptance.

Most other procedures described for the management of acute variceal bleeding, including laser and heater probe management of the esophageal varices through an endoscope, have also been abandoned as ineffective.

GASTRIC LESIONS IN PORTAL HYPERTENSION

Certain cirrhotics with upper gastrointestinal bleeding may have gastric varices or portal hypertensive gastropathy. Gastric varices are usually a direct continuation of esophageal varices.[19] In the author's experience these have usually disappeared after successful eradication of esophageal varices by repeated sclerotherapy.[49, 51]

A second variety of gastric varices are those that appear for the first time after successful eradication of varices by sclerotherapy or esophageal transection. These gastric varices may also bleed acutely, although bleeding from both forms of gastric varices has been unusual in the author's experience. When hemorrhage occurs, it can be difficult to manage. When bleeding persists, our group attempts sclerotherapy first and, if this fails, resorts to either a portosystemic shunt or a devascularization operation.

The third variety of gastric varices are isolated gastric varices associated with segmental portal hypertension caused by splenic vein thrombosis. This type is rare but can give rise to significant bleeding. It may occur in association with pancreatic carcinoma, in which case definitive management becomes irrelevant. However, in idiopathic cases and in cases in which it occurs after splenic trauma or pancreatitis, the condition can be cured by gastric devascularization and splenectomy.[22] Gastric devascularization alone may be sufficient without splenectomy but has yet to be reported.

Portal hypertensive gastropathy and the specific gastric mucosal lesions of portal hypertension have probably been underdiagnosed in the past.[24, 29, 40] These lesions, which are part of the anatomic features of portal hypertension in the esophagus and stomach,[19] have been better recognized and defined recently. Fortunately, they are rarely a cause of bleeding, and the bleeding usually stops spontaneously. If it does not, and the patient develops persistent acute bleeding, current evidence suggests that a portacaval shunt provides definitive treatment.

CONCLUSIONS

Patients with suspected esophageal variceal bleeding should be admitted to an intensive care unit and resuscitated. Emergency endoscopy is mandatory to prove, as far as is possible, that varices are the source of the bleeding. When varices are the cause of bleeding, immediate sclerotherapy at the time of the first endoscopy is advocated. The role of pharmacologic therapy to lower portal pressure has yet to be clearly defined. Either a continuous intravenous infusion of vasopressin plus nitroglycerin or an infusion of somatostatin appears to be the most effective agent. Balloon tube tamponade is highly effective in controlling active variceal bleeding when required because sclerotherapy has failed. The balloon tube should be removed and sclerotherapy performed within 6 to 12 hours. Patients require further emergency therapy to prevent recurrent bleeds. Currently, injection sclerotherapy is the most widely recommended procedure, with portosystemic shunts and transection operations being reserved for the failures of sclerotherapy. Endoscopic variceal ligation is currently under evaluation as alternative therapy. Angiographic portal decompression is a novel and minimally invasive approach that appears to be of value as a ''holding maneuver'' prior to liver transplantation but whose overall utility remains to be determined.

In most institutions where emergency injection sclerotherapy is used, either at the time of the initial emergency endoscopy or after a period of control with pharmacologic agents or balloon tube tamponade, variceal bleeding is controlled in 90 to 95 per cent of patients. However, more than one injection will be required in 30 per cent of patients and the 5 to 10 per cent of sclerotherapy failures require a more major surgical procedure such as a shunt or a transection operation. The ideal technique of injection sclerotherapy remains to be determined.

Any patient who rebleeds after two emergency sclerotherapy treatments during a single hospital admission should have the bleeding temporarily recontrolled by balloon tube tamponade and be subjected to emergency shunting or esophageal transection. An early decision about the patient's candidacy for liver transplantation should be made.

Acknowledgments: *Studies reported in this chapter were supported by grants from the South African Medical Research Council and the Staff Research Fund of the University of Cape Town. The assistance of many colleagues in the treatment and documentation of patients is gratefully acknowledged.*

References

1. Barsoum MS, Bolous FI, El-Rooby AA, et al: Tamponade and injection therapy in the management of bleeding oesophageal varices. Br J Surg 69:76, 1982.
2. Bengmark S, Borjesson B, Hoevels J, et al: Obliteration of esophageal varices by PTP. A follow-up of 43 patients. Ann Surg 190:549, 1979.
3. Bornman PC, Terblanche J, Kahn D, et al: Limitations of multiple injection sclerotherapy sessions for acute variceal bleeding. S Afr Med J 70:34, 1986.
4. Burroughs AK, Hamilton G, Phillips A, et al: A comparison of sclerotherapy with staple transection of the esophagus for the emergency control of bleeding from esophageal varices. N Engl J Med 321:857, 1989.
5. Burroughs AK, McCormick PA, Hughes MD, et al: Randomized, double-blind, placebo-controlled trial of somatostatin for variceal bleeding. Emergency control and prevention of early variceal rebleeding. Gastroenterology 99:1388, 1990.
6. Cello JP, Grendell JH, Crass RA, et al: Endoscopic sclerotherapy versus portacaval shunt in patients with severe cirrhosis and acute variceal hemorrhage. Long-term follow-up. N Engl J Med 316:11, 1987.
7. Conn HO: The varix volcano connection. Gastroenterology 79:1333, 1980.
8. Conn HO: Emergency portacaval anastomosis (EPCA): The long-awaited trial. Hepatology 5:1058, 1986.
9. Freeman JG, Cobden I, Lishman AH, et al: Controlled trial of terlipressin (glypressin) versus vasopressin in the early treatment of oesophageal varices. Lancet 2:66, 1982.
10. Graham DY, Smith JL: The course of patients after variceal hemorrhage. Gastroenterology 80:800, 1981.
11. Hassab MA: Nonshunt operations in portal hypertension without cirrhosis. Surg Gynecol Obstet 131:648, 1970.
12. Hosking SW, Doss W, El-Zeiny H, et al: Pharmacological constriction of the lower oesophageal sphincter: A simple method of arresting variceal haemorrhage. Gut 29:1098, 1988.
13. Huizinga WKJ, Angorn PA, Baker LW: Esophageal transection versus injection sclerotherapy in the management of bleeding esophageal varices in patients at high risk. Surg Gynecol Obstet 160:539, 1985.
14. Jenkins SA, Shields R, Jaser N, et al: The management of gastrointestinal haemorrhage by somatostatin after apparently successful endoscopic injection sclerotherapy for bleeding oesophageal varices. J Hepatol 12:296, 1991.
15. Johnston GW: Simplified oesophageal transection for bleeding varices. Br Med J 1:1388, 1979.
16. Kahn D, Bornman PC, Terblanche J: A 10-year prospective evaluation of balloon tube tamponade and emergency injection sclerotherapy for actively bleeding oesophageal varices. HPB Surg 1:207, 1989.
17. Keagy BA, Schwartz JA, Johnson G: Should ablative operations be used for bleeding esophageal varices? Ann Surg 203:463, 1986.
18. Kitano S, Koyanagi N, Iso Y, et al: Prevention of recurrence of esophageal varices after endoscopic injection sclerotherapy with ethanolamine oleate. Hepatology 7:810, 1987.
19. Kitano S, Terblanche J, Kahn D: Venous anatomy of the lower oesophagus in portal hypertension: Practical implications. Br J Surg 73:525, 1986.

20. Kleber G, Sauerbruch T, Fischer G, et al: Reduction of transmural oesophageal variceal pressure by metoclopramide. J Hepatol 12:362, 1991.

21. Larson AW, Cohen H, Zweiban B, et al: Acute esophageal variceal sclerotherapy. Results of a prospective randomized controlled trial. JAMA 255:497, 1986.

22. Madsen MS, Petersen TH, Sommer H: Segmental portal hypertension. Ann Surg 204:72, 1986.

23. Matory WE, Sedgwick CE, Rossi RL: Nonshunting procedures in management of bleeding esophageal varices. Surg Clin North Am 60:281, 1980.

24. McCormack TT, Sims J, Eyre-Brook I, et al: Gastric lesions in portal hypertension: Inflammatory gastritis or congestive gastropathy? Gut 26:1226, 1985.

25. McKee R. A study of octreotide in oesophageal varices. Digestion 45 (Suppl 1):60, 1990.

26. Novis BH, Duys P, Barbezat GO, et al: Fiberoptic endoscopy and the use of the Sengstaken tube in acute gastrointestinal haemorrhage in patients with portal hypertension and varices. Gut 17:258, 1976.

27. Orloff MJ, Bell RH, Hyde PV, et al: Long-term results of emergency portacaval shunt for bleeding esophageal varices in unselected patients with alcoholic cirrhosis. Ann Surg 192:325, 1980.

28. Osborne DR, Hobbs KEF: The acute treatment of haemorrhage from oesophageal varices: A comparison of oesophageal transection and staple gun anastomosis with mesocaval shunt. Br J Surg 68:734, 1981.

29. Papazian A, Braillon A, Dupas JL, et al: Portal hypertensive gastric mucosa: An endoscopic study. Gut 27:1199, 1986.

30. Paquet KJ, Feussner H: Endoscopic sclerosis and esophageal balloon tamponade in acute hemorrhage from esophagogastric varices: A prospective controlled randomized trial. Hepatology 5:580, 1985.

31. Paquet KJ, Oberhammer E: Sclerotherapy of bleeding oesophageal varices by means of endoscopy. Endoscopy 10:7, 1978.

32. Perez-Ayuso RM, Pique JM, Bosch J, et al: Propranolol in prevention of recurrent bleeding from severe portal hypertensive gastropathy in cirrhosis. Lancet 337:1431, 1991.

33. Pitcher JL: Safety and effectiveness of the modified Sengstaken-Blakemore tube: A prospective study. Gastroenterology 61:291, 1971.

34. Ready JB, Robertson AD, Rector WG. Effects of vasopressin on portal pressure during hemorrhage from esophageal varices. Gastroenterology 100:1411, 1991.

35. Reveille RM, Goff JS, Stiegmann GV, et al: Combination endoscopic variceal ligation (EVL) and low-volume endoscopic sclerotherapy (ES) for bleeding esophageal varices: A faster route to variceal eradication? [Abstract]. Gastrointest Endosc 37:243, 1991.

36. Richter GM, Noeldge G, Roessle M, et al: Transjugular intrahepatic portosystemic stent shunt (TIPS). Radiology 174:1027, 1990.

37. Ring EJ, Lake JR, Roberts JP, et al: Using transjugular intrahepatic portosystemic shunts to control variceal bleeding before liver transplantation. Ann Intern Med 116:304, 1992.

38. Saeed ZA, Michaletz PA, Winchester CB, et al: Endoscopic variceal ligation in patients who have failed endoscopic sclerotherapy. Gastrointest Endosc 36:572, 1990.

39. Sarfeh IJ, Rypins EB, Mason GR: A systematic appraisal of portacaval H-graft diameters. Clinical and hemodynamic perspectives. Ann Surg 204:356, 1986.

40. Sarfeh IJ, Tarnawski A: Gastric bleeding in portal hypertension: Inflammatory or congestive? Hepatology 6:535, 1986.

41. Spence RAJ, Johnston GW: Stapled esophageal transection for varices. Results in 100 consecutive patients. Surg Gynecol Obstet 160:323, 1985.

42. Spina GP, Santambrogio R, Opocher E, et al: Emergency portosystemic shunt in patients with variceal bleeding. Surg Gynecol Obstet 171:456, 1990.

43. Stiegmann GV, Goff JS, Michaletz-Onody PA, et al: Endoscopic sclerotherapy as compared with endoscopic ligation for bleeding esophageal varices. N Engl J Med 326:1527, 1992.

44. Sugiura M, Futagawa S: Further evaluation of the Sugiura procedure in the treatment of esophageal varices. Arch Surg 112:1317, 1977.

45. Takasaki T, Kobayashi S, Muto H, et al: Transabdominal esophageal transection by using a suture device in cases of esophageal varices. Int Surg 62:426, 1977.

46. Taranto D, Suozzo R, de Sio I, et al: Effect of metoclopramide on transmural oesophageal variceal pressure and portal blood flow in cirrhotic patients. Digestion 47:56, 1990.

47. Terblanche J, Northover JMA, Bornman P, et al: A prospective evaluation of injection sclerotherapy in the treatment of acute bleeding from esophageal varices. Surgery 85:238, 1979.

48. Terblanche J, Yakoob HI, Bornman PC, et al: Acute bleeding varices. A 5-year prospective evaluation of tamponade and sclerotherapy. Ann Surg 194:521, 1981.

49. Terblanche J, Bornman PC, Kahn D, et al: Failure of repeated injection sclerotherapy to improve long-term survival after oesophageal variceal bleeding. A five-year prospective controlled clinical trial. Lancet 12:1328, 1983.

50. Terblanche J, Burroughs AK, Hobbs KEF: Controversies in the management of bleeding esophageal varices. N Engl J Med 320:1393, 1469, 1989.

51. Terblanche J, Kahn D, Bornman PC: Long-term injection sclerotherapy treatment for esophageal varices: A 10 year prospective evaluation. Ann Surg 210:726, 1989.

52. Terblanche J, Krige JEJ, Bornman PC: The treatment of esophageal varices. Ann Rev Med 43:69, 1992.

53. Terblanche J: The surgeon's role in the management of portal hypertension. Ann Surg 209:381, 1989.

54. Terblanche J: Has sclerotherapy altered the management of patients with variceal bleeding? Am J Surg 160:37, 1990.

55. Tsai Y-T, Lee F-Y, Lin H-C, et al: Hyposensitivity to vasopressin in patients with hepatitis B–related cirrhosis during acute variceal hemorrhage. Hepatology 13:407, 1991.

56. Walker S, Stiehl A, Raedsch R, et al: Terlipressin in bleeding esophageal varices. A placebo-controlled, double-blind study. Hepatology 6:112, 1986.

57. Westaby D, Hayes PC, Gimson AES, et al: Controlled clinical trial of injection sclerotherapy for active variceal bleeding. Hepatology 9:274, 1989.

58. Zemel G, Katzen BT, Becker GJ, et al: Percutaneous transjugular portosystemic shunt. JAMA 266:390, 1991.

59. Orloff MJ, Orloff MS, Rambotti M, et al: Is portal-systemic shunt worthwhile in Child's Class C cirrhosis? Long-term results of emergency shunt in 94 patients with bleeding varices. Ann Surg 216:526, 1992.

Endoscopic Treatment of Esophageal Varices

Greg Van Stiegmann, M.D.

• • •

Endoscopic treatment of esophageal varices was first reported by Crafoord and Frenckner, two Swedish surgeons, in 1939.[1] Scattered reports of successful use of endoscopic sclerotherapy for treatment of bleeding varices, and for prevention of rebleeding, appeared during the subsequent 10 years. Enthusiasm for endoscopic treatment was strongly overshadowed by the introduction of the portacaval shunt in 1946[2] and its widespread acceptance in the 1950s and 1960s.

Interest in endoscopic sclerotherapy was dormant until the 1970s when the shortcomings of shunt and devascularization operations became better understood. This decade witnessed a rebirth of interest in endoscopic treatment, initiated primarily by surgeons employing rigid endoscopes and performing sclerotherapy with the patient under general anesthesia.

Paralleling the rekindled interest in endoscopic treatment of esophageal varices was the progressive refinement and widespread acceptance of flexible fiberoptic endoscopes, initially for diagnostic use and subsequently for therapeutic purposes including sclerotherapy. By the mid-1980s, flexible endoscopic sclerotherapy, performed in the awake, sedated patient, was accepted as the first-line treatment for patients with variceal hemorrhage. Surgeons were joined by large numbers of physician endoscopists, and these procedures, now performed in the endoscopy suite or the intensive care unit, replaced many of the various shunt and devascularization operations. New endoscopic treatment methods, including polymer injection and mechanical O ring ligation, were introduced in the mid-1980s. Currently, the results of prospective randomized trials comparing various regimens of endoscopic sclerotherapy, and comparing sclerotherapy with medical, surgical, and other forms of endoscopic treatment, are emerging. During the coming decade, better definition of the merits of endoscopic treatment, particularly as related to long-term survival and prophylactic treatment, is expected.

VARICEAL ANATOMY

Unlike shunt operations, which aim to decompress all or a portion of the portal venous system, endoscopic treatment is aimed primarily at venous channels in the distal esophagus. Variceal hemorrhage can occur throughout the gastrointestinal tract;[3, 4] however, the majority of variceal hemorrhages emanate from just above the gastroesophageal junction.[5]

Gastroesophageal varices are predominately supplied by the left gastric and short gastric veins, which arise from the portal and splenic veins.[6] In the proximal stomach, these vessels lie in the submucosa, but at or near the gastroesophageal junction they traverse the muscularis mucosa to lie superficially beneath the distal esophageal mucosa. This superficial location is maintained for a cephalad distance of from 1 to 4 cm, at which point the vessels again pass through the muscularis mucosa to continue in a cephalad direction under the relative protection of this layer. At variable distances above the gastroesophageal junction, these longitudinal vessels traverse the muscularis propria of the esophagus to join with the azygous system.[7-9] Anatomic studies[10] have demonstrated the venous anatomy of the normal lower esophagus to consist of four layers of venous channels and a series of perforating veins that join the adventitial system with the deeper veins (Fig. 102–1A and B). Further observations employing corrosion cast techniques in patients who died with portal hypertension and esophageal varices showed that all of these venous channels were markedly dilated (Fig. 102–1C). The three to five deep longitudinal intrinsic veins became the major recognizable variceal channels, and both these and the superficial venous plexus were noted to connect across the gastroesophageal junction with their counterparts in the stomach. Enlarged perforating vessels were reported present in all specimens and occurred in the area above the gastroesophageal junction. Based on these studies, Kitano and associates postulate that major variceal bleeds may occur following rupture of a large, deep intrinsic vein (varix), and that minor bleeds, which stop spontaneously, may result from rupture of branches of the superficial venous plexus or from the intraepithelial channels. They further postulate that perforating vessels may, in part, be responsible for the recurrence of variceal channels following successful eradication by sclerotherapy.[10] Such anatomic studies are basic to the complete understanding of local treatment methods such as endoscopic sclerotherapy. Newer endoscopic Doppler flow measurement techniques and endoscopic ultrasound imaging capabilities may further refine our understanding of success and failure at local control of esophageal varices.

TECHNIQUES OF SCLEROTHERAPY

The goal of endoscopic sclerotherapy is arrest of acute variceal bleeding and prevention of recurrent hemorrhage

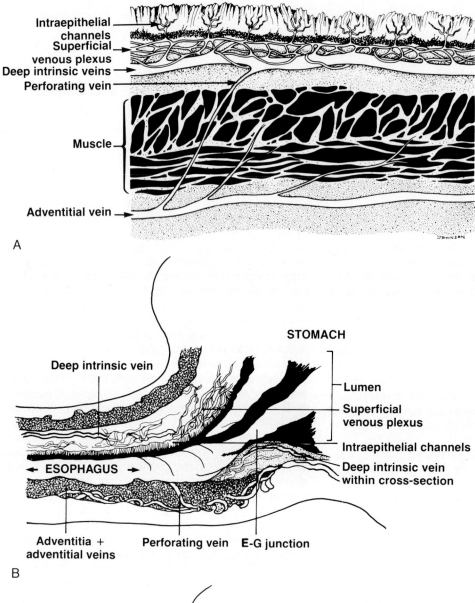

A

B

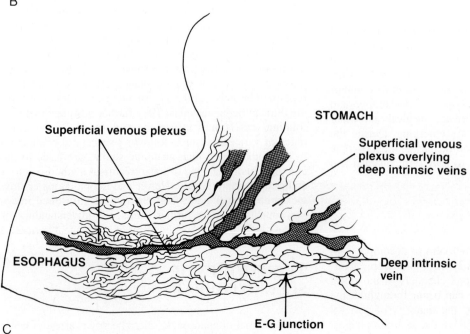

C

FIGURE 102–1. A and B, Venous anatomy of the lower esophagus. Note that the deep intrinsic and superficial venous plexuses freely communicate across the gastroesophageal junction. Perforating vessels are present at varying positions and connect the adventitial system with the deep veins. C, Distal esophagus/proximal stomach in portal hypertension. Esophageal varices consist of dilated deep intrinsic and superficial veins. Superficial veins overlying deep intrinsic veins give the endoscopic appearance of varices on varices. (A–C, From Kitano S, Terblanche J, Kahn D, et al: Venous anatomy of the lower oesophagus in portal hypertension: Practical implications. Br J Surg 73:525, 1986, by permission of Butterworth Heinemann, Ltd, Oxford, publisher.)

by eradication of distal esophageal variceal channels. This may be accomplished by injecting sclerosants directly into variceal channels (intravariceal injection) or by injection into the tissue beside the varix (paravariceal injection). Paravariceal treatment is favored by many European endoscopists[11] and is accomplished by using multiple injections of small quantities (1 ml or less) of sclerosant beside the variceal channels over the distal 5 to 10 cm of esophagus. Intravariceal injection employs 3 to 5 ml of sclerosant per varix, usually in one injection site per varix, at or near the gastroesophageal junction. Intravariceal treatment is aimed at thrombosing variceal channels whereas paravariceal injections are designed to create a tough fibrous cap over the varix to prevent bleeding. In practice, regardless of the aim of the endoscopist, it is probable that a combination of the two techniques usually results.

Sanowski reported that 44 per cent of attempted intravariceal injections, performed using a combination of 5 per cent sodium morrhuate and contrast agent and followed by serial roentgen examination, resulted in accumulation of contrast medium in the wall of the esophagus.[12] Clearance of contrast occurred in approximately 3 hours. True intravariceal injections demonstrated rapid clearance of contrast in a cephalad (42 per cent) or caudad (14 per cent) direction. These data have been corroborated in another study[13] and may explain the failure of the intravariceal technique to effect variceal thrombosis in certain situations in which variceal flow rates are high. It also points to the potential for systemic complications resulting from widespread dissemination of toxic sclerosing agents, as well as the possibility that caudad migration of the sclerosant may result in portal vein thrombosis.

Rigid Endoscopic Sclerotherapy

Rigid endoscopic sclerotherapy is performed in the operating theater with a large caliber esophagoscope and a long rigid injection needle. This author seldom employs the rigid endoscope in either the acute or the elective setting because of the necessity for general anesthesia, with its attendant risks, in this often severely compromised patient group. Young children, who will usually require general anesthesia regardless of the endoscopic technique employed, may be safely and effectively treated with a modified rigid pediatric esophagoscope, which provides the advantage of effective tamponade of the treated site following injection.[14]

Flexible Endoscopic Sclerotherapy

Flexible endoscopic sclerotherapy may be performed in the endoscopy suite or in the intensive care unit provided adequate support personnel, who are thoroughly familiar with the technique as well as with airway management, are present. Treatment of acute bleeding mandates minimal or no sedation and judicious application of topical anesthetic in order to minimize the risk of postprocedure pulmonary aspiration. Severely disoriented patients may require heavy sedation and endotracheal intubation. For prevention of aspiration in otherwise cooperative patients, an alternative is the use of an endoscopic overtube. Such tubes effectively isolate gastric secretions from the oropharynx and hypopharynx and allow repeated lavage as needed. The selection of endoscopic equipment is largely a matter of personal preference. Double-lumen therapeutic endoscopes are now widely available and may be valuable when hemorrhage is intense. However, a large (3.5 mm) working channel instrument will provide adequate clearance of secretions and blood in most situations, even with the injection needle occupying the channel.

Injection needles for flexible endoscopic sclerotherapy are produced by a number of manufacturers and are provided in both multiple-use and disposable form. Such devices consist of a flexible outer sheath into which the needle can be withdrawn to protect the working channel of the endoscope from accidental puncture (Fig. 102–2). Needles commonly range from 23 to 25 gauge in size and may be extended beyond their protective sheaths for distances of from 3.6 to 5.6 mm.[15] No prospective clinical assessment of the impact of needle size, type, or exposed length on the outcome of treatment has been performed. Because endoscopists performing sclerotherapy should, in part, judge the appropriateness of needle placement when injecting varices by the amount of resistance encountered upon injection, it is essential that they gain familiarity with this characteristic of both the specific needle and the sclerosant agent employed.

The patient is positioned in the left lateral (left side down) decubitus position, and the endoscope is introduced. If active bleeding is in progress, an attempt to localize the source is imperative, since even in patients with known esophageal varices and upper gastrointestinal hemorrhage, the likelihood of a nonvariceal site of bleeding may exceed 30 per cent.[16] If esophageal varices are present and no other potential site of bleeding is identified, variceal hemorrhage may be presumed and treated accordingly.

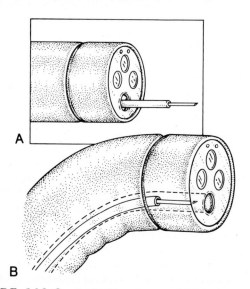

FIGURE 102–2. *A*, Flexible endoscope with injection needle protruding. The needle is passed through the working channel retracted inside its outer sheath. Care must be taken to avoid inadvertent exposure of the needle during passage through the endoscope. *B*, Retching or coughing necessitates withdrawal of the injection apparatus into the scope to prevent inadvertent laceration of esophageal varices.

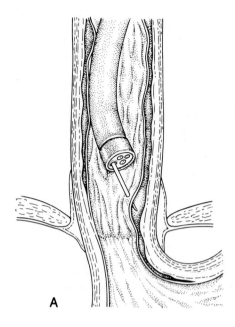

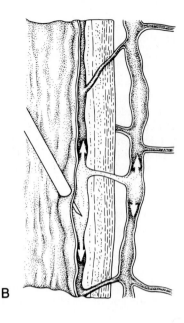

FIGURE 102–3. *A*, Flexible, freehand, endoscopic sclerosis. Sclerosing treatments are confined to the lower 5 to 10 cm of the esophagus above the gastroesophageal junction. *B*, Intravariceal injection may result in systemic dissemination of sclerosant via perforating vessels that communicate with the adventitial veins. Systemic effects may result.

This author prefers a direct intravariceal injection technique with a 23-gauge needle. Following the initial survey of the esophagus, stomach, and duodenum, the endoscope is positioned 3 to 4 cm above the gastroesophageal junction where three to five variceal channels are usually present. In the nonactively bleeding patient, injection is initiated in the most gravity-dependent portion of the esophagus, since bleeding from higher injection sites may obscure the target area. If an actively bleeding variceal site is identified, it is attacked first. The needle is plunged into the varix, and 2 to 5 ml of sclerosant is injected per variceal channel. Both the resistance sensed during the injection and the appearance of the varix as injection proceeds are important parameters. Stiff resistance to injection may indicate that the needle has been positioned in a previously thrombosed varix or, conversely, has been advanced into the esophageal wall itself. If such resistance is met, the injection should be aborted and another site selected. The varix usually slowly balloons and blanches during the course of an accurate intravariceal injection. If unusually rapid ballooning occurs, the needle may have been placed between the esophageal mucosa and the variceal wall. Continued injection in such a location can result in the development of ulceration over a nonthrombosed channel, which may cause delayed hemorrhage. Certain large variceal channels may exhibit little change in caliber or appearance during injection since the rapid intravariceal blood flow may promptly dissipate the sclerosing agent (Fig. 102–3). For this reason, injection probably should not be performed in the mid or proximal esophagus, since the toxic sclerosant may be transported rapidly into the pulmonary circulation, producing untoward effects.[17] Injection volumes should seldom exceed 5 ml per varix and may often be considerably less as patients progress, with repeated treatments, toward variceal eradication. Following completion of injection, some bleeding is common. The flexible endoscope provides some tamponade effect and should be advanced into the stomach and remain there for several minutes. During this period, the air insufflated into the stomach during the procedure is aspirated. The endoscope is withdrawn slowly to allow final inspection of the

treated sites, which usually appear gray-blue in color. If significant bleeding from a particular injection site is present, the endoscope may be positioned to effectively tamponade the bleeding and should be held in this position for 3 to 5 minutes (Fig. 102–4).

A variety of devices have been advocated to facilitate flexible endoscopic sclerotherapy. A slotted sheath that allows protrusion of the varix through the slot and, with rotation, provides compression of the just-injected varix, has been described and studied by the Kings College group.[18] A Linton tube may be placed into the stomach and the balloon inflated and drawn snugly against the gastroesophageal junction to slow variceal flow during the course

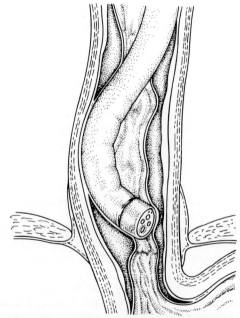

FIGURE 102–4. Persistent bleeding following injection may be treated with this maneuver. The endoscope is positioned to compress the bleeding site and tamponade is maintained for 3 to 5 minutes.

of injection.[19] A specially designed balloon may be attached over the distal end of the endoscope and employed to tamponade injection sites following treatment.[20] Similarly, balloon tamponade (Sengstaken-Blakemore) may be employed for varying lengths of time following sclerotherapy. However, there appears to be little advantage to any of these maneuvers. This author prefers straightforward free-hand injection techniques without the use of such appliances. Patients in whom bleeding cannot be adequately controlled or in whom torrential bleeding precludes flexible endoscopic injection are treated under general anesthesia with the rigid endoscope.

Recommended intervals between elective repeat sclerotherapy treatments vary widely and usually range from 1 to 3 weeks. Two prospective trials comparing 1- and 3-week injection schedules have shown no appreciable difference between such intervals with the exception of a greater frequency of recognized injection site ulcerations noted in the 1-week interval groups.[21, 22] This author believes a 10- to 14-day interval is satisfactory for most patients. High-risk patients appear to have a greater propensity for development of injection site ulceration, which may be slow to heal and may temporarily preclude repeated treatment. For this reason, a degree of flexibility in scheduling repeat injection sessions is indicated based upon individual patient characteristics. Better-risk patients are often retreated at shorter intervals.

SCLEROSANT AGENTS

Agents commonly employed in the United States include tetradecyl sodium, morrhuate sodium, ethanolamine oleate, and various mixtures of these substances with other solutions such as 50 per cent dextrose or cefazolin. Many European centers employ a solution of polidocanol (recommended only for paravariceal injection) and ethanolamine oleate for intravariceal injection. The former agent is not available in the United States.

Using a reproducible canine model of esophageal varices, Jensen found that 95 per cent ethanol, 1.5 per cent tetradecyl, and 5 per cent morrhuate were the most effective single agents for thrombosing the large dilated abdominal wall veins that develop in such animals.[23] When injected endoscopically into the esophageal varices of these animals, ulcerations developed in 90 per cent of those treated with 95 per cent alcohol, 40 per cent of those treated with 1.5 per cent tetradecyl, and 30 per cent of those to whom 5 per cent morrhuate was given. Although other animal studies have shown no difference in ulceration rates between 3 and 1.5 per cent tetradecyl,[24] clinical experience from the author's institution suggests otherwise,[25] and a clinical study comparing 3 per cent tetradecyl with 5 per cent morrhuate has further confounded matters by demonstrating a greater incidence of ulceration with morrhuate.[26] The multitude of sclerosants and sclerosant ''cocktails'' available and a lack of objective human data on their merits and shortcomings suggest that all are less than ideal.

Endoscopic sclerotherapy is an ''operator-dependent'' procedure, and it is likely that minor variations in individual technique may have more importance than the particular agent employed. It appears that the most effective thrombotic agents are also those that are most toxic to surrounding tissue. Based on these considerations and on the limited experimental data available, this author continues to recommend 5 per cent ethanolamine oleate for intravariceal treatment and would select 1.5 per cent tetradecyl sodium as an alternative.

COMPLICATIONS

Endoscopic sclerotherapy was initially greeted as a benign form of treatment for an often disastrous disease. It is now recognized that sclerotherapy is frequently accompanied by minor complications and results in an appreciable number of major problems. The overall incidence of major complications reported to occur from repeated endoscopic sclerotherapy varies from series to series and ranges from 2 to 20 per cent.[16, 27, 28]

Complications of endoscopic sclerotherapy may be categorized as early (within 24 hours) or late, and as either local or systemic. Early complications are most often directly related to the endoscopic procedure itself and include acute perforation, aspiration, and precipitation of hemorrhage. Perforation is uncommon with flexible instruments, and aspiration should seldom occur during elective treatment but appears more commonly during control of acute hemorrhage. Treatment-associated hemorrhage from varices is usually minor; however, a sudden retch or cough may result in laceration of the varix with the needle and subsequent rapid bleeding. Substernal chest pain with or without fever may occur in up to 50 per cent of patients[29] but usually persists less than 24 hours. Pain following sclerotherapy may be the result of chemical mediastinitis or esophageal spasm.[30, 31] Spasm may also account for the transient swallowing difficulty seen in some patients.

The development of unremitting substernal pain 2 to 14 days following endoscopic sclerotherapy should raise the possibility of delayed chemical necrosis of the esophageal wall. This complication is often insidious in appearance and has been reported in from 1 to 6 per cent of patients undergoing repeated sclerotherapy. It has an apparent proclivity for high-risk patients.[25] Exudative pleural effusion is present in the majority of such patients; however, effusions may also be seen in many asymptomatic patients following sclerotherapy.[29] In the presence of suspected perforation, water-soluble contrast studies should be performed to determine if a leak is present, and, if so, whether it is confined to a walled-off cavity that drains freely back into the esophagus or if a free perforation exists. Conservative management including antibiotics, nasogastric drainage, and closed tube thoracostomy may be indicated in the former situation and is often successful. Aggressive surgical drainage is indicated when free perforation is present, and survival is infrequent.

Injection site ulceration is common following endoscopic sclerotherapy and may be found in up to 94 per cent of patients who undergo repeat endoscopy within 24 hours, and in up to 80 per cent of patients who have endoscopy within 1 week following sclerotherapy.[21, 32] Small, shallow ulcerations that involve only the mucosa and submucosa are most often benign and may well be the sign of an effective injection. Large, deeper lesions that involve the muscle wall itself occur with unknown frequency and may be associated with troublesome secondary hemorrhage. The frequency of ulceration has been reported to correspond with the volume of sclerosant injected,[32] and as noted earlier, the most effective thrombotic agents appear also to be those with the greatest ulcerogenic potential.

The spectrum of ulceration associated with endoscopic sclerotherapy ranges from small, shallow lesions to esophageal wall necrosis. Damage to the underlying esophageal wall may manifest late as esophageal stenosis or a motility disorder. Esophageal stenosis may develop in up to 10 per cent of sclerotherapy patients[5] and usually responds to conservative treatment with dilatation. Esophageal motility disorders, including reduced lower esophageal sphincter pressure, have been reported in one study[33] and are consistently observed in this author's institution[34] but have not been reported in other series.[35, 36] The importance of reduced acid clearance from the postsclerotherapy esophagus is also unclear and may, in part, explain the development of some strictures.[37]

Systemic complications of sclerotherapy often present early and may be devastating. Bacteremia appears in a small percentage of sclerotherapy patients,[38] but antibiotic prophylaxis does not appear to be indicated except in patients who have prosthetic heart valves. Morrhuate sodium (5 per cent) was associated with spinal cord paralysis in a 4-year-old child who at autopsy was found to have thrombosis of the anterior spinal artery.[39] Mesenteric thrombosis has been reported in two cases following injection of a mixture of 50 per cent dextrose and tetradecyl sodium.[40] Acute respiratory distress syndrome was observed in two patients following treatment with 5 per cent morrhuate.[41] Two prospective clinical studies have shown no significant effect of sclerotherapy on pulmonary or systemic hemodynamics.[42, 43] However, experimental studies in dogs that underwent injection of ethanolamine oleate into the right atrium demonstrated deleterious effects on pulmonary hemodynamics when the sclerosant was administered in quantities of 0.25 ml/kg or more.[44]

RESULTS

Endoscopic sclerotherapy of esophageal varices was compared with medical therapy in five prospective randomized trials that assessed control of acute bleeding and in eight that assessed long-term control and follow-up. Four of five studies that compared sclerotherapy with medical management for acute treatment of variceal bleeding demonstrated no advantage for sclerotherapy in prevention of early recurrent bleeding or improved survival.[45–49] Endoscopic sclerotherapy confers little advantage early in the course of variceal hemorrhage.

Eight trials compared serial endoscopic sclerotherapy with medical management for long-term treatment.[45, 47–53] Recurrent bleeding was less in sclerotherapy-treated patients in four of the eight trials. Sclerotherapy-treated patients survived longer than medically treated patients in five trials. Soderland and associates failed to demonstrate a survival advantage in sclerotherapy patients despite a reduction in the incidence of recurrent hemorrhage in that group.[49] The Cape Town study did not demonstrate a survival advantage for sclerotherapy-treated patients but differed from the other trials because control patients received acute sclerotherapy for recurrent variceal bleeding.[52] Results from seven of these eight studies were assessed using meta-analysis methods.[54] Combined data suggested that endoscopic sclerotherapy reduced the number of deaths by up to 25 per cent. Significant nonbleeding complications associated with sclerotherapy occurred in 23 per cent of patients.

Lebrec and coworkers demonstrated that the beta-adrenoreceptor blocking agent propranolol could reduce portal pressure and prevent recurrent variceal hemorrhage in cirrhotic patients with portal hypertension.[55] This effect presumably relates to propranolol's reduction of splanchnic blood flow, most likely due to diminished cardiac output.[56] Three prospective randomized trials compared sclerotherapy with propranolol for prevention of recurrent bleeding.[57–59] Results of these trials are summarized in Table 102–1. Two of the three prospective evaluations supported the contention that propranolol may be as effective as sclerotherapy in preventing recurrent hemorrhage. All three trials showed no difference in survival for propranolol as opposed to sclerotherapy treatment. These data must be interpreted cautiously, however. All trials entered patients only after the index variceal bleed had ceased and patients were hemodynamically stable for periods of from 1 to 15 days. From 47 to 83 per cent of all patients with variceal bleeding seen during the study period were ineligible for inclusion in these trials, and only one trial included Child class C patients. Overall, 26 per cent of propranolol-treated patients required endoscopic therapy for control of recurrent hemorrhage during the course of study. Three additional trials compared the use of sclerotherapy alone with sclerotherapy combined with propranolol.[60–62] Results of these trials are also summarized in Table 102–1. These data include a more typical proportion of Child class C patients as well as a number who were actively bleeding on admission whose index hemorrhage was initially controlled with sclerotherapy. None of the studies showed a significant

Table 102–1. Results of Three Prospective Randomized Trials Comparing Sclerotherapy Alone With Propranolol Alone for Treatment of Patients Who Had Bled From Esophageal Varices and Three Prospective Randomized Trials Comparing Sclerotherapy Plus Propranolol (S + P) With Sclerotherapy Alone for Treatment of Patients With Bleeding Esophageal Varices

Author	No. Patients	Therapy	Rebled (%)	Survival (%)	Compl (%)
Flieg[58]	36	S	28	91	11
	34	P	29	85	3
Alexandrino[57]	31	S	55	66	16
	34	P	73	68	6
Westaby[59]	56	S	45	66	0
	52	P	54	55	8
Vickers[62]	35	S + P	45	63	NA
	34	S	29	73	NA
Westaby[60]	26	S + P	27	73	8
	27	S	30	74	NA
Jensen[61]	15	S + P	20	93	0
	16	S	75	94	0

S, sclerotherapy; P, propranolol; Compl, complications of therapy.
*p <.05.

Table 102-2. Results of Six Prospective Randomized Trials Comparing Endoscopic Sclerotherapy (ES) With Shunt Surgery*

Study	No. Patients	Therapy	Rebled (%)	Surgery (%)	Survival (%)
Cello[63]	24	Shunt	21	—	17
	28	ES	50	11	32
Rikkers[64]	27	Shunt	19	—	65
	30	ES	57	7	61
Teres[65]	42	Shunt	14	—	71
	48	ES	38	6	68
Warren[68]	35	Shunt	3	—	51
	36	ES	53	31	75
Spina[66]	20	Shunt	5	—	100
	20	ES	35	0	95
Planas[67]	34	Shunt	3	—	83
	35	ES	40	17	79

*All trials but Cello's were conducted in an elective or semi-elective setting, and only one showed sclerotherapy superior to shunt operation.

Surgery (%), Percent of sclerotherapy patients who required salvage operation.

*$p < .05$.

difference in survival. Based on these data, propranolol does not appear to afford an advantage over sclerotherapy when the endoscopic procedure is performed by an experienced therapeutic endoscopist, nor does propranolol appear to be a useful adjunct to endoscopic sclerotherapy.

Six prospective trials comparing sclerotherapy with operative treatment[63–68] are summarized in Table 102-2. Cello and colleagues' study was restricted to high-risk patients, and the surgical treatment used was a portacaval shunt.[63] This trial initially suggested an advantage for sclerotherapy-treated patients. However, in the final analysis, sclerotherapy was not found to be superior to emergent portacaval shunt. The remaining trials compared stable patients treated by sclerotherapy with those treated by central or selective splenorenal shunts. The Atlanta data showed that both survival and preservation of hepatic function were superior in patients initially treated with sclerotherapy despite the fact that 31 per cent of sclerotherapy-treated patients rebled and required a shunt operation.[68] In contrast, the Omaha, Barcelona, and Italian groups demonstrated no superiority of one technique over the other with regard to either survival or preservation of hepatic function.[64, 67]

PROPHYLACTIC SCLEROTHERAPY

Prevention of the first variceal bleed is the goal of prophylactic sclerotherapy. Two thirds of patients with varices never bleed; hence, preventive treatment of cirrhotics with varices who have never bled must target patients who are at high risk for bleeding.[69] Several trials have shown a reduction in mortality in sclerotherapy-treated patients who had never bled compared with a medically treated cohort.[70–72] Two of the studies cited have been criticized because of a higher than expected incidence of hemorrhage in control patients and failure to employ the best available method of treatment in control patients who did bleed. One trial consisted predominantly of patients with nonalcoholic

cirrhosis and showed a benefit with prophylactic sclerotherapy only in high-risk (Child class B and C) patients.[71] Other trials demonstrated no survival advantage for patients who received prophylactic treatment.[73–75] The Veterans' Affairs Cooperative Trial of prophylactic sclerotherapy compared with sham sclerotherapy was halted after interim analysis showed nearly twice the mortality in patients treated with sclerotherapy.[75] A recent meta-analysis concluded that prophylactic sclerotherapy resulted in a small survival benefit for patients so treated but cautioned against widespread use of prophylactic endoscopic therapy.[76] Accurate identification of patients who are at high risk for a first variceal bleed is problematic, and prophylactic sclerotherapy does not appear to be justified at this time.

ENDOSCOPIC POLYMER INJECTION

Endoscopic injection of the tissue adhesive *N*-butyl-2-cyanoacrylate (Histoacryl) or isobutyl-2-cyanoacrylate (Bucrylate) for treatment of esophageal and gastric fundal varices has been described by several European groups.[77, 78] These two agents are tissue adhesives that harden within 20 seconds in moist conditions and more rapidly in blood. The aim of polymer injection treatment is to effect more rapid control of active bleeding than is possible with sclerotherapy. The latter agent (Bucrylate) has been removed from the market because of fears that it is carcinogenic. The former agent is not available for clinical use in the United States.

Soehendra and colleagues reported use of Histoacryl in 27 patients with actively bleeding esophageal varices and in 4 with bleeding fundal varices.[79] Early rebleeding occurred seven times in four patients, and all early rebleeding episodes were controlled with repeat injections of tissue adhesive. Survival from the index hospitalization in 40 actively bleeding patients treated with tissue adhesive or polidocanol occurred in 82.5 per cent. An additional 31 patients with fundal varices were treated electively with Histoacryl injections. One or two treatment sessions resulted in elimination of such varices with no observed complications. Ramond and associates reported 49 patients treated with Bucrylate injections.[77] Fifteen patients were actively bleeding at the index treatment session, and hemorrhage was controlled in all but one. Elective repeat injections were performed with Bucrylate at varying intervals. Rebleeding occurred in 37 per cent of patients during the first 6 months of follow-up and in 42 per cent by 1 year. Survival after 6 months of follow-up was 100 per cent for Child class A, 63 per cent for Child class B, and 13 per cent for Child class C patients; survival for the entire group at 1 year was 53 per cent.

Complications associated with tissue adhesive injection appear to be similar to those observed with conventional sclerotherapy. The Hamburg group[79] reported a 6.5 per cent incidence of esophageal stenosis and the Villejuif-Clichy group[77] reported 4 per cent. The latter group attributed three deaths (6 per cent) directly to complications of

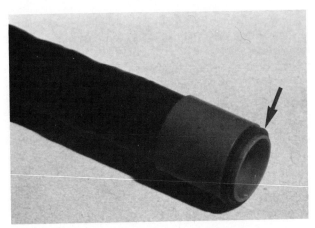

FIGURE 102–5. Endoscopic ligating device mounted on the distal end of a standard gastroscope. Note the rubber O ring (arrow) stretched over the inner cylinder.

the technique (mediastinitis) and treated three additional patients with persistent fevers successfully with antibiotics. More alarming is a brief report from Paris detailing two patients who developed strokes immediately following Bucrylate injections.[80] The neurologic injury was shown by subsequent radiologic studies to have resulted from dissemination of the tissue glue into the cerebral arterial system.

Polymer injection is effective for control of acute variceal hemorrhage from either esophageal or gastric fundal varices. Long-term treatment aimed at eradication of esophageal varices does not appear to be either significantly more promising or safer than conventional sclerotherapy.

ENDOSCOPIC VARICEAL LIGATION

Endoscopic variceal ligation of bleeding varices is performed using an endoscopic ligating device (Bard Interventional Products, Tewksbury, MA), which effects ligation of varices using small elastic O rings[81] (Figs. 102–5 to 102–7). From five to eight individual ligations are done at the initial treatment in patients with large varices. Progressively fewer ligations are required during elective retreatments as varices diminish in size and number.

In the presence of active bleeding the endoscopist approaches and directly ligates the bleeding site if identifiable. If the exact site of bleeding cannot be identified, ligation of varices commences at the gastroesophageal junction and continues as described previously until all channels in the distal esophagus are ligated at least once. Control of hemorrhage in the latter circumstance is achieved by reduction of inflow into esophageal varices.

The effects of endoscopic variceal ligation on the esophagus, stomach, and varices have been examined experimentally using the Jensen portal hypertensive canine model.[82–84] Three to 7 days following ligation of varices, slough of variceal tissue and shallow ulcerations were observed at all treatment sites. By 14 to 21 days after treatment there were minimal residual varices and no evidence of full-thickness esophageal injury. Sites of previous shallow ulcers appeared healed, and microscopy showed full-

thickness replacement of vascular structures in the submucosa with maturing scar tissue. An intense inflammatory response was present, and reepithelialization of treated sites had occurred by 21 days. Endoscopic observations in the clinical setting have paralleled those obtained from the laboratory. The shallow ulcers produced at each ligated site resulted in little risk of bleeding and, as many practitioners of sclerotherapy believe, probably represent evidence of an effective treatment. Goff and colleagues compared patients who had undergone endoscopic ligation with those treated by sclerotherapy and with untreated controls who had esophageal varices.[85] Patients treated with sclerotherapy had a greater incidence of stricture formation; however, esophageal manometric studies did not show persistent long-term differences between the three groups.

Endoscopic ligation was examined in four uncontrolled trials and is under evaluation in four prospective randomized studies comparing ligation with sclerotherapy.[86–93] The author's group studied 146 consecutive unselected patients with variceal hemorrhage who were treated with endoscopic ligation for control of acute hemorrhage and were then serially treated to achieve variceal eradication.[89] Control of active variceal hemorrhage was accomplished in 94 per cent of 33 patients who were actively bleeding at index endoscopy. Variceal obliteration was achieved in 79 per cent of the 125 patients who remained in the trial for more than 30 days with a mean of 5.5 endoscopic treatment sessions. Recurrent hemorrhage occurred in 44 per cent, and the overall survival rate in 146 patients who entered the study was 73 per cent at a mean follow-up of 15 months. A total of four treatment-related nonbleeding complications was observed.

One prospective randomized trial comparing endoscopic sclerotherapy with endoscopic ligation has been

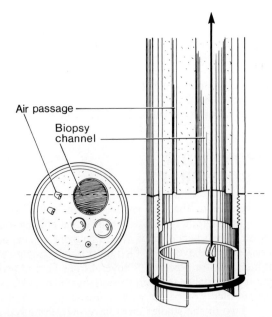

Air passage
Biopsy channel

FIGURE 102–6. Cutaway view of endoscopic ligating device showing inner and outer cylinders with trip wire attached to inner cylinder running retrograde in biopsy channel of endoscope. (From Stiegmann G, Goff J: Endoscopic esophageal varix ligation (EVL): Preliminary clinical experience. © by Am Soc for Gastrointestinal Endoscopy 34:113, 1988.)

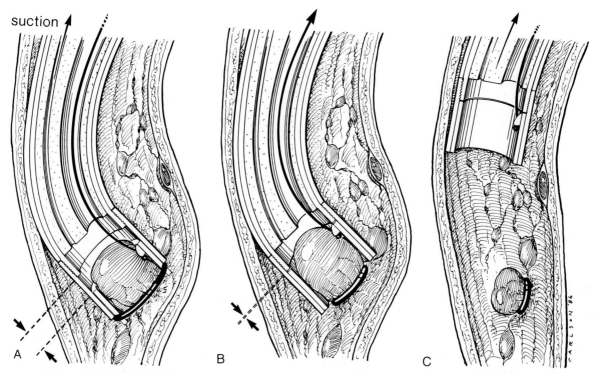

FIGURE 102–7. *A*, The endoscopist has aspirated the target inside the cylinder. An endoscopic "red out" is produced when the target fills the entire chamber. At this point the endoscopist pulls the trip wire, which moves the inner cylinder toward the endoscope *(B)*, releasing the elastic O ring securely around the base of the ensnared varix. *C*, The varix is securely ligated and the endoscope is now removed for reloading and reapplication to adjacent varices. (*A–C*, From Stiegmann G, Goff J: Endoscopic esophageal varix ligation [EVL]: Preliminary clinical experience. © by Am Soc for Gastrointestinal Endoscopy 34:113, 1988.)

completed, and three are ongoing.[87, 90, 91, 93] Data from these trials are summarized in Table 102–3. These studies support the contention that endoscopic variceal ligation is at least as effective as sclerotherapy for control of acute bleeding and prevention of recurrent hemorrhage and results in comparable or improved survival while resulting in few nonbleeding complications. The mechanical ligation technique also appears to eradicate esophageal varices with fewer

treatments than are necessary with sclerotherapy. More efficient eradication may contribute to the trend toward less recurrent variceal bleeding observed in these trials and the significant improvement in survival over sclerotherapy-treated patients seen in one trial.

ENDOSCOPIC VARICEAL LIGATION COMBINED WITH LOW-VOLUME SCLEROTHERAPY

Recurrent hemorrhage in patients treated with either sclerotherapy or ligation usually occurs before esophageal varices are eradicated. Our group postulated that combining low-volume sclerotherapy with endoscopic ligation might hasten eradication of esophageal varices. Combination treatment is performed by injecting 1 ml of sclerosant per varix intravariceally immediately cephalad to the ligation sites (Fig. 102–8). Combination therapy may result in more rapid eradication of varices because of the additive effects of mechanical stasis (ligation) and intimal damage (sclerotherapy). Use of low volumes of sclerosant may result in fewer sclerosant-related complications.

The initial experience with combination therapy consisted of 46 patients.[94] Eradication was accomplished in 76 per cent of these patients with a mean of 2.1 treatment sessions. The rebleeding rate was 30 per cent, and one death resulted from hemorrhage. Overall survival during the short follow-up period was 85 per cent. These data were recently

Table 102–3. Results From Three Ongoing and One Concluded Prospective Randomized Trials Comparing Endoscopic Ligation With Endoscopic Sclerotherapy

Study	No. Patients	Therapy	Rebled (%)	Mean No. Rx Needed to Eradicate	Survival (%)	Compl (%)
Multicenter[88]	65	ES	48	5	55	20
	64	EVL	36	4	72	2
El-Newihi[90]	19	ES	37	6*	95	68
	20	EVL	25	4*	95	25
Westaby[91]	40	ES	53	5*	NA	NA
	48	EVL	32	3*	NA	NA
Young[93]	13	ES	NA	6*	92	15
	10	EVL	NA	4*	90	0

ES, endoscopic sclerotherapy; EVL, endoscopic variceal ligation; Mean No. Rx Needed to Eradicate, mean number of treatments needed to eradicate esophageal varices; Compl, nonbleeding complications requiring active treatment.

*p <.05.

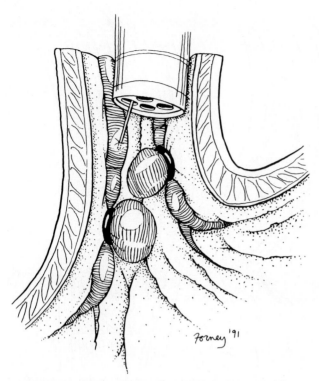

FIGURE 102–8. Combination endoscopic ligation and low-volume sclerotherapy. Individual varices are ligated at the gastroesophageal junction. Following ligation, each varix is injected with 1 ml of sclerosant at a site from 2 to 3 cm cephalad to the site of ligation. Combination therapy appears to result in more rapid eradication of varices than is possible with either endoscopic ligation or sclerotherapy alone. (From Stiegmann GV, Yamamoto M: Approaches to the endoscopic treatment of esophageal varices. World J Surg [In press].)

confirmed by a preliminary report from France, which supports the theory that more rapid eradication is possible using a combination of ligation and low-volume sclerotherapy.[95]

SUMMARY

Endoscopic treatment is accepted for control of acute bleeding and eradication of esophageal varices. Once performed with rigid endoscopes, sclerotherapy is now done using flexible endoscopes in awake patients, often as an outpatient procedure. Acute sclerotherapy does not confer a measurable survival advantage in patients with variceal bleeding, but serial treatment lowers the risk of recurrent hemorrhage and prolongs life. Primary treatment by endoscopic sclerotherapy is more effective than conventional medical management and is equal or superior to treatment with propranolol. The incidence of rebleeding, treatment-related complications, and mortality in sclerotherapy-treated patients is high, and sclerotherapy as prophylactic treatment against a first variceal bleed is not justified.

Endoscopic polymer injection is useful for control of acute bleeding, particularly from gastric fundal varices. The cyanoacrylate polymer agents are no more effective than conventional sclerotherapy for serial treatments aimed at eradicating varices and are not available for clinical use in the United States.

Endoscopic elastic band ligation eradicates varices more rapidly, causes fewer complications, and may be associated with better long-term survival than endoscopic sclerotherapy. Further trials are needed to confirm the efficacy of this new method and examine the role of endoscopic ligation in combination with low-volume sclerotherapy.

References

1. Crafoord C, Frenckner P: New surgical treatment of varicose veins of the esophagus. Acta Otolaryngol (Stockholm) 27:422, 1939.
2. Moersch HJ: Treatment of esophageal varices by injection of a sclerosing solution. JAMA 135:754, 1947.
3. Wang M, Desigan G, Dunn D: Endoscopic sclerotherapy for bleeding rectal varices: A case report. Am J Gastroenterol 80:779, 1985.
4. Ricci RL, Lee KR, Greenberger NJ: Chronic gastrointestinal bleeding from ileal varices after total proctocolectomy for ulcerative colitis correction by mesocaval shunt. Gastroenterology 78:1053, 1980.
5. Williams R, Westaby D: Endoscopic sclerotherapy for esophageal varices. Dig Dis Sci 31:108, 1986.
6. Butler H: The veins of the esophagus. Thorax 6:276, 1951.
7. Noda T: Angioarchitectural study of esophageal varices. Virchows Arch (Pathol Anat) 404:381, 1984.
8. DeCarvalho CAF: Sur l'angio-architecture veineuse de la zone de transition oesophago-gastrique et son interpretation fonctionelle. Acta Anat 64:125, 1966.
9. Spence RAJ: The venous anatomy of the lower oesophagus in normal subjects and in patients with varices: an image analysis study. Br J Surg 71:739, 1984.
10. Kitano S, Terblanche J, Kahn D, et al: Venous anatomy of the lower oesophagus in portal hypertension: Practical implications. Br J Surg 73:525, 1986.
11. Paquet KJ: Endoscopic paravariceal injection sclerotherapy of the esophagus—Indications, technique, complications, results of a period of nearly fourteen years. Gastrointest Endosc 29:310–315, 1983.
12. Sanowski RA: Venography during sclerotherapy. In Sivak MV (ed): Endoscopic Sclerotherapy of Esophageal Varices. New York, Praeger Special Studies, 1984, pp 43–47.
13. Barsoum MS, Khattar NY, Risk-Allah MA: Technical aspects of injection sclerotherapy of acute oesophageal variceal hemorrhage as seen by radiography. Br J Surg 65:588, 1978.
14. Lilly JR: Endoscopic sclerosis of esophageal varices in children. Surg Gynecol Obstet 152:513, 1981.
15. Castellana FS: Injection needles—Physical measurements and design parameters. Endoscopy Review 2:27, 1985.
16. Terblanche J, Yakoob HI, Bornman PC, et al: Acute bleeding varices—A five-year prospective evaluation of tamponade and sclerotherapy. Ann Surg 4:521, 1981.
17. Jones JG, Minty BD, Beeley JM, et al: Pulmonary epithelial permeability is immediately increased after embolization with oleic acid but not with neutral fat. Thorax 37:169, 1982.
18. Westaby D, Macdougall BRD, Melia W, et al: A prospective randomized trial of two sclerotherapy techniques for esophageal varices. Hepatology 3:681, 1983.
19. Kirkham JS, Quayle JB: Esophageal varices: Evaluation of injection sclerotherapy without general anesthesia using the flexible fiberoptic gastroscope. Ann R Coll Surg Engl 64:401, 1982.
20. Johnson AG, Simms JM, Stoddard CJ: Is there a role for injection sclerotherapy in the presence of active bleeding? In Westaby D, Macdougall BRD, Williams R (eds): Variceal Bleeding. London, Pitman, 1982, pp 159–164.
21. Westaby D, Melia WM, Macdougall BRD, et al: Injection sclerotherapy for esophageal varices: A prospective randomized trial of different treatment schedules. Gut 25:129, 1984.
22. Sarin SK, Sachdev G, Nanda R, et al: Comparison of two time schedules for endoscopic sclerotherapy: A prospective randomized controlled study. Gut 27:710, 1986.
23. Jensen DM: Evaluation of sclerosing agents in animal models. Gastrointest Endosc 29:315, 1983.

24. Blenkinsopp WK: Choice of sclerosant: An experimental study. Angiologica 7:182, 1970.
25. Perino LE, Gholson CF, Goff JS: Esophageal perforation following fiberoptic variceal sclerotherapy. J Clin Gastroint 9:286, 1987.
26. Gibbert V, Feinstat T, Burns M, et al: A comparison of the sclerosing agents sodium tetradecyl sulfate and sodium morrhuate in endoscopic injection sclerosis of esophageal varices. Gastrointest Endosc 28:147, 1982.
27. Sivak MV, Stout DJ, Skipper G: Endoscopic injection sclerosis (EIS) of esophageal varices. Gastrointest Endosc 27:52, 1981.
28. Palani CK, Abuabara S, Kraft AR, et al: Endoscopic sclerotherapy in acute variceal hemorrhage. Am J Surg 141:164, 1981.
29. Hughes RW Jr, Larson DE, Viggiano TR, et al: Endoscopic variceal sclerosis: A one-year experience. Gastrointest Endosc 28:62, 1982.
30. Gebhard RL, Ansel HJ, Silvis SE: Origin of pain during variceal sclerotherapy [Abstract]. Gastrointest Endosc 28:131, 1982.
31. Shoenut JP, Micflikier AB: Retrosternal pain subsequent to sclerotherapy. Gastrointest Endosc 32:84, 1986.
32. Sarin SK, Nanda R, Vij JC, et al: Oesophageal ulceration after sclerotherapy—A complication or an accompaniment? Endoscopy 18:44, 1986.
33. Ogle SJ, Kirk CJC, Bailey RJ, et al: Esophageal function in cirrhotic patients undergoing injection sclerotherapy for oesophageal varices. Digestion 18:178, 1978.
34. Goff JS: Personal communication.
35. Soderlund C, Thor K: Esophageal function after sclerotherapy for bleeding varices. Acta Chir Scand Suppl 524:63, 1985.
36. Reilly JJ, Schade RR, Van Thiel DS: Esophageal function after injection sclerotherapy: Pathogenesis of esophageal stricture. Am J Surg 147:85, 1984.
37. Bailey-Newton RS, Connors AF, Bacon BR: Effect of endoscopic variceal sclerotherapy on gas exchange and hemodynamics in humans. Gastroenterology 89:368, 1985.
38. Camera DS, Gruber M, Barde CJ, et al: Transient bacteremia following endoscopic injection sclerotherapy of esophageal varices. Arch Intern Med 143:1350, 1983.
39. Seidman E, Weber AM, Morin CL, et al: Spinal cord paralysis following sclerotherapy for esophageal varices. Hepatology 4:950, 1984.
40. Thatcher BS, Sivak MV, Ferguson DR, et al: Mesenteric venous thrombosis as a possible complication of endoscopic sclerotherapy: A report of two cases. Am J Gastroenterol 81:126, 1986.
41. Monroe P, Morrow CF Jr, Millen JE, et al: Acute respiratory failure after sodium morrhuate esophageal sclerotherapy. Gastroenterology 85:693, 1983.
42. Korula J, Baydur A, Sassoon C: Effects of esophageal variceal sclerotherapy (EVS) on lung function. Arch Intern Med 146:1517, 1986.
43. Bailey-Newton RS, Connors AF Jr, Bacon BR: Effect of esophageal variceal sclerotherapy (EVS) on gas exchange and hemodynamics in humans. Gastroenterol 89:363, 1985.
44. Umekita N: Experimental studies on respiratory insufficiency after endoscopic injection sclerotherapy using ethanolamine oleate. Nippon Geka Gakkai Zasshi 87:172, 1986.
45. Barsoum M, Bolous F, El-Rooby A, et al: Tamponade and injection sclerotherapy in the management of bleeding oesophageal varices. Br J Surg 69:76, 1982.
46. Larson A, Cohen H, Zweiban B, et al: Acute esophageal variceal sclerotherapy: Results of a prospective randomized controlled trial. JAMA 255:497, 1986.
47. Paquet K-J, Feussner H: Endoscopic sclerosis and esophageal balloon tamponade in acute hemorrhage from esophagogastric varices: A prospective controlled randomized trial. Hepatology 5:580, 1985.
48. The Copenhagen Esophageal Varices Study Project: Sclerotherapy after first variceal hemorrhage in cirrhosis: A randomized multicenter trial. N Engl J Med 311:1594, 1984.
49. Soderland C, Ihre T: Endoscopic sclerotherapy v. conservative management of bleeding oesophageal varices: A 5-year prospective controlled trial of emergency and long term treatment. Acta Chir Scand 151:449, 1985.
50. El-Zayadi A, el-Din SS, Kabil SM: Endoscopic sclerotherapy versus medical treatment for bleeding esophageal varices in patients with schistosomal liver disease. Gastrointest Endosc 34:314, 1988.
51. Korula J, Balart L, Radvan G, et al: A prospective, randomized, controlled trial of chronic esophageal variceal sclerotherapy. Hepatology 5:584, 1985.
52. Terblanche J, Bornman P, Kahn D, et al: Failure of repeated injection

53. sclerotherapy to improve long-term survival after oesophageal variceal bleeding: A five-year prospective controlled clinical trial. Lancet 2:1328, 1983.
53. Westaby D, Macdougall B, Williams R: Improved survival following injection sclerotherapy for esophageal varices: Final analysis of a controlled trial. Hepatology 5:827, 1985.
54. Infante-Rivard C, Esnaola S, Villeneuve JP: Role of endoscopic variceal sclerotherapy in the long-term management of variceal bleeding: A meta-analysis. Gastroenterology 96:1087, 1989.
55. Lebrec D, Corbic M, Nouel O, et al: Propranolol—A medical treatment for portal hypertension? Lancet 2:180, 1980.
56. Frohlich ED, Tarazi RC, Dustan HP, Page IH: The paradox of beta-adrenergic blockade in hypertension. Circulation 37:417, 1968.
57. Alexandrino PT, Martins Alves M, Correia JP: Propranolol or endoscopic sclerotherapy in the prevention of recurrent variceal bleeding. J Hepatol 7:175, 1988.
58. Flieg FE, Stange EF, Hunecke R, et al: Prevention of recurrent bleeding in cirrhotics with recent variceal hemorrhage: Prospective, randomized comparison of propranolol and sclerotherapy. Hepatology 7:355, 1987.
59. Westaby D, Polson RJ, Gimson AES, et al: A controlled trial of oral propranolol compared with injection sclerotherapy for the long-term management of variceal bleeding. Hepatology 11:353, 1990.
60. Westaby D, Melia W, Hegarty J, et al: Use of propranolol to reduce the rebleeding rate during injection sclerotherapy prior to variceal obliteration. Hepatology 6:673, 1986.
61. Jensen LS, Krarup N: Propranolol in prevention of rebleeding from oesophageal varices during the course of endoscopic sclerotherapy. Scand J Gastroenterol 24:339, 1989.
62. Vickers C, Rhodes J, Hillenbrand P, et al: Prospective controlled trial of propranolol and sclerotherapy for prevention of rebleeding from oesophageal varices. Gut 28:A1359, 1987.
63. Cello J, Grendell J, Crass R, et al: Endoscopic sclerotherapy versus portacaval shunt in patients with severe cirrhosis and acute variceal hemorrhage: Long-term follow-up. N Engl J Med 316:11, 1987.
64. Rikkers LF, Volentine GD, Buchi KN, et al: Shunt surgery versus endoscopic sclerotherapy for long-term treatment of variceal bleeding: Early results of a randomized trial. Ann Surg 206:261, 1987.
65. Teres J, Bordas JM, Bravo D, et al: Sclerotherapy vs. distal splenorenal shunt in the elective treatment of variceal hemorrhage: A randomized controlled trial. Hepatology 7:430, 1987.
66. Spina GP, Santambrogio R, Opocher E, et al: Distal splenorenal shunt versus endoscopic sclerotherapy in the prevention of variceal rebleeding. Ann Surg 211:178, 1990.
67. Planas R, Boix J, Broggi M, et al: Portacaval shunt versus endoscopic sclerotherapy in the elective treatment of variceal hemorrhage. Gastroenterology 100:1078, 1991.
68. Warren WD, Henderson JM, Millikan WJ, et al: Distal splenorenal shunt versus endoscopic sclerotherapy for long-term management of variceal bleeding: Preliminary report of a prospective, randomized trial. Ann Surg 203:454, 1986.
69. McCormick P, Burroughs A: Prophylaxis for variceal hemorrhage. Gastrointest Endosc Clin North Am 2:167, 1992.
70. Paquet K-J: Prophylactic endoscopic sclerosing treatment of the esophageal wall in varices—A prospective controlled trial. Endoscopy 14:4, 1982.
71. Piai G, Cipolletta L, Claar M, et al: Prophylactic sclerotherapy of high risk esophageal varices: Results of a multicentric prospective controlled trial. Hepatology 8:1495, 1988.
72. Witzel L, Wolbergs E, Merki H: Prophylactic endoscopic sclerotherapy of oesophageal varices: A prospective controlled study. Lancet 1:773, 1985.
73. De Franchis R, Primignani M, Arcidiacono P, et al: Prophylactic sclerotherapy in high-risk cirrhotics selected by endoscopic criteria. Gastroenterology 101:1087, 1991.
74. Santangelo WC, Dueno MI, Estes BL, et al: Prophylactic sclerotherapy of large esophageal varices. N Engl J Med 318:814, 1988.
75. The Veterans Affairs Cooperative Variceal Sclerotherapy Group: Prophylactic sclerotherapy for esophageal varices in men with alcoholic liver disease: A randomized, single-blind, multicenter trial. N Engl J Med 324:1779, 1991.
76. Ruiswyk JV, Byrd JC: Efficacy of prophylactic sclerotherapy for prevention of first variceal hemorrhage. Gastroenterology 102:587, 1992.
77. Ramond MJ, Valla D, Gotlib JP, et al: Obturation endoscopique des

varices oeso-gastriques par le Bucrylate. Gastroenterol Clin Biol 10:575, 1986.

78. Soehendra N, Nam VC, Grimm H, et al: Endoscopic obliteration of large esophagogastric varices with bucrylate. Endoscopy 18:25, 1986.

79. Soehendra N, Grimm H, Nam VC, et al: N-butyl-2-cyanoacrylate: A supplement to endoscopic sclerotherapy. Endoscopy 19:221, 1987.

80. See A, Florent C, Lamy P, et al: Accidents vasculaires cerebraux apres obturation endoscopique des varices oesophagiennes par l'iso-butyl-2-cyanoacrylate chez deux malades. Gastroenterol Clin Biol 10:604, 1986.

81. Stiegmann GV, Goff JS, Sun JH, et al: Technique and early clinical results of endoscopic variceal ligation (EVL). Surg Endosc 3:73, 1989.

82. Jensen DM, Machicado GA, Tapia JL: A reproducible canine model of esophageal varices. Gastroenterology 84:573, 1983.

83. Stiegmann GV, Sun JH, Hammond WS: Results of experimental endoscopic esophageal varix ligation. Am Surg 54:105, 1988.

84. Weisz N, Jensen DM, Hirabayashi K, et al: Efficacy and safety of elective endoscopic rubber band ligation versus sclerotherapy of canine esophageal or gastric varices. Gastroenterology 98:A147, 1990.

85. Goff JS, Reveille RM, Stiegmann GV: Endoscopic sclerotherapy versus endoscopic variceal ligation: Esophageal symptoms, complications, and motility. Am J Gastroenterol 83:1240, 1988.

86. Hall RJ, Lilly JR, Stiegmann GV: Endoscopic esophageal varix ligation: Technique and preliminary results in children. J Pediatr Surg 23:1222, 1988.

87. Stiegmann G, Goff J, Michaletz-Onody P, et al: Endoscopic sclerotherapy as compared with endoscopic ligation for bleeding esophageal varices. N Engl J Med 326:1527, 1992.

88. Saeed Z, Michaletz P, Winchester C, et al: Endoscopic variceal ligation in patients who have failed sclerotherapy. Gastrointest Endosc 36:572, 1990.

89. Goff JS: Endoscopic variceal ligation. Can J Gastroenterol 4:639, 1990.

90. El-Newihi H, Migicovsky B, Laine L: A prospective randomized comparison of sclerotherapy and ligation for the treatment of bleeding esophageal varices [Abstract]. Gastroenterology 100:A59, 1991.

91. Westaby D: Prevention of recurrent variceal bleeding: Endoscopic techniques. Gastrointest Endosc Clin North Am 2:121, 1992.

92. Yamamoto M, Suzuki H, Aoki T, et al: Endoscopic variceal ligation (EVL). Digest Endosc 2:269, 1990.

93. Young M, Sanowski R, Raschke R: Comparison and characterization of ulcerations induced by endoscopic ligation of esophageal varices versus endoscopic sclerotherapy [Abstract]. Gastrointest Endosc 38:285, 1992.

94. Reveille RM, Goff JS, Stiegmann GV, et al: Combination endoscopic variceal ligation (EVL) and low volume sclerotherapy (ES) for bleeding esophageal varices: A faster route to variceal eradication? [Abstract]. Gastrointest Endosc 37:243, 1991.

95. Koutsomanis D: Endoscopic variceal ligation combined with low volume sclerotherapy: A controlled study [Abstract]. Gastroenterology 102:A835, 1992.

103

Percutaneous Interventions in Portal Hypertension

Ernest J. Ring, M.D., and Ziv J. Haskal, M.D.

• • •

Since the late 1960s, a variety of fluoroscopically guided percutaneous interventions have been developed to aid in the management of patients with complications of portal hypertension. Some of these methods cause reduction in overall portal pressure; others selectively obstruct flow only to bleeding varices. Access for these therapeutic procedures has generally been accomplished by direct transhepatic portal vein catheterization or through preexisting surgical portosystemic shunts. More recently, the transjugular approach has been increasingly used as a way of entering the portal venous system through the hepatic veins. This chapter reviews the status of these procedures and discusses their current role in patient management.

TRANSHEPATIC EMBOLIZATION OF ESOPHAGEAL VARICES

In 1974, Lunderquist and Vang described a percutaneous transhepatic technique for placing catheters in the portal vein.[1] Using this method, the portal tributaries could be selectively catheterized and variceal hemorrhage treated by embolizing the bleeding varices (Fig. 103–1). Subsequent investigators found this therapy effective at controlling acute variceal bleeding, but rates of both recurrent bleeding and portal thrombosis were so high that the method had very limited clinical application.[2, 3] For example, l'Hermine and colleagues performed transhepatic variceal embolization on 400 consecutive patients and were able initially to control bleeding in 83 per cent of cases. However, bleeding recurred in 55 per cent of their patients by 6 months and in 66 per cent by 1 year.[4] In addition, portal vein thrombosis was present in 16 per cent of the patients who underwent repeat angiography. Several randomized studies have conclusively demonstrated a much greater patient survival and a lower incidence of rebleeding when varices are obliterated by endoscopic therapy; accordingly, the use of transhepatic variceal embolization has been largely abandoned as a treatment for variceal bleeding.[5, 6]

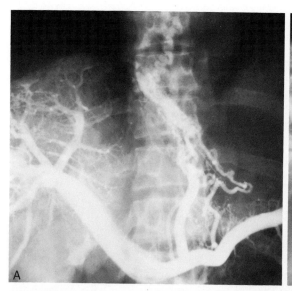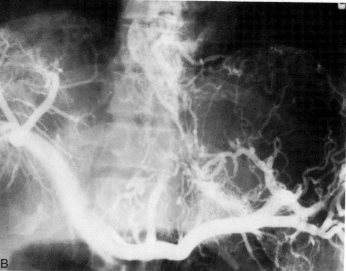

FIGURE 103-1. Recurrent variceal bleeding through collaterals following transhepatic embolization. *A,* A splenic venogram performed percutaneously via a transhepatic approach demonstrates two large veins supplying the esophageal varices. *B,* Both of the gastric veins supplying the varices were selectively catheterized and embolized. This resulted in immediate cessation of bleeding. However, 3 days later the bleeding recurred, and the portal vein was again catheterized. A repeat splenic venogram shows persistent occlusion of the gastric veins but filling of the esophageal varices through multiple short gastric collaterals.

The high incidence of portal thrombosis due to transhepatic variceal embolization is interesting, especially compared with the much lower risk of this complication after endoscopic sclerotherapy or banding of varices. Most likely, this difference is attributable to the more global nature of the venous occlusion that is produced when the occluding agent is introduced into the main coronary vein. The injected material flows into all the downstream portal-azygos venous collaterals, not just the veins associated with the submucosal gastric and esophageal varices; extensive venous obliteration results. Large mediastinal veins that are outside the esophagus and never cause bleeding are also blocked. These veins contribute so much to the outflow of the portal venous system that when they are occluded, stagnant portal vein flow results in thrombosis.

Although clearly not useful on a routine basis, transhepatic variceal embolization may still occasionally have a role in the management of specific clinical problems. Most often it is used after distal splenorenal shunt to treat the late development of encephalopathy or recurrent variceal bleeding (Fig. 103-2). With this type of shunt these problems develop when small or incompletely ligated gastric veins enlarge to become major collaterals between the high-pressure portal vein and the low-pressure splenic vein. Transhepatic catheterization and portal venography can easily identify the portal vein–splenic vein connections, and selective catheterization and embolization can be used as an alternative to reoperation to occlude them.

TRANS-SHUNT INTERVENTIONS

After portosystemic shunt surgery, it is usually not difficult to advance an angiographic catheter from the inferior vena cava across the shunt into the portal venous system to perform a variety of therapeutic interventions.

Embolization of Varices. Once a catheter has been manipulated through a shunt, it can be used to occlude flow in any persistent varices. This technique is most commonly used in patients who have undergone small, partially decompressive shunts (Fig. 103-3). Surgeons who advocate the use of small-diameter shunts to reduce the incidence of post-shunt encephalopathy recommend routine postoperative catheterization and employ transcatheter embolization if any residual varices are demonstrated.[7, 8] There is much less likelihood of complications with trans-shunt embolization than with transhepatic embolization because even small-caliber shunts provide enough outflow to avoid the development of portal vein thrombosis. Moreover, occluding competing collateral veins after a small-caliber shunt may increase the residual mesenteric venous pressure and improve portal perfusion of the liver, which might further reduce the incidence of postoperative encephalopathy.

Dilatation of Stenotic Shunts. Anastomotic stenoses are very uncommon following large-caliber portosystemic shunts. However, small-diameter shunts, particularly mesocaval shunts constructed with prosthetic grafts, occasionally develop a significant narrowing at one of the venous anastomoses. Several reports have described the use of balloon angioplasty to enlarge narrow shunt anastomoses; unfortunately, however, recurrent stenoses are common, and repeated dilatations are frequently necessary to maintain shunt patency.[9-11] Alternatively, expandible metallic stents are now available, and although experience with these devices in shunt stenoses is still too small to evaluate, the improved patency seen in other vessels suggests the possi-

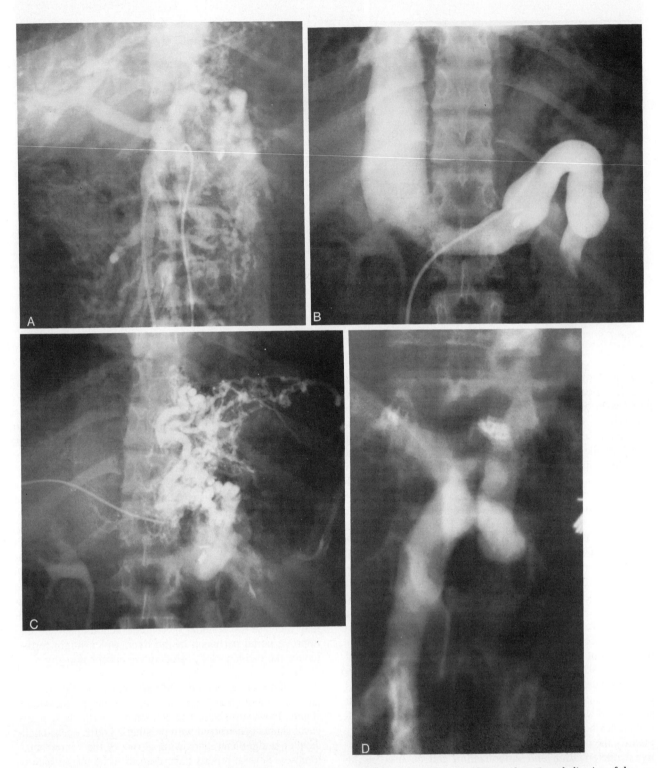

FIGURE 103–2.   Recurrent variceal bleeding following distal splenorenal shunt surgery treated by transhepatic embolization of the portal collaterals. *A*, Several years after distal splenorenal shunt surgery this patient presented with acute variceal hemorrhage. Arterial portography demonstrates large gastric varices filling from the portal vein. *B*, The shunt was catheterized through the renal vein, and a splenic venogram showed the shunt to be widely patent. *C*, The portal vein was entered transhepatically, and the gastric veins were selectively catheterized. Collaterals can be seen filling the renal vein. *D*, The collateral veins were occluded using stainless steel coil emboli, and the portal venogram was repeated. All of the connections from the high-pressure portal side of the shunt have been occluded.

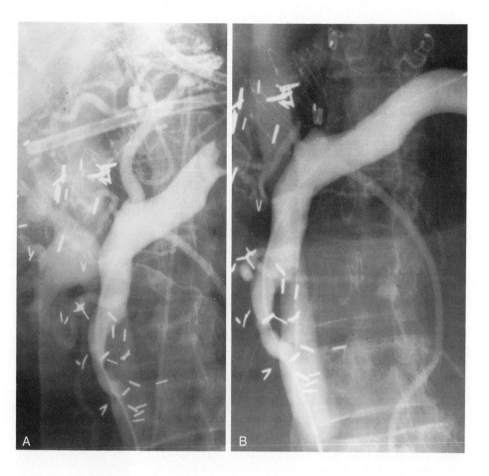

FIGURE 103–3. Transshunt catheterization and embolization for continued bleeding following a small-caliber mesocaval shunt. *A,* A catheter was advanced from the inferior vena cava through the shunt into the splenic vein. A splenic venogram demonstrates filling of the coronary vein. The mesocaval shunt is patent, but the channel is quite narrow. *B,* Following selective catheterization of the coronary vein and occlusion with ethanol and stainless steel coils, the splenic venogram was repeated. The varices no longer fill and there is improved flow through the shunt as evidenced by the increased caval opacification.

bility of a better long-term outcome than has been reported for balloon angioplasty alone.

Recanalization of Occluded Shunts. Percutaneous techniques can also be used to reopen occluded shunts but are less likely to be successful because of the added difficulty encountered in trying to advance a catheter through a shunt that is completely obstructed. Occluded portacaval shunts are particularly hard to catheterize because there is usually nothing visible angiographically to identify the site of the anastomosis. On the other hand, catheters can usually be advanced through occluded mesocaval or splenorenal shunts. The success of shunt catheterization is much greater when the procedure is attempted soon after the occlusion and the clot is still soft enough to permit passage of a guidewire readily.

Once a catheter has been advanced across an occluded shunt, patency can be reestablished in several ways. Cope reported successful use of urokinase to restore flow through occluded mesocaval shunts.[11] To avoid the risk of fibrinolytic drugs in patients at risk for bleeding, the authors have used balloon catheters to fragment and dislodge the clot from the shunt. The clot is either pushed by the balloon into a portal vein branch or an outflow varix such as the coronary vein, or it is pulled into the inferior vena cava. The resulting pulmonary embolization is not without risk, but the authors have used this approach for emergency therapy in several patients and have found that iatrogenic pulmonary emboli are surprisingly well tolerated. None of the patients developed pulmonary complications or any

clinical evidence that pulmonary embolization had occurred.

Occluding Patent Shunts. Although the incidence of encephalopathy following conventional portacaval shunt surgery varies considerably in different series, it may be as high as 60 per cent. In most cases, the symptoms are mild or episodic and are reasonably well controlled with medical therapy. Occasionally, however, the mental disturbance is so disabling that the patient is willing to forego the shunt and risk further variceal bleeding. The authors have used stainless steel coils to occlude flow through mesocaval shunts in two patients, and in both cases these were successful in blocking shunt flow.

TRANSJUGULAR INTRAHEPATIC PORTASYSTEMIC SHUNTS

In 1969, Rosch and colleagues reported a new method of decompressing the portal venous system through a percutaneously created shunt between the portal and hepatic veins.[12] In a series of dog experiments they showed the feasibility of passing a needle from the jugular vein into a hepatic vein and then advancing the needle through the liver parenchyma into a portal vein branch. They then tried to establish a functional shunt between the veins using a series of coaxial catheters. A segment of Teflon-coated catheter was then left across the parenchymal segment to try to maintain flow. No serious complications occurred and good portasystemic decompression was demonstrated in all of the dogs treated. They then began experimenting with a variety of cutting, drilling, and cryoprobe techniques to try to develop a shunt large enough for clinical use. Although they were able to create tracts as large as 10 mm in diameter, none of their experimental shunts remained patent for more than 1 or 2 weeks.

When modern balloon angioplasty catheters became available in the late 1970s, Burgener and Gutierrez used them to establish intra-hepatic shunts in dogs with portal hypertension.[13] They inflated 12- and 15-mm balloons across the parenchymal tract and achieved normalization of portal pressure in all the animals. All of their initial shunts rapidly occluded but when they repeated the dilatations at weekly intervals (up to five times), some remained patent for up to a year. In 1982, Colapinto and associates reported the first clinical use of transjugular intrahepatic portasystemic shunts (TIPS).[14] They kept a 9-mm balloon inflated across the parenchymal tract for 12 hours and were able to lower portal pressure and control variceal bleeding in 15 patients. Unfortunately, the majority of their patients rebled and died within a month, and only two patients survived for more than a year without rebleeding.

In 1985, Palmaz and colleagues began investigating the use of expandable metallic stents for TIPS and found that in dogs with artificially created portal hypertension, shunts remained patent through 48 weeks when a stent was placed in the parenchymal tract.[15] At necropsy, they found a thin smooth layer of neointima covering the stent's luminal surface. In 1987, Rosch and coworkers reported similar experimental results using Gianturco stents to perform TIPS in swine.[16] In 1990, Richter and colleagues used Palmaz stents to perform TIPS in three patients who had repeatedly failed to respond to endoscopic sclerotherapy.[17] In a follow-up article, Richter and colleagues expanded the series to include nine patients.[18] In each case, rapid decompression of portal hypertension was achieved, and bleeding was controlled. More recently, Zemel and associates reported clinical and technical success using TIPS to treat variceal bleeding in eight patients and documented continued shunt patency for up to 9 months.[19]

In 1992, the authors described their initial results with TIPS in 13 patients who developed intractable variceal bleeding while awaiting liver transplantation.[20] All of the patients had continued significant gastric or esophageal variceal bleeding despite multiple attempts at endoscopic sclerotherapy. The authors found that TIPS could be safely performed in these high-risk patients and that it effectively lowered portal pressure and controlled bleeding until the transplant could be performed. Histologic examination of the explant liver specimens revealed a neointimal lining along the luminal surface of the TIPS within 3 weeks after stent placement. The authors have continued to evaluate the role of TIPS as a bridge to transplantation but have expanded the indications to include patients who are not transplant candidates.[21] The next section describes the methods, indications, and results in over 200 of these TIPS procedures.

TIPS Method. Prior to performing TIPS, the patients are stabilized as much as possible with blood transfusions, intravenous vasopressin, and, if necessary, esophageal balloon tamponade. No special effort is made to correct coagulation factors because procedure-related bleeding is uncommon. All patients undergo complete upper endoscopy prior to the procedure to confirm the diagnosis of variceal bleeding; duplex ultrasound is performed to evaluate portal vein patency. Mesenteric angiography is performed only when ultrasound fails to demonstrate portal flow. Immediately prior to the procedure, a broad-spectrum antibiotic is administered, and intravenous sedation and analgesics are given as appropriate. The right internal jugular vein is then percutaneously punctured, and a 40-cm long 9-Fr angiographic sheath is advanced into the inferior vena cava. A curved angiographic catheter is manipulated under fluoroscopic guidance into a hepatic vein with a large enough diameter to form an adequate shunt (Fig. 103–4). The right hepatic vein is generally preferred, but TIPS can also be created from the middle and left hepatic veins.

Once the appropriate hepatic vein has been catheterized, a transjugular needle is advanced through the sheath over a rigid guidewire. The needle used by the authors for this purpose is the Colapinto biopsy needle. It is a two-part needle, composed of a curved inner 16-gauge metal needle and an outer 9-Fr catheter. Although there are other needles available for TIPS, the Colapinto is particularly well suited to this procedure. Its reversed bevel facilitates passage through the catheter around the curve at the hepatic vein–inferior vena cava junction, and its relatively large diameter

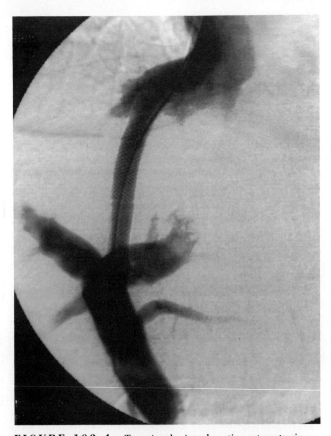

FIGURE 103–4. Transjugular intrahepatic portasystemic shunt (TIPS). A transjugular approach was used to catheterize the right hepatic vein and to pass a needle into the left portal vein. The tract was dilated and stented. A final portal venogram shows blood flow through the shunt.

allows a controlled puncture to be made even through hard, cirrhotic liver parenchyma.

The Colapinto needle is rotated anteromedially and advanced caudally out of the right hepatic vein 4 to 5 cm into the liver parenchyma. A syringe is attached, and the needle is aspirated as it is slowly withdrawn. When blood returns, contrast medium is injected to determine which vascular structure has been entered. When a portal vein branch is identified, a guidewire is passed through the needle and manipulated down the main portal vein into the splenic or mesenteric vein. The inner needle is removed, and a 5-Fr catheter is advanced into the portal venous system.

Portal venography is performed to evaluate the anatomy and determine the direction of portal flow; an initial portal pressure is recorded (Fig. 103–4). The 5-Fr catheter is then exchanged for an 8-mm angioplasty balloon catheter, which is inflated in the tract between the hepatic and portal veins. The tract is then stented with a metallic endoprosthesis and expanded to 8 mm using the angioplasty balloon. The portal venogram is repeated, and the pressure is remeasured. If portal pressure remains elevated and there is continued rapid filling of varices, the stent is further distended to its maximum 10-mm diameter (Fig. 103–5). The venogram and pressures are then repeated. If varices are still filling briskly, they are selectively catheterized and embolized. In about 10 per cent of the patients a 10-mm diameter shunt does not produce sufficient reduction in the portosystemic gradient to prevent recurrent bleeding (more than a 15-mmHg residual gradient). In these cases, the

authors have been able to further reduce portal pressure by performing a second parallel TIPS from a different hepatic vein to a portal vein branch in the opposite lobe of the liver.

At the completion of the shunt, the jugular vein catheter is usually exchanged for a shorter 8.5-Fr sheath through which fluid and blood can be administered when necessary. All patients are then observed at least overnight in an intensive care unit. Prior to discharge from the hospital a baseline duplex ultrasound examination is performed to evaluate shunt flow, and this is repeated at regular 3-month follow-up visits. As part of our proctocol, shunt venograms are performed at 1 year or whenever ultrasound examinations suggest a reduction in shunt flow.

The most difficult step in the performance of a TIPS is the portal vein puncture. To facilitate the portal entry a variety of guidance techniques have been advocated. Richter and colleagues initially placed a transhepatic catheter in the portal vein and then passed a metal stone basket through it to serve as a target.[17, 18] This proved to be not only unnecessary and time consuming (procedure times were more than 8 hours) but also massive bleeding from the transhepatic catheter entry site caused the death of one of their first patients. Others have used intraprocedural ultrasound to guide the puncture or to place a metallic coil adjacent to the portal branch to aid fluoroscopically guided punctures. The authors currently do not believe that any of these methods are sufficiently helpful to warrant their routine use and have simply directed their punctures toward an area in the liver where they expect to find the portal branches. Using this approach, they have successfully per-

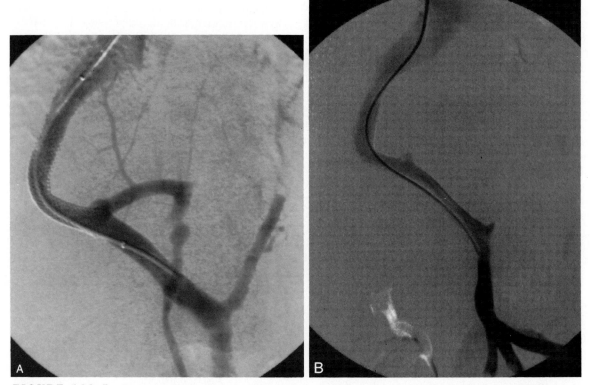

FIGURE 103–5. Increasing the diameter of a TIPS to eliminate variceal filling. *A,* Portal venography after an 8-mm TIPS shows persistent filling of the umbilical and coronary veins. *B,* The TIPS was further distended with a 10-mm balloon, and the venogram was repeated. All of the portal flow is now diverted through the TIPS.

Table 103–1. Patients Undergoing TIPS: Clinical Features

Patients	100
Age	50 (5–84)
Sex	64 males, 36 females
Prior shunt	31
Childs-Pugh classification	10 A, 35 B, 55 C
Encephalopathy	31
Ascites	78

TIPS, Transjugular intrahepatic portasystemic shunt.

Table 103–3. Indications for TIPS

Active bleeding	32
Sclerotherapy failure	(32)
Vasopressin	(27)
Balloon tamponade	(7)
Average transfusion	10.7 units
Recurrent bleeding	63
Average number of prior bleeds	3.6
Ascites	4
Hepatorenal syndrome	1

TIPS, Transjugular intrahepatic portasystemic shunt.

formed TIPS in every patient who has a patent portal vein, and the typical procedure time is about 1 hour. Although several parenchymal passes are usually required before the portal vein is entered, the low pressure in the hepatic vein at the puncture site seems to make this route much safer than other types of transhepatic procedures.

WallStents were used to form the shunts in all of the authors' cases. They prefer this stent because it is directly attached to its delivery catheter and does not require preliminary passage of a large introducer sheath. The delivery catheter is also relatively small (7 Fr) and quite flexible so that it can be introduced from almost any point of entry into the portal venous system. Once expanded, the Wall-Stent maintains a cylindric lumen even around sharp bends and follows the venous anatomy from a small peripheral portal vein branch into a more central vein that has a large enough diameter to form an adequate shunt.

Indications for TIPS. As previously mentioned, the authors' use of TIPS was initially limited to liver transplant candidates with variceal bleeding that could not be controlled by endoscopic sclerotherapy. The authors continue to use the procedure in this situation, and thus far, 21 of the patients in their series have gone on to have a liver transplant between 4 and 166 days after the procedure was performed. TIPS is particularly attractive in these patients because it lowers portal pressure and allows time for completion of the pretransplant evaluation. Relief of portal hypertension facilitates performance of the actual liver transplant. The intrahepatic location of the shunt does not complicate the transplant operation nor is it usually even encountered during removal of the liver.

Because TIPS is such a new procedure most of the data describe the technical success and the acute morbidity and mortality. These results in the authors' first 100 patients are included in Tables 103–1 to 103–4. Clearly, the 87 per cent 30-day survival and low complication rate in these high-risk patients makes TIPS an attractive alternative in a wide variety of settings. However, to determine the role of

TIPS in patients who are not transplant candidates, much more information is necessary about the shunt's long-term patency. The authors used TIPS primarily in patients considered sclerotherapy failures and have just begun a randomized study comparing TIPS with chronic sclerotherapy for long-term management of patients with bleeding. Other studies are being performed to compare TIPS with conventional surgical shunts.

Less frequent indications for TIPS may include intractable ascites, hepatorenal syndrome, and hypersplenism. The authors have performed TIPS in patients with these complications of portal hypertension who were also bleeding and noted improvement equivalent to that seen with other types of side-to-side portosystemic shunts. The authors have also used TIPS for preoperative reduction of portal hypertension in two patients with failing liver transplants to facilitate the retransplant operation.

Contraindications to TIPS. Initial experience with TIPS suggests that it is versatile, since it can be performed in almost any situation in which there is symptomatic portal hypertension requiring decompression. Cystic liver disease appears to be the only absolute contraindication to attempting TIPS. There are, however, several relative contraindications that make TIPS more difficult or more hazardous, although they do not preclude the procedure. For example, the authors have attempted to perform TIPS in 10 patients with complete occlusion of the portal vein; in seven cases they were able to establish successful shunts.[22] These included two patients with cavernous transformation of the portal vein (Fig. 103–6) and five patients with obstructing thrombus in the portal vein. The authors have also performed TIPS on two patients with Budd-Chiari syndrome who had complete obliteration of the intrahepatic hepatic veins.[23] In these cases the shunt was formed by connecting the right portal vein to a short stump of right hepatic vein near the inferior vena cava junction. TIPS has been success-

Table 103–2. Etiology of Portal Hypertension

Cirrhosis	97
Laennec's	(56)
Postnecrotic	(26)
Cryptogenic	(15)
Portal vein occlusion	10
Budd-Chiari syndrome	1
Sarcoidosis	1
Mesothelioma	1

Table 103–4. Technical Results of TIPS

Successful placement	96/100
Portal pressure reduction	11 mmHg
Final portosystemic gradient	10.7 mmHg
Shunt sizes:	22
8 mm	64
10 mm	8
8 mm and 10 mm	2
10 mm and 10 mm	

TIPS, Transjugular intrahepatic portasystemic shunt.

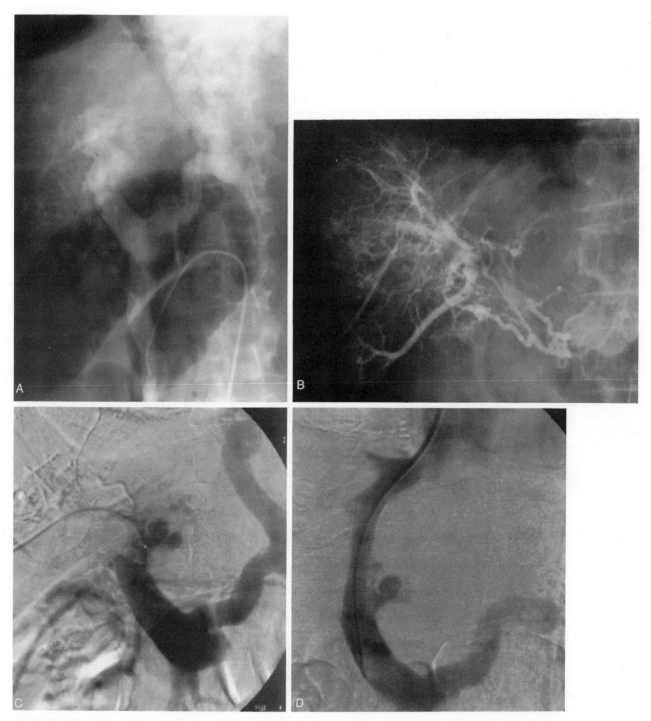

FIGURE 103–6.   TIPS for portal vein occlusion. *A*, A superior mesenteric arteriogram shows typical changes of cavernous transformation of the portal vein. *B*, A peripheral intrahepatic portal branch was catheterized transhepatically. *C*, The catheter was manipulated through the cavernous segment into the main portal vein. *D*, The tract was dilated with a balloon catheter, and the balloon was used to guide the puncture for TIPS. Following placement of the shunt, the portal venous system is decompressed, and the varices are no longer filling.

fully performed on patients with dilated bile ducts and intrahepatic tumor. Patients have also successfully undergone TIPS despite occlusion of the right internal jugular veins from a prior Leveen shunt, using either the right external jugular or the left internal jugular vein.

Unique Anatomic and Hemodynamic Considerations. Although TIPS functions hemodynamically like a side-to-side shunt, it has some unique features that may offer advantages over conventional surgical shunts. First, unlike surgical side-to-side shunts, in which the flow is generally perpendicular to the anastomosed veins, TIPS is an *in-line* shunt and flow occurs in the same direction as the main portal vein. Although the significance of this difference is unclear, it may allow improved patency compared to H-type mesocaval shunts, for example, which have manifested such a high rate of occlusion.

TIPS is also the only portosystemic shunt that flows into the suprahepatic inferior vena cava. This may be clinically important in patients who have enlargement of the caudate lobe to such an extent that there is caval compression and elevated pressure in the inferior vena cava. Although this problem appears to affect the function of surgical shunts only rarely, the authors encountered two patients in their series who had previously undergone surgical shunts that were ineffective because of elevated caval pressures. The suprahepatic venous connection also may prove important in hypercoagulable patients with Budd-Chiari syndrome who have associated caval thrombosis. In these cases, TIPS could be used as an alternative to a mesoatrial shunt.

Finally, the TIPS technique offers a unique advantage over surgical shunts because an optimal shunt size can be tailored to the hemodynamics of the individual patients. This is possible because the procedure is performed under angiographic guidance so that changes in portal pressure, flow dynamics, and variceal filling can be monitored during the procedure. Based on these changes, the diameter of the metallic stent used to support the tract can be progressively enlarged to increase the size of the shunt. Extensive surgical literature has suggested that this may be a reasonable approach because small, partially decompressive shunts appear to be just as effective as larger shunts at controlling variceal bleeding but have a much lower incidence of postshunt encephalopathy. Sarfeh and colleagues found encephalopathy rates of 9 per cent, 19 per cent, and 39 per cent in three groups of patients receiving shunts of 8-, 10-, and 12-mm or greater in diameter.[24] Johansen similarly found a 6 per cent incidence of rebleeding in patients who received small-stoma (10 to 12 mm) side-to-side portacaval shunts.[25]

By observing the pattern of flow during the TIPS procedure, the shunt size can be increased until variceal opacification begins to diminish. The veins leading to the varices can then be selectively catheterized and embolized. Using this approach, the authors created 8-mm shunts in 26 per cent of their patients and shunts of 10 mm in 64 per cent.[21] In the other 10 per cent of patients the portal pressure remained very elevated after a 10-mm shunt (mean, 19 mmHg), and the varices continued to fill briskly. Since the maximum diameter of the currently available Wallstent is only 10 mm, in order to increase the volume of shunt flow in these patients a second parallel TIPS was created from

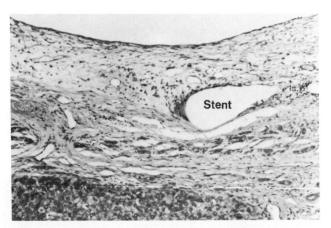

FIGURE 103–7. Histologic appearance of TIPS lining in an explant specimen 3 weeks after implantation. The stent wires have been incorporated in a maturing neointima. A one-cell thick endothelial lining has already developed.

another hepatic vein to the opposite main portal vein branch.[26] Even when a larger stent becomes available, the authors intend to continue using two small shunts instead of a single large one because dual shunts offer the potential for partial reversibility; if encephalopathy does develop, one of the shunts can be occluded with coils or balloon catheters.

It is too soon to determine the nature of the eventual impact of TIPS on the management of patients with portal hypertension. The procedure is clearly versatile and can be performed safely in most clinical settings. Procedure-related morbidity and mortality appear to be much lower than those seen with conventional surgical shunts, but the lack of evidence of durability of TIPS using present methods clearly limits its use. All centers reporting experience with the procedure have indicated that significant stenosis and occlusions develop in at least one third of their patients within 1 year.[27–29] TIPS stenoses occur at points where the layer of neointima proliferates excessively (Fig. 103–7).[30] Stenoses occur either within the parenchymal segment of the shunt or in the hepatic vein cephalad to the stent. Although these lesions are easily treated by balloon dilatation, allowing secondary or primary assisted patency to be achieved in most cases, the need for serial ultrasonographic surveillance and repeated intervention to maintain patency is clearly present. At present the authors and others limit the use of this procedure mainly to patients who are expected to undergo hepatic transplantation. However, it is likely that, as better technical methods, such as covered stents, are developed and the cause of neointimal stenosis is more clearly understood, this limitation will be overcome and TIPS will become a more durable therapy applicable to a wide variety of patients with portal hypertension.

References

1. Lunderquist A, Vang J: Transhepatic catheterization and obliteration of the coronary vein in patients with portal hypertension and esophageal varices. N Engl J Med 291:646, 1974.
2. Johnson, WC, Widrich WC, Ansell JE, et al: Control of bleeding varices by vasopressin: a prospective randomized study. Ann Surg 186:369, 1977.

3. Viamonte M, Pereiras R, Russell E, et al: Transhepatic obliteration of gastroesophageal varices: Results in acute and nonacute bleeders. AJR 129:237, 1977.

4. l'Hermine C, Chastanet P, Delemazure O, et al: Percutaneous transhepatic embolization of gastroesophageal varices: Results in 400 patients. AJR 152:755, 1989.

5. Funaro AH, Ring EJ, Freiman DB, et al: Transhepatic obliteration of esophageal varices using the stainless steel coil. AJR 133:1123, 1979.

6. Terabayashi K, Ohnishi K, Tsunoda T, et al: Prospective controlled trial of elective endoscopic sclerotherapy with percutaneous transhepatic obliteration of esophageal varices in patients with cirrhosis. Gastroenterology 93:1205, 1987.

7. Coldwell DM, Moore ADA, Ben-Menachem Y, Johansen KH: Bleeding gastroesophageal varices: Gastric vein embolization after partial portal decompression. Radiology 178:249, 1991.

8. Sarfeh IJ, Rypins EB, Fardi M, et al: Clinical implications of portal hemodynamics after small-diameter portacaval H graft. Surgery 96:223, 1984.

9. Cope C: Dilation of mesocaval shunts. Ann Radiol 29:178, 1986.

10. Soyer P, Levesque M, Zeitoun G: Treatment of mesocaval shunt stenosis with a metallic stent. AJR 158:1251, 1992.

11. Cope C: Balloon dilatation of closed mesocaval shunts. AJR 135:989, 1980.

12. Rosch J, Hanafee WN, Show H: Transjugular portal venography and radiologic portacaval shunt: An experimental study. Radiology 92:1112, 1969.

13. Burgener FA, Gutierrez OH: Nonsurgical production of intrahepatic portosystemic venous shunts in portal hypertension with the double lumen balloon catheter. ROFO 130:686, 1979.

14. Colapinto RF, Stronell RD, Gildiner M, et al: Formation of intrahepatic portosystemic shunts using a balloon dilatation catheter: Preliminary clinical experience. AJR 140:709, 1983.

15. Palmaz JC, Sibbitt RR, Reuter SR, et al: Expandable intrahepatic portacaval shunt stents: Early experience in the dog. AJR 145:821, 1985.

16. Rosch J, Uchida BT, Putnam JS, et al: Experimental intrahepatic portacaval anastomosis: Use of expandable Gianturco stents. Radiology 162:481, 1987.

17. Richter GM, Noeldge G, Palmaz JC, Roessle M: The transjugular intrahepatic portosystemic stent-shunt (TIPSS): Result of a pilot study. Cardiovasc Intervent Radiol 13:200, 1990.

18. Richter GM, Noeldge G, Palmaz JC, et al: Transjugular intrahepatic portacaval stent shunt: Preliminary clinical results. Radiology 174:1027, 1990.

19. Zemel G, Katzen BT, Becker GJ, et al: Percutaneous transjugular portosystemic shunt. JAMA 266(3):390, 1991.

20. Ring EJ, Lake JR, Roberts JP, et al: Using percutaneous intrahepatic portosystemic shunts to control variceal bleeding prior to liver transplantation. Ann Intern Med 116(4):304, 1992.

21. LaBerge JM, Ring EJ, Gordon RL, et al: Creation of transjugular intrahepatic portosystemic shunts with the Wallstent endoprosthesis: Results in 100 patients. Radiology 187:413, 1993.

22. Radosevich PM, Ring EJ, LaBerge JM, et al: Transjugular intrahepatic portosystemic shunts in patients with portal vein occlusion. Radiology 186:523, 1993.

23. Peltzer MY, Ring EJ, LaBerge JM, et al: Treatment of Budd-Chiari by a transjugular intrahepatic portosystemic shunt. J Vasc Intervent Radiol 4:263, 1993.

24. Sarfeh IJ, Rypins EB, Conroy RM, Mason GR: Portacaval H-graft: Relationships of shunt diameter, portal flow patterns and encephalopathy. Ann Surg 197:422, 1983.

25. Johansen K: Partial portal decompression for variceal hemorrhage. Am J Surg 157:479, 1989.

26. Haskal ZJ, Ring EJ, LaBerge JM, et al: Role of parallel transjugular intrahepatic portosystemic shunts in patients with persistent portal hypertension. Radiology 185:813, 1992.

27. Pernuau JM, Noeldge G, Roessle M: Intrahepatic portocaval shunt by the transjugular route, using the Palmaz stent. Presse Med 20(36):1770, 1991.

28. Boudghene F, Grange JD, Faintuch JM, et al: Intrahepatic portocaval shunt by the transjugular route. Presse Med 20(41):2108, 1991.

29. Richter GM, Noeldge G, Roessle M, Palmaz JC: Evolution and clinical introduction of TIPSS, the transjugular intrahepatic portosystemic stent-shunt. Semin Intervent Radiol 4:331, 1991.

30. LaBerge JM, Ferrell LD, Ring EJ, et al: Histopathologic study of transjugular intrahepatic portosystemic shunts. J Vasc Intervent Radiol 2:549, 1991.

104

Operative Therapy for Portal Hypertension

Kaj H. Johansen, M.D., Ph.D., and Layton F. Rikkers, M.D.

• • •

Hepatic cirrhosis is common, and a third or more of patients with advanced cirrhosis develop variceal hemorrhage secondary to the portal hypertension that may result from this condition. As is true for surgical decision making in general, operative therapy for variceal bleeding is usually reserved for circumstances in which *non*operative therapy—risk factor modification, drugs, endoscopic treatment, angiographic interventions—either have failed or are contraindicated. The other major general indication for operative therapy—prophylactic intervention to forestall a catastrophic complication of the disease—has *not* been shown to be useful in the management of portal hypertension, as discussed later.

GENERAL PERIOPERATIVE CONSIDERATIONS

Because patients with variceal hemorrhage are almost always acutely and chronically ill, with multiple medical comorbidities complicating the hospital course and the conduct of the operation itself, several perioperative management issues merit discussion.

Candidacy for Operation

As previously noted in this section (see Chapter 100), decompensated Child-Pugh class C cirrhotics tolerate anesthesia, major operation, significant blood loss, and diversion of hepatic portal perfusion poorly. Therefore, if at all possible, patients with persistent jaundice, intractable ascites, spontaneous encephalopathy, and advanced muscle wasting should be managed by endoscopy, angiographic shunt, or, when appropriate, orthotopic liver transplantation. A vigorous course of nutritional and metabolic resuscitation can frequently improve cirrhotic patients' Child-Pugh status and therefore their likelihood of surviving definitive shunt therapy.[1] Similarly, documented abstinence from alcohol for 6 to 12 months in a previously recalcitrant alcoholic cirrhotic may permit consideration of liver transplantation.[2]

An independent relative contraindication to operation is significant coagulopathy, for example, a prothrombin time longer than 16 seconds that is unresponsive to vitamin K administration. Such patients have an excessive risk of intra- and postoperative hemorrhage, and operation should be withheld. Thrombocytopenia is a usual finding in patients with variceal hemorrhage, with values commonly in the region of 60,000 or less; platelet counts can be maintained by platelet administration in the perioperative period, and successful portosystemic shunt generally reverses hypersplenism and restores platelet counts to normal levels.[3]

Children usually develop portal hypertension because of extrahepatic portal vein thrombosis;[4] their hepatic function and coagulation status are frequently normal, and their bleeding can commonly be controlled with endoscopic therapy.[5] Pediatric patients with cirrhosis, for example, as a consequence of biliary atresia, should usually be considered excellent candidates for liver transplantation. If an interval operative shunt is required, a procedure that does not invade the right upper quadrant, such as a distal splenorenal shunt or a Clatworthy or prosthetic graft mesocaval shunt, should be considered.[6]

In the Budd-Chiari syndrome, congenital or thrombotic occlusion of the hepatic veins or the suprahepatic vena cava (or both) leads to acute hepatic congestion with severe right upper quadrant pain, massive ascites, and hepatic dysfunction. It may occasionally be managed by interventional radiologic techniques, including thrombolytic therapy or balloon dilatation[7] (see Chapter 103). In most circumstances, however, such patients present subacutely and require operative therapy. Angiography, including careful examination of the inferior vena cava, is crucial in these patients. If the inferior vena cava is patent, a side-to-side portacaval shunt (converting the portal vein into an outflow tract for the congested liver) is curative.[8] Others prefer a mesocaval shunt using the internal jugular vein in order to avoid subhepatic scarring that might complicate later liver transplantation.[9] In patients in whom there is caval obstruction at or above the level of the liver, a portacaval shunt will not work. However, a mesoatrial shunt, connecting the superior mesenteric vein to the right atrial appendage as described by Cameron and Maddrey,[10] may satisfactorily decompress the portal system. Liver transplantation may be an effective management option,[9, 11, 12] although patients whose Budd-Chiari syndrome arises because of a hypercoagulable state may be at higher risk for graft malfunction because of a heightened risk of hepatic artery thrombosis.[11, 12]

Anesthetic Considerations

A panoply of special concerns accompanies the anesthetic management of cirrhotics, especially those undergoing shunts or liver transplantation.[13, 14] Because their generalized arteriovenous shunting extends to the pulmonary circulation, they may manifest significant hypoxemia.[15, 16] The presence of coagulopathy and thrombocytopenia makes consideration of conduction anesthesia imprudent in most cases. Chronic hepatocellular dysfunction results in a slowed clearance of anesthetic agents and sedatives ordinarily metabolized in the liver; cirrhosis is associated with an upregulation of benzodiazepine receptors in the brain,[17] making this family of sedative agents relatively contraindicated. Fluid and electrolyte disorders—extracellular volume excess, respiratory alkalosis, total body potassium deficiency—can be anticipated. Actively bleeding patients require maintenance of blood volume. Endotracheal intubation of patients who have recently been bleeding is fraught with the risk of aspiration of gastric contents; this problem may be made more acute when ascites results in significantly raised intra-abdominal pressure. Intraoperatively, intravenous vasopressin is commonly administered if the patient is bleeding; coronary vasoconstriction leading to myocardial ischemia (perhaps exacerbated by underlying alcoholic cardiomyopathy) may be associated with administration of this agent. Concurrent administration of nitroglycerine with vasopressin may significantly reduce the latter agent's coronary vasoconstrictive side effects.[18] These patients' hypoalbuminemia and sodium excess warrant consideration of volume restitution by the use of noncrystalloid volume replacement such as plasma, albumin, or hetastarch.

Emergency Management

Variceal hemorrhage can be torrential. Further, a small percentage of patients may have early recurrence of bleeding or continued hemorrhage despite vasopressin administration and endoscopic variceal sclerotherapy or banding. As noted in Chapter 101, virtually all such patients with early recurrent or persistent bleeding can be controlled with esophageal balloon tamponade. In fact, persistent bleeding despite these maneuvers raises the possibility of a nonvariceal bleeding source—duodenal ulcer, esophageal ulceration secondary to sclerotherapy, or Mallory-Weiss tear. In a patient whose bleeding is temporarily controlled by balloon tamponade, definitive management must be planned within the next 48 to 72 hours, by which time balloon tamponade must be discontinued (see Chapter 101).

In such a setting an angiographic shunt (transjugular intrahepatic portasystemic shunt [TIPS]) should be contemplated if available; good short-term control of bleeding in about 90 per cent of patients has been demonstrated with this method in such patients (see Chapter 103). TIPS is contraindicated in hemodynamically unstable patients: Helton and colleagues demonstrated a 56 per cent mortality, independent of Child-Pugh classification, when TIPS was attempted in patients with active bleeding who were inadequately resuscitated.[19]

Although a general anesthetic and a major operation in a hypovolemic, coagulopathic, chronically ill cirrhotic might seem fraught with an overwhelming risk of morbidity and mortality, Orloff and Bell performed emergency side-to-side portacaval shunts in more than 450 patients.[20] Although early mortality was 16 per cent in patients undergoing emergency shunt, further variceal bleeding was eliminated, and the 5-year survival exceeded 70 per cent.[20] These remarkable results are ascribed to simplified diagnosis, operation within 8 hours, and aggressive lifelong follow-up; late demise correlates with return to alcohol consumption.

If TIPS is unavailable, repeat endoscopic therapy is thought unwise (for example, because of a recent course of variceal injections or banding), and emergency shunt seems imprudent, laparotomy and staple transection of the esophagus may be the optimal approach[21] (see later discussion). Such an approach is rapid, relatively straightforward, and effective (at least in the short term), and does not significantly interfere with consideration of a shunt or liver transplantation if the patient is later a candidate for either.

Thrombosis of the Portal Vein or Its Tributaries

Patients with variceal hemorrhage due to extrahepatic portal vein thrombosis are often not considered candidates for TIPS or liver transplantation, and definitive portal decompression generally must be accomplished by splenorenal or mesocaval shunt. Because these patients' hepatic function is frequently either normal or only minimally diminished, they may have an excellent long-term prognosis.[22] Patients who suffer extrahepatic portal vein thrombosis in the presence of postnecrotic cirrhosis must be carefully screened, by serum alpha-fetoprotein levels and hepatic imaging, for an underlying hepatocellular carcinoma.[23]

Portal hypertension resulting from diffuse splanchnic venous thrombosis, arising usually as a result of a hematologic disorder,[24] may be difficult to treat. In some circumstances in which the portal, splenic, and superior mesenteric veins are diffusely thrombosed, the inferior mesenteric vein may be patent and can be anastomosed to the left renal vein, thereby effecting a durable portasystemic shunt.[25] If this option is unavailable, esophageal staple transection (or some other devascularization procedure) may be the best option.[21] In such patients, intra-abdominal variceal collaterals, for example those around the thrombosed portal vein, may be huge, but an attempt to anastomose one of these collaterals to the systemic venous circulation must be resisted; such makeshift shunts rarely remain patent.

Splenic veins may thrombose as a result of chronic pancreatic inflammation, usually secondary to alcoholic pancreatitis.[26] In such a setting, an isolated "sinistral" or "left upper quadrant" venous hypertension may occur, manifested by massive splenomegaly, hypersplenism, and gastric varices. In such cases, splenectomy will be curative. Polyvalent pneumococcal vaccine must be administered to diminish the risk of postsplenectomy sepsis.

GENERAL OPERATIVE CONSIDERATIONS

Operations for managing the hemorrhagic complications of portal hypertension can be divided into two conceptual categories: *palliative* operations, which interrupt either the bleeding varices themselves or the venous channels leading to them, or *definitive* operations, which relieve the underlying portal hypertension either by a decompressive shunt or by liver transplantation. Depending on the clinical circumstances, especially the urgency with which variceal hemorrhage must be treated and the patient's clinical status, one or another of these treatment modalities may be warranted. Indeed, the patient's status may change significantly, for better or worse, so that therapeutic options may develop or be eliminated by the passage of time and new clinical findings.

Devascularization Procedures

Direct operative attack upon bleeding esophageal and gastric varices has been a well-established therapeutic concept for well over a century. Certain approaches, such as direct oversewing of variceal columns after thoracotomy and longitudinal esophagotomy[27] or the "Boerema button,"[28] are obsolete. Certain other devascularization procedures, usually variations on a theme combining splenectomy, gastroesophageal variceal plexus ligation, and occlusion of collateral channels such as the coronary, gastroepiploic, and short gastric veins, have been performed.[29–30] Although these procedures provide acceptable short-term protection against variceal rebleeding and may avoid the accelerated liver failure and encephalopathy resulting from many portasystemic shunt procedures, medium- and long-term follow-up of such patients shows excessive rates of rebleeding. Accordingly, most of these procedures have fallen into disfavor.

An extremely aggressive devascularization procedure, performed via a staged thoracotomy and laparotomy, has been promoted by Sugiura and Futagawa;[31] although results reported by the operation's developer have been impressive, this procedure has rarely been performed on a regular basis outside Japan, and its relevance to the management of alcoholic cirrhotics seen in Western cultures has been challenged.

Del Guercio and colleagues have suggested that direct access to the portal circulation via mini-laparotomy and angiographic cannulation of the umbilical vein (through which transportal catheter embolization of coronary and short gastric veins can be accomplished) and splenic exclusion by Gelfoam or Gianturco coil embolization of the splenic artery, may be effective in halting variceal hemorrhage without requiring a major anesthetic, operation, or blood loss.[32] Although early success has again been note-worthy in these patients, experience with the technique is not widespread, and follow-up is short; like other palliative endoscopic, angiographic, and operative approaches, rede-velopment of varices and recurrent hemorrhage seems in-evitable.

The development of clinically usable surgical stapling devices led to the concept of simple, effective control of esophageal variceal hemorrhage by transection and reanas-tomosis of the terminal esophagus using the end-to-end anastomosis (EEA) stapling device.[33, 34] Early hopes that staple transection of the esophagus would prove to be a simple, rapid, and durable treatment for esophageal variceal hemorrhage have not consistently been borne out by sub-sequent clinical experience.[35] However, in experienced hands the approach may be an excellent "holding maneu-ver" while the patient is resuscitated to a state where more definitive therapy for variceal hemorrhage may be contem-plated. Staple transection of the esophagus is the initial operative approach chosen for patients with variceal bleed-ing who are considered endoscopic therapy "failures" in many major centers in Great Britain.[21, 33]

Portal Decompression

Because variceal hemorrhage results from underlying portal hypertension, reduction of portal pressure to normal physiologic levels invariably halts such bleeding. Certain procedures to increase portal systemic collaterals (for ex-ample, by transposing the spleen into the thoracic cavity[36]) are now of historic interest only. Bypassing splanchnic ve-nous outflow obstruction by connecting the hypertensive portal system to the systemic venous circulation, either di-rectly or by means of various autogenous or synthetic con-duits, has proved to be a highly effective means of halting variceal hemorrhage.

Shunt operations appear to have been performed first in animals by Eck in 1885,[37] although the first substantive investigations of the metabolic effects of portasystemic shunts were performed in the 1890s in the laboratories of Pavlov,[38] also in imperial Russia. A resurgence of interest in portasystemic shunts paralleled the beginnings of arterial reconstructive surgery in the 1940s and 1950s,[39] and such procedures, usually end-to-side or side-to-side portacaval shunts, became common therapy for patients with variceal hemorrhage in the years following World War II.

Several complicating factors became evident. A char-acteristic neuropsychiatric disorder, characterized by memory loss, altered levels of consciousness, behavioral changes, and (in its advanced stages) stupor, coma, and death, was noted to be a frequent and unpredictable result in patients who had undergone portasystemic shunt.[40] This syndrome, portasystemic encephalopathy ("hepatic coma"), remains poorly understood and has continued, in varying degrees, to plague all forms of portal decompres-sion.

Further, the nascent analytic tool of the prospective randomized clinical trial was used to investigate the effect of portasystemic shunts on survival, both in variceal bleed-ers and in cirrhotics whose varices had never bled. These studies showed that patients who survived a shunt operation

rarely bled again. However, those who had undergone a *therapeutic* shunt to treat previous variceal bleeding were found to show, at best, only nonsignificant trends toward improved survival compared to patients managed medi-cally; the sharp reduction in risk of dying from bleeding in surgically treated patients was nearly equalized by a sub-stantially increased likelihood of death from liver fail-ure.[41–44] Patients who had undergone *prophylactic* shunt to prevent an initial episode of variceal bleeding were found to do *worse* than medically managed patients.[45] (That a prophylactic operation would not be helpful to patients who had never bled from varices is not surprising in view of the fact that only a third of cirrhotics with varices ever actually bleed from them.)

More than half a century previously, Pavlov's labora-tory had demonstrated that dogs undergoing portacaval shunt become listless and anorectic, suffer premature mor-tality, and have hepatic atrophy at autopsy.[38] Extensive in-vestigations in the 1950s and 1960s, summarized most ele-gantly by Starzl and colleagues,[46] suggested that the equivalent phenomenon in humans, portasystemic enceph-alopathy, occurs because diversion of portal flow deprives the liver of a splanchnic venous factor (insulin seems a likely candidate) necessary for normal hepatocellular func-tion and regeneration. General acceptance of this "hepata-trophic theory," combined with the demonstration that therapeutic portacaval shunts only minimally improve sur-vival in prospective randomized trials, led to a significant decline in the performance of portacaval shunts and ani-mated the basic and clinical investigations leading to the concept of the "selective" portosystemic shunt.

Drapanas and colleagues theorized that a conduit from a *tributary* of the portal vein (such as the superior mesen-teric vein) to the systemic venous circulation might pre-serve prograde portal flow (and continued hepatic perfu-sion) while still effecting adequate portal decompression and protection against further variceal hemorrhage; devel-opment of the prosthetic interposition mesocaval shunt quickly followed.[47] Although mesocaval shunts have been extensively performed, their reliability is questionable; they were initially constructed using large-caliber Dacron grafts, which have an unacceptably high incidence of thrombosis (about 10 per cent per year),[48] undoubtedly because of slow flow velocity through a highly thrombogenic synthetic con-duit. Better results have recently been recorded using a small-caliber expanded polytetrafluoroethylene (ringed PTFE) interposition graft between the superior mesenteric vein and the infrarenal vena cava.[49] Interposition of autolo-gous tissue (most commonly internal jugular vein) as a mesocaval graft probably has the highest likelihood of long-term patency.[50] The underlying premise—that hepatic portal venous perfusion can be preserved by a mesocaval shunt—has *not* been borne out; such patients have a likeli-hood of postshunt complications equivalent to that of cir-rhotics undergoing standard portacaval shunt.[48]

Simultaneous decompression of the portal system while maintaining prograde portal flow is a hemodynamic impossibility. A hypothesis of more enduring value has been that of the selective shunt, most vigorously pursued in investigations of the distal splenorenal shunt by W. Dean Warren and colleagues.[51–54] Warren based his concept on the premise that portal venous perfusion of the liver could be maintained only if pressure in the portal vein remained high, to overcome the significant perisinusoidal block present in cirrhosis. On the other hand, if the gastrosplenic circulation, into which the gastroesophageal variceal plexus collateralizes via the short gastric veins, could be separated from the hypertensive portomesenteric venous system, the variceal plexus could be decompressed into the nearby left renal vein (or even the vena cava) without disturbing prograde portal venous flow to the liver. Thus, the concept of Warren's distal splenorenal shunt was developed (Fig. 104–1)—end-to-side anastomosis of the splenic vein to the left renal vein, combined with meticulous ligation of all collateral veins actually or potentially connecting the high-pressure portomesenteric and low-pressure gastrosplenic venous circuits.

Initial clinical trials of the distal splenorenal shunt appeared to bear out its theoretical rationale; despite a number of relative or absolute contraindications (active variceal hemorrhage, ascites, Child-Pugh C liver status, prior splenectomy, retrograde portal venous flow, unfavorable splenic or left renal venous anatomy), the procedure reliably protects against variceal rebleeding, and encephalopathy rates appear to be less than those associated with the standard portacaval shunt. Because the Warren shunt avoids the hepatic hilum, it is considered by many to be the optimal shunt in patients who may be a liver transplant candidate in the future. Distal splenorenal shunt became the portal decompressive approach of choice in many medical centers during the 1970s and 1980s.

Recent analyses, however, have clouded the validity of the selective shunt hypothesis. A gradual but predictable loss of selectivity of the distal splenorenal shunt,[55, 56] primarily by the development of peripancreatic venous collaterals from the high-pressure portomesenteric circulation to the splenic vein, effectively converts the initially selective shunt into a total shunt. Loss of prograde flow, or even complete thrombosis, in the portal vein can be demonstrated in up to 50 per cent of distal splenorenal shunt patients at 1-year follow-up; for unclear reasons, this appears to be much more common in alcoholic cirrhotics than in those whose liver dysfunction is caused by other disease

states.[57] Warren and coworkers responded with a technical tactic—"splenopancreatic dissociation," a complete dissection of the splenic vein out of its pancreatic bed—to combat this inexorable collateralization.[54] Although some clinical evidence supports the utility of this approach, splenopancreatic dissociation makes an already technically challenging operative procedure even more lengthy, tedious, and risky. Long-term analyses of outcomes following distal splenorenal shunt with splenopancreatic dissociation are unavailable, and it has not been definitively demonstrated that this maneuver provides durable protection against loss of selectivity of the splenorenal shunt. Prospective randomized comparisons of selective and total shunts have not demonstrated a survival advantage in patients undergoing selective shunt.[58-60]

Inokuchi and colleagues reported performance of what may be the ultimate selective portal decompression, the coronary-caval shunt.[61] This procedure reroutes the coronary vein into the intrahepatic vena cava, either by direct end-to-side anastomosis or by means of an interposed saphenous vein graft. Inokuchi and colleagues reported excellent results, with a 2.2 per cent operative mortality, 7.4 per cent variceal rebleeding, and no new encephalopathy, in 146 patients followed for a mean of 66 months. The procedure is technically challenging and has rarely been performed outside Japan.

Partial Portal Decompression. Portal perfusion is lost following total shunt (end-to-side or side-to-side portacaval shunt, central splenorenal shunt, mesocaval shunt); because resistance to flow is so much less through the shunt and into the systemic venous circulation than in the portal vein, hilar portal venous flow reverses, and the vessel becomes a venous outflow tract into the shunt. Hepatic nutrition is then maintained entirely by the hepatic artery; in fact, it has been hypothesized that a patient's ability to tolerate a total portosystemic shunt is based upon the capacity of the hepatic artery to vasodilate.[52] The possibility that prograde portal flow could be maintained by forming a smaller, higher resistance portosystemic shunt was investigated initially by Marion and associates[63] and by Bismuth and colleagues.[64]

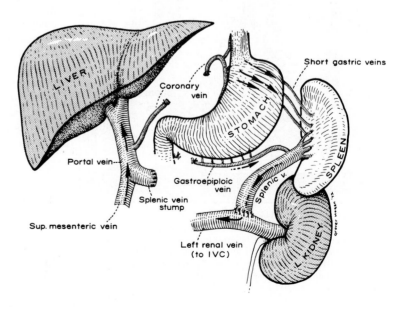

FIGURE 104–1. Conceptually, the distal splenorenal shunt of Warren and colleagues combines decompression of the esophagogastric variceal complex via the short gastric veins, the spleen, and the splenic vein into the left renal vein with maintenance of a high-pressure portomesenteric circulation. This latter state results from closure of the central end of the splenic vein as well as meticulous ligation of all potential right-to-left coronary and gastroepiploic venous collaterals.

These studies appeared to suggest no difference in rebleeding, liver failure, or encephalopathy rates in patients receiving small- or large-orifice shunts (although the shunts were constructed with interrupted sutures, and the possibility that the small-orifice shunts had dilated and become "total" was not investigated).[64]

In the early 1980s Sarfeh and colleagues introduced the concept of the small-caliber PTFE interposition portacaval graft (Fig. 104–2).[65] Although their study population was small, and initial reports suggested a substantial risk of graft thrombosis, the procedure is technically straightforward, and its protection against postshunt encephalopathy seems excellent. Sarfeh and colleagues ascribed this last favorable characteristic to maintenance of hepatic portal perfusion, which they have demonstrated angiographically and by radionuclide techniques[66] (although others' studies of PTFE interposition portacaval graft patients do not support this conclusion[67]).

In patients undergoing a direct side-to-side small-orifice portacaval shunt with postoperative duplex sonography,[68] Johansen showed consistent loss of portal perfusion of the liver *despite* the relatively high resistance of the shunt (10 mmHg portacaval pressure gradient).[69] However, an incidence of encephalopathy of only 6 per cent in these patients suggested that maintenance of first-pass portal perfusion of the liver may not be relevant to the development of postshunt encephalopathy. Studies in rats undergoing end-to-side portacaval shunt suggest an inverse relationship between splanchnic venous pressure and absorption of ammonia from the gut into the mesenteric circulation.[70] In a prospective comparison,[71] patients undergoing partial portal

decompression had a late mortality rate of 13 per cent and an encephalopathy rate of 8 per cent compared to total shunt patients' late mortality risk of 39 per cent ($p < .05$) and encephalopathy risk of 56 per cent ($p < .0001$). All patients in both groups had lost portal perfusion of the liver by postoperative duplex sonography.[68]

Whether partially decompressing portacaval shunts protects against encephalopathy and liver failure by preserving prograde portal flow[63–66] or by maintaining "physiologic" splanchnic venous pressures[67, 69, 71, 72] remains unclear. The unacceptably high incidence of postshunt complications associated with total portal decompression and the ever increasing technical complexity of the distal splenorenal shunt may result in increased enthusiasm for the concept of partial portal decompression when operative portal decompression is required.

OPERATIVE TECHNIQUES

Although this chapter is not intended to usurp the function of a surgical atlas, certain elements of surgical technique for each of the commonly performed operations for complications of portal hypertension bear emphasis. More specific details about operative techniques may be found in standard surgical compendia.

Staple Transection of the Esophagus

As previously indicated, EEA staple transection of the esophagus (Fig. 104–3) may provide effective short-term palliation in patients with persistent or recurrent esophageal variceal hemorrhage in whom definitive shunt surgery cannot or should not be attempted.

Exploration is begun through an upper midline or left subcostal incision, and the proximal stomach and lower esophagus are mobilized. The stapler is inserted in the "opened" position through a high gastrotomy into the lower esophagus, a heavy suture around the outside of the distal esophagus is tied down snugly around the shaft of the stapler, and it is then closed. Firing the device then divides and reanastomoses the distal esophagus, simultaneously interrupting all variceal columns traversing the lower esophagus.

Staple transection obviously does not treat gastric varices or portal hypertensive gastropathy; it may be rendered more difficult or impossible to perform if the esophagus is extensively edematous, inflamed, or scarred because of prior endoscopic variceal therapy. Because the vagus nerves may unavoidably be divided during esophageal transection, pyloroplasty may be warranted to prevent postoperative gastric outlet obstruction.

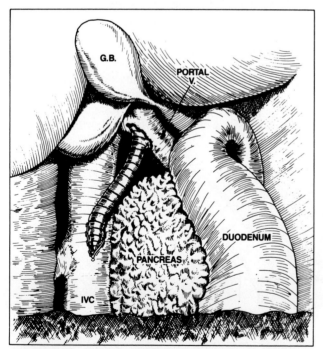

FIGURE 104–2. The portacaval H-graft shunt of Sarfeh and colleagues uses an 8- or 10-mm externally reinforced polytetrafluoroethylene (PTFE) graft interposed between the inferior vena cava *(left)* and the portal vein *(right)*. (From Sarfeh IJ, Rypins EB, Mason GR: A systematic appraisal of portacaval H-graft diameters. Clinical and hemodynamic perspectives. Ann Surg 204:356, 1986.)

Total Shunts

The goal of a total shunt is to accomplish complete portal decompression. Theoretically, such shunts should have the highest likelihood of protecting against further variceal rebleeding, and in general this is borne out; of some 1500 portacaval shunts performed by Orloff, fewer

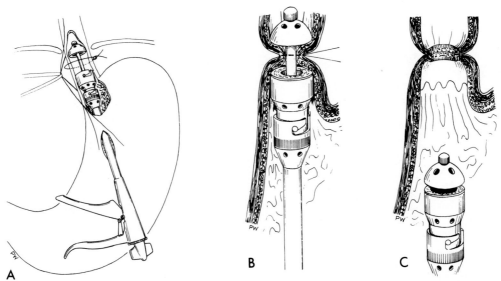

FIGURE 104–3. Esophageal transection using the end-to-end anastomosis (EEA) stapling device. *A,* Stapler introduced into the distal esophagus via a high gastrotomy. The distal esophagus is carefully dissected, and the vagus nerves are identified and preserved. *B,* A heavy monofilament suture is tied around the esophagus overlying the stapler's central rod in the "open" position. *C,* After firing, the stapler is removed, and the gastrotomy is closed in two layers. The area of esophageal transection and reanastomosis is carefully inspected, and the tissue "donut" from the stapler is checked for completeness.

than 10 (less than 0.1 per cent) have been associated with proven variceal rebleeding (MJ Orloff, personal communication). Shunt failure, when it occurs, almost always results from an attempt to use a partially or completely thrombosed portal vein in the anastomosis rather than an alternative portal decompressive procedure. Total shunts can conceptually be divided into the following categories: portacaval shunts (end-to-side or side-to-side), mesocaval shunts, and proximal (or central) splenorenal shunts.

Portacaval Shunts

The relative anatomic (Fig. 104–4) proximity of the portal vein and the inferior vena cava make direct anastomosis between the two relatively straightforward technically. The patient should be placed in a left lateral decubitus position; many surgeons find "flexing" the patient with the kidney rest or a "bean bag" facilitates exposure to the intrahepatic vena cava and portal triad. An extended right Kocher incision is made, carried laterally to the mid-axillary line; the general approach is from the lateral perspective (which allows a portacaval shunt to be completed even in the presence of adhesions from prior right upper quadrant operations). Extensive venous collaterals may be found in the subcutaneous tissue during performance of the initial incision; electrocautery proves advantageous in this situation.

Abdominal exploration generally reveals ascites, a substantially enlarged spleen, fragile portosystemic venous collaterals in the retroperitoneum and at any site of prior operative adhesions, and the cirrhotic liver in the right upper quadrant. It should be examined carefully for evidence for a concurrent hepatocellular carcinoma (especially in patients with a prior history of hepatitis).

Attention is first turned to dissection of the inferior vena cava. The vessel is exposed in its entirety from a cephalad direction, where it is dissected free from the caudate lobe (carefully dividing from one to four caudate lobe veins) to a point just below the renal veins, following a generous Kocher maneuver. There are no lumbar veins cephalad to the renal veins; however, the right adrenal vein may be large, fragile, multiple, and located at any point from the retrohepatic inferior vena cava to the right renal vein. Careful and complete mobilization of the inferior vena cava, including the central portions of the renal veins, is crucial because most of the mobilization permitting approximation of the inferior vena cava and the portal vein in the performance of a portacaval shunt is derived from careful caval dissection.

Attention is then turned to the isolation of the portal vein. The portal triad is palpated (passing a finger through the foramen of Winslow), among other reasons to ensure that there is no aberrant or replaced right hepatic artery in the lateral aspect of the structure (if one is present, it must be carefully preserved). Again, just as for the inferior vena cava, commencing the dissection cephalad near the hepatic hilum provides the best exposure to the portal vein. Incising the peritoneum overlying the portal vein, well lateral to the common bile duct, usually exposes a substantial number of enlarged lymphatic channels and nodes. Removal of a characteristic large "sentinel" lymph node generally exposes the portal vein. This vessel is then carefully dissected from its bifurcation in the hepatic hilum caudad to a site where it disappears beneath the pancreas. *Extreme* caution must be adopted in dissecting medially beneath the common bile duct: one to four large, fragile, high-pressure coronary veins may reside there, and these vessels are extremely difficult to control if inadvertently avulsed.

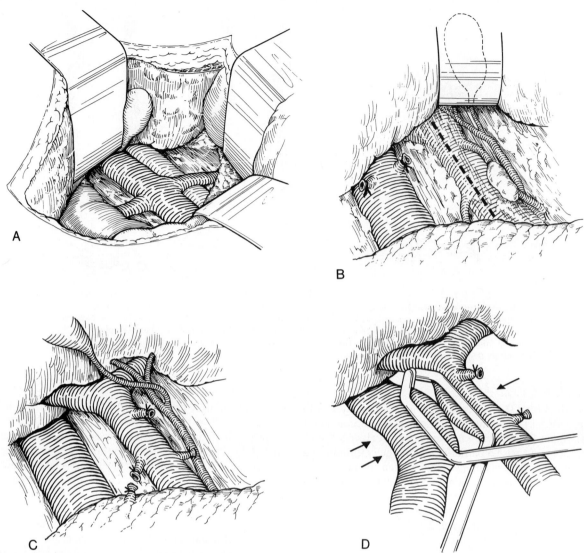

FIGURE 104–4.   Portacaval shunt. *A,* An extensive Kocher maneuver is performed to expose the infrahepatic inferior vena cava caudally to a point just below the renal veins. *B,* Exposing the portal vein. This structure is best approached by incising the peritoneum over the lateral hepatoduodenal ligament *(hatched line);* alternatively, careful dissection of a prominent, anteriorly placed lymph node may expose the portal vein. *C,* Mobilization of the portal vein by careful ligature and division of one or more medially directed coronary veins (two are depicted here) and a constant, large posterolateral portal vein tributary from the head of the pancreas. *D,* Properly mobilized inferior vena cava and portal vein can be readily apposed for side-to-side anastomosis using apposing Satinsky clamps.

Illustration continued on opposite page

An end-to-side portacaval shunt is performed by dividing the portal vein as close to the hepatic hilum as possible, preferably even by dividing the right and left portal veins just cephalad to the portal vein bifurcation. This usually permits a relatively tension-free anastomosis to the side of the infrahepatic inferior vena cava. A Satinsky or other partially occluding vascular clamp is placed on the anteromedial surface of the portal vein; a linear cavotomy equivalent to the diameter of the portal vein is made, and the portacaval anastomosis is constructed between the end of the portal vein and the inferior vena cava using a 4–0 or 5–0 monofilament suture. Pressures should be measured in the portal vein and the inferior vena cava; if total decompression is intended but the portacaval pressure gradient (portal vein pressure minus inferior vena cava pressure) exceeds 5 mmHg, the anastomosis should be dismantled and reconstructed.

The side-to-side portacaval shunt is thought by some to be technically more difficult than the end-to-side shunt because the tension between the two vessels to be anastomosed may be increased by the intervening hypertrophied caudate lobe of the liver. This in fact should rarely be a problem; *complete* dissection of an adequate length of portal vein and inferior vena cava, and resection (if necessary) of a segment of caudate lobe (using the electrocautery or individual suture ligature of bleeding parenchymal vessels) should permit a tension-free side-to-side portacaval anastomosis.

On rare occasions the gap between the portal vein and the inferior vena cava is too great for an acceptable direct

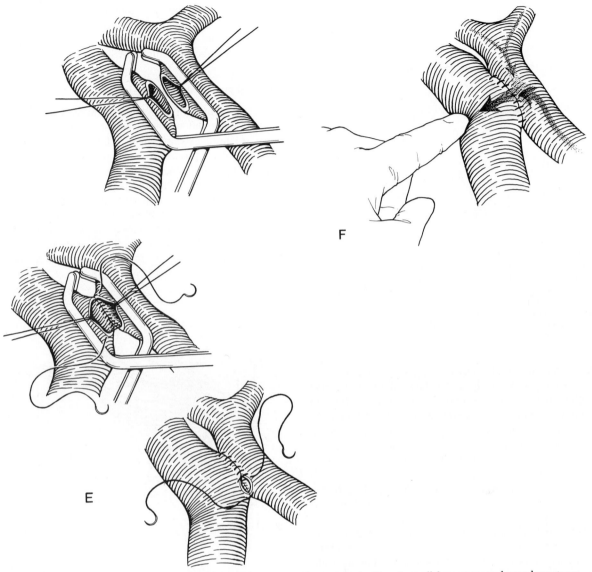

FIGURE 104–4. *Continued* *E*, Completing the portacaval anastomosis. *Top*, A parallel cavotomy and portal venotomy are carried out, and stay sutures are placed as shown. *Middle*, After starting the anastomotic suture (a 4–0 or 5–0 monofilament stitch) at the top, the posterior walls are anastomosed from within using the first "arm" of the stitch. *Bottom*, The anterior closure is accomplished from the outside using the other "arm" of the stitch. *F*, Patency of the shunt can be assessed by palpation of the inferior vena cava wall opposite the shunt; a thrill or jet is frequently noted. Pressures should be measured to ensure that portal decompression is adequate. (*A–F*, From Johansen K, Helton WS: The relief of portal hypertension. *In* Yao JST, Jamieson CW [eds]: Rob and Smith's Operative Surgery. 5th ed. London, Chapman & Hall, 1994.)

anastomosis; in this circumstance, interposition of a prosthetic vascular graft (see later) or, better, the left renal vein (divided over the aorta and anastomosed end-to-side to the portal vein), suffices.

Mesocaval Shunt

Connecting the superior mesenteric vein and the inferior vena cava was initially thought to offer the possibility of variceal decompression while simultaneously permitting continued portal perfusion of the liver.[47] This is now known not to be true; the mesocaval shunt is hemodynamically equivalent to a standard portacaval shunt (Fig. 104–5). The mesocaval shunt has also been thought by some to be tech-

nically more straightforward than other portal decompressive procedures.

The operation is usually performed through a celiotomy incision. The inferior vena cava is generally exposed by leftward visceral rotation, including a Kocher maneuver. Alternatively, the inferior vena cava can be identified by dissecting dorsally through the root of the great mesentery, just to the right of the palpable aortic pulsation. The entire infrarenal inferior vena cava is dissected down to the iliac vein confluence, including ligation and division of several lumbar vein pairs (although the dissection need not be so extensive as that needed for portacaval anastomosis).

Attention is then turned to the dissection of the superior mesenteric vein. With the transverse colon retracted

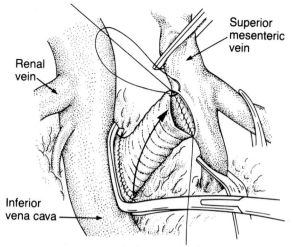

FIGURE 104–5. Mesocaval shunt. Anastomosis of a graft to the infrarenal inferior vena cava has been accomplished, and the anastomosis to the posterolateral superior mesenteric vein has been partially completed. Giving the prosthetic graft approximately a 30 per cent clockwise twist *(solid arrow over graft)* accommodates the different vectors of the superior mesenteric vein and the inferior vena cava and eliminates any risk of kinking of the graft.

cephalad and the small intestine retracted to the right, a transverse incision is made at the base of the transverse mesocolon near the ligament of Treitz. The peritoneum overlying the superior mesenteric vein is incised longitudinally (best done with electrocautery) for a distance of 5 cm, exposing the vein and several large branches. These tributaries may be ligated and divided to provide a 4- to 5-cm length of mobilized superior mesenteric vein.

An appropriately sized graft—10-, 12-, or 14-mm externally reinforced PTFE or Dacron, or internal jugular vein—is anastomosed end-to-side to the inferior vena cava. The graft is then brought ventrally around the lower portion of the duodenum in proximity to the superior mesenteric vein. The latter is clamped and rotated so that its right posterolateral aspect is anterior. A venotomy appropriate to the diameter of the graft is made, and the graft–superior mesenteric vein anastomosis is accomplished, again using monofilament vascular suture. When the clamps are removed, the graft should rest in a gentle curve below the duodenum.

In general, patency rates for mesocaval shunts have not equaled those of portacaval decompressive procedures. Dacron grafts have a thrombosis rate of more than 25 per cent.[48] Although autogenous jugular vein grafts have had excellent patency rates in several small series,[50] they have not been used widely enough for a conclusion to be drawn about their general adequacy. A similar statement can be made about externally reinforced PTFE grafts in the mesocaval position.[49]

Lower patency rates and uncertainty about the proper graft material make the indications for mesocaval shunt relatively limited. This procedure should be contemplated primarily in patients with portal vein thrombosis or in those in whom the possibility of future liver transplantation makes avoidance of a right upper quadrant shunt prudent. Relief of ascites and hypersplenism and accentuation of encephalopathy and liver decompensation are equivalent in

mesocaval shunts and other total portal decompressive procedures; the apparent lower risk of encephalopathy observed in some series probably relates to the higher likelihood of thrombosis of mesocaval shunts.[48]

Central Splenorenal Shunt

Anastomosis of the splenic vein to the left renal vein decompresses the portal system in both the central and distal splenorenal shunts (Fig. 104–6). However, conceptually the two procedures are profoundly different. The central shunt is hemodynamically equivalent to a standard portacaval shunt and cannot preserve prograde portal flow.

The central splenorenal shunt is generally performed through a midline laparotomy or a transverse left upper quadrant incision. Splenectomy is performed, and the splenic vein is dissected centrally from its intimate attachments to the back of the pancreas. The left renal vein is

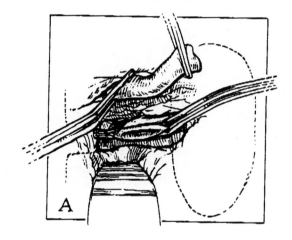

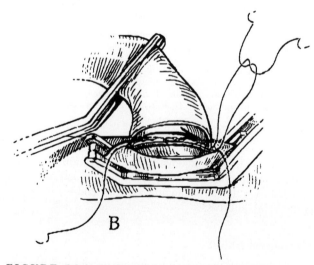

FIGURE 104–6. Proximal or central splenorenal shunt includes, after splenectomy, anastomosis of the mesenteric end of the splenic vein to the anterior-superior surface of the left renal vein *(A)*. As for other portal decompressive shunts, suture of the posterior wall of the anastomosis from within may facilitate their closure *(B)*. (*A* and *B*, From Jones RS: Portal hypertension. *In* Atlas of Liver and Biliary Surgery. Chicago, Year Book Medical, 1990, p 297. By permission of Mosby.)

exposed from beneath the pancreas and the transverse mesocolon. Gonadal or adrenal tributaries of the renal vein may be ligated and divided to free up this vessel. An end-to-side anastomosis of the splenic vein to the upper surface of the left renal vein is then accomplished, making sure that the splenic vein is not kinked acutely around the lower border of the pancreas.

Like the mesocaval shunt, the central splenorenal shunt has the advantage of effective portal decompression without involving the hilum of the liver. Notwithstanding early hopes to the contrary, this is a totally decompressing shunt, with the same risk of encephalopathy and accelerated liver failure as a portacaval shunt. This operation provides excellent treatment for hypersplenism.

Selective Shunts

Despite their excellent protection against variceal rebleeding, totally decompressing shunts may result in accelerated liver failure as well as an increased risk of portasystemic encephalopathy. Warren and colleagues designed the distal splenorenal shunt to provide isolated or "selective" decompression of the gastroesophageal variceal plexus with preservation of portal perfusion of the liver.[51–54]

Distal Splenorenal Shunt

The distal splenorenal shunt (Fig. 104–7) is generally performed through an oblique left upper quadrant incision. It is composed of two parts: anastomosis of the splenic end of the divided splenic vein to the left renal vein, and meticulous ligation and division of all potential venous collaterals between the portomesenteric and gastrosplenic venous beds.

The splenic vein is dissected away from the pancreas from above and behind (through the lesser sac) or from below the lower border of the pancreas. Initial reports suggested dissecting just enough of the splenic vein to permit its anastomosis to the left renal vein.[51] However, the subsequent finding that the low-pressure shunt attracts collaterals from the high-pressure portomesenteric circulation through the pancreatic "siphon" led to the concept of splenopancreatic dissociation—meticulous dissection, ligation, and division of *all* connections between the pancreas and the splenic vein throughout its entire length.[54] Extensive collateral ligation is performed by dividing the coronary vein (through a retrogastric approach), the gastroepiploic veins, the inferior mesenteric vein, and any other obvious potential right-to-left collateral veins.

The distal splenorenal shunt cannot be performed in patients who have previously undergone splenectomy. It is also thought to be relatively contraindicated in patients with ascites, with very poor hepatocellular function (Child-Pugh class C), or when preoperative angiography demonstrates abnormalities of the splenic or left renal veins—unfavorable anatomic displacement, diminutive vessels, or areas of thrombosis. Because the procedure (especially with the addition of splenopancreatic dissociation) is a lengthy one, it is generally not indicated as an emergency decompressive operation.

LIVER TRANSPLANTATION

Because it restores both portal pressure and hepatic functional reserve to normal, liver transplantation appears to be the ideal therapy for variceal hemorrhage. However, in contrast to the other operations described in this chapter, which are directed specifically toward the treatment of portal hypertensive bleeding, transplantation is generally considered only for patients with end-stage liver disease, one symptom of which may be variceal hemorrhage. For example, although 29 per cent of 498 adult patients receiving liver transplants at the University of Nebraska Medical Center between 1985 and 1992 had a history of variceal bleeding, only 39 (8 per cent) had bled within a month of the transplant operation. Variceal bleeding in the remaining transplant candidates had been successfully treated with either endoscopic sclerotherapy or portosystemic shunting, and the decision for transplantation had been mandated by subsequent deterioration of hepatic function rather than by bleeding. During the same time interval, 72 patients underwent nontransplant operations (shunt or esophagogastric devascularization) for the treatment of variceal hemorrhage, either emergently or electively. Thus, in a referral center for patients with chronic liver disease where sclerotherapy, shunt surgery, and liver transplantation are all readily available, nontransplant operations are still more commonly performed for definitive control of variceal hemorrhage than is liver replacement.

Even though hepatic transplantation is rarely utilized as treatment for variceal bleeding per se, the onset of variceal hemorrhage in a patient with chronic liver disease should always precipitate the following questions: Is the patient a candidate for liver transplantation? If so, should the transplant be done in the near future or later during the course of the disease? What should be done to prevent recurrent bleeding until a transplant is indicated or until a donor organ is available? Most variceal bleeders will never be transplant candidates, and even if they were, the limited donor organ supply would preclude transplantation for most of them. Individuals with noncirrhotic portal hypertension (schistosomiasis, portal vein thrombosis, splanchnic arterioportal fistulae, and idiopathic portal hypertension) generally maintain their hepatic functional reserve indefinitely and experience normal life spans if their bleeding can be successfully controlled by nontransplant strategies. In addition, a significant number of cirrhotic patients have one or more of the following absolute contraindications to liver transplantation: inoperability because of advanced dysfunction of another organ system (usually the pulmonary or cardiovascular system), intractable medical noncompliance, acquired immunodeficiency syndrome, extrahepatic malignancy, or active drug or alcohol abuse. Portal hypertensive bleeding can frequently be treated successfully in these patients by a single nontransplant therapy or a sequence of treatments (e.g., chronic endoscopic sclerotherapy, followed by a selective or partial shunt when sclerotherapy fails).

The most controversial patients are those with alcoholic cirrhosis, the single most common cause of chronic liver disease and variceal bleeding in Western industrialized countries. Several series have now demonstrated that short-

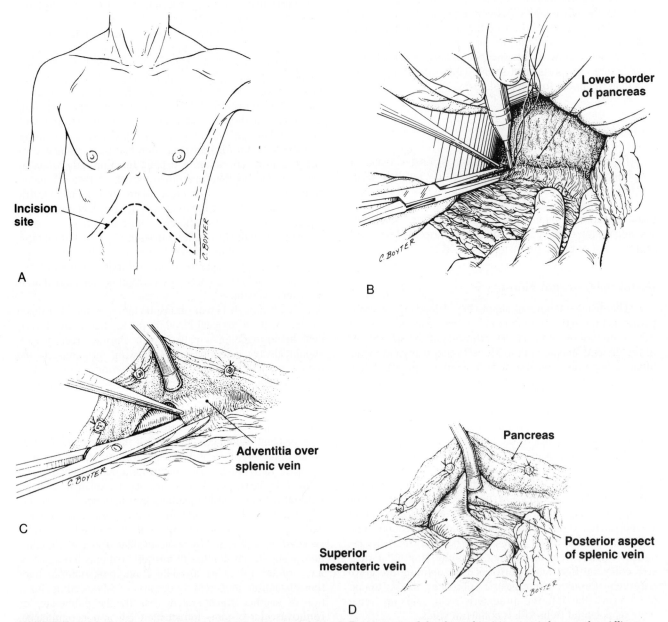

FIGURE 104–7. Steps in performing a distal splenorenal shunt. *A,* Exposure via a left subcostal incision, carried across the midline to the right side. *B,* Division of the gastrocolic omentum to expose the lower border of the pancreas. *C,* Exposure of the splenic vein caudad and dorsal to the lower border of the pancreas. *D,* Dissection of the splenic vein rightward to its junction with the superior mesenteric vein.

Illustration continued on opposite page

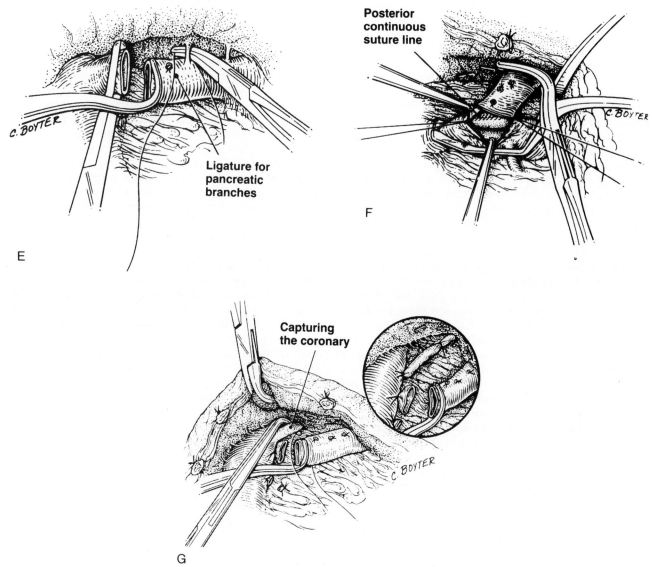

FIGURE 104–7. *Continued*   E, Division of the splenic vein and oversewing of the superior mesenteric vein side. Dissection of the splenic vein away from the pancreas, by painstaking ligation and division of multiple small fragile pancreatic venous tributaries, commences. F, After identification of the left renal vein, found dorsally and inferiorly, end-to-side anastomosis of the splenic and left renal veins is accomplished. The splenic vein may need to be shortened to avoid kinking of the shunt. G, Ligature of the coronary vein is a crucial component of the distal splenorenal shunt. It can be found exiting posteriorly from the hepatoduodenal ligament above the confluence of the splenic vein and the superior mesenteric vein. (A–G, From Warren WD, Millikan WJ: The distal splenorenal shunt. Contemp Surg 18:13, 1981.)

term results of transplantation are at least as good in patients with alcoholic cirrhosis as in those with nonalcoholic liver disease.[73, 74] When alcoholic patients are carefully selected, based on either an interval of abstinence or an alcohol prognosis scale that takes into account numerous psychosocial factors, post-transplantation recidivism rates have been less than 20 per cent.[74] Although the ethical issues surrounding expenditure of a limited resource on individuals with a self-induced disease continue to be debated,[2] it is becoming increasingly clear that a significant fraction of patients with alcoholic cirrhosis are excellent candidates for hepatic transplantation.

Once candidacy for transplantation has been established for a variceal bleeder, the timing of the operation must be determined. A key factor in such a decision is the patient's hepatic functional reserve, most commonly assessed with the Child-Pugh classification (see Chapter 100). Patients who are Child-Pugh class C should be transplanted as soon as a donor organ can be located. Additionally, individuals with Child-Pugh class A or B disease who manifest symptoms that adversely affect quality of life, such as extreme fatigue, encephalopathy, bone pain, or severe pruritus, should undergo transplantation rather than a palliative therapy directed at prevention of recurrent bleeding alone.

Most Child-Pugh class A patients should undergo nontransplant therapy for long-term control of portal hypertensive bleeding and should be monitored at 6-month or yearly intervals to assess the status of their liver disease. When it is apparent that the disease is progressive and is becoming end-stage, these individuals should then be listed for transplantation. Such patients should be treated with either chronic sclerotherapy or a portosystemic shunt, depending upon individual circumstances. Chronic endoscopic therapy is preferred for patients with ready access to medical and surgical treatment so that recurrent bleeding, if it occurs, can be treated expeditiously. Patients who reside in a rural environment, who bleed from gastric varices or portal hypertensive gastropathy, or who fail to respond to chronic endoscopic therapy are best treated with portal decompression.[75] Most of these individuals are good candidates for selective variceal decompression (distal splenorenal shunt), which offers the advantage of a lower incidence of postshunt encephalopathy. Child-Pugh class B patients should be managed on a case-by-case basis after a comprehensive evaluation of psychosocial situation, hepatic hemodynamics, and functional hepatic reserve to determine whether early or delayed transplantation is likely to produce the best overall results.

Due to the imprecisions inherent in the Child-Pugh classification,[76] quantitative tests of hepatic function such as galactose elimination capacity and aminopyrine clearance and estimation of hepatic mass by computed tomography have been used to determine the timing of hepatic transplantation in some centers. The Emory group has proposed that variceal bleeders with a galactose elimination capacity of less than 225 mg/min or a liver volume of less than 50 per cent of the predicted value should undergo transplantation rather than a shunt because their hepatic reserve is insufficient to sustain life for long without liver transplantation.[77]

Patients with variceal hemorrhage who are early trans-

plant candidates can usually be treated successfully with one or more sessions of variceal sclerosis until a donor liver becomes available. If bleeding persists or recurs repeatedly despite endoscopic therapy, portal decompression must be considered. The ideal procedure in this setting is the transjugular intrahepatic portosystemic shunt (TIPS) because it does not require surgical intervention and does not interfere with a later transplant operation.[78] TIPS is less desirable for patients who are unlikely to require transplantation for several years because the long-term reliability of this procedure is unknown.[19] If the expertise for TIPS is not available and urgent portal decompression is required to prevent exsanguination, the operative procedure selected optimally should avoid the hepatic hilum so that future transplantation is not compromised. In this situation, an interposition mesocaval shunt[50] or esophageal transection[33] is optimal.

Most evidence indicates that a prior portosystemic shunt does not significantly compromise subsequent transplantation;[79, 80] post-transplant survival rates are similar in patients with and without a prior portosystemic shunt. However, a prior shunt, especially when the portal vein is utilized, makes the transplant procedure more difficult and may increase the transfusion requirement.[80] Because they avoid the hepatic hilum, the distal splenorenal shunt and the interposition mesocaval or mesorenal shunts are probably the best alternatives for long-term and short-term bridges to transplantation, respectively.

Contemporary results from major transplantation centers demonstrate an operative mortality of 5 to 10 per cent, 1- and 2-year survival rates exceeding 80 per cent, and good-to-excellent quality of life in a significant majority of graft recipients. Because chronic graft rejection cannot yet be successfully prevented, up to one third of orthotopic liver transplant recipients may require retransplantation. Ongoing ethical debates about the suitability of liver transplantation for patients with alcoholic cirrhosis, as well as the procedure's extraordinary fiscal costs and a worsening deficit of donor organs, continue to limit this procedure's utilization for the great majority of patients with the complications of portal hypertension.

References

1. Holman JM, Rikkers LF: Success of medical and surgical management of acute variceal hemorrhage. Am J Surg 140:816, 1980.
2. Moss AH, Siegler M: Should alcoholics compete equally for liver transplantation? JAMA 2625:1295, 1991.
3. Soper NJ, Rikkers LF: Effect of operations for variceal hemorrhage on hypersplenism. Am J Surg 144:700, 1982.
4. Sherlock S: Portal hypertension in childhood. Proc R Soc Med 55:767, 1962.
5. Stellen GP, Lilly JR: Esophageal endosclerosis in children. Surgery 98:970, 1985.
6. Fonkalsrud EW: Surgical management of portal hypertension in childhood: Long-term results. Arch Surg 115:1042, 1980.
7. Yamada R, Sato M, Kawabata M, et al: Segmental obstruction of the hepatic inferior vena cava treatment by transluminal angioplasty. Radiology 149:91, 1983.
8. Orloff M, Gerard B: Long-term results of treatment of Budd-Chiari syndrome by side-to-side portacaval shunt. Surg Gynecol Obstet 168:33, 1989.
9. Bismuth H, Sherlock DJ: Portasystemic shunting versus liver transplantation for the Budd-Chiari syndrome. Ann Surg 214:581, 1991.
10. Cameron JL, Maddrey WC: Mesoatrial shunt: A new treatment for the Budd-Chiari syndrome. Ann Surg 187:42, 1978.

11. Halff G, Todo S, Tsakis A, et al: Liver transplantation for the Budd-Chiari syndrome. Ann Surg 211:43, 1990.

12. Campbell DA, Rolles K, Jamieson N, et al: Hepatic transplantation with perioperative and long-term anticoagulants as treatment for Budd-Chiari syndrome. Surg Gynecol Obstet 166:511, 1988.

13. Maza M, Prager MC: Anesthesia and the liver. *In* Miller RD (ed): Anesthesia. 3rd ed. New York, Churchill Livingstone, 1990.

14. Carmichael FJ, Lindop MJ, Farman JV: Anesthesia for hepatic transplantation: Cardiovascular and metabolic alterations in management. Anesth Analg 64:108, 1985.

15. Yao EH, Kong MC, Hsue GL, et al: Pulmonary function changes in cirrhosis of the liver. Am J Gastroenterol 82:352, 1987.

16. Krowka MJ, Cortese DA: Pulmonary aspects of chronic liver disease and liver transplantation. Mayo Clin Proc 60:407, 1985.

17. Mullen KD, Martin JV, Mendelson WB, et al: Could an endogenous benzodiazepine ligand contribute to hepatic encephalopathy? Lancet 1:457, 1988.

18. Sirinek KR, Adcock DK, Levine BA: Simultaneous infusion of nitroglycerin and nitroprusside to offset adverse effects of vasopressin during portosystemic shunting. Am J Surg 157:33, 1989.

19. Helton WS, Belshaw A, Althaus S, et al: Critical appraisal of the angiographic portacaval shunt (TIPS). Am J Surg 165:566, 1993.

20. Orloff MJ, Bell RH Jr: Long-term survival after emergency portacaval shunting for bleeding varices in patients with alcoholic cirrhosis. Am J Surg 151:176, 1986.

21. Burroughs AK, Hamilton G, Phillips A, et al: A comparison of sclerotherapy with staple transection of the esophagus for the emergency control of bleeding from esophageal varices. N Engl J Med 321:857, 1989.

22. Webb LJ, Sherlock S: The etiology, presentation and natural history of extrahepatic portal venous obstruction. Q J Med 48:627, 1979.

23. Okuda K, Ohnishi K, Kimura K, et al: Incidence of portal vein thrombosis and liver cirrhosis: An angiographic study in 708 patients. Gastroenterology 89:279, 1985.

24. Schafer AL: The hypercoagulable state. Ann Intern Med 102:814, 1985.

25. Gorini P, Johansen K: Use of the inferior mesenteric vein for portal decompression. J Cardiovasc Surg (Torino) (In press).

26. Little AG, Moossa AR: Gastrointestinal hemorrhage from left-sided portal hypertension: An unappreciated complication of pancreatitis. Am J Surg 141:153, 1981.

27. Britton RC, Crile G: Late results of transesophageal suture of bleeding esophageal varices. Surg Gynecol Obstet 117:10, 1963.

28. Boerema I: Bleeding varices of the esophagus in cirrhosis of the liver and Banti's disease. Arch Chir Neerland 1:253, 1949.

29. Hassab MA: Gastroesophageal decongestion and splenectomy in the treatment of esophageal varices in bilharzial cirrhosis: Further studies with the report of 355 operations. Surgery 61:169, 1967.

30. Peters RM, Womack NA: Surgery of vascular distortions in cirrhosis of the liver. Ann Surg 154:432, 1961.

31. Sugiura M, Futagawa S: Results of 636 esophageal transections with paraesophagogastric devascularization in the treatment of esophageal varices. J Vasc Surg 1:254, 1984.

32. Del Guercio LRM, Hodgson WJB, Morgan JC, et al: Splenic artery and coronary vein occlusion for bleeding esophageal varices. World J Surg 8:680, 1984.

33. Johnston GW: Six years' experience of esophageal varices using a circular stapling gun. Gut 23:770, 1982.

34. Wanamaker SR, Cooperman M, Carey L: Use of the EEA stapling instrument for control of bleeding esophageal varices. Surgery 94:620, 1983.

35. Durtschi M, Carrico CJ, Johansen KH: Esophageal transection fails to salvage high-risk patients with variceal bleeding. Am J Surg 150:18, 1985.

36. Foster JH, Stoney WS, Scott HW: An experimental study of thoracic transposition of the spleen: A method of portal decompression. Surgery 49:223, 1961.

37. Eck NV: On the question of ligature of the portal vein. Voen Med J 130:1, 1877 [Translated in Surg Gynecol Obstet 96:375, 1953.]

38. Pavlov IP: On a modification of the Eck fistula between the portal vein and the inferior vena cava. Arch Sci Biol 2:580, 1893.

39. Whipple AO: The problem of portal hypertension in relation to the hepatosplenopathies. Ann Surg 122:499, 1945.

40. Sherlock S, Summerskill WHJ, White LP, et al: Portosystemic encephalopathy: Neurological complications of liver disease. Lancet 2:453, 1954.

41. Jackson FC, Perrin EB, Felix WR, et al: A clinical investigation of the portacaval shunt: V. Survival analysis of the therapeutic operation. Ann Surg 174:672, 1971.

42. Resnick RH, Iber FL, Ishihara AM, et al: A controlled study of the portacaval shunt. Gastroenterology 67:843, 1974.

43. Rueff B, Degos F, Degos JD, et al: A controlled study of therapeutic portacaval shunt in alcoholic cirrhosis. Lancet 1:655, 1976.

44. Reynolds TB, Donovan AJ, Mikkelson WP, et al: Results of a 12 year randomized trial of portacaval shunt in patients with alcoholic liver disease and bleeding varices. Gastroenterology 80:1005, 1981.

45. Conn HO, Lindemuth WW, May LJ, et al: Prophylactic portacaval anastomosis: A tale of two studies. Medicine 51:27, 1972.

46. Starzl TE, Porter KA, Francavilla JA: One Hundred Years of the Hepatotrophic Controversy: Hepatotrophic Factors. CIBA Symposium. Amsterdam, Elsevier Excerpta Medica, 1978.

47. Drapanas T, LoCicero J, Dowling JB: Hemodynamics of the interposition mesocaval shunt. Ann Surg 181:523, 1975.

48. Smith RB, Warren WD, Salam AA, et al: Dacron interposition shunts for portal hypertension: An analysis of morbidity correlates. Ann Surg 192:9, 1980.

49. Paquet K-J, Mercado MA, Gad HA: Surgical procedures for bleeding esophagogastric varices when sclerotherapy fails: A prospective study. Am J Surg 160:43, 1990.

50. Stipa S, Ziparo V, Anza M, et al: A randomized controlled trial of mesentericocaval shunt with autologous jugular vein. Surg Gynecol Obstet 153:353, 1981.

51. Warren WD, Zeppa R, Fomon JJ: Selective transplenic decompression of gastroesophageal varices by distal splenorenal shunt. Arch Surg 168:437, 1967.

52. Warren WD: Control of variceal bleeding. Reassessment of rationale. Am J Surg 145:8, 1983.

53. Millikan WJ, Warren WD, Henderson JM, et al: The Emory prospective randomized trial: Selective vs. nonselective shunt to control variceal bleeding. Ten-year follow-up. Ann Surg 201:712, 1985.

54. Warren WD, Millikan WJ, Henderson JM, et al: Splenopancreatic disconnection: Improved selectivity of distal splenorenal shunt. Ann Surg 204:346, 1986.

55. Maillard GN, Flamant YM, Chandler JG: Selectivity of the distal splenorenal shunt. Surgery 86:663, 1979.

56. Belghiti J, Grenier P, Nouel O, et al: Long term loss of Warren's shunt selectivity. Angiographic demonstration. Arch Surg 116:1121, 1981.

57. Henderson JM, Millikan WJ Jr, Wright-Bacon L, et al: Hemodynamic differences between alcoholic and non-alcoholic cirrhotics following distal splenorenal shunt: Effect on survival? Ann Surg 204:346, 1983.

58. Harley HAJ, Morgan T, Redecker AG, et al: Results of a randomized trial of end-to-side portacaval shunt and distal splenorenal shunt in alcoholic liver disease and variceal bleeding. Gastroenterology 91:802, 1986.

59. Grace ND, Conn HO, Resnick RH, et al: Distal splenorenal vs. portal systemic shunts after hemorrhage from varices: A randomized controlled trial. Hepatology 8:1475, 1988.

60. Spina GP, Galeotti F, Opocher E, et al: Selective distal splenorenal shunt. Clinical results of a prospective controlled study. Am J Surg 155:564, 1988.

61. Inokuchi K, Beppu K, Koyanagi N, et al: Fifteen years experience with left gastric venous caval shunt for esophageal varices. World J Surg 8:716, 1984.

62. Burchell AR, Moreno AH, Panke WF, Nealon TF: Hepatic artery flow improvement after portacaval shunt: A single hemodynamic clinical correlate. Ann Surg 192:9, 1976.

63. Marion P, Balique JG, George M, et al: Anastomose porta-cave latero-laterale a debit minimum pour cirrhose haemorrhagique. Med Chir Dig 10:245, 1981.

64. Bismuth H, Franco D, Hepp J: Portal-systemic shunt in hepatic cirrhosis: Does the type of shunt decisively influence the clinical results? Ann Surg 179:209, 1974.

65. Sarfeh IJ, Rypins EB, Conroy RM, et al: Portacaval H-graft: Relationship of shunt diameter, portal flow patterns and encephalopathy. Ann Surg 197:422, 1988.

66. Rypins EB, Sarfeh IJ: Influence of portal hemodynamics on long-term survival of alcoholic patients after small diameter portocaval H-grafts. Am J Surg 155:152, 1988.

67. Rosemurgy AS, McAllister EW, Kearney RE: Prospective study of a prosthetic H-graft portacaval shunt. Am J Surg 161:159, 1991.

68. Helton WS, Montana M, Dwyer D, Johansen KH: Duplex sonography accurately assesses portacaval shunt patency. J Vasc Surg 8:657, 1988.

69. Johansen KH: Partial portal decompression for variceal hemorrhage. Am J Surg 157:479, 1989.

70. Johansen KH, Girod C, Lee SS, Lebrec D: Mesenteric venous stenosis reduces hyperammonemia in the portacaval-shunted rat. Eur Surg Res 22:170, 1990.

71. Johansen KH: Prospective comparison of partial versus total portal decompression for bleeding esophageal varices. Surg Gynecol Obstet 175:528, 1992.

72. Rikkers LF: Portal hemodynamics, intestinal absorption and post-shunt encephalopathy. Ann Surg 94:126, 1983.

73. Kumar S, Stauber RE, Gavaler JS, et al: Orthotopic liver transplantation for alcoholic liver disease. Hepatology 11:159, 1990.

74. Campbell DA Jr, Merion RM, McCurry KR, et al: The role of liver transplantation in the management of the patient with variceal hemorrhage. Probl Gen Surg 9:3, 1992.

75. Rikkers LF, Jin G, Burnett DA, et al: Shunt surgery versus endoscopic sclerotherapy for variceal hemorrhage: Late results of a randomized trial. Am J Surg 165:27, 1993.

76. Conn HO: A peek at the Child-Turcotte classification. Hepatology 1:673, 1981.

77. Millikan WJ, Henderson JM, Stewart MT, et al: Change in hepatic function, hemodynamics and morphology after liver transplant. Ann Surg 209:513, 1989.

78. Martin M, Zajko AB, Orons P, et al: Transjugular intrahepatic porta-systemic shunt (TIPS) in the management of variceal hemorrhage: Indications and clinical results. Surgery 114:719, 1993.

79. Langnas AN, Marujo WC, Stratta RJ, et al: Influence of a prior porta-systemic shunt on outcome after liver transplantation. Am J Gastro-enterol, 87:6, 1992.

80. Mazzaferro V, Todo S, Tzakis AG, et al: Liver transplantation in patients with previous porta-systemic shunt. Am J Surg 160:111, 1990.

Surgical Management of Renovascular Disorders

Edited by Richard H. Dean, M.D., B.A.

࿕

105

Renovascular Hypertension: An Overview

Richard H. Dean, M.D., B.A.

• • •

Although hypertension has been recognized for centuries, the importance of its identification and treatment has been appreciated only since the 1830s. Most commonly, hypertension is a silent process and is manifested only by the sequelae of acceleration in the rate of atherogenesis and the frequency of cardiovascular morbid and mortal events. Uncommonly, the hypertension may be so severe that the elevated pressure itself produces vessel wall injury and the clinical picture of malignant hypertension. Although most physicians appreciate the potentially lethal nature of this malignant variety and the importance of its control, physician apathy toward the merits of aggressive diagnostic evaluation and management of asymptomatic patients with less severe hypertension continues to limit the impact of current knowledge on population-wide success with treatment of this disorder.

Bright of Guy's Hospital, London, called attention to the association of hypertension with renal disease in 1836.[1] He observed the apparent association between hardness of the pulse, dropsy, albuminuria, and granular shrunken kidneys. This is especially remarkable because the modern sphygmomanometer was not described until 1896. Although Bright's observation stimulated much interest in the kidney, 70 years passed before Tigerstedt and Bergman, in 1897, discovered a renal pressor substance in the rabbit.[31] They called this crude extract renin. Confirmation of a renovascular source of hypertension, however, awaited Goldblatt's classic experiment.[10] In 1934, he and coworkers showed that constriction of the renal artery produced atrophy of the kidney and hypertension in the dog. After this documentation of a renovascular origin of hypertension,

many patients were treated by nephrectomy because they had hypertension and a small kidney revealed by intravenous pyelography. Curiously, there was rarely any interest in documenting a renal artery occlusive lesion in any of these patients. Dissatisfaction with the results of this form of treatment prompted Smith, in 1956, to review 575 cases treated in this manner.[26] He found only a 26 per cent rate of cure of hypertension by nephrectomy with the use of his criteria, which led him to suggest that nephrectomy should be performed only for strict urologic indications. Two years earlier, however, Freeman and associates had performed an aortic and bilateral renal artery thromboendarterectomy on a hypertensive patient, with the resultant resolution of the hypertension.[9] This was the first cure of hypertension by renal revascularization.

DeCamp and Birchall, Morris and associates, and others soon followed with additional descriptions of relief of hypertension by renal revascularization.[7, 16, 19, 23] Concomitant with the appearance of these reports, aortography began to be widely used. During the late 1950s, many centers were demonstrating renal artery stenosis aortographically in hypertensive patients and then performing either aortorenal bypass or thromboendarterectomy. Nevertheless, by 1960, it became apparent that revascularization in hypertensive individuals with renal artery stenosis was associated with reduction of blood pressure in fewer than 50 per cent. General pessimism followed regarding the merits of operative treatment of hypertension.

As this experience pointed out, the coexistence of renal artery stenosis and hypertension does not establish a causal relationship. Many normotensive patients, especially those past the age of 50, have renal artery stenosis. Obviously, special studies are required to establish the functional significance of renal artery lesions. The most recent era in the history of the operative treatment of renovascular hypertension began with the introduction of meaningful tests of split renal function by Howard and Conner and by Stamey and associates.[14, 28] Further, the work of Page and Helmer and others in the identification of the renin-angiotensin system of blood pressure control added a new dimension to physicians' understanding of renovascular hypertension.[2, 18, 24, 32] With the more recently developed accurate methods of measuring plasma renin activity, the physician can now accurately predict which renal artery lesion is producing renovascular hypertension. The author's experience has shown that if the findings of split renal function studies or renal vein renin assays are positive, a good response in blood pressure can be expected after successful surgery in more than 95 per cent of cases.[5]

However, the incidence of renovascular hypertension, the need for its identification, and the value of operative management remain poorly defined. Some centers routinely evaluate hypertensive patients for a renovascular origin of the disorder and submit suitable candidates to the appropriate interventional treatment. Other centers seldom study patients for renovascular hypertension and even more uncommonly select operative management for this form of hypertension. Several factors have led to this disparity in approaches. Among the reasons for it are the emphasis in some reports on the infrequency of a renovascular cause of hypertension, the low cost-effectiveness of diagnostic investigation, the infrequent cure of hypertension by operation, and improvements in management by drug therapy. Unfortunately, inappropriately biased collection of data and conflicting results of studies in these areas have engendered a lack of uniformity in concepts regarding the value of diagnostic study and the merits of operative treatment. In this section, diagnostic studies and methods of management of the respective causes of renovascular disease and hypertension are reviewed, with an emphasis on the current status of their value and the results of their use.

INCIDENCE

Renovascular hypertension is generally thought to affect 5 to 10 per cent of the hypertensive population. Tucker and Labarthe suggested an even lower prevalence.[33] Estimates of the prevalence of hypertension in the United States from all causes vary from 30 to 60 million people and from 10 to 15 per cent of the adult population. The incidence of renovascular hypertension is undoubtedly low indeed in this general hypertensive population if all patients with even mild hypertension are included. Because the renovascular form tends to be relatively severe, its prevalence in the large subpopulation of mildly hypertensive patients (those with an untreated diastolic blood pressure of less than 105 mmHg) is probably negligible. In contrast, however, it occurs frequently in the smaller group of severely hypertensive people. Hollifield investigated 137 patients with previously unrecognized hypertension discovered through a shopping center screening program (Table 105–1).[13] Diagnostic study of these patients included arteriography and, when appropriate, renal vein renin assays and split renal function studies. None of the 102 patients with diastolic blood pressure between 90 and 115 mmHg had renovascular hypertension. In contrast, 9 of the 35 patients (26 per cent) with diastolic blood pressure of 118 mmHg or higher did have it. Further, if these numbers are broken down according to race, the results are even more informative. In the more severely hypertensive group, none of the 13 black patients had renovascular hypertension, whereas the disorder occurred in 9 of the 22 white patients (41 per cent) in this group. Similarly, Davis and colleagues showed a 31 per cent incidence of renovascular hypertension in 85 patients initially evaluated at Vanderbilt University for malignant hypertension.[3]

In the author's experience, severe hypertension at the two extremes of life carries the highest probability of being of renovascular origin. The review by the author's group of the causes of hypertension in 74 children admitted for diagnostic evaluation over a 5-year period showed that in 78 per cent of those younger than 5 years of age, it had a correctable renovascular origin (Table 105–2).[17] Interestingly, after childhood, the age group that is next most likely to have renovascular hypertension is the elderly. In the author's experience, 33 per cent of patients over 60 years of age admitted for evaluation have had the disorder. Certainly, these elderly patients represent the more severe spectrum of hypertension, for those with less severe levels most likely would not have been referred to the author's center.

On the basis of these data, it is inappropriate to view hypertensive patients as a homogeneous group with respect to the prevalence of renovascular hypertension. Rather, the probability of finding a renovascular origin correlates with the severity of the hypertension. Accordingly, the search for the disease should be directed to the subset of patients with the more severe degree of hypertension. It must be remembered, however, that severity of hypertension is

Table 105–2. Classification of Hypertension in 74 Children

Type of Hypertension	No. of Patients			
	0–5 Years	*6–10 Years*	*11–15 Years*	*16–20 Years*
Essential	1	5	24	21
Correctable	8 (78%)	4 (44%)	5 (17%)	6 (22%)
Total	9	9	29	27

Table 105–1. Results of Screening 137 New Hypertensive Patients

Parameter	Total	With Renovascular Hypertension	Per Cent
Diastolic blood pressure			
90–115 mmHg	102	0	
>117 mmHg	35	9	26
Race			
Black	13	0	
White	22	9	41

based on its level without medication and does not take into account the difficulty of its control by drug therapy.

CHARACTERISTICS

Because of the relative infrequency of renovascular hypertension in the entire hypertensive population, many reports have focused on the value of demographic factors, physical findings, and screening tests to discriminate between it and essential hypertension as a basis for deciding to pursue further diagnostic study. Most frequently quoted among these are recent onset of hypertension, young age, lack of family history of hypertension, and presence of an abdominal bruit. The most complete study comparing the clinical characteristics of patients with renovascular hypertension and those with essential hypertension was the Cooperative Study of Renovascular Hypertension.[25] This study compared the prevalence of certain clinical characteristics in 339 patients who had essential hypertension with their prevalence in 175 patients who had renovascular hypertension secondary to atherosclerotic lesions (91 patients) or fibromuscular dysplasia (84 patients). A summary of the differential points identified in this study is presented in Table 105–3. Although several characteristics show signif-

icant differences in prevalence between the two disorders, *none* of them has sufficient discriminative value to be used to exclude patients from further diagnostic investigation for renovascular hypertension. Certainly, the finding of an epigastric bruit in a young white woman with malignant hypertension is strongly suggestive of a renovascular origin of the hypertension. However, the absence of such criteria does not exclude the presence of the disease, and such criteria should not be used to eliminate patients from further diagnostic study.

The demographic characteristics of patients with renovascular hypertension who present for operative management have evolved since the early 1960s. Of the first 122 patients with renovascular hypertension treated at Vanderbilt University Hospital, 52 per cent had a family history of hypertension, 46 per cent had no audible abdominal bruit, ages ranged from 4 months to 69 years (mean, 46 years), and duration of hypertension ranged from 2 months to 20 years (mean, 4.8 years).[8] Comparison of these data with the author's most recent experience since 1988 at Wake Forest University underscores the evolving characteristics of patients currently undergoing operation (Table 105–4).[12] Because renovascular hypertension can be secondary to any of several processes affecting the renal artery and because each of these diseases has its own clinical characteristics, it

Table 105–3.   Clinical Considerations in Hypertension and Renovascular Hypertension

	Essential Hypertension (339 cases)		Renovascular Hypertension			
			Arteriosclerotic (91 cases)		Fibromuscular (84 cases)	
	Per Cent	Years	Per Cent	Years	Per Cent	Years
History						
Average age		41		48		35
< 20 years	2		1		14	
Average duration		3.1		1.9		2.0
< 1 year	10		23		19	
> 10 years	23		12		10	
Average age at onset		35		46		33*
> 50 years	7		39		3*	
< 20 years	12		2		16*	
Sex (female)	40		34		81	
Race (black)	29		7		10	
Acceleration of hypertension	13		23		14*	
Family history						
Hypertension	67		68*		41	
Stroke	37		44*		22	
Neither of foregoing	19		30*		46	
Symptoms						
Nocturia	38		55		35	
Weakness, fatigue	32		49		42*	
Angina						
Headache						
All of foregoing	0		14		10	
Previous vascular occlusive disease	10		20		6*	
Physical examination						
Body habitus						
Obese	38		17		11	
Thin	6		13*		30	
Fundi (grades 3 and 4)	12		26		10*	
Bruit						
Abdomen	6		38		55	
Flank	1		8		20	
Abdomen or flank	7		41		57	

From Simon N, Franklin SS, Bleifer KH, et al: Clinical characteristics of renovascular hypertension. JAMA 220:1209, 1972.

Table 105–4. Comparison of Earlier Surgical Experience With Current Series

	1961–1972*	1987–1991†
Number of patients	122	200
Mean age (yr)		
NAs-RVD	33	38
As-RVD	50	62
Duration of hypertension (yr)		
NAs-RVD	4.6	11.2
As-RVD	5.1	15.0
Renal artery disease (%)		
NAs-RVD	35	21
As-RVD	65	29
Renal artery repair (%)		
Unilateral	80	60
Bilateral	20	40
Combined‡	13	32
Renal insufficiency (%)		
Not dependent on dialysis	8	65
Dependent on dialysis	0	6
Graft failure (%)	16	3
Hypertension response (%)		
NAs-RVD		
Cured	72§	43
Improved	24§	49
As-RVD		
Cured	53§	15
Improved	36§	75

*Adapted from Foster JH, Dean RH, Pinkerton JA, et al: Ten years experience with the surgical management of renovascular hypertension. Ann Surg 177:755, 1973.

†Data from Hansen KJ, Starr SM, Sands E, et al: Contemporary surgical management of renovascular disease. J Vasc Surg 16:319, 1992.

‡Combined aortic repair for occlusive or aneurysmal disease.

§Hypertension response excluding technical failures.

As-RVD, atherosclerotic renovascular disease; NAs-RVD, nonatherosclerotic renovascular disease.

is not surprising that exclusion of patients from further study because of demographic or physical findings such as age, abdominal bruit, and duration of hypertension would risk inappropriately excluding patients with renovascular hypertension. Therefore, the decision for diagnostic study should be based on the severity of hypertension. Mild hypertension has a minimal chance of being renovascular in origin. In contrast, the more severe the hypertension, the greater the probability that it is from a correctable cause. With this in mind, the author submits all patients with diastolic blood pressure above 105 mmHg who would be acceptable candidates for operation to evaluation for a correctable origin of hypertension.

DIAGNOSTIC EVALUATION

The initial general evaluation of all hypertensive patients is outlined in Table 105–5. Electrocardiography is important to gauge the extent of secondary myocardial hypertrophy or associated ischemic heart disease. Serum electrolyte and serial serum potassium determinations can effectively exclude patients with primary aldosteronism if potassium levels are greater than 3.0 mg/100 ml. One must remember, however, that hypokalemia is most often due to salt-depleting diets and previous diuretic therapy. Estimation of renal function is mandatory. Preexisting renal dis-

ease may reduce renal function and cause hypertension. Further, hypertension from any cause may produce intrarenal arteriolar nephrosclerosis and subsequent depression of renal function. Finally, when the history or physical examination findings are suggestive, assessment of the urinary 17-hydroxysteroid and 17-ketosteroid and vanillylmandelic acid levels should be performed to identify effectively the rare patient with a pheochromocytoma or a functioning adrenocortical tumor.

Identification of a noninvasive screening test that will accurately identify all patients with renovascular disease that might require interventional management remains an elusive goal. Determination of peripheral plasma renin activity, rapid-sequence intravenous pyelography, and saralasin infusion are examples of tests that have been abandoned. Isotope renography continues to be proposed as a valuable screening test, but the methods employed are continuously modified in hopes of improving the sensitivity and specificity. The newest versions of isotope renography consist of renal scanning performed before and after exercise or captopril infusion. With these methods, a test result is interpreted as positive when there is augmentation of derangements in renal perfusion after exercise or captopril infusion.[21] Although these methods have improved the specificity of isotope renography, their reliance on activation of the renin-angiotensin system leads to an unacceptable incidence of false-negative results.

The author's bias is that screening tests that image the vascular anatomy and assess the hemodynamics of renal flow are the most promising methods of widespread screening for renovascular disease. In this regard, vascular imaging using magnetic resonance imaging or positron emission tomography may hold great promise. Current expense, lack of widespread availability, and limitations of patient selection criteria prevent its application as a screening tool except in the most unusual circumstances.

Renal duplex sonography has been proposed by several investigators as a useful screening test with which candidates for arteriography can be identified. The author's group has reported its experience with duplex sonography and has evaluated the sensitivity and specificity of this method for identifying renovascular occlusive disease.[11] The study population for renal duplex sonography validity analysis consisted of 74 consecutive patients who had 77 comparative renal duplex sonographic and standard angiographic studies of the arterial anatomy to 148 kidneys. Renal duplex sonography results from 6 kidneys (4 per cent) were considered inadequate for interpretation. This study population contained 26 patients (35 per cent) with severe renal insufficiency (mean serum creatinine level, 3.6

Table 105–5.   General Evaluation of Patients With Hypertension

History and physical examination
Hemogram, SMA-12, urinalysis, urine culture, serum potassium (3 times)
Electrocardiogram and chest x-ray study
Analysis of 24-hour urine collection for creatinine clearance, electrolytes, catecholamines, vanillylmandelic acid, and 17-hydroxysteroids and 17-ketosteroids
Rapid-sequence intravenous pyelogram
Renal arteriogram

SMA-12, Sequential Multiple Analyzer (12-test serum profile).

mg/dl) and 67 individuals with hypertension (91 per cent). Fourteen patients (19 per cent) had 20 kidneys with multiple renal arteries. Renal duplex sonography correctly identified the presence of renovascular disease in 41 of 44 patients with angiographically proven lesions, and renovascular disease was not identified in any patient free of disease. When single renal arteries were present (122 kidneys), renal duplex sonography provided a 93 per cent sensitivity, a 98 per cent specificity, a 98 per cent positive predictive value, a 94 per cent negative predictive value, and an overall accuracy of 96 per cent. These results were adversely affected when kidneys with multiple (polar) renal arteries were examined. Although the end-diastolic ratio was inversely correlated with serum creatinine ($r = .30773$; $p = .009$), a low end-diastolic ratio in 35 patients submitted to renovascular reconstruction did not preclude beneficial blood pressure or renal function response. The author's group concluded from this analysis that renal duplex sonography can be a valuable screening test in the search for correctable renovascular disease causing global renal ischemia and secondary renal insufficiently (ischemic nephropathy). Renal duplex sonography does not, however, exclude polar vessel renovascular disease causing hypertension alone, nor does it predict hypertension or renal function response after correction of renovascular disease.

With these results in mind, the author's group now uses renal duplex sonography as the screening tool of choice. Nevertheless, because it does not accurately identify accessory vessels or branch vessel disease, they proceed to arteriography when hypertension is severe, is difficult to control, or is occurring in pediatric patients.

Both aortography and selective renal arteriography with multiple projections may be necessary to examine the entire renal artery adequately. Orificial lesions are best seen with aortography. Because the renal artery often arises from a posterolateral site, oblique projections are required to visualize this portion of the vessel. Finally, multiple renal arteries are seen in about 25 per cent of hypertensive patients, and each of these must be scrutinized for hidden areas of stenosis.

When an obstructive lesion is found by renal arteriography, its functional significance should be evaluated. Most centers now rely solely on renal vein renin assays to establish the diagnosis of renovascular hypertension. The pathophysiology of the disease and functional tests that examine the renin-angiotensin pressor system are discussed in the following chapter and are not detailed further here.

With the advent of renal vein renin assays, most centers have stopped using split renal function studies because of the associated discomfort, possible complications, and confusing results. However, valuable information can be obtained from these studies that is not obtained from renal vein renin assays. Information regarding the likelihood that a severely ischemic, poorly functioning kidney is viable and can have function retrieved by revascularization is one of the benefits of split renal function studies.

THERAPEUTIC OPTIONS

Identification of the optimal method of treating patients with renovascular hypertension remains an elusive goal. Advocates of drug therapy, operative management, and percutaneous transluminal angioplasty separately defend their viewpoints with selective data from the literature to strengthen the validity of their arguments. The majority of the medical community still evaluates patients for renovascular hypertension only when medications are not tolerated and hypertension remains severe and uncontrolled. The report by Hunt and Strong remains the most informative study available for assessing the comparative values of drug therapy and operation.[15] These investigators compared the results of operative treatment in 100 patients with the results of drug therapy in 114 similar patients. After 7 to 14 years of follow-up, 84 per cent of the patients who were operated on were alive, as compared with 66 per cent in the drug therapy group. Furthermore, of the 84 patients alive in the group that was operated on, 93 per cent were cured or had significantly improvement, whereas 16 (21 per cent) of the patients alive in the drug therapy group had required surgery for uncontrollable hypertension. Another 7 patients continued to have uncontrolled disease but did not undergo operative treatment. Death during follow-up was twice as common in the medically treated group. These differences were statistically significant ($p < .01$) both in patients with atherosclerotic lesions and in those with fibromuscular lesions of the renal artery.

Additional data influencing the decision for operative management of renovascular hypertension in the atherosclerotic patient are the anatomic and renal function changes that occur during drug therapy. The author's group reported the results of serial renal function studies performed on 41 patients with renovascular hypertension secondary to atherosclerotic renal artery disease who were randomly selected for nonoperative management (Table 105–6).[6] In 19 patients, serum creatinine levels increased between 25 and 120 per cent. The glomerular filtration rates dropped between 25 and 50 per cent in 12 patients. Fourteen patients (37 per cent) lost more than 10 per cent of renal length. In 4 patients (12 per cent), a significant stenosis progressed to total occlusion. Seventeen patients (41 per cent) had deterioration of renal function or loss of renal size that led to

Table 105–6. Frequency of Severe Deterioration in Parameters of Renal Function

Parameter	No. of Patients Followed Up	Mean Follow-up (mo)	Failure Event	No. Affected	Per Cent Affected
Renal length	38	33	≥ 10% decrease	14	37
Serum creatinine level	41	25	≥100% increase	2	5
Glomerular filtration rate or creatinine clearance	30	19	≥ 50% decrease	1	3

operation. One patient required removal of a previously reconstructable kidney. Of the 17 patients in whom renal function deteriorated, 15 had acceptable control of blood pressure during the period of nonoperative observation. Therefore, the author's group believes that progressive deterioration of renal function in nonoperatively treated patients with atherosclerotic renal artery stenosis and renovascular hypertension is common and occurs even in the presence of blood pressure control with drugs.

The detrimental changes that occur during drug therapy and the current excellent results of operative management argue for an aggressive attitude toward renal revascularization in the treatment of renovascular hypertension.[5] The author's indications for interventional management have been outlined in detail elsewhere.[4] Nevertheless, in brief, all patients with severe, difficult-to-control hypertension should be considered for intervention. This includes patients with complicating factors such as branch lesions and extrarenal vascular disease and patients with associated cardiovascular disease that would be improved by blood pressure reduction.

Young patients whose hypertension is moderate, who complain of no diseases, and who have an easily correctable atherosclerotic or fibromuscular main renal artery stenosis also are candidates for intervention. The chance for cure of moderate hypertension is quite good in such patients who have no complicating factors. It remains to be proved that drug control is ever as good as the complete cure of hypertension. In fact, it could be argued that reduction in the driving pressure of blood flow across the stenosis by successful drug therapy might accelerate deterioration in renal function by further reducing renal perfusion.

Finally, there is no clear evidence that age, type of lesion (whether atherosclerotic or fibromuscular), duration of hypertension, or presence of bilateral lesions by themselves has proven value as a determinant of operative risk or of the likelihood of successful management. They should not, therefore, be considered deterrents to such management.

CURRENT STATUS OF PERCUTANEOUS TRANSLUMINAL ANGIOPLASTY AND OPERATIVE MANAGEMENT

The decision regarding the initial use of percutaneous transluminal angioplasty or operation continues to be controversial. A detailed discussion of the use of percutaneous transluminal angioplasty is provided in Chapter 107. Nevertheless, a brief overview of its use is appropriate.

Experience with the liberal use of percutaneous transluminal angioplasty has helped to clarify its role as one of the therapeutic options in the treatment of renovascular hypertension, but data now accumulated argue for its selective application. In this regard, percutaneous transluminal angioplasty of nonorificial atherosclerotic lesions and medial fibrodysplastic lesions limited to the main renal artery yields results comparable to the results of operation if carried out by those experienced in this technique.[20, 22, 27, 29, 30] In contrast, the use of percutaneous transluminal angio-

plasty for the treatment of congenital lesions, of fibrodysplastic lesions involving renal artery branches, and of ostial atherosclerotic lesions is associated with inferior results and increased risk of complications. For this reason, the author believes that operation remains the initial treatment of choice for patients in these latter groups and that the decision for interventional therapy for renovascular hypertension must be individualized.

References

1. Bright R: Cases and observations illustrative of renal disease accompanied with the secretion of albuminous urine. Guy's Hosp Rep 1:388, 1836.
2. Bruan-Memendez E, Fasciolo JC, Lelois LF, et al: La substancia hipertensora de la sangre del rinon, isquemiado. Rev Soc Argent Biol 15:420, 1939.
3. Davis BA, Crook JE, Vestal RE, et al: Prevalence of renovascular hypertension in patients with grade III or IV hypertensive retinopathy. N Engl J Med 301:1273, 1979.
4. Dean RH: Indications for operative management of renovascular hypertension. J S C Med Assoc 73:523, 1977.
5. Dean RH: Operative management of renovascular hypertension. *In* Bergan JJ, Yao JST (eds): Surgery of the Aorta and Its Body Branches. New York, Grune & Stratton, 1979, p 377.
6. Dean RH, Kieffer RW, Smith BM, et al: Renovascular hypertension. Arch Surg 116:1408, 1981.
7. DeCamp PT, Birchall R: Recognition and treatment of renal arterial stenosis associated with hypertension. Surgery 43:134, 1958.
8. Foster JH, Dean RH, Pinkerton JA, et al: Ten years experience with the surgical management of renovascular hypertension. Ann Surg 177:755, 1973.
9. Freeman NE, Leeds FH, Elliott WG, et al: Thromboendarterectomy for hypertension due to renal artery occlusion. JAMA 156:1077, 1954.
10. Goldblatt H: Studies on experimental hypertension. J Exp Med 59:347, 1934.
11. Hansen KJ, Trible RW, Reavis SW, et al: Renal duplex sonography: Evaluation of clinical utility. J Vasc Surg 12:227, 1990.
12. Hansen KJ, Starr SM, Sands E, et al: Contemporary surgical management of renovascular disease. J Vasc Surg 16:319, 1992.
13. Hollifield JW: Unpublished data.
14. Howard JE, Conner TB: Use of differential renal function studies in the diagnosis of renovascular hypertension. Am J Surg 107:58, 1964.
15. Hunt JC, Strong CG: Renovascular hypertension. Mechanisms, natural history and treatment. Am J Cardiol 32:562, 1973.
16. Hurwitt ES, Seidenberg B, Haimovici H, et al: Splenorenal arterial anastomosis. Circulation 14:537, 1956.
17. Lawson JD, Boerth RK, Foster JH, et al: Diagnosis and management of renovascular hypertension in children. Arch Surg 112:1307, 1977.
18. Lentz KE, Skeggs LT Jr, Woods KR, et al: The amino acid composition of hypertensin II and its biochemical relationship to hypertensin I. J Exp Med 104:183, 1956.
19. Luke JC, Levitan BA: Revascularization of the kidney in hypertension due to renal artery stenosis. Arch Surg 79:269, 1959.
20. Martin LG, Casarella WJ, Alspaugh JP, et al: Renal artery angioplasty: Increased technical success and decreased complications in the second 100 patients. Radiology 159:631, 1986.
21. Meier GH, Sumpio B, Black HR, Gusberg RJ: Captopril renal scintigraphy—An advance in the detection and treatment of renovascular hypertension. J Vasc Surg 11:770, 1990.
22. Miller GA, Ford KK, Braun SD, et al: Percutaneous transluminal angioplasty vs surgery for renovascular hypertension. AJR 144:447, 1985.
23. Morris GC Jr, Cooley DA, Crawford ES, et al: Renal revascularization for hypertension. Clinical and physiologic studies in 32 cases. Surgery 48:95, 1960.
24. Page IH, Helmer OM: A crystalline pressor substance (angiotonin) resulting from the reaction between renin and renin activator. J Exp Med 71:29, 1940.
25. Simon N, Franklin SS, Bleifer KH, et al: Clinical characteristics of renovascular hypertension. JAMA 220:1209, 1972.
26. Smith HW: Unilateral nephrectomy in hypertensive disease. J Urol 76:685, 1956.

27. Sos TA, Pickering TG, Sniderman K, et al: Percutaneous transluminal renal angioplasty in renovascular hypertension due to atheroma or fibromuscular dysplasia. N Engl J Med 309:274, 1983.
28. Stamey TA, Nudelman IJ, Good PH, et al: Functional characteristics of renovascular hypertension. Medicine (Baltimore) 40:347, 1961.
29. Tegtmeyer CJ, Kellum CD, Ayers C: Percutaneous transluminal angioplasty of the renal artery. Results and long-term follow-up. Radiology 153:77, 1984.
30. Tegtmeyer CJ, Teates CD, Crigler N, et al: Percutaneous transluminal angioplasty in patients with renal artery stenosis. Radiology 140:323, 1981.
31. Tigerstedt R, Bergman PG: Niere und Kreislauf. Scand Arch Physiol 8:223, 1898.
32. Tobian L: Relationship of juxtaglomerular apparatus to renin and angiotensin. Circulation 25:189, 1962.
33. Tucker RM, Labarthe DR: Frequency of surgical treatment for hypertension in adults at the Mayo Clinic from 1973 through 1975. Mayo Clin Proc 52:549, 1977.

106

Pathophysiology of Renovascular Hypertension

E. Darracott Vaughan, Jr., M.D.

• • •

Renovascular hypertension is one of the most common causes of secondary hypertension; however, the exact prevalence is not well defined because it is a difficult diagnosis to make on clinical grounds alone.[13, 72] Moreover, the precise mechanisms that underlie renovascular hypertension have been more difficult to elucidate than expected. It was Goldblatt's classic studies in dogs that rekindled interest in the renin-angiotensin-aldosterone system.[23] Indeed, following the observation by Goldblatt that sustained hypertension could be produced in dogs by uninephrectomy and concurrent narrowing of the renal artery to the remaining kidney, it was assumed that excess renin secretion leading to excess angiotensin formation was the pathogenic mechanism of renovascular hypertension. With the development of precise methods of measuring plasma renin activity, however, numerous investigators demonstrated with despair that increased renin secretion was only transient in this model and that the chronic hypertensive state was characterized by normal renin levels.[1, 5, 36] Moreover, despite the early report of clinical success in patients with unilateral renal disease whose hypertension was cured by nephrectomy, Smith's encompassing review in 1956 revealed benefit in only 26 per cent of cases so treated.* Subsequently, normal plasma renin activity found in many patients with renal artery stenosis further confused the picture.[16] In the face of this dilemma, it became apparent that a better understanding of the role of the renin-angiotensin-aldosterone system in a wide variety of hypertensive disorders might allow the development of concepts that could explain the paradoxes found in clinical and experimental renal hypertension.

It now is established that the renin-angiotensin-aldosterone system (Fig. 106–1) is an integrated hormonal system that normally operates to regulate sodium and potassium balance and arterial blood pressure simultaneously.[34] Derangements have been identified in the system that appear to be involved both in the relatively uncommon syndromes of malignant hypertension, primary aldosteronism, and oral contraceptive hypertension and in the more common entity of essential hypertension. From observations in these entities, it has been possible to understand chronic hypertensive states in terms of volume and vasoconstriction abnormalities.[32] Hence, hypertension may be maintained by overfilling of the arterial system (volume hypertension), by arteriolar constriction without increased volume (vasoconstrictor hypertension), or by an inappropriate interaction of these two factors. In all three settings, there is an excess volume relative to the capacity of the arterial tree. The renin-angiotensin-aldosterone system exerts major control over these variables through both angiotensin II–induced vasoconstriction and aldosterone-induced volume expansion. Moreover, the kidneys must play a key role, not only through renin secretion but also by sustaining sodium and volume retention in excess of vascular capacity, despite increased perfusion pressure. This renal behavior could result from active vasoconstriction, aldosterone stimulation, or intrinsic renal disease.

If these concepts are carried over to renal hypertension, it is possible to speculate that there could be two forms of renal hypertension exhibiting quite different abnormalities of the renin-angiotensin-aldosterone system.

Figure 106–2 shows the system in the setting of unilateral renal arterial stenosis and a normal contralateral kidney. Following arterial stenosis, there is decreased renal blood flow and glomerular filtration rate, leading to renin release and angiotensin II formation. This response is char-

---

*See references: cure by nephrectomy, 9, 35; benefit, 60.

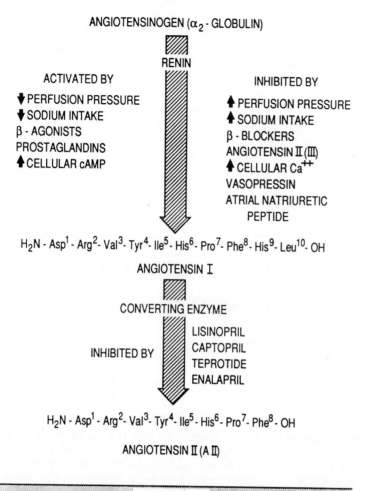

ANGIOTENSINOGEN (α_2 - GLOBULIN)

RENIN

ACTIVATED BY	INHIBITED BY
↓ PERFUSION PRESSURE	↑ PERFUSION PRESSURE
↓ SODIUM INTAKE	↑ SODIUM INTAKE
β - AGONISTS	β - BLOCKERS
PROSTAGLANDINS	ANGIOTENSIN II (III)
↑ CELLULAR cAMP	↑ CELLULAR Ca^{++}
	VASOPRESSIN
	ATRIAL NATRIURETIC
	PEPTIDE

H_2N - Asp^1 - Arg^2 - Val^3 - Tyr^4 - Ile^5 - His^6 - Pro^7 - Phe^8 - His^9 - Leu^{10} - OH

ANGIOTENSIN I

CONVERTING ENZYME

INHIBITED BY   LISINOPRIL
CAPTOPRIL
TEPROTIDE
ENALAPRIL

H_2N - Asp^1 - Arg^2 - Val^3 - Tyr^4 - Ile^5 - His^6 - Pro^7 - Phe^8 - OH

ANGIOTENSIN II (A II)

A II RECEPTOR

ACTIVATION OF RECEPTOR RESULTS IN:	A II RECEPTOR BLOCKED BY A II ANALOGUES: PROTOTYPE
1. VASOCONSTRICTION	
2. SODIUM RETENTION	(Sarcosine^1, Valine^5,
3. RELEASE OF ALDOSTERONE	Alanine^8) A II (Saralasin)
4. RELEASE OF CATECHOLAMINES	

FIGURE 106–1. The renin-angiotensin-aldosterone system. (From Vaughan ED Jr, Sosa RE: Renovascular hypertension. *In* Walsh PC, Retik AB, Stamey TA, Vaughan ED Jr [eds]: Campbell's Urology. 6th ed. Philadelphia, WB Saunders, 1992, p 2024.)

acterized by increased renin secretion from the stenotic kidney, which is manifested by an increased peripheral renin activity level when indexed against the concurrent 24-hour sodium excretion. The resultant increase in angiotensin II production leads to vasoconstriction and also to aldosterone secretion. Under increased pressure, the opposite normal kidney will suppress its renin secretion to zero. With the elevation of blood pressure, however, there is a resultant natriuresis from the opposite normal kidney. Accordingly, sodium retention, which is due either to the hemodynamic alterations in the stenotic kidney or to aldosterone secretion that would serve to feed back and shut off renin secretion, is limited. Thus, abnormal renin secretion is sustained and the patient is hypertensive primarily because of unilateral hypersecretion of renin resulting in an-

giotensin II–induced vasoconstriction. Moreover, the presence of some sodium retention enhances the angiotensin vasoconstrictor effect. These alterations in the system are characteristic of curable renovascular, renin-dependent renal hypertension.[51, 68]

In contrast, a renal artery lesion or unilateral renal parenchymal disease can occur in a situation in which there is overt or occult contralateral disease. Again, the initial events may parallel those previously described in the case of hypersecretion of renin from the stenotic kidney. With bilateral disease (or in the experimental model with the absence of the opposite kidney), however, the opposite kidney is not able to compensate for the increased sodium retention with a natriuresis. Thus, volume expansion serves to return the renin secretion to normal (manifested by a

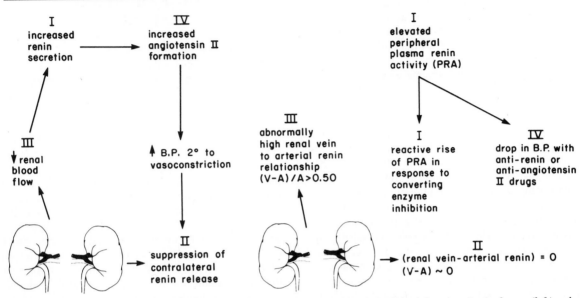

FIGURE 106–2. Characteristics of the early phase of two-kidney, one-clip Goldblatt's hypertension in the rat *(left)* and the criteria derived from the animal model that identify the patient with correctable renal hypertension *(right)*. (From Vaughan ED Jr: Renovascular hypertension. Used with permission from *Kidney International,* volume 27, page 811, 1985.)

normal peripheral plasma renin activity level), decreasing the vasoconstriction induced by angiotensin II generation but at the expense of a volume-dependent hypertension. Thus, in this setting, any alleviation of hypertension subsequent to renal revascularization would have to be due to enhancement of renal blood flow, glomerular filtration rate, and sodium excretion, rather than to elimination of overtly abnormal renin secretion. Here, only vascular repair is appropriate. Indeed, it follows that uninephrectomy might actually accelerate the hypertensive process by further decreasing the patient's capacity to excrete sodium. This situation, with bilateral renal disease and attendant volume and sodium expansion, appears to be dominant in patients with unilateral renal parenchymal disease or end-stage bilateral renal disease and in hypertensive patients with only one kidney.*

In order to validate further the existence of two different mechanisms involved in renal hypertension, considerable evidence has been derived from animal models. Two kinds of experimental Goldblatt hypertension can be produced in animals. In one, a renal artery is clamped and the opposite kidney is left in place—''two-kidney one-clip Goldblatt.'' In the second model, one renal artery is clipped and the opposite kidney is removed—''one-kidney one-clip Goldblatt.'' Although these two models are equally hypertensive, there are distinct pathophysiologic differences.

The two-kidney one-clip model is characterized by increased renin content in the clipped kidney, reduced renin

content in the contralateral kidney (contralateral renin suppression), mild sodium retention, and increased sodium and water turnover, primarily from the contralateral kidney.[25] Elevated renin levels are found in this model both initially and in the established phase (see Fig. 106–2).[45]

The synthesis of specific angiotensin II inhibitors introduced a new era in the study of experimental renal hypertension.[70] Hence, Brunner and coworkers infused the Sar[1] Ala[8] angiotensin II analogue, saralasin, intravenously in the two-kidney and one-kidney models.[7] They demonstrated that the blood pressure in the two-kidney animals was, in fact, angiotensin II–dependent because administration of the inhibitor dramatically reduced the blood pressure, although not fully to control levels. In contrast, the one-kidney animal did not exhibit a fall in blood pressure. With protracted occlusion, however, even the two-kidney animal loses its overt angiotensin dependency.[21]

The animal model at this time has been termed chronic. The rapidity with which the animal model fails to lower its blood pressure with angiotensin II blockade is dependent on the presence or absence of the opposite kidney. The chronic phase is initiated in a much more rapid fashion if the contralateral kidney is removed. The general view of this setting is that the hypertension is maintained as a result of damage to the contralateral kidney and cannot be reversed even with removal of the stenosis or removal of the ischemic kidney.[59]

In the one-kidney model, the increase in renin secretion following renal artery constriction is transient.[1, 5, 36] This initial rise is correlated with the initial rise in blood pressure, and in the short term the hypertension can be reversed either by administration of angiotensin II antago-

---

*See references: parenchymal disease, 69; end-stage bilateral disease, 56; only one kidney, 30.

nists or with angiotensin I–converting enzyme inhibitors.* Hence, in this model the initiation of hypertension is dependent on angiotensin II–induced vasoconstriction. The renin secretion is, however, suppressed to normal quite rapidly by volume expansion caused by sodium and water retention.[36] In the chronic state, the fall in blood pressure that follows unclamping is correlated with significant negative salt and water balance. Hence, in the chronic state the hypertension is maintained by volume expansion, not by demonstrably increased angiotensin levels. The interrelationship between these two mechanisms was shown by Gavras and coworkers, who demonstrated that the one-kidney one-clip sodium-restricted rat maintained angiotensin II–dependent hypertension, as shown by a striking drop in blood pressure with the angiotensin II inhibitor Sar[1] Ala[8] A II. In contrast, these same animals failed to show a response to acute angiotensin II inhibition following sodium repletion.[22]

Taken all together, the difference between the two hypertensive models during the early phase is that the one-kidney one-clip animal, with a marked reduction in renal mass and sodium-excreting ability, is initially an angiotensin II–dependent model but rapidly expands volume to sustain its blood pressure on a volume basis. One can, however, convert the one-kidney sodium-volume model to a renin (angiotensin II)–dependent model by sodium depletion. In contrast, the two-kidney Goldblatt model remains angiotensin II–dependent as long as the contralateral kidney is normal and responds to the hypertension by freely excreting sodium and water. The hypertension in this animal model is primarily a vasoconstrictor hypertension caused by the continual, unabated release of renin with angiotensin II generation. Moreover, it is this model with unilateral renal artery constriction, a normal opposite kidney, and increased renin secretion that should be analogous to the potentially curable patient with unilateral renal artery stenosis.

The information concerning the long-term models suggests that in any clinical series, there will be some hypertensive patients (albeit usually azotemic ones) who do not meet defined preoperative criteria used to predict curability but whose hypertension will nevertheless be reversed following successful revascularization. Blood pressure control could be due either to restoration of renal blood flow, glomerular filtration rate, and sodium excretion or to reversal of an at present ill-defined role of angiotensin II in the presence of a normal peripheral plasma renin activity level. The chance of cure of hypertension in these patients is, however, less than if the criteria outlined here were present. However, the primary indication for renal revascularization in these patients is for maintenance or restoration of renal function rather than solely for cure of the hypertension.[4] Moreover, nephrectomy is contraindicated in these patients if the kidney is contributing to total renal function. The determination of residual renal function in a small kidney is one of the few remaining indications for divided renal function studies using cystoscopy and ureteral catheterization.[69]

---

*See references; angiotensin II antagonists, 3, 7; enzymes inhibitors, 3, 44.

PHYSIOLOGIC STUDIES TO REVEAL THE FUNCTIONAL SIGNIFICANCE OF RENAL ARTERIAL DISEASE

Following appropriate screening studies and the demonstration of a renal arterial lesion, it remains to be proved whether the lesion is causally related to the patient's hypertension. Indeed, it is well recognized that "radiographically significant" renal arterial lesions can be found in normotensive patients.[18]

The need for accurate means to identify the potentially curable patient with renovascular hypertension is apparent when the results of a large cooperative study are reviewed. Foster and associates found that only 51 per cent of 502 patients operated on with renal arterial stenosis were cured; 15 per cent had improvement, and 34 per cent failed to show a fall in blood pressure.[19] Moreover, there was a 5.9 per cent operative mortality rate, and the "anatomic failure rate" varied from 18 to 45 per cent between institutions. More recent series, in which physiologic studies are used to select patients for corrective surgical procedures, demonstrate a considerably higher success rate.[37]

Differential Renal Function Studies

The quest for a reliable physiologic test to identify the potentially curable patient is not of recent origin. After Smith's disappointing review in 1956 of the results of nephrectomy,[60] Howard and colleagues, in 1957, made the initial clinical attempt to assess the physiologic significance of a renal arterial lesion.[12] Howard's differential renal function test was based on animal studies that had demonstrated that subsequent to the reduction in renal blood flow and glomerular filtration rate, there was increased fractional reabsorption of sodium and water in the affected kidney.[46] Subsequently, Howard and Connor established the criteria for a positive Howard test result as 60 per cent or more reduction in urine volume, 15 per cent or more reduction in urine sodium concentration, and 50 per cent or more increase in urine creatinine on the suspected side.[27] This last criterion is based on the physiologic event of increased sodium reabsorption in the hypoperfused kidney, which generates a greater osmotic gradient from cortex to medulla than found in the sodium-losing contralateral kidney. Accordingly, there is more water reabsorption, resulting in an increased concentration of nonreabsorbable solute. Because of subsequent reports of both false-positive and false-negative test results, especially in patients with segmental lesions or bilateral disease, numerous modifications of split renal function tests have been proposed.[40, 64] The physiologic basis remains the same, however.

In 1968, Maxwell and coworkers reviewed world experience and found that despite many modifications of the test, its value in identifying potentially curable patients was questionable.[40] Thus, although 83 per cent of patients with positive test results were cured or had improvement, an additional 65 per cent of patients with negative test results were also cured or had improvement by corrective surgery.

Despite these cumulative results, several groups have continued to find split renal function tests valuable; specifically, Dean and others found that the presence of hyperconcentration has accurately predicted functional accuracy following successful renal revascularization.[14, 15, 55] These tests are, however, used in a complementary manner with differential renal vein renin determinations.

An additional use of differential renal function studies has been to determine the effective renal plasma flow to the contralateral kidney in order to establish its normalcy.[63] Operative cure has, however, occurred despite a low opposite flow.[49] This observation may possibly be explained by the vasoconstrictor effect of circulating angiotensin II on the renal blood flow of the opposite kidney, giving the false impression of contralateral disease.[75] More recently, contralateral suppression of renin secretion has been used successfully to identify a normal opposite kidney.[31, 68]

Taken all together, it is generally believed that differential renal function studies are useful as an adjunctive test when the differential renal vein renin studies are not diagnostic and additional information is needed.

However, it is important to understand that these physiologic changes do occur in patients with renovascular hypertension. In fact, these changes are part of the underlying pathophysiology that explains the ability of the administration of angiotensin II–converting enzyme inhibitor to delineate between the normal kidney and a ''stenotic'' kidney as the basis of the captopril renogram (discussed later). In the kidney with renal artery stenosis and a marked reduction in glomerular filtration rate, the glomerular filtration rate drops even further as efferent arteriolar tone is reduced. In contrast, in the normal contralateral kidney, the role of angiotensin II as an afferent constrictor is removed and the renal blood flow and glomerular filtration rate go up. The net difference between the two kidneys is then apparent with the use of a scanning agent that measures glomerular filtration rate or, less accurately, renal blood flow.

Renin Determinations

As discussed previously, unilateral hypersecretion of renin with subsequent angiotensin II–induced vasoconstriction should be the hallmark of potentially curable renovascular hypertension. Under most circumstances, because the clearance rate of renin remains a constant proportion of the arterial renin level, the peripheral renin level is a reflection of the rate of renal renin secretion.[58] However, because a large percentage of patients subsequently cured exhibited a seemingly ''normal'' peripheral level preoperatively, there is considerable disenchantment with this determination.[39] This inconsistency may be explained by two factors not well appreciated. First, it is now recognized that the peripheral plasma renin activity level must be indexed against some marker of the state of sodium balance. A reliable method of accomplishing this task has been devised by Laragh and coworkers.[33] The plasma renin activity in plasma samples obtained at noon is related to the concurrent daily rate of sodium excretion ($U_{Na}V$). In normal subjects, a dynamic hyperbolic relationship exists between plasma renin activity and sodium excretion, with the renin level falling as the sodium excretion increases (Fig. 106–

3). Second, it is now apparent that essentially all diuretic and antihypertensive drugs influence the system.[33] Thus, for accurate assessment of actual renin secretion, using the peripheral plasma renin activity level indexed against sodium excretion, patients must not receive any antihypertensive and diuretic drug therapy for at least 3 weeks. Taking these factors into consideration, an abnormally high peripheral renin level in relation to the 24-hour sodium excretion indicates abnormal renin secretion.

Using the renin-sodium index, the author's group found excessive peripheral plasma renin activity in 80 per cent of patients who were subsequently cured by anatomically successful surgery.[51] Hence, hypersecretion of renin appears to be basic to curable renovascular hypertension. The problem lies in clearly defining ''normal''—a problem not yet totally resolved. If the pitfalls listed in Table 106–1 are avoided, however, the test is extremely useful. It is nevertheless also clear that some patients who are cured or who show improvement have normal peripheral plasma renin values. Hence, although the renin-sodium index is an improvement, it is not an altogether precise guide to normalcy and may not always unmask renin involvement.

An additional approach to identifying renin hypersecretion that the author's group has found useful is to evaluate the response of plasma renin activity to angiotensin II blockade. Initially, it was demonstrated that saralasin or teprotide induced increases in plasma renin activity to a greater extent in patients with renovascular hypertension than in patients with essential hypertension.[6, 11] With the availability of the oral converting enzyme inhibitor captopril, the author's group began using single oral test doses

Table 106–1. Aids to Increase the Accuracy of Determinations of Peripheral Plasma Renin Activity

Problems	Solution
''Normal'' value for plasma renin activity varies from laboratory to laboratory	Clearly understand factors that affect ''normal'' values in your laboratory: Time of sampling State of ambulation (upright posture influences plasma renin activity) State of sodium intake
Method of collecting blood samples may vary from that used for samples to establish normal range	Use identical conditions for sampling
All antihypertensive and diuretic drugs affect plasma renin activity	Stop all treatment 2 weeks before blood sampling for plasma renin activity
Plasma renin activity is inversely related to sodium intake and excretion	Collect 24-hour urine sample for sodium determination at same time you collect blood for plasma renin activity. Use sodium intake level that your laboratory uses to define their normal range*
Inferior vena cava renin is used as ''peripheral''	Obtain peripheral blood for plasma renin activity as described on a day separate from renal vein sampling

Adapted from Vaughan ED Jr: Laboratory tests in the evaluation of renal hypertension. Urol Clin North Am 6:485, 1979.

*If a new method is being established, suggest the development of a renin-sodium index.

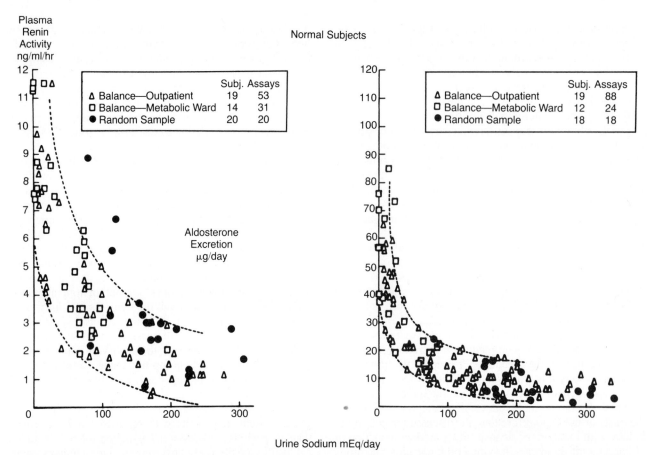

FIGURE 106–3. Relation of both renin activity in plasma samples obtained at noon and the corresponding 24-hour urinary excretion of aldosterone to the concurrent daily rate of sodium excretion. For these normal subjects, the data describe a similar dynamic hyperbolic relationship between each hormone and sodium excretion. Of note is the fact that subjects on random diets outside the hospital exhibited similar relationships, a finding that validates the use of this nomogram in studying outpatients or subjects not receiving constant diets. (From Laragh JH, Baer L, Brunner HR, et al: The renin-angiotensin-aldosterone system in pathogenesis and management of hypertensive vascular disease. *In* Laragh JH [ed]: Hypertension Manual. New York, Yorke Medical Books, 1974.)

instead of intravenous infusions. Results very similar to those obtained using the intravenous competitive antagonist saralasin or the converting enzyme inhibitor teprotide were found, including a marked rise in plasma renin activity.[10] An additional advantage was the observation that renovascular hypertensive patients being treated with a beta-adrenergic blocker still responded to oral administration of captopril with a fall in blood pressure and a rise in plasma renin activity (Fig. 106–4).

The protocol for using single oral doses of captopril to screen for renovascular hypertension is shown in Table 106–2, and current criteria for interpretation are summarized in Table 106–3. In a study of 246 hypertensive patients, the test was highly accurate in patients without renal insufficiency. The test identified all 56 patients with proven renovascular disease among 200 hypertensive patients without renal dysfunction. In this group, false-positive results occurred in only 2 of 112 patients with essential hypertension and in 6 with secondary hypertension.[47]

Numerous other studies have now been published concerning the converting enzyme inhibitors, and the majority of authors have also found them useful[17, 24, 73] in adults and in children.[74] However, others have found the test less use-

ful as a prospective screening test. Gaul and coworkers reviewed 16 studies involving 805 patients and found numerous differences in these studies, including differences in the documentation of renovascular hypertension, the methodology of captopril administration, and the definitions of a positive test result.[20]

In summary, the captopril test appears to be useful in identifying patients with renovascular hypertension, and it is safe and simple to perform. However, there is a need for standardization of the tests and a more precise definition of a positive test result, as well as for more prospective studies. In addition, a 24-hour urine collection is not necessary and the patient can remain on beta-blockade. Hence, the test is complementary to the renin-sodium index to identify renin hypersecretion.

If Bayes' theorem is applied to the most commonly used tests for identifying renovascular hypertension, it is apparent that the captopril test is the most accurate (Table 106–4).

In most patients the blood pressure also fell, so the mechanism of the reactive rise in plasma renin activity could have been due to either a systemic or a renal baroreceptor response or to inhibition of angiotensin II direct

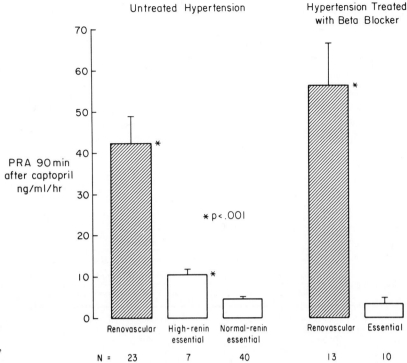

FIGURE 106–4. Levels of plasma renin activity (PRA) in renovascular and essential hypertension 90 minutes after a single dose of captopril. A marked reactive hyper-reninemia was found in the group with renovascular hypertension, whether or not they were already receiving beta-blocker therapy. (From Case DB, Atlas SA, Laragh JH: Physiologic effects and blockade. *In* Laragh JH, Bühler FR, Seldin DW [eds]: Frontiers in Hypertension Research. New York, Springer-Verlag, 1982, pp 541–550.)

feedback inhibiting renin release. This latter possibility is intriguing because this direct feedback seems to be operative in sodium-restricted normal or one-kidney one-clip hypertensive dogs.[2, 29]

Hypersecretion of renin, as determined by an elevated peripheral plasma renin level indexed against sodium secretion, is the first criterion for the diagnosis of renovascular hypertension, but its presence alone does not establish the diagnosis. A high level of peripheral plasma renin activity is found in 16 per cent of patients with essential hypertension and is characteristic of malignant hypertension.[8, 33] Hence, unilaterality of renin secretion also must be established.

The study of converting enzyme inhibitors in both the diagnosis and the treatment of renovascular hypertension led to the finding of decreased renal function in some patients.[28] Eventually, these observations led to the concept that one might be able to use a combination of converting enzyme inhibition and renography to identify kidneys with renal artery stenosis. The response of renal blood flow and glomerular filtration rate to converting enzyme inhibition in the two-kidney one-clip dog model established in the author's laboratory is shown in Figure 106–5. Infusion of enalapril produced a dramatic fall in renal blood flow and glomerular filtration rate in the kidney with renal artery stenosis, whereas renal blood flow increased in the opposite kidney. As previously stated, the mechanism involved is the loss of efferent arteriolar constriction, a mechanism maintaining glomerular filtration rate in the kidney with the stenotic main renal artery, taken together with a decrease in

Table 106–2.   Single-Dose Captopril Test

Drugs

The patient should be off all antihypertensive medicines for at least 2 weeks if possible. Otherwise, leave the patient on a beta-blocker but avoid diuretics, converting enzyme inhibitors, and nonsteroidal anti-inflammatory drugs for at least 1 week, ideally 2 weeks.

Diet

A diet with normal or high sodium content is necessary. Too low a sodium intake will produce false-positive results. If there is a question about diet, a 24-hour urine collection for sodium will closely reflect the intake.

Procedure

The patient is seated comfortably for 20 to 30 minutes before testing and is maintained in this position for the duration of the test.

Blood pressure is measured at 20, 25, and 30 minutes (three stable baseline measurements should be obtained), then blood is sampled for plasma renin activity (in a lavender top Vacutainer kept at room temperature).

A 25-mg captopril tablet is crushed (to ensure that it dissolves), and 30 ml of water is added to prepare a suspension. The patient is instructed to drink the suspension, wash the contents out twice, and drink those also.

Blood pressure and plasma renin activity are remeasured after 30 and 60 minutes.

From Muller FB, Sealey JE, Case DB, et al: The captopril test for identifying renovascular disease in hypertensive patients. Am J Med 80:633, 1986.

Table 106–3.   Single-Dose Captopril Test: Criteria That Distinguish Patients With Renovascular Hypertension From Those With Essential Hypertension

Stimulated PRA of ≥ 12 ng/ml/hr
   and
Absolute increase in PRA of ≥ 10 ng/ml/hr
   and
Per cent increase in PRA of ≥ 150%, or 400% *if* the baseline PRA <3 ng/ml/hr

From Muller FB, Sealey JE, Case DB, et al: The captopril test for identifying renovascular disease in hypertensive patients. Am J Med 80:633, 1986.
PRA, plasma renin activity.

Table 106–4.   Predictive Value of Screening Tests for Renovascular Hypertension

	Intravenous Urogram[26]	Digital Angiography[26]	Plasma Renin Activity[6, 51]	Single-Dose Captopril[47]
Sensitivity (%)	75	88	80	100
Specificity (%)	86	89	84	95
False-positive rate (%)	14	11	16	5
False-negative rate (%)	25	12	20	0
Predictive value (%)				
Prevalence 2%	9.9	14.6	9.3	29
5%	22.1	30.5	20.8	51.3
10%	37.5	48.1	35.7	69
Exclusion value (%)				
Prevalence 2%	99.4	99.7	99.5	100
5%	98.5	99.3	98.8	100
10%	96.7	98.5	97.4	100

Calculations:

$$\text{Predictive value} = \frac{\text{Sensitivity} \times \text{prevalence}}{(\text{Sensitivity} \times \text{prevalence}) + \text{false-positive rate} \times (100 - \text{prevalence})} \times 100$$

$$\text{Exclusion value} = \frac{\text{Specificity} \times (100 - \text{prevalence})}{[\text{Specificity} \times (100 - \text{prevalence}) + \text{false-negative rate}] \times \text{prevalence}} \times 100$$

From Sosa RE, Vaughan ED Jr: Renovascular hypertension. In *Gillenwater JY, Grayhack JT, Howards SS, Duckett JW (eds): Adult and Pediatric Urology. Chicago, Year Book Medical Publishers, 1987.*

afferent constriction in the opposite kidney, which leads to the increase in renal blood flow.[38, 43, 50]

Thus, although the standard isotopic renogram has not been accurate in identifying patients with renovascular hypertension, performing renography before and after the administration of captopril can enhance the diagnostic accuracy of the test. Hence, the test not only screens for renovascular hypertension but also identifies the involved kidney, which will perhaps obviate the need for renal vein renin determinations in the future. Wilcox and coworkers[73] reviewed the results of three series and concluded that the predictive value of the test did not yet approach that of renal vein renin determinations.[51]

Future advancements, including determination of both renal blood flow and glomerular filtration rate, employment of new agents and a single study, and reevaluation of response criteria, should define better the overall usefulness of the study. However, differential renal vein renin determinations currently remain the gold standard for identifying which kidney is the cause of abnormal renin secretion in a patient with renovascular hypertension.

Differential renal vein renin measurements have been used as another dimension in the clinical analysis. This approach is essential to establish the unilaterality of a renin hypersecretory state or, stated another way, to exonerate the opposite, presumably uninvolved kidney from participation in the renin hypersecretion. The physiologic basis for this requirement has been well established in animal models, in which it is clear that the opposite, uninvolved kidney undergoes endocrine suppression, so that all the circulating renin arises via hypersecretion from the "clip" kidney.[25]

Earlier studies described empirically good results from operation whenever renal vein renin levels were one and a half to two times higher from the suspect side. The inability of the simple renal vein renin ratio to recognize a lesser, although possibly significant, addition of renin by the contralateral kidney is a serious limitation to this widely accepted but arbitrarily based analysis. Failure to recognize the lack of complete contralateral suppression of renin secretion undoubtedly accounts for some surgical failures in spite of a "positive" renal vein renin ratio.[39, 52]

More recently, with the appreciation that the kidneys do not remove renin from the arterial blood, it has become desirable to subtract the arterial renin level (A) from the

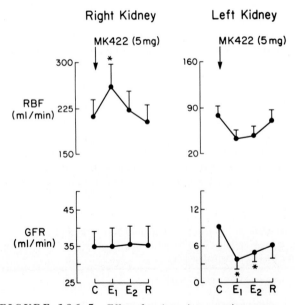

FIGURE 106–5. Effect of angiotensin-converting enzyme inhibition on renal blood flow (RBF) and glomerular filtration rate (GFR), showing a marked fall in GFR in the kidney with renal artery stenosis. 2-K, 2-kidney; 1-C, 1-clip; C, control; E, experimental periods; R, recovery. (From Vaughan ED Jr, Sosa RE: Renovascular hypertension. *In* Walsh PC, Retik AB, Stamey TA, Vaughan ED Jr [eds]: Campbell's Urology. 6th ed. Philadelphia, WB Saunders, 1992, p 2033.)

renal venous level (V) on each side.[31] With this method, the renin value (V − A) should approach zero from the uninvolved side in potentially curable patients. This contralateral suppression of renin secretion, in fact, has been shown to occur, making it a second criterion in addition to the first (an elevated peripheral renin-sodium index) for identifying unilateral hypersecretion of renin and thereby predicting curability.[66, 68] In practice, arterial renin levels need not be collected to derive the value (V − A), and an infrarenal inferior vena cava sample can be substituted because it has been shown that there is no aortic-to-caval renin difference.[58]

A third criterion is based on studies of renal vein and arterial renin relationships in patients with essential hypertension. The mean renal vein renin level has been determined to be about 25 per cent higher than the arterial renin level (Fig. 106–6).[59] Hence, a total renal increment (both kidneys) of approximately 50 per cent is necessary to maintain a given peripheral renin level. Therefore, (V − A)/A would equal 50 per cent in this setting. If only one kidney were present, the total renin secretion would drop by half and the increment from the remaining kidney would be 50

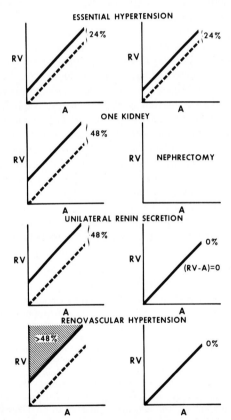

FIGURE 106–6. Renal vein (RV) renin to arterial (A) renin relationships in four theoretical settings. In essential hypertension, at all levels of renin secretion, the renal vein renin from each kidney will be 24 per cent higher than arterial renin. Following uninephrectomy and a decrease in total renin secretion, the renal vein renin from the remaining kidney will be 48 per cent higher than the arterial value. This relationship also applies if there is unilateral renin secretion without blood flow reduction. If there is renal blood flow reduction, the amount of elevation of the relationship above 48 per cent is inversely proportional to, and gives an index of, the reduction of flow. (From Vaughan ED Jr: The renin-angiotensin-aldosterone system in renal and adrenal hypertensions. *In* Devine CJ Jr, Stecker JF Jr [eds]: Urology in Practice. Boston, Little, Brown and Company, 1978.)

per cent. However, a reduction in renal blood flow also influences the renal vein renin concentration; accordingly, the value obtained is no longer a true reflection of simple secretion but is also an index of the decrease in renal blood flow shifting the renal vein arterial renin relationship upward. Therefore, the elevation of the increment above 50 per cent (in the presence of contralateral suppression) becomes an index of the severity of reduction in renal blood flow consequent to the obstructing vascular lesion.

Another warning is that a small kidney with reduced flow can have decreased renin secretion and yet have a high venous renin concentration. In this setting, the patient should have high peripheral plasma renin activity or a positive captopril test result and the addition of contralateral suppression before the isolated increased renal vein renin value can be accepted as indicating hypersecretion of renin.

Of a group of 46 patients with proven renal artery stenosis who underwent successful angioplasties, 34 had technically successful sampling.[51] Of the 34 patients with technically acceptable values, there were 23 true-positives, 0 false-positives, 3 true-negatives, and 8 false-negative results. Of the 8 patients with false-negative findings, 4 had a (V − A)/A between 40 and 48 per cent and 6 of 8 had contralateral suppression. This problem, which has been emphasized by others,[54] is due to the fact that there is a significant methodologic variability in renal vein renin determinations and the fact that the renal vein renin concentration is normally only about 25 per cent higher than the arterial input.

Therefore, it is important to realize that all of the criteria discussed must be taken as a whole and that patients with a high clinical index of suspicion of having renovascular hypertension should undergo vascular imaging even if the renal vein renin study results are negative.

The application of these physiologic relationships has led to the definition of the three criteria to identify and evaluate patients suspected of having renovascular hypertension (Table 106–5). These criteria have been applied in several retrospective analyses and have been shown to provide greater accuracy than the use of renal vein renin ratios alone.[65, 68, 70]

The author's group attempts to minimize this problem by relating the renal vein value to the inferior vena cava renin value so that it is possible to discern when the total increment from both kidneys is less than 50 per cent and it is likely that at least one of the sampling catheters was incorrectly positioned or that there is segmental disease. In this setting, either repeated sampling with segmental collections or arteriography should be performed.[57] In addition, this group again uses angiotensin blockade to enhance renin secretion. Administration of a converting enzyme inhibitor, as shown in Figure 106–7, will result in unilateral enhancement without inducing renin secretion from the normal kidney.[53] Use of the criteria described, coupled with captopril enhancement of unilateral renin secretion, when necessary, reduces the number of false-negative studies.

ANATOMIC CONFIRMATION OF THE CRITERIA

It should be noted that virtually the entire evaluation of the hypertensive patient can now be accomplished with-

Table 106–5. Renin Values for Predicting the Curability of Renovascular Hypertension

Collection of Samples (moderate sodium intake of 40–100 mEq/day)
Blood for ambulatory peripheral PRA and 24-hour urine specimen for sodium excretion under steady state conditions (i.e., not on day of arteriography)
Blood for PRA before and after converting enzyme blockade
With patient supine, blood for
    Renal vein renin from suspect kidney (V1) and inferior vena cava renin (A1)
    Renal vein renin from contralateral kidney (V2) and inferior vena cava renin (A2)
Enhancement of renin secretion by converting enzyme blockade if initial renin sampling is inconclusive

Criteria for Predicting Cure

High PRA in relation to U_{Na} V	Measurement of hypersecretion of renin
Contralateral kidney: (V2 − A2) = 0	Indicator of absence of renin secretion from contralateral kidney
Suspect kidney: (V1 − A1)/A1 = 0.50	Indicator of unilateral renin secretion
(V1 − A1)/A1 > 0.50	Measurement of reduced renal blood flow

$$\frac{(V - A)}{A} + \frac{(V - A)}{A} < 0.50 \text{ in patients with high PRA indicates:}$$

Incorrect sampling or segmental disease	Repeat with segmental sampling

PRA, plasma renin activity; U_{Na} V, 24-hour urinary sodium excretion.

out hospitalization, thus avoiding much of the expense previously believed to be too excessive to warrant evaluation.[41, 42] The author's group has performed more than 300 renal vein renin samplings in outpatients, with 100 of them accompanied by digital angiography, which is approximately 90 per cent accurate in identifying renal arterial lesions.[48] This group uses a central injection for the digital angiography, which gives better definition of the renal vas-

culature. The major error arises with branch or segmental disease involving the smaller renal vessels.

Accordingly, digital angiography can be used both to accompany renal vein sampling for renin to give anatomic definition of the renal vasculature, and to follow up patients after correction of a renovascular lesion.[61] The only caveat is to remember that digital angiography demonstrates only anatomic vascular disease, and the functional significance of the lesion must still be demonstrated.

Taken all together, screening criteria have been identified that provide great assurance that the patient with renovascular disease will be both physiologically and anatomically characterized and the success of a corrective procedure can be predicted. When these criteria have been identified, the patient is admitted to the hospital for definitive management of the offending lesion.

VALIDATION OF THE CRITERIA

In addition to seeing a favorable clinical response to renal angioplasty,[61] the author's group has also had the unique opportunity to study the effect of restoration of blood flow on renal vein renin concentration and renin secretion.[51, 71] This goal was accomplished by monitoring the immediate effect of successful angioplasty on renal vein renin secretion. Thirty minutes following angioplasty, there was a marked reduction in the renal vein renin from the previously stenotic side (Fig. 106–8). The residual ipsilateral increment of renal vein renin was approximately 50 per cent above the peripheral level, whereas contralateral renin suppression persisted. This 50 per cent increment has been predicted previously to occur in the setting of unilateral renin secretion and normal renal blood flow.[68]

Several months after angioplasty, there was a marked fall in peripheral plasma renin activity with a return to normal in most patients, indicating a reduction in renin secretion (see Fig. 106–8). Of equal interest is the restora-

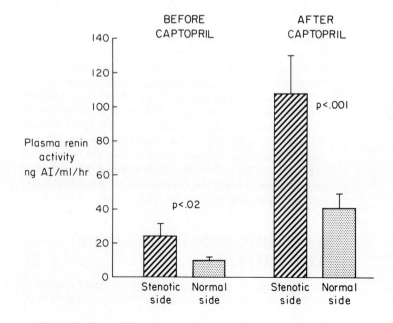

FIGURE 106–7. Renal vein renin determinations (renal vein levels only) in patients with documented renovascular hypertension before and after captopril stimulation. Captopril accentuates renin secretion from the ischemic kidney. Not shown are the inferior vena cava levels, which are the same as the levels measured from the normal side both before and after captopril stimulation. (From Vaughan ED Jr, Case DB, Pickering TG, et al: Clinical evaluation of renovascular hypertension and therapeutic decision. Urol Clin North Am 11:393, 1984.)

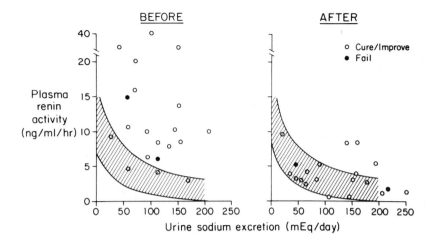

FIGURE 106–8. Effect of angioplasty on peripheral plasma renin activity indexed against 24-hour sodium excretion. *Left,* Before angioplasty. *Right,* Six months after angioplasty. The hatched area shows the normal range. (From Pickering TG, Sos TA, Vaughan ED Jr, et al: Predictive value and changes of renin secretion in hypertensive patients with unilateral renovascular disease undergoing successful renal angioplasty. Am J Med 76:398, 1984.)

tion of a bilateral renin increment of about 25 per cent above the inferior vena cava renin level (Fig. 106–9). Hence, contralateral renin suppression reversed following successful angioplasty. This 25 per cent increment from both kidneys is characteristic of the renin secretory pattern found in patients with essential hypertension.[58]

Overall, the finding that the characteristics of renovascular hypertension reverse following successful angioplasty and correction of the hypertension is strong evidence that these characteristics truly reflect the abnormal secretory behavior of renin in curable renovascular hypertension.

IDENTIFYING THE POTENTIALLY CURABLE PATIENT: A COST-EFFECTIVE APPROACH

The current approach of the author's group is outlined in Figure 106–10. All patients with fixed hypertension are potential candidates for this protocol because this group believes that nearly all patients with renovascular hypertension, when identified, can be best managed by angioplasty or revascularization. With respect to this empirical protocol, it could be argued that patients with a high index of suspi-

cion could be screened initially with a digital angiogram (especially those with positive captopril scanning findings). However, the functional significance of an anatomic lesion with respect to ischemia-induced renin release still must be established, so this group routinely begins with a determination of peripheral plasma renin activity.

In their experience, low plasma renin activity is rarely found in untreated patients with nonazotemic renal arterial disease, and the author's group therefore does not usually continue this evaluation in these patients unless they demonstrate refractoriness to treatment. Patients with high or normal plasma renin activity undergo a peripheral captopril test. The test cannot be performed if the patient is receiving long-term captopril therapy. If the test result is positive, differential renal vein sampling and digital angiography are performed together. The sampling procedure is ideally done first, and then the catheter is advanced into the superior vena cava for injection of contrast material. This combined study is performed in the radiology suite; afterward, the patient lies quietly in the hypertension unit for 2 to 4 hours before returning home.

After the diagnostic criteria have been established, the patient is briefly hospitalized for selective arteriography and percutaneous transluminal angioplasty.

FIGURE 106–9. Effect of angioplasty on renal vein renin level. Samples were taken immediately before angioplasty, 30 minutes after, and 6 months after. The higher values correspond to the ischemic kidney; the lower, to the contralateral kidney. *Asterisks* indicate a significant difference between the two kidneys, and the *dotted line* is the normal level of V − A/A (0.24). (From Pickering TG, Sos TA, Vaughan ED Jr, et al: Predictive value and changes of renin secretion in hypertensive patients with unilateral renovascular disease undergoing successful renal angioplasty. Reprinted from American Journal of Medicine: Vol. 76; 1984, pg. 398.)

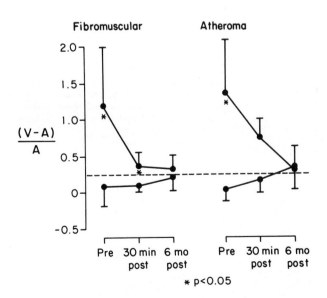

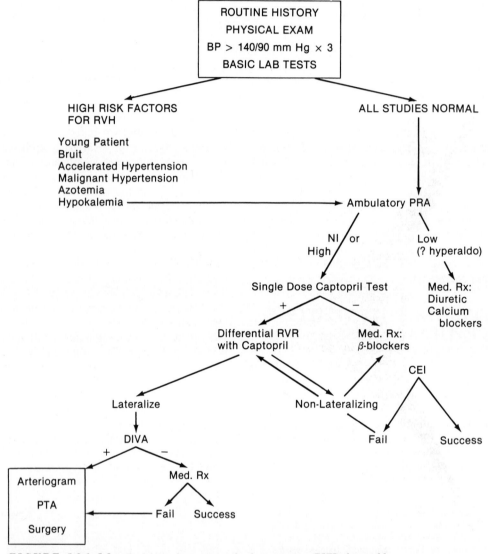

FIGURE 106–10.   Evaluation for renovascular hypertension (RVH). hyperaldo, hyperaldosteronism; BP, blood pressure; PRA, plasma renin activity; NI, normal; Rx, treatment; CEI, correcting enzyme inhibitor; RVR, renal vein renin; DIVA, digital intravenous angiography; PTA, percutaneous transluminal angioplasty. (From Sosa RE, Vaughan ED Jr: Evaluation of surgically curable hypertension. AUA Update Series, Vol II, Lesson 31. Houston, AUA Office of Education, 1983.)

The author's group continues to believe that the functional significance of a renal artery lesion must be identified before the therapeutic decision is directed toward intervention.

References

1. Ayers CR, Harris RH Jr, Lefer LG: Control of renin release in experimental hypertension. Circ Res 24–25:1, 1969.
2. Ayers CR, Katholi RE, Vaughan ED Jr, et al: Intrarenal renin-angiotensin-sodium interdependent mechanism controlling post clamp renal artery pressure and renin release in the conscious dog with chronic one-kidney Goldblatt hypertension. Circ Res 40:238, 1977.
3. Ayers CR, Vaughan ED Jr, Yancey MR, et al: Effect of sarcosine[1] alanine[8] angiotensin-II and converting enzyme inhibitor on renin release in dog acute renovascular hypertension. Circ Res 34–35:1, 1974.
4. Bedoya L, Ziegelbaum M, Vidt DG, et al: The effect of baseline renal function on the outcome following renal revascularization. Cleve Clin J Med 56:415, 1989.
5. Bianchi G, Tenconi LT, Lucca R: Effect in the conscious dog of constriction of the renal artery to a sole remaining kidney on hemodynamics, sodium balance, body fluid volume, plasma renin concentration and pressor responsiveness to angiotensin. Clin Sci 38:741, 1970.
6. Brunner HR, Gavras H, Laragh JH, et al: Angiotensin II blockade in man by Sar[1]-Ala[8]-angiotensin II for understanding and treatment of high blood pressure. Lancet 2:1045, 1973.
7. Brunner HR, Kirshman JD, Sealey JE, et al: Hypertension of renal origin: Evidence for two different mechanisms. Science 174:1344, 1971.
8. Brunner HR, Laragh JH, Baer L, et al: Essential hypertension: Renin and aldosterone, heart attack and stroke. N Engl J Med 284:441, 1972.
9. Butler AM: Chronic pyelonephritis and arterial hypertension. J Clin Invest 16:889, 1937.
10. Case DB, Atlas SA, Laragh JH: Reactive hyperreninemia to angiotensin blockade identifies renovascular hypertension. Clin Sci 57:313S, 1979.
11. Case DB, Laragh JH: Reactive hyperreninemia in renovascular hypertension after angiotensin blockade with saralasin or converting enzyme inhibitor. Ann Intern Med 91:153, 1979.
12. Connor TB, Berthrong M, Thomas WC Jr, et al: Hypertension due to unilateral renal disease with a report on a functional test helpful in diagnosis. Bull Johns Hopkins Hosp 100:241, 1957.
13. Davidson RA, Wilcox CS: Newer tests for the diagnosis of renovascular disease. JAMA 268:3353, 1992.
14. Dean RH, Foster JH: Criteria for the diagnosis of renovascular hypertension. Surgery 74:926, 1973.
15. Dean RH, Lawson JD, Hollifield JW, et al: Revascularization of the poorly functioning kidney. Surgery 85:44, 1979.
16. del Greco F, Simon NM, Goodman S, et al: Plasma renin activity in primary and secondary hypertension. Medicine 46:475, 1967.
17. Derkx FHM, Tan-Tjiong HL, Wentig GJ, et al: Captopril test for diagnosis of renal artery stenosis. In Glorioso M (ed): Renovascular Hypertension. New York, Raven Press, 1987, p 295.
18. Eyler WR, Clark MD, Garman JE, et al: Angiography of the renal areas including a comparative study of renal arterial stenosis in patients with and without hypertension. Radiology 78:879, 1962.
19. Foster JH, Maxwell MH, Franklin SS, et al: Renovascular occlusive disease: Results of operative treatment. JAMA 231:1043, 1975.
20. Gaul MK, Linn WD, Mulrow CD: Captopril-stimulated renin secretion in the diagnosis of renovascular hypertension. Am J Hypertens 2:335, 1989.
21. Gavras H, Brunner HR, Thurston H, et al: Reciprocation of renin dependency with sodium volume dependency in renal hypertension. Science 188:1316, 1975.
22. Gavras H, Brunner HR, Vaughan ED Jr, et al: Angiotensin-sodium interaction in blood pressure maintenance of renal hypertensive and normotensive rats. Science 180:1369, 1973.
23. Goldblatt H: Studies on experimental hypertension. J Exp Med 59:347, 1934.
24. Gosse P, Dupas JY, Reynaud P, et al: Captopril test in the detection of renovascular hypertension in a population with low prevalence of the disease. A prospective study. Am J Hypertens 2:191, 1989.
25. Gross F: The renin-angiotensin system in hypertension. Ann Intern Med 75:777, 1971.
26. Harvey RJ, Krumlovsky F, del Greco F, et al: Screening for renovascular hypertension. JAMA 254:388, 1985.
27. Howard JE, Connor TB: Use of differential renal function studies in the diagnosis of renovascular hypertension. Am J Surg 107:58, 1964.
28. Hricik DE, Browning PJ, Kopelman R, et al: Captopril induced functional renal insufficiency in patients with bilateral renal artery stenosis or renal artery stenosis in a solitary kidney. N Engl J Med 308:373, 1983.
29. Kimbrough HM Jr, Vaughan ED Jr, Carey RM, et al: Effect of intrarenal angiotensin II blockade on renal function in conscious dogs. Circ Res 40:174, 1977.
30. Kurtzman NA, Pillay VKG, Rogers PW, et al: Renal vascular hypertension and low plasma renin activity. Arch Intern Med 133:195, 1974.
31. Laragh JH: Curable renal hypertension—Renin, marker or cause? JAMA 218:733, 1971.
32. Laragh JH: The modern evaluation and treatment of hypertension: The causal role of the kidneys. J Urol 147:1469, 1992.
33. Laragh JH, Baer L, Brunner HR, et al: Renin, angiotensin and aldosterone system in pathogenesis and management of hypertensive vascular disease. Am J Med 52:633, 1972.
34. Laragh JH, Sealey JE: The renin-angiotensin-aldosterone system in the renal regulation of sodium, potassium, and blood pressure regulation. In Windhager EE (ed): Handbook of Physiology. New York, Oxford Press, 1991.
35. Leadbetter WF, Burkland CE: Hypertension in unilateral renal disease. J Urol 39:611, 1938.
36. Liard JF, Cowley AW, McCaa RE, et al: Renin, aldosterone, body fluid volumes, and the baroreceptor reflex in the development and reversal of Goldblatt hypertension in conscious dogs. Circ Res 34:549, 1974.
37. Libertino JA: Renovascular surgery. In Walsh PC, Retik AB, Stamey TA, Vaughan ED Jr (eds): Campbell's Urology. 6th ed. Philadelphia, WB Saunders, 1992.
38. London GM, Safar ME: Renal hemodynamics in patients with sustained essential hypertension and in patients with unilateral stenosis of the renal artery. Am J Hypertens 2:244, 1989.
39. Marks LS, Maxwell MH: Renal vein renin value and limitations in the prediction of operative results. Urol Clin North Am 2:311, 1975.
40. Maxwell MH, Lupu AN, Kaufman JJ: Individual kidney function tests in renal arterial hypertension. J Urol 100:384, 1968.
41. McNeil BJ, Adelstein SJ: Measures of clinical efficacy: The value of case finding in hypertensive renovascular disease. N Engl J Med 293:221, 1975.
42. McNeil BJ, Varady PD, Burrows BA: Measures of clinical efficacy: Cost-effectiveness calculations in the diagnosis and treatment of hypertensive renovascular disease. N Engl J Med 293:216, 1975.
43. Meier GH, Sumpio B, Black HR, et al: Captopril renal scintigraphy—An advance in the detection and treatment of renovascular hypertension. J Vasc Surg 11(6):770, 1990.
44. Miller ED Jr, Samuels AI, Haber E, et al: Inhibition of angiotensin conversion in experimental renovascular hypertension. Science 177:1108, 1972.
45. Möhring J, Möhring B, Näumann HJ, et al: Salt and water balance and renin activity in renal hypertension of rats. Am J Physiol 288:1847, 1975.
46. Mueller CB, Surtshin A, Carlin MR, et al: Glomerular and tubular influences on sodium and water excretion. Am J Physiol 165:411, 1951.
47. Muller FB, Sealey JE, Case DB, et al: The captopril test for identifying renovascular disease in hypertensive patients. Am J Med 80:633, 1986.
48. Osborne RW Jr, Goldstone J, Hillman BJ, et al: Digital video subtraction angiography: Screening technique for renovascular hypertension. Surgery 90:932, 1981.
49. Palmer JM: Prognostic value of contralateral renal plasma flow in renovascular hypertension. JAMA 217:794, 1971.
50. Pederson EB, Sorensen SS, Amdisen A, et al: Abnormal glomerular and tubular function during angiotensin converting enzyme inhibition in renovascular hypertension evaluated by lithium clearance method. Eur J Clin Invest 19:135, 1989.
51. Pickering TG, Sos TA, Vaughan ED Jr, et al: Predictive value and changes of renin secretion in hypertensive patients with unilateral

renovascular disease undergoing successful renal angioplasty. Am J Med 76:398, 1984.

52. Poutasse EF, Marks LS, Wisoff CP, et al: Renal-vein renin determinations in hypertension: Falsely negative tests. J Urol 110:371, 1973.

53. Re R, Novelline R, Escourrou MT, et al: Inhibition of angiotensin-converting enzyme for diagnosis of renal artery stenosis. N Engl J Med 298:582, 1978.

54. Russell RP: Renal hypertension. Surg Clin North Am 54:349, 1974.

55. Schaeffer AJ, Fair WR: Comparison of split function ratios with renal-vein renin ratios in patients with curable hypertension caused by unilateral renal artery stenosis. J Urol 112:697, 1974.

56. Schalekamp MA, Beevers DG, Briggs JD, et al: Hypertension in chronic renal failure: Abnormal relation between sodium and the renin-angiotensin system. Am J Med 55:379, 1973.

57. Schambelan M, Glickman M, Stockigt JR, et al: The selective renal vein renin sampling in hypertensive patients with segmental renal lesions. N Engl J Med 290:1153, 1974.

58. Sealey JE, Bühler FR, Laragh JH, Vaughan ED Jr: The physiology of renin secretion in essential hypertension: Estimation of renin secretion rate and renal plasma flow from peripheral and renal vein renin levels. Am J Med 55:391, 1973.

59. Sealey JE, Laragh JH (eds): What is the mechanism of one-kidney, one-clip hypertension and its relevance to low renin essential hypertension. Am J Hypertens Suppl 4(10 Part 2):519S, 1991.

60. Smith HW: Unilateral nephrectomy in hypertensive disease. J Urol 76:685, 1956.

61. Sos TA, Sniderman KW, Pickering TG, et al: Percutaneous transluminal renal angioplasty in renovascular hypertension due to atheroma or fibromuscular dysplasia. N Engl J Med 309:274, 1983.

62. Sosa RE, Vaughan ED Jr: Renovascular hypertension. In Gillenwater JY, Grayhack JT, Howards SS, Duckett JW (eds): Adult and Pediatric Urology. Chicago, Year Book Medical Publishers, 1987.

63. Stamey TA: Functional characteristics of renovascular hypertension with emphasis on the relationship of renal blood flow and hypertension. Circ Res 11:209, 1962.

64. Stamey TA: Renovascular Hypertension. Baltimore, Williams & Wilkins, 1963.

65. Stanley JC, Fry WJ: Surgical treatment of renovascular hypertension. Arch Surg 112:1291, 1977.

66. Stockigt JR, Noakes CA, Collins RD, et al: Renal-vein renin in various forms of renal hypertension. Lancet 1:1194, 1972.

67. Vaughan ED Jr: The renin-angiotensin-aldosterone system in renal and adrenal hypertensions. In Devine CJ Jr, Stecker JF Jr (eds): Urology in Practice. Boston, Little, Brown, 1978.

68. Vaughan ED Jr, Bühler FR, Laragh JH, et al: Renovascular hypertension: Renin measurements to indicate hypersecretion and contralateral suppression, estimate renal plasma flow, and score for surgical curability. Am J Med 55:402, 1973.

69. Vaughan ED Jr, Bühler FR, Laragh JH, et al: Hypertension and unilateral parenchymal renal disease: Evidence for abnormal vasoconstriction-volume interaction. JAMA 233:1177, 1975.

70. Vaughan ED Jr, Peach MJ (eds): Saralasin. Kidney Int 15(Suppl 9):51, 1979.

71. Vaughan ED Jr, Sos TA, Sniderman KW, et al: Renal vein renin secretory patterns before and after transluminal angioplasty in patients with renovascular hypertension: Verification of analytic criteria. In Laragh JH (ed): Frontiers in Hypertension Research. New York, Springer-Verlag, 1981.

72. Vaughan ED Jr, Sosa ER: Renovascular hypertension. In Walsh PC, Retik AB, Stamey TA, Vaughan ED Jr (eds): Campbell's Urology. 6th ed. Philadelphia, WB Saunders, 1992, p 2017.

73. Wilcox GS, Smith TP, Fredrickson ED, et al: Captopril glomerular filtration rate renogram in renovascular hypertension. Clin Nucl Med 14:1, 1989.

74. Willems CED, Shah V, Uchiyama M, et al: The captopril test: An aid to investigation of hypertension. Arch Dis Child 64:229, 1989.

75. Zimmerman BG: Involvement of angiotensin-mediated renal vasoconstriction in renal hypertension. Life Sci 13:507, 1973.

107

Radiologic Evaluation and Treatment of Renovascular Hypertension

Michael D. Dake, M.D., and Ernest J. Ring, M.D.

• • •

Renal artery disease is the most common surgically curable form of hypertension. Estimates of its prevalence vary widely (from 0.18 to 13 per cent of all hypertensive patients), but it is likely that at least 600,000 people in the United States are affected.[1-7] Despite important developments in the detection and management of renovascular disease over the last half century, the manner in which this population should be identified and treated remains controversial.

It is well established that normalizing blood pressure in hypertensive patients leads to less renal insufficiency, less myocardial injury, fewer strokes, and prolonged life expectancy.[8-10] The 1977 Joint National Committee on Detection, Evaluation, and Treatment of High Blood Pressure recommended medical therapy and discouraged extensive evaluation of newly diagnosed hypertensive patients.[11] Only in patients with clinical presentations highly suggestive of renovascular hypertension or in those whose conditions were refractory to drug therapy was an evaluation for renal artery disease recommended. More recent observations, however, indicate that although blood pressure can now be controlled more readily with the latest antihypertensive medications—particularly beta-blockers and angiotensin-converting enzyme inhibitors—both atherosclerotic disease and fibromuscular renal artery disease commonly progress and can severely compromise renal function.[12–14] Thus, the clinical challenge is to devise economical, low-risk strategies for determining which patients will benefit from renal artery revascularization procedures.

The diagnosis of physiologically significant renal artery stenosis is difficult and still can be made with absolute certainty only in retrospect, after a successful response to renal artery reconstruction or angioplasty. Renal arteriography can certainly establish the presence of renovascular disease and can usually determine the cause of renal artery stenosis. It cannot, however, determine whether the stenotic lesion is responsible for hypertension because many normotensive patients and patients with essential hypertension have renal artery lesions.[15–17]

There are no pathognomonic symptoms or physical findings that lead to a reliable clinical diagnosis. The Cooperative Study of Renovascular Hypertension investigated many potentially valuable clinical features, including an abdominal systolic-diastolic bruit, retinopathy, hypokalemia, and a family history of hypertension.[9] After reviewing the results of the study, Simon and associates concluded that there were no valid clinical indicators of renovascular hypertension.[9] Indeed, most patients with renovascular hypertension do not present with the prototypical history of a sudden onset of severe hypertension at a young age but are clinically indistinguishable from patients with essential hypertension.[18]

New understandings of endocrine mechanisms and technologic advances in radiology (computed tomography, ultrasound imaging. Doppler flow studies, digital subtraction angiography, and magnetic resonance imaging) have allowed more accurate and less invasive assessment of renovascular disease. However, the low prevalence of renovascular hypertension compared with that of essential hypertension makes any test designed for diagnosis questionable on the basis of exaggerated cost : benefit and risk : benefit ratios. Even a test of high sensitivity and specificity will have a low predictive value and result in a large number of patients with essential hypertension undergoing unnecessary, costly procedures.[18]

Until fairly recently, the decision to embark on a diagnostic work-up of renovascular hypertension was also discouraged by the rather poor outcome of many of the earlier surgical series. With improved operative technique and the potential for nonsurgical therapy with angioplasty, interest has been rekindled in identifying patients who have a great deal to gain by early diagnosis and treatment.

Once the decision is made to pursue an evaluation for renovascular hypertension, multiple imaging and physiologic tests may be used. Included in these studies are radiologic and other imaging techniques such as intravenous urography, nuclear medicine studies, digital subtraction angiography, conventional arteriography, computed tomography, magnetic resonance imaging, ultrasound imaging, and Doppler flow studies. Because of the imprecise studies available and the variability of clinical conditions, personalized work-up strategies rather than rigid diagnostic policies are necessary.

INTRAVENOUS UROGRAPHY

Abnormalities in the excretory urogram have been used for several decades as clues to renovascular disease. However, it was not until the introduction of the rapid-sequence urogram that urography became widely accepted as a screening method for renovascular hypertension.[19] This technical modification used films exposed at 1, 2, 3, and 5 minutes after contrast infusion to evaluate the parenchymal and early excretory function better.

It must be emphasized that intravenous urography does not directly image renal arterial anatomy. Rather, it relies on differences in excretory function between a normally perfused and an ischemic kidney. The three major features of renal artery stenosis demonstrated on the rapid-sequence modification of the intravenous urogram are (1) delayed appearance of contrast material in the calyces of the ischemic kidney, which reflects diminished glomerular filtration rate; (2) hyperconcentration of the contrast material within the collecting system of the underperfused kidney, which reflects increased fractional resorption of salt and water; and (3) decreased size of the ischemic kidney, which reflects reduced intrarenal blood volume and is manifested by differences in renal size in cases in which the right kidney is at least 2 cm shorter than the left or the left is at least 1.5 cm shorter than the right.[20] Identification of one or more of these features constitutes a positive study result.

Maxwell and coworkers, innovators of the rapid-sequence intravenous urogram, detected urographic abnormalities in 89 per cent of their hypertensive patients with angiographically proven renal artery stenosis.[19] Unfortunately, the efficacy of hypertensive urography as a test for renal artery stenosis varies greatly among series. In the largest angiographically controlled cooperative study, rapid-sequence urogram findings were abnormal in 78 per cent of patients with renovascular hypertension and in 11 per cent of hypertensive patients with normal arteriographic findings.[21] The predictive value for the diagnosis of renal artery stenosis from this study was 31 per cent. Bilateral and segmental renal arterial lesions accounted for a significant number of the false-negative examination findings.

Rapid-sequence intravenous urography is clearly a less than optimal screening test for renovascular hypertension. In the current work-up of hypertension, intravenous urography is used as much to exclude renal parenchymal disease as to look for signs of renovascular disease.

NUCLEAR MEDICINE STUDIES

The development of radionuclide urography as a screening procedure for renovascular hypertension closely paralleled that of intravenous urography. In 1956, Taplin and coworkers proposed that radionuclide urograms might be used to identify patients with renovascular hypertension.[22] Several other investigators applied this concept in studies that employed infusions of nonresorbable solutes such as iodine-131–iodohippurate sodium.[23–26]

The rationale for using these agents is that an underperfused kidney will accumulate a peak concentration and excrete the infused solute more slowly than the normal contralateral kidney. Radionuclide urography using iodine-131–iodohippurate sodium serves as an indirect measure of effective renal plasma flow, and its images represent radionuclide analogues of the intravenous urogram.[27] Data from several arteriographically controlled series that used iodine-131–iodohippurate sodium urograms to evaluate renovascular hypertension revealed a composite sensitivity of 74 per cent and a specificity of 77 per cent.[24–26, 28–31] More recent studies have used rapid-sequence imaging with the blood pool agent technetium-99m–diethylenetriamine penta-acetic acid (^{99m}Tc-DTPA), glucoheptonate, or similar agents in combination with traditional radionuclide urography with iodine-131–iodohippurate sodium[32–35] (Fig. 107–1). The uptake of ^{99m}Tc-DTPA by the kidneys is known to be reflective of relative glomerular filtration rates.[27] The use of ^{99m}Tc-DTPA and the introduction of computer-generated time versus tracer activity curves allow a more quantitative evaluation of renal blood flow and functional symmetry than was previously possible. Collective results from three arteriographically controlled investigations of renovascular hypertension using the combination of iodine-131–iodohippurate sodium and ^{99m}Tc-DTPA produced a composite sensitivity of 86 per cent and a specificity of 89 per cent.[32–34]

Even with the higher accuracy gained by using a combination of nuclides, the use of radionuclide urography as a screening test for patients with renal insufficiency is limited because of the test's added cost, its number of false-negative findings, and its low etiologic specificity as a result of poor anatomic detail.

The modification of isotope renography to include the use of the angiotensin-converting enzyme inhibitor captopril has significantly improved its diagnostic value.[36–40] Increased production of angiotensin II is a final result of functionally significant renal artery stenosis. This increased production of angiotensin II leads to selective vasoconstriction of the postglomerular efferent arterioles. The impact of this is to maintain glomerular capillary filtration. Therefore, when angiotensin II production is blocked by captopril, glomerular filtration drops precipitously. This phenomenon is used to compare the renal handling of technetium-99m–labeled mercaptoacetyltriglycine before and immediately after ingestion of a dose of captopril. The finding of a deterioration in renal handling of the radiotracer after captopril ingestion is indicative of the presence of a functionally significant stenosis. In comparison to the results of arteriography, this study has been reported to have a 92 per cent sensitivity, a 94 per cent specificity, a 93 per cent

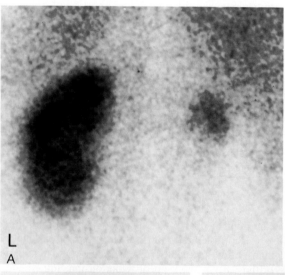

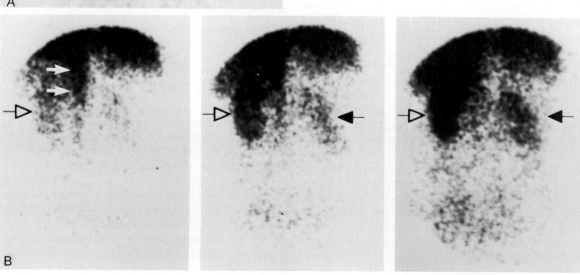

FIGURE 107–1. Radionuclide studies of renal artery stenosis. *A,* Posteriorly imaged iodine-131–iodohippurate scan demonstrates poor tracer uptake by the right kidney. This indicates a relative decrease in effective renal plasma flow to the right kidney caused by a renal artery stenosis. *B,* Three scans from a posteriorly imaged technetium-99m–diethylenetriamine penta-acetic acid study show dynamic flow to the kidneys. There is a delayed appearance of tracer and decreased radionuclide uptake by the right kidney (*black arrow*) relative to the left (*open arrow*). This blood pool agent is handled by glomerular filtration, and the unilateral delayed perfusion suggests a right renal artery stenosis (aorta, *white arrows*).

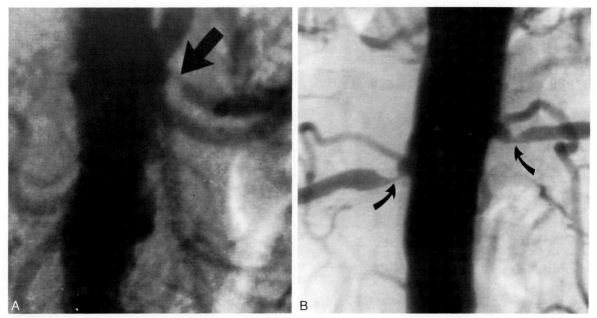

FIGURE 107–2. Comparison of intravenous and intra-arterial digital subtraction angiography (DSA). *A*, Intravenous DSA image demonstrates left renal artery stenosis (*arrow*). *B*, Intra-arterial DSA examination shows bilateral renal artery lesions (*arrows*). An intra-arterial study results in a higher quality image than that produced by intravenous DSA because contrast is injected in the specific region of interest rather than through a central venous catheter. If necessary, intra-arterial DSA may be easily combined with selective renal artery catheterization.

accuracy, a 94 per cent positive predictive value, and a 91 per cent negative predictive value.[40]

DIGITAL SUBTRACTION ANGIOGRAPHY

In general, digital subtraction angiography (DSA) refers to the visualization of vessels with the use of digital fluorographic techniques for image enhancement (Fig. 107–2). Renal DSA transfers radiographic exposures onto an image intensifier after the intravenous injection of contrast material. In order to visualize the abdominal aorta and renal arteries better, a computer subtracts the digitally reconstructed perfect contrast material enters the abdominal circulation from those containing intra-arterial dye. The contrast media can be administered intravenously or directly into an artery, much like with conventional angiography.

Intravenous DSA can be performed as an outpatient procedure using central venous catheterization following puncture of an antecubital or femoral vein.[41] It can be used in conjunction with renal vein renin sampling and for monitoring patients after anatomic correction of a renal artery lesion.[42] The main advantage of DSA is its ability to produce in many cases arterial images with less risk, discomfort, and expense than conventional arteriography. The degree of benefit depends on the angiographer's experience and on institutional billing policies.

There are several disadvantages of intravenous DSA when compared with conventional arteriography.[43–47] Patient cooperation is essential in obtaining a quality image because motion produces artifacts. Even involuntary motion, including respiratory movement, cardiovascular motion, and intestinal peristalsis, will result in misregistration

artifacts that decrease both spatial and contrast resolution.[45] For imaging the abdominal aorta and the renal arteries, intravenous administration of glucagon is frequently used to decrease peristalsis, although it is often only partially successful.[48] Compression bands and prone positioning of the patient may displace bowel gas from over the aorta and kidneys, but both of these technical aids are cumbersome and uncomfortable.[49] Despite such maneuvers, bowel gas often precludes adequate imaging of the intrarenal vessels. Another difficulty often encountered with DSA is caused by calcium in certain atherosclerotic plaques.[49] When an atherosclerotic plaque containing a large amount of calcium has encircled the vessel being imaged, the plaque can appear as an area of increased density or lucency that obscures the underlying opacified artery.

In comparison with conventional angiography, intravenous DSA has considerably worse spatial resolution.[20, 49] Although DSA can often define the anatomy and location of the main renal arteries, lack of resolution limits its ability to visualize vessels in the distal main renal artery or interlobar branches.[20] Fibromuscular dysplasia usually involves the mid-, distal, or segmental arteries, and it may be missed with intravenous DSA.[50] In addition, unexpected accessory renal arteries with significant lesions are usually overlooked.[51] Furthermore, because the intravenous injection provides global opacification, overlapping visceral vessels can obscure significant renal artery pathology.[20, 43–45, 49] With the use of multiple projections, superimposition problems can be minimized; however, these projections prolong the examination and increase the risk of contrast-induced complications. Intravenous DSA images are sometimes totally uninterpretable, especially in obese patients or in patients with diminished cardiac function.[20, 43–46]

Finally, there is a misconception that intravenous DSA

is a simple "noninvasive" examination. DSA involves placement of a catheter into the central venous system (usually the superior vena cava or the right atrium) and injection of a large volume of contrast medium. The risk of contrast-induced acute renal dysfunction rises with increasing amounts of contrast media administered and with decreasing degrees of patient hydration.[52] This danger is amplified in patients with preexisting moderate to severe renal impairment.

Despite encouraging early results with the use of DSA as a screening procedure, two studies with conventional arteriographic controls[41, 43] showed the sensitivity of intravenous DSA to be only 83 and 87 per cent, with a specificity of only 79 and 87 per cent, respectively. In addition, other reviews noted that 5 to 20 per cent of renal DSA studies performed were uninterpretable.[20, 41, 43, 44, 53–55] The high rate of technically unsatisfactory examinations and the poor resolution have been discouraging, and many centers have abandoned this method for screening purposes.

CONVENTIONAL ARTERIOGRAPHY

Conventional arteriography using either filming or digital subtraction with selective injection and magnification techniques continues to be the most reliable test for detecting renal artery disease.[56] The great reliability of modern arteriography is universally accepted. Disappointed by unreliable and inaccurate screening studies, many clinicians now regard the traditional diagnostic work-up of renovascular hypertension (determination of peripheral plasma renin activity, testing with angiotensin analogues or converting enzyme inhibitors, intravenous urography, nuclear medicine studies, renal vein renin studies, and DSA) as overly expensive, complicated, nondiagnostic, and designed to determine the need for renal arteriography. In clinical practice, arteriography is often eventually performed, regardless of prior test results.[18]

The usual angiographic technique for evaluation of renal hypertension consists of abdominal aortography and bilateral selective renal arteriography. In addition to improving visualization of the main renal artery by eliminating overlapping mesenteric vessels, selective renal arteriography helps to identify peripheral renovascular abnormalities and renal parenchymal diseases.[57]

ANGIOGRAPHIC FINDINGS IN RENOVASCULAR HYPERTENSION

The morphology of renal artery stenotic lesions is important in the natural history, clinical relevance, and response to treatment of renovascular hypertension. The vast majority of cases of renal artery disease are due to two pathologic processes: atherosclerosis and fibromuscular dysplasia.[56] Many other causes of renovascular hypertension have been reported, but they account for fewer than 10 per cent of all cases.[58] Additional causes include stenotic and nonstenotic lesions, such as renal artery aneurysm (Fig. 107–3); congenital stenosis or coarctation of the renal artery; renal artery embolus or thrombosis with secondary infarction; arteriovenous fistula; Takayasu's arteritis (Fig. 107–4); necrotizing angiitis; iatrogenic renal artery stenosis (after catheter manipulation, irradiation, or surgery) (Fig. 107–5); neurofibromatosis; aortic dissection; extrinsic compression of the renal artery by tumor, cysts, diaphragm crura, or fibrous bands; and trauma with resultant vascular pedicle injury, arteriovenous fistula, infarction, or perinephric hematoma (Page's kidney).

Because atherosclerosis and fibromuscular dysplasia account for more than 90 per cent of the cases of renovascular hypertension, a more detailed focus on these disorders follows.

Atherosclerosis is a generalized degenerative disease of major blood vessels that is the most common cause of renal artery stenosis. It is usually associated with aging and is frequently noted among individuals in their 5th decade

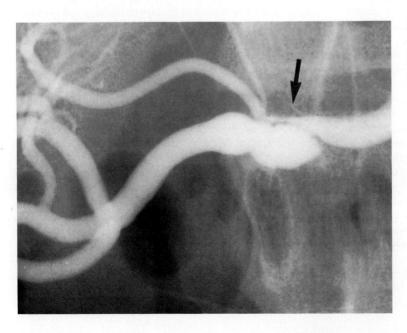

FIGURE 107–3. Renal artery dissection. A selective injection of the right renal artery demonstrates a dissection with intimal flap (*arrow*). This occurred spontaneously in a 31-year-old man with a generalized angiopathy.

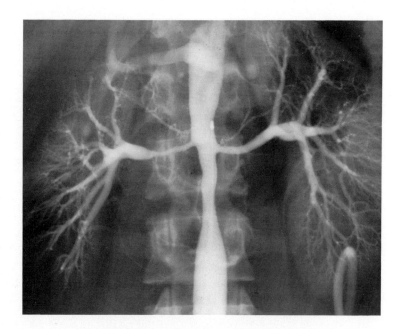

FIGURE 107–4. Takayasu's arteritis. Abdominal aortogram showing an occluded superior mesenteric artery, smooth segmental narrowing of the proximal renal arteries bilaterally, and long narrowing of the infrarenal aorta. Symmetric long segmental stenoses of the aorta or its branches are characteristic findings in Takayasu's arteritis.

or older. It affects men twice as often as women. Although some individuals present at a young age with accelerated disease, symptoms usually do not become manifest before the age of 50.[56, 59] The kidneys are frequently involved, and most often the disease affects the renal arteries on only one side; however, significant bilateral atherosclerotic stenoses are noted in 33 to 43 per cent of cases.[59–61] There is no propensity for either right-sided or left-sided involvement. The natural history of atherosclerotic renal artery disease is poorly understood. Its progression, however, appears to parallel that observed in the carotid, coronary, and peripheral arteries.[56]

Atherosclerosis usually involves the orifice or the proximal third of the renal artery with an eccentric narrow-

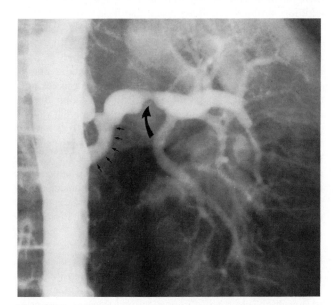

FIGURE 107–5. Postoperative stenosis after surgical revascularization. Six weeks after aortorenal bypass grafting using the left hypogastric artery (*small arrows*), an abdominal aortogram demonstrates an eccentric stenosis of the left renal artery (*large arrow*) distal to the graft. This is caused by intimal hyperplasia.

ing often associated with post-stenotic dilatation[58] (Fig. 107–6A). However, distal main renal artery and segmental artery involvement is not infrequent. Serial angiographic studies document that one third to one half of patients experience progression of their disease and that new stenoses may develop.[62, 63] If the stenosis or occlusion develops slowly, collateral circulation may be demonstrated angiographically in some patients.

With atherosclerotic renal artery disease, coexisting diffuse atherosclerosis with plaque formation in the abdominal aorta may be present (see Fig. 107–6B). If the aorta is severely involved, it may be very difficult to determine by aortography if intra-aortic plaque is compromising the origin of the renal artery. Although individuals with localized atherosclerotic lesions appear to have a better long-term survival than those with generalized disease, these differences are not well defined.

Fibromuscular dysplasia refers to a group of idiopathic fibrous and fibromuscular lesions that tend to involve central arteries that are long and straight. Commonly affected vessels include the renal, internal carotid, superior mesenteric, and external iliac arteries. Many classifications of this disorder have been proposed, but for practical purposes it is simplest to classify the disease by the specific region of the arterial wall predominantly involved. Thus, lesions are grouped into three types: (1) intimal, (2) medial, and (3) perimedial-adventitial.[64] These disorders account for approximately one third of all cases of renovascular hypertension and occur in women with a 3 : 1 preponderance to men.[58, 65] Bilateral involvement is common. In one study, it occurred in 43 per cent of cases.[66] The age of patients on detection is usually between the 2nd and 4th decades.[57] However, the disease has been identified in children as young as 6 months, and the largest reported series indicates that stenoses as a result of fibromuscular dysplasia are often found in middle-aged and older women.[57, 63, 67]

Intimal fibrodysplasia (Fig. 107–7A) accounts for about 5 per cent of fibromuscular disease.[56] It appears angiographically as a smooth concentric collar or funnel-shaped narrowing of the renal artery that is caused by a

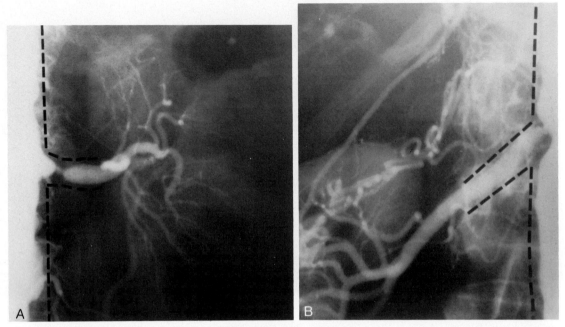

FIGURE 107–6. Renal artery stenosis caused by atherosclerotic disease. (*Dashed lines* approximate the outer wall of the aorta and the renal artery.) *A,* Abdominal aortogram demonstrates a typical atherosclerotic stenosis of the renal artery. The ostial segment is widely patent, and the narrowing is 2 to 3 mm into the renal artery. *B,* Abdominal aortogram reveals stenosis of the right renal artery caused by large aortic plaques narrowing the ostium. This type of lesion does not respond well to percutaneous transluminal angioplasty (PTA).

circumferential subintimal collagen deposit. The etiology of this process has been hypothetically linked to embryonic cell rests within the intima, intrauterine or early neonatal arterial injuries, and thrombotic sequelae of infectious diseases such as rubella.[56]

Medial fibrodysplasia (see Fig. 107–7B) is the most commonly encountered type of fibromuscular dysplasia. It accounts for 85 per cent of these lesions.[56] In medial fibrodysplasia, there are ridges of fibrous tissue and loosely deposited collagen that replace the normal smooth muscle of the media. The resultant areas of luminal narrowing alternate with multiple dilated or aneurysmal segments. These dilated segments are of greater diameter than the normal renal artery lumen.[58] Angiographically, this combination of multiple narrowed lesions with intervening normal or dilated segments produces a characteristic "string-of-beads" or corrugated appearance that is virtually pathognomonic for medial fibrodysplasia. The lesion typically involves the distal two thirds of the main renal artery and proximal segmental renal arteries.[57] Angiographically, the anatomy is best defined when films are obtained during deep inspiration (Fig. 107–8). This pattern of involvement, which spares the proximal segment of the vessel, is similar to that observed in other arteries affected by fibromuscular dysplasia. The predilection for more frequent and severe involvement of the right renal artery is an oddity shared by all types of fibromuscular dysplasia.[58, 68] Progression of medial fibroplasia in patients over the age of 40 years is considered rare.[68]

Perimedial-adventitial dysplasia (see Fig. 107–7C) accounts for 10 per cent of fibromuscular renal artery stenoses.[56] It occurs almost exclusively in women younger than 30 years.[68] Affected individuals are commonly hypertensive. Pathologically, this type of dysplasia is characterized by a concentric deposit of collagen between the media and the adventitia. The dense collar of collagen often invades these layers and produces a beaded angiographic appearance. The beads, however, do not represent aneurysms as in medial fibroplasia. In this lesion, the beads are smaller than the diameter of the normal renal artery lumen.[58] In addition, prominent collateral circulation is a very common angiographic finding in perimedial-adventitial dysplasia.[68]

Less common angiographic appearances of fibromuscular dysplasia include a web, a diaphragm-like stenosis involving only a short segment (Fig. 107–9), and a smooth segmental narrowing that mimics an atheromatous lesion.[57] Other abnormalities associated with fibromuscular disease include post-stenotic aneurysmal dilatation, medial dissection, and branch vessel aneurysms (Fig. 107–10). Although fibromuscular dysplasia may undergo remission, the limited knowledge of its natural history suggests that the disease process is progressive. Thus, it is especially important to identify patients with fibromuscular dysplasia because they are usually young and face a long course of medical therapy for a disorder that is particularly responsive to angioplasty and surgical therapy.

Significant insight into renovascular hypertension can be gained by comparing and contrasting atherosclerosis, fibromuscular dysplasia, and essential hypertension. Data from the 1972 Cooperative Study of Renovascular Hypertension highlight the differences among these disease processes.[9] Patients with atherosclerotic renovascular hypertension were older (mean age, 49.7 years) than those with stenoses caused by fibromuscular dysplasia (mean age, 34.9

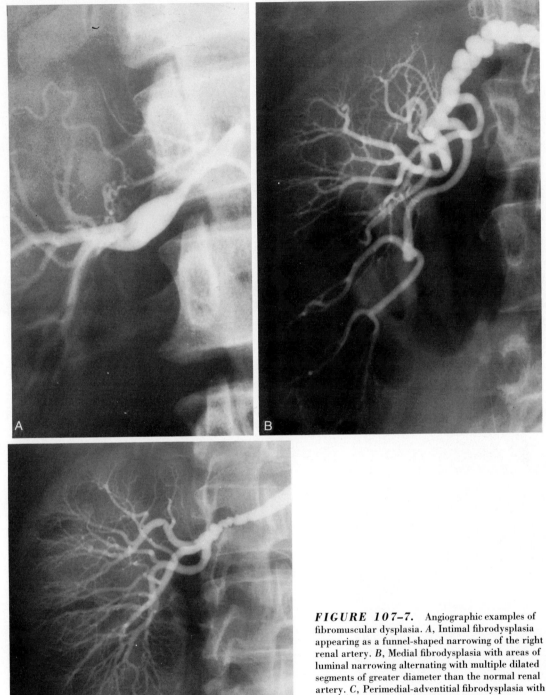

FIGURE 107-7. Angiographic examples of fibromuscular dysplasia. *A*, Intimal fibrodysplasia appearing as a funnel-shaped narrowing of the right renal artery. *B*, Medial fibrodysplasia with areas of luminal narrowing alternating with multiple dilated segments of greater diameter than the normal renal artery. *C*, Perimedial-adventitial fibrodysplasia with multiple collar-like constrictions producing the beaded appearance. The beads are smaller than the diameter of the normal lumen and do not represent aneurysms as in medial fibrodysplasia.

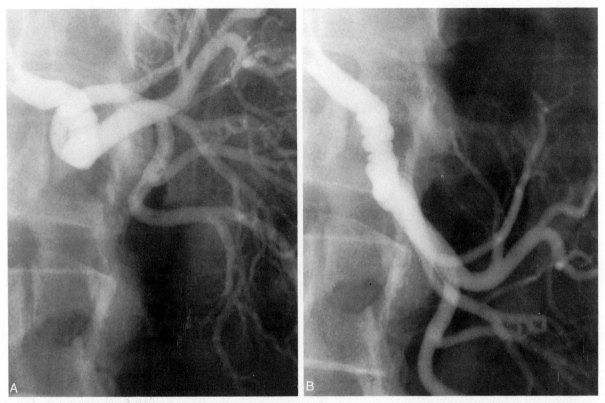

FIGURE 107–8. The value of an angiographic study performed during inspiration for evaluating fibromuscular dysplasia. *A*, Selective left renal arteriogram during expiration shows some irregularity of a coiled main renal artery. *B*, Repeated injection during inspiration unravels the renal artery and reveals the extent of fibromuscular disease.

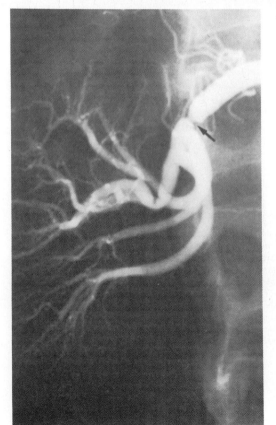

FIGURE 107–9. Fibromuscular dysplasia. A web-like stenosis (*arrow*) of the distal main right renal artery, typical of fibromuscular dysplasia.

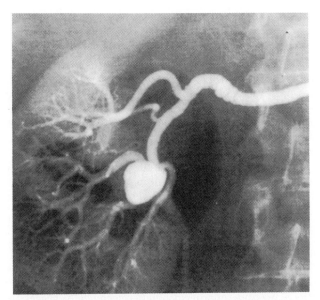

FIGURE 107-10. Fibromuscular dysplasia with an aneurysm. Selective right renal arteriogram reveals a corrugated appearance of the distal third of the main renal artery, characteristic of medial fibrodysplasia. An associated saccular aneurysm is noted at the trifurcation of lower pole branches.

years). By comparison, patients with essential hypertension had a mean age of 40.8 years. The onset of hypertension after age 50 was noted in 39 per cent of patients with atherosclerotic renovascular hypertension, as compared with 7 per cent of patients with essential hypertension and only 3 per cent of patients with fibromuscular lesions. In contrast, the onset of hypertension under age 20 was reported in only 2 per cent of patients with atherosclerotic renovascular hypertension, as opposed to 12 per cent of patients with essential hypertension and 16 per cent of those with fibromuscular dysplasia. Eighty-one per cent of patients with fibromuscular renovascular hypertension were women. Most patients with essential and atherosclerotic renovascular hypertension were men.

Accelerated hypertension was more common in atherosclerotic renovascular hypertension (23 per cent) than in essential hypertension (13 per cent) and fibromuscular renovascular hypertension (14 per cent).

COMPUTED TOMOGRAPHY, MAGNETIC RESONANCE IMAGING, AND ULTRASOUND

Technologic advances in computed tomography and magnetic resonance imaging have raised hopes that these two modalities may become clinically useful in detecting renal artery stenosis. Although improvements in image resolution and reductions in scan time have made this prospect feasible, the experience reported is only anecdotal, and more studies will be needed before the clinical value of these modalities is established.[56, 69]

More data are available on the use of ultrasound, especially Doppler velocimetry, to detect renal artery stenosis

(see Fig. 107–11 on Color Plate V). Results of four large arteriographically controlled studies suggest that analysis of velocity waveforms derived from ultrasonic techniques can accurately identify this disease.[70–73] With the use of hemodynamic criteria based on Doppler characteristics of abnormal blood velocity, the overall sensitivity of velocimetry ranged between 83 and 89 per cent and its specificity varied from 73 to 97 per cent.

Because the method is noninvasive and nonionizing and can be repeatedly performed with relatively inexpensive instruments, Doppler velocimetry may be useful in following the progression of lesions in patients known to have renovascular disease. Another advantage is its potential for determining the physiologic significance of renal artery stenosis using techniques similar to the Doppler ultrasound methods of diagnosing hemodynamically significant cerebrovascular and peripheral vascular disease.

Despite their promise, there are some disadvantages to using ultrasonic techniques. As with DSA, a certain percentage of examinations will be nondiagnostic because of factors that prevent successful scanning of the renal arteries. Conditions that decrease the probability of obtaining a good study include obesity, previous abdominal surgery with scarring, and abdominal aortic aneurysm.[71]

However, with further study and improvements in instrumentation, ultrasound may become widely used for detecting patients with renal artery stenosis.

DIAGNOSTIC STRATEGY

Many clinicians today use a dogmatic prefixed set of tests to identify the patient with potentially curable hypertension. Yet, it is clear that no single approach can offer an accurate, reliable, and cost-effective solution when applied to all clinical circumstances.

Instead, a flexible strategy based on clinical features, disease severity, response to antihypertensive drug therapy, and suspicion of renovascular disease is necessary to provide cost-effective diagnoses without unnecessary invasive procedures. More than 60 per cent of all newly diagnosed hypertensive patients will have a reduction in blood pressure following diuretic therapy.[74] Any patient with fixed hypertension whose blood pressure is not responsive to diuretics is more likely to have renin-dependent hypertension and should be considered a candidate for further evaluation. If such nonresponding patients do not exhibit distinctive clinical features and simulate having essential hypertension, noninvasive studies may be used to screen for possible renovascular hypertension. Patients suspected of having renovascular hypertension include young patients, individuals with systolic-diastolic epigastric bruits, patients with severe and accelerated hypertension, and patients whose hypertension cannot be controlled with antihypertensive drug therapy. These higher-risk categories compose about 10 per cent of the entire hypertensive population.[9] If an accurate diagnosis can be made, these individuals have the potential benefit of avoiding long-term drug therapy. Because the duration of hypertension is inversely related to the cure rate from surgery or angioplasty,[18, 75–79] screening studies with a high false-negative rate are unacceptable. Therefore, arteriographic studies should be performed on these patients even if the findings of screening tests, including DSA, are negative.

In general, when the suspicion of renovascular disease is high, conventional renal arteriography is used to rule out this disorder or to identify a lesion. Renal vein renin determinations or blood pressure response to anatomic correction determines its functional significance. When the likelihood of renovascular hypertension is lower, noninvasive studies and DSA are employed.

PERCUTANEOUS TRANSLUMINAL ANGIOPLASTY

Percutaneous transluminal angioplasty (PTA) of the renal arteries is now well established as a treatment for renovascular hypertension. The clinical efficacy and low morbidity of renal artery dilatation have been proved by several large series.[42, 75, 77–80] Technical success rates of 85 to 95 per cent have been reported.[42, 75, 77–90] These technical success rates are associated with equally high initial therapeutic success rates. Results from several studies document a marked blood pressure reduction in 80 to 90 per cent of patients who have had technically successful PTA.[42, 75, 77–90] The rate of restenosis is low, and in most patients blood pressure improvement is maintained for more than 2 years.[84, 85, 91]

The highest technical and therapeutic success rates of PTA have been in patients with fibromuscular dysplasia[92–94] (Fig. 107–12). Similar success has been achieved with fi-brotic stenoses occurring after bypass surgery[80, 93] or secondary to a diffuse arteritis.[93, 95] The efficacy of PTA in correcting other fibrotic stenoses, such as those that are due to radiation injury, is uncertain.[93, 96] Hypertension associated with renal transplant arterial stenosis at the anastomotic site has been successfully treated with PTA.[75, 95, 97–103] Limited experience with balloon dilatation of renal artery lesions associated with neurofibromatosis is discouraging. In most reported cases, the renal artery stenoses could not be dilated.[80, 93–95, 104, 105]

Dilating focal atherosclerotic lesions is only slightly less successful than PTA of fibromuscular stenoses[94] (Fig. 107–13). Diffuse atherosclerotic lesions and ostial stenoses at the aortic wall have a much lower initial success rate.[106] Nevertheless, the development of intraluminal stents has created enthusiasm regarding the potential role of these devices in combination with PTA for the treatment of orificial disease. Initial results with their use suggest that they may improve the success rate in selected patients.[107, 108] Blood pressure improvement after technically successful PTA occurs more frequently in patients with renovascular hypertension of short duration than in those with long-standing disease.[75–79]

In general, a decrease in blood pressure following PTA is associated with a marked reduction in renin secretion from the previously stenotic side.[77–79, 109] A good therapeutic response, however, has been obtained despite persistent lateralization of renal vein renin values[77–79, 109] and without a nonlateralizing pre-PTA renal vein renin profile.[77, 79, 89, 109, 110]

As with most surgical or interventional procedures, the risk of complications from PTA has decreased with experi-

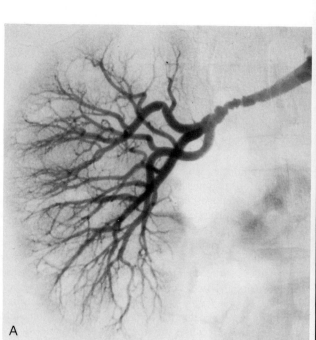

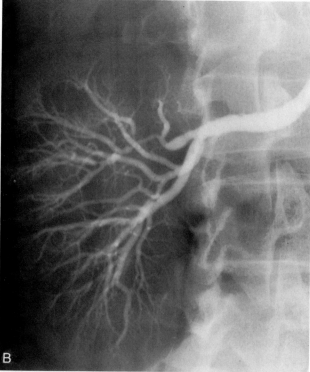

FIGURE 107–12. Angioplasty of fibromuscular dysplasia. *A,* Selective right renal arteriogram demonstrates the characteristic corrugated appearance of fibromuscular dysplasia involving the distal main renal artery. *B,* After angioplasty with an 8-mm balloon, there is a marked increase in luminal diameter.

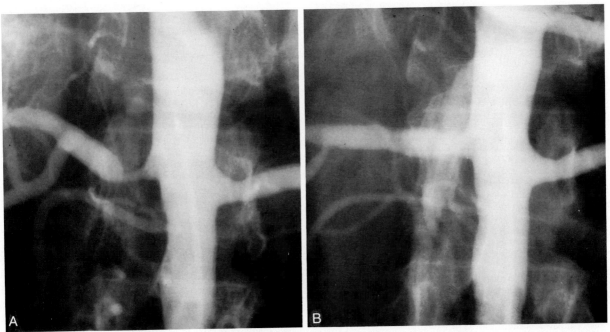

FIGURE 107–13.   PTA of a nonostial atherosclerotic renal artery stenosis. *A,* Abdominal aortogram demonstrates a typical atherosclerotic stenosis of the right renal artery. *B,* Following PTA, an excellent angiographic response is evident.

ence. Results from multiple large series suggest that PTA is a relatively low-risk procedure. Some investigators propose that the main risks are those of arteriography rather than of PTA itself.[91]

Most series report a PTA complication rate between 10 and 12 per cent.[42, 75, 77–90] The most common complications have been hematoma at the puncture site and transient worsening of renal function from the contrast load.[91, 111] Other, less common complications that require surgery in 2 to 6 per cent of all PTA cases include puncture site trauma and renal artery dissection, thrombosis, and rupture.[86, 111] Distal embolization with infarction occurs, but it is very rare.[86, 104]

In conclusion, many clinicians consider PTA the treatment of choice for renovascular hypertension caused by fibromuscular dysplasia or atherosclerotic disease involving the nonostial portion of the renal artery. PTA provides long-term benefit similar to that of surgery, but with a lower complication rate. Stenosis of the renal artery ostium is probably best treated surgically.

References

1. Tucker RM, Labarthe DR: Frequency of surgical treatment for hypertension in adults at the Mayo Clinic from 1973–1975. Mayo Clin Proc 52:549, 1977.
2. Gifford RW Jr: Epidemiology and clinical manifestations of renovascular hypertension. *In* Stanley JC, Ernst CB, Fry WJ (eds): Renovascular Hypertension. Philadelphia, WB Saunders, 1984, p 77.
3. Baldwin DS, van den Broek H, Harnes JR, et al: Renovascular hypertension in unselected patients. Arch Intern Med 120:176, 1967.
4. Bech K, Hilden T: The frequency of secondary hypertension. Acta Med Scand 197:65, 1975.
5. Wilhelmsen L, Berglund G: Prevalence of primary and secondary hypertension. Am Heart J 94:543, 1977.
6. Danielson M, Dammstrom B-G: The prevalence of secondary and curable hypertension. Acta Med Scand 209:451, 1981.
7. Kaplan NM: Hypertension. II. Prevalence, risks, and effect of therapy. Ann Intern Med 98:705, 1983.
8. Hypertension Detection and Follow-up Program Cooperative Group: Five-year findings of the Hypertension Detection and Follow-Up Program. I. Reduction in mortality of persons with high blood pressure, including mild hypertension. JAMA 242:2562, 1979.
9. Simon N, Franklin SA, Bleiter KH, et al: Cooperative Study of Renovascular Hypertension: Clinical characteristics of renovascular hypertension. JAMA 220:1209, 1972.
10. Hunt JC, Strong CG: Renovascular hypertension: Mechanisms, natural history and treatment. Am J Cardiol 32:562, 1973.
11. Report of the Joint National Committee on Detection, Evaluation, and Treatment of High Blood Pressure. A cooperative study. JAMA 237:255, 1977.
12. Meaney TF, Dustan HP, McCormack CJ: Natural history of renal arterial disease. Radiology 91:881, 1968.
13. Schreiber MJ, Pohl MA, Novick AC: The natural history of atherosclerotic and fibrous renal artery disease. Urol Clin North Am 11:383, 1984.
14. Wollenweber J, Sheps SG, David DG: Clinical course of atherosclerotic renovascular disease. Am J Cardiol 21:60, 1968.
15. Eyler WR, Clark MD, Garman JE, et al: Angiography of the renal areas including a comparative study of renal artery stenosis in patients with and without hypertension. Radiology 78:879, 1962.
16. Holley KE, Hunt JC, Brown AL, et al: Renal artery stenosis: A clinical-pathologic study in normotensive patients. Am J Med 37:14, 1964.
17. Dustan HP, Humphries AW, deWolfe VG, et al: Normal arterial pressure in patients with renal arterial stenosis. JAMA 187:1028, 1964.
18. Maxwell MH, Waks AU: Evaluation of patients with renovascular hypertension. Hypertension 6:589, 1984.
19. Maxwell MH, Gonick HC, Wiita R, et al: Use of the rapid sequence intravenous pyelogram in the diagnosis of renovascular hypertension. N Engl J Med 270:213, 1964.
20. Havey RJ, Krumlovsky F, delGreco F, et al: Screening for renovascular hypertension: Is renal digital-subtraction angiography the preferred noninvasive test? JAMA 254:388, 1985.
21. Maxwell MH, Bleifer DH, Franklin SS, et al: Cooperative study of renovascular hypertension: Demographic analysis of the study. JAMA 220:1195, 1972.
22. Taplin GV, Orsell MM Jr, Kade H, et al: The radioisotope renogram:

An external test for individual kidney function and upper urinary tract patency. J Lab Clin Med 48:886, 1956.

23. Winter CC: Renogram and other radioisotope tests in the diagnosis of renal hypertension. Am J Surg 107:43, 1964.

24. Burbank MK, Hung HC, Tauxe WN, et al: Radioisotope renography: Diagnosis of renal arterial disease in hypertensive patients. Circulation 27:328, 1963.

25. Luke RG, Briggs JD, Kennedy AC, et al: The isotope renogram in the detection and assessment of renal artery stenosis. Q J Med 35:237, 1966.

26. Foster JH, Oates JA, Rhamy RK, et al: Detection and treatment of patients with renovascular hypertension. Surgery 60:240, 1966.

27. Britton KE, Maisey MN: Renal radionuclide studies. *In* Maisey MN, Britton KE, Gilday DC (eds): Clinical Nuclear Medicine. Philadelphia, WB Saunders, 1983, p 93.

28. Giese J, Mogensen P, Munck O: Diagnostic value of renography for detection of unilateral renal or renovascular disease in hypertensive patients. Scand J Clin Lab Invest 35:307, 1975.

29. McNeil BJ, Varady PD, Burrows BA, et al: Cost-effectiveness calculations in the diagnosis and treatment of hypertensive renovascular disease. N Engl J Med 293:216, 1975.

30. Hunt JC, Strong CG, Harrison EG Jr, et al: Management of hypertension of renal origin. Am J Cardiol 26:280, 1970.

31. Buda JA, Baer L, Parra-Carillo JZ, et al: Predictability of surgical response in renovascular hypertension. Arch Surg 111:1243, 1976.

32. Arlart L, Rosenthal J, Adam WE, et al: Predictive value of radionuclide methods in the diagnosis of unilateral renovascular hypertension. Cardiovasc Radiol 1:115, 1979.

33. McAfee JG, Thomas FD, Grossman Z, et al: Diagnosis of angiotensinogenic hypertension: The complementary roles of renal scintigraphy and the saralasin infusion test. J Nucl Med 18:669, 1977.

34. Chiarini C, Espositi ED, Losinno F, et al: Renal scintigraphy versus renal vein renin activity for identifying and treatment of renovascular hypertension. Nephron 32:8, 1982.

35. Gruenwald SM, Collins LT: Renovascular hypertension. Quantitative renography as a screening test. Radiology 149:287, 1983.

36. Taylor A Jr, Martin LG: The utility of 99mTc-mercaptoacetyltriglycine in captopril renography. Am J Hypertens 4(12 Pt 2):731S, 1991.

37. Sheps SG, Blaufox MD, Nally JV Jr, Textor SC: Radionuclide scintirenography in the evaluation of patients with hypertension. American College of Cardiology position statement. J Am Coll Cardiol 21(3):838, 1993.

38. Fleishman MJ, Greenspan RL, Van Heertum RL: The additional value of visual findings in captopril-enhanced renal scintigraphy with Tc-99m MAG3. Clin Nucl Med 18(5):382, 1993.

39. Itoh K, Tsukamoto E, Kakizaki H, et al: Phase II study of Tc-99m MAG3 in patients with nephrourologic diseases. Clin Nucl Med 18(5):387, 1993.

40. Roccatello D, Picciotto G, Rabbia C, et al: Prospective study on captopril renography in hypertensive patients. Am J Nephrol 12(6):406, 1992.

41. Smith CW, Winfield AC, Price RR: Evaluation of digital venous angiography for the diagnosis of renovascular hypertension. Radiology 144:51, 1982.

42. Sos TA, Pickering TG, Sniderman K, et al: Percutaneous transluminal angioplasty in renovascular hypertension due to atheroma or fibromuscular hypertension. N Engl J Med 309:274, 1983.

43. Buonocore E, Meaney TF, Borkowski GP, et al: Digital subtraction angiography of the abdominal aorta and renal arteries: Comparison with conventional angiography. Radiology 139:281, 1981.

44. Harrington DP: Renal digital subtraction angiography. Cardiovasc Intervent Radiol 6:214, 1983.

45. Tifft CP: Renal digital subtraction angiography—A nephrologist's view: A sensitive but imperfect screening procedure for renovascular hypertension. Cardiovasc Intervent Radiol 6:231, 1983.

46. deJong TE, Appelman PT, Lampmann LE: Subtraction pitfalls in venous DSA of the renal arteries. Rofo Fortschr Geb Roentgenstr Neuen Bildgeb Verfahr 145:21, 1986.

47. Rabe FE, Smith EJ, Yune HY, et al: Limitations of digital subtraction angiography in evaluating potential renal donors. AJR 141:91, 1983.

48. Rabe FE, Yune HY, Klatte EC, et al: Efficacy of glucagon for abdominal digital angiography. AJR 139:618, 1982.

49. Neiman HL, Mintzer RA, Vogelzang RL: Digital subtraction angiography. *In* Neiman HL, Yao JST (eds): Angiography of Vascular Disease. New York, Churchill Livingstone, 1985, p 27.

50. Stanley JC, Whitehouse WM Jr: Occlusive and aneurysmal disease of the renal arterial circulation. DM 30:1, 1984.

51. Guthaner DF, Brody WR, Miller DC: Intravenous aortography after aortic dissection repair. AJR 137:1019, 1981.

52. Krumlousky FA, Simon N, Santhanam S, et al: Acute renal failure: Association with administration of radiographic contrast material. JAMA 239:125, 1978.

53. Clark RA, Alexander ES: Digital subtraction angiography of the renal arteries: Prospective comparison with conventional arteriography. Invest Radiol 18:6, 1983.

54. DeSomer FM, Auman JL, Baert AL, et al: Results of intravenous digital subtraction angiography (IVDSA) as a screening method for renovascular hypertension. Br J Radiol 57:667, 1984.

55. Jackson B, Dugdale L: Renal artery digital-subtraction angiography: An outpatient investigation for renovascular hypertension. Med J Aust 142:18, 1985.

56. NHLBI Workshop on Renovascular Disease: Summary report and recommendations. Hypertension 7:452, 1984.

57. Chuang VP, Ernst CB: Angiography for renal hypertension. *In* Neiman HL, Yao JST (eds): Angiography of Vascular Disease. New York, Churchill Livingstone, 1985, p 151.

58. Hillman BJ: Lesions causing renovascular hypertension. *In* Imaging and Hypertension. Philadelphia, WB Saunders, 1983, p 49.

59. Webb JA, Talner LB: The role of intravenous urography in hypertension. Radiol Clin North Am 17:187, 1979.

60. Bookstein JJ, Abrams HL, Buenger RE, et al: Radiologic aspects of renovascular hypertension. III. Appraisal of arteriography. JAMA 221:368, 1972.

61. Klatte EC, Worrell JA, Forster JH, et al: Diagnostic criteria of bilateral renovascular hypertension. Radiology 101:301, 1971.

62. Novick AC: Atherosclerotic renovascular disease. J Urol 126:567, 1981.

63. Stewart BH, Dustan HP, Kiser WS, et al: Correlation of angiography and natural history in evaluation of patients with renovascular hypertension. J Urol 104:231, 1970.

64. Harrison EG Jr, McCormack LJ: Pathologic classification of renal arterial disease in renovascular hypertension. Mayo Clin Proc 46:161, 1971.

65. Youngberg SP, Sheps SG, Strong CG: Fibromuscular stenosis of the renal arteries. Med Clin North Am 61:623, 1977.

66. Hunt JC, Harrison EG Jr, Kincaid OW, et al: Idiopathic fibrous and fibromuscular stenosis of the renal arteries associated with hypertension. Mayo Clin Proc 36:707, 1972.

67. Ekelund L, Gerlock J, Molin J, et al: Roentgenologic appearance of fibromuscular dysplasia. Acta Radiol Diagn 19:433, 1978.

68. Meaney TF, Baghery SAS: Radiology of renovascular hypertension. *In* Breslin DJ, Swinton NW Jr, Libertino JA, et al (eds): Renovascular Hypertension. Baltimore, Williams & Wilkins, 1982, p 78.

69. Newhouse JH, Markisz JA, Kazam E: Magnetic resonance imaging of the kidneys. Cardiovasc Intervent Radiol 8:351, 1986.

70. Avasthi PS, Boyles WF, Greene ER: Noninvasive diagnosis of renal artery stenosis by echo-Doppler velocimetry. Kidney Int 25:824, 1984.

71. Norris CS, Rittgers SE, Barnes RW: A new screening technique for renal artery occlusive disease. Curr Surg 41:83, 1984.

72. Rittgers SE, Norris CS, Barnes RW: Detection of renal artery stenosis: Experimental and clinical analysis of velocity waveforms. Ultrasound Med Biol 11:523, 1985.

73. Norris CS, Pfeiffer JS, Rittgers SE, et al: Noninvasive evaluation of renal artery stenosis and renovascular resistance: Experimental and clinical studies. J Vasc Surg 1:192, 1984.

74. Maxwell MH, Waks U, Burkhalter JF: Blood pressure response to furosemide: Initial screening test for renovascular hypertension. *In* Abstracts, Fifth Scientific Meeting of the International Society of Hypertension, Paris, 1978, p 174.

75. Tegtmeyer CJ, Dyer R, Teates CD, et al: Percutaneous transluminal dilatation of the renal arteries: Techniques and results. Radiology 135:589, 1980.

76. Weinberger MH, Yune HY, Grim CE, et al: Percutaneous transluminal angioplasty for renal artery stenosis in a solitary functioning kidney. Ann Intern Med 91:684, 1979.

77. Katzen BT, Chang J, Lukowsky GH, et al: Percutaneous transluminal

angioplasty for treatment of renovascular hypertension. Radiology 131:53, 1979.

78. Madias NE, Ball JT, Millan VG: Percutaneous transluminal renal angioplasty in the treatment of unilateral atherosclerotic renovascular hypertension. Am J Med 70:1078, 1981.

79. Kuhlman U, Vetter W, Furrer J, et al: Renovascular hypertension: Treatment by percutaneous transluminal dilatation. Ann Intern Med 92:1, 1980.

80. Schwarten DE, Yune HY, Klatte EC, et al: Clinical experience with percutaneous transluminal angioplasty (PTA) of stenotic renal arteries. Radiology 135:601, 1980.

81. Geyskes GG, Puylaert CB, Oei HY, et al: Intraluminal dilatation of renal artery stenosis. Clin Sci 57(Suppl 5):441s, 1979.

82. Freiman DB: Transluminal angioplasty of the renal arteries. Urol Clin North Am 12:737, 1985.

83. Sos TA, Pickering TG, Saddekni S, et al: The current role of renal angioplasty in the treatment of renovascular hypertension. Urol Clin North Am 11:503, 1984.

84. Kuhlmann U, Greminger P, Gruntzig A: Long-term experience in percutaneous transluminal dilatation on renal artery stenosis. Am J Med 79:692, 1985.

85. Tegtmeyer CJ, Kellum CD, Ayers C: Percutaneous transluminal angioplasty of the renal artery: Results and long-term follow-up. Radiology 153:77, 1984.

86. Martin LG, Casarella WJ, Alspaugh JP, et al: Renal artery angioplasty: Increased technical success and decreased complications in the second 100 patients. Radiology 159:631, 1986.

87. Tegtmeyer CJ, Kofler TJ, Ayers CA: Renal angioplasty: Current status. AJR 142:17, 1984.

88. Colaptino RF, Stronell RD, Harries-Jones EP, et al: Percutaneous transluminal dilatation of the renal artery: Follow-up studies on renovascular hypertension. AJR 139:727, 1982.

89. Schwarten DE: Transluminal angioplasty of renal artery stenosis: 70 experiences. AJR 135:969, 1980.

90. Tegtmeyer CJ, Teates CD, Crigler N, et al: Percutaneous transluminal angioplasty in patients with renal artery stenosis: Follow-up studies. Radiology 140:323, 1981.

91. Pickering TG, Sos TA, Laragh JH: Role of balloon dilatation in the treatment of renovascular hypertension. Am J Med 77(2A):61, 1984.

92. Tegtmeyer CJ, Elson J, Glass TA, et al: Percutaneous transluminal angioplasty: The treatment of choice for renovascular hypertension due to fibromuscular dysplasia. Radiology 143:631, 1982.

93. Saddekni S, Sniderman KW, Hilton S, et al: Percutaneous transluminal angioplasty of nonatherosclerotic lesions. AJR 135:975, 1980.

94. Miller GA, Ford KK, Braun SD, et al: Percutaneous transluminal angioplasty vs. surgery for renovascular hypertension. AJR 144:447, 1985.

95. Martin EC, Diamond NG, Casarella WJ: Percutaneous transluminal angioplasty in nonatherosclerotic disease. Radiology 135:27, 1980.

96. Guthaner DF, Schmitz L: Percutaneous transluminal angioplasty of radiation-induced arterial stenoses. Radiology 144:77, 1982.

97. Sniderman KW, Sos TA, Sprayregan S, et al: Percutaneous transluminal angioplasty in renal transplant arterial stenosis for relief of hypertension. Radiology 135:23, 1980.

98. Raynaud A, Bedrossian J, Remy P, et al: Percutaneous transluminal angioplasty of renal transplant arterial stenosis. AJR 146:853, 1986.

99. Diamond NG, Casarella WJ, Hardy MA, et al: Dilatation of critical transplant renal artery stenosis by percutaneous transluminal angioplasty. AJR 133:1167, 1979.

100. Whiteside CI, Cardella CJ, Yeung H, et al: The role of percutaneous transluminal dilatation in the treatment of transplant renal artery stenosis. Clin Nephrol 17:55, 1982.

101. Mollenkopf F, Matas A, Veith FJ, et al: Percutaneous transluminal angioplasty for transplant renal artery stenosis. Transplant Proc 15:1089, 1983.

102. Gerlock AJ, MacDonell RC, Smith CW, et al: Renal transplant arterial stenosis: Percutaneous transluminal angioplasty. AJR 140:325, 1983.

103. Curry NS, Cochran S, Barbaric ZL, et al: Interventional radiologic procedures in the renal transplant. Radiology 152:647, 1984.

104. Madias NE, Millan VG: Percutaneous transluminal renal angioplasty in the treatment of renovascular hypertension. *In* Breslin DJ, Swinton NW Jr, Libertino JA, et al (eds): Renovascular Hypertension. Baltimore, Williams & Wilkins, 1982, p 148.

105. Gardiner GA Jr, Friedman AM, Shlansky-Goldberg R: Percutaneous transluminal angioplasty: Delayed response in neurofibromatosis. Radiology 169:78, 1988.

106. Cicuto KP, McLean GK, Oleaga JA, et al: Renal artery stenosis: Anatomic classification for percutaneous transluminal angioplasty. AJR 137:599, 1981.

107. Wilms GE, Peene PT, Baert AL, et al: Renal artery stent placement with use of the Wallstent endoprosthesis. Radiology 179(2):457, 1991.

108. Joffre F, Rousseau H, Bernadet P, et al: Midterm results of renal artery stenting. Cardiovasc Intervent Radiol 15(5):313, 1992.

109. Mahler F, Krneta A, Haertel M: Treatment of renovascular hypertension by transluminal renal artery dilatation. Am J Med 70:1078, 1981.

110. Schwarten DE: Percutaneous transluminal angioplasty of the renal artery. Cardiovasc Intervent Radiol 8:197, 1980.

111. Martin LG, Price RB, Casarella WJ, et al: Percutaneous angioplasty in clinical management of renovascular hypertension: Initial and long-term results. Radiology 155:629, 1985.

108

Renal Artery Fibrodysplasia and Renovascular Hypertension

James C. Stanley, M.D., and Louis M. Messina, M.D.

. . .

Occlusive renal artery disease is the most common cause of surgically correctable hypertension. Although the precise incidence of renovascular hypertension has not been defined, its clinical importance has been clearly established. Fibrodysplastic renal artery stenoses affect less than 0.5 per cent of the general population, but these lesions are second only to arteriosclerotic disease as the most frequent cause of renovascular hypertension.

Dysplastic renal artery stenoses are a heterogeneous group of lesions affecting both pediatric and adult patients.[86] They are usually categorized according to the principal level of vessel involvement. Intimal fibroplasia, medial hyperplasia, medial fibroplasia, and perimedial dysplasia are the four most regularly encountered dysplastic renovascular lesions.[36, 82] The first two are distinctly different pathologic processes, whereas the latter two may appear as a continuum of the same disease. Developmental stenoses, exhibiting derangements of all vessel wall layers, represent yet another distinct form of renal artery dysplasia.[85]

This overview of renal artery fibrodysplasia and secondary hypertension is directed in particular to a discussion of the clinical manifestations and indications for operation, the appropriateness of drug therapy and percutaneous transluminal angioplasty, and the role of surgical therapy in the management of fibrodysplastic renovascular hypertension.

CLINICAL MANIFESTATIONS AND INDICATIONS FOR OPERATION

The prevalence of renovascular hypertension in the hypertensive population is low, and the prevalence of that caused by arterial fibrodysplasia is even lower.[49] Thus, the first decision in a reasonable management algorithm depends on recognizing the clinical clues of fibrodysplastic renovascular hypertension (Fig. 108–1).[22] Hypertension in pediatric patients that is unaccompanied by obvious renal disease and the sudden onset of diastolic hypertension of greater than 115 mmHg in women under 45 years of age are two characteristic presentations of this type of hypertension. Elevated blood pressure in this group of patients tends to be refractory to simple medical management. Furthermore, when the entire renal mass is at risk for ischemia, impaired renal function often accompanies the use of angio-

tensin-converting enzyme (ACE) inhibitors. Fibrodysplastic renovascular hypertension is rare among the black population.[43] Smoking, which has been suggested to be a causal factor in renovascular fibromuscular dysplasia,[67] was not reported to be a common finding in earlier epidemiologic surveys. Other clinical findings may be more common in patients with renovascular hypertension than in those with essential hypertension, but unfortunately they are not pathognomonic of this disease.[69] For instance, younger children and infants with renovascular hypertension frequently exhibit failure to thrive, whereas hyperkinesis, seizure disorders, cephalalgia, and fatigability often affect older children and adolescents.[16, 105] Adults with fibrodysplastic renovascular hypertension most often complain of lethargy. Abdominal bruit and hypertensive retinal arteriolar changes are also common findings in fibrodysplastic renovascular hypertension, but they are not specific enough to distinguish this disease from essential hypertension.

Certain general characteristics of pediatric and adult patients with this disease are noteworthy. In an earlier report from the University of Michigan, arterial fibrodysplastic renovascular hypertension was the basis for surgical therapy in 34 pediatric patients: 19 boys and 15 girls, with mean ages of 10.1 and 13.7 years, respectively.[88] The average duration of known hypertension in these young patients was 11.2 months. Their blood pressures averaged 175/118 mmHg without drug therapy, and although little effort was made with long-term medical therapy, their pressures did decrease with drug treatment to an average of 162/106 mmHg ($p<.01$). ACE inhibitors were not used in this early experience, and no patient was normotensive at the time surgical intervention was undertaken.

During this same period, adults undergoing surgery for fibrodysplastic renovascular hypertension at the University of Michigan included 133 women and 11 men, with mean ages of 39.1 and 30.5 years, respectively.[88] The average duration of known hypertension in this group was 42.5 months. Blood pressures without therapy averaged 206/122 mmHg, falling to 184/111 mmHg with drug treatment ($p<.01$). As was the case with pediatric patients, no adults received preoperative ACE inhibitors or were normotensive at the time of surgical therapy.

Indications for operation in the management of fibrodysplastic renovascular hypertension at the University of Michigan include demonstration of the presence of a he-

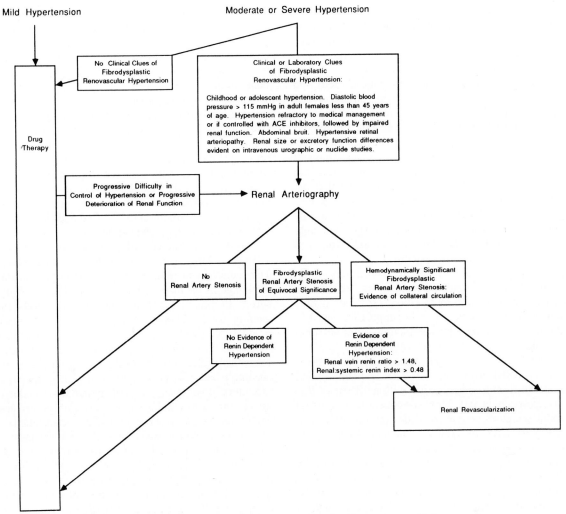

FIGURE 108–1. Management algorithm for fibrodysplastic renovascular hypertension.

modynamically significant stenotic lesion and evidence of its functional importance. In this regard, the limitations of diagnostic and prognostic studies must be clearly recognized in evaluating patients suspected of having renovascular hypertension.[84] Previously, at the authors' institution, hypertensive urography, renal scanning, renography, split renal function studies, operative renal artery pressure gradient measurements, and kidney biopsies were used as diagnostic and prognostic guides. These studies have been replaced by careful preoperative arteriographic examinations and plasma renin assays. Hypertensive urography is considered to be an invalid prognostic test because of numerous normal study results in patients proved by successful operation to have renovascular hypertension. Abnormal urographic findings in only 27 per cent of pediatric patients[81] and 48 per cent of adults with fibrodysplastic disease[102] who benefited from operative intervention confirm that it is not a sensitive screening test. Similar experiences at other centers have caused abandonment of hypertensive urography as a diagnostic study for fibrodysplastic renovascular hypertension.

Arteriographic studies have proved to be the most useful tests for assessing clinically relevant renal artery dys-

plastic occlusive disease.[79–81] Demonstration of collateral vessels as a manifestation of a hemodynamically significant stenosis has been important in this regard. The development of collateral vessels circumventing a renal artery stenosis occurs when the pressure gradient across the obstruction approaches 10 mmHg. This same gradient is generally accepted to be associated with an increased release of renin from the juxtaglomerular apparatus of the kidney. In this regard, demonstration of nonparenchymal renal artery branches functioning as collateral channels by pharmacoangiographic techniques using epinephrine and acetylcholine has been useful in defining the significance of many stenoses of equivocal clinical importance.[7] Intravenous digital subtraction angiography is not recommended for evaluating patients suspected of having fibrodysplastic renovascular hypertension because it is inadequate for demonstrating anything other than the most obvious of main renal artery lesions. Fibrodysplastic stenoses affecting segmental renal arteries are poorly demonstrated by intravenous digital subtraction angiography, and collateral vessels may be overlooked altogether by such studies. Intra-arterial digital subtraction angiography, on the other hand, often provides high enough resolution of small vessel anatomy so as to be comparable to conventional arteriography. Transabdominal duplex scanning of the renal arteries has the potential for identifying renal artery stenoses, although this technology will require further refinement to become of practical value in the routine diagnosis of fibrodysplastic disease.

Plasma renin assays become important in detecting functionally important renal ischemia when arteriography reveals a renal artery stenosis of equivocal hemodynamic significance (see Fig. 108–1). The renal vein renin ratio (RVRR), which compares renin activity in the venous effluent from the ischemic and contralateral kidneys, has not been a reliable predictive test. In part, this may reflect the frequent existence of bilateral disease or the fact that the RVRR reverts toward unity with the development of collateral vessels.[24] Although RVRRs are considered abnormal when they exceed 1.48, lower ratios occur in approximately 15 to 20 per cent of patients who are eventually found to have a renovascular cause of hypertension.[79, 83]

Determination of each kidney's renin secretory activity, expressed as a renal-systemic renin index (RSRI), has lessened errors incumbent to renin ratio determinations.[50, 83] These indices, which document renin suppression and hypersecretion, are calculated by subtracting systemic renin activity from renal vein renin activity and dividing the remainder by the systemic renin activity. Hypersecretion occurs with an RSRI of greater than 0.48, and suppression of renin release from a kidney exists with an RSRI of less than 0.24, approaching 0.0. This assessment of individual kidney renin secretory activity provides reasonable identification of both adult and pediatric patients likely to be cured or have improvement after surgery.[16, 79, 80]

Among subsequently cured patients at the University of Michigan, the effluent blood from the ischemic kidney exhibited renin activity 119 per cent more than that in the peripheral blood (RSRI, 1.19), whereas the contralateral kidney exhibited an increase of only 4 per cent over peripheral levels (RSRI, 0.04). Among patients who had subsequent improvement, there was a 123 per cent increase from the ischemic kidney (RSRI, 1.23), but more importantly, there was a 32 per cent increase from the contralateral kidney (RSRI, 0.32). The latter suggests that patients with improvement have nonsuppressed renin production from the contralateral kidney, whereas in cured patients, renin release is suppressed from the nontreated, contralateral kidney. Absolute and relative renin activities do not appear to vary between pediatric and adult patient populations with dysplastic disease.[16, 81, 95] Limited experience supports the use of ACE inhibitors as a means of enhancing the sensitivity of RVRR and RSRI data in documenting the existence of renovascular hypertension.[61, 101]

DRUG THERAPY

Improved antihypertensive drugs have facilitated the medical management of fibrodysplastic renovascular hypertension.[104, 107] The principles of drug therapy are based on understanding the pathophysiologic sequelae of renal artery stenoses. Renin-angiotensin–mediated vasoconstriction assumes greatest importance with unilateral disease in patients who have a normal contralateral kidney. Renin-angiotensin–

aldosterone–mediated sodium retention and hypervolemia are the dominant pathophysiologic changes in patients with bilateral renal artery stenoses, as well as in those with unilateral stenoses associated with contralateral parenchymal disease or renal absence due to agenesis or prior nephrectomy.

Blood pressure elevations in most patients with fibrodysplastic renovascular hypertension may be controlled with appropriate pharmacologic intervention. However, controversial issues that need to be considered regarding drug therapy include (1) the side effects of treatment, (2) limited patient compliance even in carefully structured programs, and (3) whether blood pressure control will be attended by decreased renal function, either as a direct effect of the drug or through unrecognized and insidious progression of renal artery occlusive disease.

In patients known to have renovascular hypertension, a beta-blocking agent is often the first drug administered. The reduction in renin release that occurs with the use of these agents is responsible for lowering the blood pressure.[10] Propranolol and atenolol are the drugs most frequently used, although metoprolol, nadolol, timolol, and pindolol are similar agents. High doses of these drugs may be required to control the blood pressure, although in most cases the primary effect of suppressing renin release can be accomplished with very small doses. In instances of more refractory hypertension, especially that due to bilateral renal artery stenoses or unilateral lesions with contralateral parenchymal disease, addition of a standard diuretic is advised. A thiazide, a hydrogenated thiazide, or a similar compound is recommended in this setting. In patients with impaired renal function secondary to decreased blood flow, a loop diuretic such as furosemide will provide a more effective diuretic action. ACE inhibitors are some of the more efficient agents for treating hypertension in general and renovascular hypertension in particular.[1, 11, 27, 37] Antihypertensive effects other than decreased generation of angiotensin II, such as those involving increased levels of bradykinin, occur with the use of these agents. Captopril and enalapril are currently the most commonly used ACE inhibitors. They may be supplemented with beta-blockers or diuretics in resistant hypertension. In more severe hypertension, vasodilators such minoxidil may be required. In this regard, calcium channel blockers have been used to supplement ACE inhibitors in the management of renovascular hypertension.

It is important to recognize that ACE inhibitors, when administered to patients with renovascular occlusive disease, may impair renal function.[14] ACE inhibitors decrease efferent but not afferent arteriolar resistance, thereby causing a decrease in glomerular filtration rate. This impairment in renal function by ACE inhibitors becomes especially relevant in patients who have bilateral renal artery stenoses, as well as in those with a stenosis affecting a solitary kidney or a unilateral stenosis in the presence of contralateral renal parenchymal disease.[38] In such instances, severe deterioration of glomerular filtration may occur, and the use of these agents is contraindicated. Newer ACE inhibitors may have less profound effects when the entire renal mass appears affected by fibrodysplastic renovascular disease, but this remains to be better documented.

PERCUTANEOUS TRANSLUMINAL RENAL ANGIOPLASTY

Successful percutaneous transluminal renal angioplasty was first reported by Gruntzig and colleagues.[34] This report involved the dilatation of an atherosclerotic renal artery stenosis. Percutaneous renal angioplasty was soon recognized to be effective in the treatment of fibrodysplastic lesions.[29, 31, 32, 54, 68, 97] However, many facts about this technology remain to be defined, including (1) differences in treating the various types of stenoses comprising the spectrum of renal artery dysplastic disease, (2) the durability of successful dilatation, (3) the long-term effects of dilatation on the vessel wall, (4) the incidence of dilatation-related renal and extrarenal complications, and (5) whether all stenoses can be unequivocally identified angiographically and thus ensure the completeness of the angioplasty procedure.

The mechanisms by which balloon angioplasty dilates fibrodysplastic stenoses are similar to those accompanying the dilatation of arteriosclerotic vessels. As the balloon is inflated, the vessel wall is stretched and fracturing of the intima occurs. Further dilatation of the balloon results in separation of the intima from the underlying vessel wall, with splitting of the media and stretching of the adventitia beyond its elastic recoil. The dilated vessel gradually undergoes a fibroproliferative reparative process, and a neointima is formed.

Percutaneous transluminal angioplasty is generally performed after aortography or selective renal arteriographic studies have defined the severity and extent of stenotic disease. The renal artery is usually entered with a "shepherd's crook" or "sidewinder" catheter. This catheter is then exchanged over a guidewire for a balloon catheter of the appropriate size made of polyvinylchloride or polyethylene. The balloon is positioned within the dysplastic stenosis and inflated two or three times for brief periods, at pressures ranging from 4 to 8 atm. Newer balloons may be inflated at much greater pressures, although this is not usually needed for dilating fibrodysplastic stenoses. Completion arteriography is then undertaken, and the angioplasty is considered successful when preexisting pressure gradients across a stenosis are abolished and anatomic documentation of an adequate dilatation is apparent.[71, 100]

Adult patients with fibrodysplastic renovascular hypertension benefit from transluminal balloon angioplasty in approximately 85 per cent of cases (Table 108–1). Cure rates are often lower than those reported in surgical series.[35, 98, 99] Recurrent stenoses develop in approximately 10 per cent of patients,[99] but they are usually amenable to repeated angioplasty. Failures in most reported series usually do not include cases in which lesions were not technically able to be dilated. Unfortunately, as many as 25 per cent of stenoses in patients with renal artery fibrodysplasia are not amenable to percutaneous transluminal angioplasty because of technical difficulties with vessel catheterization. The best results with transluminal renal angioplasty are obtained in adult patients with unilateral medial fibrodysplasia. Intimal fibroplasia, particularly that associated with congenital defects, is more resistant to dilatation.

The results of transluminal angioplasty for renal artery fibrodysplasia in pediatric patients are quite variable.[12] In these younger patients, this technology is best limited to treatment of mid– or distal renal artery stenoses.[91] Attempts to dilate proximal ostial lesions, especially those associated with neurofibromatosis or aortic anomalies, are unlikely to be successful.[58, 59] In one series of pediatric cases, 60 per cent of unsuccessful angioplasties resulted in nephrectomy.[105]

The precise frequency of significant complications after angioplasty is unknown, but the overall complication rate in a review of 624 procedures averaged 11 per cent (range, 2.5 to 38.5 per cent).[73] Although the variability among individual series undoubtedly reflects differing definitions of complications, untoward sequelae of angioplasty, including vessel thrombosis and perforation, are far from being rare events.[53, 99] Spasm, although usually of little con-

Table 108–1. Results of Percutaneous Transluminal Angioplasty for Renovascular Hypertension Due to Fibrodysplasia

Medical Center	No. of Patients	Postangioplasty Status*			Length of Follow-Up
		Cure (%)	Improvement (%)	Failure (%)	
New York Hospital–Cornell[70] (1978–1981)	31	52	29	19	4–40 mo; average, 16 mo
University Hospital, Zurich[51] (1978–1985)	28	50	39	11	15 mo average
University of Virginia[99] (1979–1988)	66	39	59	2	1–121 mo; average, 39 mo
Indiana University[33] (1980–1985)	26	58	35	8	1–60 mo; average, 26 mo
University Hospital, Utrecht[45] (1978–1986)	47	38	55	7	6–96 mo
Emory University[55] (1980–1983)	20	25	60	15	3–36 mo; average, 16 mo
University Hospitals, Leuven[2] (1979–1987)	19	58	21	21	6–72 mo; average, 26 mo
University Hospital, Uppsala[35] (1980–1985)	18	33	22	44	6–36 mo; average, 25 mo

*Criteria for blood pressure reponse are defined in the cited publications. Data are expressed to the nearest 1%.

sequence, may be associated with renal infarction.[45] Intimal disruption occurs more often with dilatation of the proximal renal artery, where elasticity of the vessel is greater and medial disruption is less likely, whereas medial tears are most likely with dilatation of the more distal renal artery, where vascular elasticity is less.[66] The latter becomes particularly relevant in that 25 per cent of medial dysplastic disease involves the segmental vessels. In such settings, percutaneous angioplasty is more hazardous. Reports have indicated that intimal lesions remodel slowly after dilatation and that persistent stenoses evident immediately after angioplasty may diminish with time.[96] Transluminal angioplasty is contraindicated in patients who have renal artery stenoses associated with macroaneurysms, extensive segmental disease, or dissections. In these circumstances, the frequency of angioplasty-related thromboses is unacceptably high.

Early results indicate that percutaneous transluminal renal angioplasty is useful in the management of select patients with fibrodysplastic renovascular hypertension.[65] Clearly, once a good outcome has been achieved, the results of this form of therapy appear durable.[99]

SURGICAL THERAPY

Operative Technique

Exposure is critical to the performance of successful arterial reconstructive surgery for renal artery fibrodysplastic disease. At the University of Michigan, preference is given to a supraumbilical transverse incision in which both rectus muscles are transected. The incision is extended from the opposite mid-clavicular line to the mid-axillary line on the side of the renal artery reconstruction. Transverse abdominal incisions provide a small but definite technical advantage in the handling of instruments perpendicular to the longitudinal axis of the body. During complex renovascular procedures, this advantage greatly facilitates the ease of reconstruction. Mid-line vertical incisions can also be used for renal artery reconstructions, and some surgeons maintain a strong bias for this type of transabdominal approach. After the peritoneal cavity has been entered and its contents have been explored, the intestines are displaced to the opposite side of the abdomen. In children and infants, proper exposure is more easily obtained if the intestines are eviscerated.

When right-sided reconstructions are being performed, the renal artery and vein, as well as the inferior vena cava and the aorta, are exposed by incising the lateral parietes from the hepatic flexure to the cecum and reflecting the right colon, duodenum, and pancreas medially in an extended Kocher-like maneuver. This provides excellent visualization of the mid-abdominal aorta, the vena cava, and the distal vessels of the right kidney (Fig. 108–2). Dissection of the renal artery should begin in its mid-portion just lateral to the vena cava and usually requires retraction of the renal vein superiorly. The vein should be carefully dissected from surrounding tissues, and small branches, such as those to the adrenal gland, should be ligated and transected. If the more distal renal artery is dissected first, troublesome injury to small arterial and venous branches is

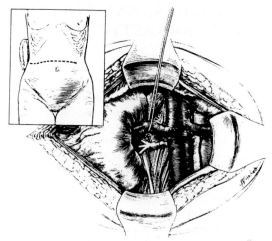

FIGURE 108–2. Operative approach through a transverse supraumbilical abdominal incision, with an extraperitoneal dissection and reflection of the colon and foregut structures providing exposure of the renal and great vessels.

more likely. In treating developmental right-sided ostial lesions, the cava may be retracted laterally and the proximal renal artery exposed near its origin.

When left-sided reconstructions are being undertaken, the renal vessels are exposed with a retroperitoneal dissection similar to that performed on the right, with reflection of the viscera, including the left colon, medially. Such a retroperitoneal approach through a transverse incision offers better visualization of the mid- and distal renal vessels than does an anterior exposure through the mesocolon at the root of the mesentery. Exposure of the left renal artery usually requires mobilization of the renal vein with ligation and transection of the gonadal branch inferiorly and the adrenal venous branches superiorly.

The infrarenal aorta is dissected about its circumference for approximately 5 cm, just below the origin of the renal arteries. A side-biting vascular clamp is used to occlude the aorta partially at this level. In some instances, total aortic occlusion is necessary. Systemic anticoagulation is accomplished by intravenous administration of heparin sodium, 150 U/kg, before the aorta is clamped. An aortotomy is created, the length of which is approximately two to three times the graft diameter. Whenever possible, the saphenous vein is harvested so that a branch is included at its caudal end. This branch is incised so that its orifice is connected to the lumen of the main trunk. The generous anastomotic circumference created by this maneuver allows a more perpendicular origin of the vein graft from the aorta (Fig. 108–3). The vein graft–aorta anastomosis is performed with 4–0 or 5–0 polypropylene suture. In certain patients, other sites of origin for renal grafts are preferable, with the common iliac, splenic, and hepatic arteries being the most frequent nonaortic vessels from which grafts may originate.[13]

The graft is then positioned for the renal anastomosis. The most direct route for right-sided aortorenal grafts is in a retrocaval position originating from a lateral aortotomy. However, some grafts will be less likely to kink when taken from an anterolateral aortotomy and carried in front of the inferior vena cava and then posterior to the renal vessels.

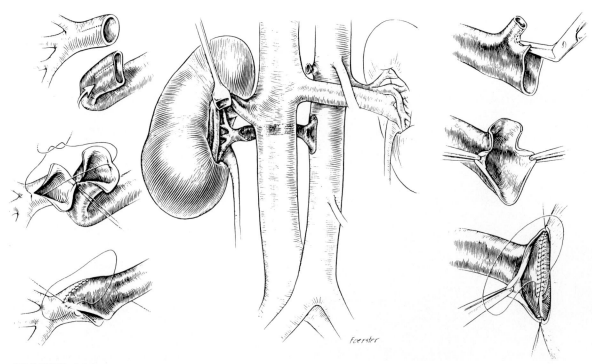

FIGURE 108–3. Technique of end-to-end graft–renal artery anastomosis following spatulation of the artery anteriorly and the graft posteriorly, and end-to-side graft–aorta anastomosis following creation of a common orifice between a branch and the central lumen of the saphenous vein.

The choice of antecaval or retrocaval graft positioning must be individualized. Grafts to the left kidney are usually positioned beneath the left renal vein. The aortic clamp should be left in place during completion of the renal anastomosis. To remove it and to place an occluding device on a vein graft might injure the latter conduit.

Attention is then directed to performing the renal anastomosis. The proximal renal artery is clamped, transected, and ligated. Before antegrade renal artery blood flow is interrupted, a sustained diuresis should be established, usually by intravenous administration of 12.5 gm of mannitol. Preformed collateral vessels usually provide enough blood flow to maintain kidney viability during renal artery occlusion. Miniature microvascular clamps, developing tensions ranging from 30 to 70 gm, are favored over conventional vascular clamps or elastic slings for occluding distal renal vessels. They have less potential for causing vessel injury, and because of their very small size, they do not obscure the operative field.

A graft–renal artery anastomosis in an end-to-end fashion is preferred over an end-to-side anastomosis. This is facilitated by spatulation of the graft posteriorly and of the renal artery anteriorly (see Fig. 108–3). This allows visualization of the artery's interior such that inclusion of intima with each stitch is easily accomplished. In adults, the anastomosis is completed with a continuous suture of 6–0 polypropylene. In pediatric patients, three or four sutures are interrupted to provide for anastomotic growth. In the case of vessels smaller than 2 mm in diameter, the anastomosis is best completed with individual interrupted sutures about the entire circumference. Spatulated anastomoses are ovoid and with healing are less likely to develop strictures (Fig. 108–4).

Direct reimplantation of the renal artery into the side of the aorta has been standard practice recently at the University of Michigan for treating orificial stenoses in pediatric patients[76] (Fig. 108–5). In these cases, the renal artery is dissected from its aortic origin to the renal hilum. The vessel is transected proximally, just beyond the orificial stenosis. After spatulation of the vessel on its anterior and posterior sides, so as to create a more generous circumference, it is anastomosed to the aorta. An aortotomy 6 to 8 mm in length is made to accommodate the renal vessel, and the anastomosis is fashioned with interrupted 6–0 or 7–0 polypropylene sutures. This type of renal revascularization avoids the use of grafts and multiple anastomoses and can be performed without the extensive mobilization of the kidney required of pelvic autotransplantation accompanying ex vivo renal artery repairs.

After the aortic and renal anastomoses or the aortic reimplantations have been completed, the vascular clamps are removed, antegrade renal blood flow is reestablished, and the heparin effect is reversed with slow intravenous administration of 1.2 mg of protamine sulfate for each 100 units of heparin previously given. Assessment of the reconstruction is undertaken with duplex scanning or by evaluating flow with a directional, continuous-wave Doppler ultrasound machine. Intraoperative arteriography is seldom necessary, but before discharge all patients should undergo postoperative arteriography to establish the adequacy of the reconstructive procedure and provide a baseline for continued graft follow-up.

In treating fibrodysplastic renovascular disease, autologous vein grafts are usually preferred for reconstructions in adults.[79] Autologous hypogastric artery grafts are favored for use in pediatric patients[72, 92] (Fig. 108–6), although some authors have advocated the use of vein with the application of an external mesh at the time of the initial operation.[6]

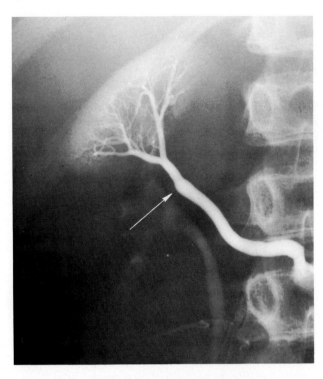

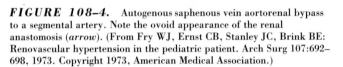

FIGURE 108–4. Autogenous saphenous vein aortorenal bypass to a segmental artery. Note the ovoid appearance of the renal anastomosis (*arrow*). (From Fry WJ, Ernst CB, Stanley JC, Brink BE: Renovascular hypertension in the pediatric patient. Arch Surg 107:692–698, 1973. Copyright 1973, American Medical Association.)

Hypogastric artery grafts may also be used in adult reconstructions.[62, 93] Vein grafts are carefully procured, gently handled, and cautiously irrigated with heparinized blood before implantation. Procurement of the hypogastric artery for use as an interposition graft proceeds in a similar manner, with care taken not to cause excessive vessel wall trauma. Synthetic grafts of fabricated Dacron or expanded polytetrafluoroethylene may also be used for main renal artery reconstructive procedures,[42, 46] but these conduits are less pliable and technically more difficult to use when revascularizations involve small dysplastic segmental vessels.

Arterial dilatation, alone or in conjunction with a bypass procedure, is sometimes used for treatment of intraparenchymal intimal and medial fibrodysplastic stenoses. After the renal artery has been exposed in a manner similar to that noted previously, the patient is systemically anticoagulated and rigid, cylindrical-tipped dilators are advanced through a transverse arteriotomy in the main renal artery (Fig. 108–7). Dilators are thoroughly lubricated with heparinized blood or a silicone solution so as to lessen intimal drag. The stenotic area is progressively dilated in increments of 0.5 mm by careful passage of increasingly larger

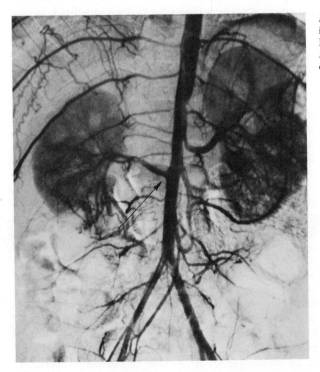

FIGURE 108–5. Renal artery–aortic reimplantation (*arrow*) in an infant who had an orificial renal artery stenosis. (From Stanley JC, Brothers TE: Surgical treatment of renovascular hypertension in children. *In* Ernst CB, Stanley JC [eds]: Current Therapy in Vascular Surgery. 2nd ed. Philadelphia, BC Decker, 1991, pp 875–880.)

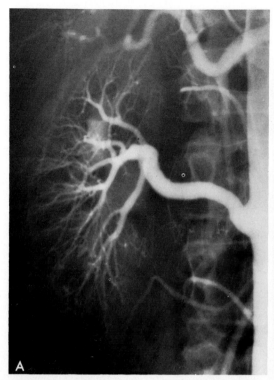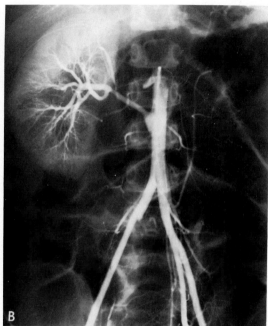

FIGURE 108–6. *A,* Autogenous saphenous vein aortorenal graft. *B,* Autogenous iliac artery aortorenal graft. Routine arteriographic documentation of early as well as late graft status is recommended. (*A,* From Stanley JC, Graham LM: Renovascular hypertension. *In* Miller DC, Roon AJ [eds]: Diagnosis and Management of Peripheral Vascular Disease. Menlo Park, CA, Addison-Wesley, 1981, pp 321–353. *B,* From Stanley JC, Fry WJ: Pediatric renal artery occlusive disease and renovascular hypertension. Etiology, diagnosis and operative treatment. Arch Surg 116:669–676, 1981. Copyright 1981, American Medical Association.)

dilators. Dilators 1.0 mm larger than the diameter of the normal proximal artery should not be used because they may disrupt the vessel wall. The role of intraluminal operative dilatation of fibrodysplastic renal artery stenoses using standard axial balloon catheters or linear extrusion balloon catheters awaits further clinical testing.

Management of stenotic disease affecting multiple renal arteries or segmental branches usually involves one of three alternative methods. The first requires separate implantations of the renal arteries into a single conduit. This is usually accomplished with a proximal end-to-side anastomosis and a distal end-to-end anastomosis to a vein graft.

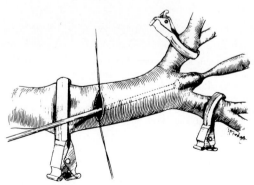

FIGURE 108–7. Technique of operative dilatation for intraparenchymal segmental stenotic disease.

If a nonreversed branching segment of saphenous vein in which the valves have been cut or a hypogastric artery with its branches is used as the bypass conduit, separate graft–renal artery anastomoses may be undertaken in an end-to-end fashion. The second method entails an in situ anastomosis of the involved arteries in a side-to-side manner, so as to form a common orifice. The vein graft is then anastomosed to the single channel created by this arterial union (Fig. 108–8). The third method involves implantation of an affected artery, beyond its diseased segment, into an adjacent normal artery in an end-to-side manner. Such an anastomosis usually involves second-order branches of the renal artery, but implantation may be undertaken into the main renal artery if the anastomosis can be fashioned without tension.

In the case of left-sided lesions in adults, an in situ splenorenal bypass offers an attractive alternative to aortorenal bypass.[44, 60] However, before undertaking a splenorenal bypass, the surgeon must document that the proximal celiac artery does not have an occlusive lesion that might perpetuate the hypertensive state after such a bypass. Splenorenal bypasses should be avoided in treating pediatric renovascular stenotic disease. Results of this approach in these younger patients have been exceedingly poor.[56, 63] This may be a reflection of the small splenic artery caliber in children but is more likely due to evolving or occult celiac artery stenoses occurring as a consequence of developmental arterial occlusive disease.[85] Surgeons should be prepared to perform ex vivo repairs with bench reconstruc-

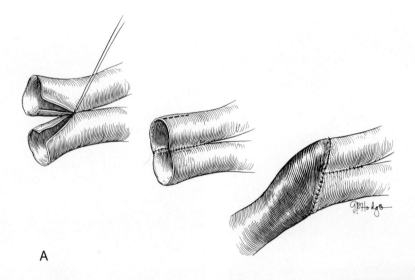

A

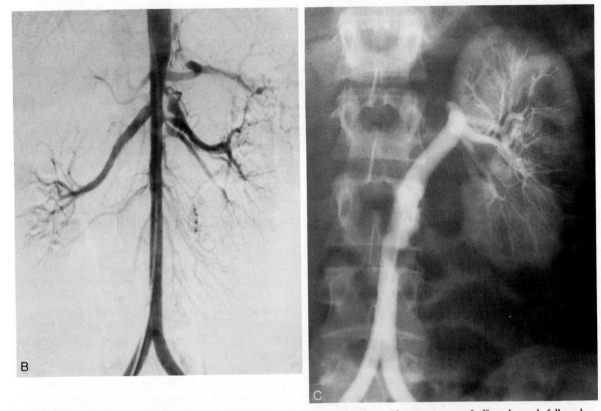

B

C

FIGURE 108–8. *A*, Revascularization of multiple renal arteries with side-to-side anastomoses of affected vessels followed by the anastomosis of a vein graft to their common orifice. *B* and *C*, Preoperative and postoperative arteriograms of this type of repair, with three vessels joined together before being anastomosed to a vein graft. (*A*, From Ernst BC, Fry WJ, Stanley JC: Surgical treatment of renovascular hypertension: Revascularization with autogenous vein. *In* Stanley JC, Ernst CB, Fry WJ [eds]: Renovascular Hypertension. Philadelphia, WB Saunders, 1984, p 284. *B* and *C*, From Stanley JC, Fry WJ: Pediatric renal artery occlusive disease and renovascular hypertension. Etiology, diagnosis and operative treatment. Arch Surg 116:669–676, 1981. Copyright 1981, American Medical Association.)

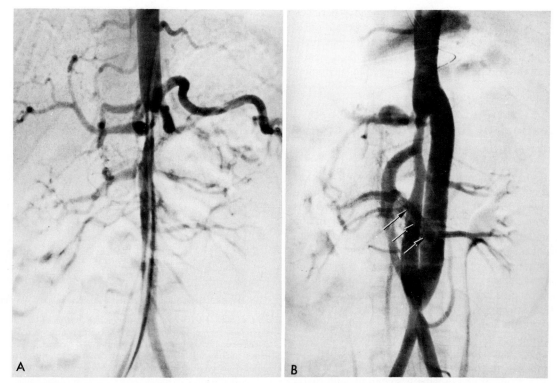

FIGURE 108–9. Complex renal reconstructive procedure for suprarenal aortic coarctation and stenosis (*arrow*) of the right superior renal artery (*A*) by thoracoabdominal bypass and saphenous vein bypass to the obstructed renal artery (*B*). (*A* and *B*, From Graham LM, Zelenock GB, Erlandson EE, et al: Abdominal aortic coarctation and segmental hypoplasia. Surgery 86:519, 1979.)

tion of diseased vessels when complex segmental renal artery fibrodysplasia exists.[3, 8, 56, 94]

Operative treatment of fibrodysplastic renovascular hypertension associated with aortic hypoplasia or coarctation is often complex (Fig. 108–9). Thoracoabdominal bypasses and local aortoplasties are the most common aortic operations, with concomitant renal artery reconstructions

performed in a standard manner.[30, 57] More recently, the authors have favored direct patch aortoplasty with the implantation of spatulated renal arteries into normal aorta[75] (Fig. 108–10). This is considered simpler, safer, and more likely to provide excellent long-term results than are complex aortic and renal reconstructions requiring the use of more graft material and multiple anastomoses. There

FIGURE 108–10. Aortoplasty (ap) of mid-abdominal aortic coarctation with a polytetrafluoroethylene patch and bilateral aortic reimplantation of renal arteries *(arrows)* in a child with suprarenal aortic coarctation and bilateral renal artery orificial stenotic disease. (From Stanley JC, Brothers TE: Midabdominal aortic coarctation and hypoplasia associated with renal artery stenosis. *In* Ernst CB, Stanley JC [eds]: Current Therapy in Vascular Surgery. 2nd ed. Philadelphia, BC Decker, 1991, pp 856–860.)

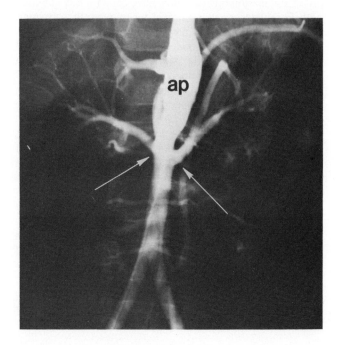

have been no operative deaths in the Michigan experience with these reconstructions, and although the reported operative mortality rate for extensive combined aortic and renal revascularization procedures approaches 8 per cent, nearly 90 per cent of the survivors have benefited from such interventions.[30]

Complications of Renal Artery Reconstructions

Specific hazards attending renovascular surgery attest to the importance of a properly planned and executed initial reconstructive procedure.[25, 89] Reoperation for complications of renal artery reconstructive surgery undertaken in the pediatric and adult fibrodysplastic groups entails nephrectomy rates of 60 and 39 per cent, respectively.[89]

Early thromboses of aortorenal, iliorenal, hepatorenal, or splenorenal bypass grafts can occur with either autologous tissue or prosthetic material. The incidence of this complication affecting aortorenal vein grafts is approximately 2 per cent, and it is slightly higher with prosthetic grafts. Thromboses of arterial autografts are even more uncommon.[52, 93] Occasionally, conduits are too small and early thromboses are more likely. Autogenous vein less than 3 mm in diameter and prosthetic materials with diameters of less than 5 mm should be avoided in reconstructing the main renal artery. However, vein or artery of smaller diameters may be satisfactory for reconstruction of segmental vessels.

Intravenous urograms, as well as isotopic renograms and renal scans, are of limited use in establishing postoperative graft patency. Relatively normal renal function and perfusion may persist in patients with acutely occluded grafts because of an extensive preexistent collateral circulation. Arteriography is essential in the diagnosis of early graft occlusion. Immediate anticoagulation and reoperation should be contemplated once this complication has been recognized.

Late anastomotic strictures have become less common with improved vascular surgical techniques. In particular, creation of a generous ovoid graft–renal artery anastomosis has lessened the likelihood of this complication. Intimal fibroplasia is a second, but poorly understood, cause of late graft stenosis. Turbulent flow causing stimulation of myointimal cells and continual deposition of a fibrin coagulum may be important contributing factors in these cases. The role of antiplatelet agents in lessening this complication remains to be defined. Other causes of late graft stenoses are well known. The deleterious long-term consequences of placing clamps on vein grafts has been documented as a cause of graft stenosis. Similarly, overzealous advancement of large dilators through stenoses or "sounding" of segmental vessels beyond the site of anastomosis may be a cause of late fibrous strictures. Late vein graft narrowings, many of inconsequential character, are not uncommon, with clinically significant stenoses encountered in 8 per cent of aortorenal vein grafts.[23, 77] Late stenoses of arterial autografts are very rare.[41, 93]

Late vein graft dilatation, documented in 20 to 44 per cent of aortorenal saphenous vein grafts, usually appears as

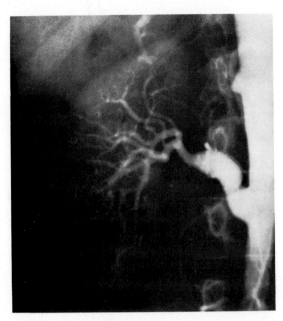

FIGURE 108–11. Aneurysmal dilatation of an autogenous saphenous vein aortorenal graft. This complication is most likely to affect pediatric patients. (From Stanley JC, Ernst CB, Fry WJ: Fate of 100 aortorenal vein grafts: Characteristics of late graft expansion, aneurysmal dilatation, and stenosis. Surgery 74:931, 1973.)

a nonprogressive, uniform increase in graft diameter.[21, 77] Marked aneurysmal changes affect approximately 2 per cent of aortorenal vein grafts in adults[77] and at least 20 per cent of vein grafts placed in pediatric patients[81] (Fig. 108–11). Other authors have reported a lower incidence of this complication.[21] The predisposition for dilatation to affect pediatric patients may reflect the precarious state of vasa vasorum in veins of younger individuals. Veins in pediatric patients are more likely to incur ischemic injury during transplantation. Expansion and aneurysmal dilatation have also been reported to occur with renovascular reconstructions using autogenous arterial segments, but the frequency of this event is much lower than that affecting veins.[21, 93] Rupture of aneurysmal aortorenal vein grafts has not been reported. However, luminal thrombus formation and distal embolization of microthrombi can occur in aneurysmal veins and may be reason to replace or plicate these dilated grafts.[87]

Results of Surgical Therapy

Benefits of operative intervention for renovascular disease and secondary hypertension are directly proportionate to the accurate identification of surgical candidates and the performance of appropriate reconstructive procedures. The Cooperative Study of Renovascular Hypertension was undertaken nearly 2 decades ago in an attempt to better define the optimal diagnostic and therapeutic management of this disease entity. The poor results in the Cooperative Study probably reflect errors in patient selection and early technical problems in the surgical management of renovascular hypertension.[26, 28] The Cooperative Study's overall results of 577 surgical procedures undertaken in 520 patients with all forms of renovascular hypertension included cure in 51 per cent, improvement in 15 per cent, failure in 34 per cent. These results certainly dampened the initial enthusiasm for renovascular reconstructions. More recent experiences from 11 active centers reporting on surgical therapy in 2460 patients with renovascular hypertension depict remarkably better overall results.[78] Furthermore, patients with fibrodysplastic lesions were more likely to have a salutory response following operative intervention than those with arteriosclerotic disease.

Fifteen institutions participated in the Cooperative Study, which documented arterial fibrodysplastic disease in 286 of the 2442 individuals evaluated.[26] Dysplastic disease was the basis for operation in 179 study patients. With the exclusion of 6 individuals who died and another 22 who had undefinable results, 151 patients were categorized with respect to outcome after either revascularization or nephrectomy. Among these patients, the eventual results included cure in 58 per cent, improvement in 13 per cent, and failure in 29 per cent. Unfortunately, a total of only 57 per cent were considered cured or improved after primary arterial reconstruction. Poor results in the cooperative study following primary arterial reconstructions reflected technical problems, with 27 of the 32 operative failures considered to be due to anatomic faults. The overall cure and improvement rate was 84 per cent when these anatomic failures were eliminated and only technically successful arterial reconstructions were considered.

More recent results of the surgical treatment of fibrodysplastic renovascular hypertension in adults document excellent outcomes regarding blood pressure control, with 90 to 95 per cent of properly selected patients being cured or improved (Table 108–2). Several other findings in current practice are noteworthy. The first relates to improved reconstructive techniques. The incidence of primary nephrectomy is much lower: it was performed in only 6 of 152 primary operative procedures at the authors' institution.[80] Second, operative mortality has approached zero in treating patients with fibrodysplastic renovascular hypertension at most major institutions. This may represent better preoperative and postoperative care or fewer intraoperative complications during arterial reconstructive procedures. Whatever the case may be, a mortality rate of 3.4 per cent, as noted for surgical treatment of fibrodysplastic patients in the Cooperative Study, would be clearly unacceptable in contemporary practice. Lastly, although renal failure accompanying fibrodysplastic renovascular disease is quite uncommon in contrast to that seen with arteriosclerotic disease, clear benefits are associated with revascularization in these cases.[19, 106]

Cumulative surgical experiences with pediatric patients reveal that they have the best outcomes of any subgroup of patients with renovascular hypertension (Table 108–3). Although the numbers of pediatric patients in most series are small, a beneficial outcome is anticipated in up to 98 per cent of children treated operatively. However, marked variances exist between centers with regard to the number of patients who undergo primary arterial reconstructions as opposed to primary nephrectomy.[16, 56, 74, 81] Improved vascular surgical techniques have allowed more individuals to be satisfactorily revascularized.[74, 81] Occasionally, vessels in infants are too small to be safely reconstructed. In these instances, drug therapy may be appropriate until the patient's arteries have achieved a size that will allow successful reconstruction.[15, 48] Certainly, microvascular and macrovascular techniques have evolved to the extent that few patients should be treated by primary nephrectomy. As is

Table 108–2. Results of Surgical Therapy for Renovascular Hypertension Due to Fibrodysplasia in Adults

| Medical Center | No. of Patients | Postoperative Status* | | | Operative Mortality Rate (%) |
		Cure (%)	Improvement (%)	Failure (%)	
University of Michigan[88] (1961–1980)	144	55	39	6	0
Baylor College of Medicine[47] (1959–1979)	113	43	24	33	0†
Cleveland Clinic[64] (1975–1984)	104	63	30	7	0
University of California, San Francisco[93] (1964–1980)	77	66	32	1.3	0
University of Essen[40] (1971–1979)	75	63	24	13	0
Mayo Clinic[39] (1965–1968)	63	66	24	10	Unknown
Vanderbilt University[18] (1977–1982)	56	77	19	1	0
University of Leiden[103] (1962–1982)	53	53	34	11	1.9
Columbia University[9] (1962–1976)	42	76	14	10	Unknown
University of Lund–Malmo General Hospital[5] (1971–1977)	40	66	24	10	0

Criteria for blood pressure response are defined in the cited publications.

†No deaths occurred in 100 isolated renal reconstructions; data on 13 patients with associated arteriosclerosis were unavailable.

Table 108–3. Results of Surgical Treatment of Renovascular Hypertension due to Fibrodysplasia in Pediatric Patients

| Medical Center | No. of Patients | No. of Primary Procedures | | No. of Secondary Procedures | Postoperative Status* | | | Operative Mortality Rate (%) |
		Arterial Reconstruction	Nephrectomy		Cure (%)	Improvement (%)	Failure (%)	
University of Michigan[81]† (1963–1980)	40	49	2	6	85	12.5	2.5	0
Cleveland Clinic								
(1955–1977)[4, 63]	27	22	11	5	59	18.5	18.5	4
(1978–1988)[56]	28	34	1	Unstated	78	18	4	Unstated
University of California, Los Angeles[90] (1967–1977)	26	19	11	7	84.5	7.5	4	4
Vanderbilt University[48]‡ (1962–1977)	21	15	8	4	68	24	8	0
University of Pennsylvania[6] (1974–1987)	17	30	0	1§	76.5	23.5	0	0
University of California, San Francisco[92] (1960–1974)	14	10	4	2	86	7	0	7

*Criteria for blood pressure response are defined in the cited publications. Data are expressed to the nearest 0.5%.

†Results include data from 6 patients treated at the University of Texas Southwestern.

‡Results include data from 4 patients with parenchymal disease treated by nephrectomy. A more recent but less detailed review includes 28 patients with cure, improvement, and failure rates of 72%, 21%, and 7%, respectively.[17]

§Two revascularized kidneys that subsequently became infarcted were not removed.

the case with operative treatment of fibrodysplastic disease in adults, operative treatment of infants and children should encompass little mortality.

The benefits of surgical treatment of renovascular hypertension due to dysplastic arterial disease become more apparent when the results are examined in specific patient subgroups from the authors' institution (Table 108–4). Patients were classified into four distinct categories: (1) pediatric patients up to 17 years of age with fibrodysplastic disease, (2) adults with fibrodysplastic disease, (3) adults with arteriosclerotic renal artery lesions *without* clinically overt extrarenal arteriosclerotic cardiovascular disease, and (4) adults with arteriosclerotic renal artery lesions *with* clinically overt extrarenal arteriosclerotic cardiovascular disease. Patients in the latter group include individuals with extracranial cerebrovascular disease manifest by stroke or transient ischemic attacks, coronary artery disease associated with angina pectoris or myocardial infarction, symptomatic peripheral artery occlusive disease, and aneurysmal disease of the abdominal aorta or its branches.

This classification becomes relevant in discussions of the operative management and the anticipated outcomes of treatment. Benefits of surgical treatment were most likely in pediatric and adult fibrodysplastic categories, in which 97 and 94 per cent of patients, respectively, were cured or improved. Responses were also excellent in adults with focal arteriosclerotic disease, 91 per cent of whom were cured or improved postoperatively. These outcomes stand in contrast to that observed in adults with clinically overt generalized arteriosclerosis, only 72 per cent of whom had a salutory response to operation and only 25 per cent of whom were considered to be cured.

Table 108–4. Results of Surgical Treatment of Renovascular Hypertension in Specific Patient Subgroups

| Patient Subgroup | No. of Patients | Postoperative Status*† | | | Operative Mortality (%) |
		Cure (%)	Improvement (%)	Failure (%)	
Fibrodysplasia					
Pediatric	34	85	12	3	0
Adult	144	55	39	6	0
Arteriosclerosis					
Focal renal artery disease	64	33	58	9	0
Overt generalized disease	71	25	47	28	8.5§

Data from the University of Michigan experience, 1961–1980, as reported in Stanley JC, Whitehouse WM Jr, Graham, LM, et al: Operative therapy of renovascular hypertension. Br J Surg 69S(Suppl):S63, 1982.

*Represents the outcome of 415 operations (346 primary, 59 secondary), including initial nephrectomy in 17 patients.

†Cure was defined as blood pressures of 150/90 mmHg or lower for a minimum of 6 months postoperatively during which no antihypertensive medications were administered (lower pressure level standards were used in evaluating pediatric patients). Improvement meant normotensive while on drug therapy or diastolic blood pressures ranging between 90 and 100 mmHg but at least 15% lower than preoperative levels. Failure meant diastolic blood pressures of greater than 90 mmHg but less than 15% lower than preoperative levels or greater than 110 mmHg.

‡Operative mortality rate includes deaths within 30 days of operation.

§Four of six deaths occurred in patients undergoing concomitant aortic reconstructive surgery.

Although some authors have stated that operative intervention for fibrodysplastic renovascular hypertension offers little long-term benefit with respect to survival,[47] data from an earlier Mayo Clinic experience revealed higher patient survival rates among individuals treated operatively than among those treated by drug therapy alone.[39] Survival benefits are not as clearly defined as control of hypertension. Surgical therapy provides very durable salutory outcomes with regard to reductions in blood pressure.[20, 88] The fact that operative intervention can be performed with a high likelihood of success and minimal risks has caused most physicians to prefer surgical treatment or percutaneous transluminal angioplasty over long-term drug therapy for fibrodysplastic renovascular hypertension.

Alternatives to operative treatment of secondary hypertension due to renal artery fibrodysplasia must be judged in light of the excellent long-term operative results currently possible, as well as an up-to-date analysis of morbidity and mortality attributed to surgical therapy. The tenet that surgical treatment is appropriate in the management of fibrodysplastic renovascular hypertension receives strong support from recent clinical experiences, in which 90 to 95 per cent of properly selected patients experienced long-term benefit from operative intervention.

References

1. Aldigier J, Plouin PF, Guyene TT, et al: Comparison of the hormonal and renal effects of captopril in severe essential and renovascular hypertension. Am J Cardiol 49:1447, 1982.
2. Baert AL, Wilms G, Amery A, et al: Percutaneous transluminal renal angioplasty: Initial results and long-term follow-up in 202 patients. Cardiovasc Intervent Radiol 13:22, 1990.
3. Belzer FO, Raczkowski A: Ex vivo renal artery reconstruction with autotransplantation. Surgery 92:642, 1982.
4. Benjamin SP, Dustan HP, Gifford RW Jr, et al: Stenosing renal artery disease in children: Clinicopathologic correlation in 20 surgically treated cases. Cleve Clin Q 43:197, 1976.
5. Bergentz SE, Ericsson BF, Husberg B: Technique and complications in the surgical treatment of renovascular hypertension. Acta Chir Scand 145:143, 1979.
6. Berkowitz HD, O'Neill JA Jr: Renovascular hypertension in children. Surgical repair with special reference to the use of reinforced vein grafts. J Vasc Surg 9:46, 1989.
7. Bookstein JJ, Walter JF, Stanley JC, Fry WJ: Pharmaco-angiographic manipulation of renal collateral blood flow. Circulation 54:328, 1976.
8. Brekke IB, Sodal G, Jakobsen A, et al: Fibromuscular renal artery disease treated by extracorporeal vascular reconstruction and renal autotransplantation: Short- and long-term results. Eur J Vasc Surg 6:471, 1992.
9. Buda JA, Baer L, Parra-Carrillo JZ, et al: Predictability of surgical response in renovascular hypertension. Arch Surg 111:1243, 1976.
10. Buhler FR, Laragh JH, Baer L, et al: Propanolol inhibition of renin secretion. N Engl J Med 287:1209, 1972.
11. Case DB, Atlas SA, Marion RM, Laragh JH: Long-term efficacy of captopril in renovascular and essential hypertension. Am J Cardiol 49:1440, 1982.
12. Chevalier RL, Tegtmeyer CJ, Gomez RA: Percutaneous transluminal angioplasty for renovascular hypertension in children. Pediatr Nephrol 1:89, 1987.
13. Chibaro EA, Libertino JA, Novick AC: Use of the hepatic circulation for renal revascularization. Ann Surg 199:406, 1984.
14. Chrysant SG, Dunn M, Marples M, DeMasters K: Severe reversible azotemia from captopril therapy. Report of three cases and review of the literature. Arch Intern Med 143:347, 1983.
15. Daniels SR, Loggie JMH, McEnery PT, Towbin RB: Clinical spectrum of intrinsic renovascular hypertension in children. Pediatrics 80:698, 1987.
16. Deal JE, Snell MF, Barratt TM, Dillon MJ: Renovascular disease in childhood. J Pediatr 121:378, 1992.
17. Dean RH: Renovascular hypertension during childhood. *In* Dean RH, O'Neil JA Jr (eds): Vascular Disorders of Childhood. Philadelphia, Lea & Febiger, 1983, pp 77–96.
18. Dean RH: Renovascular hypertension. Curr Probl Surg 22:1, 1985.
19. Dean RH, Englund R, Dupont WD, et al: Retrieval of renal function by revascularization. Study of preoperative outcome predictors. Ann Surg 202:367, 1985.
20. Dean RH, Krueger TC, Whiteneck JM, et al: Operative management of renovascular hypertension. Results after a follow-up of fifteen to twenty-three years. J Vasc Surg 1:234, 1984.
21. Dean RH, Wilson JP, Burko H, Foster JH: Saphenous vein aortorenal bypass grafts: Serial arteriographic study. Ann Surg 130:469, 1974.
22. Detection, evaluation and treatment of renovascular hypertension. Final report. Working Group on Renovascular Hypertension. Arch Intern Med 147:820, 1987.
23. Ekelund J, Gerlock J Jr, Goncharenko V, Foster J: Angiographic findings following surgical treatment for renovascular hypertension. Radiology 126:345, 1978.
24. Ernst CB, Bookstein JJ, Montie J, et al: Renal vein renin ratios and collateral vessels in renovascular hypertension. Arch Surg 104:496, 1972.
25. Foster JH, Dean RH, Pinkerton JA, Rhamy RK: Ten years experience with surgical management of renovascular hypertension. Ann Surg 177:755, 1973.
26. Foster JH, Maxwell SS, Bleifer KH, et al: Renovascular occlusive disease. Results of operative treatment. JAMA 231:1043, 1975.
27. Franklin SS, Smith RD: A comparison of enalapril plus hydrochlorothiazide with standard triple therapy in renovascular hypertension. Nephron 44(Suppl 1):73, 1986.
28. Franklin SS, Young JD Jr, Maxwell MH, et al: Operative morbidity and mortality in renovascular disease. JAMA 231:1148, 1975.
29. Geyskes GG, Puylaert CBAJ, Oei HY, Mees EJD: Follow-up study of 70 patients with renal artery stenosis treated by percutaneous transluminal dilatation. Br Med J 287:333, 1983.
30. Graham LM, Zelenock GB, Erlandson EE, et al: Abdominal aortic coarctation and segmental hypoplasia. Surgery 86:519, 1979.
31. Grim CE, Luft FC, Yune HY, et al: Percutaneous transluminal dilatation in the treatment of renal vascular hypertension. Ann Intern Med 95:439, 1981.
32. Grim CE, Yune HY, Donohue JP, et al: Unilateral renal vascular hypertension: Surgery vs dilation. Vasa 11:367, 1982.
33. Grim CE, Yune HY, Donohue JP, et al: Renal vascular hypertension. Surgery vs dilation. Nephron 44(Suppl 1):96, 1986.
34. Gruntzig A, Vetter W, Meier B, et al: Treatment of renovascular hypertension with percutaneous transluminal dilatation of a renal artery stenosis. Lancet 1:801, 1978.
35. Hagg A, Aberg H, Eriksson I, et al: Fibromuscular dysplasia of the renal artery—Management and outcome. Acta Chir Scand 153:15, 1987.
36. Harrison EG, McCormack LJ: Pathologic classification of renal artery disease in renovascular hypertension. Mayo Clin Proc 46:161, 1971.
37. Hodsman GP, Brown JJ, Cummings AMM, et al: Enalapril in treatment of hypertension with renal artery stenosis. Changes in blood pressure, renin, angiotensin I and II, renal function, and body composition. Am J Med 77:52, 1984.
38. Hricik DE, Browning PJ, Kopelman R, et al: Captopril-induced renal insufficiency in patients with bilateral renal-artery stenosis or renal-artery stenosis in a solitary kidney. N Engl J Med 308:373, 1983.
39. Hunt JC, Strong CG: Renovascular hypertension. Mechanisms, natural history and treatment. Am J Cardiol 32:562, 1973.
40. Jakubowski HD, Eigler FW, Montag H: Results of surgery in fibrodysplastic renal artery stenosis. World J Surg 5:859, 1981.
41. Kaufman JJ: Renovascular hypertension: The UCLA experience. J Urol 112:139, 1979.
42. Kaufmann JJ: Long-term results of aortorenal Dacron grafts in the treatment of renal artery stenosis. J Urol 111:298, 1974.
43. Keith TA III: Renovascular hypertension in black patients. Hypertension 4:438, 1982.
44. Khauli RB, Novick AC, Ziegelbaum M: Splenorenal bypass in the treatment of renal artery stenosis: Experience with sixty-nine cases. J Vasc Surg 2:547, 1985.
45. Klinge J, Mali WPTM, Puijlaert CBAJ, et al: Percutaneous translu-

minal renal angioplasty: Initial and long-term results. Radiology 171:501, 1989.

46. Lagneau P, Michel JB, Charrat JM: Use of polytetrafluoroethylene grafts for renal bypass. J Vasc Surg 5:738, 1987.

47. Lawrie GM, Morris GC Jr, Soussou ID, et al: Late results of reconstructive surgery for renovascular disease. Ann Surg 191:528, 1980.

48. Lawson JD, Boerth R, Foster JH, Dean RH: Diagnosis and management of renovascular hypertension in children. Arch Surg 122:1307, 1977.

49. Lewin A, Blaufox MD, Castle H, et al: Apparent prevalence of curable hypertension in the Hypertension Detection and Follow-Up Program. Arch Intern Med 145:424, 1985.

50. Luscher TF, Greminger P, Kuhlmann TJ, et al: Renal venous renin determinations in renovascular hypertension. Diagnostic and prognostic value in unilateral renal artery stenosis treated by surgery or percutaneous transluminal angioplasty. Nephron 44(Suppl 1):17, 1986.

51. Luscher TF, Keller HM, Imhof HG, et al: Fibromuscular hyperplasia: Extension of the disease and therapeutic outcome. Results of the University Hospital Zurich Cooperative Study on fibromuscular hyperplasia. Nephron 44(Suppl 1):109, 1986.

52. Lye CR, String ST, Wylie EJ, Stoney RJ: Aortorenal arterial autografts. Late observations. Arch Surg 110:1321, 1975.

53. Mahler F, Triller J, Weidmarim P, Nachbur B: Complications in percutaneous transluminal dilation of renal arteries. Nephron 44(Suppl 1):60, 1986.

54. Martin EC, Diamond NG, Casarella WJ: Percutaneous transluminal angioplasty in nonatherosclerotic disease. Radiology 135:27, 1980.

55. Martin LG, Price RB, Casarella WJ, et al: Percutaneous angioplasty in clinical management of renovascular hypertension: Initial and long-term results. Radiology 155:629, 1985.

56. Martinez A, Novick AC, Cunningham R, Goormastic M: Improved results of vascular reconstruction in pediatric and young adult patients with renovascular hypertension. J Urol 144:717, 1990.

57. Messina LM, Reilly LM, Goldstone J, et al: Middle aortic syndrome: Effectiveness and durability of complex revascularization techniques. Ann Surg 204:331, 1986.

58. Millan VG, McCauley J, Kopelman RI, Madias NE: Percutaneous transluminal renal angioplasty in nonatherosclerotic renovascular hypertension. Long-term results. Hypertension 7:668, 1985.

59. Miller GA, Ford KK, Braum SD, et al: Percutaneous transluminal angioplasty vs surgery for renovascular hypertension. AJR 144:447, 1985.

60. Moncure AC, Brewster DC, Darling RC, et al: Use of the splenic and hepatic arteries for renal revascularization. J Vasc Surg 3:196, 1986.

61. Muller FB, Sealey JF, Case DB, et al: The captopril test for identifying disease in hypertensive patients. Am J Med 80:633, 1986.

62. Novick AC, Stewart BH, Straffon RA: Autogenous arterial grafts in the treatment of renal artery stenosis. J Urol 118:919, 1977.

63. Novick AC, Straffon RA, Stewart BH, Benjamin S: Surgical treatment of renovascular hypertension in the pediatric patient. J Urol 119:794, 1978.

64. Novick AC, Ziegelbaum M, Vidt DG, et al: Trends in surgical revascularization for renal artery disease. Ten years' experience. JAMA 257:498, 1987.

65. Ramsay LE, Waller PC: Blood pressure response to percutaneous transluminal angioplasty for renovascular hypertension: An overview of published series. Br Med J 300:569, 1990.

66. Saffitz JE, Totty WG, McClennan BL, Gilua LA: Percutaneous transluminal angioplasty. Radiological-pathological correlation. Radiology 141:651, 1981.

67. Sang CN, Whelton PK, Hamper UM, et al: Etiologic factors in renovascular fibromuscular dysplasia. Hypertension 14:472, 1989.

68. Schwarten DE, Yune HY, Klatte EC, et al: Clinical experience with percutaneous transluminal angioplasty (PTA) of stenotic renal arteries. Radiology 135:601, 1980.

69. Simon N, Franklin SS, Bleifer KH, Maxwell MH: Clinical characteristics of renovascular hypertension. JAMA 220:1209, 1972.

70. Sos TA, Pickering TG, Sniderman KW, et al: Percutaneous transluminal renal angioplasty in renovascular hypertension due to atheroma or fibromuscular dysplasia. N Engl J Med 309:274, 1983.

71. Sos TA, Saddekini S, Pickering TG, Laragh JH: Technical aspects of percutaneous transluminal angioplasty in renovascular disease. Nephron 44(Suppl 1):45, 1986.

72. Stanley JC: Renal vascular disease and renovascular hypertension in children. Urol Clin North Am 11:451, 1984.

73. Stanley JC: Surgery of failed percutaneous transluminal renal artery angioplasty. In Bergan JJ, Yao JST (eds): Reoperative Arterial Surgery. Orlando, FL, Grune & Stratton, 1986, pp 441–454.

74. Stanley JC: Surgical intervention in pediatric renovascular hypertension. Child Nephrol Urol 12:167, 1992.

75. Stanley JC, Brothers TE: Midabdominal aortic coarctation and hypoplasia associated with renal artery stenosis. In Ernst CB, Stanley JC (eds): Current Therapy in Vascular Surgery. 2nd ed. Philadelphia, BC Decker, 1991, pp 856–860.

76. Stanley JC, Brothers TE: Surgical treatment of renovascular hypertension in children. In Ernst CB, Stanley JC (eds): Current Therapy in Vascular Surgery. 2nd ed. Philadelphia, BC Decker, 1991, pp 875–880.

77. Stanley JC, Ernst CB, Fry WJ: Fate of 100 aortorenal vein grafts: Characteristics of late graft expansion, aneurysmal dilatation, and stenosis. Surgery 74:931, 1973.

78. Stanley JC, Ernst CB, Fry WJ: Surgical treatment of renovascular hypertension: Results in specific patient subgroups. In Renovascular Hypertension. Philadelphia, WB Saunders, 1984, pp 363–371.

79. Stanley JC, Fry WJ: Renovascular hypertension secondary to arterial fibrodysplasia in adults. Criteria for operation and results of surgical therapy. Arch Surg 110:922, 1975.

80. Stanley JC, Fry WJ: Surgical treatment of renovascular hypertension. Arch Surg 112:1291, 1977.

81. Stanley JC, Fry WJ: Pediatric renal artery occlusive disease and renovascular hypertension. Etiology, diagnosis and operative treatment. Arch Surg 116:669, 1981.

82. Stanley JC, Gewertz BL, Bove EL, et al: Arterial fibrodysplasia. Histopathologic character and current etiologic concepts. Arch Surg 110:561, 1975.

83. Stanley JC, Gewertz BL, Fry WJ: Renal: systemic renin indices and renal vein renin ratios as prognostic indicators in remedial renovascular hypertension. J Surg Res 20:149, 1976.

84. Stanley JC, Graham LM, Whitehouse WM Jr: Limitations and errors of diagnostic and prognostic investigations in renovascular hypertension. In Bernhard VM, Towne JB (eds): Complications in Vascular Surgery. 2nd ed. Orlando, FL, Grune & Stratton, 1985, pp 213–227.

85. Stanley JC, Graham LM, Whitehouse WM Jr, et al: Developmental occlusive disease of the abdominal aorta, splanchnic and renal arteries. Am J Surg 142:190, 1981.

86. Stanley JC, Wakefield TW: Arterial fibrodysplasia. In Rutherford RB (ed): Vascular Surgery. 3rd ed. Philadelphia, WB Saunders, 1989, pp 245–265.

87. Stanley JC, Whitehouse WM Jr, Graham LM: Complications of renal revascularization. In Bernhard VM, Towne JB (eds): Complications in Vascular Surgery. New York, Grune & Stratton, 1980, pp 189–218.

88. Stanley JC, Whitehouse WM Jr, Graham LM, et al: Operative therapy of renovascular hypertension. Br J Surg 69(Suppl):S63, 1982.

89. Stanley JC, Whitehouse WM Jr, Zelenock GB, et al: Reoperation for complications of renal artery reconstructive surgery undertaken for treatment of renovascular hypertension. J Vasc Surg 2:133, 1985.

90. Stanley P, Gyepes MT, Olson DL, Gates GF: Renovascular hypertension in children and adolescents. Radiology 129:123, 1978.

91. Stanley P, Hieshima G, Mehringer M: Percutaneous transluminal angioplasty for pediatric renovascular hypertension. Radiology 153:101, 1984.

92. Stoney RJ, Cooke PA, String ST: Surgical treatment of renovascular hypertension in children. J Pediatr Surg 10:631, 1975.

93. Stoney RJ, DeLuccia N, Ehrenfeld WK, Wylie EJ: Aortorenal arterial autografts. Long-term assessment. Arch Surg 116:1416, 1981.

94. Stoney RJ, DeLuccia N, Ehrenfeld WK, Wylie EJ: Aortorenal arterial autografts. Long-term assessment. Arch Surg 116:1416, 1981.

95. Stringer DA, deBruyn R, Dillion MJ, Gordon I: Comparison of aortography, renal vein renin sampling, radionuclide scans, ultrasound and the IVU in the investigation of childhood renovascular hypertension. Br J Radiol 57:111, 1984.

96. Surur MF, Sos TA, Saddekni S, et al: Intimal fibromuscular dysplasia and Takayasu arteritis: Delayed response to percutaneous transluminal angioplasty. Radiology 157:657, 1985.

97. Tegtmeyer CJ, Elson J, Glass TA, et al: Percutaneous transluminal angioplasty: The treatment of choice for renovascular hypertension due to fibromuscular dysplasia. Radiology 143:631, 1982.

98. Tegtmeyer CJ, Kellum CD, Ayers C: Percutaneous transluminal angioplasty of the renal artery. Results and long-term follow-up. Radiology 153:77, 1984.
99. Tegtmeyer CJ, Selby JB, Hartwell GD, et al: Results and complications of angioplasty in fibromuscular disease. Circulation 83(Suppl):I-155, 1991.
100. Tegtmeyer CJ, Sos TA: Techniques of renal angioplasty. Radiology 161:577, 1986.
101. Thibonnier M, Joseph A, Sassano P, et al: Improved diagnosis of unilateral renal artery lesions after captopril administration. JAMA 251:56, 1984.
102. Thornbury JR, Stanley JC, Fryback DG: Hypertensive urogram: A nondiscriminatory test for renovascular hypertension. Am J Roentgenol 138:43, 1982.

103. vanBockel JH, van Schilfgaarde R, Felthuis W, et al: Long-term results of in situ and extracorporeal surgery for renovascular hypertension caused by fibrodysplasia. J Vasc Surg 6:355, 1987.
104. Vidt DG: Advances in the medical management of renovascular hypertension. Urol Clin North Am 11:417, 1984.
105. Watson AR, Balfe JW, Hardy BE: Renovascular hypertension in childhood: A changing perspective in management. J Pediatr 106:366, 1985.
106. Whitehouse WM Jr, Kazmers A, Zelenock GB, et al: Chronic total renal artery occlusion. Effects of treatment on secondary hypertension and renal function. Surgery 89:753, 1981.
107. Zweifler AJ, Julius S: Medical treatment of renovascular hypertension. In Stanley JC, Ernst CB, Fry WJ (eds): Renovascular Hypertension. Philadelphia, WB Saunders, 1980, p 231.

109

Evaluation and Management of Ischemic Nephropathy

Richard H. Dean, M.D., B.A., and Kimberley J. Hansen, M.D.

• • •

The usefulness of renal revascularization in controlling hypertension secondary to renal artery occlusive disease is widely recognized. Although the criteria for patient selection are still controversial, there is no denying the durable benefit derived by many patients. Alternatively, severe occlusive disease may lead to inadequate effective renal plasma flow and diminished excretory function of the kidney. Traditionally, study of the sequelae of renovascular occlusive disease has centered on the pathophysiology and management of the resultant renovascular hypertension. More recent reports, however, have emphasized the potential for simultaneous retrieval of excretory function in some patients with combined hypertension and renal insufficiency.[1-3] These observations have renewed awareness of this functional consequence of renal ischemia and have led to the coining of the term *ischemic nephropathy*. By definition, ischemic nephropathy reflects the presence of anatomically severe occlusive disease of the extraparenchymal renal artery in a patient with excretory renal insufficiency.

Two groups of patients are potential candidates for revascularization to improve renal function. The first group is represented by the patient with a normal or slightly elevated serum creatinine value who is found to have a poorly functioning or nonfunctioning kidney on diagnostic evaluation for renovascular hypertension. In this patient, overall renal function is being maintained by the contralateral normal kidney, and the clinical question is whether to remove or to revascularize the poorly functioning kidney. The second group is represented by the azotemic or dialysis-dependent patient who has extraparenchymal renovascular occlusive disease (ischemic nephropathy). In this patient, the question is whether the probability of retrieving clinically significant function or of significantly slowing the decline of function justifies the risk of operation.

The issues pertinent to management decisions in these groups are different and merit individual attention. In the succeeding sections, currently available data and considerations important in the selection of patients in these groups for renal artery reconstruction are reviewed separately.

THE NONAZOTEMIC PATIENT

Hypertension in the nonazotemic patient with renal artery occlusion and a poorly functioning or nonfunctioning kidney can be treated equally well by revascularization or nephrectomy. However, the management of hypertension as well as the retrieval of function by revascularization would be superior if both of these end-results could be predicted and assessed. The practical value of this premise is obvious when one considers that as many as 35 per cent of patients with mild contralateral occlusive lesions will progress to hemodynamically severe occlusive lesions within 5 years. When such patients have undergone nephrectomy for renovascular hypertension and their contralateral disease has progressed, global renal function is threatened and operative intervention must then be contemplated for patients who are severely azotemic and have potentially dialysis-dependent renal failure. It is also possible that the atherosclerotic occlusive disease in the remaining kidney will not develop in a manner that will be recognized appropriately or will develop at a site not amenable to surgical correction. On the other hand, a too-aggressive attitude toward revascularization of the initially poorly functioning or nonfunctioning kidney and attempted recovery of function at the lowest limits of retrievability will sometimes lead to revascularization of a kidney in which no functional response can be achieved. In this instance, primary nephrectomy would be simpler than revascularization and would be equally beneficial in the control of hypertension. Therefore, evaluation of the expected results of revascularizing poorly functioning kidneys and of the value of preoperative predictors of retrieval are important in the management of these patients.

Reports of retrieval of function in the nonazotemic patient underscore the potential value of aggressive management.[4, 5] The authors reviewed the effect of revascularization on renal function in 64 patients who had a preoperative creatinine clearance by the affected kidney of less than or equal to 15 ml/min.[6] Results of this study and the authors' subsequent experience have led them to proceed with revascularization whenever the distal vessel is identified and appears normal by arteriography. Similarly, when at least 10 per cent of total renal function is coming from the poorly functioning kidney on isotope renography, the authors will explore the distal vessel even when it is not visualized by arteriography. In about 40 per cent of such cases, the authors will find a normal distal vessel and will proceed with revascularization. Nevertheless, if atherosclerotic lesions are present at the level of the branches, they will proceed with nephrectomy.

Although Zinman and Libertino found preoperative renal biopsy to be a useful predictor of functional retrieval in their series of patients,[7] the authors of this chapter have not found it worthwhile. Having identified diffuse hyalinization of glomeruli in specimens obtained by open biopsy of selected sections of kidneys with adequate renal function and in kidneys with marked improvement in excretory function, the authors long ago abandoned the technique as misleading and potentially hazardous.

A number of factors influence the successful revascularization of poorly functioning kidneys. Although studies have not defined limits below which clinically important retrieval of function is impossible, they have identified preoperative variables that may predict a favorable response. Removal of a nonfunctioning kidney does nothing to diminish excretory function. Indeed, subsequent improvement in blood pressure control with the concomitant elimination of high-dose diuretics and other medications that might adversely affect renal function may lead to improvement in function in the remaining kidney. Nevertheless, long-term follow-up studies of renal function and renal anatomy in patients with renovascular hypertension underscore the frequently progressive nature of the disease in both the ipsilateral and the contralateral kidney.[8, 9] For this reason, the aggressive use of revascularization rather than nephrectomy in patients with characteristics favorably predicting retrieval of function should improve the long-term management of these patients. The application of predictors such as urinary hyperconcentration of nonreabsorbable solutes on split

renal function studies[6] and the identification of a disease-free distal renal artery on preoperative angiography or intraoperatively should allow a more accurate selection of the appropriate operation and thereby limit the frequency of inappropriate revascularization leading to subsequent nephrectomy.

THE AZOTEMIC PATIENT

The severely azotemic patient with renovascular occlusive disease more clearly resembles the atherosclerotic patient with end-stage disease than does the nonazotemic patient. Although retrieval of function has immediate practical significance, the hazard of aggravating renal failure to a dialysis-dependent level or of placing the patient with dialysis dependence at a potentially higher operative risk by inappropriate surgery tempers enthusiasm for a nonselective approach to the management of these patients.

Morris and associates, reporting in 1962 on eight azotemic patients with either severe bilateral renal artery occlusions or unilateral occlusive disease and an absent contralateral kidney, described a salutary effect of revascularization on both hypertension and renal function.[10] Novick and colleagues found a similar beneficial functional response to renal revascularization when bilateral lesions were corrected in azotemic patients.[11] Nevertheless, little information in the literature accurately describes the incidence, prevalence, spectrum of clinical presentations, and natural history of ischemic nephropathy. Circumstantial evidence, however, suggests that it may be a more common cause of progressive renal failure in the atherosclerotic age group than was previously recognized. In a 1986 survey, 73 per cent of patients with end-stage renal disease were in the atherosclerotic age group.[12] In a report by Mailloux and coworkers, a presumed renovascular cause of end-stage renal disease increased in frequency from 6.7 per cent for the period between 1978 and 1981 to 16.5 per cent for the period between 1982 and 1985.[13] The median age at the onset of end-stage renal disease for this group was the highest among all groups: the 7th decade of life. Each of these clinical characteristics is in concert with the demographic data on the authors' reported patient group with proven ischemic nephropathy.[14] In the authors' group, all patients had at least moderate hypertension, the mean age was 63 years, and only 14 per cent had diabetes mellitus. The authors believe these data argue that renovascular disease may be either the primary cause or a superimposed secondary accelerant of renal insufficiency in a larger proportion of patients with renal insufficiency than is commonly recognized. Using this premise as a guide, the authors currently screen all adult patients older than 50 years of age who have newly recognized renal insufficiency when hypertension of any level is a coexistent morbidity.

Renal duplex sonography is the authors' preferred method for this preliminary screening. Their experience with the use of renal duplex sonography as a screening technique was previously reported.[15] In this review, the authors found renal duplex sonography to have an overall accuracy of 96 per cent for establishing the presence or absence of main renal artery occlusive disease. Because the term *ischemic nephropathy* implies the presence of global renal ischemia, the authors believe that renal duplex sonography, when performed by an experienced technician, is an adequate method for initially screening the patient with renal insufficiency. Through preliminary screening with renal duplex sonography, the authors limit the use of arteriography in patients with renal insufficiency to those with either positive findings on renal duplex sonography or severe hypertension.

The authors have continued to rely on standard "cut film" arteriography in patients with renal insufficiency who have clinical or duplex sonographic evidence of renovascular disease. In the authors' experience, adequate assessment of the renal vasculature and the juxtarenal aorta requires multiple injections when intra-arterial digital subtraction angiography is employed. The use of a single mid-stream flush aortogram requires no more contrast material than that required for such multiple intra-arterial digital subtraction studies. Additionally, standard arteriography provides information about cortical thickness and renal length, as well as improved clarity for interpretation of the renal artery anatomy. The fact that arteriography in patients with severe renal insufficiency, especially those with concomitant diabetes mellitus, can aggravate renal failure is widely recognized. Nevertheless, the authors believe that this risk is justified in such patients who have severe or accelerated hypertension or who have positive findings on renal duplex sonography. In these circumstances, the potential benefit derived from identification and correction of a functionally significant renovascular occlusive lesion exceeds the risk of arteriography.

To improve the understanding of ischemic nephropathy, the authors undertook a retrospective review of data collected during a 42-month period from 58 consecutive patients with ischemic nephropathy who had operative treatment at the authors' center.[14] The rate of decline in their renal function during the period before intervention and the impact of surgery on their outcome were examined. Patient ages ranged from 22 to 79 years (mean, 69 years). Based on serum creatinine values, immediate preoperative estimated glomerular filtration rates (EGFRs) ranged from 0 to 46 ml/min (mean, 23.85 ± 9.76 ml/min). Eight patients were dialysis dependent or anuric at the time of operation. Patients with at least three sequential measurements for calculations of EGFR changes during the 6 months before operation (n = 50) and the first 12 months after operation (n = 32) were used to describe the preoperative rate of decline in EGFR and the impact of operation on this decrease in the operative survivors. In addition, comparative analyses were performed of data from patients with unilateral versus bilateral lesions and patients classified as having improvement in EGFR versus no improvement after operation. Comparison of the immediate preoperative EGFR with the immediate postoperative EGFR for the entire group showed significant improvement in response to operation (Fig. 109–1).

The immediate impact of operation on the EGFR when results were examined according to the site of disease and operation is summarized in Table 109–1. In this evaluation, lesions (and procedures) to solitary kidneys and procedures consisting of unilateral revascularization with contralateral nephrectomy are recorded with the bilateral group. As noted in Table 109–1, when the groups were evaluated according to the site of operation, the bilateral group experienced a significant improvement in EGFR after operation ($p = .0001$). Although four patients (33 per cent) in the unilateral group had an improvement in EGFR (a 20 per

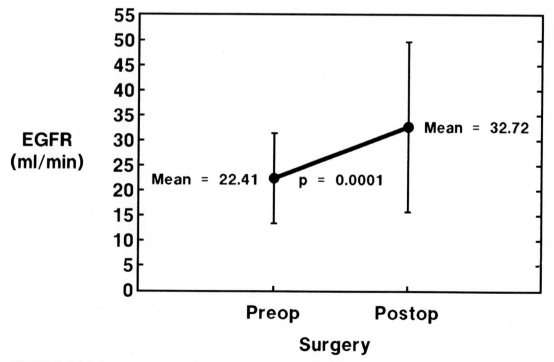

FIGURE 109–1. Comparison of the mean estimated glomerular filtration rate (EGFR) immediately before and at least 1 week after operation. The *p* value for differences is determined using the *t*-test for unpaired data. (From Dean RH, Tribble RW, Hansen KJ, et al: Evolution of renal insufficiency in ischemic nephropathy. Ann Surg 213:446, 1991.)

Table 109–1. Estimated Glomerular Filtration Rate Response Versus Site of Operation

| Operation | No. of Patients* | Estimated Glomerular Filtration Rate (ml/min)† | | p Value‡ |
		Preoperative	Postoperative	
Unilateral	12	25.94 ± 11.86	29.14 ± 14.34	.1633
Bilateral	41	21.38 ± 8.89	33.77 ± 18.39	.0001

*Operative deaths and patients who were preoperatively dialysis dependent were excluded from the analysis.
†Values are mean ± SD.
‡The p values are for the paired t-test.

cent or greater increase in EGFR) after operation (Table 109–2), no statistically significant benefit was seen when all patients with unilateral disease were collectively evaluated (see Table 109–1). The effects of surgery on each of the patients who were preoperatively dialysis dependent or anuric are summarized in Table 109–3. As noted, six of these eight patients were rendered dialysis independent by operation. Notably, all of those who received such benefit had undergone bilateral revascularization.

Figure 109–2 shows the rapid rate of change in EGFR for the entire group for the 6 months before operation and the beneficial impact of revascularization on this decline. Retrospective comparison of the rate of deterioration in EGFR before operation for the group who had improvement in EGFR by operation versus those receiving no benefit suggests that the rate of decline in GFR may have value in predicting the probability of retrieval of GFR by operation (Figs. 109–3 and 109–4). Unfortunately, the heterogenicity of individual slopes of change in EGFR prevent comment on a critical rate of decline that would predict retrieval of renal function by operation. Nevertheless, a rapidly deteriorating GFR should alert the physician to the potential presence of ischemic nephropathy and should argue for the likelihood of retrieval of function by operation when ischemic nephropathy is identified.

Renal revascularization had a beneficial impact on both the rate of decline in EGFR and the EGFR itself when data for the entire group were analyzed collectively. Nevertheless, when data were analyzed with respect to the individual subgroups, the salutary effect of operation on the rate of deterioration of EGFR was seen only in the subset that experienced an immediate improvement in EGFR by operation. This observation may have major clinical significance because the detrimental effect of renovascular occlusive disease may theoretically be from either of two causes. First, the lesion may limit renal perfusion to a degree that it affects excretory function. Second, it may be the source of microscopic atheroembolization that destroys functioning renal parenchyma. The authors' data suggest that correction of lesions causing reversible ischemia will provide both an immediate improvement in EGFR and a slowing of its rate of decline when compared with the preoperative rate of decline. Unfortunately, when the lesion was not producing significant reversible ischemia, as reflected by the absence of improvement in EGFR immediately after operation, no improvement in the rate of decline in EGFR was realized after operation. This argues that when atheroembolism is the only potentially active pathophysiologic consequence of the lesion, its correction does not lead to clinically important slowing of the rate of deterioration in renal function.

The authors' experience underscores the rapidity of the deterioration in renal function in patients with ischemic nephropathy and demonstrates the potential benefit of operation on both GFR and its rate of deterioration in a subset of patients. Nevertheless, the risk associated with operation is not inconsequential and requires comment. The authors' operative experience with this group of patients is associated with a 9 per cent operative mortality and underscores the fact that these patients are at accelerated risk for any major operative procedure. All of these patients had some degree of renal insufficiency, and 88 per cent had cardiac, cerebrovascular, or peripheral vascular manifestations of atherosclerosis. With such evidence of multi-faceted, site-specific end-organ damage in this relatively elderly population, one must question the merits of benefit afforded by a therapy that has a 9 per cent operative mortality rate and a cumulative 1-year survival rate of only 78 per cent. Nev-

Table 109–2. Change in Estimated Glomerular Filtration Rate Versus Site of Disease

| | Unilateral | | Bilateral | |
	No.	Per Cent	No.	Per Cent
Improved (≥20% increase)	4	33	27	66
No change (±19% change)	7	58	9	33
Worse (≥20% decrease)	1	9	5	12
Total	12		41	

Table 109–3. Results in the Dialysis-Dependent Group

Age (yr)	Sex	Dialysis Duration (days)	Immediate Postoperative EGFR (ml/min)	Site of Operation
51	F	11	32.7	Bilateral
63	M	32	34.6	Bilateral
65	M	6	44.5	Bilateral
59	M	30	49.0	Bilateral
76	M	10	30.7	Bilateral
61	F	0*	13.5	Bilateral
66	M	6	CD	Unilateral
75	M	54	CD	Unilateral

*The patient had developed anuria, and the operation was undertaken without dialysis.
CD, continued on dialysis; EGFR, estimated glomerular filtration rate.

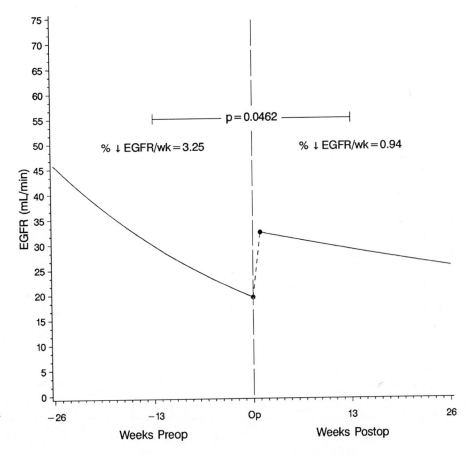

FIGURE 109–2. Percentage deterioration in EGFR per week for the entire group during the 6 months before (n = 50) and after (n = 32) operation. The immediate effect of operation on EGFR is also depicted. The *p* values for differences are determined using the *t*-test for unpaired data. Note the improvement in the slope of decline in EGFR after operation. (From Dean RH, Tribble RW, Hansen KJ, et al: Evolution of renal insufficiency in ischemic nephropathy. Ann Surg 213:446, 1991.)

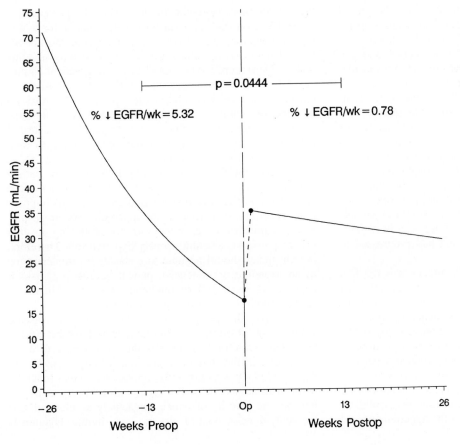

FIGURE 109–3. Percentage deterioration in EGFR per week during the 6 months before (n = 23) and after (n = 25) operation in the group of patients who had at least a 20 per cent improvement in EGFR following operation. The immediate effect of operation on EGFR in this group is also depicted. The *p* values for differences are determined using the *t*-test for unpaired data. Note the improvement in the slope of decline in EGFR after operation in this group. (From Dean RH, Tribble RW, Hansen KJ, et al: Evolution of renal insufficiency in ischemic nephropathy. Ann Surg 213:446, 1991.)

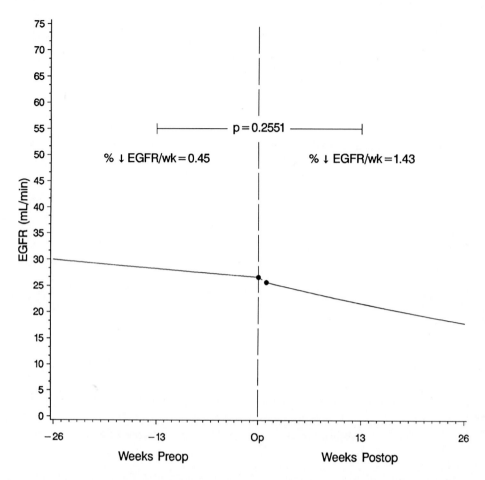

FIGURE 109-4. Percentage deterioration in EGFR per week during the 6 months before (n = 18) and after (n = 8) operation in the group of patients who had no significant immediate benefit in EGFR after operation. The *p* values for differences are determined using the *t*-test for unpaired data. Note the absence of improvement in the rate of deterioration of EGFR after operation in this group. (From Dean RH, Tribble RW, Hansen KJ, et al: Evolution of renal insufficiency in ischemic nephropathy. Ann Surg 213:446, 1991.)

ertheless, this risk and the rate of survival must be placed into context with the probability of survival without operation. In a study of the duration of survival following the institution of dialysis, Mailloux and coworkers found that end-stage renal disease caused by uncorrected renovascular disease was associated with the most rapid rate of death during follow-up.[13] In their study, patients with renovascular disease had a median survival after the initiation of dialysis of only 27 months and a 5-year survival rate of only 12 per cent. This equates with a death rate in excess of 20 per cent per year. The life table survival curve of the authors' group of patients with ischemic nephropathy suggests that if an individual survives operation and the early follow-up period, he or she is afforded an improved probability, because 2- and 3-year survival rates for these patients appear to be significantly better than those seen in patients who had not received intervention and had progressed to the point of dialysis dependence.

Finally, the authors' experience underscores the fact that not all patients with azotemia and even bilateral renal artery stenosis can be expected to benefit from revascularization. Preoperative indicators that influence the potential for functional retrieval in this group are the severity of the occlusive lesions and the type of hypertension. Functionally severe bilateral renal artery occlusions produce a particularly severe and difficult-to-control variety of hypertension. When such hypertension is present in combination with correctable bilateral stenoses or occlusions, revascularization should dramatically alleviate both the hypertension and

the concomitant azotemia. In these patients, preoperative dependence on dialysis is not a negative factor for a successful outcome, even though some physicians do not believe that such revascularization can reverse long-standing dialysis dependence. This belief has little practical significance because these patients have little to lose from revascularization. They have the greatest potential for retrieval of function with revascularization and only a minimal chance for prolonged survival without operation because of their dialysis-dependent renal failure combined with their severe, uncontrollable hypertension.

In contrast, the absence of hypertension in the patient with renovascular occlusions and azotemia should argue against the probability that revascularization will improve renal function. Such lesions are apparently not of physiologic significance because they are not producing an integral response to ischemia, namely hypertension. Therefore, the physician should hesitate to consider revascularization in an azotemic normotensive patient because the risk of aggravating renal failure outweighs the probability that function will be improved by such intervention.

Finally, the patient with chronic occlusive disease whose onset of oliguria or anuria is acute must be considered. This acute onset is usually the consequence of acute thrombosis in the stenotic artery to a solitary kidney or to the only kidney with previous significant residual function. Most of these patients will present with a history of hypertension, the severity of which has acutely accelerated, and the acute development of oliguric renal failure. Diagnostic evaluation of any patient presenting with such signs should include angiography. Although physicians were reticent in the past to perform angiography because of the nephrotoxic effect of the large amount of contrast material necessary for such an evaluation, the current use of ''one-shot'' aortography has greatly lessened the potential renal insult.

Although many physicians are tempted to react to the acute clinical presentation with immediate operation and attempted revascularization, a more carefully planned approach is superior. Because the acute event is usually at least 24 hours old and primarily represents a reduction in perfusion to below the critical level for maintaining urinary output, preoperative correction of metabolic derangements is essential to reduce the risk of surgical intervention. Thus, the patient may require several days of dialysis or the correction of other, more lethal cardiac derangements before renal revascularization can be attempted. The physician should remember that renal failure can be controlled by hemodialysis while hypertension and cardiac risk factors are decreased and that the amount of retrievable renal function is not dependent on the timing of intervention. In most of these patients, urine flow is almost instantaneous after completion of the revascularization, and the majority of patients will require no further dialysis in the immediate postoperative period.

TECHNIQUES OF OPERATIVE MANAGEMENT

Various operative techniques have been used to correct renal artery stenoses secondary to atherosclerotic disease. These techniques include thromboendarterectomy, aortorenal bypass, renal artery reimplantation, and extra-anatomic bypasses such as hepatorenal and splenorenal bypasses.

Certain measures and maneuvers are applicable in almost all renal artery operations. Early in the operation, 12.5 gm of mannitol is administered intravenously. Just before renal artery cross-clamping, 75 mg or 7500 units of heparin is given intravenously. Protamine is occasionally required to reverse the effects of heparin at the end of the reconstruction.

Exposure of the renal arteries is the most difficult aspect of renal artery surgery. A mid-line incision from xiphoid to pubis provides excellent access to either renal artery. To expose the left renal artery, the posterior peritoneum overlying the aorta is incised longitudinally, the duodenum is mobilized to the patient's right, and the left renal vein is dissected out and mobilized (Fig. 109–5). Extending the posterior peritoneal incision to the left along the inferior border of the pancreas allows an avascular plane behind the pancreas to be entered. The inferior mesenteric vein courses obliquely through the left peritoneal area; often, it is ligated and divided to facilitate this exposure. When this vein is ligated, the surgeon must be certain that it is not accompanied by an ascending branch of the inferior mesenteric artery, ligation of which might compromise colonic perfusion if there are atherosclerotic occlusions in the visceral artery. This exposure allows excellent access to the entire renal hilum on the left, which is of special significance when distal lesions are to be managed. By combining this exposure with partial division of the crura of the diaphragm as they drape around the juxtarenal aorta, the surgeon can easily perform aortic cross-clamping above the superior mesenteric artery. This is of particular value when bilateral renal artery thromboendarterectomy is chosen as the technique for renal revascularization.

The artery lies behind the left renal vein. In some cases, it is easier to retract the vein cephalad in order to expose the artery. In others, caudad retraction of the vein provides better access. Usually, the gonadal and adrenal veins that enter the renal vein must be ligated and divided to facilitate exposure of the artery. Another frequent tribu-

FIGURE 109–5. Exposure of the left renal hilum through the base of the mesentery. The adrenal and gonadal veins must be ligated and divided to give adequate visualization of the renal artery. Note the anterior accessory right renal artery. This uncommon right lower pole artery traverses anterior to the vena cava and can easily be traumatized if its presence is not recognized.

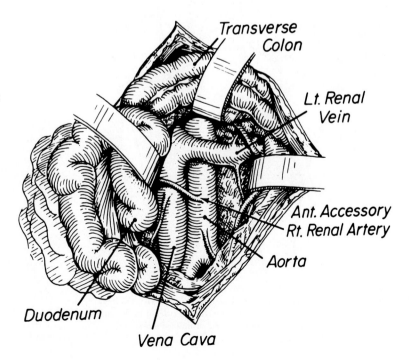

tary is the descending lumbar vein, which enters the posterior wall of the left renal vein and is easily avulsed unless special care is taken in mobilizing the renal vein. Similarly, the proximal right renal artery can be exposed through the base of the mesentery by ligating two or more pairs of lumbar veins and retracting the vena cava and the right renal vein to the patient's right (Fig. 109–6). Usually, however, the right renal artery is best exposed by medial mobilization of the duodenum and the right colon (Fig. 109–7). The right renal vein is mobilized and retracted in order to expose the artery. In some patients, an accessory right renal artery arises from the anterior wall of the aorta about 2.5 cm above the origin of the inferior mesenteric artery. This artery is unusual in that it runs anterior to the vena cava and then over to the lower pole of the right kidney, instead of running retrocavally, as the right renal artery does. The accessory vessel can be injured easily if the surgeon is unaware of its presence.

Thromboendarterectomy

In some cases of orificial atherosclerotic occlusion, thromboendarterectomy is the procedure of choice. Its use is limited in the authors' center to patients with bilateral lesions requiring correction. In this circumstance, the authors prefer to use a transverse aortotomy, with extension of the incision out both renal arteries to a point beyond the lesions. After endarterectomy has been performed under direct vision, the arteriotomy is closed with either a vein patch or a patch of synthetic material (Fig. 109–8). The authors limit the use of the longitudinal aortotomy and endarterectomy to patients with multiple renal arteries that require removal. When this is performed, close attention

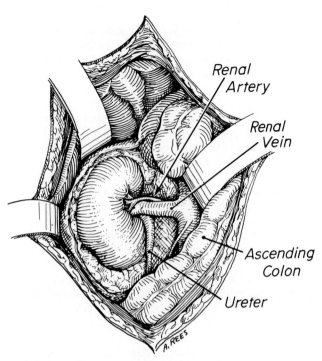

FIGURE 109–7. Exposure of the right renal artery following reflection of the duodenum and right colon to the left. The distal right renal artery and its branches are best visualized by this technique.

must be paid to the status of the end-point of endarterectomy. This technique has a higher risk of leaving a ledge of residual plaque or loose intima in the nonvisualized distal end of the endarterectomy. For this reason, the authors routinely survey the completed endarterectomy site with intraoperative duplex sonography to exclude the pres-

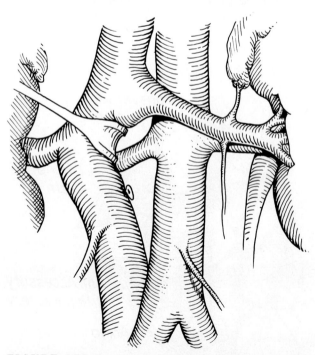

FIGURE 109–6. Exposure of the proximal right renal artery through the base of the mesentery. Two pairs of lumbar veins have been ligated and divided, and the vena cava is retracted to the right. Proximal right renal artery lesions can be visualized adequately through this approach.

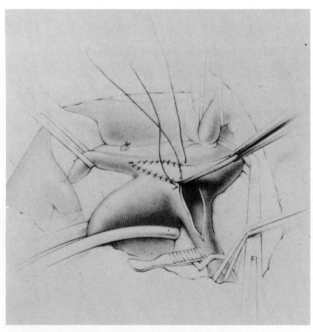

FIGURE 109–8. Incision closure after transverse aortotomy and renal artery endarterectomy showing the use of a patch to widen the orifice of the renal arteries.

ence of residual lesions. On occasion, a separate renal arteriotomy is required to manage such residual lesions.

Aortorenal Bypass Graft

Three types of graft are usually available for aortorenal bypass: autologous saphenous vein, autologous hypogastric artery, and a synthetic prosthesis. Which graft should be used depends on a number of factors. The authors prefer to use the saphenous vein. If it is small—less than 4 mm in diameter—or has been used previously, an expanded polytetrafluoroethylene prosthesis is used for patients with atherosclerotic lesions. A 6-mm polytetrafluoroethylene graft is quite satisfactory if the distal renal artery is of large caliber, as is often the case in atherosclerotic renal artery stenosis.

The side-to-end anastomosis between the renal artery and the graft is performed first. Silastic slings can be used to occlude the renal artery distally. This method of vessel occlusion is especially applicable to this procedure. In contrast to vascular clamps, these slings are essentially atraumatic to the delicate distal renal artery. The absence of clamps in the operative field is also advantageous. Further, when tension is applied to the slings, they lift the vessel out of the retroperitoneal soft tissue for more accurate visualization.

The length of the arteriotomy should be at least three times the diameter of the renal artery to guard against late suture line stenosis. A 6–0 or 7–0 monofilament polypropylene (Prolene) suture material is employed, with loupe magnification.

After the renal artery anastomosis has been completed, the occluding clamps and slings are removed from the renal artery and a small bulldog clamp is placed across the vein graft adjacent to the anastomosis. The aortic anastomosis is then done. First, an ellipse of the anterolateral aortic wall is removed, and then the anastomosis is performed. If the graft is too long, kinking of the vein and subsequent thrombosis may result. If there is any element of kinking or twisting of the graft after both anastomoses have been completed, the aortic anastomosis should be taken down and redone after appropriate shortening or reorientation of the graft. In certain instances, an end-to-end anastomosis between the graft and the renal artery provides a better reconstruction. The authors routinely employ an end-to-end renal artery anastomosis when combining aortic replacement with renal revascularization. In this circumstance, the saphenous vein is attached to the Dacron aortic graft before its insertion. After the aortic graft has been attached and flow has been restored to the distal extremity, the renal artery can be transected and attached to the end of the saphenous vein graft without interruption of aortic flow (Fig. 109–9).

Renal Artery Reimplantation

Many patients will have a somewhat redundant renal artery after it has been dissected from the surrounding retroperitoneal tissue. When the renal artery stenosis is orificial and the vessel is redundant, the renal artery can simply be transected and reimplanted, after spatulation, into the aorta at a slightly lower level. Although the authors use this

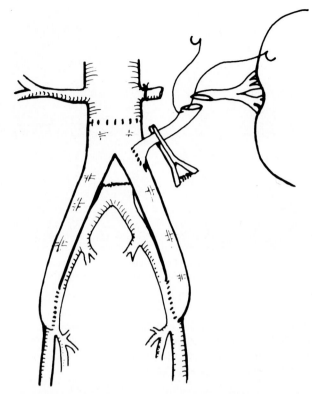

FIGURE 109–9. Method of performing concomitant aortofemoral bypass and renal artery bypass. The saphenous vein graft is attached to the Dacron graft before its insertion. With a bulldog clamp occluding the saphenous vein graft, the aortic graft is inserted. The renal artery is then transected, and an end-to-end anastomosis to the saphenous vein graft is performed.

technique most commonly in children with orificial lesions, it is also available for use in the management of atherosclerotic lesions (Fig. 109–10).

Extra-Anatomic Bypasses

Extra-anatomic procedures have received increased use and popularity as an alternative method of renal revascularization in the high-risk patient.[16] The authors do not believe that these procedures are comparable to direct reconstructions, but they are useful in a highly selective subgroup of high-risk patients.

Hepatorenal Bypass

A right subcostal incision is usually used to perform the hepatorenal bypass. The hepatoduodenal ligament is incised, and the common hepatic artery both proximal and distal to the gastroduodenal artery origin is encircled (Fig. 109–11). Next, the descending duodenum is mobilized by Kocher's maneuver, the inferior vena cava is identified, the right renal vein is identified, and the right renal artery is encircled where it is found, either immediately cephalad or caudad to the renal vein.

A greater saphenous vein graft is usually used to construct the bypass. The hepatic artery anastomosis of the vein graft can be placed at the site of the amputated stump of the gastroduodenal artery or proximal to this branch

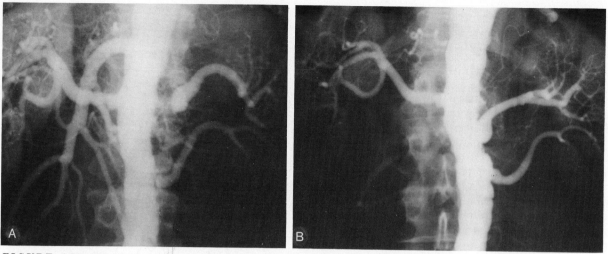

FIGURE 109–10.   Preoperative (*A*) and postoperative (*B*) arteriograms showing the appearance of the renal artery following reimplantation in a 65-year-old man with orificial occlusive disease and a redundant distal vessel.

when it must be saved as a collateral to gut perfusion. After completion of this anastomosis, the renal artery is transected and brought anterior to the vena cava for anastomosis end-to-end to the graft (Fig. 109–12).

Splenorenal Bypass

Splenorenal bypass can be performed through a midline or a left subcostal incision. The posterior pancreas is mobilized by reflecting the inferior border cephalad. When the retropancreatic plane has been entered, the splenic artery can be mobilized from the left gastroepiploic artery to the level of its branches. The left renal artery is exposed as described earlier. After the splenic artery has been completely mobilized, it is divided distally, spatulated, and anastomosed end-to-end to the transected renal artery (Fig. 109–13).

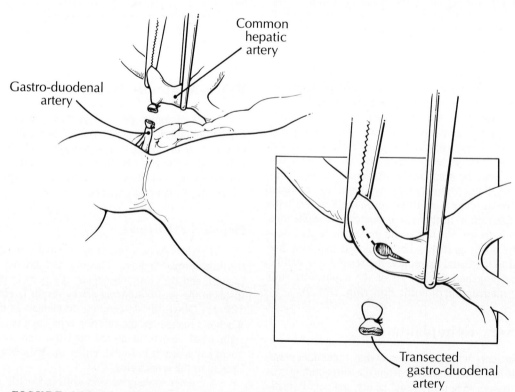

FIGURE 109–11.   Exposed common hepatic artery and the proximal gastroduodenal artery after excision of the hepatoduodenal ligament.

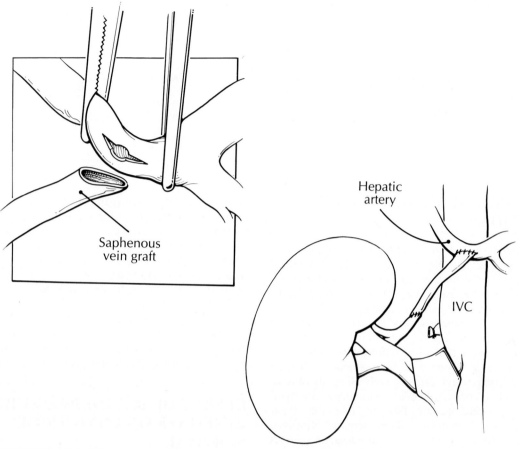

FIGURE 109–12.   Completed saphenous vein graft used as an interposition graft between the side of the hepatic artery and the distal end of the transected right renal artery. IVC, inferior vena cava.

FIGURE 109–13.   Transected splenic artery that has been anastomosed end-to-end to the transected left renal artery.

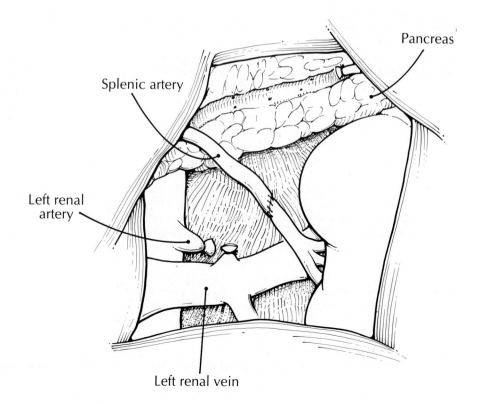

Table 109-4. Results of Operative Treatment for Atherosclerotic Disease

Center	No. of Patients	Cure (%)	Improvement (%)	Failure (%)	Operative Mortality (%)
Vanderbilt University					
Renovascular reconstruction alone[3]	126	31	62	7	1
Aortic and renal surgery[5]	50	9	72	19	12
University of Michigan					
Focal renal lesions[10]	64	33	58	9	0
Diffuse atherosclerosis[10]	71	25	47	28	8.5
Cleveland Clinic[8]	78	40	51	9	2

BLOOD PRESSURE RESPONSE TO OPERATION

Refinements in patient selection and operative technique have substantially improved the results of renal revascularization in the management of renovascular hypertension. Contemporary results of operation for atherosclerotic disease from several centers are summarized in Table 109-4. In a summary of experience by the author,[17] only one operative death occurred in a group of 126 patients who underwent procedures limited to renovascular reconstruction. Included in this group were both patients with focal renovascular disease and patients with clinically diffuse atherosclerosis. In contrast, Stanley and colleagues experienced an 8.5 per cent operative mortality rate in the treatment of 71 patients with diffuse atherosclerosis.[18] However, all but two of their operative deaths occurred in patients who had undergone combined aortic and renal artery procedures. The authors of this chapter noted a 12 per cent operative mortality rate in the treatment of 50 patients who underwent combined aortic and renovascular procedures.

Blood pressure response to operation is less dramatic in the atherosclerotic patient. The frequency of cure ranged from 25 to 40 per cent in the respective centers reviewed.[18-23] In the authors' experience, predictability of a beneficial response (cure or improvement) has been similarly high in both the fibrodysplastic (96 per cent) and the atherosclerotic (93 per cent) patient. Because many patients with atherosclerotic renovascular lesions have a background of previous mild essential hypertension and frequently have microscopic evidence of arteriolar nephrosclerosis, the infrequency of absolute cure of hypertension is not surprising. The effect of the severity of atherosclerosis on the magnitude of benefit is demonstrated in both the Vanderbilt University and the University of Michigan experiences. In the Vanderbilt series,[20] atherosclerotic disease requiring only renovascular procedures was associated with a 31 per cent cure rate and a 61 per cent improvement rate. These results fell to 9 per cent cure and 72 per cent improvement rates when combined aortic and renovascular surgery was required.[21] Similarly, the results in the University of Michigan series for the management of focal renovascular disease were cure in 33 per cent and improvement in 58 per cent. The response declined to a 25 per cent cure rate and a 47 per cent improvement rate when patients with overt generalized disease were treated in that center.[18]

From the authors' review of the Vanderbilt experience with the operative management of renovascular hypertension, 1- to 23-year follow-up sequential angiography of 198 reconstructions is available for evaluation (Table 109-5). Four saphenous vein grafts and two hypogastric autografts have undergone aneurysmal dilatation. Only one of these, a hypogastric autograft, has required replacement. The remaining five have stabilized, and the patients have remained cured of hypertension.

Although the incidence of aneurysmal degeneration is low in the authors' overall experience, all cases have occurred in children, suggesting that the saphenous vein is particularly susceptible to this phenomenon in them.

EFFECT OF BLOOD PRESSURE RESPONSE ON LONG-TERM SURVIVAL

Because the logic for the management of hypertension of any cause is to decrease long-term cardiovascular morbidity and improve event-free survival, the authors reviewed the outcome in 71 patients who had undergone operative management of renovascular hypertension from 15 to 23 years previously.[24] Complete follow-up was available in 66 of the 68 patients who survived surgery. Comparison of the initial blood pressure response to operation (1 to 6 months postoperatively) with the blood pressure status at the time of death or the current date (up to 23 years later) showed that the effect of operative treatment was maintained over the long-term follow-up (Fig. 109-14). In patients who required repeated renovascular surgery for recurrent renovascular hypertension during follow-up, the majority of the operations were performed for the management of contralateral lesions that had progressed to functional significance (i.e., produced renovascular hypertension).

Table 109-5. Sequential 1- to 23-Year Follow-Up Arteriography in 198 Reconstructions

Status	No. of Grafts	Per Cent
No adverse change	174	88.0
Aneurysmal dilatation	7	3.5
Stenosis	10	5.0
Occlusion	4	2.0
False aneurysm	3	1.5

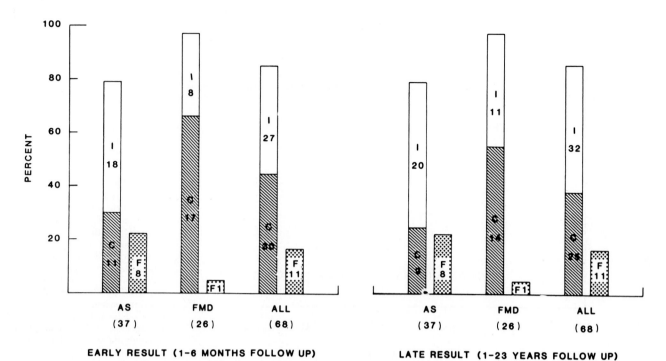

FIGURE 109-14. Initial benefit versus late blood pressure response in the respective types of lesions. (From Dean RH, Krueger TC, Whiteneck JM, et al: Operative management of renovascular hypertension: Results after a follow-up of fifteen to twenty-three years. J Vasc Surg 1:234, 1984.)

FIGURE 109-15. Kaplan-Meier life table analysis: survival by response to operation in 37 arteriosclerotic patients (deaths from cardiovascular causes). (From Dean RH, Krueger TC, Whiteneck JM, et al: Operative management of renovascular hypertension: Results after a follow-up of fifteen to twenty-three years. J Vasc Surg 1:234, 1984.)

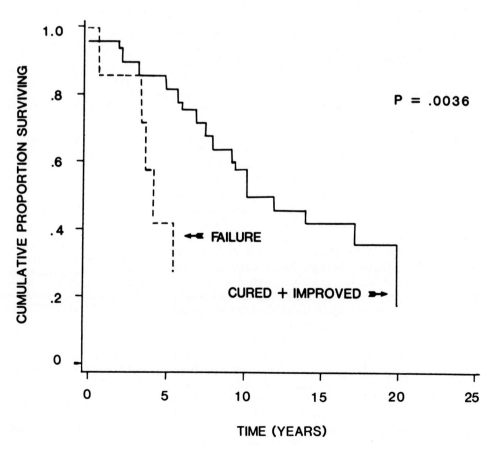

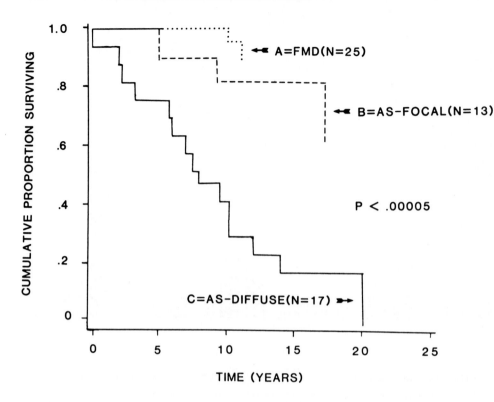

FIGURE 109–16. Kaplan-Meier life table analysis: survival of patients who benefited from operation by type and stage of disease (deaths from cardiovascular causes). FMD, fibromuscular dysplasia; AS-focal, atherosclerosis; AS-diffuse, diffuse atherosclerosis. (From Dean RH, Krueger TC, Whiteneck JM, et al: Operative management of renovascular hypertension: Results after a follow-up of fifteen to twenty-three years. J Vasc Surg 1:234, 1984.)

Assessment of the effect of blood pressure response on late survival produced results that were not surprising. Although the subgroup of nonresponders was small, they experienced a significantly more rapid death rate during follow-up than did patients who had a blood pressure response to operation (Fig. 109–15). This confirms the validity of the premise that inadequate management of renovascular hypertension leaves the patient at higher risk for early death from cardiovascular events. The presence of angiographically diffuse atherosclerosis at the time of evaluation and operation was predictive of a more rapid rate of death during follow-up (Fig. 109–16). This difference in the subsequent death rate was present even though comparison between patients with diffuse atherosclerotic disease and focal atherosclerotic disease was undertaken only in patients experiencing a significant blood pressure response. In view of the suggestion by some physicians that the presence of diffuse disease precludes a high rate of blood pressure response to operation, it is worthwhile to stress that there was no significant difference in the frequency of response between the focal atherosclerotic disease (80 per cent) and the diffuse atherosclerotic disease (77 per cent) groups in this study. In addition, although the presence of diffuse atherosclerotic disease was associated with a more rapid death rate, it does not preclude the probability of a longer survival in this subgroup than in a similar group of patients who either do not undergo operation or receive no blood pressure benefit from such intervention. Further, if one considers that diffuse atherosclerotic disease is only a later stage of focal atherosclerotic disease, it is not surprising that the end-point of clinically significant disease, namely death from cardiovascular events, arrives sooner when one begins follow-up or removes a risk factor that causes its acceleration later in its natural history.

References

1. Scobie JE, Maher ER, Hamilton G, et al: Atherosclerotic renovascular disease causing renal impairment—A case for treatment. Clin Nephrol 31:119, 1989.
2. Bengtsson U, Bergentz S-E, Norback B: Surgical treatment of renal artery stenosis with impending uremia. Clin Nephrol 2:222, 1974.
3. Novick AC, Pohl MA, Schreiber M, et al: Revascularization for preservation of renal function in patients with atherosclerotic renovascular disease. J Urol 129:907, 1983.
4. Dean RH, Lawson JD, Hollifield JW, et al: Revascularization of the poorly functioning kidney. Surgery 85:44, 1979.
5. Libertino JA, Zinman L: Revascularization of the poorly functioning and the nonfunctioning kidney. In Novick AC, Straffon RA (eds): Vascular Problems in Urologic Surgery. Philadelphia, WB Saunders, 1982, pp 173–187.
6. Dean RH, Englund R, Dupont WD, et al: Retrieval of renal function by revascularization. Study of preoperative outcome predictors. Ann Surg 202:367, 1985.
7. Zinman L, Libertino JA: Revascularization of the chronic totally occluded renal artery with restoration of renal function. J Urol 228:517, 1977.
8. Dean RH, Kieffer RW, Smith BM, et al: Renovascular hypertension: Anatomic and renal function changes during drug therapy. Arch Surg 116:1408, 1981.
9. Dean RH: Renovascular hypertension. Curr Probl Surg 22(2):6, 1985.
10. Morris GC Jr, DeBakey ME, Cooley DA: Surgical treatment of renal failure of renovascular origin. JAMA 182:609, 1962.
11. Novick AC, Pohl MA, Schreiber M, et al: Revascularization for preservation of renal function in patients with atherosclerotic renovascular disease. J Urol 129:907, 1983.
12. Annual Report. Raleigh, NC, NC Kidney Council, 1986.
13. Mailloux LU, Bellucci AG, Mossey RT, et al: Predictors of survival in patients undergoing dialysis. Am J Med 84:855, 1988.
14. Dean RH, Tribble RW, Hansen KJ, et al: Evolution of renal insufficiency in ischemic nephropathy. Ann Surg 213:446, 1991.
15. Hansen KJ, Tribble RW, Reavis SW, et al: Renal duplex sonography: Evaluation of clinical utility. J Vasc Surg 12:227, 1990.
16. Moncure AC, Brewster DC, Darling RC, et al: Use of the splenic and hepatic arteries for renal revascularization. J Vasc Surg 3:196, 1986.
17. Dean RH: Renal artery repair—Errors in patient selection. *In* Bern-

hard VM, Towne JB (eds): Complications in Vascular Surgery. New York, Grune & Stratton, 1980.
18. Stanley JC, Whitehouse WM Jr, Graham LM, et al: Operative therapy of renovascular hypertension. Br J Surg 69(Suppl):S63, 1982.
19. Bergentz S-E, Ericsson BF, Husberg B: Technique and complications in the surgical treatment of renovascular hypertension. Acta Chir Scand 145:143, 1979.
20. Dean RH: Renovascular hypertension. *In* Moore WS (ed): Vascular Surgery. A Comprehensive Review. New York, Grune & Stratton, 1983, p 433.
21. Dean RH, Keyser JE III, Dupont WD, et al: Aortic and renal vascular

disease: Factors affecting the value of combined procedures. Ann Surg 200:336, 1984.
22. Novick AC, Straffon RA, Stewart BH, et al: Diminished operative morbidity and mortality in renal revascularization. JAMA 246:749, 1981.
23. Stoney RJ, De Luccia N, Ehrenfeld WK, et al: Aortorenal arterial autografts: Long-term assessment. Arch Surg 116:1416, 1981.
24. Dean RH, Krueger TC, Whiteneck JM, et al: Operative management of renovascular hypertension: Results after a follow-up of fifteen to twenty-three years. J Vasc Surg 1:234, 1984.

110

Ex Vivo Renal Artery Reconstructions

Richard H. Dean, M.D., B.A.

• • •

Since the report by Ota and associates in 1967 of the first clinical ex vivo reconstruction to treat complex renal artery occlusion,[1] numerous authors have reported similar successes with techniques that protect the renal parenchyma during prolonged renovascular reconstructive procedures. Through the use of these techniques, lesions that were previously amenable only to nephrectomy now can be corrected and the kidneys can be salvaged. Although some surgeons report the use of ex vivo techniques and autotransplantation in nearly 50 per cent of their renovascular procedures for such lesions of fibromuscular dysplasia,[2, 3] the author's group has required its use in only approximately 5 to 10 per cent of their cases.[4] In the vast majority of these cases, in situ techniques can be safely and successfully employed.

The author's group considers ex vivo reconstructions to be indicated in two generic circumstances. First, they employ preservative infusion techniques and ex vivo reconstruction when they project that the renal ischemia time required for the procedure will exceed 45 minutes to 1 hour. Second, the author's group also uses this technique in circumstances in which dissection and exposure of small branches would be impaired if an in situ technique were attempted. Examples of situations in which they employ ex vivo techniques include in patients who require remedial procedures after failed previous branch percutaneous transluminal renal angioplasty or distal renal artery bypass; in patients with hilar arteriovenous fistulae; in patients with an aneurysm or stenoses involving multiple renal artery branches; and in patients with renal artery dissection extending into multiple branches.

TECHNIQUES OF RENAL FUNCTION PROTECTION

Renal Preservation Solutions

Most extensive laboratory studies evaluating perfusates for use in the protection of renal parenchyma during periods of total renal ischemia were begun to facilitate homologous renal transplantation. Several perfusates have been studied by Sacks and colleagues,[5] Collins and associates,[6, 7] and others.[8-10] Through these studies, solutions approximating intracellular electrolyte concentrations have been shown to be superior to solutions such as Ringer's lactate or other solutions that mimic extracellular fluid concentrations. Furthermore, perfusates that are hyperosmolar, such as Collins' solution, are also superior because of their ability to minimize the cellular swelling during and after the period of perfusion. For these reasons, the author's group employs a modified Collins solution, the composition of which is listed in Table 110–1.

Methods of renal perfusion vary among centers in which ex vivo renal artery reconstructions are performed. Complex perfusion pump systems have been developed by Belzer and coworkers[11] and by Milsten and associates[12] to allow continuous perfusion during the period of total renal ischemia. Although continuous perfusion may have comparative superiority for prolonged renal preservation during storage periods, simple intermittent flushing with the chilled preservative solutions provides equal protection during the shorter periods (2 to 3 hours) required for ex vivo dissection and complex renal artery reconstruction.

Table 110–1. Electrolyte Solution for Intermittent Flushing

Composition (gm/L)		Ionic Concentration (mEq/L)		Additives at Time of Use
Component	Amount	Electrolyte	Concentration	to 930 ml of Solution
K_2HPO_4	7.4	Potassium	115	50% dextrose, 70 ml
KH_2PO_4	2.04	Sodium	10	Heparin sodium, 2000 units
KCl	1.12	Phosphate (HPO_4^-)	85	
$NaHCO_3$	0.84	Phosphate ($H_2PO_4^-$)	15	
		Chloride	15	
		Bicarbonate	10	

Note: *Solution (electrolyte solution for kidney preservation) supplied by Travenol Labs, Inc, Deerfield, IL.*

The procedure used by the author's group for intermittent flushing is as follows: A liter of the Collins solution to be used for flushing is refrigerated overnight. Immediately before its use, the additional components are added and the liter of chilled (5 to 10°C) solution is hung on an intravenous stand so as to provide at least 2 m of gravitational perfusion pressure. Five hundred milliliters of solution is flushed through the kidney as soon as it is removed from the renal fossa. At the completion of each anastomosis, an additional 150 to 200 ml of solution is flushed through the kidney, a procedure that also allows the surgeon to examine the suture line for leaks.

Hypothermia Preservation

Potentially of greatest importance in renal function preservation techniques is the maintenance of profound renal parenchymal hypothermia during the period of total ischemia. Canine studies have shown that warm ischemia times in excess of 30 minutes are associated with increasing degrees of loss of excretory function.[13] Furthermore, more than 1 hour of warm ischemia is associated with increasing amounts of permanent loss of function. For these reasons, ex vivo perfusion of the kidney is performed with a chilled preservative solution. Although lowering the renal core temperature dramatically slows energy-dependent metabolism of the cortical cells, it also inactivates the cellular membrane sodium-potassium pump, with subsequent cellular swelling occurring as a result of salt and water entrance into the cell.[14] However, the use of flushing solutions with intracellular electrolyte composition minimizes this adverse effect of hypothermia. Because intermittent perfusion of the chilled preservative is used, surface hypothermia provides improved maintenance of constant hypothermia during ex vivo renal artery reconstruction. Many techniques for producing surface hypothermia have been described.[15, 16] The method used by the author's group consists of placing 2-L bottles of normal saline solution in an ice sluch overnight. The removed kidney is placed in a watertight plastic sheet from which excess saline solution can be suctioned away. Laparotomy pads are placed over the kidney and are kept cool and moist by a constant drip of the chilled saline solution. With the use of intermittent perfusion with chilled preservative solution and the application of continuous surface hypothermia, renal core temperatures of 10 to 15°C are maintained throughout the period of ischemia.

OPERATIVE TECHNIQUES FOR EX VIVO RECONSTRUCTION

The general aspects of patient management and operative technique for renovascular reconstruction are outlined elsewhere.[17] In all instances, the author's group uses 2.5× to 4.5× magnification and 6–0, 7–0, and even 8–0 monofilament polypropylene suture material for the anastomoses.

Three techniques for the management of the kidney during ex vivo reconstruction have been used in the author's center: (1) total renal mobilization without renal vein transection, (2) ex vivo repair with autotransplantation, and (3) ex vivo repair with replacement back to the renal fossa. A mid-line xiphoid-to-pubis incision is used for most renovascular procedures and is preferred when autotransplantation of the reconstructed kidney or combined aortic reconstruction is to be performed. An extended flank incision parallel to the lower rib margin and carried to the mid-axillary line (Fig. 110–1) currently is used when complex branch renal artery repairs alone are required. This is the preferred approach at the author's center when ex vivo reconstruction without autotransplantation is performed. In all cases of ex vivo reconstructions, the ureter is mobilized but left intact. However, an elastic sling or a noncrushing clamp is placed around the ureter to prevent continued collateral perfusion and inadvertent rewarming, as well as continued blood loss through this route during the ex vivo repair.

Complete Mobilization Without Renal Vein Transection

The technique of complete mobilization without renal vein transection is seldom used by the author's group at this time because they believe that most instances requiring perfusion and ex vivo repair are best managed by bringing the kidney onto the abdominal wall. However, occasionally this technique provides the necessary increased exposure for multiple branch repairs and allows the same capacity for surface cooling and perfusion with chilled preservative solution without the need for reattachment of the renal vein.

The flank incision most easily facilitates this exposure and technique. Total mobilization of the kidney is accomplished after the extrarenal portion of the renal artery and the renal vein have been completely mobilized from surrounding tissue. When the kidney has been mobilized, Ger-

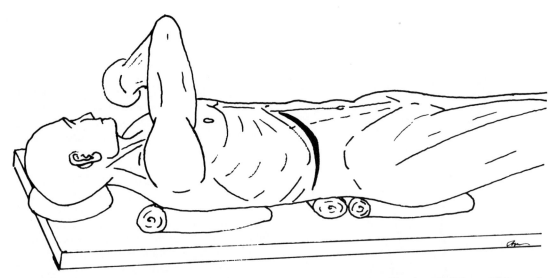

FIGURE 110–1.   Patient positioning and site of incision for the flank approach to the right kidney and the renal vasculature.

ota's capsule is entered medially and is totally lifted from around the kidney, leaving a pocket for subsequent replacement of the kidney. After aortic mobilization and graft harvesting have been completed, the mobilized ureter is looped by a silicone rubber (Silastic) sling to occlude inflow to the kidney. The kidney is then covered with moistened laparotomy pads and placed in the plastic envelope within the wound yet elevated from the renal fossa. After transection of the renal artery, the renal vein is crossclamped at its junction with the vena cava and cannulated on the renal side of the clamp with a 14-gauge catheter (Fig. 110–2). The kidney is then flushed with 500 ml of the preservative solution, with the effluent escaping the renal vein via the cannula.

As with the other ex vivo techniques, surface hypothermia is maintained by a constant drip of chilled saline solution onto the surface of the kidney. After all renal artery branches have been attached to the graft, the kidney is replaced in the renal fossa and the aortic attachment of the graft is performed in the standard fashion. At the moment of reperfusion of the kidney, the renal vein clamp and the renal vein cannula are removed, and the renal vein puncture site is closed with sutures. Finally, after suture line and retroperitoneal hemostasis has been ensured, Gerota's capsule is reapproximated to stabilize the kidney in its original position.

Ex Vivo Reconstruction With Autotransplantation

Although it was initially used as the preferred technique, the author's group now believes that autotransplantation should be limited to cases in which replacement of the kidney in the renal fossa is contraindicated. With this bias, this group now limits autotransplantation to patients in whom previous dissection of the juxtarenal aorta has led to intense scarring of the renal vein, those in whom excision of the renal vein at its junction with the vena cava is

technically ill-advised, and those in whom reanastomosis will leave a foreshortened vein.

This technique is most simply performed through a mid-line xiphoid-to-pubis incision. However, the kidney and the renal vasculature are exposed from a lateral approach, and the ascending or descending colon is mobilized medially. After complete mobilization as described in the preceding section, the renal artery and vein are transected and the kidney is transferred to the abdominal wall. Mobilization of the uterer to a point below the pelvic brim facilitates transfer of the kidney out of the abdomen without the necessity for ureteral transection. However, again an elastic sling or a noncrushing clamp is placed across the

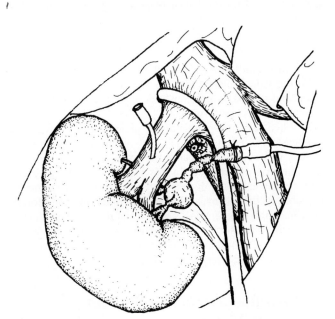

FIGURE 110–2.   Use of renal vein occlusion and proximal cannulation. Note that the kidney is completely mobilized for ex vivo reconstruction and is connected only by the occluded renal vein and ureter.

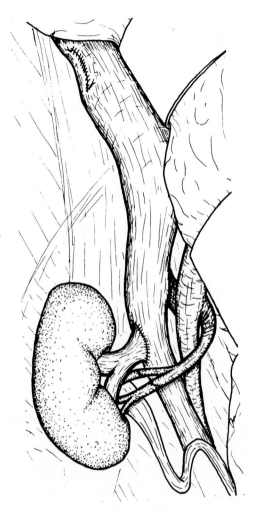

FIGURE 110–3. Autotransplanted kidney after ex vivo renal artery reconstruction. Renal vein anastomosis is performed first. Note that in this example, the hypogastric artery has been mobilized and divided at the branch level for attachment to the renal artery branches.

ureter to occlude ureteral collateral vessels to the kidney. With the kidney placed into the plastic envelope and perfused and cooled as previously described, the renal artery reconstruction is performed.

When autotransplantation is planned, the ipsilateral hypogastric artery is exposed and examined. When this vessel is normal and matches the renal artery in size, no graft material is required. In this instance, attaching renal artery branches to the distally transected hypogastric artery branches facilitates revascularization without the need for a proximal graft anastomosis. In this technique, the spatulated renal vein is anastomosed to the iliac vein before the renal artery or graft anastomosis is made to the hypogastric or the common iliac artery (Fig. 110–3).

Ex Vivo Reconstruction Without Autotransplantation

The author's group believes ex vivo reconstruction without autotransplantation to be the superior method for

most ex vivo renal artery reconstructions. Although autotransplantation of the iliac fossa has become the accepted method for reattachment of the ex vivo reconstructed renal artery, this latter technique was initially borrowed from the renal transplant surgeon without thought being given to the significant differences in the two patient populations. The reduction in the magnitude of the operative exposure, the manual palpation of the transplanted kidney, the potential use of irradiation for episodes of rejection, and the ease of removal when treatment in the case of rejection has failed are all historical and practical reasons for placing the transplanted kidney into the recipient's iliac fossa. None of these advantages applies to the patient with complex renal artery disease that requires ex vivo reconstruction. In contrast, factors most important in ex vivo renal artery reconstruction relate to improving the predictability of the permanent success of revascularization. Because many ex vivo procedures are performed in relatively young patients, durability of the operation should be measured in terms of decades. For this reason, the author's group believes that attachment of the kidney to the iliac arterial system within or below sites commonly susceptible to significant atherosclerotic occlusive disease can subject the autotransplanted kidney to disease that may reduce the permanency of success of the renovascular surgery. In addition, this group believes that the subsequent management of peripheral vascular disease may be complicated by the presence of the autotransplanted kidney. Furthermore, after the kidney has been replaced into the original renal fossa, the attachment of the renal artery graft to the aorta at a proximal infrarenal site should

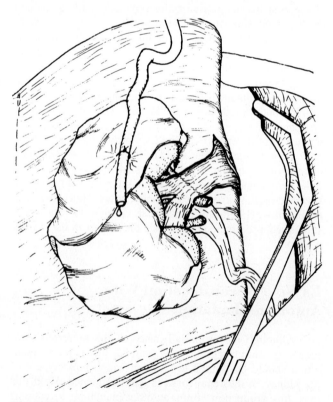

FIGURE 110–4. Placement of a partially occluding clamp on the vena cava and excision of an ellipse of vena cava wall with renal vein origin; this allows reattachment without concern for renal vein anastomotic stenosis.

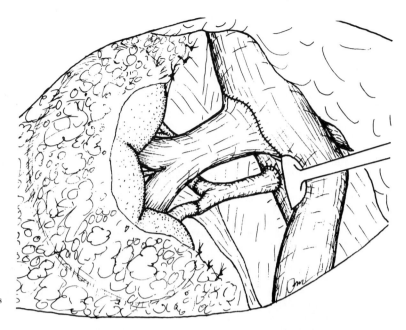

FIGURE 110–5.   Replaced kidney after the completion of ex vivo repair and repositioning of the kidney into the renal fossa. Note that Gerota's capsule is reattached to provide stability to the replaced kidney.

mimic standard aortorenal bypasses, with a high probability of technical success (greater than 97 per cent) and long-term durability (more than 90 per cent).[17]

To replace the kidney into its original site, Gerota's capsule is removed from the kidney during mobilization, as described earlier. At the point of renal vein transection, a large vascular clamp is placed to occlude the vena cava partially at the site of renal vein entrance. An ellipse of vena cava containing the renal vein origin is then excised, and the kidney is removed for ex vivo perfusion and reconstruction (Fig. 110–4). When the microvascular renal artery–graft anastomoses have been completed, the kidney is replaced into its original bed and the ellipse of vena cava is reattached (Fig. 110–5). This technique ensures that there

is no chance for renal vein anastomotic stenosis from technical error. After this, the renal artery graft is attached to the aorta in the standard manner. Figure 110–6 demonstrates the angiographic appearance of the pre- and postoperative anatomy of a 25-year-old white woman with multiple renal artery aneurysms in a solitary right kidney that was managed in this manner.

To summarize, ex vivo renal artery reconstruction, with the attendant capacity to allow extended periods of safe ischemic time for prolonged microvascular reconstructions, has expanded the role of renal revascularization and salvage in the treatment of renovascular disease and renovascular hypertension. Although the indications for this technique may vary among centers employing it, its use by

FIGURE 110–6.
Preoperative (A) and postoperative (B) arteriograms in a 25-year-old white woman who had a congenital solitary right kidney with multiple aneurysms of the right renal artery separately involving each of the branches. Ex vivo repair and replacement into the renal fossa were performed.

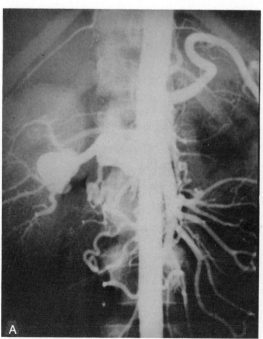
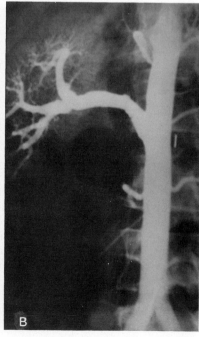

experienced surgeons has been highly successful. In view of the complexity of reconstructions using the ex vivo technique, the excellent success reported with this procedure[2-4, 18, 19] underscores the value of the added exposure and the microvascular methods employed for this operation.

References

1. Ota K, Mori S, Awane Y, Ueno A: Ex-situ repair of renal artery for renal vascular hypertension. Arch Surg 94:370, 1967.
2. Dubernard JM, Martin X, Gelet A, et al: Renal autotransplantation versus bypass techniques for renovascular hypertension. Surgery 97:529, 1985.
3. van Bockel JH, van Schilfgaarde R, Overboshch EH, et al: The influence of the surgical technique upon the short term and long term anatomic results in reconstructive operation for renovascular hypertension. Department of Surgery, University Hospital, Leiden, The Netherlands. Surg Gynecol Obstet 166(5):402, 1988.
4. Dean RH, Meacham PW, Weaver FA: Ex vivo renal artery reconstructions: Indications and techniques. J Vasc Surg 4:546, 1986.
5. Sacks SA, Petritsch PH, Kaufman JJ: Canine kidney perfusion using a new perfusate. Lancet 1:1024, 1973.
6. Collins GM, Bravo-Sugarman M, Terasakai PI: Kidney preservation for transportation. Lancet 2:1219, 1969.
7. Collins GM, Halsz NA: Forty-eight hour ice storage of kidneys: Importance of cation content. Surgery 79:432, 1976.
8. Feduska NJ, Collins GM, Amend WJ, et al: Comparative study of albumin solution and cryoprecipitated plasma for renal preservation: A preliminary report. Transplant Proc 11:472, 1979.
9. Marshall VF, Whitsell J, McGovern JH, Miscall BG: The practicality of renal autotransplantation in humans. JAMA 196:1154, 1966.
10. Clunie GJA, Murphy KJ, Lubin L, et al: Autotransplantation of the kidney in the treatment of renovascular hypertension. Surgery 69:326, 1971.
11. Belzer FO, Ashby BS, Dunphy JE: 24-hour and 72-hour preservation of canine kidneys. Lancet 2:536, 1967.
12. Milsten R, Neifield J, Koontz WW: Extracorporeal renal surgery. J Urol 112:425, 1974.
13. Ward JP: Determination of the optimum temperature for regional renal hypothermia during temporary renal ischemia. Br J Urol 47:17, 1975.
14. Cort JH, Kleinzeller A: The effect of temperature on the transport of sodium and potassium by kidney cortex slices. J Physiol 142:208, 1958.
15. Gibbons RP, Correa RJ, Cummings KB, Mason JT: Surgical management of renal lesions using in situ hypothermia and ischemia. J Urol 115:12, 1976.
16. Metzner PJ, Boyce WH: Simplified renal hypothermia: An adjunct to conservative renal surgery. Br J Urol 44:76, 1972.
17. Dean RH, Foster JH: Surgery of the renal artery. In Haimovici H (ed): Vascular Surgery: Principles and Techniques. Norwalk, CT: Appleton-Century-Crofts, 1984, pp 827–840.
18. van Bockel JH, van Schilfgaarde R, van Brummelen P, Terpstra JL: Long-term results of renal artery reconstruction with autogenous artery in patients with renovascular hypertension. Eur J Vasc Surg 3(6):515, 1989.
19. van Bockel JH, van den Akker PJ, Chang PC, et al: Extracorporeal renal artery reconstruction for renovascular hypertension. J Vasc Surg 13:101, 1991.

111

Renal Artery Aneurysms and Arteriovenous Fistulae

Charles W. Van Way III, M.D.

Renal Artery Aneurysms

Renal artery aneurysms are a diverse group of lesions. The best classification is that of Poutasse, who defined four types.[64, 65] Most common is the saccular type. Next most common is the fusiform type, which is usually associated with renal artery stenosis. Third is the dissecting aneurysm, which is rare but significant because of the direct threat it poses to the kidney. The fourth type comprises miscellaneous lesions of the intrarenal arteries.

By the mid-1960s, only about 300 cases were reported.

With the great increase in the use of aortography and renal arteriography that has occurred since then, these lesions are now known to be far more common than previously thought. Schwartz and White, using postmortem renal arteriography in 154 unselected autopsy cases, found aneurysms in 15 cases, or 9.7 per cent.[73] Erdsman reported an incidence of 0.73 per cent in 965 subjects of renal arteriography, a figure that seems to be somewhat more reasonable.[23] If the true incidence were as high as 1 per cent in patients undergoing renal arteriography, most vascular surgeons would be expected to encounter the problem several times during their careers.

TYPES OF RENAL ARTERY ANEURYSMS

Saccular Aneurysms

The saccular aneurysm is the classic renal artery aneurysm (Fig. 111–1). This lesion characteristically occurs at the bifurcation of the renal artery. Saccular aneurysms were initially thought to be congenital, but the peak incidence occurs between the ages of 40 and 60 years. It is more probable that a weakness in the artery at this point leads to a ballooning out of the artery, with secondary atherosclerotic changes and intraluminal thrombus.[65] The aneurysm wall becomes calcified, producing the characteristic radiographic finding of ring-shaped calcification in the renal hilum (Figs. 111–2 and 111–3). Saccular aneurysms do not usually exceed 5 cm in diameter, although larger ones have been reported.[63] The noncalcified aneurysms have generally been thought to be most likely to rupture, but ruptured calcified aneurysms have been reported. Poutasse suggested that calcification is often incomplete and that rupture probably results from the formation of a secondary aneurysm in a weak area of the aneurysm wall in either a calcified or a

noncalcified aneurysm.[65] Because rupture results from the progressive weakness of the wall as the aneurysm enlarges, the small lesions are relatively safe. Poutasse recommended nephrectomy or arterial reconstruction of all aneurysms 2 cm or more in diameter, especially those that are incompletely calcified or noncalcified.[65] As is discussed later, this "classic recommendation" should be modified.

Fusiform Aneurysms

Aneurysms associated with renal artery occlusive disease are usually fusiform enlargements of the renal artery distal to the stenosis. These are generally small, only 2 to 3 cm long and 1 to 2 cm in diameter, although larger ones have been reported.

The patient with fibromuscular disease of the renal artery will often show multiple aneurysms along the course of the dysplastic artery. The aneurysms are usually only a few millimeters in diameter. Fibromuscular disease characteristically produces a "string-of-beads" appearance in the renal artery, and these aneurysms are only an exaggeration of this pathologic appearance (see Chapter 108).

Dissecting Aneurysms

Dissecting aneurysm of the renal artery in association with a fibrotic lesion of the artery was described by Pou-

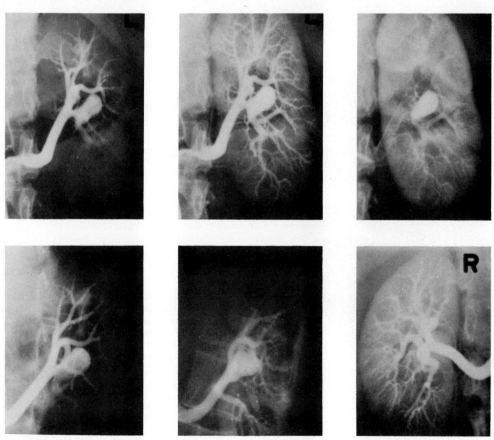

FIGURE 111–1. Saccular aneurysm of a branch of the left renal artery, with a normal right renal artery.

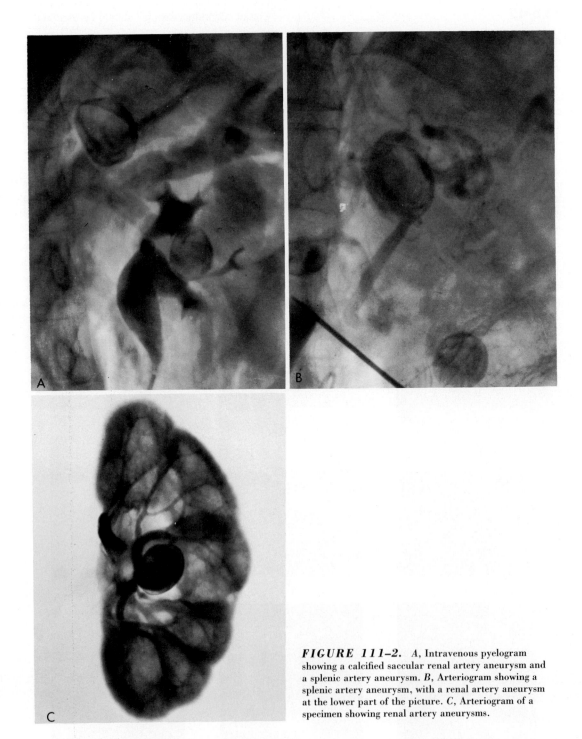

FIGURE 111–2. *A,* Intravenous pyelogram showing a calcified saccular renal artery aneurysm and a splenic artery aneurysm. *B,* Arteriogram showing a splenic artery aneurysm, with a renal artery aneurysm at the lower part of the picture. *C,* Arteriogram of a specimen showing renal artery aneurysms.

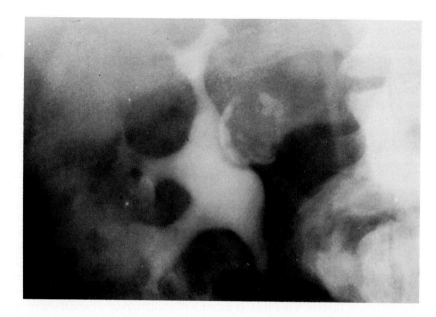

FIGURE 111–3. Calcified saccular aneurysm of the right kidney showing indentation of the collecting system by the aneurysm.

tasse in 14 of his original 57 cases, and by others.[31, 37, 50, 64] Aortic dissections can involve the renal arteries, but this particular lesion is confined to the renal artery. It is related to the mural fibroplasias of the renal artery and may be caused by a tear in the intima at the site of the mural lesion. On the other hand, it may be that mural fibrosis is caused by dissection, at least in some cases.[31, 37]

This type of aneurysm may have a characteristic clinical picture. The patient presents with flank pain resembling renal colic. The intravenous pyelogram shows nonfunction or poor function. The syndrome is quite similar to that produced by thrombosis of the artery, by embolism, or by aortic dissection. Arteriography is indicated, as is immediate operation, but reconstructive treatment is often frustrated by the extent of damage to the renal arterial tree, and nephrectomy is usually necessary.

A number of affected patients present only with hypertension, with no history of an acute episode. In these chronic cases, the dissection has presumably reentered distally, and flow to the kidney is present but impaired. There is extensive fibrosis about the site of the old dissection. Partial obstruction to the renal artery or a branch causes hypertension. In a case of mural fibroplasia and "healed" dissection, it may be impossible to tell which condition is primary and which secondary.[31, 37]

False Aneurysms

The false aneurysm (aneurysma spurium) occurs from rupture of a diseased renal artery or from trauma, with containment and later fibrous encapsulation of the resultant hematoma. These aneurysms may manifest as abdominal masses. Because the danger of rupture is great, they should be removed.

A special case of false aneurysm is aneurysm following renal transplantation. These have been said to rupture, causing not only blood loss but also loss of the transplanted kidney.[44, 57, 59] Because of the risks, these aneurysms should probably be repaired. The duplex Doppler ultrasound de-

vice can be used to diagnose such complications of renal transplantation noninvasively.[84]

Intrarenal Aneurysms

The final category of renal artery aneurysm is the intrarenal aneurysm. Such aneurysms are often multiple. They may be congenital, post-traumatic, or associated with collagen vascular disease. These lesions are closely related to intrarenal arteriovenous fistulae. For example, a "cirsoid" aneurysm reported by Gil Montero and Bagley was associated with hypertension and yielded a positive renal vein renin assay result.[28] This was probably a congenital arteriovenous fistula that closed spontaneously, leaving the aneurysm and a diminished blood supply to the lower pole.[28] Intrarenal aneurysms have mixed symptoms. They may cause hypertension by interfering with intrarenal arteries; may rupture into a calyx and cause hematuria or "clot colic" from the passage of blood clots; or may be completely asymptomatic, appearing only as arteriographic abnormalities.[6]

Aneurysms characteristically appear in polyarteritis nodosa.[33, 76, 88] These are small intrarenal aneurysms that are usually associated with renal cortical infarcts. They have been successfully treated with renal artery embolization to occlude the aneurysms and preserve function in the rest of the kidney.[69]

CLINICAL MANIFESTATIONS

Rupture

The literature shows a lack of unanimity regarding the natural history of renal artery aneurysms. Harrow and Sloane, in reviewing 169 cases in the literature up to 1959, found that of the 100 noncalcified aneurysms, 14 had ruptured.[32] McCarron and coworkers, however, reviewing 126 cases up to 1974, found only six reports of rupture, five of noncalcified aneurysms and one of a calcified aneurysm.[49] In a review of 29 patients with aneurysms, Hageman and coworkers saw no ruptures among the 19 patients with small aneurysms who were not operated on.[30] Hubert and colleagues followed up 62 patients with solitary aneurysms ranging from 0.3 to 4.0 cm in size, 67 per cent of which were calcified.[35] With follow-up periods from 1 to 17 years, no ruptures occurred. Henriksson and associates followed 34 aneurysms in 21 patients for an average of 35 months; 28 showed no change at all, and none ruptured.[34] Martin and colleagues reported that 18 patients were observed from 1 to 16 years without operation; none had rupture. All aneurysms were smaller than 26 mm; only four were larger than 15 mm.[53]

Much of the earlier literature assumed that the natural history of the renal artery aneurysm was similar to that of the more commonly encountered splenic artery aneurysm. A splenic artery aneurysm should be removed because of the danger of rupture, especially in women of childbearing age. McCarron and coworkers pointed out that in 19,600 autopsies performed at The New York Hospital, no instance of rupture of a renal artery aneurysm could be found.[49] They were able to find only one report of rupture in 33 clinical cases of renal artery aneurysm. Of 180,000 pregnancies brought to term, no instance of rupture of a renal artery aneurysm was reported. The uncertainty on this point has major implications. Although the spleen can be removed for even a relatively small risk of rupture of a splenic artery aneurysm, removal of a kidney or reconstruction of the renal artery cannot be undertaken as lightly. As is noted later, the weight of opinion is that renal artery aneurysms are an especial danger during pregnancy.

Does lithotripsy pose a risk to calcified aneurysms? Carey and Streem reported on four patients with aneurysms; one had a calcified renal artery aneurysm 5 cm from the renal stone.[5] No harm was done, and there were no sequelae at 30 months.

Hypertension

The relationship of renal artery aneurysms to hypertension is fairly well defined. With the renal vein renin assay, it is possible to determine whether or not a given aneurysm is causing hypertension. A well-studied series of 13 hypertensives with aneurysms reported on by Cummings and associates showed that 6 of 13 had evidence of renal artery stenosis.[11] Five had positive results of renal vein renin studies, and a 6th had positive split renal function results. All 6 were cured of their hypertension by arterial reconstruction or nephrectomy. Six other patients were operated on without evidence of unilateral renal ischemia; 5 had aneurysms without stenosis, and the 6th had stenosis but negative split renal function results. None was cured of hypertension. A 13th patient, operated on for the sequela of a dissecting aneurysm of the renal artery, was not hypertensive before operation.

The point of this and other studies is that if the renal vein renin assay or split renal function studies fail to demonstrate a renal cause of the hypertension, removal or reconstruction of the aneurysm will not cure the hypertension.

This point is extremely important. Renal arteriograms are usually obtained as part of an evaluation for renal disease or hypertension, and the great majority of patients with aneurysms in the more recent series have been hypertensive. Obviously, if one obtains arteriograms in patients with hypertension, one will find aneurysms in association with hypertension. In renal artery aneurysm, just as in renal artery stenosis, the relationship between the renal artery lesion and the hypertension must be determined by appropriate studies (see Chapter 105).

A contrary viewpoint has been expressed. Soussou and coworkers operated on 25 hypertensive patients with 30 renal artery aneurysms and used arterial reconstructive techniques in all but 2 patients.[80] There were no operative deaths. Three patients later required nephrectomy. Follow-up from 6 months to 19 years showed relief of hypertension in 19 of the 25 patients. Their report makes no mention of either renin or split function studies.

Although it is true that aneurysms associated with renal artery stenosis or dissecting aneurysms are much more likely to be associated with surgically correctable renal hypertension than are saccular or intrarenal aneurysms, one should not ignore the possibility that one of the latter types may be producing hypertension. Saccular aneurysms may compress a branch artery, causing renal ischemia. Intrarenal aneurysms, as in the case reported by Gil Montero and Bagley, may be associated with partial renal ischemia.[28]

Other Manifestations

Renal artery aneurysms are often associated with flank or abdominal pain. The mechanism for this is difficult to understand, except in dissecting aneurysms. Renal artery aneurysms are usually slow-growing and small. However, the association has been noted in a number of cases.

Renal artery thrombosis and obstruction can be produced by renal artery dissection or by the stenosis associated with fusiform aneurysms. The saccular aneurysm, however, although itself often partially thrombosed, is rarely if ever associated with thrombosis of the renal artery.

Obstruction of the collecting system is quite rare. The larger aneurysms are generally located in the main renal artery or its primary branches and are unlikely to be in a position to obstruct the caliceal system. Aneurysms of the intrarenal arteries are typically small, and although caliceal distortion may be seen on intravenous pyelography, obstruction does not often occur. Because hematuria is an occasional presenting symptom for intrarenal aneurysms, it may be that an aneurysm in contact with the collecting system is more likely to perforate into the collecting system than to grow and obstruct it.

INDICATIONS FOR OPERATION

There are four reasons to operate on renal artery aneurysms. The first is renal hypertension, as shown by the appropriate studies. The second is dissection. Acute dissection, as mentioned earlier, is a surgical emergency. Besides the risk to the kidney, there is the additional risk of rupture of the dissecting vessel, with consequent retroperitoneal hemorrhage. The chronic, "healed" dissection is a more difficult problem. The risk of future dissection or rupture is probably small, but operation may be required for hypertension. The third indication is rupture, which is also an emergency.

The fourth indication is the risk of rupture. This indication is controversial because the risk cannot be estimated with certainty. The decision to resect may cost the patient a functioning kidney if reconstruction is not successful, and it requires a large operation in any case. The small aneurysm, less than 2.5 cm, can be safely left alone. Aneurysms up to 4 cm have been followed for years without rupture. Mid-sized aneurysms, between 2.5 and 4 cm, should be regarded with suspicion. Aneurysms with partial calcification, or lobulations, are probably more risky than those that are heavily calcified. Aneurysms larger than 4 cm should be resected.

Pregnancy appears to increase the risk of rupture. Cohen and Shamash reviewed 18 cases of rupture during pregnancy. They believe that renal artery aneurysms are more likely to rupture during pregnancy.[9] Pliskin and coworkers reported a giant aneurysm with associated fistula diagnosed postpartum. This probably resulted from rupture of an aneurysm into the renal vein during the pregnancy.[63] Removal of any renal artery aneurysm in a woman who may become pregnant is probably indicated.

TECHNIQUE OF OPERATION

Reconstruction of the renal artery and its major branches after excision of an aneurysm at the bifurcation is considerably more difficult than aortorenal bypass of a stenotic lesion.[53, 64, 65] One has the choice between excision of the aneurysm and reconstruction of the bifurcation, and anastomosis of an aortorenal graft to the major branches of the renal artery with excision of the aneurysm and main renal artery. The first choice may be appropriate for the small saccular aneurysm, and the second is usually mandatory for the aneurysm associated with a stenosis.

An aneurysm of a polar renal artery may compress it, causing hypertension. Citarelli and coworkers reported such a case with successful excision and end-to-end anastomosis.[8]

A vein or hypogastric artery is the graft of choice. Sewing the delicate branch vessels into a Dacron graft is technically difficult. Poutasse recommended using the splenic artery as a renal artery substitute.[64, 65] If the lesion is on the left side, a direct splenorenal anastomosis can be performed safely without removal of the spleen.

Extracorporeal reconstruction is appropriate for some of these cases, as in multiple branch vessel stenosis (see Chapter 110). Perfusion is carried out through the main renal artery to preserve the kidney while the aneurysm is excised and the bifurcation is reconstructed. Use of this technique should allow reconstruction in some cases that might otherwise require nephrectomy.[30, 53] Dayton and associates reported autotransplantation of a patient's single kidney for ruptured renal artery aneurysm in the 5th month of pregnancy.[12]

With the increasing use of "bench" surgery, it has become possible to attack the variant of fibromuscular disease in which multiple stenoses and "chain-of-lakes" aneurysms are seen in the renal artery in the major branches.[17, 18] Dean and colleagues, in Nashville, managed 24 patients with extensive fibromuscular disease, 11 of whom had branch stenosis and aneurysms.[13] Their operative procedures were well tolerated, with only one operative death (see Chapter 110).

Intrarenal aneurysms may present a difficult technical problem. Kyle reported a case in which the lower third of the kidney was removed under regional hypothermia after clamping of the renal pedicle.[39] A flank approach was used.

Operative surgery is usually best for ruptured aneurysm. Nonetheless, Routh and colleagues reported a case of transcatheter thrombosis of a leaking saccular aneurysm in a high-risk elderly patient.[68] Gianturco coils and coiled guidewires, thrombin, and bucrylate were used. Flow was maintained to the distal renal artery, and the patient survived—although he died of gastrointestinal bleeding within a year.

SUMMARY

Renal artery aneurysms will continue to be recognized with increasing frequency as arteriography is more commonly performed. In the presence of demonstrable renal hypertension and in cases of dissecting renal artery aneurysm, the indications for operation are clear. The risk of rupture of a renal artery aneurysm is real but not precisely defined. Until more information becomes available on the natural history of this lesion, it is probably wise to treat aneurysms larger than 4 cm aggressively, with arterial reconstruction when possible and nephrectomy when reconstruction cannot be performed.

Renal Arteriovenous Fistulae

Renal arteriovenous fistula was first reported in 1923 by Varela,[87] but at the time of the review by Maldonado and coworkers in 1964,[51] there were only 35 cases in the English literature. McAlhaney and coworkers found 118 cases by 1971.[47] Since then, the disease has become more common and is sufficiently well known that only unique cases are now being reported.

TYPES OF RENAL ARTERIOVENOUS FISTULAE

Renal arteriovenous fistulae are usually classified by origin (Table 111–1). Postbiopsy fistulae are by far the most common, with an incidence of around 15 per cent. Other types of fistulae are uncommon.[60]

Congenital

The diagnosis of congenital fistula is made on the basis of angiographic appearance. These lesions are angiomatous or cirsoid, with multiple arteriovenous communications, and are invariably located in the renal parenchyma.

Spontaneous

The spontaneous fistula may arise from a parenchymal or hilar aneurysm that erodes into an adjacent vein, from a dissecting aneurysm of the renal artery (as shown in Figs. 111–4 and 111–5), from an inflammatory process such as chronic pyelonephritis or granulomatous disease, or from atherosclerosis.[51] Spontaneous fistulae are usually parenchymal but may be hilar. They are nearly always fed by one or at most two vessels. The diagnosis is made by excluding previous trauma, operative injury, and renal biopsy. The differentiation between congenital and spontaneous fistulae is somewhat arbitrary, being based on the characteristic angiographic appearance of congenital fistulae.

Neoplastic

Renal cell carcinoma is a vascular tumor. The existence of small vascular shunts is one of the angiographic criteria for its diagnosis. A true arteriovenous fistula probably forms when the tumor erodes into a major vein. In patients with arteriovenous fistulae, there will be a flank bruit, the early appearance of contrast medium in the renal vein on angiography, and perhaps cardiovascular manifestations.[25]

Neoplastic fistulae may produce systemic manifestations. In a review of 10 cases, including 3 of their own, Wise and associates pointed out that affected patients tend to show cardiovascular manifestations, such as cardiomegaly, diastolic hypertension, cardiac murmurs, and even congestive heart failure, and further, that these symptoms were relieved by nephrectomy.[88] Barzilai and associates reported an uncommon tumor, renal angiomyolipoma, associated with arteriovenous shunting in at least one patient.[1] Sanchez and coworkers reported a case of bleeding from an aneurysm within an angiomyolipoma, which was treated successfully with embolization using a Gianturco coil.[70] Presumably, the arteriovenous fistula arose secondary to the aneurysm.

The importance of making the diagnosis of this particular type of fistula is that it may be an indication for further treatment, especially if there are cardiovascular manifestations. Even if metastatic disease is present, the patient may be best served by nephrectomy. If there are contraindications to operation, such as extensive metastases and poor general condition, intra-arterial thrombosis of the fistula may be the best choice. Because most patients with renal cell carcinoma undergo arteriography, the diagnosis of a fistula should be made in nearly all cases.

Traumatic

Either blunt or penetrating trauma to the kidney may result in the formation of an arteriovenous fistula. A hematoma probably forms around the damaged artery and vein, and the fistula itself does not appear until the clot lyses. For this reason, it is common for such fistulae to be missed after the initial injury, only to appear years later. Traumatic fistulae are nearly always fed by a single artery and may be either parenchymal or hilar.

Postoperative

The formation of a fistula between the main renal artery and the renal vein following nephrectomy is well known, although rare.[36, 41] The use of mass ligation of the renal pedicle, especially with suture ligatures, predisposes a patient to this complication. Besides mass ligation, predisposing factors include renal tuberculosis, pyelonephritis, renal cell carcinoma, and postoperative infection.[7, 10, 24] Postoperative fistulae are typically large, producing congestive heart failure and other cardiovascular manifestations. They behave like peripheral rather than renal arteriovenous fistulae in one important respect: whereas renal arteriovenous fistulae, being typically within the renal parenchyma,

Table 111–1. Types of Renal Arteriovenous Fistulae

Congenital	Traumatic
Spontaneous	Postoperative
Neoplastic	Postbiopsy

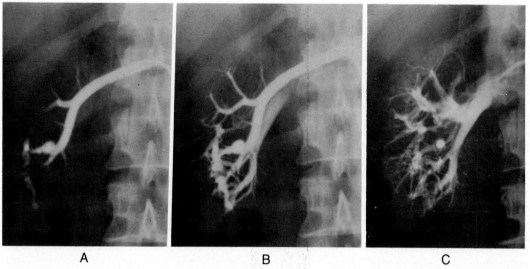

FIGURE 111–4.   Acquired right renal arteriovenous fistula. The fistula may have formed in a small saccular aneurysm in the mid-portion of the kidney. *A,* The saccular aneurysm, venous communication, and initial venous filling are seen. *B,* The renal vein fills before the arterial injection is complete. *C,* Filling of parenchymal branches is delayed.

are usually fed by only one vessel, postnephrectomy fistulae may acquire blood supply from two or more sources. The fistula in the case reported by Cummings and associates, for example, although clearly between the main renal artery and vein, had acquired a second arterial supply.[10]

Less well known, but increasingly more common, is the parenchymal arteriovenous fistula occurring after other operations on the kidney, especially nephrolithotomy and partial nephrectomy.[24, 79] The mechanism of formation is probably the same as that for the post-traumatic fistula, with intrarenal hemorrhage leading to hematoma formation, then subsequent establishment of the fistula as the clot resorbs.

Postbiopsy

The widespread use of percutaneous needle biopsy of the kidney has made possible great precision in the diagnosis of renal disease. However, one of the prices paid for this precision is postbiopsy arteriovenous fistula.

When percutaneous biopsy was first introduced, there was much concern over possible damage to the kidney. The incidence of gross hematuria was carefully studied and was found to range from 5 to 13 per cent. Usually transient, this complication nonetheless shows that vascular damage occurs occasionally.

When reports of arteriovenous fistula following renal biopsy began to appear, it was at first thought to be rare. Elkin noted only two instances of arteriovenous fistula in 600 children in whom biopsy had been performed.[22] He pointed out that conventional physical examination is not adequate for demonstration of these often small fistulae and that only routine angiography following biopsy could detect all fistulae. Ekelund and Lindholm carried out arteriography in 41 patients who had 48 needle biopsies.[20] They found that 7 patients (15 per cent) had arteriovenous fistulae but that in 5 the fistulae closed spontaneously. In a similar study of 58 hypertensive patients, Bennett and Wiener noted arteriovenous fistulae in 9 (16 per cent).[2] Ekelund and Gothlin conducted an experimental study in which rab-

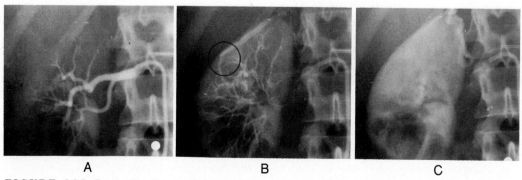

FIGURE 111–5.   Small acquired right renal arteriovenous fistula. Note the fistula between a branch of the renal artery and a capsular vein, which circumferentially traverses the upper pole of the kidney to drain into the renal vein. *A,* Initial arterial injection is normal. *B,* Early filling of a capsular vein *(circle). C,* Drainage of the enlarged capsular vein around the upper pole to the renal vein.

bit kidneys were punctured one to four times with a 0.7-mm steel cannula.[19] Six of 16 animals (38 per cent) developed arteriovenous fistulae.

There are three major factors predisposing to fistula formation after needle biopsy: nephrosclerosis of the renal vessels, hypertension, and passage of the needle through the central portion of the kidney.[2, 20, 22, 45] Little can be done about nephrosclerosis; indeed, one of the purposes of biopsy is to determine if it exits. Hypertension can, however, be controlled. Elkin recommended treatment with antihypertensive drugs before biopsy, a precaution that seems sensible. Choice of a peripheral biopsy technique is best for both diagnostic accuracy and avoidance of vessel damage. Carrying out the biopsy under radiologic control is widely accepted.

Most postbiopsy fistulae close spontaneously.[20] Therefore, one is not obligated to recommend angiography or duplex Doppler ultrasonography after all biopsies. Nevertheless, all patients undergoing needle biopsy of the kidney should be specifically examined several months later for flank bruit and other signs and symptoms of a persisting fistula.

The transplanted kidney is especially vulnerable to postbiopsy arteriovenous fistula, probably because of impaired healing and because of the frequency of biopsies.[16, 59] Morse and associates presented two cases.[56] In both cases, renal function deteriorated and hypertension became severe. One patient had therapeutic embolization combined with dilatation of a coexisting anastomotic stenosis. Function improved, and the blood pressure returned to normal. Boschiero and associates reported successful embolization in one case.[3]

CLINICAL MANIFESTATIONS

The single most reliable indication of the presence of a fistula is a flank bruit. Maldonado and coworkers reported that bruits were found in 69 per cent of 35 patients.[51] Wise and associates reported bruits in 9 of 10 patients in their review of neoplastic fistula.[88] The finding of a flank bruit, especially the typical continuous bruit, should always lead to arteriography.

Pain and hematuria each occur in about one third of patients. The mechanism for pain in renal arteriovenous fistula, as in renal artery aneurysm, is not obvious, but it is a valuable if nonspecific sign. Hematuria is somewhat easier to explain, although it also is nonspecific.

Duplex Doppler ultrasonography is the best screening test. Middleton and coworkers used the color Doppler instrument to diagnose eight patients after renal transplantation and biopsy.[54] Five of the eight fistulae closed under observation with sonography; angiography was not necessary. These authors and others have advocated the use of the color Doppler instrument for the detection of both renal arteriovenous fistulae and aneurysms.[4, 14, 54, 82, 89] Intravenous pyelography may show a mass displacing a portion of the caliceal system. Computed tomography may be used to show the lesion. Magnetic resonance angiography may be useful, although this technique is not widely available. Renal angiography is the definitive diagnostic study and is

indicated if either operative surgery or catheter embolization is contemplated.

Cardiovascular Manifestations

Any large arteriovenous fistula may produce the manifestations of high-output cardiac failure: tachycardia, cardiomegaly, and congestive heart failure. This syndrome is present with roughly half of clinically evident renal arteriovenous fistulae.[51, 83] The kidneys normally have high blood flow, with each kidney carrying about 10 per cent of the total cardiac output. One would expect cardiovascular manifestations to be present in many cases of renal arteriovenous fistula. Congestive heart failure is most common with the postnephrectomy fistula, probably because of the size of the vessels involved and the tendency for the fistula to be relatively large. Also common in the postnephrectomy fistula is a widened pulse pressure, which is characteristic of large peripheral arteriovenous fistulae.

Hypertension and Renal Ischemia

The development of diastolic hypertension in association with a fistula has been clearly documented.[24, 46] The presence of functional renal tissue distal to a fistula appears to be a requirement. The hypertension is usually alleviated after either surgical occlusion of the fistula or nephrectomy. The renal venous blood flow is considerably larger in a kidney with an arteriovenous fistula than on the other side, so that the results of the usual renal vein renin studies are not valid. An increased renin release from the involved kidney will be diluted by the increased blood flow and will not appear as an increased concentration.

Even a small fistula may result in significant ischemia of the involved kidney. Maldonado and coworkers reported on a patient in whom hypertension and congestive heart failure had progressed for 5 years after a complicated delivery in which the abdomen had been vigorously massaged.[51] A right renal arteriovenous fistula was present. The radioisotope renogram showed delayed concentration on the right. There were decreases in flow, sodium concentration, inulin clearance, and para-aminohippurate clearance on the right. Nephrectomy greatly decreased the hypertension, although the patient still required antihypertensive therapy. Lindgardh and coworkers studied four cases of postbiopsy fistula with simultaneous catheterizations of the renal artery and vein.[46] The total renal blood flow on the side of the fistula was 30 to 100 per cent greater than that on the other side, but the fistula flow was 60 to 82 per cent of the total renal blood flow. The parenchymal blood flow was smaller on the side of the fistula than on the uninvolved side in all cases. In two cases, the extraction ratios and clearances for chromium-51–edetate and para-aminohippurate were determined and were found to be lower on the side of the fistula.

The role of renin in the development of hypertension remains unclear. Moore and Phillippi reported the case of a woman with a massive right renal fistula who presented with hypertension.[55] Renal vein renin studies did not show hyper-reninemia. Split renal function study results were equal bilaterally. Nephrectomy cured the hypertension. Kirkpatrick, however, presented a case of post-traumatic arteriovenous fistula in which the patient actually developed malignant hypertension with grand mal seizures.[38] Elevated levels of plasma renin were seen in peripheral blood before the operation and in renal venous blood drawn at operation. Nephrectomy was curative in this case as well. The case reported by Maldonado and coworkers in which hypertension occurred was studied with juxtaglomerular cell counts, which were found to be significantly higher in the atrophic zone distal to the fistula than in the normal areas elsewhere in the kidney.[51] This finding supports the hypothesis that renal ischemia leading to renin release causes the hypertension seen in these patients.

There have been few experimental studies in this area. In the study of Ekelund and Gothlin, measurement of blood pressures in rabbits before and after induction of arteriovenous fistulae by simulated renal biopsy showed no hypertension in the six animals developing fistulae.[19] Lasher and Glenn created an arteriovenous fistula between the main renal artery and vein and found a mild, transient hypertension.[42] Secrest, using a similar preparation, found that three of five dogs developed hypertension.[75] These last two studies were conducted before the renin assay was widely available.

It is probably significant that in both clinical and experimental studies, cases showing hypertension tended to involve large fistulae. There have been two case reports of postbiopsy fistulae associated with hypertension, but studies of postbiopsy fistulae have failed to demonstrate hypertension in most cases.[20, 21, 46, 78] Whatever the reason for the development of hypertension, a large fistula appears to be necessary.

Rupture

Rupture of an arteriovenous fistula has been reported but is very rare. In the three reported cases, the aneurysm was calcified.[40, 71, 72] All the fistulae were, presumably, acquired. Calcification is not especially common in renal arteriovenous fistulae. It may be that calcification is a sign of weakness in the wall. On the other hand, it may be that these particular fistulae were initially calcified aneurysms that ruptured into the renal venous system to form fistulae and then ruptured into the retroperitoneal tissues. Ruptured arteriovenous fistulae produce retroperitoneal hemorrhage and must be treated with immediate operation.

Massive Hematuria

Gross or microscopic hematuria is not uncommon in arteriovenous fistulae, but massive hematuria is rare. In a case reported by Tveter and coworkers, hematuria was sufficiently massive to produce anemia.[86] The patient illustrated in Figure 111–6 also had massive hematuria and anemia. Renal biopsy may produce significant hematuria and arteriovenous fistula concurrently. Rizk and associates presented a case in which the patient required treatment by catheter embolization because of massive hematuria.[66] In such cases, however, the arteriovenous fistula is incidental to the postbiopsy hematuria. Why is mild hematuria relatively common and massive hematuria rare? Perhaps the chronic fistula is associated with an inflammatory reaction in adjacent calices that causes mild hematuria but protects against erosion of the fistula into the calix.

The diagnosis of arteriovenous fistulae on renal perfusion scanning is made by noting early visualization of the inferior vena cava. Rosen and colleagues pointed out that normal patients may occasionally (3 of 217) show visualization of the inferior vena cava in 3 to 6 seconds.[67] In renal arteriovenous fistula, visualization is coincident with peak aortic activity.

INDICATIONS FOR OPERATION

The first thing to be emphasized is that not all fistulae need to be corrected. If the fistula is uncalcified, if it does not cause hypertension, if there is no sign of increased cardiac output or congestive failure, and if there is no bleeding, then the fistula does not need to be closed. Indeed, such a fistula may have no effect whatsoever on the patient. This was shown by Starzl and coworkers in the case illustrated in Figure 111–7.[81] This angiogram was taken in an asymptomatic woman who wished to donate a kidney to her daughter. Despite the finding of a small spontaneous fistula, the kidney was transplanted and functioned well for at least 12 years.

The major indications for closure of the fistula are diastolic hypertension, increased cardiac output with or without secondary cardiomegaly or congestive heart failure, significant bleeding, and rupture. As mentioned previously, diastolic hypertension is presumed to be a direct result of the fistula. According to Nelson and coworkers, approximately 60 per cent of patients with fistulae who had nephrectomy or other surgical correction had relief of hypertension.[58] Renal vein renin studies may not be of value, as discussed earlier. It is probably best to recommend that the fistula be corrected in every patient who has significant hypertension, with the patient's general condition, the ease of pharmacologic control of the hypertension, and the condition of the opposite kidney taken into account.[47, 74]

If the fistula is large enough to produce an increase in cardiac output, it should be corrected. Even though the patient might be asymptomatic at the time of initial presentation, the chance of subsequent development of congestive heart failure is too great to allow the condition to continue unchecked. Once congestive heart failure is established, obliteration of the fistula may produce only a moderate improvement.[36] This recommendation must be modified for neoplastic fistula, in which the presence of metastatic disease may limit the patient's life expectancy. In patients with a solitary kidney, the risk to the kidney may be greater than the value of preventing future cardiac problems. In such cases, correction should be performed only for established congestive heart failure, and the asymptomatic patient should be followed up closely.

As noted, bleeding is a relatively rare indication for operation. Probably any patient with persisting gross hematuria should be considered for operation, with the other factors mentioned previously also influencing the decision.

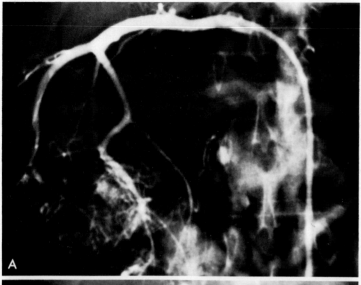

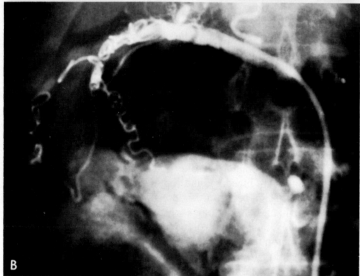

FIGURE 111–6. Use of transcatheter embolization. This 69-year-old woman presented with renal cell carcinoma, pulmonary metastases, and anemia from massive hematuria. *A*, Arteriogram shows several branches of the renal artery feeding a tumor mass; the arteriovenous fistula cannot be seen clearly at this early phase. Barium can be seen in the colon. Through the angiographic catheter, Gelfoam was injected, followed by small, medium, and then large Gianturco coils (see text). The entire procedure took approximately 30 minutes. *B*, Postembolization angiogram shows multiple coils in place and complete occlusion of the vessels feeding the tumor. The patient complained of nausea and back pain throughout the afternoon and evening but was well the next morning. Her hematuria stopped, and her hematocrit stabilized. (*A* and *B*, Courtesy of Delmar H. Knudson, M.D., Department of Radiology, Denver General Hospital.)

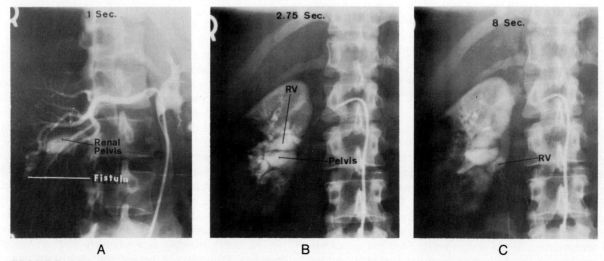

FIGURE 111–7. Right renal arteriovenous fistula found incidentally on a donor arteriogram taken before mother-to-child renal transplantation. The fistula is small and is located in the lower pole. The kidney was transplanted and functioned well in the recipient for more than 10 years. (*A–C*, Courtesy of Thomas Starzl, M.D. A version of this was previously published in Starzl TE, Vanhoutte JJ, Brown DW, et al: Radiology and organ transplantation. Radiology 95:3, 1970.)

Rupture is also rare. Obviously, any patient with a known fistula who presents in shock should undergo surgical exploration. Given the fact that the reported ruptures have all been in calcified fistulae, should all calcified fistulae be subjected to correction or nephrectomy? This question is troublesome to answer. In a patient with a normal opposite kidney and good general health, a calcified arteriovenous fistula should probably be removed.

TECHNIQUES OF OPERATION

A number of techniques are available for correction of renal arteriovenous fistulae, ranging from direct ligation of the fistula to transcatheter embolization of the feeding vessels. The choice of procedure depends on the type of fistula, its location in the kidney, the state of the other kidney, the patient's general condition, and the available expertise.

The easiest fistula to manage is the postnephrectomy fistula. It should be treated like any other peripheral fistula, with ligation of all vessels and excision of the fistula. The technique was nicely described by Cummings and associates.[10] Griffin and associates used cardiopulmonary bypass, deep hypothermia, and circulatory arrest to repair a posttraumatic fistula between the aorta and the left renal vein.[29]

Correcting fistulae associated with functioning kidneys is more difficult. Most of these are parenchymal, although a few are hilar. Four types of treatment are available: nephrectomy, resection or direct closure, arterial ligation, and transcatheter embolization.

Nephrectomy is the basic mode of therapy. If an open operation is performed, the surgeon should be prepared to carry out a nephrectomy. Any of the more conservative operations described later may be tried, but nephrectomy may become necessary. For a small and peripheral fistula, therefore, it may be best to attempt transcatheter embolization first, reserving an open operation for patients in whom the closed procedure has failed. For a larger fistula, open operation may be the only practical procedure, with nephrectomy as the alternative if the more conservative procedure fails.

Direct closure or resection of the fistula, if possible, is best. In direct closure, the branch artery feeding the vessel is ligated and the fistula is opened and occluded with sutures.[24] A polar fistula may be very adequately treated by partial nephrectomy. In a hilar fistula, it may be possible to excise the fistula and reconstruct the arterial supply to the distal portion of the kidney. Extracorporeal renal surgery as described elsewhere may be worth consideration.

Freeman and associates reported a technique of direct transluminal repair for intrarenal arteriovenous fistula in three patients.[26] The fistulae were at the upper pole, the lower pole, and the mid-portion of the kidney. In each case, the kidney was cooled and the thin shell of tissue over the fistula was incised. The vessels within the fistula were sutured with polypropylene. The parenchyma was closed with absorbable suture (see Chapter 110).

Some fistulae, such as parenchymal fistulae deep in the kidney, cannot be approached directly. *Arterial ligation* should then be considered. This takes advantage of one of the most remarkable aspects of the renal arterial tree: the renal branch arteries are end-arteries. If one can isolate the

artery leading to the fistula, simple ligation may be curative.[46, 61] This operation is best carried out from the anterior approach, through either a transverse or a long midline incision. The renal hilum should be approached as for an aortorenal bypass; the surgeon must gain control of the proximal renal artery before proceeding distally. For exposure of the branch arteries in the hilum, each artery should be occluded in turn while the surgeon listens over the kidney with a sterile stethoscope or feels the palpable bruit. The branch artery supplying the fistula is then ligated. This obviously results in a renal infarct, but because the parenchyma distal to the fistula is ischemic to begin with, the infarct should inflict no further damage. The disadvantage of this procedure is that the fistula is left in place and therefore may recur. Further, if there is an anastomotic blood supply to the infarcted area, hypertension may persist. Neither of these complications has been reported, but the procedure is relatively new.

It should be possible to embolize the feeding artery to a fistula via a catheter and thus to accomplish obliteration of the fistula without performing an operation. This challenge has been taken up with enthusiasm by vascular radiologists. A number of techniques of *transcatheter embolization* have been used, including transcatheter coagulation; the use of detachable balloons and Fogarty catheters; and embolization by autogenous clot, Gelfoam, lead shot, and Gianturco coils.* Use of the Gianturco coils, probably the best of the available methods, was introduced in 1975.[27] This method uses small spring steel coils with wool filaments protruding from one end. The basic idea of using coils is that they can be straightened to pass through catheters but resume their original shape once they have passed beyond the catheter. This is a very ingenious solution to the problem of embolizing material bigger than the catheter. With materials such as Gelfoam and autogenous blood clot, one is limited to embolizing material that is no larger than the catheter through which one is injecting. With lead shot, for example, one can embolize 1.1-mm shot through a No. 9 Fr catheter.[42] But with the Gianturco coils, one can employ a coil much larger than the catheter. Since the original publication by Gianturco and colleagues, a number of reports have documented the use of Gianturco coils in renal arteriovenous fistulae.[15, 27, 43]

The method is illustrated in Figure 111–6. The twin pitfalls of catheter embolization are too-proximal thrombosis of the vessel, leading to thrombosis of the renal artery or distal embolization, and insufficient occlusion of the vessels feeding the fistula, leading to recurrence. The technique used is first to shower the central vessels with 3- to 4-mm squares of Gelfoam through the catheter and then to place several Gianturco coils, beginning with small coils and using progressively larger ones. It is fairly universal for the patient to experience back pain and nausea in the first 24 hours after this procedure. More serious complications include necrosis of the entire kidney and infection in the portion of the kidney distal to the embolus.

Transcatheter embolization is most suitable for relatively small fistulae. It is ideally suited for the postbiopsy

---

*See references: coagulation, 48; balloons, 52; Fogarty catheters, 62, 77; autogenous clot, 66, 85; Gelfoam, 15, 69; lead shot, 66; Gianturco coils, 15, 27, 43.

fistula that fails to close spontaneously. It is also very useful in the patient with malignant renal arteriovenous fistula, in whom avoidance of operation may be desired.

SUMMARY

Renal arteriovenous fistulae can produce hypertension, high-output congestive heart failure, and bleeding. They can also be asymptomatic and innocuous. The single most common cause is percutaneous needle biopsy of the kidney. Although most such fistulae close spontaneously, those that do not constitute at least half of all symptomatic renal arteriovenous fistulae.

Operative therapy is generally required for symptomatic fistulae. Nephrectomy was the treatment of choice in the past and is still frequently used. More recent experience has emphasized the use of more conservative procedures, such as ligation of the feeding vessel, partial nephrectomy, excision of the fistula, and transcatheter embolization.

References

1. Barzilai IM, Braden GL, Ford LD, et al: Renal angiomyolipoma with arteriovenous shunting. J Urol 137:483, 1987.
2. Bennett AR, Wiener SN: Intrarenal arteriovenous fistula and aneurysm. A complication of percutaneous renal biopsy. AJR 95:372, 1965.
3. Boschiero LB, Saggin P, Galante O, et al: Renal needle biopsy of the transplant kidney: Vascular and urologic complications. Urol Int 48:130, 1992.
4. Bunchman TE, Walker HSJ III, Joyce PF, et al: Sonographic evaluation of renal artery aneurysm in childhood. Pediatr Radiol 21:312, 1991.
5. Carey SW, Streem SB: Extracorporeal shock wave lithotripsy for patients with calcified ipsilateral renal arterial or abdominal aortic aneurysms. J Urol 148:18, 1992.
6. Charron J, Belanger R, Vauclair R, et al: Renal artery aneurysm: Polyaneurysmal lesion of kidney. Urology 5:1, 1975.
7. Chew QT, Madayag MA: Postnephrectomy arteriovenous fistula. J Urol 109:456, 1973.
8. Citarelli F, Shin CS, Ippolito JJ, et al: Aneurysm of a polar renal artery. Surgery 78:660, 1975.
9. Cohen JR, Shamash FS: Ruptured renal artery aneurysms during pregnancy. J Vasc Surg 6:51, 1987.
10. Cummings KB, Jolly PC, Graber JD, et al: Arteriovenous fistula of the renal vessels: Surgical management. J Urol 144:776, 1975.
11. Cummings KB, Lecky JW, Kaufman JJ: Renal artery aneurysms and hypertension. J Urol 109:144, 1973.
12. Dayton B, Helgerson RB, Sollinger HW, Archer CW: Ruptured renal artery aneurysm in a pregnant uninephric patient: Successful ex-vivo repair and autotransplantation. Surgery 107:708, 1990.
13. Dean RH, Meachum PW, Weaver FA: Ex vivo renal artery reconstructions: Indications and techniques. J Vasc Surg 4:546, 1986.
14. Deane C, Cowan N, Giles J, et al: Arteriovenous fistulas in renal transplants: Color Doppler ultrasound observations. Urol Radiol 13:211, 1992.
15. deSouza NM, Reidy JF, Koffman CG: Arteriovenous fistulas complicating biopsy of renal allografts: Treatment of bleeding with superselective embolization. AJR 156:507, 1991.
16. Diaz-Buxo JA, Kopen DF, Donadie JV Jr: Renal allograft arteriovenous fistula following percutaneous biopsy. J Urol 112:577, 1974.
17. Dubernard JM, Martin X, Gelet A, et al: Aneurysms of the renal artery: Surgical management with special reference to extracorporeal surgery and autotransplantation. Eur Urol 11:26, 1985.
18. Dubernard JM, Martin X, Mongin D, et al: Extracorporeal replacement of the renal artery: Techniques, indications and long-term results. J Urol 33:13, 1985.
19. Ekelund L, Gothlin J: Blood pressure and intrarenal arteriovenous fistula. An experimental study in the rabbit. Scand J Urol Nephrol 7:210, 1973.
20. Ekelund L, Lindholm T: Arteriovenous fistulae following percutaneous renal biopsy. Acta Radiol 11:38, 1971.
21. Ekelund L, Gothlin J, Lindholm T, et al: Arteriovenous fistulae following renal biopsy with hypertension and haemodynamic changes. Report of a case studied by dye-dilution technique. J Urol 108:373, 1972.
22. Elkin M: Renal vascular shunts. Clin Radiol 22:156, 1971.
23. Erdsman G: Angionephrography and suprarenal angiography. Acta Radiol (Stockholm) 155(Suppl):104, 1957.
24. Eriksson L, Berglund G: Intrarenal arteriovenous fistula after nephrolithotomy. Scand J Urol Nephrol 8:73, 1974.
25. Francois G, Desveaux B, Garnier LF, et al: Arteriovenous fistula disclosing a renal cancer. Apropos of a case [in French]. Arch Mal Coeur 79:1632, 1986.
26. Freeman MB, Andriole GL, Sicard GA, et al: Transluminal repair of large intrarenal arteriovenous fistulas. J Urol 139:1292, 1988.
27. Gianturco C, Anderson JH, Wallace S: Mechanical devices for arterial occlusion. AJR 124:428, 1975.
28. Gil Montero GH, Bagley M: Renal vascular hypertension secondary to renal artery aneurysm. Urology 6:647, 1975.
29. Griffin LH Jr, Fishback ME, Galloway RF, et al: Traumatic aortorenal vein fistula: Repair using total circulatory arrest. Surgery 81:480, 1977.
30. Hageman JH, Smith RF, Szilagyi DD, et al: Aneurysms of the renal artery: Problems of prognosis and surgical management. Surgery 84:563, 1978.
31. Hare WSC, Kincaid-Smith P: Dissecting aneurysm of the renal artery. Radiology 97:255, 1970.
32. Harrow BR, Sloane JA: Aneurysm of renal artery: Report of five cases. J Urol 81:35, 1959.
33. Hekali P, Kivisaari L, Standerskjold-Nordenstam CG, et al: Renal complications of polyarteritis nodosa: CT findings. J Comput Assist Tomogr 9:333, 1985.
34. Henriksson C, Bjorkerud S, Nilson AE, et al: Natural history of renal artery aneurysm elucidated by repeated angiography and pathoanatomical studies. Eur Urol 11:244, 1985.
35. Hubert JP Jr, Pairolero PC, Kazmier FJ: Solitary renal artery aneurysm. Surgery 88:557, 1980.
36. Joseph RS, Lubell DL, Lambrew CT: Postnephrectomy arteriovenous fistula. NY State J Med 72:2209, 1972.
37. Kaufman JJ, Coulson WF, Lecky JW, et al: Primary dissecting aneurysm of renal artery: Report of a case causing reversible renal hypertension. Ann Surg 177:259, 1973.
38. Kirkpatrick JR: Traumatic arteriovenous fistula of the kidney: An unusual cause of hypertensive encephalopathy. J Trauma 15:363, 1975.
39. Kyle VN: Renal artery aneurysms. Can Med Assoc J 98:815, 1968.
40. Lacker H, Wolker W, Tellack T: Calcified intrarenal arteriovenous fistula with spontaneous rupture: A case report. J Urol 97:997, 1967.
41. Lacombe M: Renal arteriovenous fistula following nephrectomy. Urology 25:13, 1985.
42. Lasher EP Jr, Glenn F: Effects on kidney and blood pressure of artificial communication between renal artery and vein. Arch Surg 38:886, 1939.
43. Layne TA, Finck EJ, Boswell WD: Transcatheter occlusion of the arterial supply to arteriovenous fistulas with Gianturco coils. AJR 131:1027, 1978.
44. Lehr HA, Waltzer WC, Anaise D, et al: Management of a postbiopsy arterial pseudoaneurysm in a transplanted kidney: Utilization of epsilon aminocaproic acid and controlled hypotension. Transplant Proc 8:976, 1986.
45. Leonard JC, Nanney SM, Tytle T: Arteriovenous fistula secondary to renal biopsy. Clin Nucl Med 11:284, 1986.
46. Lindgardh G, Lindquist B, Lundstrom B: Renal arteriovenous fistula following puncture biopsy. Scand J Urol Nephrol 5:181, 1971.
47. McAlhaney JC Jr, Black HC, Hanback LD, et al: Renal arteriovenous fistula as a cause of hypertension. Am J Surg 122:117, 1971.
48. McAlister DS, Johnsrude I, Miller MM, et al: Occlusion of acquired renal arteriovenous fistula with transcatheter electrocoagulation. AJR 132:998, 1979.
49. McCarron JP Jr, Marshall VF, Whitsell JC II: Indications for surgery on renal artery aneurysms. J Urol 114:177, 1975.
50. McCormack LJ, Poutasse EF, Meaney TF, et al: A pathologic-arteriographic correlation of renal arterial disease. Am Heart J 72:188, 1966.

51. Maldonado JE, Sheps SG, Bernatz PE, et al: Renal arteriovenous fistula. Am J Med 37:449, 1964.

52. Marshall FF, White RI Jr, Kaufman SL, et al: Treatment of traumatic renal arteriovenous fistulas by detachable silicone balloon embolization. J Urol 122:237, 1979.

53. Martin RS III, Meacham PW, Ditesheim JA, et al: Renal artery aneurysm: Selective treatment for hypertension and prevention of rupture. J Vasc Surg 9:26, 1989.

54. Middleton WD, Kellman GM, Melson GL, Madrazo BL: Postbiopsy renal transplant arteriovenous fistulas: Color doppler US characteristics. Radiology 171:253, 1989.

55. Moore MA, Phillippi PJ: Reversible renal hypertension secondary to renal arteriovenous fistula and renal cell carcinoma. J Urol 117:246, 1977.

56. Morse SS, Sniderman KW, Strauss EB, et al: Postbiopsy renal allograft arteriovenous fistula: Therapeutic embolization. Urol Radiol 7:161, 1985.

57. Muldrije ED, Berden JH, Buskens FG, et al: False and true aneurysms of the renal artery after kidney transplantation. A report of two cases. Br J Radiol 58:896, 1985.

58. Nelson BD, Brosman SA, Goodwin WF: Renal arteriovenous fistulas. J Urol 109:779, 1973.

59. Nivani S, Christos FF, Athanasoulis A: Renal homotransplantation: Spectrum of angiographic findings of the kidney. Am J Roentgenol Radium Ther Nucl Med 113:433, 1971.

60. Norin RP, Dunn EJ, Wright CB: Renal arteriovenous fistulas: A review of etiology, diagnosis, and management. Surgery 99:114, 1986.

61. O'Connor VJ Jr, Bergan JJ: Surgical repair in a solitary kidney of a larger intrarenal arteriovenous fistula resulting from needle biopsy. J Urol 109:934, 1973.

62. Pingoud EG, Glickman MG, Pais SO: Balloon-induced thrombosis of renal arteriovenous fistula. AJR 124:605, 1980.

63. Pliskin MJ, Dresner ML, Hassell LH, et al: A giant renal artery aneurysm diagnosed post partum. J Urol 144:1459, 1990.

64. Poutasse EF: Renal artery aneurysms: Their natural history and surgery. J Urol 95:297, 1966.

65. Poutasse EF: Renal artery aneurysms. J Urol 443:113, 1975.

66. Rizk GK, Atallah NK, Bridi GI: Renal arteriovenous fistula treated by catheter embolization. Br J Radiol 46:22, 1973.

67. Rosen JM, Binkert BL, Seldin DW, et al: Scintigraphic criteria for the diagnosis of renal arteriovenous fistulas. Clin Nucl Med 11:847, 1986.

68. Routh WD, Keller FS, Gross GM: Transcatheter thrombosis of a leaking saccular aneurysm of the main renal artery with preservation of renal blood flow. AJR 154:1097, 1990.

69. Sachs D, Langevitz P, Moraq B, et al: Polyarteritis nodosa and familial Mediterranean fever. Br J Rheumatol 26:139, 1987.

70. Sanchez FW, Vujic I, Ayres RI, et al: Hemorrhagic renal angiomyo-lipoma: Superselective renal arterial embolization for preservation of renal function. Cardiovasc Intervent Radiol 8:39, 1985.

71. Sanoudos GM, Berenbaum E, Clauss RH: Ruptured renal arteriovenous fistula. JAMA 219:1581, 1972.

72. Sauter KE, Sargent JW: Spontaneous rupture of intrarenal arteriovenous fistulae: Report of a case. J Urol 83:17, 1960.

73. Schwartz CJ, White RA: Aneurysm of the renal artery. J Pathol Bacteriol 89:349, 1965.

74. Sechas MN, Plessas SN, Skalkas GD: Posttraumatic renovascular hypertension. Surgery 76:666, 1971.

75. Secrest AJ: Experimental renal arteriovenous fistula. J Urol 102:552, 1969.

76. Sellar RJ, Mackay IG, Buist TA: The incidence of microaneurysms in polyarteritis nodosa. Cardiovasc Intervent Radiol 9:123, 1986.

77. Selman SH, Zelch JV, Kursh ED: Successful treatment of a renal arteriovenous fistula with a Fogarty catheter. J Urol 122:387, 1979.

78. Smith GH, Remmers AR Jr, Dickey BM, et al: Intrarenal arteriovenous fistulae: Systemic hypertension following percutaneous renal biopsy. Nephron 5:24, 1968.

79. Snodgrass WT, Robinson MJ: Intrarenal arteriovenous fistula: A complication of partial nephrectomy. J Urol 91:135, 1964.

80. Soussou ID, Starr DS, Lawrie GM, et al: Renal artery aneurysm. Long-term relief of renovascular hypertension by *in situ* operative correction. Arch Surg 114:1410, 1979.

81. Starzl TE, Vanhoutte JJ, Brown DW, et al: Radiology and organ transplantation. Radiology 95:3, 1970.

82. Sullivan RR, Johnson MB, Lee KP, Ralls PW: Color Doppler sonographic findings in renal vascular lesions. J Ultrasound Med 10:161, 1991.

83. Takatera H, Nakamura M, Nakano E, et al: Renal arteriovenous fistula associated with a huge renal vein dilatation. J Urol 137:722, 1987.

84. Taylor KJ, Morse SS, Rigsby CM, et al: Vascular complications in renal allografts: Detection with duplex Doppler ultrasound. Radiology 162:31, 1987.

85. Tucci P, Doctor D, Diagonale A: Embolization of post-traumatic renal arteriovenous fistula. Urology 13:192, 1979.

86. Tveter KJ, Taksdal S, Mathisen W: Traumatic renal arteriovenous fistula treated by ligation and preservation of the kidney. Scand J Urol Nephrol 9:289, 1975.

87. Varela ME: Aneurisma arteriovenoso de los vaso renales y assistolia consecutiva. Rev Med Lat Am 14:3244, 1923. Cited in Nelson BD, Brosman SA, Goodwin WE: Renal arteriovenous fistulas. J Urol 109:779, 1973.

88. Wise GJ, Bosniak MA, Hudson PB: Arteriovenous fistula associated with renal cell carcinoma of the kidney. Br J Urol 39:270, 1967.

89. Yura T, Yuasa S, Ohkawa M, et al: Noninvasive detection and monitoring of renal arteriovenous fistula by color Doppler. Am J Nephrol 11:250, 1990.

112

Acute Occlusive Events Involving the Renal Vessels

Richard H. Dean, M.D., B.A.

· · ·

Most clinical considerations of renovascular disease involve elective management of secondary renovascular hypertension and retrieval of renal function in the chronically azotemic patient. Collectively less common than these considerations are the lesions producing acute ischemia to the kidney: that is, lesions that require urgent or emergent management. The most common of the latter lesions are renal artery trauma, acute embolic and thrombotic occlusion of the renal artery, and acute renal artery dissections. In some instances, urgent management may be directed toward preventing the loss of renal function or retrieving that function; in others, intervention is required to prevent death. Because each of these conditions is distinct from the others, they are addressed individually in this chapter.

RENAL ARTERY TRAUMA

Renal artery trauma is an uncommon clinical problem; it occurs in only 7 per cent of penetrating and 4 per cent of blunt abdominal and back injuries.[1, 2] Common signs and symptoms of renal trauma include flank pain and tenderness and microscopic or gross hematuria, but approximately 20 per cent of patients with significant renal injury have no hematuria.

Although life-threatening hypotension secondary to profound hypovolemic shock may abort the appropriateness of preoperative diagnostic studies, a bolus injection of contrast material followed by a "one-shot" excretory urogram is a valuable study in the patient with massive abdominal trauma. Its value is primarily in excluding the presence of major renal trauma and in proving the presence of a normally functioning contralateral kidney before exploration is undertaken in a patient with suspected renal injury who may prove to have retroperitoneal hematoma from some other cause.

When the patient's hemodynamic stability allows a more thorough preoperative assessment, standard excretory urography or contrast-enhanced abdominal computed tomography is indicated whenever major intra-abdominal blunt or penetrating trauma has occurred. If a discrepancy in the function of the two kidneys is identified, angiographic study of the renal anatomy is indicated. This empir-ical approach to the exclusion of renovascular injuries is particularly useful in patients with blunt abdominal trauma because as many as 25 per cent of renal injuries will not be readily apparent at operation.[3]

Operative management of renal artery trauma depends on several factors, among them the extent and site of the renovascular injury, the degree of associated trauma to the renal parenchyma and pelvis, and the magnitude of associated nonrenal injuries. Most commonly, if associated abdominal trauma is severe, nephrectomy of the traumatized kidney is required.[2, 4] Certainly, when a normal contralateral kidney is present, sacrificing the injured kidney while managing other complicated, potentially lethal injuries is appropriate. Occasionally, however, the renal artery lesion is the only major injury and revascularization is feasible.

In patients with injuries of the main renal artery or extrarenal branch renal arteries for whom the added risk and duration of operation are not a practical concern, operative management of the injured artery usually requires an aortorenal bypass. Occasionally, the ends of the injured vessel can be reapproximated.

Proximal control of the aorta and, if possible, of the proximal renal artery is achieved before the hematoma is entered. After the proximal and distal portions of the vessel have been isolated and the area of trauma has been débrided, the reversed saphenous vein is anastomosed end-to-end, as described elsewhere.[5] Although revascularization of even multiple branch injuries is rarely appropriate clinically, it may be required. Ex vivo repair is then appropriate because the kidney can be cooled with a renal preservative solution and the multiple branches can be repaired in a more controlled environment.

Unfortunately, the results of renal revascularization following both blunt and penetrating trauma have been disappointing. In the review by Clark and colleagues,[3] only 2 of 12 kidneys (17 per cent) undergoing successful revascularization had clinically significant retrieval of function, even though revascularization was performed between 3 and 18 hours after injury. This pessimistic view regarding the retrieval of preoperatively absent renal function reflects the experience of the author's group and tempers enthusiasm for revascularization in a patient who has had several hours of warm, total renal ischemia.

EMBOLIC RENAL ARTERY OCCLUSION

Traube is credited with the first description of embolic renal artery occlusion and secondary renal infarction.[6] These emboli gained little attention after Traube's report in 1856 until 1940, when Hoxie and Coggin reviewed 205 cases of renal artery emboli and infarction found at autopsy.[7] The uncommon nature of this lesion is apparent in their report because their cases were collected from a total autopsied population of 14,411, and in only 2 of the 205 patients had the correct diagnosis been made ante mortem. This report summarized the important clinical features of embolic occlusion of the renal artery, which include acute onset of back or flank pain, costovertebral angle tenderness, nausea and vomiting, and hematuria. Unfortunately, these symptoms reflect the consequences of the acute renal infarction, and they do not appear early, when the effects of the renal ischemia might be reversed.

More than 90 per cent of major renal artery emboli originate in the heart, and as many as 30 per cent may be bilateral.[8] The frequency of bilaterality may be lower, however, because some unilateral emboli, if they have not caused symptoms, may remain unrecognized. In contrast, major bilateral emboli will acutely affect total excretory function and lead promptly to profound azotemia.

The initial evaluation to identify acute renal ischemia secondary to renal artery embolization should include isotope renography, and if that study suggests impaired renal perfusion, renal angiography should be performed. Characteristically, renal angiography will demonstrate the proximal stump of the renal artery without showing the distal vessel or branches (Fig. 112–1). If the embolus is small or

has fragmented on impact, similar segmental branch occlusions may be seen.

Unfortunately for the viability of a functioning kidney, a variety of disorders imitate acute renal artery embolic occlusion in their presentation, and the correct diagnosis is rarely made in the first few hours after insult. In their 1984 review, Nicholas and DeMuth cited a mean delay of 4.3 days between the onset of symptoms and surgical intervention.[9]

The decision to intervene surgically and remove an occlusive renal artery embolus is dependent on the degree of associated excretory dysfunction, the site of the embolus, and the overall status of the patient. Nonoperative management with anticoagulant therapy may be preferable in the patient with distal branch emboli and in the patient with severe cardiac disease or other severe risk factors in whom contralateral renal function is satisfactory. In contrast, urgent intervention with embolectomy is preferable when the embolus is only partially occlusive or when overall renal function is threatened by bilateral emboli or an embolus in the artery to a solitary kidney. Although urgent intervention is important for reestablishing renal perfusion, the operation should be undertaken only after the patient is stabilized and after uremic acidosis and any significant abnormalities in cardiac performance and fluid and electrolyte balances are corrected. The added time consumed in correcting these risk factors only minimally increases the extent of function already irreversibly lost by the delay in diagnosis, and it significantly improves the patient's probability of survival.

A mid-line xiphoid-to-pubis incision is used to expose the renal artery and aorta, as described elsewhere.[5] Additional proximal aortic exposure for cross-clamping above the superior mesenteric artery is achieved by partially dividing the right and left diaphragmatic crura. A transverse

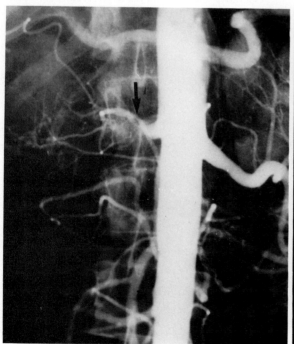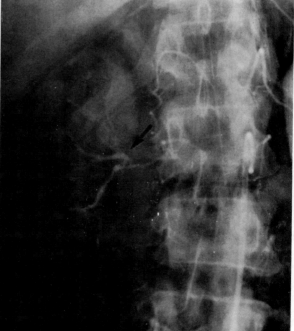

FIGURE 112–1. Arteriogram of a patient who presented with acute flank pain and a cardiac dysrhythmia. Note the abrupt occlusion of the renal artery (*arrow, left*), with a normal proximal vessel and faint opacification of the distal vessel beyond the embolus (*arrow, right*).

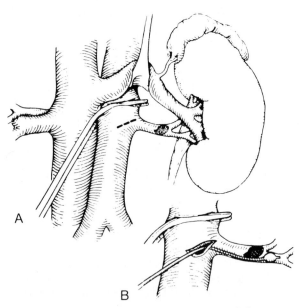

FIGURE 112–2. Technique of renal artery embolectomy. *A,* Depiction of site of aortotomy. *B,* Demonstration of passage of balloon catheter beyond this embolus.

aortotomy is performed at the level of the renal artery, and an embolectomy catheter is used to retrieve the embolus (Fig. 112–2). Primary closure of the aortotomy without a patch is usually possible. If associated atherosclerotic disease of the renal artery is identified, the incision is carried across the ostium and endarterectomy is performed. Following endarterectomy, the incision is commonly closed with a patch to ensure maintenance of a widely patent vessel.

Results of revascularization for embolic renal artery occlusion are distinctly superior to results of revascularization for traumatic renal artery occlusion. Reviewing collected cases of embolic renal artery occlusion, Lacombe found that function was salvaged in 23 of 33 kidneys (70 per cent) undergoing embolectomy;[10] in contrast to most traumatic occlusions, many of these renal artery emboli had been nonocclusive. In the absence of total occlusion, the residual patency has allowed sufficient parenchymal perfusion to maintain cellular structure and thus a viable kidney for return of function following revascularization.

Experience with local intra-arterial infusion of fibrinolytic agents suggests that it may also have a role in the management of renal artery emboli.[11] Its potential clinical value is in patients with distal branch emboli and in patients considered to be unacceptable operative risks. Its success, however, is limited to patients with emboli composed of relatively immature clot, because embolized valvular vegetations, portions of mature organized thrombi, and atheromatous debris will not respond to fibrinolytic therapy. For this reason, operative intervention with embolectomy is superior when the operative risk is acceptable and the embolus is in a retrievable location.

RENAL ARTERY DISSECTIONS

Renal artery dissections may produce clinically insignificant disturbances in renal perfusion, may create a he-

modynamically important stenosis and secondary renovascular hypertension, or may present acutely with signs of renal infarction. When a dissection does not produce acute symptoms, it goes unrecognized until the patient is evaluated angiographically for renovascular hypertension.

Acute spontaneous renal artery dissections usually occur as a complication of underlying atherosclerotic or fibromuscular dysplastic renovascular disease. In the review by Smith and associates, upper abdominal or flank pain with radiation to the epigastrium was the most common associated complaint (92 per cent), hematuria was present in 33 per cent of patients, all patients had onset of severe hypertension, and 40 per cent had acceleration of preexisting hypertension.[12]

The initial diagnostic evaluation of these complaints includes isotope renography. Once an abnormality of renal function has been noted, angiographic definition of any causative vascular lesion is required. Angiography usually demonstrates an irregular contour to the arterial lumen, with alcoves of contrast medium in the dissected false lumen and double densities reflecting opacification of the true and false lumens (Fig. 112–3). Branch vessels may have stenotic origins or may be totally occluded by the intramural hematoma. In the review by Smith and associates, 33 per cent of patients had branch renal artery involvement and 25 per cent had bilateral dissection.[12]

Because acute spontaneous dissections are recognized by their production of acute local symptoms of renal ischemia, progression of the dissection to total occlusion and permanent loss of renal function is a threat unless intervention with revascularization is performed. Like the approach to the management of other acute renal artery lesions, intervention for renal artery dissections should be emergent after control of any associated conditions that might increase the risk of intervention.

Operative intervention usually includes a branch renal artery repair. When the distal end of the dissection is limited to the main renal artery, this repair may entail only

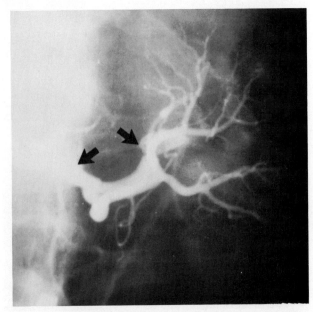

FIGURE 112–3. Arteriogram showing dual channels within the renal artery secondary to dissection of the vessel (*arrows*). Note the false channel involving the upper pole renal artery branch.

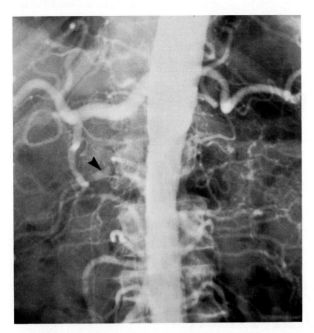

FIGURE 112–4. Arteriogram of a patient who presented with acute oliguric renal failure and uncontrolled hypertension. Note the bilateral total occlusion of the renal artery, yet opacification of the distal vessel beyond the occlusion (*arrowhead*).

extension of the arteriotomy onto an appropriate branch. However, if the dissection has extended distally to involve the origin of the renal artery branches, ex vivo preservation of the kidney during multiple branch repairs is a better procedure. For this reason, preparations for ex vivo reconstruction should be made in every instance. Details of this technique are described in Chapter 110.

ACUTE RENAL ARTERY THROMBOSIS

Acute thrombosis of a previously stenotic renal artery is usually silent or is simply a manifestation of progression of the underlying atherosclerotic lesion. In most instances, collateral perfusion to the kidney has developed to such an extent that the event is totally silent and goes unrecognized. Occasionally, however, the lesion is recognized acutely because of its adverse effect on the excretory function of a solitary kidney (Fig. 112–4) or in the only kidney with previously significant residual function. Although all patients with acute renal artery thrombosis have a history of hypertension, the acute presentation represents acceleration of the hypertension and the development of oliguric acute renal failure.

The diagnostic evaluation of any patient presenting with the constellation of symptoms suggesting acute thrombosis should include angiography. Previously, reticence to perform angiography was based on the nephrotoxic effect of the large amount of contrast material necessary. However, with the introduction of nonionic contrast agents and digital subtraction angiography, as little as 6 ml of contrast material is used, and this amount has no significant detrimental effect on any residual renal function.

Although it is tempting to react with immediate operation and attempted revascularization in these patients, a planned approach is superior. Because the acute event is usually more than 24 hours old and primarily represents a reduction in perfusion to a point below the critical level for maintenance of urinary output, attention to correcting any metabolic derangements before intervention is of the utmost importance in controlling the risk of surgical intervention. Thus, the patient may require several days of dialysis preoperatively and and even correction of potentially lethal cardiac derangements. During this period, it is reassuring to adopt the premise that the amount of retrievable renal function is not dependent on the timing of intervention.

Prediction of a salutary effect of revascularization is based on the demonstration of distally patent vessels beyond the occlusions and on the presence of bilateral disease. In a review of experience by the author's group, patients with bilateral reconstructable lesions or a lesion in the artery supplying a solitary kidney responded most dramatically to intervention.[13] In these patients, reinstitution of urine flow was almost instantaneous after completion of revascularization, and the majority required no further dialysis in the immediate postoperative period.

References

1. Lock JS, Carraway RP, Hudson HC Jr, et al: Proper management of renal artery injury from blunt trauma. South Med J 78:406, 1985.
2. Brown MF, Graham JM, Mattox KL, et al: Renovascular trauma. Am J Surg 140:802, 1980.
3. Clark DE, Georgitis JW, Ray FS: Renal arterial injuries caused by blunt trauma. Surgery 90:87, 1981.
4. Turner WW Jr, Snyder WH III, Fry WJ: Mortality and renal salvage after renovascular trauma: Review of 94 patients treated in a 20 year period. Am J Surg 146:848, 1983.
5. Dean RH: Surgery for renovascular hypertension. *In* Bergan JJ, Yao JST (eds): Operative Techniques in Vascular Surgery. New York, Grune & Stratton, 1980, pp 81–87.
6. Traube L: Über den Zusammenhang von Herz und Nieren Krankheiten. *In* Gesammelte Beiträge zur Pathologie und Physiologie. Berlin, A Hirschwald, 1856, p 77.
7. Hoxie HJ, Coggin CB: Renal infarction: Statistical study of two hundred and five cases and detailed report of an unusual case. Arch Intern Med 65:587, 1940.
8. Lessman RK, Johnson SF, Coburn JW, et al: Renal artery embolism: Clinical features and long-term follow-up of 17 cases. Ann Intern Med 89:477, 1978.
9. Nicholas GG, DeMuth WE Jr: Treatment of renal artery embolism. Arch Surg 119:278, 1984.
10. Lacombe M: Surgical versus medical treatment of renal artery embolism. J Cardiovasc Surg 18:281, 1977.
11. Fischer CP, Konnak JW, Cho KJ, et al: Renal artery emoblism: Therapy with intra-arterial streptokinase infusion. J Urol 125:402, 1981.
12. Smith BM, Holcomb GW III, Richie RE, et al: Renal artery dissection. Ann Surg 200:134, 1984.
13. Dean RH, Tribble RW, Hansen KJ, et al: Evolution of renal insufficiency in ischemic nephropathy. Ann Surg 213:446, 1991.

The Management of Extracranial Cerebrovascular Disease

Edited by Wesley S. Moore, M.D.

113

Fundamental Considerations in Cerebrovascular Disease

Wesley S. Moore, M.D.

• • •

Stroke is the third leading cause of death in the United States each year. It is the second leading cause of cardiovascular death and the most common cause of death as a result of neurologic disorders. The incidence of new stroke is approximately 160 per 100,000 population per year.[62, 67] In addition to death, the disability following cerebral infarction must be considered from the standpoint of the crippling effect on the patient as well as the socioeconomic burden on the patient, his or her family, and society. Reviews of the financial impact of stroke for calendar year 1976 were estimated to be $7.4 billion of direct and indirect cost.[2, 69]

The earliest report linking stroke with extracranial vascular disease is credited to Gowers, who in 1875 described a patient with right hemiplegia and blindness in the left eye.[40] He attributed this syndrome to an occlusion of the left carotid artery in the neck. Several similar reports soon followed.[9, 12, 43] In 1914, Hunt emphasized that extracranial carotid artery occlusive disease was a possible cause of stroke.[55] He noted that the cervical portions of the carotid arteries were not examined routinely postmortem and urged that thorough examination of this portion of the circulatory system be carried out during autopsy. Furthermore, he felt that transient cerebral ischemia was tantamount to intermittent claudication of the brain and represented a prodrome to a major stroke. In spite of these early reports, work in this field remained relatively dormant until Moniz and co-workers reported in 1937 that arteriography could be used to diagnose carotid artery occlusion.[81] Johnson and Walker reviewed 101 cases of carotid occlusion diagnosed by arteriography and advocated either carotid arterectomy or cervical ganglionectomy to relieve cerebral vasospasm, which

they believed to be a major cause of subsequent disability following the initial stroke.[59] Strully and his associates are credited with the first attempt at carotid endarterectomy of a totally occluded vessel; however, this was unsuccessful.[103] The first report of a successful surgical procedure on the extracranial carotid artery appeared in 1954. Eastcott and colleagues described their experience with a patient who had episodes of transient hemispheric cerebral ischemic attacks.[23] She was found to have an atherosclerotic lesion at the carotid bifurcation that was treated with a resection and primary anastomosis. A later publication of DeBakey[16] and one of Carrea and coworkers[10] cite operative procedures performed at an earlier date, but the report of Eastcott and colleagues must be credited as the most influential in bringing the possibility of carotid artery repair to medical attention. Vascular surgery had progressed to a point at which surgical repair of this lesion was rapidly accepted, and subsequently carotid endarterectomy has become one of the most common and successful operations performed on the vascular system.

The surgical approach to cerebrovascular disease is predicated on the relief of symptoms of cerebral dysfunction and the prevention of cerebral infarction or stroke by excision of a critical lesion in the extracranial carotid artery. There is currently a major international debate concerning the efficacy of carotid endarterectomy in stroke prevention when one considers the combination of perioperative risk and late results. An aggressive surgical approach to cerebrovascular disease can be justified only when the operation can be performed with sufficiently low rates of morbidity and mortality for the longevity and quality of survival of patients with cerebrovascular atherosclerosis to be materially altered when compared with the natural history of the disease with medical management.

EPIDEMIOLOGY AND NATURAL HISTORY OF CEREBROVASCULAR DISEASE

Knowledge of the incidence and natural history of hemispheric transient ischemic attacks (TIAs) and strokes in a given population is of paramount importance, not only in understanding the magnitude of the problem but also in designing a program of diagnosis, treatment, and prevention. The magnitude of the problem will dictate its investigative priority, and knowledge of the natural history is fundamental in evaluating and comparing the impact, if any, of various therapeutic programs.

The objective of all therapeutic intervention is to prevent cerebral infarction. Although episodes of transient cerebral ischemia may be alarming, their major significance rests as harbingers of subsequent stroke, neurologic disability, or death.

Cerebral Infarction

There is considerable variability concerning the incidence of stroke, depending on the year of reporting, geographic location, and racial and sex mix of patients. For example, there has been a steady decline in mortality from cerebrovascular disease in the United States dating back to 1915.[116] This decline in mortality may or may not translate into a true decline in stroke incidence. The reason for the decline in stroke mortality is difficult to ascertain. It may be something as simple as a more accurate diagnosis of stroke on a death certificate, or it may represent a change in the incidence of the disease. Finally, various interventions, ranging from control of hypertension to the use of aspirin antiplatelet drugs to carotid endarterectomy, must be interpreted accordingly.

There have been several population studies designed to look at stroke incidence. The Rochester, Minnesota, population study (from 1955 to 1969) emphasized the influence of advancing age on the progressive incidence of cerebral infarction.[73] The age group from 55 to 64 years had a cerebral infarction rate of 276.8 per 100,000 population per year; the age group 65 to 74 years had an incidence of 632 per 100,000 population per year; and the over-75 age group had a stroke rate of 1786.4 per 100,000 population per year. Analysis of the cerebral infarction rate divided by sex distribution indicated that in men the rate was approximately 1.5 times as great as that in women of the same age. Six months following survival from cerebral infarction, only 29 per cent of the patients in the Rochester study had normal cerebral function; 71 per cent continued to have manifestations of neurologic dysfunction. In the latter group, 4 per cent required total nursing care, 18 per cent were disabled but capable of contributing to self-care, and 10 per cent were aphasic. Of those patients who suffered a fatal stroke, 38 per cent died of the initial stroke, 10 per cent died of a subsequent stroke, and 18 per cent died from complications of coronary artery disease. The chance of a recurrent stroke within 1 year of the initial stroke was 10 per cent, and the chance of a recurrent stroke within 5 years of the initial attack was 20 per cent.

Wallace and associates studied the natural history of stroke in 188 patients in the city of Goulburn, Australia.[111] The overall incidence of stroke for all ages was 330 per 100,000 population per year. During a 24-month interval, they accumulated 158 cases of stroke, of which 101 were presumed to be due to cerebral infarction. The mortality rate of the first attack was 37 per cent, and the recurrence rate among survivors was 35 per cent. The mortality rate with the first recurrence was 35 per cent, but the mortality rate for subsequent recurrences in survivors of a first recurrence was 65 per cent.

Baker and his colleagues reported a series of 430 hospitalized patients who survived their initial cerebral infarction.[4] The mortality rate from the initial stroke was not described. However, the overall mortality rate for the 430 survivors, during the interval of study, was 40 per cent. On a life table, the mortality rate was 10 per cent per year of patients at risk. The cumulative 5-year mortality rate was 50 per cent. Twenty-three per cent of subsequent deaths were due to recurrent cerebral infarction. Of the 430 survivors of the initial stroke, 26 per cent developed a subsequent cerebral infarction and 20 per cent experienced new TIAs. Because some patients have both TIA and stroke, a combined 38 per cent were reported to develop a new neurologic event: stroke, transient cerebral ischemia, or both. Of the 113 patients who developed a new cerebral infarction, 62 per cent died.

Sacco and coworkers, reviewing the stroke data from the Framingham, Massachusetts, population, noted an alarmingly high incidence of recurrent cerebral infarction in the same anatomic region.[98] Among 394 patients surviving an initial stroke, 84 second and 27 third strokes were reported. The cumulative 5-year recurrent stroke rate in the male population was 42 per cent. Thus, the recurrent stroke rate, following an initial stroke, is approximately 9 per cent per year.

These data indicate that cerebral infarction produces significant morbidity and mortality in the United States. Of particular interest is the remarkably high rate of recurrence of cerebral infarction in patients following their first stroke, if no intervention has taken place. By and large, most of the recurrences appear to occur within the first year of the initial event. Not only is the rate of recurrence with progressive neurologic deterioration high but also the death rate with subsequent infarction is considerable.

Transient Ischemic Attacks

In order to discuss the incidence and significance of TIAs, one must define the type and anatomic distribution of the event. Those reports that combine focal neurologic events with those of global symptoms such as dizziness and vertigo cloud the issue and lead to erroneous conclusions because the natural history and prognosis of the two types of attack are quite different. Most authors agree that TIAs producing focal neurologic deficit have a more profound significance with regard to subsequent cerebral infarction.

Table 113–1. Average Annual Incidence of New Transient Ischemic Attacks in a Previously Asymptomatic Population*

Age (yr)	Rochester		Framingham		Lehigh Valley	
	Male	*Female*	*Male*	*Female*	*Male*	*Female*
45–54	21	12	56	15 ⎫		
55–64	96	50	114	49 ⎬	85	48
65–74	263	192	184	142 ⎭	244	151

Expressed in number/100,000 population.

For purposes of this discussion, therefore, TIAs are considered those that produce transient focal neurologic deficit, in either the anterior or the posterior circulation.

Because many patients with attacks of transient ischemia never reach a hospital, studies of hospital populations are not an accurate reflection of the disease. Those studies that review the overall incidence in specific communities give a far better view of the incidence and natural history of the event. There have been several such population studies, and these are cited in the text and among the references. One of the most important studies has been carried out using Rochester, Minnesota, as a population base and reported by members of the staff of the Mayo Clinic. Their reports evaluated two time intervals: 1945 to 1954 and 1955 to 1969.[73, 114] In the Rochester, Minnesota, population, the incidence of TIAs amounted to 31 patients per 100,000 population per year for all ages, with a rapidly rising incidence associated with advancing age. The incidence of new attacks in the 65- to 74-year-old age group was 200 patients per 100,000 population per year. As in the instance of cerebral infarction, there was also a higher incidence of TIAs in men than in women of the same age group at a ratio of 1.3:1. Table 113–1 compares the average annual incidence of first TIA per 100,000 population in three population studies: Rochester, Minnesota; Framingham, Massachusetts; and Lehigh Valley, Pennsylvania.

Reviewing the natural history of patients with TIA reveals somewhat conflicting data. This is due, primarily, to the lack of definition of the underlying lesion present in the patient population manifesting transient cerebral ischemia. For example, if one population has a large preponderance of patients with high-grade stenoses, composed of soft plaque with ulceration, there is likely to be a much higher subsequent stroke rate than there would be if the population consisted of a large number of patients with low-grade to medium stenoses. Nonetheless, there is considerable information to be gained by looking at some of the general population studies with regard to TIA outcome. In the Rochester, Minnesota, study, the probability of surviving free of stroke 5 years after the onset of TIA was only 64 per cent. Conversely, the incidence of stroke was 36 per cent. Fifty-one per cent of the strokes occurred within the first year following the onset of TIAs (Fig. 113–1.) In the stroke population, the authors noted that, in addition to advancing age, the three major predisposing factors for cerebral infarction were transient ischemia, hypertension, and cardiac disease.

In an excellent review of the available literature, Wiebers and Whisnant noted that of the available studies, the reported annual stroke incidence in patients with TIA ranged from 5.3 to 8.6 per cent per year for the first 5 years.

They concluded that the average annual stroke rate among TIA patients was 7 per cent per year for the first 5 years or that approximately one third of patients with TIA will suffer a stroke within 5 years of onset.[115]

Asymptomatic Lesions of the Carotid Artery

Asymptomatic, potentially critical lesions of the carotid bifurcation can be divided into two categories: preocclusive stenoses resulting in hemodynamic compromise; and large, grossly irregular or ulcerative lesions, independent of hemodynamic compromise but with the potential of releasing emboli into the cerebral circulation. In the past few years, the natural history of these lesions has been better defined as a result of several retrospective studies as well as new prospective studies.

The asymptomatic carotid stenosis was the original asymptomatic lesion to be identified as a potential cause of stroke. Stenotic lesions can now be readily identified in screening programs that utilize noninvasive testing. The natural history of these lesions, however, still remains variable and controversial. Three prospective randomized trials

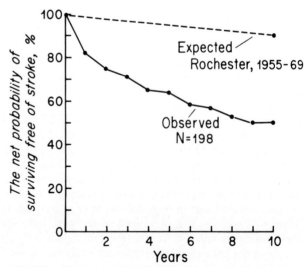

FIGURE 113–1. Conditional probability of surviving free of stroke after first transient ischemic attack (TIA), given survival. Expected survivorship is for a population of the given age and sex and is based on the stroke incidence rates of the Rochester, Minnesota, study for 1955 through 1969. (From Whisnant JP, Matsumoto N, Elveback LR: Transient cerebral ischemic attacks in a community. Rochester, Minnesota, 1955 through 1969. Mayo Clin Proc 48:194, 1973.)

were started in order to determine the efficacy (or lack thereof) of carotid endarterectomy in patients with asymptomatic, hemodynamically significant, carotid stenosis. The European study (Casanova) reported no benefit of carotid endarterectomy when compared with medical management alone. Unfortunately, the study was hampered by serious methodologic flaws in that a large number of patients in the control group were removed and operated on, but were counted as medically managed in an intent-to-treat design. Furthermore, the reasons that the patients were removed from the control group, including TIAs, were not considered treatment failures.[119] The Veterans Administration has just reported that the combined incidence of ipsilateral neurologic events (TIA plus stroke) was 8 per cent in the surgery group in contrast to 20.6 per cent in the medical group ($p < .001$). Unfortunately, the study was not designed to look for differences in stroke alone.[120] The largest of the three studies, the Asymptomatic Carotid Stenosis Study (ACAS), is supported by National Institute for Neurologic Diseases and Stroke (NINDS) and continues to randomize patients. There are not more than 1500 patients in the study.[121]

Perhaps one of the most important arguments in favor of prophylactic repair of asymptomatic lesions is based on a review of various populations of stroke patients. Careful histories from patients who have suffered a stroke reveal that only 30 to 50 per cent of patients had antecedent TIAs. That means that more than half of patients who developed stroke proceeded from an asymptomatic lesion one day to a stroke the next.

The early leaders in the aggressive surgical approach to the asymptomatic stenoses are Thompson and colleagues, who in 1978 described their experience with 138 patients who presented with asymptomatic bruit and who were followed without operation. They noted that 37 of these patients began to develop TIAs and required endarterectomy. Another 24, or 17 per cent, presented with stroke without antecedent TIA. From these data, the authors argue that the imminence of stroke is significant in the asymptomatic patient and recommended prophylactic operation when an appropriate lesion is identified.[105–107] The weakness of this argument lies in the fact that the data do not have angiographic substantiation of the nature of the lesion that was present in the patients that were being followed, nor were there noninvasive observations made to determine whether a hemodynamically significant stenosis was present. Perhaps a more impressive series was reported by Kartchner and McRae in 1977, in which they followed 147 patients who had oculoplethysmographic and phonoangiographic evidence of carotid stenosis. Without carotid operation, 17 of these 147 patients, or approximately 12 per cent, suffered an acute stroke.[64]

Two fairly new prospective studies have been reported. Roederer and colleagues studied 167 asymptomatic patients with cervical bruit using duplex scanning. They noted that progression of a lesion to compromise the lumen by 80 per cent or more carried a 35 per cent risk of stroke, TIA, or occlusion within 6 months and a 46 per cent event rate at 12 months. Further, they noted that 89 per cent of all events were preceded by a disease progression to greater than 80 per cent stenosis. This probably represents an underestimate of risk in view of the fact that 96 of the 167

patients underwent carotid endarterectomy during the study interval.[94]

The second important natural history study was carried out by Chambers and Norris. These authors have followed the natural history of 500 patients with asymptomatic carotid bruit in whom the carotid arteries were characterized by Doppler scanning. The patients were restudied every 6 months. In patients identified as having carotid stenoses in excess of 75 per cent, the neurologic event rate was 18 per cent per year and the completed stroke rate was 5 per cent per year. The completed stroke rate without antecedent TIA was 3 per cent per year.[11]

The arguments against an aggressive approach to asymptomatic carotid stenosis is best exemplified in a report by Humphries and colleagues from the Cleveland Clinic.[54] They followed 168 patients with 182 carotid stenoses for an average of 32 months and noted that 26 patients developed TIAs and underwent surgical correction, whereas only 4 patients developed a stroke before operative intervention could be considered. This report suggested that asymptomatic stenosis is a relatively benign lesion and that an imminent stroke will usually be heralded by an antecedent TIA. It is of interest that Dr. Humphries' colleagues at the Cleveland Clinic, in spite of this report, continue to advocate prophylactic operation on the asymptomatic stenosis.

In addition to the asymptomatic stenosis, the asymptomatic ulceration in the absence of concomitant stenosis has been identified as a lesion of potential stroke risk. The author's group has carried out a retrospective review of nonstenotic ulcerative lesions that were identified at the time of angiography being performed for contralateral symptomatic lesions.[82] Because it had been this group's practice not to operate on the asymptomatic ulcer, the author and his associates had the opportunity to examine the natural history of 67 patients with ulcerative lesions in 72 carotid arteries. The ulcer size was semi-quantitatively described as small (group A), medium (group B), or large (group C). In the initial series, there were 40 lesions classified as group A and 32 lesions that were combined group B and group C. The follow-up of these patients was expressed in the life table format in which the event of stroke was looked at as a function of duration of follow-up. The author's follow-up extended for approximately 7 years. In this group, only 1 patient in the small ulcer series (group A) went on to develop a stroke. There were, however, ten strokes in the group with larger ulceration, and this produced a stroke rate that averaged 12.5 per cent per year of follow-up. The report was challenged by a retrospective review carried out by Kroener and colleagues, who confirmed the benign prognosis of small ulcers in group A but could not find a significant stroke risk in group B ulcers.[66] It is of interest that their series excluded patients with the large ulcers, group C, since it had been their practice to operate routinely on those with a very large carotid ulceration. More recently, the author's group reviewed yet another series and included data from their original report. This yielded 153 asymptomatic, nonstenotic ulcerative lesions of the carotid bifurcation in 141 patients. During the course of the study, with follow-up extending up to 10 years, 3 per cent of patients in group A, 21 per cent of patients in group B, and 19 per cent of patients in group C developed hemispheric strokes without antecedent transient ischemia on the side appropriate to lesion. The interval stroke rates were 4.5 per cent per year for group B and 7.5 per cent per year for group C.[20] Because the interval stroke rate among patients with asymptomatic ulcers was comparable with the stroke rate among patients with TIA, the author and his associates have made the recommendation that prophylactic operation be carried out in patients who are good surgical candidates when they have an identifiable group B or C ulceration.

It is quite likely that the management of the asymptomatic carotid lesion will remain controversial until the results of the two prospective randomized studies are reported. As the risk of carotid endarterectomy continues to drop, however, it becomes harder to justify a nonsurgical approach to the asymptomatic lesion, particularly in those centers in whom the combined morbidity and mortality rate for operation is less than 2 per cent.

PATHOLOGY

The primary pathologic entity responsible for disease in the extracranial cerebrovascular system is atherosclerosis. This accounts for approximately 90 per cent of lesions in the extracranial system seen in the Western world. The remaining 10 per cent include such entities as fibromuscular dysplasia, arterial kinking as a result of elongation, extrinsic compression, traumatic occlusion, intimal dissection, the inflammatory angiopathies, and migraine. Radiation-induced arteriosclerotic change of the extracranial carotid artery has become a recognized entity. Other rare entities, usually involving intracranial vessels, include fibrinoid necrosis, amyloidosis, polyarteritis, allergic angiitis, Wegener's granulomatosis, granulomatous angiitis, giant cell arteritis, amphetamine-associated arteritis, infectious arteritis, and moyamoya disease.[28] Embolization of cardiac origin is a major entity, but for purposes of this presentation, it will not be considered a primary manifestation of arterial disease of the extracranial system.

Atherosclerosis

The atherosclerotic plaque consists of nodular deposition of fat, primarily cholesterol, in the arterial intima. There is an associated inflammatory response resulting in fibroblastic proliferation (Fig. 113–2). In addition, calcium salts may be precipitated in the primary fatty plaque, producing various degrees of calcification of the lesion. The lesion may enlarge as a result of progression of the atheromatous process, or it may be altered by a sudden intraplaque hemorrhage causing precipitous enlargement and possibly occlusion. With either slow or rapid enlargement, there may be a rupture of the intimal lining with discharge of degenerative atheromatous debris into the lumen of the vessel. Following such an atheromatous discharge, an open cavity remains within the central portion of the lesion. This cavity, or so-called ulcer, can be the nidus for platelet aggregation or thrombus formation or the outlet for further degenerative plaque egress (Fig. 113–3). If the aggregates within the ulcer are only loosely attached, they can be swept into the arterial bloodstream as secondary arterial emboli.

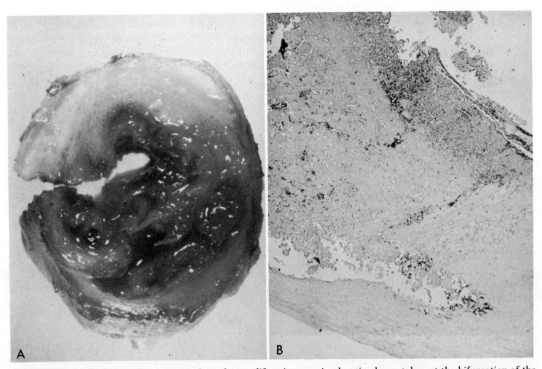

FIGURE 113–2. *A*, Cross section through a proliferative arteriosclerotic plaque taken at the bifurcation of the common carotid artery. Note the tiny lumen that remains. The material is glistening and consists primarily of cholesterol and necrotic atheromatous debris. *B*, Microscopic section at 10× magnification. The atheromatous portion of the diseased intima is at the upper part of the photograph. The small spaces or clefts distributed throughout the intimal lesion represent cholesterol crystals.

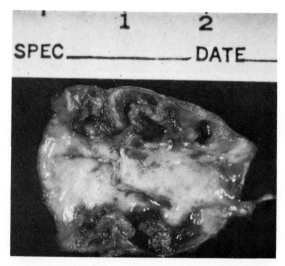

FIGURE 113–3. Atherosclerotic plaque removed from a carotid bifurcation and opened longitudinally to demonstrate the cavities, or ulcers, produced by evacuation of atheromatous debris. These ulcers continue to harbor degenerative atheromatous debris, platelet aggregate material, and thrombus.

Atheromatous lesions characteristically occur at branches or arterial bifurcations. The common sites include the points of takeoff for the branches of the aortic arch; the origins of the vertebral artery from the subclavian artery; the bifurcation of the common carotid artery and, particularly, the carotid bulb; the carotid siphon; and the origins of the anterior and middle cerebral arteries. The course of the basilar artery may also be studied with atheromatous beads, often corresponding with the origins of major

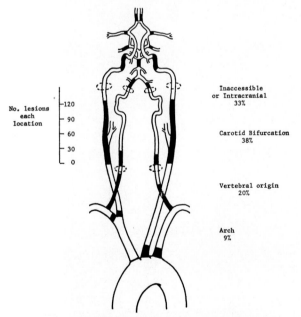

FIGURE 113–4. Location and incidence of significant atherosclerotic lesions. The length of the dark area at each location (measured against the scale at left) corresponds to the number of lesions detected by arteriography in this series. (Reprinted by permission of the Western Journal of Medicine: Blaisdell FW, Hall AD, Thomas AN, Ross SJ: Cerebrovascular occlusive disease. Experience with panarteriography in 300 consecutive cases. Calif Med 103:321, 1965.)

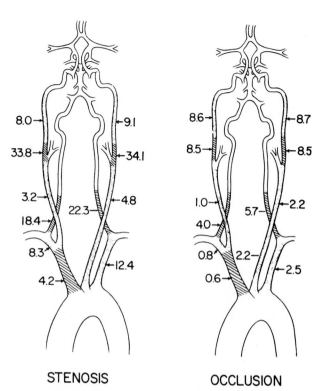

STENOSIS   OCCLUSION

FIGURE 113–5. Frequency distribution of arterial lesions at surgically accessible sites (4748 patients). (From Hass WK, Fields WS, North RR, et al: Joint study of extracranial arterial occlusion. II. Arteriography, techniques, sites, and complications. JAMA 203:961–968. Copyright 1968, American Medical Association.)

branches including the posterior cerebral arteries. All of these locations are of clinical importance, but the relative frequency of involvement of each potential site influences the frequency of occurrence of various clinical manifestations. The predilection of the carotid bifurcation for atheromatous plaquing has been extensively studied and appears to be related to arterial geometry, velocity profile, and wall shear stress.[117] The relative distribution has been studied both by angiography and at the time of autopsy (Figs. 113–4 to 113–6). Without question, the most common location of significant lesions is the carotid bifurcation. The ratio of extracranial to intracranial lesions is in excess of 2:1. Blaisdell and associates, in a review of aortocranial angiograms of 300 patients, noted that 33 per cent of lesions seen on angiography were distributed intracranially or in locations that were inaccessible to direct surgical repair.[7] The remaining 67 per cent were extracranial, with 38 per cent of all lesions located at the carotid bifurcation, 20 per cent at vertebral origins, and 9 per cent at the origin of the branches of the aortic arch. Hass and coworkers, reviewing the arteriograms of 4748 patients followed in the joint study of extracranial arterial occlusive disease, reported a similar distribution.[47]

Arterial Elongation, Tortuosity, and Kinking

Sixteen to 21 per cent of the carotid arteriograms of adults demonstrate some degree of elongation of the inter-

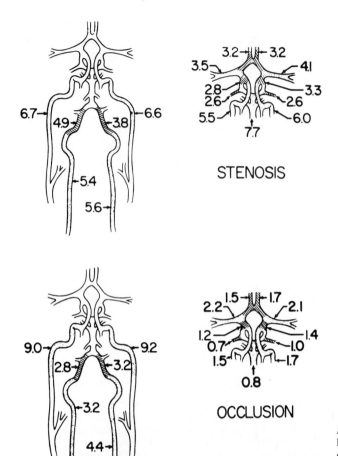

STENOSIS

OCCLUSION

FIGURE 113–6.   Frequency distribution of surgically inaccessible lesions. (From Hass WK, Fields WS, North RR, et al: Joint study of extracranial arterial occlusion. II. Arteriography, techniques, sites, and complications. JAMA 203:961–968. Copyright 1968, American Medical Association.)

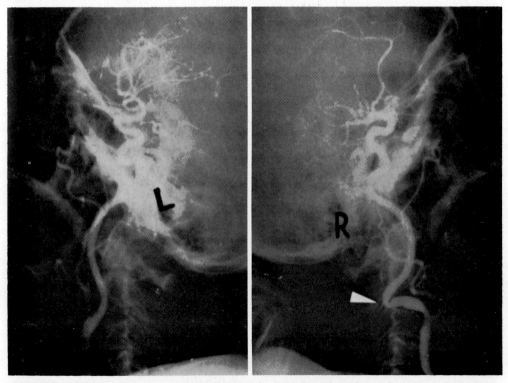

FIGURE 113–7.   Carotid arteriograms showing bilateral coiling of circular configuration at level of base of skull (*arrow* shows 360-degree coil). No aneurysmal dilatation is present in proximal segment of arteries. (From Weibel J, Fields WS: Tortuosity, coiling, and kinking of the internal carotid artery. I. Etiology and radiographic anatomy. Neurology [Minneap] 15:7, 1965.)

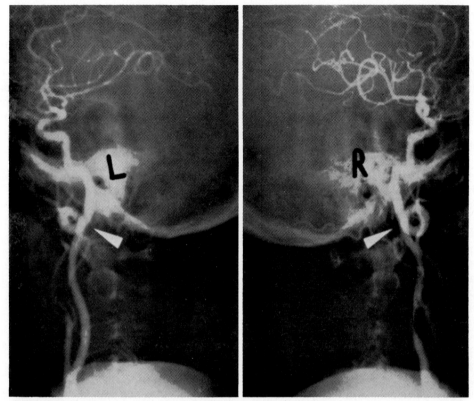

FIGURE 113–8. Carotid arteriograms demonstrating mild post-stenotic aneurysmal dilatation and kinking of the right internal carotid artery *(arrowheads)*. Left internal carotid artery has S-shaped tortuosity. (From Weibel J, Fields WS: Tortuosity, coiling, and kinking of the internal carotid artery. I. Etiology and radiographic anatomy. Neurology [Minneap] 15:7, 1965.)

nal carotid artery in its cervical portion. The extent can vary from a mild tortuosity to as much as a 360-degree coil (Fig. 113–7). On occasion, excessive redundancy of the vessel will produce kinking with apparent compromise of blood flow[91] (Fig. 113–8). These changes are attributed to either congenital or acquired factors. The carotid artery is formed from the third aortic arch and the dorsal aorta. During embryonic development, the carotid normally is redundant or kinked. As the heart descends into the thorax, the carotid artery is stretched and the redundancy is eliminated. Some redundancy may remain until further growth takes place, as evidenced by a redundancy rate as high as 43 per cent seen in arteriograms of infants.[99, 112] The acquired form of carotid redundancy is attributed to a manifestation of atherosclerosis that produces lengthening of the affected vessels leading to redundancy and, ultimately, to anatomic kinking.

Fibromuscular Dysplasia

The pathology of this entity is discussed in detail in Chapter 122.

Extrinsic Compression

Extrinsic compression of the cervical arteries carrying blood to the brain is seen most often in the vertebral arteries as they course through the bony vertebral canal. Hyperos-

toses, or bone spurs, related to the cervical transverse processes can impinge on the vertebral artery and result in compression.[3, 5, 46, 102]

Another source of external compression can be caused by neoplasms within the neck. Tumors can surround the carotid artery and invade its wall.

Radiation-Induced Carotid Stenosis

It has been long recognized experimentally that external radiation can produce an arterial injury.[71] With the increasing use of cervical radiation to treat neoplasia, we are now beginning to see patients with radiation-induced atherosclerotic change producing symptomatic carotid artery disease.[26, 75]

Postoperative Restenosis of the Carotid Artery

The pathology of this lesion is discussed in detail in Chapter 126.

Traumatic Occlusion and Spontaneous Intimal Dissection

Blunt craniocervical trauma, as a result of either a direct blow or the indirect effect of sudden head and neck extension, has been reported to produce occlusion of the internal carotid artery.[34, 35, 53, 100] Angiographic and autopsy studies suggest that the most likely mechanism for this phenomenon is a tear of the intima followed by an acute intimal dissection, resulting in an occlusion of the lumen with secondary thrombosis. Spontaneous intimal dissection in the absence of trauma can also occur (Fig. 113–9).

Inflammatory Arteriopathies

Inflammatory conditions are rare, but they should be kept in mind during the evaluation of patients with cerebrovascular symptoms. Takayasu's disease is an inflammatory arteriopathy that involves the major trunks of the aortic arch. This is most frequently seen in females and occurs with greatest frequency in Asia and the Middle East. It has also been reported with some frequency in Latin America. It is less common in North America and Europe. The lesion produces occlusion of major branches of the aortic arch with the concomitant physical findings and varying symptomatic manifestations.[60] One dramatic finding on examination is often the total absence of extremity pulses; hence, the common synonym for this condition is "pulseless disease." The central nervous system may also be involved in the systemic collagen vascular diseases, which include periarteritis nodosa, lupus erythematosus, and temporal arteritis.

Migraine

The vasospasm associated with migraine prodrome can cause transient neurologic dysfunction. The visual symptoms associated with the prodrome, the so-called scintillating scotoma, on occasion can be mistaken or misinterpreted as amaurosis fugax. There are also documented cases of permanent neurologic damage resulting from the prolonged phase of cerebral vasospastic prodrome.

PATHOGENETIC MECHANISMS OF CEREBRAL DYSFUNCTION

In addition to a knowledge of the various pathologic lesions that can affect the extracranial system, an understanding of the mechanism by which a lesion produces symptoms, either transient or permanent, is of particular importance when planning a diagnostic work-up and selecting appropriate therapy.

Lateralizing Transient Ischemic Attacks

Several theories have been proposed to explain ischemic events that are transient in nature. These have included

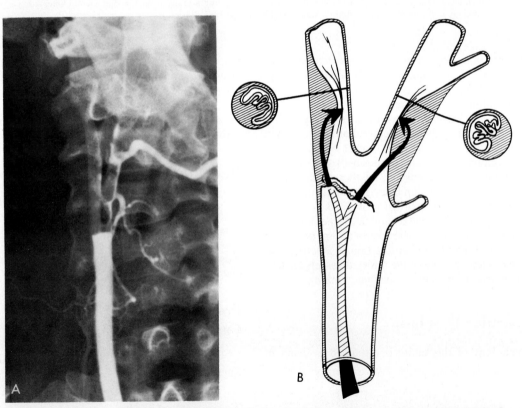

FIGURE 113–9. *A,* Right carotid arteriogram of a 32-year-old man who experienced a sudden episode of left hemiparesis. Carotid arteriography demonstrates a sharp cutoff contrast at the carotid bifurcation with faint visualization of the internal and external carotid arteries beyond. Subsequent exploration of this region revealed a spontaneous transverse intimal tear with subintimal dissection of blood and distal occlusion. *B,* Artist's concept of an intimal tear with subintimal dissection of blood and occlusion of the lumen. The insets of the internal and external carotid arteries in cross section graphically demonstrate luminal compromise by subintimal dissection.

cerebral angiospasm, mechanical reduction of cerebral blood flow secondary to a critical arterial lesion, cerebral emboli originating from arteriosclerotic plaques, cervical arterial kinking or compression, polycythemia, anemia, and the transient shunting of blood away from the brain such as is seen in the subclavian steal syndrome.[19, 77, 79] The theory of cerebral vasospasm was held to be an important mechanism in the not-too-distant past. Therapy that was advocated to treat symptoms that were due to cerebral vasospasm included carotid arterectomy or cervical sympathetic ganglionectomy.[59] Eastcott and colleagues spoke out against the vasospastic theory, stating that it would be difficult to conceive of spasm involving just those few vessels that were required to produce repetitive ischemic attacks, while the remaining cerebral vessels were left unaffected.[23] Rothenberg and Corday[95] produced experimental evidence against the angiospasm theory, and Millikan[79] pointed out that such potent vasodilators as 5 per cent carbon dioxide mixed with 95 per cent oxygen and cervical sympathectomy were not effective in preventing or treating attacks of transient cerebral ischemia. Two theories emerged as the primary explanation for transient ischemic events. These are the arterial stenotic theory (mechanical flow reduction) and the cerebral embolic theory.

During the early experience with carotid artery disease, most surgeons accepted the concept that arterial stenosis, producing reduced cerebral blood flow, represented the mechanism for transient cerebral ischemia. For example, Crawford and coworkers stated that the criterion for carotid endarterectomy should be the presence of a pressure gradient across a stenosis involving the internal carotid artery.[15] These authors measured the carotid artery pressure during operation, and if a gradient was present across a stenotic lesion, an endarterectomy was performed. If no gradient could be documented, the artery was not opened, since it was assumed that the patient's symptoms might be due to something other than a lesion in the carotid artery. On the basis of this experience, the authors stated that at least a 50 per cent stenosis, as measured in one projection of an arteriogram, was necessary to justify operation on the carotid artery. In their opinion, a gradient indicated not only decreased flow in that artery but also a decrease in total cerebral blood flow. This concept was affirmed by other investigators.[17, 18, 50] Haller and Turrell stated that cerebral ischemia as a result of carotid artery disease was purely the result of mechanical flow obstruction and that surgical treatment should be directed at relief of this obstruction.[44] They concluded that lesions that failed to produce a pressure gradient did not constitute a significant threat to the patient. The mechanical concept of transient cerebral ischemia is appealing, particularly when surgeons are used to treating stenotic or obstructive arteries in other locations. The concept of transient ischemia has been likened to intermittent claudication of the brain. However, with the advent of techniques for the measurement of cerebral blood flow, it has been determined that the cerebral perfusion rate is relatively constant. For this reason, it is difficult to understand how a constant stenosis could produce intermittent reduction in blood flow. In an attempt to explain this inconsistency, several authors suggested that TIAs may result from intermittent episodes of systemic hypotension or decreased cardiac output in patients with stenosed or occluded cerebral arteries.[14, 19, 56]

In spite of the wide acceptance of the hemodynamic theory, there appeared increasing evidence to dispute it. In 1963, Adams and associates studied cerebral blood flow in patients with carotid and vertebral artery stenoses. They found that cerebral blood flow, prior to carotid artery surgery, was normal and that endarterectomy did not produce any change or increase in hemispheric cerebral blood flow.[1] Brice and colleagues measured carotid artery blood flow at the time of ligation for intracranial aneurysm and found that blood flow was not reduced until a stenosis of 84 to 93 per cent was produced.[8] In view of these observations, those who advocate operating on an artery that is only 50 per cent stenotic would have to offer some justification other than the improvement of blood flow. Furthermore, the intermittent nature of ischemic attacks is difficult to reconcile with the presence of a constant stenosis, since there is no significant variation in the demand for cerebral blood flow. Some authors state that transient reduction in blood pressure or cardiac output associated with a stenosis may cause neurologic symptoms. Kendall and Marshall studied 37 patients who had frequent TIAs. They were unable to reproduce these symptoms with deliberately induced systemic hypotension.[65] Similar experience was reported by others.[23, 27] Russell and Cranstone noted that ophthalmic pressures did not diminish in patients with associated ischemic attacks and carotid artery stenosis.[96] When total occlusion of the internal carotid artery occurred, the ophthalmic artery pressure fell transiently, but then rapidly returned to normal levels as collateral circulation became effective. Several authors have noted that TIAs disappear at the time of carotid occlusion.[21, 97] It is unlikely that transient cerebral ischemia results from mechanical reduction of blood flow through a stenosed artery when the symptoms can be relieved by total occlusion of the same vessel. A similar phenomenon has been observed by surgeons who noted that occlusion of the common carotid artery under local anesthesia at the time of carotid endarterectomy is usually well tolerated.

Several authors have stated that hemispheric TIAs can best be explained as a manifestation of cerebral embolization.[43, 52, 79] Atheromatous plaques in the extracranial arteries can be a source of either atheromatous or platelet emboli. The fact that atheromatous plaques can be a source of emboli was first reported by Panum in 1862.[87] Flory reported a series of autopsies in which emboli from atheroma were detected in kidneys, spleen, and thyroid.[33] The presence of emboli, confirmed microscopically, produced areas of infarction in the affected organs. Although Chiari, in 1905, suggested that carotid artery lesions could produce cerebral emboli, this was not documented conclusively until 1947.[12, 78] Handler, studying embolization of atheromatous material in a series of autopsy cases, noted that there was a frequent occurrence of encephalomalacia in patients who demonstrated atheroma embolism to other parts of the body.[45] Prior support for the embolic cause of transient cerebral ischemia came from the reports of Millikan and associates in 1955 and Fisher in 1958, who noted that TIAs could be virtually eliminated if the patients were placed on anticoagulant therapy.[30, 80] In examining the ocular fundus of patients with carotid artery stenosis, Fisher described a "boxcar" effect in the retinal arteries.[31] He did not arrive at a definite explanation for this phenomenon, but suggested that it might represent embolic material in the retinal arteries and that transient cerebral ischemia might be due to the same type of embolism. Hollenhorst described a series of patients with "bright plaques" in the retinal vessels and suggested that these were cholesterol crystals from eroded atheromatous plaques.[51] Russell observed two patients presenting with transient monocular blindness, and concluded that this phenomenon was due to retinal emboli composed of friable thrombus.[97] He stated that if this observation was correct, thrombotic microemboli carried to the brain might be responsible for TIAs often associated with carotid artery disease. McBrien and coworkers performed a histologic examination of retinal vessels of a patient who had been having transient monocular blindness.[74] These authors noted that the material within the vessels was indeed microembolic and consisted of platelets, a few leukocytes, and a small quantity of lipid material. Julian and associates reported a series of patients in whom ulceration was seen in carotid plaques at the time of operation.[61] They postulated that thrombotic material within the ulcer might embolize and cause episodes of transient cerebral ischemia. Ehrenfeld and colleagues reported a series of patients with carotid stenosis and intermittent monocular blindness.[24] They found that the ocular phenomenon as well as the cerebral ischemic attacks stopped following carotid endarterectomy. Additional evidence for the embolic theory of transient cerebral ischemia comes from the fact that ischemic attacks stop abruptly when carotid stenosis progresses to occlusion, providing that the patient does not go on to have a major stroke. The cessation of TIAs presumably occurs because the route for embolic material to the brain has been obstructed, not because of the establishment of collateral circulation.[21, 96] The relationship between transient cerebral ischemia and emboli has been difficult to prove on the basis of operative results, since the criterion for operation dictates that a hemodynamically significant carotid stenosis be present before an operation is performed. After reviewing the overwhelming evidence in favor of the embolic theory, it occurred to the current author's group that the presence of a hemodynamically significant stenosis is probably not necessary for the release of embolic material.

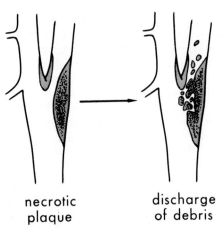

necrotic plaque   discharge of debris

FIGURE 113–10.   Graphic representation of the process by which a bulky atheromatous lesion undergoes central degeneration with subsequent discharge of atheromatous debris into the arterial lumen with embolization to the brain.

Rather, the nature of the plaque itself would be the important factor. Atherosclerotic plaques whose consistency leads to degeneration with atheromatous fragmentation or whose surface characteristics are irregular or ulcerated, thus forming a suitable nidus for platelet aggregation, are the necessary requirements for emboli. The author's group began to operate on patients with so-called nonstenotic ulcerative lesions who were experiencing hemispheric TIAs. In two subsequent publications, this group described prompt relief without recurrence of transient ischemic phenomena following removal of the low-profile or nonstenotic ulcerative lesion.[83, 84] These reports represented the first surgical series in which the lesions removed did not have associated stenosis or compromise in blood flow and in which, therefore, the relief of symptoms could be construed to be due not to the augmentation of blood flow but rather to the removal of the ulcerated plaque as a source of cerebral emboli.

From this discussion, it seems evident that the primary mechanism responsible for episodes of transient monocular or hemispheric symptoms associated with atherosclerotic lesions is cerebral emboli originating from the plaque surface. These emboli may consist of atheromatous debris, platelet aggregate material, or thrombus. Embolization may occur either at the time an atheromatous plaque ruptures

FIGURE 113–11.   An irregular or ulcerated surface on an arterial sclerotic plaque can provide a nidus for deposition of platelet aggregate material. These platelet aggregates can be dislodged into the arterial lumen and can embolize to the intracranial circulation.

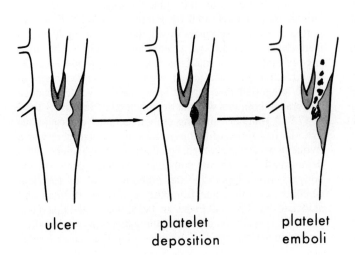

ulcer   platelet deposition   platelet emboli

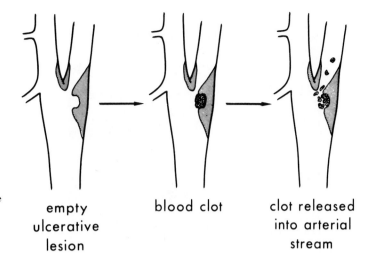

empty
ulcerative
lesion

blood clot

clot released
into arterial
stream

FIGURE 113–12. An empty ulcerative lesion can also be filled with mature thrombus material. The thrombus can be dislodged by the arterial stream or by manipulation, thus releasing clot into the arterial lumen with subsequent cerebral embolization.

into the luminal surface and dislodges atheromatous contents into the bloodstream, or from secondary platelet or thrombus aggregation within the irregularity or ulceration on the surface of the plaque (Figs. 113–10 to 113–16).

One question often posed by those who doubt the embolic theory is: "If these episodes are embolic, why is the same pattern of neurologic dysfunction frequently reproduced in a carbon-copy fashion? Shouldn't the recipient site be random if the cause is really embolization?" The answer to this question is related to the fluid mechanics associated with laminar blood flow. If the source of emboli from an ulcerated atheromatous plaque is located at one

point on the arterial wall circumference, embolic discharge into the bloodstream will inevitably be carried to the same terminal branch because of the characteristics of laminar blood flow. This phenomenon was nicely demonstrated by Millikan. During experiments on cerebral embolization, he introduced tiny metal beads through a needle placed in the internal carotid artery in monkeys. This method of introduction is analogous to a point source of atheromatous embolization. Autopsy studies of these experimental animals demonstrated that the metallic embolic beads would inevitably stack up, one behind the other, in the same cortical branch (Fig. 113–17).

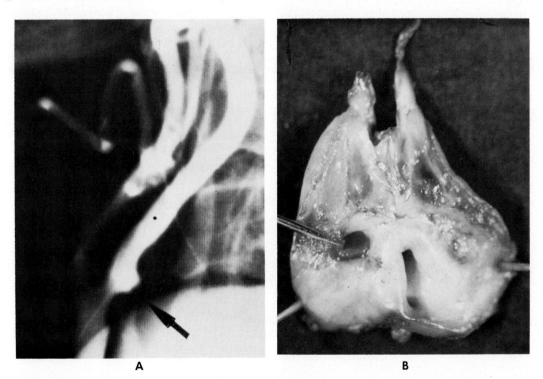

A   **B**

FIGURE 113–13. *A,* Left carotid arteriogram in a patient who was experiencing episodes of left hemispheric transient cerebral ischemia. The *arrow* points to a posterior outpouching of the internal carotid artery just beyond the bifurcation. This finding was interpreted as being an ulcerative atherosclerotic lesion. *B,* Atherosclerotic plaque that corresponds to the angiographically demonstrated lesion. It was removed from the carotid bifurcation, and the pointer indicates the ulcerative lesion containing remnants of mature thrombus.

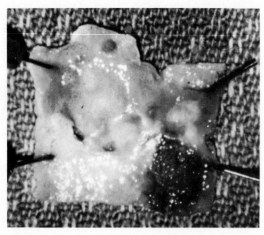

FIGURE 113–14.   Example of an atherosclerotic plaque removed from the carotid bifurcation and opened out for visualization of the luminal surface. In the lower right-hand corner, a mature thrombus is loosely adherent to a very superficial ulceration.

Lateralizing Ischemic Attacks With Concomitant Internal Carotid Occlusion

Although the majority of territorial TIAs are probably caused by emboli of arterial origin that pass through a patent internal carotid artery, we do see patients who experience these symptoms in the presence of a known and totally occluded internal carotid artery. Two possible explanations for these phenomena exist: emboli may come from collateral sources; or marginally perfused brain tissue, distal to the internal carotid artery occlusion, may temporarily fall below the minimal threshold of perfusion to maintain function. The external carotid artery is a well-recognized source of collateral blood flow and a recently recognized source of emboli. Ulcerated plaques at the carotid bifurcation can release emboli into the external carotid artery, where they pass retrograde via collateral communications to the ophthalmic artery and subsequently to the carotid siphon and into branches of the middle cerebral artery.[13, 48] Barnett and colleagues have identified the "stump" of the occluded internal carotid artery as a source of emboli to the external carotid artery.[6] This stump serves as a functional ulcer feeding emboli to a major collateral branch.

Emboli can also reach the hemisphere ipsilateral to an internal carotid artery occlusion from the opposite carotid artery or from the vertebral-basilar system.

Finally, marginally perfused brain, distal to an internal carotid artery occlusion, will be more susceptible to temporary alterations in systemic blood pressure. In this instance, the cerebral vasculature is maximally vasodilated and therefore does not have the capacity to autoregulate in response to a drop in blood pressure. There will be a direct and linear relationship between blood pressure and perfusion.

Nonlateralizing Transient Ischemic Attacks

Nonlateralizing ischemic attacks, such as dizziness, vertigo, ataxia, or syncope, may represent symptoms that are associated with brain stem or posterior circulation dysfunction. Because these attacks are often precipitated by postural changes, the mechanism is presumed to be flow-related rather than a consequence of emboli. In order to make this connection between symptoms and lesions, it is necessary to have either occlusive lesions of several extracranial vessels involving both anterior and posterior circulation or a critical lesion in the vertebral-basilar distribution with an effective anatomic disconnection between anterior and posterior blood flow.

One variant of posterior circulation ischemia occurs with the subclavian steal syndrome. The anatomic lesion

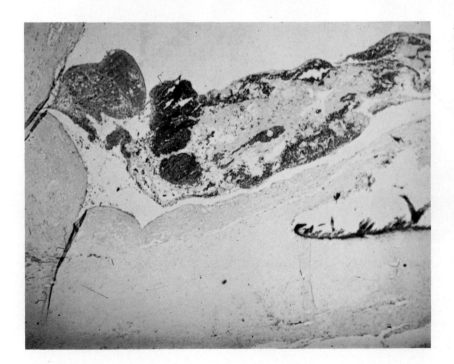

FIGURE 113–15.   Microscopic section through a superficial ulcerating atheromatous plaque. Loose fibrin platelet thrombus material is demonstrated within the ulcer crater.

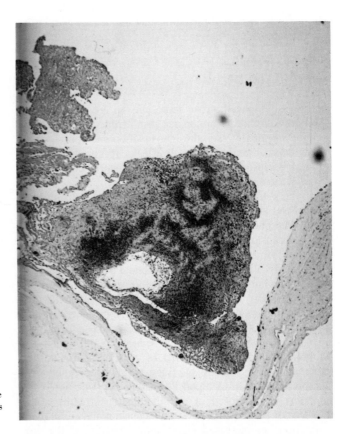

FIGURE 113–16. Microscopic section taken through a deeper ulcerating lesion of an atheromatous plaque removed from the carotid bifurcation. An organizing thrombus, only loosely attached, is seen partially filling the ulcer crater.

and the collateral circulatory response to arm ischemia have been described previously. It is easy to associate brain stem ischemic symptoms that occur with arm exercise in the presence of an ipsilateral subclavian artery occlusion; blood is diverted away from the vertebral-basilar system as a result of retrograde flow down the ipsilateral vertebral artery. This diversion occurs because the vertebral artery now functions as a collateral channel for the exercising upper extremity. However, in order for this to occur, the principal or dominant vertebral artery must be on the side of the subclavian stenosis or occlusion. If the dominant vertebral artery is on the opposite side and a smaller vertebral artery is on the side of subclavian occlusion, it is not physiologi-

cally possible for a small artery to steal sufficient quantity of blood from the posterior circulation because the opposite or dominant vertebral artery can more than make up the difference. Likewise, if the dominant vertebral artery is on the side of a total subclavian artery occlusion and the opposite vertebral is either small or absent, it is possible to have these symptoms in the absence of arm exercise because, in this instance, the subclavian artery stenosis or occlusion becomes a de facto vertebral artery stenosis or occlusion and compromises blood flow through this dominant vessel to the brain stem.[25, 76]

It is probable that emboli may occur in association with atherosclerotic plaques in the vertebral-basilar system,

FIGURE 113–17. Brain of monkey removed following experimental embolization with ball bearings. The ball bearings were introduced from a point source in the carotid artery. Note that all the ball bearings lodged in a single cortical branch. (Courtesy of Dr. Clark Millikan, Mayo Department of Neurology, Mayo Clinic.)

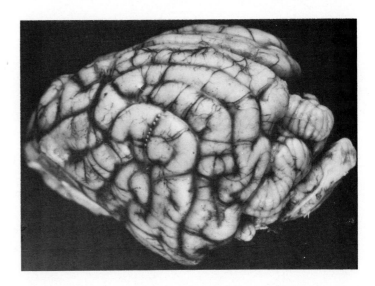

but the exact nature of the clinical consequences of such an event is not clear at present.

Completed Stroke

The completed stroke represents an area of brain infarction. Cerebral infarction can result from embolic occlusion of a critical vessel, thrombosis of an end-vessel, or an acute deprivation of blood flow as a result of proximal arterial occlusion with inadequate collateral contribution through the circle of Willis.

The mechanism of embolic occlusion of a distal cerebral vessel is essentially the same as that of a hemispheric TIA. Why one embolic event results in transient symptoms on one occasion and produces an area of cerebral infarction at a later time is the subject of considerable speculation. Presumably, the variables that operate during any one embolic event must include the size of the embolus, the nature of the embolic material, and the final location of the embolic fragment. A large embolus clearly presents a major threat of infarction, since the likelihood of subsequent fragmentation or rapid clot lysis is reduced. Similarly, if the embolic material is composed of platelet aggregates or thrombus, the chances of fragmentation or lysis with prompt restoration of blood flow are good, whereas if the embolus is composed of an atheromatous fragment, the chances of permanent end-vessel occlusion and subsequent infarction are increased significantly. Finally, if the embolus lodges in a critical location such as the internal capsule, the time during which the ischemic changes are reversible is likely to be shorter and the neurologic dysfunction that occurs with such a critical embolization is likely to be more prominent.

Evidence using computed tomography (CT) scanning and magnetic resonance imaging (MRI) also indicates that what is clinically a transient ischemic event is actually cerebral infarction in a small focal zone that is compensated for function by adjacent tissue.

It is likely that intracerebral thrombosis is caused by one of two mechanisms. The first is related to intracranial atheromatosis, with branch vessel occlusion occurring in association with a critical stenotic lesion. The second mechanism results from propagation of thrombus from the internal carotid artery distal to the proximal atheromatous stenosis. The top of the column of thrombus in the internal carotid artery can literally spill into the middle cerebral artery and cause occlusion and cerebral infarction. This mechanism has not been recognized uniformly, but it can be deduced from the sequence of events that take place with carotid thrombosis. An atheromatous lesion located at the origin of the internal carotid artery will slowly and progressively cause a reduction of blood flow as the lesion produces a further compromise of cross-sectional luminal area. Ultimately, the lesion approaches a critical compromise, following which the flow is so reduced that thrombosis will occur. When this happens, there may be no sequelae, or the patient may suffer a cerebral infarction with major neurologic deficit. Because the flow is so reduced just prior to occlusion, it is unreasonable to assume that the tiny flow through the vessel before occlusion is really that important and that the absence of this tiny flow will make the difference between live functioning brain and cerebral infarction. In some patients, when thrombosis occurs, the column of clot probably progresses up to the first major branch, such as the ophthalmic artery, and stops. In this instance, the clinical consequence of stroke is unlikely, and this sequence represents the events that occur in patients who later are found to have an asymptomatic carotid occlusion. In other patients, however, the clot may not stop at the siphon branches but may progress through the siphon to the takeoff of the middle cerebral artery. If some of this clot "spills over" or is carried by collateral blood flow, thrombotic occlusion of a major intracranial artery will occur and cerebral infarction will be the consequence, resulting in a major stroke (Fig. 113–18). This phenomenon has been demonstrated at autopsy in patients who died shortly after a critical event. If the patient lives for a consid-

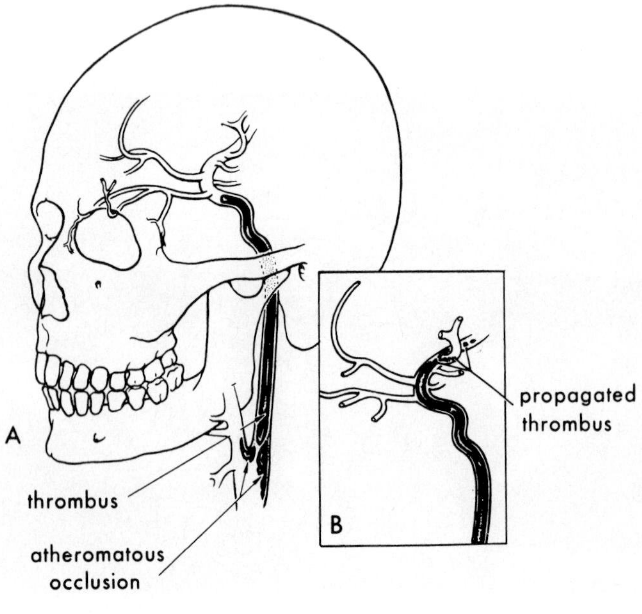

FIGURE 113–18. *A*, Artist's concept of the events following carotid occlusion. The thrombus within the internal carotid artery ascends to the first branch of that artery, the ophthalmic artery. At this point, the thrombus stops and the remaining portion of the intracranial circulation is not compromised. *B*, An alternative sequence of events in which the thrombus does not stop at the ophthalmic artery but progresses up to the terminal branches of the internal carotid artery, so that thrombus material spills over and propagates into the middle cerebral artery, producing cerebral infarction.

propagated thrombus

thrombus

atheromatous occlusion

A

B

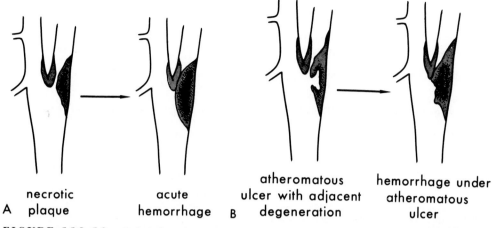

necrotic

A plaque

acute

hemorrhage **B**

atheromatous
ulcer with adjacent
degeneration

hemorrhage under
atheromatous
ulcer

FIGURE 113–19. *A,* Artist's concept of spontaneous hemorrhage within an atherosclerotic plaque resulting in sudden acute occlusion of the internal carotid artery. *B,* A similar phenomenon can occur within the depths of an atheromatous ulcer, producing acute cessation of blood flow.

erable time after the initial stroke, the propagated thrombus will usually undergo lysis back to the branches of the siphon and no clue will remain at subsequent autopsy to demonstrate the actual events that occurred.

On occasion, a modest atheromatous lesion of the internal carotid artery may undergo sudden intraplaque hemorrhage. This will produce an acute occlusion (Fig. 113–19). This precipitate event will cause an acute change in circulatory dynamics. Occlusion of this type will produce acute ischemia, and probably infarction, in the distribution of that artery. Likewise, thrombosis and propagation as described earlier may also take place with the same consequences.

Stroke-in-Evolution

The stroke-in-evolution, in contrast to a simple acute stroke, is one in which the resultant neurologic deficit progressively worsens by a series of discrete exacerbations occurring over a period of hours or days. The exact mechanism for this type of progression is unknown. There are several hypotheses that can be speculated on to explain this pattern. One might be a series of infarct-producing emboli from a bulky, friable, carotid bifurcation lesion. These emboli, occurring serially, would result in a series of events that produce a progressively worsening neurologic deficit.[38, 39] Another explanation might be a series of thromboemboli coming off the top of a thrombotic column in an occluded internal carotid artery. A third possibility might involve the dynamics of the infarct zone such as secondary thrombosis or occlusion of a neighboring vessel in the brain substance as the result of edema or expansion of the original infarct zone as a consequence of central hemorrhage, although this last mechanism is probably unlikely.

Deterioration of Intellectual Function

The relationship between intellectual dysfunction with cerebrovascular disease is a hotly debated issue among neu-

rologists. Many believe that dementia is not a manifestation of vascular disease, but others do not share this concept. The subjective responses of patients following carotid thromboendarterectomy are interesting. Patients often will report an improvement in intellectual function following successful operation, which may be manifested as improved ability to carry out mathematical operations, improved reading comprehension, better conversational ability, and so forth. The patients' observations usually are shared by their friends or relatives.[110]

If we accept the notion that intellectual abilities are a function of cerebral performance, and that reduced blood flow, either from proximal arterial occlusive disease or from distal embolization, can impair cerebral function, it is reasonable to assume that multiple thromboembolic events in the areas of the brain that are silent with regard to motor and sensory functions but are important to intellectual function may be affected adversely by decreased arterial perfusion. Areas that may be so affected include the frontal lobes. If the embolic or ischemic events persist, intellectual deterioration may result in time. The author's group has followed several such patients who, when arteriograms were finally performed, demonstrated loss of multiple branches in the distribution of the anterior cerebral artery. This group has also had experience with patients who were somnolent when first examined, being aroused with great difficulty, and in whom there were multiple extracranial stenoses or occlusions. Repair or bypass of these lesions resulted in a prompt return to normal level of consciousness and a resumption of previous intellectual function.

In evaluating the status of patients following cerebrovascular operations, the surgeon must be careful to avoid taking credit for seeming intellectual improvement as a result of the effect of operation. The patient who is told that a major occlusive lesion was removed from a critical artery going to his or her brain may, following operation, exhibit a brightness and jubilation because he or she believes that his or her brain is now going to work better. Improved intracranial function may be a sham effect of operation, but correction of multiple cerebral occlusive lesions with intellectual improvement is an undeniable observation.

References

1. Adams JE, Smith MC, Wylie EJ: Cerebral blood flow and hemodynamics in extracranial vascular disease: Effect of endarterectomy. Surgery 53:449, 1963.
2. Adelman SM: The national survey of stroke/economic impact. Stroke 12(part 2):I-69, 1981.
3. Bakay L, Leslie EV: Surgical treatment of vertebral artery insufficiency caused by cervical spondylosis. J Neurosurg 23:596, 1965.
4. Baker RN, Schwartz WS, Ramseyer JC: Prognosis among survivors of ischemic stroke. Neurology (Minneap) 18:933, 1968.
5. Balla JI, Langford KH: Vertebral artery compression in cervical spondylosis. Med J Aust 1:284, 1967.
6. Barnett HJM, Peerless SJ, Kaufmann JCE: ''Stump'' on internal carotid artery—A source for further cerebral embolic ischemia. Stroke 9:448, 1978.
7. Blaisdell FW, Hall AD, Thomas AN, et al: Cerebrovascular occlusive disease. Experience with panarteriography in 300 consecutive cases. Calif Med 103:321, 1965.
8. Brice JG, Dowsett DJ, Lowe RD: Hemodynamic effects of carotid artery stenosis. Br Med J 3:1363, 1964.
9. Cadwalader WB: Unilateral optic atrophy and contralateral hemiplegia consequent on occlusion of the cerebral vessels. JAMA 59:2248, 1912.
10. Carrea R, Molins M, Murphy G: Surgical treatment of spontaneous thrombosis of the internal carotid artery in the neck. Carotid-carotid anastomosis: Report of a case. Acta Neurol Lat Am 1:71, 1955.
11. Chambers BR, Norris JW: Outcome in patients with asymptomatic neck bruits. N Engl J Med 315:860, 1986.
12. Chiari H: Ueber das Verhalten des Teilungswinkels der Carotid communis bei der Endarteriitis chronica deformans. Verh Dtsch Ges Pathol 9:326, 1905.
13. Connolly JE, Stemmer EA: Endarterectomy of the external carotid artery. Arch Surg 106:799, 1973.
14. Corday E, Rothenberg S, Weiner SM: Cerebral vascular insufficiency: An explanation of the transient stroke. Arch Intern Med 98:683, 1956.
15. Crawford ES, DeBakey ME, Blaisdell FW, et al: Hemodynamic alterations in patients with cerebral arterial insufficiency before and after operation. Surgery 48:76, 1960.
16. DeBakey ME: Successful carotid endarterectomy for cerebrovascular insufficiency. Nineteen-year follow-up. JAMA 233:1083, 1975.
17. DeBakey ME, Crawford ES, Fields WS: Surgical treatment of patients with cerebral arterial insufficiency associated with extracranial arterial occlusive lesions. Neurology (Minneap) 11:145, 1961.
18. DeBakey ME, Crawford ES, Cooley DA, et al: Cerebral arterial insufficiency: One- to 11-year results following arterial reconstructive operation. Ann Surg 161:921, 1965.
19. Denny-Brown D: Recurrent cerebrovascular episodes. Arch Neurol 2:194, 1960.
20. Dixon S, Pais SO, Raviola C, et al: Natural history of nonstenotic asymptomatic ulcerative lesions of the carotid artery: A further analysis. Arch Surg 117:1493, 1982.
21. Drake WE Jr, Drake MAL: Clinical and angiographic correlates of cerebrovascular insufficiency. Am J Med 45:253, 1968.
22. Dyken ML: Precipitating factors, prognosis, and demography of cerebrovascular disease in an Indiana community: A review of all patients hospitalized from 1963 to 1965 with neurological examination of survivors. Stroke 1:261, 1970.
23. Eastcott HHG, Pickering GW, Robb CG: Reconstruction of internal carotid artery in a patient with intermittent attacks of hemiplegia. Lancet 2:994, 1954.
24. Ehrenfeld WK, Hoyt WF, Wylie EJ: Embolization and transient blindness from carotid atheroma. Surgical considerations. Arch Surg 93:787, 1966.
25. Eklof B, Schwartz SI: Effects of subclavian steal and compromised cephalic blood flow on cerebral circulation. Surgery 68:431, 1969.
26. Elerding SC, Fernandez RN, Grotta JC, et al: Carotid artery disease following external cervical irradiation. Ann Surg 194:609, 1981.
27. Fazekas JF, Alman RW: The role of hypotension in transitory focal cerebral ischemia. Am J Med Sci 248:567, 1964.
28. Feigin I, Budzilovich GN: The general pathology of cerebrovascular disease. In Vinken PJ, Bruyn GW (eds): Handbook of Clinical Neurology. Part I. Amsterdam, North-Holland Publishing Co, 1972.
29. Fields WS: Selection of stroke patients for arterial reconstructive surgery. Am J Surg 125:527, 1973.
30. Fisher CM: The use of anticoagulants in cerebral thrombosis. Neurology 8:311, 1958.
31. Fisher CM: Observations of the fundus oculi in transient monocular blindness. Neurology (Minneap) 9:333, 1959.
32. Fisher CM, Pritchard JE, Mathews WH: Arteriosclerosis of the carotid arteries. Circulation 6:457, 1952.
33. Flory CM: Arterial occlusions produced by emboli from eroded aortic atheromatous plaques. Am J Pathol 21:549, 1945.
34. Garg AG, Gordon DS, Taylor AR, et al: Internal carotid artery thrombosis secondary to closed craniocervical trauma. Br J Surg 55:4, 1968.
35. Gee W, Kaupp HA, McDonald KM, et al: Spontaneous dissection of internal carotid arteries. Arch Surg 115:944, 1980.
36. Gertler MM, Rusk HA, Whiter HH, et al: Ischemic cerebrovascular disease. The assessment of risk factors. Geriatrics 23:135, 1968.
37. Goldner JC, Whisnant JP, Taylor WF: Long-term prognosis of transient cerebral ischemic attacks. Stroke 2:160, 1971.
38. Goldstone J, Moore WS: Emergency carotid artery surgery in neurologically unstable patients. Arch Surg 111:1284, 1976.
39. Goldstone J, Moore WS: A new look at emergency carotid artery operations for the treatment of cerebrovascular insufficiency. Stroke 9:599, 1978.
40. Gowers WR: On a case of simultaneous embolism of central retinal and middle cerebral arteries. Lancet 2:794, 1875.
41. Grunnet ML: Cerebrovascular disease: Diabetes and cerebral atherosclerosis. Neurology (Minneap) 13:486, 1963.
42. Gunning AJ, Pickering GW, Robb-Smith AHT, et al: Mural thrombosis of the internal carotid artery and subsequent embolism. Q J Med 33:155, 1964.
43. Guthrie LG, Mayou S: Right hemiplegia and atrophy of left optic nerve. Proc R Soc Med 1:180, 1908.
44. Haller JA Jr, Turrell R: Studies on effectiveness of endarterectomy in treatment of carotid insufficiency. Arch Surg 85:637, 1962.
45. Handler FP: Clinical and pathological significance of atheromatous embolization, with emphasis on an etiology of renal hypertension. Am J Med 20:366, 1956.
46. Hardin CA, Williamson WP, Steegmann AT: Vertebral artery insufficiency produced by cervical osteoarthritic spurs. Neurology (Minneap) 10:855, 1960.
47. Hass WK, Fields WS, North RR, et al: Joint study of extracranial arterial occlusion. II. Arteriography, techniques, sites, and complications. JAMA 203:961, 1968.
48. Hertzer NR: External carotid endarterectomy. Surg Gynecol Obstet 153:186, 1981.
49. Hirst AE Jr, Gore I, Hadley GG, et al: Gross estimation of atherosclerosis in aorta, coronary, and cerebral arteries. A comparative study in Los Angeles and Southern India. Arch Pathol 69:578, 1960.
50. Hohf RP: The clinical evaluation and surgery of internal carotid insufficiency. Surg Clin North Am 47:1:71, 1967.
51. Hollenhorst RW: Significance of bright plaques in the retinal arteries. JAMA 178:23, 1961.
52. Hollenhorst RW: Vascular status of patients who have cholesterol emboli in the retina. Am J Ophthalmol 61:1159, 1966.
53. Houck WS, Jackson JR, Odom DL, et al: Occlusion of the internal carotid artery in the neck secondary to closed trauma to the head and neck: A report of two cases. Ann Surg 159:219, 1964.
54. Humphries AW, Young JR, Santilli PM, et al: Unoperated, asymptomatic significant internal carotid artery stenosis. Surgery 80:695, 1976.
55. Hunt JR: The role of the carotid arteries in the causation of vascular lesions of the brain, with remarks on certain special features of the symptomatology. Am J Med Sci 147:704, 1914.
56. Hutchinson EC, Yates PO: Caroticovertebral stenosis. Lancet 1:2, 1957.
57. Imparato AM, Riles TS, Gorstein F: The carotid bifurcation plaque: Pathologic findings associated with cerebral ischemia. Stroke 10:238, 1979.
58. Javid M: Development of carotid plaque. Am J Surg 138:224, 1979.
59. Johnson HC, Walker AE: The angiographic diagnosis of spontaneous thrombosis of internal and common carotid arteries. J Neurosurg 8:631, 1951.
60. Judge RD, Currier RD, Gracie WA, et al: Takayasu's arteritis and the aortic arch syndrome. Am J Med 32:379, 1962.

61. Julian OC, Dye WS, Javid H, et al: Ulcerative lesions of the carotid artery bifurcation. Arch Surg 86:803, 1963.
62. Kannel WB: Epidemiology of cerebrovascular disease: An epidemiologic study of cerebrovascular disease. *In* Cerebral Vascular Diseases. American Neurological Association and American Heart Association. New York and London, Grune and Stratton, 1966, pp 53–66.
63. Kannel WB, et al: Risk factors in stroke due to cerebral infarction. Stroke 2:423, 1971.
64. Kartchner MM, McRae LP: Noninvasive evaluation and management of the "asymptomatic" carotid bruit. Surgery 82:840, 1977.
65. Kendall RE, Marshall J: Role of hypertension in the genesis of transient focal cerebral ischemic attacks. Br Med J 2:344, 1963.
66. Kroener JM, Dorn PL, Shoor PM, et al: Prognosis of asymptomatic ulcerating carotid lesions. Arch Surg 115:1387, 1980.
67. Kuller LH, Cook LP, Friedman GD: Survey of stroke epidemiology studies. Stroke 3:579, 1972.
68. Landolt AM, Millikan CH: Pathogenesis of cerebral infarction secondary to mechanical carotid artery occlusion. Stroke 1:52, 1970.
69. LeNet M: Le cout des malaides cardio-vasculaires. Coeur et Santé 33(Suppl), Edition Medicale (Commission Paritaire No 55920), Paris, 1982.
70. Levin SM, Sondheimer FK: Stenosis of contralateral asymptomatic carotid artery—To operate or not? Vasc Surg 7:3, 1973.
71. Lindsay S, Entenman C, Ellis EE, Geraci CL: Aortic arteriosclerosis in the dog after localized aortic irradiation with electrons. J Circ Res 10:61, 1962.
72. Marshall J: The natural history of transient cerebrovascular ischemic attacks. Q J Med 131:309, 1964.
73. Matsumoto N, Whisnant JP, Kurland LT, et al: Natural history of stroke in Rochester, Minnesota, 1955 through 1969: An extension of a previous study, 1945 through 1954. Stroke 4:20, 1973.
74. McBrien DJ, Bradley RD, Ashton N: The nature of retinal emboli in stenosis of the internal carotid artery. Lancet 1:697, 1963.
75. McCready RA, Hyde GL, Bivins BA, et al: Radiation-induced arterial injuries. Surgery 93(2):306, 1983.
76. McLaughlin JS, Linberg E, Attar A, et al: Cerebral vascular insufficiency. Syndromes of reversed blood flow in vessels supplying the brain. Am Surg 33:317, 1967.
77. Meyer JS: Occlusive cerebrovascular disease. Pathogenesis and treatment. Am J Med 30:577, 1961.
78. Meyer WW: Cholesterinkrystallembolie kleiner Organarterien und ihre Folgen. Virchows Arch Pathol Anat 314:616, 1947.
79. Millikan CH: The pathogenesis of transient focal cerebral ischemia. Circulation 32:438, 1965.
80. Millikan CH, Siekert RG, Shick RM: Studies in cerebrovascular disease. V. The use of anticoagulant drugs in the treatment of intermittent insufficiency of the internal carotid arterial system. Proc Staff Meeting Mayo Clin 30:578, 1955.
81. Moniz E, Lima A, deLacerda R: Hemiplegies par thrombose de la carotide interne. Presse Med 45:977, 1937.
82. Moore WS, Boren C, Malone JM, et al: Natural history of nonstenotic asymptomatic ulcerative lesions of the carotid artery. Arch Surg 113:1352, 1978.
83. Moore WS, Hall AD: Ulcerated atheroma of the carotid artery. A cause of transient cerebral ischemia. Am J Surg 116:237, 1968.
84. Moore WS, Hall AD: Importance of emboli from carotid bifurcation in pathogenesis of cerebral ischemic attacks. Arch Surg 101:708, 1970.
85. Moossy J: Morphology sites and epidemiology of cerebral atherosclerosis. Res Publ Assoc Res Nerv Ment Dis 41:1, 1966.
86. Muci-Mendoza R, Arruga J, Edward WO, et al: Retinal fluorescein angiographic evidence for atheromatous microembolism. Stroke 11:154, 1980.
87. Panum PL: Experimentelle Beitrage zur Lehre von der Embolie. Virchows Arch (Pathol Anat) 25:308, 1862.
88. Parrish HM, Payne GH, Allen WC, et al: Mid-Missouri stroke survey: A preliminary report. Mo Med 63:816, 1966.
89. Paulson OB: Cerebral apoplexy (stroke) pathogenesis, pathophysiology and therapy as illustrated by regional blood flow measurements in the brain. Stroke 2:327, 1971.
90. Peterson RE, Livington KE, Escohar A: Development and distribution of gross atherosclerotic lesions at cervical carotid bifurcation. Neurology (Minneap) 10:955, 1960.
91. Quattlebaum JK Jr, Wade JS, Whiddon CM: Stroke associated with elongation and kinking of the carotid artery: Long-term follow-up. Ann Surg 177:572, 1973.
92. Rob CG: Surgical treatment of extracranial occlusive disease. *In* Dale WA (ed): Management of Arterial Occlusive Disease. Chicago, Year Book Medical Publishers, 1971.
93. Robinson RW, Cohen WD, Higano N, et al: Life-table analysis of survival after cerebral thrombosis: Ten-year experience. JAMA 169:1149, 1959.
94. Roederer GO, Langlois YE, Jager KA, et al: The natural history of carotid arterial disease in asymptomatic patients with cervical bruits. Stroke 15:605, 1984.
95. Rothenberg SF, Corday E: Etiology of the transient cerebral stroke. JAMA 164:2005, 1957.
96. Russell RW, Cranstone WI: Ophthalmodynamometry in carotid artery disease. J Neurol Neurosurg Psychiatry 24:281, 1961.
97. Russell RWR: Observations on the retinal blood-vessels in monocular blindness. Lancet 2:1422, 1961.
98. Sacco RL, Wolf PA, Kannel WB, et al: Survival and recurrence following stroke in the Framingham study. Stroke 13:290, 1982.
99. Sarkari NBS, Holmes JM, Bickerstaff ER: Neurological manifestations associated with internal carotid loops and kinks in children. J Neurol Neurosurg Psychiatry 33:194, 1970.
100. Schneider RC, Lemmen LJ: Traumatic internal carotid artery thrombosis secondary to nonpenetrating injuries to the neck: A problem in the differential diagnosis of craniocerebral trauma. J Neurosurg 9:495, 1952.
101. Schwartz CJ, Mitchell JRA: Atheroma of the carotid and vertebral arterial systems. Br Med J 4:1057, 1961.
102. Sheehan S, Bauer RB, Meyer JS: Vertebral artery compression in cervical spondylosis. Arteriographic demonstration during life of vertebral artery insufficiency due to rotation and extension of the neck. Neurology (Minneap) 10:968, 1960.
103. Strully KJ, Hurwitt ES, Blankenberg HW: Thromboendarterectomy for thrombosis of the carotid artery in the neck. J Neurosurg 10:474, 1953.
104. Thiele BL, Young JV, Chikos PM, et al: Correlation of arteriographic findings and symptoms in cerebrovascular disease. Neurology (NY) 30:1041, 1980.
105. Thompson JE, Austin DJ, Patman RD: Carotid endarterectomy for cerebrovascular insufficiency: Long-term results in 592 patients followed up to thirteen years. Ann Surg 172:663, 1970.
106. Thompson JE, Patman RD: Endarterectomy for asymptomatic carotid bruits. Surg Digest 7:9, 1972.
107. Thompson JE, Patman RD, Talkington CM: Asymptomatic carotid bruit. Ann Surg 188:308, 1978.
108. Toole JF, Janeway R, Choi K, et al: Transient ischemic attacks due to atherosclerosis. A prospective study of 160 patients. Arch Neurol 32:5, 1975.
109. Treiman RL, Foran RF, Shore EH, et al: Carotid bruit. Significance in patients undergoing an abdominal aortic operation. Arch Surg 106:803, 1973.
110. Vitale JH, Pulos SM, Okada A, et al: Relationships of psychological dimensions to impairment in a population with cerebrovascular insufficiency. J Nerv Ment Dis 158:456, 1974.
111. Wallace DC: A study of the natural history of cerebral vascular disease. Med J Aust 1:90, 1967.
112. Weibel J, Fields WS: Tortuosity, coiling, and kinking of the internal carotid artery. I. Etiology and radiographic anatomy. Neurology (Minneap) 15:7, 1965.
113. Whisnant JP: Epidemiology of stroke: Emphasis on transient cerebral ischemic attacks and hypertension. Stroke 5:68, 1974.
114. Whisnant JP, Fitzgibbons JP, Kurland LT, et al: Natural history of stroke in Rochester, Minnesota, 1945 through 1954. Stroke 2:11, 1971.
115. Wiebers DO, Whisnant JP: *In* Warlow C, Morris PJ (eds): Transient Ischemic Attacks. New York, Marcel Dekker, 1982, p 8.
116. Wolfe PA, Kannel WB, McGee DL: Epidemiology of strokes in North America. Stroke 1:19, 1986.
117. Zarins CK, Giddens DP, Bharadvaj BK, et al: Carotid bifurcation atherosclerosis: Quantitative correlation of plaque localization with flow velocity profiles and wall shear stress. J Circ Res 53:502, 1983.
118. Ziegler DK, Hassanein RS: Prognosis in patients with transient ischemic attacks. Stroke 4:666, 1973.
119. The Casanova Study Group: Carotid surgery vs. medical therapy in asymptomatic carotid stenosis. Stroke 22:1229, 1991.

120. Hobson RW II, Weiss DG, Fields WS, et al: Efficacy of carotid endarterectomy for asymptomatic carotid stenosis. N Engl J Med 328:221, 1993.

121. The Asymptomatic Carotid Artery Stenosis Group: Study design for a randomized prospective trial of carotid endarterectomy for asymptomatic atherosclerosis. Stroke 20:844, 1989.

114

Clinical Manifestations and Evaluation of Patients With Ischemic Cerebrovascular Disease

Stanley N. Cohen, M.D.

• • •

Patients presenting with a stroke syndrome need to be evaluated with a carefully taken history, general physical examination, and detailed neurologic examination. The primary goal of this clinical evaluation is to rule out nonvascular diseases that may present with the same clinical signs and symptoms as ischemic stroke. The second goal is to localize the disturbance in cerebral physiology to one vascular distribution, if possible. It is only after the disease has been properly localized, the size of the vessel involved determined, and the most probable etiology evaluated (e.g., embolic, atherosclerotic, vasculitic) that the proper treatment modality can be selected.

CLASSIFICATION OF CEREBRAL ISCHEMIC ATTACKS

There are three major categories of cerebral ischemic neurologic deficits—transient ischemic attack (TIA), resolving ischemic neurologic deficit (RIND), and ischemic infarction. A TIA is a focal area of cerebral ischemia attributable to one cerebrovascular distribution that has a brief duration and clears completely. Episodes of global ischemia, such as those associated with orthostatic hypotension, should not be considered TIAs even though they are brief and resolve completely. Such spells are due to a generalized decrease in blood flow to the brain, not to focal disease. They are not due to the same pathophysiologic mechanisms and, in general, do not carry the same prognosis. They do not require the same treatment as a TIA. The traditional definition of a TIA includes spells lasting up to 24 hours. The majority of TIAs will last from minutes up to a maximum of 4 hours.[1, 2] When a spell lasts longer than a few hours, one should be very suspicious of another disease entity that is masquerading as a TIA. Many patients will

have the bulk of their symptoms resolve relatively rapidly, while "minor" signs and symptoms will remain beyond 24 hours. Some authors have considered this a "TIA with minimum residual." This term has limited usefulness, since the "minimum residual" indicates permanent central nervous system dysfunction and indicates that the patient has had a stroke. Transient monocular blindness, also called amaurosis fugax, is considered a subset of TIA. These spells are almost invariably very brief, lasting from 1 to 30 minutes. A RIND is an ischemic deficit that lasts longer than 24 hours but clears completely within 1 week. The residual deficit beyond 24 hours indicates an area of structural damage to the brain, albeit probably small in size. A RIND has no distinct pathophysiologic or prognostic significance. A patient with a clinically diagnosed ischemic cerebral infarction will have signs and symptoms that do not clear completely. The term cerebrovascular accident (CVA) should be discarded because it lumps thrombotic, embolic, and hemorrhagic stroke into one category. It would be preferable to use the term stroke syndrome until the patient can be categorized as having ischemic or hemorrhagic stroke. A patient with a progressing stroke, or stroke-in-evolution, will show an increasing neurologic deficit over the course of time but has not yet reached the maximal potential loss (i.e., complete plegia or sensory loss). Although many patients will show stroke progression in the first few days after the initial event, progressing stroke may occur up to 2 weeks after the initial event.

CLINICAL MANIFESTATIONS OF MAJOR VESSEL OCCLUSIONS

Careful neurologic examination will help to localize the distribution of the disturbance in cerebral physiology.

No single neurologic finding will enable a precise localization to be made with certainty; however, the constellation of findings may point to the artery involved. Although occlusion of the internal carotid artery may occur asymptomatically, the presentation will depend on the adequacy of the collateral circulation.[3] If the anterior communicating artery is small and the posterior cerebral artery is fed primarily off the carotid rather than the basilar artery, carotid occlusion can result in massive infarction of the entire hemisphere. Such a patient would present with a depressed level of consciousness and contralateral hemiplegia. If sensory modalities could be tested, the patient would be found to have a hemisensory deficit and a homonymous hemianopsia. With adequate collateral supply to the anterior and posterior cerebral arteries, carotid occlusion will present with motor and sensory involvement of the arm, face, and leg, in decreasing order of severity. If the dominant hemisphere is involved, the patient may have a global aphasia. If the nondominant hemisphere is involved, the patient may have left-sided anosognosia (denial of the left-sided weakness) and neglect of the left side.

A mainstem middle cerebral artery (MCA) occlusion may present in a similar fashion.[4] In a patient with poor collateral flow, hemiplegia, hemisensory loss, hemianopsia, and a tonic gaze deviation toward the side of the lesion can be seen. The MCA occlusion can present with a decreased level of consciousness in about 25 per cent of patients.[5] If only the upper division of the MCA is involved, the infarct will involve the cortical surface of the frontal and anterior parietal lobes. The lower two thirds of the face and the arm will be primarily affected, with relative sparing of the leg. In the dominant hemisphere, the aphasia would be predominantly a motor (Broca's) aphasia. In the nondominant hemisphere, the neglect and anosognosia would be less prominent than in the more proximal arterial occlusions. Emboli traveling to the lower division of the MCA tree may leave very little evidence of weakness and sensory loss. The patient will have a visual field deficit. In the dominant hemisphere, the patient will have a fluent (Wernicke's) aphasia. An isolated nondominant parietal lobe lesion will result in abnormalities in stereognosis (the ability to recognize objects by sense of touch alone), double simultaneous stimulation, and graphesthesia (the ability to recognize figures written on the skin). A dominant hemisphere parietal occipital lesion may result in Gerstmann's syndrome, consisting of finger agnosia (inability to recognize one's own fingers), acalculia (inability to calculate), right-left disorientation, and agraphia (inability to write).[6]

A unilateral occlusion of the anterior cerebral artery (ACA) will lead to motor and sensory loss involving the contralateral foot and leg, with the greatest amount of weakness found distally.[7] Motor involvement will be greater than the deficit in the primary sensory modalities. A more extensive infarct may involve the proximal arm, with relative sparing of the face. A bilateral ACA stroke may cause paraparesis and incontinence, bladder more often than bowel. A bilateral ACA infarct can cause akinetic mutism. A patient with akinetic mutism will appear to have sleep-wake cycles. However, while awake, the patient will have little or no movement, vocalizations, or response to her or his environment. There are few long tract signs.[8] Although bilateral ACA infarction may have devastating effects, it rarely results in death.[9]

A unilateral posterior cerebral artery (PCA) infarction may result in a contralateral homonymous hemianopsia with macular sparing. The macular region is usually spared because it receives blood supply from both the MCA and the PCA. Several features will distinguish an occipital hemianopsia from a middle cerebral distribution hemianopsia. With occipital hemianopsia, the patient may complain of the visual field deficit (the patient with an MCA hemianopsia may be unaware of it, until she or he is tested), may have differing amounts of involvement in the superior and inferior quadrants, and may have preservation of optokinetic nystagmus. With bilateral PCA infarction, the patient may have bilateral homonymous hemianopsia with or without macular sparing (cortical blindness). A patient with cortical blindness (Anton's syndrome) may not admit to being blind and will confabulate when asked to name objects in the room. The patients may also have metamorphopsia (visual distortion of objects), palinopsia (persistence of an image after it has left the visual field), memory impairment, delirium, or severe sensory loss, or a combination of these.[10]

Vertebrobasilar ischemia may result in a combination of ipsilateral cranial nerve or cerebellar abnormalities with contralateral motor and sensory abnormalities on the trunk and limbs. There are numerous syndromes associated with occlusion of individual penetrating arteries off the basilar artery. The lateral medullary syndrome presents with ipsilateral facial numbness, decreased gag reflex, paralysis of the vocal cord, ataxia, and Horner's syndrome and contralateral loss of pain and temperature sensation over half the body. Patients will frequently have complaints of nausea, vomiting, vertigo, and facial pain. This syndrome has most often been associated with an occlusion of the vertebral artery, although it has also been associated with occlusion of the posterior inferior cerebellar artery. Patients with a cerebellar infarction may present with an isolated cerebellar ataxia. However, they will frequently progress to have vertigo, vomiting, nystagmus, diplopia, headache, and a decreased level of consciousness. Cerebellar hemorrhage may have the same clinical presentation. Prompt recognition of this syndrome is essential, since prompt surgical intervention can be life saving.[11, 12] Occlusion of the basilar artery can have a variable presentation including coma, quadriplegia, or a locked-in state. It may also be asymptomatic. This will depend on the portion of the basilar artery involved and the availability of collateral flow. When the occlusion occurs at the distal end of the basilar artery, presentation can be that of rostral brain stem dysfunction or posterior hemisphere dysfunction, or a combination of the two. Rostral brain stem lesions can cause eye movement and pupillary abnormalities, somnolence, and peduncular hallucinosis.[13] Peduncular hallucinosis consists of nonhorrendous, often pleasurable, colorful hallucinations.[14] Patients with lesions in the pretectal region may have vertical gaze palsy, binocular pupillary light reflex impairment (often with a light near dissociation), and convergence-retraction nystagmus.[15] It should be remembered that occurrence of isolated drop attacks, dizziness, or even true vertigo, when unaccompanied by other manifestations of vertebrobasilar ischemia, is not considered a manifestation of focal posterior circulation disease.[16]

A significant stenosis of the subclavian or innominate artery proximal to the origin of the vertebral artery may cause neurologic symptoms. This type of stenosis may result in a lower pressure in the subclavian artery than in the vertebrobasilar tree. This may produce a siphoning of blood from the basilar system, down the ipsilateral vertebral artery (a reversal of normal flow) to feed the occluded subclavian. This vascular larceny (subclavian steal syndrome) can be responsible for relative brain stem ischemia. Patients will complain of dizziness or vertigo, visual disturbances, limb claudication and paresthesias, and headache.[17, 18] On examination, the patient will have a decreased pulse in the affected limb and a supraclavicular bruit. Some patients may have their cerebrovascular symptoms reproduced with limb exercise.

Transient monocular blindness, amaurosis fugax, is caused by decreased blood flow through or embolization into the ophthalmic artery or one of its branches. Patients will usually complain of a unilateral monocular visual loss. The patient will often describe the sensation as a curtain or a shade coming across the visual field, usually from top to bottom or from bottom to top. Although these spells most commonly resolve relatively rapidly, rarely they may cause residual visual deficit.

Compromise of the small penetrating arteries of the brain will result in lacunar infarctions. These small lesions, usually measuring less than 10 mm in diameter, are found in the deep white matter of the brain. They are found most commonly in patients with diabetes or hypertension, or both. Although lacunar infarctions are most often associated with small vessel disease, they may also be associated with large vessel disease.[19, 20] Over 20 lacunar syndromes have been described.[21] The most common include pure motor stroke, pure sensory stroke, ataxic hemiparesis (crural paresis with homolateral ataxia), or clumsy hand dysarthria. Pure motor stroke is defined as a paralysis of one side of the body in the absence of sensory signs, visual field defect, or dysphasia. This syndrome is most commonly associated with a lesion in the internal capsule or the basis pontis,[22] although ischemic and hemorrhagic lesions in other locations have been reported.[23] Pure sensory stroke involving face, arm, and leg without associated neurologic findings is usually associated with a lacunar infarction in the thalamus[24, 25] but has been associated with ischemic and hemorrhagic lesions in other locations.[26] Ataxic hemiparesis has been reported with lacunar or hemorrhagic infarction of the basis pontis and the posterior limb of the internal capsule.[27–29] Of course, a lacunar infarction may also present with a sensorimotor stroke or other focal neurologic deficits, depending on which pathways are disrupted.

There are five fairly common stroke presentations that manifest in a non-stroke-like fashion.[30] The leaking aneurysm may present as a sudden severe headache with no focal neurologic deficit. The patient may have only a mild stiff neck. There may be some impairment of the level of consciousness or the quality of cognitive functioning. The cerebellar hemorrhage may present with the sudden onset of an inability to stand or walk, with the patient complaining of dizziness and repeated vomiting. The neurologic examination may show facial paresis, gaze paresis, and unilateral cerebellar ataxia. However, these findings are frequently overlooked in this acutely ill, vomiting patient who is not eager to be moved about for an examination. With an occipital infarction resulting in a homonymous hemianopsia, the patient may have little else wrong on neurologic examination and the field defect will be found only when visual field testing is performed. A nondominant parietal lobe infarction may result in little or no motor deficit. The patient may present strange behavioral abnormalities. Only careful testing will reveal the parietal lobe abnormalities discussed earlier. The patient with an isolated fluent aphasia can present with no motor deficit. Frequently, they are brought to the hospital because of behavioral abnormalities. They do not complain of their problem involving comprehension or speech.

Seizures may occur in the patient who has had a stroke. In one series of 1000 patients, 4.4 per cent had seizure within the first 2 weeks of the stroke.[31] Seizures were most common after intraparenchymal hemorrhage (15.4 per cent) and less common after cortical infarction (1.3 per cent).

CLINICAL EVALUATION

As noted previously, the most valuable tools in the evaluation of the patient presenting with cerebrovascular disease are a carefully taken history and physical examination. The majority of patients presenting with cerebrovascular disease will have hemorrhage, thrombosis, or embolism. Even in these three categories, the differential diagnosis is large. There are also a number of noncerebrovascular diseases that will have clinical presentations that may mimic cerebrovascular disease (Table 114–1).

A detailed history of the progression of the event should be taken. The speed of onset of symptoms, the localization of symptoms at the onset, and the associated neurologic and systemic symptoms may all be important. A patient with a history of a spell that began in the distal extremity and gradually marched up the arm might be suspected of having a seizure disorder rather than cerebrovascular disease. A spell that begins with a scintillating scotoma and results in a transient hemicranial throbbing headache associated with vomiting is most likely migraine. It must be remembered that ischemic and hemorrhagic infarctions may be associated with headache even in the nonmigrainous patient. If the spells are repeatedly brought on by rapid changes in body position, orthostatic hypotension should be suspected. If the spell is brought on by activities involving one arm, subclavian steal should be suspected. A history of myalgias, arthralgias, fever, rash, or weight loss would make a diagnosis of collagen vascular disease more likely. A history of recent neck trauma should make one suspicious of a traumatic carotid dissection. A hematologic disorder would be considered in a patient with a history of menorrhagia, epistaxis, bleeding gums, purpura, petechia, or intermittent dark urine.

Family history can be important. A history of family members with stroke or myocardial infarction at a young age would indicate possible familial hyperlipidemia or other causes of premature atherosclerosis. A history of a family member with multiple spontaneous abortions or severe dysmenorrhea may indicate a blood dyscrasia. A history of collagen vascular disease in a family member may be important.

The general physical examination may yield important information. Blood pressure measurements should be taken in each arm. The patient should be tested for lying and standing blood pressures. During examination of the neck, one should check for nuchal rigidity, lymphadenopathy, as well as carotid pulsations. Evidence of diabetic or hypertensive retinopathy on funduscopic examination is important in terms of risk factors for small vessel disease. The presence of a bright refractile body at a branch point in a retinal artery indicates a cholesterol embolus (Hollenhorst's plaque). A subhyaloid hemorrhage is indicative of intracranial bleeding. Cardiac examination will help to determine whether there is evidence of valvular disease (including mitral valve prolapse) or arrhythmia. Evidence of obstructive pulmonary disease would make one concerned about the possibility of polycythemia. Abnormal patterns of respiration, such as Cheyne-Stokes respirations, may be of assistance in localizing a cerebral lesion. Evidence of liver disease may make one consider problems with coagulation. Skin lesions may lead to a diagnosis of collagen vascular disease. Needle tracks would make one suspect stroke as-sociated with drug abuse. Vascular examination is important. Diminished peripheral pulsations over a major artery indicate generalized large vessel disease. Careful auscultation should be performed over the carotid arteries, subclavian arteries, and femoral arteries. Although the absence of a bruit does not rule out local stenosis in a vessel, and the presence of a bruit does not indicate significant stenosis with certainty, the finding of an arterial bruit on examination indicates vascular disease in general and is a risk factor for vascular disease.

Detailed neurologic examination is essential for all patients being evaluated for cerebrovascular disease. Careful mental status testing, looking for localizable abnormalities, can be very productive in finding focal abnormalities that would be silent on a more cursory examination. Patients should be tested for speech, praxis, calculations, right-left orientation, finger agnosia, reading, constructions, memory, and attention. To test language function, six characteristics should be tested to get a satisfactory localization of abnormality. These are fluency of spontaneous speech, comprehension of spoken language, repetition, naming, reading, and writing.[32] Right-handed adults with fluent aphasia invariably have a lesion posterior to the left central sulcus, whereas those with a nonfluent aphasia have a lesion anterior to the central sulcus. Patients with a global aphasia, who have severe impairment in all aspects of language, will have damage both anterior and posterior to the central sulcus.[33] Patients with a nonfluent aphasia will speak with great effort at a slow rate of speech using short phrases that have a high percentage of substantive words. Comprehension is most severely affected by lesions posterior to the central sulcus, but will be affected to a lesser degree by anterior aphasias. Abnormalities of calculation, right-left disorientation, and finger agnosia, when seen together, indicate a posterior lesion in the dominant hemisphere. Cranial nerve testing is most helpful in localizing problems affecting the brain stem. Although testing primary sensory modalities is important, the testing of double simultaneous stimulation, stereognosis, and graphesthesia is especially useful in assessing parietal lobe function. Motor, reflex, cerebellar, and station and gait testing should also be well tested and documented. In the patient thought to be asymptomatic or to have cleared completely, the careful neurologic examination may pick up abnormalities indicative of asymptomatic structural disease. In the patient with known structural disease, the careful documentation of the neurologic examination is essential for establishing a baseline in case of early or suspected progression.

LABORATORY EVALUATION

It has been said that the diagnostic armamentarium should be well aimed before it is fired. Cost containment is an important part of modern medical practice. However, one should not miss a treatable cause of stroke syndrome for lack of ordering an appropriate diagnostic test. There are numerous diagnostic tests that are appropriate in cerebrovascular disease, although not all tests need to be ordered on all patients. The patient must be individually evaluated and the appropriate test battery selected.

Table 114–1. Differential Diagnosis of Acute Ischemic Stroke

Diseases Within the Blood Vessels
Inflammatory
   Systemic rheumatologic diseases (systemic lupus erythematosus, rheumatoid arthritis, Sjögren's syndrome)
   Infectious (e.g., syphilis, tuberculosis, fungal, ophthalmic zoster)
   Giant cell arteritis (temporal arteritis, Takayasu's arteritis)
   Polyarteritis nodosa, allergic angiitis
   Granulomatoses (Wegener's granulomatoses, lymphatoid granulomatoses, granulomatosis angiitis)
   Drug-induced (amphetamines)
Noninflammatory
   Atherosclerotic stenosis
   Ulcerative plaque with or without stenosis
   Carotid dissection (traumatic, spontaneous)
   Lipohyalinosis
   Compression
   Fibromuscular hyperplasia
   Moyamoya
   Vasospasm (subarachnoid hemorrhage, migraine)
Hematologic Disorders
Polycythemia
Problems with coagulation
   Lupus anticoagulant
   Thrombocythemia
   Disseminated intravascular coagulation
   Pregnancy/peripartum
   Platelet disorders
Cardiac Disorders
Atrial fibrillation/flutter (with or without valvular disease)
Valvular disease (including mitral valve prolapse)
Left ventricular aneurysm
Cardiomyopathy
Atrial myxoma
Nonvascular Disease Presenting as Stroke
Brain tumor (primary or secondary)
Subdural hematoma
Hypoglycemia
Focal seizure

Blood Test

A complete blood count is useful in screening for polycythemia. In cerebrovascular disease, a highly elevated hematocrit may be hazardous because sludging may occur.[34, 35] An elevated white count may be the first indication of an underlying infection. In older patients, an erythrocyte sedimentation rate should be ordered to rule out temporal arteritis and to screen for other collagen vascular disorders. In young patients, antiphospholipid antibodies should be screened by obtaining studies for lupus anticoagulant and anticardiolipin antibody levels.[36, 37] Stroke in young patients can also be associated with deficiency in protein C or protein S.[38, 39] A platelet count, prothrombin time, and partial thromboplastin time should be ordered to screen for other forms of coagulopathy. If indicated, an antinuclear antibody test, rheumatoid factor, and Venereal Disease Research Laboratory test should also be ordered. Blood urea nitrogen and creatinine should be tested in any patient who may be undergoing a contrast-enhanced scan during their work-up. Additionally, patients with swallowing difficulties may run into problems with dehydration and can be followed with these laboratory studies. A fasting glucose, triglycerides, cholesterol, total lipids, high-density lipoprotein, and low-density lipoprotein should be ordered to evaluate the patient's risk factors.[40, 41] In young patients with no clear atherosclerotic or embolic cause for stroke, a toxicology screen for amphetamines and cocaine may identify the cause of the acute infarction.[42, 43]

Cardiologic Tests

An electrocardiogram (ECG) is important in all patients with cerebrovascular disease. New-onset ECG abnormalities are frequently seen in the setting of acute stroke.[44, 45] Because of the known high association of myocardial damage in the setting of acute stroke, serial cardiac enzymes should also be monitored.[46, 47] In patients in whom there is reason to suspect cardiac embolism or valvular disease, an echocardiogram is warranted. An echocardiogram should be performed on all patients who are under the age of 50 years presenting with a stroke syndrome of uncertain cause or when they have known coronary artery disease, prior recent myocardial infarction, cardiomyopathy, known valvular disease, or chest x-ray indicating cardiomegaly. In patients in whom an embolic source is suspected, a transesophageal echocardiogram should be performed even if the transthoracic echocardiogram is normal.[48, 49] In patients in whom arrhythmia is suspected, a Holter monitor is useful. Holter's monitoring is unlikely to find previously unsuspected atrial fibrillation.[50] However, other arrhythmias are found often enough to warrant Holter's monitoring in acute stroke patients who have otherwise unexplained strokes.[51, 52] It must be remembered that an arrhythmia alone without associated embolization is usually responsible for global ischemia and will cause diffuse cerebral symptoms rather than focal cerebral symptoms.[53]

The association of cerebrovascular disease and cardiovascular disease is well established.[54] Approximately 40 per cent of stroke patients with no symptoms of ischemic coronary artery disease will have severe stenosis in at least one coronary artery.[55, 76] Coronary artery evaluation, including exercise ECGs and resting and exercise radionuclide cardiac studies, should be undertaken on an individual basis.[56, 57] Dipyridamole-thallium myocardial imaging can be useful in diagnosing asymptomatic ischemic heart disease in stroke patients unable to perform exercise studies.[58] Stroke patients who have an abnormal ECG or clinically significant angina pectoris should be considered for coronary angiography.[59]

Cerebrospinal Fluid

The role of routine cerebrospinal fluid (CSF) examination in cerebrovascular disease is controversial.[60, 61] Certainly, it must be tested if subarachnoid hemorrhage, vasculitis, embolic infective endocarditis, or infection is suspected. In patients under the age of 40 years who do not have a clear athersclerotic or embolic cause of stroke, a lumbar puncture should be done routinely as part of the stroke work-up.[62] CSF examination is especially useful in stroke patients presenting with unexplained fever, elevated white blood cell count, stiff neck, prior unexplained headache, or a history of syphilis or lupus. In the absence of a traumatic tap, the presence of blood in the CSF is the sine qua non of intracranial bleeding. With subarachnoid hemorrhage, the white cell count and protein may be elevated and the glucose may be normal or depressed. The CSF will be xanthochromic. When the amount of blood in the subarachnoid space is small, the computed tomography (CT) scan will be negative and the lumbar puncture is the only means of making the diagnosis. In arteritis, the CSF findings are variable. The protein and the white blood cell count may be elevated with the glucose normal. If heparin is to be administered and a CT scan is not available, a lumbar puncture, unless contraindicated, should be performed to rule out intracranial bleeding. It must be remembered that heparin should not be started within 1 hour after a spinal tap in order to avoid spinal hematoma.[63]

Cerebrovascular Imaging Studies

A detailed discussion of noninvasive cerebrovascular testing appears in Chapter 116. Application of a battery of noninvasive testing is useful in identifying patients with high-grade extracranial carotid stenosis. However, these tests do not identify ulcerative plaques, may falsely call a vessel occluded, and do not give adequate information about the intracranial cerebrovascular tree. Intravenous digital subtraction angiography had held a promise of providing a low-risk method of accurate imaging of the cerebral vasculature. With increasing experience, it has been found that this technique is not "noninvasive."[64] It is inadequate in evaluating the intracranial vascular tree. Some of the early enthusiasm for this procedure in ischemic cerebrovascular disease has since waned.[65] Duplex ultrasonography may provide similar information with equal accuracy and no morbidity.[66] When done properly, transcranial Doppler studies can detect severe intracranial stenosis involving major arteries at the base of the brain.[67] Magnetic resonance angiography (MRA) is a noninvasive method of imaging both the extracranial and the intracranial vasculature.[68] The study is expensive and requires a lot of patient cooperation. The spatial resolution is not adequate for reliably detecting ulcerated plaques. With improvements in both software and hardware, this technique may play a larger role in routine evaluation of stroke patients. However, in current clinical practice, the angiogram remains the gold standard in evaluating the vascular tree in stroke patients. It is useful in identifying the etiology of the stroke in the majority of cases and has a relatively low morbidity in this setting.[69] Further detailed discussion of this is in Chapter 115.

Blood Flow and Cerebral Metabolism

Positron emission tomography (PET) scanning is a powerful tool for examining the brain and giving information regarding cerebral blood flow, oxygen utilization, and oxygen extraction.[70, 71] With this information, blood flow relative to the metabolic need in the area of interest in the brain can be determined. This is discussed in greater detail in Chapter 117. Regional cerebral blood flow can be determined by radiolabeled xenon. Single photon emission tomography can be used to assess cerebral perfusion.[72] Despite the potential wealth of information that these studies could provide, each is not widely available and is used for research applications rather than clinical purposes.[73]

Cerebral Imaging Studies

The two best methods for imaging the intracranial contents are CT and magnetic resonance imaging (MRI) of the head. Each of these techniques is discussed in greater detail in Chapter 117. At the present time, CT scanning remains the best method for identifying intraparenchymal hemorrhage and hemorrhagic infarction. MRI scanning is more sensitive for identifying small deep white matter lesions such as lacunar infarction. Cerebral imaging is essential for ruling out structural lesions that may be presenting as cerebrovascular disease. It is also needed in determining the exact localization before choosing the proper patient management.

Electroencephalography

Electroencephalography (EEG) is an excellent clinical tool for assessing the electrophysiologic activity of the brain. EEG and evoked potential testing to monitor patients during cerebrovascular surgery are controversial but may be of value in selected circumstances.[74] However, in current clinical practice, outside the operating room and in the absence of stroke-related seizures, these tests have a very limited role in the clinical evaluation of the patient with acute cerebrovascular disease. Brain mapping and other forms of computerized analysis of EEG hold a promise of being valuable tools in clinical evaluation of these patients, but right now they remain research tools.[75]

References

1. Levy DE: How transient are transient ischemic attacks? Neurology 38:674, 1988.
2. Werdelin L, Juhler M: The course of transient ischemic attacks. Neurology 38:677, 1988.
3. Countee RW, Vijayanthan T: External carotid artery in internal carotid artery occlusion. Angiographic, therapeutic and prognostic considerations. Stroke 10:450, 1979.
4. Caplan L, Babikian V, Helgason C, et al: Occlusive disease of the middle cerebral artery. Neurology 35:975, 1985.
5. Bogousslavsky J, Barnett HJM, Fox AJ, et al: Atherosclerotic disease of the middle cerebral artery. Stroke 17:1112, 1986.
6. Jewesbury ECO: Parietal lobe syndromes. *In* Vinken PJ, Bruyn GW (eds): Handbook of Clinical Neurology. Amsterdam, North-Holland, 1969, vol. 2, pp 680–699.
7. Bogousslavsky J, Regli F: Anterior cerebral artery territory infarction in the Lausanne stroke registry. Arch Neurol 47:144, 1990.
8. Plum F, Posner JB: The Diagnosis of Stupor and Coma. Philadelphia, FA Davis, 1972, pp 23–24.
9. Hung T-P, Ryu S-J: Anterior cerebral artery syndromes. *In* Vinken PJ, Bruyn GW, Klawans HL, Toole JF (eds): Handbook of Clinical Neurology. Amsterdam, Elsevier Science Publishers, 1988, vol. 53, pp 339–352.
10. Caplan LR: "Top of the basilar" syndrome. Neurology 30:72, 1980.
11. Woodhurst WB: Cerebellar infarction—Review of recent experiences. Can J Neurol Sci 7:97, 1980.
12. Brennan RW, Bergland RM: Acute cerebellar hemorrhage. Neurology 27:527, 1977.
13. Caplan LR: "Top of the basilar" syndrome. Neurology 30:72, 1980.
14. Toole JF, Cole M: Ischemic cerebrovascular disease. *In* Baker AB, Joynt RJ (eds): Clinical Neurology. Philadelphia, Harper & Row, 1985.
15. Keane J: The pretectal syndrome: 206 patients. Neurology 40:684, 1990.
16. Caplan LR: Vertebrobasilar disease. Stroke 12:111, 1981.
17. Fields WS, Lemark NA: Joint study of extracranial arterial occlusion. VII. Subclavian steal—A review of 168 cases. JAMA 222:1139, 1972.
18. Hafer CD: Subclavian steal syndrome. Arch Surg 111:1074, 1976.
19. Bogousslavsky J, Barnett HMJ, Fox AJ, et al: Atherosclerotic disease of the middle cerebral artery. Stroke 17:1112, 1986.
20. Ringelstein EB, Zeumer H, Angelou D: The pathogenesis of strokes from internal carotid artery occlusion. Diagnostic and therapeutic implications. Stroke 14:867, 1983.
21. Fisher CM: Lacunar strokes and infarcts: A review. Neurology 32:871, 1982.
22. Fisher CM, Curry HB: Pure motor hemiplegia of vascular origin. Arch Neurol 13:30, 1965.
23. Ho KL: Pure motor hemiplegia due to infarction of the cerebral peduncle. Arch Neurol 39:524, 1982.
24. Fisher CM: Thalamic pure sensory stroke: A pathologic study. Neurology 28:1141, 1978.
25. Fisher CM: Pure sensory stroke and allied conditions. Stroke 13:434, 1982.
26. Tuttle PV, Reinmuth OM: Midbrain hemorrhage producing pure sensory stroke. Arch Neurol 41:794, 1984.
27. Fisher CM, Cole M: Homolateral ataxia and crural paresis: A vascular syndrome. J Neurol Neurosurg Psychiatry 28:48, 1965.
28. Fisher CM: Ataxic hemiparesis. Arch Neurol 35:126, 1978.
29. Iragui VJ, McCutchen CB: Capsular ataxic hemiparesis. Arch Neurol 39:528, 1982.
30. Mohr JP, Kase CS, Adams RD: Cerebrovascular diseases. *In* Petersdorf RG, Adams RD, Braunwald E, et al (eds): Harrison's Principles of Internal Medicine. New York, McGraw-Hill, 1983, pp 2028–2060.
31. Kilpatrick CJ, Davis SM, Tress BM, et al: Epileptic seizures in acute stroke. Arch Neurol 47:157, 1990.
32. Cummings JL, Benson DF: Dementia: A Clinical Approach. Boston, Butterworths, 1983, pp 19–22.
33. Legatt AD, Rubin MJ, Kaplan LR, et al: Global aphasia without hemiparesis. Neurology 37:201, 1987.
34. Thomas DJ, Marshall J, Ross Russell RW, et al: Cerebral blood flow in polycythemia. Lancet 2:161, 1977.
35. Grotta JC, Manner C, Pettigrew LC, et al: Red blood cell disorders and stroke. Stroke 17:811, 1986.

36. Brey RL, Hart RG, Sherman DG, Tegeler CH: Antiphospholipid antibodies and cerebral ischemia in young people. Neurology 40:1190, 1990.

37. Nencini P, Baruffi MC, Abbate R, et al: Lupus anticoagulant and anticardiolipin antibodies in young adults with cerebral ischemia. Stroke 23:189, 1992.

38. Sacco RL, Owen J, Mohr JP, et al: Free protein S deficiency: A possible association with cerebrovascular occlusion. Stroke 20: 1657, 1989.

39. Camerlingo M, Finazzi G, Casto L, et al: Inherited protein C deficiency and nonhemorrhagic arterial stroke in young adults. Neurology 41:1371, 1991.

40. Grotta JC, Yatsu RM, Pettigrew LC, et al: Prediction of carotid stenosis progression by lipid and hematologic measurements. Neurology 39:1325, 1989.

41. Wolf PA, D'Agostino RB, Belanger AJ, Kannel WB: Probability of stroke: A risk profile from the Framingham study. Stroke 22:312, 1991.

42. Daras M, Tuchman AJ, Marks S: Central nervous system infarction related to cocaine abuse. Stroke 22:1320, 1991.

43. Levine SR, Brust JCM, Futrell N, et al: Cerebrovascular complications of the use of the ''crack'' form of alkaloidal cocaine. N Engl J Med 323:699, 1990.

44. Norris JW, Froggatt GM, Hachinski VC: Cardiac arrhythmias in acute stroke. Stroke 9:392, 1978.

45. Goldstein DS: The electrocardiogram in acute stroke: Relationship to pathophysiological type and comparison with prior tracings. Stroke 10:253, 1979.

46. Dimant J, Grob D: Electrocardiographic changes and myocardial damage in patients with acute cerebrovascular accidents. Stroke 8:448, 1977.

47. Myers MG, Norris JW, Hachinski VC, et al: Cardiac sequelae of acute stroke. Stroke 13:838, 1982.

48. Tegeler CH, Downes TR: Cardiac imaging in stroke. Stroke 22:1206, 1991.

49. Cujec B, Polasek P, Voll C, Shuaib A: Transesophageal echocardiography in the detection of potential cardiac source of embolism in stroke patients. Stroke 22:727, 1991.

50. Koudstall PJ, van Gijn J, Klootwijk APJ, et al: Holter monitoring in patients with transient and focal ischemic attacks of the brain. Stroke 17:192, 1986.

51. Abdon N-J, Zettervall O, Carlson J, et al: Is occult atrial disorder a frequent cause of non-hemorrhagic stroke? Long-term ECG in 86 patients. Stroke 13:832, 1982.

52. Rem JA, Hachinski VC, Broughner DR, et al: Value of cardiac monitoring and echocardiography in TIA and stroke patients. Stroke 16:950, 1985.

53. Reed RL, Siekert RG, Merideth J: Rarity of transient focal cerebral ischemia in cardiac dysrhythmia. JAMA 223:893, 1973.

54. Chimowitz MI, Mancini GBJ: Asymptomatic coronary artery disease in patients with stroke. Stroke 23:433, 1992.

55. Hertzer NR, Young JR, Beven EG, et al: Coronary angiography in 506 patients with extracranial cerebrovascular disease. Arch Intern Med 145:849, 1985.

56. Adams HP, Kassell NF, Mazuz H: The patient with transient ischemic attacks—Is this the time for a new therapeutic approach? Stroke 15:371, 1984.

57. DiPasquale G, Andreoli A, Pinelle G, et al: Cerebral ischemia and asymptomatic coronary artery disease: A prospective study of 83 patients. Stroke 17:1098, 1986.

58. DiPasquale G, Andreoli A, Carini G, et al: Noninvasive screening for silent ischemic heart disease in patients with cerebral ischemia: Use of dipyridamole-thallium myocardial imaging. Cerebrovasc Dis 1:31, 1991.

59. Graor RA, Hetzer NR: Management of coexistent carotid artery and coronary artery disease. Stroke 19:1441, 1988.

60. Powers WJ: Should lumbar puncture be part of the routine evaluation of patients with cerebral ischemia? Stroke 17:332, 1986.

61. Hart RG, Foster JW: In response to Dr. Powers. Stroke 17:333, 1986.

62. Caplan LR, Flamm ES, Mohr JP, et al: Lumbar puncture and stroke: A statement for physicians by a committee of the Stroke Council, American Heart Association. Circulation 75:505A, 1987.

63. Ruff RL, Dougherty JH: Complications of lumbar puncture followed by anticoagulation. Stroke 12:879, 1981.

64. Ball JB, Lukin RR, Tomsick TA, et al: Complications of intravenous digital subtraction angiography. Arch Neurol 42:969, 1985.

65. Peltz DM, Fox AJ, Vinuela F: Digital subtraction angiography: Current clinical applications. Stroke 16:528, 1985.

66. Peltz D, Rankin RN, Ferguson GG: Intravenous digital subtraction angiography and duplex ultrasonography in postoperative assessment of cartid endarterectomy. J Neurosurg 66:88, 1987.

67. Therapeutics and Technology Assessment Subcommittee, American Academy of Neurology: Assessment: Transcranial Doppler. Practice handbook. Minneapolis, American Academy of Neurology, 1989, pp 115–118.

68. Edelman RR, Mattle HP, Atkinson DJ, Hoogewoud HM: MR angiography. AJR 154:937, 1990.

69. Lisovoski F, Rousseaux P: Cerebral angiography in young people: A study of 148 patients with early cerebral angiography. J Neurol Neurosurg Psychiatry 54:576, 1991.

70. Ackerman RH, Correia JA, Alpert NM, et al: Positron imaging in ischemic stroke disease using compounds labeled with oxygen 15. Arch Neurol 38:537, 1981.

71. Powers WJ, Raichle ME: Positron emission tomography and its application to the study of cerebrovascular disease in man. Stroke 16:361, 1985.

72. Lee RGL, Hill TC, Holman BL, et al: N-isopropyl(I-123)p-iodoamphetamine brain scans with single photon emission tomography: Discordance with transmission computed tomography. Radiology 145:795, 1982.

73. Therapeutics and Technology Assessment Subcommittee, American Academy of Neurology: Assessment: Positron emission tomography (PET). Practice handbook. Minneapolis, American Academy of Neurology, 1989, pp 83–91.

74. Therapeutics and Technology Assessment Subcommittee, American Academy of Neurology: Assessment: Intraoperative neurophysiology. Practice handbook. Minneapolis, American Academy of Neurology, 1989, pp 61–64.

75. Therapeutics and Technology Assessment Subcommittee, American Academy of Neurology: Assessment: EEG brain mapping. Practice handbook. Minneapolis, American Academy of Neurology, 1989, pp 29–30.

76. Cohen SN, Hobson RW, Weiss DG, et al: Mortality associated with asymptomatic carotid stenosis: Long-term clinical evaluation. J Vasc Surg 18:1002, 1993.

Anatomy and Angiographic Diagnosis of Extracranial and Intracranial Vascular Disease

Larry-Stuart Deutsch, M.D., C.M., F.R.C.P.(C.)

• • •

ARTERIAL ANATOMY: EXTRACRANIAL AND INTRACRANIAL VASCULAR SYSTEM

The surgical approach to the treatment of cerebrovascular disease requires an understanding of the anatomic framework that begins with the aortic arch and ends with the principal intracranial arteries. Although a broader consideration of the inflow and outflow of the region is beyond the scope of this discussion, the vascular surgeon should always keep in mind the possibility that certain cerebral vascular abnormalities may actually be the result of disease conditions affecting the heart, cerebral microcirculation, or venous structures of the head and neck.

Aortic Arch and Its Branches

The normal aortic arch curves smoothly upward into the superior mediastinum, running from right to left and anterior to posterior with its apex at approximately the mid-manubrial level. It passes to the left of the trachea, arching over the pulmonary artery bifurcation and the left mainstem bronchus, descending to the left of the esophagus. The ligamentum arteriosum, a fibrous remnant of the fetal ductus arteriosus, tethers the concave undersurface of the aortic arch to the proximal left main pulmonary artery, attaching at a point usually just distal to the left subclavian artery.

In approximately 95 per cent of all patients, the aortic arch gives rise to three major branches: the innominate artery (right brachiocephalic trunk), the left common carotid artery, and the left subclavian artery (Fig. 115–1). One of the most common variants is a common ostial origin of the innominate and left common carotid arteries, which occurs in approximately 10 per cent of patients. However, a true brachiocephalic trunk of more than a few millimeters in length that then divides into innominate and left common carotid arteries is relatively rare. Separate origin of the left vertebral artery directly from the aorta proximal to the left subclavian artery is another common anatomic variant, occurring in approximately 5 per cent of patients (Fig. 115–2).

True anomalies of the aortic arch are actually rela-

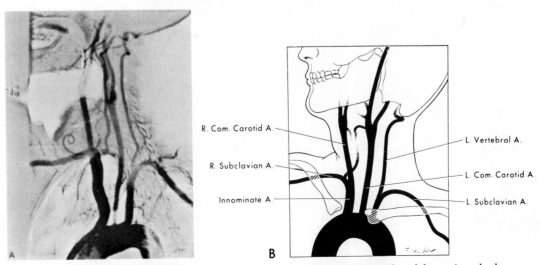

R. Com. Carotid A.

R. Subclavian A.

Innominate A.

L. Vertebral A.

L. Com. Carotid A.

L. Subclavian A.

FIGURE 115–1. *A,* An arch aortogram demonstrating the three primary branches of the aortic arch: the innominate artery, the left common carotid artery, and the left subclavian artery. *B,* Artist's concept of an arch aortogram illustrating the three primary branches of the aortic arch and their pertinent anatomic relationships.

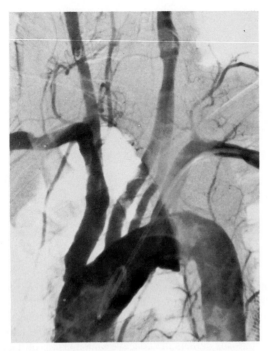

FIGURE 115–2. Arch aortogram obtained using an arterial catheter inserted via the left subclavian artery. Visualization of the primary branches of the aortic arch demonstrates that the left vertebral artery originates from the arch between the left common carotid and the left subclavian arteries.

tively rare and account for less than 2 per cent of cases in an adult patient population. Anomalies such as double aortic arch; interrupted arch; right arch, especially the mirror image branching form; and cervical arch are often associated with complex congenital heart disease or symptoms caused by pressure on the trachea or esophagus and thus require surgical correction in the neonatal or pediatric age group. Because routine surgical correction of such anomalies is relatively recent, few of these patients have reached the age group subject to the most common of adult cerebro vascular diseases, atherosclerosis. The most common aortic arch anomaly compatible with long-term survival is the aberrant right subclavian artery that originates from the proximal descending thoracic aorta and passes posterior to the esophagus (Fig. 115–3). Unless this anomaly causes dysphagia in the neonatal period, it may escape detection until the patient is examined angiographically later in life. Simple right aortic arches with normal branching, uncomplicated right arches with mirror image branching, and mirror image arch associated with thoracic situs inversus are uncommon.

Innominate Artery (Right Brachiocephalic Trunk)

The innominate artery (right brachiocephalic trunk) is the first major branch of the thoracic aorta and the largest

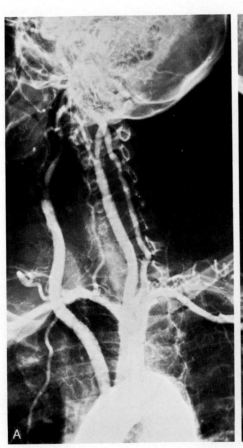
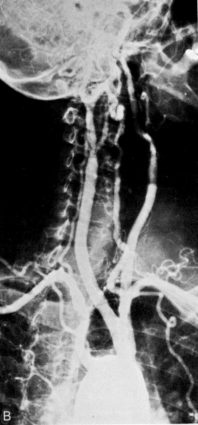

FIGURE 115–3. *A* and *B*, An arch aortogram demonstrating the first branch of the aortic arch to be an isolated right common carotid artery. An aberrant right subclavian artery originates just distal to the left subclavian artery and courses posterior to all of the other major branches of the aortic arch.

of its branches. It originates in the superior mediastinum posterior to the mid-point of the sternal manubrium and passes superiorly and posteriorly for a distance of 4 to 6 cm, then bifurcates into the right common carotid and right subclavian arteries in the root of the neck posterior to the right sternoclavicular joint. Whereas the proximal segments of the other major branches of the aortic arch are usually relatively straight, the innominate artery and the proximal segments of the right common carotid and subclavian arteries are often rather tortuous in elderly patients. Such tortuosity, especially when it involves the right subclavian artery at the base of the neck, can often mimic aneurysmal dilatation on physical examination and angiography.

Subclavian Arteries

The right subclavian artery originates from the innominate artery and arches laterally and posteriorly, passing posterior to the scalenus anterior muscle. The left subclavian artery originates directly from the aorta and is usually its third branch. It ascends vertically within the mediastinum, then arches laterally in the root of the neck to also pass posterior to the scalenus anterior muscle. Both subclavian arteries pass immediately superior to the dome of the pleura. The principal branches of the subclavian arteries arise from the segment proximal to the medial border of the scalenus anterior muscle and include the vertebral, internal mammary, thyrocervical, and costocervical arteries (Fig. 115–4). The vertebral and internal mammary arteries have a very constant relationship, originating directly opposite each other with the vertebral artery arising from the cranial surface and the internal mammary artery arising from the anteroinferior surface. The subclavian arteries then exit the neck by passing over the superior surface of the first rib posterior to the clavicle in close relationship to the lower portion of the brachial plexus. Once past the lateral aspect of the first rib, these vessels are arbitrarily renamed the axillary arteries. Although the vertebral artery is the primary subclavian branch of significance to the cerebral circulation, the other branches may become important sources of collateral supply in the setting of vertebral occlusive disease.

Common Carotid Arteries

The right common carotid artery originates from the innominate artery in the base of the neck, whereas the left common carotid artery originates directly from the aortic arch in the mediastinum. However, the anatomy of the cervical segments is virtually identical on both sides (Fig. 115–5). The common carotid arteries ascend in the neck, running anterior to the transverse processes of the cervical vertebrae and separated from them by the scalenus anterior, longus coli, and capitis muscles and by the sympathetic trunk. The common carotid artery usually bifurcates into the external and the internal carotid arteries near the superior horn of the thyroid cartilage, although there is considerable variation in the level of this bifurcation. The carotid arteries bifurcate at the same level in only 28 per cent of cases; in 50 per cent, the left bifurcation is more cranial than the right, whereas the opposite is true in the remaining 22 per cent. Throughout their cervical course, the common and internal carotid arteries are enclosed in a dense fibrous sheath, which they share with the internal jugular vein and the vagus nerve.

External Carotid Arteries

The external carotid artery is usually smaller than the internal carotid artery and originates anterior and medial to it, passing laterally to ascend just posterior to the ramus and neck of the mandible and superficial to the styloid process. It supplies the face, scalp, oronasopharynx, skull, and meninges through four major branch vessel groups: anterior branches (superior thyroid, lingual, facial, transverse facial), posterior branches (occipital and auricular), ascending branches (ascending pharyngeal), and terminal branches (superficial temporal, internal maxillary) (Fig. 115–6). These vessels are of no significance to the cerebral circulation except in the setting of carotid or vertebral artery occlusive disease, at which point they can become important sources of collateral blood supply. One of the most common collateral routes involves distal anastomoses between the pterygopalatine branches of the internal maxillary artery and the ethmoidal branches of the ophthalmic artery

FIGURE 115–4. Artist's concept of the relationships of the subclavian arteries and their primary branches.

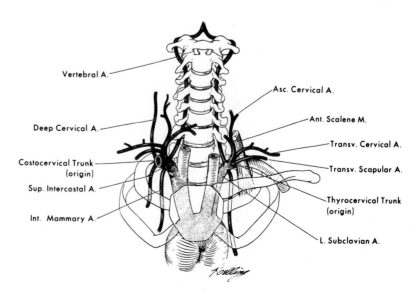

Vertebral A.

Asc. Cervical A.

Ant. Scalene M.

Deep Cervical A.

Transv. Cervical A.

Costocervical Trunk (origin)

Transv. Scapular A.

Sup. Intercostal A.

Thyrocervical Trunk (origin)

Int. Mammary A.

L. Subclavian A.

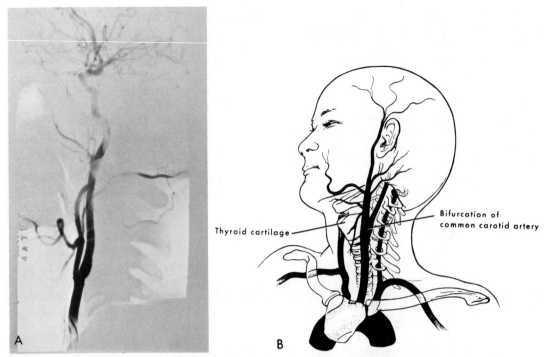

FIGURE 115–5. *A,* A selective injection of the left common carotid artery outlines the common carotid artery as it bifurcates into the internal and external carotid arteries within the mid-cervical region. *B,* Artist's concept of the bifurcation of the common carotid artery demonstrating the major anatomic relationships within the neck.

system (Fig. 115–7). Other important collateral pathways include anastomoses between orbitonasal branches of the facial artery and orbital branches of the ophthalmic artery, anastomoses between anterior branches of the superficial temporal artery and ethmoidal branches of the ophthalmic artery, and anastomoses between ascending pharyngeal branches of the external carotid artery and muscular branches of the vertebral artery.

Internal Carotid Arteries

The internal carotid artery is divided into four major segments: cervical, petrous, cavernous, and cerebral (Fig. 115–8). The cervical segment has no significant branches

and ascends in the neck immediately anterior to the transverse processes of the cervical vertebrae and their associated muscles. The internal carotid artery then enters the skull via the carotid canal, traversing the petrous portion of the temporal bone in a slightly medial direction and separated from the middle ear structures by only a thin layer of bone. The petrous segment also has no major branches, although there are small branches that anastomose with pterygopalatine branches of the internal maxillary artery, which can become sources of collateral supply in the setting of occlusive disease.

The cavernous segment of the internal carotid artery is called the carotid siphon because of its gentle S-shaped configuration as it passes through the cavernous sinus along the sella turcica toward the anterior clinoid process. Along

FIGURE 115–6. Artist's concept of the distribution of the external carotid artery with its major branches visualized.

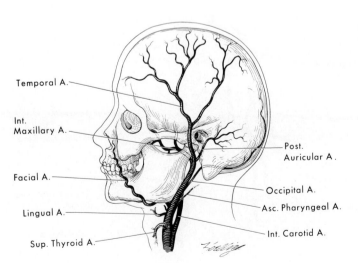

Temporal A.

Int. Maxillary A.

Facial A.

Lingual A.

Sup. Thyroid A.

Post. Auricular A.

Occipital A.

Asc. Pharyngeal A.

Int. Carotid A.

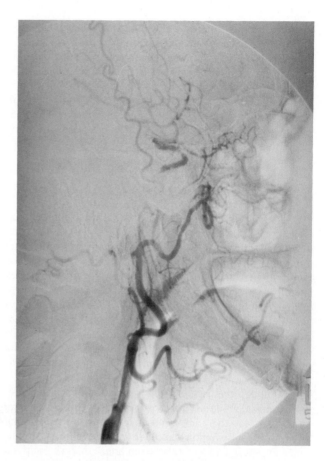

FIGURE 115-7.   Carotid angiogram (lateral view) showing occlusion of the internal carotid artery at its origin with collateral flow to the intracranial portion of the internal carotid artery system via collateral anastomoses between the pterygopalatine branches of the internal maxillary artery and the ethmoidal branches of the ophthalmic artery.

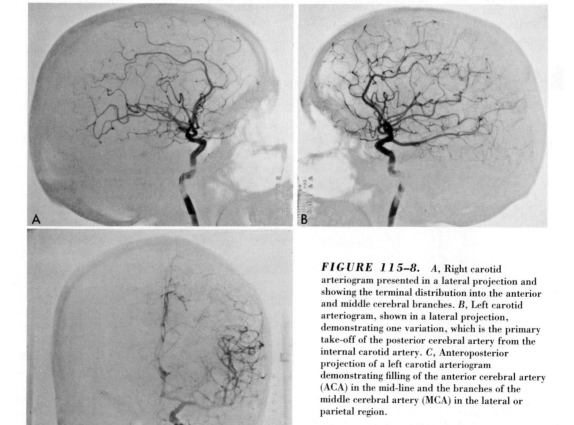

FIGURE 115-8.   *A,* Right carotid arteriogram presented in a lateral projection and showing the terminal distribution into the anterior and middle cerebral branches. *B,* Left carotid arteriogram, shown in a lateral projection, demonstrating one variation, which is the primary take-off of the posterior cerebral artery from the internal carotid artery. *C,* Anteroposterior projection of a left carotid arteriogram demonstrating filling of the anterior cerebral artery (ACA) in the mid-line and the branches of the middle cerebral artery (MCA) in the lateral or parietal region.

its course through the cavernous sinus it often indents the wall of the sphenoid sinus, sometimes separated from the sinus cavity by only dura and sinus mucosa. Although this segment has several branches, the ophthalmic artery is the cavernous segment branch of greatest clinical importance.

The cerebral segment of the internal carotid artery is relatively short. After traversing the dura mater medial to the anterior clinoid process, it passes superolaterally to divide into the anterior and middle cerebral arteries.

Vertebral Arteries

The vertebral artery is the first branch of the subclavian artery. It takes a relatively straight course, entering the transverse foramen of C6 and passing cranially through the transverse foramina of C6–C1. Because the transverse foramen of the atlas is lateral to that of the axis, it passes laterally between the axis and the atlas. It then runs posteromedially along the arch of the atlas lateral to the atlanto-occipital joint. On leaving the atlas, it turns sharply cephalad to enter the cranium via the foramen magnum. Inside the skull, the vertebral arteries pass medially along the inferior surface of the brain stem to unite into a single midline vessel, the basilar artery (Fig. 115–9).

Although the carotid arteries are of similar size bilaterally, considerable asymmetry is frequent in the vertebral system, even to the point of absence of one of the vertebral arteries. These variations are of little or no clinical significance except in cases of subclavian artery disease proximal to the vertebral origin. A moderate degree of tortuosity and smooth variation in caliber of the intracranial vertebral arteries is common even in young individuals and is also of no clinical significance.

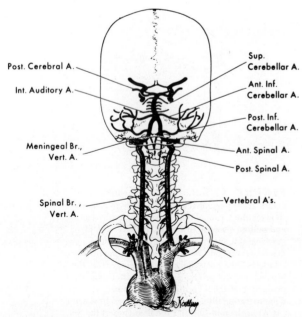

FIGURE 115–9. Artist's concept of the relationship of the vertebral arteries as they enter the root of the neck and ascend within the vertebral canal en route to joining at the brain stem to form the basilar artery. The significant cervical and cranial branches are labeled.

The cervical portion of the vertebral arteries supplies multiple small segmental branches to the spinal cord, cervical vertebrae, and adjacent muscles. The anastomotic connections between these small branches and the occipital and ascending pharyngeal branches of the external carotid artery system form potential collateral routes in the event of vertebral or carotid occlusive disease (Fig. 115–10).

The intracranial portion of the vertebral artery gives rise to the anterior and posterior spinal arteries, the penetrating medullary arteries, and the complex posterior inferior cerebellar artery, which supplies the inferior surface of the cerebellum.

Basilar Artery

The basilar artery is a relatively short mid-line vessel formed by the union of the vertebral arteries along the inferior surface of the pons. It runs along the pons, dividing into the left and right posterior cerebral arteries. In its short course, it gives rise to several important paired sets of arteries, including the anterior inferior cerebellar arteries, the internal auditory arteries, multiple small pontine arteries, and the superior cerebellar arteries (Fig. 115–11). Although these branch vessels are important sources of blood supply to the brain, they are generally beyond the practical reach of the vascular surgeon.

Middle Cerebral Artery

The middle cerebral artery (MCA) (Fig. 115–12) is generally larger in caliber than the anterior cerebral artery (ACA), and its initial segment forms a relatively straighter pathway from the internal carotid artery than the corresponding segment of the ACA. For this reason, most of the emboli originating in, or traversing, the carotid system lodge in branches of this vessel. The initial (M1) segment of the MCA is straight and runs laterally along the inferior surface of the anterior perforated substance of the brain toward the sylvian fissure, which separates the temporal lobe from the frontoparietal lobes. Numerous short, straight, vertical lenticulostriate arteries arise from this segment to supply the basal ganglia and adjacent structures. The MCA branches in the sylvian fissure, and its branches bend upward to run over the surface of the insula, then turn inferiorly again to emerge onto the cortical surface of the temporal and frontoparietal lobes. This pathway forms a characteristic upwardly convex "genu" or knee-like curvature.

Although there is considerable variation in the course of the MCA branches as they emerge from the sylvian fissure, they form three general groups: the anterior temporal artery; the anterior group, including the orbitofrontal and operculofrontal arteries; and the posterior group, including the posteroparietal, angular, and posterior temporal arteries. Although the indications for extracranial-intracranial (EC-IC) bypass procedures are still controversial, these MCA branches do provide a fortuitously convenient bypass pathway because of their accessibility on the surface of the brain and the close proximity of the overlying superficial temporal branches of the external carotid system.

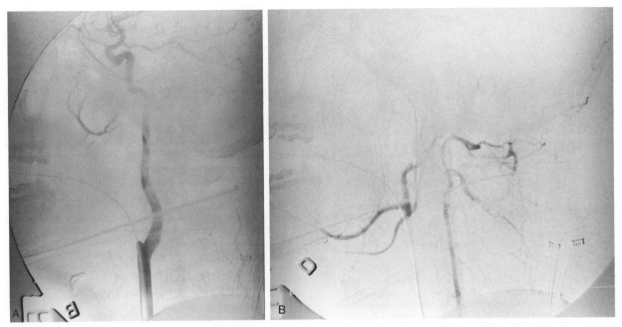

FIGURE 115-10. *A*, Carotid angiogram showing occlusion of the external carotid artery at its origin with collateral flow to the internal maxillary artery system via orbital collaterals (not shown). *B*, Vertebral angiogram showing collateral flow to the external carotid artery system via anastomoses between deep muscular branches of the vertebral artery and the ascending pharyngeal artery and similar branches communicating with the occipital artery.

Anterior Cerebral Artery

The ACA begins at the bifurcation of the internal carotid artery (Fig. 115–13). Its initial segment is the short, straight (A1) segment that runs anteromedially just above the optic chiasm. Several medial lenticulostriate arteries originate from this segment. The A1 segment communi-

cates with its opposite counterpart across the interhemispheric fissure via the short but important anterior communicating artery, the anterior component of the circle of Willis. A reciprocal size relationship between the A1 segment and the anterior communicating artery is common; a relatively hypoplastic A1 segment is usually accompanied by a large-caliber anterior communicating artery. In such cases, both ACAs are preferentially dependent on a single

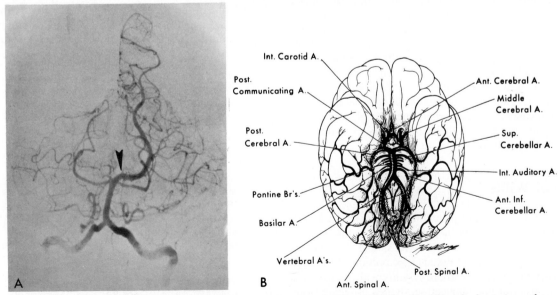

FIGURE 115-11. *A*, Vertebral-basilar arteriogram demonstrating the confluence of both vertebral arteries as they form the basilar artery running along the brain stem. Note that on the left side the basilar artery terminates in the posterior cerebral artery, but on the right side the terminal branch is the right superior cerebellar artery. This occurred because the right posterior cerebral artery originated from the carotid artery in this patient. *B*, Artist's concept of the relationship of the vertebral-basilar system to the brain stem. All of the major branches of the terminal vertebral arteries and the extent of the basilar arteries are named.

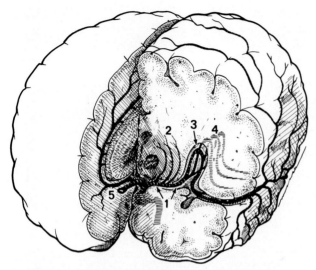

FIGURE 115–12. Artist's concept showing the relationship of the MCA to adjacent structures (the sylvian fissure has been exaggerated to emphasize that the MCA loops over the insula). *1*, M1 (horizontal) segment. The "genu" is the upward curve of the MCA branches into the sylvian fissure. *2*, Lateral lenticulostriate arteries. *3*, Sylvian fissure. *4*, MCA branches within the depths of the sylvian fissure. *5*, ACA. (From Osborn AG: Introduction to Cerebral Angiography. Hagerstown, MD, Harper & Row, 1980.)

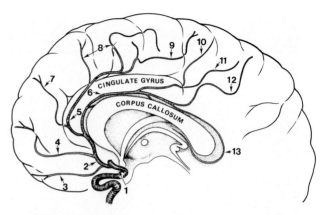

FIGURE 115–13. Artist's concept showing the relationship of the ACA to adjacent structures. *1*, A1 (horizontal) segment. *2*, ACA in front of lamina terminalis. *3*, Orbitofrontal artery. *4*, Frontopolar artery. *5*, Callosomarginal artery. *6*, Pericallosal artery. (From Osborn AG: Introduction to Cerebral Angiography. Hagerstown, MD, Harper & Row, 1980.)

internal carotid system and thus are especially sensitive to flow disturbances and other abnormalities in the corresponding carotid artery.

Beyond the origin of the anterior communicating artery, the ACA turns abruptly upward to pass around the genu of the corpus callosum. As it passes the genu, it gives rise to the pericallosal artery, which runs posteriorly along the superior surface of the corpus callosum and the callosomarginal artery, which runs along the cingulate sulcus roughly parallel to the pericallosal artery. The branches of these vessels supply the inner aspects of the frontal and parietal cortex in the interhemispheric fissure and end by passing over the superior margins of the interhemispheric fissure to supply a small band of cortical tissue along the anterior two thirds of the frontal and parietal lobes. Although the ACA and its branches are of considerable functional significance, they are largely inaccessible to the vascular surgeon because of their location deep within the interhemispheric fissure.

Circle of Willis

The circle of Willis is a unique vascular ring that encircles the diencephalon including the sella turcica and pituitary. The A1 segments of the ACAs and the anterior communicating artery form the anterior portion of the ring and connect the internal carotid systems with each other. The short posterior communicating arteries originate from the internal carotid arteries at or near the bifurcation into anterior and middle cerebral arteries. The posterior communicating arteries run posteriorly to connect with the corresponding proximal segments of the posterior cerebral arteries (PCAs), thus connecting the internal carotid system,

the anterior circulation, with the vertebral-basilar system, the posterior circulation (Fig. 115–14).

The circle of Willis, as described, effectively forms an arterial manifold that balances the inflow coming from the internal carotid and vertebral arteries with the outflow to the anterior, middle, and posterior cerebral arteries. However, only 20 per cent of patients actually have the "textbook" symmetric circle of Willis; hypoplasia of one or more components occurs in most individuals. Hypoplasia, or absence of one or both posterior communicating arteries, occurs in approximately 25 to 30 per cent of cases, thus effectively isolating the anterior and posterior circulations to a greater or lesser degree. Anomalies of the anterior communicating artery, including hypoplasia, absence, or duplication, occur in approximately 10 per cent of cases. Hypoplasia of the A1 segments occurs in approximately 25 per cent of cases, making both ACA systems preferentially dependent on a single internal carotid artery. Hypoplasia of

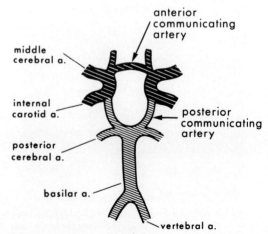

FIGURE 115–14. The classic intact circle of Willis forms a distribution manifold balancing the anterior (*dark shading*) inflow with the posterior (*light shading*) inflow; however, many variations occur and the circle is often incomplete.

the initial (P1) segment of the PCA with primary or sole flow to the PCA via an enlarged posterior communicating artery from the internal carotid artery occurs in approximately 15 to 20 per cent of cases and is termed a fetal origin. Persistence of additional fetal communications between the carotid and the vertebral-basilar systems, including the trigeminal, otic, hypoglossal, and proatlantal intersegmental arteries, also occurs but is relatively rare.

The frequency of variations in the textbook arrangement of the circle of Willis often explains seemingly paradoxical ischemic or embolic neurovascular abnormalities. Such variations are also of considerable practical clinical significance because they imply that existence of the textbook collateral routes cannot be simply assumed before surgical interventions such as carotid endarterectomy are undertaken. Adequate collateral supply must therefore be proved by preoperative angiography or intraoperative hemodynamic and/or electroencephalographic (EEG) monitoring.

ANGIOGRAPHIC DIAGNOSIS AND TREATMENT OF EXTRACRANIAL AND INTRACRANIAL VASCULAR DISEASE

Indications and Contraindications

The surgical aphorism "there is no such thing as a *little* operation" applies equally well to angiography and, indeed, to all invasive radiologic procedures. Although re-markably free of serious complications, angiography is not a simple laboratory test nor is it an inexpensive screening examination. Accordingly, the angiographer should function as a consultant specialist able to evaluate the indications and contraindications of the proposed procedure with regard to the patient's overall medical history and physical status as well as the specific details of the present illness and the proposed treatment. Furthermore, the angiographer should also be able to provide guidance in the selection of appropriate noninvasive imaging prior to, or instead of, angiography. Angiographic procedures, like surgical operations, should also be tailored to the needs of the individual patient. Thus, optimal patient care involves a consultative relationship between the angiographer and the referring physician; angiography should not be "ordered" like a routine laboratory test. Furthermore, if the proposed therapy is surgical in nature, a surgeon should be involved in the patient's care prior to angiography.

The approach to investigation and management of intracranial lesions has changed significantly since the early 1980s, largely as a result of dramatic advances in imaging technology. High-resolution x-ray computed tomography (CT) and magnetic resonance imaging (MRI) have virtually replaced angiography as primary diagnostic modalities. Conventional nuclear medicine brain scanning for the investigation of mass lesions has been all but eliminated, whereas the radioisotope cerebral perfusion study has become an essential tool in the determination of brain death (Fig. 115–15). Positron emission tomography (PET) scanning with its ability to image and quantitate regional metabolic function now offers even greater insights, although

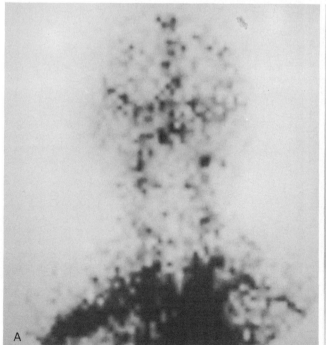 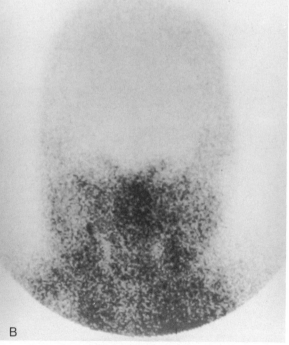

FIGURE 115–15. *A,* Normal isotope brain flow study showing filling of the internal carotid, anterior cerebral, and middle cerebral arteries. The relative paucity of flow to the facial regions is simply a reflection of preferential flow to the intracranial circulation. *B,* Abnormal isotope brain flow study with no detectable flow in the area of the anterior or middle cerebral arteries, indicating ischemic brain death associated with severe cerebral edema. Increased isotope activity in the facial regions represents increased flow in the external carotid artery branches, which fill preferentially because there is no longer any significant flow to the intracranial vessels. (*A* and *B,* Courtesy of Felix Wang, M.D., Nuclear Medicine Section, University of California Irvine Medical Center, Orange, California.)

the high cost and, for the present, limited availability make PET scanning largely a research tool.

Similarly, the approach to the investigation and management of extracranial cerebrovascular disease has also changed considerably over the past few years. Noninvasive duplex Doppler screening evaluations of the cervical carotid circulation can now be performed effectively and inexpensively using a combination of high-resolution gray-scale ultrasound imaging to delineate anatomic detail and Doppler ultrasound scanning to determine the hemodynamic significance of lesions identified by anatomic imaging. Duplex Doppler evaluations can actually be performed using relatively simple Doppler ultrasound scanners; however, many units now offer a choice of either region-by-region cursor-directed Doppler interrogation of the anatomic image with waveform display or a two-dimensional point-by-point color-encoded quantitative display of the Doppler signal superimposed on the real-time gray-scale anatomic image. Although supraorbital and transcranial Doppler ultrasound examinations provide information about the state of the intracranial portions of the carotid circulation, the circle of Willis, and some of the common collateral circulation pathways not evaluated by duplex Doppler scanning, these examinations have a far steeper learning curve and they are far more operator-dependent. Accordingly,

although they are still used in many noninvasive vascular laboratories, they have not really gained general acceptance. Similarly, oculoplethysmography, once a common examination, is still used in some centers, although it has been largely replaced by duplex Doppler scanning.

MRI is yet another noninvasive imaging technique that shows promise for use in evaluating the cerebrovascular circulation because of its inherent sensitivity to blood flow. By varying pulse sequences and signal sampling methods, images can be created that exploit various aspects of the differences between the physical properties of flowing blood and adjacent tissues. Mathematically "stacking" multiple closely spaced cross-sectional "slice" images of a body region permits three-dimensional depiction of a vessel that can then be displayed in many different formats, some of which closely resemble conventional contrast angiograms (Fig. 115–16). It is, however, important to remember that the physical basis of magnetic resonance angiography (MRA) is very different than that of conventional contrast angiography, a fact that makes experience transfer an unreliable basis for evaluation. Factors affecting MRA image quality include flow direction, velocity, vessel size, turbulence (chaotic flow), vortices (localized areas of direction reversal), boundary layer flow separation, pulsatility, elasticity, capacitance, and peripheral impedance. Vessel tortuos-

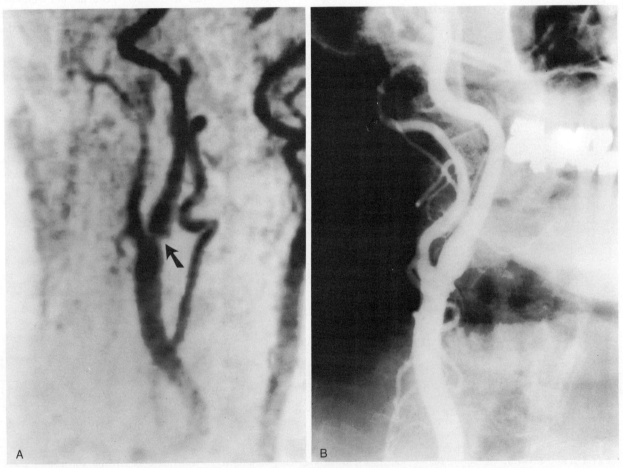

A B

FIGURE 115–16. *A,* Magnetic resonance angiogram (MRA) showing what appears to be high-grade focal stenosis at the origin of the right internal carotid artery (*arrow*). Note that the MRA is a nonselective arterial study showing all of the major arterial structures in the region of interest. *B,* Conventional selective contrast angiogram of the same vessel (performed in a slightly different obliquity) showing no evidence of a significant internal carotid artery stenosis, demonstrating that the abnormality seen on the MRA study represented an artifact rather than a true lesion. (*A* and *B,* Courtesy of William G. Bradley, M.D., Long Beach Memorial Medical Center, Long Beach, California.)

ity as well as the intravascular disturbances of flow encountered in the region of a lesion such as a carotid bifurcation stenosis include complex and unpredictable combinations of most of these flow phenomena leading to imaging artifacts that can be difficult to evaluate. Accordingly, although MRA is rapidly becoming a very sophisticated technique capable of impressive image quality, its utility as a screening technique is still unproved. Nevertheless one only has to look at the incredible progress in MRI technology achieved since the crude images of orange slices and cadaver mice abdomens shown proudly by MRI researchers in 1980 to appreciate the potential of this technology in the area of vascular imaging. MRA is very likely to become a valuable screening tool in the future; although that time may come soon, perhaps even very soon, it has not yet arrived.

The choice of noninvasive testing or angiography in the investigation and management of patients with cerebrovascular lesions depends largely on the question of lesion type, location, and symptoms. The incidence of asymptomatic intracranial central nervous system mass lesions is sufficiently low that routine noninvasive screening is rarely warranted, except in systemic conditions known to be associated with intracranial lesions such as the Osler-Weber-Rendu syndrome. Noninvasive (CT and MRI) delineation and characterization of symptomatic intracranial mass lesions are generally so reliable that angiography is used primarily as a tool in planning or administering therapy rather than as a purely diagnostic tool. In the case of surgically treatable mass lesions, mapping of the associated vascular supply and drainage is often vital to a successful outcome. Sometimes, successful surgery also requires preoperative alteration of the blood supply to the lesion by means of transcatheter embolization. In the case of intracranial lesions not amenable to surgical treatment, angiographic methods such as embolization or regional infusion of chemotherapeutic agents provide effective treatment for a number of benign and malignant lesions.

The investigation and management of purely vascular intracranial lesions (i.e., vascular malformations, aneurysms, and occlusive lesions) is quite different than in the case of mass lesions that may or may not have a significant vascular component. The true incidence of asymptomatic lesions is not well known. Furthermore, CT scanning and MRI scanning have proved far less than reliable in detection and characterization of such lesions, except in the case of large vascular malformations and giant aneurysms, which tend to behave like mass lesions. Generally, such patients do not come to medical attention until they have become symptomatic, often in a catastrophic manner associated with intracranial hemorrhage. In such patients, CT or MRI scanning is often useful as a guide to planning angiographic investigation, but prompt angiography is the definitive procedure for diagnosis and therapy planning. Depending on the location, characteristics, and size of the lesion, angiographic methods such as transcatheter embolization may even be preferable to surgical therapy.

Unlike intracranial vascular lesions, asymptomatic extracranial lesions, specifically hemodynamically significant carotid stenoses, do occur with sufficient frequency that routine noninvasive screening is reasonable in specific at-risk patient populations. The duplex Doppler scan, a bimodal ultrasound examination combining anatomic and functional imaging, permits the screening of asymptomatic patients in groups thought to be at risk for significant cervical carotid disease who might benefit from surgical intervention despite the lack of neurologic symptoms such as elderly patients about to undergo major cardiothoracic or abdominal surgery, patients with symptomatic occlusive vascular disease in the coronary or peripheral circulation, and patients with asymptomatic carotid bruits. Once identified by noninvasive testing, such lesions should generally be investigated angiographically to determine the need for further intervention and delineate the anatomic details of the lesion. Symptomatic carotid vascular disease, on the other hand, generally merits prompt angiographic investigation and surgical treatment.

Despite significant advances in noninvasive imaging, angiography is still the method of choice for definitive evaluation of vascular lesions of both the extracranial and the intracranial circulation because of the complex three-dimensional nature of the vascular system and the need for very-high-resolution images. Furthermore, angiographic methods including thrombolytic infusion, balloon angioplasty, and transcatheter embolization have become the methods of choice for treating certain lesions that are either inaccessible to the surgeon or unresponsive to conventional surgical methods. Although there is an increasing crossover between the interests of the neurosurgeon and those of the vascular surgeon in these areas, the following discussion is aimed primarily at the needs of the vascular surgeon.

The Basic Examination Plan

From the point of view of the vascular surgeon, most angiography of the cerebrovascular system is performed for the evaluation of atheromatous occlusive disease of the carotid system in the region of the carotid bifurcation, since this is the most common location of this very common disease. Nevertheless, a complete examination must allow for the possibility that the disease process may not be confined to that region and that it may not even be atheromatous in nature.

Multi-view imaging and examination of the inflow and outflow are the basic principles in the angiographic evaluation of any vascular system. Therefore, a complete examination of the cerebrovascular system from the point of view of the vascular surgeon should theoretically include delineation of the aortic arch origins of the great vessels and their major branches, the cervical and intracranial segments of the carotid and vertebral arteries, and the major intracranial branches of these vessels. This can be accomplished by first obtaining a nonselective arch aortogram in the right posterior oblique (RPO) projection to demonstrate the aortic arch origins of the great vessels and their major branches. Omission of the preliminary nonselective aortic arch angiogram is unwise when investigating patients for occlusive vascular disease, even when selective angiography of the carotid arteries is planned. Ostial disease of the principal aortic arch branch vessels is sufficiently common that failure to detect such lesions prior to selective catheterization needlessly exposes the patient to the risks of embolization associated with markedly irregular atheromatous plaques or cerebral ischemia associated with traversing high-grade

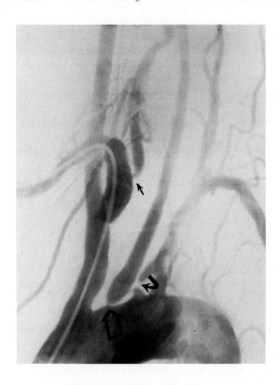

FIGURE 115–17. Arch aortogram (subtraction film). The right vertebral artery (*straight arrow*) and left common carotid artery (*open arrow*) are both stenotic. The left vertebral artery (*curved arrow*) arises from the aorta and is also stenotic. A decreased pulse in the left carotid artery was not recognized prior to this examination.

stenoses (Fig. 115–17). The aortogram also serves as a roadmap for multi-view angiography obtained by selective catheterization of the right and left common carotid arteries demonstrating the carotid arteries from the level of the bifurcation to the terminal branches of the anterior and middle cerebral arteries.

Several variations of the basic examination have gained wide acceptance. High-quality biplane oblique RPO and left posterior oblique (LPO) nonselective arch aortograms showing the cerebrovascular system from the level of the aortic arch to the level of the proximal major intracranial branches are often sufficient to evaluate the cerebrovascular system. Such examinations are usually adequate for the evaluation of atheromatous occlusive disease because significant atheromatous disease distal to the carotid siphon is relatively uncommon, although disease at that level is not uncommon. Obviously, both carotid bifurcations must be well demonstrated; otherwise, the examination should be supplemented by selective angiography of one or both carotid arteries. Disease of the vertebral-basilar system may also require supplemental selective angiography of the vertebral-basilar system with views designed to show the vertebral-basilar junction. Because the basilar artery is formed by the union of the right and left vertebral arteries, it is rarely necessary to perform selective angiography of both vertebral arteries.

RADIOGRAPHIC EQUIPMENT AND IMAGING TECHNIQUES

Specific Considerations for Cerebrovascular Angiography

Image-intensified video fluoroscopy and rapid-sequence filming devices have become standard equipment in angiographic laboratories. High-output x-ray generators and high-resolution video fluoroscopic systems have further increased the examiner's ability to visualize and manipulate small-caliber catheters even in obese patients. Unfortunately, biplane angiographic filming capability, although very desirable because of the reduction in contrast dosage and procedure time achieved by simultaneous multi-view filming, is still relatively uncommon even in many tertiary care facilities because of its expense. In fact, because of the decline in diagnostic neuroangiographic procedures occasioned by the advent of CT and MRI, older biplane units have often been replaced by newer single-plane units because this capability is less important in other areas of the body.

The most significant technical advance in cerebrovascular angiographic filming has been the development of digital fluoroscopic image processing, including both digital angiography (DA) and digital subtraction angiography (DSA). High-resolution digitized images are obtained directly from the fluoroscopic image intensifier; these images can then be manipulated by computer to enhance image contrast or subtract background detail from contrast-filled vessels. Both DA and DSA images are composed of a fixed number of pixels (picture elements), a fact that creates an important field of view versus resolution tradeoff. Because resolution is at least partially dependent on the pixel density per unit area, resolution can be improved by using the magnification modes of the image intensifier at the expense of reducing the field of view to a specific region of interest. In that manner, a given number of pixels span a smaller anatomic region, thus showing the region in greater detail.

Both DA and DSA images are available on the computer console immediately after contrast injection, unlike conventional photographic x-ray films, which require chemical processing; thus, use of either DA or DSA techniques offers greater convenience than film technique, allowing an examination to progress considerably faster. DA images, unlike those of DSA, are basically conventional fluoroscopic images recorded digitally for storage and enhancement (Fig. 115–18). DSA, on the other hand, is an image subtraction process and thus requires a much greater degree of patient cooperation than either DA or conventional unsubtracted film techniques. The basic assumption inherent in both DSA and film image subtraction is the absence of any change in the image other than the appearance of radiographic contrast material within the vascular system. Motion such as simple head and neck movement, swallowing, or breathing creates artifacts in the subtraction process. Simple translational movement artifacts can be eliminated by shifting the precontrast and postcontrast injection images relative to each other to compensate for such movements. Artifacts that are due to complex motion such as swallowing or breathing are nonuniform across the image field of view and cannot be totally eliminated by simple image shifting. When such artifacts overlie the areas of interest, they can cause significant diagnostic uncertainties. Although satisfactory results can often be obtained—even in the presence of motion artifacts—by simple correlation of the information obtained from different views, this is not always possible, especially in patients unable to cooperate with the examiner.

The appearance of a film subtraction or DSA image is dependent on the accuracy of the subtraction process as well as the lack of motion between the initial noncontrast ''mask'' image and subsequent images, which are assumed to be identical other than the presence of intravascular contrast media. Thus, in the ideal situation, all structures not containing contrast agents are eliminated from the image after film or DSA subtraction processing, leaving an image composed solely of contrast-filled vessels. In the case of film subtraction, the mask is actually a photographic reversal of an angiographic film taken prior to the injection of contrast media, made by copying that film onto a special film that accurately renders the various gray shades of an image in the mathematically opposite shades of white. When the mask film is superimposed on a film containing contrast medium, the images cancel except for the contrast-filled vessels. In the case of DSA, the mask is simply a precontrast digital image and subtraction is just a point-by-point mathematical process. In practice, however, there are slight differences between the precontrast mask and the contrast images, caused primarily by motion, that make the subtraction less than perfect, leaving faint residual images of bone and soft tissue. Although the presence of faint residual images associated with imperfections in the subtraction process might at first seem undesirable, these residual background images are actually quite useful in providing a visual frame of reference for what would otherwise be a difficult to evaluate ''disembodied'' image of a vessel. For that reason, most modern DSA systems now include the capability to subtract a variable percentage of the original image pixel values, thus leaving residual landmark images of whatever intensity the examiner desires (Fig. 115–19).

DSA provides far better contrast resolution than either DA or standard photographic x-ray film technique, making visualization of vessels possible with much less contrast material (or much more dilute material) than that required

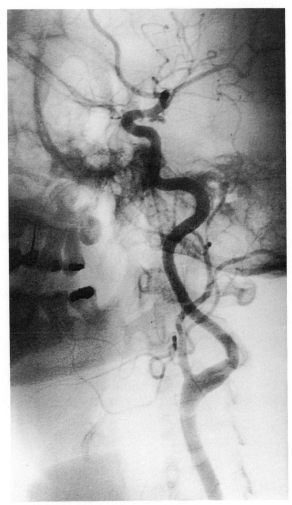

FIGURE 115–18. Digital angiography (DA) of the carotid artery. Because this is a nonsubtracted image, it is relatively immune to the sort of motion artifacts that can severely degrade a digital subtraction angiography (DSA) image. However, because it is also a digital image, the DA image can be manipulated to enhance various details using the viewing station computer system just like a DSA image. (Courtesy of Julius Grollman, M.D., Little Company of Mary Hospital, Torrance, California.)

by film technique. This fact was the basis for early efforts at intravenous DSA. Injection of contrast material through a small right atrial catheter introduced via a percutaneous antecubital venipuncture held out the promise of rapid, low-cost, low-risk outpatient angiographic carotid artery screening. However, problems with motion artifacts are much more frequent with venous injection than with arterial injection because there is a much longer period between the onset of the subjective sensations resulting from the injection and filling of the vessels of interest than there is with arterial injection. Dispersal and dilution of the contrast bolus in patients with low cardiac output also tended to degrade image quality. For these reasons, the percentage of diagnostic quality studies proved to be disappointing and the technique has been largely abandoned except in special circumstances such as the presence of severe upper and lower extremity peripheral vascular disease that limits arterial access. In addition, the advent of small-caliber (4 and 5 Fr), high-flow arterial catheters has also reduced arterial

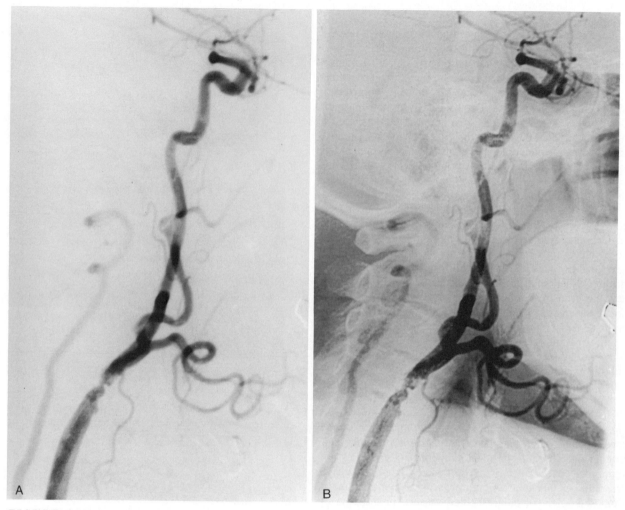

FIGURE 115–19. *A*, DSA showing a high-grade focal stenosis of the distal common carotid artery. Owing to the lack of motion artifact, background subtraction is virtually complete. Although this shows the lesion to advantage, it also makes orientation difficult. *B*, Reducing the degree of background subtraction in the same DSA image produces an image that contains useful background landmarks. (*A* and *B*, Courtesy of Julius Grollman, M.D., Little Company of Mary Hospital, Torrance, California, and Toshiba America Medical Systems, Irvine, California.)

puncture site complications so much that outpatient arterial angiography now carries little more risk than venous angiography.

Although DSA provides superior contrast resolution and both DA and DSA offer considerable convenience, standard photographic x-ray film still provides considerably better spatial resolution than either DA or DSA, even with the use of field of view limitation as described previously, and therein lies a critical tradeoff: contrast resolution versus spatial resolution. Therefore, the choice of conventional x-ray film or DA or DSA technique depends largely on the clinical situation. If nonocclusive ulcerative disease or fibromuscular dysplasia is suspected, fine detail and high resolution are essential, virtually mandating the use of conventional x-ray film methods. Also, if the patient is incapable of cooperation sufficient to avoid DSA motion artifacts, DA or conventional x-ray film methods are preferable. If, on the other hand, occlusive disease is the primary clinical suspicion and the patient is sufficiently cooperative, spatial resolution becomes a secondary issue, making the choice dependent on examiner preference and other clinical fac-

tors. Perhaps the best example of this tradeoff is the classic problem of differentiating a total occlusion from a near-total occlusion where distal flow cannot be shown with certainty on a conventional film angiogram but it can be detected on a DSA study owing to the superior contrast resolution of the DSA technique.

Technical Aspects of Cerebrovascular Angiography

Prior to the advent of selective catheterization via peripheral vascular access routes, direct puncture carotid angiography was routinely employed. The technique is simple, quick, and relatively safe, although, by definition, it limits the scope of examination, making assessment of the proximal vessel segment virtually impossible. Direct cannulation is accomplished by puncturing the common carotid artery low in the neck using a thin-walled cannula equipped with a hollow stylet. Single- or double-wall (puncture and pull-back) techniques are acceptable. Once the vessel has

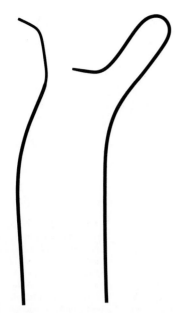

FIGURE 115–20. *Left*, Headhunter catheter—an advancement catheter. *Right*, Simmons sidewinder catheter—a withdrawal catheter.

been successfully punctured, as shown by brisk blood flow through the cannula, the cannula is advanced a short distance into the vessel over a soft-tipped guidewire. Between injections, the cannula is plugged with a blunt-tipped obturator to prevent thrombus formation in the cannula; frequent flushing and meticulous injection techniques are also essential. Numerous needle, cannula, and sheath combinations have been designed for this purpose, and most work well.

The development of small-caliber high-torque catheters that can be introduced via remote access sites (e.g., femoral, axillary, or brachial arteries) and easily manipulated into the cerebral vessels has largely supplanted direct puncture carotid angiography, as it allows the entire cerebrovascular system to be conveniently studied using a single puncture. In addition, there is usually less patient anxi-

ety associated with distal puncture than with the direct technique. A detailed discussion of the techniques and materials used for cerebrovascular angiography is beyond the scope of this text; however, just as there are strong personal preferences regarding surgical instruments among surgeons, catheter choice is often a matter of both technical and personal preference among radiologists. The development of small-caliber (4 and 5 Fr) high-flow, high-torque preshaped catheters available in a wide range of curve shapes and sizes has virtually eliminated the use of "homemade" heat-shaped polyethylene catheters once popular among neuroradiologists.

Although the variety of catheter shapes is too numerous to discuss in detail, there are two basic classes of catheter shape: advancement and withdrawal (Fig. 115–20). Advancement catheters are designed to be advanced into the vessel of choice by a combination of torque and guidewire manipulations. Withdrawal catheters, typified by the shepherd's crook–shaped Simmons sidewinder catheter, are used by advancing beyond the vessel ostium and withdrawing in order to engage the tip in the vessel ostium (Fig. 115–21). Thus, withdrawal catheters are advanced out of a vessel and withdrawn into it. The withdrawal catheters are particularly useful when the angulation of the proximal segment of the branch vessel makes direct advancement difficult. Although they are easy to use, withdrawal catheters have the disadvantage of requiring a re-forming maneuver to regain their special shape after being introduced into the vessel over a guidewire in a relatively straight configuration (Fig. 115–22). The choice of catheter shape is largely dependent on the configuration and tortuosity of the vessels to be traversed.

For reasons of simple convenience, most angiographers prefer the percutaneous femoral artery approach popularized by Dr. Sven Seldinger. However, when that approach proves to be impractical because of severe ileofemoral vascular disease, cerebral angiography can be carried out successfully via percutaneous axillary, brachial, or even translumbar catheterization. Withdrawal catheters are generally used as part of the transaxillary approach, and the right axillary artery is generally chosen because it

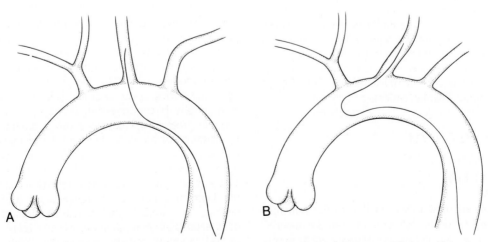

FIGURE 115–21. *A*, Headhunter catheter advanced into the left common carotid artery. *B*, Simmons sidewinder catheter withdrawn into the left common carotid artery. Note that the angulation of this vessel would have made advancement catheterization with the headhunter catheter difficult.

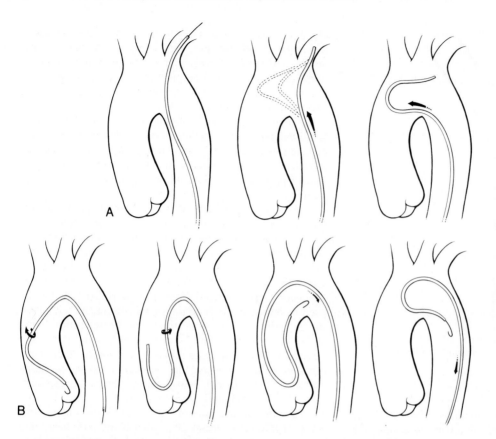

FIGURE 115–22. *A,* Simmons sidewinder catheter re-formed using the left subclavian artery as a pivot point. *B,* Catheter re-formed using the aortic valve to deflect its leading tip. Re-formation using the contralateral common iliac artery, the renal arteries, or the superior mesenteric artery can also be performed, but such maneuvers are more difficult than those shown above. (*A* and *B,* From Kadir S: Diagnostic Angiography. Philadelphia, WB Saunders, 1986.)

greatly simplifies selective catheterization of the right common carotid artery.

Numerous acceptable radiographic contrast agents are available; the ionic salts of meglumine (diatrizoate, iothalamate, and metrizoate) are well tolerated. A 60 per cent solution of meglumine iothalamate (Conray 60, Mallinkrodt Pharmaceuticals) is frequently used for selective angiography, whereas a more concentrated mixture of meglumine iothalamate (52 per cent) and sodium iothalamate (26 per cent) (Vascoray, Mallinkrodt Pharmaceuticals) is used for nonselective arch angiography because of the need to compensate for dilution in the arch. A group of nonionic and low-ionic water-soluble agents have been introduced that, although considerably more expensive, may be preferable owing to decreased neurotoxicity and nephrotoxicity. These agents include Isovue (iopamidol, Squibb Pharmaceuticals), Omnipaque (iohexol, Winthrop Pharmaceuticals), Hexabrix (ioxaglate meglumine 39.3 per cent and ioxaglate sodium 19.6 per cent, Mallinkrodt Pharmaceuticals) and Optiray (ioversol, Mallinkrodt Pharmaceuticals).

COMPLICATIONS OF CEREBROVASCULAR ANGIOGRAPHY

Most complications are associated with the puncture site or the administration of radiographic contrast material and, as such, have already been discussed elsewhere in this text. Furthermore, most of the access site complications (e.g., hematoma as a result of ineffective postwithdrawal

hemostasis or delayed puncture site bleeding and occlusion as a result of excessive postwithdrawal pressure on the vessel) can be avoided by careful technique and a refusal to delegate this important, but perhaps less enthralling, phase of the procedure to an assistant or a mechanical compression device. The occurrence of respiratory compromise due to tracheal compression or deviation associated with a cervical hematoma complicating a direct puncture carotid angiogram, once a feared complication, is now largely of historic interest owing to the virtual abandonment of direct puncture carotid angiography.

Fortunately, true neurologic complications are uncommon during cerebral angiography. The incidence of major complications (e.g., death, stroke, access site problems requiring surgical intervention) has been quoted as being approximately 0.16 per cent in one large study. Transient neurologic deficits (transient ischemic attacks, TIAs) were reported to occur with a frequency of approximately 0.9 per cent in another study. The use of systemic heparin anticoagulation during aortic arch and selective common carotid angiography is controversial. However, as is the case for surgical procedures, there is a direct relationship between the duration of the procedure and the incidence of complications. This fact is of special relevance to academic institutions where the learning needs of the house staff and the safety of the patient must be carefully balanced. Although the decision to perform the procedure is ultimately dependent on the nature of the clinical problem, the occurrence of a neurologic complication, even if relatively transient, should generally halt the angiographic study, at least until consultation with the referring physician is obtained.

Although there are varying opinions as to the level of

sedation desirable in noncerebral angiography, there is reasonable unanimity of opinion regarding the avoidance of significant sedation in most cerebrovascular angiographic procedures in order to avoid masking neurologic complications resulting from the procedure.

THE TAILORED EXAMINATION

The precise design of an angiographic study must balance the information needs of the referring physician with the risks and benefits to the patient. Broadly speaking, the clinical status of the patient is the prime determinant of how extensive or focused the study is to be. Thus, the discussion here is divided into five major subgroups of patients: symptomatic, asymptomatic, traumatized, stroke-in-evolution, and postoperative.

The Symptomatic Patient

Although there is still debate among internists, neurologists, neurosurgeons, and vascular surgeons as to the optimal modes of therapy in the symptomatic patient, there is relative unanimity of opinion as to the desirability of obtaining a definitive anatomic diagnosis. Patients with well-defined transient neurologic events thought to be ischemic or embolic in nature merit a thorough evaluation aimed at detection of disease amenable to either surgical or medical treatment.

The specific details of filming techniques, catheterization methods, and injection sites are best determined on the basis of information obtained from noninvasive testing as well as the basic history and physical examination. However, angiography limited solely to the suspect vessel is undesirable owing to the propensity for vascular occlusive disease, including atherosclerotic as well as fibromuscular dysplasia and arteritis, to occur at multiple sites. Generally, the presence of a carotid bruit and a corresponding ultrasound abnormality imply simple occlusive disease that can often be evaluated by high-quality nonselective DSA, DA, or film arch aortograms. In the absence of such findings, more detailed film angiography including selective carotid injections and additional views of suspect areas may be required to detect nonocclusive ulcerative disease that might serve as a site of thrombus formation (Fig. 115–23). In the symptomatic patient, absence of disease at the carotid bifurcation necessitates a detailed examination of the aortic arch origins as well as the intracranial vessels, particularly the region of the carotid siphon. Failure to find demonstrable anatomic disease then mandates a search for other sources of emboli, including the cardiac chambers and valves.

The finding of a seemingly occluded carotid or vertebral artery, especially on nonselective arch angiography, is a special case. Because there is a major difference in the approach to a total occlusion and to a near-total occlusion, definitive resolution of the issue is essential. In such cases, selective injection of the vessel in question should be performed with an extended filming program that provides both early and late views of the area in order to differentiate total occlusion from near-total occlusion with very slow faint antegrade filling of the distal vessel segment (Fig. 115–24) and retrograde collateral filling (Fig. 115–25). Although DSA and conventional x-ray film subtraction techniques applied to nonselective arch aortograms may be useful in evaluation of collateral filling patterns and the detection of low-volume filling distal to a near-total obstruction, they can also introduce motion artifacts that are difficult to evaluate. Selective injection presents a maximal opacification dose of undiluted contrast material to the suspect area, whereas nonselective arch angiography, of necessity, involves significant dilution of the contrast bolus (see Fig. 115–23). Once the presence of a near-total occlusion has been confirmed, consideration should be given to prompt anticoagulation because there is a definite, although not well quantified, increase in the risk of occlusion of such lesions following angiography.

Patients who have recently had a completed stroke constitute another special case of the symptomatic patient. Because surgical intervention is unlikely to be of much benefit to such patients in the immediate postevent period, angiography is also unlikely to be of much use. Indeed, because the presence of a stroke generally indicates a defect in the blood-brain barrier, the use of a neurotoxic agent such as radiographic contrast material is probably contraindicated. Little definitive data exist as to when angiography can be safely performed in the poststroke patient. The persistence of parenchymal CT contrast enhancement, which implies a defect in the blood-brain barrier, usually lasts for 6 weeks. Therefore, although the decision is based on logic rather than proof, this probably constitutes a reasonable minimal safe waiting period.

The Asymptomatic Patient

Asymptomatic patients come to medical attention as the result of abnormalities detected by either physical examination (e.g., bruits) or noninvasive screening. The differences of approach among internists, neurologists, neurosurgeons, and vascular surgeons as to the optimal modes of therapy, and even the need for therapy, in such patients are remarkable. However, there is relative unanimity of opinion as to the desirability of obtaining a definitive anatomic diagnosis in the event surgical intervention is comtemplated. Because the presence of disease of sufficient magnitude to be detectable by physical examination or noninvasive screening implies the presence of an occlusive lesion of at least moderate severity rather than a subtle irregularity of the vessel such as a superficial ulceration, high-resolution angiography is usually not required. Simple nonselective multi-view aortic arch injection DSA, DA, or conventional x-ray film angiography is usually adequate. As in the case of the symptomatic patient, however, angiography limited solely to the suspect vessel is inappropriate.

The Traumatized Patient

Angiographic examination of the patient subjected to trauma involving the extracranial or intracranial cerebral circulation, or both, constitutes an important exception to the rule of completeness, since there is usually a premium

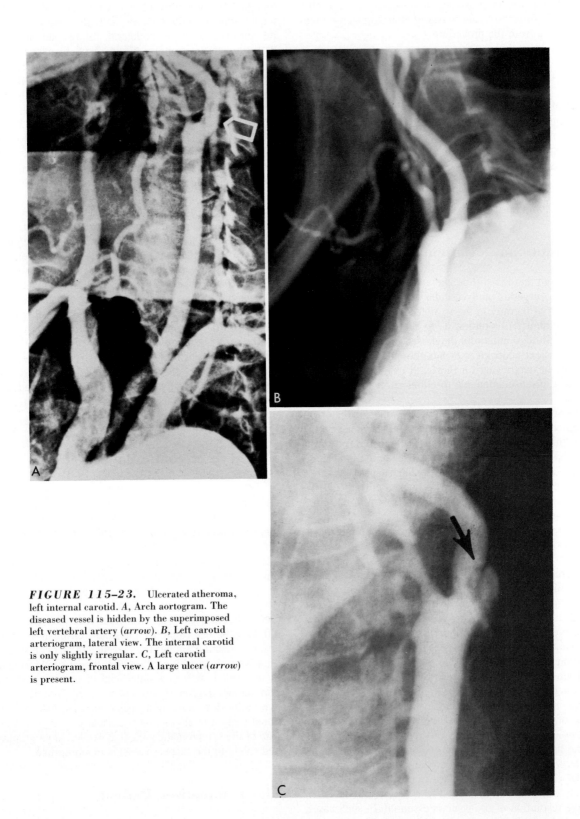

FIGURE 115–23. Ulcerated atheroma, left internal carotid. *A*, Arch aortogram. The diseased vessel is hidden by the superimposed left vertebral artery (*arrow*). *B*, Left carotid arteriogram, lateral view. The internal carotid is only slightly irregular. *C*, Left carotid arteriogram, frontal view. A large ulcer (*arrow*) is present.

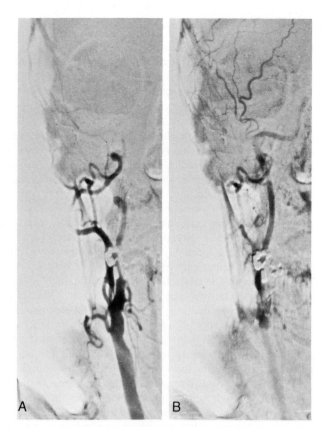

FIGURE 115–24. *A*, Early film from a right common carotid artery injection showing primarily the external carotid artery system. The proximal internal carotid artery and its high-grade ostial stenosis are actually visualized but difficult to detect (vertebral artery partly opacified by reflux flow from the common carotid to the right subclavian). *B*, Late film of the same angiogram clearly showing internal carotid artery and near-occlusive proximal stenosis.

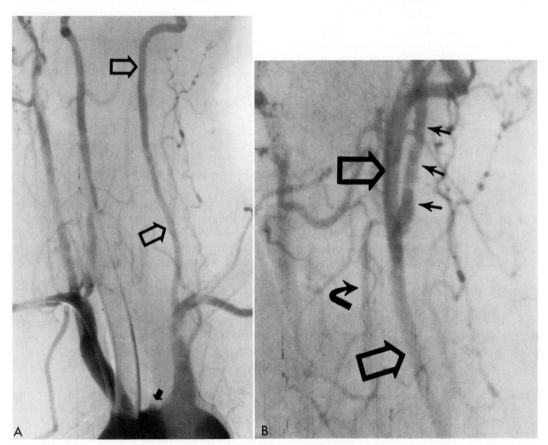

FIGURE 115–25. Occluded left common carotid artery with patent internal and external carotid branches. *A*, Arch aortogram, early film. The left common carotid is occluded (*solid arrow*). The left vertebral artery is outlined by *open arrows*. *B*, Arch aortogram, delayed film (close-up view). The vertebral artery is again outlined by *open arrows*. The internal carotid (*straight arrows*) is filled via the external carotid. The chief collateral pathway is the superior thyroid artery (*curved arrow*).

on expeditious diagnosis and treatment. Even the so-called stable patient can become perilously unstable without much advance warning. Furthermore, single-system injury is uncommon. Accordingly, the angiographer must participate in the radiologic and nonradiologic evaluation of the patient as a member of a team able to coordinate and prioritize various investigations and treatments. The need for angiographic evaluation depends on patient condition and the location and type of injury as well as the management approach of the trauma surgeons caring for the patient. Angiography of superficial facial injuries is not usually required, since physical examination is generally very accurate and surgical exploration is relatively straightforward. Deep penetrating facial injuries, on the other hand, may well require angiography for both diagnosis and treatment involving transcatheter embolization because such injuries can involve relatively inaccessible structures. Most surgeons agree as to the need for angiographic evaluation of neck injuries to zone I (angle of jaw–base of skull) and zone III (cricoid–clavicle) since these areas present significant problems in surgical exposure. The need for angiographic evaluation of injuries to zone II (cricoid–angle of jaw) is far more controversial, since this is an area relatively amenable to prompt surgical exploration. Despite the controversy, some of which is economic in nature, angiography of zone II injuries still seems like a worthwhile step in the stable patient because it can easily diagnose unsuspected vascular injuries or eliminate unnecessary explorations. In any event, however, once the role of angiography in the overall management of the patient has been determined, a goal-directed plan of study for the specific areas subjected to trauma should be formulated on the basis of the mode of injury and the areas likely to be affected by such injuries.

The most common cerebrovascular injuries of interest to the vascular surgeon that require emergency angiographic evaluation are the penetrating injuries of the neck. Although stab wounds may at first seem relatively limited in scope, it is important to remember that a small entry wound can easily hide more extensive underlying trauma. For that reason, angiographic evaluation of a stab wound should involve at least selective angiography of the cervical segments of the ipsilateral carotid or vertebral arteries, or both. If an injury is detected, views of the intracranial circulation including the contralateral supply should generally be obtained to evaluate collateral flow pathways. Knowledge of the collateral flow becomes especially important when the injury occurs in a region where surgical access is difficult, such as the zone III area just below the base of the skull, in which case ligation of an injured vessel may be preferable to repair if the collateral flow patterns permit sacrificing the vessel in question (Fig. 115–26).

The trajectory of a bullet within tissue, especially a complex area like the neck, is virtually impossible to reconstruct. Furthermore, the extent of both direct and shock wave injury is also difficult to determine simply by physical examination. If the path of injury is clearly confined to one side, ipsilateral selective angiography of the cervical segments of the carotid or vertebral arteries is usually sufficient; however, if there is any doubt as to whether the bullet crossed the mid-line, bilateral angiography should be performed. As in the case of stab wound injuries, the detection

of a cervical segment injury strongly suggests the need for delineation of the intracranial circulation and potential collateral pathways. The absence of an angiographically detectable abnormality or the presence of a minor irregularity such as localized bulging or indistinctness, which might be overlooked on routine diagnostic angiography, should be considered highly suspect in the traumatized patient, especially a bullet wound victim, and the suspect area should be carefully evaluated with additional views, selective angiography, subtraction film processing, or DSA. This is especially true if there are clinical, physical, or radiographic findings suggesting significant trauma such as hypotension or a soft tissue swelling indicating the presence of a hematoma (Fig. 115–27). Such findings should raise the examiner's "index of suspicion" as they may be the only evidence of a major vascular injury temporarily hidden by the tamponade of a precarious clot. However, additional views and selective catheterization should obviously be undertaken with considerable care, as these maneuvers may well pinpoint the injury, revealing its true significance by initiating bleeding at the injury site suddenly destabilizing the situation (Fig. 115–28). Urgent surgical intervention is required in such situations; however, simple local compression may be insufficient to stop bleeding long enough to transport the patient to the operating room. In such situations, temporary hemostasis can often be obtained very quickly by catheterizing the injured vessel with an angioplasty balloon placed across the injury site and inflated to a low pressure sufficient to provide both proximal and distal vascular control. If ligation rather than primary repair is contemplated, the same effect can also be achieved in the angiography suite by placing either coil or detachable balloon occlusive devices proximal and distal to the injury site.

Zone I injuries add a special consideration to planning the angiographic evaluation, since these injuries may actually involve intrathoracic structures such as the arch origins of the great vessels. Thus, consideration should always be given to obtaining a thoracic aortogram prior to selective catheterization in low zone I injuries. Likewise, consideration should also be given to obtaining a thoracic aortogram prior to selective angiography in the elderly patient, in whom significant unsuspected atheromatous occlusive disease may make selective catheterization of greater risk.

Direct blunt trauma to the neck and acceleration-deceleration injuries such as those sustained in motor vehicle or pedestrian-vehicle accidents presents a difficult clinical problem. If there are obvious physical signs of significant injury or neurologic signs that cannot be explained on the basis of head injury, angiography is usually indicated in the acute setting. Similarly, should the patient experience a delayed neurologic event that might be referable to vascular occlusion at the site of trauma or emboli originating from that site, prompt angiographic evaluation is also indicated.

In the case of intracranial vascular trauma, CT scanning is usually the primary evaluation modality, followed by angiography if the CT scan suggests that a salvageable situation still exists. In any event, however, diagnosis and treatment of such injuries are usually the province of the neurosurgeon rather than the vascular surgeon and, as such, are beyond the scope of this discussion.

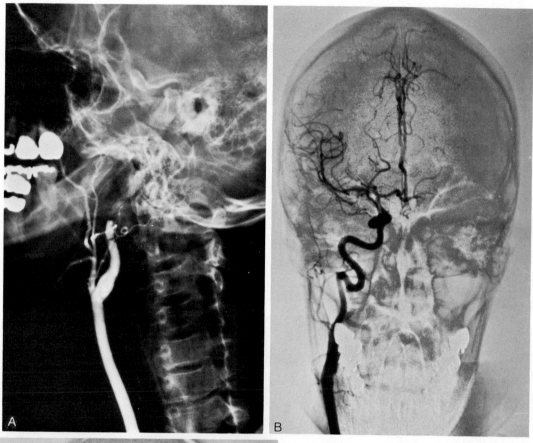

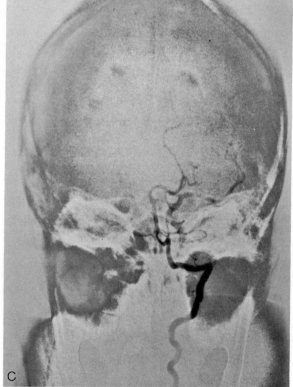

FIGURE 115–26. *A,* Selective left common carotid angiogram of a young woman stabbed in the neck just below the base of the skull during a violent rape assault. The left common carotid artery is totally occluded, but there is no evidence of extravasation. *B,* Selective right common carotid angiogram showing flow to right MCA as well as both right and left ACAs. The flow "pseudo-occlusion" of the left MCA is caused by inflow of unopacified blood to the left MCA arising from the posterior circulation. *C,* Selective left vertebral injection showing normal posterior circulation as well as supply to the left MCA. Demonstration of adequate flow from the contralateral and posterior circulations allowed safe ligation of the left internal carotid artery just below the base of the skull rather than a difficult reconstruction. (Examination of the vessel at surgery showed it to be occluded by thrombus, presumably as the result of an intimal disruption associated with violent neck motion and trauma to the vessel at the atlanto-occipital joint; no penetrating injury was found.)

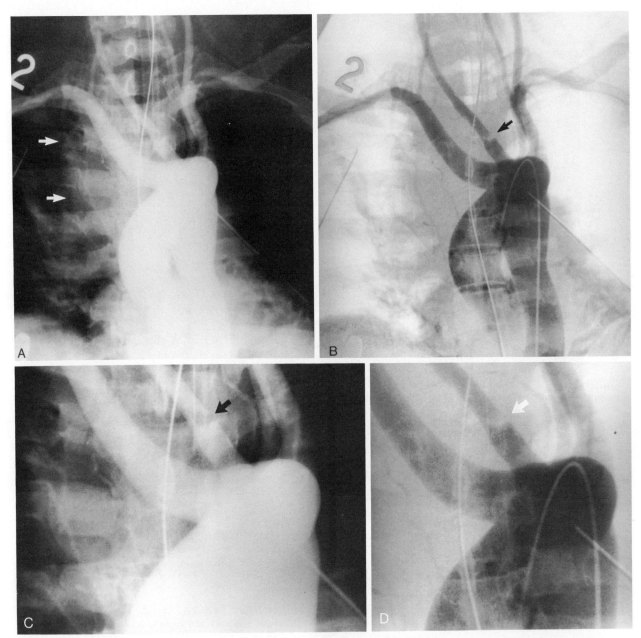

FIGURE 115–27.   *A,* Nonselective aortic arch angiogram in patient with a gunshot wound, which was initially interpreted as showing no definite evidence of a major vascular injury despite the presence of a large right superior mediastinal soft tissue density indicating the presence of a large hematoma (*arrows*). (*Note:* The aberrant right subclavian artery is a normal anatomic variant.) *B,* Film subtraction of the same angiogram revealing partial transection of the right common carotid artery (*arrow*). Although, in retrospect, this lesion may indeed have been seen on the unsubtracted angiogram, the allowance made for radiographic shadows of underlying bony structures effectively desensitized the examiner, precluding detection of this very significant injury. *C,* Unsubtracted magnification view of the same area makes the injury (*arrow*) far more obvious as does magnification film subtraction (*D*).

The Patient With Stroke-in-Evolution

The differences of approach regarding optimal modes of therapy and investigation in patients with a stroke-in-evolution are often of incredible magnitude even among colleagues within a single institution. Even definition of terms in this area is controversial. However, for the purpose of this discussion, the syndrome of crescendo TIAs, in which such events occur with ominously increasing frequency, should be considered a special and more urgent case of the symptomatic patient, as discussed previously.

The stroke-in-evolution is a far more ominous entity that consists of an ongoing neurologic event that does not appear to be transient, although it may have a waxing and waning character.

The presence of an acute cerebrovascular event-in-progress implies a major abnormality of the blood-brain barrier. Because all forms of radiographic contrast material are known to be neurotoxic, even in patients with a normal intact blood-brain barrier, angiography should be avoided unless immediate surgical or angiographic therapeutic intervention is contemplated. Furthermore, if angiography is

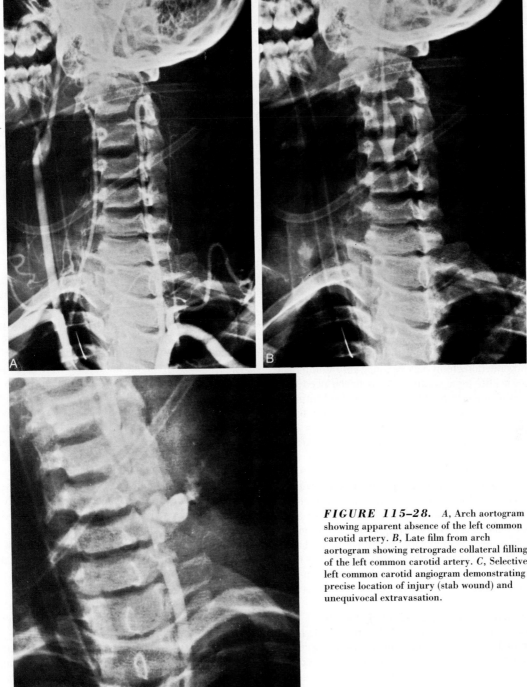

FIGURE 115–28. *A*, Arch aortogram showing apparent absence of the left common carotid artery. *B*, Late film from arch aortogram showing retrograde collateral filling of the left common carotid artery. *C*, Selective left common carotid angiogram demonstrating precise location of injury (stab wound) and unequivocal extravasation.

performed, it should be strictly limited in both scope and dosage.

Unlike the situation in the treatment of crescendo TIAs, emergency surgery has had disappointing results in the care of patients with the stroke-in-evolution syndrome, and angiography for such patients has therefore become uncommon. However, a new concept of the pathophysiology of ischemic stroke has been gaining acceptance that suggests that irreversible neurologic damage does not always occur as an all-or-nothing phenomenon. In some circumstances, a period of nonfunctioning viability seems to exist, during which restoration of flow may restore function. Thus, the stroke-in-evolution may be analogous to the situation in myocardial infarction in which a definite period of ischemic viability exists between the inciting event and ultimately irreversible infarction, during which restoration of flow will restore function and prevent infarction. German researchers at the University Hospital of Aachen, as well as a growing number of French and American investigators, have shown that localized thrombolytic infusion in cases of thrombotic (in situ or embolic) occlusion can result in restoration of neurologic function (Fig. 115–29) and that there is a premium on minimizing the time between symptom onset and flow restoration. Although such treatment is still experimental, the success reported by these investigators bodes well for the eventual acceptance of this mode of therapy.

The Postoperative Patient

Routine intraoperative ''completion angiography'' following carotid endarterectomy has become very common, although there is still some controversy as to the need for it. Irregularities of the endarterectomy margins and intimal fractures (''clamp defects'') are common and are of little clinical significance. Furthermore, such irregularities are likely to disappear with the development of neointimal healing. However, the presence of an unsuspected and potentially occlusive intimal flap or an endarterectomy that fails to traverse the area of stenosis fully is of considerable significance and therefore best detected when correction involves simply reopening an already exposed vessel and completing the endarterectomy. Although completion angiography has become commonplace, many surgeons have chosen to employ routine angioscopic evaluation, since this technique may be even more sensitive than conventional angiography in the detection of correctable technical problems.

The occurrence of an acute neurologic event in the immediate postoperative period is probably best treated by prompt reexploration when it occurs in the same vascular territory supplemented by angiography if the expected thrombus at the operative site is not found. The occurrence or recurrence of symptoms in a patient who has recently undergone carotid endarterectomy mandates angiographic evaluation of both the operative site and the downstream vascular territory subject to embolization from that area. If the surgery is not recent (more than 6 months ago), evaluation should be as thorough as in the case of a patient that has not yet had surgery because of the possibility for the development of new lesions or the exacerbation of previously mild lesions.

FUTURE TRENDS IN CEREBROVASCULAR ANGIOGRAPHY

Until fairly recently, angiography was thought of as a primarily diagnostic modality in the management of cerebrovascular disease despite rapid advances in interventional radiology elsewhere in the body. However, interventional neuroradiologic techniques, notably intracranial embolization, have also gained acceptance as a result of the poor results of surgical therapy in such cases and the relative inaccessibility of many intracranial vascular lesions. On the other hand, the excellent results and low morbidity of extracranial cerebrovascular surgery make interventional radiologic techniques such as percutaneous transluminal angioplasty (PTA) less likely to gain general acceptance in the near future except in unusual circumstances; PTA of the inaccessible intracranial vasculature is, however, slowly gaining acceptance.

In contrast to the percutaneous technique, intraoperative balloon catheter angioplasty is likely to become a relatively standard technique in management of certain carotid lesions. Intraoperative vascular control allows back-bleeding and flushing, unavailable in the nonoperative situation, thus virtually eliminating the chance of embolization. In the case of fibromuscular dysplasia, the radially directed forces involved in balloon angioplasty are far preferable to the shearing forces involved in the use of conventional rigid dilators. Rigid dilators often damage uninvolved intima while failing to disrupt the diaphragm-like lesions of fibromuscular dysplasia adequately. The angioplasty balloon, on the other hand, tends to disrupt the lesions of fibromuscular dysplasia preferentially without damaging adjacent normal intima (Fig. 115–30). This technique may also be useful in dealing with high extracranial internal carotid lesions difficult to expose by standard surgical methods and possibly even with lesions of the carotid siphon, although such uses are still experimental. Intraoperative use of balloon catheter methods is also attractive in that it adds very little to the duration of the surgery. Because the presence of an arteriotomy automatically directs the catheter into the proper vessel, passage of the catheter to the region of interest under routine intraoperative fluoroscopy using a soft-tipped guidewire can be accomplished easily and quickly. Indeed, the whole procedure can usually be accomplished within a few minutes.

As noted previously in the section discussing the angiographic management of the stroke-in-evolution, selective transcatheter infusion of thrombolytic agents may play an important role in the management of this ominous condition. Thromboembolic occlusions occurring in the region of the carotid bifurcation will probably respond readily to this approach, averting the otherwise inevitable stroke and uncovering underlying stenoses amenable to urgent but otherwise conventional surgical techniques. Intracranial thromboembolic lesions are also likely to be amenable to local

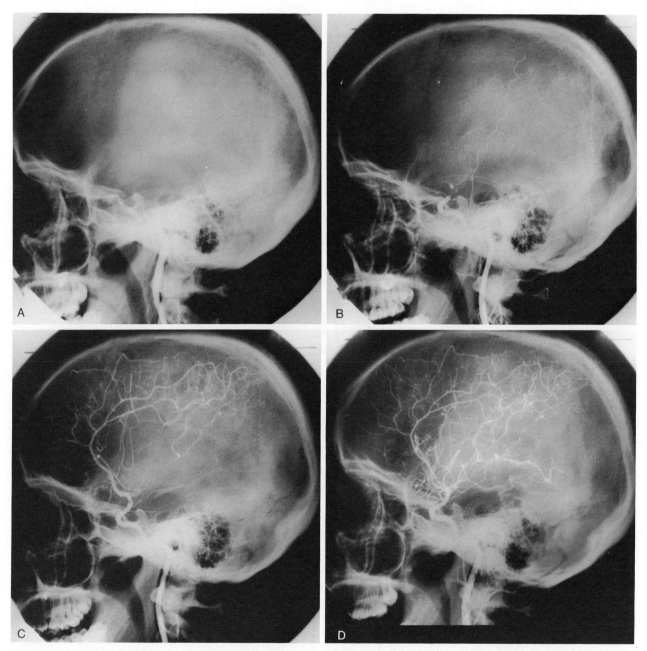

FIGURE 115–29. *A,* Angiogram showing total occlusion of the internal carotid artery at the skull base. The patient, a young woman with a prosthetic aortic valve, was in the hospital at the time of the event and had been observed to be neurologically intact less than 30 minutes before becoming densely hemiparetic and aphasic. The angiogram was performed approximately 1 hour after the event had been discovered. *B,* Selective infusion of urokinase (4000 IU/hr) in the internal carotid opened the carotid siphon, but the embolus was still virtually occlusive. *C,* After 90 minutes of infusion, the ACA was again patent and it supplied collateral flow to the MCA. The embolus was still present just distal to the carotid siphon but much smaller. Subsequent angiograms (not shown) documented complete lysis of this portion of the embolus but showed persistent occlusion of the MCA. *D,* A 2.2 Fr soft Tracker catheter was then advanced into the proximal MCA, where the infusion was continued for another 90 minutes. This resulted in restoration of antegrade flow to the MCA with the exception of some parietal lobe branches. The patient regained full sensory motor control and suffered only minimal "word grope." Within a week, she was back at work, showing no signs of neurologic impairment.

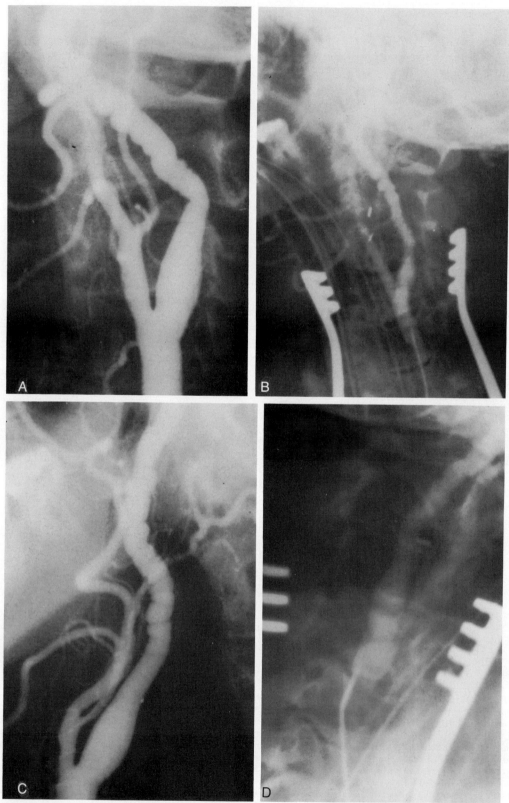

FIGURE 115–30. *A,* Preoperative left common carotid angiogram showing multiple diaphragm-like stenoses of fibromuscular dysplasia. *B,* Intraoperative completion angiogram following two attempts at dilatation using rigid DeBakey dilators, documenting the presence of residual stenoses and irregularities. *C,* Preoperative right common carotid angiogram documenting similar lesions. *D,* Intraoperative completion angiogram following dilatation using transluminal balloon angioplasty catheter, showing no significant residual stenoses.

thrombolytic infusion now that very soft, trackable 2- to 3-Fr microcatheters such as the Tracker series produced by Target Therapeutics, Inc., are available to permit superselective catheterization of clotted branches in the vertebralbasilar, middle, and anterior cerebral branches.

In addition to the procedural advances discussed, many exciting instrumentation advances are likely to have considerable impact on cerebrovascular imaging as well. Diagnostic imaging, once confined to the production and evaluation of x-ray images, has grown rapidly since the early 1980s to include many nonionizing imaging techniques. The technologies presently of greatest potential future significance to the imaging of the cerebrovascular system are MRI angiography and ultra-high-resolution video systems.

MRI, with its sensitivity to blood motion, has been used to create three-dimensional volumes of image data that can be presented in the form of projection x-ray angiograms where the same data can be viewed from any desired obliquity. If, or more likely when, this technique becomes practical, it may assume a very important role in noninvasive screening.

Ultra-high-resolution video systems are likely to eventually offer spatial resolution rivaling that of conventional film technology. As spatial resolution penalties become less important, the great power of digital technology in image manipulation will increasingly be brought to bear on cerebrovascular imaging, and indeed medical imaging of all sorts. The availability of large-capacity computer memory chips, superfast microcomputers, and ultra-high-capacity optical disk storage is critically important to this development, since the amount of pixel information contained in high-resolution images is immense. This technology has the power to unlock previously overlooked information while at the same time saving storage space and cost by reducing conventional photographic film usage. As exciting as these possibilities are, the technology is of limited utility without the ability to access and transmit these images rapidly. Although many of the technical problems involved in high-resolution digital imaging are already being successfully solved, the availability of relatively low-cost viewing devices and the ultra-high-speed data transmission technology needed to transfer such images from one place to another are still major problem areas.

References

1. Abrams HL (ed): Vascular and Interventional Radiology. Boston, Little, Brown, 1983.
2. Ben-Menachem Y: Angiography in Trauma, A Work Atlas. Philadelphia, WB Saunders, 1981.
3. Friedman SM: Visual Anatomy: Head and Neck. New York, Harper & Row, 1970.
4. Huckman MS, Shenk GI, Neems RL, et al: Transfemoral cerebral angiography versus direct percutaneous carotid and brachial arteriography: A comparison of complication rates. Radiology 132:93, 1979.
5. Kadir S: Diagnostic Angiography. Philadelphia, WB Saunders, 1986.
6. Mani RL, Eisenberg RL, McDonald EJ, et al: Complications of catheter cerebral angiography: Analysis of 5000 procedures. I. Criteria and incidence. AJR 131:861, 1978.
7. Mani RL, Eisenberg RL, McDonald EJ, et al: Complications of catheter cerebral angiography: Analysis of 5000 procedures. II. Relation of complication rates to clinical and arteriographic diagnoses. AJR 132:998, 1979.
8. Masaryk TJ, Lewin JS, Laub G: Magnetic resonance angiography. *In* Stark DD, Bradley WG (eds): Magnetic Resonance Imaging. St. Louis, The CV Mosby Company, 1988, pp 299–334.
9. McMinn RMH, Hutchings RT: Color Atlas of Human Anatomy. Chicago, Year Book Medical, 1988.
10. Osborn AG: Introduction to Cerebral Angiography. New York, Harper & Row, 1980.
11. Pelz DM, Buchan A, Fox A, et al: Intraluminal thrombus of the internal carotid arteries: Angiographic demonstration of resolution with anticoagulant therapy alone. Radiology 160:369, 1986.
12. Romanes GJ (ed): Cunningham's Manual of Practical Anatomy. London, Oxford University Press, 1986.
13. Smith DC, Smith LL, Hasso AN: Fibromuscular dysplasia of the internal carotid artery treated by operative transluminal balloon angioplasty. Radiology 155:645, 1985.
14. Thal ER: Injury to the Neck. *In* Moore EE, Mattox KL, Feliciano D (eds): Trauma. 2nd ed Norwalk, CT, Appleton & Lange, 1988, pp 305–317.
15. Vitek J, Raymon BC, Oh S: Innominate artery angioplasty. AJNR 5:113, 1984.
16. Zeumer H, Hundgen R, Ferbert EB, et al: Local intra-arterial fibrinolytic therapy in inaccessible internal carotid occlusion. Neuroradiology 26:315, 1984.
17. Zeumer H: Vascular recanalization techniques in interventional neuroradiology. J Neurol 231:287, 1985.

The Vascular Laboratory: Diagnosis and Management of Cerebrovascular Disease

J. Dennis Baker, M.D.

• • •

The initial evaluation of a patient with cerebrovascular disease is based on a careful history and physical examination, but it is not possible to evaluate the condition of the internal carotid artery fully in this manner. Until noninvasive diagnostic techniques became available, arteriography provided the only objective assessment. Since the late 1960s, extensive work on cerebrovascular diagnosis has been done in two different areas: nucleotide scanning and noninvasive physiologic measurement; however, in the past several years, magnetic resonance techniques have gained clinical application. The early noninvasive tests for detection of carotid disease were indirect methods, which assessed the effects of stenosis on the distal circulation. During recent years, however, there has been a growing trend toward direct methods, which measure flow changes at the carotid bifurcation and provide images of the vessel wall and its pathology.[6] This chapter reviews the main noninvasive techniques currently used in clinical laboratories throughout the United States.

HISTORICAL PERSPECTIVE

Periorbital Doppler Test

In the early days of noninvasive testing, a variety of methods were developed and used clinically. One of the first indirect tests was the periorbital Doppler test, originally described by Brockenbrough in 1969.[16] The method is based on detecting, in branches of the ophthalmic artery, decreased or reversed flow that is a reflection of a hemodynamically significant stenosis of the internal carotid artery. Normally, the forehead is supplied by both the internal carotid artery (via its ophthalmic branch) and the external carotid artery (via the superficial temporal artery). In the normal subject, examination with a directional ultrasonic device will show the flow coming out of the orbit toward the forehead. Compression of the superficial temporal artery removes the external carotid contribution to the forehead, and a compensatory increase in flow can be detected in the ophthalmic artery branches. In the presence of advanced internal carotid stenosis, there may be collateral flow from the forehead back through the ophthalmic artery. In this situation, flow will be reversed in frontal or supraorbital branches, as can be confirmed by superficial temporal artery

compression, which decreases or obliterates the flow signal detected in the periorbital branches.

Early work with the periorbital technique for evaluation of ophthalmic artery flow examined the flow detected in the supraorbital branch with and without compression of a superficial temporal artery. The diagnostic accuracy achieved with this technique was reported as being from 54 to 83 per cent.[36, 40] Muller advocated examining the frontal artery, and, in a comparison study, Burger and Barnes demonstrated more consistent results by using this branch than by using the supraorbital artery.[17, 46] The other modification was the inclusion of additional compression points at which collateral circulation from other external carotid branches can be evaluated. Studies of periorbital examinations in which multiple compressions were used show overall diagnostic accuracy ranging between 85 and 99 per cent.[10, 43, 56]

An advantage of the Doppler periorbital examination for the diagnosis of advanced carotid stenosis is the low cost of instrumentation. Only a directional Doppler velocity detector is needed, so patients can easily be examined outside the vascular laboratory. The primary drawback is the fact that the examination is highly operator-sensitive; its accuracy depends directly on the examiner's experience and the care applied in the specific examination. This accounts in great part for the decreased use of this method in recent years, to the point that few laboratories now use it on a regular basis.

Direct Carotid Doppler Studies

The presence of a stenosis at the origin of the internal carotid artery can be investigated by studying the flow patterns with a hand-held Doppler probe. This approach provides direct detection of the increased velocity and turbulence produced in the vicinity of the lesion rather than seeking to measure the hemodynamic consequences in distal branches, as is done with indirect tests such as the periorbital examination and ocular pneumoplethysmography. The method is technically more demanding than the periorbital examination because of the need to distinguish between the carotid branches.

The examination is performed with a continuous-wave Doppler unit with a frequency of 5 to 10 MHz. Although some experienced examiners base the test entirely on interpretation of the audio signal, most use an analog or a sonogram (spectral) display to assist in optimal probe placement as well as in interpretation of findings. The probe is gradually advanced along the course of the common carotid artery until the bulb is identified by a slight drop in peak frequency together with a somewhat muffled sound resulting from the flow separation. Beyond the bulb, it is necessary to identify each branch by its characteristic Doppler pattern. The internal carotid artery has a high flow throughout diastole as a result of the low resistance in the cerebral vessels; the flow in the external carotid drops nearly to zero in diastole, similar to the pattern seen in peripheral vessels.

A significant stenosis is identified by the pattern of increased velocity in the region of the plaque, decreasing distally. Additional information is obtained by listening for the change in the spectrum of the signal resulting from turbulence beyond a severe lesion.

A variety of quantitative methods have been developed in order to avoid pitfalls of subjective interpretation. Some groups have used ratios of Doppler-shift frequencies from the region of stenosis, and others compare frequencies from the stenosis to those from normal segments of the artery. Another approach is to estimate the degree of stenosis based on measures of turbulence defined by spectral analysis. Spectral broadening index (SBI), the latest method of measuring turbulence, was developed by Johnston and his associates.[38] A spectral analyzer determines the maximum and instantaneous mean frequencies at peak systole and calculates the parameter from the equation: SBI = (F max − F mean)/F max × 100. An index above the threshold of 55 per cent is associated with a significant carotid stenosis. This group's study has shown SBI to be superior to per cent spectral window in screening for carotid disease.

The direct Doppler examination has the advantage that it can be performed with moderately priced equipment. This method is more difficult to learn than the periorbital examination, but it yields a higher diagnostic accuracy in the hands of an experienced examiner. The greatest problems occur in the evaluation of tortuous vessels, where a sudden change in vessel orientation may produce sufficient increase in frequency to result in a false diagnosis of stenosis. Although there was enthusiastic support for this technique in the 1970s and early 1980s, it has been almost completely supplanted by other tests.

Doppler Imaging

The early work with the Doppler ultrasonic velocity detector was limited to detecting or recording flow patterns in vessels. In 1971, Hokanson and coworkers introduced a method for producing a spatial display of the course of superficial arteries.[35] The device consists of a pulsed Doppler probe attached to a position-sensing arm coupled to a storage oscilloscope. The probe is moved back and forth across the path of a superficial artery, and, whenever flow is detected, a spot is created on the oscilloscope at a point corresponding to the current position of the probe. By sweeping back and forth across the artery, it creates a two-dimensional image. Once the course of the vessel is established by this method, flow characteristics at specific points along the artery can be studied. Diagnosis is based on both the image produced and the interpretation of the Doppler velocity signal along the segment of artery studied. In the presence of stenosis, a defect will usually be seen in the contour of the two-dimensional image. In addition, increased velocity through the stenosis produces downstream turbulence.

Although Doppler imagers were used initially to screen for the presence of significant disease, it is possible to obtain an assessment of subcritical stenosis as well as a gradation of severity of advanced lesions. Experienced examiners are highly successful in distinguishing tight stenosis from occlusions.[54] The visual image, similar to a low-resolution arteriogram, provides an advantage over the direct Doppler examination in patients with tortuous vessels, permitting identification of the site from which the velocity signal is obtained. In spite of the early enthusiasm for Doppler imaging, this method has been replaced by the duplex scanner, with its advantages of real-time and high-resolution images.

CURRENT TESTS

Oculopneumoplethysmography

It has long been recognized that a hemodynamically significant stenosis of the internal carotid artery will decrease the ipsilateral ophthalmic artery pressure. For many years, ophthalmodynamometry was used to estimate ophthalmic artery pressure. A calibrated force applied to the surface of the eye increases the intraocular pressure. The pulsations in the retinal artery are observed with an ophthalmoscope while the pressure is slowly increased until all pulsations stop. The pressure at this point defines the systolic value for the ophthalmic artery pressure. The method is technically difficult to perform and has a subjective end-point, so it is difficult to make precise determinations. Inasmuch as severe carotid stenosis may produce a drop in ophthalmic artery pressure of less than 10 mmHg, a more precise method of measurement is required of a test designed to detect advanced carotid artery stenosis. In 1974, Gee and associates introduced the oculopneumoplethysmograph, a semi-automated device for measuring opthalmic artery pressure by suction ophthalmodynamometry.[28] Small suction cups applied to each eye are connected to a common vacuum source and to sensitive differential pressure transducers. Pulse tracings from each eye together with the level of suction are continually recorded on a strip chart to provide a permanent record of the examination. Suction applied to the cups distorts the shape of the eye, increasing the intraocular pressure above the systolic pressure of the ophthalmic artery, thus abolishing all pulsation of the eye. When the suction is gradually decreased, the point at which pulsation is first detected in the eye defines the systolic end-point (Fig. 116–1). The system can make highly reproducible measurements of ophthalmic artery pressure and has the advantage of measuring both eyes at the same time, avoiding potential differences as a result of making determinations sequentially of each eye.

The test is well tolerated by most patients. Subconjunctival erythema or hematoma under the area of contact with the eye cup is seen in approximately 2 per cent of those examined. Specific contraindications related to the

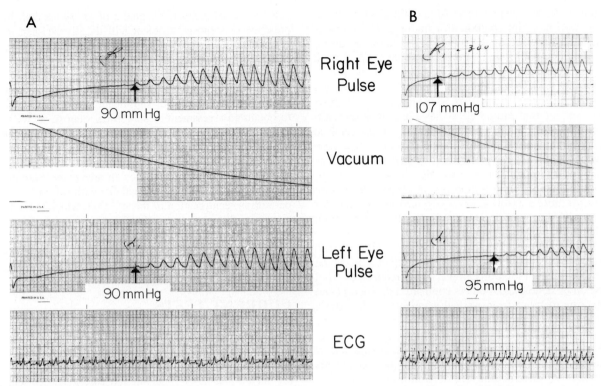

FIGURE 116–1. Oculopneumoplethysmography. *A*, Normal study: symmetric ocular pulse with ophthalmic artery pressure of 95 mmHg bilaterally. *B*, Abnormal study from patient with severe left internal carotid stenosis indicated by the 12-mmHg difference in pressures.

test include eye trauma or surgery within 6 months, any history of retinal detachment, unstable glaucoma, acute conjunctivitis, and the presence of an intraocular lens implant.

The patient is examined in the supine position. Topical ophthalmic anesthetic eye drops are put in each eye several minutes before the examination is started. The eye cups are applied to the sclera in the outer canthus. The vacuum pump is then activated, and the suction holds the cups in place. The vacuum automatically rises to 300 mmHg, then automatically decreases over a period of 30 seconds. Continuous recording of the ocular pulse waves and the vacuum level is made throughout the test. If the 300-mmHg vacuum is inadequate to obliterate the ocular pulse, the test is stopped and restarted at the 500-mmHg setting. This higher level of suction allows determination of the systolic endpoint in most hypertensive patients. The record is then analyzed by determining the level of vacuum at which the first ocular pulse is detected in each eye. By our criteria, an oculopneumoplethysmographic test result is abnormal if a difference in ophthalmic artery pressure between the two eyes of 5 mmHg or higher is found, if the difference is between 1 and 4 mmHg and the ratio of ophthalmic artery pressure to brachial artery pressure is below 0.66, or if the eye pressures are equal and the ratio is below 0.60.[7, 8] A number of clinical studies have shown an overall diagnostic accuracy ranging between 90 and 94 per cent.[7, 8, 23, 27, 41] It is important to note that all these studies used similar criteria for an abnormal test. Other studies have shown substan-

tially less accuracy, undoubtedly because they employed less sensitive criteria for the test.

In addition to diagnosis of internal carotid artery stenosis, the oculopneumoplethysmograph has been used for noninvasive measurement of internal carotid artery backpressure. This can be done by compressing the common carotid artery low on the neck and then measuring the ophthalmic artery pressure, which under this circumstance will reflect the collateral circulation. The compression should be applied and released slowly. If there is a carotid bruit low in the neck or if palpation shows the bifurcation to be abnormally low, the compression should not be performed unless an angiogram shows no significant atherosclerotic plaque in the area to be compressed. In a series of 81 patients, Gee and coworkers found that 95 per cent had less than 5-mmHg difference between the carotid backpressure measured noninvasively and the direct measurements at the time of surgery.[26] The collateral pressure has also been used to categorize the risk of stroke of an asymptomatic stenosis.[42]

Advantages of oculopneumoplethysmography include the simplicity of performing the test, mastered in a relatively short time, and the ease of interpreting the record produced. Another advantage is that the method can detect significant stenoses up to the level of the ophthalmic artery and may detect high internal carotid lesions that could be missed by direct methods. Disadvantages include the fact that the test is contraindicated in some patients with preexisting eye disease. Moreover, it is not possible to measure a systolic end-point in patients with severe hypertension, although we have encountered this problem in less than 2 per cent of all examinations conducted.

Duplex Scan

B-mode ultrasound imaging has been used since the 1960s to visualize soft tissue structures. However, vessels such as the carotid arteries could not be adequately seen until the introduction of real-time techniques, which overcame the problem of vessel wall motion. This equipment makes possible a visualization analogous to fluoroscopy. Ultrasound imaging of the carotid arteries has two major problems: (1) the inability to separate heavy wall calcification from advanced stenosis with dense calcification of the plaque, and (2) the fact that soft clot may have the same echodensity as flowing blood. In order to overcome these problems, a research team at the University of Washington developed the duplex scanner, which combines a real-time B-mode scanner with a pulse Doppler velocity detector in a single system[9] (Figs. 116–2 and 116–3).

In addition to the imaging section and the pulsed Doppler detector, scanners incorporate a spectral analyzer for measuring the flow signals. Most units include provisions for recording the real-time images on videotape and for obtaining photographs of frozen portions of the study. Although the early models could display only the image or the Doppler information, the current scanners can display both simultaneously, a feature that facilitates the examination of tortuous arteries. A manually adjusted cursor is used to measure the angle between the Doppler beam and the axis of the flow, permitting estimation of the velocity from the frequency information. Most carotid scanning is performed with high-frequency ultrasound probes (7 to 10 MHz), but lower-frequency ones are available for studies of deeper vessels.

The most recent development in duplex scanning technology was the introduction of a color-coded Doppler display. This technology permits obtaining velocity information from a matrix of sample volumes within the scan plane. The velocity at each sample point is represented as a color hue superimposed on the B-mode image. The color scanner can facilitate the examination of the carotids, especially when dealing with tortuous vessels or very eccentric stenoses; however, the benefits of this more complex system are greater for studying other parts of the body.

The initial use of the duplex scanner by Strandness and his associates focused on the interpretation of the Doppler signal, with the image being used only for accurate localization of the sampling volume.[14] Other investigators have based the diagnosis of carotid stenosis on measurements made on the scan images, with the Doppler information being used primarily to confirm the presence of flow within the vessel studied. In an initial evaluation of high-resolution scanning of 298 carotid bifurcations, Comerota and his colleagues demonstrated that the best correlation with angiography was obtained in the less severe lesions.[19] In addition, they found that accuracy also depended on the quality of the image obtained. Fifteen per cent of scans were unsuitable for diagnosis because of poor image quality. A subsequent 3-year study combining the results of three hospitals showed a similar pattern of decreased sensitivity with 70 to 99 per cent stenoses.[20] Examiner experience gained during the period of the study resulted in significant improvement in the accuracy of distinguishing tight stenosis from occlusion.

At present, most laboratories use a combination of the anatomic and the physiologic data to diagnose severity of carotid stenosis.[22, 25, 30] Experience has shown that the image provides the best assessment of early lesions, whereas the Doppler information is better for assessing severe lesions. Measurements of peak systolic and end-diastolic velocities together with qualitative assessment of spectral broadening

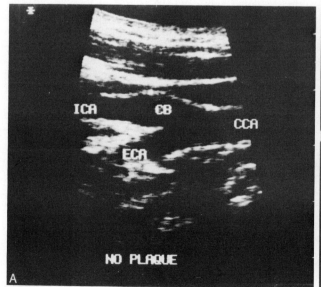
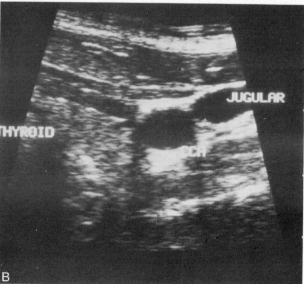

FIGURE 116–2. *A,* Typical longitudinal scan of normal carotid bifurcation. Top of scan image indicates skin level. ICA, internal carotid artery; CB, carotid bifurcation; ECA, external carotid artery; CCA, common carotid artery. *B,* Transverse scan through the bifurcation, showing the elliptical shape of the artery at this level.

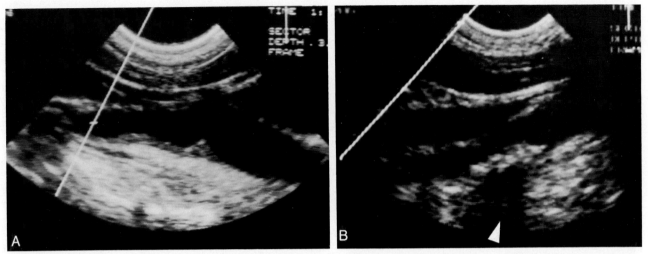

FIGURE 116–3.   *A*, Irregular plaque in the carotid bulb. *B*, Dense, calcific plaque showing ultrasound "shadowing" deep to it (*arrow*). (Courtesy of John P. Woodcock, Ph.D.)

are used to assign a category of stenosis. Table 116–1 outlines the criteria currently used by many laboratories. Even with the introduction of color duplex units, the primary diagnosis of category of stenosis remains based on the conventional Doppler spectral waveform and the gray-scale image.

Although most of the primary focus of duplex scanning has been directed at identifying the severity of stenosis, there has been a growing interest in evaluating the characteristics of the plaque itself (see Fig. 116–3). The areas of main clinical interest are (1) the composition of the plaque, especially the presence of intraplaque hemorrhage; and (2) the presence and size of ulcers. There have been a number of studies correlating the ultrasound images of plaques with histologic findings.[24, 31, 32, 48, 49, 58] A homogeneous appearance is associated with fibrous plaques, whereas a heterogeneous image indicates a complex atheroma or an intraplaque hemorrhage. High-quality scans can clearly show large ulcers as a clear-cut crater within a plaque, often with a discontinuity in the adjacent surface or an overhanging lip.[37, 48] The main problem comes in separating surface irregularity associated with complex atheroma from small ulcers. Another difficulty arises from the need to distinguish an intraplaque hemorrhage from an ul-

cer, which depends on determining whether there is a thin intimal layer covering an area of low density on the image. The improvements in resolution provided by the latest scanner designs will certainly enhance the ability to image carotid pathology, but additional studies are needed to define further the clinical significance of plaque characteristics.

The patient is usually examined supine with the head turned slightly to the opposite side. Initially, a quick survey of the carotid artery and its branches is carried out to identify tortuosity or unusual location. The common carotid is first examined in a longitudinal plane starting just above the clavicle. The artery is identified by its pulsation synchronous with the heartbeat. The transducer is moved up the neck until the bifurcation is reached, where the course of each branch is located by rotating the scan plane (see Fig. 116–2A). It is often not possible to visualize both the internal and the external branches at the same time. The scan head is rotated 90 degrees to provide a transverse or cross-sectional view, and the course of the carotid is followed from the clavicles to the mandible (see Fig. 116–2B). The two views help to locate plaques or other abnormalities. If image information is used to determine the severity of atherosclerosis, the internal diameter of normal and diseased segments can be measured on frozen images

Table 116–1.   Doppler Velocity Criteria for Internal Carotid Stenosis

ICA Stenosis	ICA Velocity	Spectrum
Normal vessel	Peak systolic velocity <125 cm/sec	No broadening
1–19%	Peak systolic velocity <125 cm/sec	Limited broadening in late systole
20–59%	Peak systolic velocity <125 cm/sec	Broadening throughout systole
60–79%	Peak systolic velocity >125 cm/sec; end-diastolic velocity <125 cm/sec	Broadening throughout systole
80–90%	End-diastolic velocity >125 cm/sec (severe stenoses may have very low velocity)	Broadening throughout systole
Occlusion	No ICA Doppler signal: flow to zero in CCA	

ICA, internal carotid artery; CCA, common carotid artery.

using electronic calipers. When plaque characterization studies are being performed, careful adjustments of the image gain settings are required to provide optimal visualization. A systematic longitudinal examination is then carried out, and Doppler velocity signals are obtained from the mid-stream position by adjusting the position of the sample volume. The correct positioning of the sample volume is determined both by listening to the audio signal and by observing the trace of the signal processor. Whenever possible, the Doppler beam is adjusted to an angle of 60 degrees or less to the axis of the artery. Greater angles result in increasing errors in the velocity estimation. Routinely, velocity recordings are made in the common carotid, the bulb, the internal carotid, and the external carotid branches. If any abnormality is noted in the signal, multiple samples are studied in the area of abnormality and as far distal as possible. Many laboratories make continuous videotape recordings of the images and of the Doppler tracing. Photographic copies of the data for inclusion in the patient's record can be made either during the examination or at a later time from the videotape.

Starting with the early duplex scan studies, excellent accuracies were obtained in identification of hemodynamically significant carotid stenoses. However, one of the reasons for choosing duplex scanning over simpler methods is the potential for differentiating the severity of stenosis, so it is important to evaluate the test on this basis. Table 116–2 summarizes a recent study from Sumner's group showing the correlation between severity of disease determined by color-coded duplex scan and by angiography.[39] The numbers on the diagonal (in boldface) indicate the cases in which the duplex scan yielded the same finding as the angiogram. The numbers off the diagonal represent cases of overestimation or underestimation. Although there is considerable overlap between mild and moderate disease, these errors do not have a substantial impact on clinical management of patients. What is important to note is the separation between moderate and severe disease and the high accuracy in identifying occluded vessels. Only 1 of 42 tight stenoses was classified as occluded by the duplex scan.

Plaque characterization and ulcer detection are recent developments, so there is less experience in these areas. Reilly obtained a 91 per cent sensitivity and 65 per cent specificity in detection of intraplaque hemorrhage by scan.[49] The false-positive results were found primarily in plaques with complex atheroma producing a heterogeneous appearance. O'Donnell and coworkers achieved a 93 per cent sensitivity and 84 per cent specificity in detection of intraplaque hemorrhage.[48] The same study found an 89 per cent sensitivity and 87 per cent specificity in detecting ulceration. Although these are excellent results in the definition of plaque characteristics, it remains to be seen whether they can be reproduced in the average noninvasive laboratory.

Some of the newer duplex scanners are designed to estimate the volume flow in a vessel. This is accomplished by increasing the sample volume so that velocities across the entire vessel are detected. A mean frequency is calculated by integrating the signal over one or more cardiac cycles. The mean Doppler-shift frequency is converted to velocity using the beam angle measured with an adjustable cursor. The vessel diameter is estimated from the image. Flow is the product of the mean velocity and the estimated cross-sectional area. Errors in the measurement of mean velocity, of angle of incidence of the Doppler beam, and of vessel diameter all contribute to the variability of flow measurements. Ackroyd, Gill, and their associates found considerable interobserver and intraobserver variability in the measurement of common carotid artery flows, so that these measurements did not improve the diagnostic accuracy of the duplex examination.[4] It is possible that internal carotid artery flow measurements may be more valuable, but they are more difficult to make.

Another area of increasing interest is the use of the duplex scanner to evaluate the vertebral artery. The scan head is placed in the supraclavicular fossa, and the proximal portion of the subclavian or the innominate artery is located. The artery is followed distally until the vertebral branch is located. Ackerstaff and associates reported an 80 per cent sensitivity and 83 per cent specificity in the detection of greater than 50 per cent stenosis of the proximal vertebral artery.[3] Unlike the situation with the carotid, spectral broadening is not a useful parameter, since the normal vertebral artery shows no spectral window, owing to its small size relative to the sample volume. The diagnosis is based primarily on velocity criteria. Bendick and Jackson have also achieved good results in identifying severe vertebral disease, but attempts to distinguish categories of stenosis have proved difficult.[12]

The experience with duplex scanning since the late 1970s has shown it to be a useful technique for determining the severity of carotid stenosis. Definition of plaque characteristics provides information not available by any other

Table 116–2. Correlation Between Severity of Carotid Stenosis Determined by Angiography and Color-Coded Duplex Screening

Duplex Scan	Angiogram				
	0–15%	*10–49%*	*50–79%*	*80–99%*	*100%*
0–15%	114	8	—	—	—
16–49%	8	47	1	—	—
50–79%	—	11	**46**	5	—
80–99%	—	—	6	**36**	—
100%	—	—	1	1	**23**

From Londrey GL, Spadone DP, Hodgson KJ, et al: Does color-flow imaging improve the accuracy of duplex carotid evaluation? J Vasc Surg 13:659, 1991.

Numbers in boldface refer to cases in which duplex scan yields the same category of stenosis as angiogram, 87% of vessels studied.

technique. One problem with the technique is the high cost of purchase and maintenance of the equipment, especially with the introduction of color duplex scanners. Increasing use of the duplex scanner for evaluating other parts of the vascular system will make it more feasible for small laboratories to buy the device. Another problem is the extensive operator experience required to obtain reliable and consistent examinations, for the duplex scan is the most demanding of all the techniques used for noninvasive cerebrovascular diagnosis.

Transcranial Doppler Studies

Although surgeons are interested in evaluating the entire internal carotid artery, the usual noninvasive methods do not assess the distal portion of the internal carotid artery. The direct methods are very accurate in identifying disease in the region of the bifurcation but may miss tight stenoses in the siphon. Oculopneumoplethysmography has the advantage of detecting advanced stenoses proximal to the ophthalmic artery but cannot evaluate disease above this level. Investigators have been interested in studying the flow in the intracranial vessels, but the skull is a formidable barrier to ultrasound. The early work was performed intraoperatively or in children with open fontanelles. Although most of the skull is too thick for satisfactory ultrasound penetration, White and coworkers demonstrated that the very thin bone in the temporal region would permit detection of Doppler signals if suitable transmitting frequencies (2 to 3 MHz) were used.[57] In 1982, Aaslid and colleagues reported the first clinical study of transcranial measurements from the cerebral arteries.[2]

The examination is performed with a 2-MHz directional, pulsed Doppler device with a probe designed to produce a narrow beam. The range-gate feature is necessary to permit selection of a specific vessel for study. With the sample volume initially set at 5 cm, the probe is placed over the temporal region above the zygomatic arch and adjusted until a Doppler signal is obtained.[1] This signal will be toward the probe and will come from the main trunk of the middle cerebral artery. Because the thinnest region of the temporal bone varies from person to person, it is necessary to move the probe along the zygomatic arch until the optimal "window" is located. The middle cerebral artery signal is similar to that of the internal carotid artery (Fig. 116–4A). With a significant proximal stenosis, there is marked attenuation of the systolic portion of the signal (Fig. 116–4B). The precommunicating portion of the anterior cerebral artery is located by maintaining the probe position and adjusting the gate until a reverse Doppler signal is located, usually at a depth of 7 to 8 cm. To find the posterior cerebral artery, the middle cerebral artery is located as a reference; the ultrasound beam is then angled posteriorly and the range increased 1.0 to 1.5 cm.

Alternate approaches are used to study other parts of the intracranial circulation. The transorbital approach provides access to the intracranial portion of the internal carotid artery, permitting detection of tight stenoses at this level.[53] The probe is placed on the closed eyelid with the beam directed through the superior orbital fissure and the optic canal. The basilar artery and the distal portions of the vertebral arteries can be detected through the foramen magnum.[5] The neck is flexed and the probe positioned at the nape in the mid-line. Flow away from the probe will be detected at 6 to 8 cm.

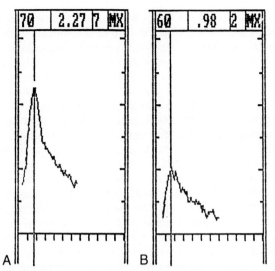

FIGURE 116–4. A, Transcranial Doppler signal from normal middle cerebral artery. B, Attenuated middle cerebral artery signal distal to tight stenosis.

The diagnosis of an internal carotid stenosis is made by comparing the signals from the two middle cerebral arteries. However, as demonstrated by Cantelmo and associates, there is probably no indication for adding evaluation of intracranial branches to duplex scanning in the routine evaluation of carotid disease.[18] Evaluation of the status of the circle of Willis and adequacy of collateral pathways can be obtained by determining the response of Doppler signals in the intracranial vessels to transient common carotid compression.[1, 5] The transcranial Doppler assessment is also a valuable tool for the neurosurgeon, for it provides a sensitive method for monitoring vasospasm. In the presence of focal spasm, there is a marked increase in the frequency of the Doppler signals with return toward normal levels as the spasm resolves.[1] These localized changes usually do not produce a detectable change in the flow pattern in the internal carotid artery, so other ultrasound techniques are of no value. Other applications under investigation include evaluation of vertebrobasilar insufficiency,[51] monitoring during carotid operations to determine changes in intracranial flow,[11, 33] and detection of emboli.[52]

Learning to perform the transcranial examination is initially difficult for technologists, since most are not familiar with the three-dimensional anatomy of the intracranial arteries. Reproducible identification of the middle cerebral artery is rapidly achieved, but reliable study of other branches requires more experience. Overall, learning the transcranial technique is comparable to learning the direct Doppler examination of the carotid bifurcation. Vessel identification may be facilitated with the use of a Doppler mapping unit[47] or a duplex scanner.[15, 34]

INDICATIONS FOR NONINVASIVE TESTING

Symptomatic Arterial Disease

Patients with clear-cut hemispheric symptoms are usually evaluated with angiography; however, the noninvasive tests may help in the choice of contrast study. In the presence of a tight stenosis, an arch injection may be adequate, whereas with mild or moderate stenosis, a selective study may be needed to provide better detail. On the other hand, the noninvasive evaluation may have a primary diagnostic role in patients with atypical or nonhemispheric symptoms when there may be no clear indication for angiography. Identification of a severe stenosis would certainly strengthen the indication for contrast studies. The other situation in which noninvasive evaluation is helpful is the case in which the patient or the primary physician is reluctant to proceed with arteriography. Demonstrating an advanced lesion can often provide a convincing reason for a full work-up.

Over the years, the question has been raised whether ultrasound tests could supplement contrast angiography as the definitive study prior to carotid endarterectomy. In 1982, Blackshear and Connar reported on four patients who had operations based on the results of Doppler imaging.[13] They pointed out that all four patients had had severe contrast reactions during previous studies, and concluded that noninvasive studies might replace angiograms in cases in which the latter were contraindicated. A year later, Sandmann and colleagues published a series of 91 operations in 74 patients who had not had angiography.[50] There have been additional reports of this practice, each advocating a cautious approach.[21, 29, 45, 55] In all cases, the authors emphasize the need for using a very experienced examiner whose previous results have been carefully validated by angiography and by operative findings.

Asymptomatic Carotid Stenosis

With the growing awareness that auscultation of the neck is an important part of the physical examination, increasing numbers of asymptomatic patients are being referred for evaluation. Some people have bruits radiating from the heart, the innominate artery, or the subclavian artery. A considerable number of the bruits are, however, found to originate from the bifurcation. The noninvasive tests permit identification of the advanced stenosis of the internal carotid artery, and further work-up depends on the individual physician's philosophy on the management of severe asymptomatic stenoses. Most investigators agree that subcritical stenoses require no further active investigation but may be followed at yearly intervals to detect progression to more advanced stenoses. The 10 per cent of patients whose isolated stenoses of the external carotid have been verified by one of the imaging techniques do not require further evaluation.

Postoperative Follow-Up

Noninvasive testing can detect internal carotid thrombosis in the early postoperative period. However, the most important use for such testing is in long-term follow-up. A number of retrospective series report the incidence of symptomatic restenosis to be between 1 and 5 per cent. Studies that have examined patients with noninvasive tests have found significant recurrence in 7 to 15 per cent. Any time postoperative monitoring is to be part of the follow-up, it is important to obtain a baseline examination soon after the operation in order to separate technical problems and early thrombosis from recurrence of a stenotic lesion.

Prospective Studies

A weakness of previous longitudinal studies of stroke is the lack of data on the status of cerebral circulation on entry into the study and the progression of atherosclerotic lesions during the follow-up period. The noninvasive tests described are ideal for inclusion in prospective studies. Stratification of subjects according to the status of the carotid artery may disclose important findings that could be masked when the entire group is analyzed.

General References

Bernstein EF (ed): Noninvasive Diagnostic Techniques in Vascular Disease. 3rd ed. St. Louis, CV Mosby, 1993.

Kempczinski RF, Yao JST (eds): Practical Noninvasive Vascular Diagnosis. 2nd ed. Chicago, Year Book Medical, 1987.

Salles-Cunha SX, Andros G: Atlas of Duplex Ultrasonography. Pasadena, CA, Appleton-Davies, 1987.

Zwiebel WJ: Introduction to Vascular Ultrasonography, 3rd ed. Philadelphia, WB Saunders, 1992.

References

1. Aaslid R: Transcranial Doppler Sonography. New York, Springer-Verlag, 1986.
2. Aaslid R, Markwalder T-M, Nornes H: Noninvasive transcranial Doppler ultrasound recording of flow velocity in basal cerebral arteries. J Neurosurg 57:769, 1982.
3. Ackerstaff RGA, Hoeneveld H, Slowikowski JM, et al: Ultrasonic duplex scanning in atherosclerotic disease of the innominate, subclavian and vertebral arteries: A comparative study with angiography. Ultrasound Med Biol 10:409, 1984.
4. Ackroyd N, Gill R, Griffiths K, et al: Quantitative common carotid artery blood flow: Prediction of internal carotid artery stenosis. J Vasc Surg 3:846, 1986.
5. Arnolds BJ, Von Reutern G-M: Transcranial Doppler sonography. Examination technique and normal reference values. Ultrasound Med Biol 12:115, 1986.
6. Baker JD: How vascular surgeons use noninvasive testing. J Vasc Surg 4:272, 1986.
7. Baker JD, Barker WF, Machleder HI: Evaluation of extracranial cerebrovascular disease with ocular pneumoplethysmography. Am J Surg 136:206, 1978.
8. Baker JD, Barker WF, Machleder HL: Ocular pneumoplethysmography in the evaluation of carotid stenosis. Circulation 62(Suppl 1):1, 1980.
9. Barber FE, Baker DW, Nation AWC, et al: Ultrasonic duplex echo-Doppler scanner. IEEE Trans Biomed Eng 21:109, 1974.
10. Barnes RW, Russell HE, Bone GE, et al: Doppler cerebrovascular examination: Improved results with refinements in technique. Stroke 8:468, 1977.
11. Bass A, Krupski WC, Schneider PA, et al: Intraoperative transcranial Doppler: Limitations of the method. J Vasc Surg 10:549, 1989.
12. Bendick PJ, Jackson VP: Evaluation of the vertebral arteries with duplex sonography. J Vasc Surg 3:523, 1986.
13. Blackshear WM, Connar RG: Carotid endarterectomy without angiography. J Cardiovasc Surg 23:477, 1982.
14. Blackshear WM, Phillips DJ, Thiele BL, et al: Detection of carotid

occlusive disease by ultrasonic imaging and pulsed Doppler spectrum analysis. Surgery 86:698, 1979.

15. Bogdahn U, Becker G, Winkler J, et al: Transcranial color-coded real-time sonography in adults. Stroke 21:1680, 1990.

16. Brockenbrough EC: Screening for the prevention of stroke: Use of Doppler flowmeter. Brochure by Alaska/Washington Regional Medical Program, 1969.

17. Burger R, Barnes RW: Choice of ophthalmic artery branch for Doppler cerebrovascular examination: Advantages of the frontal artery. Angiology 28:421, 1977.

18. Cantelmo NL, Babikian VL, Johnson WC, et al: Correlation of transcranial Doppler and noninvasive tests with angiography in the evaluation of extracranial carotid disease. J Vasc Surg 11:786, 1990.

19. Comerota AJ, Cranley JJ, Cook SE: Real-time B-mode carotid imaging in diagnosis of cerebrovascular disease. Surgery 89:718, 1981.

20. Comerota AJ, Cranley JJ, Katz ML, et al: Real-time B-mode carotid imaging—A three-year multicenter experience. J Vasc Surg 1:84, 1984.

21. Crew JR, Dean M, Johnson JM, et al: Carotid surgery without angiography. Am J Surg 148:217, 1984.

22. Dreisbach JN, Seibert CE, Smazal SF, et al: Duplex sonography in the evaluation of carotid artery disease. AJNR 4:678, 1983.

23. Eikelboom B, Riles TS, Folcarelli P, et al: Criteria for interpretation of ocular pneumoplethysmography (Gee). Arch Surg 118:1169, 1983.

24. Feeley TM, Leen EJ, Colgan MP, et al: Histologic characteristics of carotid artery plaque. J Vasc Surg 13:719, 1991.

25. Garth KE, Carroll BA, Sommer FG, et al: Duplex ultrasound scanning of the carotid arteries with velocity spectrum analysis. Radiology 147:823, 1983.

26. Gee W, Mehigan JT, Wylie EJ: Measurement of collateral cerebral hemispheric blood pressure by ocular pneumoplethysmography. Am J Surg 130:121, 1975.

27. Gee W, Oller DW, Amundsen DG, et al: The asymptomatic carotid bruit and the ocular pneumoplethysmography. Arch Surg 112:1381, 1977.

28. Gee W, Smith CA, Hinsen LE, et al: Ocular plethysmography in carotid artery disease. Med Instrum 8:244, 1974.

29. Gelabert HA, Moore WS: Carotid endarterectomy without angiography. Surg Clin North Am 70:213, 1990.

30. Glover JL, Bendick PJ, Jackson VP, et al: Duplex ultrasonography, digital subtraction angiography, and conventional angiography in assessing carotid atherosclerosis. Arch Surg 119:664, 1984.

31. Goes E, Janssens W, Maillet B, et al: Tissue characterization of atheromatous plaques: Correlation between ultrasound image and histological findings. J Clin Ultrasound 18:611, 1990.

32. Gray-Weale AC, Graham JC, Burnett JR, et al: Carotid artery atheroma: Comparison of preoperative B-mode ultrasound appearance with carotid endarterectomy specimen pathology. J Cardiovasc Surg 29:676, 1988.

33. Halsey JH, McDowell HA, Gelman S, Morawetz RB: Blood velocity in the middle cerebral artery and regional blood flow during carotid endarterectomy. Stroke 20:53, 1989.

34. Hashimoto BE, Hahrick CW: New method of adult transcranial Doppler. J Ultrasound Med 10:349, 1991.

35. Hokanson DE, Mozersky DJ, Sumner DS, et al: Ultrasonic arteriography: A new approach to arterial visualization. Biomed Eng 6:420, 1971.

36. Hyman BN: Doppler sonography. A bedside noninvasive method for assessment of carotid artery disease. Am J Ophthalmol 77:227, 1974.

37. Johnson JM, Ansel AL, Morgan S, et al: Ultrasonographic screening for evaluation and follow-up of carotid artery ulceration: A new basis for assessing risk. Am J Surg 144:614, 1982.

38. Johnston KW, Baker WH, Burnham SJ, et al: Quantitative analysis of continuous-wave Doppler spectral broadening for the diagnosis of carotid disease: Results of a multicenter study. J Vasc Surg 4:493, 1986.

39. Londrey GL, Spadone DP, Hodgson KJ, et al: Does color-flow imaging improve the accuracy of duplex carotid evaluation? J Vasc Surg 13:659, 1991.

40. Machleder HI, Barker WF: Noninvasive methods for evaluation of extracranial cerebrovascular disease. Arch Surg 112:944, 1977.

41. McDonald PT, Rich NM, Collins GJ, et al: Ocular pneumoplethysmography: Detection of carotid occlusive disease. Ann Surg 189:44, 1979.

42. Moll FL, Eikelboom BC, Vermeulen FEE, et al: Dynamics of collateral circulation in progressive asymptomatic carotid disease. J Vasc Surg 3:470, 1986.

43. Moore WS, Bean B, Burton R, et al: The use of ophthalmosonometry in the diagnosis of carotid artery stenosis. Surgery 82:107, 1977.

44. Moore DJ, Miles RD, Ohgi S, et al: Relative accuracy of the diagnostic components of noninvasive carotid arterial tests: A comparison of pulsed Doppler arteriography and spectrum analysis. J Vasc Surg 3:502, 1986.

45. Moore WS, Ziomek S, Quiñones-Baldrich WJ, et al: Can clinical evaluation and noninvasive testing substitute for arteriography in the evaluation of carotid artery disease? Ann Surg 208:91, 1988.

46. Muller HR: The diagnosis of internal carotid artery occlusion by directional Doppler sonography of the ophthalmic artery. Neurology (Minneap.) 22:816, 1972.

47. Niederkorn K, Myers LG, Nunn CL, et al: Three-dimensional transcranial Doppler blood flow mapping in patients with cerebrovascular disorders. Stroke 19:1335, 1988.

48. O'Donnell TF, Erdoes L, Mackey WC, et al: Correlation of B-mode ultrasound imaging and arteriography with pathological findings at carotid endarterectomy. Arch Surg 120:443, 1985.

49. Reilly LM: Carotid intraplaque hemorrhage: Noninvasive detection and clinical significance. *In* Bernstein EF (ed): Recent Advances in Noninvasive Diagnostic Techniques in Vascular Disease. St. Louis, CV Mosby, 1990.

50. Sandmann W, Hennerici M, Nullen H, et al: Carotid artery surgery without angiography: Risk or progress? *In* Greenhalgh RM, Rose FC (eds): Progress in Stroke Research 2. London, Pitman, 1983.

51. Schneider PA, Rossman ME, Bernstein EF, et al: Noninvasive evaluation of vertebrobasilar insufficiency. J Ultrasound Med 10:373, 1991.

52. Spencer MP, Thomas GI, Nicholls SC, Sauvage LR: Detection of middle cerebral artery emboli during carotid endarterectomy using transcranial Doppler ultrasound. Stroke 21:415, 1990.

53. Spencer MP, Whisler D: Transorbital Doppler diagnosis of intracranial arterial stenosis. Stroke 17:916, 1986.

54. Sumner DS, Russell JB, Miles RD: Pulsed-Doppler arteriography and computer-assisted imaging of the carotid bifurcation. *In* Bergan JJ, Yao JST (eds): Cerebrovascular Insufficiency. Orlando, FL, Grune & Stratton, 1983.

55. Thomas GI, Jones TW, Stavney LS, et al: Carotid endarterectomy after Doppler ultrasonographic examination without angiography. Am J Surg 151:616, 1986.

56. Towne JB, Salles-Cunha S, Bernhard VM: Periorbital ultrasound findings: Hemodynamics in patients with cerebrovascular disease. Arch Surg 114:158, 1979.

57. White DN, Curry GR, Stevenson RJ: The acoustic characteristics of the skull. Ultrasound Med Biol 3:225, 1978.

58. Wolverson MK, Bashiti HM, Peterson GJ: Ultrasonic tissue characterization of atheromatous plaques using a high-resolution real-time scanner. Ultrasound Med Biol 9:599, 1983.

COLOR PLATES

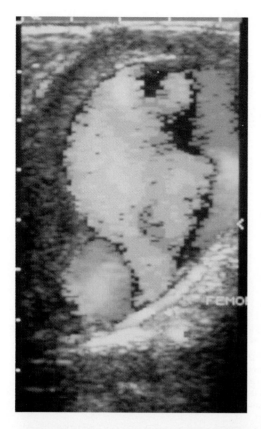

FIGURE 79–3. A color flow Doppler ultrasound image of an iatrogenic femoral false aneurysm; a jet of blood is seen flowing into the cavity during systole.

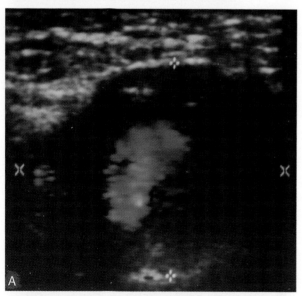

FIGURE 83–3. Duplex imaging of a left groin pseudoaneurysm in a patient with an aortobifemoral bypass. *A,* Arterial flow is demonstrated within the aneurysmal cavity.

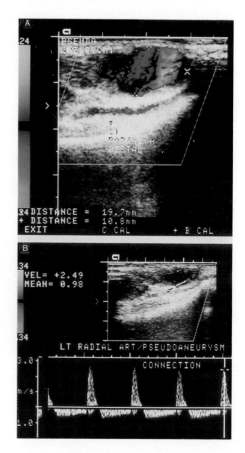

FIGURE 83–8. *A,* Duplex imaging of a left radial artery pseudoaneurysm resulting from an arterial cannula, located adjacent to the native vessel. *B,* Spectral analysis of the neck of a pseudoaneurysm shows increased peak systolic velocity and flow reversal.

Plate IV

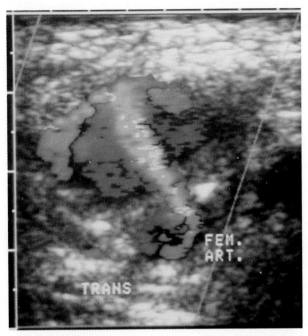

FIGURE 93–5. Color flow Doppler ultrasound image of a femoral pseudoaneurysm after femoral artery catheterization for coronary angiography.

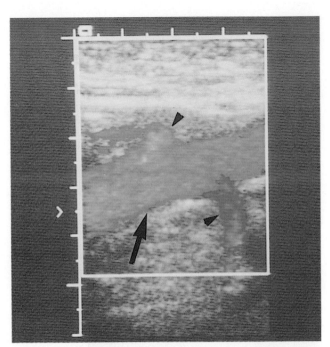

FIGURE 107–11. Ultrasound of the renal arteries. Abdominal sonogram of the aorta *(arrow)* with the left and right renal arteries *(arrowheads).* The origins and proximal segments of the renal arteries are normal. Blood flow toward the transducer is coded in red, and blood flow away from the transducer is in blue.

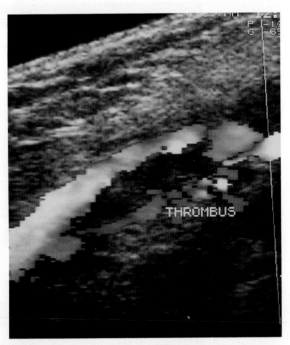

FIGURE 131–15. Color flow image of the same vein pictured in Figure 131–14. The residual lumen is filled with blue pixels outlining the thrombus.

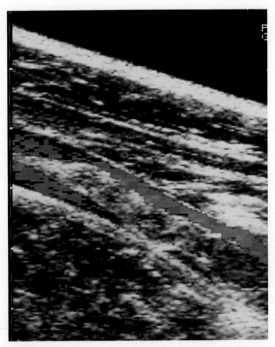

FIGURE 131–16. Color flow image of a free-floating clot in a superficial femoral vein. (From Sumner DS, Mattos MA: Diagnosis of deep venous thrombosis with real-time color and duplex scanning. *In* Bernstein EF [ed]: Vascular Diagnosis. 4th ed. St. Louis, Mosby-Year Book, 1993, pp 785–800.)

Plate V

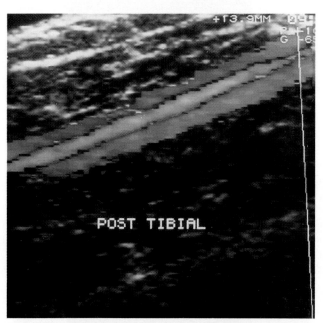

FIGURE 131–17. Venae comitantes (blue) paralleling a posterior tibial artery (red) in a normal subject. (From Sumner DS, Mattos MA: Diagnosis of deep venous thrombosis with real-time color and duplex scanning. *In* Bernstein EF [ed]: Vascular Diagnosis. 4th ed. St. Louis, Mosby-Year Book, 1993, pp 785–800.)

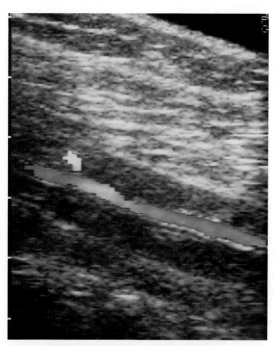

FIGURE 131–18. Total thrombotic occlusion of paired peroneal veins (no color). The peroneal artery (red) serves as an anatomic reference.

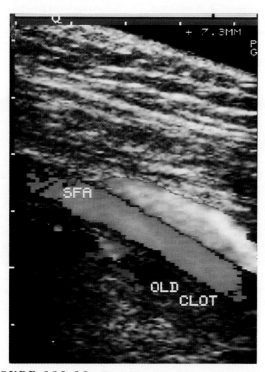

FIGURE 131–19. Paired superficial femoral veins, one of which is patent (blue) and the other of which is almost completely occluded with old thrombus. A few blue pixels in the occluded vein suggest partial recanalization. The superficial femoral artery (SFA) is filled with red pixels.

Plate VI

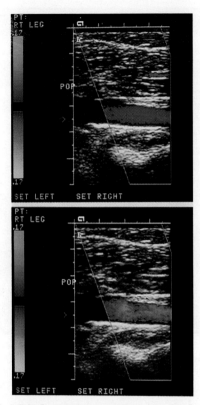

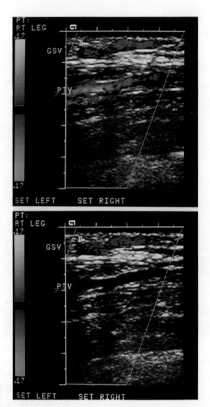

FIGURE 133–8. Real-time imaging with color flow duplex scanning allows quick assessment of venous incompetence by identifying bidirectional flow. In color flow images of an incompetent popliteal (POP) vein, blue hue *(top)* represents flow away from the transducer and red hue *(bottom)* represents flow toward the transducer (reversed flow).

FIGURE 133–9. Simultaneous color flow real-time images of the posterior tibial (PTV) and greater saphenous (GSV) veins. *Top,* Both veins show flow toward the transducer (blue hue). *Bottom,* Greater saphenous vein shows flow reversal (red hue), whereas the posterior tibial vein shows no color because flow has ceased, which implies valvular competence in the posterior tibial vein.

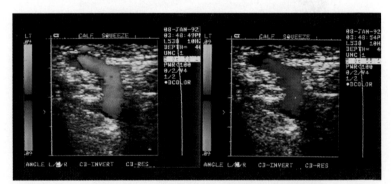

FIGURE 133–10. Color flow images of an incompetent calf perforating vein. *Right,* Transverse calf insonation demonstrating flow from the greater saphenous vein to the deep calf vein. *Left,* Flow reversal (red hue) after the release of distal calf compression.

Plate VII

Imaging in Cerebrovascular Disease

Sheldon E. Jordan, M.D., F.A.A.N., and Bradley A. Jabour, M.D.

• • •

This chapter serves as a guide to clinicians who must choose among various imaging modalities when evaluating patients with cerebrovascular disease. The options for imaging brain anatomy include computed tomography (CT) with and without intravenous iodine contrast agents,[1-3] as well as CT scans enhanced with inhaled stable xenon. Magnetic resonance imaging (MRI) scans can also be obtained for imaging brain anatomy; magnetic resonance angiography (MRA) can image flow in larger intracranial vessels.[4-7] Newer MRI techniques can image cerebral perfusion, diffusion, and metabolism of ischemic tissues.[8, 9] Positron emission tomography (PET) and single-photon emission tomography (SPECT) offer tomographic images of cerebral blood flow and/or brain metabolism.[10-15]

COMPUTED TOMOGRAPHY IN CEREBROVASCULAR DISEASE

Principles of Interpretation

A CT image of a brain slice is made of a two-dimensional matrix of small rectangular picture elements called pixels. Each two-dimensional pixel represents a small volume element of a brain slice, which is called a voxel. The whiteness or grayness of each pixel depends on the density of the corresponding tissue element. Brain tissue with excess calcium or extravascular blood will be imaged as a white pixel. With brain hemorrhage, a congregation of white pixels will appear on the two-dimensional image as a large, confluent white patch (Fig. 117–1).

Tissue elements with excess water, as in edematous brain or necrotic cystic brain, will appear as a darker gray pixel (Figs. 117–2 and 117–3). Therefore, if there is an area of edema in a slice of brain, a congregation of many darker gray pixels will appear together to form a larger patch that is grayer than the surrounding pixels representing normal brain tissue (Fig. 117–4).

Flowing intravascular blood is normally almost the same density as the surrounding brain. However, the intravenous infusion of iodinated dye increases the density of the intravascular compartment. Therefore, in postcontrast scans, arteries, veins, and dilated capillaries appear lighter on the gray scale than surrounding brain tissue.

Normally, the tight junctions of brain capillary endothelium prevent extravasation of iodinated dye into brain tissue; however, with infarcted brain tissue, capillary junctions become leaky, with the resulting extravasation of iodine dye into the extravascular compartment. Therefore, after the administration of iodinated contrast material, areas of increased density may appear in regions of brain infarction; this contrast enhancement is seen several days after an ischemic event and rarely within the first day of a vascular occlusion[3] (Fig. 117–5).

Inhaled stable xenon can also be used as a contrast agent. This agent appears to increase brain density as a function of local cerebral blood flow. Contrast enhancement

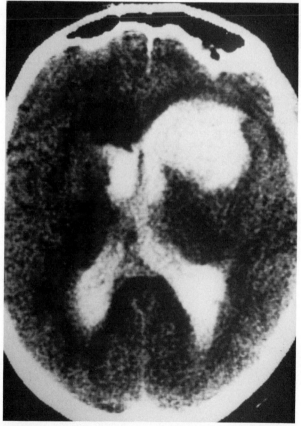

FIGURE 117–1. Acute hemorrhage in the left frontal lobe with intraventricular extension. Extravascular blood appears white, owing to its higher density compared with brain. Calcium-containing calvarial bone appears white because of its density. The air in the frontal sinuses appears as a very black space as a result of the low density of air compared with brain. The left side of the picture is the right side of the brain in this and in all subsequent images in this chapter, unless otherwise stated.

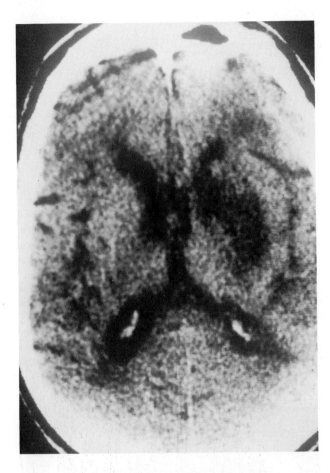

FIGURE 117–2.   Three days after left internal carotid occlusion. There is edema in the region of the internal capsule and head of the caudate with compression of the left frontal horn. Edematous brain is not typically as dark on the gray scale as cerebrospinal fluid (CSF) in the ventricles.

FIGURE 117–3.   Years after a left middle cerebral artery occlusion. Cystic encephalomalacic brain is almost as dark as the CSF within the ventricle. Note that with old, large infarctions, the underlying ventricle may enlarge as a result of loss of overlying brain tissue. The overlying gyri have become atrophic. This results in enlargement of the cortical sulci over the left convexity in this case.

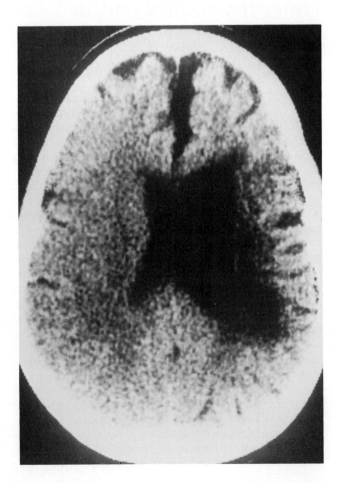

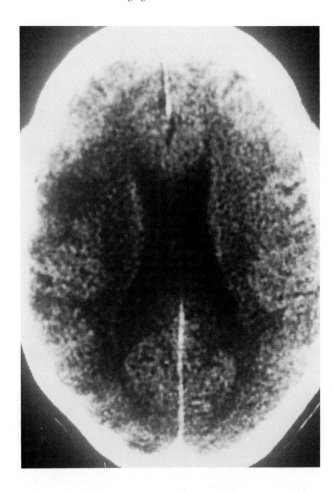

FIGURE 117–4.   After contrast enhancement within hours of
right internal carotid occlusion. The normal "blush" of the cortex is
seen on the left side. On the right side, there is a lack of the cortical
blush in the middle cerebral distribution. Also, note the effacement of
sulci on the right compared with the homologous area on the left. No
effacement of the ventricle or midline shift has occurred in spite of
the devastating nature of the patient's deficits. Even with massive
strokes, early computed tomography (CT) scans may show very
subtle abnormalities, as in this case.

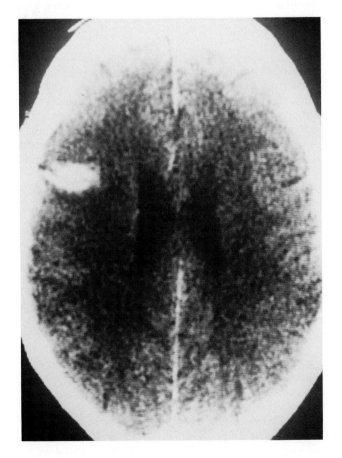

FIGURE 117–5.   Seven days after embolic occlusion of a right
frontal branch vessel. In this postcontrast scan, an enhancement of
the infarcted gyri is seen ("gyral enhancement pattern").
Presumably, this effect is due to dilatation and leakage of capillaries.

with stable xenon can be quantitated so that the local cerebral blood flow can be measured.[2]

CT Appearance of Infarction

The appearance of an infarction on a CT scan depends on both time and localization of an ischemic event. Within the first hours after vessel occlusion, brain tissue destined for ischemic necrosis may show a low density in the distribution of a vessel at risk (darker gray than normal brain). The initial low density is largely due to intracellular edema (see Fig. 117–2).

After many hours or a few days, there may be swelling of the involved brain tissue, so that the normal anatomy is distorted; for example, involved cortex may demonstrate effacement of the sulci compared with homologous sulci on the opposite side of the brain (see Fig. 117–4). The ventricles may be displaced away from the mass effect of the edematous swelling if the lesion is large and deeply situated. If there is a sudden reestablishment of blood flow to ischemic tissue, patches of low density associated with interstitial edema will develop as a result of leaks from damaged capillaries (Fig. 117–6). Blood may also extravasate

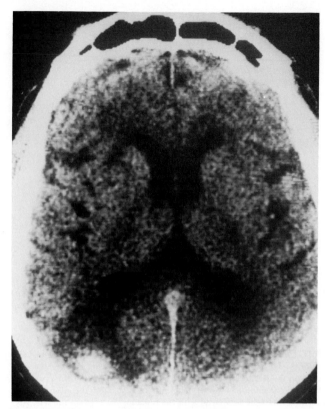

FIGURE 117–7. Five days after embolic infarction. There is a cortically based wedge-shaped hypodensity in the right parietal-occipital region. The amount of edema seen with embolic infarctions may be substantial after lysis and migration of the clot. The white area in and subjacent to the cortex represents hemorrhage within the infarction. Note the "punched-out" appearance of an old "lacunar" infarction lateral to the right frontal horn.

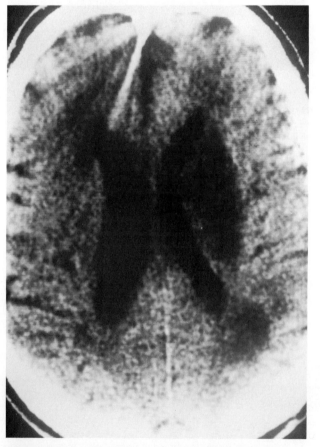

FIGURE 117–6. Several days after left internal carotid occlusion. There is a large, deep area of hypodensity. Also, note hypodensity posterolateral to the left occipital horn, which is in a border zone between the posterior cerebral distribution and the left middle cerebral distribution. The "streak" artifact arising from the frontal bone obscures detail in the frontal lobe and may be particularly troublesome in a moving, uncooperative patient.

into infarcted tissue when blood flow is suddenly restored; the latter process may produce patchy areas of increased density, particularly along cortical gyri. These changes as a result of reperfusion can be seen as embolic fragments are lysed and then migrate distally (Fig. 117–7). Similar findings can also be seen after endarterectomy for a high-grade carotid stenosis in a brain that had been chronically hypoperfused.[16]

Hemorrhage into an area of infarction is not typically seen within the first day (Fig. 117–8); however, bleeding into infarctions is seen more frequently when the scan is taken several days following the event.[17–19] Both heparin therapy and hypertension increase the chance of finding delayed hemorrhage into an infarction. It should be noted, however, that tiny amounts of increased density on CT scans, signifying petechial bleeds, are frequently seen after embolic infarction; petechial bleeds are also frequently seen in this setting when examined microscopically in a postmortem specimen.[20] Perhaps because cerebral blood flow is not typically restored in a sudden manner after thrombotic occlusion of a larger vessel, delayed hemorrhage is not as frequently seen on CT scans after thrombotic infarcts compared with the frequency of seeing delayed hemorrhage after embolic strokes.

A main concern in a patient presenting with a stroke-like event is whether there is a bleed or a mass lesion.

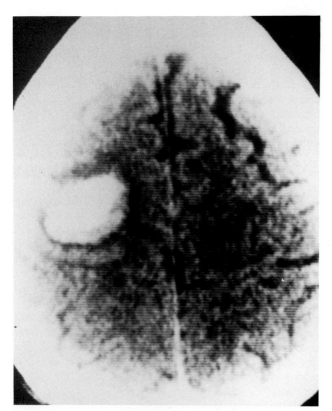

FIGURE 117–8. Within the first day of a peripheral intracranial hemorrhage, the adjacent sulci are obliterated; compare homologous areas on the opposite side. Surrounding the dense clot is a hypodense, dark gray area, presumably produced by clot retraction and, perhaps, the early development of edema.

Noncontrast CT scans are adequate tests to determine the presence or absence of hemorrhage or the presence of larger mass lesions. Because of this sensitivity and because of the rapidity and ease of obtaining noncontrast CT scans in an unstable patient, a noncontrast CT scan would appear to be the procedure of choice for the acute stroke patient. The administration of intravenous iodinated contrast material will be associated with increased complications in patients who are dehydrated, who are elderly, or who have diabetic nephropathy.[21] Contrast infusion also prolongs the time for completing the imaging; this longer examination time delays therapy and makes the patient relatively inaccessible for supportive care. If, however, high doses of contrast dye are given, particularly with a rapid injection technique, the CT scan may show an absence of the normal postcontrast blush of gray matter in an area of ischemia. In a purely nonhemorrhagic infarct, the initial noncontrast CT scan is often negative or may show an ill-defined area of low density in the vascular distribution at risk. After several days and during subsequent weeks, lower doses of intravenous contrast material will produce enhancement, particularly along the cortical gyri, as a result of a combination of capillary leakage of dye and increased tissue hypervascularity.[3, 22] Patches of contrast enhancement develop primarily along the cortical gyri and in the basal ganglia. On occasion, ring enhancement patterns or central enhancement patterns are seen in the infarction resembling postcontrast scans of tumors. However, with cerebrovascular

events, there tends to be relatively little mass effect, and also the extent of the enhancement and mass effect tends to diminish with repeated scans taken over several weeks.

Thrombotic Occlusions of Large Vessels

In order to devise a specific treatment plan, it is helpful to try to understand which vessel had become occluded and by what mechanism the occlusion occurred. For example, carotid endarterectomy may be appropriate for an 80 per cent stenosis of the internal carotid artery at the bifurcation if a small embolic infarction was detected in the ipsilateral hemisphere; however, a similar patient with multiple bilateral emboli including one in the posterior cerebral artery distribution may be suffering from cardiac embolization of the brain. In the latter case, endarterectomy of the unilateral carotid stenosis may not benefit the patient. It is hoped that in cases such as these, CT scans can help surgeons decide which vessel was responsible for the infarction. Along with other clinical facts, the scan may help determine what the mechanism of infarction might have been in a particular case. CT scanning may offer an important clue about stroke mechanism along with x-ray angiography, MRA, carotid duplex scanning, and other tests. The multiplicity, the location of an abnormality, the size of an area of hypodensity, and the contrast enhancement behavior are all helpful features to distinguish among the possibilities of large vessel thrombosis, embolism, and small vessel arteriosclerosis-related occlusions.

With acute internal carotid artery occlusion or with middle cerebral artery occlusion, a mottled hypodensity may be seen involving the cortex, basal ganglia, and subcortical white matter down to the ventricular surface. The hypodensity may take on a wedge-shaped configuration with its base on the cortex and with its apex pointing toward the ventricle. Depending on the extent of collateral supply, internal carotid artery occlusion could also be associated with a normal scan in an asymptomatic patient. If collaterals over the brain surface are adequate, internal carotid artery occlusion may present with only a deep, small, hypodense lesion in the region of the basal ganglia; this type of lesion may be indistinguishable from scans seen with lacunae that are due to occlusion of small penetrating arteries. Internal carotid artery occlusion can also be associated with hypodense lesions in the watershed zone between the distal vessels of the middle cerebral artery and the adjacent superficial territory of the posterior cerebral artery or anterior cerebral artery[23] (see Fig. 117–6).

Lacunar Infarction

Lacunar infarctions most commonly occur in the basal ganglia and internal capsule. Often these small infarcts are due to arteriosclerosis of small penetrating vessels branching off the middle cerebral artery and anterior cerebral artery. In the first 24 to 48 hours after occlusion of these smaller vessels, the CT scan may not be associated with any discernible abnormality; larger lesions may be seen after 48 hours as a slightly hypodense patch with ill-defined borders in the basal ganglia and internal capsular region. After 3 to 4 weeks, with development of cystic and encephalomalacic change, both smaller and larger lacunae will appear as punched-out hypodensities that are more sharply defined[24–27] (see Fig. 117–7).

Embolic Infarction

Embolism may arise from a carotid bifurcation atheroma or from a cardiac source; the latter would be suspected if multiple lesions of similar age are seen within different vascular distributions on a CT scan of the brain. Most often, embolic infarction appears as a peripheral wedge-shaped hypodensity based on the cortical margin with variable extension into the subcortical white matter.[28] Clots often lyse after 1 to 5 days, exposing infarcted tissue to higher perfusion pressures than were present before clot lysis. Reperfusion after clot lysis may lead to edema and petechial hemorrhage. With thrombotic infarction, reperfusion does not occur initially; therefore, thrombosis is less often associated with edema and petechial hemorrhage on noncontrast scans compared with scans of embolic infarction. With embolism, prominent postcontrast enhancement is seen following clot lysis, often following the pattern of a cortical gyrus. The enhancement may be due to a combination of hyperemia and the transudation of dye with reperfusion into damaged, weakened capillaries.[1, 29]

Intracranial Hemorrhage

Intracranial hemorrhage associated with hypertension appears as an oval-shaped mass lesion that is homogeneous and much denser than that of normal brain tissue.[30–34] Bleeds associated with hypertension often are localized in the basal ganglia and internal capsule. More peripheral hemorrhages can be seen with arteriovenous malformation; with amyloid angiopathy; with trauma; with hemorrhage into tumors; with coagulopathies; and with progressive hemorrhage into areas of infarction, as discussed previously[1] (Fig. 117–9).

Occasionally, the more deeply situated hemorrhages can rupture into the ventricles and cause acute hydrocephalus. Surrounding a hematoma, a hypodense region may be seen, typically developing after a few hours. This probably occurs as a result of clot retraction with the subsequent collection of low-density plasma into the peripheral rim. After several days, a peripherally spreading low-density area is seen as edema develops. With breakdown of hemoglobin and absorption of clot, the hematoma loses density starting at the periphery and working inward. After complete absorption of smaller hemorrhages, a small, slit-like cyst area can be left as a residual. Larger lesions will leave behind a larger area of low density as a result of encephalomalacia.

After several days, the hematoma often shows contrast enhancement around its rim; this enhancement effect tends to diminish after several weeks.

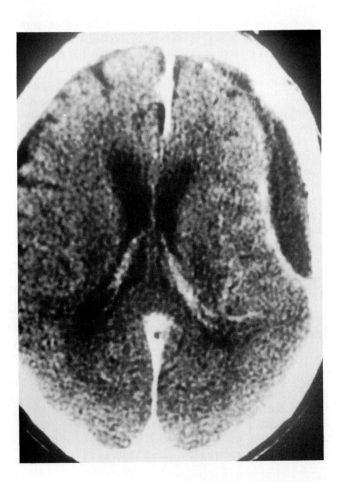

FIGURE 117–9. This patient had numerous transient episodes of right hemiparesis. The episodes continued after an otherwise successful left carotid endarterectomy. Eventually this CT scan was obtained, revealing a chronic subdural hematoma. A transient neurologic deficit may or may not have an ischemic pathophysiology. All patients presenting with transient ischemic attacks (TIAs) should have brain-imaging tests during their initial evaluation. Note that the old blood in the hematoma has become hypodense compared with brain. Blood gradually became less dense over the course of weeks or months.

Indications for CT Scans

CT scans can be obtained rapidly in relatively uncooperative and unstable patients, including those requiring ventilator support. Noncontrast CT scans are sensitive for acute hemorrhage[35] and are sufficiently sensitive for large mass lesions that might present with acute focal neurologic deficits.[21] Therefore, for an initial scanning technique, a noncontrast CT scan would seem to be a reasonable choice. Postcontrast CT scans might be helpful for evaluating patients in the days following an initial event. However, both contrast and noncontrast CT scans have definite limitations. For example, smaller infarctions along the base of the skull and in the posterior fossa may be missed with CT. Because of these limitations in selected cases, additional imaging studies might be considered.

MAGNETIC RESONANCE SCANNING IN CEREBROVASCULAR DISEASE

Principles of Interpretation

The relative brightness of a pixel for an MRI scan will depend on several characteristics of the tissue element being imaged; these characteristics include the density of hydrogen nuclei, whether the nuclei are moving or stationary (flow), and two magnetic properties of tissue called T1 and T2 relaxation.[4–7, 36–38] Scans can be generated that capitalize on tissue difference of T1, T2, hydrogen density, and flow. A scanning sequence that emphasizes tissue differences for T1 relaxation would be called a T1-weighted image; likewise, T2-weighted images can be generated.

Water produces relatively little signal (hypointensity) on T1-weighted images. Therefore, cerebrospinal fluid in the ventricles or subarachnoid spaces will appear dark on these images (Fig. 117–10). By comparison, on T2-weighted images, water appears as a bright signal (hyperintensity); therefore, on T2-weighted images, cerebrospinal fluid in the ventricles and subarachnoid spaces appears white (Fig. 117–11). Rapidly flowing blood appears as a signal void (dark area) on both T1- and T2-weighted images. Normal brain tissue generally appears as intermediate gray intensity on both T1- and T2-weighted images (Fig. 117–12).

Appearance of Abnormalities on MRI Scans

With edema, there is excess water in the parenchyma of the brain. On T1-weighted images, edematous brain will appear as a hypointense area (darker gray); however, it will not appear as hypointense as the cerebrospinal fluid within the ventricles (Fig. 117–13). On T2-weighted images, cerebrospinal fluid in the ventricles and subarachnoid spaces will appear white; similarly, water in edematous tissue will appear as a white patch (hyperintense signal). Gliotic tissue or necrotic cystic brain tissue will appear as a hyperintense

FIGURE 117–10. On T1-weighted images, the CSF within the ventricle and in the sulci appears black. Calcified bone within the skull generates very little signal, so that the calvarium appears black. The fat in the subcutaneous tissue appears white, as does the tissue within the marrow in between the tables of the skull. Normal brain tissue appears gray. In this patient, years before the magnetic resonance imaging (MRI) scan was taken, there was a large infarction as a result of a middle cerebral artery occlusion. Cystic encephalomalacic brain appears almost as dark as CSF.

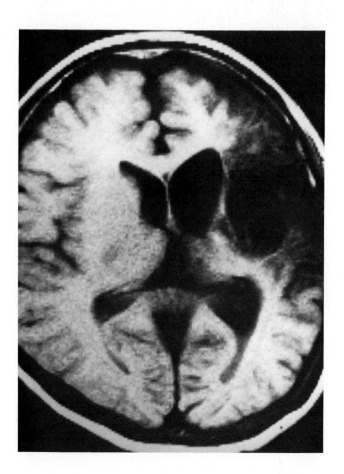

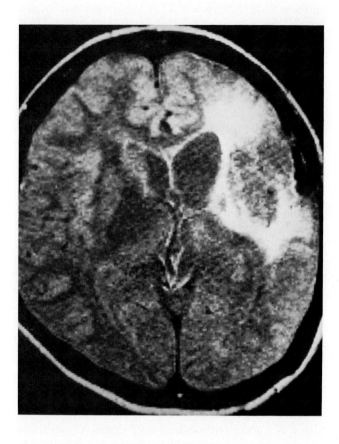

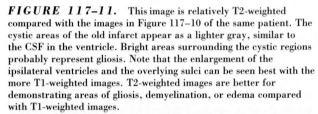

FIGURE 117–11. This image is relatively T2-weighted compared with the images in Figure 117–10 of the same patient. The cystic areas of the old infarct appear as a lighter gray, similar to the CSF in the ventricle. Bright areas surrounding the cystic regions probably represent gliosis. Note that the enlargement of the ipsilateral ventricles and the overlying sulci can be seen best with the more T1-weighted images. T2-weighted images are better for demonstrating areas of gliosis, demyelination, or edema compared with T1-weighted images.

FIGURE 117–12. Rapidly flowing arterial blood appears black in the middle cerebral, posterior cerebral, and anterior cerebral arteries, which are all identifiable in this image.

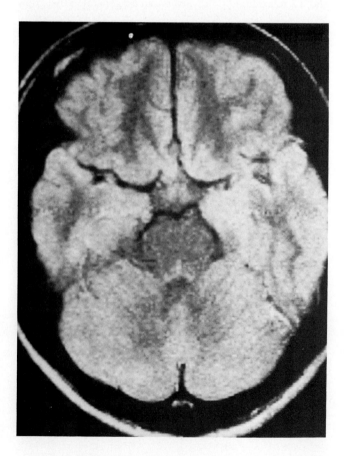

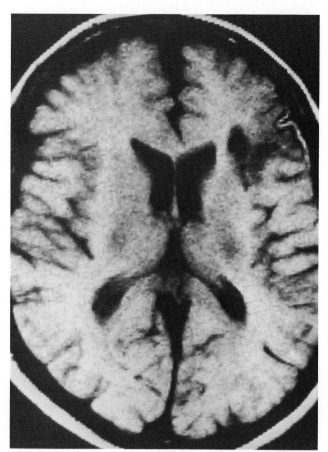

FIGURE 117–13. T1-weighted image 4 days after embolic occlusion of a left frontal branch vessel. An irregular inhomogeneous patch of low signal is present, involving a portion of the left frontal cortex and underlying subcortical region; the latter probably represents intracellular and extracellular edema. A linear bright signal area is seen following a gyral pattern, which probably represents petechial hemorrhage. The patient had a nonfluent aphasia (Broca's aphasia) as a result of a cardiac embolism to a branch vessel.

region on T2-weighted images. Probably as a result of both intracellular and interstitial edema, within 24 hours after an infarction, areas of increased signal intensity will be seen on T2-weighted images, with hypointense areas (grayer areas) on T1-weighted images (Fig. 117–14).[4] With large lesions, there may be a mass effect with local effacement of the overlying gyral pattern or displacement and compression of adjacent ventricles. With older infarctions, gliosis and cystic necrotic brain may be present with resultant hypointense areas on T1-weighted images and with hyperintense (white areas) on T2-weighted images (Fig. 117–15). Tissue loss may be suggested by focally enlarged ventricles and enlarged overlying sulci (Figs. 117–16 and 117–17).

The appearance of hemorrhage will depend on the timing of the scan after the clinical event.[39] These changes in signal intensity as a function of time appear to be related to the progressive breakdown of oxyhemoglobin to deoxyhemoglobin and subsequently into a variety of degradation products. Within the first 24 hours, blood in the middle of a hematoma will change from oxyhemoglobin to deoxyhemoglobin; this may produce a relatively low signal on T2-

weighted images and a signal that is isointense with brain tissue on T1-weighted images. This effect is seen best with higher magnetic field strengths, but it can also be seen in medium–field strength units (Fig. 117–18). After several days, the deoxyhemoglobin is degraded to methemoglobin; this is associated with a very bright signal on T1-weighted images (see Fig. 117–13). When hemosiderin forms around the periphery of a hematoma, a low signal can be seen around the rim of a hematoma on T2-weighted images (Figs. 117–19 and 117–20). Calcified areas will appear as punctate or clumpy black areas on all imaging sequences. However, finely punctate areas of calcification may not be seen on magnetic resonance scanning; the latter may be better imaged by CT scanning.

Longitudinally oriented vessels, with rapidly flowing blood, will appear as hypointense linear structures[40, 41] (see Fig. 117–12). In cross section, vessels containing rapidly flowing blood will appear as black round holes. With slowed flow or occlusion, the normally present signal void fills in; a totally occluded vessel will not have the same hypointense signal as compared with homologous patent vessels on the opposite side of the brain. Slowly flowing blood, as in superficial cortical veins, will sometimes appear as a bright linear signal in longitudinal section in T2-weighted images.[42]

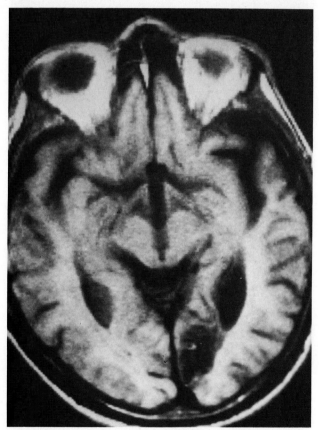

FIGURE 117–14. Two months after embolic infarction of a left posterior cerebral branch vessel. On T1-weighted images, a patch of low signal (dark area) is seen in the left occipital lobe as a result of encephalomalacia. The sulci are no longer obliterated because the edematous swelling had resolved. The subjacent occipital horn may be starting to enlarge owing to loss of overlying brain tissue.

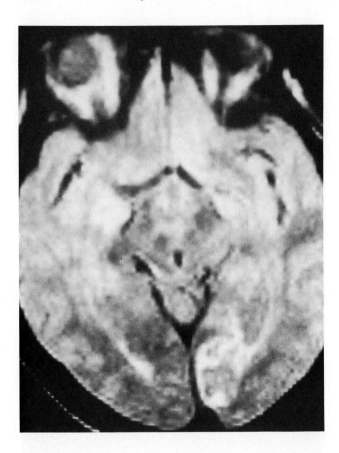

FIGURE 117–15.   Same patient as in Figure 117–14, with a T2-weighted image. The black patch seen on the T1-weighted image of Figure 117–14 now appears to be a medium gray shade, similar to the CSF within the ventricle. Surrounding this region of cystic change is a bright signal that is probably due to gliosis.

FIGURE 117–16.   Six months after an embolic infarction of the left parietal-occipital region, there appears to be a dark (low signal) area as a result of this T1-weighted image. Months after infarction, the overlying sulci and underlying ventricular spaces enlarge as necrotic tissue is removed. By contrast, acutely after infarction, edematous tissues tend to efface overlying cortex and compress subjacent ventricular spaces.

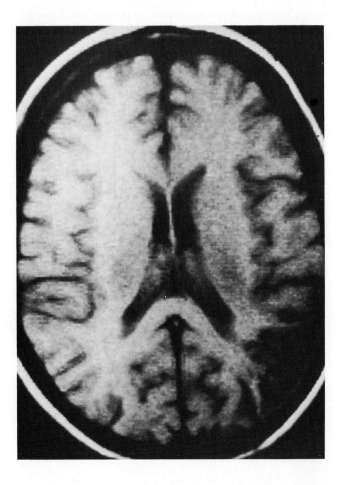

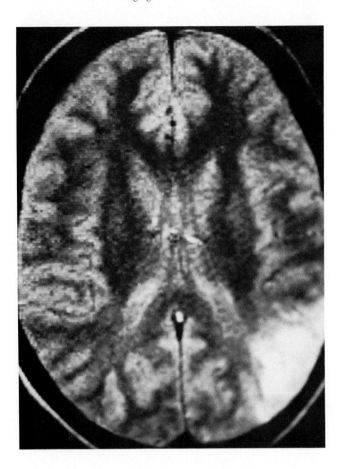

FIGURE 117–17. T2-weighted image of the same patient as in Figure 117–16. A wedge-shaped bright patch is seen in the area of old infarction. The atrophic gyral pattern is seen best on the T1-weighted images.

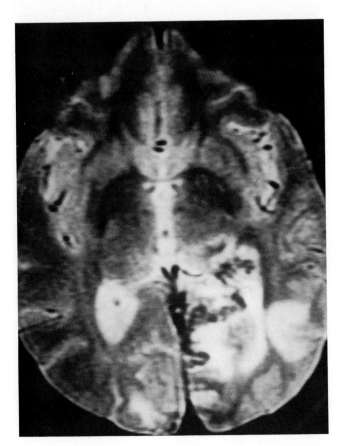

FIGURE 117–18. On T2-weighted images of this left occipital infarction, a dark linear abnormality appears to follow a gyral pattern. This abnormality probably represents petechial hemorrhage and can be seen even within the first 24–48 hours after infarction in a high-magnet-strength imaging unit.

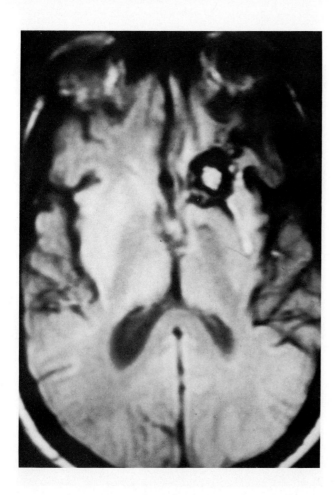

FIGURE 117–20. Same patient as in Figure 117–19, with a more T2-weighted image. Hemosiderin may appear dark on both T1-weighted and T2-weighted images.

FIGURE 117–19. The dark ring (hypointensity) in this T1-weighted image represents hemosiderin around the old hematoma of the left frontal lobe.

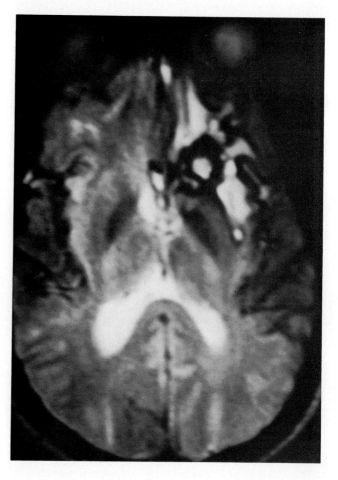

Advantages and Limitations of MRI

Using standard spin-echo imaging techniques, MRI may not be quite as accurate as CT in differentiating acute hemorrhage from infarction. However, with newer MRI techniques, as in the gradient-echo techniques, acute hemorrhage can be demonstrated. Newer techniques may also reduce the imaging times and also perhaps reduce the sensitivity for movement artifact that plagued older MRI technology. Therefore, in the coming years, it appears that MRI scanning may play more of a role for the acutely ill patient. However, the magnet room will always pose an unfavorable environment for certain metallic objects and electronic devices; therefore, patients with pacemakers or ferrometallic aneurysm clips may not be suitable for magnetic resonance scanning. Intravenous pump devices and respirators may have to be specially designed to take the magnet room environment into account. In view of these considerations, for the time being, noncontrast CT scanning appears to be a reasonable first-line imaging technique for the acute stroke patient. In the future, magnetic resonance scanning may be considered as sensitive and as safe and convenient as CT for the acutely ill patients.

CT scans may not be particularly sensitive for acute infarcts, particularly when they are small in size and located near the base of the brain or in the posterior fossa. By

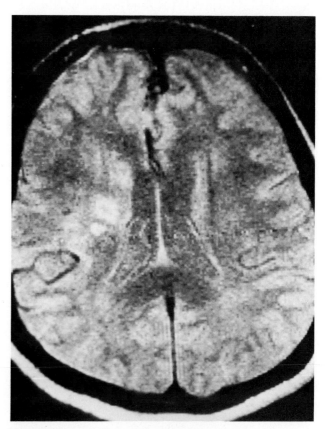

FIGURE 117–22. Same patient as in Figure 117–21, with T2-weighted images. The MRI is very sensitive for even small asymptomatic infarctions, particularly on T2-weighted images.

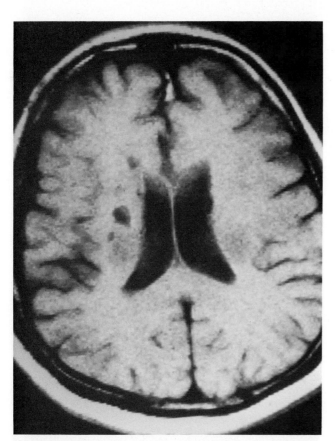

FIGURE 117–21. On T1-weighted MRI images, the old lacunar infarctions in this patient have a dark, "punched-out" appearance, similar to what is seen on CT scans in cases of this type.

contrast, magnetic resonance scanning appears to be quite sensitive even for smaller infarctions[43-48] (Figs. 117–21 to 117–24). MRI is also not plagued by the beam-hardening artifacts that obscure visualization of structures within the posterior fossa.[49] Because of these latter considerations, MRI scanning would certainly be the procedure of choice for the detection of smaller, deeply situated lesions and also for lesions in the posterior fossa. Magnetic resonance scanning also appears to be quite sensitive for detecting hemorrhage several days after an initial event; the latter technology is also compared favorably with CT in terms of sensitivity for the detection of tumors, arteriovenous malformations, and a variety of lesions that might present with an acute "stroke-like" syndrome.

Newer MRI-based techniques may be utilized for evaluating cerebral perfusion.[8] With one technique, magnetic resonance contrast is rapidly infused intravenously while MRI slices are obtained with ultrafast techniques; signal intensity at each pixel depends on perfusion from the corresponding volume of tissue. Other MRI techniques, including diffusion-weighted imaging and magnetic resonance spectroscopy,[9] may also find their way into the clinical armamentarium.

In a stable patient, magnetic resonance scanning would appear to be a reasonable technique to utilize for the further evaluation of a focal neurologic event.

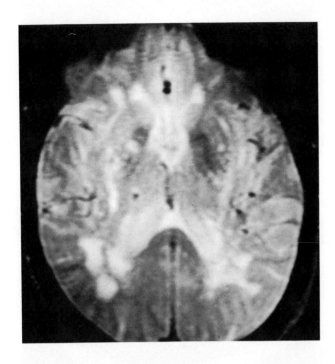

FIGURE 117–23. In elderly individuals, it may be difficult to correlate multiple, bright subcortical lesions seen on MRI with symptoms. This asymptomatic elderly individual works as a radio and television announcer.

FIGURE 117–24. This patient has multiple, cortically based lesions seen on a T2-weighted MRI image. The CT scan obtained on this patient was negative. The appearance of recent infarctions in several different vascular distributions suggests the possibility of embolization from a cardiac source in this patient with an intracardiac thrombus. Surprisingly, only the left frontal lesion was symptomatic. The great sensitivity of MRI can help elucidate the nature of a patient's problem even when other tests are negative.

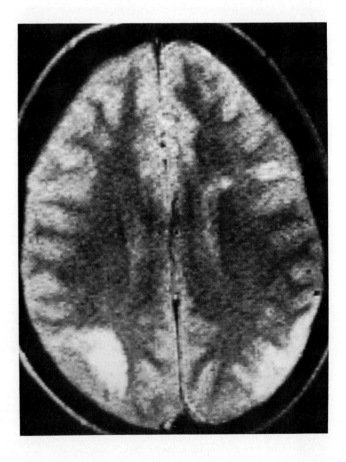

MAGNETIC RESONANCE ANGIOGRAPHY IN CEREBROVASCULAR DISEASE

Principles of Interpretation

The same MRI machine that images brain parenchyma can be used to make MRA images of extracranial and intracranial vessels.[50] One MRA technique, time-of-flight MRA (TOF-MRA), relies on the phenomenon of blood appearing as a bright signal when it flows into a stationary slice of tissue being imaged, so-called flow-related enhancement.[51]

A second main technique is called phase-contrast MRA (PC-MRA); spinning protons in stationary tissue will generate signals that have a specific phase that is determined by location along a field gradient. By contrast, in blood moving along the field gradient, spinning protons will generate signals that reflect a part of the field gradient that they were exposed to before flowing into the slice of tissue being imaged. A vascular image is generated by assigning a value of brightness to a pixel depending on the phase difference between stationary tissue in a slice being imaged and the phase of inflowing blood. The observed phase difference depends on the direction as well as the speed of moving blood as it travels through a magnetic field gradient. Different velocity-encoding gradients (VENC) can be chosen to preferentially image blood flowing at a particular velocity (Fig. 117–25). Furthermore, using two-dimensional phase-contrast techniques (2D-PC), flow direction can be depicted. The ability to preferentially image chosen flow velocities and directions is available through PC-MRA but not through TOF-MRA.[52]

Both TOF-MRA and PC-MRA techniques can acquire two-dimensional imaging slices one at a time through a vascular tree of interest, so-called 2D-TOF and 2D-PC techniques, respectively. With three-dimensional techniques, 3D-TOF and 3D-PC-MRA, whole volumes are ac-

quired simultaneously and then very thin slices of the imaged volume can be generated and displayed. Generally, 2D-MRA allows for rapid screening of very large volumes; by contrast, 3D-MRA is able to generate higher-resolution images while trading off for longer imaging times and slower throughput.

Several "tricks" can be used in order to generate MRA images that simulate conventional x-ray angiography; these techniques allow the subtraction of either arteries or veins as well as overlying stationary tissues that would overlap or obscure images of the vascular tree. One technique is to apply saturation pulses across inflowing veins so that signal from them would be suppressed, allowing arterial anatomy to be imaged without being overlapped by venous structures. For example, when imaging the carotid bifurcation in the neck, saturation pulses could be placed superior to the imaging slice in order to eliminate venous anatomy because veins in the neck flow predominantly downward in contradistinction to upward-flowing arteries.

In order to remove signal from the surrounding stationary tissues, the imaged volume is subjected to maximal-intensity projection (MIP) ray-tracing algorithms that select only the brightest pixels, which, hopefully, represent flowing blood[53] (Fig. 117–26). With targeted MIPs, selected three-dimensional segments of the vascular tree can be individually examined and rotated in any viewing angle that best displays the pathologic findings; this sort of interactive vascular imaging can be used to great advantage in imaging the carotid bifurcation in the neck or intracranial aneurysms without obscuration from overlapping vessels.[54–56]

In a manner similar to conventional x-ray angiography, vessel occlusions in MRA appear as tapered or abruptly ending branches of the vascular tree (Fig. 117–27). With MRA, areas of stenosis appear as excessively narrowed or "missing" segments of the affected vessel.

In the interpretation of MRA, one has to be aware that it is very easy to overestimate the degree of stenosis; turbulent flow distal to a point of even moderate stenosis can cause a severe drop out of MRA signal due to the produc-

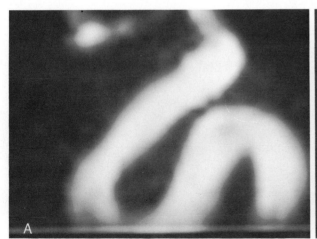
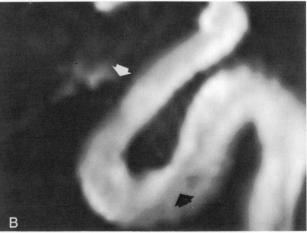

FIGURE 117–25. Magnetic resonance angiography (MRA) of the carotid siphon: three-dimensional phase-contrast (PC) versus three-dimensional time-of-flight (TOF) study. *A,* In contrast, the ophthalmic artery is not seen on this three-dimensional PC using a velocity-encoding gradient (VENC) of 40 cm/sec. This demonstrates how a vessel may fail to be visualized depending on the VENC used. *B,* This three-dimensional TOF study clearly demonstrates the ophthalmic artery (*white arrow*). Notice the loss of signal in areas where there is dephasing with change in direction of the siphon (*black arrow*).

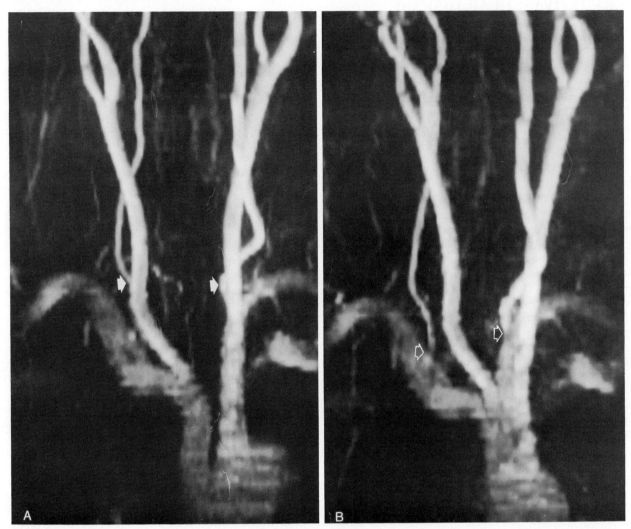

FIGURE 117–26.   MRI of cervical vessels using two-dimensional TOF: the use of interactive rotation. *A,* Anteroposterior view of this two-dimensional TOF reveals the common carotid bifurcation but conceals the origins of the vertebral arteries (*arrows*). *B,* With minimal rotation, the origin of the vertebral arteries is well displayed bilaterally (*arrows*).

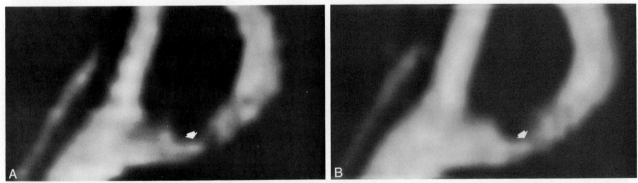

FIGURE 117–27.   Carotid narrowing: increasing resolution with higher NEX using two-dimensional TOF MRA. *A,* The narrowing in the internal carotid artery (ICA) (*arrow*) is well seen using 2 excitations (NEX). *B,* The resolution of the vessel and the atheromatous narrowing (*arrow*) are greatly improved by increasing the NEX to 4.

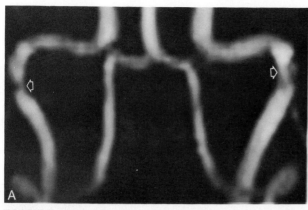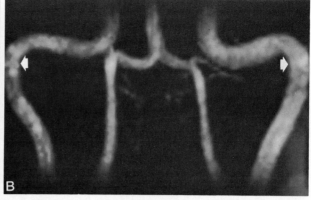

FIGURE 117–28. Flow artifacts at the skull base: two-dimensional TOF versus three-dimensional TOF. *A*, Note the narrowing in the ICA at the skull base (*arrows*), using a two-dimensional TOF technique. This must not be misinterpreted as a narrowing. *B*, The narrowing is no longer evident on this three-dimensional TOF technique (*arrows*).

tion of random phase shifts, with subsequent phase cancellation of signal within the voxels being imaged (intravoxel dephasing); this effect is particularly problematic with 2D-MRA techniques. Vortex flow distal to a stenosis also leads to loss of signal because protons within the swirling blood are excessively exposed to imaging pulses and thereby become saturated (saturation effects)[55] (Fig. 117–28).

Advantages and Limitations of MRA

Compared with conventional x-ray angiography, MRA is noninvasive and, therefore, is unassociated with contrast agent risks, embolic complications, and insertion site injuries that are encountered with the former technique. Furthermore, as an MRA is being obtained, a brain MRI can be performed in the same sitting so that the status of brain parenchyma can be evaluated. With expected enhancements in coil design and software, the imaging times may be kept to a manageable minimum. Furthermore, because the technique is reasonably accurate in depicting the vascular tree, it is considered a valuable screening test that can be used in the evaluation of patients presenting with signs and symptoms that suggest arterial stenosis or occlusion[57-60] (Fig. 117–29). However, at this time conventional x-ray angiography remains the gold standard for the accurate assessment of the degree of arterial stenosis and occlusion as well as for the depiction of smaller intracranial vessels.

MRA compares favorably with ultrasonography in the assessment of the carotid bifurcation in the neck.[57-60] In addition, MRA allows for simultaneous accurate anatomic imaging of arch vessels as well as intracranial vessels; by contrast, with ultrasound-based techniques, these areas are imaged with greater difficulty.

Several limitations and artifacts must be kept in mind when trying to apply MRA to a given patient problem or in the interpretation of results. First of all, as with MRI, MRA is difficult to use in the medically unstable or uncooperative patient. Ferromagnetic vascular clips and other implanted metallic objects preclude entry of the patient into the magnet room. Although certain metallic clips can be safely imaged, they could still distort the surrounding magnetic field and thereby seriously degrade attempts to image adja-

cent blood vessels. A variety of movement artifacts, including those associated with swallow, cough, breathing, and pulsation, can also obscure vascular anatomy.[53]

MRA can demonstrate areas of apparent stenosis that are entirely artifactual. Loss of signal with apparent disappearance or narrowing of the vascular lumen can occur because of saturation effects in a blood vessel segment that is flowing in plane with the imaging slice; this effect is characteristic of 2D-MRA. Vessels are better seen when the imaging slices are oriented transversely to the direction of blood flow. Because of magnetic susceptibility effects, the lumen of the carotid often appears to be narrowed as it courses through bone in the skull base. These effects can be partially averted with the use of 3D-MRA; however, the tradeoff is an increased imaging time.

With TOF-MRA, stationary tissues are not totally subtracted; because of this effect, bright signals from adjacent tissue may obscure vascular structures. With PC-MRA, stationary tissue can be better subtracted; however, the vessels that appear as bright signals will be confined to the velocities chosen beforehand by the imager. Signal from blood flowing above a certain range may appear to unexpectedly ''drop out''; this aliasing effect can mislead the unwary observer.

POSITRON EMISSION TOMOGRAPHY

PET is a technique that utilizes radioactive tracers to visualize the extent, intensity, and rate of biologic processes occurring within the brain.[9-12] Positron-emitting isotopes are produced for carbon, nitrogen, oxygen, and fluorine; these can be utilized to label a wide variety of metabolic substrates and drug analogues. When a positron decays, two photons are emitted 180 degrees apart; these photons are detected electronically by detectors that record only the simultaneously occurring photons 180 degrees apart (annihilation coincidence detection). Input to a ring of detectors is reconstructed to a tomographic image using techniques similar to those of CT. As the tagged substrates are transported through vessels, across membranes, or metabolized by cells, images can be formed that map the extent of

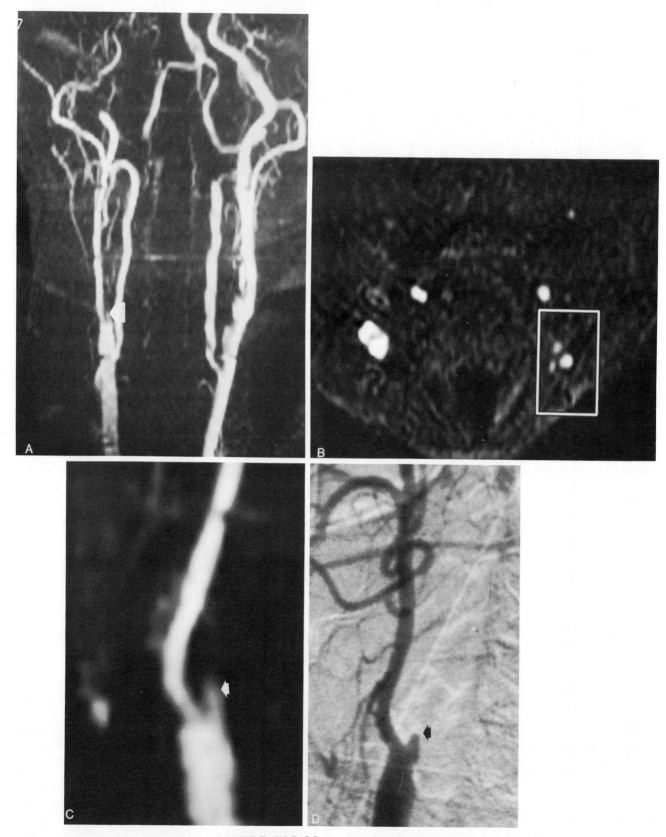

FIGURE 117–29   *See legend on opposite page*

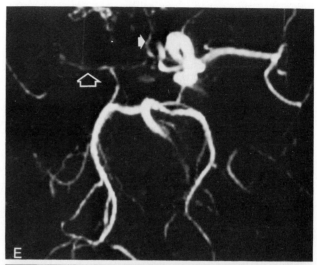

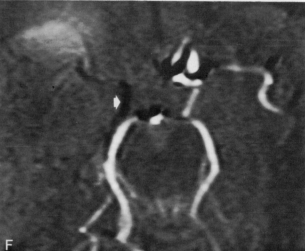

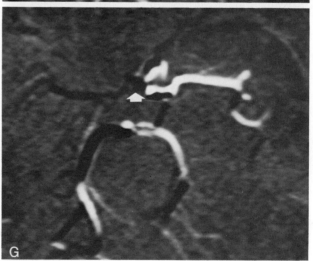

FIGURE 117–29. Occlusion of right cervical ICA: evaluation with MRA. *A,* Two-dimensional TOF MRA, skull base to common carotid artery. This screens all major cervical vessels. Overlapping vessels may obscure the occluded right ICA *(arrow)*. *B,* Targeted maximal-intensity projection (MIP) from raw data to define specific pathology. A region of interest (ROI) *(boxed area)* is placed over individual vessels (in this case, the right cervical carotid artery) and these are selectively MIPped to remove unwanted overlapping vessels. *C* and *D,* Targeted MIP of right ICA *(lateral view).* The stump of the occluded right ICA is well shown *(arrow in C)* and compares accurately with the equivalent view from the more invasive intracranial angiogram *(D) (arrow).* *E,* Three-dimensional TOF MRA of circle of Willis. MRA can also rapidly evaluate the intracranial circulation. The right ICA is occluded; however, the right middle cerebral artery *(open arrow)* and anterior cerebral artery *(closed arrow)* are patent. *F,* Two-dimensional PC MRA with anteroposterior directional flow to assess the posterior communicating artery. This directional MRA technique has the advantage of demonstrating flow direction. Anteroposterior (AP) flow is white and posteroanterior (PA) flow is black. Retrograde flow from the posterior circulation can be readily discerned on the right as evidenced by the black posterior communicating artery *(arrow).* The left posterior communicating artery maintains the more normal AP flow direction. This accounts for the maintenance of flow into the right brain in the setting of an occluded right ICA. *G,* Two-dimensional PC MRA with right-to-left flow direction to assess the anterior communicating artery. This right-to-left flow direction depicts the flow through the anterior communicating artery from left to right *(arrow)* to compensate for the occluded right ICA.

utilization and determine where processes are occurring in an abnormal or a normal fashion.

Current PET units allow rapid simultaneous acquisition of multiple slices through the brain with spatial resolution that approaches a few millimeters. However, even with improvements, it appears that PET will have a resolution for anatomic detail that is inferior to that of currently available CT scanners or MRI scanners. Tracer techniques are available for measuring cerebral blood flow, cerebral blood volume, cerebral metabolic rate for oxygen, and cerebral metabolic rate for glucose; in addition, a useful derived function is the fraction of oxygen extracted by tissue (oxygen extraction fraction).

PET in Cerebral Ischemia

Present concepts of PET suggest that a sequence of changes can be seen as cerebral perfusion is progressively reduced from a state of mild hypoperfusion to the extreme case of cerebral infarction with resultant necrosis of neural tissue.[61-64]

As local cerebral blood flow is reduced, the cerebral metabolic rate of oxygen is maintained within a relatively normal range, as is the oxygen extraction fraction; however, initially there is a local dilatation of precapillary arterioles and capillary vessels. As local flow is reduced further, the fraction of oxygen extracted from the blood increases in order to maintain the cerebral metabolic rate for oxygen. With an additional decrease in cerebral blood flow, sufficient oxygen may no longer be extracted, so that the cerebral metabolic rate for oxygen begins to fall. At this point, the cerebral metabolic rate for glucose may actually increase as a result of a switch from oxidative metabolism to glycolysis.

After tissue infarction, there may be a development of new vessels; collaterals may bring increased blood flow; previously occluded vessels may reopen. Reopening of vessels may occur, for example, after distal migration and dissolution of an embolus. In these circumstances, there may be a temporary increase of cerebral blood flow; however, infarcted tissue will have disrupted glucose and oxygen metabolism, so that oxygen utilization and extraction (oxygen extraction fraction) will not recover. This excess blood flow, in spite of reduced metabolism, is sometimes called luxury perfusion. With time, cerebral blood flow and cerebral blood volume will be relatively reduced to match the local cerebral metabolic rate for oxygen. Therefore, in a chronic infarction, the oxygen extraction fraction may return to normal.

With PET, it may be possible to identify which patients with mild stroke syndromes or transient ischemic attacks may benefit from revascularization procedures. For example, a pattern demonstrating a persistently decreased regional cerebral blood flow with relative preservation of cerebral metabolic rate of oxygen along with an increased regional oxygen extraction fraction would suggest the possibility of a hemodynamic pathogenesis for the clinical event. Patients with this type of pattern might benefit from a medical or surgical intervention that would increase cerebral blood flow further; the PET scan might suggest that the ischemic tissue is malfunctioning as a result of the

ischemia but may recover function as flow is restored. By contrast, patients with a persistently diminished cerebral metabolic rate of oxygen and a diminished oxygen extraction fraction would probably not benefit from a procedure that would increase cerebral blood flow further. The PET scan would suggest that the ischemic tissue would be nonviable even if flow could be restored. Notably, in both the cases discussed, the regional cerebral blood flow may be diminished; the ability of PET scanning to detect areas of increased oxygen extraction (relative maintenance of cerebral metabolic rate for oxygen) allows this technology to differentiate potentially viable tissue from nonviable tissue. The demonstration of reduced flow alone may not help predict which patients may benefit from a revascularization procedure.

SINGLE-PHOTON EMISSION COMPUTED TOMOGRAPHY SCANNING

In SPECT, current experience is mostly reported for two pharmaceutical agents to measure cerebral blood flow: radioactive xenon and N-isopropyl (I-123), p-iodoamphetamine (IMP). Cerebral blood flow images using a SPECT technique have a resolution on the order of over 1 cm; this is significantly less than the resolution obtainable with PET.[65] Furthermore, SPECT techniques do not measure cerebral metabolic rates for oxygen or glucose, as can be done with PET scanning. Therefore, SPECT cannot directly identify which areas may be hypometabolic but still capable of recovery of function with revascularization. Nevertheless, SPECT technology can show the localization and extent of infarcts whether such infarcts are visible or not by CT.[66] Hemodynamic responses can be measured utilizing SPECT: for example, with acetazolamide infusion.[67] This test and others may be used to identify which patients may have a reduced cerebral blood flow as a result of a compromised collateral circulation: that is, a chronic "hemodynamic insufficiency." Patients identified in this manner may possibly benefit from medical or surgical therapy aimed at increasing cerebral blood flow.

CHOOSING THE APPROPRIATE STUDY

Which study to order depends on the clinical question that needs to be answered as well as on the stability of the patient and on the age and location of a possible infarction. For acute infarctions in an uncooperative, unstable patient, the noncontrast CT scan will allow short scanning times, relative insensitivity to movement artifact, accessibility for supportive equipment, and excellent sensitivity for hemorrhage and large mass lesions. Therefore, if the main goal is to exclude acute hemorrhage or a mass lesion that may present with a stroke-like picture, a noncontrast CT study will be adequate in the initial study of most acute stroke patients.

Contrast CT scans can be obtained later if there are further questions, particularly in a somewhat more stable patient who has been hydrated and who does not have diabetic nephropathy or another relative contraindication to contrast dye infusion.

For patients who are not acutely ill, and particularly for patients who present several days after a possible ischemic event, a magnetic resonance scan would be a good choice, assuming that both T1- and T2-weighted images are obtained. The T1-weighted images will be quite sensitive to subacute hemorrhage several days after an event. T2-weighted images will show areas of edema, tissue necrosis, and gliosis in both small and larger infarctions in a manner that is more sensitive than CT scanning. MRI is better in both detection and determination of the extent of the infarction. The magnetic resonance scan is also superior to the CT scan if the suspected lesion is in the brain stem or cerebellum.

With the application of MRA to the investigation of the stroke patient, it is now possible to rapidly and noninvasively screen the entire vascular tree from the aortic arch to the intracranial circulation in the same sitting that a standard brain MRI is performed; this examination along with carotid ultrasonography can be effectively utilized to determine which patients may need conventional x-ray angiography before a surgical intervention is undertaken. There are a host of technologies available for the research evaluation of stroke-related changes in metabolism and physiology, such as PET, SPECT, and magnetic resonance–based perfusion and diffusion scanning as well as magnetic resonance spectroscopy; in the coming years, these techniques promise to clarify the cause of ischemic symptoms in patients so that therapies may be individualized.

References

1. Lee SH, Rao K, Zimmerman RA: Cranial MRI and CT. 3rd ed. New York, McGraw-Hill, 1992.
2. Wolfson SK, Gur D, Yonas H: Cerebral blood flow determination. *In* Latchaw RE (ed): Computed Tomography in the Head, Neck, and Spine. Chicago, Year Book Medical, 1985, pp 27–52.
3. Valk J: Computed Tomography and Cerebral Infarction. New York, Raven Press, 1980.
4. Brant-Zawadzki M, Weinstein P, Bartkowski H, et al: MR imaging and spectroscopy in clinical and experimental cerebral ischemia: A review. AJR 148:579, 1987.
5. Brant-Zawadzki M, Norman D (eds): Magnetic Resonance Imaging of the Central Nervous System. New York, Raven Press, 1987.
6. Wong WS, Tsuruda JS, Kortman KE, et al: Practical MRI. Rockville, MD, Aspen, 1987.
7. Mettler FA, Muroff LR, Kulkarni M (eds): Magnetic Resonance Imaging and Spectroscopy. New York, Churchill Livingstone, 1986.
8. Fisher M, Sotak CH, Minematsu K, et al: New magnetic resonance techniques for evaluating cerebrovascular diseases. Ann Neurol 32(2):115, 1992.
9. Rosen BR, Belliveau JW, Fordham JA: The role of dynamic magnetic resonance imaging in the assessment of stroke. Neuroimag Clin North Am 2(3):559, 1992.
10. Phelps ME, Mazziotta JC, Schelbert HR (eds): Position Emission Tomography and Autoradiography, Principles and Applications for the Brain and the Heart. New York, Raven Press, 1986.
11. Ackerman RH, Correia JA, Alpert NM, et al: PET studies in stroke. *In* Reivich M, Alavi A (eds): Positron Emission Tomography. New York, Liss, 1985, pp 249–262.
12. Heiss WD, Beil C, Hecholz K, et al: Atlas of Positron Emission Tomography of the Brain. Berlin, Springer-Verlag, 1985.
13. Raynaud C, Rancurel G, Samson Y, et al: Pathophysiologic study of chronic infarcts with I-123 isopropyl iodo-amphetamine (IMP): The importance of periinfarct areas. Stroke 18:21, 1987.
14. Defer G, Moretti JC, Cesaro P, et al: Early and delayed SPECT using
15. Sugiyama H, Christenson J, Olsen TS, et al: Monitoring CBF in clinical routine by dynamic single photon emission tomography (SPECT) of inhaled xenon-133. Stroke 17(6):1179, 1986.
16. Ropper A, Kehne SM: Contrast enhancement CT scan and post-endarterectomy hemorrhage. Stroke 17(5):898, 1986.
17. Hart RG, Tegeler CH: Hemorrhagic infarction on CT in the absence of anticoagulation therapy. Stroke 17(3):558, 1986.
18. Cerebral Embolism Study Group: Immediate anticoagulation of embolic stroke: Brain hemorrhage and management options. Stroke 15:779, 1984.
19. Hornig CR, Dornidorf W, Agnoli AL: Hemorrhagic cerebral infarction—A prospective study. Stroke 17(2):179, 1986.
20. Lodder J, Krijne-Kubat B, Brockman J: Cerebral hemorrhagic infarction at autopsy: Cardiac embolic cause and the relationship to the cause of death. Stroke 17(4):626, 1986.
21. Ruff RL, Dougherty JH: Evaluation of acute cerebral ischemia for anticoagulant therapy: Computed tomography or lumbar puncture. Neurology 31(6):736, 1981.
22. Ito U, Tomita H, Kito K, et al: CT enhancement after prolonged high-dose contrast infusion in the early stage of cerebral infarction. Stroke 17(3):424, 1986.
23. Bogousslausky J, Regli F: Borderzone infarctions distal to internal carotid artery occlusion: Prognostic implications. Ann Neurol 20(3):346, 1986.
24. Manelfe C, Clanet M, et al: Internal capsule: Normal anatomy and ischemic changes demonstrated by computed tomography. Am J Neuroradiol 2:149, 1981.
25. Nelson RF, Pullicino P, Kendall BE, et al: Computed tomography in patients presenting with lacunar syndrome. Stroke 11:256, 1980.
26. Donnan GA, Tress BM, Bladin PF: A prospective study of lacunar infarction using computerized tomography. Neurology 32:49, 1982.
27. Weisberg LA: Lacunar infarcts: Clinical and computed tomographic correlations. Arch Neurol 39:37, 1982.
28. Yock DH: CT demonstration of cerebral emboli. J Comput Assist Tomogr 5:190, 1981.
29. Hayman LA, Evans RA, Bastion FO, et al: Delayed high-dose contrast CT: Identifying patients at risk of massive hemorrhagic infarction. Am J Neuroradiol 2:139, 1981.
30. Weisberg LA: Computerized tomography in intracranial hemorrhage. Arch Neurol 36:422, 1979.
31. Dokinskas CA, Bilaniuk LT, Zimmerman RA, et al: Computerized tomography of intracerebral hematoma. I. Transmission CT observation on hematoma resolution. AJR 129:681, 1977.
32. Dokinskas CA, Bilaniuk LT, Zimmerman RA, et al: Computed tomography of intracerebral hematoma. II. Radionucleotide and transmission studies of perihematoma region. AJR 129:689, 1977.
33. Laster DW, Moody DM, Ball MR: Resolving intracranial hematoma: Alteration of the ''ring-sign'' with steroids. AJR 130:935, 1978.
34. Zimmerman RD, Leeds NE, Naidich TP: Ring blush with intracranial hematoma. Radiology 122:707, 1977.
35. Paxton R, Ambrose J: The EMI scanner. A brief review of the first 650 patients. Br J Radiol 47:530, 1974.
36. Bradley WG, Newton TH, Crooks LE: Physical principles of nuclear magnetic resonance. *In* Newton TH, Potts DG (eds): Advanced Imaging Techniques. San Anselmo, CA, Clavadel, 1983, pp 15–61.
37. Mills CM, De Groot J, Newton TH: Nuclear magnetic resonance imaging: The normal brain and spinal cord. *In* Newton TH, Potts DG (eds): Advanced Imaging Techniques. San Anselmo, CA, Clavadel, 1983, pp 119–158.
38. Brant-Zawadzki M: Nuclear magnetic resonance imaging: The abnormal brain and spinal cord. *In* Newton TH, Potts DG (eds): Advanced Imaging Techniques. San Anselmo, CA, Clavadel, 1983, pp 159–188.
39. Gomori JM, Grossman RI, Goldberg HI, et al: Intracranial hematomas: Imaging by high-field MR. Radiology 157:87, 1985.
40. Bradley WG, Waluch V, Lai KS, et al: The appearance of rapidly flowing blood on magnetic resonance images. AJR 143:1167, 1984.
41. Bradley WG, Waluch V: Blood flow: Magnetic resonance imaging. Radiology 154:443, 1985.
42. Waluch V, Bradley WG: NMR even echo rephasing in slow laminar flow. J Comput Assist Tomogr 8:594, 1984.
43. De Witt LD: Clinical use of nuclear magnetic imaging in stroke. Stroke 17(2):328, 1986.
44. Awad I, Modic M, Little JR, et al: Focal parenchymal lesions in

N-isopropyl p-iodoamphetamine iodine 123 in cerebral ischemia. Arch Neurol 44(7):715, 1987.

transient ischemic attacks: Correlation of computerized tomography and magnetic resonance imaging. Stroke 17(3):399, 1986.

45. De Witt LD, Kistler SP, Miller DC, et al: NMR: Neuropathologic correlation in stroke. Stroke 18:342, 1987.

46. Bryan RN, Wilcott MR, Schneiders NJ, et al: NMR evaluation of stroke: A preliminary report. Radiology 149:189, 1983.

47. Pykett IL, Buonanno FS, Brady TS, et al: True three-dimensional, NMR neuro-imaging in ischemic stroke: Correlation of NMR, x-ray CT and pathology. Stroke 14:173, 1983.

48. Sipponen JT, Kaste M, Ketmen L, et al: Serial NMR imaging in patients with cerebral infarction. J Comput Assist Tomogr 7:585, 1983.

49. Bogousslausky J, Fox AJ, Barnett HJM, et al: Clinico-topographic correlation of small vertebral basilar infarct using MRI. Stroke 17(5):929, 1986.

50. Edelmann RR, Mattle HP, Atkinson DJ, et al: MR angiography. AJR 154:937, 1990.

51. Laub G, Kaiser W: MR Angiography with gradient motion refocusing. J Comput Assist Tomogr 12:377, 1988.

52. Dumoulin CL, Souza SP, Walker MF, et al: Three-dimensional phase-contrast angiography. Magnetic Reson Med 9:139, 1989.

53. Anderson CM, Saloner D, Tsuruda JS, et al: Artifacts in maximum intensity projection display of MR angiograms. AJR 154:623, 1989.

54. Masaryk TJ, Modic MT, Ross JS, et al: Angiography of intracranial aneurysms. AJNR 10:893, 1989.

55. Rugglieri P, Laub G, Masaryk TJ, et al: Intracranial circulation: Pulse sequence considerations in three-dimensional MR angiography. Radiology 171:785, 1989.

56. Masaryk TJ, Modic MT, Ruggieri PM, et al: Three-dimensional (volume) gradient-echo imaging of the carotid bifurcation: Preliminary clinical experience. Radiology 171:801, 1989.

57. Anderson CM, Saloner D, Lee RE, et al: Assessment of carotid artery stenosis by MR angiography: Comparison with x-ray angiography and color-coded Doppler ultrasound. AJNR 13:989, 1992.

58. Mattle HP, Kent KC, Edelman RR, et al: Evaluation of the extracranial carotid arteries: Correlation of magnetic resonance angiography, duplex ultrasonography, and conventional angiography. J Vasc Surg 13:838, 1991.

59. Wilkerson DK, Keller I, Mezrich R, et al: The comparative evaluation of three-dimensional magnetic resonance imaging for carotid artery disease. J Vasc Surg 14(6):803, 1991.

60. Riles-TS, Eidelman EM, Litt AW: Original contributions: comparison of magnetic angiography, conventional angiography and duplex scanning. Stroke 23(3):341, 1992.

61. Frackowiak RSJ: PET scanning: Can it help resolve management issues in cerebral ischemic disease? Stroke 17(5):803, 1986.

62. Frackowiak RSJ: Positron tomography in ischemic cerebrovascular disease. Neurol Clin 1:183, 1983.

63. Baron JC, Bousser MG, Rey A, et al: Reversal of focal "misery-perfusion syndrome" by extra-intracranial arterial bypass in hemodynamic cerebral ischemia. Stroke 12:454, 1981.

64. Baron JC, Rougemont D, Soussaline F, et al: Local interrelationships of cerebral oxygen consumption and glucose utilization in normal subjects and in ischemic stroke patients: A positron tomography study. J Cereb Blood Flow Metabol 4:140, 1984.

65. Welch KMA, Levine SR, Ewing JR: Viewing stroke pathophysiology: An analysis of contemporary methods. Stroke 17(6):1071, 1986.

66. Defer G, Moretti JL, Cesaro P, et al: Early and delayed SPECT using N-isopropyl-p-iodoamphetamine iodine 123 in cerebral ischemia. Arch Neurol 44:715, 1987.

67. Vorstrup S, Brun B, Lassen N: Evaluation of the cerebral vasodilatory capacity by the acetazolamide test before EC-IC bypass surgery in patients with occlusion of the internal carotid artery. Stroke 17(6):1291, 1986.

118

Medical Management of Ischemic Cerebrovascular Disease

John Maher, M.B., B.Ch., B.A.O., M.R.C.P.(I.), F.R.C.P.(C.),
and Vladimir Hachinski, M.D., F.R.C.P.(C.), D.Sc. (Med.)

• • •

Stroke management has changed grudgingly but decidedly in recent years. In the not-too-distant past, patients were often treated at home; today, proper treatment necessitates hospital admission. Indeed, patients with a stroke are increasingly admitted to highly specialized stroke units, where they enter a planned research program. Clinical and animal research in cerebral ischemia has cast light on mechanisms causing neuronal death. New and improved diagnostic techniques allow a more accurate analysis to be made of the cause of a stroke. These advances are now being integrated into enhanced patient care.

An easily applied approach to the medical management of ischemic cerebrovascular disease is discussed. It starts with an assessment of the neurologic injury and its likely etiology, followed by an algorithm for ischemic stroke management. Finally, prophylactic measures to prevent stroke and vascular-related death are discussed.

DIAGNOSIS OF AN ISCHEMIC STROKE

Clinical Evaluation

The diagnosis of a stroke is still largely based on the analysis of a carefully performed history and physical examination.[1] This is integrated with neuroimaging techniques, which allow a more precise diagnosis of the type and location of a stroke.

The patient's history, including the family and social history, is invaluable in establishing a diagnosis and likely etiology of a stroke. A history of a neurologic deficit that came on suddenly is highly suggestive of a stroke. The terms *stroke* and *apoplexy* emphasize this sudden onset and draw attention to a process that acts as though the brain had been delivered a sudden blow resulting in focal, frequently devastating, dysfunction. Often, there is a history of evolution of the stroke since onset, usually over 1 to 2 hours, which is of importance for management. An ischemic episode lasting less than 24 hours, called a transient ischemic episode, needs to be differentiated from a fixed ischemic neurologic deficit because it requires no rehabilitative therapy but does necessitate urgent management if strokes are to be avoided.

Various nuances of the clinical history may indicate the likely pathogenesis of a stroke. A stroke due to a large intracerebral hemorrhage, such as into the basal ganglia, typically results in a cataclysmic neurologic deficit that reaches its maximum within minutes from onset and results in a severe headache, vomiting, stupor or coma, and a dense hemiparesis. Its onset is typically while the patient is awake and active and only rarely while the patient is asleep. Usually, there are no premonitory symptoms, and the stroke does not resolve quickly, as occasionally occurs in ischemic neurologic episodes. The alteration in the level of consciousness is due to a rapid rise in intracranial pressure. However, clinical separation of small intracerebral hemorrhages from ischemic strokes is problematic. In distinction to intracerebral hemorrhage, the archetypal embolic stroke, although also of sudden onset, tends to reach its maximum immediately from onset and frequently shows significant resolution within the first 24 hours because of fragmentation and lysis of the embolus. Of particular importance in diagnosing an embolic stroke is the existence of an identifiable source of embolus, such as atrial fibrillation or a recent myocardial infarct, in the absence of other readily identifiable causes of the stroke. Indeed, an embolic stroke may be the first sign of a myocardial infarct. An atherothrombotic stroke differs from a cardioembolic stroke in that there are frequently premonitory transient ischemic episodes. The stroke may evolve over a few hours, but a stuttering course, in which there is an intermittent stepwise deterioration of the neurologic deficit over hours or days as the clot gradually extends, is not uncommon and is particularly suggestive of a thrombotic stroke, although there are many possible causes of stroke-in-evolution. The onset is frequently during sleep. Atherothrombotic strokes are not typically associated with a rapid deterioration in the level of consciousness or with headache or vomiting.

Neurologic examination allows a more definitive separation of carotid from vertebrobasilar arterial system stroke. Carotid artery system strokes generally have signs consisting of monoparesis, hemiparesis, and hemianesthesia. There is frequently a homonymous field defect; agnosias and apraxias of different types; and if the dominant hemisphere is involved, dysphasia. Vertebrobasilar arterial system strokes generally have signs of brain stem and cerebellar dysfunction. Common features include diplopia, nystagmus, vertigo, vomiting, and truncal and limb ataxia.

A crossed deficit, which consists of ipsilateral cranial nerve involvement and contralateral long-tract signs (mainly pyramidal and spinothalamic), is characteristic of a brain stem lesion. A brain stem stroke may also have bilateral signs affecting the cranial nerves and limbs.

Fundoscopic examination allows rapid assessment of the body's smaller blood vessels and reflects the state of arterioles arising from the internal carotid artery. The fundus can be examined for changes due to hypertension, diabetes, and emboli, all of which are of interest with respect to stroke pathogenesis. Retinal emboli may cause transient monocular blindness. Emboli usually arise from an atheromatous plaque at the origin of the internal carotid artery. These emboli are most often orange-yellow cholesterol crystals (Hollenhorst's plaque), but they may be gray-white fibrin-platelet emboli. The heart's valves are occasionally the source of retinal emboli, which are typically white-colored calcium particles.

General physical examination in those with a stroke should involve paying particular attention to the cardiovascular system. The heart rate and rhythm, the blood pressure, and the body temperature should be checked. Auscultation over the extracranial vessels for bruits and over the heart for murmurs and added sounds is important, frequently guiding future investigations. Petechiae may be seen with endocarditis or a bleeding disorder. Plethora is suggestive of polycythemia, whereas pallor of the conjunctiva and skin creases is suggestive of anemia. Cyanosis with clubbing occurs in cyanotic congenital heart disease.

Neuroimaging

Neuroimaging has revolutionized the clinician's approach to the diagnosis of stroke. Computed tomography (CT) of the brain is the technique most often used in this regard. The characteristic CT appearance of a cerebral infarct is a low-density area. However, in early ischemic stroke, findings on CT of the brain are frequently negative, with positive results found in only 5 per cent of patients in the first 4 hours, in 50 per cent by 24 hours, and in 95 per cent by the 8th day.[2] Therefore, the initial diagnosis and localization of an infarct remain largely clinical. Repetition of the CT study at a later date frequently demonstrates the infarct because the quantity of tissue water rises in the infarcted area in the first few days. The main value of CT in ischemic stroke lies in its ability to rule out hemorrhagic stroke and other pathology that may masquerade as a stroke, such as a brain tumor. Unfortunately, CT is not able to rule out all pathologies that simulate an ischemic stroke, thus forcing reevaluation of the clinical symptomatology and necessitating other investigations to establish a diagnosis. Thus, for example, CT is frequently unable to distinguish lobar hemorrhage from hemorrhagic infarction, which requires a search for possible sources of embolus and an evaluation of risk factors for intracerebral hemorrhage.[3]

Magnetic resonance imaging (MRI) of the brain has been shown to be superior to CT in the detection of early ischemic infarcts, particularly those involving the brain stem and cerebellum.[4-8] It is capable of detecting ischemic changes within a few hours of stroke onset.[9-11] MR angiography is becoming increasingly sophisticated and may add significant additional information on both extra- and intracerebral vasculature. Unfortunately, a limitation of MRI is that it gives similar signals from lesions due to ischemia, demyelination, edema, and gliosis.[12] MRI is also poor at distinguishing acute hemorrhage from edema in the first few days of a stroke because both acute hemorrhage and edema give a high signal on T2-weighted images and low to isointense signals on T1-weighted images.[8, 13] Furthermore, MRI is costly, has a restricted availability, is time consuming, requires a sick patient to remain still for up to 1 hour, and frequently demonstrates lesions of uncertain significance, such as unidentified bright objects, which may confound the clinical picture.[12]

In general, although CT and MRI of the brain often localize an ischemic lesion, they seldom help in establishing an etiology. However, by dividing ischemic lesions involving medial and basal brain structures from those involving the outer cortical mantle, it is possible to gain some clue as to the likely etiology.

The medial and basal portions of the brain and brain stem, which have been called the vascular centrencephalon,[2] are supplied by penetrating arteries, which enter and supply these areas in a ventral-to-dorsal direction (Fig. 118–1). The penetrating arteries tend to supply a small volume of tissue. Therefore, disease of these vessels may cause a small cerebral infarct, called a lacunar infarct. Conditions that may result in occlusion of the penetrating arteries include intrinsic lipohyalinosis and fibrinoid degeneration, atherosclerotic occlusion of the ostium of a penetrating vessel, and occasionally an embolus. Some investigators have also argued that lacunar infarcts may be caused by severe occlusive disease, including embolus, of either intra- or extracranial arteries, with collateral circulation sparing the cortical tissue. These penetrating vessels are also the site of origin of most deep intracerebral hemorrhages. The penetrating arteries, because they arise directly from the major cerebral arteries, are exposed to high intraluminal pressure. This high intraluminal pressure, which is especially high in hypertensive persons, predisposes to fibrinoid degeneration and microaneurysm formation in the penetrating vessels and so to deep intracerebral hemorrhage.

Cortical mantle lesions are typically due to occlusive lesions, particularly embolus, to the major intracerebral arteries and their branches. These vessels, unlike those that supply the vascular centrencephalon, have a rich anastomosis. They are less prone to in situ thrombosis than the penetrating vessels. The presence of multiple infarcts scattered throughout the brain also suggests an embolic etiology. A hemorrhagic infarction also indicates a likely embolic etiology, as demonstrated by one study in which up to 60 per cent of embolic infarcts became hemorrhagic within the first 4 weeks.[14] This increased tendency for hemorrhagic infarcts to be embolic in origin has been confirmed by others.[15] Hemorrhagic infarction, however, is nonspecific, because it is also seen in up to 40 per cent of thrombotic infarcts.[12] The presence of cortical mantle watershed infarcts is indicative of a prior episode of hypotension, of extracranial arterial occlusion, or of vasospasm as occurs in subarachnoid hemorrhage. Watershed infarcts occur in arterial boundary zones, between the main cerebral and cerebellar arterial territories. They may also occur in the boundary territory between the centrencephalic vessels and the rest of the brain. A further sign that helps to identify the cause of an ischemic stroke is that reported by Gacs and coworkers, which consists of seeing an intracranial artery with a high-density signal on plain CT, the density being higher than that seen in other visualized vessels. This is of value because it suggests that the artery is occluded by clot.[16]

Other Investigations

The use of further tests is guided by clinical findings. Tests that may be considered routine in all stroke patients include a complete blood count; a blood smear; erythrocyte sedimentation rate, partial thromboplastin time, prothrombin time; electrolytes, urea, creatinine, blood glucose, and chest roentgenography. Lipid levels should be checked in patients under 65 years of age. A history of chest pain or palpitations suggests a possible cardiac basis of a stroke and prompts the need for urgent electrocardiography. Indeed, electrocardiography should be performed routinely in all stroke patients because a stroke may be the only sign of cardiac disease.

Differential Diagnosis

Not all acute focal neurologic events are due to a stroke. Common causes of confusion include Todd's paralysis, structural brain lesions such as hemorrhage into a brain tumor, and metabolic disturbances such as hypoglycemia. Several other disorders may closely mimic a transient ischemic attack or a stroke (Table 118–1).

Partial seizure activity may be followed by weakness

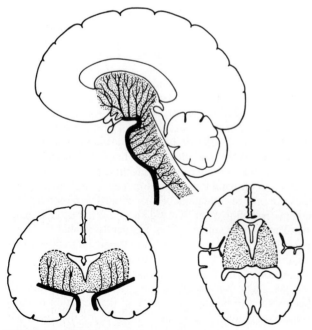

FIGURE 118–1. The vascular centrencephalon. (From Hachinski V, Norris JW: The Acute Stroke. Contemporary Neurology Series, vol. 27. Philadelphia, FA Davis, 1985.)

Table 118–1.   Causes of an Apparent Stroke-Like Deficit

Epilepsy
Intracranial space–occupying lesion
   Tumor
   Vascular malformation or aneurysm
   Subdural hematoma
   Epidural hematoma
Metabolic
   Hypoglycemia
   Hyperglycemia
   Hyponatremia
   Hypernatremia
   Uremia
   Hepatic encephalopathy
Migraine
Multiple sclerosis
Malignant hypertension
Hysteria

of the involved limb (Todd's paralysis). This is usually transient but may last for days.[17] Similarly, a partial seizure may be followed by transient aphasia or hemianopsia. The history, from the patient or a witness, is most helpful in establishing the diagnosis of a seizure-related transient focal neurologic disturbance. Electroencephalography may also be of value in Todd's paralysis because it may show transient focal slowing, which corresponds to a reduction in electrical activity of the epileptic cortex after the seizure discharge. An intracranial space–occupying lesion, such as an acute subdural or epidural hematoma or a tumor, may simulate an ischemic stroke. Neuroimaging is particularly helpful in this situation.

Metabolic disturbances may simulate or exaggerate a stroke. Metabolic disturbances of particular importance in this regard include hyper- and hypoglycemia, hyponatremia, and uremia. The stroke-like event may shift from side to side and tends to resolve and recur. Both the patient and the physician may fail to recognize hypoglycemia in the presence of a stroke-like episode if the patient has a concomitant autonomic neuropathy and so lacks the warning signs of hypoglycemia. Fortunately, hypoglycemia is usually associated with an altered level of consciousness, which should alert the physician to the possibility. A failure to recognize hypoglycemia can result in a permanent neurologic deficit, such as a hemiparesis or indeed dementia. Nonketotic hyperglycemia can also cause focal or diffuse neurologic signs. The hyperglycemia is typically accompanied by raised serum sodium and blood urea levels and increased serum osmolality. Dehydration is a useful clinical clue to the presence of hyperglycemia causing or aggravating a stroke-like episode and is usually obvious clinically. Ketotic hyperglycemia can accompany a cerebral infarct and should be thought of in any patient with a stroke who is drowsy or unconscious. For these reasons, hypo- and hyperglycemia should be ruled out by a blood glucose analysis early on in the investigation of all individuals with a stroke. Typical neurologic manifestations of hyponatremia include an alteration in mental status and seizures, but it can occasionally cause focal neurologic deficits. Advanced uremia is commonly associated with neurologic disturbance. However, the neurologic disturbances in uremia may also be due to an electrolyte disorder, hypertension, or

diabetes. Both uremic and hepatic encephalopathy may be associated with focal neurologic signs, but these are usually mild and are not persistent.

MANAGEMENT

Historical Aspects

Physicians have grappled with the management of stroke since at least the time of Hippocrates. Treatments have been many and varied. Indeed, at times the administered treatments were so bizarre that it is difficult to separate those used by the physician from those used by the quack. Hyperthermia appears to have been one of the earliest treatments for stroke. Aretaeus, a Roman, replaced hyperthermia with bloodletting as a treatment for stroke. Leeches, which have been used in medicine from at least 500 B.C. to the present, were later used as a means of facilitating phlebotomy in stroke.[18] Phlebotomy continued well into the 1850s as a treatment for stroke. At this time, phlebotomy was abandoned because anemia was recognized to be deleterious in the presence of a stroke and because a simple understanding of the circulatory system had taken root, which stressed the need for cerebral blood flow. The early 18th century saw claims by Domencio Mistichelli, a professor of medicine at the University of Pisa, that the application of a hot cautery to the foot would cure paralysis caused by a stroke, a practice that had its origin in 11th century Islamic Spain.[19] The 19th century also saw the introduction of other unproven treatments, such as the use of opium, hypnotics, and stimulants. One is reminded of the dictum *primum non nocere*—first do no harm. The late 19th and early 20th centuries established the place of rehabilitation in stroke management. Today, the greatest achievements in stroke management have come with improved understanding of the pathophysiology of stroke, accurate diagnosis, and controlled clinical trials of potential therapies.

General Management That Applies to All Stroke Patients

Assessment of Airway, Breathing, and Circulation

With stroke, as with all acute neurologic illnesses, a rapid but careful assessment should be made of the patient's *a*irway, *b*reathing, and *c*irculation. This assessment may be conveniently remembered as the "ABCs." It is of particular importance in all individuals who are helpless, have an impairment of their level of consciousness, or both. Early assessment of the adequacy of a patient's ability to protect the upper airway is essential if significant pulmonary complications are to be avoided. If the patient has impaired upper airway protective reflexes, the physician should ensure that the mouth and oropharynx are not obstructed by dentures and should clear away excessive secretions and, if present, vomit. Maintenance of an adequate circulation may require the administration of fluids if the effective circulating volume is low. Cardiac disorders, such as arrhythmias or myocardial infarction, require their own treatment.

A decision should be made early on to institute compassionate care for those patients who have suffered a massive ischemic stroke resulting in a clearly hopeless prognosis, particularly before life-supporting measures such as mechanical ventilation are instituted, because delaying this decision only prolongs suffering. Clinical features that suggest that the patient is likely to die include significant reduction in the level of consciousness, impaired central respiratory drive, decorticate posturing, and pupillary abnormalities such as a fixed, dilated pupil due to uncal herniation.[20]

Upper and Lower Respiratory Tract Difficulties

A patient's ability to maintain a clear upper airway may be assessed clinically by testing the gag and cough reflexes and the ability to swallow and by listening for dysarthria. The cough reflex can be evaluated by asking the patient to cough or, if the patient is intubated, by observing the cough reflex during suctioning. A useful way of measuring dysphagia is to observe the patient's ability to swallow his or her own saliva and, if this is accomplished, the ability to swallow a sip of water. In addition, it is worth asking about and observing for choking and apneic spells. Assessment of a patient's lower respiratory tract includes not only standard percussion and auscultation of the lungs but also observation of the respiratory rate and pattern. Rarely, the neural drive to the inspiratory and expiratory muscles is disrupted by a stroke. This occurs particularly with low brain stem strokes. Failure of the respiratory muscles typically causes tachypnea, tachycardia, and fluctuations in blood pressure.[21] Failure of the inspiratory muscles is also indicated by excessive use of the accessory muscles of respiration and by paradoxical motion of the chest wall and abdomen. Paradoxical respiratory motion, whereby the chest wall and abdomen move in opposite directions, indicates severe impairment of the inspiratory muscles.[22] Plum showed that simply by asking a patient to count slowly aloud to 20, at a rate of two numbers per second, one can get a rough idea of the patient's vital capacity and respiratory status.[23] If a patient can count only to 15, the vital capacity is approximately 1.5 L and the patient's respiratory status is probably borderline, indicating the need for quantitative assessment of respiratory function, such as measurement of the arterial blood gases and the vital capacity or respiratory pressures. In general, if there is significant impairment of the mechanisms that protect the upper airway or of ventilation, early elective intubation is preferred to emergency intubation if aspiration and hypoxia are to be avoided. Hypoxia is common after stroke,[24] especially in patients with preexisting pulmonary disease, and all patients with a significant stroke should have their arterial blood gases checked because hypoxia may aggravate the neurologic deficit.

Aspiration, atelectasis, and hypostatic pneumonia are common in stroke,[25] particularly in the presence of dysphagia, impaired gag and cough reflexes, or an altered level of consciousness. Inappropriate feeding techniques, such as too early introduction of solid feeds in dysphagic individuals, also predisposes to aspiration. The risk of aspiration should not be underestimated. Like deep venous thrombosis, aspiration is frequently silent. Whether silent or not, aspiration often results in pneumonia, a complication known to frequently cause death in acute stroke. Pneumonia is most often seen in the 2nd to 4th weeks after cerebral infarction.[26] As already stated, intubation and ventilation may be required for those who fail to protect their airways or have inadequate oxygenation. Occasionally, a tracheostomy is needed in patients who have damaged their lower brain stems or have severe supranuclear palsy that has caused prolonged impairment of their ability to protect the upper airway. Frequent chest physiotherapy, including incentive spirometry, and early mobilization aid in expectorating secretions and avoiding hypoventilation of basal alveoli and thus help to prevent hypostatic pneumonia.

Neurogenic pulmonary edema is a rare but well described complication of massive cerebral infarcts. It is characterized by hypoxia, tachypnea, and the presence of diffuse pulmonary infiltrates due to pulmonary edema. However, left ventricular failure and adult respiratory syndrome (shock lung) from sepsis are much commoner causes of severe hypoxia and pulmonary infiltrates in ischemic stroke. Whether raised intracranial pressure is a prerequisite for the formation of neurogenic pulmonary edema is uncertain.[27] Initially, there is a normal or slightly raised pulmonary capillary wedge pressure (less than 18 mmHg), best measured with a Swan-Ganz catheter.[28] The pulmonary edematous fluid is high in protein.[28] This is in contrast to left ventricular failure, from which it must be distinguished, in which there is a high pulmonary capillary wedge pressure (greater than 25 mmHg) and edematous fluid with a low protein content. Treatment is complex and requires cooperation between the neurointensivist and the anesthetist.

Cardiac Difficulties

The heart is frequently involved in stroke: it may either be the cause of the stroke or be affected by cerebral influences. Management of cardioembolic stroke is dealt with later in this chapter, in the section on anticoagulation in acute ischemic stroke. Impairment of cardiac function, such as cardiac failure, arrhythmias, or hypotension, may adversely affect outcome and require specific treatment. Ischemic stroke may cause electrocardiographic changes and myocardial cell injury, although these are most commonly seen in subarachnoid hemorrhage. Neurogenic heart disease can be divided into arrhythmias and repolarization changes, frequently suggestive of anterolateral or inferolateral subendocardial infarction or ischemia.[29]

Fluids

The administration of fluids in stroke patients requires caution. Oral fluid intake, if safe, is most desirable. If the gag and cough reflexes are adequate but the patient is dysphagic, fluids may be administered through a nasogastric tube or intravenously. In the recent past, it was believed that patients with a stroke should be fluid restricted so as to avoid raised intracranial pressure. In addition, persons with an acute stroke are frequently dehydrated on arrival at the hospital emergency department. However, evidence has suggested that fluid restriction may of itself be harmful, in that decreasing the intravascular volume may impair cerebral perfusion by causing hypotension[30] and increased blood viscosity[31] and so aggravate ischemic injury. There is also evidence that isotonic fluids do not aggravate raised intracranial pressure, provided that the serum sodium level is maintained within the normal range. Therefore, the fluid of choice in stroke is one that is isotonic, such as normal saline. A fluid intake-and-output chart is very helpful in ensuring adequacy of fluid intake. Usually, an intake of 2 L of fluid per day is adequate. Central venous pressure and pulmonary artery catheters may be of value in achieving optimal intravascular volume, without causing pulmonary edema, in those with significant cardiac dysfunction. Hyponatremia in the first few days after a stroke is most often due to the administration of excessive free water rather than to the syndrome of inappropriate antidiuretic hormone secretion. Hyperglycemia in acute stroke is associated with an adverse prognosis. Intravenous fluids containing glucose are thus probably best avoided. Insulin should be administered if hyperglycemia and ketosis occur with a stroke. Whether the transient hyperglycemia, unaccompanied by ketosis, that may occur with a stroke needs treatment is unknown. A focal neurologic deficit due to hypoglycemia should be rapidly treated with 50 ml of 50 per cent glucose followed by a 5 to 10 per cent dextrose infusion.

Nutrition

In general, it is best not to feed individuals for the first 24 to 48 hours if they have a progressive stroke, an impaired level of consciousness, or poor upper airway protection because they are at high risk for aspiration. Approximately 1000 calories per day is an adequate caloric intake in acute stroke. As with fluid intake, if the patient is dysphagic but has adequate cough and gag reflexes, liquidized food may be administered through a nasogastric tube; if this is not possible, nutrition must be intravenous. However, prolonged nasogastric feeding is often unnecessary. An absent gag reflex is not an absolute contraindication to normal oral feeding but does suggest the need for careful evaluation of the safety of oral feeding. This is best assessed by use of the modified barium swallow, which allows a fluoroscopic evaluation of the swallowing reflex. Supervised puréed meals may be started if the results of this test suggest that swallowing is adequate. Occasionally, a gastrostomy or preferably a jejunostomy tube is required if dysphagia is prolonged and there is inadequate upper airway protective mechanisms, as may occur with a brain stem infarct. The use of these feeding tubes is usually not considered until it is clear that a patient's swallowing difficulty is going to persist beyond the short term, which is usually considered to be 3 to 4 weeks from stroke onset.

Deep Venous Thrombosis and Pulmonary Embolism

Deep venous thrombosis (DVT) occurs in up to 50 per cent of patients with a stroke causing leg paralysis.[32] Pulmonary embolism (PE) may be the first sign of DVT because DVT is frequently subclinical. PE accounts for 13 per cent of stroke deaths. Anticoagulation with low-dose heparin, 5000 units twice daily, is of benefit in the prevention of DVT and is generally harmless.[33, 34] Other measures used in the prophylaxis of DVT include the use of elastic stockings, intermittent leg compression, and early mobilization. Anticoagulation should be instituted in the presence of either DVT or PE, provided that the ischemic stroke is not hemorrhagic. If the stroke is hemorrhagic, the use of an intracaval filter is indicated to prevent further PE.

Bed Sores and Contractures

Attention should be directed to pressure points, particularly in the unconscious patient or in the presence of a dense paralysis or limb anesthesia. Measures such as avoiding prolonged contact with wet or soiled bed clothing, turning the patient frequently, placing a pillow under the elbows and between the knees, and using sheepskin boots and a special mattress are frequently essential if bed sores are to be avoided. Both active and passive physiotherapy will prevent the development of contractures, a disability that can significantly hinder rehabilitation. Shoulder subluxation or dislocation is not an uncommon complication in stroke patients with upper limb involvement and may be due to improper handling of a patient or to improper positioning of the limb. Physiotherapy to the shoulder girdle, the use of an armpit roll and a shoulder sling, and awareness of the complication help to prevent this complication.

Bladder and Bowel Dysfunction

Urinary incontinence is common after a stroke. It is due to a combination of urinary retention, immobility, confusion, and dysphasia. Wet bed linen predisposes the patient to skin breakdown, besides being aesthetically unpleasing. Urinary incontinence should be treated with a Foley catheter in women but, if possible, with an external condom catheter in men. If a condom catheter is to be used, a check should be made with intermittent catheterization that there is not a large amount of postvoiding residual urine because this predisposes to urinary tract infection. If the postvoiding residual urine volume is significant (more than 100 ml), the use of an indwelling Foley catheter or intermittent catheterization is indicated. Indwelling urinary catheters predispose to urinary tract infection; therefore, they should not be used without adequate reason, and their use should be discontinued promptly once the patient has regained urinary continence. Indeed, patients frequently become continent within a few days of their stroke. Constipation and impaction easily occur in stroke patients, especially if they are drowsy or obtunded and have a poor fluid intake. Treatment includes a high-fiber diet and the administration of stool softeners. Rarely, a cecostomy is required for colonic pseudo-obstruction.

Seizures

Seizures are treated in the usual way, with anticonvulsants such as diazepam or lorazepam followed by phenytoin. Most seizures are partial motor seizures. Seizures are more common with embolic than with thrombotic cerebral infarcts.[35] Seizures may occur in the early or late phases following a stroke. A check should be made for other possible causative factors, such as hyponatremia. Seizures should be vigorously treated in acute ischemic stroke because uncontrolled seizure activity may increase neuronal damage.[36]

Depression

Depression is common after a stroke,[37] although precise determination of its incidence is difficult because these patients are acutely ill, patients with severe aphasia or confusion cannot be assessed, and there is a lack of data on the frequency of depression in an age-matched control population. Depression may significantly hinder rehabilitation. The depression tends to respond to the usual antidepressant medications, such as amitriptyline or nortriptyline.[38]

Fever

Hyperthermia, even if mild, has been shown in both animal experiments and humans to enhance ischemic brain damage.[39–41] Indeed, Hindfelt suggested that a rise in temperature of only 0.5°C was associated with a significantly worse stroke outcome and that the cause of the fever was of little or no relevance.[41] Therefore, the authors recommend that fever, even if mild, be treated vigorously in acute stroke. Fever may be due to stroke. However, the physician should check for other causes such as lung infection, urinary tract infection, and deep venous thrombosis. Pyrexia of unknown origin obligates a search for infective endocarditis, encephalitis, meningitis, brain abscess, temporal arteritis, and a connective tissue disease such as systemic lupus erythematosus or polyarteritis nodosa.

Specific Management in Ischemic Stroke

Treatment of Arterial Hypertension

Hypertension is very common after an acute ischemic stroke, having been noted by Wallace and Levy to affect 84 per cent of patients in the first 24 hours after admission (supine blood pressure greater than 150/90).[42] However, treatment of arterial hypertension in acute stroke is controversial. To understand this controversy, it is necessary first to understand the relationship of blood pressure (BP) and cerebral blood flow. Autoregulation has been defined by Johnson as "the intrinsic tendency of an organ to maintain constant blood flow despite changes in arterial perfusion pressure."[43] Autoregulation applies to the brain, heart, kidneys, liver, and skeletal muscles. The relationship between cerebral blood flow and mean arterial pressure in normotensive and hypertensive individuals is illustrated in Figure 118–2.[44] Normotensive and hypertensive persons maintain a relatively constant blood flow of about 50 to 60 ml/100 gm/min over a wide range of mean arterial BP (usually between 55 and 125 mmHg). However, in contrast to normtensive persons, hypertensive persons maintain a constant cerebral blood flow over a higher range of mean BP, as indicated by a shift to the right of the autoregulatory curve. This need of hypertensive persons for a higher range of mean arterial BP to maintain an adequate cerebral blood flow is thought to be due to the impaired ability of small arteries and arterioles to fully dilate, presumably because of structural changes in the vessel wall caused by the hypertension.[44–46] One consequence of this is that loss of cerebral autoregulation occurs at higher levels of mean arterial BP in hypertensive persons. Thus, the same mean arterial BP may be inadequate to maintain a constant cerebral blood flow in a hypertensive individual and yet be high enough in a normotensive individual to cause hypertensive encephalopathy. This situation is rendered even more complex in a patient with a stroke. A cerebral infarct can be considered as a central area of irreversibly damaged tissue surrounded by a zone of hypoperfusion in which neuronal function is impaired but potentially salvageable. This zone of hypoperfusion has been called the "ischemic penumbra."[47] The area of brain affected by a stroke, including the ischemic penumbra, is devoid of autoregulation, its blood flow being proportional to the BP.[48] Thus, antihypertensive therapy in acute stroke, particularly in those known to be previously

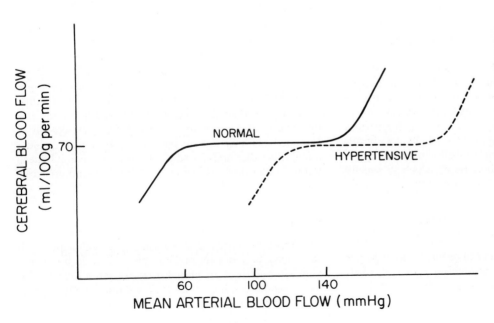

FIGURE 118–2.
Relationship between cerebral blood flow and mean arterial pressure in normotensive and hypertensive persons. Hypertensive persons have a shift to the right of their autoregulatory curve. (From Humphrey PRD: Clinical relevance of measurements of cerebral blood flow. Br J Hosp Med 26:235, 1981.)

hypertensive, by decreasing the BP and thus the blood flow to the ischemic penumbra, is associated with a significant risk of extending the area of infarction. Hypertension after stroke may also reflect an attempt by an ischemic brain stem to maintain blood flow to this vital area in the setting of raised intracranial pressure (ICP). Manipulation of BP in this setting may cause neurologic deterioration in the absence of treatment of raised ICP. Antihypertensive therapy may also cause "watershed" infarction by decreasing blood flow to the boundary zones between major arterial territories or facilitate thrombus formation by decreasing blood flow at the site of thrombus formation.[49–51] Other complications attributed to a too rapid reduction in BP include syncope, optic neuropathy, paraplegia, seizures, and death.[52–54]

Notwithstanding the previously mentioned potential hazards of antihypertensive therapy in stroke, it is evident that hypertension, particularly if marked, may be associated with a significant detrimental effect. Hypertension, if sufficiently high, may injure the blood-brain barrier and so cause vasogenic edema.[55] This tendency for hypertension to cause vasogenic edema may be especially likely in cerebral infarction, in which there is frequently damage to the blood-brain barrier.[56] Owing to loss of autoregulation, collateral blood flow to the ischemic penumbra depends on the difference between the local ICP and the local mean arterial pressure.[57] Hypertension-induced edema, by raising the pressure in an area of cerebral infarction, may interfere with collateral blood flow to the ischemic penumbra, thereby resulting in a larger stroke.[58–62] Hypertension may also be considered detrimental in acute ischemic stroke when it is associated with hypertensive encephalopathy or aortic dissection and when it causes end-organ failure, such as cardiac failure or myocardial ischemia.

Clearly, the need exists for a common ground in dealing with hypertension in acute ischemic infarction. Because several variables are involved in poststroke hypertension, each patient's situation should be considered separately. Factors to be considered include the level of BP, whether the patient was previously normo- or hypertensive, the area involved by the stroke, the cerebral perfusion pressure (mean arterial pressure minus ICP), and whether other end-organs are being actively damaged by the hypertension. It must also be recognized that two thirds of persons with hypertension after a stroke will be normotensive within 10 days of stroke onset.[42] In view of the frequent accounts of serious adverse effects resulting from a rapid reduction in BP, it is evident that if BP is to be lowered in acute stroke, it should in general be lowered slowly during the first 24 hours. Furthermore, BP should be lowered less in patients who are known to be hypertensive or who have signs of hypertension because of their need for a higher range of mean arterial pressure to maintain cerebral blood flow. Signs indicative of long-standing hypertension include retinal changes and evidence of left ventricular hypertrophy rather than admission BP. Cautious intervention is of the essence because even a small dose of antihypertensive medication can cause a precipitous drop in blood pressure.[51] One approach is to use a modified version of the treatment plan proposed by Brott and Reed (Table 118–2).[100] Intravenous antihypertensive therapy may be given if the systolic BP is greater than 230 mmHg or the diastolic BP is

Table 118–2. Treatment of Poststroke Hypertension

Treat if:
Diastolic BP > 120 mmHg and/or systolic BP > 230 mmHg with intravenous therapy, e.g.:
  Labetalol, 20 mg IV over 1–2 minutes; the labetalol dose may be repeated or doubled every 10–20 minutes to a maximal dose of 300 mg or until BP is satisfactory
  Propranolol in doses of 1 mg IV is an alternative
  With patients whose conditions are resistant or those who have contraindications to beta-blockade, such as patients with asthma, cardiac failure, and cardiac conduction defects, alternatives such as sodium nitroprusside, diazoxide, or nifedipine may be considered
  Lesser degrees of hypertension may be treated with oral antihypertensives, e.g., nifedipine, 10 mg 6–8 hourly or labetalol, 200–300 mg 8–12 hourly

In the first 24 hours after stroke onset, aim for:
In previously normotensive patients, a systolic BP of 160–170 mmHg and a diastolic BP of 95–100 mmHg
In previously hypertensive patients, a systolic BP of 180–185 mmHg and a diastolic BP of 105–110 mmHg

BP, blood pressure; IV, intravenously.

greater than 120 mmHg. Readings should be checked and therapy withheld until hypertension is confirmed on two occasions 5 minutes apart if the diastolic BP is greater than 140 mmHg, or 30 minutes apart if the diastolic BP is greater than 120 mmHg but less than 140 mmHg or the systolic BP is greater than 230 mmHg. Stroke-related hypertension is frequently associated with elevated catecholamine levels and high sympathetic nervous system activity, so it seems reasonable to use the combined alpha- and beta-adrenoreceptor antagonist labetalol or a beta-blocker such as propranolol.[63] Alternatives include sodium nitroprusside, nifedipine, and diazoxide. However, because of intense sympathetic activity, poststroke hypertension may be refractory to vasodilator therapy. Furthermore, vasodilator therapy may raise ICP by causing intracranial vasodilatation in the absence of a fall in systemic arterial BP. However, these agents frequently work well after initial sympathetic blockade. Drugs with sedative effects, such as clonidine and methyldopa, should be avoided because they make assessment of neurologic deterioration more difficult. Acute treatment of hypertension associated with an ischemic stroke also seems warranted when there is significant end-organ failure, such as fresh retinal hemorrhages, hypertensive encephalopathy, or cardiac failure, or with aortic dissection. If the patient's stroke progresses after BP reduction, antihypertensive therapy should be suspended, at least in the short term. In the long term, after discharge from the hospital, all hypertensive persons should be vigorously treated, although their BP can be reduced slowly over weeks. Monitoring of ICP may be indicated in poststroke patients in whom assessment of the optimal mean arterial pressure is complex because of the presence of probable raised ICP from a large stroke.

Treatment of Intracranial Hypertension in Acute Stroke

Cerebral edema has been reported to be the probable cause of neurologic deterioration in 7 to 20 per cent of patients with large hemispheric strokes.[64, 65] Cerebral edema following an ischemic stroke is usually at its maximum 2 to 5 days after stroke onset.[66] The physician dealing with a poststroke patient who has cerebral edema must determine if measures are needed to reduce ICP. Consideration of ICP requires that attention be directed toward the physiologic principles underlying ICP and the relationship of ICP to cerebral blood flow.

The skull is a rigid structure with a fixed volume. Its contents can be regarded as consisting of three compartments, namely neural tissue, cerebrospinal fluid, and cerebral blood, all of which are minimally compressible. The Monro-Kellie hypothesis defines the relationship of these three compartments with ICP as follows: because each compartment is minimally compressible and because the skull volume is fixed, an increase in any one compartment requires a compensatory decrease in the other compartments if ICP is not to rise.[67, 68] This hypothesis explains the rise in ICP that occurs in some individuals with a stroke and also provides a theoretical basis for therapeutic intervention for raised ICP. In acute cerebral infarction, the volume of the neural tissue may rise because of edema. This rise in the volume of the brain tends to cause a rise in ICP if the volumes of the cerebrospinal fluid and cerebral blood do not fall. Likewise, therapy aimed at treating raised ICP must result in a reduction in the volume of the cerebrospinal fluid, circulating blood, intracerebral free water, or cerebral tissue.

The importance of raised ICP in cerebral infarction can be further recognized on consideration of the interaction of ICP with cerebral perfusion pressure:

$$\text{Cerebral Perfusion Pressure} = \text{Mean Arterial BP} - \text{ICP}$$

A rise in ICP, by negating the difference between mean arterial pressure and ICP, will compromise the cerebral perfusion pressure and so result in global cerebral ischemia. This construct also emphasizes the complexities involved in manipulating BP in acute stroke. The normal ICP is generally less than 10 mmHg. The minimal cerebral perfusion pressure required to prevent ischemic cerebral injury in a normotensive person is approximately 50 mmHg.

The precise indications for ICP monitoring have not been established in acute ischemic stroke. This is particularly so because no clinical trial of raised ICP has been shown to improve outcome in ischemic stroke, even though persistently elevated ICP is associated with a poor outcome or death.[69] ICP monitoring does, however, aid in the neurologic examination of comatose patients with massive cerebral infarcts, and most clinicians agree that it helps determine the optimal treatment strategy for raised ICP and allows precise monitoring of the response to the various therapeutic interventions. In view of these issues, patient selection is clearly of prime importance. Factors to be considered before aggressive treatment of intracranial hypertension is started should include the age of the patient (younger stroke patients tend to have a better prognosis), the supposed outcome, the likely degree of intracranial hypertension (based on clinical assessment and neuroradiologic findings), and the patient's clinical course. Drowsiness is one of the earliest signs of possible raised ICP, although it may also be due to drugs, sepsis, or stroke

progression. In this respect, the Glasgow Coma Scale allows quantitative assessment of the level of consciousness and is the most useful clinical indicator of probable raised ICP. A score of less than 7 in adults and 5 in children, at least in head trauma, is usually indicative of significantly raised ICP. Other signs that may be seen early on in raised ICP include pupillary abnormalities, an altered respiratory pattern, and papilledema in adults and bulging of the fontanelles in infants. Unfortunately, these signs are of limited value because they do not always correlate with the presence of raised ICP and they frequently do not allow for easy, accurate continued assessment. However, deterioration in any of these signs is of prime importance, indicating the need for urgent investigation for raised ICP and management in an intensive care environment with appropriate monitoring techniques. Some contraindications to ICP monitoring include a bleeding disorder, scalp or calvarial sepsis, and lack of familiarity with the technique.[70]

Once it has been decided to monitor the ICP, the question arises as to the type of intracranial device best suited to each patient. The oldest and perhaps most useful monitor in this situation is the intraventricular catheter because it allows not only measurement of the ICP but also removal of small volumes of cerebrospinal fluid, which is a very effective method of reducing ICP. Intraventricular catheterization is effective in obstructive hydrocephalus associated with both supratentorial infarcts and cerebellar infarcts. With a large cerebral hemisphere infarct with raised ICP, the intraventricular catheter should be placed ipsilateral to the infarct in order to avoid subfalcial herniation. Further discussion of ICP monitoring devices is inappropriate here but may be found in the report of Lehman.[70]

Treatment of raised ICP of less than 15 mmHg usually consists of measures such as elevation of the head to 30 to 45 degrees, avoidance of neck vein compression, fluid restriction with maintainance of a normal serum sodium level, avoidance of hypotonic intravenous fluids, and treatment of any hyperthermia or significant systemic hypertension. ICP of greater than 15 mmHg generally requires more aggressive treatment, such as hyperventilation, avoidance of positive pressure ventilation, and administration of diuretics. More controversial treatments of raised ICP in ischemic stroke include corticosteroid use, barbiturate coma, and possibly even heroic measures such as surgical decompression, all of which first necessitate an urgent review of the patient's clinical condition, including a repeated CT brain scan, so as to determine if new complications have developed (Table 118–3).

Most persons with mild to moderate intracranial hypertension hyperventilate spontaneously. However, mechanical hyperventilation should be considered if there is evidence of significantly raised ICP, particularly if it is associated with impairment in the level of consciousness, and the person's arterial blood gas measurement fails to reveal hypocarbia. The ventilatory rate should be increased until the P_{CO_2} is 25 to 30 mmHg, while normal oxygenation and oxygen saturation of blood are maintained. The P_{CO_2} should not be lowered below 20 mmHg because it fails to lower the ICP further and may result in dangerous alkalosis. Hyperventilation should be continued until the raised ICP has resolved because premature discontinuation of hyperventilation may result in a rebound rise in the ICP. High

Table 118–3.   Treatment of Raised Intracranial Pressure

Elevate head 30–45 dgrees
Avoid compression of neck veins

Hyperventilate (PCO_2 of 25–30 mmHg)
Avoid positive pressure ventilation

Avoid hypotonic fluids; maintain normal serum sodium level
Mannitol 20%, 1 gm/kg IV, followed by 0.25–0.5 gm/kg $\geq$ 4
   hourly if ICP > 30 mmHg (serum osmolarity < 320 mOsm/L)
Furosemide, 0.5 mg/kg IV, followed by 0.25 mg/kg IV
   $\geq$ 1 hourly if ICP > 30 mmHg (serum osmolarity < 320
   mOsm/L)

Drainage of some cerebrospinal fluid with an intraventricular
   catheter
Surgical decompression

Dexamethasone, 10 mg IV, followed by 4–10 mg 4–6 hourly
Barbiturate coma

ICP, intracranial pressure; IV, intravenously.

levels of positive end-expiratory pressure should be avoided, although low levels of 5 to 10 mmHg can usually be tolerated with impunity. Cautious, gentle suctioning of the airway should be used because airway suctioning may be associated with a dangerous rise in the ICP.

It is usual to combine hyperventilation with diuretic therapy. Osmotic diuretics may be used alone or with loop diuretics. Loop diuretics may act synergistically with osmotic diuretics, and if given before mannitol, they help to prevent any rise in intravascular volume, and thus ICP caused by rapid infusion of osmotic diuretics, which tends to occur particularly in young children. The serum osmolarity should not be allowed to rise above 320 mOsm, and serum electrolytes should be kept in the normal range. All other intravenous fluids should be isotonic. In general, it is desirable to monitor continuously the central venous and pulmonary arterial pressure because these measures aid in fluid administration and maintenance of an optimal cardiac index.

Administration of corticosteroids is controversial in stroke, with several studies having failed to show a benefit.[71-73] Barbiturate coma may also be used to reduce raised ICP in stroke, but again this has not been shown to improve outcome. A ''burst-suppression'' pattern on electroencephalography indicates that an adequate dose of barbiturate is being administered. Likewise, surgical decompression is very rarely indicated in ischemic stroke because it has not been shown to improve outcome. However, decompression may be life saving in the case of cerebellar infarction with obstructive hydrocephalus, although ventricular catheterization frequently suffices. In addition, hemicraniectomy, in young patients with nondominant-hemisphere strokes at risk for fatal brain stem compression, may be life saving and permit a good outcome.[31]

Anticoagulation in Acute Ischemic Stroke

Anticoagulants are occasionally prescribed for stroke-in-progress or to prevent recurrent stroke. Typically, heparin is the initial therapy; it is later replaced by warfarin. However, the use of these agents is not without contro-

versy.[74] When anticoagulation is being considered in a patient with an ischemic stroke, it is of value to decide if the patient has a completed stroke or a stroke-in-progress and if the stroke arose due to a cardiac embolus.

A *completed stroke* is one that has reached its maximal severity. However, a physician seeing a patient with a stroke for the first time frequently has difficulty deciding if the stroke has reached its maximal severity because this decision is usually based on the presence of maximal deficit or on a period of observation during which the patient's condition has not deteriorated. Nevertheless, once it is evident that a person has a completed stroke, it now appears that anticoagulant therapy is of no benefit. Indeed, in several studies patients with a completed stroke who were anticoagulated fared worse.[75-78]

A *stroke-in-progress* is one in which the focal neurologic deficit increases, due to neurologic causes, in the acute stroke phase. Royden and Millikan reported progression of 26 per cent of carotid territory strokes and 54 per cent of vertebrobasilar strokes.[79] However, more recent reports have suggested that progression may be as frequent, if not more so, in the carotid system.[80, 81] In general, most carotid system strokes may progress for 48 hours and those in the vertebrobasilar system for 96 hours, although much longer times have occasionally been documented.[82] Several studies have attempted to attenuate ischemic neuronal damage in patients with stroke-in-progress with the use of anticoagulants. Four studies in the 1960s reported benefit from anticoagulation in stroke-in-progress. However, they had significant methodologic flaws in that only two trials were randomized, patient numbers were small, and all trials lacked CT brain imaging and so would have been unable to rule out pathologies that might simulate ischemic stroke, such as intracerebral hemorrhage.[83-87] A more recent study has failed to confirm a beneficial effect from anticoagulating persons with stroke-in-progress. Duke and associates performed a randomized, double-blind, placebo-controlled trial of intravenous heparin for the prevention of stroke progression in 225 patients with acute partial noncardioembolic stroke in either the carotid or the vertebrovasilar system who were treated within 48 hours of stroke onset. These investigators found no significant difference in progression between treated and control groups, with 16 per cent of treated patients having progression compared with 19 per cent of controls.[88] In this study, many patients were entered between 24 and 48 hours after stroke onset. Given that the time for therapeutic intervention in acute stroke is believed to be not more than 12 to 24 hours,[89-92] possibly many patients were treated too late after stroke onset, thus limiting the deductions that can be drawn from this study. Furthermore, because only 225 patients were enrolled in the study, it is still possible that a significant treatment benefit may have been missed. Thus, a type 2 error (false-negative) may have occurred.

Overall, there are few data to suggest a beneficial effect from anticoagulation for stroke-in-progress, but in view of the limitations of the previously performed studies, a beneficial effect has not been ruled out. This lack of data to support a beneficial effect of anticoagulation may also be partly explained by the recent understanding of the diverse pathogenesis of stroke-in-progress. Stroke-in-progress is now recognized to result not only from increasing stenosis of the involved artery or obstruction of collateral flow to the ischemic penumbra by extension of the thrombus but also from multiple other causes, such as local brain edema in the area of cerebral infarction or raised ICP, hemorrhage into an infarct, brain herniation, and systemic disturbances such as infection, hypoxia, hypotension, acid-base disturbances, electrolyte and water abnormalities, and heart, lung, kidney, or gastrointestinal complications.[82, 93] However, despite recognition of the multiple causes of stroke-in-progress, the difficulty remains that at the patient's bedside, it is often very difficult to ascertain which of these factors is responsible for the patient's decline.

A further limitation to the use of anticoagulation for stroke-in-progress is the potential for serious side effects. Spontaneous intracranial or systemic hemorrhage is the most serious complication. Haley and coworkers reported bleeding complications in 5 of 36 patients (13.9 per cent) with stroke-in-progress who were treated with heparin,[81] a rate that is similar to that reported in other series.[94, 95] Intracerebral hemorrhage is most likely to occur with embolic stroke, large cerebral infarcts, markedly elevated blood pressure, excessive anticoagulation, or heparin-induced thrombocytopenia.[95, 96] Thrombosis induced by heparin, which is not always associated with thrombocytopenia, is another worrisome complication, and although apparently rare, is being increasingly reported.[97-99] Relative or absolute contraindications to anticoagulation include marked hypertension, hemorrhagic cerebral infarction, bleeding diathesis, active peptic ulcer disease, absence of brain imaging, and septic brain embolus.

In view of the advantages and disadvantages of anticoagulation in stroke-in-progress, the prudent course in this situation may be first to eliminate those factors, other than thrombus enlargement, that may be responsible for the clinical deterioration, such as raised ICP, intracerebral hemorrhage, fever, and the other systemic disturbances previously outlined. The authors recommend anticoagulation only after elimination of as many of these factors as is possible and practical and provided that the stroke is less than 24 hours old, there is clear progression of the stroke, the stroke is submaximal in severity, and there is no contraindication to anticoagulation. Heparin should be adjusted to maintain the partial thromboplastin time between 1.5 and 2.0 times control. Warfarin should replace heparin after 48 hours of therapy.

Cardioembolic stroke is associated with a 10 to 20 per cent risk of stroke recurrence within 2 to 4 weeks of the first stroke.[100-104] Additionally, cardiac embolism is a frequent cause of ischemic stroke, accounting for 13 to 34 per cent of all ischemic strokes.[104, 105] Cardiac emboli to the brain lodge usually in branches of the middle cerebral artery, less often in the vertebrobasilar arterial tree, and only rarely in the anterior cerebral artery. Cardiac embolism should be suspected if there is a cardiac source of embolus and a lack of alternative sources of thromboembolism. Investigations that help to identify a cardiac source of embolus include echocardiography (both transthoracic and transesophageal) and electrocardiography. CT or MRI evidence of hemorrhagic transformation of a cerebral infarct is suggestive of an embolic stroke but not diagnostic.[15] Brain imaging that shows multiple widespread infarcts involving more than one vascular distribution is also helpful in that it

Table 118–4.   Cardiac Sources of Embolism

Arrhythmias
Particularly atrial fibrillation

Valvular Abnormalities
Rheumatic heart disease
Prosthetic valvular disease
Infective endocarditis
Marantic endocarditis
Mitral valve prolapse
Libman-Sacks endocarditis
Mitral annulus calcification

Heart Chamber or Wall Abnormalities
Dyskinesia of the wall
Aneurysm of the wall
Myocardial infarction with thrombus
Cardiomyopathy
Septal defects with right-to-left shunts
Atrial myxoma

suggests a cardiac source of the stroke. Cerebral angiography may also suggest embolic stroke if there is distal occlusion or if on repeated angiography the occlusion has disappeared. There are many potential sources of cardiac embolus, but the two commonest in the developed world are myocardial infarction and atrial fibrillation (Table 118–4).

Surprisingly, no clear consensus exists on the indications for anticoagulation following an acute cardioembolic stroke.[106] This is due to a lack of appropriate large, prospective, randomized, controlled studies. Some studies have suggested that anticoagulation may reduce the risk of stroke recurrence,[101, 103, 107, 108] but the risks entailed in immediate anticoagulation may outweigh the benefits. This danger of hemorrhagic conversion of an embolic infarct, with associated clinical worsening, is probably best managed by attempting to eliminate those at increased risk for hemorrhagic conversion. Patients with large, aseptic cardioembolic brain infarcts who are anticoagulated are more likely to have symptomatic hemorrhagic conversion of their infarct.[101, 102] It should also be borne in mind that caution is warranted when anticoagulation is being considered in patient's with a profound stroke because they may be more likely to have an earlier CT brain scan, which may not identify infarcts that are fated to undergo hemorrhagic conversion.[96] Therefore, in accordance with the Cerebral Embolism Study Group,[101, 102, 104] the authors recommend anticoagulating normotensive patients with a small to moderate-sized stroke at 24 hours and those with large infarcts at 5 to 7 days, provided there is no evidence of hemorrhagic conversion of the infarct on brain imaging. The general contraindications to anticoagulation, as outlined in the section on stroke-in-progress, must also be borne in mind. Heparin administration should be by constant infusion because bolus administration has been associated with a higher rate of hemorrhagic conversion.[109] A loading dose of heparin is probably best avoided, and once anticoagulation with warfarin has been established, heparin should be stopped. The authors recommend low-dose warfarin (prothrombin time of 1.2 to 1.5 times control) as this level of anticoagulation was as effective as higher levels in the Boston Area Trial and had a lower incidence of serious hemorrhage (1.9 per cent in the warfarin group and 1 per cent in the control group).[110] Long-term anticoagulation may be continued in those with persistence of moderate to high cardiac risk factors, such as atrial fibrillation with coexisting cardiovascular disease. Whether patients with low cardiac risk factors for stroke recurrence, such as mitral valve prolapse in a person younger than 60 years of age, should be continued on long-term anticoagulation or on antiplatelet therapy is controversial. In the case of hemorrhagic cardioembolic infarction, the authors recommend waiting 6 weeks before commencing anticoagulation because this time should allow the previously damaged vasculature to be replaced.[111] The authors do not recommend anticoagulation of septic cardioembolic infarcts because of the risk of mycotic aneurysm formation and subsequent rupture and because warfarin has not been shown to have a protective effect.[112, 113]

EXPERIMENTAL THERAPY IN ACUTE ISCHEMIC STROKE

Much has been published on the pathophysiology of ischemic stroke and the so-called therapeutic window, a period in the first few hours after a stroke during which therapy may limit infarct size. However, despite promising results in animal experiments, no treatment of acute focal ischemic injury is of proven value in humans. Studies that have aimed at attenuating ischemic neuronal injury can basically be divided into those that attempt to enhance blood flow to the ischemic area before the onset of neuronal death and those that attempt to modify the harmful biochemical changes that result in the death of ischemic neurons (Table 118–5).

Three therapies that have attempted to improve blood flow to the area of cerebral ischemia include thrombolysis, hemodilution, and induced hypertension. Thrombolytic therapy has been shown to reduce mortality in acute myocardial infarction by limiting infarct size through clot lysis and has been associated with a low incidence (1.14 per cent) of stroke.[114–117] Despite these encouraging results in myocardial infarction, early trials of thrombolysis in cerebral infarction were discouraging, with frequent death due to intracerebral hemorrhage.[118–120] No randomized trial has yet been performed with any thrombolytic agent. Hemodi-

Table 118–5. Experimental Therapies in Acute Stroke

Augment Blood Flow to Ischemic Penumbra
Thrombolysis
Hemodilution
Induced hypertension

Limit Damaging Biochemical Changes
Hypothermia
Barbiturates
Calcium antagonists
Excitatory neurotransmitter antagonists
Inhibit cerebral lactic acidosis
GM_1 gangliosides
Cytidine-5′-diphosphocholine
Naftidrofuryl
Antioxidants and free radical scavengers

lution has failed to show any benefit in several randomized studies.[121–123] Drug-induced hypertension has not reached acceptance because of lack of benefit and concerns about the induction of intracerebral hemorrhage or cardiac dysfunction.[124]

Developments in stroke pathophysiology have stressed the dangers of high concentrations of excitatory neurotransmitters, calcium, and free radicals in the ischemic penumbra. These developments have opened up a whole new strategy aimed at attenuating ischemic neuronal injury. If successful, they will make stroke a true medical emergency and will give renewed importance to the acute stroke unit. Of these therapies, mild hypothermia and the use of excitatory neurotransmitter antagonists are some of the most promising, but they await critical review.

REHABILITATION AFTER ISCHEMIC STROKE

Rehabilitation should start in earnest once the acute medical illness has past. Although there is no evidence that rehabilitation improves neuronal function, it should help to prevent complications related to the stroke and aid in the adaptation to various disabilities.[125] This should start with assessment of the patient's disabilities; most importantly, this includes assessment of the patient's ability to perform activities of daily living, but it also includes evaluation of higher cognitive functioning, communication, affect, and motor impairment. These clinical features can be used to predict prognosis, albeit crudely, and so help to better direct limited resources. Urinary incontinence may be especially useful in this regard because it is predictive of a poor outcome or death when it is present for more than 1 or 2 days after a stroke.[125] Patients should be mobilized early because this speeds recovery[126] and reduces the risk of complications such as pneumonia and pulmonary emboli. Psychological support should be provided for both the patient and the family, with due attention given to the possibility of poststroke depression. Good nursing care is of particular importance if complications such as bed sores, contractures, shoulder pain, and subluxation are to be avoided. Nursing assistance is also important in the provision of adequate fluid, nutrition, and psychological support and in the management of urinary and fecal incontinence. Physical, occupational, and speech therapists should be involved when appropriate. Aids should be provided if there is a need for and demonstrated benefit from such. Long-term follow-up and support are easily overlooked but are important if the patient is to maintain recovery.

PROPHYLAXIS IN ISCHEMIC CEREBROVASCULAR DISEASE

Surgical Intervention

Atherosclerotic stenosis of the bifurcation of the common carotid artery is by far the commonest cause of large vessel atherothrombotic stroke.[127] Patients who have suffered a nondisabling ischemic stroke or a transient ischemic episode should be investigated for carotid stenosis. Carotid endarterectomy should be recommended if cerebral angiography demonstrates a 70 to 99 per cent stenosis of the carotid artery appropriate to the side of the patient's symptoms and if the patient is medically fit for surgery, because it has been shown to be highly effective in preventing subsequent ipsilateral strokes, with an overall rate of stroke and death of only 2.1 per cent.[128, 129] The study of Eagle and Boucher provides useful information that helps to identify patients at high risk for cardiac complications with noncardiac surgery, such as carotid endarterectomy, who should be managed conservatively.[130]

Medical Intervention

Preventive medical therapy for atherothrombotic stroke consists of the use of aspirin, ticlopidine, and anticoagulants.

Antiplatelet Therapy

Several studies have demonstrated a beneficial effect of aspirin and ticlopidine in stroke prophylaxis following a transient ischemic attack or minor stroke.[131-135] However, studies are lacking on the benefits of immediate antiplatelet therapy in acute ischemic stroke.

Aspirin's proposed mechanism of action is inhibition of platelet aggregation and thus impairment of thrombus formation in the arterial tree. This inhibition of platelet aggregation is mainly achieved by interfering with the synthesis of cyclooxygenase in platelets, which prevents production of thromboxane, a compound that normally enhances platelet aggregation. However, in a probable dose-dependent reaction, it also inhibits production of prostacyclin by endothelial cells, which normally inhibits platelet aggregation. This double-sided effect of aspirin has resulted in confusion and in clinical trials aimed at stroke prevention in which the daily dose of aspirin administered has varied from 50 to 1500 mg. The Canadian trial demonstrated a clear benefit with 1300 mg/day of aspirin.[136] Aspirin conferred a risk reduction in vascular death or stroke of 31 per cent, although the benefit was restricted to men. This may be at least partly explained by the small number of women in the trial. This controversy about the benefit of aspirin in women continues, despite many other studies. The United Kingdom Transient Ischaemic Attack Aspirin Trial showed a benefit from aspirin, at a dose of 300 to 1200 mg/day.[137] Studies using lower doses of aspirin have also suggested a benefit after stroke or transient ischemic attack. The Swedish trial randomized 1360 patients with transient ischemic attack, retinal artery occlusion, or minor stroke (improvement to almost normal function within 3 weeks of the stroke) to receive 75 mg of aspirin daily or placebo.[132] The aspirin-treated patients had a 16 to 20 per cent reduction in the long-term risk of stroke, myocardial infarction, and death; both men and women benefited. This benefit is smaller than that with higher doses of aspirin. Therefore, low-dose aspirin may be beneficial, but the benefit may not be as great as that with high-dose aspirin. In view of this controversy, the authors recommend a dose of 1300 mg/day of enteric-coated aspirin, a dose with definite proven benefit, which can be adjusted downward if the patient develops side effects. It should be noted that despite several trials, antiplatelet drugs such as dipyridamole[138-141] and sulfinpyrazone[136] have no proven benefit.

Ticlopidine also acts by inhibiting platelet aggregation. It achieves this by inhibiting adenosine diphosphate activation of platelets and reducing the availability of fibrinogen receptors on the platelet membrane. It also prolongs the bleeding time two- to five-fold. It reaches its maximal activity within 3 to 5 days. Like aspirin, ticlopidine reduces mortality and nonfatal myocardial infarction in unstable angina pectoris.[142] Ticlopidine has been shown in several studies to be beneficial in stroke prevention, and it indeed appears to be superior to aspirin in stroke prophylaxis, particularly in women.[131, 134, 135] However, ticlopidine has a propensity for potentially serious side effects, such as neutropenia or thrombocytopenia.[131, 134, 135] Other frequent side effects are abdominal discomfort and diarrhea, which occasionally can be so severe as to necessitate discontinuation of the drug, at least temporarily, or dose reduction. Rash can also occur. Therefore, ticlopidine is best reserved for patients intolerant to aspirin or those who continue to have symptoms on aspirin. The authors consider a further stroke or transient ischemic episode a definite aspirin failure, provided the patient has been on aspirin for several days. Because approximately 0.5 per cent of patients get serious neutropenia, particularly in the early months of treatment, patients should have their full blood count checked every 2 weeks for the first 3 months. After this time, a check of the white blood cell count is not indicated unless the patient has an infection, such as a sore throat. Ticlopidine should not be combined with aspirin.

Anticoagulation Therapy

Indications for anticoagulation in stroke-in-progress and cardioembolic stroke have already been discussed. Anticoagulation with either heparin or warfarin for prevention of stroke is controversial.

Biller and coworkers performed the only randomized trial of *heparin* versus aspirin in patients who had developed transient ischemic attacks in the preceding 7 days.[143] One of 27 patients treated with heparin and 4 of 28 patients treated with aspirin developed a stroke (a nonsignificant difference). Therefore, insufficient data are available, particularly given the advent of ticlopidine, to allow heparin to be recommended for stroke prevention after transient ischemic attacks, even if crescendo in nature, or completed stroke.

Oral anticoagulants have been used to prevent stroke in transient ischemic attacks and ischemic stroke irrespective of the etiology of the attack. Their use in the prevention of stroke recurrence has been discussed. Further discussion is based on the use of oral anticoagulants as primary stroke prevention for those with heart disease and those with cerebrovascular disease.

Warfarin has long been accepted as being of value in stroke prevention in patients with rheumatic heart disease and atrial fibrillation. More recently, trials have looked at the value of warfarin in primary stroke prevention in nonrheumatic atrial fibrillation.[110, 144-146] They showed that warfarin was of benefit in patients with atrial fibrillation who had at least one of the following risk factors: history of hypertension, recent congestive cardiac failure, previous thromboembolic event, left ventricular dysfunction, and left atrial enlargement. As previously discussed, low-dose warfarin (prothrombin time of 1.2 to 1.5 times control) was shown to be as effective as higher levels.[110] How aspirin compares to warfarin in these circumstances is unknown, but it may suffice in patients with low-risk atrial fibrillation. Aspirin may be as effective as warfarin in stroke prevention in acute myocardial infarction.[147]

The value of warfarin in the primary prevention of noncardiogenic ischemic cerebrovascular attacks is questionable, and the authors do not recommend its routine use in view of the potential side effects.

Control of Risk Factors

No discussion on stroke prophylaxis would be complete without emphasizing the necessity of managing stroke risk factors. These risk factors include hypertension, atherosclerosis, heart disease, smoking, serum cholesterol, obesity, plasma fibrinogen, diabetes, oral contraceptive use, diet, and alcohol use.[148] Of these, control of hypertension and cessation of smoking are the most important. Even treatment of isolated systolic hypertension (160 mmHg or higher), over an average of 4.5 years in men and women 60 years of age or older, has been shown to reduce stroke by 36 per cent and to have other favorable cardiovascular effects.[149]

CONCLUSION

Ischemic cerebrovascular disease management has changed dramatically in recent years. With the advent of new experimental therapies, it is likely stroke will come to be regarded by the public as a brain attack, similar to a heart attack, requiring emergency treatment.

For the doctor caring for patients who have cerebrovascular disease, management must start with primary stroke prophylaxis. However, once an ischemic stroke has occurred, management should no longer be just "wait and see" but rather good medical management, proper handling of difficult problems such as hypertension in acute stroke, and early attention to secondary stroke prophylaxis.

References

1. Toole JF, Truscott BL, Anderson WW, et al: Medical and surgical management of stroke. Stroke 4:273, 1973.
2. Hachinski V, Norris JW: The Acute Stroke. Contemporary Neurology Series. Philadelphia, FA Davis, 1985, p 27.
3. Kase CS, Williams JP, Wyatt DA, et al: Lobar intracerebral hematomas. Clinical and CT analysis of 22 cases. Neurology 32:1146, 1982.
4. Kistler JP, Buonanno FS, De Witt LD, et al: Vertebral-basilar posterior cerebral territory stroke: Delineation by proton nuclear magnetic resonance imaging. Stroke 15:417, 1984.
5. Pykett IK, Buonanno FS, Brady RJ, et al: True three-dimensional nuclear magnetic resonance neuroimaging in ischemic stroke: Correlation of NMR, x-ray CT and pathology. Stroke 14:173, 1983.
6. Sipponen JT: Use of techniques: Visualization of brain infarction with nuclear magnetic resonance imaging. Neuroradiology 26:387, 1984.
7. Bryan RN, Willcott MR, Schneiders NJ, et al: Nuclear magnetic resonance evaluation of stroke: A preliminary report. Radiology 149:189, 1983.
8. Kertsez A, Black SE, Nicholson L, et al: The sensitivity and specificity of MRI in stroke. Neurology 37:1580, 1987.
9. Brant-Zawadzki M, Solomon M, Newton TH, et al: Basic principles of magnetic resonance imaging in cerebral ischemia and initial clinical experience. Neuroradiology 27:517, 1985.
10. Brant-Zawadzki M, Pereira B, Weistein P: MR imaging of acute experimental ischemia in cats. Annu J Neuroradiol 7:7, 1986.
11. Unger EC, Gado MH, Fulling KF, et al: Acute cerebral ischemia in monkeys: An experimental study using MR imaging. Radiology 162:789, 1987.
12. Mazziotta JC, Gilman S: Clinical Brain Imaging: Principles and Applications. Contemporary Neurology Series. Philadelphia, FA Davis, 1992, p 39.
13. Lenzi GL, Di Piero V, Zanette E, et al: How to assess acute cerebral ischemia. Cerebrovasc Brain Metab Rev 3(3):179, 1991.
14. Hornig CR, Dorndof W, Agnoli AL: Hemorrhagic cerebral infarction: A prospective study. Stroke 17:179, 1986.
15. Hakim AM, Ryder-Cooke A, Melanson D: Sequential computerized tomographic appearance of stroke. Stroke 14:893, 1983.
16. Gacs G, Fox AF, Barnett HJ, et al: CT visualization of intracranial arterial thromboembolism. Stroke 14:756, 1983.
17. Todd RB: Clinical Lectures on Paralysis, Diseases of the Brain and Other Afflictions of the Nervous System. London, John Churchill, 1854.
18. Kennedy JM: Blood-sucking leeches discovering new niches as a microsurgery aid. Los Angeles Times as reported in the Houston Chronicle, June 29, 1987.
19. Garrison FG: History of Neurology. Revised and enlarged by McHenry LC Jr. Springfield, IL, Charles C Thomas, 1969.
20. Marshall J, Thomas DJ: Vascular disease. *In* Asbury AK, McKhann GM, McDonald WI (eds): Diseases of the Nervous System, Clinical Neurobiology. Philadelphia, Ardmore Medical Books, 1986, p 1101.
21. Cohen CA: Clinical manifestations of inspiratory muscle fatigue. Am J Med 73:308, 1982.
22. Newsom Davis J, Goidman M, Loh L, et al: Diaphragmatic function and alveolar hypoventilation. Q J Med (New Series XLV) 177:87, 1976.
23. Plum F: *In* Bean WB (ed): Monographs in Medicine. Series 1. Baltimore, Williams & Wilkins, 1952, p 225.
24. Walshaw MJ, Pearson MG: Hypoxia in patients with acute hemiplegia. Br Med J 1:15, 1984.
25. Kaldor A, Berlin I: Pneumonia, stroke and laterality. Lancet 1:843, 1981.
26. Silver F, Norris JW, Lewis A, et al: Early mortality following stroke: A prospective review. Stroke 15:494, 1985.
27. Ducker TB: Increased intracranial pressure and pulmonary edema. I. Clinical study of 11 patients. J Neurosurg 28:112, 1986.
28. Malik AB: Mechanisms of neurogenic pulmonary edema. Circ Res 57:1, 1985.
29. Samuels MA: Cardiopulmonary aspects of neurological catastrophes. *In* Ropper AH, Kennedy SF (eds): Neurological and Neurosurgical Intensive Care. Rockville, MD, Aspen Publishers, 1988, p 99.
30. Wechsler LR: Therapy for acute ischemic stroke. *In* Ropper AH, Kennedy SF (eds): Neurological and Neurosurgical Intensive Care. Rockville, MD, Aspen Publishers, 1988, p 201.
31. Thomas DJ, du Boulay GH, Marshall J, et al: Cerebral blood flow in polycythemia. Lancet 2:161, 1977.
32. Warlow CP, Ogston D, Douglas AS: Deep vein thrombosis of the legs after strokes. 1. Incidence and predisposing factors. Br Med J 1:1178, 1976.
33. Gelmers HJ: Effects of low-dose subcutaneous heparin on occurrence of deep venous thrombosis in patients with ischemic stroke. Acta Neurol Scand 61(5):313, 1980.
34. McCarthy ST, Robertson D, Turner JJ, et al: Low-dose heparin as prophylaxis against deep-venous thrombosis after acute stroke. Lancet 2:800, 1977.
35. Black SE, Hachinski VC, Norris JW: Seizures after stroke [Abstract]. Can J Neurol Sci 9:291, 1982.
36. Collins RC, Olney JW, Lothman EW: Metabolic and pathologic consequences of focal seizures. *In* Ward AA Jr, Penry JK, Purpura D (eds): Epilepsy. New York, Raven Press, 1983, p 87.
37. Robinson RG, Starr LB, Price TR: A two year longitudinal study of

mood disorders following stroke. Prevalence and duration at six months' follow-up. Br J Psychiatry 44:256, 1984.

38. Lipsey RJ, Robinson RG, Pearlson GD, et al: Nortriptyline treatment of post-stroke depression: A double-blind study. Lancet 1:297, 1984.

39. Busto R, Dietrich WD, Globus MY, et al: Small difference in intraischemic brain temperature critically determine the extent of ischemic neuronal injury. J Cerebral Blood Flow Metab 7:729, 1987.

40. Minamisawa H, Smith M-J, Siesjö BK: The effect of mild hyperthermia and hypothermia on brain damage following 5, 10, and 15 minutes of forebrain ischemia. Ann Neurol 28:26, 1990.

41. Hindfelt B: The prognostic significance of subfebrility and fever in ischemic cerebral infarction. Acta Neurol Scand 53:72, 1976.

42. Wallace JD, Levy LL: Blood pressure after stroke. JAMA 246:2177, 1981.

43. Johnson PC: Review of previous studies and current theories of autoregulation. Circ Res 15(Suppl 1): 2, 1964.

44. Humphrey PRD: Clinical relevance of measurements of cerebral blood flow. Br J Hosp Med 26:233, 1981.

45. Strandgaard S: Autoregulation of cerebral blood flow in hypertensive patients. The modifying influence of prolonged antihypertensive treatment on the tolerance of acute, drug-induced hypotension. Circulation 53:720, 1976.

46. Strandgaard S: Autoregulation of cerebral circulation in hypertension. Acta Neurol Scand 57(Suppl 1):1, 1978.

47. Astrup J, Siesjo BK, Symon L: Thresholds in cerebral ischemia: The ischemic penumbra. Stroke 12:723, 1981.

48. Fieschi C, Angoli A, Battistini N, et al: Derangement of regional blood flow and of its regulatory mechanisms in acute cerebrovascular lesions. Neurology 18:1166, 1968.

49. Mustard JF, Rowsell HC: Factors influencing thrombus formation in vivo. Am J Med 33:621, 1962.

50. Graham DI: Ischemic brain damage of cerebral perfusion failure type after treatment of severe hypertension. Br Med J 4:739, 1975.

51. Britton M, de Faire U, Heimers C: Hazards of therapy for excessive hypertension in acute stroke. Acta Med Scand 297:253, 1980.

52. Hass JA, Streeten DHP, Kim RC, et al: Death from cerebral hypoperfusion during nitroprusside treatment of acute angiotensin-dependent hypertension. Am J Med 75:1071, 1983.

53. Hulse JA, Taylor DSI, Dillon MJ: Blindness and severe paraplegia in severe childhood hypertension. Lancet 2:553, 1979.

54. Ledingham JGG, Rajagopalan B: Cerebral complications in the treatment of accelerated hypertension. Q J Med 48:25, 1979.

55. Lassen NA, Agnoli A: The upper limit of autoregulation of cerebral blood flow—On the pathogenesis of acute hypertensive encephalopathy. Scan J Clin Lab Invest 30:113, 1973.

56. Kogure K, Bustro R, Scheinberg P: The role of hydrostatic pressure in ischemic brain edema. Ann Neurol 9:273, 1981.

57. Meyer JS, Shimazu K, Fukuuchi Y, et al: Impaired neurogenic cerebrovasculature control and dysautoregulation after stroke. Stroke 4:169, 1973.

58. O'Brien MD: Ischemic cerebral edema: A review. Stroke 10:623, 1979.

59. Katzman R, Clasen R, Klatzo I, et al: Brain edema in stroke. Stroke 8:512, 1977.

60. Johansson B, Li CL, Olssen Y, et al: The effect of acute arterial hypertension on the blood brain barrier to protein tracers. Acta Neuropathol 16:117, 1970.

61. Matakas F, Waechter R, Eibs G: Relation between cerebral perfusion pressure and arterial pressure in cerebral edema. Lancet 1:684, 1972.

62. Johnston IH, Rowan JO, Park DM, et al: Raised intracranial pressure and cerebral blood flow. V. Effects of episodic intracranial pressure waves in primates. J Neurol Neurosurg Psychiatry 38:1076, 1975.

63. Myers MG, Norris JW, Hachinski VC, et al: Plasma noradrenaline in stroke. Stroke 12:200, 1981.

64. Ng LKY, Nimmannitya J: Massive cerebral infarction with severe brain swelling. Stroke 1:158, 1970.

65. Plum F: Brain swelling and edema in cerebral vascular disease. Res Publ Assoc Res Nerv Ment Dis 41:318, 1961.

66. Ropper AH, Shafran B: Brain edema after stroke. Arch Neurol 41:26, 1984.

67. Monro A: Observations on the Structure and Function of the Nervous System. London, Creech and Johnson, 1973.

68. Kellie G: An account of the appearances observed in the dissection of the three individuals presumed to have perished in the storm of the 3rd and whose bodies were discovered in the vicinity of Leith on the morning of the 4th November 1821 with some reflections on the pathology of the brain. Trans Med Chir Sci (Edinb) 1:84, 1824.

69. Ropper AH, Shafran B: Brain edema after stroke. Arch Neurol 41:26, 1984.

70. Lehman LB: Intracranial pressure monitoring and treatment: A contemporary view. Ann Emerg Med 19:295, 1990.

71. Mulley G, Wilcox RG, Mitchell JRA: Dexamethasone in acute stroke. Br Med J 2:994, 1978.

72. Tellez H, Bauer R: Dexamethasone as treatment in cerebrovascular diseases. 2. A controlled study in acute cerebral infarction. Stroke 4:547, 1973.

73. Norris JW: Steroid therapy in acute cerebral infarction. Arch Neurol 33:69, 1976.

74. Marsh EE, Adams HP, Biller J, et al: Use of antithrombotic drugs in the treatment of ischemic stroke: A survey of neurologists in practice in the United States. Neurology 39:1631, 1989.

75. Genton E, Barnett HJM, Fields WS, et al: Report of the Joint Committee for Stroke Resources. XIV. Cerebral ischemia: The role of thrombosis and antithrombotic therapy. Stroke 8:148, 1977.

76. Weksler BB, Lewin M: Anticoagulation in cerebral ischemia. Stroke 14:658, 1983.

77. Dyken ML: Anticoagulant and platelet-antiaggregating therapy in stroke and threatened stroke. Neurol Clin 1:223, 1983.

78. Miller VT, Hart RG: Heparin anticoagulation in acute brain ischemia. Stroke 19:403, 1988.

79. Royden JH, Millikan CH: Temporal profile (clinical course) of acute carotid system cerebral infarction. Stroke 7:64, 1976.

80. Dávalos A, Cendra E, Teruel J, et al: Deteriorating ischemic stroke: Risk factors and prognosis. Neurology 40:1865, 1990.

81. Haley EC, Kassell NF, Torner JC: Failure of heparin to prevent progression in progressing ischemic infarction. Stroke 19(1):10, 1988.

82. Gautier JC: Stroke-in-progression. Stroke 16(4):729, 1985.

83. Beyers JA, Easton JD: Therapy of ischemic cerebrovascular disease. Ann Intern Med 93:742, 1980.

84. Fisher CM: Anticoagulant therapy in cerebral thrombosis. Neurology (Minneap) 11:119, 1961.

85. Carter AB: Anticoagulant therapy in progressive stroke. Br Med J 2:70, 1961.

86. Baker RN, Broward JA, Fang HC, et al: Anticoagulant therapy in cerebral infarction. Neurology (Minneap) 12:823, 1962.

87. Millikan CH: Anticoagulant therapy in cerebrovascular disease. In Millikan CH, Siekert RG, Wisnant JP (eds): Cerebral Vascular Diseases. Fourth Princeton Conference. New York, Grune & Stratton, 1965, p 183.

88. Duke RJ, Bloch RF, Turpie AGG, et al: Intravenous heparin for the prevention of stroke progression in acute partial stroke: A randomized controlled trial. Ann Intern Med 105:825, 1986.

89. Sundt TM Jr, Grant WC, Garcia JH: Restoration of middle cerebral artery flow in experimental infarction. J Neurosurg 31:311, 1969.

90. Crowell RM, Olsson Y, Klatzo I, et al: Temporary occlusion of the middle cerebral artery in the monkey: Clinical and pathological observations. Stroke 1:439, 1970.

91. Heiss WD: Pathophysiology of ischemic stroke as determined by PET. Stroke 21(Suppl 1):2, 1990.

92. Wise RJS, Bernardi S, Frackowiak RSJ, et al: Serial observations on the pathophysiology of acute stroke. Brain 106:197, 1983.

93. Silver FL, Norris JW, Lewis AJ, et al: Early mortality following stroke: A prospective review. Stroke 15:492, 1984.

94. Putman SF, Adams HP: Usefulness of heparin in initial management of patients with recent transient ischemic attacks. Arch Neurol 42:960, 1985.

95. Ramirez-Lassepas M, Quinones MR: Heparin therapy for stroke: Hemorrhagic complications and risk factors for intracerebral hemorrhage. Neurology 34:114, 1984.

96. Cerebral Embolism Study Group: Cardioembolic stroke, early anticoagulation, and brain hemorrhage. Arch Intern Med 147:636, 1987.

97. Atkinson JLD, Sundt TM, Kazmier FJ, et al: Heparin-induced thrombocytopenia and thrombosis in ischemic stroke. Mayo Clin Proc 63:353, 1988.

98. Phelan BK: Heparin-associated thrombosis without thrombocytopenia. Ann Intern Med 99:637, 1983.

99. Arthur CK, Isbister JP, Aspery EM: The heparin induced thrombosis-thrombocytopenia syndrome (H.I.T.T.S): A review. Pathology 17:82, 1985.

100. Brott T, Reed RL: Intensive care for acute stroke in the community hospital setting. The first 24 hours. Stroke 20:694, 1989.
101. Cerebral Embolism Study Group: Immediate anticoagulation of embolic stroke: A randomized trial. Stroke 14:668, 1983.
102. Cerebral Embolism Study Group: Immediate anticoagulation of embolic stroke: Brain hemorrhage and management options. Stroke 15:779, 1984.
103. Hart RG, Coull BM, Hart D: Early recurrent embolism associated with nonvalvular atrial fibrillation. Stroke 14(5):688, 1983.
104. Cerebral Embolism Task Force: Cardiogenic brain embolism: The second report of the Cerebral Embolism Task Force. Arch Neurol 46:727, 1989.
105. Stroke Prevention in Atrial Fibrillation Investigators: Preliminary report of the Stroke Prevention in Atrial Fibrillation Investigators: Preliminary report of the Stroke Prevention in Atrial Fibrillation Study. N Engl J Med 322:863, 1990.
106. Easton JD, Sherman DG: Management of cerebral embolism of cardiac origin. Stroke 2:433, 1980.
107. Koller RL: Recurrent embolic cerebral infarction and anticoagulation. Neurology 32:283, 1982.
108. Furlan AJ, Cavalier SJ, Hobbs RE, et al: Hemorrhage and anticoagulation after nonseptic embolic brain infarction. Neurology 32:280, 1982.
109. Calandre L, Ortego JF, Berbejo F, et al: Cerebral embolism and anticoagulation. Arch Neurol 41:1152, 1984.
110. Boston Area Anticoagulation Trial for Atrial Fibrillation Investigators: The effect of low-dose warfarin on the risk of stroke in patients with non-rheumatic atrial fibrillation. N Engl J Med 323:1505, 1990.
111. Yatsu FM, Hart RG, Mohr JP, et al: Anticoagulation of embolic stroke of cardiac origin: An update. Neurology 38:314, 1988.
112. Paschalis C, Pugsley W, John R, et al: Rate of cerebral embolic events in relation to antibiotic and anticoagulant therapy in patients with bacterial endocarditis. Eur Neurol 30:87, 1990.
113. Davenport J, Hart RG: Prosthetic valve endocarditis 1976–1987. Antibiotics, anticoagulation and stroke. Stroke 21:993, 1990.
114. Gruppo Italiano per lo Studio della nell'Infarto Miocardico (GISSI): Effectiveness of intravenous thrombolytic treatment in acute myocardial infarction. Lancet 1:397, 1986.
115. ISIS-2 (Second International Study of Infarct Survival) Collaborative Group: Randomised trial of intravenous streptokinase, oral aspirin, both, or neither among 17187 cases of suspected acute myocardial infarction: ISIS-2. Lancet 2:349, 1988.
116. AIMS Trial Study Group: Long-term effects of intravenous anistreplase in acute myocardial infarction: Final report of the AIMS study. Lancet 335:427, 1990.
117. Wilcox RG, von der Lippe G, Olsson CG, et al: Trials for tissue plasminogen activator for mortality reduction in acute myocardial infarction: Anglo-Scandinavian Study of Early Thrombolysis (ASSET). Lancet 2:525, 1988.
118. Meyer JS, Gilroy J, Barnhart MI, et al: Therapeutic thrombolysis in cerebral thromboembolism: Randomized evaluation of intravenous streptokinase. *In* Siekert RG, Whisnant JP (eds): Cerebral Vascular Diseases. New York, Grune & Stratton, 1963, p 200.
119. Fletcher AP, Alkjaersing N, Lew M: A pilot study of urokinase therapy in cerebral infarction. Stroke 7:135, 1976.
120. Hanaway J, Torack R, Fletcher AP, et al: Intracranial bleeding associated with urokinase therapy for acute ischemic hemispheral stroke. Stroke 7:143, 1976.
121. Scandinavian Stroke Study Group: Multicenter trial of hemodilution in acute ischemic stroke. I. Results in the total patient population. Stroke 18:691, 1987.
122. Italian Acute Stroke Study Group: Hemodilution in acute stroke: Result of the Italian Hemodilution Trial. Lancet 1:318, 1988.
123. Hemodilution in Stroke Study Group: Hypervolemic hemodilution treatment of acute stroke. Results of a randomized multicenter trial using pentastarch. Stroke 20:317, 1989.
124. Michenfelder JD, Milde JH: Failure of prolonged hypocapnia, hypothermia, or hypertension to favorably alter acute stroke in primates. Stroke 8:87, 1977.
125. Wade DT, Langton Hewer R: Rehabilitation after stroke. *In* Vinken PJ, Bruyn GW, Klawans HL (eds): Handbook of Clinical Neurology, Vascular Diseases. Part III. New York, Elsevier Science Publishing Company, 1989, p 233.
126. Hamrin E: Early activation in stroke: Does it make a difference? Scand J Rehabil Med 14:101, 1982.
127. Kistler JP, Buonanno FS, Gress DR: Carotid endarterectomy—Specific therapy based on pathophysiology. N Engl J Med 325:505, 1991.
128. North American Symptomatic Carotid Endarterectomy Trial Collaborators: Beneficial effect of carotid endarterectomy in symptomatic patients with high-grade carotid stenosis. N Engl J Med 325:445, 1991.
129. European Carotid Surgery Trialists' Collaborative Group: MRC European Carotid Surgery Trial: Interim results for symptomatic patients with severe (70–99%) or with mild (0–29%) carotid stenosis. Lancet 337:1235, 1991.
130. Eagle KA, Boucher CA: Cardiac risk of noncardiac surgery. N Engl J Med 321:1330, 1989.
131. Grotta JC, Norris JW, Kamm B, and the TASS Baseline and Angiographic Data Subgroup: Prevention of Stroke with ticlopidine: Who benefits most? Neurology 42:111, 1992.
132. The SALT Collaborative Group: Swedish Aspirin Low-Dose Trial (SALT) of 75 mg aspirin as secondary prophylaxis after cerebrovascular ischemic events. Lancet 338:1345, 1991.
133. Antiplatelet Trialists' collaboration. Secondary prevention of vascular death by prolonged antiplatelet treatment. Br Med J 296:320, 1988.
134. Gent M, Blakely JA, Easton JD, et al: The Canadian American Ticlopidine Study (CATS) in thromboembolic stroke. Lancet 1:1215, 1989.
135. Hass WK, Easton JD, Adams HP, et al: A randomized trial comparing ticlopidine hydrochloride with ASA for prevention of stroke in high-risk patients. N Engl J Med 321(8):501, 1989.
136. Canadian Cooperative Study Group: A randomized trial of aspirin and sulfinpyrazone in threatened stroke. N Engl J Med 299:53, 1987.
137. UK-TIA Study Group: United Kingdom Transient Ischaemic Attack (UK-TIA) Aspirin Trial: Interim results. Br Med J 296:316, 1988.
138. Acheson J, Danta G, Hutchinson EC: Controlled trial of dipyridamole in cerebral vascular disease. Br Med J 76:614, 1969.
139. Bousser MG, Eschwege E, Haguenau M, et al: "AICLA" controlled trial of aspirin and dipyridamole in the secondary prevention of atherothrombotic cerebral ischemia. Stroke 14:5, 1983.
140. American-Canadian Co-Operative Study Group: Persantine Aspirin Trial in Cerebral Ischemia. II. Endpoint results. Stroke 16:406, 1985.
141. Matias-Guiu J, Davalos A, Pico M, et al: Low-dose acetylsalicylic acid (ASA) plus dipyridamole versus dipyridamole alone in the prevention of stroke in patients with reversible ischemic attacks. Acta Neurol Scand 76:413, 1987.
142. Balsano F, Rizzon P, Violi F, et al: Antiplatelet treatment with ticlopidine in unstable angina. A controlled multicenter clinical trial. Circulation 82:17, 1990.
143. Biller J, Bruno A, Adams HP, et al: A randomized trial of aspirin or heparin in hospitalized patients with recent transient ischemic attacks. A pilot study. Stroke 20:441, 1989.
144. Stroke Prevention in Atrial Fibrillation Investigators: Preliminary report of the Stroke Prevention in Atrial Fibrillation Study. N Engl J Med 322:863, 1990.
145. Petersen P, Boysen G, Godtfredsen J, et al: The Copenhagen AFASAK Study. Placebo-controlled, randomised trial of warfarin and aspirin for prevention of thromboembolic complications in chronic atrial fibrillation. Lancet 28:175, 1989.
146. Stroke Prevention in Atrial Fibrillation Investigators: Stroke Prevention in Atrial Fibrillation Study: Final result. Circulation 84:527, 1991.
147. Kouvaras G, Chonopoulos G, Soufras G, et al: The effect of long-term antithrombotic treatment on left ventricular thrombi in patients after an acute myocardial infarction. Am Heart J 119:73, 1990.
148. Marmot MG, Poulter NR: Primary prevention of stroke. Lancet 339:344, 1992.
149. SHEP Cooperative Research Group: Prevention of stroke by antihypertensive drug treatment in older persons with isolated systolic hypertension. Final results of the Systolic Hypertension in the Elderly Program (SHEP). JAMA 265:3255, 1991.

119

Indications and Surgical Technique for Repair of Extracranial Occlusive Lesions

Wesley S. Moore, M.D.

• • •

The primary objective of surgery for extracranial lesions involving the cerebrovascular system is the prevention of stroke. Operation is justified to the extent that surgery alters the natural history of the disease and represents a safe and more effective therapeutic alternative to anticoagulant or antiplatelet medical management.

Although the symptomatic manifestations of various lesions can be frightening and certainly annoying, opinions differ as to whether transient ischemic attacks (TIAs) produce structural damage. For these reasons, prevention or relief of TIAs is viewed as an important secondary objective.

Selecting patients for operation requires the identification of specific patient subsets that are at high risk for stroke.

INDICATIONS FOR OPERATIVE REPAIR OF LESIONS OF THE EXTRACRANIAL ARTERIAL TREE

Indications for operation can be derived from three sources: retrospective reviews; prospective randomized trials; and position/consensus statements.

Indications Based on Retrospective Reviews

Reports that document the natural history of disease, usually subdivided by symptomatic status, are compared with reports concerning immediate and long-term results of operation. If operative results, including 30-day morbidity/mortality, and long-term reduction of monocular and neurologic symptoms, including stroke, are less with operation than with medical management, then operation can be justifiably indicated. The weakness of this approach includes the fact that the combinations of symptom, character of lesion, and operative risk are analyzed in their various permutations. The following is an analysis of operative indications by symptomatic status.

Transient Ischemic Attacks

Hemispheric or monocular TIAs have been the most readily accepted indications for carotid endarterectomy, when associated with an appropriate lesion.

Most of the early natural history studies were performed without characterization of the underlying lesion. In spite of that, it is safe to say that the stroke risk in the untreated patient with TIAs is approximately 10 per cent within the first year of symptom onset and continues at the rate of about 6 per cent per year, declining after 3 years.[24, 61] In contrast, the stroke risk in the hemisphere ipsilateral to carotid endarterectomy in the same patient group falls to less than 1 per cent per year.[4, 15, 21, 26, 28, 37, 56, 59] Providing that carotid endarterectomy, in an individual surgeon's experience, can be performed with a low stroke morbidity and mortality, TIAs become a compelling indication for operation.

Stroke With Recovery

Because many patients who suffer stroke are fortunate to have the event be only mildly disabling and often go on to complete or near-complete recovery, this group of patients needs to be carefully evaluated to determine the presence of a lesion that places such patients at risk for recurrent stroke. Studies that have evaluated the natural history of this group of patients suggests that the annual recurrent stroke rate is approximately 9 per cent per year.[2, 20, 52, 54] Antiplatelet drugs have been ineffective in reducing this recurrence rate.[30] On the other hand, carotid endarterectomy has successfully lowered the recurrent stroke rate to under 2 per cent per year.[40, 53, 57, 67]

This group of patients requires careful assessment to determine the presence of a continuing unstable lesion. For example, a patient who has suffered a left hemisphere stroke and has recovered and is found to have a high-grade stenosis involving the left internal carotid artery is at high risk for subsequent stroke in the distribution of that artery. On the other hand, if the same patient is found to have a total occlusion of that artery, carotid endarterectomy is no longer practically feasible.

Review of operative experience involving patients in this category reveals that the operative morbidity and mortality rates will be higher in this group of patients; therefore, they require special management, which will be described in the section under Operative Technique.

The judgment as to whether a patient who has made an incomplete recovery from a prior stroke is a candidate for carotid endarterectomy requires considerable experience. Generally speaking, the patient who has been devastated by a stroke is not a candidate for carotid endarterectomy. On the other hand, the patient who has had a mild stroke with complete or near-complete recovery would be an excellent candidate. The decision for operation in the in-between categories depends on a variety of factors, including how much neurologic function the patient has left to lose, his or her general functional status, and his or her life expectancy.

Stroke-in-Evolution

The patient with stroke-in-evolution represents the highest risk for either medical or surgical management. Appropriately timed and appropriately performed carotid endarterectomy in the patient who is carefully selected will yield a dramatic improvement over the natural history of the disease. On the other hand, the risk of mortality and the risk of a major stroke are high in this group of patients. Operation on these patients should be performed only by those teams that have had considerable experience in managing this category of patient and can accept the added risk in order to achieve an important benefit.[22, 70]

Global Ischemia

Patients who present with symptoms of global cerebral ischemia most often have these symptoms on the basis of decreased cardiac output secondary to arrhythmia or myocardial ischemia. There will be a few patients who have multiple lesions involving the extracranial arteries who will also manifest global ischemia and who will benefit from correction of one or more of these lesions.[33]

Subclavian Steal Syndrome

Although there are many patients who will demonstrate an anatomic subclavian steal syndrome by angiography, only a few will actually have symptoms, as a manifestation of extremity exercise ipsilateral to the side of subclavian artery stenosis or occlusion. Those patients who fall into the latter category or those who have a dominant vertebral artery on the side of the proximal subclavian lesion may well be candidates for reperfusion of the subclavian-vertebral system.[3]

Progressive Intellectual Dysfunction

Progressive intellectual dysfunction represents an extremely controversial indication for carotid endarterectomy. Nonetheless, there are many anecdotal cases that document the effect of carotid artery disease on intellectual function. This can come about either as a compromise in blood flow or as a summating effect of multiple emboli to centers of the brain responsible for intellectual function, independent of motor or sensory findings. In properly selected patients, intervention by carotid endarterectomy may improve intellectual function or prevent its further deterioration.

Asymptomatic Carotid Stenosis

Asymptomatic carotid stenosis is one of the most common indications for carotid endarterectomy. It is also probably the most controversial. In the past few years, several publications have provided surgeons with a considerable amount of natural history data that were not previously available. It is now safe to state that the risk of stroke in patients with a carotid artery stenosis in excess of 75 per cent is about 3 to 5 per cent per year of follow-up. The majority of these strokes will occur without warning symptoms.[8, 41] Several centers have recommended that patients with carotid stenoses in excess of 75 per cent, and who are otherwise in satisfactory medical condition and have a reasonable expectancy for longevity, undergo prophylactic operation, providing that the operation, in the hands of the individual surgeon, can be performed safely.[27, 42] It is recommended that an operative morbidity and mortality rate for this indication be less than 3 per cent.

The average late stroke rate in the distribution of the operated artery is 0.3 per cent per year.[74] We have recently reviewed our own 10-year experience at the University of California at Los Angeles. There were no late strokes in the distribution of the operated artery, with a mean follow-up of 54 months.[65]

Asymptomatic Ulceration

Patients who are found to have ulcerative lesions of the carotid artery, by angiography, have been shown to have an increased risk of subsequent stroke when treated expectantly. This risk rises progressively as the size and complexity of the ulceration increase.

Retrospective natural history studies have divided ulcers into three categories: A, B, and C.[47] Reports have attempted to quantitate the A, B, and C ulcers.[17] This can be done by looking at an unmagnified lateral projection of a carotid arteriogram. If the product of the length and depth of the ulcer is obtained, an A ulcer is one that is 10 mm^2 or less; a B ulcer is one that varies from 10 to 40 mm^2; and a C ulcer is one that exceeds 40 mm^2 and/or is cavernous or compound.

Retrospective natural history studies suggest that the stroke rate in the asymptomatic A ulcer is insignificant. The stroke rate in the asymptomatic B ulcer is approximately 4.5 per cent per year. The stroke rate in the asymptomatic C ulcer exceeds 7.5 per cent per year.[17] For this reason, we have recommended that when a C ulcer is identified on an arteriogram in a patient who is an acceptable surgical risk, prophylactic carotid endarterectomy be performed. The decision as to whether to operate on the patient with a B ulcer is dependent on the experience of the operating team and the individual conviction of the importance of this lesion. There is no place for surgery on the asymptomatic A ulcer.

Indications Based on Prospective Randomized Trials

Symptomatic Patients

Three prospective randomized trials have provided definitive data concerning indications for carotid endarterectomy.[64, 69, 73] Patients with hemispheric or monocular TIAs or prior mild stroke with a 70 per cent or greater stenosis have clear indications for carotid endarterectomy. Patients with crescendo TIAs in the presence of a 50 per cent or greater stenosis benefit from operation. Symptomatic patients with stenoses less than 30 per cent showed no benefit from operation in one study.[64] Symptomatic patients with stenoses ranging from 30 to 69 per cent are still being evaluated in two randomized trials.[64, 73]

Asymptomatic Patients

Two prospective randomized trials are completed and their results published. The Casanova Study Group concluded that there was no benefit to be derived from carotid endarterectomy in the asymptomatic patient.[63] However, the study was seriously flawed in design and methods of analysis. High-risk patients were excluded and 118 of 206 patients (57 per cent) randomized to medicine were systematically withdrawn as they became high-risk and were treated surgically. However, in an intent-to-treat analysis, they were counted as if they were treated medically. Therefore, no conclusions can be drawn from this study. The Veterans Affairs Cooperative Study has reported definitive results.[66] Carotid endarterectomy plus aspirin was more effective than aspirin alone in reducing the combined incidence of TIAs and stroke in patients with asymptomatic stenosis of 50 per cent or more, which was the study's hypothesis. The number of patients randomized was insufficient to make a definitive statement about stroke prevention alone, although the trend was clearly in favor of operation.

The Asymptomatic Carotid Atherosclerosis Study (ACAS) has just finished entering more than 1500 patients into a randomized protocol and is currently in the follow-up phase. As the largest study to date, it is anticipated that definitive results will be forthcoming.[62]

Consensus Statements Affecting Indications

Several organizations have published position papers or consensus statements based on the collective opinion of recognized experts. These include an ad hoc committee report from the Joint Council of the two national vascular societies[71] and the Rand Corporation.[68] Most recently, the American Heart Association convened a consensus conference and its report is currently in preparation. Table 119–1 summarizes the current indications for carotid endarterectomy and compares the recommendations from retrospective reviews, the Rand panel, the Joint Council position statement, and the prospective randomized trials.[72]

CONTRAINDICATIONS TO OPERATIVE REPAIR

An aggressive surgical approach is contraindicated if the general condition of the patient includes a serious illness that will materially shorten the normal life expectancy. In addition to this general reservation, there are patients with specific neurologic complications that prohibit operation or make its postponement advisable. These include the

Table 119–1. Current Indications for Carotid Endarterectomy

Patients	Source of Recommendation			
	Retrospective Data Analysis	*Rand Panel*	*Joint Council**	*Randomized Trials*
Symptomatic				
Single focal TIA (>70% stenosis)	Yes	Yes	Yes	Yes
Multiple focal TIAs with				
>70% stenosis	Yes	Yes	Yes	Yes
>50% stenosis with ulceration	Yes	Yes	Yes	NA
50% to 69% stenosis†	Yes	Yes	Yes	NA
30% to 49% stenosis†	Yes	Yes	Yes	NA
<30% stenosis with or without ulcer†	Yes	Yes	Yes	No
Previous stroke (mild), ipsilateral				
>70% stenosis	Yes	Yes	Yes	Yes
>50% with large ulcer	Yes	Yes	Yes	NA
30 to 69% with and without ulcer	Yes	Yes	Yes	NA
Evolving stroke				
>70% stenosis	Yes	Yes	Yes	NA
Global symptoms				
>70% carotid stenosis with uncorrectable vertebrobasilar disease	Yes	Yes	Yes	NA
Asymptomatic				
>70% stenosis with contralateral occlusion or high-grade stenosis	Yes	Yes	Yes	NA
>70% unilateral stenosis	Yes	No	Yes	NA
Large ulcer with >50% stenosis	Yes	No	NA	NA

Reprinted by permission of the Western Journal of Medicine, from Moore WS: Carotid endarterectomy for prevention of stroke. 1993, July, 159:37–43.
Key: *NA, not available; TIA, transient ischemic attack.*
*Joint Council of the Society for Vascular Surgery and the International Society for Cardiovascular Surgery (North American Chapter).
†Patients on aspirin therapy.

patient who presents acutely with a major stroke and has not yet begun to recover. A similar patient is one who has had a major stroke in the past and is so devastated by neurologic dysfunction or altered level of consciousness as to make operation inadvisable.

During early experience with carotid surgery, emergency operation for acute stroke was relatively common.[51] However, emergency thromboendarterectomy in an acutely occluded carotid artery frequently resulted in a conversion of an ischemic cerebral infarction to a hemorrhagic cerebral infarction, resulting in death. These findings were particularly dramatized in the first randomized cooperative study involving operation for carotid artery disease.[6] In addition, a premature surgical approach to a diseased but open internal carotid artery, prior to neurologic recovery, often resulted in an exacerbation of the neurologic deficit. Most surgical experience dictates that it is better to wait for the patient to reach a plateau of recovery before proceeding with elective repair.

OPERATIVE TECHNIQUE

Surgery of the Carotid Bifurcation

Anesthesia and Positioning of the Patient

Operations on the carotid bifurcation were originally, and are often still, performed with the patient under local or cervical block anesthesia. Local anesthesia has the advantage of allowing the surgeon to evaluate the patient's cerebral tolerance to trial carotid clamping. When the carotid clamp is temporarily applied, the patient is asked to speak and move the extremities of the appropriate side as evidence of adequate cerebral circulation to support brain function during the time required to remove the lesion. For this reason, a number of surgeons continue to advocate local anesthesia as the anesthetic technique of choice. There are disadvantages of local anesthesia, primarily related to patient anxiety. If the patient becomes restless or agitated, this will also disturb the surgical team. Finally, when a difficult lesion is encountered, extended operating time may exceed the forbearance of the average patient under local anesthesia.

General anesthesia has three major advantages. First, the anesthesiologist has better control over the patient's airway and ventilatory mechanics. Second, halogenated anesthetic agents have been shown to increase cerebral blood flow and, at the same time, decrease cerebral metabolic demand.[9] This combined effect may increase tolerance to temporary carotid artery clamping. Finally, the sleeping, anesthetized patient can undergo comfortably whatever exacting procedure is required without disturbing the operating field and the surgical team.

Positioning the patient is an important aspect of preparing for a carotid endarterectomy. The patient is placed supine on the operating table with the neck slightly hyperextended. This may be accomplished by placing a folded sheet under the shoulders. Excessive hypertension actually makes exposure more difficult by tightening the sternocleidomastoid muscle and by restricting the mobility of the common carotid artery and carotid bifurcation. Once the head is extended, it is then gently turned to the side opposite that of operation. Many patients in the age group appropriate for carotid artery disease may have a significant degree of cervical arthritis. Care must be taken to avoid neck injury with rotation. If the patient's blood pressure is stable, flexing the operating table and introducing a 10-degree reverse Trendelenburg inclination will bring the patient's neck into best perspective, reducing venous pressure and minimizing incisional bleeding (Fig. 119–1).

Two incisions have been employed for exposure of the carotid bifurcation. The first is a vertical incision parallel to the anterior border of the sternocleidomastoid muscle along a line connecting the sternal-clavicular junction with the mastoid process. Its exact length and placement along this imaginary line are decided by noting the position of the carotid bifurcation and the extent of the lesion on the lateral projection of the carotid arteriogram (Fig. 119–2). The incision is deepened through the platysmal layer in order to gain access to the investing fascia in the interval between the sternocleidomastoid muscle and the trachea. The author prefers this incision because it parallels the carotid artery. If the surgeon needs to gain additional exposure of the proximal or distal part of the vessel, simple extension of the incision is all that is required.

The second incision employed for exposure of the carotid bifurcation is oblique and is placed in one of the skin creases over the side of the neck (Fig. 119–3). It is deepened through the platysma, and then the subplatysmal space between the sternocleidomastoid muscle and the trachea is mobilized. The advantage of this incision is that it may produce a more cosmetically acceptable scar than that resulting from the vertical incision. The disadvantages are that it is necessary to raise skin flaps and it is more difficult to gain additional proximal or distal arterial exposure because the direction of the incision is oblique to the direction of the artery.

Following exposure, the investing fascia is incised along the anterior border of the sternocleidomastoid muscle, and the muscle is then mobilized to expose the underlying carotid sheath (Fig. 119–4). The latter is incised low on the neck, and the dissection is directed along the medial aspect of the internal jugular vein. The vein is retracted laterally to expose the common carotid artery (Fig. 119–5). The vagus nerve is usually the most posterior occupant of the carotid sheath, but occasionally it may spiral to take an anterior position at the point where the sheath is opened. This anomaly should be anticipated, and care should be taken to avoid injuring the nerve when the sheath is initially incised. The medial aspect of the jugular vein is exposed until the common facial vein is seen coursing obliquely across the common carotid artery and draining into the jugular vein. The common facial vein is a constant landmark for the carotid bifurcation and represents the venous analogue of the external carotid artery. The vein is mobilized, ligated, and divided (Fig. 119–6). Once the vein is divided, the carotid artery can be appropriately visualized. The common carotid artery is mobilized circumferentially and encircled with an umbilical tape. The periarterial dissection continues superiorly to expose the carotid bifurcation. As soon as the bifurcation is identified, 1 to 2 ml of 1 per cent lidocaine is injected into the tissues between the external and the internal carotid arteries to block the nerves

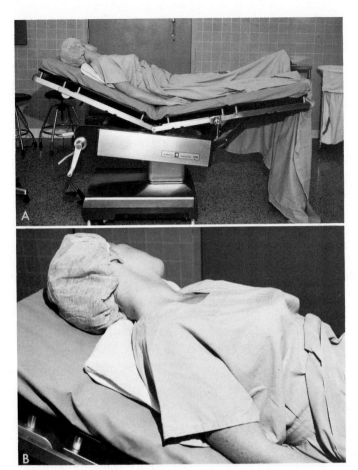

FIGURE 119–1.   *A,* The optimal operating table adjustment for carotid bifurcation endarterectomy. The table is flexed approximately 20 degrees in the reverse Trendelenburg position in order to bring the patient into a semirecumbent position. *B,* The neck is mildly hyperextended by introducing a folded sheet under the patient's shoulders. Finally, the patient's head is turned to the side opposite the operation. The neck on the side of operation is now exposed to best surgical advantage.

to the carotid body and carotid sinus. Failure to do this may permit a reflex vagal response that will result in a sinus bradycardia. Particular care must be taken during this part of the dissection to avoid undue manipulation or palpation of the carotid bifurcation and bulb of the internal carotid artery. Because this is the location of the atheromatous lesion and because the lesion may be quite friable or contain thrombotic or atheromatous debris, manipulation may cause dislodgment with subsequent cerebral embolization and stroke. The internal carotid artery is mobilized to a point well above the palpable atheromatous lesion where it

is unquestionably soft and not diseased (Fig. 119–7). The same is done for the external carotid artery, taking care not to injure the superior thyroid branch. In patients with a high carotid bifurcation or a lesion that goes relatively far up the internal carotid artery, additional exposure can be obtained by carefully dividing the tissues in the crotch formed by the internal and the external carotid arteries. This maneuver should be performed between clamps because, on occasion, the ascending pharyngeal artery can be located in this po-

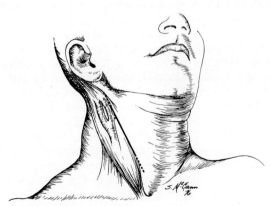

FIGURE 119–2.   Placement of a vertical incision along the anterior border of the sternocleidomastoid muscle in relationship to the underlying carotid artery bifurcation.

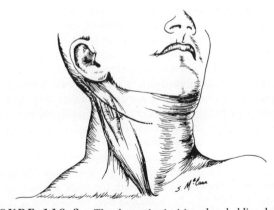

FIGURE 119–3.   The alternative incision placed obliquely in a skin crease over the carotid bifurcation. The dissection is carried down through the platysma, and subplatysmal flaps are developed in the superior and inferior aspects of the incision to convert the exposure of the carotid bifurcation to a vertical approach.

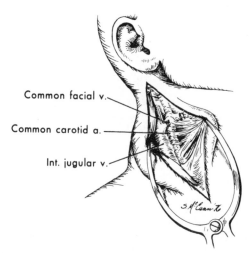

FIGURE 119–4. The relationship of the internal jugular vein and common carotid artery within the carotid sheath. The major tributary to the internal jugular vein at this level is the common facial vein. Division of the common facial vein consistently gives access to the carotid bifurcation.

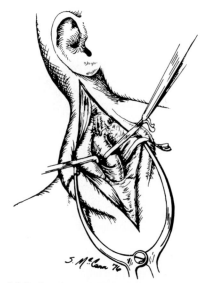

FIGURE 119–6. The mobilized common carotid artery with the surrounding umbilical tape. The dissection toward the internal and external carotid arteries has begun.

sition. The tissues in this crotch often act as a suspensory ligament of the carotid bifurcation and, once divided, will allow the bifurcation to drop down, making further mobilization of the internal carotid artery possible.

The twelfth cranial nerve should always be identified when the internal carotid artery is mobilized. It passes obliquely through the upper portion of the field, just superior to the bulb of the carotid artery, on its way to innervate the tongue (Fig. 119–8). Injury to this nerve causes a lateral deviation of the tongue toward the side of operation when the patient attempts to extrude the tongue. This also produces difficulty with initiation of swallowing. Should additional exposure of the internal carotid artery be necessary, mobilization and division of the posterior belly of the digastric muscle may be required (Fig. 119–9).

Determination of Cerebral Tolerance to Carotid Cross-Clamping

Once the carotid bifurcation is exposed, but before endarterectomy can be started, a decision must be made regarding the method of maintaining cerebral blood flow during carotid occlusion. Several options are available to the surgeon. The time-honored technique for determining the safety of temporary carotid clamping is trial occlusion under local anesthesia. The common, external, and internal carotid arteries are occluded for 3 minutes. During this time, the patient is asked to talk and move the arm and leg on the side affected by the carotid lesion. If there is no evidence of weakness or disturbance of consciousness, the intracranial circulation is judged to be adequate and operation can proceed without additional circulatory support. In the author's experience, adequate cerebral circulation is found in approximately 85 to 90 per cent of patients tested.

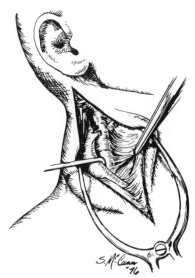

FIGURE 119–5. Following mobilization of its anteromedial aspect, the internal jugular vein is retracted laterally, giving clear exposure to the underlying common carotid artery.

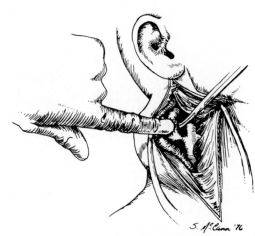

FIGURE 119–7. The internal carotid artery is mobilized well above the diseased intima. This fact is confirmed by careful palpation of the relatively normal internal carotid artery against the surface of the right-angle clamp.

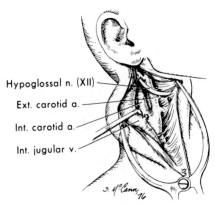

FIGURE 119-8. The relationship of the twelfth cranial nerve to the upper extent of the dissection of the carotid bifurcation.

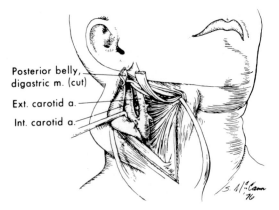

FIGURE 119-9. When the carotid bifurcation is high or when the lesion extends for an unusual distance up the internal carotid artery, additional distal exposure of the internal carotid artery can be obtained by division of the posterior belly of the digastric muscle.

In the 10 to 15 per cent in whom circulation is inadequate, an internal shunt must be employed. Local anesthesia and trial occlusion constitute a very satisfactory technique. However, if the surgeon prefers general anesthesia, an alternative method for determining the safety of temporary carotid occlusion must be employed. Many surgeons who use general anesthesia prefer to insert an internal shunt routinely. This does not identify selectively the individual patient who requires such circulatory support, but it has the advantage of "playing it safe" by providing additional flow to all patients.[58] The disadvantage of this technique is that the presence of an internal shunt makes the performance of endarterectomy somewhat more cumbersome. It also compromises precise visualization of distal end-point and introduces the potential complications inherent in the use of the shunt. These complications include scuffing or disruption of the distal intima during shunt insertion and the possible introduction of air or thrombotic emboli through the shunt when flow is started (Fig. 119–10). In a personal series, patients operated on without a shunt had a postoperative neurologic complication rate of 1.5 per cent, whereas those in whom a shunt was employed had a neurologic complication rate of 5 per cent. Because of this experience, it is the preference of the author and his colleagues to reserve the use of an internal shunt for those selected few patients with inadequate collateral circulation in whom it is clearly indicated and justified. The author and associates would prefer not to expose the remaining majority of patients (85 per cent in the author's series) to the small but finite increased risk of shunt use when there is no need to provide the additional cerebral blood flow.

The next question is how to identify the patient with inadequate collateral blood flow while employing general anesthesia. Several methods have been tried, such as the measurement of ipsilateral jugular venous oxygen tension.[38] The hypothesis on which this test is based states that patients with adequate collateral blood flow would have a higher oxygen tension in the venous blood draining from that segment than those patients with inadequate blood flow. This test was proved to be inexact because, owing to the anatomy of the venous-sinus system, the venous drainage from the brain is a mixture of blood from both hemispheres.[36] Another method suggested for determining the

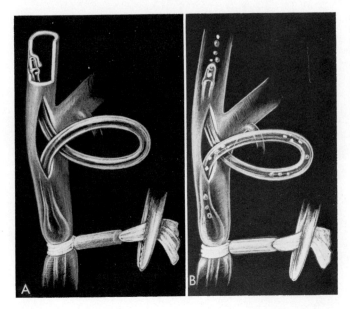

FIGURE 119-10. Two potential complications of internal shunt insertion. *A*, If the tip of the shunt is not carefully placed in the internal carotid artery, it is possible to scuff or elevate a flap of distal intima. *B*, Unless care is taken to evacuate air from the shunt or from the blind portion of the common carotid artery, it is possible to introduce air bubbles as cerebral emboli. Also, scuffing of an atherosclerotic plaque by the proximal portion of the shunt may scoop up atheromatous debris, which may also embolize to the distal cerebral circulation.

adequacy of flow is electroencephalographic monitoring during operation. Initial experience with this technique was disappointing, owing to the effect of general anesthesia on electroencephalographic tracing.[23] However, more recently, the technique was reintroduced and has now become a standard method by which adequacy of cerebral blood flow is monitored.[1, 59] This test is somewhat cumbersome because of the instrumentation involved as well as the expertise needed to interpret the electroencephalographic tracing. Nonetheless, several centers use it with enthusiasm and with excellent results.

Many surgeons have noted that patients who tolerate carotid cross-clamping also have excellent back-bleeding from the internal carotid artery through the arteriotomy when the clamps are released. Some investigators have used this observation to determine the adequacy of collateral blood flow and shunt requirement. This method can work in the hands of the experienced surgeon who has developed the ability to judge backflow; however, it is a qualitative rather than a quantitative observation, and as such cannot be taught.

Recognizing the validity of the observation of backflow, the author and his colleagues, in 1966, set about to develop a method of quantitation. The results of this clinical research have led to the introduction of the *internal carotid artery back pressure determination* as a means of estimating collateral cerebral blood flow. These investigators reasoned that a relationship existed between the intracranial collateral blood flow and perfusion pressure. Measurement of the back pressure down the proximally clamped internal carotid artery is an indirect measurement of the perfusion pressure that is present on the ipsilateral side of the circle of Willis (Fig. 119–11). The author and associates initially validated the technique by measuring back pressure in a series of 36 patients undergoing 48 carotid thromboendarterectomies under local anesthesia. The patients' conscious response to trial occlusion was correlated with the measured value of internal carotid artery back pressure. Forty-three of the 48 carotid arteries tested had back pressures that ranged from 25 to 88 mmHg. In each instance, the patient maintained full motor and intellectual function. Three patients were intolerant of trial occlusion, and their internal carotid artery back pressure ranged from 12 to 24 mmHg. These observations lead the investigators to conclude that 25 mmHg under ambient conditions of P_{CO_2} and the patient's normal blood pressure was the minimal safe level. All patients with back pressures below 25 mmHg required an internal shunt, and the carotid arteries of those with pressures above 25 mmHg could be occluded temporarily without additional cerebral circulatory support.[43] The author and colleagues subsequently validated these findings under general anesthesia but have also identified one group of patients who constitute an exception to the back pressure criteria—those who have had a previous cerebral infarction. The investigators noted an increased incidence of patients experiencing a temporary exacerbation of neurologic deficit when a shunt was not used. The author and associates postulate that patients with a previous cerebral infarction have a surrounding zone of relative ischemia that is being perfused through collateral channels, the so-called ischemic penumbra. These collateral channels have a variably higher resistance to flow; therefore, this group of patients will have

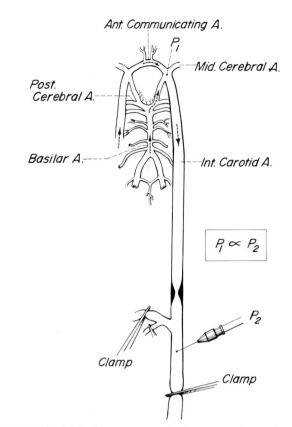

FIGURE 119–11. Pathways of collateral circulation about the circle of Willis. Perfusion pressure at middle cerebral artery (P_1). Internal carotid back pressure as measured at bifurcation (P_2). Being a closed, unbranched fluid system, P_2 is proportional to P_1. (From Moore WS, Hall AD: Carotid artery back pressure. Arch Surg 99:702–710, 1969. Copyright 1969, American Medical Association.)

a greater perfusion pressure requirement to maintain flow to the ischemic penumbra than those with normal circulatory patterns.[46] In patients with prior cerebral infarction, in the author's opinion, shunts should be routinely used regardless of the measured back pressure. The internal shunt is indicated for all patients with a prior history of cerebral infarction, as well as those with a back pressure less than 25 mmHg. Patients undergoing operations for TIAs or asymptomatic carotid stenosis in whom the back pressure is greater than 25 mmHg do not require a shunt. Using these criteria, the investigators then carried out a series of 172 carotid endarterectomies in 153 patients with a 0.6 per cent overall neurologic morbidity rate that included postoperative TIAs as well as infarction. In 74 per cent of cases, the operation can be performed without an internal shunt, whereas 26 per cent require internal shunt support.[34]

The technique for measuring internal carotid back pressure is quite simple and has been validated by others.[25, 32] After mobilizing the carotid bifurcation, 10,000 units of heparin is administered intravenously. A 22-gauge needle is bent at a 45-degree angle and is connected via rigid pressure tubing to a pressure transducer. The bent portion of the needle is then inserted into the common carotid artery so that it rests in a position that is axial to the artery and does not impinge on the posterior wall. Systemic arterial pressure is measured and compared with radial artery pressure. The common carotid artery, proximal to the needle, is then clamped. A second clamp is placed on the external carotid artery. This leaves the needle in continuity with a static column of blood that is open to the internal carotid artery. Even though the needle is placed proximal to the carotid stenosis, pressure will equalize on both sides of the carotid stenosis because there is no blood flow. The residual pressure or internal carotid artery back pressure is then recorded (Fig. 119–12).

In an effort to reduce the need for internal shunt further, investigation was conducted into possible methods of increasing cerebral blood flow during carotid surgery. The methods attempted include inducing arterial hypertension and manipulating arterial PCO_2.[19, 35, 60] Increasing arterial blood pressure by use of vasopressor drugs will increase perfusion pressure in collateral channels and presumably increase collateral blood flow. There is, however, a price to be paid for this benefit in the form of increasing afterload on the myocardium. Because most of these patients have associated coronary artery disease, the net result probably will be increased myocardial damage. The author and his colleagues would much prefer to use an internal shunt in a few more patients rather than run the risk of increasing incidence of myocardial infarction. Increasing PCO_2 (hypercapnia) has been shown to be an effective means of inducing cerebral vasodilatation.[31, 50] For this reason, many surgeons employ hypercapnia in order to provide a possible increase in cerebral blood flow during carotid occlusion. However, there is considerable evidence in the literature to suggest that the cerebral vasculature in areas of decreased cerebral perfusion is already maximally dilated. The use of

hypercapnia not only will fail to increase cerebral blood flow where it is needed, but also, in producing cerebral vasodilatation in the opposite hemisphere, will cause a redistribution of blood flow with a reduction of the collateral contribution from the normally perfused hemisphere. Because of this possibility, some investigators have suggested that the reverse approach be employed, i.e., a reduction of PCO_2 (hypocapnia), in order to cause cerebral vasoconstriction on the normally perfused side so that collateral redistribution will be from the normal to the ischemic side. The experimental data in the literature are contradictory, and the information they provide is inadequate to base a conclusion about the relative merits of hypocapnia versus hypercapnia. Because the back pressure data originally were obtained using normocapnia, the author and associates prefer to continue using normocapnia in order to avoid confusing the interpretation of back pressure values.

Internal Shunt Placement

A shunt is a valuable surgical adjunct that, properly used, can reduce the incidence of neurologic complications in those patients who depend on continued flow through the carotid artery that is undergoing repair. However, an improperly placed shunt can be the source of several complications that may lead to permanent neurologic damage. Once it has been decided to use an internal shunt, the operating surgeon should take a few minutes to describe the technique to the team and make certain that the proper shunt and appropriate instruments are immediately available in order to minimize ischemia time between carotid clamping and shunt placement. The author prefers to use the Javid shunt because of the appropriate diameter, length, and smooth finish of the ends to be inserted into the artery (Fig. 119–13). The author also prefers to hold the shunt in place with a modified Rumel tourniquet, fashioned by drawing the umbilical tape used to encircle the common and internal carotid arteries through a short segment of rubber tubing, and "snugging down" on the rubber tube clamp in order to draw the umbilical sling firmly around the internal shunt within the artery (Fig. 119–14). A longitudinal arteriotomy is begun on the posterior lateral part of the common carotid artery, well proximal to the lesion. The arteriotomy is extended through the lesion, into the carotid bulb, and beyond into the internal carotid artery as far as necessary to clear the obvious diseased intima. The distal end of the shunt is placed in the internal carotid artery, which is then allowed to back-bleed and fill the shunt with blood. The proximal part of the shunt is passed into the common carotid artery. This passage is made with the shunt actively back-bleeding in order to dissipate any air from the common carotid segment. Several insertions and withdrawals of the shunt may be required to flush all of the air out of the blind segment. The shunt is then clamped, the tourniquet about the shunt within the common carotid artery is tightened, and the clamp on the common carotid artery is released. At this point, the clamp on the shunt tubing is slowly opened and the translucent tubing is carefully observed for air bubbles and atheromatous debris. If no bubbles or debris is seen, the shunt is fully opened and the operation can proceed. The complications of an internal shunt include scuffing of the distal arterial intima, emboli-

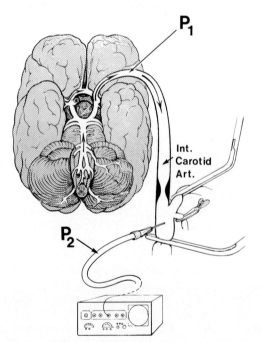

FIGURE 119–12. Relationship of middle cerebral to internal carotid perfusion pressure is represented. With common and external carotid arteries clamped, back pressure distal to internal carotid artery is in direct continuity with middle cerebral artery. Therefore, P_2 is essentially equal to P_1. (From Moore WS, Yee JM, Hall AD: Collateral cerebral blood pressure. An index of tolerance to temporary carotid occlusion. Arch Surg 106:520–523, 1973. Copyright 1973, American Medical Association.)

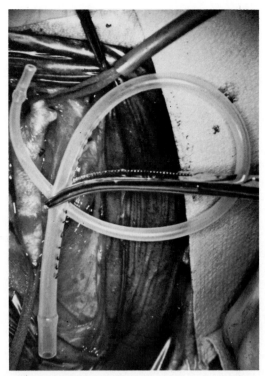

FIGURE 119–13.   A Javid shunt prior to placement. The author's group prefers this type of inlying shunt because its size is appropriate to provide maximal flow, and the proximal and distal diameter expansions reduce the possibility of inadvertent displacement while the shunt is functioning.

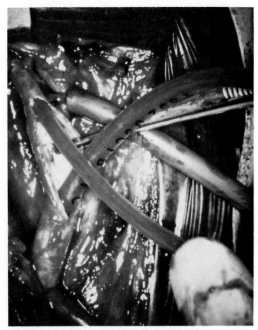

FIGURE 119–14.   A functioning shunt in place. The shunt is held in position by a proximal and distal sling tourniquet.

zation of atheromatous debris or air, and poor distal end-point management (Fig. 119–15).

Scuffing of the intima can be minimized by using the polyethylene shunt tubing with a smooth, rounded tip specifically manufactured for this purpose. Atheroma embolization can be avoided by making an arteriotomy large enough to prevent scooping up of atheromatous debris at the time the proximal portion of the shunt is inserted into

the common carotid artery. Air emboli can be prevented by careful evacuation of the air at the time of shunt insertion. Problems with distal end-point management can be reduced by opening the internal carotid artery as far as necessary to ensure direct visualization of a smooth end-point (Fig. 119–16). Another technique of shunting has been described in which the distal end of the shunt is placed in the external rather than the internal carotid artery.[39] This method will augment, to a variable degree, cerebral collateral blood flow through the external carotid artery–ophthalmic artery–internal carotid artery route, which has the advantage of keeping the shunt out of the internal carotid artery and reducing the problems with distal end-point management (Fig. 119–17).

FIGURE 119–15.   The three potential complications of an internal shunt. *A*, Scuffing of the distal intima. *B*, Embolization of air or atherothrombotic debris. *C*, Poor visualization of the distal end-point so that an intimal flap is left, producing the risk of subsequent thromboembolic complications.

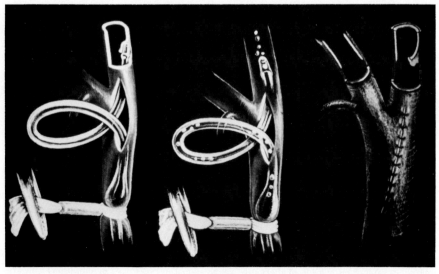

A   B   C

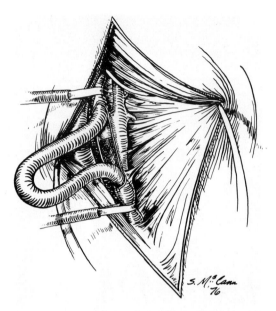

FIGURE 119–16.   Appearance of the carotid bifurcation with the shunt in place following bifurcation endarterectomy. The distal portion of the arteriotomy extends far enough up the internal carotid artery to permit direct visualization of the distal end-point.

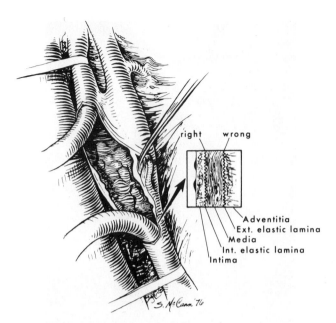

FIGURE 119–18.   The proper endarterectomy dissection plane. The optimal plane lies between the diseased intima and the media at the level of the internal elastic lamina.

Bifurcation Endarterectomy

One of the most critical details of endarterectomy is the selection of an appropriate endarterectomy plane. The optimal plane of dissection lies between the diseased intima and the circular fibers of the arterial media (Fig. 119–18). A carotid endarterectomy performed in this plane allows for a smooth distal tapering of end-point. It is very easy to get into the plane between the arterial media and the adventitia. Although this is an easily dissectible plane, obtaining a smooth tapering end-point is more difficult because of the increased thickness of the relatively normal intima and media at the termination point of dissection in the internal carotid artery. Because of this thickness, there is often a

shelf or a step-up in the internal carotid artery, which may require the use of sutures to tack down the end-point. The author believes that it is disadvantageous to use tacking sutures and would prefer to achieve a smooth, tapered end-point that occurs naturally within a proper dissection plane. Once the proper plane is established in the common carotid artery, dissection is continued with a dissector circumferentially about the artery. The circumferential dissection is completed with a right-angle clamp, making it possible to identify the same dissection plane on the opposite side of the artery (Fig. 119–19). The atheromatous lesion is then

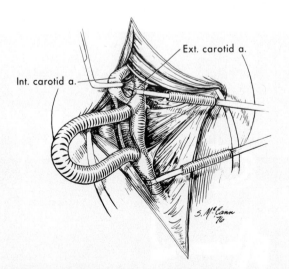

FIGURE 119–17.   Technique of placing the distal end of the shunt in the external carotid artery to provide free access to the internal carotid artery. This is an alternative way to minimize problems with end-point management.

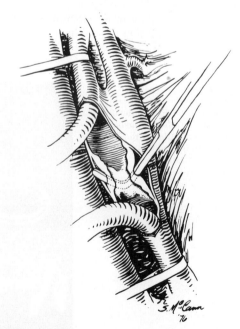

FIGURE 119–19.   Technique of completing circumferential mobilization of the atheromatous lesion by utilizing the closed jaws of a right-angle clamp.

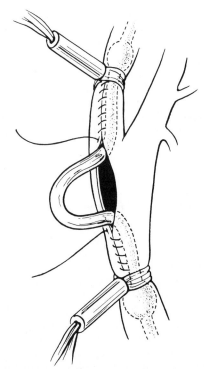

FIGURE 119-20. Partial closure of the arteriotomy with a suture beginning at each end. The arteriotomy is closed as far as the emergence of the internal shunt will permit.

sharply divided at its most proximal limit in the common carotid artery. The circumferential dissection is then carried to the external carotid artery, where a core of diseased intima is carefully developed by eversion of the artery and then gently removed. The final and most important part of the dissection can now proceed up the internal carotid artery. Care should be taken to advance equal distances circumferentially up the internal carotid artery. The specimen will suddenly become free at a point where the intima becomes relatively normal, leaving a smooth, tapering endpoint. The intimectomized surface of the carotid bifurcation is then generously irrigated with heparinized saline solution, and any loose bits of debris or tiny strips of media are carefully removed. The proximal and distal end-points in the internal and external carotid arteries are irrigated under direct vision in order to make certain that there are no floating intimal flaps. A free edge of intima that floats is gently picked at with the tip of a fine clamp. This part of the operation must not be hurried. If the patient has adequate collateral circulation, increased clamp time is not a problem. If collateral circulation is inadequate, a shunt should have been employed so that the operation can be done in a careful, unhurried fashion.

Once the endarterectomy is complete, the next step is closure. If a shunt was not employed, a careful primary closure can be performed with 6-0 polypropylene suture. Tiny, closely placed, continuous stitches will restore the normal contour of the artery without narrowing. If the arteriotomy was carried high up on a small or attenuated internal carotid artery, closure with a patch of vein or prosthetic material is desirable. In the author's experience, the need for a patch is unusual. However, reports concerning recurrent carotid stenosis suggest that the use of a patch in patients with small arteries, particularly women, will minimize both early and late recurrence of stenosis.[29] If an internal shunt was employed, the closure is somewhat encumbered and the technique must be modified. The author prefers to start a suture line at the distal portion of the arteriotomy on the internal carotid artery and carry it down to the common carotid artery. A second suture is then started proximally and is continued as far as the emergence of the plastic shunt will permit. The loop of the internal shunt will then emerge between the two sutures (Fig. 119-20). The shunt is then removed, each vessel is carefully flushed, and a partially occluding pediatric vascular clamp is applied to approximate the remaining open portion of the arteriotomy. Flow is restored initially to the external carotid artery in order to flush any possible residual air or debris into that vessel. Flow is then restored to the internal carotid artery, and final closure of the arteriotomy can be made by approximating the tissue held in place with the pediatric vascular clamp (Fig. 119-21).

Endarterectomy of an external carotid artery stenosis, in the presence of a totally occluded internal carotid artery, can be performed in the same manner as a carotid bifurcation endarterectomy.[10] In this instance, the arteriotomy extends from the common carotid artery onto the external carotid artery (Fig. 119-22). It may be more convenient to detach the occluded internal carotid artery, in which case the arteriotomy passes through the opening left by this detachment. This has the advantage of eliminating the stump of the internal carotid artery at the time of arteriotomy closure.

Several techniques are available for the correction of coiling, kinking, or tortuosity of the internal carotid artery.[49] These include resection of a segment of the internal carotid artery, reimplantation of the internal carotid artery in a more proximal location, and resection of a segment of the

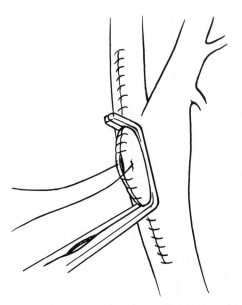

FIGURE 119-21. Application of a partially occluding pediatric vascular clamp permits restoration of blood flow to the internal and external carotid arteries while the final portion of the arteriotomy closure is completed after removal of the internal shunt.

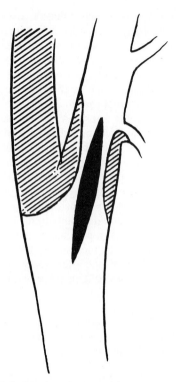

FIGURE 119–22. An endarterectomy of the external carotid artery can be carried out through an arteriotomy and begins on the common carotid artery and extends through the stenotic lesion in the external carotid artery. Because the internal carotid artery is totally occluded, the lesion in this vessel can be ignored.

common carotid artery (Fig. 119–23). If an arteriosclerotic lesion is present in the carotid bifurcation, a thromboendarterectomy must be performed in combination with one of the shortening procedures.

Verification of the Technical Result

In contrast to peripheral vascular surgery, the surgeon who performs carotid endarterectomy has one chance to get it right. For this reason, it is helpful to have some objective means of verifying the technical result of carotid endarterectomy. The most direct method is a completion angiogram. Other techniques include visualization with intraoperative B-mode ultrasound and waveform analysis with continuous Doppler ultrasound.

The technique of operative completion angiography is both simple and effective. A 20-gauge needle is bent at a 45-degree angle so as to allow the needle to be placed into the artery and for it to lie axial to the direction of the artery and minimize the risk of a subintimal injection. A 10-ml syringe is filled with angiographic contrast material and is connected to the needle with flexible tubing. A film is placed beneath the patient's head and neck either in a sterile cassette holder or slid into the film slot of the operating table. A portable x-ray machine can be used, and the 10 ml of contrast material is rapidly injected at the time the film is exposed. This will yield an excellent quality of image of the carotid bifurcation and the cervical carotid artery. The

anatomic result of operation can thus be verified. Any defect or intimal flap in the internal carotid artery can be corrected before a thromboembolic complication occurs. Likewise, if an unsatisfactory end-point of the external carotid artery appears, it is the author's recommendation this be corrected as well. If the angiographic appearance is satisfactory, the heparin can be reversed with protamine prior to closure. The author and colleagues calculate the dose of protamine as 1.25 mg of protamine per 100 units of residual heparin calculated on a heparin half-life of 1 hour.

Surgery of the Vertebral Artery

The clinical manifestations, indications, technique, and results of surgical repair of the vertebral artery are covered in detail in Chapter 120. For the sake of continuity, a brief discourse concerning the reconstruction of orificial lesions of the vertebral artery is presented in this section.

Most lesions involving the vertebral artery are really atheromatous plaques of the subclavian artery that encroach on the lumen of the vertebral artery origin. This area is best exposed through a supraclavicular incision centered over the clavicular head of the sternocleidomastoid muscle. The incision is deepened through the platysmal layer, and the clavicular head of the sternocleidomastoid muscle is divided. The scalene fat pad is dissected along its inferior margin and retracted superiorly together with the omohyoid muscle. The anterior scalene muscle is identified, and the phrenic nerve lies obliquely along this muscle. The phrenic nerve is mobilized, and the anterior scalene muscle is divided. The subclavian artery is now identified. The vessel is mobilized circumferentially, and an umbilical sling is applied. Mobilization of the subclavian artery continues proximally. At a point where the subclavian artery arches toward the mediastinum, the vertebral artery will be identified on the superior portion of the subclavian artery and the internal mammary artery identified on the inferior margin, opposite the takeoff of the vertebral artery. The vertebral artery branch can be mobilized carefully, and the proximal subclavian artery is dissected as far proximal as possible. The atherosclerotic plaque, encroaching on the vertebral artery orifice, can be handled in one of two ways. If the plaque primarily involves the orifice and does not extend into the artery itself, a most satisfactory technique is a transsubclavian artery endarterectomy. The subclavian artery is clamped proximally and distally, and a longitudinal incision is made along its anterior-inferior aspect approximately 3 mm from the vertebral artery. A thromboendarterectomy plane is established in the subclavian artery, and a circular intimal button is developed around the vertebral artery orifice (Fig. 119–24). The atheromatous lesion is then carefully cored out to achieve a clean distal end-point (Fig. 119–25). The area is flushed with saline solution, the artery is back-bled, and closure of the subclavian arterotomy is accomplished with a simple running suture of 6–0 polypropylene (Fig. 119–26). Following obtaining a completion angiogram, the wound is closed in layers. If the lesion extends up the vertebral artery for a short distance or if it was not possible to achieve a clean end-point with trans-

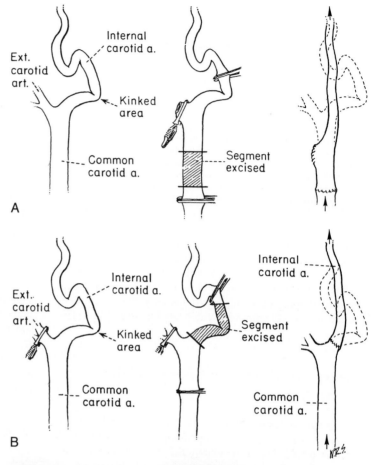

A

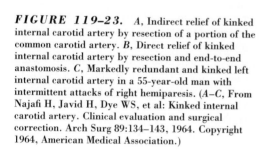

FIGURE 119–23. *A*, Indirect relief of kinked internal carotid artery by resection of a portion of the common carotid artery. *B*, Direct relief of kinked internal carotid artery by resection and end-to-end anastomosis. *C*, Markedly redundant and kinked left internal carotid artery in a 55-year-old man with intermittent attacks of right hemiparesis. (*A–C*, From Najafi H, Javid H, Dye WS, et al: Kinked internal carotid artery. Clinical evaluation and surgical correction. Arch Surg 89:134–143, 1964. Copyright 1964, American Medical Association.)

B

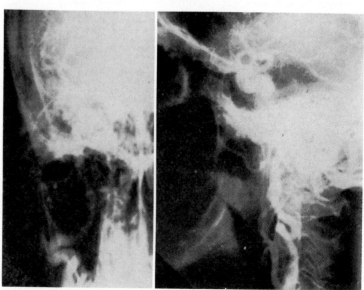

C

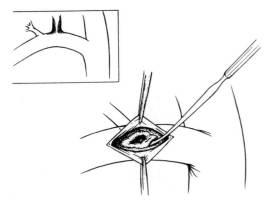

FIGURE 119–24. The trans-subclavian approach to vertebral artery endarterectomy. The inset demonstrates the vertebral artery stenosis in profile, emphasizing that the origin of the lesion is within the subclavian artery. A longitudinal arteriotomy is made on the posteroinferior aspect of the subclavian artery opposite the vertebral artery orifice. An endarterectomy is started at the base of the vertebral artery plaque within the subclavian artery.

subclavian endarterectomy, a direct vertebral thromboendarterectomy can be accomplished through a vertical arteriotomy extending from the subclavian artery through the vertebral artery orifice and up to a point distal to the atheromatous lesion. Following endarterectomy, the arteriotomy should be closed with vein patch angioplasty (Fig. 119–27).

Surgery of Occlusive Lesions of the Aortic Arch

Occlusive lesions at the level of the aortic arch account for fewer than 10 per cent of operations on the extracranial vascular tree. Early in the experience with cerebrovascular surgery, these lesions were repaired by a transthoracic or transmediastinal approach.[11, 14, 18] These approaches utilized either endarterectomy of the affected vessel or bypass graft. These operations were associated with significant morbidity and mortality rates. More recently, techniques have been described that enabled the surgeon to revascularize a branch of the aortic arch without entering either the thorax or the mediastinum to expose its proximal extent.[45]

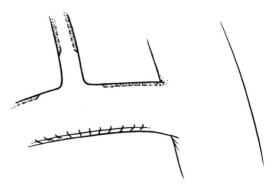

FIGURE 119–26. The final appearance following trans-subclavian endarterectomy leaving a widely patent vertebral artery and showing the closure of the subclavian arteriotomy.

Stenoses or Occlusion of the Subclavian Artery

Lesions of the subclavian artery can be repaired in one of four ways. The first is a bypass graft from the ipsilateral common carotid artery to the subclavian artery distal to the site of an occlusive lesion. The second, and most preferable, technique is transposition of the subclavian artery to the side of the common carotid artery. The third technique is a subcutaneous bypass graft extending from the opposite, unaffected axillary artery to the axillary artery distal to the subclavian lesion.[5, 12, 48] The fourth method employs a mediastinal approach to the subclavian artery, with repair by either thromboendarterectomy or bypass graft from the ascending aorta to a point distal to the obstructing lesion.

The carotid-subclavian bypass is best performed through a supraclavicular approach to the subclavian artery.

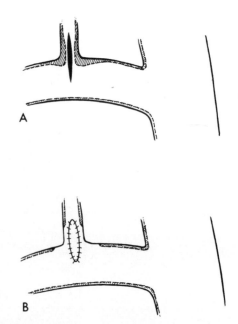

FIGURE 119–27. *A,* Technique of direct vertebral artery thromboendarterectomy through a vertical arteriotomy incision. *B,* Following endarterectomy, the arteriotomy in the vertebral artery is closed with a vein patch.

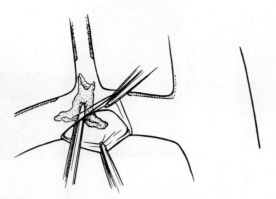

FIGURE 119–25. Separation of the atheromatous core from the distal intima within the vertebral artery and its dislocation into the subclavian artery as it is removed.

Once the subclavian artery is mobilized, the common carotid artery is easily exposed through the same incision. The sternocleidomastoid muscle is mobilized along its posterior extent in order to visualize the carotid sheath, which is opened, and the common carotid artery is mobilized for a short distance. An 8-mm Dacron graft or a 6-mm polytetrafluoroethylene (PTFE) graft can be used for bypass. The patient is systemically anticoagulated with 5000 units of heparin. The back pressure from the proximally clamped common carotid artery is measured. If the collateral back pressure or residual pressure is greater than 25 mmHg, a second distal clamp is applied to the common carotid artery. A longitudinal incision is made and an anastomosis is constructed between the end of the graft and the side of the common carotid artery. After appropriate flushing of the graft, a clamp is placed on the proximal portion of the graft and carotid artery blood flow is restored. The distal graft is then brought to the side of the subclavian artery at a convenient location and an end-to-side anastomosis is constructed in a similar manner (Fig. 119–28). The wound is closed in layers, and the operation is complete. If carotid back pressure is less than 25 mmHg, a carotid shunt can be used and subsequently withdrawn through the graft on completion of the anastomosis.

Subclavian artery transposition has three advantages. It is an autogenous reconstruction, has only one anastomosis, and carries the best long-term patency. The common carotid and subclavian arteries are exposed and mobilized as described previously. The subclavian artery must be mobilized well proximal to the vertebral and internal mammary arteries, which are both carefully preserved. The subclavian artery is then divided proximally and the proximal stump is oversewn. The distal end, proximal to the vertebral artery, is then sutured end-to-side to the common carotid artery.

The axillary-axillary bypass is an alternative procedure to the carotid-subclavian bypass. Both axillary arteries are exposed through infraclavicular incisions. The wound is deepened through the fascia. The sternal and clavicular portions of the pectoralis major muscle are split to expose the insertion of the pectoralis minor muscle. This muscle may be divided to provide additional access to the axillary artery (Fig. 119–29). A bypass graft is sutured end-to-side to the donor axillary artery, brought subcutaneously across the sternum, and anastomosed end-to-side to the recipient axillary artery (Fig. 119–30). The advantage of this technique over subclavian-carotid bypass is that temporary interruption of common carotid artery blood flow is avoided.

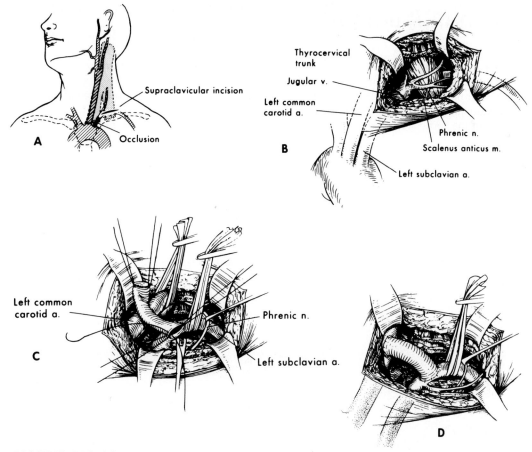

FIGURE 119–28. *A,* Placement of the supraclavicular incision. It is centered over the clavicular head of the sternocleidomastoid muscle. *B,* After division of the clavicular head of the sternocleidomastoid muscle, the relationships of the phrenic nerve, scalenus anticus, and subclavian artery are demonstrated. *C,* After mobilization of the carotid and subclavian arteries, preparation is made for a graft connection. *D,* Completion of the subclavian-carotid artery bypass is demonstrated and points out the close proximity of the two arteries and the short length of graft that is required. (*A–D,* From Moore WS, Malone JM, Goldstone J: Extrathoracic repair of branch occlusions of the aortic arch. Am J Surg 132:249, 1976.)

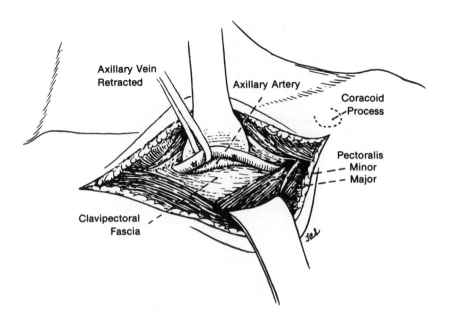

FIGURE 119–29. Surgical exposure of the axillary artery. (From Mozersky DJ, Sumner DS, Barnes RW, Strandness DE: Subclavian revascularization by means of a subcutaneous axillary-axillary graft. Arch Surg 106:20–23, 1973. Copyright 1973, American Medical Association.)

The disadvantages are that it requires two incisions, utilizes a longer graft, and is somewhat less cosmetically acceptable because the graft passes subcutaneously over the sternum.

Common Carotid Artery Occlusive Lesions

The primary cause for an occlusion of the common carotid artery is an atheromatous plaque involving its bifurcation with retrograde thrombosis. The thrombus will extend down to the innominate artery bifurcation on the right side, or to the level of the aortic arch on the left side. Some common carotid artery occlusions are due to lesions that begin at the level of the aortic arch and produce an antegrade thrombosis. Finally, there are a few occlusions of the common carotid artery that are due to lesions in its midportion with both antegrade and retrograde propagation (Fig. 119–31).

Occlusions produced by retrograde thrombosis can be treated by late retrograde thrombectomy in combination with bifurcation endarterectomy.[44] Occlusions produced by more proximal lesions can be bypassed with a subclavian-to-carotid bypass or a carotid-to-carotid bypass. The author approaches these lesions by initially exposing the carotid bifurcation in the usual manner. A bulky atheromatous

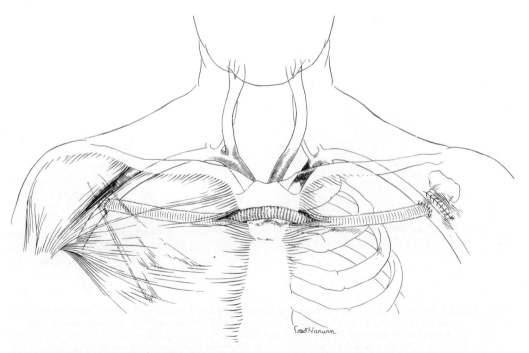

FIGURE 119–30. Diagrammatic representation of placement of the axillary-axillary graft. (From Snider RL, Porter JM, Eidemiller LR: Axillary-axillary artery bypass for the correction of subclavian artery occlusive disease. Ann Surg 180:888, 1974.)

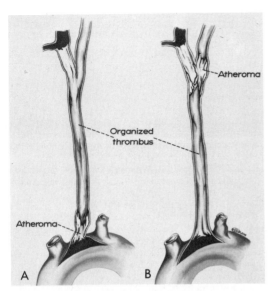

FIGURE 119–31. Occlusion of the common carotid artery can be produced by an atheromatous lesion at the origin of the common carotid artery *(A)* with antegrade thrombosis to involve the carotid bifurcation or, more commonly, by an atheromatous lesion at the common carotid bifurcation *(B)* with retrograde thrombosis down to the level of the aortic arch.

intact intima of the common carotid artery. The organized thrombotic cord can be mobilized circumferentially and then divided at a convenient portion within the arteriotomy. A smooth loop endarterectomy stripper can be used to develop the plane between thrombus and intima in a retrograde fashion. Usually, several gentle passes will free the thrombus down to the level of the aortic arch or innominate bifurcation and will allow the thrombotic cord to be pushed out of the arteriotomy by pulsatile blood flow. A clamp is then applied to the common carotid artery, once inflow is established. A standard bifurcation endarterectomy is then performed. If the internal carotid artery is occluded, it should be removed in order to avoid a blind stump that may serve as a source of further emboli. The arteriotomy is closed, and flow is restored to the external carotid artery (Fig. 119–32).

If the lesion that produced common carotid artery occlusion is located at a more proximal location or if the thrombotic cord cannot be removed by retrograde thrombectomy, a subclavian-carotid bypass can be performed in a manner identical to that described for a carotid-subclavian bypass. If a lesion is also present in the ipsilateral subclavian artery, a bypass graft in the opposite common carotid artery can be used for inflow.

plaque at the carotid bifurcation will confirm the mechanism of carotid artery occlusion to be retrograde clot propagation. The internal carotid artery may be kept open by flow between the internal and the external carotid arteries. If the internal carotid artery is occluded, one can depend on the external carotid artery to be patent beyond the superior thyroid branch. An arteriotomy should be made on the common carotid artery, proximal to the atheromatous lesion. By carefully opening the vessel, one can identify a plane that exists between the organized thrombus and the

Occlusive Lesions of the Innominate Artery

Lesions of the innominate artery are best treated directly through a median sternotomy. This can be achieved with either an open endarterectomy or a bypass graft from the ascending aorta to the innominate artery bifurcation.[13]

If the patient's general condition is so poor as to prohibit a median sternotomy, occlusive lesions of the innominate artery can be treated by a carotid-carotid bypass (Fig. 119–33). Alternative methods include left subclavian–to–right carotid bypass, subclavian-subclavian bypass, or axillary-axillary arterial bypass.

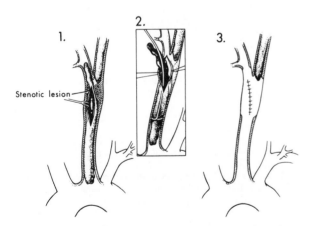

FIGURE 119–32. *Step 1*, An arteriotomy is made in the common carotid artery to begin separating the organized thrombus from the arterial wall. *Step 2*, A flexible wire loop stripper is passed over the organized thrombus in order to free its entire length. *Step 3*, After removal of the occlusive arteriosclerotic plaque at the carotid bifurcation, the outflow of the external carotid artery is restored and the arteriotomy is closed. (From Moore WS, Malone JM, Goldstone MD: Extrathoracic repair of branch occlusions of the aortic arch. Am J Surg 132:249, 1976.)

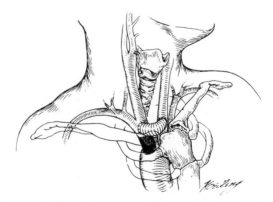

FIGURE 119–33. Bypass graft from the left carotid to the right carotid artery as a means of bypassing an innominate artery occlusion. (From Moore WS, Malone JM, Goldstone J: Extrathoracic repair of branch occlusions of the aortic arch. Am J Surg 132:249, 1976.)

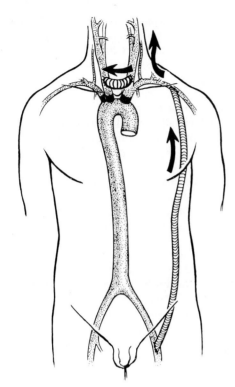

FIGURE 119–34. Artist's concept of subcutaneous bypass grafts from the right femoral to the right axillary arteries in combination with a graft from the right carotid to left carotid arteries. (From Moore WS, Malone JM, Goldstone J: Extrathoracic repair of branch occlusions of the aortic arch. Am J Surg 132:249, 1976.)

Occlusive Lesions of All Three Arch Vessels

It is rare for a patient to present with occlusive lesions involving all three major arch trunks. When this occurs, the patient is at high risk for major complications associated either with the natural history of the disease or with revascularization. The temptation to carry out a total revascularization at one operative procedure should be avoided. These patients have lost autoregulatory control of the cerebral circulation. A total revascularization places the patient at high risk for intracerebral hemorrhage as a result of hyperperfusion syndrome. In general, it is much better to stage the reconstruction of patients with this complex series of lesions, using either a direct or an extrathoracic approach. A direct approach would consist of an aortoinnominate bypass or innominate endarterectomy. This then establishes reperfusion of the right carotid and right subclavian systems. If subsequent revascularization is required, this can be achieved by various combinations of extrathoracic repair such as carotid-carotid bypass, or axillary-axillary bypass in combination with subclavian-carotid bypass.

If the patient is an unsuitable candidate for a mediastinal approach, revascularization can be carried out using a femoral-axillary bypass, providing there is an intact aortofemoral system.[45, 55] A subcutaneous bypass from the femoral artery to the right axillary artery will establish blood flow to the right vertebral and right carotid arteries through

retrograde perfusion. If necessary, a subsequent right carotid-to-left carotid artery bypass can be added to complete the extrathoracic revascularization of the arch vessels (Fig. 119–34).

References

1. Baker JD, Gluecklich B, Watson CW, et al: An evaluation of electroencephalographic monitoring for carotid study. Surgery 78:787, 1975.
2. Baker RN, Schwart WS, Ramseyer JC: Prognosis among survivors of ischemic stroke. Neurology 18:933, 1968.
3. Barner HB, Rittenhouse EA, Willman VL: Carotid-subclavian bypass for "subclavian steal syndrome." J Thorac Cardiovasc Surg 55:773, 1968.
4. Bernstein EF, Humber PB, Collins GM, et al: Life expectancy and late stroke following carotid endarterectomy. Ann Surg 198:80, 1983.
5. Bergan JJ, Dean RH, Yao JS: Use of the axillary artery in complex cerebral revascularization. Surgery 77:338, 1975.
6. Blaisdell FW, Clauss RH, Galbraith JG, et al: Joint study of extracranial artery occlusion. IV. A review of surgical considerations. JAMA 209:1889, 1969.
7. Blaisdell FW, Lim RJ Jr, Hall AD: Technical result of carotid endarterectomy. Arteriographic assessment. Am J Surg 114:239, 1967.
8. Chambers BR, Norris JW: Outcome in patients with asymptomatic neck bruits. N Engl J Med 315:860, 1986.
9. Christensen MS, Hoedi-Rasmussen K, Lassen NA: Cerebral vasodilatation by halothane anesthesia in man and its potentiation by hypotension and hypercapnia. Br J Anaesth 39:927, 1967.
10. Connolly JE, Stemmer EA: Endarterectomy of the external carotid artery. Its importance in the surgical management of extracranial cerebrovascular occlusive disease. Surgery 106:799, 1973.
11. Crawford ES, DeBakey ME, Morris GC Jr, et al: Surgical treatment of occlusion of the innominate, common carotid, and subclavian arteries: A 10-year experience. Surgery 65:17, 1969.
12. Dardik H, Dardik I: Axillo-axillary bypass with cephalic vein for correction of subclavian steal syndrome. Surgery 76:143, 1974.
13. Davis JB, Grove WJ, Julian OC: Thrombotic occlusion of the branches of the aortic arch, Martorell's syndrome: Report of a case treated surgically. Ann Surg 144:124, 1956.
14. DeBakey ME, Crawford ES, Cooley DA, et al: Surgical considerations of occlusive disease of the innominate, carotid subclavian, and vertebral arteries. Ann Surg 149:690, 1959.
15. DeWeese JA, Rob CG, Satran R, et al: Results of carotid endarterectomy for transient ischemic attacks five years later. Ann Surg 178:258, 1973.
16. Diethrich EB, Garrett HE, Ameriso J, et al: Occlusive disease of the common carotid and subclavian arteries treated by carotid-subclavian bypass. Analysis of 125 cases. Am J Surg 113:800, 1967.
17. Dixon S, Pais SO, Raviola C, et al: Natural history of nonstenotic asymptomatic ulcerative lesions of the carotid artery. Arch Surg 117:1493, 1982.
18. Ehrenfeld WK, Chapman ED, Wylie EJ: Management of occlusive lesions of the branches of the aortic arch. Am J Surg 118:236, 1969.
19. Ehrenfeld WK, Hamilton FN, Larson CP Jr, et al: Effect of CO_2 and systemic hypertension on downstream cerebral arterial pressure during carotid endarterectomy. Surgery 67:87, 1970.
20. Enger E, Boyesen S: Long-term anticoagulant therapy in patients with cerebral infarction: A controlled clinical study. Acta Med Scand 178(Suppl 438):1, 1965.
21. Eriksson SE, Link H, Alm A, et al: Results from eighty-eight consecutive prophylactic carotid endarterectomies in cerebral infarction and transitory ischemic attacks. Acta Neurol Scand 63:209, 1981.
22. Goldstone J, Moore WS: Emergency carotid artery surgery in neurologically unstable patients. Arch Surg 111:1284, 1976.
23. Harris EJ, Brown WH, Pavy RN, et al: Continuous electroencephalographic monitoring during carotid artery endarterectomy. Surgery 62:441, 1967.
24. Hass WK, Jonas S: Caution falling rock zone: An analysis of the medical and surgical management of threatened stroke. Proc Inst Med Chicago 33:80, 1980.
25. Hays RJ, Levinson SA, Wylie EJ: Intraoperative measurement of carotid back pressure as a guide to operative management for carotid endarterectomy. Surgery 72:953, 1972.

26. Hertzer NR, Arison R: Cumulative stroke and survival ten years after carotid endarterectomy. J Vasc Surg 2:661, 1985.

27. Hertzer NR, Flanagan RA Jr, O'Hara PJ, et al: Surgical versus non-operative treatment of asymptomatic carotid stenosis. Ann Surg 204:163, 1986.

28. Hertzer NR, Flanagan RA Jr, O'Hara PJ, et al: Surgical versus non-operative treatment of symptomatic carotid stenosis. Ann Surg 204:154, 1986.

29. Hertzer NR, Beven EG, O'Hara PJ, et al: A prospective study of vein patch angioplasty during carotid endarterectomy. Ann Surg 206:628, 1987.

30. High-dose acetylsalicylic acid after cerebral infarction. A Swedish Cooperative Study. Stroke 18:325, 1987.

31. Homi J, Humphries AW, Young JR, et al: Hypercarbic anesthesia in cerebrovascular surgery. Surgery 59:57, 1966.

32. Hughes RK, Bustos M, Byrne JP Jr.: Internal carotid artery pressures. A guide for use of shunt during carotid repair. Arch Surg 109:494, 1974.

33. Humphries AW, Young JR, Beven EG, et al: Relief of vertebrobasilar symptoms by carotid endarterectomy. Surgery 57:48, 1965.

34. Hunter GC, Sieffert G, Malone JM, et al: The accuracy of carotid back pressure as an index for shunt requirement: A reappraisal. Stroke 13:319, 1982.

35. Larson CP: Anesthesia and control of the cerebral circulation. *In* Wylie EJ, Ehrenfeld WK (eds): Extracranial Occlusive Cerebrovascular Disease. Philadelphia, WB Saunders, 1970.

36. Larson CP, Ehrenfeld WK, Wade JG, et al: Jugular venous oxygen saturation as an index of adequacy of cerebral oxygenation. Surgery 62:31, 1967.

37. Lord RSA: Later survival after carotid endarterectomy for transient ischemic attacks. J Vasc Surg 1:512, 1984.

38. Lyons C, Clark LC Jr, McDowell H, et al: Cerebral venous oxygen content during carotid thrombointimectomy. Ann Surg 106:561, 1964.

39. Machleder HI, Barker WF: External carotid artery shunting during carotid endarterectomy. Arch Surg 108:785, 1974.

40. McCullough JL, Mentzer RM, Harman PK, et al: Carotid endarterectomy after a completed stroke: Reduction in long neurologic deterioration. J Vasc Surg 2:7, 1985.

41. Meissner I, Wiebers DO, Whisnant JP, et al: The natural history of asymptomatic carotid artery occlusive lesions. JAMA 258:2704, 1987.

42. Moneta GL, Taylor DC, Nicholls SC, et al: Operative versus nonoperative management of asymptomatic high-grade internal carotid artery stenosis: Improved results with endarterectomy. Stroke 18:1005, 1987.

43. Moore WS, Hall AD: Carotid artery back pressure. Arch Surg 99:702, 1969.

44. Moore WS, Blaisdell FW, Hall AD: Retrograde thrombectomy for chronic occlusion of the common carotid artery. Arch Surg 95:664, 1967.

45. Moore WS, Malone JM, Goldstone J: Extrathoracic repair of branch occlusions of the aortic arch. Am J Surg 132:249, 1976.

46. Moore WS, Yee JM, Hall AD: Collateral cerebral blood pressure. An index of tolerance to temporary carotid occlusion. Arch Surg 106:520, 1973.

47. Moore WS, Boren C, Malone JM, et al: Natural history of nonstenotic asymptomatic ulcerative lesions of the carotid artery. Arch Surg 113:1352, 1978.

48. Mozersky DJ, Barnes RW, Sumner DS, et al: The hemodynamics of the axillary-axillary bypass. Surg Gynecol Obstet 135:925, 1972.

49. Najafi H, Javid H, Dye WS, et al: Kinked internal carotid artery. Clinical evaluation and surgical correction. Arch Surg 89:134, 1964.

50. Pistolese GR, Citone G, Faraglia V: Effects of hypercapnia on cerebral blood flow during the clamping of the carotid arteries in surgical management of cerebrovascular insufficiency. Neurology (Minneap) 21:95, 1971.

51. Rob CG: Operation for acute completed stroke due to thrombosis of the internal carotid artery. Surgery 65:862, 1969.

52. Robinson RW, Demirel M, LeBeau RJ: Natural history of cerebral thrombosis: Nine- to nineteen-year follow-up. J Chronic Dis 21:221, 1968.

53. Rubin JR, Goldstone J, McIntyre KE, et al: The value of carotid endarterectomy in reducing the morbidity and mortality of recurrent stroke. J Vasc Surg 4:443, 1986.

54. Sacco RL, Wolf PA, Kannel WB, et al: Survival and recurrence following stroke, the Framingham Study. Stroke 13:290, 1982.

55. Sproul G: Femoral-axillary bypass for cerebrovascular insufficiency. Arch Surg 103:746, 1971.

56. Stewart G, Ross-Russell RW, Browse NL: The long-term results of carotid endarterectomy for transient ischemic attacks. J Vasc Surg 4:600, 1986.

57. Takolander RJ, Bergentz SE, Ericsson BF: Carotid artery surgery in patients with minor stroke. Br J Surg 70:13, 1982.

58. Thompson JE: Cerebral protection during carotid endarterectomy. JAMA 202:1046, 1967.

59. Trojaborg W, Boysen G: Relation between EEG, regional cerebral blood flow and internal carotid artery pressure during carotid endarterectomy. Electroencephalogr Clin Neurophysiol 34:61, 1973.

60. Waltz AG: Effect of blood pressure on blood flow in ischemic and in nonischemic cerebral cortex. Neurology (Minneap) 18:613, 1968.

61. Whisnant JP, Matsumoto M, Elveback LR: The effect of anticoagulant therapy on the prognosis of patients with transient cerebral ischemic attacks in a community. Rochester, Minnesota 1965–1969. Mayo Clin Proc 48:844, 1973.

62. The Asymptomatic Carotid Artery Stenosis Group: Study design for randomized prospective trial of carotid endarterectomy for asymptomatic atherosclerosis. Stroke 20:844, 1989.

63. The Casanova Study Group: Carotid surgery versus medical therapy for asymptomatic carotid stenosis. Stroke 22:1229, 1991.

64. European Carotid Surgery Trialists' Collaborative Group: MRC European Carotid Surgery Trial: Interim results for symptomatic patients with severe (70–99%) or with mild (0–29%) carotid stenosis. Lancet 337:1235, 1991.

65. Freischlag JA, Hanna D, Moore WS: Improved prognosis for asymptomatic carotid stenosis with prophylactic carotid endarterectomy. Stroke 23:479, 1992.

66. Hobson RW II, Weiss DG, Fields WS, et al: Efficacy of carotid endarterectomy for asymptomatic carotid stenosis. N Engl J Med 328:221, 1993.

67. Makhoul RG, Moore WS, Colburn MD, et al: Benefit of carotid endarterectomy following prior stroke. J Vasc Surg (In press).

68. Matchar DB, Goldstein LB, McCory DC, et al: Carotid Endarterectomy: A Literature Review and Ratings of Appropriateness and Necessity. Santa Monica, CA: Rand Corporation, 1992.

69. Mayberg MR, Wilson SE, Yatsu F, et al, for the Veterans Affairs Cooperative Studies Program 309 Trialist Group: Carotid endarterectomy and prevention of cerebral ischemia in symptomatic carotid stenosis. JAMA 266:3289, 1991.

70. Mentzer RN, Finkelmeir BA, Crosby LK, Wellons MA Jr: Emergency carotid endarterectomy for fluctuating neurologic deficits. Surgery 89:60, 1981.

71. Moore WS, Mohr JP, Najafi H, et al: Carotid endarterectomy: Practice guidelines. J Vasc Surg 15:469, 1992.

72. Moore WS: Carotid endarterectomy for prevention of stroke. West J Med 159:37, 1993.

73. North American Symptomatic Carotid Endarterectomy Trial Collaborators: Beneficial effect of carotid endarterectomy in symptomatic patients with high-grade carotid stenosis. N Engl J Med 325:445, 1991.

74. Thompson JE: Carotid endarterectomy for asymptomatic carotid stenosis: An update. J Vasc Surg 13:669, 1991.

Vertebrobasilar Ischemia: Indications, Techniques, and Results of Surgical Repair

Ramon Berguer, M.D., Ph.D.

• • •

INDICATIONS

Direct surgery on the vertebral artery (VA) to correct stenosis or occlusion may be considered under three sets of circumstances: (1) in patients with vertebrobasilar ischemia (VBI), in order to increase blood flow to the basilar territory or to prevent embolization; (2) in patients with extensive and severe extracranial disease and symptoms from it, in order to increase total brain inflow; and (3) in association with carotid surgery in patients who are symptomatic, presumably from their carotid disease, but who have a dominant and severely diseased VA on the same side of the carotid lesion.

VBI may be due to microembolization from the heart or from the arteries leading to the basilar artery. These patients may present with transient ischemic attacks (TIAs) or infarctions in the territory supplied by the basilar artery. The importance of the *embolic* mechanism as a cause of vertebrobasilar symptoms has only recently been emphasized.[1, 2] This new information is derived from autopsy studies, from the availability of magnetic resonance imaging (MRI), which can identify small infarcts in the brain stem and cerebellum (previously not seen by computed tomography [CT] scanning), and from selective arteriograms showing the emb) source in the subclavian or vertebral arteries. Patients with embD VBI develop multiple infarcts in the brain stem, cerebellum, and, occasionally, posterior cerebral artery territory and have a poor prognosis with regard to stroke.

A second mechanism better recognized and probably more frequent is *hemodynamic* TIAs in the territory of the basilar artery because of the lack of appropriate inflow from the VA and inadequate compensation from the carotid territory. Neurodynamic VBI, manifesting as TIAs, is usually secondary to stenosis or occlusion of the VA. The majority of these lesions are atherosclerotic plaques. The VA, however, is also compressed extrinsically by osteophytes adjacent to the VA canal. It is essential in patients with neurodynamic VBI to rule out the common systemic causes of VBI before advising arteriography. In the later years of life, VA stenosis is a frequent arteriographic finding and dizziness is also a common symptom. The presence of both in a patient cannot be assumed to be a cause-and-effect relationship. Commonly found systemic causes of VBI are orthostatic hypotension, inappropriate antihypertensive therapy, arrhythmias and malfunction of pacemakers, anemia, brain tumor, and subclavian steal.

The work-up of patients with VBI should include a number of specific steps. The precise situation under which symptoms occur should be ascertained. Symptoms often appear on standing in older individuals with poor sympathetic control of their venous tone causing excessive pooling of blood in the veins of the leg. This is particularly common in patients with diabetes who have abolished sympathetic reflexes. We arbitrarily use a 20-mmHg systolic pressure drop on standing as the criterion for a diagnosis of orthostatic hypotension. However, the presence of orthostatic hypotension does not necessarily exclude a patient from further work-up. A systemic drop in blood pressure, even of less than 20 mmHg, may represent a critical reduction in flow in a vertebrobasilar system already impaired by stenosing disease and be the trigger mechanism for VBI.

Patients may relate symptoms to head turning or extension. Symptoms may appear only when turning the head to one side. The mechanism here is extrinsic compression of the VA, often the dominant or the only remaining one, by arthritic bone spurs.[3] To differentiate this mechanism from VBI secondary to labyrinthine disorders that may appear with head or body rotation, the author tries to reproduce the symptoms by turning the head slowly while observing the patient's response and then repeating the maneuver, but this time in a brisk fashion. In labyrinthine disease, the sudden inertial changes result in immediate symptoms and often marked nystagmus. In vertebral compression, it takes a few seconds before the patient fears for her or his balance. The demonstration of extrinsic compression of the VA, usually by osteophytes, may require an arteriogram, done with the patient sitting up, by means of bilateral brachial injections or with the patient in Trendelenburg's position with the head against a block if the femoral route is used. These maneuvers are to be added to the standard rotation and extension required to bring about symptoms and to demonstrate the extrinsic compression. The reason for these positional requirements is that the weight of the head acting on the cervical spine changes its curvature and decreases the distance between C1 and C7.

This longitudinal compression of the spine often enhances the external compression effects caused by osteophytic spurs.[4]

A CT scan is mandatory to rule out tumors and to assess the integrity of the brain. Unsuspected hemispheric infarction may be found, but brain stem infarctions are often missed because they tend to be smaller in size and the resolution of the CT scan in this area is poor. We use MRI routinely in patients who are candidates for vertebral arterial reconstruction to ascertain whether infarctions have taken place in the vertebrobasilar territory. Antihypertensive drugs can also cause hemodynamic VBI, particularly if taken in excess of need, by decreasing the main perfusion pressure and/or inducing severe orthostatic hypotension.

A 24-hour electrocardiogram (ECG) is taken in all patients being evaluated for hemodynamic VBI. Sometimes patients with VBI secondary to arrhythmias will recognize the association of palpitations with the appearance of VBI symptoms, the latter being secondary to decreased cardiac output resulting from the arrhythmia.

Physical examination will alert the physician to the possibility of a subclavian steal in patients with brachial pressure differences greater than 25 mmHg or with absent pulses in one arm. The diagnosis of reversal of VA flow can be made accurately by noninvasive methods.[5]

Any systemic mechanism that decreases the mean pressure of the basilar artery may be responsible for the syndrome of VBI. These individuals may or may not have concomitant VA stenosis or occlusion. In some patients, the cause of the drop in mean arterial pressure can be corrected by readjustment of their antihypertensive medication, by antiarrhythmic drugs, or by insertion of a pacemaker. In patients with orthostatic hypotension, the problem may not respond to the medical treatment and only the reconstruction of a diseased or occluded VA will render the patient asymptomatic in the face of persistent oscillations of blood pressure secondary to poor sympathetic venous tone control. Rheologic factors such as increased viscosity (polycythemia) or decreased oxygen-carrying capacity (anemia) may increase or cause VBI in patients with severe VA occlusive disease.

The second set of indications refers to patients who have extensive extracranial disease with one or both internal carotid arteries occluded and who have global manifestations of cerebrovascular ischemia. In these patients the carotid arteries may be occluded or involved with severe siphon stenosis, making a direct revascularization via the internal carotid arteries impossible. In these individuals, in whom the VAs are the main source of blood supply to the brain but are severely diseased or occluded, reconstruction of the VAs may offer the best hope for reestablishment of an adequate blood inflow to the brain. In this group, the presence of good-size posterior communicating arteries increases the likelihood of success.

A third group of indications is more controversial and concerns those patients with severe carotid lesions who have severe disease of the origin of the dominant or single VA on the same side of the planned carotid operation. In these patients, the author's group repairs the diseased VA at the time of the carotid operation. The principle on which this additional operation is justified is the same that supports repair of a severe renal artery lesion in the course of an abdominal aortic reconstruction. The carotid and the vertebral operation are performed through the same incision, and the additional dissection to expose the VA is of minor extent. Patients undergoing concomitant internal carotid and VA repair experience greater morbidity than those undergoing isolated carotid artery or VA repair.

In VA reconstructions done for hemodynamic symptoms and in those performed concomitantly with a carotid operation, only severely stenosed (greater than 75 per cent luminal loss) and clearly dominant or single VAs are operated on. From the point of view of anatomic criteria, it is assumed that a hypoplastic VA ending in a posterior-inferior cerebellar artery is equivalent to an occluded VA. In patients with emboligenous lesions in one vertebral (or subclavian) artery the source of the embolus is corrected regardless of the status of the opposite VA.

ARTERIOGRAPHIC EVALUATION

The arteriographic study of VA pathology requires specific positions and projections to evaluate the vertebrobasilar system from its origin to the top of the basilar artery. The VA is divided into four segments, each one with specific radiologic and pathologic features (Fig. 120–1).

Arteriographic exploration begins with an arch view, which will determine the presence or absence of VA on each side, and will indicate whether one VA is dominant

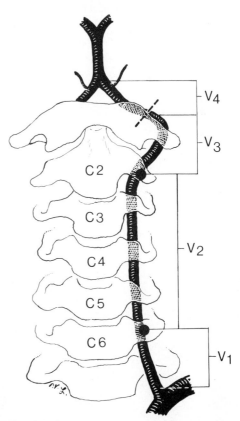

FIGURE 120–1. The four segments of the vertebral artery (VA). (From Berguer R: Surgical management of the vertebral artery. *In* Moore WS [ed]: Surgery for Cerebrovascular Disease [Chapter 60]. Reproduced by permission of Churchill Livingstone, Inc, New York, 1986.)

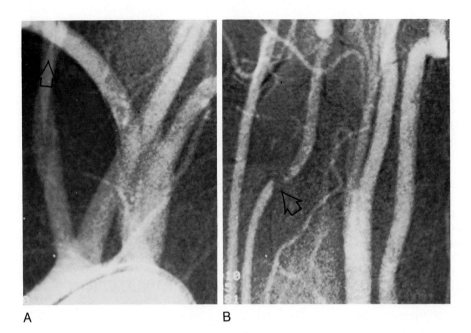

A   B

FIGURE 120–2. Arch injection in a 33-year-old woman with vertebrobasilar ischemia. *A,* The right VA and the right external carotid artery arise from a long common right carotid trunk *(arrow).* The right internal carotid is congenitally absent. The right subclavian arises as the last branch of the aorta. *B,* The right VA, which has an anomalous origin, enters the spine at a high level (C4) and is severely compressed *(arrow)* at this level on head rotation.

(generally the left) and whether one of the VAs has an abnormal origin. The most common anomaly of origin is the left VA taking origin from the arch (6 per cent). A much rarer anomaly is the right VA taking origin from the innominate or right common carotid artery (Fig. 120–2). The arch views are obtained in at least two projections: right and left posterior obliques. Usually these two views display well the *first segment* (V1) of the VA from its origin to the transverse process of C6.

The most common atherosclerotic lesion of the VA is a severe stenosis of its origin. This lesion may be missed in standard arch views because of superimposition of the subclavian artery over the first segment of the VA. Additional oblique projections may be needed until the subclavian artery is "thrown off" and a clear view of the origin can be obtained (Fig. 120–3). Sometimes, even if the origin is hidden by the superimposed subclavian artery, the poststenotic dilatation or the first centimeter or two of the VA

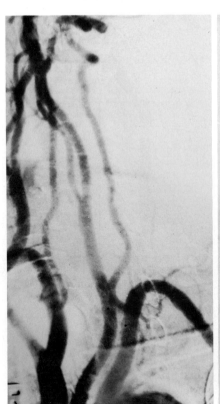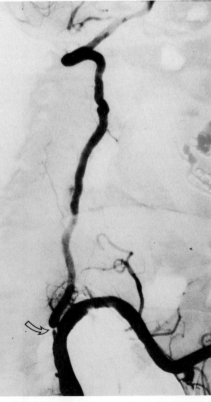

FIGURE 120–3. A severe stenosis *(arrow)* of a dominant left VA seen only after additional oblique rotation of the patient *(right).* (From Berguer R: Role of vertebral artery surgery after carotid endarterectomy. *In* Bergan JJ, Yao JST [eds]: Reoperative Arterial Surgery. Orlando, FL, Grune & Stratton, 1986, pp 555–564.)

will alert one to the hidden stenosis. Redundancy and kinks are common, but only the most severe kinks associated with post-stenotic dilatations have hemodynamic significance.

The evaluation of the *second segment* (V2) of the VA, from C6 to the top of the transverse process of C2, can usually be performed during the arch views but is completed during the selective subclavian injections. The point of entry of the artery in the spine should be determined, and an abnormally low entry at the level of C7 should be noted. This finding implies a short V1 segment of the VA, which may have inadequate length to permit its transposition to the common carotid artery. The level of entry into the spine is best determined in unsubtracted films. Extrinsic compression by musculotendinous structures is more common in a VA with abnormal level of entry into the spine (see Fig. 120–2). This is due to the sharp angulation resulting from the abnormal level of entry. The most common pathology of the V2 segment, where the VA is attached to the periostium of the vertebral foramina, is extrinsic compression of the VA by osteophytes.[3] In patients with symptoms prompted by neck rotation, the V2 segment must be evaluated with arteriograms taken with the neck in right or left rotation. The VA may be perfectly normal in one projection and be occluded in the other by extrinsic compression (Fig. 120–4). The compression agent may be bone (usually an osteophyte) or tendon (usually the longus colli). Because of their fixation to the foramina and the close relationship to its surrounding venous plexus, the V2 and V3 segments are the usual site of traumatic or spontaneous arteriovenous fistulae. The VA may tear completely or incompletely (internal rupture) as a consequence of stretch injury following extreme rotation or hyperextension of the neck.

The *third segment* (V3) extends from the top of the transverse process of C2 to the atlanto-occipital membrane at the base of the skull. The most common, although rare, pathology of this segment is a dissection of the VA, usually secondary to fibromuscular dysplasia and/or trauma to the artery from subluxation of the top two vertebrae (Fig. 120–5). This may result in stenosis or aneurysmal dilatation. A fact important to the surgeon is that when the VA is occluded proximally it usually reconstitutes at the V3 segment via the occipital connection, a collateral linking the occipital artery with the VA at this level (Fig. 120–6). It is because of this collateral that the distal (V3 + V4) vertebral and basilar arteries usually remain patent in spite of a proximal VA occlusion.

The *fourth segment* (V4) is the second most common site for atherosclerotic involvement of the VA (Fig. 120–7). Finally, the basilar artery should be clearly seen in lateral or oblique projections. Subtracted views are needed to eliminate the temporal bone density in the lateral projection. In the Towne projection, the artery is foreshortened and therefore the resolution is poor. Advanced atheromatous disease of the basilar artery contraindicates reconstruction of VA lesions.

SURGICAL TECHNIQUES

With some exceptions, most reconstructions of the VA attempt to relieve either an orificial stenosis (V1 segment)

FIGURE 120–4. A patient with a single VA showing minimal extrinsic compression *(A)* when the neck is rotated to the right and occlusion *(B)* when the neck is rotated to the left. (From Berguer R: Surgical management of the vertebral artery. *In* Moore WS [ed]: Surgery for Cerebrovascular Disease [Chapter 60]. Reproduced by permission of Churchill Livingstone, Inc, New York, 1986.)

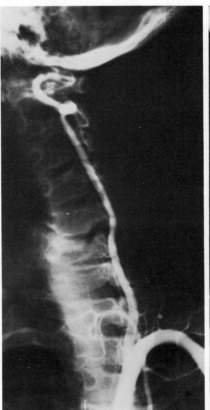

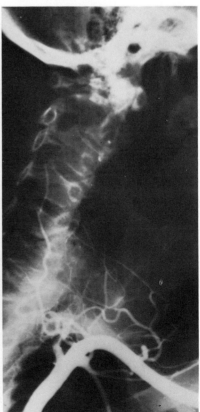

A   B

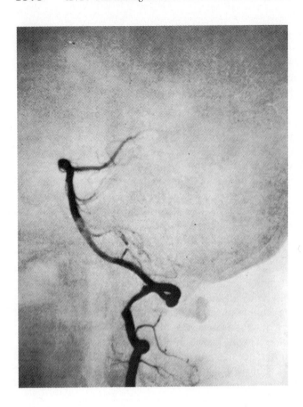

FIGURE 120–5.   Intramural dissection of the VA at the V3 segment in a 40-year-old woman with Klippel-Feil syndrome and subluxation of the atlantoaxial joint.

FIGURE 120–6.   The distal vertebral and basilar artery being fed by an occipital collateral in a patient with proximal VA occlusion.

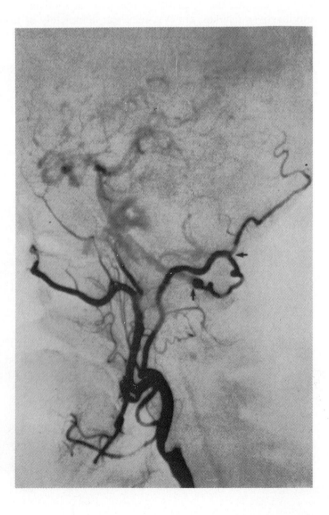

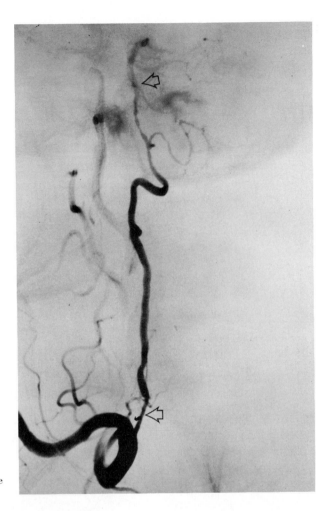

FIGURE 120-7. Arteriogram showing atheromatous disease of the V1 and V4 segments of the VA and of the basilar artery.

or disease/occlusion of its intraspinal course (V2 segment).[6] Less common problems are severe and fixed kinks at its origin and dissection of the V3 segment, secondary to trauma or fibromuscular dysplasia, or both.

Although in the 1970s we advocated the correction of proximal VA disease by subclavian-vertebral bypass,[7, 8] we seldom use this technique nowadays, reserving it for uncommon anatomic circumstances, such as a contralateral carotid occlusion that increases the risk of clamping the only carotid supply during the transposition operation or a short V1 segment, when the artery enters the foramen transversarium of C7, that leaves inadequate length to transpose the VA to the common carotid artery. For disease involving the origin of the VA, the author's group routinely performs a transposition of this vessel into the common carotid artery, the latter being a better, more durable, and more accessible artery than the subclavian. This procedure involves only one anastomosis and requires no vein graft.

For disease involving any level above the transverse process of C6, the author's group routinely carries the reconstruction up to the C2–C1 level (V3 segment). This is usually accomplished by a common carotid to distal VA bypass,[9–12] although other techniques (see discussion later) may be indicated in specific circumstances. Bypasses above the level of C1 are technically demanding and seldom required. There is no reason to approach the VA for reconstruction in its V2 portion, where the exposure is far inferior to that obtained in the V3 segment. In addition,

reconstruction of the VA above the level of C2 bypasses most potential areas of extrinsic compression by osteophytes.

Transposition of the VA Into the Common Carotid Artery

If the VA operation is performed as an isolated procedure, the incision is supraclavicular, slightly curved upward approaching the VA between the heads of the sternocleidomastoid muscle (Fig. 120–8). The jugular vein and vagus nerve are retracted laterally with soft, malleable neurosurgical retractors, and the carotid sheath is entered dissecting the carotid artery proximally as far as possible with the surgeon temporarily at the head of the patient looking down into the mediastinum. After the carotid artery is mobilized, one can see the sympathetic chain running behind and parallel to it. First, the surgeon identifies the thoracic duct and divides it between ligatures, avoiding any transfixion sutures, which may result in lymph leaks. The proximal end of the thoracic duct is ligated twice. Additional lymph ducts, if found, are ligated and divided. The entire dissection must be confined medial to the prescalene fat pad with its underlying scalenus anticus muscle and phrenic nerve. These latter structures are left undissected lateral to the field. The inferior thyroid artery generally runs transversely across the field and it is ligated in continuity and divided.

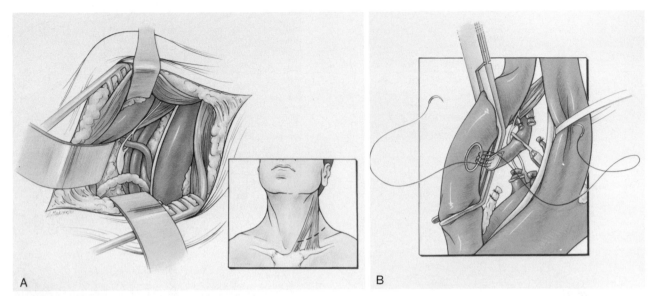

FIGURE 120–8. *A,* Access to the proximal VA between the sternocleidomastoid muscle bellies. *B,* Transposition of the proximal VA to the posterior wall of the common carotid artery. *(A and B,* From Berguer R, Kieffer E: Surgery of the Arteries to the Head. New York, Springer-Verlag, 1992.)

The vertebral vein is next identified emerging from the angle formed by the longus colli and scalenus anticus at the top and overlying the VA and the subclavian artery below. Unlike its sister artery, the vertebral vein has branches. It is also ligated in continuity and divided: below the vertebral vein lies the VA. It is important to identify and follow the sympathetic chain, carefully preserving it. The VA is looped and dissected up to the tendon of the longus colli and below to its origin in the subclavian artery. In order to preserve the sympathetic trunks and the stellate or intermediate ganglia resting on the artery, it may be necessary to isolate and loop the VA above and below these structures.

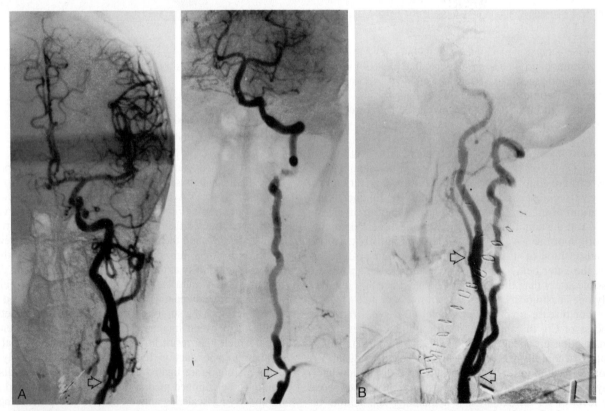

FIGURE 120–9. *A,* Arteriogram in a patient with left hemispheric transient symptoms showing carotid and vertebral (dominant) arterial stenoses. *B,* Arteriogram obtained 2 days after left carotid endarterectomy and reimplantation of the left VA into the left common carotid artery.

The VA is freed from the sympathetic trunk resting on its anterior surface without damaging the trunk or the interganglionic connections.

Once the artery is fully exposed, an appropriate site for reimplantation in the common carotid artery is selected and is cleared of adventitia. The patient is given systemic heparin (to obtain an accelerated coagulation time of 300 seconds), and the distal portion of the V1 segment of the VA is clamped below the edge of the longus colli with a Heifitz clip placed vertically to indicate the orientation of the artery and to avoid axial twisting during its anastomosis. The proximal VA, immediately above the stenosis at its origin, is occluded with a large hemoclip, cut above it, and further secured by a transfixing 6–0 polypropylene suture. The artery may then be pulled from under the overlying sympathetic trunk and brought to the proximity of the common carotid artery. A skin marker may be used to identify the spot in the carotid artery where the surgeon judges that the VA can be anastomosed without tension or redundancy. The distal free end of the VA is spatulated for anastomosis. The carotid artery is then cross-clamped. With the surgeon using a 5.2-mm aortic punch, an elliptical defect of approximately 5 × 7 mm is created in its posterolateral wall. The anastomosis is performed in open fashion with continuous 6–0 or 7–0 polypropylene, avoiding any tension on the VA, which tears easily. During suturing, the common carotid is brought down to the VA free end. Before completion of the anastomosis, the suture slack is retrieved with a nerve hook; the vessels are back-bled into the wound; the suture is tied; and flow is reestablished, first into the VA and then into the distal common carotid artery. A suction drain is left in the neck and is brought through a separate stab wound, to be removed after 12 hours. The wound is closed by approximating the platysma and the skin edges.

When a simultaneous carotid endarterectomy is planned (Fig. 120–9), the VA is approached through the standard carotid incision prolonged down to the head of the clavicle. In this approach, the sternocleidomastoid is lateral and the field is a bit narrower than when approaching the VA between the heads of the sternocleidomastoid. The remaining steps of the operation are as described previously.

Distal VA Reconstruction

Various techniques can be applied to revascularize the VA in its V3 segment between the transverse processes of C1 and C2. Access to the VA at this level is the same for all techniques.[11-13]

The incision is anterior to the sternocleidomastoid, the same as in a carotid operation, and is carried to immediately below the earlobe (Fig. 120–10). The dissection proceeds between the jugular vein and the medial edge of the sternocleidomastoid to identify the spinal accessory nerve. The nerve is gently held by a Silastic loop and followed distally as it joins the jugular vein and crosses in front of the transverse process of C1, which can be distinctly felt by the operator's finger. This requires freeing and retracting the digastric muscle upward. With the C1 process identified, the surgeon can feel the C2 transverse process, which is not as clear a landmark. The next step involves the identification of the levator scapulae, and this is best done by remov-

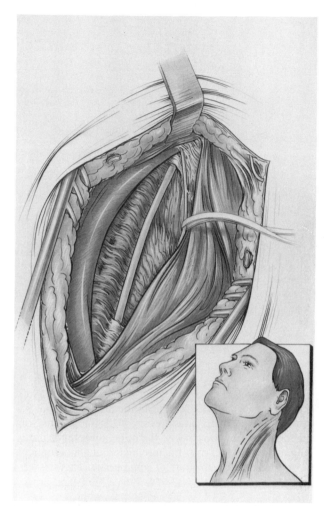

FIGURE 120–10. Retrojugular approach and isolation of the spinal accessory nerve. (From Berguer R, Kieffer E: Surgery of the Arteries to the Head. New York, Springer-Verlag, 1992.)

ing the fibrofatty tissue overlying it. With the anterior edge of the levator scapulae identified, the surgeon searches for the anterior ramus of C2. Using the C2 ramus as a guide, a right-angle clamp is slid over it elevating the levator scapulae, which is cut (Fig. 120–11). The proximal stump of the levator is excised up to the level of its insertion at the C1 transverse process to improve exposure. The C2 ramus divides into three branches immediately after crossing the VA. The artery runs below, in contact with the nerve and perpendicular to it. The surgeon cuts the ramus (Fig. 120–12) before its branching; underneath it, the VA can be seen. The dissection of the artery at this level must be accomplished with magnification (×3.5). The artery is freed from the surrounding veins always present, and this is done with extreme care because hemorrhage is tedious to control at this level. In addition to loop magnification, fine instruments and fine-pointed scissors, such as Jameson, are needed. Before looping the artery, one must make sure that the occipital collateral feeding the VA does not enter the back of the artery at the level at which one is working, where it may be torn by the right-angle clamp while the surgeon is trying to encircle the artery (Fig. 120–13). Once the VA is slung, the distal common carotid artery is dis-

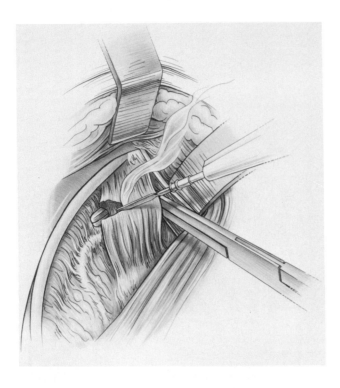

FIGURE 120–11.   Dividing the levator scapula over the C2 ramus. The vagus, internal jugular vein, and internal carotid artery are anterior to the muscle. (From Berguer R, Kieffer E: Surgery of the Arteries to the Head. New York, Springer-Verlag, 1992.)

sected and prepared to receive a saphenous vein graft. There is no need to dissect the bifurcation. The spot selected for the proximal anastomosis of the saphenous vein graft should not be too close to the bifurcation, since cross-clamping at this level may fracture underlying atheroma.

A saphenous vein graft of appropriate length is ob-

tained and prepared. A valveless segment facilitates back-bleeding of the VA after completion of the distal anastomosis. The patient is given IV heparin to obtain an accelerated coagulation time of 300 seconds. With gentle traction placed on the loop, the VA is elevated and occluded with a special J clamp that will isolate this segment

FIGURE 120–12.   Dividing the anterior ramus of C2 to expose the underlying VA running perpendicular to the former. (From Berguer R, Kieffer E: Surgery of the Arteries to the Head. New York, Springer-Verlag, 1992.)

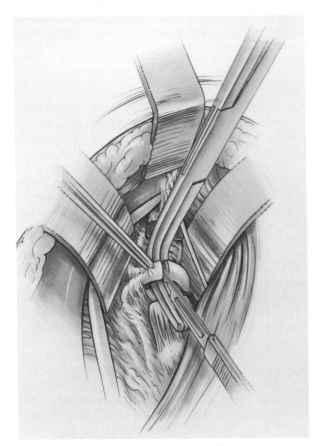

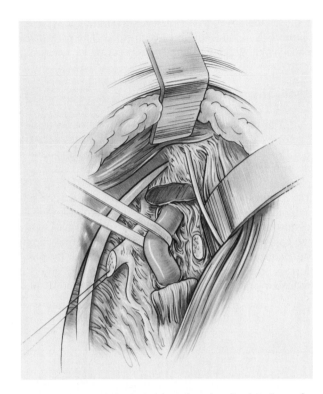

FIGURE 120–13. After the vertebral venous plexus is dissected away, the VA is slung with a Silastic loop for clamping and anastomosis. (From Berguer R, Kieffer E: Surgery of the Arteries to the Head. New York, Springer-Verlag, 1992.)

for an end-to-side anastomosis. The VA is opened longitudinally with a coronary knife for a length adequate to accommodate the spatulated end of the vein graft. The end-to-side anastomosis is done with continuous 8–0 polypropylene. The distal anastomosis is tested by backflow, and if satisfactory a Heifitz clip is placed in the vein graft proximal to the anastomosis resuming flow through the VA. The

FIGURE 120–14. A completed common carotid artery to distal VA bypass using saphenous vein. (From Berguer R, Kieffer E: Surgery of the Arteries to the Head. New York, Springer-Verlag, 1992.)

proximal end of the graft is passed under the jugular vein and into the side of the common carotid artery. The common carotid artery is then cross-clamped, an elliptical arteriostomy is made in its posterior wall with a 5.2-mm aortic punch, and the proximal vein graft is anastomosed end-to-side to the common carotid artery with continuous 6–0 polypropylene (Fig. 120–14). Prior to completing the anas-

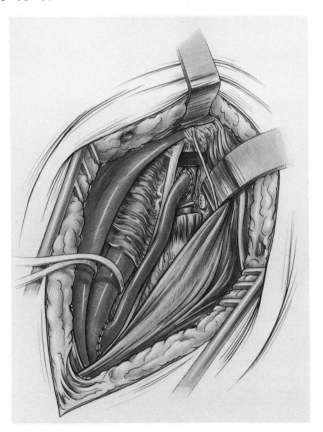

tomosis, the three vessels are back-bled into the wound, the suture is tied, and flow is reestablished. The proximal VA is occluded with a clip immediately below the anastomosis.

Variations on Technique

The distal VA may also be revascularized using the external carotid artery either directly by means of a transposition of the latter vessel into the VA or by anastomosing the proximal end of the graft to it. The transposition of the external carotid to the distal VA (Figs. 120–15 and 120–16) requires a carotid bifurcation free of disease and a long external carotid artery trunk. External carotid arteries that divide early often have branches that are too small to match the caliber of the VA. If the trunk of the external carotid is of adequate size for a length sufficient to reach the VA, the former is skeletonized, dividing all its branches, and is then rotated over the internal carotid artery and under the jugular

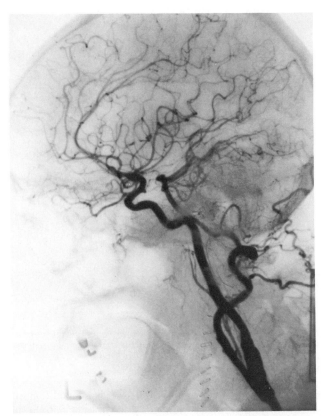

FIGURE 120–16. Arteriogram of a transposition of the external carotid artery to the distal VA. This patient had a previous internal carotid endarterectomy. (From Berguer R, Kieffer E: Surgery of the Arteries to the Head. New York, Springer-Verlag, 1992.)

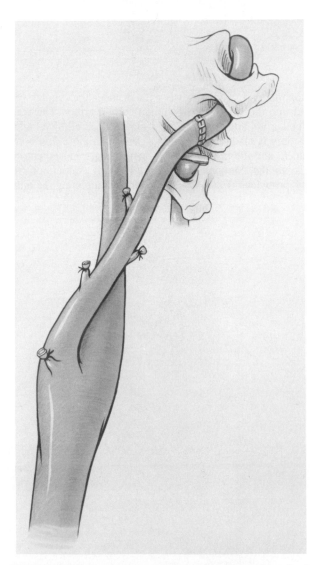

FIGURE 120–15. Transposition of external carotid to distal vertebral artery. (From Berguer R, Kieffer E: Surgery of the Arteries to the Head. New York, Springer-Verlag, 1992.)

vein to be anastomosed end-to-side to the distal VA at C1–C2 level. Following this anastomosis, the proximal VA, immediately below the anastomosis, is permanently occluded with a clip.

A patient may have a segment of saphenous vein that is of appropriate size but of a length insufficient to breach the distance between the common carotid artery and the distal VA. In this case, the proximal external carotid artery can be used as the inflow source for the vein graft by either an end-to-end or an end-to-side proximal anastomosis. Either one of these techniques is a potential solution in those cases where the opposite internal carotid artery is occluded and one may wish to avoid clamping of the common carotid supplying the only patent internal carotid artery. If a vein bypass graft is used between the external carotid artery and the distal VA, it should be placed with the proper amount of tension and checked with the neck rotated back to the neutral position to avoid redundancy or kinking.

In patients under 35 years of age, the cause of VA occlusion (segments V1, V2) is usually trauma (subluxation, injury), fibromuscular dysplasia, or deliberate ligation (during Blalock-Taussig procedure) (Fig. 120–17). These patients usually have intact internal carotids and collaterals to the distal VA fed by an enlarged external carotid branch (occipital). The collaterals are nevertheless too small to provide an adequate flow rate into the basilar system. Under

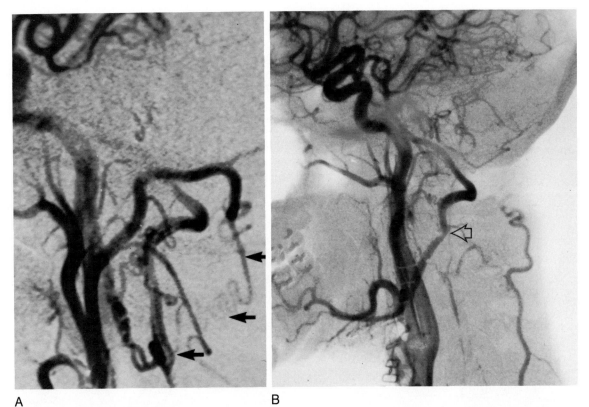

FIGURE 120–17. *A*, Occlusion of the proximal VA (bilaterally) in a young patient with congenital heart disease who underwent bilateral Blalock-Taussig procedures with ligation of both proximal VAs. *B*, Postoperative arteriogram showing an occipital to distal VA anastomosis.

these circumstances, when the occipital artery is enlarged, a reasonable size match can generally be obtained by direct anastomosis of this branch to the distal VA (Fig. 120–18). This solution is also a consideration in patients who do not have an adequate saphenous vein. However, if the patient is over 40 years of age, one should ascertain that the origin of the external carotid artery is not involved by atheroma.

These small arterioarterial anastomoses involve vessels of 2 to 3 mm in caliber and are generally done with ×3.5 loupe magnification and 8–0 polypropylene suture.

Another method of revascularization of the distal VA is the transposition of this vessel into the distal cervical internal carotid artery at the point where the latter ascends in front of the transverse process of C1 (Fig. 120–19). It is a technique that may be used in patients with inadequate saphenous veins or where the external carotid cannot be used because of either peculiar anatomy or disease in the carotid bifurcation. This is a straightforward end-to-side anastomosis between the distal VA and the distal cervical internal carotid artery. This procedure should not be done in patients with contralateral internal carotid artery occlusion where the risk of cerebral ischemia during the anastomosis would be prohibitive.

RESULTS

The author's group's experience with reconstruction of the VA comprises 233 reconstructions, of which 176 were proximal and 57 were distal operations. Thirty-five

VA reconstructions were performed in combination with another operation, usually an internal carotid endarterectomy. Among patients undergoing simultaneous carotid-vertebral reconstructions, 85 per cent had symptoms attributed to either the carotid or the VA lesion and 15 per cent had reconstruction of the VA incidental to a carotid operation for asymptomatic stenosis.

The most common complication in proximal VA operations is a partial, and usually temporary, Horner syndrome which was noted in 22 per cent of patients. Its incidence has decreased with efforts to preserve all sympathetic fibers around the VA.

A lymphocele was a frequent complication in the author's group's earlier experience when we did not routinely isolate and doubly ligate the main thoracic and accessory ducts. One patient developed a large tension lymphocele, which required drainage and produced greater than 3000 ml of lymph per day. A reoperation was required for a more proximal ligation of the thoracic duct. If any lymph leakage is noted during the procedure, the author's group makes every effort to control it. Even though most lymphoceles recede after gastrointestinal rest, aspiration, and pressure dressings, they are an annoying complication to the patient and substantially lengthen the postoperative care.

Only 1 patient had bleeding requiring reoperation. The cause was the VA stump on the subclavian artery, which had been occluded only with a large hemoclip and eventually became dislodged. A transfixion suture is routinely used distal to the hemoclip to avoid this problem. There were 4 cases of thrombosis among the proximal VA opera-

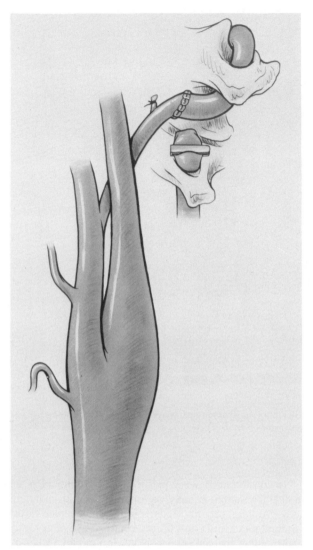

FIGURE 120–18. Transposition of the occipital artery to the distal VA. (From Berguer R, Kieffer E: Surgery of the Arteries to the Head. New York, Springer-Verlag, 1992.)

83 per cent, whereas 17 per cent were neurologically unchanged. Since the latter group had patent reconstructions, it is obvious that the anatomic lesion operated on the VA was not the etiology of their problem. The rate for cure or substantial improvement among distal VA reconstructions is 78 per cent.

Initial patency rates have been lower for distal VA reconstructions, with most failures occurring early in the author's group's experience with this technique. We have learned after 3 failed cases that there is a specific situation in which a distal VA reconstruction should not be attempted. This situation involves individuals with ipsilateral (or bilateral) internal carotid occlusion, severe external carotid stenosis, and bilateral VA occlusion. These patients have an occipital collateral feeding the VA at the level of C2. In these 3 instances, the external carotid artery was repaired by means of angioplasty to increase periorbital flow to the terminal portion of an occluded internal carotid artery. In addition, we performed a bypass to the distal VA to increase basilar artery inflow. In all 3 instances, the external carotid artery remained patent and the distal VA

tions. In 3 cases, the operation performed had been an interposition vein graft between the common carotid and the distal portion of the V1 segment of the VA. The reason to choose an interposition graft was a short V1. Interposition grafts tend to kink in the depths of the neck when placed between the common carotid and the fixed distal portion of the V1 segment of the VA. Direct reimplantation is obviously a better solution.

Immediate and long-term patency has been excellent in proximal VA reconstructions. The only cases of thrombosis have been early and were due to either technical imperfections at the anastomosis (1 case) or the choice of an interposition vein graft (2 cases).

The life expectancy of patients undergoing VA reconstructions is good. The survival rate at 5 years is 90 per cent and at 10 years 79 per cent.

The secondary patency rate (at 10 years) is 90 per cent for proximal and 82 per cent for distal VA reconstructions.

Among patients undergoing proximal VA reconstruction alone, their cure or substantial improvement rate was

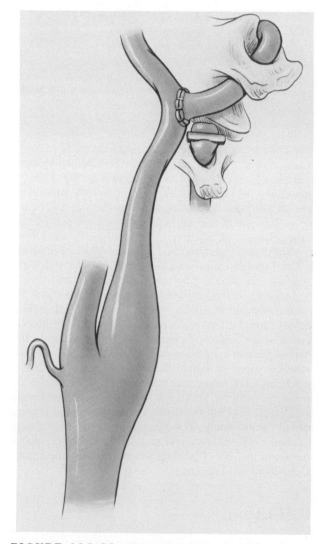

FIGURE 120–19. Transposition of the distal VA to the cervical internal carotid artery. (From Berguer R, Kieffer E: Surgery of the Arteries to the Head. New York, Springer-Verlag, 1992.)

bypass occluded within 3 days of the operation. At reexploration the reason was obvious: the bypass flow rate after thrombectomy was inadequate (25 to 35 ml/min). However, if the external carotid artery was temporarily clamped, the flow rate through the bypass increased to greater than 75 ml/min. It was evident that the occipital connection, now with a better head of pressure after an external carotid endarterectomy, competed with the vertebral bypass supplying flow to the distal VA. The distal bypass was unnecessary because the external carotid angioplasty would have sufficed. This is evident in the fact that all 3 patients were symptom-free after failed thrombectomy of the distal bypass but with patent external carotid angioplasty. Simultaneous angioplasty of an external carotid artery and ipsilateral distal vertebral bypass should not be performed.

There were 3 additional cases of thrombosis in the distal VA bypass series. In 2 of them, the distal VA to which the anastomosis was made was hypoplastic, measuring less than 2 mm. In one case, the artery was involved by arteritis; in the other, the flow rate after completion of the anastomosis was 35 ml/min, a figure that seemed inadequate. It is likely that the technical quality of the anastomoses in these 2 cases was not adequate. The remaining failed graft thrombosed immediately after the operation. It was reexplored, and no technical problem was found. The

graft has remained patent after thrombectomy. To date, no late thrombosis has been found in distal VA reconstructions. However, vein grafts to the distal portion of the VA may develop intimal hyperplasia as they do elsewhere. To date, the author's group has only 1 case of intimal hyperplasia 1 year after implantation (Fig. 120–20). The vein graft was removed and replaced without complications.

There were 32 patients undergoing combined carotid and VA reconstruction. In this group, the death/stroke rate was 6.9 per cent, considerably higher than that seen for patients undergoing operations on the VA alone. This subgroup have often multiple extracranial lesions, and the ensuing loss of autoregulation makes them more susceptible to a revascularization syndrome following reperfusion of their internal carotid artery and VA.

The reconstruction of the proximal VA alone has been a safe procedure with a good outcome. The only morbidity and mortality noted among patients undergoing proximal vertebral reconstructions were in the group that underwent combined carotid and vertebral operations. The central neurologic morbidity and mortality of the 140 patients who had pure but proximal VA reconstruction was zero.

On the other hand, distal VA reconstructions are technically more demanding and carry a higher risk for early occlusion and death.

Some of the immediate postoperative thromboses in

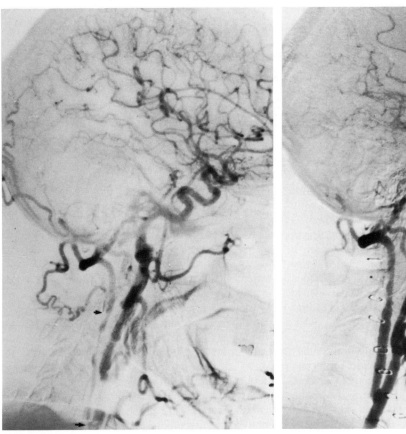
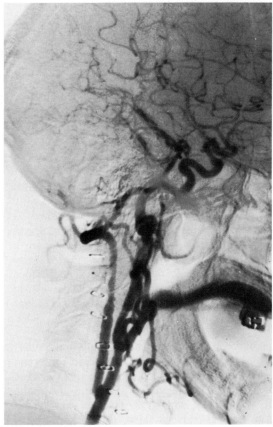

A   B

FIGURE 120–20. *A,* Fibromuscular dysplasia severely stenosing a 12-month-old common carotid artery to distal VA bypass graft *(arrows)*. *B,* Postoperative appearance after resection of the stenosed vein graft and reinsertion of a new one.

this series were due to competitive flow from the external carotid artery, a problem we now avoid. Likewise, one of the deaths in distal VA reconstruction followed a gentle thrombectomy above the level of C1 that resulted in an intradural perforation with a massive subarachnoid hemorrhage and death. Thrombectomy above the level of C1 is no longer considered a safe maneuver.

In terms of cure of clinical symptoms, approximately one fifth of the patients undergoing distal VA repair failed to improve. We need better selection criteria to improve on the clinical results of these operations.

References

1. Caplan LR, Tettenborn B: Embolism in the posterior circulation. *In* Berguer R, Caplan LR (eds): Vertebrobasilar Arterial Disease. St. Louis, Quality Medical, 1992, pp 52–65.
2. Pessin MS: Posterior cerebral artery disease and occipital ischemia. *In* Berguer R, Caplan LR (eds): Vertebrobasilar Arterial Disease. St. Louis, Quality Medical, 1992, pp 66–75.
3. Bauer RB: Mechanical compression of the vertebral arteries. *In* Berguer R, Bauer RB (eds): Vertebrobasilar Arterial Occlusive Disease: Medical and Surgical Management. New York, Raven Press, 1984, pp 45–71.
4. Ruotolo C, Hazan H, Rancurel G, Kieffer E: Dynamic arteriography. *In* Berguer R, Caplan LR (eds): Vertebrobasilar Arterial Disease. St. Louis, Quality Medical, 1992, pp 116–123.
5. Berguer R, Higgins RF, Nelson R: Noninvasive diagnosis of reversal of vertebral artery flow. N Engl J Med 302:1349, 1980.
6. Berguer R, Kieffer E: Surgery of the Arteries to the Head. New York, Springer-Verlag, 1992.
7. Berguer R, Andaya LV, Bauer RB: Vertebral artery bypass. Arch Surg 111:976, 1976.
8. Berguer R, Bauer RB: Vertebral artery reconstruction: A successful technique in selected patients. Ann Surg 193:441, 1981.
9. Edwards WH, Mulherin JL Jr: The surgical approach to significant stenosis of vertebral and subclavian arteries. Surgery 87:20, 1980.
10. Malone JM, Moore WS, Hamilton R, et al: Combined carotid-vertebral vascular disease. Arch Surg 115:783, 1980.
11. Roon AJ, Ehrenfeld WK, Cooke PB, et al: Vertebral artery reconstruction. Am J Surg 138:29, 1979.
12. Berguer R: Distal vertebral artery bypass: Technique, the occipital connection and potential uses. J Vasc Surg 2:621, 1985.
13. Kieffer E, Rancurel G, Richart T: Reconstruction of the distal cervical vertebral artery. *In* Berguer R, Bauer RB (eds): Vertebrobasilar Arterial Occlusive Disease: Medical and Surgical Management. New York, Raven Press, 1984, pp 265–289.

121

Coiling and Kinking of the Carotid Artery

Ronald W. Busuttil, M.D., Ph.D., Leslie Memsic, M.D., and David S. Thomas, M.D.

• • •

Since the introduction of safe angiography for diagnosis of cerebrovascular disease, abnormal configurations and elongations of the carotid arteries have been readily identified. However, the potential for these tortuosities to produce cerebral ischemia has been debated at length, and widely divergent opinions have been expressed. Since a symptomatic kinked carotid artery was first successfully repaired surgically in 1951, extensive clinical experience with this entity has accumulated and has provided evidence that strongly supports a causal relationship between redundancy of the carotid artery and symptoms of cerebral ischemia.[17]

The carotid coil is found most frequently in the internal carotid, but occasionally in the common carotid, and consists chiefly of an elongation of the artery in a fixed space, which results in redundancy and tortuosity of the vessel. This redundancy, which may occur in the sagittal, transverse, or coronal plane, usually assumes an S shape, but single and even double complete loops have been described (Fig. 121–1). The carotid kink is a variant of the carotid coil in which the elongation becomes acutely angu-

lated and is often associated with atherosclerotic plaque or stenosis of the vessel (Fig. 121–2).

HISTORICAL BACKGROUND

As early as 1741, anatomists described elongated distorted carotid arteries in autopsy specimens.[19] As death was usually due to other causes, little significance was ascribed to these abnormalities. However, the redundant or kinked carotid artery became a serious threat to the unwary otolaryngologist who performed a tonsillectomy or adenoidectomy or lanced a peritonsillar abscess.[2, 5, 10, 12] In these situations, an aberrant artery could be injured, and such injury frequently resulted in fatal hemorrhage.

It was not until the 1950s that redundant and kinked carotid arteries were proposed as possible sources of hemodynamic or embolic derangements leading to brain ischemia.[17] However, agreement regarding the potential for these tortuous carotid arteries to produce cerebral symptoms is not universal. Angiographic and autopsy studies

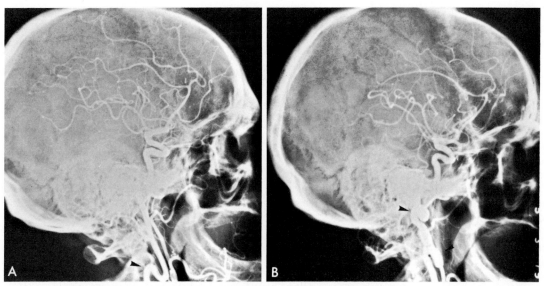

FIGURE 121–1. *A,* S-shaped internal carotid coil. *B,* Two complete internal carotid loops.

indicate that carotid redundancy is not uncommon, and that persons exhibiting such anatomy, for the most part, are asymptomatic and require no therapy.[8] However, a growing body of clinical experience suggests that, although perhaps the majority of carotid kinks are incidental findings with no clinical significance, a subset of patients with carotid artery kinks manifest cerebral ischemic symptoms as a direct consequence of carotid angulation.

The first successful surgical relief of cerebral ischemia caused by a kinked carotid artery was reported by Riser and associates in 1951.[17] In their patient, an elongated carotid artery was straightened by affixing the artery to the sheath of the sternocleidomastoid muscle. Five years later, Hsu and Kistin reported the first direct surgical repair of a kinked carotid artery, and, in 1959, Quattlebaum and coworkers published their experience with three cases successfully treated by resection and reanastomosis of the common carotid artery.[9, 15] With the advent of a reliable, safe technique for carotid endarterectomy and a better understanding of the potential of kinks to produce transient ischemic attacks and stroke, a more aggressive surgical approach to this lesion has been adopted.

REDUNDANCY OF THE CAROTID ARTERIES

Incidence

The incidence of angulated carotid arteries in the general population is unknown. Random anatomic studies in patients who have died of other causes suggest a 30 per cent incidence.[2] Angiographic reviews indicate that redundant carotid arteries occur in 10 to 43 per cent of patients studied, with kinking occurring in 4 to 16 per cent.[1, 12, 22] Redundant carotid arteries have been reported to occur in patients of all ages, including fetuses, with the overall average age being 55 years. The ratio of males:females is equal in angulated internal carotid arteries, but women outnumber men 4:1 for common carotid artery kinking.

The incidence of symptomatic carotid elongation is even more difficult to estimate, but it appears to be small but significant. In a series by Weibel and Fields, 52 of 88 patients with unilateral or bilateral coiling of the internal carotid artery presented with cerebrovascular symptoms.[23] Of these, only 11 per cent (10 patients) were felt to be symptomatic as a result of the coil itself. Because no stenosis of the coil was noted in 9 patients, a direct correlation could be made between cerebral vascular ischemia and coiling in only one of the 88 patients, or 1.1 per cent. Other

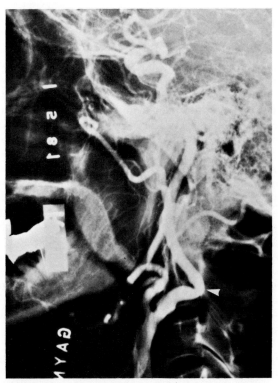

FIGURE 121–2. Internal carotid kink with associated bifurcation atheroma. External carotid artery is also elongated.

authors conclude similarly that symptoms rarely occur when coiling is present unless atherosclerotic occlusive disease is also present in the carotid arteries or in the vertebrobasilar system.

In a series of 65 patients in whom unilateral or bilateral kinking of the internal carotid was present, 51 per cent (33 patients) experienced some degree of cerebrovascular insufficiency.[23] However, work-up revealed that neurologic symptoms were not always related to the degree of angulation itself but rather to the presence of atheroma in the kinked segment. Symptoms of cerebrovascular insufficiency appeared to be directly related to the stenosis at the level of the kinking in only 10 of 33 patients, representing 18 per cent of the total number of patients found to have kinking of the internal carotid artery.

Several other factors, such as variation in blood pressure, alterations in head and neck positions, and extracranial or intracranial occlusive diseases, contribute significantly to the production of cerebral symptoms. In 60 patients found to have severe carotid kinking (angle less than 30 degrees) on angiogram in the study by Metz and associates, 14 (23 per cent) had had a significant cerebrovascular accident (stroke, 8; single transient ischemic attack [TIA], 2; recurrent TIA, 4).[13] In a series by Harrison and Davalos, 46 of 424 (19 per cent) patients evaluated by arteriography for cerebrovascular disease were found to have symptoms attributable to tortuosity of the carotid artery.[6] All of these studies are skewed by the fact that only patients who have come to angiography are included in the statistical analysis.

The lesions have been surgically corrected in patients from the age of 9.5 months to 93 years; the mean age is 57 years. However, carotid kinks compose a small portion of those operations performed for symptomatic carotid occlusive disease. Najafi and colleagues reported a 5 per cent incidence of kinking in a series of 308 patients undergoing carotid procedures.[14] Vannix and associates[22] noted 15 instances of kinking in their series of 312 carotid reconstructions (4.8 per cent), and a review of the UCLA experience over the last 13 years reveals only 10 of 670 carotid operations performed for symptomatic carotid kinks, for an incidence of 1.4 per cent.

Etiology

The etiology of carotid coils and kinks is multi-factorial and involves both embryologic and developmental aberrations and degenerative processes associated with atherosclerosis. The carotid coils seen in fetuses, infants, and children appear to be of developmental origin. Embryologically, the carotid artery arises from the third aortic arch and the dorsal aorta. During fetal maturation, the carotid artery straightens as the fetal heart and great vessels descend into the thorax. Should the descent of the heart not keep pace with the growth of the spine, however, the result is a redundancy of the carotid artery in the fixed cervical area. This discrepancy between the growth rate of the vascular system and that of skeletal spine undoubtedly plays an important role in the pathogenesis of the elongated carotid artery in children. Approximately 50 per cent of children with carotid elongation have it bilaterally, and it is at times associated with other vascular anomalies such as aortic coarctation.

On the other hand, bilaterally occurring carotid elongations exist in only 25 per cent of adult patients. The kinked carotid in the adult clearly falls within the pathologic spectrum of atherosclerotic degeneration and is marked by familiar stigmata of the disease. These include a frequent association with hypertension and peripheral vascular occlusive disease. Although kinks can be found in carotid arteries not affected by atherosclerosis, there is often concomitant intimal ulceration and plaque deposition, and occasionally aneurysm formation. The elongated carotid seen in the adult has a weak, inelastic wall and is quite friable, which at times makes surgical repair technically demanding.

Because the origin and boundaries of the carotid artery are fixed, there is a predisposition to elongation secondary to hemodynamic lateral forces. Proximally, the common carotid is tethered to the immobile subclavian artery, and distally the external carotid is fixed by its nutritive branches and the internal carotid by the base of the skull. Fibrous bands arising in response to atherosclerotic inflammation further fix the proximal common carotid and its bifurcation, leaving the proximal internal carotid available for preferential elongation and tortuosity in response to decreasing elasticity. In most cases, atherosclerotic plaques are found proximal to internal carotid kinks. Hypertension appears to be associated with elongation of the common carotid but affects fewer than 50 per cent of patients with elongation of the internal carotid. In an extensive angiographic review by Metz and associates, no association between severity of the kinking and either high blood pressure or increasing age was noted.[13]

Symptoms

Although carotid coils not associated with atherosclerosis have been implicated as sources of cerebral ischemia on occasion, especially in children,[18] it is the acutely angled carotid kink that is most commonly responsible for neurologic symptoms in patients with elongated carotid arteries. The carotid kink may produce symptoms from either reduction in flow or dislodgment of fibrin and platelet emboli.[19] Although flow reduction may occur as the kink becomes more acutely angulated as a result of either further elongation or atheromatous build-up, the most common causative mechanism is axial twisting when the patient turns his or her head to the side.[16] In most cases, ipsilateral rotation results in the greatest reduction in flow, but contralateral rotation, neck flexion, and extension also exaggerate the kink and markedly reduce flow.[20] In certain circumstances, head turning will produce total occlusion of an otherwise patent but redundant artery. A history of either focal neurologic deficit or vertebrobasilar insufficiency that is incited by head motion should arouse suspicion that there is a carotid kink.

The spectrum of ischemic symptoms produced by the carotid kink is the same as that produced by carotid ulceration or stenosis. Patients with unilateral kinks may present with amaurosis fugax, intermittent hemiparesis, aphasia, or stroke. Bilateral kinks are often associated with syncope, vertigo, global ischemia, and derangements of posterior circulation. Carotid angulation in children has been associated with learning disabilities as well as focal and grand mal seizures.

Diagnosis

There are no pathognomonic signs of the carotid kink to be found on physical examination. In rare cases, a prominent pulsation suggestive of a carotid aneurysm can be palpated in the neck. This mass is often accentuated when the head is turned and frequently (if the kink involves the internal carotid artery) is best palpated intraorally in the tonsillar fossa.[19] Seldom, with the head in the neutral position, will a bruit or thrill be present unless there is concomitant atherosclerotic stenosis. However, when auscultation is performed with the head turned to either side, a bruit may become audible.

Noninvasive oculoplethysmography has been helpful in identifying kinked carotid arteries that are hemodynamically significant. When performed with the patient's head in various positions, including right and left rotation, extension, and flexion as well as neutral, it may unmask a reduction in carotid blood flow. There is one report of an abnormal oculoplethysmogram that correlated with a decreased flow as measured intraoperatively during positional testing.[20] Although such positional testing is helpful in identifying hemodynamically significant kinking, the true incidence of false-positive oculoplethysmograms has not been adequately established, and thus this test must be corroborated by angiography.

Technetium-pertechnetate cerebral perfusion scans have demonstrated decreased hemispheric flow on the same side as the angulation; more recently, regional cerebral blood flow studies have been used to assess the relationship between kinks and cerebral ischemia.[8, 11, 21]

Electroencephalography has been of little value in the evaluation of angulation of the internal carotid artery, although electroencephalographic changes during head rotation have been described.[7, 18, 20]

The definitive diagnosis of carotid coils and kinks is by extracranial and intracranial angiography. Complete evaluation of the carotid kink dictates multiple views taken in flexion, extension, and right and left rotation. Careful attention must be paid to diagnosing concurrent atherosclerotic intimal plaques and ulcers, which are often present and may be responsible for the patient's symptoms.

Natural History and Indications for Surgery

Carotid coils and kinks have been well defined only for the last 35 years. Most patients in whom the diagnosis is made have symptoms of cerebrovascular insufficiency that have led to angiography. No large group of asymptomatic patients with carotid coils has been followed without therapy to define the natural history of this lesion. There are anecdotal reports of coiled carotid arteries found at autopsy of patients who died of noncerebral causes, suggesting that those with asymptomatic coils without athero-

sclerosis, plaques, or kinking may be safely followed. In the symptomatic patient with a carotid coil, surgical therapy is justified once a careful medical evaluation has excluded cardiac arrhythmias, hypertension, positional hypotension, cerebral tumors, or other causes of intermittent cerebral ischemia.

As mentioned previously, the carotid kink must be viewed with more caution. Certainly, any patient with focal hemispheric ischemic symptoms who has a kink demonstrated on angiography should undergo surgical repair. In this situation, surgical repair is advocated even in the absence of demonstrable atherosclerotic disease. If the primary symptoms are global, before surgical correction of the kink is recommended the following criteria should be fulfilled: (1) exclusion of an intracranial lesion, (2) control of hypertension, (3) reproduction of symptoms with head rotation, and (4) angiographic demonstration of a kink that causes a 50 per cent luminal stenosis or an angle of less than 60 degrees between contiguous segments.[13] The criteria for selection of surgical therapy for patients with "vertebrobasilar insufficiency" and for those with a demonstrable carotid kink are similar.

Available information is inadequate to formulate a precise algorithm for the management of the asymptomatic patient who has a kinked carotid demonstrated during angiography for an unrelated condition. In this situation, it would seem prudent to recommend prophylactic surgical repair if the kink reduces vessel diameter more than 50 per cent. Lesser degrees of narrowing should be treated expectantly, but the patient should be followed with periodic oculoplethysmograms. If they suggest a hemodynamic stenosis, repeated angiography should be performed. In those patients who present with global or focal symptoms and are found to have bilateral carotid kinks, a case can be made to repair both lesions in a staged procedure if the lesions fit the aforementioned criteria. Some authors, however, report resolution of symptoms with correction of one side only.[3]

Surgical Therapy

The objectives of surgical therapy are elimination of the carotid kink, disposal of any associated plaque, and restoration of normal vascular continuity. An integral part of all procedures is meticulous dissection of all fibrous

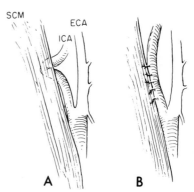

FIGURE 21–3. *A* and *B*, Elongation of internal carotid artery (ICA) by pexis to sternocleidomastoid muscle (SCM). ECA, external carotid artery.

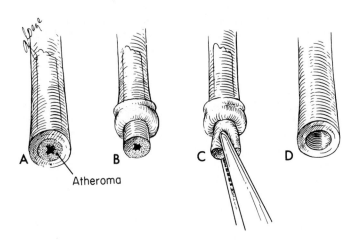

Atheroma

FIGURE 121–4. *A–D*, Eversion endarterectomy of ICA during shortening procedure.

bands and complete mobilization of the arteries, particularly the high internal carotid. Complete lysis of fibrous bands surrounding the artery affords a widening of the angle of kinking and allows a more accurate assessment of the redundant length.[11, 19]

The earliest surgical correction was nonresectional; the artery was affixed to the fascia on the underside of the sternocleidomastoid muscle (Fig. 121–3).[17] This procedure reduces the kink by realigning the vessel in a more vertical plane. Today, this method is of mainly historical interest and is used only as a last resort in an extremely poor-risk patient with friable vessels and short redundancy, and when it is certain that no atherosclerotic plaque exists. Its advantages are lack of interruption of cerebral blood flow and short operating time under local anesthesia. Other nonresection techniques have been advocated as well, but in practice these are rarely, if ever, applied. These methods include lysis of adhesions, which may be a rare cause of carotid angulation from an inflammatory source, and bypass.[4] In the bypass procedure, flow across the angulated segment is rerouted through a vein graft or fabric prosthesis. Such bypasses are found to have a high rate of postoperative occlusion and have generally been abandoned.

Many techniques have been used to correct the redundancy by partial resection of the common or internal carotid artery.[11, 15, 16, 22] All the resective procedures may be combined with carotid endarterectomy, which can be easily performed by utilizing the eversion technique (Fig. 121–4). The preferred procedure is to remove a segment of normal proximal common carotid or carotid bifurcation. Traction is

placed on the internal carotid artery until the kink is straightened, and reanastomosis of the cut ends of the vessels is then accomplished. This procedure often necessitates ligation of the external carotid artery, unless it too is redundant. By resection of the common carotid artery, the surgeon can place the anastomosis in the relatively firm, normal common carotid rather than in the flimsy, friable internal carotid, which holds sutures poorly. The main disadvantages of this technique, which are minor, are loss of the potential collateral vessels from the external carotid and possible disruption of carotid sinus nerves (Fig. 121–5).

The more anatomic procedure involves primary resection of the kinked portion of the internal carotid artery and reanastomosis with or without a patch angioplasty. As just mentioned, one disadvantage of this technique is the use of a smaller, more friable internal carotid, and another is the anatomic difficulty when the kink is in close proximity to the base of the skull (Fig. 121–6). An alternative method involves no resection but only transplantation of the origin of the internal carotid artery. The internal carotid artery is detached from the carotid bifurcation and reanastomosed more proximally to either the anterior or the lateral surface of the common carotid. Exact placement must be determined at the time of operation by rotating the patient's head to make certain the new location will not produce a new kink (Fig. 121–7).

The surgeon must be familiar with the various types of repair because the anatomic relationships, as determined at operation, will dictate the type of repair needed. Although local anesthesia has been recommended by Quattle-

Ext. carotid a.

Int. carotid a.

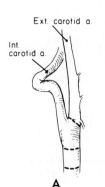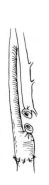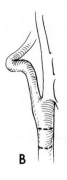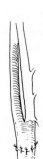

A   B

FIGURE 121–5. *A and B*, Resection of common carotid artery with reanastomosis. If ECA is also redundant, as shown in Figure 121–2, it may not require ligation.

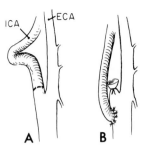

FIGURE 121–6. *A and B, Resection and reanastomosis of ICA.*

baum and coworkers, general anesthesia is preferable because of the extensive dissection required for adequate internal carotid mobilization at the base of the skull.[16] Both techniques can be used quite safely, however. The use of internal carotid shunts during repair should be selective. The principles governing the indications for shunting are the same as those previously discussed for general atherosclerotic bifurcation lesions of the carotid. In the repair of a carotid kink, the internal shunt offers the added advantage of stenting the anastomosis for ease of repair. However, extra care must be taken when inserting the shunt, and the artery must be fully mobilized and straightened prior to shunt insertion lest initial damage occur.

Implemented by the various techniques already outlined, collective experience with patients with focal hemispheric ischemia secondary to carotid kinks has been excellent. More than 80 per cent of patients have been relieved of symptoms, with approximately 5 per cent mortality and intraoperative stroke rate.[4, 7, 16, 20, 22] Patients with less specific symptoms, as would be expected, had a lesser percentage of satisfactory results.

SUMMARY

Carotid coils and kinks arise from both developmental and degenerative changes in the extracranial carotid vasculature. Coils are usually innocuous unless accompanied by deposition of atherosclerotic plaque. Kinks frequently produce cerebral symptoms with or without associated atherosclerosis. The pathogenic mechanism for cerebral ischemia is either an axial distortion that reduces luminal diameter or dislodgment of fibrin and platelet emboli. The carotid kink

must be highly suspect when the patient presents with cerebrovascular ischemia related to positional head change. Arteriography is the definitive means for diagnosis, although oculoplethysmography during changes of head position may be helpful. Generally, patients with coils or loops should be treated nonoperatively, and excellent results can be expected. The asymptomatic patient with a kink should also be treated nonoperatively unless the kink has demonstrated hemodynamic significance. Symptomatic patients with carotid kinks are candidates for surgical reconstruction.

References

1. Bauer R, Sheehan S, Meyer JS: Arteriographic study of cerebrovascular disease. Arch Neurol 4:119, 1961.
2. Cairney J: Tortuosity of the cervical segment of the internal carotid artery. J Anat 59:87, 1924.
3. Daskalakis MK: Coiling of the carotid arteries. S Med J 80(3):387, 1987.
4. Derrick JR, Kirksey TD, Estess M, et al: Kinking of the carotid arteries. Clinical considerations. Am Surg 32:503, 1966.
5. Fisher AGT: Sigmoid tortuosity of the internal carotid artery and its relation to tonsil and pharynx. Lancet 2:128, 1915.
6. Harrison JH, Davalos PA: Cerebral ischemia. Surgical procedure in cases due to tortuosity and buckling of the cervical vessels. Arch Surg 84:85, 1962.
7. Henly WW, Cooley DA, Gordon WB, et al: Tortuosity of the internal carotid artery. Report of seven cases treated surgically. Postgrad Med 31:133, 1962.
8. Herrschaft P, Duus P, Glenn F, et al: Preoperative and postoperative cerebral flow in patients with carotid artery stenoses. In Lanfitt TW, McHenry LCM Jr, Reivich M (eds): Cerebral Circulation and Metabolism. New York, Springer-Verlag, 1975, pp 276–282.
9. Hsu I, Kistin AD: Buckling of the great vessels. Arch Intern Med 98:712, 1956.
10. Jackson JL: Tortuosity of the internal carotid artery and its relation to tonsillectomy. Can Med Assoc J 29:475, 1933.
11. Leipzig TJ, Dohrmann GJ: The tortuous or kinked carotid artery: Pathogenesis and clinical considerations. Surg Neurol 25:478, 1986.
12. McKenzie W, Woolf CI: Carotid abnormalities and adenoid surgery. J Laryngol Otol 73:596, 1959.
13. Metz H, Murray-Leslie RM, Bannister RG, et al: Kinking of the internal carotid artery in relation to cerebrovascular disease. Lancet 1:424, 1961.
14. Najafi H, Javid H, Dye WS: Kinked internal carotid artery. Arch Surg 89:135, 1964.
15. Quattlebaum JK Jr, Upson ET, Neville RL: Stroke associated with elongation and kinking of the internal carotid artery. Ann Surg 150:824, 1959.
16. Quattlebaum JK Jr, Wade JS, Whiddon CM: Stroke associated with elongation and kinking of the carotid artery. Long-term follow-up. Ann Surg 177:572, 1973.
17. Riser MM, Géraud J, Ducoudray J, et al: Dolicho-carotide interne avec syndrome vertigineux. Rev Neurol (Paris) 85:145, 1951.
18. Sarkari NBS, Holmes JM, Bickerstaff ER: Neurological manifestation associated with internal carotid loops and kinks in children. J Neurol Neurosurg Psychiat 33:194, 1970.
19. Schechter DC: Dolichocarotid syndrome. Cerebral ischemia related to cervical carotid artery redundancy with kinking. I and II. NY State J Med 79:1391, 1542, 1979.
20. Stanton PE Jr, McClusky DA Jr, Lamis PA: Hemodynamic assessment and surgical correction of kinking of the internal carotid artery. Surgery 84:793, 1978.
21. Trackler RT, Mikulicich AG: Diminished cerebral perfusion resulting from kinking of the internal carotid artery. J Nucl Med 15:634, 1974.
22. Vannix RS, Joergenson FJ, Carter R: Kinking of the internal carotid artery. Clinical significance and surgical management. Am J Surg 134:82, 1977.
23. Weibel J, Fields WS: Tortuosity, coiling, and kinking of the internal carotid artery: Relationship of morphological variation to cerebrovascular insufficiency. Neurology 15:462, 1965.

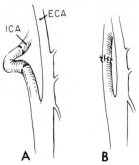

FIGURE 121–7. *A and B, Transection and reimplantation of ICA.*

Extracranial Fibromuscular Arterial Dysplasia

Robert B. Rutherford, M.D.

• • •

Fibrodysplasia of extracranial cerebral arteries is not common, yet the internal carotid artery is second only to the renal artery as a site of predilection. It is found in less than 1 per cent (0.25 per cent,[1] 0.68 per cent[2]) of consecutive cerebral arteriograms. The nature of this unusual nonatheromatous, noninflammatory arterial disease is still not totally clear. It appears to be a degenerative process that primarily involves long, unbranched segments of middle-sized arteries, e.g., the renal, internal carotid, external iliac, splenic and hepatic arteries (in order of frequency of involvement).[3, 4] Although this disease is fully described in Chapter 14, certain aspects pertinent to its involvement of the extracranial cerebral arteries are summarized here. Of the at least four distinct types, the internal carotid artery (like the renal) is predominantly involved with medial fibroplasia, the so-called string of beads lesion (Fig. 122–1). In one large series,[1] this type was seen in 89 per cent, with a fusiform narrowing in 7 per cent and an eccentric septum-like lesion in 4 per cent. Except for the latter lesion, the involvement tends to be located much higher than arteriosclerosis, in the middle and even upper thirds of the internal carotid artery. Characteristically, the artery tends to be elongated and is even kinked on occasion. On average, these lesions are bilateral in over one half of cases, with a range of 39 to 86 per cent being reported.[1, 3, 5] Close to 90 per cent of patients are women in most series.[3, 5–8] Patients with internal carotid involvement present about 10 years later than those with renal involvement. In one series, 78 per cent were in the 5th, 6th, or 7th decade of life.[6] It is possible that the later presentation relates to the fact that internal carotid lesions tend to be asymptomatic, whereas renal artery lesions are detected earlier because they cause hypertension and taking the blood pressure is a more routine part of physical examination than listening for carotid bruits.

ASSOCIATED LESIONS

There are four lesions found frequently enough in association with carotid fibromuscular dysplasia (FMD) to complicate its management, particularly in assigning treatment priorities. *First,* because of the older age of these patients, associated atheromatous disease of the carotid artery is seen in as many as 20 per cent of individuals.[9] This sometimes creates difficulties in assigning blame for symp-

toms and deciding on the appropriate surgical technique. *Second,* vertebral arterial involvement is seen in 7 to 19 per cent of those with carotid FMD lesions,[6] and, occasionally, it is found as an unexpected isolated finding. Fortunately, it is rarely responsible for symptoms and thus does not usually complicate the management of the internal carotid le-

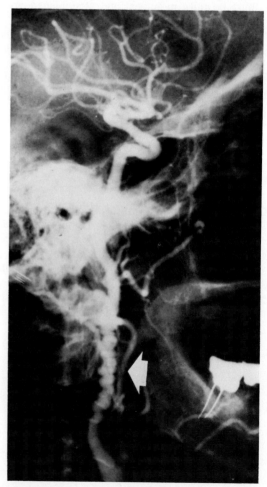

FIGURE 122–1. Carotid arteriogram demonstrating the classic appearance of fibromuscular dysplasia *(arrow)* in the usual location opposite the C1–C3 vertebral bodies and intervening discs. Note low bifurcation and long internal carotid artery.

sion. *Third,* intracranial aneurysms, another expression of the dysplastic process, are found in at least 10 per cent[6] and as many as 51 per cent[5] of patients with internal carotid FMD (average, about 20 per cent). Not only do these pose an independent threat (of rupture and subarachnoid hemorrhage) but their natural history could potentially be aggravated by relieving a proximal stenosis. *Finally,* the coexistence of renal artery FMD, in 25 to 50 per cent, creates a problem not so much with treatment priorities as with the correct sequence. These aspects are discussed later in this chapter.

CLINICAL PRESENTATION AND NATURAL HISTORY

Most reported series document the clinical presentation of carotid FMD but do not allow precise delineation of its natural history because they are naturally skewed toward symptomatic lesions. In two articles on this entity, Patman and coworkers[10] and Stewart and associates[11] flatly insist that these lesions should not be operated on until their natural history is defined! This advice is quite impractical. There is no way to define the natural history of these relatively *rare* lesions without a practical method of detecting asymptomatic lesions. At the moment, asymptomatic lesions are usually detected by either the chance auscultation of a bruit, which is unlikely because the lesion is usually located so high in the internal carotid, or incidental discovery by cerebral angiography performed for other reasons. To recommend following all lesions detected clinically, by whatever means, would not be ethical because a significant proportion of them will present with serious symptoms (see later). A major multi-center cooperative study, in which half the symptomatic and half the asymptomatic lesions are prospectively randomized to treatment, might be a more acceptable approach, but, having just been through a number of extremely expensive carotid endarterectomy trials, it seems extremely unlikely that a similar effort for carotid FMD could gain funding or, if funded, could gather sufficient data to allow meaningful conclusions in less than 10 years.

Thus, we must deal with the clinical data at hand and extrapolate. If nothing else, they show that these lesions are not innocuous. In the University of California, San Francisco, experience, reported by Effeney,[3] 41 per cent presented with transient ischemic attacks (TIAs) (23 per cent amaurosis fugax), 22 per cent with completed strokes (2 per cent temporary stroke), 31 per cent with nonlateralizing symptoms, and 6 per cent with miscellaneous other features (e.g., asymptomatic bruits). Nine per cent were left with a significant permanent neurologic deficit. In this same series, 77 per cent had bruits and 37 per cent were hypertensive. Other reported series, by Starr and coworkers[12] and Collins and associates,[13] were remarkably similar in presenting symptoms. In Stewart and associates' series,[11] consisting of 49 angiographically documented cases, 29 per cent presented with TIAs, 22 per cent were asymptomatic, and 12 per cent had suffered stroke. However, half of the latter were secondary to hemorrhages from intracranial aneu-

rysms and, thus, only 6 per cent had ischemic strokes. In So and colleagues' more recent report,[6] 18 of 32 patients (58 per cent) presented with the sudden onset of focal symptoms. Half of these (9 of 18) had cerebral infarcts (29 per cent of the total), 8 had hemispheric TIAs, and 1 had amaurosis fugax. In contrast, only 3 of 37 patients (8 per cent) in the Karolinska experience reported by Mettinger and Ericson[5] had suffered a stroke. However, a significant portion of these cases were asymptomatic patients whose lesion was detected incidentally on cerebral angiography. Finally, in one series of 79 patients, most of whom were found to have this lesion incidentally on cerebral angiogram (0.6 per cent of the total), only 3 patients (4 per cent) *subsequently* suffered a cerebral ischemic event during an average follow-up of 5 years.[7] This is as close to a natural history study of asymptomatic lesions as any reported in the literature.

To summarize, although more than half of the patients in "surgical" series presented with cerebral ischemic events, half of which resulted in infarct, only about 10 per cent of the total ended up disabled by significant neurologic deficits. Looked at prospectively rather than retrospectively, fewer than 10 per cent of patients with such lesions will go on to develop new neurologic symptoms.[4, 5, 7] If one considers only incidentally discovered, asymptomatic lesions (including those with relatively minor degrees of narrowing), this risk may appear to be reduced even further (e.g., 5 per cent). Nevertheless, two series have shown that about a third of these lesions will demonstrate significant angiographic progression with time.[4, 6] Importantly, none of these studies has followed expectantly a significant number of either symptomatic lesions or *high-grade* asymptomatic stenoses, where the risk of stroke could be expected to be much higher.

One other aspect is occasionally brought up in considering the threat posed by carotid FMD: its possible role in producing spontaneous dissection of the carotid artery. This often catastrophic event is said to be responsible for 4 per cent of strokes and is claimed to be associated with fibrodysplasia in at least 15 per cent of cases.[14] It is difficult to understand how this latter figure is arrived at, with so little crossover existing between the literature on these two entities. Even though carotid FMD often leads the list of suggested underlying etiologies in reported series of spontaneous dissections, it cannot be said with any conviction that this adds significantly to the threat posed by an asymptomatic lesion. It should be pointed out that, although fibrodysplasia may be involved to a degree in both, the two appear to be quite separate expressions of the dysplastic process, with spontaneous dissection characteristically occurring in younger males. To the author's knowledge, there are no recorded cases of a typical internal carotid FMD lesion later presenting with a classic "spontaneous" dissection, although occasional progression to focal occlusion does occur. Again, prospective studies are unlikely to solve this dilemma, and although careful postmortem examination of the carotid arteries of all patients dying following spontaneous carotid dissection might ultimately supply a definitive answer, such an undertaking would be arduous and time-consuming and likely to succeed only in a very controlled medical environment.

DIAGNOSTIC EVALUATION

It goes without saying that these patients require a careful history plus a neurologic examination, and those with focal or diffuse neurologic symptoms suggesting cerebral ischemic events obviously deserve a brain scan (computed tomography [CT] or magnetic resonance imaging [MRI]) and complete cerebral angiography. However, the latter cannot be routinely recommended for asymptomatic patients with carotid bruits or those with documented renal FMD lesions. A duplex scan can be obtained, but these FMD lesions are often so high that they cannot always be readily demonstrated by this approach and may only be suspected by indirect noninvasive tests such as oculoplethysmography (OPG) or periorbital Doppler examination. Eventually, three-dimensional CT scans or magnetic resonance angiography may solve this dilemma. Intracranial Doppler examination would also be helpful in some cases, but, at this writing, these last three diagnostic modalities are not widely available, and established indirect tests will continue to be employed. In this regard, a positive OPG or periorbital Doppler examination can also be used to gauge the hemodynamic significance of a bruit-causing lesion, the former usually being positive with over 60 per cent stenosis, the latter with 80 per cent or greater stenosis. Furthermore, the former can be performed in those suspected of kinking with the patient's head and neck in the particular positions known to be associated with symptoms. These tests are therefore still useful, particularly in evaluating asymptomatic patients or those with global symptoms (e.g., syncopal attacks) for operation, for one would only consider patients with hemodynamically significant lesions in these settings, and the hemodynamic significance of a string-of-beads lesion is difficult to determine from angiograms, particularly if there is redundancy or kinking.

Suffice it to say, this is not a lesion one treats simply because it exists or for innocuous or vague symptoms (e.g., dizziness or tinnitus). One must convince oneself (and others) that the lesion was or is capable of producing significant symptoms. For this reason, the described noninvasive testing *and* angiography will usually both be required, unless the patient has clear-cut focal symptoms.

TREATMENT

It must be apparent from the previous attempt to characterize fibrodysplasia of the internal carotid artery that complexities frequently arise in dealing with these lesions, and a number of questions need to be answered before deciding on appropriate management. For example, what symptoms can be attributed to these lesions (particularly in the face of associated atherosclerotic changes)? What is the natural history of these lesions (i.e., how frequently do they progress and become symptomatic)? If they do not infrequently progress, should very narrow but asymptomatic stenoses or tight septa be surgically treated? How does contralateral involvement modify one's approach? What are the relative importances of proximal internal carotid fibrodysplasia and distal intracranial aneurysms when they coexist on the same side and to what extent does one compro-

mise the treatment of the other? If there is renal involvement with hypertension, what is the appropriate treatment sequence? Should percutaneous balloon angioplasty, popular in dealing with similar renal artery disease, be applied to internal carotid lesions? And, finally, what is the best approach when surgical intervention is indicated?

INDICATIONS FOR INTERVENTION

Based on these observations, and the relative safety and effectiveness of surgical intervention (see later), operative management would seem appropriate for (1) lesions causing focal ischemic events (hemispheric or ocular), (2) lesions causing *documented* episodes of cerebral hypoperfusion (rare), and (3) asymptomatic *critical* stenoses in otherwise healthy patients with either bilateral disease (worst side only) or with documented defects in collateral circulation pathways (e.g., circle of Willis or vertebrobasilar system).

The first indication requires little elaboration, assuming the responsible arterial segment has not progressed to occlusion, because it can be assumed that the lesion has not only already declared itself but also remains a significant threat. Hypoperfusion events, on the other hand, are more problematic. Without significant defects in the circle of Willis, it is unlikely for an uncomplicated *unilateral* carotid FMD lesion to cause transient cerebral hypoperfusion. Nevertheless, this *can* occur. One explanation is that these segments are often redundant so that kinking could be responsible for these symptoms. More likely, such a patient will be one in whom associated hypertension has been overmedicated and this is the explanation for the transient dizziness. Therefore, true syncopal attacks in a patient with a significantly narrowed FMD lesion and with *stable* blood pressure and no other explanation for symptoms deserve further consideration, particularly in those patients with bilateral disease, with tight unilateral stenoses with poor intracranial collaterals, or with associated kinking. However, these same specific settings also deserve consideration in asymptomatic patients, and the key to proper patient selection here lies in the diagnostic assessment of both hemodynamic significance and operative risk.

SURGICAL TREATMENT

The usual fibrodysplastic lesion encountered in the internal carotid artery, like its renal counterpart, responds nicely to gentle dilatation. Surgical dilatation has been largely replaced by percutaneous transluminal balloon dilatation for renal lesions, but this approach is contraindicated for carotid lesions for these reasons: (1) embolism, which occurs to some degree in close to 10 per cent of percutaneous transluminal angioplasty (PTA), may be discounted as being of little clinical consequence in lower extremity PTAs and tolerable in view of the advantages of percutaneous treatment over a major abdominal operation for renal lesions, but it would be disastrous if it occurred in the carotid artery distribution; (2) most carotid lesions for which intervention is justified will have already presented with embolic cerebral ischemic events making them more at risk for this complication, whereas most renal lesions create symptoms by renal hypoperfusion with secondary hypertension; (3) surgical dilatation of the carotid lesion is a simple, safe operation—considerably safer than carotid endarterectomy, if proper technique is used.

The operation performed is basically the same as originally described by Morris and colleagues,[8] although a number of subtle refinements have been added to eliminate some problems encountered in early experiences. Exposure is initially gained much as for carotid endarterectomy except that, although the bifurcation is characteristically located *lower* than usual in these cases, one needs *higher* internal carotid exposure to ensure that safe dilatation is carried out under direct vision. In the usual procedure, an incision is made along the anterior border of the sternocleidomastoid muscle along its middle and upper thirds. Dissection is carried just anterior to this muscle, and then just anterior to the underlying internal jugular vein for the length of the incision, thereby avoiding the ''vascular'' lymphatic plexus and nodes directly overlying the carotid bifurcation. Division of the common facial vein will normally lead to ready exposure of the carotid bifurcation. The common and external carotid (and the superior thyroid) arteries are controlled with tapes after anesthetizing the sinus nerve, and then dissection is carried upward along the posterior aspect of the internal carotid in the space between it and the internal jugular vein, avoiding the hypoglossal nerve, the location of which is usually betrayed by following upward along the course of the ansa hypoglossi to where the two merge. Often, a small artery and vein hook around those nerves at this point, and these must be carefully divided to allow nerve retraction and further upward dissection. In high lesions, the posterior belly of the digastric muscle may need to be divided, but subluxation of the mandible is rarely required. The normal arterial segment above the highest point of involvement will be apparent by inspection, and the internal carotid is encircled at this point by a double-looped Silastic tape. Care is taken not to manipulate the intervening segment of the internal carotid artery as it is gently exposed throughout its length. Stump pressures or electroencephalographic (EEG) monitoring are *not* ordinarily needed for this brief procedure, but may be indicated if there is evidence of poor collateral circulation on noninvasive testing and/or angiography, and a more extensive procedure, such as the correction of redundancy, is planned. Except in such unusual circumstances, an indwelling shunt is an unnecessary complication.

Although heparin might not be absolutely necessary in the usual brief operation, the author not only prefers to give 100 U/kg of heparin prior to interrupting flow but also administers a single 500-ml unit of dextran 40, at 25 ml/hr, during the immediate postoperative period, beginning at the time of operation. This provides protection against early deposition of thrombotic material on the inner surfaces of the arteriotomy and the fractured septae. The common carotid artery is cross-clamped proximally 5 minutes after heparin administration and the external carotid is controlled with a Rumel tourniquet. In many cases, traction on one or the other, or both, of these will straighten out the internal carotid artery. If not, this can usually be achieved by trac-

tion on a simple Silastic ''sling'' placed around the internal carotid just above the bifurcation. After this essential step, a short arteriotomy is made in the internal carotid at the base of the bulb. Graduated ''coronary'' dilators, dipped in sterile silicone lubricant, are then gently passed up the straightened internal carotid artery, beginning with a 1.5-mm diameter probe and progressing up to a 3.5-mm, or, occasionally, a 4.0-mm diameter probe (Fig. 122–2). There is usually a series of ''giving'' sensations felt as each septal stenosis is gently fractured for the first time, but this is not felt thereafter. The procedure is terminated after the segment has been seen to be gently stretched to full diameter throughout its course. It is important not to exceed this gentle stretching and thus not to proceed beyond a 4-mm diameter dilator. These dysplastic arteries are friable and easily split, another reason not to employ *blind* balloon dilatation. However, blind dilatation with probes is just as bad. The upper limits of the disease must be fully exposed. If not, as in lesions that extend into the upper third of the internal carotid, preparations for fluoroscopic imaging must be made and transluminal balloon dilatation is used instead. Some prefer the latter as a routine, but, in the author's opinion, it is too time-consuming and expensive for the usual case. Copious back-bleeding following each passage of the dilators prevents embolism, and the arteriotomy can then be quickly closed with a simple running suture of 5–0 or 6–0 Prolene. Careful interrogation of the entire segment with a Doppler probe or duplex scanner after restoration of flow assures patency without turbulence or residual defect.

Occasionally, if there is significant associated bifurcation atherosclerosis (and confusion regarding which is responsible for the ischemic attacks), a concomitant endarterectomy may need to be carried out, in which case the initial arteriotomy will be *longitudinal*. If there is severe elongation and kinking, such that the latter cannot be ruled out as a cause of hypoperfusion episodes (particularly position-related syncope), an oblique arteriotomy, initially placed anteriorly at the base of the carotid bulb at the bifurcation,

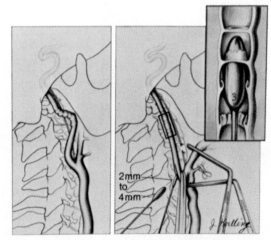

FIGURE 122–2. Drawing illustrating the main features of the operative technique. Straightening of the carotid artery from the preoperative state shown on the left and gentle graduated dilatation from 2 to 4 mm. *Inset,* The mechanism of rupture of the stenotic membranes. (From Effeney D, Ehrenfeld WK, Stoney RJ, Wylie EJ: Fibromuscular dysplasia of the internal carotid artery. World J Surg 3:179, 1979.)

can be extended circumferentially after completing the dilatation and then carried longitudinally down the common carotid artery allowing the internal carotid to be translocated downward until it is straightened out and anastomosed at this lower position. Otherwise, a short transverse arteriotomy is preferred and used in the vast majority of the cases.

Results of Surgical Dilatation

Although no operation is without risk, this procedure should come as close as any carotid operation to achieving that ultimate goal. Perforation, which occurred only once early in the 150 dilatations reported by Effeney,[3] should not occur with gentle dilatation that stops at a 3.5- or 4.0-mm diameter probe *if* this is carried out under direct vision. This same author also reported 1 asymptomatic late occlusion, 2 recurrent stenoses, and 2 late strokes in this large, well-followed series, attesting to both the safety and the durability of this procedure. Follow-up angiography is not routinely obtained but nearly always demonstrates an essentially normal lumen (Fig. 122–3). In a modern series, the mortality and permanent neurologic morbidity rates should be negligible, and the patient is normally discharged from the hospital within 48 hours.

EFFECTS OF ASSOCIATED LESIONS ON MANAGEMENT

Intracranial aneurysms, when associated with fibromuscular disease of the internal carotid artery in the neck, are felt by most to be another (albeit separate) expression of the dysplastic process. In every fourth to eighth patient,[4] this coexistence of lesions requires special consideration. In one series,[5] intracranial aneurysms were equally responsible for symptoms, although in most other reports they produced only one quarter to one third of the rate of neurologic symptoms caused by the cervical carotid lesion. In So and colleagues series,[6] five of seven intracranial aneurysms had ruptured, and in Mettinger and Ericson's report,[5] in which 51 per cent of patients had intracranial aneurysms, nearly all were the presenting lesion (mostly with subarachnoid hemorrhage). Even though these data are obviously very skewed, these intracranial lesions cannot simply be ignored. Rather, they should be treated on their own individual merits (e.g., size, presenting symptoms, coexistence of hypertension), just as should the cervical fibrodysplastic lesions, with the primary attention being directed toward the most threatening or symptomatic lesion. Suffice it to say, the mere presence of a small, asymptomatic intracranial aneurysm should not dissuade the vascular surgeon from operating on a threatening cervical lesion.

Renal FMD with hypertension may be an associated finding in one quarter to one half of the cases.[4] It should also be treated on its own merits. It presents more of a threat in those patients with intracranial aneurysms than in those with the cervical carotid string-of-beads lesion. In the former instance, the hypertension should obviously be controlled first, before attack on the aneurysm (and, in most cases, this can be initially accomplished by balloon dilatation); but in the latter instance, concern has been expressed

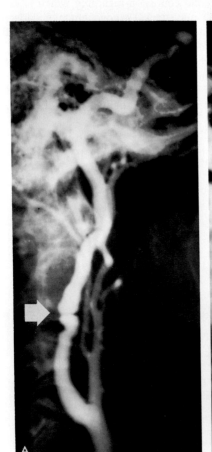
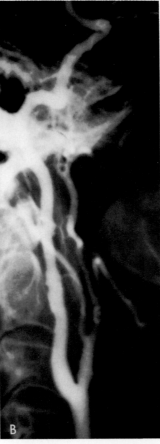

FIGURE 122–3. *A,* Preoperative right carotid arteriogram showing a localized zone of fibromuscular dysplasia characterized by an intraluminal diaphragm *(arrow). B,* Postoperative right carotid arteriogram following graduated intraluminal dilatation. The carotid lumen is now widely patent.

that prior correction of hypertension may make a tight internal carotid stenosis more likely to produce interval symptoms. The author would discount this fear on the grounds that most of the serious symptoms from these carotid lesions are thromboembolic not hemodynamic, and it is better to perform a carotid operation on a normotensive patient (or one taking little or no hypertensive medication) than the reverse.

SUMMARY

As Stanley and Wakefield[4] have said, ''Controversy exists beyond the simple assertion that certain [of these] lesions can cause cerebral ischemia symptoms.'' However, this controversy, and the degree of predictive uncertainty it expresses, should not be grounds for therapeutic nihilism. It is possible to develop a logical, selective management approach based on the much that is known and apply it to individual patients based on *their* clinical findings, *their* operative risk and longevity outlook, and the experience and skill of *their* surgeon. To summarize, half the patients will present with cerebral ischemic events, less than half of these will have suffered infarcts, and only half of the latter will be left with significant neurologic deficits (i.e., around 10 per cent of the total). The natural history of incidentally found lesions is even more benign, with one third showing angiographic progression but less than one tenth ultimately producing cerebral ischemic symptoms. Nevertheless, surgical dilatation of these lesions is very safe and effective, and any surgeon who obtains excellent results with carotid endarterectomy can expect even better results with this procedure. Under these circumstances, it is appropriate to operate on lesions producing focal hemispheric or ocular ischemic events or on critical stenoses that—in lieu of contralateral involvement, limited collateral connections, or position-induced changes—are capable of producing hypoperfusion symptoms because, if they progress, such lesions are more likely to produce permanent neurologic damage. An aggressive posture with asymptomatic lesions, however, can only be justified for unusually threatening combinations of lesions (e.g., operating on one of two severe bilateral stenoses). Associated intracranial aneurysms should be dealt with on their own merits and should not be allowed to compromise valid indications for operation on the cervical lesion. PTA is strongly discouraged because of the small but definite risks of thromboembolic events, dissections, or tears.

References

1. Osborn AG, Anderson RE: Angiographic spectrum of cervical and intracranial fibromuscular dysplasia. Stroke 8:617, 1977.
2. Houser OW, Baker HL: Fibrovascular dysplasia and other uncommon diseases of the cervical carotid artery: Angiographic aspects. AJR 104:201, 1968.
3. Effeney DJ: Surgery for fibromuscular dysplasia of the carotid artery: Indications, technique, and results. *In* Moore WS (ed): Surgery for Cerebrovascular Disease. New York, Churchill Livingstone, 1987, pp 525–533.
4. Stanley JC, Wakefield TW: Arterial fibrodysplasia. *In* Rutherford RB (ed): Vascular Surgery. 3rd ed. Philadelphia, WB Saunders, 1990, pp 245–265.
5. Mettinger KL, Ericson K: Fibromuscular dysplasia and the brain. I. Observations on angiographic, clinical and genetic characteristics. Stroke 13:46, 1982.
6. So EL, Toole JF, Dalal P, et al: Cephalic fibromuscular dysplasia in 32 patients: Clinical findings and radiologic features. Arch Neurol 38:619, 1981.
7. Corrin LS, Sandok BA, Houser OW: Cerebral ischemic events in patients with carotid artery fibromuscular dysplasia. Arch Neurol 38:616, 1981.
8. Morris GC Jr, Lechter A, DeBakey ME: Surgical treatment of fibromuscular disease of the carotid arteries. Arch Surg 96:636, 1968.
9. Effeney DJ, Ehrenfeld WK: Extracranial fibromuscular disease. *In* Rutherford RB (ed): Vascular Surgery. 3rd ed. Philadelphia, WB Saunders, 1990, pp 1412–1417.
10. Patman RD, Thompson JE, Talkington CM, et al: Natural history of fibromuscular dysplasia of the carotid artery [Abstract]. Stroke 2:135, 1980.
11. Stewart MT, Moritz MW, Smith RB, et al: The natural history of carotid fibromuscular dysplasia. J Vasc Surg 3:305, 1986.
12. Starr DS, Lawrie GM, Morris GC: Fibromuscular disease of carotid arteries: Long-term results of graduated internal dilatation. Stroke 12:196, 1981.
13. Collins GJ, Rich NM, Clagett GP, et al: Fibromuscular dysplasia of the internal carotid arteries: Clinical experience and follow-up. Ann Surg 194:89, 1981.
14. Hart RG, Easton JD: Dissections of cervical and cerebral arteries. Neurol Clin 1:155, 1983.

123

Aneurysms of the Extracranial Carotid Artery

Jerry Goldstone, M.D.

• • •

Occlusive and ulcerated atherosclerotic lesions of the cervical carotid arteries are extremely common. Aneurysms of these vessels are rare, particularly in comparison with the frequency of aneurysms involving the *intracranial* carotid arteries and their branches and the frequency of aneurysms that occur throughout the rest of the arterial system. From 1927 to 1947, only 5 cases of carotid aneurysm were encountered at the Hospital of the University of Pennsylvania, and Reid noted only 12 cases in a 30-year survey at the Johns Hopkins Hospital through 1922.[33, 53] The largest reported series from a single institution, that of McCollum and associates at Baylor University, consisted of only 37 aneurysms treated over a 21-year period during which approximately 8500 operations for arterial aneurysms of all types were performed in the same institution.[39] Similarly, only 6 extracranial carotid aneurysms were repaired by Painter and associates at the Cleveland Clinic over a 7-year

interval during which more than 1500 patients were treated for carotid occlusive disease.[48] Because of their rarity, it is impossible to define the true incidence of these aneurysms or to determine whether they are increasing in frequency; however, with the widespread use of angiography and duplex ultrasound they clearly are being recognized more often than before. This is borne out by two reports from the Mayo Clinic. The first included 6 carotid aneurysms identified between 1936 and 1963[52] and the second included 25 aneurysms treated from 1950 to 1990.[6] Although rare, extracranial carotid aneurysms are common enough to be considered in the differential diagnosis of a mass in the neck or posterior pharynx. Aneurysms of the intracranial carotid arteries are much more common, but are the concern of neurosurgeons, who must deal with the complications of the effects of local pressure on nerves and brain tissue and of hemorrhage from rupture.

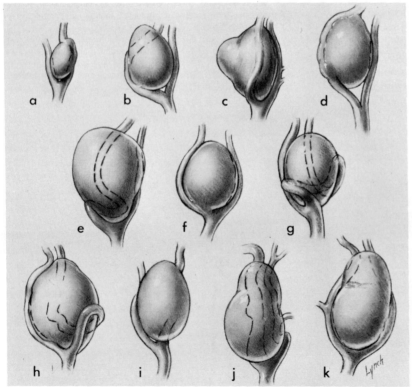

FIGURE 123–1. Artist's depiction of aneurysms of the extracranial internal carotid artery, showing variations in size and configuration. (From Alexander E Jr, Wigser SM, Davis CH: Bilateral extracranial aneurysms of the internal carotid artery. J Neurosurg 25:437, 1966.)

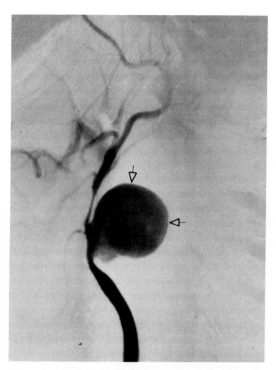

FIGURE 123–2. Left carotid arteriogram showing a 3.5 by 4.0 cm aneurysm arising from left carotid artery adjacent to common carotid bifurcation. The left internal carotid is occluded. (From Margolis MT, Stein RL, Newton TH: Extracranial aneurysms of the internal carotid artery. Neuroradiology 4:78, 1972.)

LOCATION

The common carotid artery, particularly at its bifurcation, is the most frequently reported site of aneurysm formation in the extracranial carotid system; the internal carotid is the next most common; and the external carotid the least common location (Figs. 123–1 to 123–9).[1, 54, 56, 57] Location varies with etiology, and the relative proportion

of the various causes of these aneurysms is changing. For example, atherosclerotic aneurysms usually occur at or near the carotid bifurcation, whereas those caused by blunt trauma usually involve the high cervical portion of the internal carotid artery.

NATURAL HISTORY

The natural history of extracranial carotid aneurysms is uncertain because these lesions are so rare and because no single institution has a large clinical experience with them. Thus, only estimates of natural history can be made, based on multiple case reports, small series, and collected reviews. Unfortunately, most of these include aneurysms of all types, and results have not always been correlated with specific causes, so that information regarding specific etiologies is even more fragmentary. Furthermore, because these reports describe only those aneurysms that required medical attention, it is impossible to determine the number that were never detected. Routine autopsy studies suggest that it is small. Nevertheless, the information that is available suggests that the natural history of these lesions is generally unfavorable. Winslow's 1926 report revealed a 71 per cent mortality rate in 35 untreated patients from rupture, thrombosis, or embolism, compared with a 30 per cent mortality rate in those patients who underwent proximal carotid ligation, the only surgical treatment available at that time.[67] More contemporary reviews have substantiated this poor prognosis[32, 55, 59] and have emphasized the high incidence of neurologic symptoms. For example, Zwolak and coworkers reported a stroke rate of 50 per cent for atherosclerotic aneurysms followed up without surgery.[69] An especially high incidence of complications and death with mycotic and postsurgical pseudoaneurysms is documented in recent reviews and case reports.[21, 25, 31] Conversely, some small, high cervical traumatic aneurysms remain stable or even become smaller when observed for long periods (see Fig. 123–9). Therapy must therefore be individualized, with the major objective being prevention of severe neurologic com-

FIGURE 123–3. Left common carotid arteriogram showing a 1.8 by 2.0 cm aneurysm of the left internal carotid extending up to the base of the skull, associated with stenosis of the origin of the internal artery *(closed arrows)*. *A,* Lateral projection. *B,* Anteroposterior projection. (From Margolis MT, Stein RL, Newton TH: Extracranial aneurysms of the internal carotid artery. Neuroradiology 4:78, 1972.)

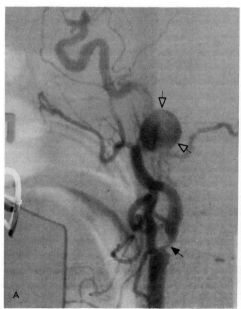
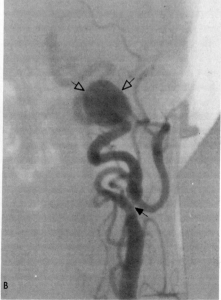

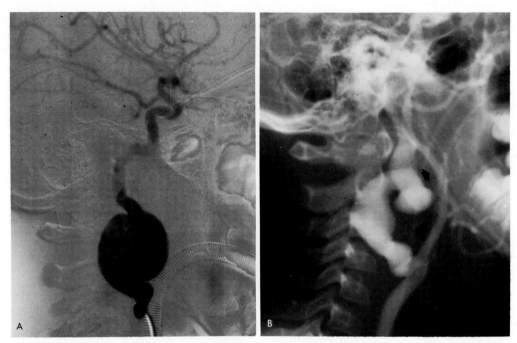

FIGURE 123-4. Right internal carotid arteriogram demonstrating fusiform aneurysm and looping of the proximal right internal carotid artery. (From Margolis MT, Stein RL, Newton TH: Extracranial aneurysms of the internal carotid artery. Neuroradiology 4:78, 1972.)

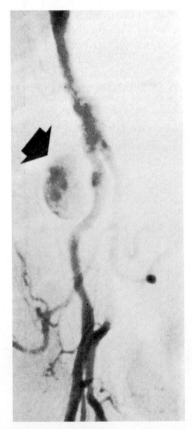

FIGURE 123-5. Left carotid arteriogram showing false aneurysm adjacent to carotid endarterectomy site *(arrow)*. (From Ehrenfeld WK, Hays RJ: False aneurysm after carotid endarterectomy. Arch Surg 104:288, 1972. Copyright 1972, American Medical Association.)

plications in atherosclerotic aneurysms and hemorrhage and thrombosis from mycotic aneurysms.[46]

ETIOLOGY

There are many causes of extracranial carotid aneurysms, and the relative frequency of each has changed over the years. Syphilis, tuberculosis, and other local infections were the most common etiologic factors 50 years ago, but they are rare today. Instead, atherosclerosis, trauma, and previous carotid surgery cause the majority of extracranial carotid aneurysms.

ATHEROSCLEROSIS

Atherosclerosis is now the most frequently reported cause, accounting for up to 70 per cent of the aneurysms in more recently published series.[13, 17, 19, 43, 48, 66, 69] The histologic features of these aneurysms are typically atherosclerotic, with disruption of the internal elastic lamina and thinning of the media. Grossly, these aneurysms tend to be fusiform rather than saccular and are most commonly located at the bifurcation of the common carotid artery or the proximal internal carotid artery. Those not involving the carotid bifurcation are frequently saccular. Most affected patients have severe arterial hypertension, but only about 14 to 25 per cent have other arterial aneurysms. Most bilateral, nontraumatic, extracranial carotid aneurysms are atherosclerotic.

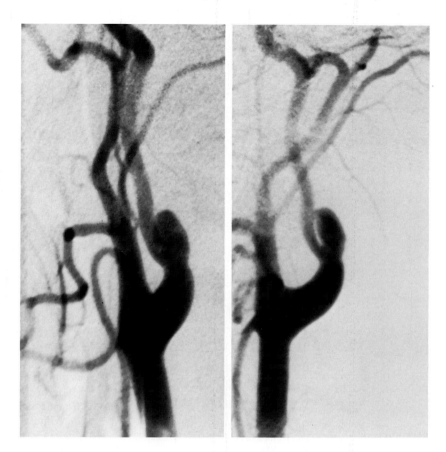

FIGURE 123–6. Left carotid arteriogram showing dissecting aneurysm of proximal internal carotid artery caused by arteriographic catheter injury.

FIGURE 123–7. Left carotid arteriogram (lateral view) showing traumatic internal carotid pseudoaneurysm involving typical location in distal internal carotid artery.

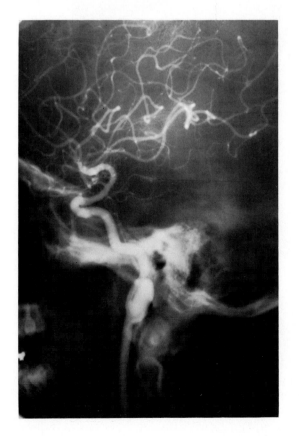

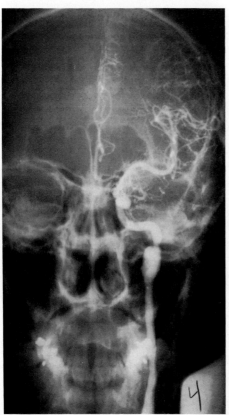

FIGURE 123–8. Left carotid arteriogram (anteroposterior view) of same patient as in Figure 123–7.

TRAUMA

Another major and increasingly frequent cause of carotid aneurysms is trauma,[15, 20, 37] both penetrating and blunt trauma. The resulting transmural carotid disruption leads to the formation of false aneurysm, or pseudoaneurysm.

Penetrating Trauma

Penetrating wounds involving the carotid arteries can lead to two important late sequelae: arteriovenous fistula (aneurysm) and false aneurysm. Arteriovenous fistula is much more common, as noted by Elkin and Shumaker.[20] In their review of World War II injuries, 48 arteriovenous aneurysms of the extracranial carotid system were encountered, compared with 13 false aneurysms.[20] Earlier reports, including that of Winslow, indicated a higher incidence of false aneurysm, probably because the causative injuries were produced by low-velocity, low-energy–releasing missiles or by penetrating hand-driven weapons.[67] The decreased number of such cases reported since the mid-1930s may be due to the high initial mortality rate associated with neck wounds produced by modern high-velocity weapons when they involve the region of the internal carotid artery. Such injuries to an area so closely related anatomically to the base of the skull are often lethal. In the Vietnam conflict, nearly all the patients who survived to be treated for carotid injuries were wounded by relatively low-velocity fragments from land mines, rockets, mortars, or grenades.

Direct carotid puncture for arteriography also can re-

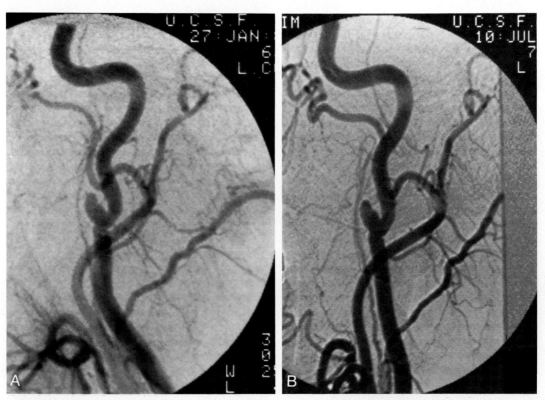

FIGURE 123–9. A, Left carotid arteriogram showing traumatic pseudoaneurysm of distal internal carotid artery. B, Left carotid arteriogram of same patient, 6 months later, showing no change in size of aneurysm.

sult in the formation of a false carotid aneurysm, but this technique is now rarely used for cerebral angiography.

Nonpenetrating Trauma

Blunt or nonpenetrating trauma, although more often the cause of thrombosis of the injured vessel, can be associated with the development of false aneurysms. Blunt injury of the carotid artery produces a spectrum of abnormalities, including spasm, intimal and medial tears, and partial or complete severance of the vessel.[65] Carotid false aneurysms are formed by the same sequence of events as false aneurysms elsewhere. Disruption of the continuity of the arterial wall is required to produce any false aneurysm. This results in formation of a periarterial hematoma that is contained by fascial planes. The center of the hematoma becomes a cavity composed of blood and laminated thrombus communicating with the arterial lumen. A fibrotic reaction is initiated in the surrounding tissues that assists in containing the aneurysm.

Hyperextension and rotation of the neck can cause compression of the distal extracranial internal carotid artery on the transverse process of the atlas, producing disruption of the wall and subsequent aneurysm formation, or intimal fracture and dissection or thrombosis.[54, 60] Similarly, the extreme displacement of the tissues of the neck that can occur during motor vehicle accidents and other trauma may stretch and/or disrupt the artery at its points of fixation to bone at the base of the skull. The styloid process has been implicated in the pathophysiology of these blunt carotid injuries because it rotates with the skull on the dens, whereas the artery moves with the cervical spine.[61] In addition, when mandibular fracture is associated with blunt cervical trauma, bone fragments may penetrate the arterial wall, with subsequent development of one or more false aneurysms. Most of these blunt injuries are located high in the neck near the base of the skull, making them difficult to approach surgically, in contrast to carotid aneurysms that are due to penetrating trauma, which most often involve the common carotid artery.

SURGERY

False aneurysms can also occur after carotid bifurcation endarterectomy for cerebrovascular insufficiency.[8, 13, 28, 45] About 50 per cent of the reported cases have followed endarterectomy in which a synthetic patch was used. These pseudoaneurysms have been attributed to the presence of infection or suture failure. However, pseudoaneurysms can also occur when a vein patch is used as well as after endarterectomy with primary closure. Although the incidence is low, significant morbidity is associated with these pseudoaneurysms. Surgical trauma to the carotid artery during tonsillectomy or drainage of a peritonsillar abscess can also lead to pseudoaneurysm formation.

SYPHILIS

Prior to World War II, syphilis was the most common cause of extracranial carotid aneurysms. In fact, Kirby and associates, in their 1949 review, stated that ''at least 90 per cent of all aneurysms of the common carotid artery are due to syphilis.''[33] This change in etiology reflects the decreasing incidence of syphilitic arteritis and the increasing percentage of older people with atherosclerosis in the population. However, mycotic aneurysms caused by other organisms still occur.

INFECTION

Prior to the development of antibiotics, most carotid aneurysms resulted from local cervical or pharyngeal infections.[59, 67] During the 19th century, children were frequently seen during streptococcal epidemics with profuse oropharyngeal bleeding from infective aneurysms of the internal carotid artery. Cervical carotid aneurysms may protrude into the posterolateral pharyngeal wall through the relatively thin pharyngeal constrictor muscles. In these situations, the true nature of these *mycotic* aneurysms was often not discovered until an unsuspecting physician drained a ''peritonsillar abscess'' only to be met with a gush of blood. *Staphylococcus aureus* has been the most frequent organism responsible for mycotic carotid aneurysms in recent years, but *Escherichia coli*, *Klebsiella*, *Corynebacterium* species, *Proteus mirabilis*, and *Yersinia enterocolitica* have also been reported. *Salmonella* species, which are a frequent pathogen in other arterial mycotic aneurysms, are very uncommon in this location.[12, 21, 25, 31] The presence of a pulsatile neck mass associated with fever and pain should strongly suggest the diagnosis of a mycotic carotid artery aneurysm. Sources of infection include septicemia with involvement of the vasa vasorum, septic emboli within the lumen, and direct extension of infection from contiguous sites. This is obviously not a common problem today, although heroin addicts are especially prone to these nonsyphilitic infectious aneurysms.[36, 39, 53]

DISSECTION

Dissection of the extracranial internal carotid artery can occur after penetrating or blunt injuries to the neck, inadvertent intraoperative trauma, percutaneous or catheter angiography, and occasionally spontaneously without obvious cause.[4, 18, 22, 23, 27, 40, 42, 47, 68] The typical angiographic findings of dissection include a tapered narrowing in the upper cervical internal carotid artery (''string sign'') as well as a localized saccular aneurysm or cylindrical dilatation in the dissected segment. The vertebral artery can also be affected by dissection. These dissecting aneurysms develop as a result of a break in the intima followed by hemorrhage into the media, which enlarges the vessel wall and reduces the caliber of the true lumen. If the hemorrhage dissects into the plane between the media and the adventitia, an aneurysm forms. About 30 per cent of carotid dissections are associated with aneurysm formation. These lesions are often associated with hemicrania and Horner's syndrome in addition to transient or fixed neurologic deficits.

MISCELLANEOUS CAUSES

Other well-documented but even less common causes of carotid aneurysm include cystic medial necrosis, Marfan's syndrome, idiopathic medial arteriopathy, and fibromuscular dysplasia.[5, 35, 41, 55, 63, 64] Several carotid aneurysms have been thought to be congenital because of their occurrence early in life, bilaterality, their saccular shape, the presence of a defect in the media of the vessel similar to the "berry" type of intracranial aneurysm, and the absence of pathologic or clinical features characteristic of other entities.[26, 44] Carotid aneurysm should be in the differential diagnosis of a painless neck mass in a young adult.[11]

CLINICAL FEATURES

Pulsatile Mass

The symptoms of extracranial carotid aneurysms vary according to the location, size, and etiology of the aneurysm. Small internal carotid aneurysms may be asymptomatic, but most cervical carotid aneurysms are identified by the finding of a pulsating mass in the neck just below the angle of the mandible. Systolic bruits are present in many of these patients, especially the elderly, but there is often no evidence of other atherosclerotic lesions. These aneurysms may be painful, and/or tender, or asymptomatic. They are occasionally recognized as a pulsating tumor of the tonsillar fossa or pharynx, with little or no manifestation of their presence externally in the neck. Shipley's classic paper emphasized that aneurysms of the internal carotid present inwardly into the throat, whereas those of the common carotid present outwardly in the neck.[59] The absence of cervical swelling in the former is attributed to the dense, deep cervical fascia and muscles attached to the styloid process anteriorly and the cervical vertebrae posteriorly that crowd the gradually dilating aneurysm inward toward the tonsillar fossa, where the thin superior pharyngeal constrictor muscle and mucous membrane offer only minimal resistance.[59] The level at which the common carotid bifurcates also influences the point of appearance, for with a low bifurcation even an internal carotid aneurysm is likely to be visible and palpable externally in the neck.

Because aneurysms that arise at or proximal to the carotid bifurcation are readily palpable, they usually pose no diagnostic difficulty, but those arising from the internal carotid near the base of the skull can and do cause diagnostic problems. A chronic unilateral swelling of the posterior pharynx should be suspect, especially when other physical signs are lacking, bizarre, or atypical. Otolaryngologists often are the first to see these lesions. A high index of suspicion will lead to angiography, which is nearly always diagnostic when an aneurysm is present.[11]

Most patients with extracranial carotid aneurysms are symptomatic. Although larger lesions tend to produce the most severe symptoms, even small carotid aneurysms can be very symptomatic.

Pain

Overall, pain probably has been the most common symptom.[32] It was prominent in 40 per cent of patients in a reported series from the Mayo Clinic.[6] Some patients have aching in the neck, retro-orbital pressure, or throbbing headaches. Glossopharyngeal compression can account for auricular pain, and radiation into the occipital area also occurs.

Dysphagia

The mass of an aneurysm can cause compression of adjacent structures. Dysphagia secondary to the bulk of the lesion or to compression of the nerve supply to the pharynx has been a frequent symptom.

Cranial Nerve Compression

Aneurysms arising near the carotid canal may compress other nerves and produce severe recurrent facial pain, fifth and sixth cranial nerve palsies, deafness, and occasionally a Horner syndrome. Vagal compression may cause hoarseness. Oculosympathetic paresis and intermittent fascial pain (Raeder's paratrigeminal syndrome) have been caused in some cases by a carotid aneurysm at the base of the skull.[34]

Central Nervous System Dysfunction

Reports indicate that central neurologic deficits are the most common symptoms produced by carotid aneurysms.[54] This reflects the high percentage of atherosclerotic aneurysms in recent series.[6, 14, 50, 51] These lesions tend to produce either transient or permanent cerebral ischemic episodes occurring in about 40 per cent of patients. Transient neurologic deficits occur about twice as often as permanent deficits.[43, 66, 69] Most are due to embolization of thrombotic material emanating from the aneurysmal wall, but some are caused by diminished flow when a large aneurysm compresses the internal carotid artery when the head is turned to certain positions. Occasionally, concomitant carotid bifurcation occlusive disease accounts for episodes of transient cerebral ischemia.

Hemorrhage

Hemorrhage is now a rare manifestation of carotid aneurysm. In older reports, many of these aneurysms were first noticed because of hemorrhage from the pharynx, ear, or nose. Bleeding of this type is usually from an internal carotid artery aneurysm or from infected false aneurysms after carotid endarterectomy. If rupture occurs into the oropharynx, the bleeding can be massive and can lead to suffocation and death. Most fatalities have usually been preceded by repeated episodes of hemorrhage that were improperly recognized or treated. Mycotic aneurysms are especially prone to rupture and bleed.[46]

DIFFERENTIAL DIAGNOSIS

The most frequently encountered lesion that must be distinguished from an extracranial carotid aneurysm is a kinked carotid artery.[33, 49] This usually involves the common carotid artery, producing a pulsatile mass at the base of the neck, typically on the right side, in obese, hypertensive, elderly women. It has been referred to by Bergan and Hoehn as "evanescent cervical pseudoaneurysm."[3] It is much more common than bona fide aneurysms in this location, from which it can be readily distinguished by the characteristic location and by the nature of the pulsation, which is parallel to the long axis of the vessel, whereas the pulsation of an aneurysm is expansile at right angles to the axis of the parent vessel. Soft tissue x-rays of the neck may reveal linear calcification in an atherosclerotic aneurysm, but not in a tortuous artery. Duplex ultrasound should be able to define the lesion.

Redundant length also causes sigmoid curves, loops, and coils of the internal carotid artery higher in the neck. These usually are discovered by angiography because their high cervical location renders them nonpalpable.

A prominent carotid bifurcation in a patient with a thin neck can also be mistaken for a carotid aneurysm, as are carotid body tumors, enlarged lymph nodes, branchial cleft cysts, and cystic hygromas. Careful physical examination should identify these entities correctly, but more objective modalities are useful in order to be certain.

Ultrasound (B-mode with or without Doppler) should establish the correct diagnosis of those aneurysms low enough in the neck to be evaluated with this technique. Extracranial carotid aneurysms can also be demonstrated by computed tomography (CT).[17] The CT anatomy of the neck, nasopharynx, and parapharyngeal spaces is well known, and carotid aneurysms deforming these areas should be clearly differentiated from other mass lesions, particularly if bolus contrast injection and dynamic scanning are employed. Magnetic resonance imaging is equally effective and may be the method of choice, when dissection is the suspected etiology, owing to its unique ability to identify old blood in the dissection plane.

Even if the diagnosis of extracranial carotid aneurysm is made by one of the imaging techniques described, angiography is necessary to obtain the detailed vascular anatomy necessary for the planning of surgery, and should be performed in virtually all patients in whom an aneurysm is suspected and cannot be excluded by other diagnostic methods.[38] Early experience with magnetic resonance angiography (MRA) indicates that it may also provide definitive diagnostic information (See Chapter 6). As they do with aneurysms in other locations, angiograms may underestimate the size of carotid aneurysms as a result of the presence of mural thrombus. High-quality, detailed views of both carotids and both vertebral arteries as well as the intracranial vessels are essential for adequate angiographic evaluation.

TREATMENT

The treatment of extracranial carotid aneurysms has evolved with the specialty of vascular surgery. The choice of treatment depends on the size, location, and etiology of the lesion in question and must be individualized. As noted previously, some small, traumatic, distal internal carotid aneurysms have been shown to remain stable or even shrink when observed for a long period, whereas mycotic aneurysms have a significantly poorer prognosis.[9]

For most patients, the primary objective of treatment is the prevention of permanent neurologic deficits that arise from atheroemboli or thromboemboli. This can best be accomplished by resection of the aneurysm and restoration of arterial continuity. Unfortunately, this is not always possible.

Ligation

In 1552, Ambroise Paré published the first account of operative ligation of the common carotid artery to control massive hemorrhage from a laceration of the artery. His patient developed aphasia and a contralateral monoplegia. In 1805, Astley Cooper performed the first common carotid ligation for an aneurysm of the artery. This patient developed hemiplegia on the 8th postoperative day, and died 13 days later. Cooper later accomplished the first successful treatment of a cervical carotid aneurysm by proximal ligation, and this, coupled occasionally with distal ligation and extirpation, remained the procedure of choice until Matas developed the technique of endoaneurysmorrhaphy. In 1926, Winslow was able to report that the death rate from cervical carotid aneurysms had decreased from 71 per cent with conservative therapy to 30 per cent following ligation, and in 1951 ligation was still recommended as the treatment of choice in spite of the unpredictability of the outcome.[67] Modifications, such as the use of partially constricting bands rather than complete occlusion, were used by some surgeons to lessen the danger of cerebral ischemia. Kirby and coworkers pointed out the dangers of such procedures, and made an unsuccessful attempt to resect a syphilitic carotid aneurysm in 1949.[33] The subsequent development of reconstructive vascular techniques has eliminated ligation as a procedure of choice. Ligation now should be limited to those aneurysms of the internal carotid that extend so far distally toward the base of the skull that distal control of the vessel cannot be obtained. In this situation, resection with arterial reconstruction is impossible. Ligation of the vessel also may be necessary if rupture has occurred, especially if infection is the cause.

Ligation results in thrombosis from the level of the interruption up to the origin of the first major intracranial collateral, usually the ophthalmic artery, thereby obliterating the aneurysm. Of patients so treated, however, 30 to 60 per cent develop neurologic deficits, and half of these die.[7, 33] Gradual carotid occlusion with devices such as the Selverstone clamp has not eliminated this problem, which may be the result of acute cerebrovascular insufficiency as a result of inadequate collateral circulation. In an effort to avoid this complication, numerous techniques have been developed for determining preoperatively the adequacy of cerebral collateral circulation. The carotid compression tests (Matas' test, and the like) have all proved unreliable, as has the observation of intracerebral cross-filling seen on angiography. Intraoperative measurement of the backpressure in the temporarily occluded internal carotid artery has been shown by Moore and associates and by others to be an excellent predictor of tolerance of temporary carotid occlusion in patients with occlusive disease, and it can be applied similarly to patients with aneurysms. The oculopneumoplethysmograph (OPG-Gee) when used with carotid compression also can be used to determine the internal carotid backpressure, and has the advantage of providing this information preoperatively.[24] Alternatively, carotid backpressure can be measured at the time of angiography by using a catheter with an inflatable balloon proximal to a measuring port. Both methods correlate closely with carotid backpressure measured intraoperatively. A carotid backpressure in excess of 60 to 70 mmHg suggests the presence of sufficient collateral cerebral perfusion to enable a patient to withstand carotid ligation without development of an ischemic neurologic deficit.

Careful analysis of the results of carotid ligation reveals a substantial number of patients who develop hemiplegia hours to days after the procedure. Because this most probably represents propagation of thrombus into the branches of the internal carotid artery rather than acute cerebrovascular insufficiency, heparin anticoagulation should be maintained for 7 to 10 days when carotid ligation is performed. When carotid ligation is required but collateral cerebral perfusion is found to be inadequate, consideration should be given to a superficial temporal–to–middle cerebral artery bypass procedure, which is available in many neurosurgical centers in order to minimize the risks of irreversible cerebral ischemia.

Wrapping

External wrapping of the aneurysm, as suggested by Thompson and Austin, is an alternative to ligation when resection is not feasible.[62] These authors used fascia lata, but prosthetic materials seem equally well suited. Wrapping will control the expansion of the aneurysm and limit the risk of rupture, but it cannot be relied on to reduce the more significant risks of embolism or thrombosis. Obviously, this method is inappropriate for infected aneurysms.

Endoaneurysmorrhaphy

This technique, originally described by Matas, has largely been replaced by more modern reconstructive vascular techniques. It still is useful, however, for fusiform aneurysms that are unresectable because they extend to the base of the skull. The endoaneurysmorrhaphy can be performed over an internal shunt wedged into the carotid foramen to control back-bleeding. Some saccular aneurysms are also treatable by localized arterial repair, and several mycotic aneurysms have been treated by a modification of this technique employing débridement of the arterial wall and patch angioplasty.[25, 31]

Resection

Resection of the aneurysm with restoration of flow is the preferred method of treatment. It is indicated for accessible lesions of the common carotid and proximal third of the internal carotid artery. More distal lesions usually present difficulties in gaining distal control, and other methods

often must be employed. A small saccular aneurysm with a narrow neck can be managed by aneurysmectomy and primary closure or patch angioplasty. Fusiform lesions and saccular lesions with large necks are not suitable for this type of local repair. They should be resected, and arterial continuity reestablished. The first report of resection of a carotid aneurysm with primary anastomosis was that of Shea and associates in 1955, although the first successful procedure of this type was performed by Dimtza in 1952.[16, 58] Beall and associates performed the first prosthetic graft replacement for this lesion in 1959.[2] In subsequent years, there have been numerous reports of successful carotid aneurysm resection with reestablishment of arterial continuity, and this should be the objective of all such procedures. Redundancy of the carotid vessels allows resection and primary anastomosis to be performed in over 50 per cent of cases, especially when the aneurysm is small. Anastomosis of the proximal external carotid artery to the more distal internal carotid artery has been successfully used to bridge an internal carotid defect resulting from aneurysm excision. An interrupted suture technique diminishes the likelihood of anastomotic narrowing. When inadequate length of vessels precludes primary anastomosis, interposition grafts must be utilized. Prosthetic and autogenous (artery or vein) grafts have been used with equally good results, although an autogenous conduit is preferable whenever infection is a possibility. Large aneurysms and aneurysms involving the most distal internal carotid artery are especially challenging technically. Exposure of the upper end of the internal carotid may be enhanced by several maneuvers, including division of the sternocleidomastoid muscle from its mastoid attachment and elevation or resection of the parotid gland; division of the digastric muscle; removal of the styloid process; and the use of intraluminal balloons (usually as an intraluminal shunt) to control distal internal carotid back-bleeding. Subluxation of the mandible by any of several techniques can increase the width of exposure of the distal field at the base of the skull by approximately 1 cm.[10, 14, 50] Nearly equal advantage can be gained by using a nasotracheal rather than an endotracheal tube for administration of general anesthesia.

Complete excision of large lesions risks injury to cranial nerves, including the facial, vagus, spinal accessory, hypoglossal, and glossopharyngeal. Profound disturbances in swallowing can occur as a result of injury to pharyngeal muscular branches arising from the vagus, superior laryngeal, and glossopharyngeal nerves. Although these are usually temporary deficits, they can be severely disturbing to affected patients and the cause of considerable postoperative morbidity. In order to minimize these problems, extreme care must be used when dissecting these structures and a bipolar cautery should be employed for hemostasis. Extreme care must also be paid to gentle handling of the aneurysm itself in order to prevent dislodgment and downstream embolization of mural thrombus.

Methods of cerebral protection during the period of carotid occlusion required for repair of carotid aneurysms are the same as those used during bifurcation endarterectomy for occlusive disease. Some surgeons employ electroencephalographic monitoring and/or cerebral blood flow measurements.[43, 61] Others selectively use an internal shunt based on backpressure criteria. Routine shunting is advocated by many surgeons because of the longer time required for this type of carotid reconstruction compared with that required for endarterectomy. The shunt may also be helpful by serving as a stent during construction of the anastomoses. Hypothermia, induced hypertension, and hypercapnia or hypocapnia appear to be unnecessary and confusing.

With modern vascular surgical techniques, correction of the uncommon extracranial carotid aneurysms should be accomplished with a high rate of success and a low rate of neurologic complications, thus approaching the excellent results now being obtained in the surgical treatment of extracranial occlusive arterial disease.

Endovascular Therapy

Higashida and Hieshima and their colleagues have treated several high-cervical true and pseudoaneurysms with intravascular detachable silicone balloons and platinum coils inserted via a transfemoral route.[29, 30] This has been used as the definitive treatment with obliteration of the aneurysm and preservation of cervical carotid patency in a small number of patients. In several other patients with acute pseudoaneurysms that were due to trauma or tumor erosion, these investigators obliterated the aneurysm by trapping it between two balloons, one placed in the cavernous carotid artery below the ophthalmic artery but beyond the inferolateral and meningohypophyseal trunk, and a second one placed just proximal to the aneurysm. Test occlusion to document tolerance to carotid occlusion is obviously mandatory prior to permanent occlusion. Although there have been neurologic complications from this form of therapy, the long-term results have been encouraging, and this procedure should be considered in the treatment of carefully selected patients with these difficult and dangerous aneurysms. The introduction of endoluminal stents and stented grafts may soon lead to further advances in this field.

References

1. Agrifoglio M, Rona P, Spirito R, et al: External carotid artery aneurysms. J Cardiovasc Surg 30:942, 1989.
2. Beall AC, Crawford ES, Cooley DA, et al: Extracranial aneurysms of the carotid artery. Report of seven cases. Postgrad Med 32:93, 1962.
3. Bergan JJ, Hoehn JG: Evanescent cervical pseudoaneurysms. Ann Surg 162:213, 1965.
4. Biller J, Hingtgen WL, Adams HP Jr, et al: Cervicocephalic arterial dissections. A ten-year experience. Arch Neurol 43:1234, 1986.
5. Bour P, Taghavi I, Bracard S, et al: Aneurysms of the extracranial internal carotid artery due to fibromuscular dysplasia: Results of surgical management. Ann Vasc Surg 6:205, 1992.
6. Bower TC, Pairolero PC, Hallett JW Jr, et al: Brachiocephalic aneurysm: The case for early recognition and repair. Ann Vasc Surg 5:125, 1991.
7. Brackett CE Jr: The complications of carotid artery ligation in the neck. J Neurosurg 10:91, 1953.
8. Buscaglia LC, Moore WS, Hall AD: False aneurysm after carotid endarterectomy. JAMA 209:1529, 1969.
9. Busuttil RW, Davidson RK, Foley KT, et al: Selective management of extracranial carotid artery aneurysms. Am J Surg 140:85, 1980.
10. Carrel T, Bauer E, von Segesser L, et al: Surgical management of extracranial carotid-artery aneurysms: Analysis of 6 cases. Cerebrovasc Dis 1:49, 1991.
11. Cunningham MJ, Rueger RG, Rothfus WE: Extracranial carotid artery aneurysm: An unusual neck mass in a young adult. Ann Otol Rhinol Laryngol 6:327, 1989.

12. Dawson KJ, Stansby G, Novell JR, Hamilton G: Mycotic aneurysm of the cervical carotid artery due to *Salmonella enteritidis*. Eur J Vasc Surg 6:327, 1992.
13. Dehn TCB, Taylor GW: Extracranial carotid artery aneurysms. Ann R Coll Surg Engl 66:247, 1984.
14. de Jong KP, Zondervan PE, van Urk H: Extracranial carotid artery aneurysms. Eur J Vasc Surg 3:557, 1989.
15. Deysine M, Adiga R, Wilder JR: Traumatic false aneurysm of the cervical internal carotid artery. Surgery 66:1004, 1969.
16. Dimtza A: Aneurysms of the carotid arteries. Report of two cases. Angiology 7:218, 1956.
17. Duvall ER, Gupta KL, Vitek JJ, et al: CT demonstration of extracranial carotid artery aneurysms. J Comput Assist Tomogr 10(3):404, 1986.
18. Ehrenfeld WK, Wylie EJ: Spontaneous dissection of the internal carotid artery. Arch Surg 111:1294, 1976.
19. Ekestrom S, Bergdahl L, Huttunen H: Extracranial carotid and vertebral artery aneurysms. Scan J Thorac Cardiovasc Surg 17:135, 1983.
20. Elkin DC, Shumaker HB Jr: Surgery in World War II (US Army). *In* Vascular Surgery. Washington, DC, Office of the Surgeon General, Department of the Army, 1955.
21. Ferguson LJ, Fell G, Buxton B, Royle JP: Mycotic cervical carotid aneurysm. Br J Surg 71:245, 1984.
22. Fisher CM, Ojemann RG, Roberson GH: Spontaneous dissection of cervicocerebral arteries. J Can Sci Neurol 5:9, 1978.
23. Friedman WA, Day AK, Guisling RG, et al: Cervical carotid dissecting aneurysms. Neurosurgery 7:207, 1980.
24. Gee W, Mehigan JT, Wylie EJ: Measurement of collateral cerebral hemispheric blood pressure by ocular pneumoplethysmography. Am J Surg 130:121, 1975.
25. Grossi RJ, Onofrey D, Tvetenstrand C, Blumenthal J: Mycotic carotid aneurysm. J Vasc Surg 6:81, 1987.
26. Hammon JW Jr, Silver D, Young WF Jr: Congenital aneurysm of the extracranial carotid arteries. Ann Surg 176:777, 1972.
27. Hart RG, Easton JD: Dissections of cervical and cerebral arteries. Neurol Clin 1:155, 1983.
28. Hejhal L, Hejhal J, Firt P, et al: Aneurysms following endarterectomy associated with patch graft angioplasty. J Cardiovasc Surg 15:620, 1974.
29. Higashida RT, Hieshima GB, Halbach VV, et al: Cervical carotid artery aneurysms and pseudoaneurysms. Acta Radiol 369:591, 1986.
30. Higashida RT, Hieshima GB, Halbach VV, et al: Intravascular detachable balloon embolization of intracranial aneurysms. Acta Radiol 369:594, 1986.
31. Jebara VA, Acar C, Dervanian P, et al: Mycotic aneurysms of the carotid arteries—Case report and review of the literature. J Vasc Surg 14:215, 1991.
32. Kaupp HA, Haid SP, Gurayj MN, et al: Aneurysms of the extracranial carotid artery. Surgery 72:946, 1972.
33. Kirby CK, Johnson J, Donald JG: Aneurysm of the common carotid artery. Ann Surg 130:913, 1949.
34. Lane RJ, Weisman RA: Carotid artery aneurysms: An otolaryngologic perspective. Laryngoscope 90:987, 1980.
35. Latter DA, Ricci MA, Forbes RDC, Graham AM: Internal carotid artery aneurysm and Marfan's syndrome. Can J Surg 32:463, 1989.
36. Ledgerwood AM, Luca CE: Mycotic aneurysm of the carotid artery. Arch Surg 109:496, 1974.
37. Magnan PE, Branchereau A, Cannoni M: Traumatic aneurysms of the internal carotid artery at the base of the skull: Two cases treated surgically. J Cardiovasc Surg 33:372, 1992.
38. Margolis MT, Stein RL, Newton TH: Extracranial aneurysms of the internal carotid artery. Neuroradiology 4:78, 1972.
39. McCollum CH, Wheeler WG, Noon GP, et al: Aneurysms of the extracranial carotid artery. Twenty-one years' experience. Am J Surg 137:196, 1979.
40. McNeill DH Jr, Driesbach J, Marsden RJ: Spontaneous dissection of the internal carotid artery. Its conservative management with heparin sodium. Arch Neurol 37:54, 1980.
41. Miyauchi M, Shionoya S: Aneurysm of the extracranial internal carotid artery caused by fibromuscular dysplasia. Eur J Vasc Surg 5:587, 1991.
42. Mokri B, Sundt TM Jr, Houser OW: Spontaneous internal carotid dissection, hemicrania, and Horner's syndrome. Arch Neurol 36:677, 1979.
43. Mokri B, Piepgras DG, Sundt TM, et al: Extracranial internal carotid artery aneurysms. Mayo Clin Proc 57:310, 1982.

44. Moosa HH, Higgins R, Shapiro SP, Harrison AM: Isolated extracranial internal carotid artery aneurysm in a 22-year-old patient. Contemp Surg 40:40, 1992.
45. Motte S, Wautrecht JC, Bellens B, et al: Infected false aneurysm following carotid endarterectomy with vein patch angioplasty. J Cardiovasc Surg 28:734, 1987.
46. Nicholson ML, Horrocks M: Leaking carotid artery aneurysm. Eur J Vasc Surg 2:197, 1988.
47. O'Connell BK, Towfighi J, Brennan RW, et al: Dissecting aneurysms of head and neck. Neurology 35:993, 1985.
48. Painter TA, Hertzer NR, Beven EG, et al: Extracranial carotid aneurysms: Report of six cases and review of the literature. J Vasc Surg 2:312, 1985.
49. Perdue GD, Barreca JP, Smith RB III, et al: The significance of elongation and angulation of the carotid artery: A negative view. Surgery 77:45, 1975.
50. Petrovic P, Avramov S, Pfau J, et al: Surgical management of extracranial carotid artery aneurysms. Ann Vasc Surg 5:506, 1991.
51. Pratschke E, Schafer K, Reimer J, et al: Extracranial aneurysms of the carotid artery. Thorac Cardiovasc Surg 28:354, 1980.
52. Raphael HA, Bernatz PE, Spittell JA Jr: Cervical carotid aneurysms: Treatment by excision and restoration of arterial continuity. Am J Surg 105:771, 1963.
53. Reid MR: Aneurysms in the Johns Hopkins Hospital. Arch Surg 12:1, 1926.
54. Rhodes EL, Stanley JC, Hoffman GL, et al: Aneurysms of extracranial carotid arteries. Arch Surg 111:339, 1976.
55. Rittenhouse EA, Radke HM, Sumner DS: Carotid artery aneurysm. Arch Surg 105:786, 1972.
56. Schechter DC: Cervical carotid aneurysms. I. NY State J Med 79:892, 1979.
57. Schechter DC: Cervical carotid aneurysms. II. NY State J Med 79:1042, 1979.
58. Shea PC, Glass LG, Reid WA, et al: Anastomosis of common and internal carotid arteries following excision of mycotic aneurysm. Surgery 37:829, 1955.
59. Shipley AM, Winslow N, Walker WW: Aneurysm in the cervical portion of the internal carotid artery. An analytical study of the cases recorded in the literature between August 1, 1925, and July 31, 1936. Report of two new cases. Ann Surg 105:673, 1937.
60. Stonebridge PA, Clason AE, Jenkins AM: Traumatic aneurysm of the extracranial internal carotid artery due to hyperextension of the neck. Eur J Vasc Surg 4:423, 1990.
61. Sundt TM Jr, Pearson BW, Piepgras DG, et al: Surgical management of aneurysms of the distal extracranial internal carotid artery. J Neurosurg 64:169, 1986.
62. Thompson JE, Austin DJ: Surgical management of cervical carotid aneurysms. Arch Surg 74:80, 1957.
63. Un-Sup K, Friedman EW, Werther LJ, et al: Carotid artery aneurysm associated with nonbacterial suppurative arteritis. Arch Surg 106:865, 1973.
64. Webb JC, Barker WF: Aneurysms of the extracranial internal carotid artery. Arch Surg 99:501, 1969.
65. Welling RE, Kakkasseril JS, Peschiera J: Pseudoaneurysm of the cervical internal carotid artery secondary to blunt trauma. J Trauma 25:1108, 1985.
66. Welling RE, Taha A, Goel T, et al: Extracranial carotid artery aneurysms. Surgery 93:319, 1983.
67. Winslow N: Extracranial aneurysm of the internal carotid artery. Arch Surg 13:689, 1926.
68. Zelenock GB, Kazmers A, Whitehouse WM, et al: Extracranial internal carotid artery dissections. Arch Surg 117:425, 1982.
69. Zwolak RM, Whitehouse WM, Knake JE, et al: Atherosclerotic extracranial carotid artery aneurysms. J Vasc Surg 1:415, 1984.

124

Extracranial-Intracranial Bypass: Current Status

Neil A. Martin, M.D., Martin Holland, M.D., and John Frazee, M.D.

• • •

C. Miller Fisher suggested in 1951 that surgeons should seek a practical means for connecting the extracranial and intracranial circulation to supply blood to the brain when it loses its normal source.[13] Until the 1960s, however, the microsurgical techniques for such anastomoses were not available. Microvascular surgery performed under the microscope was first described by Jacobsen, and the first experimental microvascular studies in neurosurgery were done in 1962.[10, 24, 54] The first extracranial-intracranial (EC-IC) bypass was performed by Donaghy and Yasargil in 1967.[10] They fashioned an anastomosis of the superficial temporal artery to the middle cerebral artery. Since the original description of this procedure, there have been several refinements in technique, including the use of saphenous vein graft from external carotid artery, subclavian artery, or proximal superficial temporal artery to provide a high-flow conduit;[47] anastomosis to proximal middle cerebral artery branches in the sylvian fissure to provide a larger-diameter distal anastomosis;[9] use of the occipital or middle meningeal artery when the superficial temporal artery is inadequate;[35, 41] and development of bypass procedures for posterior circulation revascularization.[23, 41, 45]

RATIONALE AND EARLY EXPERIENCE

The EC-IC bypass procedure was developed to provide additional blood supply to areas of the brain rendered ischemic by cerebrovascular occlusive disease that was not amenable to direct surgery (e.g., endarterectomy). This procedure was initially intended to treat patients with internal carotid artery occlusion or intracranial occlusive lesions such as siphon stenosis or middle cerebral artery occlusion or stenosis. The vascular conduit from the extracranial to the intracranial circulation is designed to circumvent the occlusive lesion and improve the collateral circulation in hypoperfused or ischemic regions, thereby preventing transient ischemic attacks (TIAs) or frank cerebral infarction.

Cerebral ischemia may have a hemodynamic mechanism, related to reduced cerebral perfusion pressure secondary to occlusion of major vessels, or an embolic mechanism, with the emboli originating from proximal arterial atherosclerotic lesions (artery-to-artery embolization).[19] Proponents of EC-IC bypass surgery argued that it might be beneficial in patients with either mechanism of ischemia. In the case of hemodynamic impairment, the bypass provides an additional source of collateral circulation and improves cerebral perfusion pressure. In patients with an embolic mechanism, the bypass provides a sufficient increase in perfusion to promote the disintegration and passage of emboli.

Several clinical studies have documented long-term resolution of ischemic symptoms following EC-IC bypass and have suggested that EC-IC bypass had the capacity to reduce long-term stroke risk.[5, 6, 8, 17, 27, 30, 41, 50, 51, 55, 56] A number of clinical physiologic studies have demonstrated that the bypass procedure results in improved cerebral blood flow in previously underperfused areas.[1, 2, 4, 7, 18, 21, 28, 29, 32, 34, 39, 42, 44, 52] However, definitive testing of the safety and efficacy of EC-IC bypass was not completed until the performance of the EC-IC Bypass Study.

THE EC-IC BYPASS STUDY

In order to test the ability of the EC-IC bypass to reduce the rate of subsequent stroke among patients with symptomatic, inaccessible atherosclerotic lesions of the internal carotid or middle cerebral arteries, an international multi-center randomized study was initiated in 1977.[12] This was a clinical trial designed to determine whether anastomosis of the superficial temporal artery to the middle artery decreased the rate of stroke and stroke-related death among patients with symptomatic atherosclerotic disease. Patients were eligible for the trial if, within 3 months before entry, they had one or more TIAs or minor completed strokes in the carotid distribution, and one of the following ipsilateral lesions:

1. Occlusion of the internal carotid artery;
2. Stenosis of the internal carotid artery at or above the C2 vertebral body (at a location inaccessible to carotid endarterectomy); or
3. Stenosis or occlusion of the middle cerebral artery.

Patients were randomly assigned either to the best medical care (aspirin 325 mg 4 times a day) or to the same regimen with the addition of bypass surgery. The patients were followed for an average of 55.8 months. The primary end-points were fatal or nonfatal stroke. Secondary events analyzed included ipsilateral stroke, death from any cause, and functional status. In this study, 1377 patients were randomly assigned to best medical care (714) or to surgery (663).

The level of surgical proficiency in this study was high. The surgical mortality rate was 0.6 per cent, and the major stroke morbidity rate was 2.5 per cent. The bypass patency rate, angiographically confirmed, was 96 per cent.

The outcomes of the medical and surgical groups were compared during a follow-up period that averaged almost 5 years. The primary conclusion of the study was that EC-IC bypass did not reduce the incidence of stroke or death. In fact, owing to perioperative morbidity and mortality, nonfatal and fatal stroke occurred slightly more frequently and earlier in the patients who were operated on. Separate analysis of patients with a variety of different angiographic lesions, including bilateral carotid occlusion and middle cerebral artery occlusion (two circumstances in which EC-IC bypass might be expected to have the greatest benefit) did not identify any subgroup that benefitted from surgery. Notably, the group of patients with severe middle cerebral artery stenosis had a significantly worse outcome when treated with the bypass than when treated medically. Presumably, in these cases, the bypass actually caused some strokes by precipitating proximal middle cerebral artery occlusion, by reducing the pressure gradient and creating stasis at the stenotic region.

AFTERMATH OF THE EC-IC BYPASS STUDY

A number of clinicians have criticized the EC-IC study.[3, 45] Apparently, without knowledge of the principal investigators of the trial study, a significant number of patients had bypass surgery outside of the trial at the participating medical centers. Furthermore, the low stroke rate of the medically treated groups in the trial suggested that lower stroke-risk patients were selected for randomization and inclusion. These facts raised the concern that, by some unknown selection criteria, high stroke-risk patients who were most in need of cerebral blood flow augmentation were identified, not submitted for trial inclusion, and operated on outside the trial. According to this hypothetical scenario, only relatively stable, low-risk patients were entered into the trial for randomization. If this were the case, and the patients most likely to benefit from surgery were not included in the trial, then the trial would not have tested fairly the effect of surgical treatment. These and other criticisms have been addressed by the EC-IC study group. They asserted that, although a number of patients may have been treated surgically outside of the study, there was no evidence that these patients were in any way clinically unique, or that there existed, at the time of the study, any selection criteria by which high-risk patients could be identified. They insisted that enough patients in each of the various clinical and angiographic subgroups were included, so that the study group was sufficiently representative of the relevant overall patient population and that, therefore, the study results were valid. Most clinicians have now come to accept the findings of the EC-IC Bypass Study as valid, at least as regards the types of patients with the specific clinical and radiographic features that were evaluated.[45]

Since the completion and publication of the EC-IC bypass study, there has been a profound reduction in the number of such surgical procedures performed. One larger center described performing as many as 70 such cases annually before the publication of the study, and performing only about 4 EC-IC bypasses for occlusive cerebrovascular disease annually in recent years.[45]

INDICATIONS FOR EC-IC BYPASS NOT STUDIED BY THE BYPASS STUDY

It is critically important to appreciate that the bypass study did not address all of the clinical circumstances in which EC-IC anastomosis might be beneficial. Several clinical categories of occlusive cerebrovascular disease were not specifically studied. These categories include patients with chronic low-perfusion syndromes, ischemic ocular syndromes, moyamoya disease, and vertebrobasilar insufficiency.[25, 35, 45] Although further study is required to define authoritatively the place of EC-IC bypass in the treatment of patients with these disorders, bypass surgery is currently in clinical use for selected patients with no effective therapeutic alternative.

CURRENT INDICATIONS FOR EC-IC BYPASS

It is the authors' view, and that of many clinicians treating patients with cerebrovascular disorders, that there remain certain valid indications for EC-IC bypass.[3, 35, 45] These include

1. Patients with persistent or progressive ischemic symptoms due to occlusive cerebrovascular disease that are refractory to maximal medical therapy, and who have demonstrated cerebral hemodynamic insufficiency.

2. Patients requiring therapeutic carotid occlusion who fail temporary balloon test occlusion.

Medically Refractory Cerebral Ischemia Due to Cerebral Hemodynamic Insufficiency

The EC-IC Bypass Study did not include patients who had failed a trial of maximal medical therapy (i.e., antithrombotic therapy). It is likely that the failure of antithrombotic therapy in some of these patients is due to the fact that their TIAs have a hemodynamic rather than an embolic mechanism.[26, 36, 40, 45] It may be possible, using physiologic testing methods, to define the subgroup of symptomatic patients who have a hemodynamic mechanism for their symptoms, and who are at highest risk for subsequent stroke. If so, these tests should prove useful in identifying the patients who might benefit from EC-IC bypass.

Physiologic Identification of Cerebral Hemodynamic Insufficiency

The pathogenesis of stroke is variable. Most strokes are due to cerebral embolization, from the heart or from proximal atherosclerotic lesions. A minority of patients, however, develop TIAs, or completed infarction due to low cerebral perfusion pressure. This is the hemodynamic mechanism for stroke. The low cerebral blood flow in "hemodynamic cases" is due to the combination of severe occlusive disease involving the major cerebral vessels and inadequate collateral circulation through the circle of Willis or through leptomeningeal collateral pathways. It has been proposed that patients with this pathophysiologic circumstance form the group that will benefit from procedures designed to improve cerebral blood flow (carotid endarterectomy for severe carotid stenosis, EC-IC bypass for carotid occlusion) and that may not benefit from antithrombotic therapy.[11, 26, 45]

The EC-IC Bypass Study selected patients based on clinical and angiographic criteria.[12] The study made no attempt to identify "hemodynamic cases" using physiologic studies. Several investigators have proposed that hemodynamic insufficiency can be identified by a variety of types of studies of cerebral blood flow (single-photon emission tomography [SPECT], positron emission tomography [PET], xenon-computed tomography [CT], transcranial Doppler [TCD]).[2, 11, 16, 18, 26, 37, 48, 53] The most promising clinical reports have focused on the measurement of the capacity of the cerebral vasculature to react to various vasodilating stimuli (CO_2, acetazolamide [Diamox]).[11, 26, 48] The value of these studies in determining hemodynamic insufficiency rests on the proposal that the resistance arteries are maximally dilated when cerebral perfusion pressure is critically reduced by occlusive disease. Under these circumstances, the ability of the cerebral vasculature to dilate further is compromised, and cerebral blood flow does not rise in response to a vasodilating stimulus. When there is severe focal compromise of cerebrovascular reactivity, a cerebral "steal" may be observed. Steal occurs when an increase in cerebral blood flow in normally perfused brain regions, resulting from a vasodilating stimulus, diverts blood flow from hypoperfused nonreactive areas. This has been described as a cerebral stress test. The study is carried out by performing cerebral blood flow measurements before and after the administration of acetazolamide. An inability to demonstrate appropriately increased cerebral blood flow or the demonstration of steal after the administration of acetazolamide constitutes a positive test. Several groups have used this test in studying patients who were candidates for EC-IC bypass.[11, 48]

Durham and associates tested cerebrovascular reactivity using xenon-CT cerebral blood flow mapping with acetazolamide stimulation in a number of medically treated patients with occlusive disease.[11] They found that patients with normal or only slightly impaired cerebrovascular reactivity had a low risk of future stroke during a mean follow-up of 18 months. However, 9 of 23 patients (39 per cent) who demonstrated a cerebral steal after the administration of acetazolamide developed a stroke during follow-up. This difference, which was statistically significant, suggests that patients with hemodynamic insufficiency, as demonstrated by the acetazolamide/cerebral blood flow evaluation, identifies patients who are at high risk for stroke. Presumably, such patients form the group most likely to benefit from surgical augmentation of cerebral blood flow.

Ringelstein and others have extensively studied patients with occlusive vascular disease employing TCD techniques.[26, 40] TCD measurements of middle cerebral artery velocity responses to changes in arterial CO_2, or to acetazolamide infusion, have been used to estimate cerebrovascular reactivity. These groups have demonstrated a relationship between the severity of angiographically defined cerebrovascular occlusive disease and impaired cerebrovascular reactivity. These studies have also retrospectively identified an association between impaired cerebrovascular reserve and the incidence of hemodynamic (watershed) stroke.[40] A study by Kleiser and Widder, published in 1992, evaluated prospectively the relationship between abnormal CO_2 reactivity measured by TCD and stroke risk.[26] They found that less than 10 per cent of the patients with adequate CO_2 reactivity developed ischemic symptoms during a follow-up period of more than 3 years. However, among patients with diminished or exhausted cerebrovascular reserve, more than 32 per cent suffered an ischemic event (4 TIAs, 8 strokes). The results of Durham and associates' and Kleiser and Widder's studies suggest that physiologic testing of cerebrovascular reserve can identify the rather select subgroup of patients with occlusive cerebrovascular disease who have a substantially increased risk of hemodynamic stroke.[11, 26] Patients who continue to have ischemic symptoms despite maximal medical therapy, and who have physiologic demonstration of impaired cerebrovascular reserve, appear to be a group at high risk for stroke. These patients, in whom alternative therapeutic options have been exhausted, form a group of patients in whom EC-IC bypass is a viable and perhaps the only alternative.[45]

MANAGEMENT ALGORITHM

The use of physiologic methods for selecting patients for EC-IC bypass can be integrated into an evaluation-treatment algorithm[45] (Fig. 124–1). Patients with cerebral ischemic symptoms are evaluated first with a cranial CT or magnetic resonance imaging (MRI) scan to rule out intracranial lesions that might cause symptoms similar to TIAs (e.g., subdural hematoma, tumor, arteriovenous malformation). A medical and cardiac evaluation should be performed to rule out hematologic disorders that may cause TIAs and to assess for the presence of cardiac arrhythmias or valvular disorders that may cause cerebral embolism. If these investigations are negative, the cervical and intracranial vessels are studied using duplex ultrasonography, TCD, and, in most cases, angiography. If severe stenosis at the carotid bifurcation is identified, carotid endarterectomy is recommended. If internal carotid artery occlusion is accompanied by a large or irregular stump, with or without external carotid stenosis, a stumpectomy and external carotid endarterectomy should be performed. If patients have symptoms due to an inaccessible internal carotid artery stenosis, internal carotid artery occlusion, or intracranial occlusive lesion, they are treated with aspirin (or possibly warfarin [Coumadin] if symptoms continue despite aspirin treatment). Persistence of symptoms despite antithrombotic treatment should prompt the performance of physiologic

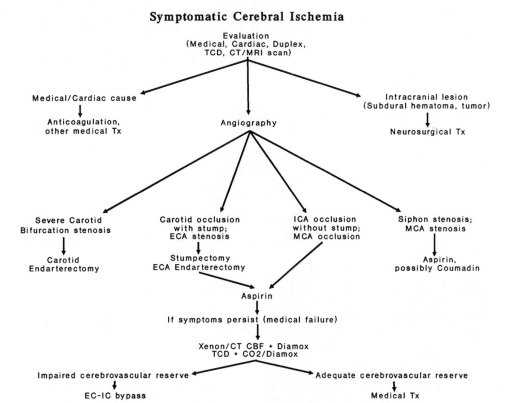

FIGURE 124–1. Management algorithm for patients with symptomatic cerebral ischemia. (Modified from Spetzler R, Hadley, M: Extracranial-intracranial bypass grafting: An update. *In* Wilkins R, Rengachary S [eds]: Neurosurgery Update II. Vascular, Spinal, Pediatric, and Functional Neurosurgery. New York, McGraw-Hill, 1991, p 197. Reproduced with permission of McGraw-Hill.)

studies of cerebrovascular reserve (TCD with CO_2 or acetazolamide activation, or xenon-CT cerebral blood flow study with acetazolamide activation) in order to assess for hemodynamic cerebrovascular insufficiency. Only those patients who are refractory to maximal medical therapy, and who have documented hemodynamic insufficiency, are considered for EC-IC bypass (Fig. 124–2).

Therapeutic Carotid Occlusion for Aneurysms or Tumors

The treatment of skull base tumors that have invaded the carotid artery may require occlusion and resection of the involved artery. Certain internal carotid artery aneurysms that are not amenable to direct surgical repair require therapeutic carotid occlusion.[15, 20, 22, 43, 49] Carotid artery occlusion cannot be carried out without causing injurious cerebral ischemia if, in the individual patient, the cerebral

collateral circulation is inadequate. The adequacy of the cerebral collateral circulation is tested, prior to permanent carotid occlusion, by temporary balloon occlusion performed under local anesthesia. When the patient develops ischemic neurologic symptoms during 20 to 30 minutes of trial occlusion, it is clear that the patient will not tolerate *permanent* carotid occlusion. Some patients who clinically tolerate a trial period of carotid occlusion nevertheless develop delayed stroke after permanent carotid occlusion. Several investigators have advocated the measurement of cerebral blood flow during test occlusion as a technique to identify the patients who are at risk for delayed stroke.[43] When test occlusion is accompanied by ischemic symptoms, or by a profound drop in cerebral blood flow, it is apparent that the collateral circulation is inadequate to accommodate permanent carotid occlusion. In these cases, EC-IC bypass provides the needed source of collateral circulation. This application of EC-IC bypass, not addressed whatsoever in the bypass study, is perhaps the most prevalent current indication for this procedure[45] (Fig. 124–3).

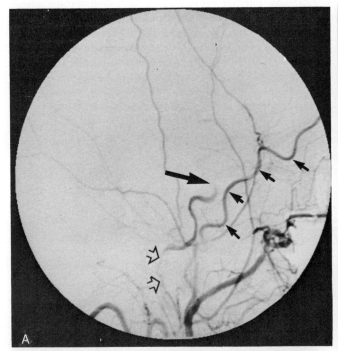

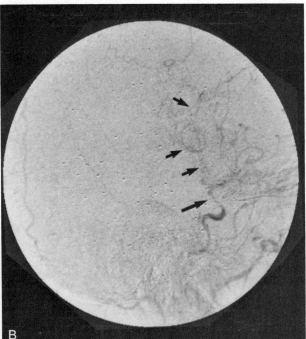

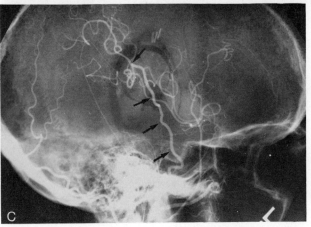

FIGURE 124–2. This 67-year-old man with a long history of cigarette smoking, hypertension, and diabetes mellitus developed recurrent left hemisphere transient ischemic attacks (TIAs) that did not cease with either aspirin or warfarin (Coumadin) antithrombotic therapy. *A,* The lateral projection of the left common carotid angiogram demonstrates markedly slow flow in the internal carotid artery due to severe diffuse narrowing that extends to the skull base *(open arrows),* with near-complete occlusion of the supraclinoid region *(large arrow).* The frontal branch of the superficial temporal artery (STA) is identified by the *small arrows. B,* A later phase of the left common carotid injection demonstrates the severe stenosis of the supraclinoid internal carotid artery *(large arrow),* and very poor filling of the middle cerebral vessels *(small arrows). C,* Lateral projection of a selective left external carotid angiogram after performance of an extracranial-intracranial (EC-IC) bypass between the frontal branch of the STA and a parietal branch of the middle cerebral artery (MCA) *(arrows).* The *upper arrow* demonstrates the site of anastomosis between the STA artery and the MCA.

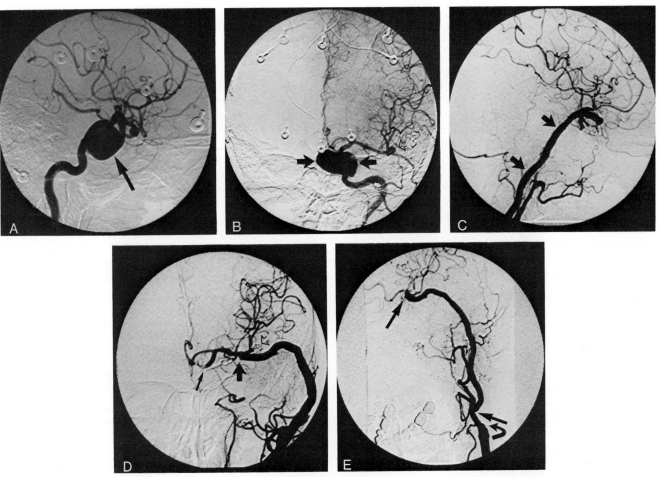

FIGURE 124–3.   This patient presented with severe left retro-orbital pain and diplopia due to a left sixth cranial nerve palsy. The lateral *(A)* and anteroposterior (AP) *(B)* views of the internal carotid angiogram demonstrate a giant intracavernous aneurysm *(arrows)*. Because the patient did not tolerate a trial of temporary occlusion of the left internal carotid artery (she developed aphasia and right hemiparesis), permanent balloon occlusion of the left carotid artery was not an option for treatment of this unclippable aneurysm. The patient was treated with a saphenous vein graft bypass from the left external carotid artery (end-to-side) to the left proximal MCA (end-to-side). The lateral *(C)* and AP *(D)* views of the common carotid artery angiogram demonstrate the saphenous vein graft *(large arrows)*. Note on the AP view *(D)*, the distal site of internal carotid artery occlusion *(small arrow)*, and the site of clipping of a small MCA aneurysm, also seen on *B* *(open arrow)*. A view of the left common carotid artery injection that includes both the carotid bifurcation and the intracranial circulation *(E)* demonstrates occlusion of the internal carotid artery *(curved arrow)*, and the proximal and distal anastomosis of the vein graft *(straight arrows)*.

SURGICAL PROCEDURE

Preoperative Evaluation

The history and neurologic examination are of major importance in selecting patients who should undergo an EC-IC bypass operation. Careful neurologic examination, immediately prior to surgery, provides a necessary baseline for postoperative comparison. Cardiac evaluation, including electrocardiography, is also mandatory because of the prevalence of cardiovascular disease in patients with cerebrovascular symptoms. CT or MRI of the brain is essential in order to rule out disorders that may cause symptoms mimicking TIAs or stroke (subdural hematoma, tumors, vascular malformations). Angiography is the definitive anatomic examination and should include both carotid circulations (including the external carotid artery circulation) and the vertebrobasilar circulation. The angiographic examination is designed to identify occlusive lesions, collateral pathways, and potential donor and recipient bypass vessels. In many cases, TCD and cerebral blood flow evaluations are employed to assess cerebrovascular hemodynamic adequacy.

Anesthesia

Anesthetic considerations are of prime importance in minimizing the risk of perioperative complications. These patients have compromised cerebral circulation, and meticulous care must be taken to maintain the normal cerebral hemodynamic status. The surgical procedures are performed under general anesthesia with maintenance of normotension, normocapnia, and optimal oxygenation. Intraoperative monitoring of the electroencephalogram (EEG) and of somatosensory evoked potentials allows continuous analysis of the functional status of the cerebral cortex.

Before temporary occlusion of the cerebral recipient vessel, cerebral protection is maximized by the administration of barbiturates (thiopental, 1 to 3 mg/kg initially) in order to achieve a pattern of burst suppression on the

EEG.[46, 47] This ensures that barbiturate administration has achieved the optimal level of cerebral metabolic suppression to provide protection of the brain during the period of temporary arterial occlusion. In many cases, the administration of barbiturates causes mild hypotension, and pressors are employed to maintain a normal level of blood pressure.

The patient does not receive systemic heparinization during the procedure, but the donor and recipient vessels are irrigated thoroughly with heparinized saline. The patients are placed preoperatively and continued postoperatively on aspirin.[45]

Superficial Temporal Artery–to–Middle Cerebral Artery Bypass

The patient is placed in the supine position with the head rotated to bring the temporal region on the symptomatic side almost horizontal.[14] The operative area is shaved,

and the superficial temporal artery branches are identified with a Doppler probe and marked. The largest superficial temporal artery branch (which in most cases is the posterior branch) as identified on the preoperative angiogram is selected as the donor vessel.

A linear incision is made over the course of the superficial temporal artery branch[35, 45] (Fig. 124–4). Local anesthesia is not used. The incision is superficial, dividing only the dermis and the epidermis. The superficial temporal artery branch is then exposed with careful subcutaneous dissection. Once the artery is identified, it is separated from the subcutaneous tissue using a curved hemostat. The skin overlying the vessel is then elevated with the hemostat and divided with a No. 15 blade. The dissection proceeds proximally and distally until the artery has been exposed from the level of the zygomatic arch to a level just above the superior temporal line. This generally provides an adequate length (10 to 12 cm) for performance of the anastomosis. After completing the cutdown over the superficial temporal

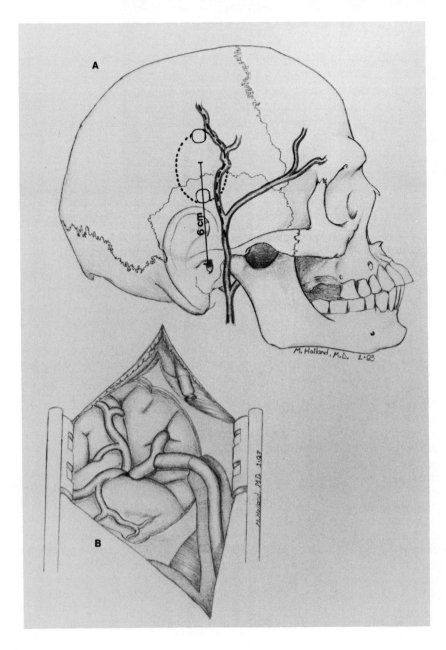

FIGURE 124–4. *A*, The incision has been made over the parietal branch of the STA. The length of the incision should expose enough artery for the anastomosis to be done under no tension. The craniotomy is centered around Chater's point, 6 cm superior to the external auditory canal. This exposes the posterior end of the sylvian fissure where several moderate-sized end arteries exit, offering a choice of anastomotic sites. *B*, The figure shows the parietal branch of the STA anastomosed to one of the arteries exiting the sylvian fissure. Notice the smooth curve that the STA branch takes on its way intracranially.

artery, small scalp flaps are developed on either side of the superficial temporal artery branch. The adventitia on either side of the branch, approximately 1.5 to 2.0 mm from the artery, is then cauterized using the bipolar coagulator, and divided with a No. 15 blade or tenotomy scissors. The adventitia is divided to the level of the temporalis muscle. The final step is to separate the adventitial cuff from the underlying temporalis fascia. Side branches from the superficial temporal artery are carefully coagulated more than 1 mm away from the main trunk of the vessel and divided. The superficial temporal artery is left in continuity at this stage, so that it continues to be perfused.

If the parietal branch of the superficial temporal artery has been selected, the cutdown incision over the artery can be employed for the craniotomy. The craniotomy is centered at a point 6 cm above the external auditory meatus (Chater's point).[5] This point lies over the posterior aspect of the sylvian fissure, where several large middle cerebral artery branches emerge from the fissure to reach the cortical surface. This area offers the widest choice of potential recipient branches.

The superficial temporal artery is retracted forward, and the temporalis muscle incised vertically. Anterior and posterior temporal muscle flaps are developed. A small circular or oval craniotomy flap is fashioned with the power drill and craniotome. Meticulous hemostasis is obtained with the use of bipolar coagulation and dural tacking sutures. The dura is opened to expose the posterior sylvian fissure. The arachnoid is opened carefully over the largest suitable middle cerebral artery branch, which should be 1.0 mm or more in diameter. A 1-cm length of the vessel is prepared to receive the anastomosis. Arachnoid stripped from the middle cerebral artery branch and tiny perforating arterial branches originating from the segment to be isolated are coagulated and cut.

At this point, the superficial temporal artery graft is prepared. The artery is occluded proximally using a temporary aneurysm clip and distally using a permanent hemostatic clip. The distal end of the superficial temporal artery, for a distance of 5 mm, is dissected free of adventitia. The artery is then divided on an angle in order to "fishmouth" the tip. This results in substantial enlargement of the arterial orifice, which should be 1.5 to 2.0 times the diameter of the recipient vessel. The vessel is then irrigated several times using a blunt needle with heparinized saline (10 U heparin/ml saline).

The superficial temporal artery orifice is then brought in proximity to the middle cerebral artery branch. It is important that there be enough length of the superficial temporal artery, so that it assumes a gentle curving course when it is approximated to the middle cerebral artery. Tension or stretching of the superficial temporal artery must be avoided. At this point, the patient is given barbiturates to provide cerebral protection during the period of middle cerebral artery occlusion. The middle cerebral artery branch is occluded proximally and distally using small, low-pressure temporary arterial clips. A linear arteriotomy is made along the middle cerebral artery branch for a length equivalent to the longest diameter of the superficial temporal artery orifice (Fig. 124–5). None of the middle cerebral artery wall is excised, as this simply reduces the final caliber of the anastomosis.

Fixation sutures (9–0 or 10–0 nylon on an atraumatic

needle) are placed at the proximal and distal corners of the anastomosis. The front and back walls are closed with interrupted 10–0 monofilament sutures. After the corner stitches, the next two sutures are placed midway along the arteriotomy on the back and the front walls. This tends to hold the arteriotomy open and minimizes the chance of catching the opposite wall of the middle cerebral artery when placing the remainder of the interrupted sutures. The back wall (that which is more awkward to expose) is sutured first. The front wall is then closed. Generally between 5 and 7 interrupted sutures are required for each wall of the anastomosis[14] (see Fig. 124–5).

The performance of the anastomosis takes place under frequent heparinized saline irrigation to clear blood from the suture site. After completion of the anastomosis, the clips are first removed from the middle cerebral artery branch. It is not uncommon to observe a brief period of oozing from the anastomosis. This rapidly ceases with gentle irrigation using nonheparinized saline. After leakage has stopped, the temporary clip is removed from the superficial temporal artery. If the anastomosis is widely patent and nonstenotic, the superficial temporal artery and the recipient segment of the middle cerebral artery should begin pulsating vigorously. The adequacy of flow through the superficial temporal artery can be confirmed using a sterile Doppler probe. Saline irrigation of the anastomotic site should result in the cessation of any bleeding that occurs when the superficial temporal artery is opened. If bleeding continues, temporary clips should be reapplied to the superficial temporal artery and the middle cerebral artery so that an additional suture can be applied to the site of leakage.

Once the temporary clips have been removed, barbiturate administration can be stopped. The base of the bone flap is trimmed to provide a channel through which the superficial temporal artery can travel without compression. The bone flap is then tied or wired into place. The dura is only loosely approximated, taking care not to compromise the superficial temporal artery. The temporalis muscle is loosely reapproximated, again to avoid constricting the superficial temporal artery. The scalp is closed using galeal/subcutaneous sutures and staples. A local dressing is applied.

If the frontal branch of the superficial temporal artery is selected, the vessel is dissected from the scalp using the cutdown technique. A second, vertically oriented incision above the ear is required to expose the craniotomy site at Chater's point. The cutdown incision over the frontal branch and the vertical incision over the craniotomy site are not connected. After performance of the craniotomy and exposure of the middle cerebral artery branches, the superficial temporal artery can be passed from the anterior incision to the posterior incision through the subgaleal plane. This tunnel is prepared by blunt dissection between the galea and the temporalis fascia. It is important to avoid twisting or kinking the superficial temporal artery during its passage from one incision to the other.

Saphenous Vein Graft Bypass

Long Vein Graft

Under certain circumstances, a saphenous vein graft should be employed for the EC-IC bypass.[35, 49] Vein grafts

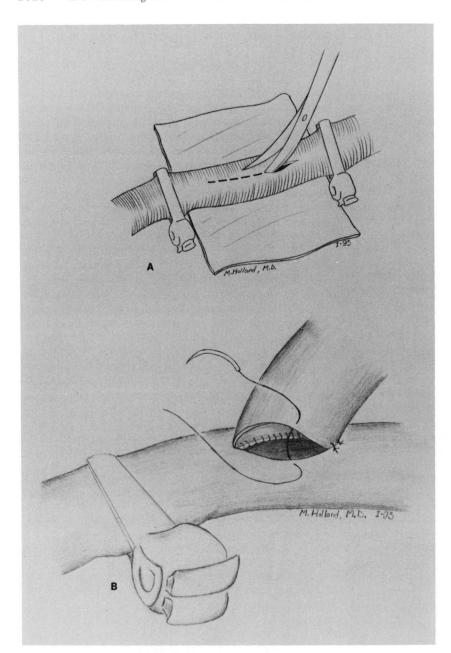

FIGURE 124–5. *A*, After the cortical branch is cleared of connective tissue, two small temporary microclips are placed on either side of the future anastomotic site to isolate the vessel. Furthermore, a piece of glove rubber is placed deep to the vessel to provide a more stable working surface and to protect the underlying brain. A linear incision is made lengthwise on the recipient vessel, long enough to accept the mouth of the donor vessel. *B*, The anastomosis is carried out using 9–0 suture for both incisional apices. The remainder of the anastomosis is performed with interrupted 10–0 sutures, first on one half of the suture line, then on the other.

are generally used when the superficial temporal artery is inadequate or has been sacrificed by prior surgery, or when treatment of a tumor or aneurysm requires therapeutic occlusion of the internal carotid artery, with immediate high-flow restoration of the hemispheric blood supply. The saphenous vein graft is generally connected to the external carotid artery, but may be anastomosed to the common carotid artery or the subclavian artery if necessary. The distal anastomosis may be fashioned to a superficial middle cerebral artery branch or to a larger, more proximal middle cerebral artery branch in the sylvian fissure (Fig. 124–6). The authors' preference has been to perform an end-to-side anastomosis between the vein graft and the external carotid artery and an end-to-side anastomosis between the vein graft and an M2 or a large M3 branch of the middle cerebral artery (just distal to the middle cerebral artery bifurcation) in the sylvian fissure. This provides a high-flow, large-

caliber conduit that is capable of supplying the entire cerebral hemisphere immediately.

The surgical procedure involves two surgical teams.[35, 49] One team first isolates the cervical carotid arteries and then performs a craniotomy to expose the middle cerebral artery branches in the sylvian fissure or on the cortical surface. The second surgical team isolates the saphenous vein from the medial malleolus proximally for a distance of about 15 cm. Side branches of the saphenous vein are ligated with 3–0 or 4–0 silk, and the vein is isolated along with a small amount of adventitial tissue. The vein is left in place, in continuity, until immediately before it is to be used for the bypass. This avoids a prolonged period of endothelial ischemia, which may compromise viability of the vein. It is important to emphasize that great care is taken in isolating the vein, in order to avoid trauma that may result in thrombosis of the bypass.

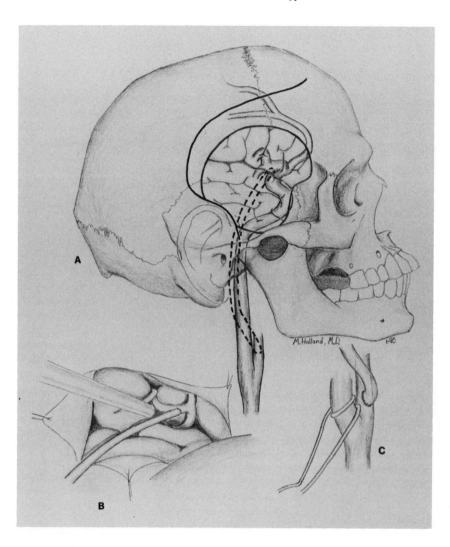

FIGURE 124–6. *A,* This shows the course of the saphenous vein graft from the external carotid artery near the carotid bulb to the sylvian fissure at the M2 segment of the MCA. *B,* The sylvian fissure is opened, exposing the MCA, and the distal anastomosis is made to one of the proximal M2 branches. *C,* Finally, the proximal end of the vein graft is anastomosed to the proximal external carotid in an end-to-side fashion.

Once the extracranial carotid artery and the recipient middle cerebral artery branch have been isolated and prepared, the vein is ligated proximally and distally and excised. The vein is flushed with cool heparinized saline. It is important to avoid high-pressure overdistention of the vein, which may cause damage to the endothelium or wall. Any side branches that leak during irrigation of the vein may be oversewn with 7–0 Prolene.

Before excising the vein, it is important that the alignment of the vein be marked. A pen marking on the superficial surface of the vein may be employed. Alternatively, one can pass a 5–0 Prolene suture through the superficial layer of the adventitia. The marking or the adventitial suture is used to ensure that the vein does not become torqued or twisted as it is positioned for the bypass.

The vein graft is passed from the cervical incision to the cranial incision (see Fig. 124–6). A large, curved clamp is passed from the cranial incision behind the zygomatic arch toward the surgeon's finger positioned in the cervical incision deep to the parotid gland. The clamp is used to grasp a large (20 Fr) chest tube and to pull the tube through this tunnel. Using a shunt-passing instrument a 0 silk suture is passed through the chest tube. The vein is brought to the cervical incision and oriented so that flow occurs in the direction of the valves (the segment of the vein that was harvested from the region of the medial malleolus is used

for the proximal anastomosis). The suture is tied to the end of the saphenous vein graft that is to be connected to the middle cerebral artery and the vein is pulled through the chest tube. The registration line (or suture) on the surface of the vein is watched carefully so as to avoid twisting. After passage of the vein through the chest tube, the chest tube is pulled from the subcutaneous tunnel leaving the vein graft in place. The vein graft is then filled with cool heparinized saline and occluded proximally and distally with temporary aneurysm clips.

The authors have found it much easier to perform the intracranial anastomosis first, as suggested by Sundt and coworkers.[49] This allows the surgeon to take advantage of a certain amount of slack in the vein graft, which can be helpful when exposing and suturing the back and front walls of the anastomosis. The terminal 10 mm of the vein graft is trimmed of adventitia. The orifice of the vein graft is fish-mouthed or beveled to create an orifice of approximately 5 to 6 mm in diameter. A suitable length of middle cerebral artery is occluded between temporary aneurysm clips, and a linear arteriotomy made in the middle cerebral branch. The vein graft is fixed to the middle cerebral artery branch using two corner tacking sutures of 8–0 or 9–0 monofilament nylon. The front and back walls are closed with interrupted sutures, or alternatively, the corner tacking sutures can be used to fashion a running closure of the anastomosis. After completion of the vein to middle cerebral artery anastomosis, flow is restored through the middle cerebral artery by removing the aneurysm clips. The temporary clip remains, at this point, on the distal end of the vein graft. The authors have not employed systemic heparinization, but the anastomotic site is continuously flushed during suturing with heparinized saline. As with superficial temporal artery to middle cerebral artery grafts, barbiturates are administered while the middle cerebral artery branch is occluded.

The vein graft is then gently pulled into the cervical incision to remove slack and redundancy. A 1.5-cm length of the external carotid artery is occluded between temporary clips, and a 8- to 10-mm linear arteriotomy is made. Again systemic heparinization is not employed, but the anastomotic site is irrigated with heparinized saline. The proximal end of the vein graft is trimmed of its adventitia and fish-mouthed to enlarge the orifice as described previously. Prolene sutures (7–0) are used to tack the vein graft to the external carotid arteriotomy and to fashion a running closure of the front and back walls. After completion of this end-to-side anastomosis, the temporary clips are removed from the external carotid artery, and subsequently from the vein graft, which has remained filled with heparinized saline. Leakage of blood from the anastomotic sites generally stops rapidly under irrigation with nonheparinized saline. If the proximal and distal anastomoses are widely patent, a bounding pulse should be visible and palpable in the vein graft. The craniotomy is closed with care to avoid compromising the vein graft by the closure of the dura or temporalis muscle. The cervical incision is closed in routine fashion.

Short Vein Graft

A short saphenous vein interposition graft can be placed between the superficial temporal artery trunk at the zygomatic arch and a branch of the middle cerebral artery.[31] This procedure is useful when only a short segment of acceptable saphenous vein is available or when, for one reason or another, the cervical external carotid artery cannot be used as the site of the proximal anastomosis. The superficial temporal artery trunk is dissected from the subcutaneous tissue just anterior to the ear at the level of the zygomatic arch. The artery at this point is somewhat larger in caliber than it is more distally over the temporal region.

As in the case of the long saphenous vein, the distal middle cerebral artery anastomosis is performed first. Subsequently, an end-to-side anastomosis is performed between the vein graft and the superficial temporal artery trunk. For this procedure, the vein graft need be only 5 to 8 cm in length.

Occipital Artery–to–Middle Cerebral Artery Graft

In cases in which the superficial temporal artery is inadequate for the bypass, or when bypass to more posteriorly located middle cerebral artery branches is desirable, the occipital artery can be used as the donor vessel.[35] The cutdown technique is again used. The occipital artery is

often more tortuous and, behind the mastoid, traverses several muscle planes. This makes isolation of the occipital artery somewhat more complex and tedious. If a sufficiently long unbranched segment of the occipital artery is available, however, it can provide an excellent EC-IC bypass.

Superficial Temporal Artery On-Lay Procedure (Encephaloduroarteriosynangiosis)

In certain cases of severe occlusive cerebrovascular disease or in the entity of moyamoya disease, there may be no adequate middle cerebral artery recipient branch. In such cases, the superficial temporal artery, left in continuity along with an associated cuff of adventitia, can be laid on the pial surface of the brain, which has been denuded of arachnoid.[33] The edges of a linear dural incision are sutured to the superficial temporal artery adventitial tissue. Although there is no direct arterial anastomosis, with time, spontaneous arterial connections form between the superficial temporal artery graft and small vessels on the pial surface. The degree of angiographic filling of cortical vessels can be quite remarkable using this procedure.

POSTOPERATIVE MANAGEMENT

After completion of the anastomosis, normal arterial pressure is maintained. Care is taken to avoid postoperative dehydration, and the patient is given aspirin (325 mg daily) to avoid postoperative graft thrombosis. Postoperative complications include continuing TIAs, stroke, intracerebral hemorrhage, and subdural hematoma.[38] New postoperative neurologic deficit or postoperative TIAs require investigation with cranial CT scanning and angiography.

RESULTS

The patency rate for superficial temporal artery to middle cerebral artery grafts has been approximately 95 per cent. The perioperative rate of stroke and/or death has been in the range of 3 to 4 per cent.[12] In the authors' experience, no superficial temporal artery to middle cerebral artery graft has occluded postoperatively, and the minor stroke rate has been approximately 3 per cent. No patient had a major disabling stroke, and there have been no perioperative deaths. Saphenous vein graft patency has been approximately 85 per cent, with a slightly higher perioperative morbidity and mortality.[49]

SUMMARY

EC-IC arterial bypass, using scalp arteries or vein interposition grafts, can be performed with high patency and low morbidity rates. Although the EC-IC Bypass Study demonstrated that most patients with symptomatic carotid occlusion or other inaccessible cerebrovascular atherosclerotic lesions are not benefitted by bypass surgery, certain clinical indications for this procedure remain valid. The strongest current indications for EC-IC bypass are

1. Continuing TIAs, refractory to maximal antithrombotic therapy, due to cerebral hemodynamic insufficiency; or

2. Requirement for therapeutic carotid occlusion in a patient with inadequate cerebral collateral circulation.

References

1. Ausman JI, Latchaw RW, Lee MC, Ramirez-Lassepas M: Results of multiple angiographic studies on cerebral revascularization patients. *In* Schmiedek P, Gratzl O, Spetzler R, et al (eds): Microsurgery for Stroke. New York, Springer-Verlag, 1977.
2. Austin G, Hayward W, Laffin D: Use of cerebral blood flow for selection and monitoring of patients. *In* Austin GM (ed): Microneurosurgical Anastomosis for Cerebral Ischemia. Springfield, IL, Charles C. Thomas, 1976, pp 327–338.
3. Awad IA, Spetzler RF: Extracranial-intracranial arterial bypass surgery: A critical analysis in light of the International Cooperative Study. Neurosurgery 19(4):655, 1986.
4. Carter LP, Hadley MN, Spetzler RF: Regional cortical blood flow during extracranial-intracranial bypass. *In* Spetzler RF, Carter LP, Selman WR, et al (eds): Cerebral Revascularization for Stroke. New York: Thieme-Stratton, 1985, pp 136–142.
5. Chater NL: Patient selection and results of extra-to-intracranial anastomosis in selected cases of cerebrovascular disease. Clin Neurosurg 23:287, 1976.
6. Chater N, Popp J: Microsurgical vascular bypass for occlusive cerebrovascular disease. Review of 100 cases. Surg Neurol 6:114, 1976.
7. Crowell RM: Electromagnetic flow studies of superficial temporal artery to middle cerebral artery bypass graft. *In* Austin CM (ed): Microneurosurgical Anastomosis for Cerebral Ischemia. Springfield, IL, Charles C. Thomas, 1976, pp 116–124.
8. Day AL: EC-IC bypass for MCA obstruction. *In* Spetzler RF, Carter LP, Selman WR, et al (eds): Cerebral Revascularization for Stroke. New York, Thieme-Stratton, 1985, pp 458–466.
9. Diaz FG, Umansky F, Mehta B, et al: Cerebral revascularization to a main limb of the middle cerebral artery in the sylvian fissure: An alternative approach to conventional anastomosis. J Neurosurg 63:21, 1985.
10. Donaghy RMP, Yasargil MG: Microvascular Surgery. St. Louis: CV Mosby, 1967.
11. Durham SR, Smith HA, Rutigliano MJ, Yonas H: Assessment of cerebral vasoreactivity and stroke risk using Xe CT acetazolamide challenge [Abstract]. Stroke 22:138, 1991.
12. The EC-IC Bypass Study Group. Failure of extracranial-intracranial arterial bypass to reduce the risk of ischemic stroke: Results of an international randomized trial. N Engl J Med 313:1191, 1985.
13. Fisher M: Occlusion of the internal carotid artery. Arch Neurol Psychiatry 65:346, 1951.
14. Fox JL, Albin MS, Bader DC, et al: Microsurgical treatment of neurovascular disease. I. Personnel, equipment, extracranial-intracranial anastomosis. Neurosurgery 3:285, 1978.
15. Gelber BR, Sundt TM: Treatment of intracavernous and giant carotid aneurysms by combined internal carotid ligation and extra- to intracranial bypass. J Neurosurg 52:1, 1980.
16. Gibbs JM, Leeders KL, Wiser RJS, Jones T: Evaluation of cerebral perfusion in patients with carotid artery occlusion. Lancet 2:310, 1984.
17. Gratzl O, Schmiedek P, Spetzler R, et al: Clinical experience with extracranial-intracranial arterial anastomosis in 65 cases. J Neurosurg 44:313, 1976.
18. Grubb RL Jr, Ratcheson RA, Raichle MD, et al: Regional cerebral blood flow and oxygen utilization in superficial temporal middle cerebral artery anastomosis patients. J Neurosurg 50:733, 1979.
19. Haas WK, Fields WS, North RR, et al: Joint study of extracranial arterial occlusion. Arteriography, techniques, sites and complications. JAMA 203:961, 1968.
20. Hadley MN, Spetzler RF, Martin NA, et al: Middle cerebral artery aneurysm due to *Nocardia asteroides*: Case report of aneurysm excision and extracranial-intracranial bypass. Neurosurgery 22:923, 1988.
21. Heilbrun MP, Reichman OH, Anderson RE, Roberts TW: Regional cerebral blood flow studies following middle cerebral artery anastomosis. J Neurosurg 43:706, 1975.
22. Hopkins LN, Grand W: Extracranial-intracranial arterial bypass in the treatment of aneurysms of the carotid and middle cerebral arteries. Neurosurgery 5:21, 1979.
23. Hopkins L, Martin N, Hadley M, et al: Vertebrobasilar insufficiency. 2. Microsurgical treatment of intracranial vertebrobasilar disease. J Neurosurg 66:662, 1987.
24. Jacobsen JH II, Suarez E: Microsurgery in anastomosis of small vessels. Surg Forum 11:243, 1960.
25. Karasawa J, Kikuchi H, Faruse S, et al: Treatment of moyamoya disease with STA-MCA anastomosis. J Neurosurg 49:679, 1978.
26. Kleiser B, Widder B: Course of carotid occlusions with impaired cerebrovascular reactivity. Stroke 23:171, 1992.
27. Latchaw RE, Ausman JI, Lee MC: Superficial temporal-middle cerebral artery bypass. J Neurosurg 51:455, 1979.
28. Latchaw RE, Ausman JI, Lee MC: STA-MCA anastomosis: Detailed analysis of pre- and postoperative angiography. *In* Ischemia. New York, Springer-Verlag, 1981.
29. Laurent JP, Lawner PM, O'Connor M. Reversal of intracerebral steal by STA-MCA anastomosis. J Neurosurg 57:629, 1982.
30. Lee MC, Ausman JI, Geiger JD, et al: Superficial temporal to middle cerebral artery anastomosis. Clinical outcome in patients with ischemia or infarction in internal carotid artery distribution. Arch Neurol 36:1, 1979.
31. Little J, Furlan A, Bryerton B: Short vein grafts for cerebral revascularization. J Neurosurg 59:384, 1983.
32. Little JR, Yamamoto VL, Feindel W, et al: Superficial temporal artery to middle cerebral artery anastomosis. Intraoperative evaluation by fluorescein angiography and xenon-133 clearance. J Neurosurg 50:560, 1979.
33. Matsushima Y, Fukai N, Tanaka K, et al: A new surgical treatment of moyamoya disease in children: A preliminary report. Surg Neurol 15:313, 1980.
34. Morawetz RB, Halsey JH Jr, Wills EL, et al: The use of STA-MCA bypass in the evaluation of rCBF. *In* Peerless SJ, McCormick CW (eds): Microsurgery for Cerebral Ischemia. New York, Springer-Verlag, 1981, pp 46–55.
35. Ojemann R, Heros R, Crowell R: Surgical Management of Cerebrovascular Disease, Baltimore, Williams & Wilkins, 1988, pp 83–120.
36. Powers WJ, Raichle ME: Positron emission tomography and its application to the study of cerebrovascular disease in man. Stroke 16:361, 1985.
37. Powers WJ, Tempel LW, Grubb RL Jr: Influence of cerebral hemodynamics on stroke risk: One-year follow-up of 30 medically treated patients. Ann Neurol 25:325, 1989.
38. Reichman OH: Complications of cerebral revascularization. Clin Neurosurg 23:313, 1976.
39. Reichman OH: Estimation of flow through STA bypass graft. *In* Fein JM, Reichman OH (eds): Microvascular Anastomosis for Cerebral Ischemia. Berlin, Springer-Verlag, 1978, pp 220–240.
40. Ringelstein EB, Sievers C, Ecker S, et al: Noninvasive assessment of CO_2-induced cerebral vasomotor response in normal individuals and patients with internal carotid artery occlusions. Stroke 19:963, 1988.
41. Samson DS, Boone S: Extracranial-intracranial (EC-IC) arterial bypass: Past performance and current concepts. Neurosurgery 3:79, 1978.
42. Schmiedek P, Gratzl O, Spetzler R, et al: Selection of patients for extracranial-intracranial bypass surgery based on rCBF measurements. J Neurosurg 44:303, 1976.
43. Spetzler RF, Carter LP: Revascularization and aneurysm surgery: Current status. Neurosurgery 66:648, 1985.
44. Spetzler RF, Chater N: Microvascular bypass surgery. 2. Physiological studies. J Neurol 45:508, 1976.
45. Spetzler R, Hadley M: Extracranial-intracranial bypass grafting: An update. *In* Wilkins R, Rengachary S (eds): Neurosurgery Update II. Vascular, Spinal, Pediatric, and Functional Neurosurgery. New York, McGraw-Hill, 1991, p 197.
46. Spetzler RF, Martin NA, Hadley MN, et al: Microsurgical endarterectomy under barbiturate cerebral protection: A prospective study. J Neurosurg 65:63, 1986.
47. Spetzler RF, Selman WR, Roski RA, et al: Cerebral revascularization during barbiturate coma in primates and humans. Surg Neurol 17:111, 1982.
48. Sullivan HG, Kingsbury TB IV, Morgan ME, et al: The rCBF response to Diamox in normal subjects and cerebrovascular disease patients. J Neurosurg 67:525, 1987.

49. Sundt TM Jr, Piepgras DG, Marsh ME, et al: Saphenous vein bypass grafts for giant aneurysms and intracranial occlusive disease. J Neurosurg 65:439, 1986.
50. Sundt TM Jr, Siekert RG, Piepgras DG, et al: Bypass surgery for vascular disease of the carotid system. Mayo Clin Proc 51:677, 1976.
51. Sundt TM Jr, Whisnant JP, Fode NC, et al: Results, complications, and follow-up of 415 bypass operations for occlusive disease of the carotid system. Mayo Clin Proc 60:230, 1985.
52. Vilagy MI, Rowed DW, Hachinski VC, et al: rCBF measurements in patients with STA-MCA shunts. *In* Peerless SJ, McCormick CW (eds): Microsurgery for Cerebral Ischemia. New York, Springer-Verlag, 1978, pp 56–58.

53. Widder B: The Doppler CO_2 test to exclude patients not in need of extracranial-intracranial bypass surgery. J Neurol Neurosurg Psychiatry 28:449, 1965.
54. Yasargil MG: Microsurgery Applied to Neurosurgery. Stuttgart, Georg Thieme Verlag, 1968.
55. Yasargil MG, Yonekawa YL: Results of microsurgical extracranial-intracranial bypass in the treatment of cerebral ischemia. Neurosurgery 1:22, 1977.
56. Yonekawa Y, Yasargil MG: Extra-intracranial arterial anastomosis: Clinical and technical aspects and results. Advances and Technical Standards in Neurosurgery. Wien, New York, Springer-Verlag, 1976, vol. 3, pp 47–48.

125

Management of Uncommon Lesions Affecting the Extracranial Vessels

Earl D. Cottrell, M.D., and Louis L. Smith, M.D.

• • •

Most discussions of the management of extracranial cerebrovascular disease focus on the more common atherosclerotic occlusive processes; however, there are several other pathologic conditions with which the physician dealing with vascular diseases must be familiar. Most vascular surgeons deal with only an occasional patient with these diseases; large studies are, therefore, not available for reference, and the management of these disorders must be based on the experience of several specialists. The compilation of these many reports provides the vascular surgeon with a valuable reference when an uncommon extracranial lesion is encountered. Several relatively uncommon extracranial processes such as vertebral-basilar insufficiency, coiling and kinking of the carotid artery, extracranial carotid aneurysms, and extracranial fibromuscular diseases are dealt with in other chapters of this text. This chapter focuses on the management of the uncommon incidence of carotid body dysfunction; carotid body tumors; carotid artery involvement by malignant diseases; irradiation-induced diseases; carotid artery infections; vascular inflammatory processes, such as Takayasu's arteritis and temporal arteritis; and carotid artery dissection.

THE DYSFUNCTIONAL CAROTID BODY

The carotid body is thought to originate in the third brachial arch, derive its cells from the neural crest, and migrate with the autonomic nervous system to develop in the adventitia of the common carotid artery. It is usually a minute oval structure 0.1 to 0.5 cm in diameter and generally located on the posterior aspect of the carotid bifurcation, but it may also lie on adjacent arteries. The blood supply is largely from a small vessel from the carotid bifurcation and the branches of the external carotid artery. The carotid body is innervated by afferent branches from the glossopharyngeal and vagus nerves and the cervical sympathetic ganglia.[1] There is specialized chemoreceptor tissue in the carotid body, which is only partly understood, that plays a complex homeostatic role in the control of arterial blood gases and pH. This type of tissue is also found in association with the jugular bulb, the middle ear, the aortic body, and the ganglion nodosum of the vagus nerve.

The carotid sinus also has a baroreceptor function, providing impulses from stretch receptors that travel along the sinus nerve of Hering and glossopharyngeal nerve (IX) and synapse with the cardioinhibitory and vasomotor centers in the medulla. The efferent fibers, which are carried in the vagus nerve, innervate the cardiac pacemakers, and the sympathetic nerves innervate the muscle fibers of the peripheral vasculature. Abnormalities of these complicated feedback mechanisms can cause heart rate and blood pressure decreases, and chronic conditions of hypoxemia may cause chemoreceptor imbalance.

Carotid sinus syndrome (CSS) has been defined as syncope secondary to carotid sinus hypersensitivity. CSS occurs in elderly patients, is more common in males, and is associated with atherosclerosis, diabetes, hypertension, and coronary artery disease.[2, 3] CSS must be distinguished from the more common etiologies of syncope, both cardiovascu-

Table 125–1. Causes of Syncope

Cause	Number of Patients	Per Cent
Cardiovascular	**58**	**28.5**
Dysrhythmia	43	
TIA	3	
Subclavian steal	2	
CSS	1	
Other	9	
Noncardiovascular	**49**	**24.0**
Vasovagal	24	
Orthostatic	14	
Other	11	
Unknown	**97**	**47.5**

Adapted from Kapoor WN, Karpf M, Wieand S, et al: A prospective evaluation and follow-up of patients with syncope. New Engl J Med 309:197, 1983.
Key: *TIA, transient ischemic attack; CSS, carotid sinus syndrome.*

lar and noncardiovascular (Table 125–1). Routine tests such as complete blood count (CBC), blood glucose, electrocardiography (ECG), Holter monitoring, carotid duplex scan, and transcranial Doppler evaluation provide useful information but electroencephalography (EEG), glucose tolerance tests, and computed tomography (CT) scans of the head are rarely helpful.[4] CSS is unique in that direct carotid massage or pressure produces the symptoms. This may be due to heart rate–independent factors as well as heart rate–dependent factors.[5] Right-sided hypersensitivity is more frequent than left-sided. Thirty per cent of patients identify a prodrome before syncope and 30 per cent have retrograde amnesia. In about half of the patients, syncope is precipitated by head movement.[6] Attempts at altering medications that block compensatory heart rate increases may be helpful in some patients, but those medications are usually necessary. In the recent past, carotid body denervation was advocated because of medical and pacemaker failures.[7, 8] Evidence now shows that these patients have excellent results when cardiac pacers are implanted, and that carotid body denervation is rarely, if ever, warranted.[9]

In an attempt to control carbon dioxide retention and asthma, some surgeons performed bilateral carotid body excision following the reported success in 65 per cent of 3914 patients in a report by Nakayama.[10] Since chemoreceptor tissue exists elsewhere, partial excision would be expected to be of little benefit. Indeed, further studies demonstrated the deleterious effects and this procedure has been abandoned.[11]

CAROTID BODY TUMORS (PARAGANGLIOMAS)

The only pathologic lesion to involve the carotid body is a tumor. Even so, carotid body tumors are rare, accounting for less than 0.5 per cent of all tumors. In the past, this neoplasm has been named chemodectoma or glomus caroticum. These are misnomers because no tumor arises from carotid sinus tissue and carotid body tumors contain no smooth muscle. The correct term for this tumor is a paraganglioma, since it develops from epithelioid cells derived from the neural crest that migrated in close association with autonomic ganglion cells. Histochemically, this has been

confirmed by the presence of multiple neuropeptide hormones as well as the neuron-specific enolase, a glycolytic enzyme.[12]

Paragangliomas can occur in the middle ear; larynx; vagus nerve; aortic arch; and within abdominal viscera, including liver, bladder, and duodenum. An exhaustive review of these interesting and unusual tumors appears in an Armed Forces Institute of Pathology fascicle that reviews the nomenclature and pathology of paragangliomas in detail.[13]

Symptoms and Findings

Initially, carotid body tumors produce no symptoms, but eventually at least 75 per cent of patients develop nonspecific symptoms such as enlarging neck mass (73 per cent); headache or neck pain (35 per cent); dizziness, tinnitus, hoarseness (8 per cent); dysphagia (8 per cent); and syncope. The patient sometimes notices a swelling below the angle of the mandible, or the tumor is discovered on a routine examination and is noted to be pulsatile but not expansile. This is in contrast to aneurysms, which are both expansile and pulsatile. A carotid body tumor can be moved side to side but not up and down. Neck bruits at the carotid bifurcation have been present in up to 25 per cent of patients.[14] Unfortunately, the failure to make the diagnosis still occurs, and nearly 25 per cent of paragangliomas are first recognized by a surprised surgeon who attempts to perform biopsy on a very vascular neck mass, suspecting it as a lymph node.

Malignancy defined by metastasis occurs in approximately 5 to 10 per cent of the cases and generally involves only the regional lymph nodes, but it can also involve lungs, liver, kidney, pancreas, thyroid, heart, and bone. Tumor of the carotid body can be spontaneous, familial, or induced by living at high altitudes.[15, 16] Sprong and Kirby[17] in 1949 reported 9 of 11 siblings in one family with carotid body tumors. More recently, Shedd and coworkers[18] have reported carotid body tumors in four related patients aged 27 to 50 years. Two of these patients had bilateral tumors, and a 32 per cent bilaterality incidence is reported in familial patterns[19] following an autosomal dominant mechanism for transmission.[20] In collected series, 8 per cent of the carotid body tumors were bilateral.[21] Younger patients with familial, bilateral, or multiple paragangliomas are prone to aggressive tumors.[22] In general, the tumors increase in size progressively and the risk of neurovascular deficits increases significantly with tumor size.

Diagnostic Studies

The diagnostic evaluation of paragangliomas is to confirm the diagnosis, evaluate the extent, identify involvement of adjacent nerves, discover any neuroendocrine activity, and consider embolization preoperatively. A carotid body tumor can be diagnosed by ultrasound, CT, or magnetic resonance imaging (MRI). Color-flow duplex sonography can easily delineate a hypervascular mass nestled in the carotid bifurcation and is now the most widely utilized noninvasive method.[23] Additionally, duplex scanning can sometimes demonstrate the blood supply from the external carotid artery. Duplex scanning may also be utilized in the screening of familial carotid body tumors as well as sequential follow-up of nonoperatively managed tumors. CT or MRI scanning is helpful in detecting multiple paragangliomas as well as determining extension to the base of the skull.

Arteriography was once the diagnostic tool of choice for demonstrating a hypervascular mass arising in the crotch of the carotid bifurcation (Fig. 125–1). It still is essential in identifying those large tumors that may be easily embolized as a preparatory step for surgical excision. Although feared, the risk of stroke during embolization has been low to nonexistent,[24, 25] and it has the advantage of decreasing blood loss, decreasing tumor size, and thus facilitating resection of very large tumors that would have been difficult, if not impossible, to resect safely. Embolization can only be regarded as a temporary preoperative technique because the tumor can acquire new blood supply and continue to enlarge if not excised.[26, 27]

Since approximately 10 per cent of cervical paragangliomas are associated with cranial nerve deficits, these nerves must be assessed carefully before operative intervention. This assessment includes indirect laryngoscopy to document vocal cord movement and a careful neurologic examination. Neuroendocrine hypersecretory activity is rare and present in only 5 per cent of patients.[28] The patients who have such activity almost always have other paragangliomas. These patients experience headaches, palpitations,

hypertension, photophobia, diaphoresis, and dysrhythmias. Catecholamine screening is advised in patients with these symptoms or in patients with familial, bilateral, or extracervical paragangliomas.

Surgical Management

Once a paraganglioma is discovered, surgical excision is the treatment of choice unless a particular patient has a specific contraindication such as terminal illness, extreme age, or high anesthetic or operative risk.[29] Radiation therapy has been utilized and is of only anecdotal benefit, since the tumor is felt to be radioresistant.[30–32] This concept has been challenged recently where there was complete response in 23 per cent, partial response in 54 per cent, and no response in the other 23 per cent of patients treated with radiotherapy.[33] Adjuvant radiotherapy after partial resection is likewise of questionable benefit,[19, 34] since most of the tumors continue to demonstrate progressive enlargement. The surgical removal of a carotid body tumor, however, requires skill and a keen understanding of vascular surgical techniques.[35]

Despite the surgical challenge involved in the removal of these tumors, the fact remains that surgical excision is the only curative therapy. Therefore, a carefully planned operative approach is essential to ensure complete tumor removal and minimize perioperative morbidity. Nasotracheal intubation allows greater upward displacement of the

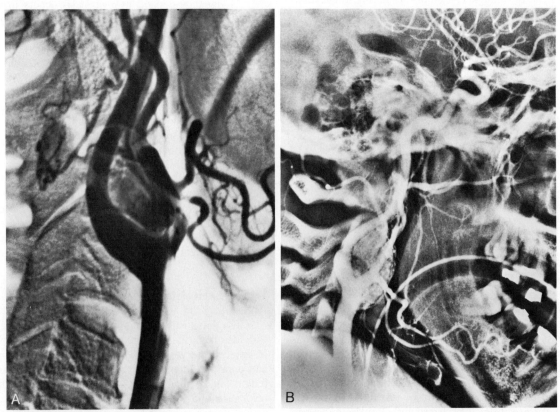

FIGURE 125–1. *A,* Subtraction selective carotid angiogram demonstrating a paraganglioma with the characteristic widening of the bifurcation—the so-called saddle deformity. *B,* Selective carotid angiogram demonstrating the vascularity of a carotid bifurcation paraganglioma.

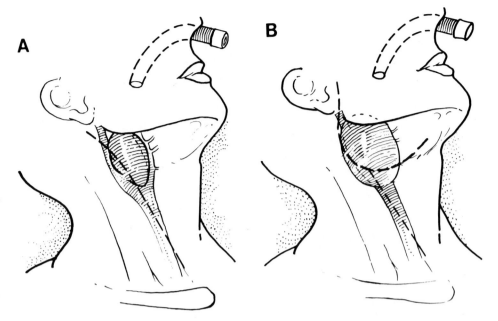

FIGURE 125–2. Neck incisions for carotid body tumor resection. A nasotracheal tube allows greater displacement of the floor of the mouth during retraction and dissection beneath the mandible. *A*, Incision for small tumor (<3 to 4 cm, Shamblin I). *B*, Incision for medium and large tumors (>4 to 5 cm, Shamblin II and III). (From Hallett JW: Carotid body tumor resection. *In* Bergen JJ, Yao JST [eds]: Techniques in Arterial Surgery. Philadelphia, WB Saunders, 1990, pp 214–222.)

floor of the mouth during retraction and dissection beneath the mandible. If preoperative evaluation suggests the necessity for high exposure of the internal carotid artery, subluxation of the ipsilateral mandible is performed.[36] A saphenous donor vein site should be prepared, since complicated arterial reconstruction is required in approximately 25 per cent of cases. Carotid shunts should also be available if clamping of the internal carotid artery is necessary and back pressure is low. Small tumors (less than 3 to 4 cm in diameter) can be approached by an anterior sternocleidomastoid incision; however, large tumors are more easily excised with a modified T-radical neck incision (Fig. 125–2). Cranial nerve preservation is best achieved by careful meticulous dissection around the tumor. Bipolar electrocautery helps to minimize heat injury to adjacent nerves. Some reports have mistakenly recommended a subadventitial dissection plane. This will lead to a weakened wall, predisposing the patient to intraoperative hemorrhage and/or postoperative carotid blowout. Therefore, the dissection is carried out in a periadventitial plane in the so-called white line described by Gordon-Taylor.[37] This white line is actually the most superficial adventitial layer. The most difficult area of dissection is the carotid bifurcation where the tumor is densely adherent and carotid injury is most likely. Temporary carotid clamping in the presence of an adequate backpressure and heparinization can make dissection easier and safer. In very large tumors (greater than 5 or 6 cm), ligation of the external carotid artery and its branches can decrease tumor size and bleeding, facilitating removal of the tumor (Fig. 125–3). Postoperatively, patients should be drained with closed suction and monitored in an intensive care setting for 6 to 12 hours, since pharyngeal swelling and hematoma may compromise the airway.

Shamblin and associates[38] have classified carotid body tumors in accordance with their gross relationship with the carotid vessels (Fig. 125–4). These three classifications are helpful in that they relate to the degree of difficulty with the operative resection of the tumors. Type I tumors account for 26 per cent of cases and are localized tumors that are easily removed. Type II tumors are adherent tumors that partially surround the carotid vessels. They make up 46 per cent of tumors and are removed with moderate difficulty. Type III tumors are 27 per cent of cases and are adherent tumors that completely surround the carotid vessels. These tumors are removed with extreme difficulty, generally require resection of the internal carotid with vein graft interposition,[39] and are associated with a high complication rate. Nearly all of the 3 per cent perioperative strokes and most of the 20 to 40 per cent incidence of cranial nerve dysfunction occur in this last group.

Early and accurate diagnosis of carotid body tumors will allow surgical intervention sooner in these relentlessly

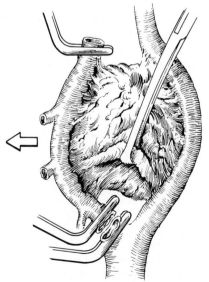

FIGURE 125–3. Resection of an external carotid artery segment to reduce bleeding during the surgical removal of a carotid body tumor. (From Krupski WC, Effeney DJ, Ehrenfeld WK, Stoney RJ: Cervical chemodectoma: Technical considerations and management options. Am J Surg 144:215, 1982.)

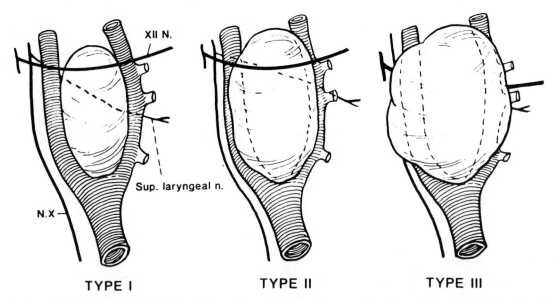

FIGURE 125–4. Difficulty of surgical resection of carotid body tumors, based on Shamblin classification. Type I tumors are well localized and easily resected, type II tumors adhere to and partially surround carotid vessels, and type III tumors surround carotid arteries. (From Nora JD, Hallett JW Jr, O'Brien PC, et al: Surgical resection of carotid body tumors: Long-term survival, recurrence, and metastasis. Mayo Clin Proc 63:348, 1988. By permission.)

slow-growing tumors. Newer noninvasive methods such as color-flow ultrasonography, CT, and MRI will allow for better confirmation and evaluation of extent of these tumors when the clinician suspects their presence. Arteriography remains useful in preoperative planning and embolization of large tumors. Although surgery is the treatment of choice, careful observation and possibly radiation can be employed in those cases unable to be resected, with survival for long periods.[40]

Nearly 95 per cent of carotid body tumors can be completely resected with a rare mortality (2 per cent). Perioperative stroke affects only 2 to 3 per cent. The greatest danger remains cranial nerve dysfunction, which can occur in up to 40 per cent, with one half of these temporary and the other half permanent. Survival of patients after carotid body tumor resection is equivalent to that of sex- and age-matched controls. Metastatic disease develops in only 2 per cent of patients and only 6 per cent develop recurrence after complete resection.[41]

CAROTID INVOLVEMENT WITH MALIGNANT DISEASE

The management of the extracranial carotid vessels when they are involved with malignancy requires adequate preoperative assessment, planning, and intraoperative flexibility to ensure durable and adequate perfusion to the cerebral tissue. Although often advocated, carotid ligation without reconstruction can result in a stroke incidence of 23 to 50 per cent and a mortality rate of 14 to 64 per cent.[22, 42, 43] Attention to thorough preoperative evaluation and intraoperative detail can decrease the stroke and mortality incidences significantly.[44, 45]

Preoperative Evaluation

Many malignant tumors of the head and neck present with primary or metastatic involvement of structures in close proximity to the carotid artery. Fortunately, there is actual invasion of the carotid in only 5 per cent of these patients.[46] Angiography cannot distinguish involvement, since it gives only a luminal projection. Narrowing of the contrast column can indicate external compression rather than invasion, and a normal appearance can falsely mislead the surgeon to believe that there is no vessel wall involvement. Angiography can, however, give data on collateral blood flow, existing carotid disease, anatomy, and, in some cases, can measure a stump pressure by a double lumen balloon.[47] Transcranial Doppler has also been reported to give valuable collateral information.[48] CT scans can determine the proximity of lesions to carotid, but fail to diagnose invasion. MRI promises to be the most helpful, as it may be the best way to visualize tissue planes as well as give anatomic data in multiple projections. Eventually, MRI may even be able to image the carotid vessels, data currently available only by arteriography.

Intraoperative Management

Often, carotid involvement can only be assessed at the time of the operation. Sometimes, even when the carotid is not actually involved, the dissection strips the vessel of its strongest layer, the adventitia. In these cases, as well as those of carotid invasion, a saphenous vein interposition graft is advised. This was first reported by Conley in 1953 when he encountered tumor invasion of the carotid.[49] The graft should be assessed intraoperatively following reconstruction angiography, angioscopy, or duplex scanning and any technical errors corrected.

If reconstruction is impossible and the carotid stump systolic pressure is greater than 70 mmHg, carotid ligation can generally be tolerated.[50] Patients with pressures less than this, however, have significant neurologic morbidity. Many of the patients suffering stroke after carotid ligation develop delayed neurologic symptoms.[41, 42, 50] The mechanism of these delayed strokes appears to be thromboembolic, with late propagation of thrombus up the internal carotid into the low-flow intracerebral circulation. Therefore, when possible, after a required ligation of the internal carotid artery, the patient should remain on heparin for 7 to 10 days. A mean backpressure less than 25 mmHg is an absolute indication for shunting while performing a graft. In difficult situations, an extracranial-intracranial bypass may be required. In contrast to the low stroke rates for atherosclerotic disease, carotid reconstruction in these patients has high stroke rates ranging from 7 to 20 per cent.[45, 49, 51, 52]

Following tumor excision and carotid reconstruction, adequate tissue coverage is mandatory to prevent life-threatening complications. Often, an advancement flap is all that is necessary. Rotation flaps using pectoralis, trapezius, or levator scapulae muscles can easily be performed.[53–55] If necessary, free tissue transfer grafts may be the only solution.[56]

Postoperative Surveillance

Those patients receiving preoperative or postoperative irradiation are subject to all of the injury explained in the next section. Additionally, the combination of irradiation injury, wound infection, or salivary leaks can predispose to breakdown and carotid rupture. The grafts themselves can easily be followed with duplex scanning for evaluation of any progressive stenoses.

CAROTID IRRADIATION ARTERITIS

Following successful resection of head and neck tumors, most patients undergo some radiotherapy. As with all treatment modalities, irradiation is not always benign and can cause numerous regional adverse tissue reactions. Most of these reactions to irradiation involve tissue perfusion concerns secondary to vessel changes. Small vessels, when irradiated, develop plaque-like thickening of the intima due to collection of fluid with foam cells and hyaline material between the endothelium and the internal elastic membrane.[57] These plaques narrow the lumen and decrease perfusion to local tissue.

Fonkalsrud and associates divide the changes that occur in irradiated arteries into acute and chronic phases based on observations in a canine model.[58] Within 48 hours of a 10-day course of 4000 cGy total dose, endothelial injury was manifested by nuclear disruption, cell sloughing, and deposition of fibrin. The media was minimally affected, and

the adventitia demonstrated only mild fibrosis and hemorrhage. Following 2 to 3 weeks, the endothelium began to regenerate, and the media and adventitia developed marked areas of necrosis and hemorrhage. After 4 months, the endothelial surface was thickened and irregular, the media and adventitia continued to develop fibrosis, and the regeneration of the endothelium combined with the fibrosis of the media and adventitia narrowed the lumen.

The described early pathologic changes secondary to irradiation predispose the vessel to thrombus formation and lipid accumulation. This intimal cell injury model parallels many studies designed to investigate arteriosclerosis. Indeed, a high-cholesterol diet administered after irradiation accelerates the atheromatous changes.[59–61] Similar early changes have been described after combined irradiation and hypertension.[62] Later pathologic changes to the media and adventitia are responsible for the total vessel involvement and this may be secondary to injury to the vasa vasora.

Irradiation damage to a large artery was first reported in humans in 1959 by Thomas and Forbus in a 21-year-old man who had received radiation for the treatment of lymphoma.[63] The irradiated arch had fibrotic changes in the intima, media, and adventitia with obliteration of the vasa vasora. Numerous reports have since been published indicating injury to most arterial systems. In the neck, the common carotid artery seems to have a greater propensity for these changes and atherosclerosis is accelerated in those patients with hypercholesterolemia.[64] Clinical irradiation-induced occlusive lesions have been described as appearing in three pathologic patterns.[65] The first pattern consists of intimal damage resulting in mural thrombosis and occurs within the first 5 years of the irradiation. The second pattern is evident within 10 years and is manifested by fibrotic occlusion. Periarterial fibrosis and accelerated atherosclerosis is common after approximately 20 years.

Clinically and angiographically, these lesions are often indistinguishable from atherosclerosis. Even so, there are some identifying factors. Often, there is diffuse narrowing rather than focal areas of atherosclerosis. Symptomatic patients generally present at an earlier age with irradiation-induced disease and are less likely to have associated coronary or other vascular disease, since irradiation injuries are localized to the irradiated areas.[64, 66]

Diagnosis of Irradiation Carotid Arteritis

All patients who have survived more than 5 years after cervical irradiation should be sequentially evaluated by duplex scanning for evidence of carotid stenosis. Recent data showed that 30 per cent of these patients had moderate or severe lesions compared with only 5.6 per cent in nonirradiated age-matched controls, and 9.4 per cent of the irradiated patients were symptomatic.[67] Symptomatic patients should undergo further testing with arteriography to evaluate the extent of the arteritis and develop a plan for reconstruction including vascular assessment of possible rotational flaps.

Management of Symptomatic Carotid Arteritis

In any symptomatic patient who has received prior irradiation to the neck, it is wise to consider and plan for the technical difficulties associated with the exposure and correction of the involved arterial segments. The tissue surrounding the artery is also injured, making it dense, fibrotic, and adherent to the damaged adventitia. The transmural radiation damage obliterates the normal cleavage planes in the vessel wall, rendering endarterectomy impossible.[64] Therefore, bypass grafting of diseased segments is the preferred treatment. Sometimes, reversed saphenous interposition grafts are possible, but many times extra-anatomic grafts or bypass grafts originating in the ascending aorta are required to avoid diseased segments. Autogenous vein grafts are preferable to avoid the increased rates of infection associated with synthetic material. Following vascular repair, it is essential to have good tissue coverage and this may require a rotation or advancement flap.

Patients presenting with symptomatic carotid stenoses after irradiation therapy may also have routine underlying atherosclerosis, which was developing prior to irradiation. In the patients who present with symptoms within 5 years of irradiation, this is often the case. These patients generally can undergo routine endarterectomy, taking into consideration the need to proceed with care through the irradiated tissues. It may be advisable to patch these patients to help prevent any future stenoses in the irradiated vessel.[68] As is the case with irradiation arteritis, preoperative and operative planning must take into consideration the need for viable tissue closure without tension, as discussed in the preceding section.

CAROTID ARTERY INFECTIONS

Patients developing carotid artery infections following head and neck surgery or endarterectomy often need rapid evaluation and creative approaches to achieve minimal neurologic morbidity. Although rare, hematogenous dissemination can also be a source for carotid artery infection.[69] Patients who rupture their carotid artery suffer a 40 per cent incidence of permanent neurologic complications and a 30 per cent mortality rate in spite of rapid and prompt treatment.[70] Contributing factors are wound infections, salivary leaks, skin or flap necrosis, and radiation. Carotid blowouts have an incidence of 3 per cent in patients after head and neck resection for cancer.[71] Many times a minor "sentinel bleed" precedes massive exsanguination, and if it occurs, prompt and definitive operative intervention is required.

Patients presenting with wound infections, flap necrosis, painful pulsatile erythematous masses, or minor bleeding from the neck require a prompt, directed surgical approach. Wound and blood cultures direct antibiotic selection, although definitive operative treatment should not be postponed pending these results. Angiography is useful in identifying possible vessel involvement as well as documenting collateral circulation. If carotid ligation is necessary, ligation when shock is present significantly increases the likelihood of stroke or death. If feasible, or if the carotid stump pressure is below 70 mmHg, extra-anatomic autogenous saphenous bypass grafts should be employed.[72] Ideally, these should avoid the direct area of infection and so an axillary to carotid bypass tunneling beneath the clavicle and routed laterally is ideal. Subclavian to carotid or carotid to carotid bypasses can also be utilized in selected circumstances. The involved carotid should be ligated proximally through a short transverse incision in uninvolved tissue to prevent further rupture, as recommended by Porto and associates.[73] Utilizing these principles, the neurologic morbidity and mortality can be decreased in these difficult to manage situations.

TAKAYASU'S ARTERITIS

Takayasu's disease (pulseless disease, occlusive thromboaortopathy, aortic arch arteritis, or aortitis syndrome) is an arteriopathy of unknown etiology that affects the aorta and its major branches. This disease was first described in a young female with visual impairment and absent carotid pulses by the Japanese ophthalmologist Takayasu in 1908.[74] The disease was originally thought to occur only in Asians, but now is known to occur in all races and nationalities. The disease can be present in all age groups; however, it most commonly affects women in the 2nd and 3rd decades of life. Although this autoimmune disease primarily affects the aorta, cerebral ischemia is considered one of the most life-threatening complications.[75]

Symptoms and Findings

The early phase of Takayasu's arteritis is difficult to diagnose because the symptoms of headache, malaise, arthralgia, myalgia, and fever are nonspecific. As the disease progresses, many years may pass before arterial obstruction occurs. In the chronic stage, the fever is absent, pulses are diminished or absent, and retinopathy is evident. Secondary complications, including hypertension, aneurysm formation, aortic valvular insufficiency, and cerebral vascular symptoms, may occur. Other diseases that must be considered in the differential diagnosis are arteriosclerosis, fibromuscular dysplasia, Behçet's disease, coarctation of the aorta, and giant cell arteritis.

The histologic pictures of both Takayasu's disease and giant cell arteritis are identical and have led some to suggest that they are different manifestations of the same disease. The absence of giant cells and marked intimal involvement in some Takayasu's specimens, and the findings of medial necrosis surrounded by inflammatory cells and numerous foreign body giant cells near the internal elastic lamina with minimal intimal involvement in some giant cell arteritis patients, have led some investigators to mistakenly report these as diagnostic differences.[76, 77] Giant cells are not a consistent microscopic feature in either of the disease processes and their presence is not essential to the diagnosis of either.[78, 79] Both Takayasu's and giant cell arteritis have three different histologic patterns. In nonspecific inflammation, the entire arterial wall is infiltrated with neutrophils, lymphocytes, and eosinophila. In granulomatous arteritis, Langhans' giant cells are present in the media, there is smooth muscle necrosis, and disruption of the internal elastic membrane is often observed. In the fibrosis stage, the vessel lumen is occluded with acellular fibrous tissue. Both forms of arteritis can produce skip lesions, once thought to be a feature of only Takayasu's disease.[80]

Universally accepted criteria for the clinical diagnosis of Takayasu's disease have not been established. Ueno and colleagues as well as Lupi-Herrera and coworkers have outlined a classification based on the anatomic involvement[81, 82] (Fig. 125–5) as determined by arteriography, which is essential to determine the extent of the disease (Fig. 125–6). There is roughly a 20 to 40 per cent incidence of both type I disease, which involves the aortic arch and its branches, and type II, which involves the distal thoracic and visceral abdominal aorta. Most patients, 50 to 65 per cent, have type III, which is both aortic arch and abdominal aortic involvement. Only 10 per cent have angiographically demonstrated type IV (pulmonary artery) involvement. Ishikawa, a long-term student of this disease, has assembled criteria for the diagnosis of the disease based on data concerning 96 Japanese patients with the disease.[83] The diagnostic criteria include one obligatory criterion (age 40 years or less at diagnosis or at onset of characteristic signs and symptoms of 1 month's duration); two major criteria (left and right subclavian artery lesions); and nine minor criteria (elevated erythrocyte sedimentation rate [ESR]; common carotid tenderness; hypertension; aortic regurgitation; and lesions of the pulmonary artery, left midcommon carotid artery, distal brachiocephalic trunk, descending thoracic aorta, and abdominal aorta). These criteria were fulfilled in 60 of the 64 patients with active disease and 21 of the 32 patients with inactive disease, producing an overall sensitivity of 84 per cent. In addition to the obligatory criteria, the presence of two major criteria, or one major plus two or more minor criteria, or four or more minor criteria suggested the high possibility of the presence of Takayasu's

disease. These criteria allow the clinician to make an early diagnosis as well as follow the effectiveness of therapy.

In addition to following clinical criteria, these patients need arteriography to document the initial extent and progression of the disease. Careful documentation of arterial involvement may require serial arteriography to determine progress and extent of disease. Recent evidence has shown duplex ultrasonography to be useful in the detection and follow-up of carotid lesions in Takayasu's disease.[84–86] The characteristic finding of a "macaroni sign," which is diffuse circumferential vessel thickening in the common carotid, can be utilized in following carotid progression and may decrease the frequency for which angiograms are needed.

Nonsurgical Treatment

Takayasu's disease is a systemic disease and so systemic treatment is indicated in the active phases of the disease, but the effectiveness of available treatments is not well defined. Even so, it is generally agreed that corticosteroids should be administered in initial daily doses of 40 to 50 mg prednisone, and the steroids tapered in response to improving clinical symptoms and laboratory signs of inflammation. Many patients can eventually discontinue steroid therapy, whereas, for others, prolonged courses of greater than 5 years are necessary. In patients without any response to corticosteroids after 3 months, cyclophosphamide therapy is also added.

The effectiveness of medical treatments is debatable. Some authors report that up to 50 per cent of patients with absent pulses have return of those pulses after several months of steroid therapy.[87] Angiographic improvement after corticosteroid treatment has also been demonstrated.[88]

FIGURE 125–5. Diagram showing the location of disease in the anatomic classification of Takayasu's arteritis.

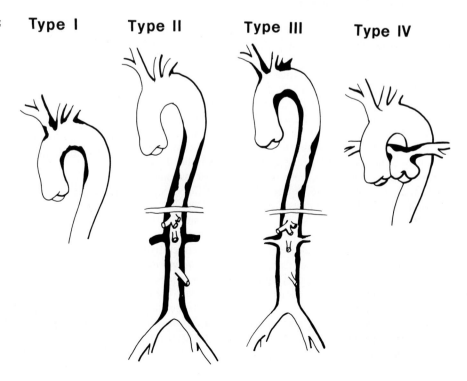

Type I   Type II   Type III   Type IV

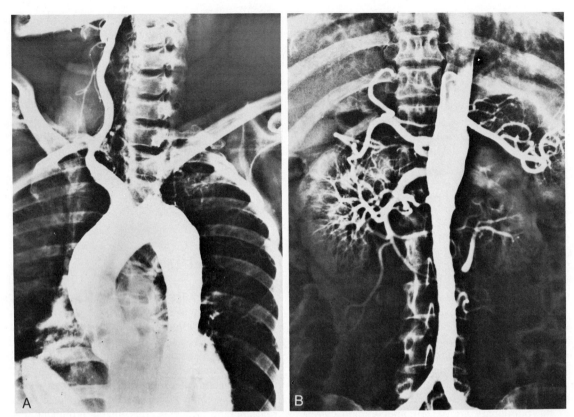

FIGURE 125–6. *A*, Arch angiogram from a patient with Takayasu's arteritis demonstrating smooth stenosis of the terminal brachiocephalic artery and complete obliteration of the left common and subclavian arteries. *B*, Abdominal aortogram from a patient with Takayasu's arteritis showing the characteristic smooth stenosis at the origin of the renal arteries and the distal aorta.

Multiple other studies document no improvement and actual angiographic progression while on corticosteroids.[89–91]

Operative Treatment

Up to one third of patients with chronic advanced disease will require surgery for palliation or prevention of ischemic complications. However, multiple questions such as timing, efficacy, and durability remain unanswered concerning arterial reconstructive procedures in patients with Takayasu's disease. Where possible, operative intervention should be avoided during the active phase of the disease. Ideally, the patients should not be taking corticosteroids or cyclophosphamide, but many times the cessation of this treatment is not possible. In these cases, clinical and laboratory findings should indicate that the disease is under control. Since the disease process involves all layers of vessel walls, endarterectomy or patch angioplasty is not recommended. Additionally, no suture lines should be placed in diseased segments in order to avoid false aneurysms and stenoses,[92, 93] and therefore, recent preoperative angiography is required to carefully select uninvolved areas. As a result, it is generally agreed that bypass procedures are the operations of choice for patients with Takayasu's occlusive lesions.[89, 90, 92, 94, 95] Since the disease may progress, the planned bypass should avoid anastomoses in areas of arteries that are presently normal, but are known to be frequently involved.

Life-threatening conditions, such as uncontrolled hypertension, chronic intestinal ischemia, and cerebrovascular symptoms of transient ischemic attacks or global ischemia, warrant prompt surgical intervention. Since stroke is a common cerebrovascular presentation in patients with Takayasu's disease,[95] prophylactic surgical repair is indicated in patients with hemodynamically significant stenoses of either the innominate or the carotid arteries. The ascending aorta is the preferred site for proximal anastomosis, since the subclavian arteries are, or could be at a later date, diseased. This approach will help decrease the incidences of anastomotic strictures and false aneurysms. Little information is available detailing the late results of carotid artery reconstruction, although strokes occur rarely, even in patients with failed reconstructions.

Results

The natural history of Takayasu's arteritis is variable but may be very severe. Clinical flare-ups are common and unpredictable, and, therefore, the patients must be followed closely. Patients who experience systemic hypertension, retinopathy, aneurysms, and aortic valve incompetence have a poor prognosis. The presence of one or more of these symptoms indicates a 30 per cent 5-year mortality rate. Whether surgical intervention decreases the mortality rate is not confirmed at this time; however, it seems reasonable to attempt palliation in patients with quiescent disease. Additionally, significant carotid lesions warrant prophylactic bypass. Close careful follow-up is required, since anastomotic aneurysms and stenoses occur.

TEMPORAL ARTERITIS

Temporal arteritis (giant cell arteritis, Horton's arteritis) is a disease of older (90 per cent are over 60 years of age), predominantly females (51 to 79 per cent of patients).[96] The disease has been reported in African-Americans,[97] but is more prevalent in northern areas and people of Scandinavian ancestry.[98] Even with the voluminous literature regarding temporal arteritis, it is still poorly understood. Two case reports published in 1932 are considered the first definite descriptions of temporal arteritis. In reality, there is a report written between 940 and 1010 by the ophthalmologist Ali Ibn Isa from Baghdad, which was translated into English in 1936.[99] The etiology of temporal arteritis remains unclear, but its association with polymyalgia rheumatica, response to corticosteroids, and genetic predisposition suggest an autoimmune disorder.[100] There may also be a link between temporal arteritis and degenerative vascular disease, with smoking being a causative factor.[101] Autopsy studies have shown large artery vasculitic involvement, including carotid, axillary, brachial, aortic, and mesenteric arteries. However, the majority of symptoms associated with temporal arteritis result from the gradual occlusion of branches of the carotid and vertebral arteries.[102]

Signs and Symptoms

The clinical presentation of temporal arteritis begins with a low-grade fever, malaise, myalgia, and headache. These flu-like symptoms of the early phase last from 1 to 3 weeks and are followed by jaw claudication (50 per cent of patients), polymyalgia rheumatica, muscular pain of the shoulder and hip regions (50 per cent of patients), and pain and/or erythema of the temporal artery in 45 to 60 per cent of patients.[103] Ocular complications occur 1 to 6 months after the prodromal period and are the most dreaded manifestations of temporal arteritis. These can range from corneal ulcerations, ocular edema, cataracts, ptosis, blurred vision, nystagmus, photophobia, diplopia, and amaurosis fugax to unilateral or bilateral blindness, which occurs in 7 to 60 per cent.[104] Fortunately, increased awareness of this disease has reduced the incidence of blindness to less than 10 per cent.[105] Visual loss is often rapid and can progress from slight blurring to blindness within 24 hours. Severe arteritis can lead to ischemic attacks or stroke in 7 per cent of patients.[105, 106] Interestingly, the extracranial vessels can be extensively involved, but since the intracranial vessels lack an internal elastic lamina, they are spared.[107]

Critical to the diagnosis and management of patients with temporal arteritis is the laboratory finding of an inflammatory process. An ESR is almost always elevated and provides a good method of following the activity of the disease. Occasionally, if the patients are taking anti-inflammatory agents for the musculoskeletal symptoms, the ESR may be suppressed and is elevated when these agents are withheld. Other laboratory findings can include mild normocytic anemia, mild thrombocytosis, leukocytosis, elevation of prothrombin time, and mild elevations of liver function tests.

Temporal artery biopsy is required in all patients in whom the possibility of temporal arteritis exists. It probably should be mandatory in all patients with polymyalgia rheumatica because of the strong association with temporal arteritis. If the artery is grossly involved, a short 2- to 3-cm segment is all that is necessary; however, when possible, a longer segment can be useful for diagnosis. If the result from the first side is negative, as it is in 10 to 15 per cent of cases, a similar segment from the contralateral side should be provided.[108, 109] The entire segment must be examined, as many times the disease is focal and segmental.

In those patients with extracranial vascular manifestations, arteriography is obtained. The typical lesions are multiple, long taperings followed by post-stenotic dilatation. Most commonly involved are the subclavian-brachial-axillary system, profunda and superficial femoral arteries, and unusually the calf, forearm, coronaries, visceral, cerebral, vertebral, and carotid arteries. Dissections and aneurysms of the ascending or descending thoracic aorta can occur in these patients. Angiography helps define the extent of the disease as well as monitor efficacy of treatment.

Treatment

Steroids are the mainstay of treatment for temporal arteritis. When the disease is suspected, based on clinical symptoms, corticosteroids are started at once. Appropriate blood studies and temporal artery biopsy can then be obtained. There is no reason to delay the institution of steroids, since the tissue remains diagnostic for several weeks, and if the biopsy is negative, the steroids can be discontinued.

Patients who present with visual symptoms should be hospitalized, intravenous steroids are begun with 100 mg of hydrocortisone every 12 hours, oral prednisone is started at 60 mg/day, and patients are given heparin empirically for 1 week to decrease the possibility of secondary thrombosis. When visual symptoms cease, intravenous steroids are stopped, and oral prednisone is decreased to 45 mg/day for 1 month. During treatment, symptoms, ESR, and other laboratory tests are monitored. These generally return to normal in 2 weeks. Then the prednisone is decreased by 5-mg increments every 10 to 14 days. Once the level of 10 mg/day is reached, further tapering is achieved in 1-mg per week increments. If the ESR rises significantly, the dose is increased by 10 mg/day for 3 to 4 weeks. In the absence of visual symptoms, prednisone is started at 60 mg/day and the preceding regimen followed. Most patients require only a single course of therapy, but in about 10 to 15 per cent, the therapy will need to be extended more than a year. Relapse rates are reported at 61 per cent, 38 per cent, and 43 per cent for 1, 2, and 3 years, respectively, of steroid therapy.[110] Alternate-day steroids have proved inadequate for disease suppression.[111] Patients should be reassessed after treatment at 3-month intervals for a year and then at 6-month intervals for another year. It is rare for a patient to have a relapse after 2 disease-free years.

Surgical intervention is generally unwarranted except for the rare cases of limb-limiting claudication, aortic valvular incompetence, aneurysms, and the rare aortic dissection. Carotid reconstructions are almost never required.[112] Significant stenotic lesions with limiting symptoms and arterial inflammation can be halted or even reversed by corticosteroid therapy. Amaurosis fugax associated with temporal arteritis responds well to steroid therapy.[113] If at all possible, necessary surgery should wait for the quiescent stage. In the very unusual case in which bypass grafts are required, occlusion rates are higher when the grafts are placed during the active phase of the disease.[113]

CAROTID ARTERY DISSECTIONS

The exact incidence of extracranial internal carotid artery dissection is unknown. It was once thought to be quite rare, but increased awareness combined with noninvasive evaluations utilizing ultrasound and magnetic resonance have demonstrated a more frequent occurrence. Even so, it probably still remains undiagnosed in a number of patients with and without precerebral neurologic events, since it can spontaneously resolve.[114] The accurate diagnosis combined with appropriate management can result in a favorable outcome.

There are three main mechanisms for carotid artery dissections: spontaneous dissection, iatrogenic dissection, and those secondary to trauma. By definition, spontaneous dissection occurs in the absence of known etiologic factors, with the first reported case in 1959.[115] Recent reports have shown that 30 of 1200, 2.5 per cent, patients with a primary stroke demonstrated spontaneous dissection of the internal carotid artery.[116] The dissection generally starts in the proximal 2 to 4 cm of the internal carotid artery and extends for variable distances. Although often reported as spontaneous, a multitude of factors can predispose a carotid artery to dissections. Hypertension is found to be present in at least 50 per cent of patients. Fibromuscular dysplasia, Marfan's syndrome, syphilis, arteriopathies, and even oral contraceptives have been implicated as possible etiologies.[117–124] Overt or unrecognized trauma probably plays some role in the development of most dissections, since a truly "spontaneous" intimal or intramural tear is unlikely. In 1982, Zelenock and coworkers[125] described two mechanisms of injury leading to dissection caused by blunt trauma. A stretch-traction-rotation injury (Fig. 125–7) produces an intimal tear of the internal carotid artery as it crosses the transverse process at C2 or C3. This can then progress to an intramural dissection or to total occlusion of the artery. The other described mechanism is direct crushing of the carotid artery between a cervical transverse process and the angle of the mandible, which can result in a mural hematoma and/or intimal dissection. Additional mechanisms described include direct blows to the neck, basilar skull fractures, and intraoral trauma. Operative and autopsy

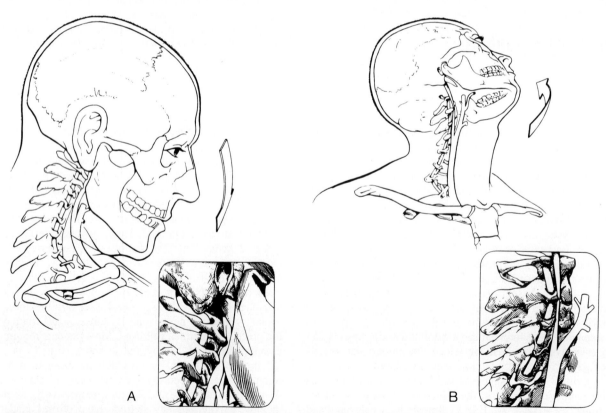

FIGURE 125–7. *A,* Flexion of the neck with compression injury to the internal carotid artery between the angle of the mandible and the upper cervical vertebrae resulting in intimal disruption and dissection. *B,* Extension with rotation of the neck producing a stretch injury of the internal carotid artery over the upper cervical vertebrae resulting in intimal disruption and dissection. (From Zelenock GB, Kazmers A, Whitehouse WM Jr, et al: Extracranial internal carotid artery dissections. Arch Surg 117:425, 1982. Copyright 1982, American Medical Association.)

specimens have shown dissections into all layers of the blood vessels. Histologic examinations of spontaneous dissections show fragmented smooth muscle cells and internal elastic membranes as well as deficient elastic membranes.[124] Often the contralateral carotid shows evidence of fibromuscular dysplasia in spontaneous dissections,[123] or there are simultaneous bilateral dissections,[122] indicating an underlying process. The net result of the dissection is a narrowing of the vessel, a decrease in cerebral perfusion, and formation of a thrombus, which can provide a source for emboli.

Symptoms and Findings

No specific symptoms or clinical findings are diagnostic for an internal carotid dissection, and, indeed, many patients may be completely asymptomatic and never discovered. The mean age for spontaneous dissections is about 45 years[126] (range, 4 to 68 years[121, 127]) with traumatic dissections presenting at earlier ages. The most commonly reported symptom is an ipsilateral headache. The headache is generally of sudden onset, severe, and localized to forehead and adjacent areas. Neck pain is usually limited to the ipsilateral neck near the angle of the mandible, and tenderness may be elicited by palpation. This pain has been reported to precede neurologic symptoms in many cases by up to 24 hours.[116, 118, 128] Approximately 50 to 75 per cent of the patients present with some type of ischemic symptoms, either a stroke or a transient ischemic attack.[116, 118, 126] Other commonly reported symptoms are Horner's syndrome, bruits, syncope, pulsatile tinnitus, blurred or lost vision,[129] and cranial nerve dysfunction (IX, X, or XII).[130, 131] Since cerebral ischemic symptoms are often delayed and are preceded by ipsilateral neck pain in the majority of patients, there exists a window of opportunity to make the diagnosis and possibly prevent irreversible neurologic damage.

The gold standard for diagnosis remains angiography, although many noninvasive tests may be useful for diagnosis and follow-up. As previously mentioned, the dissection generally begins between 2 and 4 cm distal to the bifurcation and commonly extends to the petrous bone. This pattern results in a narrowing of the lumen and the classic string sign is often present. An intimal flap as well as a double lumen may also be present. Fusiform aneurysmal dilatation can be observed in the involved segment. CT has been able to diagnose dissection as well as provide additional information as to wall thickness, extent of dissection, and possible aneurysm formation.[132] MRI offers many of the advantages of CT without the exposure to contrast media. It may even eventually replace angiography, since it can provide flow determinations as well as give the information obtained by CT. The application of duplex sonography and transcranial Doppler in diagnosing dissections has not been well established, but they may be extremely useful in following the patients with dissection.[133, 134] The characteristic high-resistance pattern associated with internal carotid artery dissection may allow duplex scanning to be advantageous for screening;[135] however, for now, arteriography remains the most accurate and reliable diagnostic test for carotid dissection diagnosis.

Treatment

Originally, the management of spontaneous dissection of the internal carotid artery was considered surgical. When explored, the diseased arterial segment was replaced, dilated, or ligated if the stump pressures were high enough. Following this approach, Ehrenfeld and Wylie produced a significant study in their management of 14 patients with internal carotid dissections.[124] There was a high incidence of stroke including those patients with interposition grafts, and in fact, only 2 of the 7 vessels subjected to more than simple exploration remained patent. In the patients without exploration, the results were found to be significantly better. Five of the 6 carotids treated with heparin alone spontaneously healed, and only 1 went on to total occlusion. These observations have led many to emphasize the relatively benign nature of internal carotid dissection.[118, 127, 136] This is also in error, since these studies excluded patients with massive infarcts on presentation.[116] The mortality rate is reported as high as 23 per cent, and, in general, significant long-term neurologic morbidity rates are as high as 30 per cent.[115–117, 124, 137, 138] Thus, the mere fact that most patients survive their occurrence of a carotid dissection does not equate with this being a benign condition.

Even so, over 85 per cent of carotids will improve angiographically with expectant observation. Recanalization and normalization of arteries documented to have had spontaneous dissection have been repeatedly confirmed in multiple studies by duplex, transcranial Doppler studies, ophthalmoplethysmography, and angiographic follow-up.[116, 118, 139] Although angiographic improvement has been documented in the absence of anticoagulation, it seems wise to institute heparin therapy after diagnosis for 10 to 12 days and then warfarin (Coumadin) for 3 to 6 months.[122] This should decrease the incidence of thrombosis and may allow for more complete and rapid recanalization. Obviously, if there is a massive or hemorrhagic infarct, anticoagulation would be unwise and antiplatelet therapy could be instituted. One report documented normalization of the carotid in 16 days on antiplatelet therapy alone,[140] although full anticoagulation should be the preferred regimen. Patients with spontaneous carotid dissections should be followed with repeat ultrasonography, transcranial Doppler examination, ophthalmoplethysmography, or MRI. If progressive stenosis is documented or neurologic symptoms persist or worsen despite anticoagulation, then operative repair may be indicated.

Although the primary recommendation for treatment currently appears to be anticoagulation, an occasional patient may present with a lesion that may warrant surgical intervention. Surgical intervention is offered to those patients with recurrent symptoms of cerebral ischemia despite anticoagulation in the hope of preventing irreversible neurologic or retinal damage. The decision to replace the diseased artery with a primary graft or to ligate the internal carotid artery is often not an easy one.

Attempting to repair the usual dissection that progresses to the base of the skull is fraught with difficulties, including possible injury to cranial nerves IX, X, XI, and XII; stroke; and the definite possibility that the double lumen is not reconstructible. In these patients with high internal carotid artery dissections, arterial ligation can be employed if the stump pressure is greater than 70 mmHg.[50] When the patient has recurring symptoms despite anticoagulation and the stump pressure is low, ligation plus extracranial-intracranial bypass should be considered.[141] This procedure will also treat low-flow situations from carotid dissection. The multi-center study that demonstrated poor results from these bypasses did not address this unusual situation.[142] Young patients with short, easily reconstructible segments demonstrating recurring symptoms may be best approached with surgery. Patients who present with traumatic dissection and subintimal injury confined to the approachable extracranial internal carotid artery can be easily treated with surgical repair consisting of vein graft interposition or external carotid artery transposition.

The management goal of this condition must be to improve on the 30 per cent morbidity, and this can only be achieved by prompt arteriographic diagnosis after the initial clinical suspicion, and then only with the institution of prompt therapy, which in most instances is anticoagulation.

CONCLUSIONS

There are some general guidelines to the management of unusual and difficult extracranial vascular lesions. The maintenance of cerebral perfusion through a patent internal carotid vessel is preferable, when possible. However, occasionally this is not achievable. In these cases, a carotid stump pressure greater than 70 mmHg indicates that the patient will usually tolerate carotid ligation without neurologic sequelae. Even so, it is important in these instances to maintain optimal intravascular hemodynamics, and, if possible, heparinization may prevent thrombus propagation into the intracranial vessels. Since many of the discussed disease processes involve adjacent vessels, thromboendarterectomy is not possible, and extra-anatomic bypass grafts such as axillo-carotid, carotid-carotid, subclavian-carotid, extracranial-intracranial, and aortic grafts are required to maintain cerebral perfusion and avoid terminal or debilitating neurologic events.

Bibliography

1. Eyzaguirre C, Zapata P: Perspectives in carotid body research. J Appl Physiol 57:931, 1984.
2. Schellack J, Fulenwider JT, Olson RA, et al: The carotid sinus syndrome. A frequently overlooked cause of syncope in the elderly. J Vasc Surg 4:376, 1986.
3. Weidemann G, Grotz J, Bewermeyer H, et al: High-resolution real-time ultrasound of the carotid bifurcation in patients with hyperactive carotid sinus syndrome. J Neurol 232:318, 1985.
4. Kapoor WN, Karpf M, Maher Y, et al: Syncope of unknown origin. The need for a more cost-effective approach to its diagnostic evaluation. JAMA 247:2687, 1982.
5. Griebenow R, Krämer L, Steffen HM, et al: Quantification of the heart rate–independent vasodepressor component in carotid sinus syndrome. Klin Wochenschr 67:1132, 1989.
6. Kenny RA, Traynor G: Carotid sinus syndrome—Clinical characteristic in elderly patients. Age Ageing 20:449, 1991.
7. Almquist A, Gornick C, Benson DW Jr, et al: Carotid sinus hypersensitivity: Evaluation of the vasodepressor component. Circulation 71:927, 1985.
8. Cheng LH, Norris CW: Surgical management of the carotid sinus syndrome. Arch Otolaryngol 97:395, 1973.
9. Brignole M, Menozzi C, Lolli G, et al: Long-term outcome of pace and non-paced patients with severe carotid sinus syndrome. Am J Cardiol 69:1039, 1992.
10. Nakayama K. Surgical removal of the carotid body for bronchial asthma. Dis Chest 40:595, 1961.
11. Wood JB, Frankland AW, Eastcott HHG: Bilateral removal of carotid bodies for asthma. Thorax 20:570, 1965.
12. Warren WH, Caldarelli DD, Javid H, et al: Neuroendocrine markers in paragangliomas of the head and neck. Ann Otol Rhinol Laryngol 94:555, 1985.
13. Glenner GG, Grimley PM: Atlas of Tumor Pathology. 2nd ser, fasc 9. Washington, DC, Armed Forces Institute of Pathology, 1974.
14. Javid H, Chawla SK, Dye WS, et al: Carotid body tumor. Resection or reflection. Arch Surg 111:344, 1976.
15. Pacheco-Ojeda L, Durango E, Rodriquez C, et al: Carotid body tumors at high altitudes: Quito, Ecuador, 1987. World J Surg 12:856, 1988.
16. Thevenuet A: Carotid body tumors: Invited commentary. World J Surg 12:860, 1988.
17. Sprong DH Jr, Kirby FG: Familial carotid body tumors. Report of nine cases in eleven siblings. Ann West Med Surg 3:241, 1949.
18. Shedd DP, Arias JD, Glunk RP: Familial occurrence of carotid body tumors. Head Neck 12:496, 1990.
19. Farr HW: Carotid body tumors: A 40-year study. CA 30:260, 1980.
20. Grufferman S, Gillman MW, Pasternak LR, et al: Familial carotid body tumors. Case report and epidemiologic review. Cancer 46:2166, 1980.
21. Smith LL, Ajalat GM: Tumor of the carotid body: Diagnosis, prognosis, and surgical treatment. In Moore WS (ed): Cerebral Vascular Disease. New York, Churchill Livingstone, 1987.
22. Nora JD, Hallett JW, O'Brien PC, et al: Surgical resection of carotid body tumors: Long-term survival, recurrence, and metastasis. Mayo Clin Proc 63:348, 1988.
23. Worsey MJ, Laborde AL, Bower T, et al: An evaluation of color duplex scanning in the primary diagnosis and management of carotid body tumors. Ann Vasc Surg 6:90, 1992.
24. Smith RF, Shetty PC, Reddy DJ: Surgical treatment of carotid paragangliomas presenting unusual technical difficulties: The value of preoperative embolization. J Vasc Surg 7:631, 1988.
25. Robison JG, Shagets FW, Beckett WC, et al: A multidisciplinary approach to reducing morbidity and operative blood loss during resection of carotid body tumor. Surg Gynecol Obstet 168:166, 1989.
26. Lasjaunias P, Menu Y, Bonnel D, Doyon D: Nonchromaffin paragangliomas of the head and neck: Diagnostic and therapeutic angiography in 9 cases explored from 1977 to 1980. J Neuroradiol 8:281, 1981.
27. Hekster REM, Luyendijk W, Matrical B: Transfemoral catheter embolization: A method of treatment of glomus jugulare tumors. Neuroradiology 5:208, 1973.
28. Hallett JW, Nora JD, Hollier LH, et al: Trends in neurovascular complications of surgical management for carotid body and cervical paragangliomas: A fifty-year experience with 153 tumors. J Vasc Surg 7:284, 1988.
29. Keating JF, Miller GA, Keaveny TV: Carotid body tumours: Report of six cases and a review of management. J R Coll Surg Edinb 35:172, 1990.
30. Chambers RG, Mahoney WD: Carotid body tumors. Am J Surg 116:554, 1968.
31. Dent TL, Thompson NW, Fry WJ: Carotid body tumors. Surgery 80:365, 1976.
32. Hewitt RI, Ichinose H, Weichert RF III, Drapanas T: Chemodectomas. Surgery 71:175, 1972.
33. Valdagni R, Amichetti M: Radiation therapy of carotid body tumors. Am J Clin Oncol 13:45, 1990.
34. Lack EE, Cubilla AL, Woodruff JM, Farr HN: Paragangliomas of the head and neck region: A clinical study of 69 patients. Cancer 39:397, 1977.
35. Martin HE: Surgery of Head and Neck Tumors. New York, PB Hoeber, 1957.
36. Dossa C, Shepard AD, Wolford DG, et al: Distal internal carotid exposure: A simplified technique for temporary mandibular subluxation. J Vasc Surg 12:319, 1990.
37. Gordon-Taylor G: On carotid body tumors. Br J Surg 28:163, 1940.
38. Shamblin WR, ReMine WH, Sheps SG, et al: Carotid body tumor

(chemodectoma), clinicopathologic analysis of ninety cases. Am J Surg 122:732, 1971.

39. Rosen IB, Palmer JA, Goldberg M, et al: Vascular problems associated with carotid body tumors. Am J Surg 142:459, 1981.

40. McCabe DP, Vaccaro PS, James AG: Treatment of carotid body tumors. J Cardiovasc Surg Torino 31:356, 1990.

41. Moore OS, Karlan M, Sigler L: Factors influencing the safety of carotid ligation. Am J Surg 118:666, 1969.

42. Moore O, Baker HW: Carotid artery ligation in surgery of the head and neck. Cancer 8:712, 1955.

43. Martinez SA, Oller DW, Gee W, et al: Elective carotid artery resection. Arch Otolaryngol 101:744, 1975.

44. Urken M, Biller HF, Haimov M, et al: Carotid artery resection and bypass for neck carcinoma. Laryngoscope 98:181, 1988.

45. Olcott CN, Fee WE, Enzmann DR, et al: Planned approach to the management of malignant invasion of the carotid artery. Am J Surg 142:123, 1981.

46. Kennedy JT, Krause CJ, Loevy S: The importance of tumor attachment to the carotid artery. Arch Otolaryngol 103:70, 1977.

47. Olcott CN, Fee WE, Enzmann DR, et al: Planned approach to the management of malignant invasion of the carotid artery. Am J Surg 142:123, 1981.

48. Lindegaard KF, Bakke CJ, Grolimund P, et al: Assessment of intracranial hemodynamics in carotid artery disease by transcranial Doppler ultrasound. J Neurosurg 63:890, 1985.

49. Conley JJ: Free autogenous grafts to the internal and common carotid arteries in the treatment of tumors of the neck. Ann Surg 137:205, 1953.

50. Ehrenfeld WK, Stoney RJ, Wylie EJ: Relation of carotid stump pressure to safety of carotid ligation. Surgery 93:299, 1983.

51. Atkinson DP, Jacobs LA, Weaver AW: Elective carotid resection for squamous cell carcinomas of the head and neck. Am J Surg 148:483, 1984.

52. Lore JM, Boulos EJ: Resection and reconstruction of the carotid artery in metastatic squamous cell carcinoma. Am J Surg 142:437, 1981.

53. Staley CJ: A muscle cover for the carotid artery after radical neck dissection. Am J Surg 102:815, 1961.

54. McCready RA, Miller SK, Hamarer RC, et al: What is the role of arterial resection in the management of advanced cervical cancer? J Vasc Surg 10:274, 1989.

55. Biller HF, Urken M, Haimov M, et al: Carotid artery resection and bypass for neck carcinoma. Laryngoscope 98:181, 1988.

56. Hardesty RA, Jones NF, Swartz WM, et al: Microsurgery for macrodefects: Microvascular free-tissue transfer for massive defects of the head and neck. Am J Surg 154:300, 1987.

57. Sheehan JF: Foam cell plaques in the interna elastica of irradiated small arteries. Arch Pathol 37:297, 1944.

58. Fonkalsrud EW, Sanchez M, Zerubavel R, et al: Serial changes in arterial structure following radiation therapy. Surg Gynecol Obstet 145:389, 1977.

59. McCready RA, Hyde GL, Bivins BA, et al: Radiation-induced arterial injuries. Surgery 93:306, 1982.

60. Gold H: Production of atherosclerosis in the rat. Effect of x-ray and high-fat diet. Arch Pathol 8:497, 1961.

61. Vesselinovitch D, Wiseler RW: Experimental production of atherosclerosis in mice. 2. Effects of atherogenic and high-fat diet on vascular changes in chronically and acutely irradiated mice. J Atheros Res 8:497, 1968.

62. Asscher AW, Wilson C, Anson SG: Sensitization of blood vessels to hypertensive damage by x-radiation. Lancet 1:583, 1961.

63. Thomas E, Forbus WB: Irradiation injury to the aorta and lung. Arch Pathol 67:256, 1959.

64. Loftus CM, Biller J, Hart MN, et al: Management of radiation-induced accelerated carotid atherosclerosis. Arch Neurol 44:711, 1987.

65. Butler MS, Lane RHS, Webster JHH. Irradiation injury to large arteries. Br J Surg 67:314, 1980.

66. Eldering SC, Fernandez RN, Grotta JC, et al: Carotid artery disease following cervical irradiation. Ann Surg 194:609, 1981.

67. Moritz MW, Higgins RF, Jacobs JR: Duplex imaging and incidence of carotid radiation injury after high-dose radiotherapy for tumors of the head and neck. Arch Surg 125:1181, 1990.

68. Hurley JJ, Nordestgaard AG, Woods JJ: Carotid endarterectomy with

69. vein patch angioplasty for radiation-induced symptomatic atherosclerosis. J Vasc Surg 14:419, 1991.

69. Killeen JD, Smith LL: Management of contiguous malignancy, radiation damage, and infection involving the carotid artery. Semin Vasc Surg 4:123, 1991.

70. Razack MS, Sako K: Carotid artery hemorrhage of ligation in head and neck cancer. J Surg Oncol 19:189, 1982.

71. Ketcham AS, Hoyle RC: Spontaneous carotid artery hemorrhage after head and neck surgery. Am J Surg 110:649, 1965.

72. Bole PV, Babu S, Clauss RH: Planned extraanatomical cerebral revascularization for carotid artery ligation. Surgery 83:440, 1978.

73. Porto DP, Adams G, Foster C: Emergency management of carotid artery rupture. Am J Otolaryngol 7:213, 1986.

74. Takayasu M: Patient who has peculiar changes in retina central vessels. Act Soc Opth Jap 12:554, 1908.

75. Isikawa K: Survival and morbidity after diagnosis of occlusive thromboaortopathy (Takayasu's disease). Am J Cardiol 47:1026, 1981.

76. Scully RE, Mark EJ, McNeeley BU: Case records of the Massachusetts General Hospital. New Engl J Med 305:1519, 1981.

77. Cupps TR, Fauci AS: Giant cell arteritis. *In* Smith LH (ed): Major Problems in Internal Medicine: The Vasculitides. Philadelphia, WB Saunders, 1981.

78. Hunder GG: Giant cell arteritis and polymyalgia rheumatica, *In* Kelly WN, Ruddy S, Sledge CB (eds): Textbook of Rheumatology. 3rd ed. Philadelphia, WB Saunders, 1989, pp 1200–1208.

79. Vinijchaikul K: Primary arteritis of the aorta and its main branches (Takayasu's arteriopathy): A clinicopathologic autopsy study of eight cases. Am J Med 43:15, 1967.

80. Klein RG, Campbell RJ, Hunder GG, et al: Skip lesions in temporal arteritis. Mayo Clin Proc 51:504, 1976.

81. Ueno A, Awane Y, Wakabayashi A, et al: Successfully operated obliterative brachiocephalic arteritis (Takayasu's) associated with elongated coarctation. Jpn Heart J 93:94, 1977.

82. Lupi-Herrera E, Sanchez GT, Horwitz S, et al: Pulmonary artery involvement in Takayasu's arteritis. Chest 63:69, 1975.

83. Ishikawa K: Diagnostic approach and proposed criteria for the clinical diagnosis of Takayasu's arteriopathy. J Am Coll Cardiol 12:964, 1988.

84. Maed H, Handa N, Matsumoto M, et al: Carotid lesions detected by B-mode ultrasonography in Takayasu's arteritis: "Macaroni sign" as an indicator of the disease. Ultrasound Med Biol 17:695, 1991.

85. Buckley A, Southwood T, Culham G, et al: The role of ultrasound in evaluation of Takayasu's arteritis. J Rheumatol 18:1073, 1991.

86. Bond JR, Charboneau JW, Stanson AW: Takayasu's arteritis. Carotid duplex sonographic appearance, including color Doppler imaging. J Ultrasound Med 9:625, 1990.

87. Hall S, Barr W, Lie JT, et al: Takayasu arteritis: A study of 32 North American patients. Medicine 64:89, 1985.

88. Ishikawa K, Yonekawa Y: Regression of carotid stenoses after corticosteroid therapy in occlusive thromboaortopathy (Takayasu's disease). Stroke 18:677, 1987.

89. Weaver FA, Yellin AE, Campen DH: Surgical procedures in the management of Takayasu's arteritis. J Vasc Surg 12:429, 1990.

90. Sise MJ, Connihan CM, Shackford SR: The clinical spectrum of Takayasu's arteritis. Surgery 104:905, 1988.

91. Shelhamer JH, Volkman DJ, Parillo JE, et al: Takayasu's arteritis and its therapy. Ann Intern Med 103:121, 1985.

92. Kieffer E, Bahnini A: Aortic lesions in Takayasu's disease. *In* Bergan JJ, Yao JST (eds): Aortic Surgery. Philadelphia, WB Saunders, 1989, pp 111–147.

93. Pokrovsky AV, Sultanaliev TA, Spiridonov AA: Surgical treatment of vasorenal hypertension in nonspecific aorto-arteritis (Takayasu's disease). J Cardiovasc Surg 24:111, 1983.

94. Takagi A, Tada Y, Sato O, et al: Surgical treatment for Takayasu's arteritis: A long-term follow-up study. J Cardiovasc Surg 30:553, 1989.

95. Giordano JM, Leavitt RY, Hoffman G, et al: Experience with surgical treatment of Takayasu's disease. Surgery 109:252, 1991.

96. Huston KA, Hunder GG, Lie JT, et al: Temporal arteritis: A 25-year epidemiologic, clinical, and pathologic study. Ann Intern Med 88:162, 1978.

97. Love DC, Rapkin J, Lesser GR, et al: Temporal arteritis in blacks. Ann Intern Med 105:387, 1986.

98. Bengtsson BA, Malmvall BE: The epidemiology of giant cell arteritis including temporal arteritis and polymyalgia rheumatica—incidences of different presentations and eye complications. Arthritis Rheum 24:899, 1981.

99. Henriet JP, Marin J, Gosselin J, et al: The history of temporal arteritis or ten centuries of fascinating adventure. J Mal Vasc 14:93, 1989.

100. Allen NB, Studenski SA: Polymyalgia rheumatica and temporal arteritis. Med Clin North Am 70:369, 1986.

101. Machado EBV, Gabriel SE, Beard CM, et al: A population-based case-control study of temporal arteritis: Evidence for an association between temporal arteritis and degenerative vascular disease? Int J Epidemiol 18:836, 1989.

102. Klein RG, Hunder GG, Stanson AW, et al: Large artery involvement in giant cell (temporal arteritis). Ann Intern Med 83:806, 1975.

103. Joyce JW: The giant cell arteritides: Diagnosis and the role of surgery. J Vasc Surg 3:827, 1986.

104. Goodman BW Jr: Temporal arteritis. Am J Med 67:839, 1979.

105. Caselli RJ, Hunder GG, Whisnant JP: Neurologic disease in biopsy-proven giant cell (temporal) arteritis. Neurology 38:352, 1988.

106. Save-Soderberg J, Malmvall BE, Anderson R, et al: Giant cell arteritis as a cause of death. JAMA 255:493, 1986.

107. Reich KA, Giansiracusa DF, Strongwater SL: Neurologic manifestations of giant cell arteritis. Am J Med 89:67, 1990.

108. Fauchald P, Rygvold O, Sytese N: Temporal arteritis polymyalgia rheumatica: Clinical and biopsy findings. Ann Intern Med 77:845, 1972.

109. Hall S, Persellin S, Lie JT, et al: The therapeutic impact of temporal artery biopsy. Lancet 2:1217, 1983.

110. Bengtsson BA, Malmvall BE: Giant cell arteritis. Acta Med Scand (Suppl) 658:1, 1982.

111. Hunder GG, Sheps SG, Allen GL, et al: Daily and alternate-day corticosteroid regimens in treatment of giant cell arteritis. Comparison in a prospective study. Ann Intern Med 82:613, 1975.

112. Forner GS, Thiele BL: Giant cell arteritis involving the carotid artery. Surgery 95:759, 1984.

113. Joyce JW, Hollier LH: The giant cell arteritides: Temporal and Takayasu's arteritis. In Bergan JJ, Yao JST (eds): Evaluation and Treatment of Upper and Lower Extremity Circulatory Disorders. Philadelphia, WB Saunders, 1984, pp 465–482.

114. Budmiger H, Bollinger A: Dissection of the internal carotid artery: A frequently missed diagnosis? Case report and review of the literature. VaSA 17:219, 1988.

115. Anderson RM, Schechter MM: A case of spontaneous dissecting aneurysms of the internal carotid artery. J Neurol Neurosurg Psychiatry 22:195, 1959.

116. Bogousslavsky J, Despland PA, Regli F: Spontaneous carotid dissection with acute stroke. Arch Neurol 44:137, 1987.

117. Brown OL, Armitage JL: Spontaneous dissecting aneurysms of the cervical internal carotid artery. AJR 118:648, 1973.

118. Mokri B, Sundt TM Jr, Houser OW, et al: Spontaneous dissection of the cervical internal carotid artery. Ann Neurol 19:126, 1986.

119. Ringel SP, Harrison SH, Norenberg MD, et al: Fibromuscular dysplasia: Multiple "spontaneous" dissecting aneurysms of the major cervical arteries. Ann Neurol 1:301, 1977.

120. Andersen CA, Collins GJ Jr, Rich NM, et al: Spontaneous dissection of the internal carotid artery associated with fibromuscular dysplasia. Am Surg 46:263, 1980.

121. O'Dwyer JA, Moscow N, Trevor R, et al: Spontaneous dissection of the carotid artery. Radiology 137:379, 1980.

122. Milandre L, Perot S, Salamon G, et al: Spontaneous dissection of both extracranial internal carotid arteries. Neuroradiology 31:435, 1989.

123. Garcia-Merino JA, Gutierrez JA, Lopez-Lozano JJ, et al: Double lumen dissecting aneurysms of the internal carotid artery in fibromuscular dysplasia. Case Report. Stroke 14:815, 1983.

124. Ehrenfeld WK, Wylie EJ: Spontaneous dissection of the internal carotid artery. Arch Surg 111:1294, 1976.

125. Zelenock GB, Kazmers A, Whitehouse WM Jr, et al: Extracranial internal carotid artery dissections. Arch Surg 117:425, 1982.

126. Hart RG, Easton JD: Dissection of cervical and cerebral arteries. Neurol Clin 1:155, 1983.

127. Friedman WA, Day AL, Quisling RG, et al: Cervical carotid dissecting aneurysms. Neurosurgery 7:207, 1980.

128. Fisher CM: The headache and pain of spontaneous carotid dissection. Headache 22:60, 1982.

129. Galetta SL, Leahey A, Nichols CW, Raps EC: Orbital ischemia, ophthalmoparesis, and carotid dissection. J Clin Neurol Ophthalmol 11:284, 1991.

130. Lieschke GJ, Davis S, Tress BM, Ebeling P: Spontaneous internal carotid dissection presenting as hypoglossal nerve palsy. Stroke 19:1151, 1988.

131. Waespe W, Niesper J, Imhof HG, Valavanis A: Lower cranial nerve palsies due to internal carotid dissection. Stroke 19:1561, 1988.

132. Petro GR, Witwe GA, Cacyorin ED, et al: Spontaneous dissection of the cervical internal carotid artery: Correlation of arteriography, CT, and pathology. AJR 148:393, 1987.

133. Mullges W, Ringelstein EB, Leibold M: Noninvasive diagnosis of internal carotid artery dissections. J Neurol Neurosurg Psychiatry 55:98, 1992.

134. Early TF, Gregory RT, Wheeler JR, et al: Spontaneous carotid dissection: Duplex scanning in diagnosis and management. J Vasc Surg 14:391, 1991.

135. Hennerici M, Steinke W, Rautenberg W: High-resistance Doppler flow pattern in extracranial carotid dissection. Arch Neurol 46:670, 1989.

136. Fischer CM, Ojemann RG, Roberson GH: Spontaneous dissection of cervicocerebral arteries. Can J Neurol 5:9, 1978.

137. Bostrom K, Lilieqist B: Primary dissecting aneurysm of the extracranial part of the internal carotid and vertebral arteries. Neurology 17:179, 1967.

138. Ojemann RG, Fisher CM, Rich JC: Spontaneous dissecting aneurysm of the internal carotid artery. Stroke 3:434, 1972.

139. Gee W, Kaupp HA, McDonald KM, et al: Spontaneous dissection of internal carotid arteries: Spontaneous resolution documented by serial ocular pneumoplethysmography. Arch Surg 115:944, 1980.

140. Pozzati E, Gaist G, Poppi M: Resolution of occlusion in spontaneously dissected carotid arteries: Report of two cases. J Neurosurg 56:857, 1982.

141. Miyamoto S, Kikuchi H, Karasawa J, et al: Surgical treatment for spontaneous carotid dissection with impending stroke. Case report. J Neurosurg 61:382, 1984.

142. The EC-IC Bypass Study Group: Failure of extracranial-intracranial bypass to reduce the risk of ischemic stroke. Results of an international randomized trial. New Engl J Med 313:1191, 1985.

126

Postoperative Management and Complications Following Carotid Endarterectomy

Norman R. Hertzer, M.D.

• • •

Few critical procedures are tolerated as well as uncomplicated extracranial reconstruction. Carotid endarterectomy accounts for the vast majority of all cerebrovascular operations and usually causes a minimum of discomfort or disability before normal activity is resumed after a brief hospital convalescence. Because of its historic success in the prevention of subsequent strokes in patients who had appropriate bifurcation lesions associated with either transient ischemic attacks (TIAs) or mild completed deficits, surgical indications at many centers inevitably were extended to include candidates having severe but asymptomatic carotid stenosis. Accordingly, carotid endarterectomy became perhaps the most common peripheral vascular procedure performed in the United States during the 1980s. Employing information from the National Center for Health Statistics, Rutkow and Ernst[127] calculated that 95,000 patients underwent carotid endarterectomy in 1983, a figure that was 76 per cent higher than the 54,000 estimated in 1979. At the same time carotid reconstruction accounted for 8489 (26 per cent) of the 32,852 operations entered into the computer registry of the Cleveland Vascular Society (unpublished data) and represented 47 per cent of the major arterial procedures reported from 1978 through 1981.[69]

The effectiveness of carotid endarterectomy in selected patients with high-grade stenosis has long been accepted within the surgical community, but it eventually became a controversial issue in the medical literature as well as in the lay press. Citing the sheer number of operations being performed, the absence of concurrent control groups, and early morbidity rates that often appeared to be excessive or curiously outdated, several neurologists implied only a few years ago that extracranial reconstruction should be abandoned unless its merit were confirmed by prospectively randomized clinical trials.[13, 84, 160]

Some of this criticism has been deflected by disclosures that surgical treatment has proved to be superior to nonoperative management among symptomatic patients having at least 70 per cent carotid stenosis in the North American Symptomatic Carotid Endarterectomy Trial (NASCET)[98] and the European Carotid Surgery Trial.[54] It must be recognized, however, that neither of these studies might have reached the same conclusions if they had been associated with prohibitive risks for perioperative stroke.

Moreover, those risks must be reduced still further to justify "prophylactic" intervention in the prospective trials addressing asymptomatic carotid stenosis, which have yet to be reported.

Whatever their future influence on public policy, serious perioperative complications are devastating to the individual patient, and both Toole and coworkers[150] and Chambers and Norris[27, 28] have demonstrated that they substantially compromise the overall long-term benefit of surgical treatment. The point is clear: There is no higher priority in the field of vascular surgery than the safety of carotid endarterectomy.

POSTOPERATIVE MANAGEMENT

Although the elements of appropriate postoperative care may differ from one center to the next, the following approach has proved to be satisfactory at the Cleveland Clinic. Patients remain for at least 8 hours in an intensive nursing area following carotid reconstruction, irrespective of whether the operation was performed under general, regional, or local anesthesia. In this setting, complications such as wound bleeding or hematoma formation, hypoxia, labile blood pressure, and abrupt neurologic deterioration may be recognized more promptly than might be the case on a conventional hospital ward. After a general anesthetic is administered, a roentgenogram of the chest is obtained with portable equipment as soon as the patient is transferred from the operating room in order to confirm the correct position of the endotracheal tube and the absence of atelectasis. The hemoglobin, hematocrit, and serum electrolyte values also are measured because many patients who undergo carotid endarterectomy are aged or require maintenance antihypertensive medication and may experience either hemodilution or hypokalemia during the administration of intravenous fluids. Coronary artery disease is prevalent among patients with carotid atherosclerosis, and a routine electrocardiogram is performed to exclude the possibility of myocardial ischemia. Patients who are recognized to have coronary involvement receive either sublingual or cutaneous nitroglycerin compounds until oral medication is resumed. Transient premature ventricular contractions are not uncommon and usually respond to potassium supplementation or the parenteral infusion of lidocaine hydrochloride.

An adequate neurologic examination is necessary to evaluate extremity strength, fine hand movements, articulate speech, visual acuity, and mentation. Provided that the lumen of the external carotid artery was not obliterated during bifurcation endarterectomy, the presence of a normal superficial temporal pulse indicates patency of the common carotid artery but does not reflect the status of the internal carotid. The neurologic evaluation is repeated frequently during the initial postoperative period by the nursing staff, and any new deficit is reported immediately to the responsible surgeon. Transient hypertension or hypotension is not unusual after carotid endarterectomy and manipulation of the sinus nerve mechanism, and because extreme fluctuations in systemic blood pressure may provoke either cerebral hemorrhage or carotid thrombosis, a percutaneous radial or brachial artery catheter is used for continuous monitoring until all parameters have been stable for several hours.

Nothing is given by mouth until the day following carotid reconstruction, since sudden neurologic deterioration or wound bleeding occasionally requires an urgent reoperation. Prophylactic antibiotics probably are superfluous unless prosthetic material was employed during the original procedure or an early reoperation is required. However, in an attempt to prevent platelet aggregation that may cause either internal carotid thrombosis or cerebral embolization, aspirin is given by rectal suppository in the recovery unit and is continued orally in a dosage of 5 to 10 grains twice daily for at least the first postoperative month. Edwards and colleagues[49] found that the preoperative use of antiplatelet agents reduced the incidence of post-endarterectomy internal carotid occlusion from 3.1 per cent to only 0.3 per cent. Nevertheless, an earlier study by French and Rewcastle[59] suggested that endothelial regeneration at the site of carotid endarterectomy is reasonably complete within an interval of 4 to 6 weeks.

Provided that all parameters are satisfactory after several hours of observation, the patient is transferred to a regular nursing unit where full activity is encouraged during the 3 or 4 days of hospital convalescence. An outpatient examination is performed approximately a month later in order to assess the neurologic results, the presence and quality of cervical pulses and residual bruits, and wound healing. Unless the patient is to have additional cardiovascular or other surgical procedures in the interim, an annual evaluation is scheduled, which probably should include noninvasive cerebrovascular testing or objective carotid imaging to detect asymptomatic progression of other extracranial lesions or recurrent stenosis on the operated side. Finally, and perhaps most importantly, the patient is instructed to report any unexpected neurologic symptoms as soon as they occur.

Wound Complications

Cervical Hematoma

Considering that carotid reconstruction ordinarily is performed under full heparin anticoagulation and that many, if not most, surgical candidates have received preoperative antiplatelet therapy, the incidence of postoperative wound bleeding is surprisingly low. Reoperations for hemostasis following carotid endarterectomy were required in only 0.7 per cent of a personal experience with 1022 patients reported by Thompson[148] and in 1.5 per cent of a 3-year series of 917 operations at the Cleveland Clinic.[72] Sodium heparin may be predictably reversed with protamine sulfate at the conclusion of the original procedure, but because sodium warfarin (Coumadin) derivatives initiate a sustained elevation of the prothrombin time, formal oral anticoagulation should be corrected preoperatively with vitamin K and, if necessary, with fresh frozen plasma. Aspirin, dipyridamole, and related compounds are so ubiquitous among cerebrovascular patients that they probably are responsible for most troublesome blood loss. Capillary bleeding caused by these agents rarely may require platelet transfusions, but patience and conventional measures usually are sufficient because the standard approach to the carotid bifurcation through an incision parallel to the anterior border of the sternocleidomastoid muscle is relatively avascular. Although opinions may differ, a retrospective review of 697 carotid endarterectomies conducted by Treiman and associates[155] has indicated that wound hematomas may occur less frequently when systemic heparin is reversed with protamine sulfate at the conclusion of the operation (1.8 per cent) than when it is not (6.5 per cent).

It is axiomatic that the best method to obtain hemostasis after an operation is to maintain it throughout the preliminary dissection. Nevertheless, postoperative bleeding from the edges of the incision sometimes occurs and may be controlled by light compression or the addition of a few superficial sutures incorporating the skin and the underlying platysma muscle. Cervical hematomas often are discovered after Valsalva's maneuvers at the time the endotracheal tube is removed, a feature implicating transient arterial hypertension and venous distention as contributing factors. For this reason, fine sutures are preferable to simple ligation for control of the facial vein and branches of the external carotid artery that may be divided to permit mobilization of the hypoglossal nerve. If an autogenous vein patch is applied to the arteriotomy, its branches should be transfixed with sutures or incorporated into the anastomosis. Low-molecular-weight dextran is administered to selected patients at the Cleveland Clinic in order to prevent immediate platelet aggregation when a subadventitial endarterectomy plane is entered during the removal of a deeply ulcerated plaque, but this precaution seems to cause no more bleeding than antiplatelet therapy alone.

A pliable vacuum drain customarily is employed to detect continued bleeding during the first postoperative hours and to prevent the accumulation of a hematoma large enough to produce deviation of the trachea and airway obstruction. However, even if ventilation is not impaired, a large cervical hematoma is undesirable because it may compress the internal carotid artery and adjacent cranial nerves, establish a potential nidus for infection, and foster a draining wound that is both uncomfortable and cosmetically unsatisfactory. Therefore, such a problem should be corrected by an elective reoperation on the same day as the original procedure. The incision should be completely opened in order to evacuate the hematoma and to obtain adequate hemostasis. The wound may be irrigated with a dilute antibiotic solution prior to primary closure, and a brief course of intravenous antibiotics also seems to be appropriate if wound exploration has been necessary for any reason.

Infection and False Aneurysm

Postoperative cervical infections almost never occur because the neck represents a clean surgical field with abundant circulation, and only anecdotal reports of carotid false aneurysms have been described. Thompson[148] had encountered a single wound infection (0.09 per cent) prior to 1979, and each of the seven false aneurysms (0.6 per cent) in his series involved a prosthetic patch applied with silk suture several years earlier. Although Ott and associates[103] have employed routine Dacron patch angioplasty during carotid endarterectomy without mycotic complications, any infection in the presence of prosthetic material could have disastrous consequences. The use of autogenous tissue has theoretical advantages in this respect, and provided that the local arterial supply is sufficient to heal a harvesting incision, a patch of saphenous vein may instead be removed from the lower leg with preservation of the proximal vein for subsequent coronary or lower extremity revascularization. Spontaneous rupture of an ankle vein patch is not impossible even in the absence of infection (Fig. 126–1), but this unpredictable catastrophe appears to be limited to fewer than 1 per cent of patients.[72, 101]

Infected false aneurysms occurred after only 4 (0.15 per cent) of 2651 carotid reconstructions at the Cleveland Clinic from 1977 through 1984.[67] Because of suppuration and degeneration of the arterial wall, multiple ligation of

the common, internal, and external carotid arteries was the only alternative in 1 patient, who subsequently experienced TIA in the ipsilateral cerebral hemisphere before these events were controlled with oral anticoagulation. The remaining 3 patients underwent vein patch angioplasty of their false aneurysms in conjunction with systemic antibiotics. Each developed a recurrent false aneurysm that required carotid ligation, but none sustained a postoperative stroke. During the same study period, a chronic infection in a Dacron patch performed at another center was treated successfully by resection of the carotid bifurcation and an interposition vein graft to the distal cervical segment of the internal carotid artery. These limited examples suggest that infected false aneurysms usually require multiple ligation unless it is feasible to excise the septic arterial wall and replace it with an uncontaminated autogenous graft.

Hypertension and Hypotension

Postoperative hypertension or hypotension may be caused by alterations in intravascular volume, peripheral vasoconstriction, or cardiac dysfunction following any major operation. However, they appear to be especially common after carotid endarterectomy, and this observation has generated considerable interest in the possible contribution of the carotid sinus mechanism because of its perceived importance in blood pressure regulation and its proximity to the carotid bifurcation. As illustrated in Figure 126–2, specialized neurons located in the adventitia of the carotid bulb monitor systemic blood pressure and respond to sustained elevations by initiating a reflex arc to the upper brain stem that is mediated by the sinus nerve of Hering, a branch

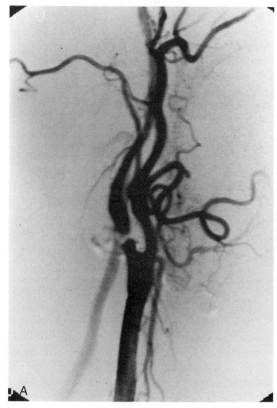

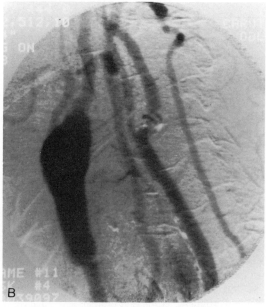

FIGURE 126–1. Preoperative (A) and postoperative (B) angiograms in a patient who sustained an acute false aneurysm 1 week after carotid endarterectomy and patch angioplasty using a segment of saphenous vein harvested from the ankle. The patch appears dilated on the postoperative study and ruptured centrally on the following day.

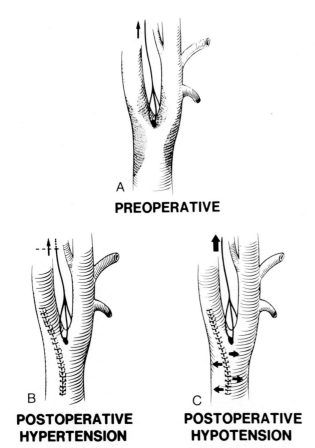

PREOPERATIVE

POSTOPERATIVE HYPERTENSION

POSTOPERATIVE HYPOTENSION

B

C

FIGURE 126–2. Schematic representation of the possible influence of the carotid sinus mechanism on blood pressure fluctuations at the time of bifurcation endarterectomy. (From Hertzer NR: Nonstroke complications of carotid endarterectomy. *In* Bernhard VM, Towne J [eds]: Complications in Vascular Surgery. 2nd ed. Orlando, FL, Grune & Stratton, 1985.)

of the glossopharyngeal nerve.[66, 67] Compensatory bradycardia and a reduction in blood pressure normally occur under these circumstances, but there is evidence that interruption of this negative-feedback system by injury to the sinus nerve during carotid endarterectomy may actually encourage a hypertensive response by simulating a hypotensive episode, particularly after bilateral carotid reconstruction has been performed.[20, 23, 133] Conversely, Angell-James and Lumley[3] also have postulated that the excision of a calcified, nondistensible atheroma may instead cause reflex hypotension in some patients by restoring compliance to the bifurcation and reactivating a dormant baroreceptor mechanism.

It is important to recognize the theoretical role of the sinus nerve in the etiology of abrupt changes in blood pressure because unanticipated bradycardia and hypotension during surgical exposure of the carotid bifurcation often may be corrected by infiltrating the sinus with local anesthetic.[3, 23] Nevertheless, Wade and colleagues[159] discovered that baroreceptor function may disappear entirely with advancing age, and Towne and Bernhard[152] were unable to demonstrate that either preservation or transection of the sinus nerve had any real influence on postoperative blood pressure in the clinical setting. Because a consistent causal relationship between sinus nerve activity and perioperative

blood pressure has not been established, other factors also deserve consideration. Davies and Cronin[41] found no correlation between preoperative and postoperative blood pressure, but both Bove and coworkers[20] and Towne and Bernhard[152] calculated that hypertensive patients had a statistically significant risk for severe postoperative hypertension, especially if preoperative medical control was inadequate. Moreover, Ranson and associates[115] concluded that an unsuspected deficit in intravascular volume was the critical feature of postoperative hypotension and that reflex bradycardia was a predictable complication only in the presence of hypovolemia. Tarlov and coworkers[144] later restated this principle and reduced their incidence of postoperative hypotension from 54 per cent to 18 per cent by using colloid infusions to maintain adequate central venous pressures. Within the past few years, elegant studies by other investigators have suggested that postoperative hypertension may be related to the systemic release of either renin or norepinephrine from obscure intracranial sources that remain poorly understood.[1, 137]

Irrespective of their etiology, extreme fluctuations in postoperative blood pressure have been associated with an increase in surgical strokes and mortality.[20, 115, 120, 133, 152] Bove and colleagues[20] encountered postoperative hypertension in 19 per cent and hypotension in 28 per cent of 100 consecutive patients and found that neurologic deficits involved 9 per cent of these two subsets, in comparison with none of those who remained normotensive. Similarly, Towne and Bernhard[152] reported operative strokes in 10 per cent of their patients who developed postoperative hypertension, compared with 3 per cent of those who did not. There are conflicting data concerning whether patients who require bilateral carotid reconstruction have a specific risk for hypertensive neurologic complications following the second operation if it is performed too soon after the first. In a small series of 56 patients described by Schroeder and associates,[134] hypertension occurred in 48 per cent when the procedures were less than 3 weeks apart and in only 8 per cent when the interval was longer. However, there was no conclusive correlation between hypertension and neurologic deficits even though the stroke rate was 20 per cent after the contralateral operations in this study, and another investigation by Satiani and coworkers[132] suggested that the staging interval had no influence on the complication rate in patients with bilateral carotid disease.

Management

Considering this accumulated experience, either hypertension or hypotension should be prevented when possible and treated judiciously when it does occur. Chronic hypertension must be under medical control even if the operation is postponed in order to obtain it.[107] By the same token, preoperative rehydration with parenteral fluids may be necessary for aged patients receiving maintenance diuretic management. Although any precise definition of hypertension or hypotension is arbitrary, blood pressure generally should be supported at preoperative levels following carotid endarterectomy. At the present time, pharmacologic treatment is initiated at the Cleveland Clinic if the postoperative systolic blood pressure exceeds 180 mmHg or falls below 100 mmHg in patients who previously were normotensive. It must be remembered, however, that precipitous manipulation of the blood pressure may itself be associated with a potential risk for either myocardial infarction or stroke.[120, 133]

Sodium nitroprusside is an effective peripheral vasodilator that provides responsive control of hypertension when titrated with a mechanical infusion pump in a dosage of 50 mg per 250 to 500 ml of 5 per cent dextrose in water (D5/W). Postoperative hypotension occurring in conjunction with bradycardia may resolve once the heart rate has been stimulated with a single intravenous bolus of 0.5 to 1.0 mg of atropine sulfate. Hypovolemia should be corrected before the use of vasoconstrictor agents if additional treatment is necessary, but provided such traditional parameters as urine volume and central venous pressure are satisfactory, low blood pressure may be reversed by the continuous infusion of dopamine hydrochloride in a dosage of 200 to 400 mg per 250 ml of D5/W. In conjunction with their hypothesis that postoperative hypertension may be associated with the intracranial production of norepinephrine, Ahn and coworkers[1] also collected anecdotal evidence that it might be prevented by the administration of sympatholytic agents (e.g., clonidine).

Postoperative blood pressure complications nearly always are transient, and most patients who experience them may be withdrawn from acute pharmacologic intervention within a matter of hours. The critical aspect of both hypertension and hypotension is their recognition and management before other related complications occur.

Cranial Nerve Dysfunction

Although the stroke rate and operative mortality associated with carotid endarterectomy have been thoroughly documented for many years, the incidence of iatrogenic injury to cranial nerves near the bifurcation has received relatively little attention. Case reports and retrospective clinical investigations have suggested that symptomatic cranial nerve dysfunction is uncommon and involves the hypoglossal nerve in 5 to 8 per cent of patients and all other cranial nerves in fewer than 2 per cent.[8, 94, 115] Nevertheless,

other reports have demonstrated that the diagnosis of cranial nerve injury is more likely to be established by prospective studies, especially when they are performed in conjunction with objective postoperative testing. In a review of carotid reconstruction at three university, Veterans Administration, and community hospitals, Krupski and colleagues[90] described at least transient injuries to the vagus or recurrent laryngeal nerves in 8 per cent of patients, the hypoglossal nerve in 4 per cent, and the marginal mandibular branch of the facial nerve in 2 per cent. Evans,[55] Liapis,[92] and their associates encountered early postoperative dysfunction of the vagus or recurrent laryngeal nerves in 15 per cent and the hypoglossal nerve in 6 per cent, but they also found that as many as 35 per cent of patients had integrated motor deficits that could be detected by speech pathologists. Functional impairment was almost always temporary, however, and only a few of these patients still had persistent deficits as soon as 6 weeks later. Others have made the same observation.[131]

Direct otolaryngologic examinations were conducted after 450 consecutive carotid procedures at the Cleveland Clinic (Table 126-1).[67, 74] Sixty (13 per cent) of these patients had a total of 72 cranial nerve injuries, corresponding to the vagus or recurrent laryngeal nerve in approximately 7 per cent, the hypoglossal nerve in 6 per cent, and the marginal mandibular and the superior laryngeal nerves each in 2 per cent. Perhaps the most important feature of this study is the fact that 24 (33 per cent) of these injuries were asymptomatic and would not have been obvious without formal evaluation. Because simultaneous dysfunction of both recurrent laryngeal or hypoglossal nerves could have disastrous consequences, the tongue should be entirely normal, and the integrity of the larynx should be established by direct inspection during the staging interval between operations in patients who require bilateral carotid endarterectomy. If either the tongue or the vocal cord is impaired, the contralateral procedure should be postponed until cranial nerve dysfunction has resolved unless there are compelling reasons to do otherwise.

As indicated in Table 126-1, 55 (76 per cent) of the 72 iatrogenic injuries in this series were reassessed by ad-

Table 126-1. Cranial Nerve Dysfunction After Carotid Endarterectomy*

| | Cranial Nerves | | | | | | | |
| | *Recurrent Laryngeal* | | *Hypoglossal* | | *Marginal Mandibular* | | *Superior Laryngeal* | |
Postoperative Dysfunction	No.	Per Cent	No.	Per Cent	No.	Per Cent	No.	Per Cent
Early Incidence								
Symptomatic	21	4.7	16	3.6	8	1.8	3	0.7
Asymptomatic	9	2.0	10	2.2	0	—	5	1.1
Total	30	6.7	26	5.8	8	1.8	8	1.8
Late Results								
Follow-up examinations	24	80	20	77	7	88	4	50
Recovery								
Complete	20	83	17	85	6	86	2	50
Mean interval (mo)	3		2		3		2	
Incomplete	4	17	3	15	2	14	2	50
Maximal interval (mo)	14		12		9		2	

*Early incidence and late results of cranial nerve dysfunction following 450 carotid endarterectomies at the Cleveland Clinic.[67, 74]

ditional examinations. Complete functional recovery occurred in most patients within 3 months after their operations, a finding that suggests that blunt trauma probably is responsible for the majority of cranial nerve complications. Temporary dysfunction may be unavoidable in some patients who have anomalous nerves or require exposure of the internal carotid artery near the base of the skull, but every surgeon who performs carotid endarterectomy should be familiar with the normal anatomy of cranial nerves depicted in Figure 126–3.

The Vagus Nerve

The vagus nerve usually pursues a course posterior or slightly lateral to the common carotid and internal carotid arteries, but it occasionally must be reflected from an anomalous anterior position in order to expose the carotid bifurcation. The recurrent laryngeal nerve customarily takes its origin from the vagus within the mediastinum and loops around the subclavian artery on the right side and the aortic arch on the left before entering the tracheoesophageal groove posterior to the thyroid gland, but it may rarely rise from the vagus near the carotid bifurcation and cross behind the common carotid artery to enter the larynx. It is conceivable that the blades of self-retaining retractors that are placed too deep in the wound may engage the recurrent laryngeal nerve where it is concealed by strap muscles behind the trachea, but because recurrent laryngeal dysfunction is the only clinical manifestation of unilateral vagal injury, most vocal cord complications probably are instead caused by direct trauma to the vagus nerve itself. Irrespective of whether the vagus is stretched within the carotid sheath or injured by forceps, electrocautery, or the application of arterial clamps, paralysis of the ipsilateral vocal cord in the paramedian position results in hoarseness and the loss of an effective cough mechanism. Although these symptoms customarily resolve within several weeks, synthetic material may be injected into the cord to return it to the midline if the symptoms persist beyond 6 to 12 months.

The Hypoglossal Nerve

The hypoglossal nerve descends into the neck in a relatively constant position medial to the internal carotid artery and jugular vein before crossing anterior to the external carotid artery to enter the base of the tongue. With the exception of patients who have especially low carotid bifurcations, the hypoglossal nerve is a surgical landmark that may interfere with adequate exposure of the internal carotid artery because it is tethered in place by the ansa hypoglossi, by the small artery and vein to the sternocleidomastoid muscle, and often by the occipital artery as well as the posterior belly of the digastric muscle. Any or all of these structures may be divided in order to elevate the hypoglossal nerve from the internal carotid artery, since the nerve is more likely to be injured by excessive retraction than by appropriate steps to mobilize it.[81, 148] Trauma to the hypoglossal nerve causes deviation of the tongue to the ipsilateral side, inarticulate speech, and clumsy mastication.

The Superior Laryngeal Nerve

The superior laryngeal nerve arises from the vagus near the jugular foramen and passes diagonally behind the internal and external carotid arteries before supplying sensation to the mucosa of the larynx as well as innervation to the cricothyroid muscle and the inferior pharyngeal constrictor. Either the motor or the sensory branch may be lacerated during dissection near the superior thyroid artery, and because the main trunk of the nerve is hidden by the carotid sinus, it may also be injured by the vascular clamp applied to the internal carotid artery. Voice fatigue and the loss of high-pitch phonation are the principal manifestations of superior laryngeal trauma, but the impairment is relatively minor in patients who are neither vocalists nor public speakers.

The Marginal Mandibular Nerve

The marginal mandibular branch of the facial nerve emerges from the anterior border of the parotid gland and

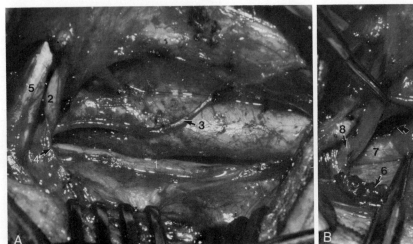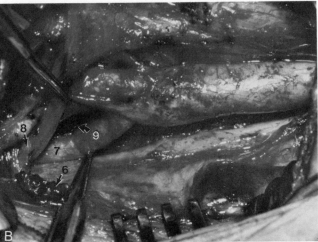

FIGURE 126–3. Surgical exposure of the carotid bifurcation. *A*, The vagus *(1)* and hypoglossal *(2)* nerves, the ansa hypoglossi *(3)*, the sternocleidomastoid (SCM) artery and vein *(4)*, and the digastric muscle *(5)*. *B*, The ansa, the SCM artery and vein, and the posterior belly of the digastric muscle *(6)* have been divided to isolate the distal internal carotid *(7)*, but it was not necessary to sacrifice the occipital artery *(8)*. The superior laryngeal nerve is hidden from view *(9)*.

extends across the masseter muscle and the ramus of the mandible before entering the perioral muscles in the lower lip. Although it lies between the platysma and the deep cervical fascia and is not visible within the surgical field, the nerve is drawn downward by rotation of the head to the opposite side. Unless the incision has been extended on a line posterior to the tragus, the nerve may be injured by retraction used to facilitate the exposure of a high carotid bifurcation. This example of blunt trauma imposes little functional disability and almost always is transient, but the inexperienced observer may sometimes misinterpret drooping at the corner of the mouth as representing an atypical stroke.

The Glossopharyngeal Nerve

Motor filaments of the glossopharyngeal nerve cross the distal cervical segment of the internal carotid artery to innervate the middle pharyngeal constrictor and the tensor muscle of the soft palate. Although glossopharyngeal trauma is unlikely unless the internal carotid lesion is exceedingly high, its symptoms are among the most serious of all cranial nerve deficits. Solid food becomes difficult to swallow because of middle constrictor paralysis. Oral fluids are tolerated even more poorly because of nasopharyngeal reflux, and because simultaneous vagal dysfunction is not uncommon, they may be aspirated into the airway as a result of ipsilateral vocal cord palsy. Under these circumstances, intravenous hyperalimentation or enteric tube feeding may be required for at least a short period of time. Because both the pharynx and the palate receive multiple motor fibers from the injured nerve as well as from the opposite side, nutritional support usually may be discontinued after 2 to 3 weeks with the anticipation that complete functional recovery will occur within the following month. Nevertheless, preservation of the glossopharyngeal nerve may well be one of the most important features of mandibular subluxation and detachment of the styloid process to enhance exposure of the internal carotid artery near the base of the skull.[123, 130]

Other Cervical Nerves

Tucker and associates[156] encountered 4 injuries to the spinal accessory nerve in a series of 850 carotid endarterectomies (0.5 per cent), but they were able to collect only 3 other examples of this complication during their review of the previous literature. Horner's syndrome may occur if the superior cervical sympathetic chain is transected during mobilization of the internal carotid artery above the level of the digastric muscle, but this injury is also so rare as to be anecdotal.[158] However, virtually every patient who has an incision parallel to the anterior margin of the sternocleidomastoid muscle experiences temporary sensory loss caused by injury to cutaneous nerves entering the neck and lower mandible. The greater auricular nerve emerges from behind the superior border of the sternocleidomastoid to supply the skin of the scalp and the external ear. Blunt trauma from retractor blades at the upper extent of a standard incision may result in painful paresthesias in the distribution of this nerve that are particularly troublesome.

Operative Stroke

Carotid endarterectomy must be associated with a low incidence of iatrogenic stroke if it is to be considered a reasonable alternative to nonoperative management of cerebrovascular disease. Considerable improvements have been made in this respect since the Joint Study of Extracranial Arterial Occlusion reported an overall early mortality of 8 per cent and determined that fatal complications occurred in 42 per cent of patients who had sustained completed strokes within the 2 weeks preceding their operations prior to 1969.[14, 56] At the present time, the combined morbidity and mortality for carotid reconstruction is well below 5 per cent at most experienced centers, largely because of refinements in patient selection and surgical technique.[66] In recognition of this progress, a subcommittee of the American Heart Association stated in 1989 that the 30-day mortality rate for all carotid endarterectomies should not exceed 2 per cent and established acceptable risks for perioperative stroke according to discrete surgical indications (asymptomatic stenosis, less than 3 per cent; previous TIA, less than 5 per cent; prior ischemic infarction, less than 7 per cent; recurrent carotid stenosis, less than 10 per cent).[15] Nevertheless, the collective results of surgeons who occasionally undertake carotid endarterectomy often fail to meet these standards and have provoked speculation concerning the safety of the operation throughout the United States.[21, 47] However unjustified, such criticism cannot be easily dismissed until the success of carotid reconstruction has been documented at every hospital in which it is performed.

Incidence

Table 126–2 contains a summary of early results for carotid endarterectomy in 25 large and/or academic series reported since 1980. Most of these series include a representative distribution of symptomatic and asymptomatic patients, but the surgical indications in the NASCET and the European Trial were of course limited to previous TIA or mild stroke with good functional recovery, and the Veterans Administration Cooperative Study was restricted to patients having asymptomatic stenosis.

Although a regional anesthetic permits continuous assessment of the neurologic status and has been associated with excellent outcome at several centers, general inhalation anesthesia is more widely used because it reduces the cerebral oxygen requirement and provides complete control of ventilation as well as a comfortable setting for both the patient and the surgical team. Every conceivable approach has been employed to determine the indications for carotid shunting, including test clamping, measurement of internal carotid back pressure, and operative electroencephalography (EEG) or cortical blood flow studies. None of these methods has an absolute correlation with stroke risk, however, and Thompson[148] long maintained that routine shunting was the safest and most expeditious alternative. Conceding a number of differences in intraoperative management, results from the 22 nonrandomized series in Table 126–2 are reasonably similar and suggest that an overall stroke and mortality rate of 4 per cent or less represents the

Table 126–2. Representative Results of Carotid Endarterectomy Reported in Large and/or Academic Series Since 1980

Series	Year	No.	Anesthesia and Cerebral Monitoring	Carotid Shunt	Neurologic Complications			Mortality (%)
					TIA (%)	Stroke (%)	Total (%)	
Ott et al[103]	1980	309	General	None	1.9	1.3	3.2	0.6
White et al[161]	1980	252	General, back pressure	87%	2.0	2.0	4.0	2.0
Whitney et al[162]	1980	1197	General	None	1.2	2.3	3.5	1.8
Bardin et al[11]	1982	456	General, back pressure	75%	4.2	2.6	6.8	0.9
Cranley[36]	1982	882	NA	NA	2.1	1.0	3.1	1.1
Imparato et al[82]	1982	956	Regional, test clamp	8%	NA	NA	2.4	NA
Peitzman et al[109]	1982	314	Regional (80%), test clamp	8%	0.6	3.2	3.8	1.9
Steed et al[138]	1982	345	Regional, test clamp	None	4.3	1.7	6.1	NA
Towne and Bernhard[153]	1982	312	General	83%	2.2	2.9	5.1	0.6
Rosenthal et al[125]	1983	818	General, EEG (28%)	39%	2.7	1.8	4.5	NA
Whittemore et al[163]	1983	219	General, EEG	16%	1.4	0.9	2.2	2.2
Baker et al[10]	1984	940	General, back pressure	None	2.2	2.4	4.7	0.6
Cleveland Vascular Registry[69]	1984	2646	Mixed	NA	NA	2.5	NA	1.2
Ouriel et al[105]	1984	402	General, EEG (35%)	17%	3.2	3.2	6.5	NA
Sachs et al[128]	1984	557	General	All	2.2	2.3	4.5	0.7
Green et al[62]	1985	562	General, EEG	18%	NA	2.7	NA	NA
Fode et al[58]	1986	2535	Mixed	NA	NA	4.2	NA	1.8
Sundt et al[142]	1986	1935	General, EEG	42%	1.8	1.8	3.6	1.3
Toronto Study Group[151]	1986	358	Mixed	NA	5.0	4.5	9.5	1.4
Cleveland Clinic[72]	1987	917	General	All	0.8	1.9	2.7	0.5
Cleveland Vascular Registry[126]	1988	8535	Mixed	NA	NA	2.1	NA	1.6
Edwards et al[48]	1989	3028	General	97%	1.3	1.0	2.3	1.5
VA Cooperative Study[154]	1990	211	General	NA	NA	2.4	NA	1.9
NASCET[98] (70–99% stenosis)	1991	328	Mixed	NA	NA	5.5	NA	0.6
European Trial[54] (70–99% stenosis)	1991	435	Mixed	NA	NA	6.9	NA	0.9

Key: *NA, data not available; EEG, operative electroencephalography; TIA, transient ischemic attack.*

contemporary standard of excellence with respect to early outcome following carotid endarterectomy.

In another large collected series of 22 publications from 1977 to 1984, sufficient data were available to make a number of comparisons regarding the influence of surgical indications, contralateral carotid disease, choice of anesthesia, and shunt protection on stroke risk (Table 126–3).[66] Permanent iatrogenic strokes occurred in 1.6 per cent of patients with asymptomatic carotid stenosis, compared with 2.5 per cent of those who had previous neurologic symptoms, and they were twice as common in patients having a history of prior strokes (3.9 per cent) as in the group whose preoperative symptoms had been limited to TIAs (1.8 per cent). Of 2589 patients for whom the angiographic status of the contralateral carotid system was designated, operative strokes occurred in 6.1 per cent of those with recognized internal carotid occlusion, in comparison with 1.1 per cent of all others. Permanent deficits occurred in conjunction with general anesthesia in 2.2 per cent, with local or regional anesthesia in 1.3 per cent, and with shunting or nonshunting in 1.9 per cent and 1.8 per cent, respectively.

These figures cannot be interpreted to imply that shunts are unnecessary, since selective shunting was used for patients who had specific indications for cerebral protection throughout most of the reference studies. In a series of 940 operations performed without shunts, Baker and associates[10] found that the stroke rate was significantly higher among patients who had low back pressure as well as contralateral carotid occlusion (11 per cent) than in those having only one (2.8 per cent) or neither (0.9 per cent) of these risk factors. Greene and coworkers[62] described ischemic EEG changes after carotid clamping in 37 per cent of pa-

tients who had contralateral internal carotid occlusion or a history of previous stroke, and Graham and associates[61] reported that an abnormal operative EEG was as much as 20 times more common in such patients than in all others.

Table 126–3. Specific Considerations Concerning the Incidence of Permanent Stroke After Carotid Endarterectomy

Specific Considerations	Composite Results of Representative Series		
	Data Available (No.)	Permanent Operative Strokes	
		No.	%
Total	14,606	323	2.2
Surgical Indications			
Asymptomatic carotid stenosis	1784	29	1.6
Previous neurologic symptoms	7712	194	2.5
Transient ischemia	3288	58	1.8
Prior strokes	933	36	3.9
Contralateral Carotid Status			
Patent	2276	26	1.1
Occluded	313	19	6.1
Anesthetic Management			
General	7494	163	2.2
Local or regional	447	6	1.3
Cerebral Protection			
Shunt	1973	37	1.9
No shunt	4479	80	1.8

From Hertzer NR: Early complications of carotid endarterectomy. In Moore WS (ed): Cerebrovascular Disease. New York, Churchill Livingstone, 1987. By permission.

Sundt and coworkers[142] have followed an elegant protocol for intraoperative assessment with both EEG and cerebral blood flow measurements, and they still concluded that shunting was warranted in 42 per cent of their patients. The perpetual controversy concerning shunts probably will not be resolved in the foreseeable future, but it appears to be related to *when* (rather than *whether*) they should be used.

Community Hospital Results

Most operations in the United States are performed at community hospitals, and Table 126–4 contains a summary of results for carotid reconstruction in this generally unreported sector from 1975 to 1989. Although the safety of carotid endarterectomy in several series was comparable with that at referral centers, Easton and Sherman[47] in southern Illinois and Brott and Thalinger[21] in Cincinnati calculated excessive complication rates from pooled community data that galvanized opposition to surgical treatment at the time of their publication. Each of these two studies included a substantial number of patients with preoperative strokes as their indication for operation, and both were collected retrospectively from many surgeons with undesignated training and limited personal experience in extracranial reconstruction. Taylor and Porter[145] subsequently reviewed the surgical literature and found that the perioperative stroke rate was twice as high among patients with a history of previous strokes who were reported in community surveys rather than in large individual series. All of these data suggest that, at least in some areas, patients having acute or profound neurologic deficits still are being selected for surgical treatment. Although Piotrowski and associates[112] have suggested that an arbitrary delay of 6 weeks or longer is not always necessary before carotid endarterectomy may be performed safely following a completed stroke, they strongly emphasized that patients must attain a stable neurologic plateau before earlier intervention can be seriously considered.

Additional information from the same two hospitals

participating in one of these investigations now is available and indicates that unsatisfactory results may be improved provided that they are discovered in the first place. While studying a related issue, Moore and associates[95] incidentally reported the 510 consecutive carotid procedures that followed the 228 operations described by Easton and Sherman in 1977. Prior stroke declined as an indication for carotid endarterectomy from 43 per cent in the earlier series to 19 per cent thereafter, and there also were impressive reductions in the operative stroke rate (from 14 per cent to 5.3 per cent) and mortality (from 6.6 per cent to 1.6 per cent). According to the prospective computer registry of peripheral vascular operations in northeastern Ohio, surgeons who are trained in arterial reconstruction and maintain an active interest in their field can perform carotid endarterectomy with exemplary success.[69, 126] Other community series have failed to demonstrate that specialty training influences the neurologic outcome, usually because their results were either universally good or consistently poor among all participating surgeons.[22, 87, 90, 136] In any event, data from southern Illinois are important because they illustrate so clearly that the recognition of unfavorable trends is essential to their solution.

Management

Postoperative neurologic deficits may be caused by atheromatous embolization during the surgical exposure, by clamp ischemia, by delayed platelet emboli or thrombosis, and rarely by cerebral hemorrhage occurring several days after the procedure. Thus, the patient who develops an ischemic event following carotid endarterectomy may have sustained: (1) an embolic TIA that will resolve without treatment, (2) an embolic stroke for which reoperation is contraindicated, or (3) a stroke-in-evolution caused by thrombosis at the endarterectomy site, which may improve dramatically if prompt thrombectomy of the internal carotid artery is performed. The cause of neurologic complications is not always immediately obvious, but the patency of the carotid bifurcation should be documented by urgent nonin-

Table 126–4. Results of Carotid Endarterectomy Reported From Community Hospitals

Series	Year	No.	Anesthesia and Cerebral Monitoring	Carotid Shunt	Neurologic Complications			Mortality (%)
					TIA (%)	*Stroke* (%)	*Total* (%)	
Nunn[99]	1975	234	General	97%	0.9	4.7	5.6	5.1
Easton and Sherman[47]	1977	228	NA	NA	NA	14	NA	6.6
Prioleau et al[114]	1977	317	NA	56%	NA	NA	11	3.2
Gundlach and Swenson[63]	1979	119	General	All	2.5	0.8	3.4	0.8
Haynes and Dempsey[65]	1979	276	General	All	2.5	1.1	3.6	1.1
Carmichael[26]	1980	445	General	1%	0.9	1.6	2.5	0.2
Brott and Thalinger[21]	1984	431	Mixed	NA	4.8	7.9	12.7	2.8
Moore et al[95]	1984	510	General, back pressure or EEG (33%)	75%	2.0	5.3	7.3	1.6
Slavish et al[136]	1984	743	General	All	3.5	1.8	5.3	2.7
Krupski et al[90]	1985	100	General, back pressure	54%	1.0	3.0	4.0	NA
Cafferata and Gainey[22]	1986	390	Mixed	74%	NA	8.5	NA	3.1
Kempczinski et al[87]	1986	750	Mixed	34%	NA	5.1	NA	2.3
Kirshner et al[88]	1989	1035	Mixed	25%	2.3	4.3	6.7	1.4
Richardson and Main[119]	1989	1039	Mixed	NA	NA	3.6	NA	3.1

Key: *NA, data not available; EEG, operative electroencephalography; TIA, transient ischemic attack.*

vasive testing, objective imaging, or cervical exploration whenever such complications occur.

A number of reports indicate that preoperative cerebral infarction is more common than would be suspected on clinical grounds, that infarcts discovered on computed scans often are associated with ulcerated lesions of the carotid bifurcation, and that atheromatous ulcers in turn have a higher risk for postoperative stroke than nonulcerated lesions.[16, 60, 70, 169] Although intraoperative neurologic deficits are recognized only after recovery from general anesthesia, Jernigan and coworkers[83] and Rosenthal and colleagues[125] employed regional anesthesia and found that most of these events appeared to be embolic because they occurred in alert patients either during carotid manipulation or at the time flow was restored after an uneventful period of clamp occlusion. The severity of the postoperative symptoms and the circumstances encountered during the original operation inevitably influence the decision whether a patient who awakens with a neurologic deficit should undergo immediate reoperation, carotid angiography, or close observation alone. For example, surgical exploration may be completely appropriate in the presence of a dense postoperative hemiparesis when there is a predictable risk of technical complications after a tedious reconstruction. Conversely, nonoperative assessment of the internal carotid artery may be the most that is necessary for a patient who is found to have a mild early deficit following routine endarterectomy of symptomatic, grossly ulcerated carotid disease.

According to experience at a number of centers, however, the majority of perioperative neurologic complications actually occur after a lucent interval during which functional recovery is satisfactory.[106, 138, 151, 162] Because it is difficult to attribute such delayed events to surgical manipulation or clamping, other contributing factors must also be considered. Carotid thrombosis and cerebral hemorrhage are the most serious of these, and, at least in some cases, they may be anticipated in time to avoid irreversible consequences.

Carotid Thrombosis

The incidence of postoperative internal carotid thrombosis has been reported to range from 2 to 18 per cent in scattered prospective studies employing hemodynamic testing or objective imaging.[2, 71, 102] Although occlusion rates almost certainly differ from one hospital and even one surgeon to the next, several reports have recommended the use of selective or routine operative angiography in an attempt to eliminate technical complications.[19, 35, 96] More recently, others have found that Doppler ultrasonography is a convenient method for intraoperative assessment that detects residual internal carotid lesions in 4 to 8 per cent of patients.[12, 46, 57, 135] Using this approach, Zierler and colleagues[167] discovered fresh thrombus or iatrogenic defects that actually required correction during 5 per cent of their operations.

In order to discourage platelet aggregation, aspirin therapy (5 grains twice daily) is administered empirically on the preoperative evening and for at least the first month after carotid reconstruction at the Cleveland Clinic. In addition, an infusion of low-molecular-weight dextran (35 to 50 ml per hour) is begun prior to closure of the arteriotomy and is continued until the following day in selected patients who have atheromatous ulceration extending into a deep endarterectomy plane. Both of these precautions are based on the principle that platelet inhibition must precede their "first pass" across the endarterectomy surface to be effective.[66] In a total of 366 patients, Edwards and associates[49] calculated that this type of antiplatelet therapy was associated with significant improvement in the incidence of perioperative stroke and carotid thrombosis in comparison with a nonrandomized control group.

Because relatively few examples of early carotid thrombosis have been reported from any single center, it is difficult to determine even from collected data whether patients who develop delayed postoperative deficits should undergo either preliminary investigation of internal carotid patency (Fig. 126–4) or immediate surgical exploration. Rosenthal and associates[125] and Perdue[110] have estimated that reoperations are indicated in only 20 per cent of patients who sustain cerebral ischemia related to carotid endarterectomy, and there is no convincing evidence that the hour or so that is necessary to perform intravenous or conventional angiography in an adequate hospital setting influences the eventual outcome in those who do have carotid thrombosis. Nevertheless, it is reasonable to return patients suspected of having this correctable complication directly to the operating room, and any decision *not* to perform a reoperation in the presence of a delayed neurologic event should be supported by some objective confirmation that the internal carotid artery has remained patent. The surgical management of postendarterectomy thrombosis is illustrated in Figure 126–5.[108] Retrograde internal carotid bleeding may be restored by removal of platelet thrombus from the bifurcation, but if a balloon embolectomy catheter is used to retrieve propagated clot, it should be introduced cautiously in order not to cause a cavernous sinus fistula.[51, 85] After a shunt has been inserted to reestablish cerebral blood flow, the distal intima may be secured with tacking sutures prior to closure of the arteriotomy with a patch of saphenous vein.

Eleven (0.4 per cent) of the 2651 patients who had carotid endarterectomy at the Cleveland Clinic from 1977 to 1984 required early reoperations because of symptomatic thrombosis of the internal carotid artery. Table 126–5 presents the results of urgent surgical treatment in these 11 patients as well as in 30 others already described in the literature.[108] All reoperations were performed within 4 hours after perioperative deficits were discovered, and the interval between the original procedure and the onset of symptoms was available for 36 of the 41 patients. Because only 4 patients recovered from their initial anesthetics with discrete deficits, some period of normal neurologic function was witnessed after endarterectomy in the remaining 32 (88 per cent). Substantial improvement occurred in 61 per cent of the composite series after thrombectomy, approximately half of whom had complete recovery, whereas neurologic function was unchanged in another 22 per cent. The overall mortality rate was 17 per cent, but a limited delay in intervention did not appear to compromise the outcome. This accumulated experience suggests that decisive surgical management is the preferred approach to postendarterectomy thrombosis and is not associated with a higher mor-

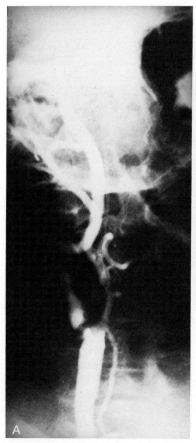

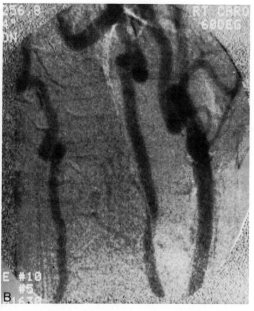

FIGURE 126–4. Preoperative (*A*) and postoperative (*B*) angiograms demonstrating an early occlusion of the right carotid system following proximal endarterectomy of a kinked internal carotid artery. An acute neurologic deficit improved after urgent thrombectomy, kink resection, and vein patch angioplasty. (From Painter TA, Hertzer NR, O'Hara PJ, et al: Symptomatic internal carotid thrombosis after carotid endarterectomy. J Vasc Surg 5:445, 1987.)

FIGURE 126–5. Technical features of urgent carotid reoperations. *A*, Careful thrombectomy. *B*, Immediate shunting. *C*, Removal of loose debris and suture fixation of the distal intima. *D*, Vein patch angioplasty. (From Painter TA, Hertzer NR, O'Hara PJ, et al: Symptomatic internal carotid thrombosis after carotid endarterectomy. J Vasc Surg 5:445, 1987.)

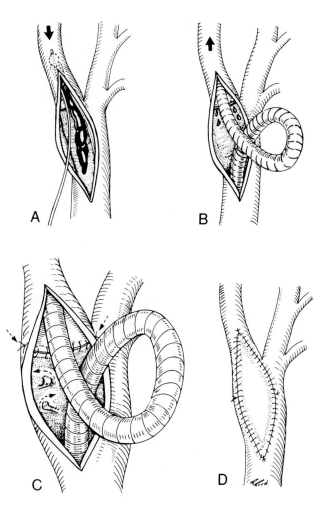

Table 126–5.   Urgent Thrombectomy in the Management of Symptomatic Internal Carotid Occlusion After Carotid Endarterectomy

| | | Postocclusion Neurologic Deficit | | | | | |
| | | Improved | | Unchanged | | Mortality | |
Eligible Patients	No.	No.	%	No.	%	No.	%
Collected series	41	25	61	9	22	7	17
Documented Surgical Delay							
<2 hours after symptoms	22	14	63	5	23	3	14
2–4 hours after symptoms	7	5	72	1	14	1	14

From Painter TA, Hertzer NR, O'Hara PJ, et al: Symptomatic internal carotid thrombosis after carotid endarterectomy. J Vasc Surg 5:445, 1987.

tality rate than might be anticipated with expectant care alone.

Cerebral Hemorrhage

Cerebral hemorrhage is the most lethal neurologic complication that can occur after any type of extracranial reconstruction (Fig. 126–6). This rare, irreversible catastrophe usually occurs several days postoperatively, and because little can then be done to improve its prognosis, selected patients warrant close surveillance and even prophylactic treatment because of their risk of having a fragile intracranial capillary bed. Caplan and coworkers[25] implicated hypertension as the principal etiologic feature of hemorrhagic infarction, but others have also described additional contributing factors, such as the correction of severe internal carotid stenosis at the time of the original procedure, diffuse cerebrovascular disease with contralateral carotid occlusion, and the administration of anticoagulants.[64, 113] Excruciating unilateral headache may be a harbinger of both focal seizure activity and cerebral hemorrhage in patients who required carotid endarterectomy for high-grade lesions associated with previous strokes.[117, 143, 164, 165]

All of these observations suggest that cerebral edema, and ultimately hemorrhage, may be caused by regional overperfusion of a recipient capillary network accustomed to a state of relatively low blood flow. It is difficult to draw absolute conclusions concerning such an unusual syndrome, but patients who exhibit any evidence of cerebral edema clearly should be kept under close observation and probably should receive empirical management in an attempt to prevent subsequent motor seizures or intracranial bleeding. Bed rest, fluid restriction, and maintenance of the blood pressure at a level slightly lower than normal are appropriate precautions, and either formal anticoagulation or antiplatelet therapy seems to be contraindicated. Like the swollen limb after extremity revascularization, the morbidity of cerebral edema undoubtedly declines as the integrity of the capillary bed is restored.[66]

Carotid Patch Angioplasty

Throughout their extensive experience, Imparato and colleagues[82] and Sundt and associates[141] have encouraged the use of patch angioplasty to complement carotid endarterectomy. Stewart and coworkers[139] have since found that patch closure was associated with better early patency than primary arterial repair after intimal resection in animal models, and patching also has eliminated operative strokes and thrombosis in several other clinical reports.[4, 44, 86] The merit of patch angioplasty was reconfirmed in a series of 801 consecutive patients who underwent 917 primary carotid endarterectomies at the Cleveland Clinic.[72] Conventional arteriotomy closure was performed during 483 operations in this 3-year study, whereas a patch of saphenous vein (usually harvested from the lower leg) was employed in 434. Otherwise, preoperative risk factors, surgical management, and antiplatelet therapy were equivalent in the patch and nonpatch groups, and the immediate technical result was documented by intravenous digital subtraction angiography in a total of 715 patients (89 per cent). As presented in Table 126–6, ischemic strokes or internal carotid thrombosis each occurred in approximately 2 per cent of the entire series. Nevertheless, both the stroke rate (0.7 per cent versus 3.1 per cent; $p = .0084$, Fisher exact test) and the incidence of postoperative thrombosis (0.5 per cent versus 3.1 per cent; $p = .0027$) were significantly lower in the patched cohort.

Although it conserves the greater saphenous system for future coronary bypass or extremity revascularization, a distal vein patch may occasionally lack the tensile strength of a segment excised from the groin. Urgent replacement was necessary for 3 (0.6 per cent) of the initial 434 vein patches at the Cleveland Clinic (see Table 126–6), and a total of 8 central patch ruptures (0.5 per cent) have occurred in the overall series of 1691 patients who received vein patch angioplasty during carotid endarterectomy at this center from 1983 to 1990.[101] All of these complications occurred within 5 days of the primary procedure (including 4 during the first 24 hours) and involved ankle vein segments, a feature that also has been noted by Riles and associates.[121] Archie and Green[6] subsequently confirmed in vitro that the hoop strength of small veins is substantially less than that of large veins, irrespective of the level at which they are harvested, and that the experimental bursting pressure for vein patches of similar size appears to be less in women than in men. These composite data suggest that, at least in women, autogenous carotid patches should be constructed using the greater saphenous vein in the upper thigh in order to avoid the low but serious risk of early postoperative rupture.

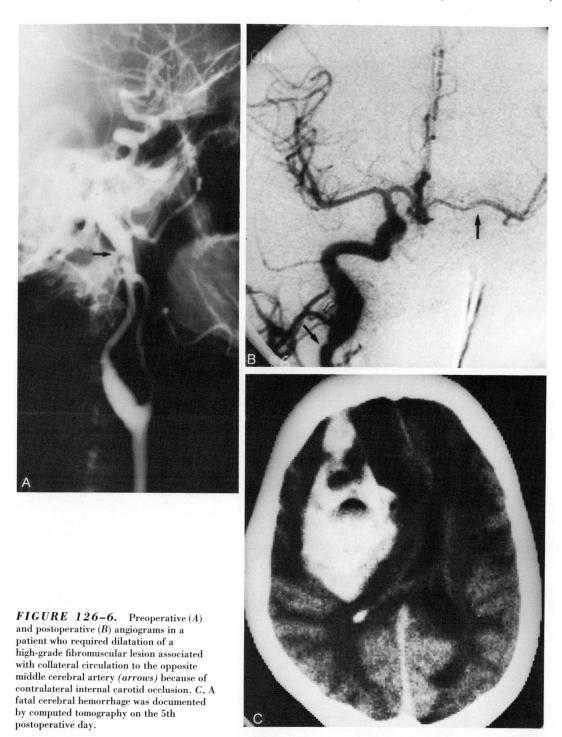

FIGURE 126-6. Preoperative (A) and postoperative (B) angiograms in a patient who required dilatation of a high-grade fibromuscular lesion associated with collateral circulation to the opposite middle cerebral artery *(arrows)* because of contralateral internal carotid occlusion. C, A fatal cerebral hemorrhage was documented by computed tomography on the 5th postoperative day.

Recurrent Carotid Stenosis

Although its true incidence and clinical implications still are controversial, recurrent stenosis can occur at virtually any interval following carotid endarterectomy (Fig. 126–7). Early complications (intimal flaps or perioperative occlusions) may eventually be misinterpreted as representing recurrent disease unless immediate surgical results are assessed by objective testing, but most recurrent lesions undoubtedly are caused by either of two etiologic factors: myointimal hyperplasia, a collagenous proliferation of the

medial layer of the arterial wall that appears to be more prevalent in women and usually is discovered within the first 3 postoperative years; or secondary atherosclerosis, occurring later in the follow-up period and more closely associated with smoking and hyperlipidemia.[31, 34, 40, 43, 77, 100, 116, 118, 140, 166] As indicated in Figure 126–8, the essential features of recurrent stenosis in a series of 65 late carotid reoperations at the Cleveland Clinic were consistent with those originally described by Stoney and String[140] several years earlier.[40] Hyperplastic recurrences generally were asymptomatic and were suspected on the basis of routine

Table 126–6.   Vein Patch Angioplasty During Carotid Endarterectomy*

Related Complications	Routine Closure No.	Routine Closure %	Patch Angioplasty No.	Patch Angioplasty %	Total No.	Total %
Perioperative Period						
Total procedures	483	100	434	100	917	100
Neurologic events	19	3.9	8	1.8	27	2.9
Transient deficits	3	0.6	4	0.9	7	0.8
Completed strokes	15	3.1	3	0.7	18	2.0
Hemorrhagic infarcts	1	0.2	1	0.2	2	0.2
Carotid thrombosis	15	3.1	2	0.5	17	1.9
Symptomatic	9	1.9	0	—	9	1.0
Asymptomatic	6	1.2	2	0.5	8	0.9
Miscellaneous						
Cervical hematoma	7	1.4	7	1.6	14	1.5
Patch disruption	—	—	3	0.7	—	—
Late Interval (Mean, 21 mo)						
Reoperations for recurrent stenosis	7	1.4	3	0.7	10	1.1
Objective imaging	146	31	186	43	332	36
Documented internal carotid defects	21	14	9	4.8	30	9.0
<70% diameter	11	7.5	5	2.7	16	4.8
≥70% diameter	8	5.5	2	1.1	10	3.0
Occlusion	2	1.4	2	1.1	4	1.2

From Hertzer NR, Beven EG, O'Hara PJ, Krewjewski LP: A prospective study of vein patch angioplasty during carotid endarterectomy. Three-year results for 801 patients and 917 operations. Ann Surg 206:628, 1987.

*Perioperative and late results of a prospective study of vein patch angioplasty during carotid endarterectomy at the Cleveland Clinic.

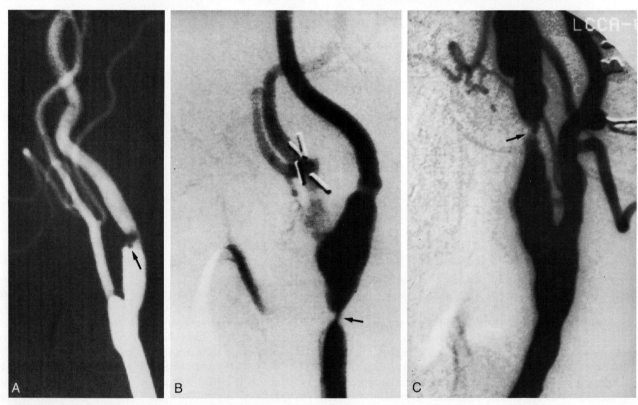

FIGURE 126–7.   The similar angiographic features of different sources for recurrent carotid stenosis. *A*, An intimal flap *(arrow)* 1 month after the original endarterectomy. *B*, A hyperplastic lesion *(arrow)* discovered at 8 months. *C*, New atherosclerosis *(arrow)* in the 8th postoperative year.

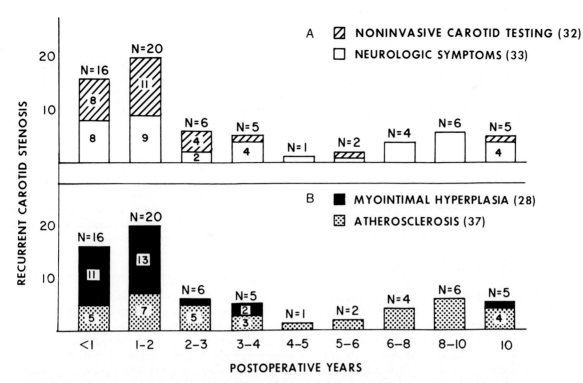

FIGURE 126–8. The interval preceding reoperations for recurrent carotid stenosis at the Cleveland Clinic, according to the method of detection (A) and the histologic diagnosis (B). (From Das MB, Hertzer NR, Ratliff NB, et al: Recurrent carotid stenosis. A five-year series of 65 reoperations. Ann Surg 202:28, 1985.)

noninvasive studies, whereas atherosclerotic lesions commonly were demonstrated by angiography after the onset of neurologic events. The mean recurrence interval for myointimal hyperplasia in this series was 21 months, compared with 57 months for atherosclerosis ($p = .0007$).

Because of the uncertain natural history of asymptomatic carotid stenosis, the possibility of recurrence has been cited as a relative contraindication to its surgical treatment.[32, 168] As a practical matter, however, the data necessary to establish this conclusion are highly contradictory (Table 126–7). The crude incidence of serious recurrent disease has been estimated to be only 1 to 4 per cent among large, retrospective series in which follow-up angiography traditionally was restricted to patients who were

Table 126–7. Recurrent Carotid Stenosis*

Series	Original Operations	Maximum Follow-up (Yr)	Recurrent Carotid Stenosis		
			Incidence (%)	Asymptomatic (%)	Reoperation (%)
Clinical Assessment					
Cossman et al[34]	361	2	3.6	–	3.6
Piepgras et al[111]	1992	12	1.7	NA	1.7
Stoney and String[140]	1654	13	1.5	0.1	1.5
Cleveland Clinic[40, 77]	1250	13	1.2	0.2	1.2
	2742	14	2.1	NA	2.1
Noninvasive Testing					
Baker et al[9]	133	4	9.7	8.3	2.6
Cantelmo et al[24]	199	8	12.1	7.5	2.0
Colgan et al[32]	80	4	12.5	11.2	NA
Kremen et al[89]	173	12	9.8	8.1	2.3
O'Donnell et al[100]	276	15	12.3	9.8	1.4
Thomas et al[147]	257	5	14.8	13.2	2.3
Turnipseed et al[157]	80	3	8.8	8.8	NA
Zbornikova et al[166]	113	9	23.9	21.2	NA
Zierler et al[168]	89	4	14.6	5.6	NA

Representative data concerning recurrent carotid stenosis detected by clinical assessment or prospective noninvasive testing.

Key: *NA, data not available.*

found to have new neurologic symptoms or cervical bruits. Since the introduction of noninvasive cerebrovascular testing, a number of reports have suggested that recurrent lesions instead occur in as many as 9 to 24 per cent of operated arteries and that the merit of carotid endarterectomy should be reconsidered on this basis. However, it should be noted from the information provided in Table 126–7 that all reoperation rates were less than 4 per cent, irrespective of whether objective studies were employed and that the vast majority of patients with evidence of recurrent stenosis on noninvasive examinations have remained asymptomatic. The unexpected results of objective tests clearly cannot be disregarded, but Zierler and colleagues[168] have described regression of recurrent lesions in 9 (41 per cent) of their 22 patients, an observation implying that at least some of the changes detected by Doppler ultrasonography may represent a normal sequence of arterial remodeling that simply was never documented before scanning was available.

Therefore, it seems likely that the actual incidence of recurrent stenosis probably strikes a balance between the figures generated from large series having incomplete follow-up and those provided by prospective noninvasive testing without angiographic confirmation. Moreover, the data in Table 126–8 illustrate that several considerations may influence the perceived recurrence rate even within a single study. Late clinical information was obtained during a mean postoperative interval of 22 months for a total of 232 patients who underwent carotid endarterectomy (270 arteries) at the Cleveland Clinic in 1980 to 1981, and a subset of this group (113 patients, 129 arteries) subsequently was reassessed by intravenous digital angiography.[29] Five-year survival and the incidence of stroke, reoperation, and at least 30 per cent recurrent stenosis were calculated using both crude and cumulative methods. There were few late strokes employing either approach, but the recurrence rate

could arbitrarily be expressed throughout a wide range of 3 per cent (reoperations in the entire series) to 34 per cent (measurable defects on objective imaging). There were no strokes related to any of the recognized recurrences even though remedial procedures were performed only for lesions associated with severe (70 to 90 per cent) stenosis. In the final analysis, the clinical significance of mild to moderate recurrent stenosis identified by noninvasive testing currently is unknown. Cook and associates[33] found in their experience that the incidence of subsequent neurologic symptoms was not substantially different, irrespective of whether recurrent stenosis did (14 per cent) or did not occur (6.5 per cent). For this reason, they have questioned the merit of long-term postoperative surveillance using duplex scanning, a clinical dilemma that assumes even greater importance in an era of cost containment in health care.

Management

Unless there are compelling reasons to do otherwise, the management of recurrent stenosis probably should be determined by the same judicious principles that are applicable to primary carotid disease. Hyperplastic stenosis tends to be asymptomatic, possibly because its smooth, firm surface discourages cerebral embolization.[100] Accordingly, early recurrences of intermediate severity should be treated with empirical antiplatelet therapy while their progress is monitored by serial objective studies. Although some investigators might disagree, elective reoperation seems to be appropriate if high-grade stenosis occurs, especially if the contralateral internal carotid artery is occluded. Because late atherosclerotic lesions often are symptomatic by the time they are discovered, a conventional approach to their diagnosis and surgical correction appears to be completely justified. Although the risk for at least temporary cranial nerve dysfunction is slightly higher (approximately 10 per

Table 126–8. Differences in Results of Carotid Endarterectomy*

| | Assessment Criteria | | | |
| | Clinical Examination | | Objective Imaging | |
Late Results	No.	%	No.	%
Patients	232	100	113	100
Mortality				
Crude	23	9.9	5	4.4
Cumulative	23	24	5	9.6
Stroke				
Crude	5	2.2	3	2.7
Cumulative	5	5.0	3	4.2
Arteries	270	100	129	100
Reoperations				
Crude	8	3.0	8	6.2
Cumulative	8	7.7	8	12
Recurrent stenosis (≥30% diameter)				
Crude	18	6.7	18	14
Cumulative	18	21	18	34

From Civil ID, O'Hara PJ, Hertzer NR, et al: Late patency of the carotid artery after endarterectomy. Problems of definition, follow-up methodology and data analysis. J Vasc Surg 8:79, 1988.

*Differences in calculated results that correspond to the ways in which data are manipulated in a single series of patients receiving carotid endarterectomy at the Cleveland Clinic.

cent) following carotid reoperations, the incidence of major neurologic complications has not exceeded 3 per cent at experienced centers.[40, 111]

From a technical standpoint, reoperations are performed using a vertical incision parallel to the anterior border of the sternocleidomastoid muscle, and sharp dissection is maintained within the plane of avascular scar tissue that leads directly to the bifurcation. The proximal common carotid may be isolated easily once the old arteriotomy has been identified as a landmark, but care must be taken not to injure the vagus nerve in this area. Dissection of the internal carotid usually is begun along its lateral aspect in order to reflect the hypoglossal nerve medially, and tethering structures (the sternocleidomastoid artery and vein, digastric muscle, and occipital artery) may be divided to facilitate access to the distal artery. Patch angioplasty should always be performed in conjunction with reoperations, and if formal endarterectomy of hyperplastic stenosis proves to be difficult, the application of a vein patch alone may be the best option. Interposition grafts are rarely necessary, but they represent yet another alternative, especially in the setting of multiple recurrences.[50] Because of the extended period of clamp ischemia during most reoperations, temporary shunting warrants serious consideration.

Carotid Patch Angioplasty

Further recurrent stenosis very rarely occurs following reoperations performed with patch angioplasty, an observation that indirectly supports the opinion long expressed by Sundt,[111, 141] Imparato[82] and their associates that primary patching should routinely be performed in order to prevent this complication. Furthermore, other investigators have encountered no serious recurrences with the use of either venous or autogenous patches in small series of patients studied by objective imaging during a maximal follow-up interval of approximately 3 years.[4, 44, 86] As indicated in Table 126–6, recurrent lesions (greater than or equal to 30 per cent diameter) have been discovered by intravenous angiography in only 4.8 per cent of patients receiving vein patch angioplasty at the Cleveland Clinic, compared with 14 per cent of those who underwent standard arteriotomy closure ($p = .0137$). Cumulative data for all 332 arteries evaluated by objective imaging in this investigation are illustrated in Figure 126–9.[72] Actuarial 3-year recurrence rates were 9 per cent and 31 per cent ($p = .0066$) for the patch and nonpatch groups, respectively, and this distinction (3.7 per cent versus 39 per cent) was especially significant ($p = .0019$) when the original surgical indication was asymptomatic carotid stenosis.[39, 91] Although few reoperations have been necessary in either cohort, these results suggest that patching may enhance the long-term outcome of carotid endarterectomy.

Several prospective studies employing duplex scanning also have implied that recurrent carotid stenosis is approximately twice as common in women as in men, and both Eikelboom and Ten Holter and their associates[52, 146] have recommended the use of vein patch angioplasty as a means to reduce the incidence of this complication in patients of either sex (Table 126–9). There currently is no consensus concerning the perceived benefit of patch angioplasty, however, since other published reports have failed

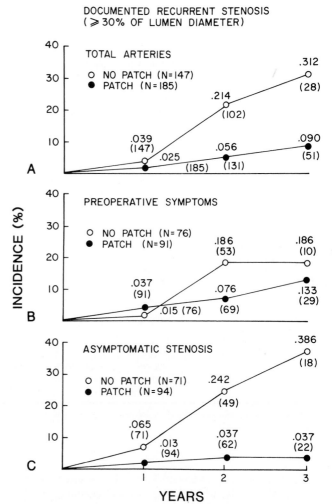

FIGURE 126–9. The cumulative incidence of recurrent carotid defects (≥30 per cent diameter) documented by noninvasive imaging in a prospective study of vein patch angioplasty at the Cleveland Clinic. *A*, All arteries eligible for objective assessment. *B*, Original operations for symptomatic disease. *C*, Original operations for asymptomatic stenosis. (From Hertzer NR, Beven EG, O'Hara PJ, Krajewski LP: A prospective study of vein patch angioplasty during carotid endarterectomy. Three-year results for 801 patients and 917 operations. Ann Surg 206:628, 1987.)

to confirm that it is associated with a reduction in the risks for either early postoperative thrombosis or late recurrent stenosis.[30, 38, 124] Clagett and coworkers[30] conducted a prospectively randomized investigation and concluded that recurrent disease during a 4-year follow-up period actually was more common (13 per cent) when patches were used than was the case following primary closure (1.7 per cent). Nevertheless, it should be noted that just 1 woman was included in this series of 136 patients, and the randomization process was initiated only after the intraoperative exclusion of 30 patients who required "obligatory" vein patching because of the small size of their internal carotid arteries or subadventitial penetration of their atherosclerotic plaques. Rosenthal and colleagues[124] calculated no significant differences in the 5-year cumulative incidence of severe restenosis among patients who received vein patch angioplasty, synthetic patches, or primary closure (3.5 per cent, 10 to 14 per cent, and 9.6 per cent, respectively), but

Table 126–9. Recurrent Stenosis: Selected Comparisons*

Series (Yr)	Length of Follow-Up	Data Analysis	Men		Women		Total	
			No.	Recurrent Stenosis	No.	Recurrent Stenosis	No.	Recurrent Stenosis
NONRANDOMIZED								
Thomas et al[147] (1984)	20 mo (mean)	Crude	161	14 (9%)	96	24 (25%)	257	38 (15%)
Ouriel and Green[104] (1987)	17 mo (mean)	Crude	61	5 (8%)	41	12 (29%)	102	17 (17%)
Sanders et al[129] (1987)	24 mo	Crude	72	3 (4%)	27	4 (15%)	99	7 (7%)
Bernstein et al[18] (1990)	42 mo (mean)	Crude	311	25 (8%)	173	24 (14%)	484	49 (10%)
Atnip et al[7] (1990)	35 mo (mean)	Crude	128	10 (8%)	56	1 (2%)	184	11 (6%)
Total			733	57 (8%)	393	65 (17%)	1126	122 (11%)
RANDOMIZED								
Eikelboom et al[52] (1988)	12 mo Primary closure	Crude	37	4 (11%)	11	6 (55%)	48	15 (31%)
	Patch angioplasty		43	2 (5%)	14	0	57	2 (4%)
Ten Holter et al[146] (1990)	36 mo Primary closure	Cumulative	124	17%	45	27%	169	NA
	Patch angioplasty		118	8%	47	7%	165	NA

*Representative data concerning the incidence of recurrent stenosis following carotid endarterectomy.
Key: NA, data not available.

vein patching was associated with a similar low recurrence rate in this study, which had previously encouraged others to advocate its routine use.

Both Archie[5] and Lord and associates[93] have noted that an element of dilatation predictably occurs in saphenous vein patches. Since this feature could eventually foster the accumulation of laminated thrombus within the carotid bifurcation, it must be anticipated by tailoring the width of the patch to no more than 5 mm at the time it is applied. On balance, although some of the data concerning carotid patching is contradictory, it appears to deserve wider consideration than it has traditionally been accorded.

Cardiac Mortality

Largely because of a concomitant reduction in the incidence of profound perioperative stroke, the early mortality of carotid reconstruction has steadily declined since 1969 when Bauer and colleagues[14] reported an operative risk of 8.4 per cent for the Joint Study of Extracranial Arterial Occlusion. The material summarized in Table 126–2 indicates that fatal complications at present occur in fewer than 2 per cent of patients, and the operative mortality was only 1.2 per cent for 2646 procedures performed at 28 northeastern Ohio hospitals by 36 vascular surgeons participating in a computer registry from 1978 to 1981.[69] Unless the stroke rate is high, most operative deaths are caused by incidental coronary artery disease (CAD). Riles and co-workers[120] found that 5 per cent of all patients suspected of

having CAD sustained perioperative myocardial infarctions despite the use of local or regional anesthesia, and other investigators have shown that surgical mortality may be correlated with predictable cardiac risk factors.[42, 53] In a series of 1546 carotid operations in 1238 patients, Ennix and associates[53] reported that the early mortality rate was 1.5 per cent for patients who had no indications of ischemic heart disease, 3 per cent for those with angina pectoris who also received simultaneous myocardial revascularization, and a surprising 18 per cent for those with angina who underwent carotid endarterectomy alone.

Although operative mortality may be limited by conservative patient selection and appropriate anesthetic precautions, neither of these measures appear to influence the impact of associated CAD on the long-term survival of patients having cerebrovascular disease. Fatal neurologic events are uncommon irrespective of whether medical or surgical treatment is advised, and several clinical studies have demonstrated that cardiac disease is the leading cause of late death after carotid reconstruction, especially in those who already have had completed strokes.[11, 17, 45, 149] Most patients who require carotid endarterectomy eventually die of myocardial infarctions, and the overall 5-year postoperative survival rate has remained constant at approximately 70 per cent for nearly two decades.[42, 68]

Crawford and colleagues[37] first demonstrated that the risk of peripheral vascular and other major procedures performed after previous coronary bypass was no higher than would be expected in patients who had no evidence of CAD. The mortality rate of subsequent operations was only

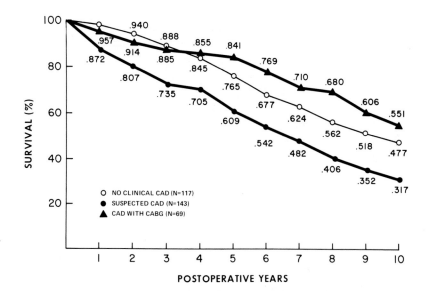

FIGURE 126–10. Cumulative 10-year survival after carotid endarterectomy at the Cleveland Clinic (1969–1973), according to conventional indications for associated coronary artery disease (CAD) and incidental coronary artery bypass grafting (CABG). (From Hertzer NR, Arison R: Cumulative stroke and survival ten years after carotid endarterectomy. J Vasc Surg 2:661, 1985.)

1.1 per cent in this retrospective series of 358 patients, and fewer than 5 per cent experienced fatal myocardial infarctions within the next 5 years. Figure 126–10 illustrates similar data for a total of 329 patients during a minimal follow-up period of 10 years after successful carotid endarterectomy at the Cleveland Clinic.[68] Ten-year survival (55 per cent) in patients who incidentally underwent coronary bypass was equivalent to that (48 per cent) for patients who had no preoperative indications of CAD and was superior to survival (32 per cent) among patients who were suspected of having CAD on clinical grounds ($p = .0001$). The 5-year cumulative cardiac mortality in these three subsets was 7 per cent, 8 per cent, and 20 per cent ($p = .009$), respectively. Furthermore, the 5-year survival rate (84 per cent) for the 69 patients making up the coronary bypass subset in this study was virtually identical to the figure (83 per cent) for 331 others who received combined carotid and coronary operations at this center during the following 8 years.[76]

Management

Obviously, the recognition of serious coronary disease is a prerequisite to its treatment. In an attempt to determine the incidence of severe CAD associated with a foreseeable risk of future myocardial infarction, coronary angiography was obtained in a series of 1000 candidates for elective vascular reconstruction at the Cleveland Clinic.[73] The angiographic results for 295 patients who were investigated primarily because of extracranial disease are presented in Table 126–10. According to a classification defined in earlier reports, 26 per cent of those under consideration for carotid endarterectomy also were found to warrant myocardial revascularization.[73, 78] Severe, correctable CAD was identified in 33 per cent of patients who had clinical indications of coronary involvement, but it also was present in 17 per cent of those who did not. Although no comparable angiographic studies are available, Rokey and associates[122] discovered nonspecific evidence of associated CAD in 29 (58 per cent) of 50 patients with prior TIA or strokes who underwent thallium myocardial imaging and exercise angiocardiography. It is reasonable to conclude from a comparison of these results with those in Table 126–10 that coronary bypass is not necessary for every patient suspected of having CAD on the basis of noninvasive testing. Nevertheless, associated coronary disease is an important influence on the surgical risk and late survival of patients who require carotid endarterectomy, and objective cardiac screening

Table 126–10. Results of Coronary Angiography*

| | Clinical Indications of Coronary Disease | | | | | |
| | None | | Suspected | | Total | |
Angiographic Classification	No.	%	No.	%	No.	%
Normal coronary arteries	19	15	8	5	27	9
Mild to moderate CAD	63	50	31	18	94	32
Advanced but compensated CAD	21	17	59	35	80	27
Severe, correctable CAD	22	17	55	33	77	26
Severe, inoperable CAD	1	1	16	9	17	6

From Hertzer NR, Beven EG, Young JR, et al: Coronary artery disease in peripheral vascular patients. A classification of 1000 coronary angiograms and results of surgical management. Ann Surg 199:223, 1984.

*Results of coronary angiography in a prospective series of 295 patients presenting with extracranial cerebrovascular disease at the Cleveland Clinic.

Key: *CAD, coronary artery disease.*

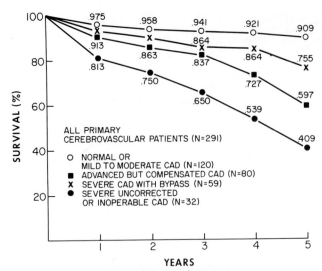

FIGURE 126–11. Cumulative 5-year survival in a prospective series of patients who presented to the Cleveland Clinic with primary extracranial lesions but also underwent survey coronary angiography and selective myocardial revascularization.[73, 79, 80]

should be a consideration at least in those with a positive history or ischemic electrocardiographic changes.

Myocardial revascularization was performed in 62 of the 77 patients with severe, correctable CAD in the Cleveland Clinic study (see Table 126–9). Three (4.8 per cent) had fatal complications after staged vascular procedures, and actuarial survival (including the risk of coronary bypass itself) for the remaining 59 is illustrated in Figure 126–11.

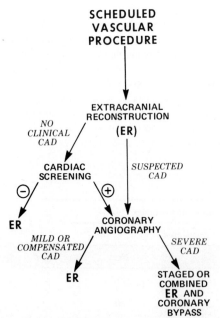

FIGURE 126–12. Algorithm depicting the current approach to associated coronary artery disease (CAD) in patients under consideration for extracranial reconstruction at the Cleveland Clinic. (From Hertzer NR, Young JR, Beven EG, et al: Coronary angiography in 506 patients with extracranial cerebrovascular disease. Arch Intern Med 145:849–852, 1985. Copyright 1985, American Medical Association.)

The 5-year survival rate of 75 per cent in the bypass subset was surpassed only by patients having normal coronary arteries or mild to moderate CAD (91 per cent), and it was superior to the cumulative figure of 41 per cent calculated for 32 others who had severe, uncorrected, or inoperable coronary lesions ($p = .0015$). In addition, the late results for all 1000 patients in this series indicate that 5-year survival after bypass exceeds 80 per cent in selected nondiabetic men presenting with peripheral vascular disease.[79, 80] Because of these data, candidates for carotid endarterectomy at this center currently are evaluated according to the algorithm depicted in Figure 126–12.[78] The staging sequence of carotid and coronary procedures remains controversial.[75] Nevertheless, this approach generally is consistent with the thoughtful recommendations made by Nicolaides and associates[97] and is based on the accepted principle that stroke-free *survival* is the measure by which the benefit of carotid endarterectomy is determined.

References

1. Ahn SS, Marcus DR, Moore WS: Postcarotid endarterectomy hypertension: Association with elevated cranial norepinephine. J Vasc Surg 9:351, 1989.
2. van Alphen HAM, Polman CH: Carotid endarterectomy: How does it work? A clinical and angiographic evaluation. Stroke 17:1251, 1986.
3. Angell-James JE, Lumley JSP: The effects of carotid endarterectomy on the mechanical properties of the carotid sinus and carotid sinus nerve activity in atherosclerotic patients. Br J Surg 61:805, 1974.
4. Archie JP: Prevention of early restenosis and thrombosis-occlusion after carotid endarterectomy by saphenous vein patch angioplasty. Stroke 17:901, 1986.
5. Archie JP Jr: Early and late geometric changes after carotid endarterectomy patch reconstruction. J Vasc Surg 14:258, 1991.
6. Archie JP Jr, Green JJ Jr: Saphenous vein rupture pressure, rupture stress, and carotid endarterectomy vein patch reconstruction. Surgery 107:389, 1990.
7. Atnip RG, Wengrovitz M, Gifford RRM, et al: A rational approach to recurrent carotid stenosis. J Vasc Surg 11:511, 1990.
8. Bageant TE, Tondini D, Lysons D: Bilateral hypoglossal-nerve palsy following a second carotid endarterectomy. Anesthesiology 43:595, 1975.
9. Baker WH, Hayes AC, Mahler D, Littooy FN: Durability of carotid endarterectomy. Surgery 94:112, 1983.
10. Baker WH, Littooy FN, Hayes AC, et al: Carotid endarterectomy without a shunt: The control series. J Vasc Surg 1:50, 1984.
11. Bardin JA, Bernstein EF, Humber PB, et al: Is carotid endarterectomy beneficial in prevention of recurrent stroke? Arch Surg 117:1401, 1982.
12. Barnes RW, Nix ML, Nichols BT, Wingo JP: Recurrent versus residual carotid stenosis. Incidence detected by Doppler ultrasound. Ann Surg 203:652, 1986.
13. Barnett HJM, Plum F, Walton JN: Carotid endarterectomy—An expression of concern. Stroke 15:941, 1984.
14. Bauer RB, Meyer JS, Fields WS, et al: Joint Study of Extracranial Arterial Occlusion. III. Progress report of controlled study of long-term survival in patients with and without operation. JAMA 208:509, 1969.
15. Beebe HG, Clagett GP, DeWeese JA, et al: Assessing risk associated with carotid endarterectomy. Circulation 79:472, 1989.
16. Berguer R, Sieggreen MY, Lazo A, Hodakowski GT: The silent brain infarct in carotid surgery. J Vasc Surg 3:442, 1986.
17. Bernstein EF, Humber PB, Collins GM, et al: Life expectancy and late stroke following carotid endarterectomy. Ann Surg 198:80, 1983.
18. Bernstein EF, Torem S, Dilley RB: Does carotid restenosis predict an increased risk of late symptoms, stroke, or death? Ann Surg 212:629, 1990.
19. Blaisdell FW, Lim R Jr, Hall AD: Technical result of carotid endarterectomy. Arteriographic assessment. Am J Surg 114:239, 1967.

20. Bove EL, Fry WJ, Gross WS, Stanley JC: Hypotension and hypertension as consequences of baroreceptor dysfunction following carotid endarterectomy. Surgery 85:633, 1979.

21. Brott T, Thalinger K: The practice of carotid endarterectomy in a large metropolitan area. Stroke 15:950, 1984.

22. Cafferata HT, Gainey MD: Carotid endarterectomy in the community hospital. A continuing controversy. J Cardiovasc Surg 27:557, 1986.

23. Cafferata HT, Merchant RF, DePalma RG: Avoidance of postcarotid endarterectomy hypertension. Ann Surg 196:465, 1982.

24. Cantelmo NL, Cutler BS, Wheeler HB, et al: Noninvasive detection of carotid stenosis following endarterectomy. Arch Surg 116:1005, 1981.

25. Caplan LR, Skillman J, Ojemann R, Fields WS: Intracerebral hemorrhage following carotid endarterectomy: A hypertensive complication? Stroke 9:457, 1978.

26. Carmichael JD: Carotid surgery in the community hospital—467 consecutive operations. Arch Surg 115:937, 1980.

27. Chambers BR, Norris JW: The case against surgery for asymptomatic carotid stenosis. Stroke 15:964, 1984.

28. Chambers BR, Norris JW: Outcome in patients with asymptomatic neck bruits. N Engl J Med 315:860, 1986.

29. Civil ID, O'Hara PJ, Hertzer NR, et al: Late patency of the carotid artery after endarterectomy. Problems of definition, follow-up methodology and data analysis. J Vasc Surg 8:79, 1988.

30. Clagett GP, Patterson CB, Fisher DF Jr, et al: Vein patch versus primary closure for carotid endarterectomy. A randomized prospective study in a selected group of patients. J Vasc Surg 9:213, 1989.

31. Clagett GP, Rich NM, McDonald PT, et al: Etiologic factors for recurrent carotid artery stenosis. Surgery 93:313, 1982.

32. Colgan MP, Kingston V, Shanik G: Stenosis following carotid endarterectomy. Arch Surg 119:1033, 1984.

33. Cook JM, Thompson BW, Barnes RW: Is routine duplex examination after carotid endarterectomy justified? J Vasc Surg 12:334, 1990.

34. Cossman D, Callow AD, Stein A, Matsumoto G: Early restenosis after carotid endarterectomy. Arch Surg 113:275, 1978.

35. Courbier MD, Jausseran JM, Reggi M, et al: Routine intraoperative carotid angiography: Its impact on operative morbidity and carotid restenosis. J Vasc Surg 3:343, 1986.

36. Cranley JJ: Presidential address: Stroke—A perspective. Surgery 91:537, 1982.

37. Crawford ES, Morris GC Jr, Howell JF, et al: Operative risk in patients with previous coronary artery bypass. Ann Thorac Surg 26:215, 1978.

38. Curley S, Edwards WS, Jacob TP: Recurrent carotid stenosis after autologous tissue patching. J Vasc Surg 6:350, 1987.

39. Cutler SJ, Ederer F: Maximum utilization of the life table method in analyzing survival. J Chronic Dis 8:699, 1958.

40. Das MB, Hertzer NR, Ratliff NB, et al: Recurrent carotid stenosis. A five-year series of 65 reoperations. Ann Surg 202:28, 1985.

41. Davies MJ, Cronin KD: Post-carotid endarterectomy hypertension. Anaesth Intens Care 8:190, 1980.

42. DeBakey ME, Crawford ES, Cooley DA, et al: Cerebral arterial insufficiency: One- to 11-year results following arterial reconstructive operation. Ann Surg 161:921, 1965.

43. DePalma RG, Chidi CC, Sternfeld WC, Koletsky S: Pathogenesis and prevention of trauma-provoked atheromas. Surgery 82:429, 1977.

44. Deriu GP, Ballotta E, Bonavina L, et al: The rationale for patch-graft angioplasty after carotid endarterectomy: Early and long-term follow-up. Stroke 15:972, 1984.

45. DeWeese JA, Rob CG, Satran R, et al: Results of carotid endarterectomies for transient ischemic attacks—Five years later. Ann Surg 178:258, 1973.

46. Dilley RB, Bernstein EF: A comparison of B-mode real-time imaging and arteriography in the intraoperative assessment of carotid endarterectomy. J Vasc Surg 4:457, 1986.

47. Easton JD, Sherman DG: Stroke and mortality rate in carotid endarterectomy: 228 consecutive operations. Stroke 8:565, 1977.

48. Edwards WH, Edwards WH Jr, Jenkins JM, Mulherin JL Jr: Analysis of a decade of carotid reconstructive operations. J Cardiovasc Surg 1989.

49. Edwards WH, Edwards WH Jr, Mulherin JL Jr, Jenkins JM: The role of antiplatelet drugs in carotid reconstructive surgery. Ann Surg 201:765, 1984.

50. Edwards WH Jr, Edwards WH Sr, Mulherin JL Jr, Martin RS III: Recurrent carotid artery stenosis. Resection with autogenous vein replacement. Ann Surg 209:662, 1989.

51. Eggers F, Lukin R, Chambers AA, et al: Iatrogenic carotid cavernous fistula following Fogarty catheter thromboendarterectomy. J Neurosurg 51:543, 1979.

52. Eikelboom BC, Ackerstaff RGA, Hoeneveld H, et al: Benefits of carotid patching: A randomized study. J Vasc Surg 7:240, 1988.

53. Ennix CL Jr, Lawrie GM, Morris GC Jr, et al: Improved results of carotid endarterectomy in patients with symptomatic coronary disease: An analysis of 1,546 consecutive carotid operations. Stroke 10:122, 1979.

54. European Carotid Surgery Trialists' Collaborative Group: MRC European Carotid Surgery Trial: Interim results for symptomatic patients with severe (70–99%) or with mild (0–29%) carotid stenosis. Lancet 337:1235, 1991.

55. Evans WE, Mendelowitz DS, Liapis CW, Florence CL: Motor speech deficit following carotid endarterectomy. Ann Surg 196:461, 1982.

56. Fields WS, Maslenikov V, Meyer JS, et al: Joint Study of Extracranial Arterial Occlusion. V. Progress report of prognosis following surgery or nonsurgical treatment of transient cerebral ischemic attacks and cervical carotid artery lesions. JAMA 211:1993, 1970.

57. Flanigan DP, Douglas DJ, Machi J, et al: Intraoperative ultrasonic imaging of the carotid artery during carotid endarterectomy. Surgery 100:893, 1986.

58. Fode NC, Sundt TM Jr, Robertson JT, et al: Multicenter retrospective review of results and complications of carotid endarterectomy in 1981. Stroke 17:370, 1986.

59. French BN, Rewcastle NB: Sequential morphological changes at the site of carotid endarterectomy. J Neurosurg 41:745, 1974.

60. Graber JN, Vollman RW, Johnson WC, et al: Stroke after carotid endarterectomy: Risk as predicted by preoperative computerized tomography. Am J Surg 147:492, 1984.

61. Graham AM, Gewertz BL, Zarins CK: Predicting cerebral ischemia during carotid endarterectomy. Arch Surg 121:595, 1986.

62. Green RM, Messick WJ, Ricotta JJ, et al: Benefits, shortcomings, and costs of EEG monitoring. Ann Surg 201:785, 1985.

63. Gundlach WJ, Swenson WM: Carotid endarterectomy in a community hospital. Surg Gynecol Obstet 148:720, 1979.

64. Hafner DH, Smith RB, King OW, et al: Massive intracerebral hemorrhage following carotid endarterectomy. Arch Surg 122:305, 1987.

65. Haynes DC, Dempsey RL: Carotid endarterectomy. Review of 276 cases in a community hospital. Ann Surg 189:758, 1979.

66. Hertzer NR: Early complications of carotid endarterectomy. *In* Moore WS (ed): Cerebrovascular Disease. New York, Churchill-Livingstone, 1987.

67. Hertzer NR: Non-stroke complications of carotid endarterectomy. *In* Bernhard VM, Towne J (eds): Complications in Vascular Surgery. 2nd ed. Orlando, FL, Grune & Stratton, 1985.

68. Hertzer NR, Arison R: Cumulative stroke and survival ten years after carotid endarterectomy. J Vasc Surg 2:661, 1985.

69. Hertzer NR, Avellone JC, Farrell CJ, et al: The risk of vascular surgery in a metropolitan community. J Vasc Surg 1:13, 1984.

70. Hertzer NR, Beven EG, Greenstreet RL, Humphries AW: Internal carotid back pressure, intraoperative shunting, ulcerated atheromata, and the incidence of stroke during carotid endarterectomy. Surgery 83:306, 1978.

71. Hertzer NR, Beven EG, Modic MT, et al: Early patency of the carotid artery after endarterectomy: Digital subtraction angiography after two hundred sixty-two operations. Surgery 92:1049, 1982.

72. Hertzer NR, Beven EG, O'Hara PJ, Krajewski LP: A prospective study of vein patch angioplasty during carotid endarterectomy. Three-year results for 801 patients and 917 operations. Ann Surg 206:628, 1987.

73. Hertzer NR, Beven EG, Young JR, et al: Coronary artery disease in peripheral vascular patients. A classification of 1000 coronary angiograms and results of surgical management. Ann Surg 199:223, 1984.

74. Hertzer NR, Feldman BJ, Beven EG, Tucker HM: A prospective study of the incidence of injury to the cranial nerves during carotid endarterectomy. Surg Gynecol Obstet 151:781, 1980.

75. Hertzer NR, Loop FD, Beven EG, et al: Surgical staging for simultaneous coronary and carotid disease: A study including prospective randomization. J Vasc Surg 9:455, 1989.

76. Hertzer NR, Loop FD, Taylor PC, Beven EG: Combined myocardial revascularization and carotid endarterectomy: Operative and late results in 331 patients. J Thorac Cardiovasc Surg 85:577, 1983.

77. Hertzer NR, Martinez BD, Benjamin SP, Beven EG: Recurrent stenosis after carotid endarterectomy. Surg Gynecol Obstet 149:360, 1979.

78. Hertzer NR, Young JR, Beven EG, et al: Coronary angiography in 506 patients with extracranial cerebrovascular disease. Arch Intern Med 145:849, 1985.

79. Hertzer NR, Young JR, Beven EG, et al: Late results of coronary bypass in patients with peripheral vascular disease. I. Five-year survival according to age and clinical cardiac status. Cleve Clin Q 53:133, 1986.

80. Hertzer NR, Young JR, Beven EG, et al: Late results of coronary bypass in patients with peripheral vascular disease. II. Five-year survival according to sex, hypertension, and diabetes. Cleve Clin J Med 54:15, 1987.

81. Imparato AM, Bracco A, Kim GE, Bergmann L: The hypoglossal nerve in carotid arterial reconstructions. Stroke 3:576, 1972.

82. Imparato AM, Ramirez A, Riles T, Mintzer R: Cerebral protection in carotid surgery. Arch Surg 117:1073, 1982.

83. Jernigan WR, Fulton RL, Hamman JL, et al: The efficacy of routine completion operative angiography in reducing the incidence of perioperative stroke associated with carotid endarterectomy. Surgery 96:831, 1984.

84. Jonas S: IMPS (intact months of patient survival): An analysis of the results of carotid endarterectomy. Stroke 17:1329, 1986.

85. Kakkasseril JS, Tomsick TA, Arbaugh JA, Cranley JJ: Carotid cavernous fistula following Fogarty catheter thrombectomy. Arch Surg 119:1095, 1984.

86. Katz MM, Jones GT, Degenhardt J, et al: The use of patch angioplasty to alter the incidence of carotid restenosis following thromboendarterectomy. J Cardiovasc Surg 28:2, 1987.

87. Kempczinski RF, Brott TG, Labutta RJ: The influence of surgical specialty and caseload on the results of carotid endarterectomy. J Vasc Surg 3:911, 1986.

88. Kirshner DL, O'Brien MS, Ricotta JJ: Risk factors in a community experience with carotid endarterectomy. J Vasc Surg 10:178, 1989.

89. Kremen JE, Gee W, Kaupp HA, McDonald KM: Restenosis or occlusion after carotid endarterectomy. A survey with ocular pneumoplethysmography. Arch Surg 114:608, 1979.

90. Krupski WC, Effeney DJ, Goldstone J, et al: Carotid endarterectomy in a metropolitan community: Comparison of results from three institutions. Surgery 98:492, 1985.

91. Lee ET, Desu MM: A computer program for comparing K samples with right-censored data. Comput Programs Biomed 2:315, 1972.

92. Liapis CD, Satiani B, Florance CL, Evans WE: Motor speech malfunction following carotid endarterectomy. Surgery 89:56, 1981.

93. Lord RSA, Raj B, Stary DL, et al: Comparison of saphenous vein patch, polytetrafluoroethylene patch, and direct arteriotomy closure after carotid endarterectomy. I. Perioperative results. J Vasc Surg 9:521 1989.

94. Matsumoto GH, Cossman D, Callow AD: Hazards and safeguards during carotid endarterectomy. Technical considerations. Am J Surg 133:458, 1977.

95. Moore DJ, Modi JR, Finch WT, Sumner DS: Influence of the contralateral carotid artery on neurologic complications following carotid endarterectomy. J Vasc Surg 1:409, 1984.

96. Moore WS, Martello JY, Quinones-Baldrich WJ, Ahn SS: Etiologic importance of the intimal flap of the external carotid artery in the development of postcarotid endarterectomy stroke. Stroke 21:1497, 1990.

97. Nicolaides AN, Salmasi AM, Sonecha TN: How should we investigate the arteriopath for coexisting lesions. J Cardiovasc Surg 27:515, 1986.

98. North American Symptomatic Carotid Endarterectomy Trial Collaborators: Beneficial effect of carotid endarterectomy in symptomatic patients with high-grade carotid stenosis. N Engl J Med 325:445, 1991.

99. Nunn DB: Carotid endarterectomy: An analysis of 234 operative cases. Ann Surg 182:733, 1975.

100. O'Donnell TF Jr, Callow AD, Scott G, et al: Ultrasound characteristics of recurrent carotid disease: Hypothesis explaining the low incidence of symptomatic recurrence. J Vasc Surg 2:26, 1985.

101. O'Hara PJ, Hertzer NR, Krajewski LP, Beven EG: Saphenous vein patch rupture after carotid endarterectomy. J Vasc Surg 15:504, 1992.

102. Ortega G, Gee W, Kaupp HA, McDonald KM: Postendarterectomy carotid occlusion. Surgery 90:1093, 1981.

103. Ott DA, Cooley DA, Chapa L, Coelho A: Carotid endarterectomy without temporary intraluminal shunt. Study of 309 consecutive operations. Ann Surg 191:708, 1980.

104. Ouriel K, Green RM: Clinical and technical factors influencing recurrent carotid stenosis and occlusion after endarterectomy. J Vasc Surg 5:702, 1987.

105. Ouriel K, May AG, Ricotta JJ, et al: Carotid endarterectomy for nonhemispheric symptoms: Predictors of success. J Vasc Surg 1:339, 1984.

106. Owens ML, Atkinson JB, Wilson SE: Recurrent transient ischemic attacks after carotid endarterectomy. Arch Surg 115:482, 1980.

107. Owens ML, Wilson SE: Prevention of neurologic complications of carotid endarterectomy. Arch Surg 117:551, 1982.

108. Painter TA, Hertzer NR, O'Hara PJ, et al: Symptomatic internal carotid thrombosis after carotid endarterectomy. J Vasc Surg 5:445, 1987.

109. Peitzman AB, Webster M, Loubeau JM, et al: Carotid endarterectomy under regional (conductive) anesthesia. Ann Surg 196:59, 1982.

110. Perdue GD: Management of postendarterectomy neurologic deficits. Arch Surg 117:1079, 1982.

111. Piepgras DG, Sundt TM Jr, Marsh WR, et al: Recurrent carotid stenosis. Results and complications of 57 operations. Ann Surg 203:205, 1986.

112. Piotrowski JJ, Bernhard VM, Rubin JR, et al: Timing of carotid endarterectomy after acute stroke. J Vasc Surg 11:45, 1990.

113. Pomposelli FB, Lamparello PJ, Riles TS, et al: Intracranial hemorrhage after carotid endarterectomy. J Vasc Surg 7:8, 1988.

114. Prioleau WH Jr, Aiken AF, Hairston P: Carotid endarterectomy: Neurologic complications as related to surgical techniques. Ann Surg 185:678, 1977.

115. Ranson JHC, Imparato AM, Clauss RH, et al: Factors in the mortality and morbidity associated with surgical treatment of cerebrovascular insufficiency. Circulation 39(Suppl 1):I-269, 1969.

116. Rapp JH, Qvarfordt P, Krupski WC, et al: Hypercholesterolemia and early restenosis after carotid endarterectomy. Surgery 101:277, 1987.

117. Reigel MM, Hollier LH, Sundt TM Jr, et al: Cerebral hyperperfusion syndrome: A cause of neurologic dysfunction after carotid endarterectomy. J Vasc Surg 5:628, 1987.

118. Reilly LM, Okuhn SP, Rapp JH, et al: Recurrent carotid stenosis: A consequence of local or systemic factors? The influence of unrepaired technical defects. J Vasc Surg 11:448, 1990.

119. Richardson JD, Main KA: Carotid endarterectomy in the elderly population: A statewide experience. J Vasc Surg 9:65, 1989.

120. Riles TS, Kopelman I, Imparato AM: Myocardial infarction following carotid endarterectomy: A review of 683 operations. Surgery 85:249, 1979.

121. Riles TS, Lamparello PJ, Giangola G, Imparato AM: Rupture of the vein patch: A rare complication of carotid endarterectomy. Surgery 107:10, 1990.

122. Rokey R, Rolak LA, Harati H, et al: Coronary artery disease in patients with cerebrovascular disease: A prospective study. Ann Neurol 16:50, 1984.

123. Rosenbloom M, Friedman SG, Lamparello PJ, et al: Glossopharyngeal nerve injury complicating carotid endarterectomy. J Vasc Surg 5:468, 1987.

124. Rosenthal D, Archie JP Jr, Garcia-Rinaldi R, et al: Carotid patch angioplasty: Immediate and long-term results. J Vasc Surg 12:326, 1990.

125. Rosenthal D, Zeichner WD, Lamis PA, Stanton PE Jr: Neurologic deficit after carotid endarterectomy: Pathogenesis and management. Surgery 94:776, 1983.

126. Rubin JR Jr, Pitluk HC, King TA, et al: Carotid endarterectomy in a metropolitan community: The early results after 8635 operations. J Vasc Surg 7:256, 1988.

127. Rutkow IM, Ernst CB: An analysis of vascular surgical manpower

requirements and vascular surgical rates in the United States. J Vasc Surg 3:75, 1986.

128. Sachs SM, Fulenwider JT, Smith RB, et al: Does contralateral carotid occlusion influence neurologic fate of carotid endarterectomy? Surgery 96:839, 1984.

129. Sanders EACM, Hoeneveld H, Eikelboom BC, et al: Residual lesions and early recurrent stenosis after carotid endarterectomy. J Vasc Surg 5:731, 1987.

130. Sandmann W, Hennerici M, Aulich A, et al: Progress in carotid artery surgery at the base of the skull. J Vasc Surg 1:734, 1984.

131. Sanella NA, Tober RL, Cipro RP, et al: Vocal cord paralysis following carotid endarterectomy: The paradox of return of function. Ann Vasc Surg 4:42, 1990.

132. Satiani B, Liapis C, Pflug B, et al: Role of staging in bilateral carotid endarterectomy. Surgery 84:784, 1978.

133. Satiani B, Vasko JS, Evans WE: Hypertension following carotid endarterectomy. Surg Neurol 11:357, 1979.

134. Schroeder T, Sillesen H, Engell HC: Staged bilateral carotid endarterectomy. J Vasc Surg 3:355, 1986.

135. Seifert KB, Blackshear WM Jr: Continuous-wave Doppler in the intraoperative assessment of carotid endarterectomy. J Vasc Surg 2:817, 1985.

136. Slavish LG, Nicholas GG, Gee W: Review of a community hospital experience with carotid endarterectomy. Stroke 15:956, 1984.

137. Smith BL: Hypertension following carotid endarterectomy. The role of cerebral renin production. J Vasc Surg 1:623, 1984.

138. Steed DL, Peitzman AB, Grundy BL, Webster MW: Causes of stroke in carotid endarterectomy. Surgery 92:634, 1982.

139. Stewart GW, Bandyk DF, Kaebnick HW, et al: Influence of vein-patch angioplasty on carotid endarterectomy healing. Arch Surg 122:364, 1987.

140. Stoney RJ, String SJ: Recurrent carotid stenosis. Surgery 80:705, 1976.

141. Sundt TM, Houser OW, Whisnant JP, Fode NC: Correlation of postoperative and two-year follow-up angiography with neurologic function in 99 carotid endarterectomies in 86 consecutive patients. Ann Surg 203:90, 1986.

142. Sundt TM Jr, Sharbrough FW, Marsh WR, et al: The risk-benefit ratio of intraoperative shunting during carotid endarterectomy. Relevancy to operative and postoperative results and complications. Ann Surg 203:196, 1986.

143. Sundt TM Jr, Sharbourgh FW, Piepgras DG, et al: Correlation of cerebral blood flow and electroencephalographic changes during carotid endarterectomy with results of surgery and hemodynamics of cerebral ischemia. Mayo Clin Proc 56:533, 1981.

144. Tarlov E, Schmidek H, Scott RM, et al: Reflex hypotension following carotid endarterectomy: Mechanism and management. J Neurosurg 39:323, 1973.

145. Taylor LM, Porter JM: Basic data related to carotid endarterectomy. Ann Vasc Surg 1:262, 1986.

146. Ten Holter JBM, Ackerstaff RGA, Schwartzenberg GWST, et al: The impact of vein patch angioplasty on long-term surgical outcome after carotid endarterectomy. J Cardiovasc Surg 31:58, 1990.

147. Thomas M, Otis SM, Rush M, et al: Recurrent carotid artery stenosis following endarterectomy. Ann Surg 200:74, 1984.

148. Thompson JE: Complications of carotid endarterectomy and their prevention. World J Surg 3:155, 1979.

149. Thompson JE, Austin DJ, Patman RD: Carotid endarterectomy for cerebrovascular insufficiency: Long-term results in 592 patients followed up to thirteen years. Ann Surg 172:663, 1970.

150. Toole JF, Yuson CP, Janeway R, et al: Transient ischemic attacks: A prospective study of 225 patients. Neurology 28:746, 1978.

151. Toronto Cerebrovascular Study Group: Risks of carotid endarterectomy. Stroke 17:848, 1986.

152. Towne JB, Bernhard VM: The relationship of postoperative hypertension to complications following carotid endarterectomy. Surgery 88:375, 1980.

153. Towne JB, Bernhard VM: Neurologic deficit following carotid endarterectomy. Surg Gynecol Obstet 154:849, 1982.

154. Towne JB, Weiss DG, Hobson RW II: First phase report of cooperative Veterans Administration asymptomatic carotid stenosis study—Operative morbidity and mortality. J Vasc Surg 11:252, 1990.

155. Treiman RL, Cossman DV, Foran RF, et al: The influence of neutralizing heparin after carotid endarterectomy on postoperative stroke and wound hematoma. J Vasc Surg 12:440, 1990.

156. Tucker JA, Gee W, Nicholas GG, et al: Accessory nerve injury during carotid endarterectomy. J Vasc Surg 5:440, 1987.

157. Turnipseed WD, Berkoff HA, Crummy A: Postoperative occlusion after carotid endarterectomy. Arch Surg 115:573, 1980.

158. Verta MJ Jr, Applebaum EL, McClusky DA, et al: Cranial nerve injury during carotid endarterectomy. Ann Surg 185:192, 1977.

159. Wade JG, Larson CP Jr, Hickey RF, et al: Effect of carotid endarterectomy on carotid chemoreceptor and baroreceptor function in man. Ann Surg 185:192, 1977.

160. Warlow C: Carotid endarterectomy: Does it work? Stroke 15:1068, 1984.

161. White JS, Sirinek KR, Root HD, Rogers W: Morbidity and mortality of carotid endarterectomy. Arch Surg 116:409, 1981.

162. Whitney DG, Kahn EM, Estes JW, Jones CE: Carotid artery surgery without a temporary indwelling shunt. Arch Surg 115:1393, 1980.

163. Whittemore AD, Kauffman JL, Kohler TR, Mannick JA: Routine electroencephalographic (EEG) monitoring during carotid endarterectomy. Ann Surg 197:707, 1983.

164. Wilkinson JT, Adams HP Jr, Wright CB: Convulsions after carotid endarterectomy. JAMA 244:1827, 1980.

165. Youkey JR, Clagett GP, Jaffin JH, et al: Focal motor seizures complicating carotid endarterectomy. Arch Surg 119:1080, 1984.

166. Zbornikova V, Elfstrom J, Lassvik C, et al: Restenosis and occlusion after carotid surgery assessed by duplex scanning and digital subtraction angiography. Stroke 17:1137, 1986.

167. Zierler RE, Bandyk DF, Thiele BL: Intraoperative assessment of carotid endarterectomy. J Vasc Surg 1:73, 1984.

168. Zierler RE, Bandyk DF, Thiele BL, Strandness E Jr: Carotid artery stenosis following endarterectomy. Arch Surg 117:1408, 1982.

169. Zukowski AJ, Nicolaides AN, Lewis RT, et al: The correlation between carotid plaque ulceration and cerebral infarction seen on CT scan. J Vasc Surg 1:782, 1984.

127

Results of Medical and Surgical Therapy for Extracranial Arterial Occlusive Disease

William J. Quiñones-Baldrich, M.D., and Wesley S. Moore, M.D.

• • •

Therapy for extracranial arterial occlusive disease is aimed primarily at the prevention of stroke. In this effort, control of important risk factors such as hypertension, diabetes, and cigarette smoking is paramount, regardless of whether surgical intervention is involved. It is evident that operations aimed at reducing stroke risk will be most effective when accompanied by risk factor control. Thus, medical and surgical therapy cannot be completely separated.

In this chapter, the authors attempt to summarize the available information on the results of operative and nonoperative therapy for extracranial arterial occlusive disease. Important new information is available from prospective randomized clinical studies that have attempted to determine the role of operative and nonoperative treatments in the management of these patients. Combined with available retrospective data, clinicians can now recommend specific therapy that has been shown to be effective in particular clinical presentations. Thus, the often difficult decision of whether to recommend an operation in the overall plan to reduce stroke risk in a particular patient has been in many instances simplified.

SURGICAL THERAPY

Surgical therapy for extracranial arterial occlusive disease may be divided into three distinct categories, depending on the location and the reconstruction required to remove or bypass an offending lesion. Lesions in the carotid bifurcation amenable to endarterectomy are the most common and by far represent the largest experience. Vertebral artery and aortic arch lesions often require more extensive reconstruction. In this chapter, discussion of surgical results is limited to endarterectomy and reconstructions of the carotid bifurcation.

Carotid Endarterectomy— Retrospective Studies

The immediate and long-term results of carotid endarterectomy are summarized in Table 127–1 according to the indication for operation. It is evident that both early and long-term results vary with the indication for the procedure and are related to the extent of neurologic dysfunction prior to operation.

The mortality rate for operation during the acute phase of cerebral infarction, as reported in the Joint Study of Extracranial Arterial Disease, was 42 per cent.[5] This rate is unacceptably high, confirming the view that operations for acute stroke are generally contraindicated. In that same series, however, the mortality rate for patients without neurologic deficit prior to operation was 2 per cent. Patients with cerebral infarction whose recovery time exceeded 2 weeks prior to operation had a mortality rate of 5 per cent. These data were pooled from several contributing institutions and covered a period from 1961 to 1968, an era relatively early in the development of surgical technique; some current series are reporting considerably lower mortality rates. DeWeese and coworkers described a postoperative mortality rate of less than 1 per cent in a series of 103 patients.[17] Thompson and associates reported a mortality rate of 1.4 per cent in patients whose indication for operation was transient ischemic attacks (TIAs).[58] The authors have reviewed data from their own series of 379 operations for all indications. There were 4 deaths in patients operated on for completed stroke, for a 1 per cent overall mortality rate. Two asymptomatic and 3 symptomatic patients suffered perioperative strokes, for an overall incidence of 1.3 per cent.[15]

Asymptomatic patients with significant lesions at the carotid bifurcation have the lowest perioperative morbidity and mortality, averaging a combined risk of 1 to 3 per cent. On the other hand, patients whose indication for operation is a previous completed stroke have the highest perioperative risk, with a combined perioperative morbidity and mortality rate averaging to 5 to 9 per cent. Patients with TIAs fall into an intermediate category, with an average perioperative morbidity and mortality ranging between 3 and 6 per cent. Therefore, intervention in the asymptomatic stage may be preferable, provided that a "high-risk" lesion is identified. To delay intervention for such lesions not only risks stroke as the first symptom but also increases the risk of surgical intervention if such were performed once the patient becomes symptomatic.

Controversies surrounding carotid endarterectomy

Table 127–1. Results of Carotid Endarterectomy According to Indication for Operation

Indication	Author	No. of Patients	Follow-up	Operative Morbidity (%)	Operative Mortality (%)	Recurrent TIAs (Ipsilateral) (%)	Stroke Ipsilateral (G) (%)	Stroke Contralateral (%)
Asymptomatic	Thompson	132	55.1 mo	1.2	0	0.75	4.7(A)	NS
	Sergeant	43	64.8 mo	2.3	2.3	0	0	0
	Moore	72	6–180 mo	0	0	2.7	5.6(B)	2.7
	Bernstein	87(C)	43 mo	NS(D)	0	NS	6.3(E)	NS
	Hertzer	126	10–14 yr	NS	NS	NS	9.0*	7.0
TIA	Lord	266	30–144 mo	2.6	1.1	NS	0.4	1.1
	Bernstein	370(H)	12–132 mo	NS	0	19.5(I)	5.2	NS
	DeWeese	103	60 mo minimum	6.0	0.97	18.4(F)	7.7	10.6
	Thompson	293	To 156 mo	2.7	1.4	16.3	4.7	0.6
	Takolander	142	5 yr actuarial	4.9	1.8	14.7	6.5	4.0
	Hertzer	123	10–14 yr	NS	NS	NS	6.0*	9.0*
Stroke	Thompson	217	Up to 156 mo	5.0	7.4(J)		8.2	NS
	Eriksson	55	21 mo avg	3.7	3.7		3.8	NS
	Bardin	127	56 mo avg	3.9	3.1		20.0	NS
	Takolander	60	5 yr actuarial	4.9	5.9	11.6(E)	10.0	NS
	McCullough	59	41 mo avg	3.4	1.7		3.3	NS
	Hertzer	80	10–14 yr	NS	NS	NS	6.0*	13.0
	Rubin	95	6–72 mo	1.8	1.8	NS	0	2.2

Key: *NS Not specified.*
*   Does not include perioperative strokes.*
A   Side of stroke not specified; three strokes were fatal.
B   Two patients suffered transient postoperative deficits with complete recovery.
C   Number of procedures; exact number of patients not specified.
D   Perioperative stroke rate of 3% in the entire series of 370 patients.
E   Side of neurologic event not specified; risk of stroke at 5 years by life table analysis.

F   Includes patients with nonterritorial symptoms.
G   Includes operative morbidity.
H   Total number of patients in series, including TIA patients.
I   Territory affected not specified.
J   Includes operations for acute strokes.

have centered around reports in which surgical morbidity and mortality have been as high as 21 per cent.[20] This unacceptable rate is frequently quoted by opponents to surgical therapy. Clearly, when one of every five patients undergoing endarterectomy is predicted to have an undesirable result, surgical intervention should not be recommended. However, the facts are that acceptable morbidity and mortality rates are frequently achieved by institutions with a large experience and individual surgeons in the community with a specialty interest in cerebrovascular disease. This underscores the importance of internal review to establish the actual and thus predicted morbidity and mortality rates of carotid endarterectomy when performed by the individual surgeon prior to recommending the procedure. Two reports from the same community have documented the importance of this type of review. Whereas a 24.7 per cent combined morbidity and mortality rate for carotid endarterectomy was reported in 1977, a more recent review noted a combined risk of 5 per cent.[41]

The importance of a low perioperative morbidity and mortality cannot be overemphasized. This factor alone can negate the long-term benefits of the procedure. The lower the morbidity and mortality rates of the procedure for a given indication, the sooner the beneficial effects of the operation are realized in the population under study.[13]

Long-term results of carotid endarterectomy with follow-up longer than 10 years are available. With few exceptions, little variability is seen among reports that take into account the indication for operation and side of symptoms on follow-up. This suggests that the information is reliable in estimating the natural history of patients following endarterectomy.

Thompson and colleagues reviewed their series of 592 patients who had cerebrovascular insufficiency treated with carotid endarterectomy and were followed for up to 13 years.[57] Their operative mortality rate for the last 476 consecutive operations was 1.47 per cent, and the permanent neurologic morbidity rate was 2.7 per cent. The overall late mortality rate on follow-up was 30 per cent, half of the deaths being due to cardiac events and only 3.9 per cent secondary to stroke. Of those patients who had a preoperative stroke as an indication for surgery, 88.9 per cent were normal or improved at follow-up. Of those patients who had TIAs preoperatively, 81 per cent had no further attacks and only 7 patients (3.3 per cent) experienced permanent deficits. Two of these 7 suffered stroke in the side that had not been operated on.

In a separate report, Thompson and his associates reviewed their experience with 132 patients undergoing 167 carotid endarterectomies for asymptomatic lesions in the carotid arteries.[58] There were no operative deaths, and permanent neurologic deficits occurred in 2 patients (1.2 per cent). Long-term follow-up (mean duration, 55.1 months) showed that 90.9 per cent of the patients remained asymptomatic. Six patients (4.5 per cent) had TIAs, 5 from the untreated side. Strokes occurred in 4.6 per cent. In comparison, in a parallel, nonrandomized series of 138 patients who had asymptomatic lesions and were not operated on for various reasons, long-term follow-up revealed that 55.8 per cent remained asymptomatic, 26.8 per cent developed transient ischemia, and 17.4 per cent suffered strokes. This was a retrospective nonrandomized analysis, and although the difference is striking, no firm conclusions should be drawn.

Sergeant and coworkers followed 141 patients after endarterectomy for up to 16 years.[52] In the asymptomatic group (43 patients), with an average follow-up of 5.4 years, there were no deaths and one stroke referable to the contralateral carotid artery. Those with a contralateral carotid occlusion who were symptomatic preoperatively (25 patients) were followed for an average of 7.3 years after endarterectomy on the nonoccluded side. Two strokes occurred in this group. There were 70 patients with symptomatic stenosis who had operations on the symptomatic side. After 7.2 years, 6 had neurologic deficits, 5 of them referable to the side of operation, a stroke rate of 7.1 per cent.

Bernstein and colleagues reported a series of 456 carotid endarterectomies followed from 1 to 11 years with an average follow-up period of 45.3 months.[6] The incidences of TIAs and strokes were different, depending on the preoperative indications for the operation. Asymptomatic patients with carotid bruits had a 1.6 per cent incidence of transient ischemia and a 3.2 per cent incidence of stroke on late follow-up. Those patients operated on because of transient ischemia had a 19.5 per cent and a 5.2 per cent incidence of new attacks or strokes, respectively. Those with prior stroke had an incidence of ischemic attacks of 7.9 per cent, and 11.0 per cent developed stroke. This trend is also evident in other series, as shown in Table 127–1.

Field reported his experience with 400 carotid endarterectomies after which the patients were followed for 2 years.[23] Late stroke occurred in less than 1 per cent, and stroke frequency was less than 2 per cent per year.

Riles and colleagues compared 146 patients who underwent unilateral carotid endarterectomy (the contralateral carotid artery was patent and nonstenotic) with 86 patients who, during the same interval, underwent bilateral carotid endarterectomy.[50] Both groups were followed during a 5-year period (mean follow-up, 4.3 years). There was no significant difference between the groups with respect to age, sex, neurologic status, or associated diseases, and all received maintenance antiplatelet therapy postoperatively. During follow-up, 17 new strokes occurred in the first group, of which only 6 involved the hemisphere ipsilateral to the endarterectomy. In the second group, there were 4 strokes. The cumulative stroke rates at 5 years by the life table method were 17.6 per cent and 5.6 per cent, respectively. This difference achieved statistical significance ($p < .05$).

Hertzer and Arison analyzed their experience with 329 patients followed a minimum of 10 years following carotid endarterectomy.[34] One hundred twenty-six patients operated on for asymptomatic lesions had a stroke incidence of 9 per cent in the ipsilateral hemisphere (average, less than 1 per cent per year). Two hundred three patients operated on because of completed stroke or TIAs had a late ipsilateral stroke incidence of 6 per cent (again, less than 1 per cent per year of follow-up). The overall ipsilateral stroke risk was 10 per cent at 10 years. Late strokes were most common among hypertensive patients (31 per cent), patients whose indication for endarterectomy was stroke (31 per cent), and patients with uncorrected contralateral stenosis

(42 per cent). The last-named group had a contralateral late stroke incidence of 36 per cent, compared with 8 per cent in patients who underwent elective bilateral carotid endarterectomy.

Two other reports from the Cleveland Clinic attempted to compare surgical versus nonoperative therapy in a parallel, contemporary population referred to that institution for digital angiography.[35, 36] Although not a randomized series, all patients had intravenous digital angiography documenting a greater than 50 per cent carotid stenosis; these patients had no history of prior cerebrovascular operations, and follow-up was complete. Of 290 asymptomatic patients, 195 received medical or no therapy and 95 underwent prophylactic endarterectomy. Five-year stroke incidence was 15 per cent in the medical group versus 14 per cent in the surgical group. However, when groups were compared according to the degree of stenosis, patients with greater than 70 per cent stenosis had a 24 to 33 per cent 5-year stroke incidence with nonoperative therapy versus 7 to 12 per cent for the same cohort after endarterectomy. Patients with greater than 50 per cent bilateral stenosis also did better when subjected to bilateral endarterectomy (4 per cent versus 20 per cent 5-year stroke incidence).

Two hundred eleven symptomatic patients were similarly analyzed in a separate report.[35] Of these, 126 were treated nonoperatively and 85 underwent carotid endarterectomy. In patients with greater than 70 per cent stenosis treated medically, the 5-year incidence of stroke was 31 per cent, compared with 7 per cent in similar patients treated surgically. This was a statistically significant difference. Symptomatic patients with greater than 50 per cent bilateral stenosis also fared better after endarterectomy (3 per cent versus 28 per cent 5-year stroke incidence).

Controversy has existed as to the outcome of patients with completed stroke undergoing carotid endarterectomy because of conflicting information available from retrospective studies. Bardin and colleagues[4] reported their experience with 127 patients undergoing carotid endarterectomy after a completed stroke. A cumulative stroke incidence of 20 per cent at 5 years and a combined perioperative morbidity and mortality rate of 7 per cent were reported. Almost one third of patients died or suffered a stroke as a result of or in spite of carotid endarterectomy. Based on the natural history after a completed cerebral infarct, one would estimate a risk of recurrent stroke of approximately 6 to 12 per cent per year. Patients in the series by Bardin and colleagues did as well as the lowest estimate for the natural history of the disease. In contrast, Rubin and associates reported no ipsilateral stroke in 95 patients followed from 6 to 72 months after carotid endarterectomy for a history of completed cerebral infarction.[51] Operative morbidity and mortality was 2.7 per cent, which yielded a 0.64 per cent per year stroke risk. This is in agreement with most other retrospective reports, as seen in Table 127–1.

A group of 123 patients treated for asymptomatic carotid stenosis undergoing 141 carotid endarterectomies has recently been reported. All patients had greater than 75 per cent carotid stenosis or significant ulceration as an indication for the operation. No perioperative deaths were noted and only 2 postoperative strokes, 1 in a cerebellar distribution and 1 in the middle cerebral artery distribution, for a perioperative stroke risk of 1.4 per cent. Importantly, during the course of follow-up ranging from 3 to 10 years (mean, 56.6 months), no patient suffered a stroke in the hemisphere ipsilateral to the carotid endarterectomy. One patient developed an ipsilateral transient ischemic attack 24 months after surgery that was associated with recurrent carotid restenosis. Carotid restenosis occurred in 2.8 per cent of the entire series.[27]

From all the foregoing discussion, it is evident that carotid endarterectomy is an effective means of permanently reducing the risk of subsequent stroke in patients with symptomatic and/or high-risk carotid bifurcation lesions. The benefits of endarterectomy are realized within the first year of follow-up when the perioperative morbidity and mortality rates of the procedure are 1 to 3 per cent for asymptomatic patients, 3 to 5 per cent for symptomatic patients without cerebral infarction, and 5 to 9 per cent for patients following a completed stroke.

Including perioperative morbidity, asymptomatic patients with high-risk carotid lesions have an estimated stroke risk of 1.5 per cent per year following carotid endarterectomy. This compares favorably with the natural history estimates of 4 to 5 per cent per year. Currently, no data are available for the results of specific medical therapy for these lesions.

Patients with TIAs have an estimated stroke risk of 2 per cent per year following carotid endarterectomy. Natural history studies estimate a risk without therapy of 10 per cent the first year and 6 per cent per year thereafter. Antiplatelet therapy reduces this risk to an estimated 5 per cent per year of follow-up. Within 6 months of endarterectomy, the reduction in stroke risk with surgical therapy is realized.

Natural history studies of patients with completed strokes suggests significant risk for a second cerebral infarction, estimated between 6 and 12 per cent per year. Stroke victims who are candidates for endarterectomy have the highest perioperative morbidity and mortality, ranging from 5 to 9 per cent. If we assume a 10 per cent morbidity and mortality from the procedure and add the estimated 10 per cent stroke risk over the subsequent 5 years, the resulting 4 per cent per year stroke risk is a reduction even when compared with the lower estimates of the natural history or with medically treated patients.

In summary, carotid endarterectomy is a safe and effective procedure that significantly lowers the stroke risk in patients with significant extracranial occlusive disease. Patients need to be properly selected, taking into account the natural history of their condition, life expectancy, indication for the operation, and perioperative morbidity and mortality rates achieved by the individual surgeon. Decisions based on sound clinical judgment will ensure that the benefits of the procedure will be fully realized.

Carotid Endarterectomy for Acute Stroke

One of the more difficult clinical situations faced by vascular surgeons performing operative therapy for extracranial arterial occlusive disease is the decision of whether to recommend intervention during the acute phase following a cerebral infarct. Early in the history of carotid endarterectomy, several reports suggested a high risk of converting an ischemic cerebral infarction to a hemorrhagic cerebral infarction in patients during an acute stroke. Thus,

it was felt that carotid endarterectomy was contraindicated in the presence of an acute cerebral infarction. It is evident, however, that many of these reports included patients being operated on with massive cerebral infarction and in an obtunded state, patients in whom an attempt was made to open an internal carotid artery several days to weeks after thrombosis, and patients operated on while unstable (many of them with severe hypertension with poor control).

More recent evidence suggests improved results if carotid artery surgery is delayed for at least 5 weeks following the acute event. Patients undergoing early operation had an 18 per cent incidence of new postoperative neurologic deficits, as opposed to patients in whom there was a 5-week waiting interval in which no morbidity or mortality was seen. The authors concluded that waiting at least 5 weeks following the acute event was preferable.[30] Dosick and associates, however, noted a 21 per cent incidence of recurrent stroke during the 4- to 6-week observation interval. This led the authors to select their patients on the basis of computed tomography (CT) scans, proceeding with surgery if the CT scan showed no evidence of intracranial bleeding. One hundred ten patients undergoing carotid endarterectomy following an acute stroke with negative CT scan, had no perioperative neurologic morbidity and no mortality.[18] A similar experience was reported in 28 patients with small, fixed neurologic deficits undergoing endarterectomy an average of 11 days from the onset of symptoms. Only 1 postoperative death was reported in this small group of patients, and no new perioperative neurologic deficits were seen. Early endarterectomy was recommended in a select group of patients with limited cerebral infarcts.[64]

In general, surgical intervention during the acute phase of a stroke is contraindicated. If the patient has a dense neurologic deficit, loss of consciousness, or cardiovascular instability, surgery is contraindicated. If, however, the patient has a mild to moderate deficit, is fully conscious and otherwise stable, carotid endarterectomy of the responsible lesion may be undertaken soon after the patient has reached a plateau in her or his recovery. This may take days or weeks after the onset of the initial event. Although for most patients with an acute cerebral infarction, medical management is the therapy of choice, selected patients with identified high-risk lesions are best treated with carotid endarterectomy as soon as they have reached a stable condition in their recovery.

Stroke-in-evolution is a variation of acute stroke in which the initial deficit is followed by varying degrees of resolution, with worsening deficit in a progressing or stuttering fashion. Medical management for these patients includes heparin anticoagulation once intracranial hemorrhage has been excluded by imaging techniques. In spite of treatment, however, the prognosis in this group of patients is extremely poor. Excellent results have been reported in patients presenting with stroke-in-evolution treated surgically.[31, 40] Operation, however, carries a high risk and should only be undertaken by experienced surgeons.

Mentzer and colleagues reported 17 patients with stroke-in-evolution operated emergently. Seventy per cent had complete recovery, 24 per cent remain unchanged, and none were worse after endarterectomy.[40] There was 1 death (6 per cent mortality). This compared favorably to a parallel group of 20 patients with stroke-in-evolution treated medically. Mortality in the medical group was 15 per cent, with 66 per cent of the remaining patients having permanent moderate to severe neurologic deficits. In a review of the literature, 55 per cent of patients having emergency carotid endarterectomy for stroke-in-evolution showed improvement, 25 per cent showed no change, and 10 per cent were worse after surgery. Mortality ranged around 10 per cent.

Patients presenting with stroke-in-evolution should be thoroughly evaluated with CT scan to exclude intracranial hemorrhage. Once a high-risk carotid lesion has been identified in a patient with either crescendo TIAs or stroke-in-evolution, properly performed carotid endarterectomy carries the best prognosis in terms of neurologic recovery. The patient and the family should be aware, however, that the procedure carries the highest mortality for all indications of carotid endarterectomy, and a small percentage of patients will worsen their neurologic condition around the time of surgery.

External Carotid Endarterectomy

The importance of the external carotid artery (ECA) as a major collateral to cerebral circulation has been demonstrated by several investigators.[39, 53, 65] This collateral pathway gains clinical significance in the presence of an ipsilateral internal carotid occlusion. Hemispheric symptoms may arise secondary to the presence of a stenosis at the origin of the ECA, which may represent either a hemodynamic compromise or an embolic source. Emboli may also originate from the cul de sac created by an occluded internal carotid stump. In addition, repair of an ECA stenosis may be indicated in highly selected patients who may be candidates for extracranial-to-intracranial bypass.

O'Hara and colleagues[48] reported their experience with 42 ECA endarterectomies in 37 patients. Patch angioplasty and/or shunting during the procedure was utilized in approximately two thirds of the cases. Thirty procedures were limited to primary ECA revascularization, whereas 12 procedures were reoperations or required complementary subclavian or intracranial bypass (extended procedure). A significant difference in perioperative morbidity and mortality was seen between these two groups. Four patients (33 per cent) in the extended procedure group suffered perioperative ipsilateral hemispheric strokes, versus none in the limited procedure group. Three late strokes, 1 ipsilateral and 2 contralateral at 4, 16, and 33 months, respectively, were seen following ECA revascularization. Five additional patients required further therapy (anticoagulation, reoperation, or bypass) for recurrent symptoms. The author of this report cautioned as to the risks of extended procedures and recommended careful patient selection for this approach.

In a review of 36 patients undergoing ECA revascularization, Halstuk and associates[32] reported a 13.8 per cent operative stroke rate and a 2.7 per cent mortality rate. In addition, 14.2 per cent of patients suffered a late stroke on follow-up. The combination of bilateral carotid occlusion and preoperative fixed neurologic deficit was found to predict the highest perioperative morbidity (37 per cent). A literature review was included in this report. In 126 reported patients, overall perioperative neurologic morbidity was 14.3 per cent.

In a collective review of the literature, Gertler and

Cambria found 23 series reporting cases in which external carotid artery reconstruction was undertaken.[29] Two hundred eighteen cases were available for analysis. There were 195 external carotid endarterectomies and 23 external carotid artery bypasses. Resolution of symptoms was seen in 83 per cent of patients, with another 7 per cent showing improvement. Perioperative mortality was 3 per cent, with a 5 per cent perioperative neurologic morbidity. Factors found to increase morbidity and mortality included a highly diseased contralateral carotid artery, and symptomatic patients with internal carotid artery occlusion. The best results were obtained when surgery was performed to relieve specific hemispheric or retinal symptoms, as opposed to nonspecific neurologic complaints or previous stroke. Disease in the vertebral arteries had no impact on outcome.

External carotid revascularization is an attractive procedure, as it is technically simple. However, a multitude of risk factors are present in patients who are candidates for this procedure. The presence of a fixed neurologic deficit, bilateral carotid occlusion, and/or severe intracranial disease may significantly increase the morbidity of external carotid revascularization. A full trial of medical therapy may be warranted in these cases. When indicated, it seems prudent to limit the procedure to the external carotid repair, allowing several weeks of recovery before proceeding with additional reconstructions.

MEDICAL THERAPY

Anticoagulation

Two randomized controlled studies were designed to evaluate the effect of warfarin (Coumadin) anticoagulation in the treatment of patients with extracranial arterial occlusive disease.[3, 49] Both studies demonstrated that the incidence of hemispheric TIAs could be reduced with anticoagulants. However, incidence of subsequent cerebral infarction was not altered. Moreover, the mortality rate among patients treated with warfarin was higher, presumably because of the hemorrhagic complications.

In a retrospective study performed in Rochester, Minnesota, regarding the use of anticoagulants in cases of cerebral ischemia, a reduction in the stroke rate was observed when treated and untreated groups were compared.[63] However, the net probability of having a stroke within 5 years remained around 20 per cent for those patients given anticoagulants. This figure compares favorably with the risk for untreated control subjects (40 per cent), but is significant when compared with that for patients who undergo surgical therapy.

Two reports from Sweden have also shown some reduction in development of transient ischemia and stroke in patients treated with anticoagulants. Link and associates observed an increased incidence of stroke when anticoagulants were discontinued and therefore recommended long-term therapy.[38] However, Torrent and Anderson noted a higher mortality rate among stroke patients treated with anticoagulants; unacceptably serious bleeding complications were seen in this group— related to lengthy treatment, high blood pressure, or insufficient compliance by the patient.[59]

It is reasonable to conclude that the risk of stroke or TIA, although reduced with anticoagulant therapy, remains high when compared with that achieved by surgical management. The need for long-term administration of anticoagulant therapy with its concomitant greater risk of complications makes such treatment less desirable. Its use in extracranial arterial occlusive disease should be reserved for situations in which surgery is not feasible.

Antiplatelet Therapy

Antiplatelet therapy has been advocated for managing patients with extracranial arteriosclerotic occlusive disease. At present, six double-blind randomized prospective studies have compared the use of platelet antiaggregants with placebo in the treatment of patients who have cerebral ischemia secondary to this entity. From 1971 to 1976, the Canadian Cooperative Study Group assembled a study population of 585 patients with evidence of cerebral ischemia of extracranial origin.[10] Roughly 65 per cent had ischemic events referable to the carotid territory, 25 per cent had symptoms of vertebral-basilar insufficiency, and 10 per cent had both. These patients were randomly allocated to one of four regimens, taken four times a day and consisting of a 250-mg capsule of sulfinpyrazone plus placebo; a placebo tablet plus 325 mg of aspirin; both active drugs; or two placebos only. Follow-up from 12 to 57 months revealed no statistically significant reduction in TIAs, stroke, or death for patients receiving sulfinpyrazone. Aspirin reduced the risk of continuing ischemic episodes, stroke, or death by 19 per cent. When the data for male patients only were analyzed, the reduction was even higher. No statistically significant differences in stroke or death rates were found among female patients taking any of the four regimens.

It is important to note that almost as many patients were excluded from the study as were admitted, and this raises questions about whether the randomized group represents patients with transient ischemia in general. Considering these data literally, the probability of stroke in men taking aspirin was in excess of 5 per cent per year and in women higher than 8 per cent per year. The extracranial occlusive disease study indicated that the probability of stroke was about 3.5 per cent per year after surgery, but if surgical morbidity was excluded, it was less than 2 per cent per year.[62] The combined rate for death and morbidity was about 8 per cent; as mentioned earlier, this is high compared with current standards.

In 1972, a double-blind randomized prospective trial of aspirin versus placebo was started and continued for 37 months.[25] Patients were assigned to medical therapy on the basis of a clinical decision by the participating neurologist. About 50 per cent of them had operable lesions in the extracranial territory. Each patient allocated to the aspirin regimen received 10 grains daily. Analysis of the first 6 months of follow-up revealed a statistically significant differential in favor of aspirin when death, cerebral or retinal infarction, and TIAs were grouped together. When each group was considered separately, however, the difference did not achieve statistical significance.

Those patients for whom a decision was made to proceed with endarterectomy were also assigned to a randomized double-blind trial of aspirin during the postoperative period. The results of this trial constitute a separate report.[26] In this surgical group, life table analysis of the aforementioned end-points at 24 months did not reveal a statistically significant difference in favor of aspirin. However, when deaths that were not stroke-related were eliminated, a significant difference in favor of aspirin emerged. A favorable trend was also noted when the occurrence of ischemic episodes during the first 6 months of follow-up was taken into consideration. All patients in the placebo group reaching an absolute end-point during the first 24 months (8 individuals) had brain infarcts, whereas only 2 of 8 patients reaching such an end-point in the aspirin group suffered a neurologic event.

These last two studies reveal a favorable influence of aspirin in the treatment of extracranial occlusive disease. In the first, aspirin was the principal form of therapy, but in the latter it was used as an adjunct to surgical treatment. In the surgical treatment group, the absolute level of cases in which the outcome was unfavorable was about half that for those treated medically only (11.3 per cent versus 19.2 per cent). This differential may reflect the independent favorable effect of surgery.

In 1980, the Danish cooperative study of aspirin in the prevention of stroke in patients with reversible cerebral ischemic attacks was completed. Two hundred three patients with TIAs were treated with 1000 mg per day of aspirin (n = 101) or placebo (n = 102) in a prospective randomized protocol with an average follow-up of 25 months. Comparable groups were achieved in regard to age, sex, and risk factors. No statistically significant differences were found between the treatment groups as to primary end-points, stroke or death (aspirin, 20.8 per cent; placebo, 16.7 per cent). The incidence of recurrent TIAs was not reduced by aspirin. A trend toward fewer myocardial infarctions was noted in the aspirin group. Thus, no favorable influence could be demonstrated in regard to aspirin as therapy for patients with TIAs. Because the sample size was small, no definite conclusions could be drawn. The study has been criticized, owing to possible type II statistical error.[19]

The AICLA (French) controlled trial of aspirin and dipyridamole in the secondary prevention of strokes in patients with extracranial arterial occlusive disease completed randomization in 1978.[8] Follow-up was carried to 3 years. Six hundred four patients were randomized, most of whom had completed strokes (84 per cent). Drug regimens were aspirin, 330 mg po t.i.d.; placebo; or aspirin, 330 mg po t.i.d., and dipyridamole, 75 mg po t.i.d. Notably, patients with "tight" carotid stenosis were excluded from the trial, as were women under 50 years of age. Using fatal and nonfatal stroke as end-points, a favorable difference in the aspirin and aspirin-dipyridamole group was noted, with an approximate 60 per cent risk reduction at 3 years in the treated groups (10.5 per cent versus 18 per cent). New ischemic strokes occurred more often in a territory other than that of the entry episode. Because of some of the exclusion criteria in this study, it is questionable whether these results can be applied to patients with significant lesions at the carotid bifurcation. Nevertheless, the study demonstrates a favorable influence of antiplatelet therapy on cerebrovascular disease in general.

Between November 1978 and December 1982, the American-Canadian Cooperative Study Group randomized 890 patients with TIAs into two groups, each receiving either aspirin (1300 mg per day) alone or aspirin (1300 mg per day) and dipyridamole (300 mg per day).[1] Follow-up ranged from 1 to 5 years. Nearly identical results were seen regarding end-point (stroke, retinal infarction, or death) rates. The investigators concluded that the addition of dipyridamole to aspirin therapy was of no additional benefit. Interestingly, the cumulative risk of stroke or retinal infarction in both groups was about 20 per cent at 4 years, or 5 per cent per year of follow-up. This is similar to that observed by other investigators with antiplatelet therapy in patients with TIAs.

A Swedish cooperative study comparing high-dose acetylsalicylic acid versus placebo in the treatment of patients with cerebral infarction was reported in 1987.[55] Five hundred five patients with symptomatic carotid disease were randomized within 3 weeks of the event to receive aspirin 1.5 gm/day or placebo. Patients were followed for 2 years. There was no difference in stroke recurrence rate in the aspirin and the placebo groups, respectively, nor was there any significant difference in the rate of recurrent stroke or death. The risk of TIA or myocardial infarction was not reduced in the aspirin group. No prophylactic effect of high-dose aspirin after cerebral infarction could be demonstrated in this trial.

In a meta-analysis of all randomized controlled trials comparing aspirin with placebo in the treatment of symptomatic patients with cerebrovascular disease, aspirin was found to have a nonsignificant reduction of stroke rate of 15 per cent compared with placebo. When aspirin was combined with sulfinpyrazone or dipyridamole, by meta-analysis evaluation, a 39 per cent reduction of stroke was observed, however, with a concomitant 350 per cent increase in gastrointestinal hemorrhage or peptic ulcer. A trend toward reduction of stroke was seen in men for any regimen containing aspirin. Multiple biases, however, suggest that the benefit of aspirin in combination with other therapy is not established. A decrease in the incidence of stroke by aspirin therapy, alone or in combination, could not be established.[56]

Other antiplatelet agents have been evaluated in their role as part of the medical management of patients with symptomatic carotid disease. Ticlopidine is a strong platelet antiaggregant that functions primarily as an inhibitor of adenosine diphosphate pathway of platelet aggregation.[22] Ticlopidine inhibits most of the known stimuli to platelet aggregation and, in difference to aspirin, does not block the production of thromboxane or the production of prostacyclin by platelets or endothelial cells, respectively. Ticlopidine alters the function of the platelet for its life span. The results of the Ticlopidine-Aspirin Stroke Study were reported in 1989.[33] Three thousand sixty-nine patients with recent transient or mild persistent focal cerebral or retinal ischemia were randomized and followed for 2 to 6 years. The 3-year event rate for nonfatal stroke or death from any cause was 17 per cent for ticlopidine and 19 per cent for aspirin; a 12 per cent risk reduction by ticlopidine. The rates of fatal and nonfatal stroke at 3 years were 10 per cent for ticlopidine and 13 per cent for aspirin; a 21 per cent risk reduction with ticlopidine. There was a significant incidence of diarrhea in patients treated with ticlopidine (20 per cent) and a small, but important, incidence of neutropenia, which appeared reversible on discontinuation of the drug. A significantly increased level of cholesterol was noted in patients treated with ticlopidine. The study group concluded that ticlopidine was somewhat more effective than aspirin in preventing strokes, although the risk of side effects was greater. The Canadian-American Ticlopidine Study was also reported in 1989.[28] One thousand seventy-two patients were entered into the study 1 week to 4 months after having a cerebral infarct. They were treated with either 250 mg twice daily of ticlopidine, or placebo. After 3 years of follow-up, there was a 30.2 per cent risk reduction of stroke in patients treated with ticlopidine. The drug was equally effective in both men and women. Neutropenia was seen in 1 per cent of patients treated with ticlopidine and required discontinuation of treatment. The beneficial effects of ticlopidine as an antiplatelet agent was suggested.

Failures of antiplatelet therapy in the treatment of symptomatic carotid artery disease have been reported.[11] Some caution must be used in following patients receiving platelet antiaggregants as primary therapy for this disease. Partial disappearance of their symptoms should be considered a failure, and alternative modes of treatment should be considered. Patients who experience complete disappearance of their ischemic events should be monitored by noninvasive cerebral vascular studies. It is important to remember that progression of the disease is not significantly altered by these drugs, although the warning signs of such progression may be eliminated. In a review of 27 cases of aspirin failure in which urgent operations were required, it was found that 12 of the 27 surgical specimens showed fresh hemorrhage in the atherosclerotic plaque.[11] Whether this was induced or aggravated by aspirin cannot be concluded. This incidence of fresh hemorrhage in endarterectomy specimens appears to be high when compared with findings in elective cases.

MEDICAL THERAPY VERSUS CAROTID ENDARTERECTOMY— PROSPECTIVE RANDOMIZED STUDIES

One of the most important advances in the knowledge of cerebrovascular disease has been realized through the efforts of study groups carrying prospective randomized trials comparing carotid artery endarterectomy to medical therapy. For this purpose, patients have been divided into two main groups: (1) asymptomatic and (2) symptomatic patients with documented carotid bifurcation lesions. The available information is presented, focusing on these two groups of patients.

Asymptomatic Patients

Three prospective randomized studies have been designed to answer the question of whether surgical removal of an asymptomatic stenosis of the internal carotid artery can prevent the occurrence of stroke and represent a risk reduction procedure for patients with significant asymptomatic carotid lesions. In 1986, the Veterans Administration Cooperative Study on Asymptomatic Carotid Stenosis was launched as a multi-center cooperative study to determine the role of carotid endarterectomy in the treatment of asymptomatic carotid stenosis.[61] Their primary objective was to compare the incidence of TIAs, stroke, and death in previously asymptomatic patients with arteriographically confirmed internal carotid stenosis greater than 50 per cent. These patients were randomly allocated to receive carotid endarterectomy and aspirin therapy versus aspirin therapy alone. The results of this randomized trial were published in 1993.[66] A total of 44 men with asymptomatic carotid stenosis were randomized. Two hundred and eleven patients were treated with aspirin plus carotid endarterectomy, whereas 233 patients were treated with optimal medical therapy. Mean follow-up was 47.9 months. The combined incidence of ipsilateral neurologic (TIA and stroke) events was 8 per cent in the surgical group and 20.6 per cent in the medical group, for a statistically significant difference. The incidence of ipsilateral stroke alone was 4.7 per cent in the surgical group and 9.4 per cent in the medical group. Combining the analysis for stroke and death for the first 30 postoperative days showed no significant differences. The study group concluded that carotid endarterectomy reduced the overall incidence of ipsilateral neurologic events in a selected group of male patients with asymptomatic carotid stenosis. When the analysis combined stroke and death, however, a significant difference could not be demonstrated.

A second effort under the National Institutes of Health was launched in 1988.[2] The Asymptomatic Carotid Atherosclerosis Study was designed to determine whether the addition of carotid endarterectomy to aspirin plus risk factor modification affects the incidence of ipsilateral TIA, amaurosis fugax, and retinal and cerebral infarction in patients with asymptomatic, hemodynamically significant carotid stenosis. Randomization has been completed, and patients continue to be monitored.

The only prospective randomized study comparing carotid surgery versus medical therapy in asymptomatic carotid stenosis that has been completed and the results published is that of the Casanova Study Group.[12] The Carotid Artery Stenosis with Asymptomatic Narrowing: Operation Versus Aspirin, was a multi-center trial in 460 patients with asymptomatic internal carotid artery stenosis ranging from 50 to 90 per cent. Angiography was performed in all patients. Two hundred six patients with unilateral and bilateral stenosis had surgery unilaterally or bilaterally, respectively. These were compared with 160 patients with unilateral stenosis who had no initial surgery. Importantly, those patients in the medical group who had bilateral stenosis had surgery on the more affected side. Surgery in the medically treated group was performed if the stenosis progressed to greater than 90 per cent, if bilateral internal carotid artery stenosis greater than 50 per cent developed, or if the patient had TIAs in the region supplied by the randomized internal carotid artery, together with any stenosis greater than 50 per cent. All patients in this study received 330 mg of aspirin and 75 mg of dipyridamole three times a day. Minimal follow-up was 3 years. Importantly, in this group of patients, 334 carotid endarterectomies were performed, in-

cluding 118 carotid endarterectomies in the medically treated group. Other violations of protocol occurred, with 12 violations of entry criteria and 72 patients in whom surgery was not performed according to protocol. In addition, it must be emphasized that patients with greater than 90 per cent stenosis were excluded from randomization. Statistical analysis found no significant difference in the number of neurologic deficits and deaths between the two groups. The multiple flaws in this study, some of which have been cited previously, suggest that determination of the role of carotid endarterectomy in the management of asymptomatic patients will have to await the results of other prospective randomized clinical trials.

Symptomatic Patients

The first prospective randomized multi-institutional study of extracranial arterial occlusive disease was initiated in 1959.[5] The Joint Study of Extracranial Arterial Occlusion randomized 1225 patients, with 621 operated on with carotid endarterectomy and 604 treated according to what the individual's participating institution considered the best medical therapy. In many but by no means in all instances, medical therapy included anticoagulation with warfarin (Coumadin). Comparison of cerebrovascular symptoms, associated diseases, and angiographic patterns of disease revealed that the two groups were remarkably matched. Analysis of mortality rates, according to the patient's clinical presentation and the angiographic pattern of disease, revealed significant differences between the medical and the surgical groups. Survival up to 42 months in the surgically treated group was better in patients with unilateral carotid stenosis who were either experiencing TIAs or had cerebral infarction with minimal residual deficits (Fig. 127–1). Survival in the medical group was better in patients who suffered a major stroke with moderate to severe residual deficits. Neurologic morbidity during follow-up as long as 42 months was evaluated in 316 patients identified as having hemispheric TIAs without residual deficit as an indication for admission to the study. This group included patients

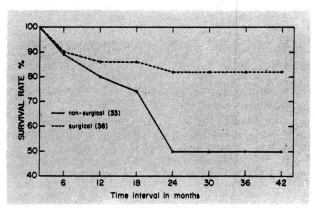

FIGURE 127–1. Cumulative survival rates in class 2 patients who had unilateral carotid artery stenosis and no other surgically accessible lesion. (From Bauer RB, Meyer JS, Fields WS, et al: Joint study of extracranial arterial occlusion. III. Progress report of controlled study of long-term survival in patients with and without operation. JAMA 208:509–518, 1969. Copyright 1969, American Medical Association.)

with unilateral carotid stenosis, bilateral carotid stenosis, and unilateral carotid stenosis with contralateral occlusion. In all three categories, the incidence of subsequent attacks of transient ischemia or cerebral infarction was lower in the surgically treated group. Either disorder occurring in a surgical patient usually affected the side contralateral to the operation, as opposed to those in the nonsurgical group in whom a subsequent ischemic attack or infarction tended to occur in the distribution of the artery that was asymptomatic at the time of randomization. These differences were found to be statistically significant. It is important to emphasize that the surgical data included the combined postoperative morbidity and mortality rate of around 8 per cent. This figure is considered to be high by today's standards and suggests that a current comparison might be more favorable to the surgically treated group.

The role of carotid endarterectomy in the management of symptomatic patients with a demonstrable carotid artery lesion has been prospectively evaluated in three recent randomized clinical trials. The European Carotid Surgery Trialists Collaborative Group randomized 2518 patients over 10 years to be treated with either carotid endarterectomy or with medical management alone.[21] These patients were stratified into mild (0 to 29 per cent), moderate (30 to 69 per cent), and severe (70 to 99 per cent) degree of stenosis in the randomized artery. The results are available for both the mild and the severe group. For 778 patients with severe (70 to 99 per cent) stenosis, there was a total risk of perioperative death and stroke and ipsilateral ischemic stroke on follow-up of 12 per cent, compared with 21.9 per cent of patients treated medically. Among the patients with severe stenosis, only 3.7 per cent had disabling strokes, compared with an 8.4 per cent in patients treated medically. A total 3-year risk of any disabling or fatal stroke in the surgical group was 6 per cent, compared with 11 per cent in the control group. Patients in the mild carotid stenosis category (0 to 29 per cent) had a very small 3-year risk of ipsilateral ischemic stroke, even in the absence of surgery, so that the surgical risks were not outweighed by its benefits.

In the United States, two prospective clinical trials were initiated at around the same time. The North American Symptomatic Carotid Endarterectomy Trial (NASCET) was conducted at 50 clinical centers throughout the United States and Canada, stratifying patients into 30 to 69 per cent degree of carotid stenosis and 70 to 99 per cent degree of carotid stenosis who had evidence of symptoms (either TIAs or stroke) within 3 months of randomization.[47] The results of patients in the moderate degree of carotid stenosis category are not available, and this is an ongoing study. The results of the 659 patients in the 70 to 99 per cent category, however, were reported in August of 1991 following a medical alert recommending that symptomatic patients with hemispheric or retinal TIA and an ipsilateral carotid stenosis greater than 70 per cent should be considered for carotid endarterectomy (Fig. 127–2). In their study, the cumulative risk of any ipsilateral stroke at 2 years was 26 per cent in the 331 medically treated patients and 9 per cent in the 328 surgically treated patients, with an absolute risk reduction of 17.3 per cent. For fatal ipsilateral stroke, the corresponding estimates were 13.1 per cent in the medical group and 2.5 per cent in the surgically treated group.

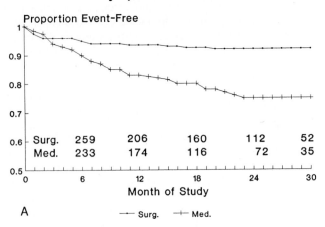

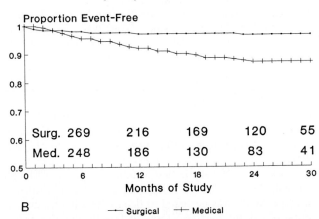

FIGURE 127–2.   Results of the North American Symptomatic Carotid Endarterectomy Trial (NASCET). *A*, Kaplan-Meier curve comparing medical and surgical event-free with respect to any ipsilateral stroke. *B*, Kaplan-Meier curve of event-free proportion of the same groups with respect to major ipsilateral stroke after randomization.

Carotid endarterectomy was found to be highly beneficial to patients with recent hemispheric and retinal TIAs or nondisabling strokes and ipsilateral high-grade stenosis of the internal carotid artery.[46] Because of the results of the NASCET trial the Veterans Administration trial has been discontinued, with the results of the limited enrollment in this trial also supporting the results reported by both NASCET and the European Trialist's Group.

PRACTICE GUIDELINES

Based on the available retrospective and prospective information, in regard to the role of carotid artery in the treatment of extracranial arterial occlusive disease, the Joint Council of the Society for Vascular Surgery and the North American Chapter of the International Society for Cardiovascular Surgery have published practice guidelines for the performance of carotid endarterectomy.[45] Importantly, it is noted that nearly one half of the strokes in the United States appear in the distribution of the carotid artery and may be related to carotid bifurcation disease.[42] The extent that carotid endarterectomy can be performed with minimal morbidity and mortality in patients who are at risk of suffering a stroke will dictate the appropriateness of this intervention.

Patient selection should be based on the symptomatic status of the patient, the nature of the lesion and, perhaps most importantly, a combination of both. Risk factor control is of paramount importance, regardless of whether endarterectomy is recommended.

Patients with a prior stroke with minimal residual deficit should be considered candidates for carotid endarterectomy as long as the surgeon can perform the operation with a morbidity and mortality rate that does not exceed 7 per cent. Lesions that are in the distribution of the affected hemisphere are appropriate for operation if they are high-grade stenosis (greater than 70 per cent), or low-profile plaques with large ulceration, or moderate stenosis with plaque of mixed consistency. Medical therapy should be recommended in patients who are at particularly high risk for operation or have a poor prognosis with limited longevity. Patients with a severe neurologic deficit that has not improved over a period of observation should not be considered candidates for carotid endarterectomy, especially if loss of consciousness is present. Patients with a hemispheric stroke who are shown to have a minimal lesion in the appropriate carotid bifurcation without overt ulceration or significant softness of the plaque consistency may well have had the stroke secondary to factors other than the carotid disease.

Asymptomatic patients with carotid artery stenosis of at least 75 per cent, who are otherwise reasonably healthy and have a life expectancy greater than 5 years, should be considered candidates for prophylactic carotid endarterectomy as long as the surgeon can perform the operation with a morbidity and mortality less than 3 per cent. The results of the ongoing prospective randomized clinical trials in asymptomatic patients may alter or confirm this recommendation. In the interval, based on retrospective information, this recommendation appears reasonable. Evidence that the lesion has progressed in severity over an interval of observation or that the consistency of the plaque has changed to a mixed or soft material will increase the risk of the lesion and therefore make the recommendation for operation more compelling. Patients with lesser degrees of stenosis but CT scan evidence of silent embolization in the same anatomic distribution may also be considered candidates for operation.

It is important to emphasize that patients who undergo successful carotid endarterectomy remain at a higher risk of stroke than age-adjusted controls and therefore should be monitored closely for the rest of their lives. There appears to be enough evidence to support prescribing a postoperative regimen of antiplatelet therapy in these patients. As surgeons have learned in the management of malignant disease, a combined approach of surgery followed by chemotherapy, in this case antiplatelet drugs, seems to offer the best chance of preventing neurologic events in patients with extracranial arterial occlusive disease. Control of risk factors (e.g., hypertension and cigarette smoking) should be part of any medical or surgical therapeutic plan. Only then will the full benefits of any intervention be realized and neurologic function preserved in patients with cerebrovascular disease.

References

1. The American-Canadian Cooperative Study Group: Persantine-aspirin trial in cerebral ischemia. II. End-point results. Stroke 16:406, 1985.
2. The Asymptomatic Carotid Atherosclerosis Study Group: Study design for randomized prospective trial of carotid endarterectomy for asymptomatic atherosclerosis. Stroke 20:844, 1989.
3. Baker RN, Schwartz WS, Rose AS: Transient ischemic strokes: A report of a study of anticoagulant therapy. Neurology (Minneap) 16:841, 1964.
4. Bardin JA, Bernstein EF, Humber PB, et al: Is carotid endarterectomy beneficial in the prevention of recurrent stroke? Arch Surg 117:1401, 1982.
5. Bauer RB, Meyer JS, Fields WS, et al: Joint study of extracranial arterial occlusion. III. Progress report of controlled study of long-term survival in patients with and without operation. JAMA 208:509, 1969.
6. Bernstein EF, et al: Influence of preoperative factors on late neurologic events after carotid endarterectomy. International Vascular Symposium Program and Abstracts. New York, Macmillan Publishers, 1981, p 460.
7. Bouchard JP, Fabia J, Simard D, et al: Carotid endarterectomy: Survival rate of 227 patients. Can Med Assoc J 113:949, 1975.
8. Bousser MG, Eschwege E, Haguenau M, et al: "AICLA" controlled trial of aspirin and dipyridamole in the secondary prevention of atherothrombotic cerebral ischemia. Stroke 14:5, 1983.
9. Byer JA, Easton JD: Transient cerebral ischemia: Review of surgical results. Prog Cardiovasc Dis 27:389, 1980.
10. The Canadian Cooperative Study Group: A randomized trial of aspirin and sulfinpyrazone in threatened strokes. N Engl J Med 299:53, 1978.
11. Carson SN, Demling RH, Esquivel CD: Aspirin failure in symptomatic arteriosclerotic carotid artery disease. Surgery 90:1084, 1981.
12. The Casanova Study Group: Carotid surgery versus medical therapy in asymptomatic carotid stenosis. Stroke 22:583, 1991.
13. Chambers BR, Norris JW: The case against surgery for asymptomatic carotid stenosis. Stroke 15:964, 1984.
14. Chung WB: Long-term results of carotid surgery for cerebrovascular insufficiency. Am J Surg 128:262, 1974.
15. Data on file, UCLA Computerized Vascular Registry, Los Angeles, CA, 1987.
16. DeBakey ME, Crawford ES, Cooley DA, et al: Cerebral arterial insufficiency: One- to 11-year results following arterial reconstructive operation. Ann Surg 161:921, 1965.
17. DeWeese JA, Rob CG, Satran R, et al: Results of carotid endarterectomies for transient ischemic attacks—Five years later. Ann Surg 178:258, 1973.
18. Dosick SM, Whalen RC, Gale SS, Brown OW: Carotid endarterectomy in the stroke patient: Computerized axial tomography to determine timing. J Vasc Surg 2:214, 1985.
19. Dyken ML: Transient ischemic attacks and aspirin, stroke and death; negative studies and type II error. [Editorial] Stroke 14:2, 1983.
20. Easton JD, Sherman DG: Stroke and mortality rate in carotid endarterectomy: 228 consecutive operations. Stroke 8:565, 1977.
21. European Carotid Surgery Trialists' Collaborative Group: MRC European Carotid Surgery Trial: Interim results for symptomatic patients with severe (70–99%) or with mild (0–29%) carotid stenosis. Lancet 337:1235, 1991.
22. Feliste R, Delebassee D, Simon MF, et al: Broad spectrum antiplatelet activity of ticlopidine and PCR 4099 involves the suppression of the effects of released ADP. Thromb Res 48:403, 1987.
23. Field PL: Effective stroke prevention with carotid endarterectomy: A series of 400 cases with two-year follow-up. International Vascular Symposium Program and Abstracts. New York, Macmillan Publishers, 1981, p 528.
24. Fields WS: Role of antiplatelet agents in cerebrovascular disease. Drugs 18:150, 1979.
25. Fields WS, Lemak NA, Frankowski RF, et al: Controlled trial of aspirin in cerebral ischemia. Stroke 8:301, 1977.
26. Fields WS, Lemak NA, Frankowski RF, Hardy RJ: Controlled trial of aspirin in cerebral ischemia. II. Surgical group. Stroke 9:309, 1978.
27. Freischlag JA, Hanna D, Moore WS: Improved prognosis for asymptomatic carotid stenosis with prophylactic carotid endarterectomy. Stroke 23:479, 1992.

28. Gent M, Blakely JA, Easton JD, et al: The Canadian-American Ticlopidine Study (CATS) in thromboembolic stroke. Lancet 1:1215, June 3, 1989.

29. Gertler JP, Cambria RP: The role of external carotid endarterectomy in the treatment of ipsilateral internal carotid occlusion: Collective review. J Vasc Surg 6:158, 1987.

30. Giordano JM, Trout HH III, Kozloff L, DePalma RG: Timing of carotid artery endarterectomy after stroke. J Vasc Surg 2:250, 1985.

31. Goldstone J, Moore WS: Emergency carotid artery surgery in neurologically unstable patients. Arch Surg 111:1284, 1976.

32. Halstuk KS, Baker WH, Littooy FN: External carotid endarterectomy. J Vasc Surg 1:398, 1984.

33. Hass WK, Easton JD, Adams HP, et al, for the Ticlopidine-Aspirin Stroke Study Group: A randomized trial comparing ticlopidine hydrochloride with aspirin for the prevention of stroke in high-risk patients. N Engl J Med 321:501, 1989.

34. Hertzer NR, Arison R: Cumulative stroke and survival ten years after carotid endarterectomy. J Vasc Surg 2:661, 1985.

35. Hertzer NR, Flanagan RA, Beven EG, O'Hara PJ: Surgical versus nonoperative treatment of symptomatic carotid stenosis: 211 patients documented by intravenous angiography. Ann Surg 204:154, 1986.

36. Hertzer NR, Flanagan RA, Beven EG, O'Hara PJ: Surgical versus nonoperative treatment of asymptomatic carotid stenosis: 290 patients documented by intravenous angiography. Ann Surg 204:163, 1986.

37. Lees CS, Hertzer NR: Postoperative stroke and late neurologic complications after carotid endarterectomy. Arch Surg 116:1561, 1981.

38. Link H, Lebram G, Johannson I, Radberg C: Prognosis in patients with infarction and TIA in carotid territory during and after anticoagulant therapy. Stroke 10:529, 1979.

39. Machleder HI, Barker WF: External carotid artery shunting during carotid endarterectomy: Evidence for feasibility. Arch Surg 108:785, 1974.

40. Mentzer RM Jr, Finkelmeier BA, Crosby IK, Wellons HA Jr: Emergency carotid endarterectomy for fluctuating neurologic deficits. Surgery 89:60, 1981.

41. Modi JR, Finch WT, Sumner DS: Update of carotid endarterectomy in two community hospitals: Springfield revisited. Stroke 14:128, 1983.

42. Mohr JP, Caplan LR, Melski JW, et al: The Harvard Cooperative Stroke Registry: A prospective registry. Neurology 28:754, 1978.

43. Moore WS, Boren C, Malone JM, Goldstone J: Asymptomatic carotid stenosis: Immediate and long-term results after prophylactic endarterectomy. Am J Surg 138:228, 1979.

44. Moore WS, Boren C, Malone JM, et al: Natural history of nonstenotic asymptomatic ulcerative lesions of the carotid arteries. Arch Surg 113:1352, 1978.

45. Moore WS, Mohr JP, Najafi H, et al: Carotid endarterectomy: Practice guidelines. Report of the Ad Hoc Committee to the Joint Council of the Society for Vascular Surgery and the North American Chapter of the International Society for Cardiovascular Surgery. J Vasc Surg 15:469, 1992.

46. North American Symptomatic Carotid Endarterectomy Trial Collaborators: Beneficial effect of carotid endarterectomy in symptomatic patients with high-grade carotid stenosis. N Engl J Med 325:445, 1991.

47. North American Symptomatic Carotid Endarterectomy Trial (NAS-CET) Steering Committee: North American Symptomatic Carotid Endarterectomy Trial: Methods, patient characteristics, and progress. Stroke 22:611, 1991.

48. O'Hara PJ, Hertzer NR, Beven EG: External carotid revascularization: Review of a 10-year experience. J Vasc Surg 2:709, 1985.

49. Report of the Veterans Administration Cooperative Study of Arteriosclerosis: An evaluation of anticoagulant therapy in the treatment of cerebrovascular disease. II. Neurology (Minneap) 11:132, 1961.

50. Riles TS, Imparato AM, Mintaer R, Baumann FS: Comparison of results of bilateral and unilateral carotid endarterectomy five years after surgery. Surgery 91:258, 1982.

51. Rubin JR, Goldstone J, McIntyre KE, et al: The value of carotid endarterectomy in reducing the morbidity and mortality of recurrent stroke. J Vasc Surg 4:443, 1986.

52. Sergeant PT, Derom F, Berzsenyi G, et al: Carotid endarterectomy for cerebrovascular insufficiency: Long-term follow-up of 141 patients followed up to 16 years. Acta Chir Belg 79:309, 1980.

53. Schuler JJ, Flanigan B, DeBord JR, et al: The treatment of cerebral ischemia by external carotid artery revascularization. Arch Surg 118:567, 1983.

54. Sorensen BS, Pedersen H, Marquartsen J, et al: Acetylsalicylic acid in the prevention of stroke in patients with reversible cerebral ischemic attacks. A Danish Cooperative Study. Stroke 14:15, 1983.

55. A Swedish Cooperative Study: High-dose acetylsalicylic acid after cerebral infarction. Stroke 18:325, 1987.

56. Sze PC, Reitman D, Pincus MM, et al: Antiplatelet agents in the secondary prevention of stroke: Meta-analysis of the randomized control trials. Stroke 19:436, 1988.

57. Thompson JE, Austen DJ, Patman RD: Carotid endarterectomy for cerebrovascular insufficiency: Long-term results in 592 patients followed up to 13 years. Ann Surg 172:663, 1970.

58. Thompson JE, Patman RD, Talkington CM: Asymptomatic carotid bruit: Long-term outcome of patients having endarterectomy compared with unoperated controls. Ann Surg 188:308, 1978.

59. Torrent A, Anderson B: The outcome of patients with transient ischemic attacks and stroke treated with anticoagulants. Acta Med Scand 208:359, 1980.

60. Tytus JS, MacLean JB, Hill LD: Prognosis in patients with transient ischemic attacks after endarterectomy. Am Surg 36:623, 1970.

61. The Veterans Administration Cooperative Study: Role of carotid endarterectomy in asymptomatic carotid stenosis. Stroke 17:534, 1986.

62. Whisnant JP: The Canadian trial of aspirin and sulfinpyrazone in threatened strokes. Am Heart J 99:129, 1980.

63. Whisnant JP, Matsumoto N, Elvergack LR: The effect of anticoagulant therapy on the prognosis of patients with transient cerebral ischemic attacks in a community: Rochester, Minnesota, 1955 through 1969. Mayo Clin Proc 48:844, 1973.

64. Whitney DG, Kahn EM, Estes JW, Jones CE: Carotid artery surgery without a temporary indwelling shunt: 1917 consecutive procedures. Arch Surg 115:1393, 1980.

65. Zarins CK, DelBaccaro EJ, Johns L, et al: Increased cerebral blood flow after external carotid artery revascularization. Surgery 89:730, 1981.

66. Hobson RW II, Weiss DG, Fields WS, et al: Efficacy of carotid endarterectomy for asymptomatic carotid stenosis. N Engl J Med 328:221, 1993.

The Management of Venous Disorders

Edited by George Johnson, Jr., M.D.

128

Introduction and General Considerations

George Johnson, Jr., M.D.

• • •

Venous disease has long plagued the human race, as documented in the Ebers papyrus from the 9th year of the reign of Amenophis I (1550 B.C.).[1] Hippocrates observed "that it was better not to stand in the case of an ulcer on the leg."[2] The ancient Greeks brought replicas of legs with varicose veins to the priests of Aesculapius to ask for relief.[3] In A.D. 400 the Arabs gave a vivid and succinct description of the "modern therapy" for varicose veins: "cut skin, expose varix, insert probe under it . . . pull out varix and cut."[4]

In the 1800s, John Gay recognized that varicose veins were not the only cause of lower extremity ulceration.[5] In the 20th century, the textile industry developed the process of circular knitting using elastic fibers, which led to compression stocking therapy.[6] Later, Conrad Jobst recognized the benefits of graded compression, as used in modern compression therapy.[7] Linton proposed the ablation of the incompetent perforator vein, a procedure that is still in vogue.[8]

As the pathophysiology of chronic venous insufficiency has been better understood, attempts have been made to correct this disease by developing procedures that bypass obstructed segments of veins with vessels containing appropriate valves. Thus, the femorofemoral bypass procedures developed by Palma and Esperon[9] and popularized by Dale and Harris[10] and the saphenofemoral vein graft bypassing the superficial femoral vein, as reported by Queral and Anneous,[11] have evolved. Kistner and Sparkuhl,[12] Raju and Fredericks,[13] and Taheri and coworkers[14] are among those who have contributed to the management of valvular insufficiency by transfer, reconstruction, or transplantation of venous valves.

Although great advances have been made in the operative treatment of arterial diseases since the late 1950s, venous diseases continue to incapacitate patients and to cause death despite intense interest and continuing efforts on the part of vascular surgeons to develop surgical methods of treatment. The management of most venous problems is still primarily nonoperative. Nevertheless, there is now a definite role for surgery in the management of many of these disorders, and the indications for operative intervention have become clear; newer techniques may further expand the indications for surgery.

Most pathologic conditions found in the venous system develop in the lower extremity. With the evolution of humans to the upright position, blood from the leg must be returned to the heart against gravity, without organs specifically developed for this purpose. The delicate valves that are found throughout the venous system in the extremities are apparently an evolutionary adaptation to the erect posture. They break up a column of blood from ankle to atrium that if unopposed would potentially exert a gravitational force at the ankle of 110 to 120 mmHg (depending on the distance from the ankle to the diaphragm). If one were to stand completely relaxed and motionless for several minutes, venous pressures in this range would develop in the veins at the ankles. Even modest motion, however, such as shifting weight, contracts the calf muscles, forcing blood toward the heart in the valved venous system. The description of this mechanism by Gunnar Bauer in 1950 has not been improved on:*

> When the calf muscles contract within their narrow fascial sheath, all the blood assembled in the deep vein trunks is forcibly squeezed out and poured into the popliteal and femoral veins. When, after a few moments, the muscles relax, this blood cannot flow back down into the lower leg because of the valves in the main trunk. The calf muscles thus act as a sort of peripheral heart or as an additional pump apparatus

---

*From Angiology, The Journal of Vascular Diseases, Volume 1:1, 1950. Reproduced with permission of the copyright owner: Westminster Publications, Inc., Roslyn, New York (U.S.A.). All rights reserved.

put in to speed up the fluid flow in the most distant parts of the tubing system, in which the blood streams tend to become too slow because of the width of the vascular bed.[15]

Regular, rhythmic motion, such as walking, "pumps" the venous blood upward and reduces the ankle venous pressure to between 0 and 30 mmHg.[16] Without a competent venomuscular pumping mechanism, we would all have swollen legs and petechial hemorrhages by day's end. In fact, in patients with paralysis, severe arthritis, or fusion of the ankle, these problems can exist without occlusion or valvular incompetence of the deep venous system. Once blood is in the abdomen, above the competent valves of the leg, its return to the heart is further aided by movement of the diaphragm. With descent of the diaphragm, blood in the iliac veins and the vena cava is subjected to increasing intra-abdominal pressure. Refilling occurs during the expiratory phase of respiration, when the diaphragm relaxes.

Superficial veins of the lower extremity are not surrounded by skeletal muscle, as are the deep veins, and thus do not empty by muscular compression. The walls, however, are thicker and contain more smooth muscle, so they have a more developed intrinsic system for emptying. When the saphenous vein ascending the leg and the communicating veins penetrating to the deep venous system have competent valves, blood readily empties into the central circulation and returns to the heart. With incompetent valves, various degrees of venous stasis develop, the sequelae of which are discussed in subsequent chapters.

Anatomically, physiologically, and pathologically, the venous system of the lower extremity can be divided into three parts: the greater and lesser saphenous subsystem, the communicating vein subsystem, and the deep vein subsystem. The pathologic process of each system has an influence on the pathophysiology of the other systems. A proximal deep venous thrombosis, for example, hinders the cephalad flow of blood from the deep venous system, and when the ambulatory "peripheral heart" functions, a strain is placed on the communicating valves to remain competent. Valvular incompetence of the superficial subsystem leads to more blood being carried by the deep venous subsystem, with up to 25 per cent of the blood flow returning through the saphenofemoral junction. Although this abnormality may lead to an increased flow, there is no evidence that high pressure, stasis, or a higher incidence of thrombosis occurs in the deep subsystem.

Burnand and coworkers defined distinct venous pressure patterns in relation to the anatomic distribution of disease.[17] Thus, depending on the subsystem involved, distinctly different phlebographic and venous patterns can be identified. The division is helpful in identifying the exact pathologic condition when selecting surgical alternatives. The hemodynamics of the venous system are further discussed in the chapters on chronic venous insufficiency.

The treatment of varicose veins unassociated with deep venous occlusion, whether by operation or injection, is most beneficial and should be undertaken when the symptoms warrant such intervention. Leaving the competent saphenous system and removing only the varicose veins is now commonplace and can be performed as a simple outpatient procedure through small incisions. This has revolutionized the therapy for varicose veins. It is inter-esting to note that the reported number of inpatient operations (high ligation and stripping of the greater saphenous system) has markedly decreased. There were 62,000 performed in the United States in nonfederal hospitals in 1979,[18] whereas only 27,000 were performed in 1989.[19] Sclerotherapy has become increasingly popular, especially for the small varicose veins.

The report on "dysplastic collagen fibrils" in varicose veins, as described by Staubesand and Fischer,[20] is fascinating and raises questions about whether this condition is primary or secondary to the hemodynamic disorders just described.

The frequent use of indwelling venous catheters has revolutionized the management of the critically ill patient but has also created new problems. When such a catheter is properly used, complications should be minimal, but when they do occur, the physician must be prepared to deal with them in an appropriate manner. Thrombosis and bleeding from a major vein are complications associated with the increasing use of indwelling venous catheters.

Therapy for thrombosis of the deep venous system continues to be a challenge to the internist as well as the surgeon. Several years ago, a consensus report from the National Institutes of Health addressed prophylaxis and concluded that any high-risk patient undergoing operative therapy should have minidose heparin, 5000 units subcutaneously every 8 to 12 hours.[21] Although other means of prophylaxis, such as intermittent compression boots, have been shown to be effective, all patients at high risk for deep vein thrombosis should receive some form of prophylaxis. Although significant inroads have been made in the fields of diagnosis and treatment, well-monitored heparin therapy, rather than surgery, is currently the mainstay of treatment for deep venous thrombosis, as well as for first-episode pulmonary emboli. Heparin therapy may lessen the prolonged illness that frequently occurs after deep venous occlusion, but it may also decrease the necessity for inferior vena caval interruption. Thrombectomy for deep venous occlusion, vena caval interruption for recurrent emboli, and embolectomy for massive pulmonary emboli are now being carried out with clearer indications.

Chronic venous insufficiency continues to plague modern society. The use of the Unna boot remains one of the first phases of therapy for the ulceration due to chronic venous insufficiency. Operative therapy, as is discussed in this section, continues to be advocated for some patients with recalcitrant symptoms or ulcers.

European investigators have been studying the molecular and cellular aspects of chronic venous insufficiency. Although this has not received a great deal of attention in the United States, it bears watching. Drug therapy for the pathology associated with chronic venous insufficiency is an attractive alternative. Finally, just as heparin is the mainstay of treatment for acute venous thromboembolism, the effectiveness of elastic compression and leg elevation for chronic venous insufficiency must be kept firmly in mind in considering surgical intervention for chronic symptoms.

References

1. Ghanlioungui P: The House of Life, Magic and Medical Science in Ancient Egypt. Amsterdam, BM Israel, 1973, p 33.

2. Adams F: The Genuine Works of Hippocrates. Baltimore, Williams & Wilkins, 1939, p 333.
3. Bettmann O: A Pictorial History of Medicine. Springfield, IL, Charles C Thomas, 1956, p 16.
4. Kamal H: Encyclopaedia of Islamic Medicine. Cairo, General Egyptian Book Organization, 1975, p 724.
5. Dodd H, Cockett FB: The Pathology and Surgery of the Veins of the Lower Limb. Edinburgh, Churchill Livingstone, 1976, p 246.
6. Johnson G: The role of elastic support in venous problems. *In* Bergan JJ, Yao JST (eds): Surgery of the Veins. Orlando, FL, Grune & Stratton, 1985, p 541.
7. Bergan JJ: Conrad Jobst and the development of pressure gradient therapy for venous disease. *In* Bergan JJ, Yao JST (eds): Surgery of the Veins. Orlando, FL, Grune & Stratton, 1985, p 529.
8. Linton RR: Atlas of Vascular Surgery. Philadelphia, WB Saunders, 1973, p 72.
9. Palma EC, Esperon R: Vein transplants and grafts in the surgical treatment of the post-phlebitic syndrome. J Cardiovasc Surg (Torino) 1:94, 1960.
10. Dale WA, Harris J: Cross-over vein grafts for iliac and femoral venous occlusion. Ann Surg 168:319, 1968.
11. Queral L, Anneous MO: Claudication treated by distal superficial femoral-to-greater saphenous vein bypass. J Vasc Surg 2:870, 1985.
12. Kistner RL, Sparkuhl MD: Surgical treatment in acute and chronic venous disease. Surgery 85:31, 1979.
13. Raju S, Fredericks RK: Late hemodynamic sequelae of deep venous thrombosis. J Vasc Surg 4:73, 1986.
14. Taheri SA, Lazar L, Elias S, et al: Surgical treatment of postphlebitic syndrome with vein valve transplant. Am J Surg 144:221, 1982.
15. Bauer G: Pathophysiology and treatment of the lower leg stasis syndrome. Angiology 1:1, 1950.
16. DeCamp PT, Ward JA, Ochsner A: Ambulatory venous pressure studies in postphlebitic and other disease states. Surgery 29:365, 1951.
17. Burnand KG, O'Donnell TF, Thomas ML, Browse NL: The relative importance of incompetent communicating veins in the production of varicose veins and venous ulcers. Surgery 81:9, 1977.
18. US Department of Health and Human Services, Public Health Service, Office of Health Research, Statistics, and Technology, National Center for Health Statistics. Detailed Diagnoses and Surgical Procedures for Patients Discharged From Short-Stay Hospitals, United States, 1979. Washington, DC, US Government Printing Office, 1982.
19. Graves EJ: Detailed diagnoses and procedures, National Hospital Discharge Survey, 1989. National Center for Health Statistics. Vital Health Stat 13:108, 1991.
20. Staubesand J, Fischer N: The ultrastructural characteristics of abnormal collagen fibrils in various organs. Connect Tissue Res 7:213, 1980.
21. Prevention of venous thrombosis and pulmonary embolism. Consensus Conference. JAMA 256:744, 1986.

129

Hemodynamics and Pathophysiology of Venous Disease

David S. Sumner, M.D.

• • •

The pathophysiology of venous disease is, in many respects, more complex than that of its arterial counterpart. With the exception of aneurysm formation, obstruction is responsible for virtually all the physiologic aberrations characteristic of arterial disease. Venous pathophysiology, on the other hand, involves both obstruction and valvular insufficiency. Moreover, the disability from venous disease includes not only regional problems but also those that result from the escape of thrombi into the pulmonary circulation. Together with the copious network of venous collaterals, the low pressure within the veins, the collapsible nature of the venous wall, and the intermittency of venous flow, these features provide a real challenge to the student of venous pathophysiology.

Despite these complexities, there is a growing body of sound information concerning venous physiology. Much of the progress in recent years has been due to the development of duplex scanning, which permits continued visualization of venous flow patterns; to the introduction of electromagnetic and Doppler flowmeters, which provide dynamic flow data; to the perfection of sensitive pressure transducers with high-frequency response; and to the use of newer plethysmographic methods.

The initial portion of this chapter is devoted to a brief review of basic venous hemodynamics. In the latter portion, pathophysiologic changes produced by venous obstruction and valvular incompetence are discussed.

NORMAL VENOUS HEMODYNAMICS

In order to understand pressure-flow phenomena in veins, it is necessary to review the effects of gravity on venous pressure, venous pressure-volume relationships, and the peculiarities associated with flow through collapsible tubes.

Venous Pressure

As discussed in Chapter 3, intravascular pressure is composed of dynamic pressure produced by the contraction of the left ventricle, hydrostatic pressure produced by the weight of the column of blood, and static filling pressure that is related to the elasticity of the vascular wall. Because this last pressure is probably less than 2 cm H$_2$O, it can be neglected for most purposes.[42]

Unlike in the arterial system, in which dynamic pressures are high, the dynamic component within the venous system is moderately low, hovering around 15 to 20 mmHg in the venules and falling to 0 to 6 mmHg in the right atrium. Consequently, in any position other than the horizontal, the hydrostatic pressure may greatly exceed the dynamic pressure. For practical purposes, hydrostatic pressure at any point below the right atrium can be estimated by measuring the distance from that point to the "phlebostatic axis." As described by Winsor and Burch, the phlebostatic axis is a point lying midway between the anterior and posterior surfaces of the trunk on a line passing transversely through the thorax at the level of the fourth costosternal junction.[160] For example, in a 6-foot-tall individual, the venous pressure at the ankle would be increased by 102 mmHg in the standing position (see Eq. 3.1):

$$\text{Hydrostatic pressure (mmHg)} =$$
$$\frac{1.056 \text{ gm cm}^{-3} \times 980 \text{ cm sec}^{-2} \times 131 \text{ cm}}{1333 \text{ dyne mmHg}^{-1}} =$$
$$102 \text{ mmHg}$$

If the pressure in the ankle veins were 15 mmHg in a supine position, it would be 15 + 102 = 117 mmHg in the standing position (Fig. 129–1). The intra-arterial pressure would increase by a similar amount.

Because there is an increased intravenous pressure, dilatation of the dependent veins occurs. This allows blood to accumulate in the veins of the leg. When a typical individual is tilted from a supine to an upright position, about 250 ml of blood is shifted to each leg.[121] This could produce syncope were it not for the effect of the muscle pump mechanism that ordinarily is operative in the upright position, as described later. Active venous constriction does not occur as a reflex response to orthostasis.[125]

At wrist level in the raised arm of an upright individual, the hydrostatic component would be decreased by about 50 mmHg. If venous pressure at the wrist were 15 mmHg in the supine position, the pressure at wrist level might be expected to fall below atmospheric pressure (15 mmHg − 50 mmHg = −35 mmHg). Obviously, this is impossible, because the combined effect of the tissue pressure (5 mmHg) and the atmospheric pressure would collapse the veins. Thus, venous pressure in a portion of the body above the heart cannot fall below tissue pressure (cf. Fig. 129–1).

Venous Pressure-Volume Relationships

Veins are collapsible tubes. This feature is responsible for the great variation in venous capacity that is possible with little change in venous pressure—a property that adapts veins to their unique role as the major storage facility for blood.

Transmural pressure is the difference in pressure between the intraluminal pressure acting to expand the vein and the tissue pressure acting from the outside to collapse the vein. When venous transmural pressure is increased from 0 to 15 mmHg, the volume of the vein may increase by more than 250 per cent.[99] This vast change in volume is due largely to the fact that the cross section of the venous lumen, which is elliptical at low transmural pressures, becomes circular at higher transmural pressures (Fig. 129–2).

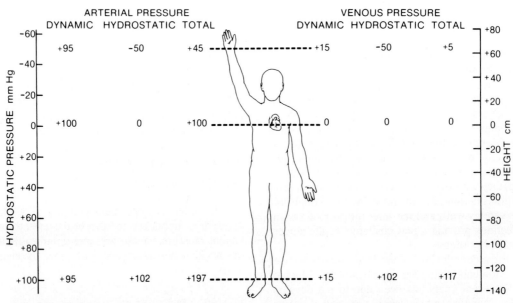

FIGURE 129–1. Effect of standing position on venous and arterial pressures. Zero pressure is at the level of the right atrium. Dynamic pressure represents that produced by the contraction of the left ventricle. If the subject were horizontal, the total intravascular pressure would closely approximate the dynamic pressure because there would be little hydrostatic effect.

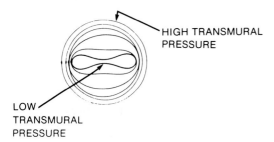

FIGURE 129–2. Cross section of venous lumen at various transmural pressures. At low pressure, the wall collapses into an elliptical configuration; at higher pressures, it becomes circular. Note that the wall also stretches with increasing pressure. (Adapted from Moreno AH, Katz AI, Gold LD, Reddy RV: Mechanics of distention of dog veins and other thin-walled tubular structures. Circ Res 27:1069, 1970. By permission of the American Heart Association, Inc.)

Little increase in pressure is required to convert a low-volume elliptical tube into a high-volume circular tube, but much more pressure is required to stretch the venous wall once the circular configuration has been reached. In fact, veins are as stiff as arteries when subjected to arterial pressure (Fig. 129–3).[9, 86, 99, 141]

Venous Blood Flow

Like fluid in all hydraulic systems, blood in the veins is propelled from one point to another by an energy gradient and is impeded by multiple factors that constitute resistance to flow. According to Bernoulli's principle, total fluid energy at any point in the venous system consists of the sum of the hydrostatic pressure, the gravitational potential energy, the kinetic energy, and the dynamic pressure produced by contraction of the left ventricle and the surrounding skeletal muscles (see Eq. 3.4). Because hydrostatic pressure and gravitational potential energy are equivalent but have opposite signs, they usually cancel each other; therefore, for most purposes it is sufficient to consider dynamic pressure as the driving force. For example, in the upright individual pictured in Figure 129–1, the energy gradient returning blood from the ankle to the heart is 15 mmHg (the dynamic pressure gradient), not 117 mmHg (the sum of the hydrostatic and dynamic pressures at the ankle). The situation is somewhat different in the raised arm. At wrist level, the pressure is only 5 mmHg (the

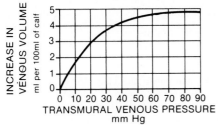

FIGURE 129–3. Relationship of venous volume to transmural pressure. Note that the veins are very compliant at low pressure but quite stiff at high pressure.

minimal value necessary to prevent collapse by tissue pressure), but the gradient returning blood to the heart is equivalent to about 50 mmHg because of the positive gravitational positional energy. In other words, blood in the elevated arm essentially "falls" back to the heart. As will be discussed later, a similar situation prevails in the legs when venous valves are incompetent.

Although veins are commonly considered to be low-resistance conduits, the energy gradient from the venules to the right atrium is equal to that from the left ventricle to the arterioles, approximately 15 mmHg. Because veins transport the same amount of blood as arteries and have a potential cross-sectional area three or four times as large, this seems somewhat incongruous. Veins, however, are seldom completely distended. The elliptical cross section assumed in their usual, partially collapsed state offers far more resistance than a circular cross section. As veins distend, their resistance falls markedly, allowing increases in blood flow to be accommodated with little increase in the energy gradient.

In the arterial system, pressure, vascular volume, and flow usually change in the same direction. In veins, the opposite frequently occurs: venous pressure and venous volume may decrease as flow increases and may increase as flow decreases or reverses (Fig. 129–4). This apparent paradox is explained by the fact that in the resting state, the peripheral venous pressure (P_{pv}) tends to remain relatively constant, whereas the central venous pressure (P_{cv}) fluctuates. When the central venous pressure falls, the pressure gradient across the intervening segment increases and—provided that the venous resistance (R_v) does not change appreciably—flow (Q_v) increases. At the same time, the pressure in the venous segment, which must lie somewhere between the peripheral and central pressures, will fall. Because venous volume is a function of venous pressure, the volume of the segment will also fall. In contrast, when the central venous pressure rises, pressure and volume increase while flow ceases or reverses. During exercise, however, contraction of the skeletal muscles momentarily increases peripheral pressure, and venous flow, pressure, and volume are simultaneously augmented.

Effect of Cardiac Contraction

The mechanism just described explains how venous flow and pressure are influenced by events occurring in the right side of the heart during the various phases of the cardiac cycle. As shown in Figure 129–5, contraction of the right atrium elevates central venous pressure and causes a transient reversal of venous blood flow. During ventricular systole, the atrium relaxes, venous flow increases, and venous pressure falls. Flow then decreases during diastole until the pressure differential across the tricuspid valve causes the valve to open. At this point, there is again a brief increase in flow, which is followed by a gradual decline to zero. Although these cardiac-induced flow and pressure pulsations are most easily perceived in the jugular veins, they may be detected with the Doppler flowmeter in the arm veins of resting subjects (Fig. 129–6). Cardiac pulsations are less evident in leg veins, where they tend to be obscured by the large fluctuations in flow produced by respiratory activity. In cases of congestive heart failure, the

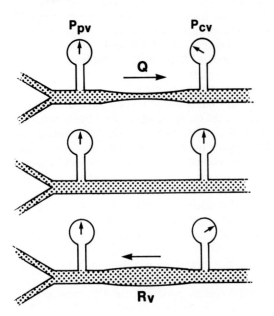

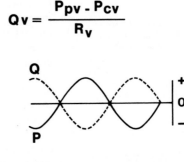

$$Qv = \frac{P_{pv} - P_{cv}}{R_v}$$

FIGURE 129-4. Relationship of flow (Q_v) in a venous segment to venous resistance (R_v), peripheral venous pressure (P_{pv}), and central venous pressure (P_{cv}). As flow increases, the vein collapses and pressure (P) in the mid-portion of the venous segment decreases. As flow decreases, the opposite occurs: pressure increases and the vein expands. Increasing pressure is indicated by a clockwise movement of the arrows on the meters. (From Sumner DS: Applied physiology in venous problems. *In* Bergan JJ, Yao JST [eds]: Surgery of the Veins. Orlando, FL, Grune & Stratton, 1985, pp 3–23.)

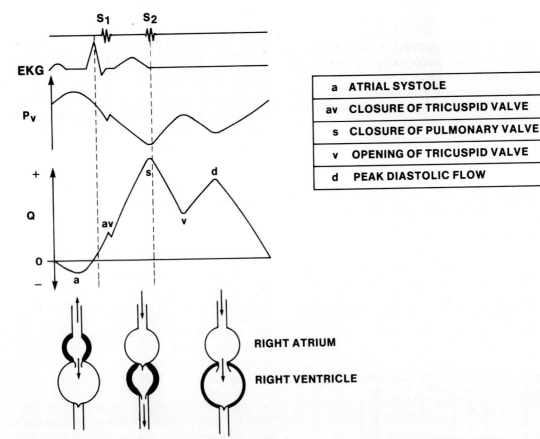

a	ATRIAL SYSTOLE
av	CLOSURE OF TRICUSPID VALVE
s	CLOSURE OF PULMONARY VALVE
v	OPENING OF TRICUSPID VALVE
d	PEAK DIASTOLIC FLOW

FIGURE 129-5. Effect of cardiac contraction on venous pressure (P_v) and venous blood flow (Q). *Vertical dashed lines* define the period of ventricular systole. First and second heart sounds are indicated by S_1 and S_2, respectively. (From Sumner DS: Applied physiology in venous problems. *In* Bergan JJ, Yao JST [eds]: Surgery of the Veins. Orlando, FL, Grune & Stratton, 1985, pp 3–23.)

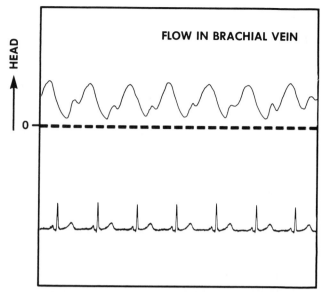

FIGURE 129–6. Doppler recordings of flow in a brachial vein demonstrating pulsations imposed by cardiac contraction. (From Sumner DS: Noninvasive vascular laboratory assessment. *In* Machleder HI [ed]: Vascular Disorders of the Upper Extremity. 2nd ed. Mt. Kisco, NY, Futura Publishing Company, 1989, pp 9–57.)

increased central venous pressure overcomes the respiratory effects, and cardiac pulsations become a prominent feature of the venous flow pattern in the lower extremities.

Flow Through Collapsible Tubes

The collapsible nature of the venous wall is responsible for a peculiar pressure-flow relationship unique to the venous system.[52, 66, 87, 88] These relationships are clarified by the model illustrated in Figure 129–7a. In this figure, the

energy (15 cmH$_2$O) driving blood back to the heart is represented by an elevated fluid reservoir. The collapsible tube passes through a closed container that has a certain pressure—in this case, 5 cmH$_2$O. The end of the tube, representing the right atrium, is open to the atmosphere at baseline level, giving an outflow pressure of 0 cmH$_2$O.

Pressure in the collapsible tube must rise until it slightly exceeds that within the closed container for the tube to open enough to permit fluid to flow through the system. Thus, flow through the tube depends on the gradient 15 cmH$_2$O − 5 cmH$_2$O = 10 cmH$_2$O, rather than on the gradient across the entire length of the tube, which would be 15 cmH$_2$O. It is evident that elevating the driving pressure will linearly increase the pressure gradient and, within limits, will have the same effect on flow (see Fig. 129–7b). On the other hand, changes in outflow pressure will have no effect on flow unless the outflow pressure rises above the pressure in the closed container, at which point the collapsible tube will remain distended (see Fig. 129–7c). Further increases in outflow pressure will decrease the pressure gradient (which now depends on the difference between the driving pressure and the outflow pressure). As a result, flow through the system decreases as the outflow pressure rises above the pressure in the closed container. Clearly, increasing the pressure within the container while the driving and outflow pressures are maintained at constant levels will decrease flow (see Fig. 129–7d).

Effect of Respiration

Respiration has a major effect on patterns of venous flow. In a supine subject, the abdominal cavity corresponds to the "closed container" through which the collapsible inferior vena cava must pass (Fig. 129–8). Thus, the pressure gradient driving blood centrally from the legs is the venous pressure in the legs minus the intra-abdominal pres-

FIGURE 129–7. (a) Model illustrating "collapsible tube" phenomenon. (b) Effect of elevating the driving pressure while maintaining container pressure and outflow pressure constant. (c) Effect of elevating outflow pressure while maintaining driving pressure and container pressure constant. (d) Effect of elevating container pressure while maintaining driving pressure and outflow pressure constant.

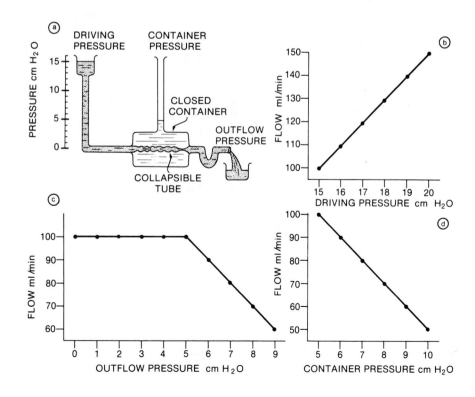

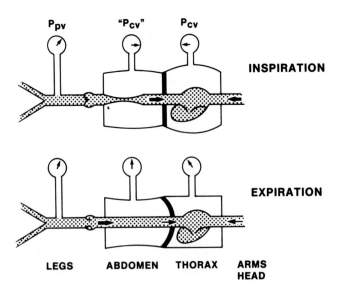

FIGURE 129-8. Effect of respiration on venous blood from the lower extremity, upper abdomen, and brachiocephalic area. Intra-abdominal pressure ("P$_{cv}$") increases during inspiration and decreases during expiration. (From Sumner DS: Applied physiology in venous problems. *In* Bergan JJ, Yao JST [eds]: Surgery of the Veins. Orlando, FL, Grune & Stratton, 1985, pp 3–23.)

sure. When the subject inspires, the diaphragm descends, thereby increasing intra-abdominal pressure. This has the effect of decreasing the pressure gradient and of decreasing blood flow during inspiration. Often, the rise in abdominal pressure is sufficient to cause venous outflow from the legs to cease momentarily (see Fig. 131–1). During expiration, the diaphragm relaxes, intra-abdominal pressure falls, the inferior vena cava expands, and blood trapped in the leg veins flows cephalad into the abdomen.

These patterns are so marked and so consistent that they constitute an important indicator of normal venous flow. Variations produced by venous obstruction are helpful in the noninvasive detection of venous thrombosis with the Doppler flowmeter and the phleborrheograph (see Chapter 131).

In considering flow from the upper extremities or from the head and neck, the high-pressure "closed container" becomes the extrathoracic tissue pressure and the "outflow" becomes the intrathoracic venous pressure (see Fig. 129–8). Because the latter ordinarily is lower than the former, respiratory movements have relatively less effect on outflow from the arms and cephalic regions. In general, venous flow increases during inspiration as the intrathoracic pressure falls and decreases during expiration as the pressure rises (see Fig. 131–2).

As one would predict from the closed container model (see Fig. 129–7), peripheral venous pressures do not reflect the central venous pressure accurately unless the latter is elevated. In cases of congestive heart failure, tricuspid insufficiency, or pulmonary hypertension, central pressures rise above tissue pressures and even above abdominal pressures, permitting events of the right side of the heart to be reflected in the peripheral venous flow pattern. As previously discussed, conditions that cause elevated central venous pressure result in a pulsatile flow pattern far distally in the veins of both the upper and the lower extremities.

VENOUS FUNCTION

The primary and most obvious function of the venous system is to return blood to the heart from the capillary beds. In addition, veins play the predominant role in regulating vascular capacity. They also serve as a part of the peripheral pump mechanism, which assists the heart in the transport of blood during exercise. Together with the capillaries, they contribute to the thermoregulatory system of the body.

These vital functions all depend on certain peculiarities of venous anatomy and wall structure, and on the presence of venous valves.

Anatomy and Wall Structures

Unlike arteries, veins are divided into a superficial and a deep system. Superficial veins are large, relatively thick walled, muscular structures that lie just under the skin. Among the superficial veins are the greater and lesser saphenous veins of the leg, the cephalic and basilic veins of the arm, and the external jugular veins of the neck. The deep veins, on the other hand, are thin walled and less muscular. They accompany arteries—often as venae comitantes—and bear the same names as the arteries they parallel. The cross-sectional area of these veins is roughly three times that of the adjacent artery.[34]

Within the skeletal muscles are large, very thin walled veins that are sometimes referred to as sinusoids. As part of the "bellows" of the muscle pump mechanism, they serve a particularly important function during exercise. The soleal sinusoids empty into the posterior tibial vein, and the gastrocnemius sinusoids usually drain into the popliteal.

In addition to the foregoing, perforating veins connect the deep and superficial systems. Of particular interest to the surgeon are a series of about six medial calf perforators that join the posterior tibial vein to the greater saphenous system through a network of superficial veins known as the "posterior arch vein."[134] Other perforators connect the peroneal vein with superficial tributaries of the saphenous vein. Posteriorly, a series of small perforating veins connects the superficial system with the intramuscular veins; these in turn are united at various levels with the posterior tibial vein. Thus, an indirect connection between the superficial and deep systems is provided via the large intramuscular veins.

Perhaps the most important anatomic feature of veins is the presence of valves (Fig. 129–9). Each of these delicate but extremely strong bicuspid structures lies at the base of a segment of vein that is expanded into a sinus. This arrangement permits the valves to open widely without coming into contact with the wall, thus permitting rapid closure when flow begins to reverse (within 0.5 seconds).[91, 151]

There are approximately 9 to 11 valves in the anterior tibial vein, 9 to 19 in the posterior tibial, 7 in the peroneal, 1 in the popliteal, and 3 in the superficial femoral vein. In two thirds of the femoral veins, a valve is present at the upper end within 1 cm of the inguinal ligament. About one quarter of the external iliac veins and one tenth of the

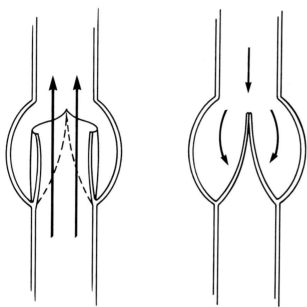

FIGURE 129-9. Representation of a longitudinal section through a venous valve demonstrating the role of sinuses in facilitating opening and closing of valve cusps. (From Sumner DS: Applied physiology in venous problems. *In* Bergan JJ, Yao JST [eds]: Surgery of the Veins. Orlando, FL, Grune & Stratton, 1985, pp 3–23.)

internal iliac veins have a valve.[76] The common iliac vein usually has no valves. Superficial veins have fewer valves—approximately 7 to 9 in the greater and lesser saphenous veins.[15, 57, 82] Valves are present in venules as small as 0.15 mm in diameter.

In all areas of the legs and arms, valve cusps are oriented to direct flow centrally and to prevent reflux. Although the classic teaching is that valves in perforating veins permit blood to flow only from the superficial to the deep venous system, studies have suggested that outward flow occurs in about one fifth of normal limbs under certain conditions.[126] There is also some controversy about the direction of flow in the perforating veins of the foot. Although previous investigators maintained that the foot is unique in that flow is directed from the deep to the superficial veins,[69, 74] studies by Koslow and DeWeese have suggested that the direction is consistent with that in other segments of the leg (i.e., from superficial to deep).[73]

During the course of the day, there may be some deterioration in valve function, even in normal extremities. About one fifth of otherwise normal legs show evidence of venous reflux after 5 or more hours of upright activity, presumably as a result of venous distention rendering the valves partially incompetent.[19]

Muscle Pump

The return of blood from the legs to the heart against the force of gravity is facilitated by the muscle pump mechanism. The muscles of the leg act as the power source, and the veins as the bellows. Although the superficial veins participate, the deep veins and the intramuscular sinusoids play the major role. The presence of competent valves is necessary to ensure that the pump functions efficiently.

In the motionless, upright subject, veins simply collect blood from capillaries and transport it passively to the heart, with the energy being supplied totally by left ventricular contraction. Because the venous valves are all open, the column of blood in the veins extends uninterrupted to the right atrium, and the venous pressure at any level equals the sum of the dynamic and hydrostatic pressures (Fig. 129–10A). During exercise, skeletal muscle contraction compresses the intramuscular and surrounding veins, raises venous pressure, and forces blood cephalad toward the heart. Closure of valves below the site of compression prevents retrograde flow (see Fig. 129–10B). On relaxation, the pressure gradient reverses: the valves above the site of compression close, precluding reflux, and the veins remain partially collapsed until they are refilled by inflow from the capillaries. Blood in the partially empty veins is now segregated into short compartments a few centimeters long, within which pressure is diminished in accordance with the venous pressure-volume compliance curve (see Figs. 129–3 and 129–10C).[116] (This segregation is seldom visible phlebographically because veins—even at the upper end of each compartment—remain partially filled. Figure 129–10C presents an exaggerated picture to emphasize the reduction in venous pressure.) After a few strong muscular contractions (such as in walking or running), venous pressure at the ankle or foot falls to very low levels in normal limbs, often below 20 mmHg (Fig. 129–11).[64, 65, 113, 139, 141] The level reached during exercise is commonly referred to as the "ambulatory venous pressure."

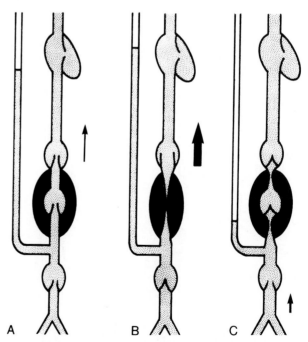

FIGURE 129-10. Operation of the muscle pump. *A*, Resting. *B*, Muscle contraction. *C*, Muscle relaxation. Venous pressure in the distal leg is indicated by the length of the hydrostatic column. (*A–C*, From Sumner DS: Applied physiology in venous disease. *In* Sakaguchi S [ed]: Advances in Phlebology. London, John Libbey and Company, 1987, pp 5–16. Reprinted by permission.)

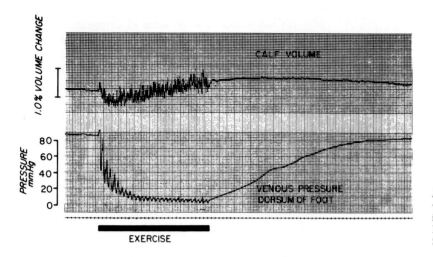

FIGURE 129–11. Effect of exercise on venous pressure at foot level in a subject 5 feet 8 inches tall. (From Strandness DE Jr, Sumner DS: Hemodynamics for Surgeons. New York, Grune & Stratton, 1975.)

Valves at the top of each segregated compartment remain closed until the venous pressure just below the valve rises to exceed the pressure at the lower end of the compartment immediately above. Thus, the pressure at the lower end of each compartment usually exceeds the length of the hydrostatic column defined by valve closure.[116] With continued venous refilling, the hydrostatic column is reestablished all the way to the heart.

The muscle pump mechanism is most highly developed in the calf, where the voluminous soleal and gastrocnemial sinusoids compose the major part of the bellows. Contraction of the calf muscles generates pressure in excess of 200 mmHg, a level high enough to compress the intramuscular veins even in the standing position.[81] Because of the strong fascial investment of these muscles, the intermuscular veins (posterior tibial, anterior tibial, and peroneal) are subjected to similar pressures. Much of the force is also transmitted to the surrounding superficial veins through the connective tissues. Thus, all the veins of the lower leg—both superficial and deep—participate to a greater or lesser degree in the pumping action. All transmit blood centrally with each muscular contraction (Fig. 129–12).[139]

Although pressure in the deep veins exceeds that in the superficial veins during muscle contraction, valves in the perforating veins prevent flow from the deep to the superficial system.[8] Valves also prevent the displacement of blood distally toward the foot in the tibial veins. When the muscles relax, the venous sinusoids are refilled by means of capillary inflow and by flow from the distal deep veins of the leg. Some inflow from superficial to deep veins also occurs, but the magnitude of this flow is less than formerly thought (see Fig. 129–12).[4, 139, 141] Studies suggest that the upward flow of blood in the leg may be initiated by compression of the plantar plexus of veins lying between the deep and superficial intrinsic muscles of the foot. This blood is discharged into the deep veins of the calf, thus priming the muscle pump.[73] The events during normal walking are synchronized in the following order: (1) dorsiflexion of the foot empties the distal calf veins, (2) weight bearing empties the foot, and (3) plantar flexion empties the proximal calf veins.[53]

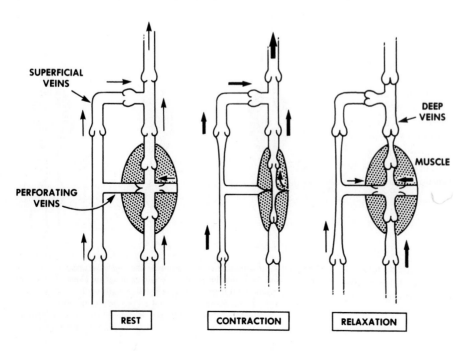

FIGURE 129–12. Dynamics of venous blood flow in response to calf muscle contraction in a normal limb. (From Sumner DS: Venous dynamics—Varicosities. Clin Obstet Gynecol 24:743, 1981.)

Effects of Venous Pressure Reduction

Reduction of venous pressure facilitates flow through the capillary bed of exercising muscles in the following manner. The total pressure in the peripheral arteries equals the sum of the hydrostatic pressure and the pressure generated by the left ventricle. For example, at the arteriolar end of a calf muscle capillary, the total pressure might be 102 mmHg (hydrostatic pressure) plus 95 mmHg (mean dynamic pressure), or 197 mmHg (see Fig. 129–1). During quiet standing, the venous pressure would be 102 mmHg (hydrostatic pressure) plus 15 mmHg (dynamic pressure), or 117 mmHg. This gives a pressure gradient across the muscle arterioles and capillaries of 197 minus 117, or 80 mmHg. With muscle contraction, however, the venous pressure will be reduced to 20 mmHg or less. Under these circumstances, the pressure gradient rises to 197 minus 20, or 177 mmHg. Together with the reduction in arteriolar resistance that accompanies exercise, this simple method of increasing the pressure gradient affords a remarkably effective way of augmenting muscle perfusion. Indeed, as much as 30 per cent of the energy required to circulate blood during strenuous exercise may be furnished by the muscle pump, which in a sense acts as a "peripheral heart."[139]

Aside from augmenting blood flow to exercising muscles, the muscle pump, by reducing venous pressure, acts to decrease the volume of blood sequestered in dependent parts of the body. Owing to the orthostatic elevation of hydrostatic pressure, assumption of a vertical position increases the volume of each leg by about 250 ml. In fact, as mentioned previously, the quantity of blood accumulating in the legs during quiet standing may be sufficient to precipitate syncope. By translocating blood from the peripheral to the central veins, the muscle pump also serves to enhance cardiac function, particularly during exercise.

In addition, reduction of venous pressure decreases the rate of edema formation in the dependent parts of the lower extremities. According to the Starling concept, most of the fluid escaping from the arteriolar end of a capillary is returned to the circulation at the venular end (Fig. 129–13).[21, 75, 138, 144] Any excess is removed by lymphatics. The forces acting to drive fluid out of the capillary are the capillary pressure, P_c, and the osmotic pressure of the interstitial fluid, π_{IF}. Acting to return fluid to the circulation are the interstitial fluid pressure, P_{IF}, and the osmotic pressure of the blood, π_c. Therefore, the net pressure P, moving fluid out of the capillary, is:

$$P = P_c + \pi_{IF} - P_{IF} - \pi_c \qquad (129.1)$$

As shown in Figure 129–13, the mean capillary pressure of +25 mmHg is exactly balanced by the sum of the other pressures ($\pi_{IF} - P_{IF} - \pi_c = +5 - 5 - 25 = -25$ mmHg).* Thus, in the supine position, there is little or no net pressure gradient across the capillary wall. However, this equilibrium is disturbed in the dependent parts of an upright individual. For example, if the mean capillary pressure, P_c, is assumed to be 25 mmHg at ankle level in a supine subject, it would rise to about 127 mmHg (25 + 102) in the standing subject (see Fig. 129–1). This creates a pressure gradient of $127 - 25 = 102$ mmHg across the capillary wall and encourages the outflow of fluid into the interstitial spaces. The escape of fluid continues until interstitial pressure, P_{IF}, rises sufficiently to balance the high intracapillary pressure. (The rate of fluid transfer is controlled by capillary surface area and permeability.[89]) Because the capacity of lymphatics is rapidly exceeded, a great deal of edema fluid must accumulate before a new equilibrium can be established.[58, 144]

Fortunately, if venous valvular function is normal, slight to moderate calf muscle activity will reduce the venous pressure markedly. In turn, mean capillary pressure will fall and the rate of edema formation will decrease. Together with arteriolar constriction, which occurs in response to standing, this mechanism keeps edema formation to a minimum.

In summary, the muscle pump serves several important functions: it assists the heart in circulating blood during exercise, increases central blood volume, relieves venous congestion in the legs, decreases peripheral edema, and facilitates flow through exercising muscles. Although these are not vital functions, their absence creates significant disability.

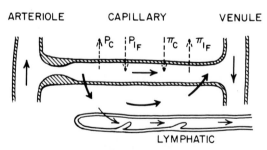

ARTERIOLE	CAPILLARY	VENULE

LYMPHATIC

Pressures (mm. Hg)

	Arteriolar	Mean capillary	Venular
P_C	35	25	15
P_{IF}	5	5	5
π_C	25	25	25
π_{IF}	5	5	5
P	+10	0	–10

FIGURE 129–13. Fluid exchange in the capillary bed. *Solid arrows* indicate the direction of fluid flow. *Dashed arrows* show the direction of pressure gradients. (From Strandness DE Jr, Sumner DS: Hemodynamics for Surgeons. New York, Grune & Stratton, 1975.)

---

*The magnitude of the interstitial fluid pressure (P_{IF}) has been the subject of considerable debate.[21, 144] Although originally P_{IF} was thought to range between +1 and +5 mmHg, most of the current evidence suggests that it is actually subatmospheric, on the order of −2 to −7 mmHg. Substituting these negative values for P_{IF} in Equation 129.1 gives a value of +13 to +18 for the intravascular pressure at the mid-point of the capillary (P_c). Thus, some of the numbers in Figure 129–13 and in the accompanying text will be changed; however, the basic concepts of transcapillary fluid exchange remain the same.

Total tissue pressure is the sum of the interstitial fluid pressure and the "solid tissue pressure" that is exerted by collagen and ground substance. If the structural elements responsible for solid tissue pressure are compressed, the solid tissue pressure will be positive. Consequently, total tissue pressure commonly ranges between +1 and +5 mmHg. It is this total tissue pressure that determines the transmural pressure across the capillaries and veins, as illustrated in Figure 129–1. Total tissue pressure and interstitial fluid pressure become equal when edema develops.

Control of Venous Capacity

About 75 per cent of the blood in the body is contained within the venous system. Even so, the total potential venous volume is far from filled. This means that some veins are always partially or completely collapsed. In a state of partial collapse, great fluctuations in venous volume are possible with little change in transmural pressure. This flexibility allows the normal venous reservoir to accept transfusions, intravenous fluids, and blood loss over wide ranges without changing the central venous pressure appreciably. Only when venous pressures are high and veins are filled will excess fluid result in large rises in central venous pressure. Similarly, a nearly empty system may be critically sensitive to sudden blood loss.

Venous capacity is affected not only by fluctuations in transmural pressure but also by the contractile state of the smooth muscle in the venous wall. When transmural pressures are low and veins have collapsed into an elliptical cross section, venomotor tone has little effect on venous capacity. On the other hand, when veins are filled sufficiently to assume a circular cross section, venomotor tone plays an important role in regulating venous volume.[107]

Unlike arterioles, which are very sensitive to the local chemical environment, venules and veins are controlled almost exclusively by sympathetic adrenergic activity. Also unlike arterioles and arteries, which are almost always partially constricted, the resting tone of veins is minimal under comfortable environmental conditions. Veins within skeletal muscles are devoid of sympathetic innervation, and cutaneous veins are primarily thermoregulatory.[84, 155] Peripheral veins contract more intensely to sympathetic stimuli than the more centrally located veins.

As a rule, veins constrict in response to stimuli that cause an increase in cardiac output.[132] Simultaneously, there usually is a decrease in total peripheral resistance. Because the systemic resistance to blood flow is largely controlled by arterioles, wall tension in veins must increase in conjunction with a decrease in arteriolar tone. Often this disparity of action is related to the vasodilator effect of the local chemical environment on the arterioles that overpowers the systemic adrenergic activity, but sometimes adrenergic activity is directly responsible for simultaneous arteriolar constriction and dilatation of the capacitance vessels.[25]

Among the stimuli known to produce venous constriction are pain, emotion, hyperventilation, deep breathing, the Valsalva maneuver, and muscular exercise.[133] The decrease in venous volume that occurs after a deep breath provides a convenient method for assessing the integrity of the sympathetic nerve supply to an extremity. As shown in Figure 65–7, the volume of a finger or toe, measured plethysmographically, will decrease promptly after a deep breath if the sympathetic nerves are intact.

By reducing the peripheral venous volume, venoconstriction during exercise assists the muscular pump mechanism in transferring blood to the central circulation, where it is required to maintain the increased cardiac output. Moreover, the reduced caliber of the veins serves to accelerate venous return. Although venoconstriction increases the hemodynamic resistance of the veins slightly, this effect is more than offset by the accompanying arteriolar dilata-

tion. The intramuscular sinusoids, which are devoid of sympathetic innervation, do not constrict with exercise.[133] Constriction of these veins would not be beneficial because they constitute the major bellows of the muscle pump.

Following hemorrhage, veins constrict both passively, in response to a decreased transmural pressure, and actively, as a result of increased venous tone. With prolonged shock, venoconstriction may give way to dilatation.

Cold causes veins to constrict both directly and as a general reflex response.[152] Although veins do not dilate in response to heat, heat negates the venoconstrictor response to deep breathing, exercise, or other such stimuli. The venous system is particularly important in the regulation of body temperature because superficial veins lie just under the skin, allowing easy transmission of heat from the interior of the body to the skin surface. Within this system, blood flow is slow, giving ample opportunity for the escape of heat. When conservation of heat becomes necessary, the superficial veins constrict, causing venous return to be diverted to the deep veins that lie in close proximity to the arteries. Not only is the distance to the skin surface increased by this reflex, but also the anatomic arrangement of the deep arteries and veins results in a countercurrent exchange of heat from artery to vein, thus further conserving heat from the interior of the body.

Curiously, venous constriction occurring in response to standing is at best slight and transient and is probably the result of emotional stimuli.[125] Teleologically, leg veins would be expected to constrict in the upright position in order to prevent dependent pooling of blood. Although reflex arteriolar constriction provides some protection against gravitationally induced fluid shifts, the major protection is provided by the muscle pump.

Veins constrict in response to epinephrine, norepinephrine, phenylephrine, serotonin, and histamine, and they dilate in response to phenoxybenzamine, phentolamine, reserpine, guanethidine, nitroglycerin, nitroprusside, barbiturates, and many anesthetic agents. Administration of isoproterenol sometimes appears to cause constriction, but at other times it results in dilatation.

ACUTE VENOUS THROMBOSIS AND THROMBOPHLEBITIS

Most venous thrombi are so limited in extent that they produce no recognizable clinical symptoms or signs and no overt physiologic defects. Many become evident only when pulmonary emboli appear; others cause pain and tenderness as a result of a local inflammatory reaction. When venous obstruction becomes sufficiently extensive, however, physiologic aberrations appear. The resulting changes, which are all related to an elevation in peripheral venous pressure, include venous congestion and edema. Rarely, shock results from fluid leaking into tissue spaces. In severe cases, the blockage may be so complete that ischemia occurs.

The magnitude of the peripheral venous pressure, P_{pv}, is related to the central venous pressure, P_{cv}; to the blood flow through the part, Q_v; and to the hemodynamic resistance of the intervening veins, R_v (Fig. 129–14):

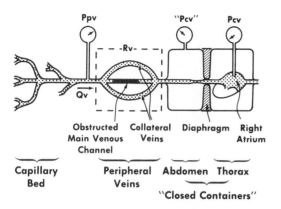

FIGURE 129–14. Major factors involved in venous return from the legs. See text for discussion. P_{pv}, peripheral venous pressure; "P_{cv}," intra-abdominal pressure; P_{cv}, central venous pressure; R_v, peripheral venous resistance; Q_v, venous flow.

$$P_{pv} - P_{cv} = Q_v R_v$$
$$\textit{or} \qquad\qquad (129.2)$$
$$P_{pv} = Q_v R_v + P_{cv}$$

This equation indicates that the peripheral venous pressure will rise when the central venous pressure rises. Ordinarily, central venous pressure is quite low, lower in fact than the intra-abdominal pressure. Therefore, in the usual case of a supine subject, P_{cv} can be taken to represent the intra-abdominal pressure. This is a manifestation of the collapsible tube phenomenon, in which the abdomen acts as a closed container and the intra-abdominal pressure determines the pressure at the central end of the venous segment (see Fig. 129–7). As discussed earlier in this chapter, the inspiratory descent of the diaphragm increases intra-abdominal pressure (P_{cv}), decreases blood flow temporarily, and then increases the peripheral pressure, P_{pv}, as blood flow rises to its preinspiratory level (Fig. 129–15). In congestive heart failure, pulmonary hypertension, or tricuspid insufficiency,

pressure in the right atrium may exceed intra-abdominal pressure; under these circumstances, peripheral venous pressure reflects central venous pressure.

An increase in blood flow (Q_v) can elevate the peripheral venous pressure. These increases are usually relatively minor and temporary, occurring, for example, during exercise. Because the venous resistance, R_v, normally is so low, little rise in peripheral venous pressure occurs (Eq. 129.2).

Thus, most significant increases in peripheral venous pressure are related to an increased hemodynamic resistance of the veins, R_v. Exercise may increase or decrease this resistance, depending on the adequacy of the venous valves or collateral channels. Unless a decrease in venous resistance accompanies exercise, the increased flow will result in an elevated peripheral venous pressure (Eq. 129.2).

Venous resistance depends on the location of the obstructed venous segments, the length of the obstructions, and the number of veins involved. The immediate effect of an acute venous thrombosis depends on the adequacy of the preexisting collateral channels. A thrombus that blocks large exit or reentry collateral veins will elevate the venous resistance more than one that occurs in an isolated venous segment. For example, a thrombus developing in the common femoral vein, where it blocks not only the superficial femoral vein but also reentry of the profunda femoris and saphenous veins (two of the major collaterals from the lower leg), will be more devastating than one isolated to the superficial femoral vein. Similarly, an extensive iliac vein thrombus that blocks cross-pelvic collaterals and the ascending lumbar vein is more restrictive than a thrombus confined to a small segment of the iliac vein. Other critical areas include the suprarenal inferior vena cava, the hepatic and portal veins, the right renal vein, the subclavian veins, and the superior vena cava.

In limbs with clinically "silent" deep venous thrombosis, it is doubtful that there is any perceptible elevation of venous pressure.[46] Measured at foot level, the average venous pressure in limbs of supine patients with acute phlebitis was found by Husni and colleagues to be 17 mmHg.[67] This was roughly 2.5 times that in normal limbs or in limbs with primary varicose veins (Table 129–1). There was essentially no difference in foot venous pressures between normal subjects and patients with acute phlebitis when they were standing quietly. This reflects the overwhelming contribution of the hydrostatic component, which tends to mask the slight pressure differences produced by the increased venous outflow resistance. On ambulation, however, the venous pressure in normal limbs dropped to about 40 per

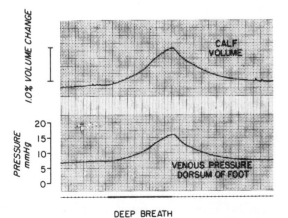

DEEP BREATH

FIGURE 129–15. Effect of a deep breath on the peripheral venous pressure and volume of the lower extremity. The simultaneous increase in pressure and venous volume is caused by a temporary increase in intra-abdominal pressure that interferes with venous outflow from the leg. Volume change was measured with a mercury strain-gauge. (From Strandness DE Jr, Sumner DS: Hemodynamics for Surgeons. New York, Grune & Stratton, 1975.)

Table 129–1. Venous Pressure at Foot Level

	Pressure (mmHg)*		
	Supine	*Standing*	*Ambulatory*
Control	7 ± 1	90 ± 7	35 ± 9
Varicose veins	7 ± 1	87 ± 5	56 ± 11
Acute phlebitis	17 ± 7	93 ± 4	90 ± 18
Postphlebitic	12 ± 5	90 ± 4	84 ± 16

Adapted from Husni EA, Ximenes JO, Goyette EM: Elastic support of the lower limbs in hospital patients—A critical study. JAMA 214:1456, 1970.
*Values are mean ± SD.

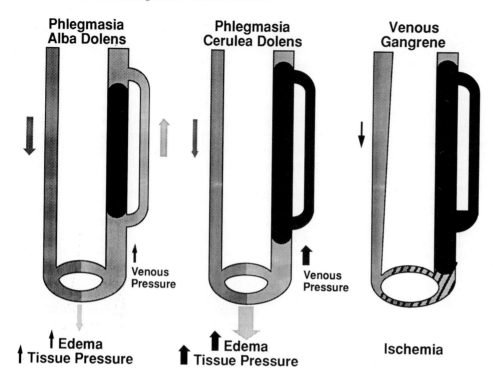

Phlegmasia Alba Dolens

Venous Pressure

↑ Edema
Tissue Pressure

Phlegmasia Cerulea Dolens

Venous Pressure

Edema
Tissue Pressure

Venous Gangrene

Ischemia

FIGURE 129–16. Pathophysiology of increasing severity of venous obstruction. In each diagram, arterial inflow is shown on the left and venous outflow on the right. *Black areas* indicate the location and extent of thrombus, which is confined to the major venous channels in phlegmasia alba dolens, involves collateral veins as well in phlegmasia cerulea dolens, and extends to the small veins and capillaries in venous gangrene. *Arrow size* indicates the magnitude of arterial and venous flow, venous and tissue pressure, and edema.

cent of the pre-exercise value but changed little in the limbs with acute phlebitis (see Table 129–1).

DeWeese and Rogoff found that venous pressures at foot level in supine patients ranged from 8 to 18 mmHg when clots were confined to the popliteal or below-knee veins.[41] Pressures were 20 to 51 mmHg when the clots were in the superficial femoral vein, and they were 32 to 83 mmHg (average, 50 mmHg) in the limbs with iliofemoral thrombosis. Similar values were reported by Ellwood and Lee.[46]

All veins subjected to increased transmural pressure dilate according to the venous pressure-volume curve and become less compliant, as shown in Figure 129–3. Superficial veins become more prominent, providing an excellent diagnostic sign of deep venous thrombosis. Sometimes this dilatation can so stretch the venous wall that valves fail to coapt properly, resulting in venous insufficiency. Reflux is, however, seldom an impressive finding in acute phlebitis.[124]

Another clinically very important result of increased venous pressure is the concomitant increase in mean capillary pressure. This upsets the Starling equilibrium (see Eq. 129.1), leading to the formation of edema. Even subclinical venous thrombi may produce minor swelling that can be detected by careful measurements of limb circumference. In fact, tenderness over the involved veins and unilateral limb swelling are the best clinical signs of acute venous thrombosis.

The degree of swelling is proportional to the elevation in venous pressure. DeWeese and Rogoff found swelling in only 70 per cent of limbs with popliteal or below-knee thrombosis, and in almost all cases this was less than 1 cm at the ankle.[41] On the other hand, swelling was present in 86 per cent of patients with femoral vein thrombosis and in all patients with iliofemoral thrombosis. The increase in circumference exceeded 1.0 cm at the ankle, 2.0 cm at the

calf, and 3.0 cm at the thigh in limbs with iliofemoral thrombosis.

Edema formation reaches truly massive proportions in phlegmasia cerulea dolens. In this dreaded condition, which is characterized by near-total thrombosis of all the veins in the involved extremity, together with ipsilateral iliac vein occlusion and obstruction of pelvic collateral veins, fluid loss may reach 6 to 10 L within 5 to 10 days.[60] This massive fluid loss reflects the tremendous elevation in venous pressure, which may reach 16 to 17 times normal values within 6 hours.[136] With the rapid formation of edema, tissue pressures attain values of 25 to 48 mmHg in 1 or 2 days.[23, 136]

Shock caused by fluid loss occurs in about one third of these patients.[22] In addition, a profound circulatory insufficiency develops, characterized by agonizing pain, cyanosis, decreased tissue temperature, absence of pulses, and often gangrene. The exact mechanism of this ischemia is uncertain, but it probably involves shock, increased venous outflow resistance, possible narrowing of the resistance vessels in response to the increased interstitial pressure, and edema (Fig. 129–16).[123, 141]

PRIMARY VARICOSE VEINS

Varicosities of the lower limb that develop spontaneously in the absence of deep venous thrombosis are referred to as "primary varicose veins." The greater saphenous vein and its tributaries are involved most frequently. Only about 12 per cent of primary varicosities are associated with the lesser saphenous system.[100]

The etiology of primary varicose veins remains uncertain. Theories include pressure exerted by incompetent perforating veins,[49] increased venous distensibility,[32, 44, 45, 119, 163]

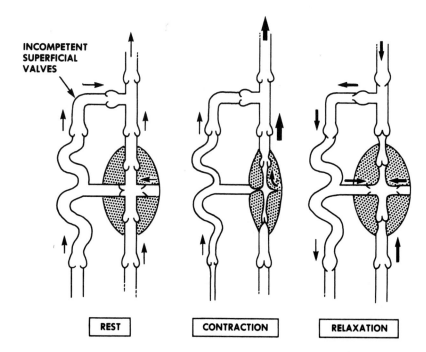

INCOMPETENT
SUPERFICIAL
VALVES

REST   CONTRACTION   RELAXATION

FIGURE 129-17. Primary varicose veins. Dynamics of venous blood flow in response to calf muscle contraction. During relaxation, flow is reversed in the saphenous vein and circular motion is established through the perforating veins. (From Sumner DS: Venous dynamics—Varicosities. Clin Obstet Gynecol 24:743, 1981.)

and increased blood flow through arteriovenous communications.[127, 128] Preexisting abnormalities of smooth muscle and endothelial cells in vein walls may also contribute to the formation of varicosities.[79] Although these factors undoubtedly play a role, much of the evidence seems to favor progressive descending valvular incompetence in response to congenital absence or incompetence of the common femoral and iliac valves.[50, 80, 83, 117] Under these circumstances, the saphenofemoral valve (lacking protection not only from hydrostatic pressure but also from episodic pressure increases caused by straining or coughing) becomes incompetent as the vein stretches. Once this valve becomes incompetent, the pressure is transmitted to the next lower valve in the saphenous vein, and so on down the leg. Finally, valves in the tributary veins also lose their competence. These subcutaneous veins then elongate, become tortuous, and present as typical varicosities.

Regardless of the etiology, the essential physiologic defect in varicose veins is venous valvular incompetence. Although the valve leaflets appear to be normal, they fail to coapt properly, perhaps because of the abnormally distensible nature of the venous wall.[35, 45, 147, 163] In the typical case, the iliofemoral valves, as well as all the valves in the greater saphenous vein, are either absent or incompetent.[50, 83, 117] Below the femoral level, deep venous valves remain competent.

In the supine position or during quiet standing, blood flow in varicose veins is quite sluggish but is directed in the normal cephalad direction (Figs. 129–17 and 129–18).[141] In addition, the pressure at ankle level is no different from that in limbs without venous incompetence (see Table 129–1).[67] However, when the upright subject with varicose veins begins to walk or otherwise contract the leg muscles, a different picture emerges. In this situation, blood flow reverses, flowing distally and quite rapidly toward the feet, as shown in Figures 129–17 and 129–18.[20, 50] Moreover, the fall in superficial venous pressure is much less than is normally seen (cf. Table 129–1).[67, 80, 114]

In response to calf muscle contraction, deep venous pressure drops markedly as a result of the effect of the muscle pump on the normally valved deep veins. Varicose veins also are partially emptied by the muscle contraction, but because of the lack of valvular protection, pressure within these superficial veins experiences only a moderate fall. Therefore, during calf muscle relaxation, a pressure gradient develops that causes blood to flow from the superficial system into the deep system via the perforating veins.[6] As a result, a "private circulation" or circular movement

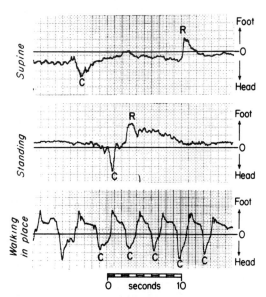

FIGURE 129-18. Blood flow in the greater saphenous vein in a patient with varicose veins. Calf muscle contraction (C) causes blood to flow toward the heart, whereas calf muscle relaxation (R) causes blood to reflux down the leg toward the feet. In the standing position, reflux flow greatly exceeds forward flow. Recordings were made with the Doppler probe pointed cephalad. (From Strandness DE Jr, Sumner DS: Hemodynamics for Surgeons. New York, Grune & Stratton, 1975.)

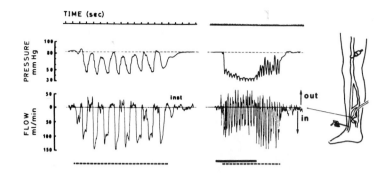

FIGURE 129–19. Flow in an incompetent perforating vein in an erect patient with varicose veins. During walking *(dashed lines)*, flow is directed "in," that is, from the superficial to the deep veins. Pressure in the greater saphenous vein is only slightly reduced. Occluding the greater saphenous vein with a "sling" ligature *(solid line)* causes flow in the perforator to seesaw "in" and "out" and causes the saphenous vein pressure to drop in a nearly normal fashion. (From Bjordal RI: Simultaneous pressure and flow recordings in varicose veins of the lower extremity. A hemodynamic study of venous dysfunction. Acta Chir Scand 136:309, 1970. Reprinted by permission.)

of blood is established in the exercising leg (see Fig. 129–17).[96] Blood pumped through the deep veins of the calf and thigh reaches the common femoral vein, where a portion reverses direction to flow distally down the functionally valveless saphenous vein. On reaching the lower parts of the leg, this blood returns to the deep system through the perforating veins, thereby completing the parasitic circuit (Fig. 129–19). During exercise, as much as one fifth to one quarter of the total femoral outflow may be involved in this circular motion.[20]

Surprisingly, this circular motion seems to have little effect on exercise tolerance.[5] Coupled with the chronically increased superficial venous pressure, however, it results in progressive distention and elongation of the superficial tributaries of the saphenous vein, producing unsightly varicosities.[137] Clinically, the increased pressure probably contributes to the heaviness and tightness of the lower leg experienced by some patients with varicose veins. Interstitial tissue pressures have been measured in patients with primary varicose veins and have been found to be raised.[112] Although superficial ulcers develop in response to the elevated tissue and venous pressures, they are never as severe as those associated with deep venous insufficiency and perforator incompetence.

Compressing the site of the leak—that is, the saphenofemoral junction—prevents reflux flow during exercise and

permits the muscle pump to return venous pressure to near-normal levels, as shown in Figure 129–19.[80, 154] This forms the physiologic basis for high ligation and stripping of varicose veins, the most effective means of treatment.[29] Elastic stockings afford similar protection.[67] The external pressure exerted by the stockings may force the venous valve cusps to come into contact, thereby restoring venous competence.[31]

CHRONIC VENOUS INSUFFICIENCY AND THE POSTPHLEBITIC SYNDROME

Physiologic abnormalities in chronic venous insufficiency consist of both venous outflow obstruction and valvular incompetence (Fig. 129–20). In the individual case, one or the other of the abnormalities may predominate.

As a rule, the obstruction that follows acute venous thrombosis tends to decrease with time. Some of the thrombi will be completely dissolved by the action of thrombolysins; others will become organized and recanalized to a variable extent. Most important, however, is the progressive enlargement of collateral venous channels, which carry an increasingly large proportion of the venous outflow. The overall effect of these processes is to reduce

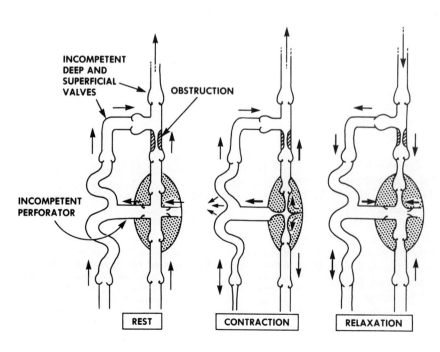

FIGURE 129–20. Chronic venous insufficiency, deep venous incompetence, and secondary varicose veins. Dynamics of venous blood flow in response to calf muscle contraction in a postphlebitic limb with residual deep venous obstruction, incompetent perforating veins, and secondary varicose veins. Note the to-and-fro motion of blood in incompetent perforating veins. (From Sumner DS: Venous dynamics—Varicosities. Clin Obstet Gynecol 24:743, 1981.)

venous resistance. Maximal venous outflow studies suggest that the average venous resistance in postphlebitic limbs is about 1.2 to 1.6 times normal. On the other hand, the resistance of postphlebitic limbs is only 0.3 to 0.6 that of limbs with acute thrombosis.[10, 12, 36, 59, 124] At rest, in the supine position, these small elevations in venous resistance usually cause the venous pressure to be elevated by only a few millimeters of mercury at ankle level.[67, 103] Ordinarily, no pressure elevation can be detected in the quietly standing individual (see Table 129–1).[40, 67]

Venous obstruction tends to subside with time, but venous valvular incompetence increases and is accompanied by progressive hemodynamic deterioration.[72, 90, 157] Organization of thrombi destroys the venous valves to a variable extent, leaving them incompetent.[43] The small high-resistance channels of recanalized veins, of course, are valveless. Dilatation of collateral veins and the remaining residual channels often prevents their valves from approximating, thus further aggravating the degree of venous incompetence. Plethysmographic studies all show that venous reflux is significantly increased in postphlebitic limbs and that most of the reflux occurs via deep veins rather than via dilated superficial veins.[11, 30, 124]

It is during exercise that the physiologic aberrations introduced by valvular incompetence and residual obstruction become most evident (cf. Fig. 129–20). When the calf muscles contract, blood is propelled up the leg in both the superficial and deep veins, much as it is in normal limbs. The temporary increase in flow exaggerates the effect of even a slight elevation of venous resistance and may actually cause the peripheral venous pressure to rise above resting levels during the phase of active muscle contraction (see Eq. 129–2). If the perforating veins are incompetent (which they often are), blood at high pressure is forced through these veins into the recipient subcutaneous veins. This in turn produces a local increase in capillary pressure.

When the muscles relax, incompetent valves allow blood to reflux down the leg, rapidly refilling the empty

Table 129–2. Change in Radioactivity of Leg Pumping Against Gravity (45-Degree Dependency)*

	Normal	Chronic Deep Venous Insufficiency
Number of legs	21	13
Degree of change (%)	− 20.5 (± 6.1)	− 10.2 (± 4.8)†
Time required (sec)	5.3 (± 2.0)	12.7 (± 7.9)†
Rate of change (%/sec)	−4.6 (± 2.1)	−0.9 (± 0.5)†

From Rutherford JB, Reddy CMK, Walker FG, Wagner HN Jr: A new quantitative method of assessing the functional status of the leg veins. Am J Surg 122:594, 1971.

Values are mean ± SD.

†Degree of significance of difference from normal: p <.001.

veins. (Reflux flow rates in limbs with stasis changes average 30 ml/sec and may reach 50 ml/sec.[153]) The hydrostatic column is reestablished, and peripheral venous pressure rises rapidly between contractions. As a result, the ability of the calf muscle pump to reduce ambulatory venous pressure is severely impaired (Fig. 129–21).[40, 63, 67, 154] The importance of the deep venous valves is illustrated by the fact that exercise induces a greater drop in venous pressure in limbs with isolated superficial venous incompetence than it does in limbs with chronic venous insufficiency (see Table 129–1). If, in addition to valvular incompetence, there is a significant element of venous obstruction, there will be almost no drop in venous pressure, and in some cases it may even rise.[7, 40, 63, 103] Because ambulatory venous pressure is the parameter that most closely reflects the hemodynamic function of the venous circulation, it is recognized as the gold standard for all tests of venous pathophysiology (see Chapter 133).

Owing to the rapid reflux of blood that occurs in the interval between calf muscle contractions and to the increased outflow resistance (which, when present, limits the quantity of blood displaced with each contraction), evacuation of the calf veins with exercise is less complete in limbs with chronic venous insufficiency than it is in normal limbs. The dependent veins, therefore, are perpetually in a state of partial congestion. Because the veins that constitute the bellows of the muscle pump are primed with an increased volume of blood, the amplitude of the pressure swing that accompanies each contraction of the calf muscle tends to be exaggerated in proportion to the severity of the postphlebitic process.[63, 64] In multi-level disease, the pressure swing may be two or three times that observed in normal limbs.

The efficiency of the venous pump is well demonstrated by radionuclide methods for estimating changes in local blood volume.[122] As shown in Table 129–2, limbs with chronic deep venous insufficiency are able to pump blood from the calf at only about one fifth the normal rate. After exercise, the volume reduction is approximately half that achieved in normal limbs. Air plethysmographic studies of limbs with venous valvular incompetence also confirm that an increased amount of blood is left in the calf after exercise. In accordance with the venous pressure-volume compliance curve (see Fig. 129–3), the quantity of blood remaining in the calf after a series of calf contractions divided by that present at rest in the dependent extremity

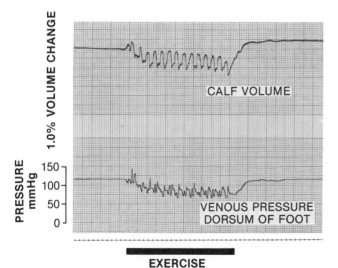

FIGURE 129–21. Effect of exercise on calf volume and venous pressure in a patient with chronic venous insufficiency. (From Strandness DE Jr, Sumner DS: Hemodynamics for Surgeons. New York, Grune & Stratton, 1975.)

(residual volume fraction) correlates well with the increased ambulatory venous pressure.[31, 157]

Adverse Effects of Venous Hypertension

Patients with proximal deep venous obstruction sometimes complain of a deep "bursting-type" pain in the leg during exercise. This pain, which has been called "venous claudication," is explained by the increased venous pressure and congestion that occur in response to the combination of exercise-induced hyperemia and increased outflow resistance.[148] The distal deep veins in these limbs are often radiologically normal, and valvular insufficiency is not a prominent feature.

In most patients with chronic venous insufficiency, symptoms related to valvular incompetence predominate. Clinically, the most significant functional abnormality is the inability of the venous pump mechanism to provide relief from orthostatic venous hypertension. Because pressure in the capillaries must exceed that in the venules and veins, capillaries in distal parts of legs with chronic venous insufficiency are chronically exposed to a high pressure when the patient is in an upright position. The elevated capillary pressure upsets the delicate balance between the intravascular and interstitial fluid and osmotic pressures, thereby increasing the rate at which fluid passes through the capillary wall (see Fig. 129–13). As long as the patient remains upright, edema continues to accumulate in the dependent parts of the lower extremity until tissue pressures rise sufficiently to restore the equilibrium. Because tissues are relatively compliant at low interstitial pressures, the limb may become quite edematous before a stable state is reached.[58]

Persistent venous hypertension causes elongation and dilatation of the cutaneous and subcutaneous capillaries and venules.[24, 47, 51] Blood flow in these dilated and engorged vessels is sluggish compared with that in normal skin.[2] The capillaries become hyperpermeable, permitting protein-rich fluid and red blood cells to escape into the subcutaneous tissues.* As the proteins become organized and the red blood cells disintegrate, the tissues become fibrotic and hyperpigmented, producing a condition known as lipodermatosclerosis.[27] Diffusion of oxygen into the tissues is restricted by the pericapillary accumulation of fibrinogen, causing localized hypoxia and malnutrition.[27, 48, 51] Venous hypertension also leads to leukocyte entrapment (neutrophils or T-lymphocytes and macrophages) in the dependent leg of patients with chronic venous insufficiency and may contribute to lipodermatosclerosis by acting as a source of oxygen free radicals and proteolytic enzymes.[146, 158, 159] Acting on this substrate, trauma (even a mild, often unrecognized injury) may lead to the death of tissue and the development of a chronic ulcer.

The frequency with which severe stasis changes and ulcers occur is related to the ambulatory venous pressure. Nicolaides and associates showed that the incidence of ulceration in limbs with ambulatory venous pressures exceeding 80 mmHg is about 80 per cent.[104, 105] On the other hand, ulcers seldom develop in limbs with ambulatory venous pressures of less than 30 or 40 mmHg (Table 129–3). Unless measures are taken to counteract edema formation, 50 per cent of limbs with edema present 1 year after an acute deep venous thrombosis will become ulcerated within 10 years.[14]

Stasis changes (induration, dermatitis, hyperpigmentation, and ulceration) are limited to the "gaiter area" of the leg, where hydrostatic pressures are high, and are typically worse on the medial aspect of the ankle just above and posterior to the medial malleolus. This distribution suggests that incompetent perforating veins connecting the deep system to the posterior arch vein play a major role in the etiology of stasis changes.[7, 33, 78] Although the precise mechanism remains controversial, the direct transmission of high-pressure impulses from deep veins to fragile superficial veins through incompetent perforators probably exacerbates the sequence of events described previously, leading to localized tissue hypoxia and nutritional deficits.[47, 141] The descriptive term *ankle blowout syndrome* was coined to emphasize the importance of incompetent perforating veins to the genesis of venous stasis changes.[33] Whatever the mechanism, ligation of incompetent perforating veins appears to decrease the likelihood that stasis ulcers, once they are healed, will recur.

Distribution of Valvular Incompetence: Relationship to Stasis Changes and Therapeutic Implications

The large number of valves in the infrapopliteal veins and the relative paucity of valves above the knee suggest that these structures have evolved to protect against hydrostatic forces imposed by the assumption of an upright posture. Certainly, the distribution of valves coincides with the hydrostatic pressure to which the veins are subjected. The concentration of valves in the lower leg also implies that they are of major importance to the muscle pump mechanism. Unlike venous pressure at the ankle, pressure in the popliteal veins falls very little with exercise and is essentially the same in postphlebitic limbs, in limbs with varicose

Table 129–3. Relationship Between Ambulatory Venous Pressure and the Incidence of Stasis Ulceration

Ambulatory Venous Pressure (mmHg)	Incidence of Ulcers (%)
≤ 45	0
45–49	5
50–59	15
60–69	50
70–79	75
≥ 80	80

Data from Nicolaides AN: Noninvasive assessment of primary and secondary varicose veins. In Bernstein EF (ed): Noninvasive Diagnostic Techniques in Vascular Disease. 2nd ed. St. Louis, CV Mosby, 1982, pp 575–586.

---

*A recent study, however, was unable to demonstrate that capillaries in the calves of patients with lipodermatosclerosis were more permeable than those in normal limbs.[131]

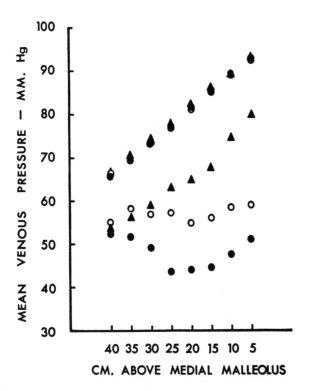

FIGURE 129-22. Pressure in the greater saphenous vein at 5-cm intervals down the leg, starting at the knee (40 cm) and ending at the ankle (5 cm). Symbols indicate normal limbs *(closed circles)*, limbs with minimal saphenous varices *(open circles)*, and limbs with gross saphenous varices *(triangles)*. Pressures at all anatomic levels are superimposed at rest *(upper points)*. Ambulatory venous pressures *(lower points)* are identical at the knee but are quite different at the ankle. (From Ludbrook J: Valvular defect in primary varicose veins, cause or effect? Lancet 2:1289, 1963. Reprinted by permission.)

veins, and in normal limbs (Fig. 129–22).[6, 65, 80] Moreover, venous refilling times (a measure of reflux) are often normal in patients with competent distal valves, despite the presence of popliteal venous valvular incompetence.[120] These and similar observations prompted earlier investigators to speculate that the absence of valves in the deep system above the knee may be less detrimental to venous function than the absence of valves below the knee.[6, 65]

Clinical findings and physiologic measurements are compatible with this thesis. Strandness and coworkers prospectively followed up a series of patients to investigate the long-term effects of deep venous thrombosis.[140] They found that 40 per cent of limbs with distal venous incompetence developed stasis pigmentation, whereas only 8 per cent of limbs with competent distal valves showed signs of chronic venous insufficiency. Moore and associates used Doppler ultrasonography to determine the distribution of incompetent valves in patients with symptoms and signs of chronic venous insufficiency.[98] Two thirds of limbs with severe stasis changes (ulcers, pigmentation, and induration) had incompetent valves below the knee (Fig. 129–23). In 23 per cent, the incompetence was limited to the infrapopliteal veins. Only 5 per cent had isolated incompetence of the proximal (superficial femoral or common femoral) veins, but another 9 per cent had incompetence limited to the proximal deep veins and saphenous veins. Almost identical findings were reported by Bruins-Slot and coworkers.[26]

Using duplex ultrasonography, van Bemmelen and colleagues found incompetence of the popliteal or the posterior tibial veins in 84 per cent of limbs with active or healed venous ulceration.[150] Although 60 per cent of limbs with no history of ulceration but a history of deep venous thrombosis had reflux in the popliteal veins, only 20 per cent had incompetence of the posterior tibial veins. In none of the patients with varicose veins and no history of stasis ulceration were the popliteal or below-knee veins incompetent. Approximately 80 per cent of the limbs in all three groups had incompetence of the common femoral or superficial femoral veins. Thus, there appeared to be a strong relationship between clinical manifestations of chronic venous insufficiency and the presence of distal venous valvular incompetence but no relationship with the presence of proximal venous valvular reflux.

Although in the experience of a number of investigators, incompetence confined to the superficial veins is relatively uncommon in patients with manifestations of chronic venous insufficiency (see Fig. 129–23),[98, 101, 120] superficial venous incompetence has been reported to be present in 17 to 78 per cent of limbs with concomitant deep venous insufficiency.[94, 98, 115] In most cases, these secondary varicose veins are probably not directly responsible for the adverse effects of chronic venous insufficiency. This interpretation, however, remains controversial because other investigators have found isolated superficial venous incompetence in 17 to 53 per cent of limbs with stasis ulceration.[61, 130] However, patients with massive, long-standing varicose veins are often asymptomatic and have normal skin and soft, pliable subcutaneous tissues in the gaiter area. This in itself is a strong argument against the theory that superficial venous incompetence alone is sufficient to cause stasis changes.

In a series of postphlebitic limbs, Shull and colleagues observed that elevated ambulatory venous pressure and stasis ulceration were closely associated with incompetence of the popliteal vein.[135] Popliteal vein incompetence was present in 75 per cent of limbs with stasis ulceration in a study reported by Hanrahan and associates.[61] Lindner and

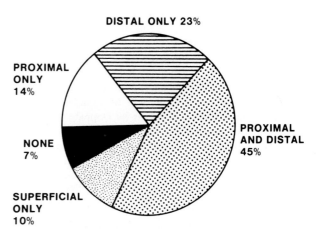

FIGURE 129-23. Distribution of venous valvular incompetence in limbs with stasis ulcers and pigmentation. (From Sumner DS: Pathophysiology of chronic venous insufficiency. Semin Vasc Surg 1:66, 1988.)

Table 129–4.   Postexercise Venous Recovery Time Versus Distribution of Deep Venous Valvular Incompetence

Location of Incompetent Valves*	Recovery Time (sec)†	Interpretation
Distal only	16.4 ± 14.0	Abnormal
Distal and proximal	14.1 ± 8.7	Abnormal
Proximal only	43.5 ± 26.8	Normal
No valvular incompetence	42.8 ± 22.4	Normal

Data from Gooley NA, Sumner DS: Relationship of venous reflux to the site of venous valvular incompetence: Implications for venous reconstructive surgery. J Vasc Surg 7:50, 1988.

  Distal: popliteal and below-knee veins; proximal: common and superficial femoral veins.

  †*Values are mean ± SD.*

coworkers found abnormal ambulatory venous pressures and shortened venous recovery times* in postphlebitic limbs with popliteal or posterior tibial venous incompetence.[77] Competence or incompetence of the superficial femoral veins bore no relationship either to clinical signs or to hemodynamic abnormalities. These observations were substantiated by Gooley and Sumner.[56] Whereas the postexercise recovery times of limbs with isolated proximal venous incompetence were delayed (greater than 20 seconds), indicating that most had normal venous dynamics, the postexercise recovery times of limbs with incompetence limited to the below-knee veins or with both proximal and distal incompetence tended to be quite short (less than 20 seconds), suggesting the presence of significant reflux (Table 129–4). Although shortened recovery times were also observed when incompetence was limited to the saphenous veins, the venous dynamics in these limbs were normalized by the application of a tourniquet. As expected, rapid recovery times were associated with the most marked stasis changes (Table 129–5). Pearce and associates, in a similar study, found venous refilling times to be abnormal in limbs with calf vein disease, despite the presence of competent femoral valves.[111] They concluded that the ''postphlebitic syndrome is chiefly a result of diseased popliteal and calf veins.'' More recently, Rosfors and colleagues, using Doppler studies, plethysmography, and foot volumetry, found the function of valves in the distal deep veins at ankle level to be clinically more important that that of valves within the popliteal or proximal calf veins in determining the stage of chronic venous insufficiency.[120]

In contrast, isolated proximal venous valvular incompetence appears to be a relatively benign condition. About 15 per cent of normal limbs and the majority of limbs with primary saphenous varicosities will be found to have incompetent common femoral valves by Doppler ultrasonography; however, cutaneous manifestations of venous insufficiency are rarely seen.[50, 117] Furthermore, venous reflux to the popliteal level may be seen during retrograde phlebography in clinically normal limbs.[145]

A mechanism explaining how the location of venous

valvular incompetence may affect ambulatory venous pressure is proposed in Figure 129–24. In normal limbs and in limbs with competent distal but incompetent proximal valves, venous pressures at the ankle are low after exercise because the column of blood extends only to the first competent valve, which will be located well below the knee.* However, when the proximal valves are competent but the distal valves are incompetent, the postexercise column is relatively long, extending almost the entire length of the leg. Consequently, ambulatory venous pressures are high, and in the event that the perforating veins are also incompetent, the superficial veins are rapidly refilled, even though their valves may remain competent. When both proximal and distal valves are incompetent, the ankle veins are subjected to the weight of an uninterrupted column of blood extending to the heart, there is little reduction in ambulatory venous pressure, and reflux into the superficial system via incompetent perforating veins is accelerated. Although superficial veins in limbs with superficial venous incompetence are rapidly refilled following exercise, external compression or removal of the saphenous veins will relieve venous hypertension as long as the deep valves are competent.

Because venous valvular incompetence is ultimately responsible for stasis changes in the skin and subcutaneous tissues, it seems logical that restoration of normal valve function should correct the pathophysiologic abnormalities and afford the optimal treatment for this disease. Superficial femoral venous valvuloplasty, transposition of a competent segment of vein into the proximal deep venous system, and autotransplantation of valve-containing venous segments into the superficial femoral or popliteal vein are among the ingenious operations that have been devised for this purpose (see Chapter 139). The rationale for all of these procedures is based on the assumption that a single competent valve placed at or above the popliteal level in an otherwise incompetent system will alleviate ambulatory venous hypertension and allow ulcers to heal. Although clinical results have been encouraging, it is difficult to determine whether the beneficial effects are due to the surgical reconstruction or to ancillary measures, such as better skin care, elastic support, saphenous vein stripping, or perforator ligation. Few studies provide objective evidence of improved venous dynamics.[38, 70, 109, 115, 129, 143, 156] Some tests of venous function may improve, whereas others do not. O'Donnell and colleagues, for example, found that venous emptying and refilling times (both measurements of valvular function) remained abnormal and unchanged following successful valve transplantation to the popliteal area.[109] Although Gillespie and associates found that popliteal vein transplantation lessened (but did not normalize) the rate of venous reflux, the volume of blood ejected with calf contraction and that remaining in the calf after contraction were essen-

---

*Because venous volume depends on venous pressure (see Fig. 129–3), postexercise plethysmographic tracings are roughly correlated with ambulatory venous pressure, and the time required for both the venous volume and the venous pressure to return to baseline levels after cessation of exercise is almost identical.[1, 106]

---

*As pointed out earlier in this chapter, this is admittedly an oversimplification, because venous pressure in each segregated compartment is determined not only by the length of the hydrostatic column but also by venous compliance and the residual content of blood.[116] Therefore, pressures at the lower end of each compartment may correspond to a hydrostatic column that extends several centimeters above the closed valve located at the proximal end of the compartment. The message, however, is unaltered by this simplification.

Table 129–5. Postexercise Venous Recovery Time Versus Clinical Signs in Postphlebitic Limbs

Signs	Recovery Time (sec)*	Limbs Abnormal (%)
Ulcer, pigmentation	10 ± 7	87
Edema only	26 ± 23	48
None	37 ± 24	27
Varicose veins		
Present	21 ± 19	68
Absent	39 ± 25	21

Data from Gooley NA, Sumner DS: Relationship of venous reflux to the site of venous valvular incompetence: Implications for venous reconstructive surgery. J Vasc Surg 7:50, 1988.

Values are mean ± SD.

tially unchanged.[54] These results, together with the evidence that the manifestations of chronic venous insufficiency are largely related to distal deep venous incompetence, raise questions regarding the actual efficacy of proximal venous valvular reconstruction.

On the basis of the analysis depicted in Figure 129–24, restoration of proximal venous valvular function would be unnecessary in limbs with competent distal valves and would afford little relief from ambulatory venous hypertension in limbs with concomitant distal venous incompetence. Stripping of incompetent superficial veins would be effective only when the distal deep veins are competent.[29, 39, 61, 94] On the other hand, simple measures, such as the use of elastic stockings or Unna boots, often prevent the development or progression of stasis changes.[31, 93]

Although elastic compression stockings are acknowledged to be quite effective in preventing and treating the cutaneous and subcutaneous manifestations of chronic venous insufficiency, the mechanism of their action remains obscure. That they reduce edema by increasing interstitial fluid pressure (see Eq. 129.1) is well substantiated;[102] but edema alone, although obviously contributory, is not sufficient to cause stasis ulcers. Patients with chronic edema due to congestive heart failure and patients with lymphedema do not develop these skin changes.[28] One theory is that stockings compress distal veins, decrease their volume, assist venous return, and reduce ambulatory venous pressure.[31] The time required for veins to refill after partial evacuation may also be prolonged.[110] Other investigators, however, have been unable to demonstrate that stockings have any effect on ambulatory venous pressure or venous reflux, even when they are clinically effective.[92]

PREGNANCY

When a woman in the third trimester of pregnancy lies on her back, the enlarged uterus tends to compress the inferior vena cava and the common iliac veins.[71, 142] As a result, venous pressure is increased in the legs and venous flow patterns become less responsive to respiration.[68, 95] Interference with venous return reduces cardiac output, sometimes to the extent that hypotension develops.[149] All these effects are relieved by turning the patient to her side, which allows the uterus to roll away from the pelvic veins.

Early in pregnancy, well before the uterus enlarges

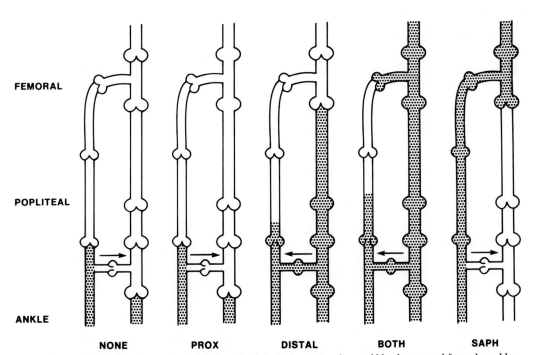

FIGURE 129–24. Comparison of the length of the hydrostatic column of blood measured from the ankle after exercise *(stippled area)* in limbs with no valvular incompetence (none), incompetence limited to the proximal deep veins (prox), incompetence limited to the distal deep veins (distal), incompetence of both proximal and distal deep veins (both), and incompetence limited to the superficial veins (saph). In each diagram, saphenous veins are on the left and deep veins are on the right. *Arrows* indicate the direction of flow in perforating veins. (From Gooley NA, Sumner DS: Relationship of venous reflux to the site of venous valvular incompetence: Implications for venous reconstructive surgery. J Vasc Surg 7:50, 1988.)

significantly, humoral factors cause the veins to become more compliant.[13] Together with the increased venous pressure that occurs later in gestation, these cause significant venous distention. Because of these factors, the velocity of blood flow in the leg veins gradually decreases as pregnancy progresses.

Although pregnancy does not cause varicose veins, the increased pressure and venous distensibility exaggerate predisposing factors. Consequently, varicose veins often first appear during pregnancy and become more severe with subsequent pregnancies. In addition, the sluggish venous flow probably contributes to the development of deep venous thrombosis.

SURGICAL VENOUS INTERRUPTION

Experimentally, ligation of the inferior vena cava causes transient decreases in cardiac output and blood pressure as a result of acute pooling of blood distal to the ligature.[17, 62] Ordinarily, these changes are short-lived because of the rapid dilatation of preexisting venous collaterals.[16] Similarly, vena caval ligation usually is well tolerated in humans.[108] However, hypotension, oliguria, and death are occasionally reported in patients with limited cardiac reserve.[55]

Ligation of the inferior vena cava causes an immediate rise in pressure distal to the ligature. In one study, this rise averaged about 13 mmHg. Plication (or clipping), however, raised the venous pressure by only 1 mmHg.[97] Consequently, acute complications of plication are usually less than with ligation because there is less interference with venous return.[3, 97] Filters of the Greenfield variety, on the other hand, cause little or no obstruction unless they become occluded with a large embolus.

Chronic effects of venous interruption are similar to the sequelae seen in postphlebitic limbs. They are all due to the physiologic effects of venous obstruction. There is no appreciable difference in the incidence of these complications between vena caval ligation and plication procedures, averaging about 15 per cent in both. Although plication causes fewer immediate effects than ligation, about 35 per cent of the plications eventually become occluded.[18] However, complications are probably less related to the vena caval obstruction than they are to preexisting venous thrombosis in the lower limbs.

Objective studies of vena caval ligation have shown that peripheral venous pressures may remain elevated for several months, despite collateral development.[17, 37] This obstruction has little effect in the resting state, but it may cause significant pressure elevations during exercise.[40] Venous outflow studies show that plication also causes some physiologic obstruction.[85]

Ligation of the femoral vein causes a prompt rise in peripheral venous pressure and a significant decrease in femoral artery flow (Fig. 129–25).[161] Although most of this initial resistance to blood flow can be attributed to an increase in venous outflow resistance, an appreciable portion may be due to reflex constriction of arterioles.[141, 162] This information may be pertinent to the treatment of combined

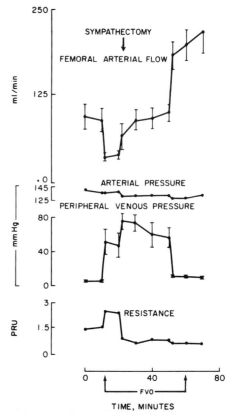

FIGURE 129–25.   Effect of femoral vein occlusion (FVO) followed by lumbar sympathectomy on hemodynamics in the canine hindlimb. Peripheral venous pressure was measured from the saphenous vein. Note that occlusion results in a fall in femoral arterial blood flow, a prompt rise in peripheral venous pressure, and a rise in total limb resistance (PRU). Sympathectomy increases femoral flow without changing the peripheral venous pressure appreciably, suggesting that the resistance change occurred primarily in the arterioles or venules rather than in the larger venous collaterals. (From Wright CB, Sayre JT, Casterline PI, Swan KG: Hemodynamic effects of sympathectomy in canine femoral venous occlusion. Surgery 74:405, 1973.)

trauma to arteries and veins. Although collateral development rapidly alleviates much of the venous outflow obstruction, in the initial period following reconstructive surgery the patency of the arterial repair may be jeopardized if the accompanying vein is ligated.[118]

Selected References

Alexander RS: The peripheral venous system. *In* Hamilton WF, Dow P (eds): Handbook of Physiology. Washington, DC, American Physiological Society, 1963, vol. II, pp 1075–1098.

Bergan JJ, Goldman MP (eds): Varicose Veins and Telangiectasias. St. Louis, Quality Medical Publishing, 1993.

Bergan JJ, Yao JST: Venous Disorders. Philadelphia, WB Saunders, 1991.

Browse NL, Burnand KG, Thomas ML: Diseases of the Veins: Pathology, Diagnosis and Treatment. London, Edward Arnold, 1988.

Dodd H, Cockett FB: The Pathology and Surgery of the Veins of the Lower Limb. 2nd ed. Edinburgh, Churchill Livingstone, 1976.

Gauer OH, Thron HL: Postural changes in the circulation. *In* Hamilton WF, Dow P (eds): Handbook of Physiology. Washington, DC, American Physiological Society, 1963, vol. III, pp 2409–2439.

Gottlob R, May R: Venous Valves: Morphology, Function, Radiology, Surgery. Wien, Springer-Verlag, 1986.

Guyton AC: Venous return. *In* Hamilton WF, Dow P (eds): Handbook of Physiology. Washington, DC, American Physiological Society, 1963, vol. II, pp 1099–1133.

Guyton AC, Taylor AE, Granger HJ: Circulatory Physiology II: Dynamics and Control of the Body Fluids. Philadelphia, WB Saunders, 1975.

Johnson HD, Pflug J: The Swollen Leg: Causes and Treatment. Philadelphia, JB Lippincott, 1975.

Ludbrook J: Aspects of Venous Function in the Lower Limbs. Springfield, IL, Charles C Thomas, 1966.

Shepherd JT: Role of the veins in the circulation. Circulation 33:484, 1966.

Strandness DE Jr, Sumner DS: Hemodynamics for Surgeons. New York, Grune & Stratton, 1975.

Strandness DE Jr, Thiele BL: Selected Topics in Venous Disorders. Pathophysiology, Diagnosis, and Treatment. Mount Kisco, NY, Futura Publishing, 1981.

References

1. Abramowitz HB, Queral LA, Flinn WR, et al: The use of photoplethysmography in the assessment of venous insufficiency: A comparison to venous pressure measurements. Surgery 86:434, 1979.
2. Abu-Own AA, Scurr JH, Coleridge Smith PD: Assessment of microangiopathy of the skin in chronic venous insufficiency by laser Doppler fluxmetry [Abstract]. J Vasc Surg 17:429, 1993.
3. Adams JT, Feingold BE, DeWeese JA: Comparative evaluation of ligation and partial interruption of the inferior vena cava. Arch Surg 103:272, 1971.
4. Almén T, Nylander G: Serial phlebography of the normal lower leg during muscular contraction and relaxation. Acta Radiol 57:264, 1962.
5. Arenander E: Hemodynamic effects of varicose veins and results of radical surgery. Acta Chir Scand 260(Suppl):1, 1960.
6. Arnoldi CC: Venous pressure in patients with valvular incompetence of the veins of the lower limb. Acta Chir Scand 132:628, 1966.
7. Arnoldi CC, Linderholm H: On the pathogenesis of the venous leg ulcer. Acta Chir Scand 134:427, 1968.
8. Arnoldi CC, Linderholm H: Venous blood pressures in the lower limb at rest and during exercise in patients with idiopathic dysfunction of the venous pump of the calf. Acta Chir Scand 135:601, 1969.
9. Attinger EO: Wall properties of veins. IEEE Trans Biomed Eng 16:253, 1969.
10. Barnes RW, Collicott PE, Mozersky DJ, et al: Noninvasive quantitation of maximum venous outflow in acute thrombophlebitis. Surgery 72:971, 1972.
11. Barnes RW, Collicott PE, Mozersky DJ, et al: Noninvasive quantitation of venous reflux in the postphlebitic syndrome. Surg Gynecol Obstet 136:769, 1973.
12. Barnes RW, Collicott PE, Mozersky DJ, et al: Noninvasive quantitation of venous hemodynamics in postphlebitic syndrome. Arch Surg 107:807, 1973.
13. Barwin BN, Roddie IC: Venous distensibility during pregnancy determined by graded venous congestion. Am J Obstet Gynecol 125:921, 1976.
14. Bauer A: A roentgenological and clinical study of the sequels of thrombosis. Acta Chir Scand 86(Suppl 74):1, 1942.
15. Beecher HK, Field ME, Krogh A: The effect of walking on the venous pressure at the ankle. Skand Arch Physiol 73:133, 1936.
16. Beltz WR, Condon RE: Influence of level of ligation on the results of vena caval interruption. Surg Gynecol Obstet 133:257, 1971.
17. Benavides J, Noon R: Experimental evaluation of inferior vena cava procedures to prevent pulmonary embolism. Ann Surg 166:195, 1967.
18. Bernstein EF: The place of venous interruption in the treatment of pulmonary thromboembolism. *In* Moser KM, Stein M (eds): Pulmonary Thromboembolism. Chicago, Year Book Medical Publishers, 1973, pp 312–323.
19. Bishara RA, Sigel B, Rocco K, et al: Deterioration of venous function in normal lower extremities during daily activity. J Vasc Surg 3:700, 1986.
20. Bjordal RI: Simultaneous pressure and flow recordings in varicose veins of the lower extremity. A hemodynamic study of venous dysfunction. Acta Chir Scand 136:309, 1970.
21. Brace RA: Progress toward resolving the controversy of positive vs. negative interstitial fluid pressure. Circ Res 49:281, 1981.
22. Brockman SK, Vasko JS: Phlegmasia cerulea dolens. Surg Gynecol Obstet 121:1347, 1965.
23. Brockman SK, Vasko JS: The pathologic physiology of phlegmasia cerulea dolens. Surgery 59:997, 1966.
24. Browse NL: The pathogenesis of venous ulceration: A hypothesis. J Vasc Surg 7:468, 1988.
25. Browse NL, Shepherd JT: Differences in response of veins and resistance vessels in limbs to same stimulus. Am J Physiol 211:1241, 1966.
26. Bruins-Slot H, Vermeiden I, van Dam R: The detection of deep venous incompetence in 980 legs using the Doppler in combination with a spectral analyser. Presented at the Second International Vascular Symposium, London, 1986, abstract 511.2.
27. Burnand KG, Whimster I, Naidoo A, et al: Pericapillary fibrin in the ulcer-bearing skin of the leg: The cause of lipodermatosclerosis and venous ulcerations. Br Med J 285:1071, 1982.
28. Chant ADB: Hypothesis: Why venous oedema causes ulcers and lymphoedema does not. Eur J Vasc Surg 6:427, 1992.
29. Christopoulos D, Nicolaides AN, Galloway JMD, Wilkinson A: Objective noninvasive evaluation of venous surgical results. J Vasc Surg 8:683, 1988.
30. Christopoulos D, Nicolaides AN, Szendro G: Venous reflux: Quantification and correlation with the clinical severity of chronic venous disease. Br J Surg 75:352, 1988.
31. Christopoulos DG, Nicolaides AN, Szendro G, et al: Air-plethysmography and the effect of elastic compression on venous hemodynamics of the leg. J Vasc Surg 5:148, 1987.
32. Clarke GH, Vasdekis SN, Hobbs JT, Nicolaides AN: Venous wall function in the pathogenesis of varicose veins. Surgery 111:402, 1992.
33. Cockett FB, Jones DEE: The ankle blowout syndrome, a new approach to the varicose ulcer problem. Lancet 1:17, 1953.
34. Conrad MC: Functional Anatomy of the Circulation to the Extremities. Chicago, Year Book Medical Publishers, 1971.
35. Cotton LT: Varicose veins, gross anatomy and development. Br J Surg 48:549, 1961.
36. Dahn I, Eiriksson E: Plethysmographic diagnosis of deep venous thrombosis of the leg. Acta Chir Scand 398(Suppl):33, 1968.
37. Dale WA: Ligation of the inferior cava for thromboembolism. Surgery 43:24, 1958.
38. Dalsing MC, Lalka SG, Unthank JL, et al: Venous valvular insufficiency: Influence of a single venous valve (native and experimental). J Vasc Surg 14:576, 1991.
39. Darke SG, Penfold C: Venous ulceration and saphenous ligation. Eur J Vasc Surg 6:4, 1992.
40. DeCamp PT, Schramel RJ, Roy CJ, et al: Ambulatory venous pressure determinations in postphlebitic and related syndromes. Surgery 29:44, 1951.
41. DeWeese JA, Rogoff SM: Phlebographic patterns of acute deep venous thrombosis of the leg. Surgery 53:99, 1963.
42. Duomarco JL, Rimini R: Venous pressure of man in space. Aerosp Med 41:175, 1970.
43. Edwards EA, Edwards JE: The effect of thrombophlebitis on the venous valve. Surg Gynecol Obstet 65:310, 1937.
44. Edwards JE, Edwards EA: The saphenous valves in varicose veins. Am Heart J 19:338, 1940.
45. Eiriksson E, Dahn L: Plethysmographic studies of venous distensibility in patients with varicose veins. Acta Chir Scand 398 (Suppl):19, 1968.
46. Ellwood RA, Lee WB: Pedal venous pressure: Correlation with presence and site of deep-venous abnormalities. Radiology 131:73, 1979.
47. Fagrell B: Local microcirculation in chronic venous incompetence and leg ulcers. Vasc Surg 13:217, 1979.
48. Falanga V, Moosa HH, Nemeth AJ, et al: Dermal pericapillary fibrin in venous disease and venous ulceration. Arch Dermatol 123:620, 1987.
49. Fegan WG, Kline AL: The cause of varicosity in superficial veins of the lower limb. Br J Surg 59:798, 1972.
50. Folse R: The influence of femoral vein dynamics on the development of varicose veins. Surgery 68:974, 1970.
51. Franzeck UK, Bollinger A, Huch R, et al: Transcutaneous oxygen tension and capillary morphologic characteristics and density in patients with chronic venous incompetence. Circulation 70:806, 1984.
52. Fry DL, Thomas LJ, Greenfield JC Jr: Flow in collapsible tubes. *In* Patel DJ, Vaishnav RN (eds): Basic Hemodynamics and Its Role in

Disease Processes. Baltimore, University Park Press, 1980, pp 407–424.

53. Gardner AMN, Fox RH: The return of blood to the heart: Venous pumps in health and disease. London, John Libbey Eurotext, 1989.

54. Gillespie DL, Cordts PR, Hartono C, et al: The role of air plethysmography in monitoring results of venous surgery. J Vasc Surg 16:674, 1992.

55. Gazzaniga AB, Cahill JL, Replogle RL, Tilney NL: Changes in blood volume and renal function following ligation of the inferior vena cava. Surgery 62:417, 1967.

56. Gooley NA, Sumner DS: Relationship of venous reflux to the site of venous valvular incompetence: Implications for venous reconstructive surgery. J Vasc Surg 7:50, 1988.

57. Greenfield ADM: The venous system in cardiovascular functions. *In* Luisada AA (ed): Cardiovascular Functions. New York, McGraw-Hill, 1962.

58. Guyton AC: Interstitial fluid pressure. II. Pressure-volume curves of interstitial space. Circ Res 16:452, 1965.

59. Hallböök T, Göthlin J: Strain gauge plethysmography and phlebography in diagnosis of deep venous thrombosis. Acta Chir Scand 137:37, 1971.

60. Haller JA Jr: Effects of deep femoral thrombophlebitis on the circulation of the lower extremities. Circulation 27:693, 1963.

61. Hanrahan LM, Araki CT, Rodriguez AA, et al: Distribution of valvular incompetence in patients with venous stasis ulceration. J Vasc Surg 13:805, 1991.

62. Harsanyi PG, Ruis-Garriga J, Moser KM: Acute hemodynamic consequences of ligation of the inferior vena cava. J Thorac Cardiovasc Surg 57:442, 1969.

63. Hjelmstedt Å: Pressure decrease in the dorsal pedal veins on walking in persons with and without thrombosis. Acta Chir Scand 134:531, 1968.

64. Hjelmstedt Å: The pressure in the veins of the dorsum of the foot in quiet standing and during exercise in limbs without signs of venous disorder. Acta Chir Scand 134:235, 1968.

65. Höjensgård IC, Stürup H: Static and dynamic pressures in superficial and deep veins of the lower extremity in man. Acta Physiol Scand 27:49, 1952.

66. Holt JP: Flow through collapsible tubes and through in situ veins. IEEE Trans Biomed Eng 16:274, 1969.

67. Husni EA, Ximenes JO, Goyette EM: Elastic support of the lower limbs in hospital patients—A critical study. JAMA 214:1456, 1970.

68. Ikard RW, Ueland K, Folse R: Lower limb venous dynamics in pregnant women. Surg Gynecol Obstet 132:483, 1971.

69. Jacobsen BH: The venous drainage of the foot. Surg Gynecol Obstet 131:22, 1970.

70. Johnson ND, Queral LA, Flinn WR, et al: Late objective assessment of venous valve surgery. Arch Surg 116:1461, 1981.

71. Kerr MG, Scott DB, Samuel E: Studies of the inferior vena cava in late pregnancy. Br Med J 1:532, 1964.

72. Killewich LA, Bedford GR, Beach KW, Strandness DE Jr: Spontaneous lysis of deep venous thrombi: Rate and outcome. J Vasc Surg 9:89, 1989.

73. Koslow AR, DeWeese JA: Anatomical and mechanical aspects of a plantar venous plexus. Presented at the Jobst Symposium on Current Issues in Venous Disease, Chicago, 1988.

74. Kuster G, Lofgren CP, Hollinshead WH: Anatomy of the veins of the foot. Surg Gynecol Obstet 127:817, 1968.

75. Landis EM, Pappenheimer JR: Exchange of substances through capillary walls. *In* Hamilton WF, Dow P (eds): Handbook of Physiology. Washington DC, American Physiological Society, 1963, vol. II, pp 961–1034.

76. LePage PA, Salander JM, Villavicencio JL: The pathology, valvular anatomy, and management of the internal iliac venous insufficiency syndrome. Presented at the Jobst Symposium on Current Issues in Venous Disease, Chicago, 1988.

77. Lindner DJ, Edwards JM, Phinney ES, et al: Long-term hemodynamic and clinical sequelae of lower extremity deep vein thrombosis. J Vasc Surg 4:436, 1986.

78. Linton RR: Post-thrombotic ulceration of the lower extremity: Its etiology and surgical treatment. Ann Surg 138:415, 1953.

79. Lowell RC, Gloviczki P, Miller VM: In vitro evaluation of endothelial and smooth muscle function of primary varicose veins. J Vasc Surg 16:679, 1992.

80. Ludbrook J: Valvular defect in primary varicose veins, cause or effect? Lancet 2:1289, 1963.

81. Ludbrook J: The musculovenous pumps of the human lower limb. Am Heart J 71:635, 1966.

82. Ludbrook J: Aspects of Venous Function in the Lower Limbs. Springfield, IL, Charles C Thomas, 1966.

83. Ludbrook J, Beale G: Femoral venous valves in relation to varicose veins. Lancet 1:79, 1962.

84. Ludbrook J, Loughlin J: Regulation of volume in postarteriolar vessels of the lower limb. Am Heart J 67:493, 1964.

85. Ludbrook J, Westcott E: Venous outflow obstruction of the lower limb following plication of the inferior vena cava. Surg Gynecol Obstet 127:1017, 1968.

86. Lye CR, Sumner DS, Hokanson DE, Strandness DE Jr: The transcutaneous measurement of the elastic properties of the human saphenous vein femoropopliteal bypass graft. Surg Gynecol Obstet 141:891, 1975.

87. Lyon CK, Scott JB, Wang CY: Flow through collapsible tubes at low Reynolds numbers. Circ Res 47:68, 1980.

88. Lyon CK, Scott JB, Anderson DK, Wang CY: Flow through collapsible tubes at high Reynolds numbers. Circ Res 49:988, 1981.

89. Mani R: Venous haemodynamics—A consideration of macro- and microvascular effects. Proc Inst Mech Eng [H] 206:109, 1992.

90. Markel A, Manzo RA, Bergelin RO, Strandness DE Jr: Valvular reflux after deep vein thrombosis: Incidence and time of occurrence. J Vasc Surg 15:377, 1992.

91. Masuda EM, Kistner RL: Prospective comparison of duplex scanning and descending venography in the assessment of venous insufficiency. Am J Surg 164:254, 1992.

92. Mayberry JC, Moneta GL, De Frang RD, Porter JM: The influence of elastic compression stockings on deep venous hemodynamics. J Vasc Surg 13:91, 1991.

93. Mayberry JC, Moneta GL, Taylor LM Jr, Porter JM: Fifteen-year results of ambulatory compression therapy for chronic venous ulcers. Surgery 109:575, 1991.

94. McEnroe CS, O'Donnell TF Jr, Mackey WC: Correlation of clinical findings with venous hemodynamics in 386 patients with chronic venous insufficiency. Am J Surg 156:148, 1988.

95. McLennan CE: Antecubital and femoral venous pressure in normal and toxemic pregnancy. Am J Obstet Gynecol 45:568, 1943.

96. McPheeters HO, Merkert CE, Lundblad RA: The mechanics of the reverse flow in varicose veins as proved by blood pressure readings. Surg Gynecol Obstet 55:298, 1932.

97. Miles RM: Prevention of pulmonary embolism by the use of a plastic vena caval clip. Ann Surg 163:192, 1966.

98. Moore DJ, Himmel PD, Sumner DS: Distribution of venous valvular incompetence in patients with the postphlebitic syndrome. J Vasc Surg 3:49, 1986.

99. Moreno AH, Katz AI, Gold LD, Reddy RV: Mechanics of distention of dog veins and other thinwalled tubular structures. Circ Res 27:1069, 1970.

100. Myers TT: Varicose veins. *In* Allen EV, Barker NW, Hines EA Jr (eds): Peripheral Vascular Disease. Philadelphia, WB Saunders, 1962, pp 636–658.

101. Neglén P, Raju S: A rational approach to detection of significant reflux with duplex Doppler scanning and air plethysmography. J Vasc Surg 17:590, 1993.

102. Nehler MR, Moneta GL, Woodward DM, et al: Perimalleolar interstitial pressure effects of elastic compression stockings [Abstract]. J Vasc Surg 17:431, 1993.

103. Negus D, Cockett FD: Femoral vein pressures in postphlebitic iliac vein obstruction. Br J Surg 54:522, 1967.

104. Nicolaides AN: Noninvasive assessment of primary and secondary varicose veins. *In* Bernstein EF (ed): Noninvasive Diagnostic Techniques in Vascular Disease. 2nd ed. St. Louis, CV Mosby, 1982, pp 575–586.

105. Nicolaides AN, Hussein MK, Szendro G, et al: The relation of venous ulceration with ambulatory venous pressure measurements. J Vasc Surg 17:414, 1993.

106. Nicolaides AN, Miles C: Photoplethysmography in the assessment of venous insufficiency. J Vasc Surg 5:405, 1987.

107. Öberg B: The relationship between active constriction and passive recoil of the veins at various distending pressures. Acta Physiol Scand 71:233, 1967.

108. Ochsner A, Ochsner JL, Sanders HS: Prevention of pulmonary embolism by caval ligation. Ann Surg 171:923, 1970.

109. O'Donnell TF, Mackey WC, Shephard AD, et al: Clinical, hemodynamic, and anatomic follow-up of direct venous reconstruction. Arch Surg 122:474, 1987.

110. O'Donnell TF, Rosenthal DA, Callow AD, Ledig BL: Effect of elastic compression on venous hemodynamics in postphlebitic limbs. JAMA 242:2766, 1979.

111. Pearce WH, Ricco J-B, Queral LA, et al: Hemodynamic assessment of venous problems. Surgery 93:715, 1983.

112. Pflug JJ, Zubac DP, Kersten DR, Alexander NDE: The resting interstitial tissue pressure in primary varicose veins. J Vasc Surg 11:411, 1990.

113. Pollack AA, Wood EH: Venous pressure in the saphenous vein at the ankle in man during exercise and changes in posture. J Appl Physiol 1:649, 1949.

114. Pollack AA, Taylor BE, Myers TT, Wood EH: The effect of exercise and body position on the venous pressures at the ankle in patients having venous valvular defects. J Clin Invest 28:559, 1949.

115. Raju S, Fredericks R: Valve reconstruction procedures for nonobstructive venous insufficiency: Rationale, techniques, and results in 107 procedures with two- to eight-year follow-up. J Vasc Surg 71:301, 1988.

116. Raju S, Fredericks R, Lishman P, et al: Observations on the calf pump mechanism: Determinants of postexercise pressure. J Vasc Surg 17:459, 1993.

117. Reagan B, Folse R: Lower limb venous dynamics in normal persons and children of patients with varicose veins. Surg Gynecol Obstet 132:15, 1971.

118. Rich NM, Hobson RW II, Wright CB, Fedde CW: Repair of lower extremity venous trauma: A more aggressive approach required. J Trauma 14:639, 1974.

119. Rose SS, Ahmed A: Some thoughts on the aetiology of varicose veins. J Cardiovasc Surg 27:534, 1986.

120. Rosfors S, Lamke L-O, Nordström E, Bygdeman S: Severity and location of venous valvular insufficiency: The importance of distal valve function. Acta Chir Scand 156:689, 1990.

121. Rushmer RF: Effects of posture. In Cardiovascular Dynamics. 3rd ed. Philadelphia, WB Saunders, 1970, pp 192–219.

122. Rutherford RB, Reddy CMK, Walker FG, Wagner HN Jr: A new quantitative method of assessing the functional status of the leg veins. Am J Surg 122:594, 1971.

123. Saffle JR, Maxwell JG, Warden GD, et al: Measurement of intramuscular pressure in the management of massive venous occlusion. Surgery 89:394, 1981.

124. Sakaguchi S, Ishitobi K, Kameda T: Functional segmental plethysmography with mercury strain gauge. Angiology 23:127, 1972.

125. Samueloff SL, Browse NL, Shepherd JT: Response of capacity vessels in human limbs to head up tilt and suction on lower body. J Appl Physiol 21:47, 1966.

126. Sarin S, Scurr JH, Coleridge Smith PD: Medial calf perforators in venous disease: The significance of outward flow. J Vasc Surg 16:40, 1992.

127. Schalin L: Arteriovenous communications to varicose veins in the lower extremities studied by dynamic angiography. Acta Chir Scand 146:397, 1980.

128. Schalin L: Arteriovenous communications in varicose veins localized by thermography and identified by operative microscopy. Acta Chir Scand 147:409, 1981.

129. Schanzer H, Pierce EC II: A rational approach to surgery of the chronic venous stasis syndrome. Ann Surg 195:25, 1982.

130. Shami SK, Sarin S, Cheatle TR, et al: Venous ulcers and the superficial venous system. J Vasc Surg 17:487, 1993.

131. Shami SK, Scurr JH, Coleridge Smith PD: Capillary filtration in venous disease [Abstract]. J Vasc Surg 17:444, 1993.

132. Shepherd JT: Role of the veins in the circulation. Circulation 33:484, 1966.

133. Shepherd JT: Reflex control of the venous system. In Bergan JJ, Yao JST (eds): Venous Problems. Chicago, Year Book Medical Publishers, 1978, pp 5–23.

134. Sherman RS Sr: Varicose veins: Anatomy, reevaluation of Trendelenburg tests, and an operative procedure. Surg Clin North Am 44:1369, 1964.

135. Shull KS, Nicolaides AN, Fernandes é Fernandes J, et al: Significance of popliteal reflux in relation to ambulatory venous pressure and ulceration. Arch Surg 114:1304, 1979.

136. Snyder MA, Adams JT, Schwartz SI: Hemodynamics of phlegmasia cerulea dolens. Surg Gynecol Obstet 125:342, 1967.

137. Somerville JJF, Byrne PJ, Fegan WG: Analysis of flow patterns in venous insufficiency. Br J Surg 61:40, 1974.

138. Starling EH: On the absorption of fluids from the connective tissue spaces. J Physiol 19:312, 1896.

139. Stegall HF: Muscle pumping in the dependent leg. Circ Res 19:180, 1966.

140. Strandness DE Jr, Langlois Y, Cramer M, et al: Long-term sequelae of acute venous thrombosis. JAMA 250:1289, 1983.

141. Strandness DE Jr, Sumner DS: Hemodynamics for Surgeons. New York, Grune & Stratton, 1975.

142. Sumner DS: Venous dynamics—Varicosities. Clin Obstet Gynecol 24:743, 1981.

143. Taheri SA, Heffner R, Meenaghan MA, et al: Technique and results of venous valve transplantation. In Bergan JJ, Yao JST (eds): Surgery of the Veins. Orlando, FL, Grune & Stratton, 1985, pp 219–231.

144. Taylor AE: Capillary fluid filtration, Starling forces and lymph flow. Circ Res 49:557, 1981.

145. Thomas ML, Keeling FP, Ackroyd JS: Descending phlebography: A comparison of three methods and an assessment of the normal range of deep vein reflux. J Cardiovasc Surg 27:27, 1986.

146. Thomas PRS, Nash GB, Dormandy JA: White cell accumulation in dependent legs of patients with venous hypertension: A possible mechanism for trophic changes in the skin. Br Med J 296:1693, 1988.

147. Thulesius O: Elastizität und Klappenfunktion peripherer Venen bei primärer Varikosis. Phlebol Proktol 8:97, 1979.

148. Tripolitis AJ, Milligan EB, Bodily KC, Strandness DE Jr: The physiology of venous claudication. Am J Surg 139:447, 1980.

149. Ueland K: Pregnancy and cardiovascular disease. Med Clin North Am 61:17, 1977.

150. van Bemmelen PS, Bedford G, Beach K, Strandness DE Jr: Status of the valves in the superficial and deep venous system in chronic venous disease. Surgery 109:730, 1991.

151. van Bemmelen PS, Bedford G, Beach K, Strandness DE: Quantitative segmental evaluation of venous reflux with duplex ultrasound scanning. J Vasc Surg 10:425, 1989.

152. Vanhoutte PM, Shepherd JT: Thermosensitivity and veins. J Physiol (Paris) 63:449, 1970.

153. Vasdekis SN, Clarke GH, Nicolaides AN: Quantification of venous reflux by means of duplex scanning. J Vasc Surg 10:670, 1989.

154. Warren R, White EA, Belcher CD: Venous pressures in the saphenous system in normal, varicose, and postphlebitic extremities. Surgery 26:435, 1949.

155. Webb-Peploe MM, Shepherd JT: Response of large hindlimb veins of the dog to sympathetic nerve stimulation. Am J Physiol 215:299, 1968.

156. Welch HJ, McLaughlin RL, O'Donnell TF Jr: Femoral vein valvuloplasty: Intraoperative angioscopic evaluation and hemodynamic improvement. J Vasc Surg 16:694, 1992.

157. Welkie JF, Comerota AJ, Katz ML, et al: Hemodynamic deterioration in chronic venous disease. J Vasc Surg 16:733, 1992.

158. Whiston RJ, Hallett MB, Lane IF, Harding KG: Lower limb neutrophil oxygen radical production in increased venous hypertension [Abstract]. J Vasc Surg 17:445, 1993.

159. Wilkinson LS, Bunker C, Edwards JCW, et al: Leukocytes: Their role in the etiopathogenesis of skin damage in venous disease. J Vasc Surg 17:669, 1993.

160. Winsor T, Burch GE: Phlebostatic axis and phlebostatic level, reference level for venous pressure measurements in man. Proc Soc Exp Biol 58:165, 1945.

161. Wright CB, Swan KG: Hemodynamics of venous occlusion in the canine hindlimb. Surgery 73:141, 1973.

162. Wright CB, Sayre JT, Casterline PI, Swan KG: Hemodynamic effects of sympathectomy in canine femoral venous occlusion. Surgery 74:405, 1973.

163. Zoster T, Cronin RFP: Venous distensibility in patients with varicose veins. Can Med Assoc J 4:1293, 1966.

130

Superficial Venous Thrombosis

George Johnson, Jr., M.D.

• • •

Thrombosis or thrombophlebitis of the superficial venous system receives little attention in textbooks of surgery and medicine. It is frequently encountered, however, and at times can cause significant incapacitation. It is usually a benign, self-limiting disease but can be recurrent and doggedly persistent. Although the etiology is frequently obscure, superficial venous thrombosis is most often associated with one of the components of Virchow's triad: intimal damage (which can result from trauma, infection, or inflammation), stasis, or changes in the blood constituents (presumably causing changes in coagulability).

A relationship between oral contraceptive use and superficial thrombophlebitis is suspected but has not been definitively established.

TYPES OF SUPERFICIAL VENOUS THROMBOSIS

Traumatic Thrombophlebitis

Superficial venous thrombosis following an injury usually occurs in an extremity, manifesting as a tender cord along the course of a vein juxtaposing the area of trauma. Ecchymosis may be present, indicating extravasation of blood associated with injury to the vein.

Thrombophlebitis frequently occurs at the site of an intravenous infusion as a result of the drugs being given or of the intraluminal catheter or cannula itself. This is by far the most common type of thrombophlebitis encountered. Usually, redness and pain signal its presence while the infusion is being given, but thrombosis may manifest as a small lump days or weeks after the infusion apparatus has been removed and may take months to completely resolve.

The features of the iatrogenic form of traumatic ("chemical") phlebitis deliberately produced by sclerotherapy are discussed in Chapter 137.

Thrombophlebitis in a Varicose Vein

Superficial thrombophlebitis frequently occurs in varicose veins. It may extend up and down the saphenous vein or may remain confined to a cluster of tributary varicosities away from the main saphenous vein. Although it may follow trauma to a varix, it often appears to occur without antecedent cause. Thrombophlebitis develops as a tender, hard "knot" in a previously noted varicose vein and is frequently surrounded by erythema. At times, significant bleeding may occur as the reaction extends through the vein wall and skin. It is frequently seen in varicose veins surrounding venous stasis ulcers.

Thrombophlebitis as the Result of an Infection

In 1932, DeTakats suggested that dormant infection in varicose veins was a factor in the development of thrombophlebitis occurring at operation or after injection treatments, trauma, or exposure to radiation therapy.[1] Altemeier and colleagues suggested that the presence of L-forms and other atypical bacterial forms in the blood may play an important etiologic role in the disease.[2]

Septic phlebitis usually occurs in association with the long-term use of an intravenous cannula inserted for the administration of fluid or medications.

Suppurative thrombophlebitis is a more serious, even lethal complication of intravenous cannulation and therapy and is characterized by purulence within the vein. It is frequently associated with septicemia.

Migratory Thrombophlebitis

Migratory thrombophlebitis was first described by Jadioux in 1845 as an entity characterized by repeated thrombosis developing in superficial veins at varying sites but most commonly in the lower extremity.[3] Although numerous etiologic factors have been proposed, none has been confirmed. The association of carcinoma was first reported by Trousseau in 1856.[3] Sproul noted migratory thrombophlebitis to be especially prevalent with carcinoma of the tail of the pancreas.[4]

Phlebitis occurs in diseases associated with vasculitis, such as polyarteritis nodosa (periarteritis nodosa) and Buerger's disease. Buerger noted phlebitis in 8 of 19 patients,[5] and Shionoya reported it in 43 per cent of the 255 patients he followed up.[6]

Thrombophlebitis of the Superficial Veins of the Breast and the Anterior Chest Wall (Mondor's Disease)

Mondor's disease is a rare condition. The thrombophlebitis is usually located in the anterolateral aspect of the upper portion of the breast or in the region extending from the lower portion of the breast across the submammary fold toward the costal margin and the epigastrium. A characteristic finding is a tender, cord-like structure that may best be demonstrated by tensing the skin, as by elevating the arm.[3] The cause is unknown, but a search for malignancy is indicated.

DIAGNOSIS

Diagnosis of the condition is usually not difficult. The patient complains of pain associated with a cord-like structure or knot along the course of a vein. The accompanying inflammatory reaction frequently gives rise to redness along the course of the vein.

Duplex scanning will document the clot in the superficial vein and give the clinician information about extension into the deep venous system. Lutter and associates reported that 12 per cent of 186 patients with superficial thrombophlebitis of the great saphenous vein above the knee had extension into the deep venous system.[7]

Venography is not necessary to confirm the diagnosis; in fact, it may actually make the symptoms worse. At times it is useful in excluding the diagnosis of deep venous thrombosis, but duplex scanning can also accomplish this.

TREATMENT

The treatment of superficial venous thrombosis depends on its etiology, extent, and symptoms. Duplex scanning gives an accurate appraisal of the extent of disease and thus allows more rational therapy.

For the superficial, localized, mildly tender area of thrombophlebitis that occurs in a varicose vein, treatment with mild analgesics, such as aspirin, and the use of some type of elastic support are usually sufficient. Patients are encouraged to continue their usual daily activities.[8] If extensive varicosities are present or if symptoms persist, phlebectomy of the involved segment may be indicated.

More severe thrombophlebitis, as indicated by the degree of pain and redness and the extent of the abnormality, should be treated by bed rest with elevation of the extremity and the application of massive hot, wet compresses. The latter measure seems to be more effective when a large bulky dressing, including a blanket and plastic sheeting, followed by hot water bottles, is used. The immobilization is probably as beneficial as the moist heat. Long-leg, heavy-gauge elastic stockings or elastic (Ace) bandages are indicated when the patient becomes ambulatory. Antibiotics are usually not necessary unless the process is suppurative. In persistent cases or even as early definitive therapy, excision of the inflammatory process is effective. The wounds usually heal well with primary closure; the inflammatory process is nonbacterial and localized and is completely removed.

Some anti-inflammatory drugs may be of benefit. Phenylbutazone, salicylates, indomethacin, and ibuprofen have been reported to be effective. The salicylates, ibuprofen, and dipyridamole have been used as antithrombotic agents, but their effectiveness has not been documented in this setting. Because thrombophlebitis is primarily due to inflammation and fibrin clot, antithrombotic or anti–platelet-aggregating agents would seem to have little value. Anticoagulants are not indicated unless the process extends into the deep venous system.

Because thrombophlebitis tends to recur if the vein has not been excised, it is usually advisable to instruct the patient in ways to prevent stasis in the vein. The use of elastic stockings may be indicated, especially if the patient is going to stand in an upright position for long periods. Slight elevation of the foot of the bed and avoidance of long periods of standing in an upright position or inactivity are recommended. Migratory thrombophlebitis, especially without good cause, may well be an indication for a more detailed evaluation of the gastrointestinal tract in search of a malignant lesion and a more extensive work-up for antithrombin III, protein C, or protein S abnormalities.

With persistence or spread of the process, the thrombophlebitic vein should be excised.[8] This is especially true for the greater saphenous vein if the process extends upward toward the femoral vein in the groin.

Duplex scanning may demonstrate more extension into the deep veins than was originally thought to occur. In the deep veins of the thigh, anticoagulation with heparin, if not excision, is indicated if this occurs.

If the thrombophlebitis is associated with a cannula or a catheter, the device should be immediately removed and cultured. If the patient is septic, appropriate antibiotics should be given. If suppurative thrombophlebitis is suspected, immediate and complete excision of all of the involved veins is indicated. The wound is packed open for secondary closure or skin grafting at a later date. The use of appropriate systemic antibiotics is always indicated.

If the suppurative process involves one of the deep veins, aggressive antimicrobial and anticoagulant therapy will be necessary (see Chapter 134).

PROGNOSIS

The prognosis is usually good. Superficial phlebitis is rarely associated with pulmonary embolism, although it can occur, particularly if the process extends into a deep vein. There does not seem to be a great tendency for those with superficial venous thrombosis to develop deep venous thrombosis; however, duplex scanning may prove this assumption wrong. Superficial venous thrombosis, on the other hand, does occur frequently in association with deep venous thrombosis, especially in patients with ulceration around the ankle.

The patient should be told to expect the disease process to persist for 3 to 4 weeks or longer. If it occurs in the lower extremity in association with varicose veins, it has a high likelihood of recurrence unless excision is performed.

References

1. DeTakats G: "Resting infection" in varicose veins, its diagnosis and treatment. Am J Med Sci 184:57, 1932.
2. Altemeier WA, Hill EO, Fullen WD: Acute and recurrent thromboembolic disease: A new concept of etiology. Ann Surg 170:547, 1969.
3. Glasser ST: Principles of Peripheral Vascular Surgery. Philadelphia, FA Davis, 1959.

4. Sproul EE: Carcinoma and venous thrombosis: Frequency of association of carcinoma in body or tail of pancreas with multiple venous thrombosis. Am J Cancer 34:566, 1938.
5. Buerger L: The veins in thromboangiitis obliterans: With particular reference to arteriovenous anastomosis as a cure for the condition. JAMA 52:1319, 1909.
6. Shionoya S: Buerger's Disease: Pathology, Diagnosis and Treatment. Nagoya, Japan, University of Nagoya Press, 1990.
7. Lutter KS, Kerr TM, Roedersheimer LR, et al: Superficial thrombophlebitis diagnosed by duplex scanning. Surgery 110:42, 1991.
8. Cranley JJ: Thrombophlebitis in obstetrics and gynecology. *In* Rakel RE (ed): Conn's Current Therapy. Philadelphia, WB Saunders, 1984.

131

Diagnosis of Deep Venous Thrombosis

David S. Sumner, M.D.

• • •

It is fair to say that the clinical diagnosis of acute deep venous thrombosis (DVT) is hardly more accurate than tossing a coin.[71, 150] In other words, exclusive reliance on the history and physical examination is likely to lead to a 50 per cent incidence of false-positive or false-negative diagnoses. Careful phlebographic studies have shown that only 46 to 62 per cent of patients with clinically diagnosed DVT actually have thrombi in their veins.[18, 71, 116, 214, 220, 260] When signs and symptoms are minimal, 66 to 84 per cent of the diagnoses may be wrong.[116, 260] On the other hand, no symptoms at all may be evident in 52 to 69 per cent of limbs with thrombi proved by positive findings on iodine-125–fibrinogen uptake studies.[152, 168] According to Coon and Willis, only 19 per cent of thrombi found at autopsy were suspected before death.[64]

There are a number of reasons for the lack of clinical diagnostic accuracy. First, the history is often poor, the complaints are vague, and the symptoms are non-specific.[116] Physical signs may be quite subtle and frequently are mimicked by other pathologic conditions. Second, venous obstruction is not as readily detected as arterial obstruction, which usually can be recognized by simple palpation of the peripheral pulses. Because venous flow is nonpulsatile, venous pressure is low and the venous wall is easily compressed; palpation is seldom of value unless the involved vein is superficial enough to allow the obstructing thrombus to be felt. Moreover, venous collaterals are so extensive that isolated thrombi often produce no perceptible disturbance of the outflow of blood; no swelling appears to alert the clinician to the presence of a clot.

Although many thrombi in small veins may have little immediate clinical significance, silent thrombi in larger veins are potentially very dangerous. These thrombi must be identified if pulmonary emboli are to be prevented and if the disability from chronic venous insufficiency is to be avoided. Even those clots that are confined to veins below the knee may be responsible for the development of chronic venous stasis syndromes.[290] Equally distressing is the fact that a number of patients may be treated for nonexistent DVT or pulmonary embolism. In a study of the practice of consultants in Scotland, Prentice and colleagues found that 47 per cent of those responding to a questionnaire based their diagnosis of DVT solely on clinical observation.[237] Similarly, 33 per cent employed clinical methods alone for the diagnosis of pulmonary embolism. No figures are available, but hundreds of patients must endure unnecessary insertion of vena caval filters every year in the United States, and thousands more must be treated unnecessarily with anticoagulants. Neither of these treatment modalities is devoid of complications. The fact that both patient and physician may be deluded as to the correct diagnosis is also important. Fear of recurrent thrombosis, leg ulceration, and pulmonary embolism often persists in the misdiagnosed patient, even to the point of producing a postphlebitic psychoneurosis.[268]

Clearly, every effort should be made to improve the clinical diagnosis of DVT. In all cases in which the diagnosis is suspected, an objective diagnostic technique should be employed. It seems likely that this message has been gradually accepted by the medical community. The development of accurate noninvasive tests has made objective diagnosis less formidable than it was in the past, when phlebography was the only available diagnostic method. The author and his colleagues were encouraged to find that the practice in their hospitals changed radically over a 10-year period. Whereas in 1973 only 24 per cent of patients discharged from the hospital with the diagnosis of DVT had had the diagnosis confirmed by objective methods, by 1983 the proportion had risen to 97 per cent.[112] During this same period, the number of patients treated for DVT more than doubled, suggesting that cases previously overlooked by clinical assessment alone were being identified.

In a survey of 16 short-stay hospitals located in central Massachusetts, Anderson and Wheeler found that 95 per cent of patients discharged between July 1, 1988 and December 31, 1989 with the diagnosis of DVT had undergone

one or more objective diagnostic tests for venous thrombosis; however, 10 per cent of those discharged with the diagnosis of DVT either had undergone no testing or had had negative test results.[10] Thus, even in medically sophisticated communities, some patients continue to be treated without benefit of objective diagnosis.

CLINICAL EVALUATION

Despite the fallibility of the clinical diagnosis of DVT, certain symptoms and signs, associated conditions, and predisposing factors in the patient's history alert the physician to the possible presence of the disease. Identification of patients in whom DVT is suspected or likely is a necessary first step in the diagnostic process.

Symptoms and Signs

DVT is often asymptomatic, but it may cause pain in the calf, thigh, or inguinal region—not in the toes or foot. Likewise, in the upper extremity, pain is confined to the arm; the hand is spared. Only a rough correlation exists between the extent and location of the thrombotic process and the area in which pain occurs. Although pain is usually confined to the calf when clots are isolated to the infrapopliteal veins, when the more proximal veins are involved, pain may be felt at any level and may be diffuse throughout the leg. Symptoms are rarely severe, are often dull or mild, and may be described as an ache, cramp, or tight sensation. Although the onset may be relatively acute, patients seldom recall a specific time. Usually, discomfort develops gradually and worsens over the next few days. Once pain appears, it is present continuously but may fluctuate in intensity. Pain tends to be exacerbated by activity and is frequently alleviated by bed rest and elevation of the leg.

Limbs should be examined to identify points of tenderness. This is best accomplished with the patient's knee flexed to relieve tension in the calf muscles. In cases of DVT, there may be tenderness on deep palpation between the heads of the gastrocnemius muscle. Other patients may have tenderness over the posterior tibial, popliteal, superficial femoral, or common femoral veins, or in the arm, over the brachial or axillary veins. A palpable tender "cord" with localized inflammation is indicative of superficial thrombophlebitis; deep veins are seldom felt. *Homans' sign*, originally defined as a limitation in dorsiflexion of the foot caused by irritability of the soleus and gastrocnemius muscles but now popularly defined as pain in the calf with dorsiflexion, is mentioned only to be condemned. This sign not only is insensitive to the presence of DVT but is also very nonspecific, occurring in many patients who have been on bed rest. Homans himself disowned the sign as being unreliable.[44]

In some patients, swelling of the legs or arms is the principal or only complaint. Unilateral swelling (or asymmetric swelling) suggests venous obstruction and is one of the best signs of DVT. Bilaterally symmetric edema is more likely to be caused by a systemic problem, such as congestive heart failure, but can occur in cases of inferior vena caval obstruction. Depending on the location and extent of

the thrombotic process, swelling may be mild and not easily detected or severe and visually obvious. Pitting edema at the ankle level is the most common presentation and may be the only manifestation of DVT when clots are confined to the infrapopliteal veins. When there is extensive intramuscular venous thrombosis, the calf muscles may become turgid, a change in consistency most apparent when the knee is flexed. Normal relaxed calf muscles are soft and "floppy." Edema of both the foot and the calf suggests extension to the popliteal or superficial femoral vein, and swelling of the entire leg implies iliofemoral venous thrombosis. A comparison of limb circumference measurements is often helpful in detecting subtle degrees of swelling. Ordinarily, circumferences measured at the same level in the two limbs should differ by no more than a centimeter.

Because hydrostatic pressure has a major influence on the rate of fluid accumulation, patients on bed rest may have little swelling despite the presence of venous obstruction. Edema due to acute venous thrombosis usually decreases when the limb is elevated and increases when the limb is dependent. Swelling may persist for weeks or months after the initial episode and may never disappear entirely. Easily pitting edema suggests that the swelling is reversible and of relatively short duration.

Venous collaterals are often visible through the skin of the groin and lower abdomen in patients with iliofemoral venous thrombosis or over the shoulder and beneath the clavicle when the axillary or subclavian veins are involved. Otherwise, superficial venous distention is a relatively uncommon and nonspecific sign of acute DVT.

Most limbs with acute DVT are nearly normal in color or have a faintly cyanotic discoloration caused by congestion of the cutaneous veins. *Phlegmasia alba dolens* (turgid, white, painful leg) is characterized by diffuse swelling of the entire extremity, pallor, and moderate pain. In combination with tenderness over the common femoral vein and visible collaterals in the groin, this constellation of findings is almost diagnostic of iliofemoral venous thrombosis. Because the condition was initially described in postpartum patients and was mistakenly attributed by physicians in the 18th century to suppression of lactation and the accumulation of milk in the blood vessels of the leg, it was called "milk leg," a designation that persists to this day.[7, 326]

Phlegmasia cerulea dolens (turgid, blue, painful leg) is the term applied to deeply cyanotic, severely painful, markedly swollen limbs in which most of the major deep and superficial veins are obstructed with thrombus. In the lower extremity, the iliac, common femoral, superficial femoral, popliteal, tibial, and greater saphenous veins and their tributaries may all be involved. Multiple petechiae are frequently present; pedal pulses may be reduced or absent; and compartment pressures are elevated (see Chapter 129). Phlegmasia cerulea dolens may represent progression of phlegmasia alba dolens, or it can appear de novo. Patients may be in shock owing to entrapment of blood in the leg and massive loss of fluid into the interstitium. In more severe cases, hemorrhagic bullae form; the distal tissues become ischemic; and gangrene (often of the "wet" variety) develops. The mortality rate is high (especially in patients with venous gangrene), and patients who survive frequently require amputations. Despite the presence of ischemia and the absence of peripheral pulses, phlegmasia cerulea dolens is easily differentiated from acute arterial obstruction and is one form of venous thrombosis in which an accurate diagnosis can be made clinically. Fortunately, venous ischemic syndromes are rare, occurring in only 2 to 10 per cent of patients with DVT.[117]

Clinical History and Predisposing Conditions

Although DVT often occurs without any apparent antecedent event or precipitating factor, its incidence is known to be increased in a number of commonly encountered situations. Because of increased blood coagulability, decreased fibrinolytic activity, and immobility, venous thrombosis is frequent following major operations and trauma. Patients undergoing total hip and knee arthroplasties are especially vulnerable. Postoperative venous thrombosis occurs more often after abdominal operations than after less severe, extracavitary soft tissue procedures. Malignancy, advanced age, heart failure, a history of venous thrombosis, bed rest, and obesity are other conditions that predispose to DVT. The risk is also increased during the postpartum period and in women using oral contraceptives. Antithrombin III, protein C, and protein S deficiencies are relatively rare causes of DVT. In some patients, a recent long airplane, bus, or automobile trip may be the instigating event. The presence of any of these risk factors serves to heighten the suspicion that symptoms and signs may be due to DVT.

Differential Diagnosis

Table 131–1 lists some of the conditions that may mimic DVT. Because venous thrombosis can coexist with any of these problems, objective testing for venous thrombosis may be required even when an alternative diagnosis appears likely. Only after DVT has been excluded is it entirely safe to attribute leg pain or swelling to another cause. Not infrequently, symptoms and signs remain unex-

Table 131–1. Conditions That May Mimic Acute Deep Venous Thrombosis

Muscle strain or blunt trauma
Ruptured muscle with subfascial hematoma
Spontaneous hemorrhage or hematoma
Ruptured synovial cysts (Baker's cysts)
Arthritis, synovitis, or myositis
Cellulitis, lymphangitis, or inflammatory lymphedema
Superficial thrombophlebitis
Arterial insufficiency
Pregnancy or oral contraceptive use
Lymphedema
Lipedema
Chronic venous insufficiency or venous reflux syndromes
Extrinsic venous compression: lymphadenopathy, tumors, lymphomas, hematomas, abscesses, right iliac artery
Systemic edema: congestive heart failure, metabolic, nephrotic syndrome, post–arterial reconstruction
Dependency or leg immobilization (casts)
Arteriovenous fistula

plained. In these cases, the discomfort is probably due to excessive or unaccustomed muscle activity.

There are often clues to the proper diagnosis. Ecchymoses may appear posterior to the medial malleolus several days after the patient has suffered a painful tear of the gastrocnemius muscle. Spontaneous hemorrhage or hematoma occurs primarily in patients taking anticoagulants. Pain in the knee joint that is exacerbated by motion suggests arthritis, especially when other joints are affected. Patients with ruptured Baker's cysts may also give a history of arthritis. Limbs with cellulitis are warm, erythematous, and tender, and limbs with lymphangitis typically have red streaks along the course of inflamed lymphatics. Patients with these conditions are usually febrile and have an elevated white blood cell count. A site of entry for bacteria may be identified, such as a crack between the toes. As mentioned earlier, a palpable, tender, inflamed cord coinciding with the location of a superficial vein is practically diagnostic of superficial thrombophlebitis. (Perhaps one sixth of patients with above-knee superficial venous thrombosis also have involvement of the deep system.[283]

Except in cases of phlegmasia cerulea dolens, arterial insufficiency should seldom be confused with venous thrombosis; even then, the presentation and physical signs are distinctive. Occasionally, pregnant women or women taking estrogen-containing contraceptives may experience leg pain in the absence of DVT (possibly due to venous dilatation or muscle cramps). Unilateral leg swelling may be caused by compression of the iliac vein by a gravid uterus.

Woody edema suggests chronic lymphatic obstruction, but lymphedema of recent onset (such as that following peripheral arterial reconstruction) may be pitting and impossible to distinguish from the edema of acute DVT. Tissues in the gaiter area of patients with chronic venous insufficiency (postphlebitic syndrome) are usually firm, and hard plaques of fibrotic tissue may be palpated. Some older obese women complain of tender swollen legs in the absence of pitting edema. For want of a better term, this has been called "lipedema." Why the condition is painful is not known, but it is not related to venous or lymphatic disease.

Swelling caused by tumors, hematomas, or other masses that compress adjacent deep veins may be impossible to differentiate clinically from that caused by acute DVT. Rarely, compression of the left iliac vein by the right iliac artery may be responsible for intermittent or chronic swelling of the left leg. Bilateral edema suggests a systemic cause, such as congestive heart failure, protein deficiency, or the nephrotic syndrome. Lastly, patients who sit most of the day with their legs dependent, patients with paralyzed lower extremities, and patients whose limbs have been immobilized in a plaster cast may develop edema resembling that of acute DVT.

Landfeld and associates identified five independent clinical correlates of proximal DVT: swelling above the knee, swelling below the knee, recent immobility, cancer, and fever.[169] If none of these findings were present, phlebographic findings were positive in only 5 per cent of patients with suspected DVT; however, if two or more were present, DVT was found in 42 per cent.

OBJECTIVE DIAGNOSTIC METHODS

Since the mid-1960s, many semi-invasive and noninvasive techniques have been devised to supplement or replace phlebography in the objective diagnosis of DVT (Table 131–2). Early physiologic methods, such as Doppler ultrasonography, impedance phlebography, and phleborheography, have been extensively studied and their accuracy in diagnosing clots in above-knee veins has been well established. These tests, however, were limited in their ability to detect below-knee thrombi, often overlooked nonocclusive clots and thrombi in duplicated veins, provided little information about the precise location and extent of the clots, and were unable to access the age or chronicity of the thrombotic process or the degree of recanalization. Moreover, they did not distinguish between venous obstruction caused by extrinsic compression and that due to intraluminal clotting. Another well-studied method, the iodine-125–labeled fibrinogen uptake test, proved to be quite sensitive for detecting asymptomatic clots developing in calf veins, but false-positive errors were common. Furthermore, the test was relatively insensitive to established thrombi, was inaccurate above the knee, and often required a day or two before positive results were evident. Although the fibrinogen uptake test was popular for a time in England, it was never widely used in the United States. Owing to the risk of transmission of blood-borne diseases, labeled fibrinogen is no longer commercially available.

Talbot's demonstration in 1982 that B-mode ultrasonography could be used to diagnose DVT represented a major breakthrough.[309] With this device, both occlusive and nonocclusive clots could be visualized and their location and extent determined. Other investigators found that duplex scanning, which combines B-mode imaging and Doppler ultrasonography, had significant advantages. Assessment of flow patterns with Doppler ultrasonography supplements the anatomic information obtained with B-mode imaging, thereby assisting in the recognition of hypoechogenic thrombi and thrombi in poorly visualized veins. In turn, B-mode imaging helps in the selection and identification of veins to be interrogated with Doppler ultrasonography. Technologic advances in the latter part of the 1980s added a real-time color flow map to the conventional duplex image. By providing instantaneous flow information over an extended length of vein, color facilitates the scanning process (especially below the knee) and aids in the recognition of partially occluding clots.

Requirements of the "ideal" test for DVT are listed in Table 131–3. Clearly, none of the methods currently available fulfills all of these criteria; all (including phlebography) have their limitations and peculiar advantages. Duplex and color flow scanning, however, come the closest to meeting these requirements and are now generally accepted as the noninvasive methods of choice for the diagnosis of DVT. Nonetheless, various circumstances may dictate the use of one of the other modalities. If the limitations of the physiologic tests are recognized, their use remains acceptable for certain purposes.

Phlebography

Contrast phlebography (venography) remains the gold standard against which all other techniques must be evaluated. When properly performed, it is highly sensitive and specific for the presence of venous clots in all of the major veins of the leg and arm. However, phlebography also has drawbacks. Compared with arteriography, phlebography is more difficult to perform and the resulting studies are less easily interpreted.[336] Observers may disagree about the presence of a thrombus in as many as 10 per cent of examinations.[191, 266] Attesting to these problems are the multitude of phlebographic techniques that have been de-

Table 131–2. Comparison of Objective Tests for Diagnosing Venous Disease

	Deep Venous Thrombosis				Superficial Venous Thrombosis	Valvular Incompetence
	Proximal		Calf			
Test	SENSITIVITY	SPECIFICITY	SENSITIVITY	SPECIFICITY		
Invasive						
X-ray phlebography	+	+	+	+	+	+/−
Semi-invasive						
Radionuclide phlebography	+	+	−	−	−	−
Iodine-125–fibrinogen uptake	+/−	+/−	+	+/−	−	−
Noninvasive						
Doppler ultrasonography	+	+	+/−	+/−	+	+
Strain-gauge plethysmography	+	+	−	−	−	+
Impedance plethysmography	+	+	−	−	−	−
Pulse volume recorder	+/−	+/−	−	−	−	−
Phleborheography	+	+	+/−	+/−	−	+/−
Light reflection rheography	?+	?+/−	?+	?+/−	−	+
Magnetic resonance imaging	?+	?+	?+/−	?+/−	−	−
Thermography	?+	?+	?+	?+	+/−	−
B-mode, duplex, and color flow scanning	+	+	+	+	+	+

+, good results reported; +/−, fair results reported; −, poor results reported or not suitable; ?, few reports, insufficient information.

Table 131–3.   Requirements of the "Ideal" Test for Diagnosing Deep Venous Thrombosis

The Test Should Be
1. Accurate (high sensitivity, specificity, and predictive value)
2. Safe, and should cause minimal discomfort
3. Rapidly performed and easily interpreted, and should provide an immediate diagnosis
4. Convenient, portable, widely applicable, repeatable, and inexpensive

The Test Should Be Able To
1. Detect clots in the leg (both above and below the knee), in the pelvis and abdomen, and in the upper extremity
2. Detect clots in both the deep and superficial veins
3. Detect clots in nonaxial deep veins (the internal iliac, profunda femoris, and intramuscular veins of the calf)
4. Determine the precise location and extent of the thrombotic process
5. Identify nonocclusive clots and clots with a free-floating tail
6. Access the age and chronicity of clots and the extent of recanalization
7. Detect clot propagation and lysis
8. Identify extrinsic compression by hematomas, tumors, cysts, enlarged lymph nodes, and abscesses
9. Assess valvular incompetence and identify incompetent valves

vised.[85, 214, 239, 310] Multiple injections are sometimes necessary, and various technical modifications employing tourniquets, tilt tables, calf compression, Valsalva maneuvers, and calf muscle contraction are required to fill all the venous channels. Particularly difficult to demonstrate are the intramuscular sinusoids, the profunda femoris vein, and the internal iliac vein—all areas that may harbor thrombi. (Visualization of the common and external iliac veins and the inferior vena cava is also often inadequate unless the contrast medium is injected into the femoral vein.) Moreover, phlebography requires special equipment and is best performed in the radiology suite. The studies may be costly and time consuming and are often painful. In addition, a small number of patients (fewer than 10 per cent) will develop thrombophlebitis as a direct result of the contrast medium itself.[5, 6, 18] All of these factors may make the physician somewhat reluctant to order phlebograms, especially when the index of suspicion is low. They virtually preclude the use of phlebography for routine follow-up studies or for prospective surveys of patients at high risk for developing venous thrombosis.

Like arteriography, phlebography provides little physiologic information. It gives no objective data on the severity of the venous obstruction beyond that which can be surmised from the extent and location of the thrombotic process. This sort of information is important to the clinical scientist who wishes to document the course of the disease and to the physician who wants to evaluate the results of his or her therapeutic endeavors.

Because of these drawbacks, an increasing number of clinicians advocate using noninvasive tests as the initial diagnostic method in patients in whom DVT is suspected. In particular, duplex or color flow scanning is being used more often as the initial method or as a backup for other tests.[35, 201] If, however, the results of any of these tests are equivocal or otherwise unsatisfactory, the clinician should not hesitate to obtain phlebographic confirmation.

The techniques, interpretation, accuracy, and complications of phlebography are discussed in detail in Chapter 132.

Doppler Ultrasonography

Of the many instruments currently employed for the diagnosis of DVT, none is more convenient to use or more readily available than the Doppler velocity detector. With this device, diagnosis of venous disease depends on the recognition of distorted flow patterns or the absence of flow in the larger veins.[297] As with the stethoscope, a moderate degree of interpretive skill is required, and proficiency can be gained only with practice. This requirement, together with the possibility that nonocclusive thrombi may be overlooked, constitutes a relative drawback to the use of the "Doppler." Although the profunda femoris vein and the venous sinusoids of the soleus and gastrocnemius muscles cannot be examined and the anterior tibial and peroneal veins are difficult to examine, most of the deep and superficial veins of the legs and arms are easily accessible to the ultrasonic beam. When Doppler ultrasonography is combined with B-mode imaging (as in duplex scanning), many of these limitations and drawbacks are eliminated.

Doppler ultrasonography has the following advantages: (1) it is a reasonably accurate method for detecting thrombi in those veins that are the sources of fatal pulmonary emboli; (2) incompetence of deep, superficial, and perforating veins can be recognized; (3) it is totally noninvasive, painless, and safe; (4) studies can be accomplished rapidly in almost any patient at the bedside and can be repeated as frequently as necessary; and (5) the equipment is rugged, inexpensive, and portable.

Technique

Although a pocket-type instrument is often adequate, in many cases it is helpful to have the added information provided by one of the more complex direction-sensing devices or by duplex scanning. The signal can easily be recorded for documentation, but for most purposes, the audible signal is all that is necessary. Because lower-frequency sound has greater penetrating power, instruments with frequencies of about 5 MHz are preferred by most investigators for studying the deep veins. In the author's experience, however, the more superficial veins, such as the saphenous and posterior tibial, are best examined with a 10-MHz probe.

Studies are performed with the patient in a supine position with his or her head resting on a pillow. It is usually advantageous to elevate the head of the bed a few degrees to ensure complete filling of the veins of the legs. A moderate amount of external rotation at the hip and flexion of the knee facilitates access to the veins and relieves muscle tension. In all studies, it is most important that the legs be relaxed to prevent venous compression, which, if present, will distort flow patterns and lead to false-positive interpretations. Similarly, all constrictive clothing should be removed.

The Doppler probe is coupled to the skin with ultrasonic gel. No pressure should be applied to the skin when the superficial veins are being examined, and only a modest amount of pressure should be used when the deep veins are studied. Because venous pressure is so low, excessive probe pressure may collapse the underlying veins. For optimum

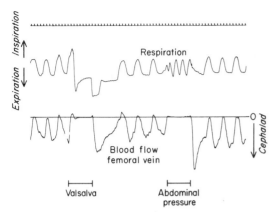

FIGURE 131–1. Flow pattern in a normal common femoral vein recorded with a direction-sensing ultrasonic flow detector. Simultaneous respiratory movements are shown in the upper tracing. Flow increases with expiration and decreases with inspiration. Note that a Valsalva maneuver causes flow to cease without producing retrograde flow. (From Strandness DE Jr, Sumner DS: Hemodynamics for Surgeons. New York, Grune & Stratton, 1975.)

signal reception, the ultrasonic beam should intersect the vein at an acute angle. In most areas of the limbs, this can be accomplished by holding the probe at a 45-degree angle to the skin; however, in the popliteal space, where the vein moves away from the skin toward the adductor hiatus, the optimum angle may approach 90 degrees.

Normal Venous Flow Patterns

Normal venous signals are low pitched, contain a wide spectrum of frequencies, and sound much like a windstorm. In the legs of a supine subject, the signal is phasic with respiration, decreasing with inspiration and increasing with expiration (Fig. 131–1). With each inspiration, the descent of the diaphragm causes the intra-abdominal pressure to rise, compressing the inferior vena cava and decreasing venous outflow from the legs. With expiration, the intra-abdominal pressure falls, and venous outflow again occurs (see Chapter 129). Ordinarily, these phasic changes can be detected in all the major veins of the leg down to and including the posterior tibial veins and saphenous veins at

the ankle. Finding a phasic signal virtually assures the observer that all the venous channels proximal to the position of the Doppler probe are patent—or at least functionally patent.

Respiratory variation is sometimes less noticeable in females. It may even have an opposite phasic relationship in subjects who tend to breathe thoracically. In these individuals, flow increases during inspiration and decreases during expiration. Venous flow in the arms is also phasic with respiration, but it usually increases with inspiration and decreases with expiration (Fig. 131–2). This same pattern may be seen in the legs when the subject is in an upright position.[175] Owing to gravitational effects, veins tend to remain dilated in upright subjects, with the result that venous flow patterns are directly responsive to changes in intrathoracic pressure.

Smaller pulsations attributable to the contraction of the right atrium are superimposed on the phasic changes that are due to respiration. These waves travel retrograde from the heart to the periphery. Although they can be heard and recorded in normal individuals (especially in the arm veins; see Fig. 131–2), they are most striking when the venous pressure is elevated.[216, 243] Markedly pulsatile venous flow is characteristic of patients with congestive heart failure or tricuspid insufficiency.

As shown in Figure 131–1, when the normal supine subject performs a Valsalva maneuver, there is usually no reflux of blood down the veins of the leg, despite the sudden marked increase in abdominal pressure. Sometimes, however, small amounts of blood may pass down the leg before the iliofemoral valve or valves have a chance to close. Unless the expiratory effort is maintained for a prolonged period, no venous outflow will be detected at the common femoral level. On release of the Valsalva maneuver, a sudden surge of blood rushes up the leg veins to fill the void in the inferior vena cava. These effects can be detected as far peripherally as the ankle.

Venous flow can be augmented by various maneuvers. Squeezing the hand into a fist or plantar flexing the foot will evacuate the forearm and calf veins, respectively (see Fig. 131–2). A more convenient method is to compress the calf or forearm manually. Only a very gentle squeeze is required. When venous valves are normal, compressing the limb proximal to the position of the Doppler probe will

FIGURE 131–2. Flow pattern in a normal brachial vein. Pulsations coinciding with the cardiac cycle are prominent. Note that flow increases with both quiet inspiration and slow deep inspiration. Rapid deep inspiration, however, may collapse the subclavian vein at the thoracic outlet and decrease flow. Flow is augmented by squeezing the hand or forearm. (From Sumner DS: Noninvasive vascular laboratory assessment. *In* Machleder HJ [ed]: Vascular Disorders of the Upper Extremity. 2nd ed. Mount Kisco, NY, Futura Publishing, 1989, pp 9–57.)

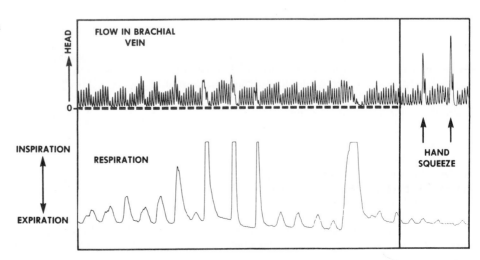

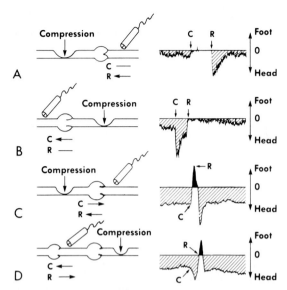

FIGURE 131–3. Venous flow responses to augmentation maneuvers. *A* and *B*, Normal response. *C* and *D*, Abnormal responses typical of venous valvular incompetence. Because the Doppler probe was pointed cephalad, flow toward the head (antegrade) is indicated by a downward deflection of the tracing; flow toward the foot (retrograde) is indicated by an upward deflection. C, compression; R, release of compression.

cause venous flow to cease. On release of the compression, the trapped blood will rush past the probe (see Fig. 131–3*A*). If the limb is squeezed distal to the probe, there will be a copious, "easy" flow of blood. With release of the compression, flow will cease momentarily until the veins have had a chance to refill from capillary inflow (see Fig. 131–3*B*).

Venous Obstruction

If the ultrasonic beam is directed into a completely obstructed venous segment where there is no flow, no audible signal will be received (Fig. 131–4*B*). When the probe is over a patent vein but peripheral to an obstruction, the flow signal will be "continuous," showing little phasic variation with respiration (see Fig. 131–4*C*). It will not be interrupted by a deep breath. Even a Valsalva maneuver may not completely stop flow. This flow pattern is frequently observed in the common femoral vein when there is an obstruction of the iliac vein or the inferior vena cava.

The continuous flow pattern is explained by the high venous pressure that develops peripheral to an obstruction. Because of this high peripheral pressure, mild variations in venous outflow resistance produced by changes in intra-abdominal pressure have little effect on the pressure gradient that controls the rate of venous flow.

When the probe is positioned proximal or cephalad to a venous obstruction, venous flow may be either relatively normal or reduced in volume, depending on the adequacy of the collateral inflow. Compression of the limb peripheral to the site of obstruction will produce little or no augmentation of venous flow in a vein cephalad to the obstruction (see Fig. 131–4*D*). Unfortunately, this test may not always be reliable because it depends on the amount of blood moved by the compression and the functional capacity of

existing collateral channels. Comparison with the response at a similar level on the opposite limb is necessary to avoid misinterpretation.

Venous Valvular Incompetence

Venous valves may be congenitally incompetent or may become incompetent as a result of venous distention or valvular destruction. Scarring and retraction of the delicate valve cusps accompany resolution of a venous thrombosis. Because valvular incompetence is a hallmark of the postphlebitic limb, it is important to recognize the presence of incompetent valves even when the Doppler survey is being undertaken primarily to detect obstruction. Finding incompetent valves in the deep veins below the common femoral level should alert the examiner to the possibility that any venous obstruction found in the same limb might be chronic rather than acute.

Valvular incompetence can be identified in several ways. At the common femoral level, it is convenient to use the Valsalva maneuver. As discussed previously, the Valsalva maneuver normally produces little or no reflux of abdominal venous blood into the common femoral vein, but when the iliofemoral valves are absent or incompetent, an audible rush of blood toward the probe can be detected or a surge of retrograde flow can be recorded.[243] The retrograde flow continues down the limb until a competent valve is encountered and may be detected as far peripherally as the posterior tibial or ankle saphenous vein when all the intervening valves are incompetent.

Gentle compression of the leg in the vicinity of incompetent valves will force blood to flow both antegrade and retrograde. When the compression is released, the collapsed veins are refilled from above by blood refluxing down the leg and from below by blood flowing up the leg. As a result, an augmented Doppler signal is detected both during

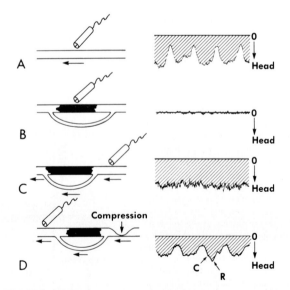

FIGURE 131–4. Changes in venous flow pattern produced by an obstructing thrombus. *A*, No obstruction, normal flow pattern. *B*, Probe over the obstruction. *C*, Probe distal to the obstruction. *D*, Lack of augmentation when the vein is obstructed distal to the probe. The Doppler probe is pointed cephalad; flow in the normal antegrade direction produces a downward deflection of the tracing.

compression and release. This seesaw flow pattern is easily distinguished from the normal response to limb compression (see Fig. 131–3). Depending on the location of the probe relative to the incompetent valve and the site of limb compression, the initial signal may be toward or away from the probe; the signal on release will have the opposite orientation. By placing the probe over the superficial femoral, popliteal, posterior tibial, and saphenous veins and compressing the limb both above and below the site of probe application, the examiner can determine the competency of the veins in the segment under investigation. Studies should be performed with the patient supine and then repeated with the patient standing. Having the patient shift his or her weight from one leg to another is another way of revealing reflux flow.

If the study is being performed for symptoms suggestive of acute DVT, Valsalva maneuvers and vigorous limb compression should be avoided in order to minimize the risk of dislodging a clot that might embolize to the lungs.

Evaluating Patients With Suspected Acute Deep Venous Thrombosis

In cases of suspected acute venous thrombosis, the emphasis should be on the recognition of venous obstruction rather than valvular incompetence. Thus, the examiner is primarily concerned with *absence* of flow in a particular vein, presence of a *continuous* flow pattern, *lack of augmentation* of the flow signal with distal compression, and *excessive flow* in superficial veins.

Because changes in venous dynamics are sometimes subtle, it is mandatory that an orderly, careful study be performed. The common femoral, superficial femoral, popliteal, posterior tibial, and saphenous veins are examined—usually in that order. It is important to compare the signal from the same vein in the opposite limb before moving to the next level. Repeated comparisons will frequently bring out slight differences in flow patterns that might not be apparent initially.

At each level, the first step is to determine the presence or absence of a spontaneous flow signal. Because collateral venous channels are often present, it is necessary for the examiner to be absolutely certain that he or she is studying the vein in question; otherwise, erroneous interpretations are inevitable. This is best accomplished by first identifying the adjacent artery and then moving the probe in the appropriate direction to find the vein of the same name. Ordinarily, the probe need only be moved very slightly, usually less than 1 cm. Merely shifting the skin or tilting the probe should suffice in most instances. When venous flow is first encountered, the arterial signal should still be audible in the background. Many errors can be avoided by adhering to this procedure. A better venous signal, with little arterial interference, can then be obtained by further adjustment of the probe.

If, at this stage, doubt remains about the identity of the vein, the signal may be traced up or down the limb. Whereas major veins are relatively straight, occupying a well-prescribed course, collateral channels tend to veer off from the normal pathway and are difficult to follow. The use of a duplex or color flow scanner will obviate many of

these difficulties by providing positive identification of the veins being studied.

When the probe is in the correct position, the absence of a spontaneous venous signal usually indicates obstruction of the underlying vein. If spontaneous flow is not immediately detected, the examiner should forego the temptation to augment the signal by squeezing the leg distal to the probe. Not only is this maneuver potentially dangerous in patients in whom there is a possibility of pulmonary embolism, but also it may lead to erroneous conclusions. By increasing the velocity of flow in adjacent collateral veins or in residual venous channels, a forceful squeeze can give rise to confusing signals that lead the examiner to suspect that the underlying vein is patent when in reality it is obstructed. With a little patience, spontaneous flow signals can be obtained from all patent deep veins of the leg. A possible exception to this rule is the posterior tibial vein at the ankle. Occasionally, the velocity of flow in this vein is below the threshold of the ultrasonic flowmeter. In these cases, a gentle foot squeeze will produce a free flow of blood if the posterior tibial vein is patent. In the author's experience, however, spontaneous signals are present in 87 per cent of posterior tibial veins, provided that the foot is warm, the leg is relaxed, and no pressure is applied with the probe.[302]

If the vein beneath the probe is patent, the second step in the examination is to assess the quality of the flow signal. A phasic flow pattern, easily interrupted by a deep breath, indicates that all proximal veins are functionally patent. On the other hand, a continuous flow pattern—especially one that persists with a deep breath—is highly suggestive of proximal obstruction. Valsalva maneuvers are not performed in patients with suspected pulmonary embolism, for fear of dislodging additional thrombi.

Augmentation maneuvers constitute the third step in the examination. As pointed out earlier, the patency of major veins distal to the probe can sometimes be assessed with this procedure. Although some investigators rely heavily on augmentation maneuvers, in the author's opinion augmented signals are not dependable and should be interpreted cautiously. The generated signal depends on the force and rapidity with which the leg is squeezed, the volume of blood in the area being squeezed, the anatomic configuration of the part, and the distance of the probe from the area being squeezed. Even when the major deep veins are obstructed between the probe and the site being squeezed, a forceful squeeze may produce a deceptively good flow signal, leading the examiner to conclude that the deep veins are patent. Flow in this case passes up the leg via collateral channels to reach the vein underlying the probe, as shown in Figure 131–4D.

As a final step, flow in the superficial veins should be assessed. The examination should include the saphenous vein at the ankle and lower thigh and any visible superficial veins in the region of the groin. When the deep veins are occluded, the velocity of flow in the ipsilateral superficial veins is often greatly increased in comparison with that in comparable veins of the contralateral extremity. In the author's experience, this is a most reliable secondary sign of DVT. It is particularly helpful in diagnosing venous thrombosis below the knee, where flow patterns in the posterior tibial vein may be difficult to evaluate.

Superficial Venous Thrombosis

Superficial and deep venous thrombosis may coexist. Although the diagnosis of superficial venous thrombosis can usually be made on physical examination, trauma, fat necrosis, cellulitis, vasculitis, and lymphangitis may produce similar signs. Absence of a venous signal in the area of inflammation or over the tender palpable cord is presumptive evidence of superficial venous thrombosis, provided it is known that a vein passes through the involved area.[34] If venous flow is detected, one of the other alternative diagnoses must be considered. Arterial signals are often detected in the adjacent hyperemic tissues. Because of their characteristic pulsatility, arterial signals are easily distinguished from signals of venous origin and therefore should cause no confusion.

When the greater saphenous vein in the thigh is involved, it is important to examine the flow pattern in the common femoral vein to rule out propagation of clot into the deep venous system at this level.

Upper Extremity Venous Thrombosis

Recognition of venous thrombosis in the tributaries of the superior vena cava is somewhat more difficult than it is in the lower extremity. Despite the presence of thrombi, a rich system of collateral channels serves to maintain adequate venous flow. Moreover, the prominent pulsations characteristic of upper extremity venous flow and the variable responses to respiration compound the problem (cf. Fig. 131–2). Nevertheless, thrombi can usually be detected in the brachial, axillary, or subclavian veins if careful attention is paid to lack of respiratory variation, impaired augmentation, and the presence of continuous flow.[286, 313] Increased flow in superficial veins such as the cephalic, the external jugular, and the subcutaneous veins around the shoulder girdle helps to confirm the diagnosis. Impaired flow in the internal jugular vein indicates thrombosis of the innominate vein, which not infrequently accompanies obstruction of the more peripheral veins of the upper extremity. Again, as in the leg, it is mandatory to compare the signals from one arm with those from the other; otherwise, subtle changes in the venous flow pattern may be overlooked.

Recurrent Deep Venous Thrombosis

Previous thrombophlebitis, with its residue of occluded and recanalized veins and dilated collateral channels, makes recognition of acute recurrent venous thrombosis difficult.[33] Unless the patient has been followed carefully, it may be impossible to differentiate between an old and a new clot. Because this information is seldom available, other diagnostic methods are usually needed in patients in whom a diagnosis of recurrent thrombophlebitis is seriously considered.

The post-thrombotic condition itself is easily diagnosed with the Doppler technique. When the examination reveals incompetent valves in deep veins other than the common femoral vein (which may be congenitally incompetent) or when prominent veins that occupy a circuitous

course differing from that of normal veins are detected, it is quite likely that venous obstruction may be chronic rather than acute. Because of extensive collateral development, confusing signals may be detected in the vicinity of a chronically clotted vein. In such cases, the inexperienced examiner may conclude that the vein is patent when, in fact, it is occluded.

Sources of Error

Table 131–4 lists the major pitfalls encountered in using Doppler ultrasonography to diagnose DVT. Some of these have been alluded to previously. (Many errors in this list can be avoided by using Doppler ultrasonography in conjunction with duplex scanning.)

Inaccessible Veins

Like other flow-dependent methods, Doppler ultrasonography can detect only those thrombi that involve the major deep veins existing in continuity from the ankle (or wrist) to the heart. Isolated thrombi within tributaries, such as the internal iliac, profunda femoris, gastrocnemial, and soleal veins, will escape recognition. Because isolated internal iliac thrombi occur in fewer than 6 per cent of limbs with venous thrombosis and isolated profunda femoris thrombi are found in about 1 per cent of such limbs, the false-negative incidence related to missing clots in these areas is relatively low.[86, 275]

The problem is more serious in the calf. Isolated calf vein thrombi occur in 20 to 46 per cent of limbs with DVT. Because the posterior tibial vein (the only calf vein that can be studied reliably with the Doppler technique) is involved in only 60 per cent of limbs with infrapopliteal thrombosis, the estimated incidence of false-negative studies should range from 8 to 18 per cent.[86, 212] Unfortunately, the peroneal veins, which are involved in 81 per cent of limbs with calf vein thrombosis, are prohibitively difficult to examine. Although it may be possible to detect flow in the anterior tibial vein, the additional effort required is seldom justified because this vein is rarely the site of isolated thrombi.[86] As mentioned previously, increased flow in the superficial veins of the calf is an important secondary sign of venous thrombosis in this area. Appreciation of this sign will decrease the incidence of false-negative errors.

Table 131–4. Sources of Error in Doppler Ultrasonographic Study for Acute Venous Thrombophlebitis

Thromboses below the knee
Previous thrombophlebitis
Nonocclusive thrombi
Poor sound transmission
Excessive pressure on the transducer
Severe congestive heart failure
Hyperemia due to inflammation
Severe vasoconstriction
External compression (ascites, tumors, knee
  surgery, ruptured popliteal cysts, hematoma)
Pregnancy
Inexperience

Nonocclusive Thrombi

Inasmuch as the Doppler flowmeter detects the presence or absence of flow and only roughly measures its quantity, long, narrow, nonocclusive thrombi originating in venous valvular sinuses may be overlooked. Until these clots become securely attached to the endothelial surface, they may break away to cause pulmonary emboli. Failure to recognize such clots constitutes a potentially serious indictment of the Doppler technique. Although the majority of thrombi developing in high-risk asymptomatic patients may be nonocclusive,[188] according to Diener,[86] only 5.4 per cent of those found in acutely symptomatic patients are of this variety. In fact, most reviews suggest that nonocclusive clots in veins above the knee are responsible for few false-negative errors,[13, 89, 121, 194, 302] and those that are sufficiently large may even be detected.[31, 87, 132, 165] It is disturbing, nonetheless, to reflect on the fact that Doppler survey results are positive in only 23 to 61 per cent of patients with documented pulmonary emboli.[11, 27, 51] Because approximately 90 per cent of these emboli originate in leg veins, clots are either being missed or, having broken away, are leaving only small, nondetectable residues.

Venous Collaterals and Duplicated Veins

Enlarged collateral veins may be mistaken for a neighboring deep vein, which may be occluded. This error is especially apt to occur in the groin, where collaterals bypassing an occluded common femoral vein are often well developed and lie close to the common femoral artery. Careful examination techniques, as described earlier in this chapter, will usually differentiate between collateral and main channel flow.

Because the major deep veins of the calf are duplicated, clots isolated to one of the venae comitantes will escape detection. Similarly, duplications of the popliteal or superficial femoral veins are occasionally responsible for false-negative errors.

Extrinsic Compression

External compression at the popliteal level may distort the flow pattern in the popliteal and posterior tibial veins, leading to a false-positive interpretation.[165, 242] Knee surgery, ruptured popliteal cysts, and local hematomas from disrupted muscle bellies are the main offenders. When these diagnoses are suspected, finding a normal superficial femoral venous signal suggests extrinsic compression rather than thrombosis. Compression of the inferior vena cava or the pelvic veins by tumors or ascites can produce a continuous signal in the common femoral vein, mimicking the findings associated with iliac vein thrombosis.[165] In most cases of iliac vein thrombosis, however, the common femoral vein is also occluded.

Because the gravid uterus may compress the vena cava and the iliac veins, false-positive results may be obtained in pregnant women near term.[165, 242] Abnormal flow patterns observed with the patient in the supine position usually revert to normal when the woman is turned on her side and the uppermost limb is examined. Because this maneuver relieves pressure on the venous outflow, persistence of an abnormal signal in the uppermost limb implies intrinsic obstruction.

Other Sources of Error

Sound transmission through edematous or very obese legs, through hematoma, and through scar tissue is often poor, and due allowances must be made when these conditions prevail in order to avoid false-positive interpretations. Superficial veins, such as the saphenous and posterior tibial veins (at the ankle), are easily compressed by pressure from the probe, and even deep veins may be compressed when the pressure exerted is excessive. Collapse of the underlying veins under these circumstances gives a false impression of venous occlusion. When superficial veins are examined, the probe should not actually touch the skin but should be coupled to the skin through an acoustic gel.[302] The probe should just barely indent the skin when deep veins are examined.

Confusing flow patterns may occur in some generalized and local conditions. In patients suffering from congestive heart failure or tricuspid insufficiency, the veins within the abdominal cavity may remain distended throughout the respiratory cycle despite periodic fluctuations of abdominal pressure. The signal will not vary with respiration as it normally does but will display pulsations coinciding with the retrograde transmission of pressure waves from the heart.[165, 242] Hyperemia associated with inflammatory processes may produce such high rates of flow that the signal becomes nearly continuous.[165] These findings should seldom be confused with the continuous flow signal heard distal to a proximal venous occlusion. The excessively large volume of flow and physical findings typical of inflammation make differentiation easy.

Lack of a venous signal can be due to sluggish flow caused by vasoconstriction or to compression caused by muscle contraction. Keeping the patient warm and relaxed will minimize these effects. Arterial obstruction seldom has an adverse effect on venous flow patterns.

Inexperience is perhaps the most common cause of error.[31, 194] Although the Doppler examination is conceptually simple, in practice it requires concentration, interest, some knowledge of anatomy and physiology, and well-developed interpretive skills. Careless, hasty examinations will inevitably produce many false-positive and false-negative results.

Accuracy

The reported accuracy of the Doppler device for detecting DVT is summarized in Table 131–5. Few of the studies included in this table were prospective, and in most, phlebography, which served as the gold standard, was performed at the discretion of the referring physician. This approach tends to increase the relative number of positive examination results, creating a selection bias that may have made the figures appear better than they would have been had the studies included all patients who presented with suspected DVT. The wide variation in reported accuracy is not easily explained but is probably a function of the different populations that were studied and the different techniques that were employed. Results seemed to be worse

Table 131–5.   Accuracy of Doppler Survey for Diagnosing Deep Venous Thrombosis, Both Above and Below the Knee (Summary of 24 Reports)

	No. of Studies	Accuracy (%)				
		SENS	SPEC	PPV	NPV	ACC
Range	32–271	31–100	59–100	50–100	50–100	49–96
Median	119	78	89	83	87	87
Mean ± SD	130 ± 76	77 ± 19	87 ± 10	81 ± 12	85 ± 13	83 ± 12
Cumulative	3130	77	90	82	88	86
		$\frac{866}{1121}$	$\frac{1814}{2009}$	$\frac{866}{1061}$	$\frac{118}{2069}$	$\frac{2680}{3130}$

Data from references 13, 31, 40, 89, 104, 121, 132, 148, 150, 179, 187, 190, 194, 200, 211, 223, 245, 272, 277, 291, 302, 335, 337, and 340.
SENS, sensitivity; SPEC, specificity; PPV, positive predictive value; NPV, negative predictive value; ACC, overall accuracy.

Table 131–6.   Accuracy of Doppler Survey for Diagnosing Deep Venous Thrombosis, Above the Knee Only (Summary of 12 Reports)

	No. of Studies	Accuracy (%)				
		SENS	SPEC	PPV	NPV	ACC
Range	46–222	74–100	67–99	50–98	89–100	76–97
Median	119	93	93	84	96	92
Mean ± SD	127 ± 52	90 ± 8	90 ± 8	80 ± 15	96 ± 4	91 ± 6
Cumulative	1522	89	91	80	95	90
		$\frac{396}{443}$	$\frac{981}{1079}$	$\frac{396}{494}$	$\frac{981}{1028}$	$\frac{1377}{1522}$

Data from references 14, 31, 104, 121, 132, 173, 187, 194, 223, 245, 302, and 337.
SENS, sensitivity; SPEC, specificity; PPV, positive predictive value; NPV, negative predictive value; ACC, overall accuracy.

Table 131–7.   Accuracy of Doppler Survey for Diagnosing Deep Venous Thrombosis

	Phlebography			
Doppler	Negative	Positive (Above Knee)	Positive (Below Knee)	Total
Negative	104	2	3	109
Positive	17	34	32	83
Total	121	36	35	192

Sensitivity			Predictive value		
Overall:	66/71	= 93%	Positive:	66/83	= 80%
Above knee:	34/36	= 94%	Negative:	104/109	= 95%
Below knee:	32/35	= 91%	Overall accuracy:	170/192	= 89%
Specificity:	104/121	= 86%			

Data from Sumner DS, Lambeth A: Reliability of Doppler ultrasound in the diagnosis of acute venous thrombosis both above and below the knee. Am J Surg 138:205, 1979.

when the examinations were limited to the more proximal veins and when augmented rather than spontaneous signals were emphasized.[281] The relatively low cumulative sensitivity (77 per cent) reflects the inclusion of both above-knee and below-knee venous thromboses in the study population. In all reports, most false-negative errors represent a failure to detect below-knee thrombi. When only thrombi involving above-knee veins are considered, the average reported sensitivity is around 90 per cent and the negative predictive value is about 95 per cent (Table 131–6). In other words, only 5 per cent of limbs with negative Doppler study results had phlebographic findings that were positive for proximal venous thrombi.

Results of a study from the author's laboratory, in which the complete survey methods advocated in this chapter were used, are shown in Table 131–7.[302] Ninety-four per cent of proximal venous thrombi and 91 per cent of isolated below-knee thrombi were detected by this approach, for an overall sensitivity of 93 per cent. The specificity was 86 per cent. The author and his colleagues are content to sacrifice specificity and positive predictive value in order to maintain a high sensitivity and negative predictive value. Suspected infrapopliteal disease not confirmed phlebographically accounted for the majority of false-positive errors (13 of 17). Similar results have been reported by Barnes and associates, whose examination techniques are practically identical to those the author employs.[31, 32] For identifying and ruling out below-knee thrombosis, their accuracy was as follows: sensitivity, 94 per cent; specificity, 78 per cent; positive predictive value, 68 per cent; and negative predictive value, 97 per cent. These data suggest that the Doppler survey can be used to rule out most serious calf vein thrombi in symptomatic patients; however, positive results may require phlebographic confirmation.

Much less information is available concerning the accuracy of Doppler ultrasonography for diagnosing thromboses of the upper extremity. Although an accuracy of 100 per cent was reported by Gray and associates,[114] Sottiurai and coworkers found a specificity of only 50 per cent and a sensitivity of 89 per cent.[286] Both series, however, were small, and further confirmation is required.

Venous Occlusion Plethysmography

Thrombi occluding the major veins of the leg decrease venous compliance and increase venous outflow resistance. Plethysmographic methods for diagnosing DVT depend on recognition of these physiologic effects. All plethysmographs measure the same thing—volume change (specifically of the calf)—and any of the various types can be used, including impedance plethysmographs, air plethysmographs, and mercury- or indium-gallium–filled strain-gauges (see Chapter 4). The most popular of these, however, is the impedance plethysmograph. Indeed, before the advent of duplex scanning, impedance plethysmography was the most widely used and most thoroughly investigated noninvasive test for DVT.

Clots involving veins above the knee are detected with a high degree of accuracy; studies can be performed on most patients, both in the clinic and at the bedside; the test is totally noninvasive and can be repeated as frequently as necessary; the techniques are standardized and require little training to master; and the instrumentation is rugged, portable, and relatively inexpensive—all significant advantages. The main disadvantage of impedance plethysmography is its insensitivity to calf vein thrombi.

Rationale

When a pneumatic cuff wrapped around the thigh of a supine patient is inflated to a pressure of 50 mmHg, venous outflow is impeded. Because the arterial inflow is unaffected, blood accumulates in the veins distal to the cuff until the peripheral venous pressure rises to equal the congesting pressure. In normal limbs, the preocclusion venous pressure is 10 mmHg or less. Consequently, raising the venous pressure to 50 mmHg causes the calf volume to increase by 2 or 3 per cent (Fig. 131–5).[25] The increase in volume is measured by a plethysmograph placed around the calf. In contrast, when the peripheral venous pressure is already elevated owing to venous obstruction, raising the venous pressure to 50 mmHg causes considerably less change in calf volume (see Fig. 131–5).[119] Expansion of the calf is reduced, not only because the pressure increment is less but also because the pressure-volume curve is in the "stiff" area, where venous volume is relatively insensitive to pressure change. Thus, impaired calf volume expansion (also called venous capacitance) suggests venous thrombosis. Measurement of calf volume change in response to venous congestion was one of the earliest plethysmographic tests for DVT. Although the mean volume change observed in normal limbs is statistically different from that observed in limbs with DVT, overlapping values degrade the sensitivity and specificity of the test (Fig. 131–6).

Venous resistance can be estimated by noting the rate at which the calf volume decreases when the congesting pressure is rapidly released (Fig. 131–7). Because the pressure in the peripheral veins (P_{pv}) rises to equal that in the thigh cuff and because the central venous pressure (P_{cv}) is quite low (almost zero) and relatively constant, a standardized pressure gradient ($P_{pv} - P_{cv}$) is established. Under

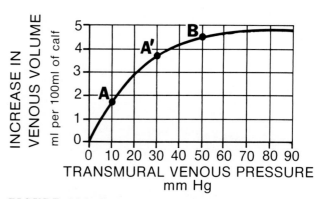

FIGURE 131–5. Calf venous pressure-volume curve. Pressure in the normal limb is low (A), but it is elevated in the limb with acute deep venous thrombosis (A'). Inflating the thigh cuff to 50 mmHg increases the volume of normal limb by almost 3 per cent (A to B); however, in the abnormal limb, the volume increase is less than 1 per cent (A' to B). (From Sumner DS: Diagnosis of deep vein thrombosis by strain-gauge plethysmography. *In* Bernstein EF [ed]: Vascular Diagnosis. 4th ed. St. Louis, CV Mosby, 1993, pp 811–819.)

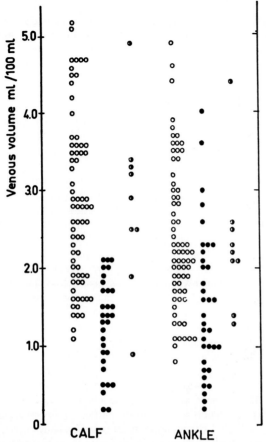

FIGURE 131–6. Calf and ankle volume expansion in response to a congesting pressure of 50 mmHg. Normal limbs are depicted by *open circles*; limbs with acute deep venous thrombosis (DVT), *closed circles*; postphlebitic limbs, *half-closed circles*. (From Hallböök T, Göthlin J: Strain-gauge plethysmography and phlebography in diagnosis of deep venous thrombosis. Acta Chir Scand 137:37, 1971.)

these conditions, the initial rate of calf volume decrease, the maximal venous outflow (Q_o), is roughly inversely proportional to venous resistance (R_v):[292, 298]

$$Q_0 = (P_{pv} - P_{cv})/R_v \approx P_{pv}/R_v \qquad (131.1)$$

On the basis of published values for maximal venous outflow (MVO), the venous resistance in limbs with acute DVT appears to be about three to five times normal.[24, 25, 79, 119, 255] Thus, MVO is a better diagnostic test than venous compliance.

Because the venous outflow curve decreases in slope as the calf volume decreases, MVO may be difficult to measure. This has led to the practice of measuring the quantity of outflow at a specific time (usually 2 or 3 seconds) after cuff release (see Fig. 131–7). The 2- or 3-second outflow, however, not only is a function of venous resistance but also depends on the compliance of the venous wall. Timed outflow, therefore, is not strictly analogous to MVO.

Although a discussion of the complex interaction of the factors that determine the shape of the venous outflow curve is beyond the scope of this text, it is intuitively evident that, given a constant venous resistance, the rate of outflow will decrease as the peripheral venous pressure falls following cuff release. Perhaps less evident is the fact that the peripheral venous pressure also depends on the venous compliance and on the volume of blood in the veins (which decreases progressively following cuff release) (Fig. 131–8). Thus, the amount of blood leaving the calf within a specific time can be approximated by the following equation:[9, 292, 298]

$$\Delta V_t = V_o(1 - e^{-(E/R_V)t}) \qquad (131.2)$$

In this equation, ΔV_t is the decrease in calf volume at a specific time, t; V_o is the maximal volume expansion or venous capacitance before cuff release; E is the elastic

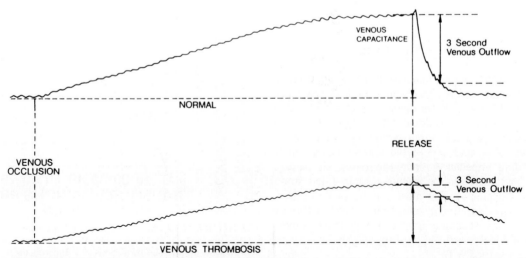

FIGURE 131–7. Typical impedance plethysmography tracings. The 3-second venous outflow is markedly reduced with recent DVT. (From Wheeler HB, Anderson FA Jr: Diagnosis of deep vein thrombosis by impedance plethysmography. *In* Bernstein EF [ed]: Vascular Diagnosis. 4th ed. St. Louis, CV Mosby, 1993, pp 820–829.)

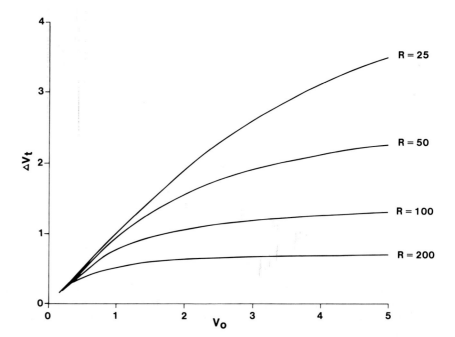

FIGURE 131–8.
Relationship of 3-second venous outflow (ΔV_t) to maximum calf volume expansion (V_o) at various levels of venous resistance (R). Values are based on equation 131–2. (From Sumner DS: Applied physiology in venous problems. *In* Bergan JJ, Yao JST [eds]: Surgery of the Veins. Orlando, FL, Grune & Stratton, 1985, pp 3–23.)

modulus of the venous wall (pressure/volume), the reciprocal of compliance; and e is the base of the natural logarithm. Because venous compliance varies with the state of venous distention, increasing as the venous volume decreases, E varies continuously during the period following cuff release; therefore, Equation 131.2 is an oversimplification.[305] Nonetheless, it emphasizes that the timed outflow, ΔV_t, increases as the maximal volume expansion or venous capacitance, V_o, increases—provided that the venous resistance remains constant (see Fig. 131–8). At higher resistances, however, the slope of the line $\Delta V_t = f(V_o)$ becomes almost horizontal. In other words, the separation between the lines increases as V_o increases. These relationships have been confirmed experimentally and provide a theoretical basis for the discriminant line shown in Figure 131–9.[145] It follows that diagnostic accuracy should be improved by plotting the timed venous outflow against the venous capacitance and by measuring venous outflow when venous capacitance is maximal.

FIGURE 131–9. Impedance plethysmographic results displayed as a graph of 3-second venous outflow plotted as a function of venous capacitance (rise vs fall). A *diagonal line* accurately divides patients with normal venograms from those with recent proximal DVT. (From Hull R, van Aken WG, Hirsh J, et al: Impedance plethysmography using the occlusive cuff technique in the diagnosis of venous thrombosis. Circulation 53:696, 1976. Reprinted by permission of the American Heart Association, Inc.)

Impedance Plethysmography

With the patient lying supine, the leg being examined is elevated 20 to 30 degrees to facilitate venous drainage.[327] A pillow is placed under the calf and heel, the knee is flexed about 10 to 20 degrees, and the leg is externally rotated slightly at the hip (Fig. 131–10). These measures are taken to ensure that the extremity is relaxed and that there is no compression of the popliteal vein by the posterior border of the tibia. An 8-inch-wide pneumatic cuff is wrapped around the thigh, and a set of two electrodes is placed on the calf. After the instrument has been electrically balanced, the cuff is inflated to about 50 to 70 cmH₂O (37 to 51 mmHg). The pressure is maintained until a plateau is reached; then the cuff is rapidly deflated (see Fig. 131–7). Measurements are made of the rise of the tracing from the baseline (venous capacitance) and the fall from the peak value that occurs within 3 seconds of cuff release (3-second venous outflow).[146, 329] These measurements are then plotted

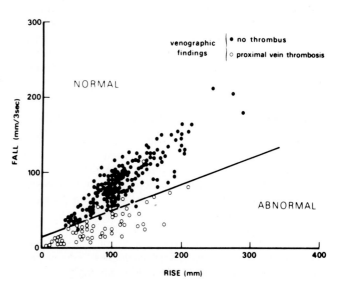

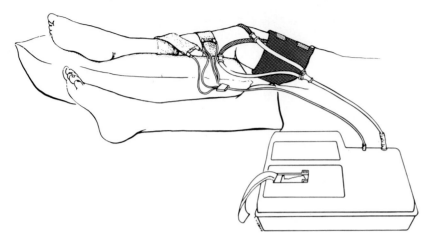

FIGURE 131-10. Impedance plethysmography measures venous volume changes in the calf in response to temporary venous obstruction produced by a pneumatic cuff on the thigh. (Reproduced with permission from Wheeler HB, Anderson FA Jr: Impedance plethysmography. *In* Kempczinski RF, Yao JST [eds]: Practical Noninvasive Vascular Diagnosis, 2nd edition. Copyright © 1987 by Year Book Medical Publishers, Inc, Chicago.)

on a graph in which the vertical axis represents the "fall," or venous outflow, and the horizontal axis represents the "rise," or venous capacitance (see Fig. 131–9).[146] If the point described by these two parameters lies above the experimentally determined discriminant line, the test finding is considered to be negative for DVT. On the other hand, if the point lies below the discriminant line, the test should be repeated, with a longer period of occlusion (120 seconds) to ensure that venous capacitance is maximal. The test is considered positive when, after repeated periods of cuff inflation, the point continues to fall below the discriminant line.

Hull and coworkers advocate a five-test sequence with occlusion times of 45, 45, 120, 45, and 120 seconds, respectively.[145] In phlebographically normal limbs, they found that 76 per cent of the initial test results fell in the normal area but that 20 per cent were falsely positive. With repeated testing, these abnormal points became normal, as the venous wall stretched and the venous capacitance improved. In other words, the points followed a line similar to that designated R = 25 in Figure 131–8. Although 82 per cent of limbs with proximal DVT had test results that were abnormal initially and remained so on repeated testing, in 10 per cent the initial test result fell above the discriminant line and would have been considered normal had no further tests been performed. When the venous capacitance was increased with repeated and prolonged cuff occlusion, the subsequent test results fell in the abnormal area, with the points roughly following a line similar to R = 100 or R = 200 in Figure 131–8. Thus, repeated testing improves both sensitivity and specificity.

Studies in Postphlebitic Limbs

Occlusions of the major deep veins may not be detected in postphlebitic limbs when venous collaterals are well developed. Positive study results in patients with a history of DVT are frequently hard to interpret. It is reasonable to assume that an abnormal test result in a patient in whom recent study results were normal represents recurrent DVT. Abnormal test results, however, may merely reflect residual obstruction from prior episodes of venous thrombosis. Venous volume excursions, analogous to the respiratory waves obtained with Doppler ultrasonography, are usu-

ally present in postphlebitic limbs but are absent in limbs with recent clots.[327] These excursions are best observed when the legs are flat or slightly below heart level. If the tracing rises appreciably with a deep inspiration or with a Valsalva maneuver, the obstruction is likely to be chronic rather than acute.

Sources of Error

Like the Doppler survey, impedance plethysmography will detect only those thrombi that obstruct the major outflow veins of the leg. Clots in tributary veins, such as the profunda femoris and the internal iliac veins, do not impede venous outflow. Impedance plethysmography is even less sensitive than Doppler ultrasonography to the presence of clots confined to the calf veins, with results being positive in only about 20 per cent of such limbs. Small, nonocclusive thrombi will also be missed.

Contraction of the leg muscles in nervous patients who are unable to relax interferes with venous outflow. False-positive results may also be due to extrinsic compression from popliteal cysts, tumors, or other extravascular masses. Elevation of the central venous pressure (P_{cv}) in patients with congestive heart failure decreases the pressure gradient driving blood out of the leg (see Eq. 131.1), thereby decreasing venous outflow. Reduced arterial inflow in patients with severe peripheral arterial obstructive disease and in patients with low cardiac outputs restricts venous filling and may lead to false-positive interpretations. Vasoconstriction may have a similarly adverse effect. It is usually possible, however, to overcome the effects of decreased arterial inflow by repeated testing, by employing longer periods of congestion, by applying local heat, or by having the patient exercise the calf just before the measurements are taken.

When the gravid uterus compresses the iliac veins or the inferior vena cava, having the patient lie on the opposite side from that being tested and internally rotating rather than externally rotating the thigh will usually relieve the obstruction.

Limitations

Impedance plethysmography cannot be performed when bandages, casts, or skeletal traction preclude the

Table 131–8.   Accuracy of Impedance Plethysmography for Diagnosing Above-Knee Deep Venous Thrombosis (Summary of 19 Reports)

	No. of Studies	Accuracy (%)				
		SENS	*SPEC*	*PPV*	*NPV*	*ACC*
Range	15–530	70–100	40–100	29–100	67–100	61–100
Median	98	93	94	84	98	94
Mean ± SD	154 ± 154	92 ± 8	88 ± 17	81 ± 19	94 ± 8	90 ± 9
Cumulative	2933	92	93	85	96	93
		824	1898	824	1898	2722
		893	2040	966	1967	2923

Data from references 53, 60, 65, 104, 107, 115, 123, 125, 140, 142, 145–147, 176, 225, 229, 327, 341, and 342.
SENS, sensitivity; SPEC, specificity; PPV, positive predictive value; NPV, negative predictive value; ACC, overall accuracy.

application of either the calf electrodes or the thigh cuff. Patients who are uncooperative, who have muscular twitches or spasms, or who are unable to relax as a result of confusion or pain may be impossible to study. The procedure may also be difficult in excessively obese patients, simply because of mechanical problems; in patients with severe edema, which reduces the electrical impedance, making it hard to balance the instrument; and in patients with respiratory problems that prevent them from lying flat. Therefore, the limitations imposed on impedance plethysmography are somewhat more restrictive than those that affect the application of Doppler ultrasonography.

Accuracy

An emphasis on sequential testing and prolonged occlusion times has made impedance plethysmography a precise, reproducible, and accurate method of detecting acute thrombosis of the popliteal and more proximal veins. No other noninvasive modality has undergone more thorough or rigorous validation. As indicated in Table 131–8, the cumulative sensitivity derived from 19 reports is 92 per cent and the specificity is 93 per cent. The positive and negative predictive values are 85 per cent and 96 per cent, respectively. The apparent accuracy, therefore, is slightly greater than that of the Doppler survey for similar patients.

However, it should be noted that the majority of the studies (1726 of 2933, 59 per cent) from which the data in

Table 131–8 were derived emanated from two laboratories with a special interest in impedance plethysmography. The experience of other investigators has been less satisfactory. Comerota and associates reported a sensitivity of 83 per cent and a specificity of 81 per cent for detecting proximal venous thrombosis with the impedance plethysmograph in a prospective study of patients in whom there was a clinical suspicion of the disease.[60] In asymptomatic patients who were believed to be at high risk for developing DVT, the sensitivity was only 32 per cent, but the specificity was a respectable 90 per cent. Patterson and colleagues, in a study of patients with suspected DVT, reported a specificity of 45 per cent and a positive predictive value of only 48 per cent.[225] They concluded that the high false-positive rate of impedance plethysmography precludes treatment based on this modality alone.

Strain-Gauge Plethysmography

Mercury or indium-gallium strain-gauges are sensitive and highly accurate instruments for detecting volume changes in the calf (see Chapter 4). They are more easily calibrated than the impedance plethysmograph but are more delicate and somewhat more cumbersome to use.

The position of the patient is identical to that used for impedance plethysmography, and the examination procedure is similar (Fig. 131–11). A contoured cuff measuring 22 × 71 cm is wrapped around the thigh. It is quite important that the tubes leading to the cuff have a large diameter (3/8-inch inside diameter) to permit rapid deflation. Tripolitis and associates showed that the apparent rate of venous outflow is highly sensitive to the rate at which the cuff deflates.[315] The length of the unstretched gauge should be about 90 per cent of the circumference of the calf. When stretched around the calf, the gauge should exert enough tension to ensure good contact with the skin but should not be tight enough to compress the underlying veins. During venous occlusion, the cuff is inflated to 50 mmHg and is allowed to remain inflated for about 2 minutes or until the tracing reaches a stable plateau.

Calf expansion (venous capacitance) is determined by comparing the rise of the curve from baseline with a 1.0 per cent electrical calibration signal and is reported in terms of per cent volume increase or as milliliters per 100 milliliters of calf volume.[131] Maximal venous outflow (MVO) is determined by drawing a tangent to the initial part of the downslope of the volume curve, beginning at the point at

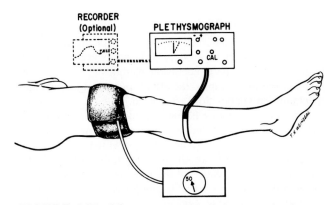

FIGURE 131–11. Venous outflow plethysmography. A mercury strain-gauge applied to the calf is used to record volume changes produced by inflating the thigh cuff to 50 mmHg. Volume changes can be recorded on a strip chart or directly from the plethysmograph.

which pressure is released.[24, 79, 119] Alternatively, outflow can be measured by noting the volume decrease 2 seconds after cuff deflation.[26] Both values are expressed in terms of milliliters of outflow per 100 milliliters of calf volume per minute.

Calf volume expansion averages around 2 to 3 per cent in normal limbs and is usually less than 2 per cent in limbs with acute DVT.[25, 119] As discussed previously, the extensive overlapping of results precludes the use of calf volume expansion as a single diagnostic test. MVO provides better differentiation. Barnes and associates found that this measurement was 91 per cent sensitive and 88 per cent specific when an MVO of 20 ml/100 ml/min was used as the dividing line between normal and abnormal limbs.[24] AbuRahma and Osborne, adopting the same criterion, reported a sensitivity of 96 per cent and a specificity of 98 per cent.[1] (When limbs with the postphlebitic syndrome were included, the specificity dropped to 78 per cent.) With the 2-second outflow method, Barnes and coworkers recorded mean values of 45 ± 18 ml/100 ml/min in normal volunteers (range, 20 to 91 ml/100 ml/min).[26] Mean 2-second outflows for limbs with acute DVT were as follows: iliofemoral, 13 ± 7 ml/100 ml/min; femoropopliteal, 11 ± 4 ml/100 ml/min; and calf vein, 20 ± 16 ml/100 ml/min. When 20 ml/100 ml/min was used as the dividing line, the sensitivity of the 2-second outflow was 90 per cent for detecting thrombi above the knee and 66 per cent for thrombi confined to the below-knee veins. The overall specificity was 81 per cent. Failure to diagnose isolated calf vein thrombi accounted for 13 of their 16 false-negative errors.

Tripolitis and coworkers observed a consistent decline in both venous capacitance and venous outflow in postoperative patients after a few days of bed rest.[316] Because there was no evidence of venous thrombosis in these patients, it is likely that the decreased outflow was not caused by an increased venous resistance but rather by a change in venous elasticity (see Eq. 131.2). These findings again support the argument for considering both venous capacitance and outflow when a patient is being tested for DVT. Cramer and colleagues devised a graph for plotting venous capacitance against venous outflow with a discriminant line appropriate for strain-gauge studies.[68] Initial results in a small number of patients yielded a sensitivity of 100 per cent and a specificity of 92 per cent.

There are few reports concerning the use of strain-gauge plethysmography in the evaluation of upper extremity DVT. In a small study, Zufferey and associates found the mean MVO in arms with acute DVT (79 ± 30 ml/100 ml/min) to be significantly ($p<.05$) less than that in normal arms (162 ± 52 ml/100 ml/min) and suggested that 110 ml/100 ml/min be adopted as the lower limit of normal.[339]

Strain-gauge plethysmography is subject to the same limitations and same sources of error that apply to impedance plethysmography.

Air Plethysmography

The air-filled plethysmograph designed by Raines and known as the ''pulse volume recorder'' has been applied to the diagnosis of venous thrombosis (see Chapter 4).[241] It is used in much the same way as the strain-gauge plethysmo-

graph. One pneumatic cuff, which serves as the volume sensor, is placed around the calf and inflated with 10 cc of air to ensure contact with the leg. The occlusion cuff, which is placed around the thigh, is inflated to 50 mmHg, and venous capacitance and MVO are measured.

Various methods of interpreting the results have been proposed. Nicholas and associates used a 50 per cent decrease in the volume of entrapped blood over a 2-second period as the dividing line between a normal and an abnormal study result.[211] With this criterion, a sensitivity of 91 per cent and a specificity of 78 per cent were obtained.[211] Hanel and coworkers, using a 1-second, 50-mm outflow (measured from the recording paper), reported a sensitivity and specificity of only 77 per cent and 62 per cent, respectively. Neither shifting the criterion nor adding the venous capacitance measurement improved the results.[121] Other investigators have employed the criteria proposed by Raines, which involve calculating a ''venous score'' based on the 1-second outflow, the venous capacitance, a ratio of the venous capacitances of the two legs, the presence or absence of respiratory variations in limb volume, and Doppler ultrasonographic findings.[241] The higher the score, the more likely the patient is to have DVT. Although there has been some variation in the scores selected to divide normal from abnormal results, scores of 4 or less are commonly assumed to exclude thrombosis, scores of 5 to 7 are in the uncertain area, and scores greater than 8 imply venous obstruction. On the basis of this method of interpretation, reported sensitivities have ranged from 44 to 92 per cent; specificities, from 61 to 93 per cent; and overall accuracies, from 70 to 93 per cent.[133, 253, 269, 272, 293] In several of these studies, the contribution of Doppler sonography to the diagnosis was not clearly distinguished from that made by air plethysmography alone. On the basis of their results, Hanel and coworkers no longer employ the pulse volume recorder for venous diagnosis,[121] and other investigators have questioned whether it significantly improves the results over those obtained with the Doppler apparatus alone.[133, 272]

Without benefit of studies comparing air plethysmography with other noninvasive tests in the same patients, it is not possible to assess its accuracy reliably; however, it appears to be somewhat less accurate than either impedance plethysmography or Doppler ultrasonography.

Phleborheography

Although phleborheography is a plethysmographic test, it is based on an entirely different concept from that which governs venous occlusion methods.[70, 72, 73] As with Doppler ultrasonography, the effects of respiration and augmentation on venous flow are sensed.

To ensure venous filling, the patient is studied lying supine, with the bed tilted 10 degrees foot down (Fig. 131-12). Pneumatic cuffs designed to sense volume changes are placed around the thorax, the mid-thigh, the upper calf, the mid-calf, the lower calf, and the foot. The cuffs at foot and lower calf levels also serve as compression devices. When functioning as sensing devices, the cuffs are inflated to a pressure of 10 mmHg. There are three operational modes. In the first, all cuffs on the thigh and leg serve as volume sensors while the foot cuff is inflated three times in rapid succession to 100 mmHg. In the second mode, the mid-calf

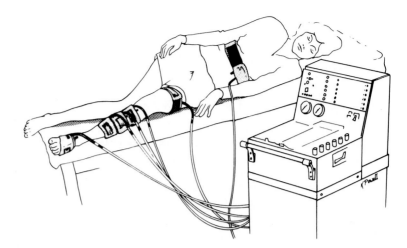

FIGURE 131–12. Phleborheography employs six pneumatic cuffs to measure venous volume changes in response to respiration or temporary external compression of the foot or calf.

cuff is inflated three times to 50 mmHg and the remaining cuffs are used to record volume changes. The last mode is similar to the second except that the compression cuff is moved to the ankle.

Phasic changes coinciding with respiration are normally observed in the recordings obtained from the thigh and calf (Fig. 131–13). These so-called respiratory waves are analogous to the phasic variations in flow detected with the Doppler device. With inspiration, the descent of the diaphragm raises intra-abdominal pressure, temporarily impeding outflow from the lower extremities. Blood backs up in the leg veins, and the limb volume increases. With expiration, the process is reversed. Diminution or absence of these waves signifies the presence of deep venous obstruction.

When the foot is compressed, a bolus of blood is forced centrally. If there is no proximal venous obstruction, blood flows freely out of the leg, causing little change in venous pressure or venous volume (see Fig. 131–13). Venous obstruction, on the other hand, prevents the free egress of blood; venous pressure rises temporarily, and venous volume increases. Compression of the calf simulates the

action of the calf muscle pump; consequently, the foot volume normally decreases while the volume of the more proximal parts of the limb remains unchanged. Absence of a change in foot volume during calf compression is therefore indicative of venous obstruction.

To summarize, a normal phleborheographic study must demonstrate well-defined respiratory waves and no rise in the baseline of thigh, leg, and calf tracings during compression of the lower calf or foot.[70] An abnormal study is characterized by the absence of respiratory waves and a rise in the baseline of the limb tracings with foot or calf compression. Abnormal foot emptying is suggestive, but not diagnostic, of deep venous obstruction.

Upper Extremity Studies

To study the upper extremity, cuffs are placed on the upper arm, on the upper and middle forearm, and at the wrist.[72] The wrist cuff is used for compression, and the other cuffs serve as volume sensors. Because of the extensive collateral network around the shoulder, respiratory waves may persist in the arm despite proximal venous

FIGURE 131–13. Phleborheographic tracings from normal limbs and from limbs with deep venous obstruction. Time is on the abscissa, and volume changes are on the ordinate. In the normal tracings, limb volume at all levels varies with respiration. Respiratory waves are absent in the abnormal limbs. Foot compression has no effect on leg volume in the normal limb but causes an increase in volume in the abnormal one. Lower calf compression decreases foot volume in the normal limb but has a negligible effect on the foot volume in the abnormal limb. (From Cranley JJ, Canos AJ, Sull WJ, Grass AM: Phleborheographic technique for diagnosis of deep venous thrombosis of the lower extremities. Surg Gynecol Obstet 141:331, 1975. Reprinted by permission of Surgery, Gynecology & Obstetrics.)

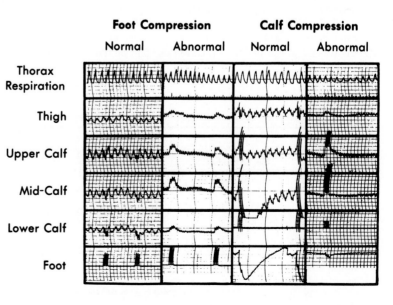

obstruction.[286, 296] In most cases, therefore, diagnosis of upper extremity venous obstruction must be based only on a rise in the baseline of the arm and forearm tracing with wrist compression.

Chronic Occlusion and Recurrent Venous Thrombosis

Because collateral development reduces venous resistance, phleborheography results are often negative in limbs with chronic occlusions. After an episode of acute venous thrombosis, respiratory waves gradually reappear, often becoming quite large in the postphlebitic limb.[70] As a result, it may be difficult to recognize the presence of a recurrent venous thrombosis.

Sources of Error

Phleborheographic studies are subject to the same sources of error that plague other physiologic tests. False-positive study results are usually due to extrinsic compression by tumor masses, tense muscles, or bony prominences. Flexing the knee, changing the position of the leg, and adopting measures to ensure relaxation of the patient will avoid many of these problems. Respiratory waves, which may be diminished when the patient is supine, can often be improved by having the patient lie on the left side—a maneuver that apparently shifts the weight of the viscera away from the inferior vena cava.[72] For similar reasons, pregnant patients are best studied when they are lying on their side. Even when these maneuvers were used, Nicholas and coworkers found false-positive phleborheographic tracings in 9 of 25 women who were examined during each trimester of pregnancy and in the early postpartum period.[210]

Small clots in the infrapopliteal veins cannot be detected. Cranley reported a 26 per cent false-negative rate for detecting clots isolated to this area.[70] Similarly, nonocclusive clots may be missed.

Interpretation of phleborheographic tracings is somewhat subjective and requires far more skill and experience than is required to interpret the results of impedance plethysmography. Technicians must be trained to recognize abnormal patterns and to attempt to correct any possible artifacts related to the patient's position or state of relaxation.

Accuracy

When the examination is performed properly and the tracings are interpreted skillfully by competent personnel, phleborheography is a reliable method of diagnosing DVT. Table 131–9 summarizes the results of nine investigations that compared phleborheographic interpretations with phlebographic findings in symptomatic patients. Median and cumulative values are similar to those obtained with impedance plethysmography. In a prospective study of patients with symptoms or signs suggestive of DVT, Comerota and associates found that phleborheography detected above-knee thrombi with a sensitivity of 92 per cent; however, only 16 per cent of below-knee thrombi were detected.[60] The specificity was 81 per cent. Sensitivity was markedly reduced in asymptomatic patients under surveillance for the development of DVT (33 per cent for above-knee and 22 per cent for below-knee thrombi). The specificity in this group of patients was 94 per cent. Subsequently, these same investigators reported a sensitivity of only 29 per cent for detecting above-knee thrombi and of 0.0 per cent for detecting below-knee thrombi developing in asymptomatic patients undergoing total joint replacement.[59]

The accuracy of the phleborheograph for investigating upper extremity venous thrombosis has been less thoroughly studied. Sottiurai and coworkers and Sullivan and colleagues reported sensitivities of 84 and 88 per cent and specificities of 75 and 92 per cent, respectively, in symptomatic arms.[286, 296]

Because the examination itself is more cumbersome and time consuming than impedance plethysmography or Doppler surveys, phleborheography was never as popular as the other hemodynamic tests and is now rarely used. Even the developers of phleborheography have shifted their allegiance to duplex scanning.[73, 103]

Light Reflection Rheography

Light reflection rheography is a promising new plethysmographic method for diagnosing DVT in symptomatic patients.[17, 311] Like photoplethysmography (see Chapter 4), light reflection rheography measures the quantity of blood in the dermal venous plexus. Because infrared light emitted by diodes incorporated in the probe is absorbed by red blood cells, the intensity of light reflected back to the probe

Table 131–9. Accuracy of Phleborheography for Diagnosing Deep Venous Thrombosis (Summary of 9 Reports)*

| | No. of Studies | Accuracy (%) | | | | |
		SENS	SPEC	PPV	NPV	ACC
Range	24–709	69–100	79–100	59–100	69–100	75–96
Median	65	90	95	91	94	93
Mean ± SD	159 ± 215	86 ± 10	91 ± 8	88 ± 12	89 ± 12	89 ± 7
Cumulative	1432	89	91	87	93	91
		495	801	495	801	1296
		556	876	570	862	1432

Data from references 48, 54, 56, 57, 59, 60, 97, 288, and 294.
Includes some below-knee thrombi.
SENS, sensitivity; SPEC, specificity; PPV, positive predictive value; NPV, negative predictive value; ACC, overall accuracy.

is inversely proportional to the number of red blood cells present in the underlying tissue. The sensor is attached to the medial surface of the calf about 10 cm above the malleolus. After resting for 5 minutes in a sitting position with their legs dependent, patients are asked to perform 10 dorsiflexions of the foot. In normal subjects, contraction of the calf muscles decreases tissue blood content and results in a well-defined increase in light reflectivity (indicated by a distinct rise in the tracing). When the venous outflow is obstructed, exercise of the calf muscle fails to empty the venous plexus and little or no increase in light reflectivity occurs.

Thomas and coworkers reported that light reflection rheography had a sensitivity of 92 per cent and a specificity of 84 per cent for detecting or ruling out DVT in patients with clinically suspected DVT who were referred for phlebography.[311] The positive and negative predictive values were 84 and 92 per cent, respectively. Unlike other plethysmographic tests, light reflection rheography detected isolated calf vein thrombosis with a sensitivity equal to that attained for proximal DVT. Arora and associates, in a similar study, reported a positive predictive value of 79 per cent and a negative predictive value of 97 per cent.[17]

Light reflection rheography has the advantages of being a simple and rapid method of excluding DVT. Because the positive predictive value is relatively low, a positive result requires corroboration by phlebography or ultrasonic scanning. If the initial favorable results are substantiated by further study, light reflection rheography may have a role as a screening test in symptomatic patients.

Ultrasonic Scanning

B-mode, duplex, and color-coded duplex scanning are now widely recognized as the most versatile and accurate of the noninvasive tests for DVT.[35, 59, 225, 309] With these instruments, it is possible not only to detect the presence of thrombi but also to determine which veins are involved. Nonocclusive clots and clots with free-floating tails are readily identified and easily distinguished from those that are completely obstructive or adherent to the venous wall.[20, 39, 103] Extrinsic compression that is due to hematomas, lymphadenopathy, or tumor masses can be differentiated from intrinsic obstruction, and conditions such as intramuscular bleeding and popliteal cysts can be diagnosed even in the presence of concomitant DVT.[3, 16, 81, 196] With sufficient persistence, most of the below-knee veins can be studied individually, including the posterior tibial, anterior tibial, and peroneal veins.[156, 232, 250, 318] Even the intramuscular veins (soleal and gastrocnemius) may be visualized.[103, 195] In addition, the profunda femoris vein, iliac veins, and inferior vena cava can be examined.[95, 103, 262] Both the greater and lesser saphenous veins are easily studied, and enlarged perforating and collateral veins may be detected. Clot morphology and echogenicity can be used to differentiate old from new thrombi. Finally, valvular function can be evaluated and incompetent valves identified.[156, 259] Thus, B-mode imaging and duplex scanning—at least conceptually—overcome many of the limitations of Doppler ultrasonography and the various plethysmographic techniques.

Compared with contrast phlebography, ultrasonic imaging has the advantage of being totally noninvasive and of revealing tributary veins that are seldom visualized adequately on the routine roentgenographic study. Furthermore, ultrasonic imaging is ideally suited for studying the natural history of DVT and for evaluating the results of therapy.[94, 159, 164, 181, 185, 195, 289, 319] It may be the only noninvasive technique accurate enough to be used for surveillance purposes in high-risk patients.[30, 59, 188, 217, 332]

At present, the main drawbacks to ultrasonic scanning appear to be the time required for a thorough examination, the need for skilled technicians and experienced interpreters, and the expense of the instrumentation.

Technique

A wide variety of real-time B-mode and duplex instruments have been employed. Both sector scanners and linear array devices are in use. Transducer frequencies vary from 3.5 to 10 MHz; the lower frequencies are required for deeper structures, whereas the higher frequencies are more suitable for shallow work. For most applications, the 5- and 7.5-MHz transducers are adequate. Although some investigators are content to do without Doppler support, relying on the image alone, the ability of duplex instruments to evaluate vessels for the presence of flow and to assess the flow pattern is perceived by most to be a significant advantage.[156, 160] The use of real-time color-coded flow-mapping devices accelerates the examination process by facilitating the identification of veins and by immediately demonstrating the presence or absence of flow.[106, 251, 304] These devices are particularly useful below the knee, where venous channels are small and difficult to follow.[232, 251, 304, 318]

To ensure venous filling, the common femoral, superficial femoral, profunda femoris, anterior tibial, posterior tibial, and greater saphenous veins are examined with the patient lying supine in a reversed Trendelenburg position at a 10- to 15-degree foot-down tilt.[58, 156] The legs are slightly flexed at the hip and knee and externally rotated at the hip. The popliteal vein may be evaluated with the patient prone, the ankles supported by a pillow, or with the patient lying in a lateral decubitus position.[295] These positions are also useful for imaging the lesser saphenous, soleal, and proximal peroneal and posterior tibial veins.[58, 156] Other portions of the infrapopliteal veins may be examined with the patient supine and the knee bent to relax the calf muscles. Some investigators prefer to study the calf veins with the patient sitting with the foot resting on a low stool or on the examiner's knee.[95, 250]

Beginning proximally over the common femoral vein (or the inferior vena cava) and moving distally, the examiner images the veins both transversely and longitudinally at increments of 1 to 3 cm.[58, 95, 319] Transverse views help localize the vein and are useful for determining compressibility. Longitudinal scans provide confirmation of the transverse images and are useful for assessing clot morphology and density, for locating small nonocclusive clots or those confined to a valve cusp, and for evaluating valve function.[58] The time-gain control is adjusted so that the lumen of an adjacent artery is free of echoes.[3, 240] It is important to apply the probe to the skin with only a slight amount of pressure.

Although a complete study usually takes about 20 to 30 minutes, it may require 1 hour. Imaging the calf veins often proves to be the most time-consuming part of the examination. An abbreviated study, limited to the common femoral, superficial femoral, and popliteal veins, has been advocated by a number of investigators, who feel that this approach will identify most thrombi of clinical significance.[12, 75, 174, 240, 320, 322] Others believe that scanning of the calf veins is worthwhile and should be part of the routine examination.[251, 304]

The upper extremity and cervical veins are studied with the patient supine, either lying flat or in a slight Trendelenburg position.[295] Accessible veins include the internal jugular vein in the neck; the subclavian vein in the deltopectoral triangle; and the axillary, brachial, radial, ulnar, cephalic, and basilic veins in the arm.[58] Although the proximal subclavian and distal innominate veins can be visualized with a supraclavicular approach, it is not possible to study the proximal innominate vein or the superior vena cava. Because veins in the thoracic inlet cannot be compressed, Doppler flow studies and color flow imaging are helpful adjuncts in this area.[163]

Interpretation

The diagnostic criteria originally proposed by Talbot and further developed by Cranley and others have proved to be reliable.[95, 103, 156, 295, 309] Normal veins have thin walls, appear to be "empty," and collapse completely when light pressure is applied with the probe.[74] Diameter changes coinciding with respiration and, to a lesser extent, with the cardiac cycle may be observed.[95, 103] Valsalva maneuvers, coughing, proximal limb compression, and downward tilting all tend to increase the diameter of normal veins.[12, 103] Owing perhaps to rouleau formation, blood flow often produces visible echoes during low-flow states when acceleration or deceleration occurs.[103, 279, 280] Under ideal conditions, valve motion may be seen.[58, 95, 259, 295]

Actual visualization of a clot is the most specific sign of venous thrombosis (Fig. 131–14).[58, 95, 156] Unfortunately, fresh clots are sometimes difficult to see because their acoustic properties are similar to those of blood. Although Elias and coworkers estimate that 90 per cent of clots are visible,[95] other investigators report visible clots in only about 50 per cent of thrombosed veins.[75, 240] A second valuable sign of venous thrombosis is the inability to collapse the vein completely with probe pressure.[156, 295, 309] Some authors consider the response to compression to be the most sensitive and specific method of identifying or ruling out venous thrombosis.[12, 75, 240] Several important venous segments, however, are resistant to compression even when no clot is present. These include the thoracic inlet veins, the subclavian vein beneath the clavicle, the profunda femoris vein at its junction with the common femoral vein, and the superficial femoral vein within the adductor hiatus.[58, 103, 163, 240]

Failure of the diameter to change with quiet respiration or a Valsalva maneuver, an indirect indication of thrombosis, may be helpful in assessing veins that are not easily compressed but ordinarily adds little to the diagnosis.[3] Although the presence of visible blood flow implies patency, its absence is not specific for thrombosis.[103]

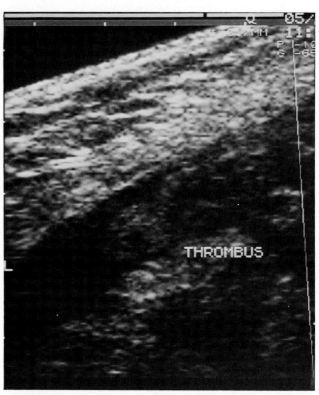

FIGURE 131–14. Real-time B-mode image of a popliteal vein showing a partially occluding thrombus.

The duplex scanner permits blood flow to be assessed in any visible vein. After placing the pulsed Doppler sample volume in the area of interest, the examiner can either interpret the audible signal or record the spectrum for future reference. The criteria for interpreting flow patterns are identical to those employed when the hand-held Doppler device is used. Evaluation of venous flow signals is particularly helpful for distinguishing veins from arteries, for examining veins without visible clot, and for indirectly predicting patency or obstruction in veins above or below the site of examination. Failure to detect blood flow is diagnostic of venous obstruction even though the vein appears normal on the B-mode scan, a not infrequent occurrence in acutely thrombosed veins with hypoechogenic clots. A continuous flow pattern implies obstruction of the venous channel above the site being studied. For example, finding continuous flow at the common femoral level strongly suggests involvement of the iliac vein (which because of technical factors may be difficult to visualize). Similarly, absence of phasic flow in the axillary vein or the distal subclavian vein should alert the examiner to the presence of obstruction of the proximal subclavian vein—another site not readily seen with the B-mode scanner. Indeed, Killewich and associates found the presence or absence of phasic flow to be the most sensitive (92 per cent) and specific (92 per cent) criterion for establishing the diagnosis of DVT with the duplex scanner.[160] In the series of limbs that were studied, clot visualization, although quite specific (92 per cent), had a sensitivity of only 50 per cent. Compressibility, on the other hand, was neither very sensitive (79 per cent) nor specific (67 per cent).

When real-time color-coded flow-mapping devices are

used, the presence or absence of flow is immediately apparent (see Fig. 131–15 on Color Plate V).[106, 218, 304] The Doppler shift signal is coded both for flow direction (blue or red) and for velocity (color saturation). Colors are assigned so that venous flow will be predominately blue and arterial flow will be red. An increased velocity is indicated by a lighter color. Although "spontaneous" flow that varies with respiration is usually visible in normal popliteal and femoral veins, augmentation may be necessary to visualize flow in the infrapopliteal veins. Absence of blue-colored pixels (after augmentation) in a structure paralleling an artery and having the B-mode characteristics of a vein is virtually diagnostic of venous thrombosis. Partial obstruction is indicated by a contracted color flow image or by flow on either side of a central filling defect (see Fig. 131–15 on Color Plate V). Free-floating clots appear as structures waving about in a stream of blue pixels (see Fig. 131–16 on Color Plate V).

The use of color has many advantages. Blood vessels are rapidly identified and clearly differentiated from nonvascular structures; veins are readily distinguished from arteries; and flow is visible over an extended region and simultaneously in multiple vessels. Thus, color not only facilitates longitudinal tracking of veins and the identification of veins in cross-sectional views but also decreases and often obviates the need to assess venous compressibility and to evaluate Doppler flow patterns. Color also facilitates the evaluation of calf veins, which because of their length, small diameters, and complex anatomy are difficult to examine with conventional duplex scanning (see Figs. 131–17 and 131–18 on Color Plate VI). It has proved to be especially helpful for identifying parallel channels in duplicated veins and for detecting hypoechogenic and nonocclusive thrombi (see Fig. 131–19 on Color Plate VI). These advantages translate into a more accurate, more complete, less demanding, and more expeditious examination.

Distinguishing Acute From Chronic Venous Thrombosis

Various characteristics of the B-mode image can be used to estimate the duration of the thrombotic process.[156, 250] Fresh clots have an acoustic density only slightly greater than that of flowing blood and may be practically invisible. They tend to have a homogeneous appearance and, if not totally occlusive, have a smooth surface. Recently formed thrombi are soft and partially compressible. When the entire lumen is filled with an acute thrombus, the diameter of the vein may be increased.[95, 103] Clot retraction begins within a few hours of onset, leaving a thin gap between the vein wall and the thrombus—analogous to the "railroad-track sign" seen in phlebography.[156] Finding a clot with a limited attachment to the vein wall and a free-floating tail is always indicative of an acute process (see Fig. 131–16 on Color Plate V).[95, 103]

Shortly after a thrombus has formed, there is a period of decreasing echogenicity, after which the clot becomes progressively more reflective.[55, 227, 250] An organized thrombus may even have an acoustic density approaching that of a calcified arterial plaque.[103] Older clots typically have a heterogeneous texture, may appear to be striped, have an

irregular surface, and are tightly adherent to the venous wall.[95, 156] Aging clots contract, become quite firm, and are totally noncompressible. The diameter of a chronically involved vein is frequently reduced, and its wall appears to be thickened. Although collaterals may develop within a few days following a venous occlusion, the presence of large, tortuous collateral veins suggests a long-standing process.[58, 103] Thickened, contracted, rigid valve cusps, frozen in the open position or adherent to the vein wall, are indicative of chronic venous insufficiency.[103, 259] Reflux may be noted with the Doppler attachment and may be "seen" with the color-coded flow-mapping device.[308] With this instrument, venous valvular incompetence is indicated by a blue-to-red color change occurring during a Valsalva maneuver or in response to proximal or distal limb compression. Trickles of color through an echogenic thrombus reveal recanalization, typical of chronically thrombosed veins.[303, 304] Enlarged incompetent perforating veins may also be seen.

Both acute and chronic thrombi are often present in the same limb.[156] In fact, Rollins and associates found ultrasonic evidence of chronic thrombi in 48 (76 per cent) of 63 limbs with acute venous thrombosis.[250] Only 13 per cent of the patients in this study gave a history of previous DVT.

Other Causes of Limb Swelling or Pain

Hematomas and popliteal cysts, which often simulate acute DVT, are readily identified with B-mode scanning. Hematomas present in the calf or thigh as somewhat elliptical, hypoechogenic areas, surrounded by muscle. Layering of the thrombus within the hematoma may be observed. With time, their extent and acoustic density tend to decrease.[16] Popliteal cysts are sharply demarcated, echo-free, oblong structures that originate behind the flexion crease of the knee and extend distally into the upper calf.[16, 196] They usually lie medial to the popliteal vessels, from which they are distinctly separated; the majority appear to communicate with the joint space. In a series of patients with symptoms suggestive of DVT, Aronen and colleagues found that 10 per cent had hematomas and 8 per cent had popliteal cysts.[16] Other investigators, using B-mode ultrasonography, have reported the frequent occurrence of hematomas and popliteal cysts in patients being scanned for acute DVT.[3, 81] Less commonly, venous thrombosis and popliteal cysts are detected concurrently.[16, 196]

In addition, B-mode scans can identify other causes of venous obstruction, including enlarged lymph nodes, tumor masses, and aneurysms. Color is an especially valuable adjunct because it clearly differentiates between aneurysms and hematomas and between vascular and nonvascular structures.

Errors and Limitations

Clot visualization can be quite subjective.[12] Sometimes it is hard to tell whether echoes arising from the venous lumen represent clots or reverberation artifacts. Adjusting the time-gain control to eliminate all artifacts may suppress low-level echoes from fresh thrombi.[240] Moreover, as discussed earlier in this chapter, fresh clot is often anechogenic. Not infrequently, when small vessels are being studied, arteries and other structures may be mistaken for veins. Use of the Doppler apparatus to confirm the presence or absence of flow and the character of the flow pattern will avoid most of these errors. By graphically displaying the pattern of flow, color-assisted scanning provides the same information as Doppler flow interrogation, with less effort and equal accuracy. When color is properly used, the identity of the vessel being studied is seldom in question and the degree of clot echogenicity makes little difference (see Fig. 131–14; see also Fig. 131–15 on Color Plate V).[303, 304]

Veins lying proximal to the inguinal ligament may be difficult to image because of their depth or the presence of bowel gas.[295] Using a low-frequency probe (3.5 MHz) and having the patient fast for 6 hours may diminish this problem.[170] However, many elderly patients are chronically flatulent, and it may be necessary to rely on indirect studies of flow patterns in the common femoral veins to determine patency of the iliac veins. Fortunately, obstruction of the iliac vein is often accompanied by thrombosis of the common femoral vein. Color, which facilitates the imaging of iliac veins, decreases the need for indirect flow assessment.[262] Other relatively difficult areas include the subclavian vein beneath the clavicle and the superficial femoral vein in the adductor canal.[3, 103, 163] In one study, conventional duplex scanning failed to detect 6 of 14 (43 per cent) partial occlusions and 5 of 11 (45 per cent) short total occlusions of the subclavian vein.[118] The inability to compress normal veins in the adductor canal region can lead to false-positive errors unless this limitation is recognized.[160, 333] Duplication of the superficial femoral and popliteal veins is not uncommon. False-negative results can occur when a patent vein is found paralleling an occluded channel. With conventional duplex scanning, frequent cross-sectional views and evaluation of venous compressibility in both veins are required to avoid this error. Color scanning, by displaying both channels simultaneously, decreases the likelihood that a thrombus in a parallel vein will be overlooked (see Fig. 131–19 on Color Plate VI).[304]

Because of their small size, complicated anatomy, and depth, calf veins are less easily examined than thigh veins; consequently, full visualization may be inordinately time consuming and frustrating. Although highly experienced sonographers are able to evaluate the anterior tibial, posterior tibial, and peroneal veins in about 90 per cent and the soleal veins in 50 per cent of legs subjected to B-mode and conventional duplex scanning, most examiners will not achieve a comparable success rate.[103, 170] Wright and co-workers found that 35 per cent of erroneous or equivocal duplex scanning results reported in the literature were related to problems encountered in diagnosing isolated calf vein thrombosis,[333] and in several series, failure to detect infrapopliteal thrombi accounted for all false-negative errors.[160, 208, 333]

As mentioned previously, color flow mapping facilitates the identification of calf veins and makes it easier to evaluate their patency. Polak and associates found that all normal peroneal and posterior tibial veins and 55 per cent of normal anterior tibial veins could be visualized when flow was augmented by gentle limb compression.[232] Likewise, van Bemmelen and colleagues were able to image all paired calf veins from the knee to the ankle in 30 normal subjects.[318] Although extensive thromboses of the calf veins are reliably detected, short, nonocclusive clots limited to the calf veins are frequently overlooked, especially when the color image is suboptimal.[188, 251]

Other factors that may interfere with the examination include muscle spasm or contraction, gross edema, and excess obesity.[3, 95] Studies are compromised when the patient is apprehensive, agitated, combative, or in pain, and a complete examination may not be possible in limbs with fresh surgical wounds or when casts, traction, or splints limit access to underlying veins. Errors have been made in pregnant patients, owing to the obstructive flow pattern produced by uterine compression and to the apparent incompressibility of the common femoral vein.[171] Rotating the patient to her side will usually permit a correct diagnosis to be made.

Accuracy depends on the quality of the study. The necessary skills are not easily or quickly acquired. In order to derive the most information from the examination and to interpret the results correctly, both the technologist performing the test and the physician who reads the videotapes must be well grounded in the anatomy, physiology, and pathophysiology of venous disease and must be thoroughly acquainted with ultrasonic imaging and Doppler signal analysis.[58, 218]

Probe compression as a method of diagnosing DVT carries the very slight risk of dislodging a fresh clot.[240] One report described the disappearance of a free-floating clot during compression of the common femoral vein and the immediate occurrence of a pulmonary embolus.[271] The use of color flow patterns rather than compression to diagnose fresh nonocclusive thrombosis should enable examiners to avoid this hazard.

Accuracy

Table 131–10 lists the results of 21 studies in which phlebography was used to determine the accuracy of B-mode or duplex scanning for detecting DVT in symptomatic patients. On the basis of these data, it appears that ultrasonic scanning is somewhat more accurate than other commonly used noninvasive tests (cf. Tables 131–5, 131–8, and 131–9). Moreover, the range of reported values is less with duplex and B-mode scanning than it is with other tests, suggesting that scanning provides more consistent results. If 10 prospective studies and 3 with incomplete data are excluded, only 6 per cent (490 of 7811) of limbs undergoing B-mode or duplex scanning for suspected DVT were also subjected to phlebography. The reasons for performing phlebography were not clearly enunciated in many of the reports, but confirmation of positive scan findings appeared to be the justification for many of the phlebograms. Selection, therefore, may have biased some of the results in favor of an improved accuracy. Nonetheless, the overall accuracy (96 ± 2 per cent) reported in the 10 prospective investigations is impressive.

Initial reports comparing the results of color flow imaging and phlebography in patients with clinically suspected DVT of the proximal veins have suggested that this modality is at least as accurate as conventional duplex scanning and is perhaps even more accurate (Table 131–11).

Table 131–10. Accuracy of B-Mode and Duplex Imaging for Diagnosing Deep Venous Thrombosis

Study	No. of Extremities	Sensitivity (%)	Specificity (%)	Positive Predictive Value (%)	Negative Predictive Value (%)	Overall Accuracy (%)
Oliver, 1985[221]	28	88 (7/8)	95 (19/20)	88 (7/8)	95 (19/20)	93 (26/28)
Raghavendra et al, 1986[240]	20*	100 (14/14)	100 (6/6)	100 (14/14)	100 (6/6)	100 (20/20)
Dauzat et al, 1986[81]	145	94 (94/100)	100 (45/45)	100 (94/94)	88 (45/51)	96 (139/145)
Appelman et al, 1987[12]	110*†	96 (48/50)	97 (58/60)	96 (48/50)	97 (58/60)	96 (106/110)
Cronan et al, 1987[75]	51*†	89 (25/28)	100 (23/23)	100 (25/25)	88 (23/26)	94 (48/51)
Aitkin and Godden, 1987[23]	42*†	94 (15/16)	100 (26/26)	100 (15/15)	96 (26/27)	98 (41/42)
Elias et al, 1987[95]	847†	98 (325/333)	94 (483/514)	91 (325/356)	98 (483/491)	95 (808/847)
Vogel et al, 1987[322]	53*†	95 (19/20)	100 (33/33)	100 (19/19)	97 (33/34)	98 (52/53)
Karkow et al, 1987[156]	75	96 (44/46)	90 (26/29)	94 (44/47)	93 (26/28)	93 (70/75)
Rollins et al, 1988[250]	46	100 (40/40)	100 (6/6)	100 (40/40)	100 (6/6)	100 (46/46)
Cronan et al, 1988[74]	62	95 (42/44)	89 (16/18)	95 (42/44)	89 (16/18)	94 (58/62)
Killewich et al, 1989[160]	50	92 (35/38)	92 (11/12)	97 (35/36)	79 (11/14)	92 (46/50)
Patterson et al, 1989[225]	64	89 (24/27)	92 (34/37)	89 (24/27)	92 (34/37)	91 (58/64)
Lensing et al, 1989[174]	220†	91 (70/77)	99 (142/143)	99 (70/71)	95 (142/149)	96 (212/220)
Mantoni, 1989[184]	85*†	97 (34/35)	96 (48/50)	94 (34/36)	98 (48/49)	97 (82/85)
Mussurakis et al, 1990[208]	94†	83 (30/36)	100 (58/58)	100 (30/30)	91 (58/64)	94 (88/94)
Fletcher et al, 1990[105]	44*†	100 (14/14)	97 (29/30)	93 (14/15)	100 (29/29)	98 (43/44)
Comerota et al, 1990[59]	72	98 (43/44)	86 (24/28)	92 (43/47)	96 (24/25)	93 (67/72)
Wright et al, 1990[333]	71	91 (31/34)	95 (35/37)	94 (31/33)	92 (35/38)	93 (66/71)
van Ramshorst et al, 1991[320]	120*†	91 (58/64)	95 (53/56)	95 (58/61)	90 (53/59)	93 (111/120)
Montefusco et al, 1993[202]	268	100 (87/87)	100 (181/181)	100 (87/87)	100 (181/181)	100 (268/268)
Cumulative	2567	95 (1099/1155)	96 (1356/1412)	95 (1099/1155)	96 (1356/1412)	96 (2455/2567)
Range	20–847	83–100	86–100	88–100	79–100	91–100
Median	71	95	97	96	95	95
Mean ± SD	122 ± 177	94 ± 5	96 ± 4	96 ± 4	94 ± 5	95 ± 3

Modified from Sumner DS, Mattos MA: Diagnosis of deep venous thrombosis with real-time color and duplex scanning. In Bernstein EF (ed): Vascular Diagnosis. 4th ed. St. Louis, Mosby–Year Book, 1993, pp 785–800.

*Infrapopliteal veins were not studied or were not included in the analysis.

†Prospective studies.

Abdominal and Pelvic Veins

Unlike other noninvasive tests, which provide only indirect evidence of thrombosis above the inguinal ligament, ultrasonic scanning can be used to detect thrombosis of the inferior vena cava by direct examination. In a prospective study, Elias and coworkers found that clot was present in the inferior vena cava in 47 of 241 limbs (19.5 per cent) with DVT. Three of the 47 clots were suprarenal.[95] These figures emphasize the importance of surveying the intra-abdominal veins. Compared with phlebography, duplex scanning was 100 per cent sensitive and 99 per cent specific for detecting thrombosis of the inferior vena cava.[96] Sarpa and associates were able to obtain adequate color flow images of iliac veins in only 61 per cent of patients

with suspected DVT.[262] Of the patients with positive scan findings anywhere in the leg, 11 per cent had iliac vein thrombosis, and in 5 per cent the thrombosis was confined to the iliac veins. There were no false-negative or false-positive results in 18 patients who also underwent phlebography.

Calf Veins

Most of the studies listed in Table 131–10 included below-knee thrombi in their data analysis. Few, however, directly addressed the issue of accuracy in this area. Rollins and associates, in a meticulous investigation of 46 limbs with suspected DVT, found that the anatomic extent of

Table 131–11. Accuracy of Color-Coded Duplex Imaging for Diagnosing Symptomatic Deep Venous Thrombosis in Femoropopliteal Veins

Study	No. of Extremities	Sensitivity (%)	Specificity (%)	Positive Predictive Value (%)	Negative Predictive Value (%)	Overall Accuracy (%)
Persson et al, 1989[226]	23	100 (15/15)	100 (8/8)	100 (15/15)	100 (8/8)	100 (23/23)
Foley et al, 1989[106]	47*	89 (17/19)	100 (28/28)	100 (17/17)	93 (28/30)	98 (45/47)
Schindler et al, 1990[270]	94	98 (54/55)	100 (39/39)	100 (54/54)	98 (39/40)	99 (93/94)
Rose et al, 1990[251]	75	96 (25/26)	100 (49/49)	100 (25/25)	98 (49/50)	99 (74/75)
Mattos et al, 1992[188]	77†	100 (32/32)	98 (44/45)	97 (32/33)	100 (44/44)	99 (76/77)

Modified from Sumner DS, Mattos MA: Diagnosis of deep venous thrombosis with real-time color and duplex scanning. In Bernstein EF (ed): Vascular Diagnosis. 4th ed. St. Louis, Mosby–Year Book, 1993, pp 785–800.

*100% accuracy for the femoral vein segment.

†Above-knee popliteal veins only.

Table 131–12.   Accuracy of B-Mode and Duplex Imaging for Diagnosing Symptomatic Calf Vein Thrombosis

Study	Modality	Sensitivity (%)	Specificity (%)	Positive Predictive Value (%)	Negative Predictive Value (%)
Dauzat et al, 1986[81]	B-mode	63 (5/8)	100 (45/45)	100 (5/5)	94 (45/48)
Elias et al, 1987[95]	Duplex	91 (84/92)	96 (483/501)	82 (84/102)	98 (483/491)
Fletcher et al, 1990[105]	Duplex	85 (11/13)	83 (25/30)	69 (11/16)	93 (25/27)
Mitchell et al, 1991[201]	Duplex	81 (17/21)	89 (25/28)	85 (17/20)	86 (25/29)

Modified from Sumner DS, Mattos MA: Diagnosis of deep venous thrombosis with real-time color and duplex scanning. In Bernstein EF (ed): Vascular Diagnosis. 4th ed. St. Louis, Mosby–Year Book, 1993, pp 785–800.

thrombi detected with B-mode scanning and that disclosed by phlebography corresponded within ± 1.5 cm in 84 per cent of the anterior tibial, 86 per cent of the posterior tibial, 93 per cent of the peroneal, and 92 per cent of the popliteal veins.[250] Results of below-knee studies from other laboratories using conventional and color-coded duplex scanning in the investigation of suspected DVT are listed in Tables 131–12 and 131–13.

As discussed previously, accuracy in the infrapopliteal area is highly dependent on the quality of the scan and the extent of the thrombotic process. For example, Rose and colleagues reported a rather unimpressive overall sensitivity of 73 per cent and a somewhat disappointing specificity of 86 per cent in their study of below-knee DVT (see Table 131–13), but in a subset of 44 limbs in which color images were technically adequate, the sensitivity (95 per cent), specificity (100 per cent), positive predictive value (100 per cent), and negative predictive value (96 per cent) were excellent.[251] However, when scans were judged to be suboptimal or when clots were confined to isolated segments of the below-knee vein, both the sensitivity and specificity suffered.

Upper Extremity Veins

There is little information on the accuracy of duplex scanning in the upper extremity. Although it is reasonable to assume that results in this area should be comparable to those in the lower extremity,[158] the sensitivity for detecting subclavian vein thrombosis in one report was disappointingly low (56 per cent).[118] The specificity and the positive

predictive value, however, were 100 per cent. Knudson and associates, using color flow imaging, reported a sensitivity of 78 per cent, a specificity of 92 per cent, a positive predictive value of 88 per cent, and a negative predictive value of 86 per cent in a series of 22 patients with suspected thrombosis of the upper extremity or thoracic inlet veins.[163] In this study, the two false-negative results occurred in patients with proximal subclavian thromboses. Extrinsic compression was responsible for the single false-positive result. Grassi and Polak reported no positive or negative errors in a follow-up study of 13 patients with effort thrombosis who were examined with color duplex imaging and phlebography.[113]

Comment on Accuracy

Because ultrasonic imaging is highly accurate in symptomatic patients for detecting venous thrombi above the knee and is promising below the knee, a number of enthusiasts have proposed that this modality replace phlebography as the gold standard—and in terms of actual day-to-day practice, some laboratories have already done so.[58, 95, 156, 170] Whether this step is justified is a question that can be answered only by further work.

Surveillance

The results of conventional and color-coded duplex scanning in surveillance studies of high-risk asymptomatic patients are discussed later in this chapter.

Table 131–13.   Accuracy of Color-Coded Duplex Imaging for Diagnosing Symptomatic Deep Venous Thrombosis in Tibioperoneal Veins

Study	No. of Extremities	Sensitivity (%)	Specificity (%)	Positive Predictive Value (%)	Negative Predictive Value (%)	Overall Accuracy (%)
Foley et al, 1989[106]	16	100 (4/4)	100 (12/12)	100 (4/4)	100 (12/12)	100 (16/16)
Mattos et al, 1992[188]	75	94 (31/33)	81 (34/42)	80 (31/39)	94 (34/36)	87 (65/75)
Rose et al, 1990[251]	74	73 (22/30)	86 (38/44)	79 (22/28)	83 (38/46)	81 (60/74)
Technical adequacy						
Adequate*	44	95 (19/20)	100 (24/24)	100 (19/19)	96 (24/25)	98 (43/44)
Inadequate	30	30 (3/10)	70 (14/20)	33 (3/9)	67 (14/21)	57 (17/30)
Extent						
Not isolated	25	86 (18/21)	75 (3/4)	95 (18/19)	50 (3/6)	84 (21/25)
Isolated†	49	44 (4/9)	88 (35/40)	44 (4/9)	88 (35/40)	80 (39/49)

Modified from Sumner DS, Mattos MA: Diagnosis of deep venous thrombosis with real-time color and duplex scanning. In Bernstein EF (ed): Vascular Diagnosis. 4th ed. St. Louis, Mosby–Year Book, 1993, pp 785–800.

*The tibioperoneal trunk and all portions of the posterior tibial and peroneal veins were visualized.

†Clots were confined to calf veins (no above-knee thrombus).

Computed Tomography and Magnetic Resonance Imaging

Contrast-enhanced computed tomograms may be useful for diagnosing venous thrombosis in pelvic and abdominal veins. Like phlebography, computed tomography has the disadvantage of requiring the intravenous administration of an iodinated contrast medium. Computed tomography is usually employed to determine the cause of leg swelling or to evaluate a soft tissue mass and is rarely used as the primary method of diagnosing DVT. It is very useful for investigating intra-abdominal venous abnormalities, especially as they relate to aneurysm resection.[110]

Magnetic resonance imaging (MRI), on the other hand, is totally noninvasive, and unlike ultrasonic scanning, it has the advantage of being relatively operator independent and of providing a hard-copy record for subsequent review. Other advantages include its ability to image both extremities simultaneously and its ability to examine veins in the pelvis, abdomen, and thorax unencumbered by the presence of gaseous interfaces. MRI shares with ultrasound the ability to distinguish between extrinsic venous compression and venous thrombosis and to identify cysts, hematomas, tumors, and other masses that may be responsible for venous obstruction or leg swelling.

Both spin-echo and limited-flip-angle gradient-echo imaging methods have been used, and each has its advocates.[99, 234, 287, 323] With spin-echo imaging, rapidly flowing blood produces a "flow void;" thus, under proper conditions, the lumen of a patent vein will be devoid of signals. Acutely thrombosed veins are distended, are completely filled with signals, and have blurred wall margins due to perivascular edema.[99] A bright image surrounded by a concentric signal void is indicative of a recent thrombus that has retracted away from the wall, leaving a rim of flowing blood.[126] Chronic thrombosis is distinguished by the presence of collateral veins, a lumen partially filled with signals, and evidence of recanalization. In contrast, the gradient-echo method displays flowing blood as a "bright" image.[323] Signals, therefore, are decreased or absent in the lumen of a completely occluded vein. When a clot retracts from the vessel wall, a central core composed of low or absent signals is surrounded by high-intensity signals produced by blood flowing around the thrombus.[287] Enhancement of the entire lumen confirms venous patency. Studies with both methods require about 30 minutes to 1 hour to complete.

A number of artifacts may interfere with the interpretation of MR images. Spin-echo images are most reliable when velocity is high and when flow is perpendicular to the imaging plane (transverse image).[323] Slowly moving blood in small veins or during the inspiratory phase of respiration can mimic the appearance of a clot, and turbulence and changes in the direction of flow may also produce confusing signals. Gradient-echo imaging is more rapid than spin-echo imaging, can be used in the coronal and sagittal planes, and appears to be less prone to flow artifacts.[234] MR venograms (analogous to MR arteriograms) can be obtained by manipulation of the gradient-echo technique.[323]

Few studies correlating the accuracy of MRI with phlebography are available. Erdman and associates reported a sensitivity of 90 per cent and a specificity of 100 per cent for spin-echo imaging of the upper and lower extremities in a series of 36 patients, 30 of whom had phlebographic findings that were positive for DVT.[99] Gradient-echo studies of leg veins were found to be equally accurate (sensitivity, 100 per cent; specificity, 93 per cent) by Spritzer and colleagues in 26 patients, 12 of whom had DVT.[287] One study of 10 patients suggested that MRI is as accurate as phlebography for detecting calf vein thrombi and that it has the additional advantage of identifying causes of calf pain in patients in whom no clots are found.[324]

Although MRI has been shown to be accurate in the diagnosis of superior vena caval and jugular vein thrombosis,[122] Haire and coworkers reported less favorable results in patients with catheter-induced subclavian vein thromboses.[118] Six of 22 patients with negative MRI findings had partial occlusion of the subclavian vein, and 1 had a short total occlusion, for a negative predictive value of only 68 per cent. Carpenter and coworkers, using two-dimensional time-of-flight techniques, found that MR venography had a sensitivity of 100 per cent and a specificity of 99 per cent when compared with phlebography of the popliteal vein to the inferior vena cava in patients with suspected DVT.[49] Hypogastric and profunda femoris veins, which were not seen on any of the phlebograms, were visualized in 84 and 90 per cent of the MR venography studies, respectively.

The spatial resolution of MRI is far superior to that obtained with radionuclide phlebography but is inferior to that of duplex scanning or conventional contrast phlebography. Although small veins, such as those in the calf, can be seen with MRI, its relatively poor resolution, together with the difficulties encountered in the registration of low-flow velocities, makes it a poor choice for the evaluation of DVT in small veins. Moreover, MRI is expensive, cumbersome, and time consuming, and it is not as readily available as other diagnostic modalities. At present, the role of MRI in venous diagnosis remains unclear.[323] It appears to be useful for demonstrating the proximal extent of thrombosis when the major veins of the leg are involved, for investigating abdominal and thoracic vein thrombosis, and for evaluating patients who are poor candidates for phlebography, either because of renal failure or allergies to contrast media.[99, 287] It may also help differentiate acute from chronic venous thrombosis.[99] Nonetheless, MRI is in its infancy, and future technologic advances may define an increasing role for this versatile instrument in the investigation of venous disorders. Some enthusiasts have suggested that MR venography may eventually replace contrast phlebography.[49]

Iodine-125–Fibrinogen Uptake

That radionuclide-labeled fibrinogen circulating in the bloodstream is incorporated into developing thrombi was first demonstrated in 1960 by Hobbs and Davies.[130] This provided the rationale for the development of the iodine-125–fibrinogen uptake test (FUT) as a method of diagnosing acute DVT.[19, 209] By 1970, Kakkar and coworkers had simplified the test, making it practical for screening large numbers of patients at the bedside.[155] There followed a decade of activity in which the FUT proved to be very valuable as a research tool for defining the natural history of DVT and for evaluating the efficacy of various prophylactic measures designed to reduce the incidence of the disease. Although the technique proved to be very sensitive for detecting developing calf vein thrombi,[36, 152, 162, 168] it had some glaring defects, including a lack of sensitivity to pelvic vein thrombosis and reduced sensitivity to thrombosis in the thigh, an inability to detect established thrombi, frequent false-positive results,[265] and the necessity of having to wait 18 to 72 hours before a positive diagnosis could be made.[69, 129] Consequently, the FUT is not suited for the routine diagnosis of clinically suspected DVT.[144] It can be useful, however, for detecting acute recurrent venous thrombosis and for identifying calf vein thrombi when the results of physiologically based noninvasive tests are negative.[136, 142] Unfortunately, owing to the risk of blood-borne infection, radionuclide-labeled fibrinogen is no longer commercially available in the United States. The following discussion, therefore, is largely of historical interest.

Methods and Interpretation

To prevent uptake of radioactive iodine by the thyroid, potassium iodide is administered orally 24 hours before the injection of the iodine-125–labeled fibrinogen, or sodium iodide is given intravenously 1 hour before the tracer is injected (Fig. 131–20). Oral potassium iodide is continued for 14 days. The study is initiated with the injection of 100 μCi of iodine-125–labeled human fibrinogen, obtained from hepatitis-free donors. If necessary, the injection can be repeated after 7 days. Patients are scanned with their legs elevated 15 to 45 degrees to minimize pooling of blood in the calf veins. A scintillation detector coupled with a scaler-timer or a rate meter is used to scan the legs, beginning at the inguinal ligament and continuing at 2- to 3-inch intervals down the thigh along the course of the superficial femoral vein. Below the knee, scanning is continued at

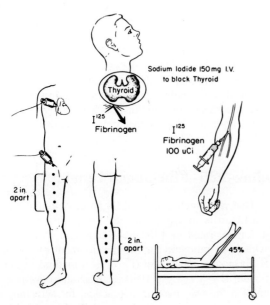

FIGURE 131–20. Outline of the fibrinogen uptake test.

similar intervals posteriorly from the popliteal fossa to the ankle. Readings are recorded as a percentage of the count obtained over the precordium. Recordings are made 1 to 4 hours after injection and are then repeated every 24 hours.

Test results are considered to be positive if the count relative to the precordial activity at any point is 20 per cent or more higher than that recorded over the same point on the previous day, over adjacent points on the same leg, or over a corresponding point of the opposite leg. Venous thrombosis is diagnosed if the abnormality persists for more than 24 hours.

Errors and Limitations

Any condition that leads to an accumulation of fibrinogen, fibrin, or fibrin degradation products can produce a false-positive result. The list includes hematomas, fractures, burns, surgical incisions, cellulitis, ulcers, arthritis, vasculitis, gross edema, superficial thrombophlebitis, and even varicose veins—all conditions that are frequently confused with or may coexist with calf vein thrombosis.[42, 168, 205] False-negative results can occur in limbs with older clots that are not actively incorporating fibrinogen and in limbs of patients receiving anticoagulants.[42, 45, 152, 233]

Because the background count is increased over the bladder (which accumulates radioactive urine) and over the large vessels of the upper thigh and pelvis, the FUT is insensitive to thrombi developing in the pelvis, is inaccurate over the upper thigh, and is only moderately sensitive over the lower thigh.[42, 124, 152, 189, 224, 267] Failure to detect potentially dangerous thrombi in these locations constitutes the major limitation of the FUT.[189] The need to wait for 24 to 48 hours (sometimes 72 hours) before a definitive diagnosis can be made is a significant drawback that severely compromises the clinical value of the test.

Administration of iodine-125–labeled fibrinogen is contraindicated in pregnancy and during lactation because the isotope crosses the placental barrier and is secreted in the milk. To avoid an accumulation of radioactive iodine in the thyroid gland, patients under the age of 40 probably should not be studied. As mentioned earlier, there is a small risk of transmitting hepatitis and other blood-borne diseases.

Accuracy

Representative data defining the accuracy of the FUT compared with phlebography are listed in Tables 131–14 and 131–15. The high sensitivity of the test for detecting early postoperative calf vein thromboses is reflected in the data from reports surveying patients undergoing major abdominal surgery. Sensitivities are considerably worse in limbs of patients undergoing hip operations, owing to the tendency for these patients to develop thrombosis in the proximal thigh veins, where the FUT is inaccurate. Comerota and associates found that the FUT was 81 per cent sensitive for detecting developing calf vein thrombi and 63 per cent sensitive for thrombi in the thighs of patients who had total joint replacements.[60] In a similar group of patients, Paiement and colleagues found that FUT results were positive in only 14 per cent of limbs with thrombosis of the thigh veins.[224] They concluded that the FUT, even in com-

Table 131–14.   Accuracy of Iodine-125–Labeled Fibrinogen Uptake Test for Diagnosing Deep Venous Thrombosis (Surveillance Studies)

Study	No. of Extremities	Sensitivity (%)	Specificity (%)	Positive Predictive Value (%)	Negative Predictive Value (%)	Overall Accuracy (%)
Abdominal Surgery						
Lambie et al, 1970[168]	62	95 (40/42)	80 (16/20)	91 (40/44)	89 (16/18)	90 (56/62)
Tsapogas et al, 1971[317]	95	92 (11/12)	100 (83/83)	100 (11/11)	99 (83/84)	99 (94/95)
Kakkar, 1972[152]	88	94 (32/34)	93 (50/54)	89 (32/36)	96 (50/52)	93 (82/88)
Hip Surgery						
Harris et al, 1975[124]	142	49 (25/51)	96 (87/91)	86 (25/29)	77 (87/113)	79 (112/142)
Sautter et al, 1979[267]	146	58 (29/50)	70 (67/96)	100 (29/29)	76 (67/88)	66 (96/146)
LeMoine and Moser, 1980[172]	42	100 (9/9)	94 (31/33)	81 (9/11)	100 (31/31)	95 (40/42)
Lindblad et al, 1987[177]	93	79 (15/19)*	90 (67/74)	68 (15/22)	94 (67/71)	88 (82/93)
Paiement et al, 1988[224]	937	59 (78/133)†	96 (769/804)	69 (78/113)	93 (769/824)	90 (847/937)
Comerota et al, 1988[60]	111	73 (41/56)	71 (39/55)	72 (41/57)	72 (39/54)	72 (80/111)

*Positive findings in the thigh of the operated limb were excluded.
†Calf thrombi only.

bination with impedance plethysmography, is not an effective screening method—a conclusion reached independently by Cruickshank and associates, who found this combination of tests to be only 50 per cent sensitive for detecting DVT in patients after hip surgery.[77]

When the FUT is used diagnostically to rule in or out DVT in symptomatic limbs, the results are inferior to those reported for Doppler ultrasonography, plethysmography, and ultrasonic imaging (see Table 131–15). Using the FUT in combination with impedance plethysmography, Hull and coworkers reported a sensitivity of 90 per cent for detecting DVT in symptomatic limbs; however, only 24 of 114 thrombi (21 per cent) were detected by the FUT alone.[142] Of the 78 thigh vein thromboses, the FUT detected only 4 (5 per cent). These and similar observations led Hull and associates to conclude that "125I-fibrinogen leg scanning should never be used as the only diagnostic test in clinically suspected deep venous thrombosis."[144]

Radionuclide Phlebography

Radionuclide phlebography provides images of the larger veins of the legs and pelvis that resemble conventional contrast phlebograms. The procedure is minimally invasive, can be performed rapidly, causes little discomfort, uses a nonirritating injectate, exposes the patient to less radiation than conventional phlebography, may be repeated within 24 hours or less, and may be coupled with a perfusion lung scan. The equipment required, although expensive and sophisticated, is available in most modern hospitals. Although veins are much less clearly defined with radio-

nuclide phlebography than they are with conventional x-ray studies or with ultrasonic imaging, the reported accuracy has been good, especially when the test is used to study veins of the upper thigh and pelvis. However, small thrombi within calf veins are easily missed, partially occluding clots cannot be distinguished from those that totally occlude the vessel, and extrinsic compression cannot be distinguished from intrinsic obstruction.

Technique and Interpretation

With the patient lying supine, 1.0 to 2.0 mCi of technetium-99m–labeled macroaggregated albumin or microspheres is injected through scalp vein needles inserted into a dorsal vein of both feet (Fig. 131–21).[37, 254, 334] Tourniquets are applied to the ankles to direct the flow of the tracer into the deep veins, and radioactive markers are affixed to the knee and pubis for orientation purposes. Following injection of the radionuclide, its course up the leg is monitored with the diverging collimator of a gamma camera (dynamic imaging). Images are recorded on Polaroid film and on videotape. Repeated scans are obtained after the tourniquets have been removed. In order to detect residual radioactivity, the legs are again studied after a period of 5 to 10 minutes (static imaging). At the end of the venous examination, a perfusion lung scan may be obtained.[66, 98, 254, 321, 334]

Although unbound sodium pertechnetate can be used, it is not captured in the lung and therefore cannot be used for pulmonary scanning.[29, 151] Recirculation of the isotope has the further disadvantage of increasing the background radioactivity.

Calf veins are not seen as discrete images but appear

Table 131–15.   Accuracy of Iodine-125–Labeled Fibrinogen Uptake Test for Diagnosing Deep Venous Thrombosis (Symptomatic Patients)

Study	No. of Extremities	Sensitivity (%)	Specificity (%)	Positive Predictive Value (%)	Negative Predictive Value (%)	Overall Accuracy (%)
Browse et al, 1971[45]	195	71 (46/65)	85 (110/130)	70 (46/66)	85 (110/129)	80 (156/195)
Kakkar, 1972[152]	102	83 (62/74)	54 (15/28)	83 (62/75)	56 (15/27)	75 (77/102)
Moser et al, 1977[206]	42	70 (16/23)	79 (15/19)	80 (16/20)	68 (15/22)	74 (31/42)
Hull et al, 1981[142]	274	21 (24/114)	97 (155/160)	83 (24/29)	63 (155/245)	65 (179/274)

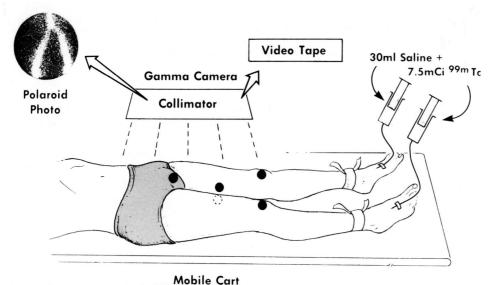

Video Tape

Gamma Camera

Collimator

Polaroid Photo

30ml Saline + 7.5mCi ^{99m}Tc

Mobile Cart

FIGURE 131–21. Method for performing radionuclide phlebography. *Closed circles* indicate the locations of radioactive markers.

as a broad area of radioactivity. The popliteal, femoral, and iliac veins are represented by a well-defined continuous column of radioactivity that converges in the pelvis with the column from the opposite side to form an image of the inferior vena cava (Fig. 131–22). Owing to the admixture of nonlabeled blood from the internal iliac veins, the common iliac veins are typically less densely radioactive than those located below. Venous obstruction is indicated by (1) areas of nonfilling along the course of the major deep veins, (2) visualization of collateral channels (which may be quite striking, particularly in the pelvis), (3) slow ascent of the isotope, and (4) residual "hot spots" observed on the delayed scan (Fig. 131–23). An important secondary sign that is highly suggestive of deep venous occlusion is the appearance of radioactivity in the superficial veins before it appears in the deep veins.[66]

Hot spots must be interpreted cautiously because they may be seen in 10 to 15 per cent of normal extremities, most commonly in the calf.[66, 98, 254] In limbs without thromboses, they are thought to represent areas of sluggish flow, as might occur in the soleal sinusoids, beneath valve cusps, or in varicose veins. However, those persisting after muscle contraction are suggestive of venous obstruction.[98] Al-

though it was initially theorized that the labeled microspheres were adherent to the clot, the mechanism of hot spots is now thought to be due to accumulation of the isotope below sites of venous obstruction.[37, 321]

Accuracy

There have been relatively few studies comparing the findings of radionuclide and conventional x-ray phlebography. Henkin and associates[127] and Yao and coworkers[334] reported overall correlations of 89 to 96 per cent in two early studies. Later reports substantiated these observations (Table 131–16). It is clear—particularly from the work of Bentley and associates—that accuracy tends to be much better in the thigh and pelvis than it is in the calf.[37] If the calf is excluded, the overall accuracy appears to be similar to that reported for other diagnostic tests.

Although radionuclide phlebography is undoubtedly a reasonably good method for diagnosing DVT, it has few advantages compared with other, simpler methods. It may, however, have a limited role when, after conventional x-ray studies or other tests have been performed, the status of the pelvic veins remains uncertain or when the physician

Normal Isotope Phlebogram

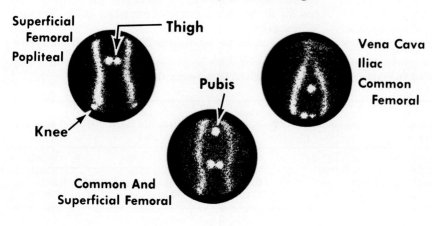

Superficial Femoral

Popliteal

Thigh

Knee

Pubis

Common And Superficial Femoral

Vena Cava

Iliac

Common Femoral

FIGURE 131–22. Normal radionuclide phlebograms. Circles of radioactivity represent the locations of markers. Note the dilution of activity in the common iliac veins and the inferior vena cava.

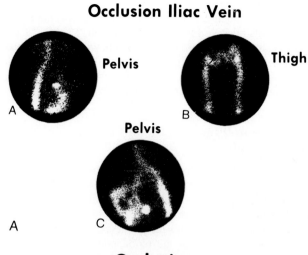

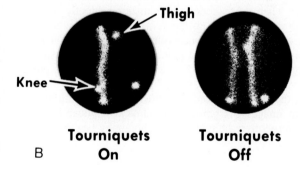

FIGURE 131–23. Abnormal radionuclide phlebograms. *A*, Three examples of iliac vein occlusion: no image of the left iliac vein. (A), cross-pelvic collaterals. (B), and right iliac venous thrombosis with extensive ipsilateral collateral development. (C). *B*, With tourniquets in place, there is no visualization of veins in the left thigh; with tourniquets removed, the left saphenous vein is seen, but there is no evident radioactivity from the deep veins.

Table 131–16. Accuracy of Radionuclide Phlebography for Diagnosing Deep Venous Thrombosis

Study	No. of Extremities	Sensitivity (%)	Specificity (%)	Positive Predictive Value (%)	Negative Predictive Value (%)	Overall Accuracy (%)
Calf						
Vlahos et al, 1976[321]	98	94 (34/36)	95 (59/62)	92 (34/37)	97 (59/61)	95 (93/98)
Bentley et al, 1979[37]	200	66 (59/89)	71 (79/111)	65 (59/91)	72 (79/109)	69 (138/200)
Thigh						
Vlahos et al, 1976[321]	98	100 (24/24)	96 (71/74)	89 (24/27)	100 (71/71)	97 (95/98)
Bentley et al, 1979[37]	200	75 (18/24)	99 (174/176)	90 (18/20)	97 (174/180)	96 (192/200)
Pelvis						
Bentley et al, 1979[37]	200	100 (17/17)	100 (183/183)	100 (17/17)	100 (183/183)	100 (200/200)
Overall						
Cordoba et al, 1977[66]	44	100 (34/34)	80 (8/10)	94 (34/36)	100 (8/8)	95 (42/44)
Ennis and Elmes, 1977[98]	154	90 (52/58)	99 (95/96)	98 (52/53)	94 (95/101)	95 (147/154)
Ryo et al, 1977[254]	47	89 (16/18)	90 (26/29)	84 (16/19)	93 (26/28)	89 (42/47)
Bentley et al, 1979[37]	200	73 (68/93)	70 (75/107)	68 (68/100)	75 (75/100)	72 (143/200)

believes that a concomitant lung scan is desirable. According to several reports, when examinations are extended to include perfusion scans, 24 to 58 per cent of patients with positive radionuclide phlebographic findings also have lung scan results positive for pulmonary emboli.[66, 98, 254, 334] Conversely, in 10 to 41 per cent of patients with indeterminate or intermediate-probability lung scan findings, radionuclide phlebographic results are positive for DVT, thus obviating the need for pulmonary arteriography.[126]

Technetium-99m–Red Blood Cell Phlebography

Another form of radionuclide phlebography employs red blood cells labeled with technetium-99m.[180, 222, 338] The ability to image leg veins by injecting the tracer into an easily cannulated arm vein rather than directly into a foot vein is an advantage of this technique. Although the isotope is distributed throughout the blood pool, veins are selectively visualized because their capacity is considerably larger than that of the neighboring arteries. Another possible advantage is that unlike in studies conducted with free technetium-99m or technetium-99m–labeled albumin, the image is persistent. Venous definition, however, seems to be better when the isotope is administered directly into a foot vein and its course up the veins is followed with the gamma camera.[222] Zorba and colleagues reported that the test, compared with contrast phlebography, had a sensitivity, specificity, positive predictive value, and negative predictive value of 90, 93, 77, and 97 per cent, respectively.[338] Most of the errors involved false-positive interpretations of calf vein images. At present, the clinical applicability of technetium-99m–red blood cell phlebography has not been established.[126]

Thrombus Scintigraphy

Several still largely experimental methods of detecting DVT should be mentioned. These are based on the static imaging of thrombi that accumulate isotope-labeled constituents. The labeled marker is injected intravenously, and the patient is then scanned with a gamma camera after an appropriate period. An advantage of these methods over iodine-125–fibrinogen uptake studies is that the results may be available within minutes to hours of the injection.

The technetium-99m–plasmin test may be interpreted with a scintillation counter and rate meter (much like the FUT) or with a gamma camera, which affords some localization. Readings are made 5 to 30 minutes after injection. Sensitivities exceeding 90 per cent are commonly reported, but specificities tend to be low (around 50 per cent).[15, 67, 78, 182] Another disadvantage is that positive results may be obtained for up to 6 months after an acute episode of DVT, making the test unreliable for detecting recurrent disease.[91, 167] One study has shown that the test lacks sufficient sensitivity or specificity to be used as a screening method in patients undergoing hip surgery.[52]

Indium-111–labeled platelets accumulate on venous thrombi as well as on atherosclerotic plaques. Although gamma camera images can become positive in 4 hours after injection, delayed images 24 hours later should be obtained if the result of the initial study is negative or equivocal.[274] Clots must be less than 6 hours old to be labeled consistently. Thus, the test is more suited to surveillance than to diagnostic studies.[50] Because heparin inhibits the accretion of platelets by thrombi, false-negative results may occur in patients receiving anticoagulation.[101, 102] Twenty-four hour sensitivities and specificities exceeding 90 per cent have been reported both for screening and for the diagnosis of symptomatic venous thrombosis.[82, 101, 274] In a prospective study, however, Ezekowitz and coworkers found that indium-labeled platelets detected only 10 per cent of phlebographically demonstrated thrombi in calf veins, 18 per cent in popliteal veins and 61 per cent in thigh veins of patients with clinically suspected DVT.[100] Impedance plethysmography and duplex scanning were far more sensitive.

Technetium-99m–labeled streptokinase and urokinase produce scintigraphic images within 1 hour after injection and may be used to visualize established thrombi that are not actively incorporating fibrinogen.[157, 199] Iodine-123–labeled fibrinogen scintigraphy avoids some of the limitations of iodine-125–labeled fibrinogen (although it still requires thyroid blockade). Unlike the FUT, it is accurate in the upper thigh and pelvic regions, where both sensitivities and specificities greater than 90 per cent have been reported.[84] Studies must be delayed for 4 to 8 hours and are more reliable at 24 hours. Radionuclide-labeled monoclonal antibodies specific for human fibrin and for the platelet surface have been investigated as possible new tests for detecting venous thrombi.[228, 252] These and other scintigraphic tests for DVT are reviewed and compared in an article by Chaudhuri and colleagues.[50]

Thermography

Thermography can be used to detect and (to some extent) to localize acute deep venous thromboses, which typically raise the temperature of the overlying skin by 0.5°C to more than 1.2°C. The temperature elevation has been attributed to increased arterial blood flow secondary to the release of vasoactive amines from the site of the venous thrombus. Thus, thermography detects a hyperemic response in the neighboring tissues. Most thermographic systems employ a scanning camera with an infrared detector and a display unit, but simpler, less expensive devices are available and liquid crystals can even be used.[52, 62, 215, 261] The number of reports is limited. Some reports suggest that thermography is quite accurate in both the calf and thigh regions (sensitivities and specificities above 90 per cent), provided that no other heat-producing lesion is present.[38, 62] Several authors have noted good sensitivities (above 90 per cent) but poor specificities (in the 50 to 60 per cent range);[215, 261] others have noted fair sensitivities and specificities (75 to 85 per cent).[246, 284] Unacceptably low specificities (20 per cent) have also been reported.[120] False-positive results would be expected in limbs with traumatic injuries, hematomas, infection, arthritis, ruptured Baker's cysts, Paget's disease, osteomyelitis, varicose veins, superficial thrombophlebitis, or bone tumors. False-negative findings occur in association with small calf vein thrombi and clots that are no longer fresh (2 to 13 days old).

At present, with the ready availability of other, equally simple and more consistently accurate methods of detecting DVT, the role of thermography seems to be limited.

APPLICATIONS

The diagnostic approach to DVT varies according to the clinical presentation of the patient, the nature of the information being sought, the urgency of the situation, and the availability of diagnostic tests and of personnel skilled in their use.

Clinically Suspected Acute Deep Venous Thrombosis

Patients with unexplained acute limb swelling, calf pain, or tenderness along the course of a major deep vein are possible candidates for the diagnosis of acute DVT. It is well known, however, that in about half of these patients, the symptoms and signs arise from another cause (see Table 131–1). Despite this impressive list of alternative diagnoses, in an appreciable number of limbs in which DVT has been excluded, the diagnosis remains obscure. Confounding the problem in the individual patient is the frequent association of DVT with any of the conditions listed in Table 131–1.

Although phlebograms could be obtained in every suspected case, phlebography—as pointed out earlier in this chapter—is expensive, is time consuming, must be performed in the radiology suite, is often painful, and carries a small (but very real) risk of causing DVT. Except for research purposes and in hospitals in which no other diagnostic modalities are available, this approach is not practical. Moreover, because of the reluctance on the part of many physicians to obtain phlebograms, especially in patients with minimal symptoms, there is the risk of missing potentially serious thromboses or, in patients with more striking clinical manifestations, of diagnosing thrombosis when in reality the symptoms are due to some other cause. For these reasons, noninvasive testing is advocated as the initial objective study in all patients suspected of having acute DVT, provided that the vascular laboratory personnel are skilled in the required techniques.

Cost:benefit analysis has shown that failure to treat suspected DVT is at least twice as expensive as treating all such cases with anticoagulants.[22] Treating patients on the basis of clinical assessment alone is only half as cost-effective as using contrast phlebography to establish the diagnosis before treatment. The cost-effectiveness of noninvasive testing is comparable to or somewhat less than that of routine outpatient phlebography, but noninvasive testing has the advantage of sparing the patient the discomfort and risks of unnecessary phlebography. Certainly, outpatient noninvasive testing is far more cost-effective than admitting the patient for phlebography.[141]

Initial Diagnostic Evaluation

The initial evaluation may be carried out with any of the noninvasive methods that have been proved to be accurate in published clinical trials. These include *Doppler ultrasonography, impedance plethysmography, phleborheography, and duplex ultrasonic imaging.* Air and strain-gauge plethysmography are probably also acceptable. Even if iodine-125–fibrinogen were still available, the FUT, which is insensitive to proximal venous thrombi and is subject to false-positive interpretations, should not be relied on for the diagnosis of acute DVT.[143] Thermography, in the author's opinion, is too inaccurate to be used, and the multiple tests that employ scintigraphy have no established track record and are rarely available. Radionuclide phlebography may be an alternative when concomitant pulmonary scanning is needed, but it offers no particular advantage over the more routine tests and is best reserved for special situations. The role of MRI remains to be determined. In choosing which of the noninvasive tests to employ, the individual laboratory must be guided by personal experience. Because of their versatility and superior accuracy, conventional duplex and color flow scanning are generally considered to be the methods of choice. Physiologic tests, however, remain useful for screening purposes and are a satisfactory alternative when ultrasonic imaging cannot be performed. Compared with ultrasonic scanning, physiologic tests are more easily and rapidly performed, require less training, are less expensive, and are more likely to be available—all significant advantages, especially in busy laboratories where duplex scanners are often tied up with other studies.

Physiologic Tests

The algorithm in Figure 131–24 outlines an approach to the diagnosis of acute DVT based on physiologic testing. When the results are clearly positive and there is no reason to suspect extrinsic compression (or other conditions known to produce a false-positive result), appropriate treatment can be instituted without further study. When the examiner is satisfied that the results are definitely normal and is confident that involvement of the popliteal and more proximal veins has been excluded, no further diagnostic tests need be undertaken. If, on the other hand, the results of the initial test are equivocal or if there is reason to suspect extrinsic compression or calf vein thrombosis, further studies are necessary.

Conventional x-ray phlebography is a direct and widely available way of arriving at a definitive diagnosis in cases in which the results of physiologic studies are indeterminate, but ultrasonic scanning (in good hands) seems to be as good in many circumstances and better in some. For example, in cases in which obstruction is due to extrinsic compression, ultrasonography—unlike arteriography—may reveal the nature of the obstructive process (e.g., lymphadenopathy or hematoma). In addition, when iliac vein obstruction is suspected, ultrasonic scanning (or isotope phlebography) may be more informative than an ascending phlebogram obtained by injecting contrast into the foot. Adequate phlebographic visualization of the iliac veins often requires a separate injection of contrast into the femoral veins.

How to proceed when the result of the initial physiologic test is negative is a question that has not been completely resolved. Between 70 and 90 per cent of patients referred to vascular laboratories for evaluation of suspected

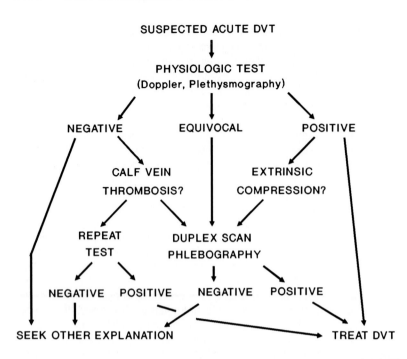

SUSPECTED ACUTE DVT

PHYSIOLOGIC TEST
(Doppler, Plethysmography)

NEGATIVE   EQUIVOCAL   POSITIVE

CALF VEIN   EXTRINSIC
THROMBOSIS?   COMPRESSION?

REPEAT   DUPLEX SCAN
TEST   PHLEBOGRAPHY

NEGATIVE   POSITIVE   NEGATIVE   POSITIVE

SEEK OTHER EXPLANATION   TREAT DVT

FIGURE 131–24. Algorithm depicting a diagnostic approach to suspected acute DVT based on physiologic tests.

venous disease have negative physiologic test results.[134, 137, 288, 330] Approximately 15 per cent of symptomatic patients with negative impedance plethysmographic findings and 10 per cent of patients with negative Doppler survey findings have phlebographically demonstrable calf vein thromboses.[60, 140, 300] Far fewer patients (4 to 5 per cent) with negative studies have thromboses above the knee (see Tables 131–6 and 131–8). If, as shown in one limb of the algorithm (Fig. 131–24), the physician decides not to perform additional tests on patients with clearly negative noninvasive findings and elects to withhold anticoagulant therapy, the deep venous thromboses present in at least 15 per cent of these patients will remain untreated. Most of these thromboses, however, will be confined to the calf veins and may therefore not constitute a major hazard.

Wheeler and colleagues demonstrated the safety of withholding anticoagulant therapy on the basis of a single negative physiologic test result.[328] They followed a large series of patients with suspected DVT who, because the impedance plethysmographic findings were normal, were not treated with anticoagulants. Only 1 per cent suffered a pulmonary embolus (none fatal), and only 0.4 per cent returned with subsequent symptoms of DVT. Negative phleborheographic findings have also been shown to virtually eliminate the possibility of clinically significant venous disease; only 1 of 593 patients followed up by Stallworth and associates developed a pulmonary embolus, and only 3 developed postphlebitic swelling.[288] Again, none of the emboli were fatal. In the author's laboratory, a negative Doppler survey result appears to be fairly reliable, ruling out all but 2 per cent of acute proximal venous thrombi and all but 3 per cent of major calf vein thrombi.[302] The author and his colleagues know of no instance of pulmonary embolism in patients with negative Doppler study findings who were not anticoagulated.

To reduce the likelihood of a serious false-negative error, Hull and associates recommend serial studies in symptomatic patients with negative plethysmographic findings.[137] Examinations are repeated on days 3, 5 to 7, 10,

and 14. If, during this time, impedance plethysmographic findings become positive, a diagnosis of DVT is made and the patient is begun on anticoagulants. Because the impedance plethysmograph is insensitive to thrombi localized to the calf veins, a positive study result suggests propagation into the popliteal or more proximal veins. During the period of diagnostic surveillance, Hull and associates found that plethysmographic findings became positive in only 2.6 per cent of patients whose results were initially negative.[137] Patients with negative studies, many of whom probably had calf vein thrombosis, were not treated, yet none died of a pulmonary embolus during follow-up, and only 1.9 per cent developed venous thromboembolism. The results of a similar investigation conducted by Huisman and associates in Holland confirmed these observations.[134]

Despite the relative safety of using serial tests to rule out clot propagation in patients with negative physiologic test findings, it is reassuring and probably more cost-effective to use phlebography or ultrasonic scanning to confirm the absence of thrombosis in patients in whom there is a strong suspicion of calf vein involvement (see Fig. 131–24).

The combined use of two tests, such as Doppler ultrasonography and plethysmography, that are primarily sensitive to proximal venous thrombosis has been advocated by some investigators as the initial screening procedure.[104, 245] Although this approach will increase sensitivity (provided that the study result is considered to be positive if either of the individual test results is positive), there will usually be some loss of specificity (more false-positive diagnoses).[299] When the results of the two tests coincide, the diagnosis is virtually assured.[104] In the author's opinion, there is little justification for the routine use of two tests.

Ultrasonic Imaging

An algorithm outlining the use of duplex scanning or color flow imaging for diagnosing acute DVT is illustrated in Figure 131–25.[304] Because of the high positive predictive value of these tests in the femoropopliteal segment (see

Tables 131–10 and 131–11), no further studies are required when a thrombosis is demonstrated in the above-knee veins, and treatment for DVT can be instituted based solely on the results of the scan. Although a negative study finding effectively rules out proximal DVT (see Tables 131–10 and 131–11), the reliability of both positive and negative results below the knee depends on the technical adequacy of the test (see Tables 131–12 and 131–13)—a judgment that is best made by the technologist performing the examination. If visualization of the calf veins is adequate and no clots are detected, no further studies are necessary, and some other cause for the patient's complaints must be sought.[263] Likewise, when clots are definitely identified in the infrapopliteal veins, the patient can be anticoagulated, or if the physician's policy is not to treat isolated calf vein thrombosis, scanning can be repeated over the next week or so to detect propagation into the popliteal or superficial femoral vein. However, when scan results are equivocal, visualization is imperfect, or the study is compromised in some other way, phlebography should be performed or scanning should be repeated in an effort to obtain a definitive study or to rule out proximal propagation.

Even when no thrombi are detected, the scan may provide an explanation for the patient's complaints. Conditions frequently confused with calf vein thrombosis, such as popliteal cysts and hematomas developing in response to a torn muscle, are readily identified. Tumors, enlarged lymph nodes, and other masses that compress proximal veins are also easily identified. Another advantage of ultrasonic imaging is that unlike physiologic tests, it differentiates between occlusive and nonocclusive clots and provides detailed anatomic information about the location, extent, and chronicity of the thrombotic process—information that is required if the disease process is to be classified according to the criteria proposed by the Subcommittee on Reporting Standards in Venous Disease.[235] The information obtained may also affect therapeutic decisions. For example, recognition of a free-floating clot in a proximal vein may serve as an impetus to insert a filter.[20, 39, 219] Moreover,

the potential ability of scanning to locate the proximal extent of a clot may be helpful when vena caval interruption or filter insertion is contemplated.[90, 213]

It should be evident from the preceding discussion that ultrasonic imaging is uniquely suitable both for initial testing of patients with suspected acute DVT and as a backup for physiologic testing (see Fig. 131–24). When duplex scanning can be used as the initial diagnostic modality, further studies are seldom required. The only drawbacks to its universal use are the time required for each study, the need for expert technologists, and the expense of the instruments. Unless the laboratory is especially well endowed, other demands placed on the imager may curtail its routine use as the primary diagnostic modality.

Limiting the scan to the popliteal and more proximal veins—an approach favored by some investigators—simplifies and accelerates the examination but sacrifices one of the unique advantages of imaging, the identification of calf vein thrombi. Twenty to 40 per cent of clots responsible for symptomatic DVT are isolated to the infrapopliteal veins and would not be detected by this approach.[164, 188, 212, 249, 250] Although remarkably few of these isolated clots become symptomatic in the immediate follow-up period (as shown by the results of physiologic testing), it is by no means certain that calf vein thrombi are entirely benign.[181, 230] About 20 per cent propagate into the popliteal or more proximal veins;[153, 164, 181, 285] even those that remain isolated may occasionally be responsible for pulmonary emboli;[181, 197, 204] and perhaps a significant number may serve as the nidus for subsequent, more extensive, thrombosis.[250] Moreover, there is evidence that valvular destruction caused by calf vein thrombi may play a major role in the development of chronic venous insufficiency.[154, 159, 186, 203, 273, 290] Therefore, now that noninvasive methods are available for detecting infrapopliteal thrombi, it seems logical to incorporate the study of calf veins in the routine examination of patients with suspected DVT (see Fig. 131–25). Color flow imaging simplifies what may be a tedious process with conventional duplex scanning, making it feasible to conduct

FIGURE 131–25. Algorithm depicting a diagnostic approach to suspected acute DVT based on duplex scanning. AK, above knee; BK, below knee

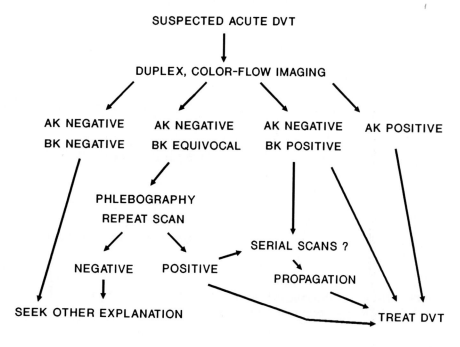

a thorough study rapidly and with minimal effort.[251, 304] In the author's opinion, there is no longer any valid reason to neglect the infrapopliteal veins.

Acute Recurrent Deep Venous Thrombosis

The patient with a history of DVT who returns with acute swelling or pain in the leg, suggesting a recurrent episode of thrombosis, presents a difficult diagnostic problem. Only about 20 to 30 per cent of these individuals actually have the disease; the remainder have symptoms arising from chronic venous insufficiency or from any of the causes listed in Table 131–1.[33, 135, 136] Some merely have "thromboneurosis," their symptoms being manifestations of a morbid fear of thromboembolism.[268] Included in this group are patients who never actually had DVT.

An approach to the diagnosis of acute recurrent DVT is illustrated in Figure 131–26. Similar algorithms have been published by Barnes[23] and by Hull and associates.[144] The patient is initially screened with Doppler ultrasonography, plethysmography, or ultrasonic imaging (B-mode or duplex). Because venous reflux is easily recognized with Doppler ultrasonography or with duplex scanning, these modalities are preferred over impedance plethysmography, which is not readily adapted to the detection of venous incompetence. Moreover, in limbs with well-developed collaterals, plethysmographic results may be normal despite the presence of chronic obstruction.

Noninvasive studies in patients in whom recurrent DVT is suspected may have negative results, reveal valvular incompetence only, or detect venous obstruction (with or without concomitant valvular incompetence). Provided studies are technically adequate and complete, negative duplex examination findings effectively exclude recurrent disease in patients with a history of DVT (see Fig. 131–26).[76] Negative findings with the use of hand-held Doppler instruments or with plethysmography are usually reliable but must be interpreted more cautiously, as outlined in Figure 131–24.

Although incompetence of the deep venous valves is usually indicative of a previous (often unrecognized) thrombotic event, in the absence of demonstrable venous obstruction, incompetence alone is not indicative of recurrent disease. In questionable cases, radionuclide scanning can be performed, but the yield of positive results will be small in limbs with or without valvular incompetence and no evidence of venous obstruction. (Fewer than 10 per cent of such limbs had positive findings in the study of Hull and coworkers.[136])

In the absence of extrinsic compression, venous obstruction is indicative of a thrombotic process—either old or new (see Fig. 131–26). If the patient has been followed up closely in the vascular laboratory, it may be possible to identify a change in the noninvasive findings consistent with the development of a new clot. In this event, no other diagnostic tests are required. Huisman and colleagues obtained phlebographic confirmation of recurrent DVT in 85 per cent of patients with a documented history of DVT in whom impedance plethysmographic findings reverted to an abnormal status.[135] Jay and associates found that impedance plethysmographic findings returned to normal within 3 months in 60 per cent of patients following an episode of extensive proximal DVT;[149] Huisman and colleagues, using the same modality, found that 95 per cent of the study results were normal at 12 months;[135] and Killewich and coworkers, using ultrasonic duplex scanning, noted that 93

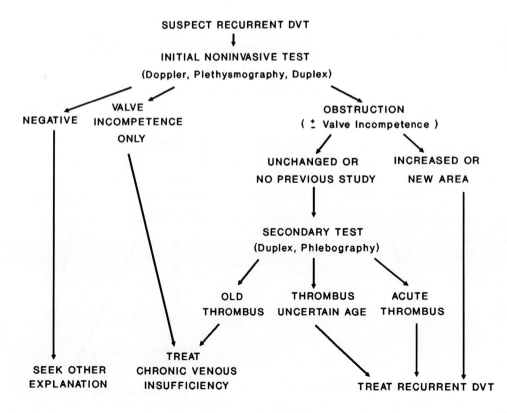

FIGURE 131–26.
Algorithm depicting a diagnostic approach to suspected recurrent DVT.

per cent of clots had lysed by 30 days.[159] Others reported that positive duplex scan findings returned to normal in 47 to 73 per cent of limbs with acute DVT after an average interval of 12 to 14 months.[76, 184] Thus, the presence of obstructed veins in a symptomatic patient with a history of DVT who has never been examined before must be considered presumptive evidence of recurrent acute disease until proved otherwise. These patients and patients in whom the noninvasive findings are abnormal but are unchanged from those of a previous examination should undergo secondary testing, either with contrast phlebography or duplex scanning. Clearly, the use of duplex scanning as the initial diagnostic test, rather than simple Doppler surveys or plethysmography, is advantageous under these circumstances.

Although phlebography has long been considered the gold standard for the identification of recurrent disease, extensive collateral development and recanalization may make phlebographic findings difficult to interpret. There may be nothing to distinguish an acute thrombus from preexisting chronic disease.[248] As described earlier in this chapter, B-mode ultrasonography has the potential advantage of being able to estimate the age of clots based on their echogenicity, compressibility, degree of retraction, and adherence to the venous wall.[103, 250] Color flow duplex scanning has the additional advantage of detecting recanalized flow channels in occluded veins, thereby establishing the chronicity of the obstructing thrombus.

If fresh clots are identified, the patient should be anticoagulated. A problem arises when the age of the thrombus is uncertain. In this event, radionuclide tests, if available, may be used to determine whether the thrombotic process is active or quiescent. Anticoagulants are begun when these tests are abnormal or when there is any question of clot activity; otherwise, the patient is treated for chronic venous insufficiency. In the study by Hull and coworkers, approximately 80 per cent of patients with symptoms of recurrent DVT who had abnormal impedance plethysmographic findings required anticoagulation.[136]

Because the risk of death from pulmonary embolism is high in patients with recurrent DVT, it is better to err on the side of treatment.[144] Few mistakes will be made if all patients in whom the results of noninvasive tests are positive for obstruction are anticoagulated and if treatment is withheld from those with normal test results or with findings limited to valvular incompetence.

Surveillance

The iodine-125–fibrinogen uptake test was instrumental in alerting surgeons to the astonishing frequency with which clots form in leg veins of patients during the perioperative period. Between 10 and 40 per cent of patients over the age of 40 undergoing major abdominal or thoracic surgery will develop calf vein thrombosis; 2 to 8 per cent, proximal venous thrombosis; 1 to 8 per cent, clinically evident pulmonary embolism; and 0.1 to 0.4 per cent, a fatal pulmonary embolus.[257] In high-risk patients and those undergoing orthopedic surgery of the lower limbs, the incidence of calf vein thrombosis and proximal venous thrombosis jumps to 40 to 80 per cent and 10 to 20 per cent, respectively. Five to 10 per cent of patients in this category

experience a pulmonary embolus, and 1 to 5 per cent die as a result of pulmonary embolism.[257] Until they embolize, the vast majority of these thrombi are completely asymptomatic.

There are three ways of dealing with this problem: (1) wait until the patient develops signs and symptoms of phlebitis or pulmonary embolism and then proceed with the appropriate diagnostic and therapeutic measures; (2) survey all patients, both preoperatively and postoperatively, treating those thrombi that are detected before they cause serious complications; or (3) institute prophylactic treatment in all moderate- or high-risk patients undergoing operation. Although the second approach (surveillance) is intellectually appealing and effective, it is logistically difficult; is costly in terms of time, personnel, and money; and depending on the technique employed, unnecessarily subjects many patients who would not suffer a pulmonary embolus to full anticoagulant therapy with its inherent risk of bleeding complications.[128, 152, 256, 282] Of the three approaches, the third (prophylaxis) is probably the most cost-effective.[256] The first approach (no prophylaxis, no surveillance), although still practiced by many surgeons, not only is costly (because of the substantial diagnostic and therapeutic expenses associated with clinical thromboembolism) but also does nothing to decrease the risk of a fatal embolism.[61]

Most of the early prospective studies used the iodine-125–fibrinogen uptake test (FUT) to detect thrombi forming in the perioperative period. Because many of these thrombi were small and were located below the knee, most had no immediate clinical significance. Whether to treat or not to treat below-knee clots disclosed by this method remains a matter of some controversy.[46, 88, 178, 330] Because the primary goal of surveillance is to detect potentially lethal clots, the test employed for this purpose must be sensitive to thrombi developing in iliofemoral veins, from which most fatal pulmonary emboli arise. Because the FUT was less accurate above the knee and was unsuited for examining veins of the proximal thigh or pelvis, it fell short of being the ideal method for prospective surveillance. To overcome these problems, it was necessary to follow the pattern of radioactivity over an extended period. If propagation was demonstrated by an increased uptake of labeled fibrinogen in the thigh (as happened in 20 per cent of cases), anticoagulation was indicated.[43, 153, 238]

When used for postoperative surveillance, the FUT had an unacceptably high false-positive and false-negative rate, especially in patients undergoing hip replacement.[60, 124, 205, 224, 244, 265, 267] Detection of proximal venous thrombosis in orthopedic patients is critically important because they have a higher incidence (about 25 per cent) of proximal vein thrombi than do general surgical patients, in whom early clots tend to be concentrated below the knee. One must conclude that the FUT should be considered a research tool best suited for studying the development of postoperative thrombi and for evaluating the efficacy of prophylactic measures designed to prevent their occurrence. An immense literature attests to its early contributions to research in this area.

Plethysmography, which is insensitive to below-knee thrombi, is established as an accurate method for detecting disease above the knee in symptomatic patients; however, plethysmography may miss nonocclusive free-floating clots—the very clots that are most likely to embolize.[219] In two early studies of patients undergoing elective hip surgery, impedance plethysmography identified 70 to 77 per cent of proximal venous thrombi.[123, 147] More recently, Comerota and associates reported that impedance plethysmography, when used for perioperative surveillance of patients undergoing joint replacement, had a sensitivity of only 32 per cent for thrombi developing above the knee.[60] The sensitivity of phleborheography in the same area was equally poor: 33 per cent. Seventy-seven per cent of the above-knee clots were nonocclusive; therefore, they did not alter venous hemodynamics sufficiently to be detected. An even lower sensitivity (19 per cent for all clots and 24 per cent for proximal DVT) was reported by Agnelli and co-workers, who used serial impedance plethysmography in a prospective study of asymptomatic patients scheduled for hip surgery.[2]

By combining plethysmography and iodine-125–fibrinogen scanning, Comerota and associates attained a higher detection rate of 70 per cent for above-knee thrombi;[60] however, Paiement and colleagues, in a similar study of patients undergoing hip replacement, found that the combination raised the sensitivity for venous thrombi in the thigh only slightly, from 12 to 23 per cent.[224] They concluded that either test alone or both together were ineffective as a screening method. Although investigators at McMaster University now share a similar opinion,[77] in their earlier studies they were encouraged to find that the concomitant use of these two modalities improved the positive predictive value for DVT in patients undergoing hip surgery.[139] This strategy, however, was of little benefit in general surgical patients, in whom postoperative venous thromboses were largely confined to the infrapopliteal veins.

Doppler ultrasonography, because of its ready availability and portability, would appear to be ideally suited for postoperative surveillance. Like plethysmography, however, it may overlook nonocclusive thrombi; in addition, although clots involving the posterior tibial vein may be detected, clots confined to the other below-knee veins will be missed. Moreover, the interpretation of Doppler signals is subjective, and the expertise required to obtain consistently reliable results exceeds that required by either impedance plethysmography or the FUT. Investigators using the Doppler apparatus to screen surgical patients prospectively reported a 2 to 5 per cent incidence of DVT developing in the postoperative period.[21, 244, 278] Because these figures are far below those usually reported with the FUT, many infrapopliteal thrombi were undoubtedly missed. In a prospective study of patients—some symptomatic but most of whom were undergoing joint replacement—Nix and associates found that Doppler ultrasonography detected only 68 per cent of phlebographically demonstrable thrombi developing in the femoropopliteal segment.[217] Thus, Doppler ultrasonography, although possibly somewhat better than plethysmography, also appears to be inadequate when used for surveillance.

Because of its ability to visualize nonocclusive free-floating clots, clots of limited extent isolated to short segments of vein, and clots confined to one of a pair of parallel venous channels, duplex scanning is emerging as the method of choice for surveillance purposes. As shown in Table 131–17, the reported sensitivity of duplex scanning for detecting thrombi developing in femoropopliteal veins of high-risk postarthroplasty patients ranged from 83 to 100 per cent when studies incorporated the full potential of the instrument. When, however, clots were identified only on the basis of incomplete venous compressibility, the sensitivity appeared to suffer, as illustrated by one study in which

Table 131–17.   Accuracy of Duplex Imaging for Diagnosing Asymptomatic Deep Venous Thrombosis in Postoperative Surveillance Studies

Study	No. of Extremities	Sensitivity (%)	Specificity (%)	Positive Predictive Value (%)	Negative Predictive Value (%)	Overall Accuracy (%)
Total Limb						
Barnes et al, 1989[30]	153*	34 (10/29)	95 (118/124)	63 (10/16)	86 (118/137)	84 (128/153)
Woolson et al, 1990[332]	150*	63 (17/27)	100 (123/123)	100 (17/17)	92 (123/133)	93 (140/150)
Comerota et al, 1990[59]	38	89 (8/9)	100 (29/29)	100 (8/8)	97 (29/30)	97 (37/38)
Ginsberg et al, 1991[109]	247‡	26 (16/61)	99 (184/186)	89 (16/18)	80 (184/229)	81 (200/247)
Above Knee						
Barnes et al, 1989[30]	153	83 (10/12)	96 (135/141)	63 (10/16)	99 (135/137)	95 (145/153)
Froehlich et al, 1989[108]	40	100 (5/5)	97 (34/35)	83 (5/6)	100 (34/34)	98 (39/40)
Woolson et al, 1990[332]	150	89 (17/19)	100 (131/131)	100 (17/17)	97 (131/133)	99 (148/150)
Comerota et al, 1990[59]	36	100 (7/7)	100 (29/29)	100 (7/7)	100 (29/29)	100 (36/36)
White et al, 1990[331]	32	92 (11/12)	100 (20/20)	100 (11/11)	95 (20/21)	97 (31/32)
Ginsberg et al, 1991[109]	247‡	52 (10/21)	97 (219/226)	61 (11/18)	96 (219/229)	93 (230/247)
Below Knee						
Comerota et al, 1990[59]	31	50 (1/2)	100 (29/29)	100 (1/1)	97 (29/30)	97 (30/31)
Ginsberg et al, 1991[109]	223‡§	5 (2/37)	99 (184/186)	50 (2/4)	84 (184/219)	83 (186/223)
Mattos et al, 1992[188]	92†	79 (19/24)	97 (66/68)	90 (19/21)	93 (66/71)	92 (85/92)

Modified from Sumner DS, Mattos MA: Diagnosis of deep venous thrombosis with real-time color and duplex scanning. In Bernstein EF (ed): Vascular Diagnosis. 4th ed. St. Louis, Mosby–Year Book, 1993, pp 785–800.

*Calf veins were not studied.
†Color flow scans.
‡Compression studies only.
§Isolated calf veins only.

the reported sensitivity was only 52 per cent.[109] In these reports, the predictive value of a positive study result varied from 61 to 100 per cent. Specificities and negative predictive values approached 100 per cent.

Relatively little information is available about the accuracy of duplex scanning for detecting clots developing in calf veins during the postoperative period (see Table 131–17). Surveying the calf is a particularly challenging problem for the technologist, not only because of the large number of small (usually duplicated) veins that are in jeopardy and their complex anatomy but also because nascent thrombi are often isolated to short venous segments. Surveillance studies, therefore, are much more difficult than diagnostic studies conducted in the same area because asymptomatic calf vein thrombi are less extensive and are more frequently isolated than their symptomatic counterparts. The initial experience with color flow imaging suggests that this modality may overcome some of the difficulties encountered with conventional duplex scanning. In a phlebographically controlled study, Mattos and associates reported a sensitivity of 79 per cent and a specificity of 97 per cent for detecting or ruling out calf vein thrombi when color duplex scanning was used to survey postarthroplasty patients (see Table 131–17).[188] The positive and negative predictive values were 90 and 93 per cent, respectively. These results are especially encouraging because more than 90 per cent of the clots were isolated to the below-knee veins and 89 per cent were nonoccluding.

Restricting scans to the more easily examined proximal veins, as is the practice of some investigators, invariably reduces the overall sensitivity of the test (see Table 131–17). For example, in a series of postarthroplasty patients studied by Barnes and coworkers, clots were isolated to calf veins in 17 of the 29 limbs (59 per cent) in which thrombi were demonstrated phlebographically.[30] Because calf veins were not scanned, the overall sensitivity was only 34 per cent. Similarly, in Woolson and colleagues' study of postarthroplasty patients, 30 per cent of the phlebographically detected thrombi were confined to the infrapopliteal veins.[332] Although the above-knee sensitivity was a respectable 89 per cent, the decision to limit scanning to the proximal veins reduced the total limb sensitivity to 63 per cent. This policy would have an even more adverse effect on overall sensitivity if it were applied to patients undergoing major abdominal operations, in whom thrombi are more likely to be confined to calf veins and less likely to develop in the proximal veins than they are in patients undergoing orthopedic procedures. It follows that serial scanning should be considered in all high-risk patients with negative above-knee study findings when the infrapopliteal veins have not been examined.

Role of Surveillance

The ideal method for surveillance should be noninvasive, transportable, easily performed, widely applicable, and inexpensive; above all, it should be capable of detecting both proximal and distal thrombi and of identifying those thrombi that are most likely to embolize. Although no method currently available satisfies all these requirements, duplex and color flow scanning come the closest. A negative scan rules out the more dangerous proximal venous

thrombi, and a good-quality positive study predicts the presence of thrombi with reasonable accuracy. Results with color below the knee are also promising.

Imaging, however, is time consuming, technically demanding, and expensive, and its widespread application would quickly exhaust the facilities of most hospitals. Phlebography, which is equally accurate, suffers from the same limitations and also subjects patients to the risk of contrast-induced venous thrombosis. Combining several noninvasive methods to improve sensitivity is impractical because of the time required and the additional expense. Moreover, even when results are unequivocally negative, the possibility remains that thrombi may form in the days and weeks after the study has been completed.[314, 331] Serial studies would be required as long as the patient remains in jeopardy. This problem is particularly pertinent to the surveillance of other high-risk patients (e.g., patients with a history of thromboembolism, elderly bedridden patients, and those with congestive heart failure, carcinoma, paraplegia, and other chronic medical diseases), who unlike patients undergoing operations or suffering a traumatic injury, remain permanently at risk. Therefore, the role of surveillance in clinical practice remains unclear.[8, 41]

Likewise, routine prophylaxis, the alternative to surveillance, is not the ideal answer because it does not afford complete protection after abdominal operations and is even less effective following orthopedic procedures. Routine prophylaxis of other high-risk patients is simply not practical. Perhaps further study will identify certain groups in whom surveillance for DVT is the most cost-effective approach. Until then, the primary role of surveillance will continue to be that of an essential research tool for the clinical investigator.

Pulmonary Embolism

Because the majority (perhaps 90 per cent) of pulmonary emboli arise from the deep veins of the pelvis and leg,[192, 275] detection of thrombi in these veins plays an adjunctive role in the diagnosis of pulmonary embolism.[27, 138, 206, 264, 276]

Pulmonary embolism continues to be both overdiagnosed and underdiagnosed.[80, 247] The test most frequently used to diagnose pulmonary embolism is the perfusion lung scan. This test is highly sensitive but not very specific.[231] Although a negative lung scan finding usually rules out pulmonary embolism, a positive scan finding is associated with angiographically proven pulmonary embolism in only about 25 per cent of cases (range, 17 to 66 per cent).[51, 111, 193, 198, 207, 236, 307, 312] A ''high-probability'' perfusion scan (one showing multiple segmental or lobar defects) increases the positive predictive value to 50 to 80 per cent. On the other hand, pulmonary emboli are found in an appreciable number of patients (8 to 40 per cent) with ''low-probability'' scans (those showing subsegmental or nonsegmental defects).[51, 138, 193, 198, 207] Specificity can be improved by adding a ventilation scan. Reported figures suggest that pulmonary embolism is present in about 90 per cent of cases in which there is a high-probability perfusion scan and a ventilation-perfusion mismatch.[51, 138, 193, 198, 207, 231] A ventilation-perfusion match, however, does not rule out pulmonary embolism.[138]

On the basis of these data, it is probably reasonable to assume that there are no pulmonary emboli when perfusion scan findings are negative and that emboli are present when there is a high-probability perfusion scan coupled with a normal or nonmatching ventilation scan.[231] Approximately two thirds of positive perfusion scan results must be considered to be equivocal.[138] In these patients, pulmonary angiography should be performed to establish the diagnosis. It is in this group that phlebography or noninvasive testing may be of assistance in permitting a reduction in the number of angiograms.

Although fewer than 10 per cent of patients dying of pulmonary embolism have clinical manifestations of DVT,[63] phlebographically demonstrable clots are present in 47 to 87 per cent of patients in whom the diagnosis of pulmonary embolism has been made.[47, 67, 260, 325] In a prospective study of patients with angiographically confirmed pulmonary emboli, 70 per cent had DVT on phlebography.[138] A truly remarkable (and unduplicated) association between the findings on pulmonary angiography and those seen on impedance plethysmography was reported by Sasahara and colleagues.[264] In patients with suspected pulmonary embolism, 90 per cent of those with positive leg plethysmographic findings had angiographically diagnosed pulmonary emboli, and 90 per cent of those with negative plethysmographic findings had negative angiographic findings. Impedance plethysmographic results were positive in 70 per cent of the patients with positive pulmonary angiographic results in the prospective study reported on by Hull and colleagues.[138] Other authors reported positive Doppler examination findings in 49 to 61 per cent of patients in whom pulmonary emboli were diagnosed.[11, 27] In contrast, Cheely and coworkers found abnormal Doppler flow patterns in the legs of only 23 per cent of patients with angiographically demonstrated pulmonary emboli.[51] Similarly, only 7 of 16 patients (44 per cent) with angiographically proven pulmonary emboli had leg vein thrombi demonstrated by color flow duplex scanning in the study reported on by Killewich and coworkers.[161] Thus, despite the high sensitivity of this modality, most patients with pulmonary emboli had negative noninvasive findings.

It is quite possible that the incidence of positive noninvasive and phlebographic findings is spuriously low in some of the published reports because the diagnosis of pulmonary embolism was not confirmed by pulmonary angiography but was based on clinical judgment or perfusion scans alone. The explanation is more difficult in studies that were angiographically controlled. In some of the limbs in which phlebographic findings were negative, the thrombus responsible for the pulmonary embolus may have been localized to a segment of the venous tree that is difficult to visualize (e.g., the soleal sinusoids, profunda femoris vein, or internal iliac vein). In other cases, it is reasonable to postulate that most of the thrombus had already broken off and floated downstream to the lungs by the time that phlebography was performed, leaving only a small residual in a valve cusp. Finally, an unknown number may have originated in the brachiocephalic circulation, renal veins, or right atrium. Plethysmographic and Doppler findings may also be negative when the responsible clot is nonocclusive or is located below the knee. Duplex and B-mode scans should, of course, detect most of these clots.

Clearly, a negative phlebographic or noninvasive study finding does not rule out the possibility of a pulmonary embolism, but a positive study result does reinforce the diagnosis.[27, 138, 264] At any rate, the therapeutic approach is clarified because anticoagulant therapy is indicated for the thrombotic process in the legs whether or not a pulmonary embolus is actually present. Barnes[23] and Hull and associates[143] have incorporated noninvasive testing (or phlebography) into algorithms proposed for the diagnosis of pulmonary embolism.[23, 143] Patients presenting with symptoms suggestive of massive pulmonary embolism should undergo immediate pulmonary angiography; all others should be referred for a ventilation-perfusion lung scan. If the scan result is normal, no further diagnostic tests need be performed and another diagnosis should be sought. If the perfusion scan shows multiple segmental or lobar defects and there is a clear ventilation-perfusion mismatch (high-probability study), it can be assumed that the patient has a pulmonary embolism. All other patients should undergo a noninvasive or phlebographic study of the leg veins. When the leg study result is positive, the patient may be treated as if he or she had a pulmonary embolus. If the test result is negative, pulmonary angiography should be performed. (An argument, however, can be made for performing pulmonary angiography even in patients whose study findings are positive for DVT, because a confirmed diagnosis of pulmonary embolism may affect the decision to place a vena caval filter.[161])

On the other hand, examination of the leg veins may also be indicated in patients in whom the diagnosis of pulmonary embolism has been firmly established. Demonstration of a residual clot (especially one that is free-floating) in the leg veins is important when the patient is being considered for placement of a vena caval filter.[39, 51, 90, 213]

Monitoring Venous Therapy and Follow-Up of Venous Thrombotic Disease

Objective monitoring of the results of venous therapy not only is pertinent to the individual case but also is important for assaying the efficacy of treatment modalities. Only in this way can rational decisions be made about whether to adopt a new method, discard an old method, or seek improvements in a basically effective technique. Although phlebography depicts morphologic results accurately, it is invasive and provides little functional information. Noninvasive tests have the advantage of furnishing information pertinent to the physiologic evaluation of residual venous obstruction and to the development of venous valvular incompetence.

Doppler ultrasonography, plethysmography, radionuclide phlebography, and duplex scanning have been used to assess the results of thrombolytic therapy.[4, 37, 56, 93, 154, 166, 289] Applications include determining the immediate efficacy of therapy and, based on the extent of the physiologic or anatomic changes, deciding whether to continue or discontinue infusing the thrombolytic agent;[56, 166, 289] predicting the likely outcome from duplex estimation of the age of the thrombus;[93] and on follow-up, evaluating the functional results.[4, 154, 273] In one study, in which plethysmographic testing was used, 83 per cent of limbs treated with streptokinase showed venous outflow obstruction and 72 per cent had developed venous incompetence at a mean follow-up of 29 months.[4] Similarly, noninvasive studies have been used to assess the immediate anatomic and long-term functional results of venous thrombectomy.[28, 92, 119, 306] On follow-up, three groups reported anatomic obstruction in 39, 50, and 53 per cent of the operated limbs; functional obstruction in 0, 17, and 71 per cent; and venous reflux in 0, 50, and 71 per cent, respectively.[28, 92, 306] Patency of veins in the lower limb after ligation or plication of the inferior vena cava can be ascertained by Doppler ultrasonography, isotope phlebography, or duplex scanning. A high incidence of functional obstruction has been observed in these cases.[83, 301] Duplex scanning can also be used to determine the location of vena caval filters and to disclose the presence of clot within or below the filter.

Few clinicians have made serious attempts to document the natural history of DVT objectively. In a prospective study of patients who were followed up with noninvasive testing after having been treated for acute DVT, Strandness and associates found that 40 per cent of limbs with abnormal Doppler findings in the below-knee veins developed stasis pigmentation, compared with only 8 per cent of those in which the distal veins were normal.[290] Kakkar and Lawrence prospectively followed 153 patients for 2 years from the onset of DVT and found that plethysmographic evidence of venous obstruction correlated well with the phlebographic distribution of disease.[154] Despite anticoagulation with heparin or aggressive thrombolytic therapy, 60 per cent of limbs with thrombi confined to the below-knee veins and 87 per cent with combined calf and iliofemoral thromboses had moderate to severe hemodynamic abnormalities. Other investigators, using noninvasive techniques to follow patients treated with anticoagulants for DVT, have also reported the persistence of venous obstruction and valvular incompetence in a large proportion of limbs.[183, 185, 258]

Duplex ultrasonic scanning was used by researchers at the University of Washington to follow prospectively the rate at which clots lysed (or retracted) and the rate of development of venous valvular incompetence. By 7 days, lysis of clot was noted in some venous segments in 44 per cent of the limbs with acute DVT, and almost all affected limbs demonstrated lysis by 30 days.[159] After 90 days, only 14 per cent of the originally thrombosed segments continued to obstruct venous flow. Within 1 week of the initial diagnostic study, 17 per cent of limbs with acute DVT demonstrated reflux in one or more venous segments, and by 1 year, two thirds of the limbs had incompetent valves.[186]

Propagation of isolated calf vein thrombi to the popliteal or thigh veins has been documented in 15 to 48 per cent of limbs studied serially with duplex scanning.[164, 181, 285] Duplex scanning has also been used to monitor the natural history of free-floating thrombi found in the popliteal or more proximal veins. During follow-up (limited to the acute period), about 50 per cent of the free-floating clots reported in three studies became attached to the venous wall, 7 to 14 per cent propagated, and 11 to 47 per cent decreased in size or disappeared, either as a result of lysis or emboliza-

tion.[20, 39, 289] Associated pulmonary emboli were noted in 13 to 26 per cent of these patients, but some of the emboli were discovered before the legs were scanned. Thus, the true potential for embolization of free-floating thrombi remains to be determined.

Duplex scanning clearly adds a new dimension to the prospective study of venous thrombosis. Coupled with other noninvasive modalities better suited to the objective measurement of venous obstruction and incompetence, this modality, with its unique ability to visualize clot morphology and valvular structure, promises to enhance our understanding of the natural history of venous disease.

References

1. AbuRahma AF, Osborne L: A combined study of the strain gauge plethysmography and I-125 fibrinogen leg scan in the differentiation of deep vein thrombosis and postphlebitic syndrome. Am Surg 50:585, 1984.
2. Agnelli G, Cosmi B, Ranucci V, et al: Impedance plethysmography in the diagnosis of asymptomatic deep vein thrombosis in hip surgery: A venography-controlled study. Arch Intern Med 151:2167, 1991.
3. Aitken AGF, Godden DJ: Real-time ultrasound diagnosis of deep vein thrombosis: A comparison with venography. Clin Radiol 38:309, 1987.
4. Albrechtsson U, Anderson J, Einarsson E, et al: Streptokinase treatment of deep venous thrombosis and the postthrombotic syndrome. Arch Surg 116:33, 1981.
5. Albrechtsson U, Olsson CG: Thrombotic side-effects of lower-limb phlebography. Lancet 1:723, 1976.
6. Albrechtsson U, Olsson CG: Thrombosis following phlebography with ionic and non-ionic contrast media. Acta Radiol [Diagn] (Stockh) 20:46, 1979.
7. Allen EV, Barker NW, Hines EA Jr: Venous thrombosis, thrombophlebitis, and pulmonary embolism. In Peripheral Vascular Diseases. 3rd ed. Philadelphia, WB Saunders, 1962, pp 559–623.
8. Anderson FA Jr: Duplex ultrasound surveillance for asymptomatic DVT. J Vasc Technol 15:15, 1991.
9. Anderson FA Jr, Durgin WW, Wheeler HB: Interpretation of venous occlusion plethysmography using a nonlinear model. Med Biol Eng Comput 24:379, 1986.
10. Anderson FA Jr, Wheeler HB: Physician practices in the management of venous thromboembolism: A community-wide survey. J Vasc Surg 16:707, 1992.
11. Alexander RH, Folse R, Pizzorno J, Conn R: Thrombophlebitis and thromboembolism: Results of a prospective study. Ann Surg 180:883, 1974.
12. Appelman PT, De Jong TE, Lampmann LE: Deep venous thrombosis of the leg: US findings. Radiology 163:743, 1987.
13. Appleberg M: The diagnosis of deep vein thrombosis in the lower limbs by means of the transcutaneous Doppler ultrasound method. S Afr Med J 50:953, 1976.
14. Archie JP Jr, McDaniel DN, Dean VH, et al: Doppler ultrasound evaluation for lower extremity deep venous thrombosis in a community hospital. N C Med J 50:457, 1989.
15. Aronen HJ, Korppi-Tommola T, Suoranta HT, et al: 99mTc-plasmin test in deep vein thrombosis of the leg. Eur J Nucl Med 10:10, 1985.
16. Aronen HJ, Pamila M, Suoranta HT, et al: Sonography in differential diagnosis of deep venous thrombosis of the leg. Acta Radiol 28:457, 1987.
17. Arora S, Lam DJK, Negus DN, Gusberg RJ: Light reflection rheography: A simple noninvasive screening test for deep venous thrombosis [Abstract]. J Vasc Surg 17:430, 1993.
18. Athanasoulis CA: Phlebography for the diagnosis of deep leg vein thrombosis. In Fratantoni J, Wessler S. (eds): Prophylactic Therapy of Deep Vein Thrombosis and Pulmonary Embolism. 1975, pp 62–76. DHEW publication (NIH) 76-866.
19. Atkins P, Hawkins LA: Detection of venous thrombosis in the legs. Lancet 2:1217, 1965.
20. Baldridge ED, Martin MA, Welling RE: Clinical significance of free-floating venous thrombi. J Vasc Surg 11:62, 1990.

21. Barnes RW: Prospective screening for deep vein thrombosis in high risk patients. Am J Surg 134:187, 1977.

22. Barnes RW: Cost/benefit analysis of noninvasive testing for venous thromboembolism. *In* Bernstein EF (ed): Noninvasive Diagnostic Techniques in Vascular Disease. 2nd ed. St. Louis, CV Mosby, 1982, pp 570–574.

23. Barnes RW: Algorithms for diagnosis and therapy of venous thromboembolism. *In* Bernstein EF (ed): Noninvasive Diagnostic Techniques in Vascular Disease. 3rd ed. St. Louis, CV Mosby, 1985, pp 797–804.

24. Barnes RW, Collicott PE, Mozersky DJ, et al: Noninvasive quantitation of maximum venous outflow in acute thrombophlebitis. Surgery 72:971, 1972.

25. Barnes RW, Collicott PE, Sumner DS, et al: Noninvasive quantitation of venous hemodynamics in postphlebitic syndrome. Arch Surg 107:807, 1973.

26. Barnes RW, Hokanson DE, Wu KK, et al: Detection of deep vein thrombosis with an automatic electrically calibrated strain gauge plethysmograph. Surgery 82:219, 1977.

27. Barnes RW, Kinkead LR, Wu KK, et al: Venous thrombosis in suspected pulmonary embolism: Incidence detectable by Doppler ultrasound. Thromb Haemost 36:150, 1976.

28. Barnes RW, Miller EV: Late venous hemodynamics following thrombectomy for iliofemoral venous thrombosis. Vasc Surg 12:288, 1978.

29. Barnes RW, McDonald GB, Hamilton GW, et al: Radionuclide venography for rapid dynamic evaluation of venous disease. Surgery 73:706, 1973.

30. Barnes RW, Nix ML, Barnes CL, et al: Perioperative asymptomatic venous thrombosis: Role of duplex scanning versus venography. J Vasc Surg 9:251, 1989.

31. Barnes RW, Russell HE, Wilson MR: Doppler Ultrasonic Evaluation of Venous Disease. 2nd ed. Iowa City, University of Iowa Press, 1975, pp 1–251.

32. Barnes RW, Russell HE, Wu KK, et al: Accuracy of Doppler ultrasound in clinically suspected venous thrombosis in the calf. Surg Gynecol Obstet 143:425, 1976.

33. Barnes RW, Turley DG, Quereshi GD, et al: Objective diagnosis of recurrent deep vein thrombosis. Thromb Haemost 46:168, 1981.

34. Barnes RW, Wu KK, Hoak JC: Differentiation of superficial thrombophlebitis from lymphangitis by Doppler ultrasound. Surg Gynecol Obstet 143:23, 1976.

35. Becker DM, Philbrick JT, Abbitt PL: Real-time ultrasonography for the diagnosis of lower extremity deep venous thrombosis. The wave of the future? Arch Intern Med 149:1731, 1989.

36. Becker J: The diagnosis of venous thrombosis in the legs using I-labelled fibrinogen: An experimental and clinical study. Acta Chir Scand 138:667, 1972.

37. Bentley PG, Hill PL, deHass HA, et al: Radionuclide venography in the management of proximal venous occlusion. A comparison with contrast venography. Br J Radiol 52:289, 1979.

38. Bergquist D, Efsing HO, Hallböök T: Thermography, a noninvasive method for diagnosis of deep venous thrombosis. Arch Surg 112:600, 1977.

39. Berry RE, George JE, Shaver WA: Free-floating deep venous thrombosis. A retrospective analysis. Ann Surg 211:719, 1990.

40. Bolton JP, Hoffman VJ: Incidence of early post-operative iliofemoral thrombosis. Br Med J 1:247, 1975.

41. Borris LC, Christiansen HM, Lassen MR, et al: Real-time B-mode ultrasonography in the diagnosis of postoperative deep vein thrombosis in non-symptomatic high-risk patients. Eur J Vasc Surg 4:473, 1990.

42. Browse NL: The ¹²⁵I-fibrinogen uptake test. Arch Surg 104:160, 1972.

43. Browse NL: The problems of deep vein thrombosis. Am Heart J 84:149, 1972.

44. Browse NL, Burnand KG, Thomas ML: Diseases of the Veins: Pathology, Diagnosis, and Treatment. London, Edward Arnold, 1988.

45. Browse NL, Clapham WF, Croft DN, et al: Diagnosis of established deep vein thrombosis with the ¹²⁵I-fibrinogen uptake test. Br Med J 4:325, 1971.

46. Browse NL, Clemenson G: Sequelae of an ¹²⁵I-fibrinogen detected thrombus. Br Med J 2:468, 1974.

47. Browse NL, Thomas ML: Source of nonlethal pulmonary emboli. Lancet 1:258, 1974.

48. Bynum LJ Jr, Wilson JE, Crotty CM, et al: Noninvasive diagnosis of deep venous thrombosis by phleborheography. Ann Intern Med 89:162, 1978.

49. Carpenter JP, Holland GA, Baum RA, Cope C: Magnetic resonance venography for the detection of deep venous thrombosis: Comparison with contrast venography and duplex Doppler ultrasonography [Abstract]. J Vasc Surg 17: 425, 1993.

50. Chaudhuri TK, Fink S, Farpour A: Physiologic considerations in imaging of lower extremity venous thrombosis. Am J Physiol Imaging 6:90, 1991.

51. Cheely R, McCartney WH, Perry JR, et al: The role of noninvasive tests versus pulmonary angiography in the diagnosis of pulmonary embolism. Am J Med 70:17, 1981.

52. Christensen AW, Wille-Jørgensen P, Kj RL: Contact thermography, ⁹⁹ᵐTc-plasmin scintimetry and ⁹⁹ᵐTc-plasmin scintigraphy as screening methods for deep venous thrombosis following major hip surgery. Thromb Haemost 58:831, 1987.

53. Clarke-Pearson DL, Creasman WT: Diagnosis of deep venous thrombosis in obstetrics and gynecology by impedance phlebography. Obstet Gynecol 58:52, 1981.

54. Classen JH, Richardson JB, Koontz C: A three-year experience with phleborheography: A noninvasive technique for the diagnosis of deep venous thrombosis. Ann Surg 195:800, 1982.

55. Coelho JC, Siegel B, Ryva JC, et al: B-mode sonography of blood clots. J Clin Ultrasound 10:323, 1982.

56. Comerota AJ: An overview of thrombolytic therapy for venous thromboembolism. *In* Comerota AJ (ed): Thrombolytic Therapy. Orlando, FL, Grune & Stratton, 1988, pp 65–89.

57. Comerota AJ, Cranley JJ, Cook SE, et al: Phleborheography—Results of a ten-year experience. Surgery 91:573, 1982.

58. Comerota AJ, Katz ML: The diagnosis of acute deep venous thrombosis by duplex venous imaging. Semin Vasc Surg 1:32, 1988.

59. Comerota AJ, Katz ML, Greenwald LL, et al: Venous duplex imaging: Should it replace hemodynamic tests for deep venous thrombosis? J Vasc Surg 11:53, 1990.

60. Comerota AJ, Katz ML, Grossi RJ, et al: The comparative value of noninvasive testing for diagnosis and surveillance of deep venous thrombosis. J Vasc Surg 7:40, 1988.

61. Conti S, Daschbach M: Venous thromboembolism prophylaxis: A survey of its use in the United States. Arch Surg 117:1036, 1982.

62. Cooke ED, Pilcher MF: Deep vein thrombosis: Preclinical diagnosis by thermography. Br J Surg 61:971, 1974.

63. Coon WW: The spectrum of pulmonary embolism. Arch Surg 111:398, 1976.

64. Coon WW, Willis PW: Deep venous thrombosis and pulmonary embolism. Prediction, prevention, and treatment. Am J Cardiol 4:611, 1959.

65. Cooperman N, Martin EW Jr, Satiani B, et al: Detection of deep venous thrombosis by impedance plethysmography. Am J Surg 137:252, 1979.

66. Cordoba SA, Figueras CN, Garcia FR: Scintiscanning in venous thrombosis of the lower extremities. Surg Gynecol Obstet 145:533, 1977.

67. Corrigan TP, Fossard DP, Spindler J, et al: Phlebography in the management of pulmonary embolism. Br J Surg 61:484, 1974.

68. Cramer M, Beach KW, Strandness DE Jr: The detection of proximal deep vein thrombosis by strain gauge plethysmography through the use of an outflow/capacitance discriminant line. Bruit 7(12):17, 1983.

69. Cranley JJ: Invited commentary of Hirsh J, Hull R: Comparative value of tests for the diagnosis of venous thrombosis. World J Surg 2:36, 1978.

70. Cranley JJ: Phleborheography. *In* Kempczinski RE, Yao JST (eds): Practical Noninvasive Diagnosis. 2nd ed. Chicago, Year Book Medical Publishers, 1987, pp 438–463.

71. Cranley JJ, Canos AJ, Sull WJ: The diagnosis of deep venous thrombosis. Arch Surg 111:34, 1976.

72. Cranley JJ, Hyland LJ, Comerota AJ: Diagnosis of deep venous thrombosis of the lower extremity by phleborheography. *In* Bernstein EF (ed): Noninvasive Diagnostic Techniques in Vascular Disease. 2nd ed. St. Louis, CV Mosby, 1982, pp 459–467.

73. Cranley JJ, Canos AJ, Sull WJ, Grass AM: Phleborheographic technique for diagnosis of deep venous thrombosis of the lower extremities. Surg Gynecol Obstet 141:331, 1975.

74. Cronan JJ, Dorfman GS, Grusmark J: Lower-extremity deep venous thrombosis: Further experience with and refinements of US assessment. Radiology 168:101, 1988.

75. Cronan JJ, Dorfman GS, Scola FH, et al: Deep venous thrombosis: US assessment using vein compression. Radiology 162:191, 1987.

76. Cronan JJ, Leen V: Recurrent deep venous thrombosis: Limitations of US. Radiology 170:739, 1989.

77. Cruickshank MK, Levine MN, Hirsh J, et al: An evaluation of impedance plethysmography and ^{125}I-fibrinogen leg scanning in patients following hip surgery. Thromb Haemost 62:830, 1989.

78. Dahlborn M, Ahlborg G, Soderborg B, et al: Gamma camera detection of ^{99m}Tc-plasmin in the diagnosis of deep-vein thrombosis. Eur J Nucl Med 9:499, 1984.

79. Dahn I, Eiriksson E: Plethysmographic diagnosis of deep venous thrombosis of the leg. Acta Chir Scand Suppl 398:33, 1968.

80. Dalen JE, Alpert JS: Natural history of pulmonary embolism. Prog Cardiovasc Dis 17:259, 1975.

81. Dauzat MM, Laroche J-P, Charras C, et al: Real-time B-mode ultrasonography for better specificity in the noninvasive diagnosis of deep venous thrombosis. J Ultrasound Med 5:625, 1986.

82. Davis HH, Siegel BA, Sherman L: Scintigraphy with ^{111}In-labelled autologous platelets in venous thromboembolism. Radiology 136:203, 1980.

83. DeMeester TR, Rutherford RB, Blazek JV, Zuidema GD: Plication of the inferior vena cava for thromboembolism. Surgery 62:56, 1967.

84. DeNardo SJ, Bogren HG, DeNardo GL: Detection of thrombophlebitis in the lower extremities: A regional comparison of ^{123}I-fibrinogen scintigraphy and contrast venography. AJR 145:1045, 1985.

85. DeWeese JA, Rogoff SM: Phlebographic patterns of acute deep venous thrombosis of the leg. Surgery 53:99, 1963.

86. Diener L: Origin and distribution of venous thrombi studied by postmortem intraosseous phlebography. *In* Nicolaides AN (ed): Thromboembolism: Etiology, Advances in Prevention and Management. Baltimore, University Park Press, 1975, pp 149–166.

87. Doig RL, Browse NL: Rapid propagation of thrombus in deep vein thrombosis. Br Med J 4:210, 1971.

88. Doouss TW: The clinical significance of venous thrombosis of the calf. Br J Surg 63:377, 1976.

89. Dosick SM, Blakemore WS: The role of Doppler ultrasound in acute deep vein thrombosis. Am J Surg 136:265, 1978.

90. Dow JD: Retrograde phlebography in major pulmonary embolism. Lancet 2:407, 1973.

91. Edenbrandt CM, Hedner U, Nilsson J, et al: Return to normal of ^{99m}Tc-plasmin test after deep venous thrombosis and its relationship to vessel wall fibrinolysis. Eur J Nucl Med 12:197, 1986.

92. Einarsson E, Albrechtsson U, Eklof B, et al: Follow-up evaluation of venous morphologic factors and function after thrombectomy and temporary arteriovenous fistula in thrombosis of iliofemoral vein. Surg Gynecol Obstet 163:111, 1986.

93. Elias A, Bouvier JL, Le Corff G, et al: A new therapeutic approach of deep vein thrombosis using ultrasound imaging and Doppler. *In* Boccalon H (ed): Angiologie: Strategie du Diagnostic et de la Therapeutique (Supplement). London, Paris, John Libbey Eurotext, 1988, pp 113–115.

94. Elias A, Bouvier JL, Le Corff G, et al: A new therapeutic approach of deep venous thrombosis using ultrasound imaging and Doppler. *In* Boccalon H (ed): Angiologie: Strategie du Diagnostic et de la Therapeutique (Supplement). London, Paris, John Libbey Eurotext, 1988, pp 113–115.

95. Elias A, Le Corff G, Bouvier JL, et al: Value of real time ultrasound imaging in the diagnosis of deep vein thrombosis of the lower limbs. Int Angiol 6:175, 1987.

96. Elias A, Le Corff G, Bouvier JL, et al: Detection of inferior vena cava thrombosis using duplex scanning. Diagnostic value. *In* Boccalon H (ed): Angiologie: Strategie du Diagnostic et de la Therapeutique (Supplement). London, Paris, John Libbey Eurotext, 1988, pp 109–111.

97. Elliott JP, Hageman JH, Belanger AC, et al: Phleborheography: A correlative study with venography. Henry Ford Hosp Med J 28:189, 1980.

98. Ennis JT, Elmes RJ: Radionuclide venography in the diagnosis of deep vein thrombosis. Radiology 125:441, 1977.

99. Erdman WA, Jayson HT, Redman HC, et al: Deep venous thrombosis of extremities: Role of MR imaging in the diagnosis. Radiology 174:425, 1990.

100. Ezekowitz MD, Migliaccio F, Farlow D, et al: Comparison of platelet scintigraphy, impedance plethysmography, gray scale and color flow duplex ultrasound and venography for the diagnosis of venous thrombosis. Prog Clin Biol Res 355:23, 1990.

101. Ezekowitz MD, Pope CF, Sostman HD, et al: Indium-111 platelet scintigraphy for the diagnosis of acute venous thrombosis. Circulation 73:668, 1986.

102. Fedullo PF, Moser KM, Moser KS, et al: Indium-111–labeled platelets: Effect of heparin on uptake by venous thrombi and relationship to the activated partial thromboplastin time. Circulation 66:632, 1982.

103. Flanagan LD, Sullivan ED, Cranley JJ: Venous imaging of the extremities using real-time B-mode ultrasound. *In* Bergan JJ, Yao JST (eds): Surgery of the Veins. Orlando, FL, Grune & Stratton, 1985, pp 89–98.

104. Flanigan DP, Goodreau JJ, Burnham SJ, et al: Vascular-laboratory diagnosis of clinically suspected acute deep-vein thrombosis. Lancet 2:331, 1978.

105. Fletcher JP, Kershaw LZ, Barker DS, et al: Ultrasound diagnosis of lower limb deep venous thrombosis. Med J Aust 153:453, 1990.

106. Foley WD, Middleton WD, Lawson TL, et al: Color Doppler ultrasound imaging of lower-extremity venous disease. AJR 152:371, 1989.

107. Foti MEG, Gurewich V: Fibrin degradation products and impedance plethysmography. Measurements in the diagnosis of acute deep vein thrombosis. Arch Intern Med 140:903, 1980.

108. Froehlich JA, Dorfman GS, Cronan JJ, et al: Compression ultrasonography for the detection of deep venous thrombosis in patients who have a fracture of the hip. A prospective study. J Bone Joint Surg 71A:249, 1989.

109. Ginsberg JS, Caco CC, Brill-Edwards PA, et al: Venous thrombosis in patients who have undergone major hip or knee surgery: Detection with compression US and impedance plethysmography. Radiology 181:651, 1991.

110. Gomes MN, Choyke PL: Assessment of major venous anomalies by computerized tomography. J Cardiovasc Surg 31:621, 1990.

111. Goodall RJR, Greenfield LJ: Clinical correlations in the diagnosis of pulmonary embolism. Ann Surg 191:219, 1980.

112. Gooley NA, Sumner DS: Deep venous thrombosis (DVT): Diagnostic practice in two midwestern community hospitals. Second International Vascular Symposium, London, 1986, Abstract S9.5.

113. Grassi CJ, Polak JF: Axillary and subclavian venous thrombosis: Follow-up evaluation with color Doppler flow US and venography. Radiology 175:651, 1990.

114. Gray B, Williams LR, Flanigan DP, et al: Upper extremity deep venous thrombosis: Diagnosis by Doppler ultrasound and impedance plethysmography. Bruit 7:30, 1983.

115. Gross WS, Burney RE: Therapeutic and economic implications of emergency department evaluation for venous thrombosis. JACEP, 8:110, 1979.

116. Haeger K: Problems of acute deep venous thrombosis. I. The interpretation of signs and symptoms. Angiology 20:219, 1969.

117. Haimovici H: Ischemic venous thrombosis: Phlegmasia cerulea dolens and venous gangrene. *In* Vascular Emergencies. New York, Appleton-Century-Crofts, 1982, pp 589–608.

118. Haire WD, Lynch TG, Lund GB, et al: Limitations of magnetic resonance imaging and ultrasound-directed (duplex) scanning in the diagnosis of subclavian vein thrombosis. J Vasc Surg 13:391, 1991.

119. Hallböök T, Göthlin J: Strain gauge plethysmography and phlebography in diagnosis of deep venous thrombosis. Acta Chir Scand 137:37, 1971.

120. Hamberg O, Madsen G, Hansen PB, et al: Segmental mean temperature differences in the diagnosis of acute venous thrombosis in the legs. Scand J Clin Lab Invest 47:191, 1987.

121. Hanel KC, Abbott WM, Reidy NC, et al: The role of two noninvasive tests in deep venous thrombosis. Ann Surg 194:725, 1981.

122. Hansen ME, Spritzer CE, Sostman HD: Assessing the patency of mediastinal and thoracic inlet veins: Value of MR imaging. AJR 155:1177, 1990.

123. Harris WH, Athanasoulis C, Waltman AC, et al: Cuff impedance phlebography and ^{125}I-fibrinogen scanning versus roentgenographic phlebography for diagnosis of thrombophlebitis following hip surgery. J Bone Joint Surg 58A:939, 1976.

124. Harris WH, Salzman EW, Athanasoulis C, et al: Comparison of ^{125}I-fibrinogen count scanning with phlebography for detection of venous thrombi after elective hip surgery. N Engl J Med 292:665, 1975.

125. Harris WH, Waltman AC, Athanasoulis C, et al: The accuracy of the in vivo diagnosis of deep vein thrombosis in patients with prior venous thromboembolic disease or severe varicose veins. Thromb Res 21:137, 1981.

126. Hayt DB, Binkert BL: An overview of noninvasive methods of deep vein thrombosis detection. Clin Imaging 14:179, 1990.

127. Henkin RE, Yao JST, Quinn JL III, Bergan JJ: Radionuclide venography (RNV) in lower extremity venous disease. J Nucl Med 15:171, 1974.

128. Hirsh J: Venous thromboembolism, diagnosis, treatment, and prevention. Hosp Pract 10:53, 1975.

129. Hirsh J, Hull R: Comparative value of tests for the diagnosis of venous thrombosis. World J Surg 2:27, 1978.

130. Hobbs JT, Davies JWL: Detection of deep venous thrombosis with ^{131}I-labelled fibrinogen in the rabbit. Lancet 2:134, 1960.

131. Hokanson DE, Sumner DS, Strandness DE Jr: An electrically calibrated plethysmograph for direct measurement of limb blood flow. IEEE Trans Biomed Eng 22(1):25, 1975.

132. Holmes MCG: Deep venous thrombosis of the lower limbs diagnosed by ultrasound. Med J Aust 1:427, 1973.

133. Howe HR Jr, Hansen KJ, Plonk GW Jr: Expanded criteria for the diagnosis of deep venous thrombosis. Use of the pulse volume recorder and Doppler ultrasonography. Arch Surg 119:1167, 1984.

134. Huisman MV, Buller HR, ten Cate JW, et al: Serial impedance plethysmography for suspected deep venous thrombosis in outpatients. The Amsterdam general practitioner study. N Engl J Med 314:823, 1986.

135. Huisman MV, Buller HR, ten Cate JW: Utility of impedance plethysmography in the diagnosis of recurrent deep-vein thrombosis. Arch Intern Med 148:681, 1988.

136. Hull RD, Carter CJ, Jay RM, et al: The diagnosis of acute, recurrent, deep-vein thrombosis: A diagnostic challenge. Circulation 67:901, 1983.

137. Hull RD, Hirsh J, Carter CJ, et al: Diagnostic efficacy of impedance plethysmography for clinically suspected deep-vein thrombosis. A randomized trial. Ann Intern Med 102:21, 1985.

138. Hull R, Hirsh J, Carter C, et al: Pulmonary angiography, ventilation lung scanning, and venography for clinically suspected pulmonary embolism with abnormal perfusion lung scan. Ann Intern Med 98:891, 1983.

139. Hull R, Hirsh J, Powers P, et al: The value of adding impedance plethysmography to ^{125}I-fibrinogen leg scanning for the detection of deep vein thrombosis in high risk surgical patients: A comparative study between patients undergoing general surgery and hip surgery. Thromb Res 15:227, 1979.

140. Hull R, Hirsh J, Sackett DL, et al: Combined use of leg scanning and impedance plethysmography in suspected venous thrombosis, an alternative to venography. N Engl J Med 296:1497, 1977.

141. Hull R, Hirsh J, Sackett DL, Stoddart G: Cost effectiveness of clinical diagnosis, venography, and noninvasive testing in patients with symptomatic deep-vein thrombosis. N Engl J Med 304:1561, 1981.

142. Hull R, Hirsh J, Sackett DL, et al: Replacement of venography in suspected venous thrombosis by impedance plethysmography and ^{125}I-fibrinogen leg scanning. Ann Intern Med 94:12, 1981.

143. Hull RD, Raskob GE, Hirsh J: Practical approaches to the diagnosis of pulmonary embolism. In Hirsh J (ed): Venous Thrombosis and Pulmonary Embolism, Diagnostic Methods. Edinburgh, Churchill Livingstone, 1987, pp 161–174.

144. Hull RD, Raskob GE, Hirsh J: Practical approaches to the diagnosis of venous thrombosis. In Hirsh J (ed): Venous Thrombosis and Pulmonary Embolism, Diagnostic Methods. Edinburgh, Churchill Livingstone, 1987, pp 103–119.

145. Hull R, Taylor DW, Hirsh J, et al: Impedance plethysmography: The relationship between venous filling and sensitivity and specificity for proximal vein thrombosis. Circulation 58:898, 1978.

146. Hull R, van Aken WG, Hirsh J, et al: Impedance plethysmography using the occlusive cuff technique in the diagnosis of venous thrombosis. Circulation 53:696, 1976.

147. Hume M, Kuriakose TX, Jamieson J, et al: Extent of leg vein thrombosis determined by impedance and ^{125}I-fibrinogen. Am J Surg 129:455, 1975.

148. Jaques PF, Rickey WA, Ely CA, et al: Doppler ultrasonic screening prior to venography for deep venous thrombosis. AJR 129:451, 1977.

149. Jay R, Hull R, Carter C, et al: Outcome of abnormal impedance plethysmography results in patients with proximal-vein thrombosis: Frequency of return to normal. Thromb Res 36:259, 1984.

150. Johnson WC: Evaluation of newer techniques for the diagnosis of venous thrombosis. J Surg Res 16:473, 1974.

151. Johnson WC, Patten DH, Widrich WC, et al: Technetium-99m isotope venography. Am J Surg 124:424, 1974.

152. Kakkar V: The diagnosis of deep vein thrombosis using the ^{125}I-fibrinogen test. Arch Surg 104:152, 1972.

153. Kakkar VV, Howe CT, Flanc C, Clarke MB: Natural history of postoperative deep-vein thrombosis. Lancet 2:230, 1969.

154. Kakkar VV, Lawrence D: Hemodynamic and clinical assessment after therapy for acute deep vein thrombosis: A prospective study. Am J Surg 150(4A):54, 1985.

155. Kakkar VV, Nicolaides AN, Renney JTG, et al: ^{125}I-labelled fibrinogen test adapted for routine screening of deep vein thrombosis. Lancet 1:540, 1970.

156. Karkow WS, Ruoff BA, Cranley JJ: B-mode venous imaging. In Kempczinski RF, Yao JST (eds): Practical Noninvasive Vascular Diagnosis. 2nd ed. Chicago, Year Book Medical Publishers, 1987, pp 464–485.

157. Kempi V, Van der Linden W, Von Scheele C: Diagnosis of deep vein thrombosis with ^{99m}Tc-streptokinase: A clinical comparison with phlebography. Br Med J 4:748, 1974.

158. Kerr TM, Lutter KS, Moeller DM, et al: Upper extremity venous thrombosis diagnosed by duplex scanning. Am J Surg 160:202, 1990.

159. Killewich LA, Bedford GR, Beach KW, et al: Spontaneous lysis of deep venous thrombi: Rate and outcome. J Vasc Surg 9:89, 1989.

160. Killewich LA, Bedford GR, Beach KW, Strandness DE Jr: Diagnosis of deep venous thrombosis: A prospective study comparing duplex scanning to contrast venography. Circulation 79:810, 1989.

161. Killewich LA, Nunnelee JD, Auer AI: Value of lower extremity venous duplex examination in the diagnosis of pulmonary embolism. J Vasc Surg 17:934, 1993.

162. Kiviniitty K, Kauppila A, Taskinew PJ, et al: Examination of postoperative thrombosis by means of fibrinogen-I-125. Fortschr Geb Roentgenstr Nuklearmed 115:803, 1971.

163. Knudson GJ, Wiedmeyer DA, Erickson SJ, et al: Color Doppler sonographic imaging in the assessment of upper-extremity deep venous thrombosis. AJR 154:399, 1990.

164. Krupski WC, Bass A, Dilley RB, et al: Propagation of deep venous thrombosis identified by duplex ultrasonography. J Vasc Surg 12:467, 1990.

165. Kupper C, Shugart R, Burnham S: Errors of Doppler ultrasound in diagnosis of deep venous thrombosis. Bruit 3(2):15, 1979.

166. Kupper CA, White GC, Burnham SJ: Streptokinase therapy for deep vein thrombosis: The role of noninvasive testing. Bruit 6(6):17, 1982.

167. Lagerstedt C, Olsson C-G, Fagher B, Öqvist B: ^{99m}Tc plasmin in 394 consecutive patients with suspected deep venous thrombosis. Eur J Nucl Med 15:771, 1989.

168. Lambie JM, Mahaffy RG, Barber DC, et al: Diagnostic accuracy in venous thrombosis. Br Med J 2:142, 1970.

169. Landfeld CS, McGuire E, Cohen AM: Clinical findings associated with acute proximal deep venous thrombosis: A basis for quantifying clinical judgment. Am J Med 88:382, 1990.

170. Langsfeld M, Hershey FB, Thorpe L, et al: Duplex B-mode imaging for the diagnosis of deep venous thrombosis. Arch Surg 122:587, 1987.

171. Langsfeld M, Hurley JJ, Thorpe LE, et al: Real-time venous imaging in pregnancy: A case report illustrating the potential pitfalls in diagnosing deep venous thrombosis. Bruit 10:244, 1986.

172. LeMoine JR, Moser KM: Leg scanning with radioisotope-labeled fibrinogen in patients undergoing hip surgery. Comparison with contrast phlebography and lung scans. JAMA 243:2035, 1980.

173. Lensing AWA, Levi MM, Büller HR, et al: Diagnosis of deep-vein thrombosis using an objective Doppler method. Ann Intern Med 113:9, 1990.

174. Lensing AWA, Pradoni P, Brandjes D, et al: Detection of deep-vein thrombosis by real-time B-mode ultransonography. N Engl J Med 320:342, 1989.

175. Lewis J, Hobbs J, Yao J: Normal and abnormal femoral vein velocities. In Roberts C (ed): Blood Flow Measurement. London, Sector Publishing, 1972, pp 48–52.

176. Liapis CD, Bhagwan S, Kuhns M, et al: Value of impedance plethysmography in suspected venous disease of the lower extremity. Angiology 31:522, 1980.

177. Lindblad B, Bergqvist D, Fredin H, et al: The accuracy of 125-I–radioactive uptake test for detection of deep venous thrombosis using

different labelled proteins (fibrinogen, albumin) and compared to phlebography in hip surgery patients. Vasa 16:251, 1987.

178. Lindhagen A, Bergqvist D, Hallbook T, et al: Venous function in the leg after postoperative thrombosis diagnosed with ^{125}I-fibrinogen uptake test. Ann Surg 197:215, 1983.

179. Lindqvist R: Ultrasound as a complementary diagnostic method in deep vein thrombosis of the leg. Acta Med Scand 201:435, 1977.

180. Lisbona R, Derbekyan V, Novales-Dias JA, et al: Tc-99m red blood cell venography in deep venous thrombosis of the lower limb. An overview. Clin Nucl Med 10:208, 1985.

181. Lohr JM, Kerr TM, Lutter KS, et al: Lower extremity calf thrombosis: To treat or not to treat. J Vasc Surg 14:618, 1991.

182. Luckers AEG, Luth WJ, Teule GJJ, et al: Diagnosis of deep venous thrombosis with ^{99m}Tc plasmin using gamma camera. Eur J Nucl Med 9:282, 1984.

183. Mahler DK, Foldes MS, Hayes AC, et al: Followup of old deep venous thrombosis by Doppler ultrasound and strain gauge plethysmography. Bruit 6(6):30, 1982.

184. Mantoni M: Diagnosis of deep venous thrombosis by duplex sonography. Acta Radiol 30:575, 1989.

185. Mantoni M: Deep venous thrombosis: Longitudinal study with duplex US. Radiology 179:271, 1991.

186. Markel A, Manzo RA, Bergelin RO, Strandness DE Jr: Valvular reflux after deep vein thrombosis: Incidence and time of occurrence. J Vasc Surg 15:377, 1992.

187. Maryniak O, Nicholson CG: Doppler ultrasonography for detection of deep vein thrombosis in lower extremities. Arch Phys Med Rehabil 60:277, 1979.

188. Mattos MA, Londrey GL, Leutz DW, et al: Color-flow duplex scanning for the surveillance and diagnosis of acute deep venous thrombosis. J Vasc Surg 15:366, 1992.

189. Mavor GE, Walker MG, Dhall DP, et al: Peripheral venous scanning with I[125]-tagged fibrinogen. Lancet 1:661, 1972.

190. McCaffrey J, Williams O, Stathis M: Diagnosis of deep venous thrombosis using a Doppler ultrasonic technique. Surg Gynecol Obstet 140:740, 1975.

191. McLachlan MSF, Thomson JG, Taylor DW, et al: Observer variation in the interpretation of lower limb venograms. AJR 132:227, 1979.

192. McLachlin J, Paterson JC: Some basic observations on venous thrombosis and pulmonary embolism. Surg Gynecol Obstet 93:1, 1951.

193. McNeil BJ: A diagnostic strategy using ventilation-perfusion studies in patients suspect for pulmonary embolism. J Nucl Med 17:613, 1976.

194. Meadway J, Nicolaides AN, Walker CJ, et al: Value of Doppler ultrasound in diagnosis of clinically suspected deep vein thrombosis. Br Med J 4:552, 1975.

195. Meibers DJ, Baldridge ED, Ruoff BA, et al: The significance of calf muscle venous thrombosis. J Vasc Technol 12:143, 1988.

196. Meibers DJ, Stedje KG, Ruoff BA, et al: B-mode scan characteristics of Baker's cysts. J Vasc Technol 11:125, 1987.

197. Menzoian JO, Sequeira JC, Doyle JE, et al: Therapeutic and clinical course of deep vein thrombosis. Am J Surg 146:581, 1983.

198. Menzoian JO, Williams L: Is pulmonary angiography essential for the diagnosis of acute pulmonary embolism? Am J Surg 137:543, 1979.

199. Millar WT, Smith JFB: Localisation of deep-venous thrombosis using technetium-99m–labelled urokinase. Lancet 2:695, 1974.

200. Milne RM, Gunn AA, Griffiths JMT, Ruckley CV: Post-operative deep venous thrombosis. A comparison of diagnostic techniques. Lancet 2:445, 1971.

201. Mitchell DC, Grasty MS, Stebbings WSL, et al: Comparison of duplex ultrasonography and venography in the diagnosis of deep venous thrombosis. Br J Surg 78:611, 1991.

202. Montefusco-von Kleist CM, Bakal CW, Sprayregen S, et al: Comparison of duplex ultrasonography and ascending contrast venography in the diagnosis of venous thrombosis. Vasc Surg 27:350, 1993.

203. Moore DJ, Himmel PD, Sumner DS: Distribution of venous valvular incompetence in patients with the postphlebitic syndrome. J Vasc Surg 3:49, 1986.

204. Moreno-Cabral R, Kistner RL, Nordyke RA: Importance of calf vein thrombophlebitis. Surgery 80:735, 1976.

205. Morris GK, Mitchell JRA: Evaluation of ^{125}I-fibrinogen test for venous thrombosis in patients with hip fractures: A comparison between isotope scanning and necropsy findings. Br Med J 1:264, 1977.

206. Moser KM, Brach BB, Dolan GF: Clinically suspected deep venous thrombosis of the lower extremities. A comparison of venography, impedance plethysmography, and radiolabeled fibrinogen. JAMA 237:2195, 1977.

207. Moses DC, Silver TM, Bookstein JJ: The complementary roles of chest radiography, lung scanning, and selective pulmonary angiography in the diagnosis of pulmonary embolism. Circulation 49:179, 1974.

208. Mussurakis S, Papaioannou S, Voros D, Vrakatselis T: Compression ultrasonography as a reliable imaging monitor in deep venous thrombosis. Surg Gynecol Obstet 171:233, 1990.

209. Negus D, Pinto DJ, Le Quesne LP, et al: ^{125}I-labelled fibrinogen in the diagnosis of deep vein thrombosis and its correlation with phlebography. Br J Surg 55:835, 1968.

210. Nicholas GG, Lorenz RP, Botti JJ, et al: The frequent occurrence of false-positive results in phleborheography during pregnancy. Surg Gynecol Obstet 161:133, 1985.

211. Nicholas GG, Miller FJ, DeMuth WE Jr, et al: Clinical vascular laboratory diagnosis of deep venous thrombosis. Ann Surg 186:213, 1977.

212. Nicolaides AN, O'Connell JD: Origin and distribution of thrombi in patients presenting with clinical deep venous thrombosis. *In* Nicolaides AN (ed): Thromboembolism: Etiology, Advances in Prevention and Management. Baltimore, University Park Press, 1975, pp 167–180.

213. Nicolaides AN, Lewis JD: The management of deep venous thrombosis. *In* Nicolaides AN (ed): Thromboembolism: Etiology, Advances in Prevention and Management. Baltimore, University Park Press, 1975, pp 269–286.

214. Nicolaides AN, Kakkar VV, Field ES, Renney JTG: The origin of deep venous thrombosis: A venographic study. Br J Radiol 44:653, 1971.

215. Nilsson E, Sunden P, Zetterquist S: Leg temperature profiles with a simplified thermographic technique in the diagnosis of acute venous thromboses. Scand J Clin Lab Invest 39:171, 1979.

216. Nippa JH, Alexander RH, Rolse R: Pulse wave velocity in human veins. J Appl Physiol 30:558, 1971.

217. Nix ML, Nelson CL, Harmon B, et al: Duplex venous scanning: Image vs. Doppler accuracy. J Vasc Technol 12:121, 1989.

218. Nix ML, Troillett RD: The use of color in venous duplex examination. J Vasc Technol 15:123, 1991.

219. Norris CS, Greenfield LJ, Herrmann JB: Free-floating iliofemoral thrombus: A risk of pulmonary embolism. Arch Surg 120:806, 1985.

220. O'Donnell TF, Abbott WM, Athanasoulis CA, et al: Diagnosis of deep venous thrombosis in the outpatient by venography. Surg Gynecol Obstet 150:69, 1980.

221. Oliver MA: Duplex scanning in venous disease. Bruit 9:206, 1985.

222. Oster ZH, Atkins HL, Trivedi M: Radionuclide venography vs Tc-99m-RBC equilibrium angiography: A comparative paired study. Eur J Nucl Med 13:174, 1987.

223. Ouriel K, Whitehouse WM Jr, Zarins CK: Combined use of Doppler ultrasound and phlebography in suspected deep venous thrombosis. Surg Gynecol Obstet 159:242, 1984.

224. Paiement G, Wessinger SJ, Waltman AC, et al: Surveillance of deep venous thrombosis in asymptomatic total hip replacement patients. Impedance phlebography and fibrinogen scanning versus roentgenographic phlebography. Am J Surg 155:400, 1988.

225. Patterson RB, Fowl RJ, Keller JD, et al: The limitations of impedance plethysmography in the diagnosis of acute deep venous thrombosis. J Vasc Surg 9:725, 1989.

226. Persson AV, Jones C, Zide R, Jewell ER: Use of triplex scanner in diagnosis of deep venous thrombosis. Arch Surg 124:593, 1989.

227. Peter DJ, Flanagan LD, Cranley JJ: Analysis of blood clot echogenicity. J Clin Ultrasound 14:111, 1986.

228. Peters AM, Lavender JP, Needham SG, et al: Imaging thrombus with radiolabelled monoclonal antibody to platelets. Br Med J 293:1525, 1986.

229. Peters SHA, Jonker JJG, de Boer AC, et al: Home diagnosis of deep venous thrombosis with impedance plethysmography. Thromb Haemost 48:134, 1982.

230. Philbrick JT, Becker DM: Calf deep venous thrombosis: A wolf in sheep's clothing? Arch Intern Med 148:2131, 1988.

231. PIOPED Investigators: Value of the ventilation/perfusion scan in acute pulmonary embolism. Results of the prospective investigation of pulmonary embolism diagnosis (PIOPED). JAMA 263:2753, 1990.

232. Polak JF, Culter SS, O'Leary DH: Deep veins of the calf: Assessment with color Doppler flow imaging. Radiology 171:481, 1989.

233. Pollack EW, Webber MM, Barker WF, et al: Autologous ^{125}I-fibrinogen uptake test in the detection and management of venous thrombosis. Arch Surg 109:48, 1974.

234. Pope CF, Dietz MJ, Ezekowitz MD, Gore JC: Technical variables influencing the detection of acute vein thrombosis by magnetic resonance imaging. Magn Reson Imaging 9:379, 1991.

235. Porter JM, Rutherford RB, Clagett GP, et al: Reporting standards in venous disease. J Vasc Surg 8:172, 1988.

236. Poulose K, Reba RC, Gilday DL, et al: Diagnosis of pulmonary embolism. A correlative study of the clinical scan, and angiographic findings. Br Med J 3:67, 1970.

237. Prentice AG, Lowe GDO, Forbes CD: Diagnosis and treatment of venous thromboembolism by consultants in Scotland. Br Med J 285:630, 1982.

238. Provan JL, Thomson C: Natural history of thrombophlebitis and its relationship to pulmonary embolism. Can J Surg 16:284, 1973.

239. Rabinov K, Paulin S: Roentgen diagnosis of venous thrombosis in the leg. Arch Surg 104:134, 1972.

240. Raghavendra BN, Horii SC, Hilton S, et al: Deep venous thrombosis: Detection by probe compression of veins. J Ultrasound Med 5:89, 1986.

241. Raines JK, Jaffrin MY, Rao S: A noninvasive pressure-pulse recorder: Development and rationale. Med Instrum 7:245, 1973.

242. Ramirez C, Box M, Gottesman L: Characteristics of extrinsic compression noted in plethysmographic and Doppler techniques for deep venous thrombosis. Bruit 4(9):42, 1980.

243. Reagan B, Folse R: Lower limb venous dynamics in normal persons and children of patients with varicose veins. Surg Gynecol Obstet 132:15, 1971.

244. Reilly MK, McCabe CJ, Abbott WM, et al: Deep venous thrombophlebitis following aortoiliac reconstructive surgery. Arch Surg 117:1210, 1982.

245. Richards KL, Armstrong JD, Tikoff G, et al: Noninvasive diagnosis of deep venous thrombosis. Arch Intern Med 136:1091, 1976.

246. Ritchie WGM, Soulen RL, Lapayowker MS: Thermographic diagnosis of deep venous thrombosis. Radiology 131:341, 1979.

247. Robin ED: Overdiagnosis and overtreatment of pulmonary embolism: The emperor may have no clothes. Ann Intern Med 87:775, 1977.

248. Rollins DL, Semrow C, Calligaro K, et al: Diagnosis of recurrent deep venous thrombosis using B-mode ultrasonic imaging. Phlebology 1:181, 1986.

249. Rollins DL, Semrow CM, Friedell ML, et al: Origin of deep vein thrombi in an ambulatory population. Am J Surg 156:122, 1988.

250. Rollins DL, Semrow CM, Friedell ML, et al: Progress in the diagnosis of deep venous thrombosis: The efficacy of real-time B-mode ultrasonic imaging. J Vasc Surg 7:638, 1988.

251. Rose SC, Zwiebel WJ, Nelson BD, et al: Symptomatic lower extremity deep venous thrombosis: Accuracy, limitations, and role of color duplex flow imaging in diagnosis. Radiology 175:639, 1990.

252. Rosebrough SF, Kudryk B, Grossman ZD, et al: Radioimmunoimaging of venous thrombi using iodine-131 monoclonal antibody. Radiology 156:515, 1985.

253. Russell JC, Becker DR: The noninvasive venous vascular laboratory: A prospective analysis. Arch Surg 118:1024, 1983.

254. Ryo UY, Gazi M, Srikantaswamy S, et al: Radionuclide venography: Correlation with contrast venography. J Nucl Med 18:11, 1977.

255. Sakaguchi S, Ishitobi K, Kameda T: Functional segmental plethysmography with mercury strain gauge. Angiology 23:127, 1972.

256. Salzman EW, Davies GC: Prophylaxis of venous thromboembolism. Analysis of cost effectiveness. Ann Surg 191:207, 1980.

257. Salzman EW, Hirsh J: Prevention of venous thromboembolism. *In* Colman RW, Hirsh J, Marder VJ, Salzman EW (eds): Hemostasis and Thrombosis: Basic Principles and Clinical Practice. Philadelphia, JB Lippincott, 1982, pp 986–999.

258. Sandager G, Bartel P, Blackburn D, et al: Venous hemodynamics after acute deep venous thrombosis. Bruit 6(9):25, 1982.

259. Sandager G, Williams LR, McCarthy WJ, et al: Assessment of venous valve function by duplex scan. Bruit 10:238, 1986.

260. Sanders RJ, Glaser JL: Clinical uses of venography. Angiology 20:388, 1969.

261. Sandler DA, Martin JF: Liquid crystal thermography as a screening test for deep venous thrombosis. Lancet 1:665, 1985.

262. Sarpa MS, Messina LM, Smith M, et al: Reliability of venous duplex scanning to image the iliac veins and to diagnose iliac vein thrombosis in patients suspected of having acute deep venous thrombosis. J Vasc Technol 15:299, 1991.

263. Sarpa MS, Messina LM, Villemure P, et al: Significance of a negative duplex scan in patients suspected of having acute deep venous thrombosis of the lower extremity. J Vasc Technol 13:224, 1989.

264. Sasahara AA, Sharma GVRK, Parisi AF: New developments in the detection and prevention of venous thromboembolism. Am J Cardiol 43:1214, 1979.

265. Satiani B, Tetalman MC, Van Aman M, Evans WE: Deep vein thrombosis following aortic surgery: Prospective evaluation of I^{125} fibrinogen and impedance plethysmography. Am Surg 45:507, 1979.

266. Sauerbrei E, Thomson JG, McLachlan MSF, Musial J: Observer variation in lower limb venography. J Can Assoc Radiol 31:28, 1981.

267. Sautter RD, Larson DE, Bhattacharyya SK, et al: The limited utility of fibrinogen I-125 leg scanning. Arch Intern Med 139:148, 1979.

268. Schatz IJ: The emotional aspects of thrombophlebitis. Geriatrics 17:815, 1962.

269. Schiff MJ, Feinberg AW, Naidich JB: Noninvasive venous examinations as a screening test for pulmonary embolism. Arch Intern Med 147:505, 1987.

270. Schindler JM, Kaiser M, Gerber A, et al: Colour coded duplex sonography in suspected deep vein thrombosis of the leg. Br Med J 301:1369, 1990.

271. Schroder WB, Bealer JF: Venous duplex ultrasonography causing acute pulmonary embolism: A brief report. J Vasc Surg 15:1082, 1992.

272. Schroeder PJ, Dunn E: Mechanical plethysmography and Doppler ultrasound: Diagnosis of deep-vein thrombosis. Arch Surg 117:300, 1982.

273. Schulman S, Granqvist S, Juhlin-Dannfelt A, Lockner D: Long-term sequelae of calf vein thrombosis treated with heparin or low-dose streptokinase. Acta Med Scand 219:349, 1986.

274. Seabold JE, Conrad GR, Ponto JA, et al: Deep venous thrombophlebitis: Detection with 4-hour versus 24-hour platelet scintigraphy. Radiology 165:355, 1987.

275. Sevitt S, Gallagher N: Venous thrombosis and pulmonary embolism. A clinico-pathological study in injured and burned patients. Br J Surg 48:475, 1961.

276. Sharma GVRK, Tow DE, Parisi AF, et al: Diagnosis of pulmonary embolism. Annu Rev Med 28:159, 1977.

277. Sigel B, Felix WR Jr, Popky GK, et al: Diagnosis of lower limb venous thrombosis by Doppler ultrasound technique. Arch Surg 104:174, 1972.

278. Sigel B, Ipsen J, Felix WR: The epidemiology of lower extremity deep venous thrombosis in surgical patients. Ann Surg 179:278, 1974.

279. Sigel B, Machi J, Beitler JC, et al: Variable ultrasound echogenicity in flowing blood. Science 218:1321, 1982.

280. Sigel B, Machi J, Beitler JC, Justin JR: Red cell aggregation as a cause of blood flow echogenicity. Radiology 148:799, 1983.

281. Sigel B, Popky GL, Mapp EM, et al: Evaluation of Doppler ultrasound examination. Its use in diagnosis of lower extremity venous disease. Arch Surg 100:535, 1970.

282. Skillman JJ: Postoperative deep vein thrombosis and pulmonary embolism. A selective review and personal viewpoint. Surgery 75:114, 1974.

283. Skillman JJ, Kent KC, Porter DH, Kim D: Simultaneous occurrence of superficial and deep thrombophlebitis in the lower extremity. J Vasc Surg 11:818, 1990.

284. Soini IH: Thermography in suspected deep venous thrombosis of lower leg. Eur J Radiol 5:281, 1985.

285. Solis MM, Ranval TJ, Nix L, et al: Is anticoagulation indicated for asymptomatic postoperative calf vein thrombosis? J Vasc Surg 16:414, 1992.

286. Sottiurai VS, Towner K, McDonnell AE, et al: Diagnosis of upper extremity deep venous thrombosis using noninvasive technique. Surgery 91:582, 1982.

287. Spritzer CE, Sostman HD, Wilkes DC, Coleman RE: Deep venous thrombosis: Experience with gradient-echo MR imaging in 66 patients. Radiology 177:235, 1990.

288. Stallworth JM, Plong GW Jr, Horne JB: Negative phleborheography: Clinical followup in 593 patients. Arch Surg 116:795, 1981.

289. Stedje KG, Hannan LJ, Karkow WS, et al: Assessing the results of

heparin and streptokinase therapy of deep venous thrombosis using sequential real-time B-mode ultrasound scans. Bruit 9:197, 1985.

290. Strandness DE Jr, Langlois Y, Cramer M, et al: Long-term sequelae of acute venous thrombosis. JAMA 250:1289, 1983.

291. Strandness DE Jr. Sumner DS: Ultrasonic velocity detector in the diagnosis of thrombophlebitis. Arch Surg 104:180, 1972.

292. Strandness DE Jr, Sumner DS: Hemodynamics for Surgeons. New York, Grune & Stratton, 1975.

293. Sufian S: Noninvasive vascular laboratory diagnosis of deep venous thrombosis. Am Surg 47:254, 1981.

294. Sull WJ: Diagnosis of thrombophlebitis in the lower extremity. Mo Med 75:552, 1978.

295. Sullivan ED, Peter DJ, Cranley JJ: Real-time B-mode venous ultrasound. J Vasc Surg 1:465, 1984.

296. Sullivan ED, Reece CI, Cranley JJ: Phleborheography of the upper extremity. Arch Surg 118:1134, 1983.

297. Sumner DS: Diagnosis of venous thrombosis by Doppler ultrasound. *In* Bergan JJ, Yao JST (eds): Venous Problems. Chicago, Year Book Medical Publishers, 1978, pp 159–185.

298. Sumner DS: Applied physiology in venous problems. *In* Bergan JJ, Yao JST (eds):Surgery of the Veins. Orlando, FL, Grune & Stratton, 1985, pp 3–23.

299. Sumner DS: Evaluation of noninvasive testing procedures: Data analysis and interpretation. *In* Bernstein EF (ed): Noninvasive Diagnostic Techniques in Vascular Disease. 3rd ed. St. Louis, CV Mosby, 1985, pp 861–889.

300. Sumner DS: Doppler ultrasound. *In* Hirsh J (ed): Venous Thrombosis and Pulmonary Embolism, Diagnostic Methods. Edinburgh, Churchill Livingstone, 1987, pp 54–76.

301. Sumner DS, Baker DW, Strandness DE Jr: The ultrasonic velocity detector in a clinical study of venous disease. Arch Surg 97:75, 1968.

302. Sumner DS, Lambeth A: Reliability of Doppler ultrasound in the diagnosis of acute venous thrombosis both above and below the knee. Am J Surg 138:205, 1979.

303. Sumner DS, Londrey GL, Spadone DP, et al: Study of deep venous thrombosis in high-risk patients using color flow Doppler. *In* Bergan JJ, Yao JST (eds): Venous Disorders. Philadelphia, WB Saunders, 1991, pp 63–76.

304. Sumner DS, Mattos MA, Londrey GL, et al: Clinical application of color Doppler in venous problems. *In* Yao JST, Pearce WH (eds): Technologies in Vascular Surgery. Philadelphia, WB Saunders, 1992, pp 185–200.

305. Sumner DS, Rabinovitch E, Lambeth A: The effect of venous capacitance on venous outflow. Second International Vascular Symposium, London, 1986, Abstract S11.4.

306. Swedenborg, J, Hagglof R, Jacobsson H, et al: Results of surgical treatment for iliofemoral venous thrombosis. Br J Surg 73:871, 1986.

307. Symbas PN, Harlaftis N, Gonzalez AC: Diagnosis of pulmonary embolism: Correlation of value of perfusion lung scan and pulmonary arteriography in selecting patients for inferior vena cava interruption. Am Surg 44:137, 1978.

308. Szendro G, Nicolaides AN, Zukowski AJ, et al: Duplex scanning in the assessment of venous incompetence. J Vasc Surg 4:237, 1986.

309. Talbot SR: Use of real-time imaging in identifying deep venous obstruction: A preliminary report. Bruit 6(6):41, 1982.

310. Thomas ML: Phlebography. Arch Surg 104:145, 1972.

311. Thomas PRS, Butler CM, Bowman J, et al: Light reflection rheography: An effective non-invasive technique for screening patients with suspected deep venous thrombosis. Br J Surg 78:207, 1991.

312. Tow DE, Simon AL: Comparison of lung scanning and pulmonary angiography in the detection and follow-up of pulmonary embolism: The urokinase–pulmonary embolism trial experience. Prog Cardiovasc Dis 17:239, 1975.

313. Towner KM, McDonnell AE, Turcotte JK, et al: Noninvasive assessment of upper extremity deep venous obstructions. Bruit 5:21, 1981.

314. Tremaine MD, Choroszy CJ, Menking SA: Deep vein thrombosis in the total hip arthroplasty patient after hospital discharge. J Vasc Technol 16:23, 1992.

315. Tripolitis AJ, Blackshear WM Jr, Bodily KC, et al: The influence of limb elevation, examination technique, and outflow system design on venous plethysmography. Angiology 31:154, 1980.

316. Tripolitis AJ, et al: Venous capacitance and outflow in the postoperative patient. Ann Surg 190:634, 1979.

317. Tsapogas MJ, Goussous H, Peabody RA, et al: Postoperative venous thrombosis and effectiveness of prophylactic measures. Arch Surg 103:561, 1971.

318. van Bemmelen PS, Bedford G, Strandness DE: Visualization of calf veins by color flow imaging. Ultrasound Med Biol 16:15, 1990.

319. van Ramshorst B, Legemate DA, Verzijlbergen JF, et al: Duplex scanning in the diagnosis and follow-up of DVT. *In* Boccalon H (ed): Angiologie: Strategie du Diagnostic et de la Therapeutique. London, Paris, John Libbey Eurotext, 1988, pp 457–460.

320. van Ramshorst B, Legemate DA, Verzijlberggen JF, et al: Duplex scanning in the diagnosis of acute deep vein thrombosis of the lower extremity. Eur J Vasc Surg 5:255, 1991.

321. Vlahos L, MacDonald AF, Causer DA: Combination of isotope venography and lung scanning. Br J Radiol 49:840, 1976.

322. Vogel P, Laing FC, Jeffrey RB Jr, et al: Deep venous thrombosis of the lower extremity: US evaluation. Radiology 163:747, 1987.

323. Vogelzang RL, Fitzgerald SW: Magnetic resonance imaging of venous disorders. *In* Yao JST, Pearce WH (eds): Technologies in Vascular Surgery. Philadelphia, WB Saunders, 1992, pp 106–125.

324. Vukov LF, Berquist TH, King BF: Magnetic resonance imaging for calf deep venous thrombophlebitis. Ann Emerg Med 20:497, 1991.

325. Walker MG: The natural history of venous thrombo-embolism. Br J Surg 59:54, 1972.

326. Warren R: Behavior of venous thrombi. Historical observations. Arch Surg 115:1151, 1980.

327. Wheeler HB, Anderson FA Jr: Impedance plethysmography. *In* Kempczinski RF, Yao JST (eds): Practical Noninvasive Vascular Diagnosis. 2nd ed. Chicago, Year Book Medical Publishers, 1987, pp 407–437.

328. Wheeler HB, Anderson FA Jr, Cardullo PA, et al: Suspected deep vein thrombosis. Management by impedance plethysmography. Arch Surg 117:1206, 1982.

329. Wheeler HB, O'Donnell JA, Anderson FA Jr, et al: Occlusive impedance phlebography: A diagnostic procedure for venous thrombosis and pulmonary embolism. Prog Cardiovasc Dis 17:199, 1974.

330. Wheeler HB, O'Donnell JA, Anderson FA, et al: Bedside screening for venous thrombosis using occlusive impedance plethysmography. Angiology 26:199, 1975.

331. White RH, Goulet JA, Bray TJ, et al: Deep-vein thrombosis after fracture of the pelvis: Assessment with serial duplex-ultrasound screening. J Bone Joint Surg 72A:495, 1990.

332. Woolson ST, McCrory DW, Walter JF, et al: B-mode ultrasound scanning in the detection of proximal venous thrombosis after total hip replacement. J Bone Joint Surg 72A:983, 1990.

333. Wright DJ, Shepard AD, McPharlin M, Ernst CB: Pitfalls in lower extremity venous duplex scanning. J Vasc Surg 11:675, 1990.

334. Yao JST, Henkin RE, Conn J Jr, et al: Combined isotope venography and lung scanning. Arch Surg 107:146, 1973.

335. Yao JST, Gourmos C, Hobbs JT: Detection of proximal-vein thrombosis by Doppler ultrasound flow-detection method. Lancet 1:1, 1972.

336. Zachrisson BE, Jansen H: Phlebographic signs in fresh postoperative venous thrombosis of the lower extremity. Acta Radiol 14:82, 1973.

337. Zielinsky A, Hull R, Hirsh J, et al: Comparative study of Doppler ultrasound and impedance plethysmography in the diagnosis of symptomatic and asymptomatic deep vein thrombosis [Abstract 453]. Circulation 58(Suppl II): 117, 1978.

338. Zorba J, Schier D, Posmituck G: Clinical value of blood pool radionuclide venography. AJR 146:1051, 1986.

339. Zufferey P, Pararas C, Monti M, Depairon M: Assessment of acute and old deep venous thrombosis in upper extremity by venous strain gauge plethysmography. Vasa 21:263, 1992.

340. Evans DS: The early diagnosis of deep vein thrombosis by ultrasound. Br J Surg 57:726, 1970.

341. Todd JW, Frisbie JH, Rossier AB, et al: Deep venous thrombosis in acute spinal cord injury: A comparison of ^{125}I-fibrinogen leg scanning, impedance plethysmography and venography. Paraplegia 14:50, 1976.

342. Toy PCTY, Schrier SL: Occlusive impedance plethysmography. A noninvasive method of diagnosis of proximal deep vein thrombosis. West J Med 90:89, 1978.

132

Venography

Steven C. Rose, M.D.

• • •

Contrast venography has generally become accepted as the gold standard for diagnosis of most extremity venous disease. Unfortunately, venography entails significant patient discomfort and a low but defined risk of potentially serious complications related to the injection of contrast material. Technologic developments have resulted in alternative, noninvasive techniques for the evaluation of venous disease. Examples include color flow duplex imaging and magnetic resonance angiography, which are pain-free and virtually risk-free. Contrast venography is now usually reserved for situations in which the noninvasive imaging modalities either are unavailable or are unable to fully answer the clinical questions.

HISTORICAL PERSPECTIVE

Contrast venography was initially described in 1923 by Berberich and Hirsch.[1] For decades, clinical acceptance of contrast venography was tempered by suboptimal diagnostic results. An incomplete understanding of normal and pathologic venous blood flow patterns contributed to technically inadequate examinations and to misinterpretation of radiographic findings. In 1972, the beginning of the modern era of venography was marked by the back-to-back articles of Rabinov and Paulin[2] and Thomas.[3] The fundamental techniques for ascending contrast venography described by these authors have largely been retained by most contemporary diagnosticians. Hull and coworkers[4] and Ramsey[5] showed that both the morbidity and the expense of venography are significantly less than those of routine anticoagulation when venography is uniformly used in patients with clinically suspected deep venous thrombosis (DVT).

VALIDATION

Although venography has been widely accepted as the diagnostic standard for the evaluation of extremity venous disease, particularly acute DVT, direct validation of this technique is sparse. Venous thrombosis is a dynamic disease that is treated medically; thus, the opportunity for pathologic correlation (at autopsy or after limb amputation) is uncommon. The validity of venographic abnormalities that are diagnostic of venous thrombosis is shown by Lund and associates, who used bilateral intraosseous venography (in which the veins are filled by contrast medium injected via a needle introduced into the trabecular bone of the calcaneus) to examine 100 cadavers for DVT.[6] Pathologic correlation yielded a sensitivity of 86 per cent and a specificity of 95 per cent. The validity of venographic findings negative for DVT was documented by Hull and colleagues.[7] These authors withheld anticoagulant therapy in 160 consecutive patients who were suspected clinically of having lower extremity DVT but who had negative venographic findings. Clinical follow-up of these patients yielded only 2 (1.3 per cent) with documented DVT; both cases occurred within 5 days of venography, and they may have been due to contrast-induced phlebitis. Indirect support for the validity of contrast venography in the diagnosis of acute DVT is provided by the innumerable works that correlate venography (the reference modality) with various noninvasive techniques (the modality being investigated). Nevertheless, interobserver variation in interpretation does occur. Several reports have indicated that under the best of circumstances (experienced interpreters using standardized venographic technique and mutually agreed on diagnostic criteria in patients clinically suspected of harboring DVT), observers will disagree about the presence or absence of thrombus in approximately 10 to 30 per cent of examinations.[8–10] Interobserver variability is less for negative study findings (2 per cent) than for positive study findings (30 per cent), presumably because of disagreement regarding small thrombi.[10]

LOWER EXTREMITY VENOGRAPHY

Acute Deep Venous Thrombosis

Acute lower extremity DVT is both common and serious. Treatment of DVT, depending on the location, extent, and patient risk factors, is generally either long-term anticoagulation or placement of an inferior vena cava filter. Because both treatment modalities carry significant risk of morbidity (primarily hemorrhage due to anticoagulation and inferior vena cava thrombosis due to an indwelling caval filter), it is imperative that DVT be proved with certainty to be either present or absent.

Venous Anatomy

The venous drainage of the foot may be characterized as a valveless system with profuse intercommunication between the multiple superficial and deep veins. In general, contrast medium injected into one portion (e.g., a vein on the dorsum of the foot) will be redistributed to most portions of the deep drainage system, particularly if a tight tourniquet is applied near the ankle (Fig. 132–1).

In the calf, the paired branches of the anterior tibial, peroneal, and posterior tibial veins typically flank the arteries of the same name until they join to form common trunks proximally (Fig. 132–2). These anterior tibial, peroneal, and posterior tibial venous trunks usually coalesce below the knee joint to form a single popliteal vein. Many variant patterns of infrapopliteal venous coalescence have been described. In 36 to 40 per cent of persons, this coalescence occurs proximal (cephalad) to the knee joint, in which case the popliteal vein is duplicated (Fig. 132–3).[11, 12] Large-caliber saccular venous channels, termed the soleal sinuses, drain from the muscles that bear the same name into either the peroneal or posterior tibial veins (Fig. 132–4). As the soleal muscles contract during exercise, blood is propelled centrally. Normally, blood flow in the deep venous system is unidirectional because of the presence of multiple venous valves. In nonambulatory patients, stasis of blood within the soleal sinuses occurs. As a result of such stasis, DVT commonly originates within the soleal sinuses.[13–15] Although the soleal sinuses usually opacify dur-

ing routine ascending venography, tight tourniquets applied to the upper calf or the lower thigh (for retrograde filling of the soleal sinuses) may occasionally be necessary.[14] The veins that drain the gastrocnemius muscles drain into the popliteal vein or veins and do not seem to function as a "peripheral pump" to return blood centrally (see Fig. 132–4).

The superficial femoral vein is typically single, but it is duplicated (or even triplicated) in 18 to 38 per cent of persons (Fig. 132–5).[11, 12] In some cases, femoral venous duplication may be a continuation of a duplicated popliteal system. Blood from within the deep femoral vein is not usually opacified with contrast medium because this vein primarily drains the thigh musculature.[16, 17] However, communicating channels between the deep femoral veins and the superficial femoral or popliteal veins occur in up to 86 per cent of people, which may in turn permit deep femoral vein opacification (Fig. 132–6).[18] The common femoral and the external and common iliac veins are normally visualized on good-quality standard ascending venograms. The left common iliac vein may be compressed between the right common iliac artery and the sacrum, a condition termed the May-Thurner syndrome (Fig. 132–7).[19] The internal iliac (hypogastric) veins are typically not identified unless there has been retrograde filling in a patient who has performed

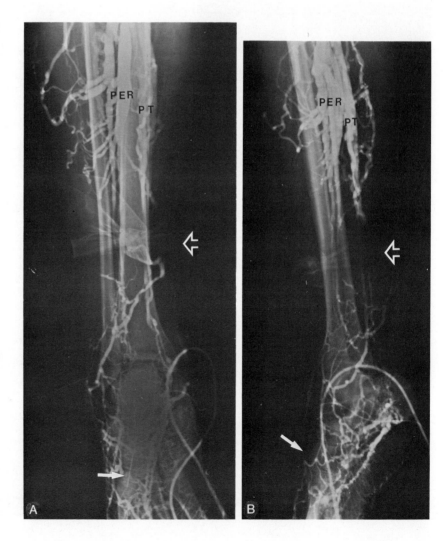

FIGURE 132–1. Foot vein injection of contrast fills the calf deep venous system. Anteroposterior (*A*) and lateral (*B*) views of the right distal calf and foot; the injection site of contrast medium is in a dorsal foot vein (*arrows*). Contrast fills the intercommunicating, valveless foot venous system. A tourniquet (*arrowheads*) preferentially drives contrast medium into the deep veins of the calf. PT, posterior tibial veins; PER, peroneal veins.

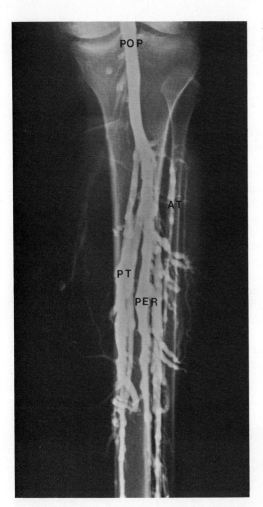

FIGURE 132-2.   Conduit veins of the calf; anteroposterior view of the normal calf veins. AT, anterior tibial veins; POP, popliteal vein.

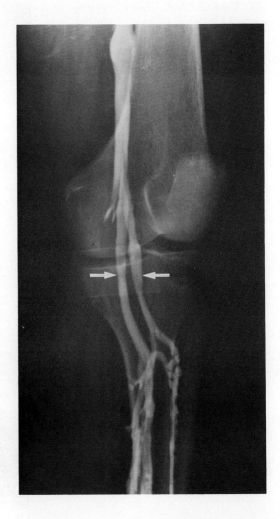

FIGURE 132-3.   Duplicated popliteal vein. Near-lateral view at the knee. Incomplete fusion of the calf conduit veins results in two popliteal veins (*arrows*) until fusion occurs above the knee joint.

FIGURE 132–4. Muscular veins of the calf. Anteroposterior (*A*) and lateral (*B*) views of the calf. The soleal sinuses (S) communicate with the peroneal and posterior tibial veins centrally (*arrows*) and often distally (*arrowheads*). The soleal sinuses are capacious reservoirs that drain the deep soleal musculature. The gastrocnemius veins (G) drain the more cephalad and superficial gastrocnemius muscles and empty into the popliteal vein or veins near the knee joint.

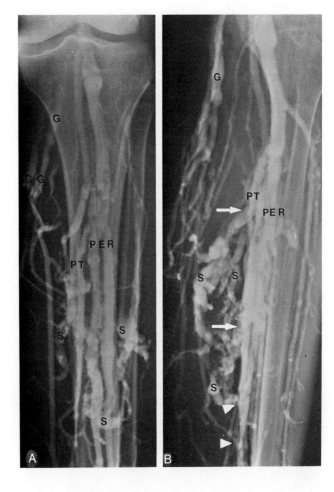

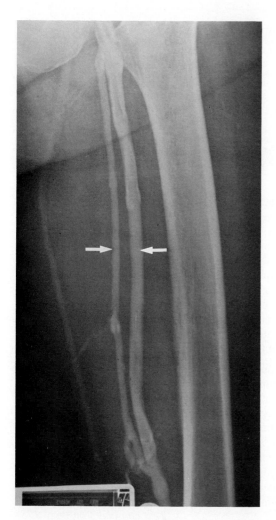

FIGURE 132–5. Duplicated superficial femoral vein. Anteroposterior view of the thigh. The superficial femoral vein has duplicated lumina (*arrows*) extending from just above the adductor canal segment almost to the femoral bifurcation.

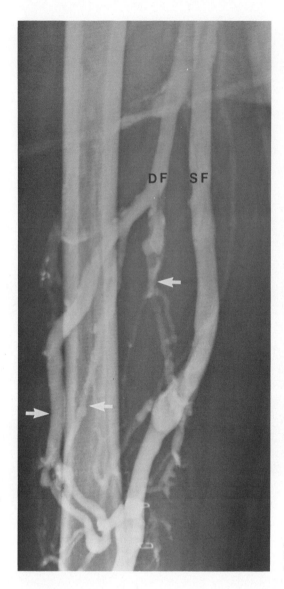

DF   SF

FIGURE 132–6.   Communicating channels at the adductor canal level (*arrows*) between the superficial femoral vein (SF) and the deep femoral vein (DF); anteroposterior view of the thigh.

a vigorous Valsalva maneuver, or in cases in which the internal iliac veins act as collateral channels because of common iliac, external iliac, or common femoral vein occlusion (Fig. 132–8).[17]

The superficial venous system is located in the subcutaneous tissues and is dominated by the greater saphenous vein, which courses from the superficial dorsal venous arch and the medial marginal vein of the foot to join the common femoral vein centrally (Fig. 132–9). The lesser saphenous vein originates from the lateral portion of the superficial dorsal venous arch near the lateral malleolus and runs posteriorly in the calf to enter the popliteal vein or veins centrally (Fig. 132–10). Perforating veins communicate between the superficial and deep venous systems; flow is normally unidirectional from the superficial toward the deep system because of the presence of competent valves.

Ascending Venographic Technique

The fundamentals of present-day venographic technique were published by Rabinov and Paulin in 1972.[2]

Water-soluble contrast medium is injected into a vein on the dorsum of the foot. The patient is positioned semi-upright in order to obtain complete venous filling. To avoid extrinsic compression of the vein by muscular contraction, the extremity being examined is not allowed to bear weight. No tourniquets are applied in Rabinov and Paulin's technique. Fluoroscopy is used to monitor filling of the venous system by contrast medium. Spot radiographs are obtained once the venous segments have been sufficiently filled.

Technical modifications that this author has found useful include the following:

1. Routinely apply a tight tourniquet just above the ankle to minimize the amount of contrast medium delivered to the superficial venous system (Fig. 132–11) and to prove competency of the valves of the perforating veins.

2. Obtain calf radiographs in the lateral (best separation of the anterior tibial, soleal, and gastrocnemius veins) and anteroposterior views and with 15 degrees of internal rotation (best separation of the tibia from the fibula and of the peroneal from the posterior tibial veins) (Fig. 132–12).

3. Repeat the calf examination after the ankle tourni-

Text continued on page 1753

FIGURE 132–7. May-Thurner syndrome. *A,* Anteroposterior pelvic digital subtraction angiogram. Injection of contrast medium into the left iliac vein catheter demonstrates an abrupt, transverse occlusion (*arrowheads*) of the central left iliac vein with transpelvic collateral veins draining into the right iliac system. There is an incidental small thrombus in the left internal iliac vein (*arrow*). *B,* Anteroposterior pelvic digital subtraction angiogram. Injection of contrast agent into the right iliac vein proves the normalcy of the right common iliac vein and the inferior vena cava. *C,* Computed tomogram at the level of the proximal common iliac arteries (A) after simultaneous injection of contrast into both iliac veins (V) illustrates the compression of the proximal left common iliac vein (*arrow*) between the crossing right iliac artery and the sacrum. Incidentally seen is contrast in both ureters (lateral to the iliac arteries and veins).

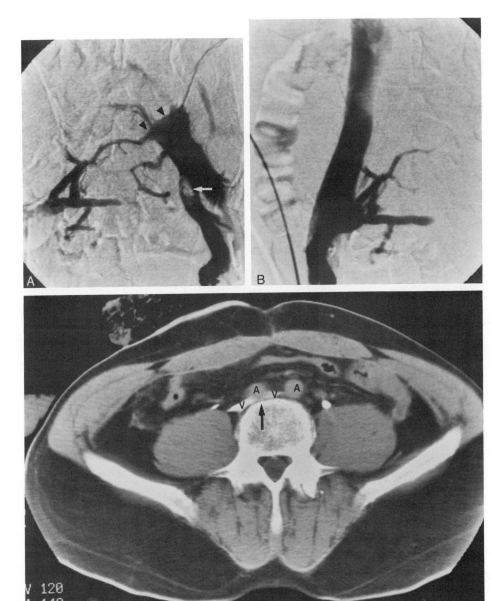

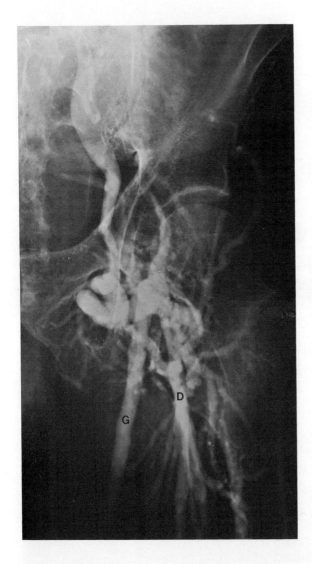

FIGURE 132–8. Opacification of the internal iliac vein. Anteroposterior radiograph centered at the groin. The left superficial femoral, common femoral, and external iliac veins have been chronically thrombosed. Contrast from the patent left deep femoral (D) and greater saphenous (G) veins drains via multiple pelvic collateral veins into the left internal iliac (I) and common iliac veins.

FIGURE 132–9. Greater saphenous vein. Anteroposterior views of the calf (*A*), distal thigh (*B*), and groin (*C*). The greater saphenous vein arises from the medial marginal (MM) vein of the foot, courses medially along the length of the lower extremity, and drains into the common femoral (CF) vein at the saphenofemoral junction (*black arrow*). Nonopacified flow from the deep femoral vein is imaged as a relative filling defect within the otherwise opacified common femoral vein. Of note, communicating channels (*white arrowheads*) at the level of the adductor canal may be a cause of recurrent varices following saphenous vein ligation centrally.

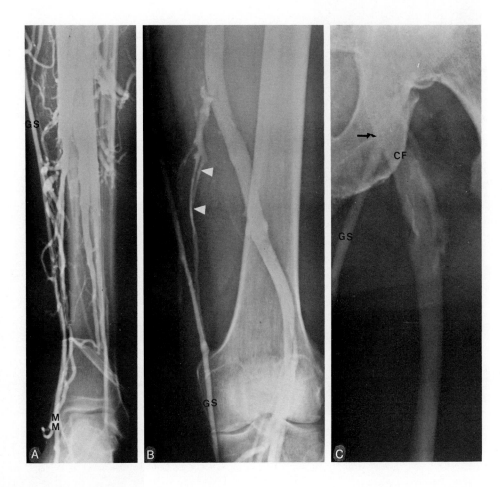

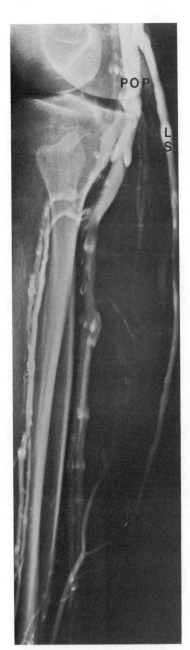

FIGURE 132–10.   Lesser saphenous vein. Lateral radiograph of the calf. After arising from the superficial dorsal venous arch in the foot, the lesser saphenous (LS) vein courses in the subcutaneous tissue of the posterior aspect of the calf to drain into the popliteal vein (POP) (duplicated in this patient) above the knee joint.

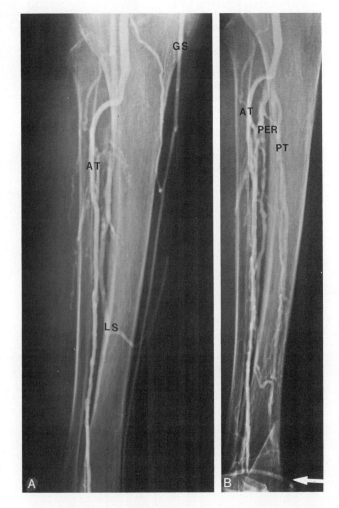

FIGURE 132–11.   Improved visualization of the deep venous system with the tourniquet technique. Anteroposterior calf radiographs with no tourniquets (*A*) and after application of a tight tourniquet (*B*) just above the ankle (*arrow*). In the former, contrast fills only the greater saphenous, lesser saphenous, and anterior tibial veins. After the tourniquet is applied, the saphenous veins do not fill, whereas the posterior tibial, peroneal, and anterior tibial (AT) veins are opacified.

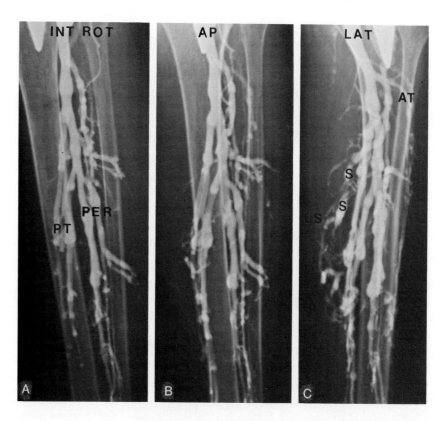

FIGURE 132–12. Value of multiple views in the calf. Series of exposures with the calf in 15 degrees of internal rotation (*A*), which separates the tibia from the fibula and the posterior tibial from the peroneal veins, and anteroposterior (*B*) and lateral (*C*) views, which best separate the anterior tibial (AT) veins, soleal sinuses (S), lesser saphenous vein, and gastrocnemius veins (nonopacified in this patient).

quet has been released (not uncommonly, normal anterior tibial veins, and occasionally normal posterior tibial veins, may not be visualized because of tourniquet compression) (Fig. 132–13).

4. Optimize iliac venous opacification by manually compressing the common femoral veins, returning the patient to a horizontal position, having the patient sustain a Valsalva maneuver, elevating the lower extremity, and releasing manual pressure on the femoral vein so as to release the opacified venous blood suddenly into the iliac veins.

On occasion, the location of venous access may need to be altered to complete filling of the calf trifurcation veins (e.g., the cannula may need to be replaced into a medial foot vein in order to fill the posterior tibial vein more completely). A tight tourniquet placed just below or above the patella may help to opacify the soleal sinuses by promoting retrograde filling.[14]

Fluoroscopic observation or repeated radiography may help to differentiate thrombus from a filling defect in the contrast column caused by the inflow of nonopacified blood (Fig. 132–14).

It is recommended that a plastic cannula (e.g., Angiocath, Deseret Medical, Sandy, UT) be used for venous access to minimize the likelihood of contrast extravasation and skin slough. Gothlin found at least a threefold decrease in contrast medium extravasation when a Teflon cannula was used compared with a steel needle.[20] In patients with significant lower extremity edema, elevation of the leg, compression with an elastic bandage, and application of heat (e.g., towels soaked with hot water) may improve the likelihood of successful venous access. On occasion, ultrasonography or transillumination may be helpful in identifying the veins.[21, 22]

Complications

Although contrast venography is relatively safe, potentially serious complications due to injection of contrast medium do occur. The frequency of idiosyncratic allergic-like reactions following intravenous injection of ionic contrast medium is 5 to 8 per cent for mild reactions (e.g., urticaria) and approximately 0.1 per cent for serious or major reactions (e.g., laryngospasm, bronchospasm, or anaphylactoid reactions).[23–25] The cited incidence of fatalities approximates 1 in 40,000.[23] Contrast reactions are more frequent in patients with an atopic history (4-fold increase), a history of prior contrast reactions (11-fold increase), and prior heart disease (5-fold increase).[23] The incidence of contrast reactions has been shown to be lower when nonionic contrast medium is employed (its use decreases severe contrast reactions 4.5- to 5.5-fold).[25, 26] In patients with a history of a contrast medium reaction, pretreatment with a short course of steroids (e.g., prednisone, 25 mg orally 1, 7, and 13 hours before contrast injection) and the use of a nonionic contrast medium are indicated.[24, 26] Additionally, some investigators recommend the use of agents to block histamine release (e.g., cimetidine, 300 mg intravenously, and diphenhydramine, 25 to 50 mg intramuscularly or intravenously) in selected cases.[24]

The frequency of contrast-induced nephrotoxicity depends on whether risk factors are present. Known risk factors include preexistent renal disease, hypovolemia, congestive heart failure, insulin-dependent diabetes, advanced age, and high volumes of administered contrast medium.[27–29] The use of nonionic contrast medium has not been proved to lower the risk of contrast-induced nephrotoxicity.[30] Preventive measures include optimized patient hydration and

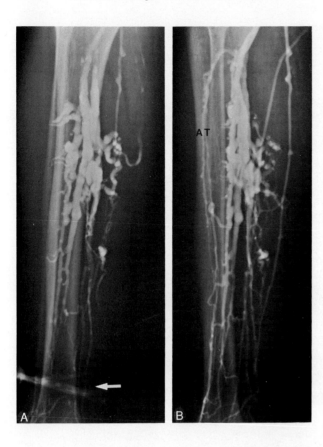

FIGURE 132–13. Impact of the tourniquet technique on anterior tibial vein opacification. Lateral calf radiographs with a tight ankle tourniquet (*A*; *arrow*) and without an ankle tourniquet (*B*). The anterior tibial veins are opacified only after the tourniquet has been released.

cardiac function, as well as judicious use of contrast material.

Injection of contrast medium may precipitate de novo venous thrombosis, probably because of injury involving the venous endothelium.[31] The incidence of radiolabeled-fibrinogen uptake test results converting from negative to positive after contrast venography ranges from 29 to 39 per cent.[32–35] The incidence of postphlebographic DVT that is clinically symptomatic and venographically proven is lower (2 to 13 per cent).[35–37] Postphlebographic thrombophlebitis may be diminished by using less-concentrated contrast medium. Bettman and associates found a rate of venographically proven postphlebography DVT of 13 per cent when they used 60 per cent sodium methylglucamine diatrizoate, as opposed to only 3 per cent when a 45 per cent concentration was used.[35] Several investigators have found no significant difference between nonionic and ionic contrast media of comparable concentration with respect to the incidence of postphlebographic DVT.[36, 37] Additionally, the incidence of contrast-induced DVT may be reduced by the infusion of heparinized saline (e.g., 1000 units of heparin in 250 ml of saline) through the venous access site before termination of the procedure.[38] Cerulea phlegmasia dolens is a rare limb-threatening and potentially life-threatening situation in which both the deep venous system and much of the superficial venous system are thrombotically occluded.[39] Because venography could cause thrombosis of the few remaining patent veins and further embarrass lower extremity perfusion and drainage, venography may be contraindicated when this diagnosis is suspected, particularly when the diagnosis is so readily made by noninvasive testing.

If contrast medium extravasates into the subcutaneous tissues, skin slough may occur (Fig. 132–15).[24, 40–42] Most likely, tissue necrosis is related to the volume and the osmolarity of the contrast agents. Localized erythema occurs within 12 to 24 hours. Bullae form within 24 to 48 hours, followed by skin loss that may require months to heal. In patients with poor arterial blood supply, the likelihood of eventual spontaneous healing is lower.[40, 42] Measures to prevent contrast medium extravasation include passage of the aforementioned plastic cannula well into the venous lumen and visual inspection for both blood return during aspiration and the absence of injection site swelling during contrast infusion. If the patient complains of injection site pain, the infusion should be terminated. Multiple initial treatment options have been described; they include application of heat, application of cold, elevation, aspiration of contrast medium, injection of saline (theoretically to dilute the contrast agent), and injection of hyaluronidase (theoretically to reduce the extent of skin necrosis by enzymatically breaking down connective tissue mucoprotein hyaluronic acid).[24] None of these modalities has been proved effective. Eventual skin grafting may be required.

Although manipulation of the lower extremity theoretically could result in pulmonary embolism, this complication is rare.[43] Nonetheless, massage of the lower extremity to improve iliac vein visualization should be discouraged.

Interpretation

Radiographic findings diagnostic of acute DVT include (1) a central filling defect within the column of con-

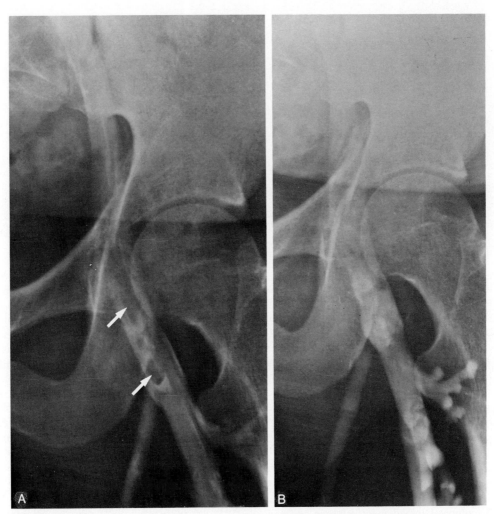

FIGURE 132–14.   Filling defect caused by inflow of nonopacified blood. Anteroposterior
radiographs of the left groin. *A*, Nonopacified blood entering from the deep femoral and other muscular
veins creates a stream-like filling defect (*arrows*) in the common femoral vein. *B*, Second radiograph
obtained several minutes later was taken while the patient sustained a Valsalva maneuver (note the
retrograde filling of the deep femoral vein). The inflow artifact is much less evident and has changed
morphology.

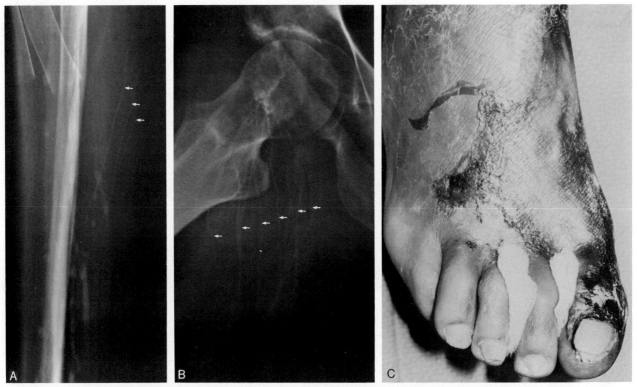

FIGURE 132–15.   Contrast-induced skin slough. Lateral view of the calf (A) and anteroposterior view of the groin (B) demonstrate lymphatic filling (*arrows*) from contrast extravasated during contrast venography. Photograph of the foot (C) 3 days later illustrates necrosis of the skin over the dorsum of the foot at the site of contrast extravasation.

trast medium (the "tram-track" sign) on at least two films (Fig. 132–16) and (2) nonvisualization of a venous segment that is not due to technical factors, especially if a filling defect is noted at either end of the occluded segment (a "trailing edge") and collateral venous channels are of small caliber (Fig. 132–17).[2, 44, 45] Technical factors that may cause artifactual venous nonopacification include the following:

1. A tight ankle tourniquet may impair filling of either the anterior or the posterior tibial veins.

2. A cannula placed along the medial aspect of the foot may not fill the anterior tibial veins, whereas a cannula placed laterally may not fill the posterior tibial veins.

3. Contraction of the soleal, gastrocnemius, or other muscles (e.g., if the patient is not truly non–weight bearing) may extrinsically compress the adjacent veins; in addition, nonpacified blood expelled from the soleal sinuses may wash contrast out of the posterior tibial, peroneal, and popliteal veins (Fig. 132–18).

4. The film may not be exposed during maximal venous filling if fluoroscopic monitoring is not performed.

Filling defects in the contrast column may also be caused by the inadvertent introduction of air bubbles (Fig. 132–19) or by the inflow of nonopacified blood from a branch vein. These diagnostic pitfalls can be correctly identified visually by fluoroscopic monitoring, repeated filming (inflow defects change appearance, whereas thrombi do not), or retrograde filling of central branch veins with a Valsalva maneuver (Fig. 132–20; see also Fig. 132–14). Overlapping densities, such as opacified veins or bone cor-

tex, can mimic a filling defect ("pseudo–tram-track" sign), especially in the calf (Fig. 132–21).

The natural history of DVT is variable. In approximately 12 per cent (calf vein DVT) to 67 per cent (femoral vein DVT) of patients, the occluded venous segment will remain occluded and the collateral veins will enlarge with the passage of time (Fig. 132–22; see also Fig. 132–8).[44] Partial recanalization may be expected in approximately one half of cases; it is manifest venographically by the presence of a narrow central lumen with irregular margins and webs (Fig. 132–23). In the remaining limbs, the venous recanalization is complete and may be manifest as (1) normal venographic findings, (2) a normal-caliber venous channel with subtle irregularity of the wall (Fig. 132–24) (presumably focal intimal hyperplasia), or (3) short, thickened, incompetent venous valves (see Fig. 132–23). Although several investigators have noted that venous pressure is often elevated in the presence of either acute or chronic thrombotic occlusion, this finding is of limited diagnostic value.[46]

Chronic Venous Insufficiency

Chronic venous insufficiency (chronic venous stasis) is a common disorder of adulthood. Tailoring treatment to correct a patient's chronic venous insufficiency requires definition of the cause or causes of venous stasis (e.g., valvular incompetence), the location (e.g., the superficial femoral vein), and the severity (e.g., Kistner grades). Venography has an important role in defining the pathologic anatomy.

Text continued on page 1761

FIGURE 132–16.   Tram-track sign. Anteroposterior radiograph over the knee. Contrast medium outlines the nonadherent filling defect (*arrows*) that represents acute deep venous thrombosis of the calf conduit, popliteal, and superficial femoral veins.

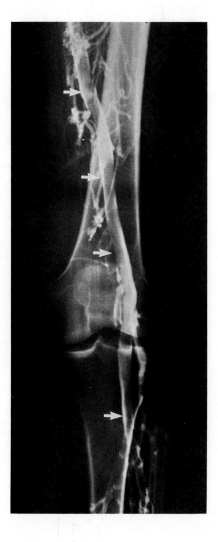

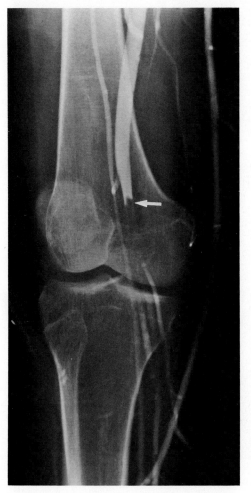

FIGURE 132–17.   Nonvisualized segment due to acute deep venous thrombosis. Externally rotated radiograph over the knee. There is no opacification of the calf conduit veins and most of the popliteal vein despite adequate filling of the collateral superficial veins (which are not enlarged) and the proximal portions of the popliteal vein. The filling defect in the distalmost portion of the opacified popliteal vein (*arrow*) represents a ''trailing edge'' of nonattached thrombus extending from the remainder of thrombus that is adherent to the vein wall.

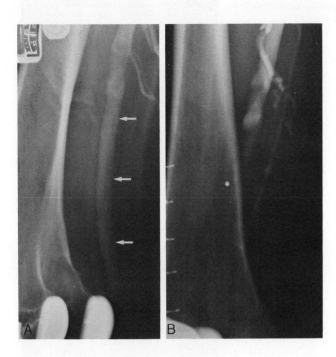

FIGURE 132–18. Artifactual nonopacification. Radiographs over the distal right thigh. The initial, lateral radiograph (*A*) confirms that the proximal popliteal vein and the portion of the superficial femoral vein that traverses the adductor canal are patent and normal (*arrows*). On the subsequent anteroposterior radiograph (*B*), the patient tensed the thigh musculature, which extrinsically compressed the popliteal and distal superficial femoral veins (note the tapered distal end to the contrast column) and expelled contrast from the adductor canal segment.

FIGURE 132–19. Air bubbles. Anteroposterior films taken a few seconds apart. Multiple rounded filling defects (*arrows*) initially in the distal peroneal vein (*A*) move centrally at the time of the second exposure (*B*).

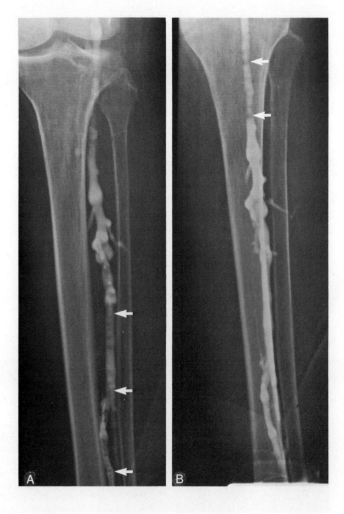

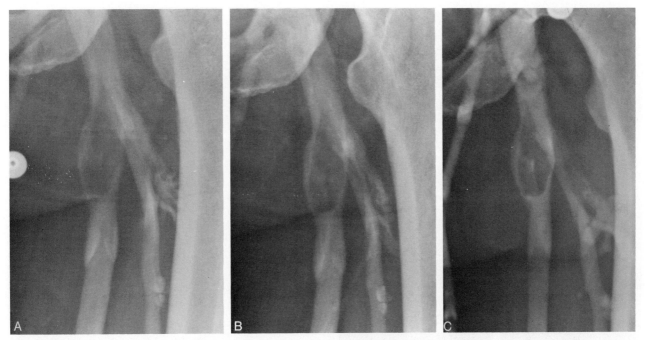

FIGURE 132–20.   Constancy of thrombotic filling defects. The filling defect caused by acute thrombus localized to the region of the femoral vein bifurcation does not change appearance whether the patient is at rest (*A*), sustains a Valsalva maneuver (*B*), or has the lower extremity raised to optimize venous opacification (*C*). Additionally, the thrombus has caused the affected vein to expand in caliber.

FIGURE 132–21.
Pseudo–tram-track sign. *A*, Anteroposterior view of the distal calf. A longitudinal dark stripe (*arrows*) that mimics the appearance of a thrombotic filling defect is in fact caused by superimposed opacities including the tibial cortex and overlapping normal, opacified veins. *B*, An externally rotated radiograph confirms the normalcy of the distal peroneal veins.

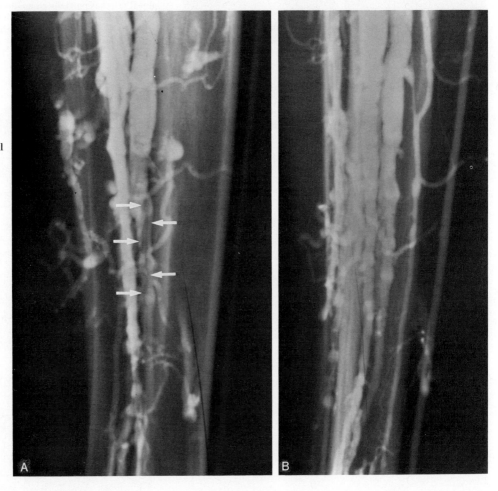

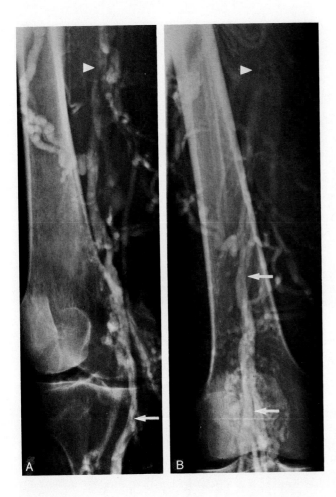

FIGURE 132–22.   Chronic thrombotic occlusion. Lateral (*A*) and anteroposterior (*B*) radiographs of the distal right thigh. The popliteal vein has partially recanalized with multiple webs (*arrows*) and an irregular lumen. The superficial femoral vein is occluded in the mid-thigh (*arrowheads*), with venous drainage provided by multiple enlarged collateral veins.

FIGURE 132–23.   Sequelae of prior venous thrombosis: webs and damaged valves. Lateral (*A*) and anteroposterior (*B*) radiographs just above the knee. Recanalization of prior thrombosis has left both transverse and string-like longitudinal webs (*arrowheads*). In addition, valve cusps have been shortened, thickened, and deformed (*arrows*).

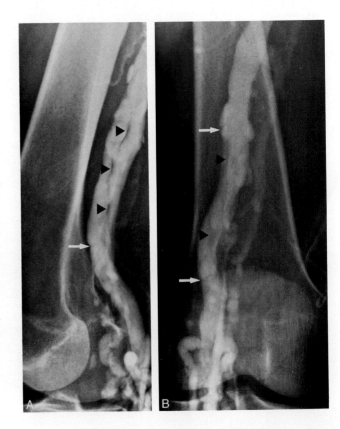

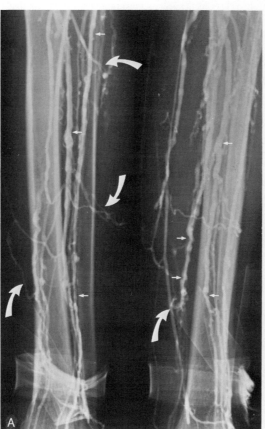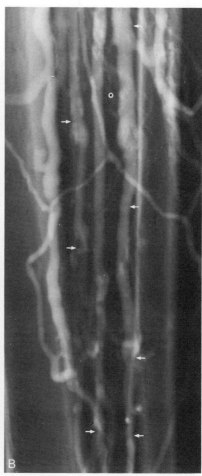

FIGURE 132–24.
Residual of prior venous thrombosis: luminal irregularity and incompetent perforating veins. *A,* Anteroposterior (*left*) and lateral (*right*) radiographs of the calf. *B,* Enlargement of the distal calf. The lumina of the calf conduit veins are patent but manifest undulating margins (*small arrows*) indicative of wall thickening caused by prior thrombus that has subsequently recanalized. Although the ankle tourniquet is not optimally tightened, there is reversed flow in multiple perforating veins (*large arrows*), indicating incompetent valves in these veins.

Role and Modifications of Ascending Venography

Ascending venography may be used to diagnose or exclude chronic venous thrombosis as the underlying cause of chronic venous insufficiency. If the proximal deep venous system is obstructed, stripping of the saphenous vein would be contraindicated because it provides the primary route of venous drainage. Incompetence of the perforating veins is proved by the demonstration of venous flow from the deep venous system to the superficial system (Fig. 132–25).[47] Such a pattern of flow may be identified by placement of a tight tourniquet at the level of the ankle: opacification of the superficial system does not normally occur if the valves in the perforating veins are patent. Additionally, during fluoroscopic monitoring of the venous filling, the specific incompetent perforating veins near an ulcer may be identified. Marking the skin at the site of the offending perforating veins allows the surgeon to ligate the targeted perforating veins with minimal soft tissue dissection.

Descending Venography

Because the normal progression of venous opacification with ascending venography is from peripheral to central, this technique is not useful for detecting incompetent femoral vein valves (reversal of femoral venous flow).[48] Alternatively, in descending venography, contrast medium (which is heavier than blood) is delivered into the common femoral vein, and either gravity or a Valsalva maneuver is used to detect reversed (central to peripheral) blood flow.[48–50] The primary role of descending venography is the detection and quantification of reversed flow, as well as the localization of incompetent valves in the superficial femoral vein before valve transplantation or repair.

Descending venography can be performed either from an ipsilateral femoral vein puncture, with a short end-hole catheter placed so that the tip is located in the distal external iliac vein, or from a contralateral femoral vein puncture, with an angiographic catheter that is passed via the iliocaval junction and has its tip located in the common femoral vein of the leg to be studied. The radiographic table is tilted to an approximately 60 degree reverse Trendelenburg position (head up) (Fig. 132–26).[49] Under fluoroscopic observation, a 60 per cent radiographic contrast medium is slowly injected by hand. Typical volumes required to fill the veins range from 30 to 100 ml. The most distal extent of contrast migration is documented with a spot radiograph, both while the patient is breathing normally and after performing a Valsalva maneuver.

Kistner published a grading scale for quantification of the severity of femoral venous reflux:[51] grade 0 is no incompetence (no contrast refluxes into the superficial femoral

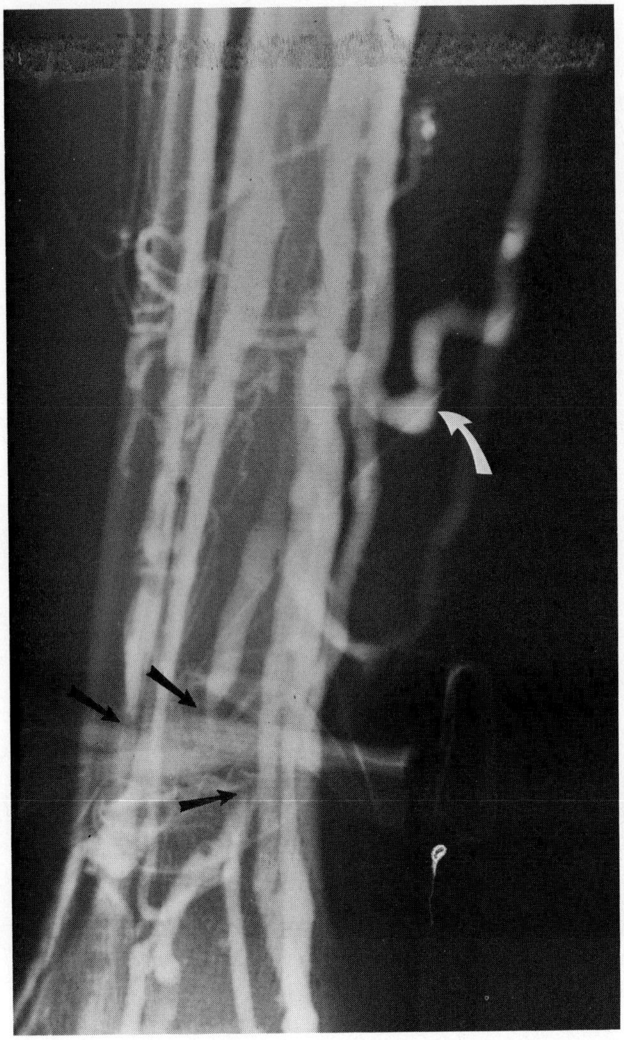

FIGURE 132–25. Incompetent perforating veins. Anteroposterior radiograph of the distal calf. A tight tourniquet located just above the ankle (*black arrows*) occludes nearly all antegrade flow in the superficial veins while preserving flow in the deep conduit veins. Opacification of the superficial veins above the tourniquet occurs by reversed flow (reflux) in the perforating veins (*white arrow*).

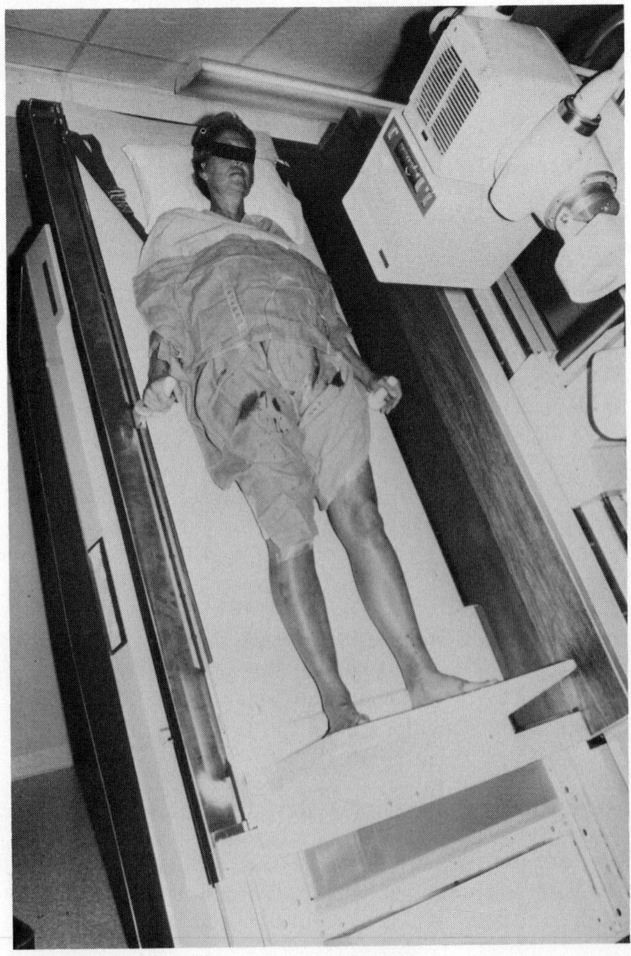

FIGURE 132–26. Descending venography. An angiographic catheter has been inserted into the right femoral vein and fluoroscopically advanced up the right iliac veins and down the left iliac veins so that the tip is located in the left external iliac vein. The sterile field has been taped to the skin. The radiographic table has been tilted to a near-upright position. Contrast medium injected by hand will be fluoroscopically monitored for distal migration and documented by radiographic spot films.

vein); grade 1 is minimal incompetence (contrast refluxes into the superficial femoral vein, but only to the level of the proximal thigh); grade 2 is mild incompetence (contrast refluxes into the popliteal vein to the level of the knee) (Fig. 132–27); grade 3 is moderate incompetence (contrast refluxes into the infrageniculate popliteal vein and possibly into the proximal paired calf trifurcation veins); and grade 4 is severe incompetence (contrast refluxes to the level of the distal calf or ankle). Most authors believe that femoral venous reflux determined by descending venography must be at least of grade 2 to be clinically significant.[49–51] Descending venography has also been shown to demonstrate incompetence of the greater saphenous vein.[52] Because the treatment of varicose veins associated with saphenous vein reflux may include proximal saphenous vein ligation, whereas no such treatment is indicated with primary varicose veins, this distinction is important.

Varicography

After either saphenous vein stripping or proximal ligation, varicose veins may recur. Depiction of the venous anatomy (e.g., duplicated greater saphenous veins or anomalous communications) and delineation of residual incompetent perforating veins are typically obtained with ascending venography. Some authors have reported that direct injection of low-osmolarity contrast agents into each of the variceal groups provides complementary information before repeated operative ablation. Varicography may delineate dilated perforating veins that are in the mid-thigh or that communicate with the gastrocnemius veins.[47, 53, 54]

Saphenography

The greater saphenous vein is a common conduit material for vascular bypass grafts, especially for coronary artery bypass and for femoropopliteal or femorotibial artery bypass. Although preoperative imaging of the donor saphenous vein is not routinely performed, direct injection of low-osmolarity contrast into the saphenous vein may be used to prove that the vein is suitable for harvesting.[55] In order to fill the saphenous vein optimally, no tourniquets are used. Abnormalities that may affect the suitability of the saphenous vein for harvest include small caliber, dupli-

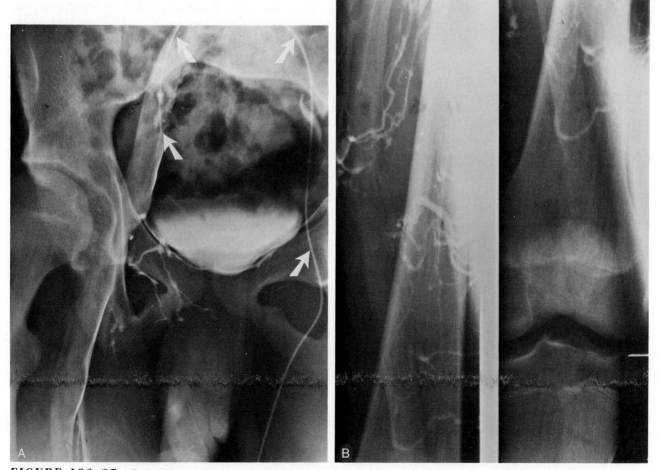

FIGURE 132–27. Descending venogram with valvular incompetence. Anteroposterior radiographs of the pelvis (*A*) and the right thigh and knee (*B*). The catheter (*arrows*) is inserted via the left femoral vein and placed such that the tip is within the right external iliac vein. With the patient in a steep reverse Trendelenburg position and breathing normally, contrast descends to the level of the popliteal vein, indicating common and superficial femoral valvular incompetence of at least Kistner grade 2. Because no significant contrast descends down either the deep femoral or the saphenous veins, the valves in these venous systems are competent.

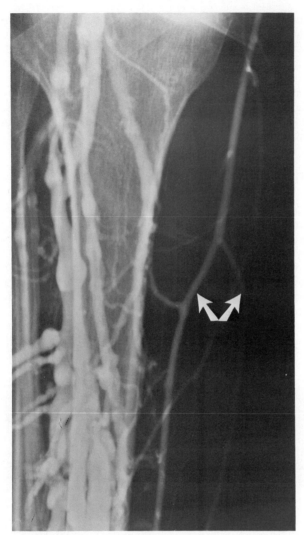

FIGURE 132–28.   Duplicated greater saphenous vein (*arrows*). Ascending venogram; anteroposterior view of the proximal right calf.

cated segments (Fig. 132–28), and absence or damage caused by prior surgical harvesting or stripping. Because of the theoretical risk of contrast-induced endothelial injury, many centers use duplex imaging to "map" the saphenous vein preoperatively.

UPPER EXTREMITY VENOGRAPHY

Clinical Perspective

Although pulmonary emboli infrequently originate from upper extremity veins, obstruction of venous drainage from the upper extremity is an increasingly common problem.[56, 57] Typically, the obstruction is located in the central veins (the axillary, subclavian, and innominate veins, and central portions of the internal jugular vein). Etiologies include extrinsic compression in the thoracic inlet; intimal hyperplasia and superimposed thrombosis related to current or past chronic indwelling central venous

lines or peripheral hemodialysis vascular access sites, or both; and less commonly, central venous invasion by tumor. The clinical issues are usually twofold: (1) diagnosis of the cause and treatment for relief of the patient's arm swelling and discomfort and (2) improvement of central venous flow in order to preserve central venous access (e.g., for total parenteral nutrition or transvenous cardiac pacemaker leads) or function of peripheral hemodialysis access sites. In obstructive upper extremity venous disease, unlike in venous obstruction of the lower extremity, transcatheter techniques (e.g., fibrinolysis, transluminal angioplasty, and the insertion of expandable metallic stents) are commonly employed.

Techniques

Most upper extremity venography is performed in an angiography suite with rapid film changer or digital subtraction angiographic (DSA) capability. Because gravity is not necessary to obtain adequate venous filling, the patient is supine. With the use of a plastic cannula, venous access is made into an antecubital vein, preferably the basilic vein (medial). If antecubital access is not obtainable, a peripheral hand vein can be accessed. A diagnostic study may often be obtained with contrast medium injected peripherally, particularly if DSA image acquisition is used. At the very least, a peripheral venous injection will allow fluoroscopic opacification of the antecubital veins in order to provide a target for venipuncture. Approximately 20- to 30-ml boluses of either 43 or 60 per cent strength contrast medium are hand injected. Serial filming is performed in the region of interest, typically at 1- to 2-second intervals. In most cases, DSA acquisition is diagnostically sufficient so that the contrast medium can be diluted by approximately one half.[58] Contrast injected at or distal to the antecubital fossa will usually spontaneously fill the deep arm and central veins such that a tourniquet is unnecessary unless the cephalic vein is selectively catheterized. The upper extremity is positioned with at least 30 degrees of abduction. If the arm is in complete adduction, the musculature of the shoulder girdle can cause extrinsic compression of the axillary vein or central portions of the brachial vein (Fig. 132–29).

In many cases (e.g., venous obstruction related to a central venous line or suspected thoracic inlet syndrome), the examination may be focused on the region medial to the shoulder, including both the mediastinum and the base of the neck. In patients with suspected superior vena cava involvement, contrast medium should be simultaneously injected into the antecubital veins bilaterally, with serial filming over the upper chest (Fig. 132–30). If the initial venogram in the neutral position shows normal findings in patients with suspected thoracic inlet obstruction (Paget-Schroetter syndrome), a repeated examination should be performed with the patient placed in a provocative maneuver (Fig. 132–31). Provocative maneuvers include the Adson maneuver (neck extended and head turned toward the side being studied while holding full inspiration), the Wright maneuver (head turned away from the side being studied, with the arm abducted fully and laterally rotated), and the costoclavicular maneuver (shoulders pulled dorsally and caudally).[59]

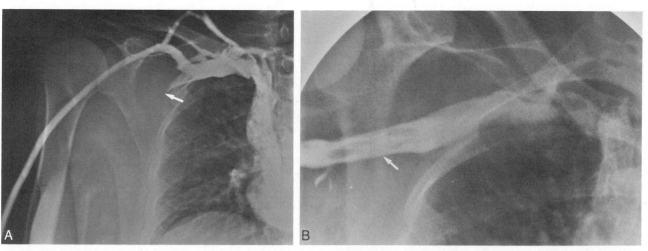

FIGURE 132–29.   Artifactual nonopacification of the brachial vein. Anteroposterior radiographs of the right shoulder with the arm adducted (A) and then abducted (B). The brachial vein (*arrow*) does not opacify because of compression by the shoulder musculature when the arm is adducted. A repeated study with the arm abducted confirms normalcy (*arrow*). (A and B, Courtesy of Antoinette S. Gomes, M.D.)

FIGURE 132–30.   Normal central thoracic veins. Anteroposterior digital subtraction angiogram centered over the upper chest. Simultaneous hand injection of contrast medium into the antecubital veins bilaterally provides diagnostically adequate images of the superior vena cava and the innominate and subclavian veins (all normal in this patient). Incidental indwelling right internal jugular central line is present.

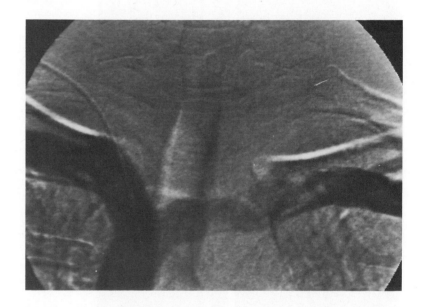

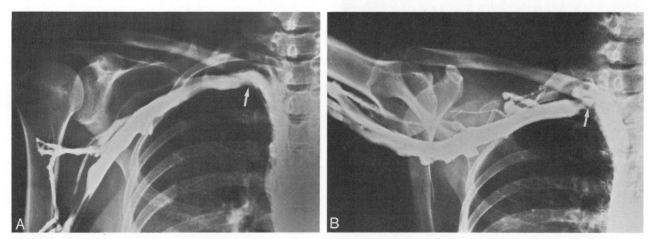

FIGURE 132–31.   Thoracic outlet syndrome. Anteroposterior views of the right shoulder and chest. A, With the arm adducted (note the compression of the basilic and brachial veins), the subclavian vein caliber is normal as the vein passes between the first rib and the clavicle (*arrow*). B, Alternatively, when the arm is abducted and externally rotated, with the head turned to the left (Wright's maneuver), the subclavian vein is markedly narrowed (*arrow*).

Evaluation of hemodialysis vascular access sites requires technical modifications. All such vascular access sites must be routinely evaluated from the peripheral artery-graft or artery-vein anastomosis to the superior vena cava centrally. Vascular access with a dialysis needle or a plastic cannula is obtained either within the graft or in the enlarged venous segment downstream (central) from the arterial anastomosis (i.e., wherever the needles are usually placed for dialysis). In view of the high pressure and flow velocities within the vascular access site, a "biphasic" examination is necessary in order to study the peripheral portions of the fistula (Fig. 132–32). Specifically, a blood pressure cuff is placed over the upper arm and inflated to a suprasystolic pressure in order to occlude arterial inflow. Contrast medium is hand injected, and serial radiographs (either conventional film or DSA) are obtained. When contrast has flowed retrograde into the arterial system (identified directly during DSA acquisition, or by the patient reporting a sensation of heat or pain in the hand), the blood pressure cuff is deflated while filming is continued for several seconds in order to evaluate the venous outflow. Because flow is central (downstream) from the vascular access site, the blood pressure cuff does not need to be inflated for the remainder of the study. An alternate method of arteriovenous shunt evaluation involves injection of contrast medium directly into the brachial artery.[60] Vascular stenosis or occlusion may occur anywhere between the arterial anastomosis and the superior vena cava.[60–63] In order to examine

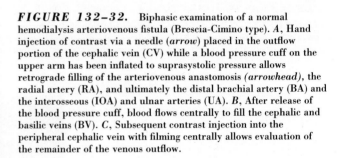

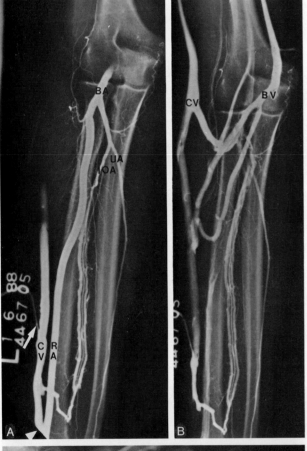

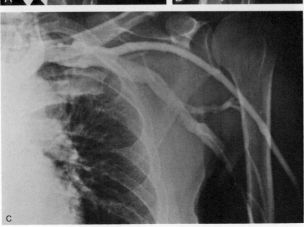

FIGURE 132–32. Biphasic examination of a normal hemodialysis arteriovenous fistula (Brescia-Cimino type). *A*, Hand injection of contrast via a needle *(arrow)* placed in the outflow portion of the cephalic vein (CV) while a blood pressure cuff on the upper arm has been inflated to suprasystolic pressure allows retrograde filling of the arteriovenous anastomosis *(arrowhead)*, the radial artery (RA), and ultimately the distal brachial artery (BA) and the interosseous (IOA) and ulnar arteries (UA). *B*, After release of the blood pressure cuff, blood flows centrally to fill the cephalic and basilic veins (BV). *C*, Subsequent contrast injection into the peripheral cephalic vein with filming centrally allows evaluation of the remainder of the venous outflow.

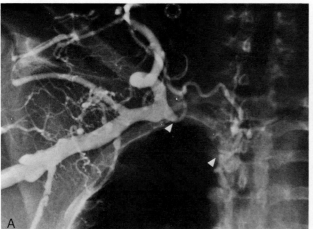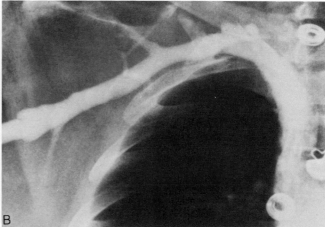

FIGURE 132–33. Subclavian vein occlusion. *A,* Anteroposterior radiograph of the right shoulder and chest in a patient with a peripheral hemodialysis access site and recent onset of right upper extremity swelling and elevated hemodialysis venous return pressures (240 mmHg). The subclavian vein is occluded (*between tips of arrowheads*). Numerous collateral veins provide venous drainage; the innominate vein is reconstituted at the level of the *more central arrowhead.* The occluded segment was probed with the reversed end of a heavy-duty guidewire. The occluded segment was very firm and most likely represented intimal hyperplasia. *B,* Subsequent balloon dilatation restored both an angiographically and a functionally normal lumen.

the entire length of venous outflow, multiple overlapping fields of view are necessary, each with a separate injection of contrast medium.

Interpretation

Central venous obstruction is usually manifest directly as either narrowing or occlusion of the lumen and indirectly by the presence of collateral draining veins (Fig. 132–33). Unless a fixed intraluminal filling defect (tram-track sign) is present, it may be impossible to distinguish narrowing or occlusion caused by intimal hyperplasia from that caused by thrombus. In some cases, it may be warranted to attempt passage of a guidewire or to perform a therapeutic trial of transcatheter local thrombolysis (see Fig. 132–33). Assessment of collateral veins provides important corroborative hemodynamic information. If collateral veins are identified but no site of central venous obstruction has been identified, one must suspect that an obstruction is present but somehow obscured, such that views in other projections are warranted. If an apparent narrowing is identified venographically but is not associated with collateral veins, the hemodynamic significance of the narrowing is suspect. Venous narrowing related to thoracic inlet compression is often eccentric, primarily occurring along the inferior margin of the subclavian vein as it courses over the first rib, and it is typically worsened by one of the aforementioned provocative maneuvers (see Fig. 132–31).

Diagnostic difficulties caused by the inflow of non-opacified blood simulating either thrombus or a stenosis are most evident where the external and internal jugular veins join the subclavian vein (Fig. 132–34). The characteristic location, changing morphology, and absence of collateral veins are usually diagnostic.

In patients with indwelling central lines, the intraluminal filling defect caused by thrombus may be subtle, surrounding the catheter like a stocking (Fig. 132–35).[64]

Gentle hand injection of contrast medium via the indwelling catheter lumen will frequently confirm the presence of a fibrin sheath enveloping the catheter. Often, contrast medium fills the surrounding pocket and is not washed away quickly. Additionally, in patients presenting with malfunction of indwelling central lines, radiographic inspection of the catheter is mandated to exclude kinks or malposition of the tip into a tributary vein.

Closed-System Venography

Vascular malformations with a venous but no arteriocapillary component and some hemangiomas will not be opacified by arteriography. Delineation of the feeding veins as well as of the full extent of the angiodysplasia can be

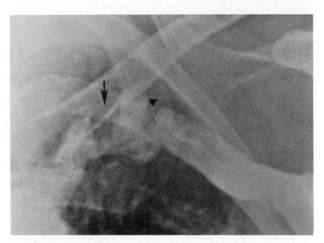

FIGURE 132–34. Jugular vein inflow artifacts. Anteroposterior exposure of the left side of the chest after contrast injection of an antecubital vein. Filling defects within the opacified subclavian vein represent inflow of nonopacified blood from the internal jugular (*arrow*) and external jugular (*arrowhead*) veins.

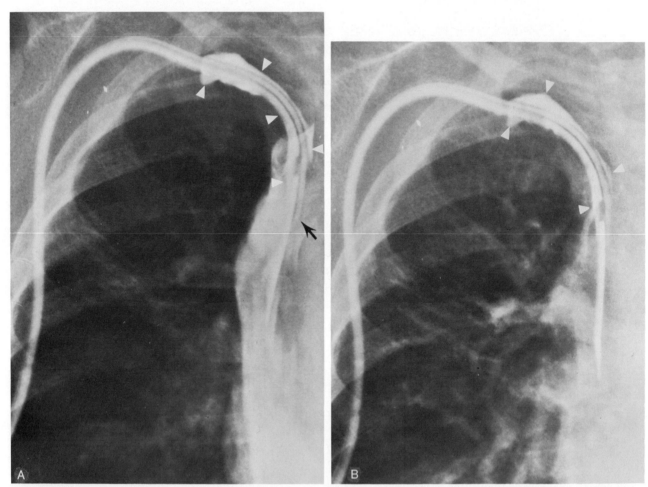

FIGURE 132–35.   Fibrin sheath on a central line. *A,* Anteroposterior radiograph of the right side of the chest after hand injection of contrast into a malfunctioning double-lumen hemodialysis catheter. Blood flow rates were insufficient for timely hemodialysis when blood was aspirated from the lumen with the upstream end-hole (*black arrow*). When contrast is injected via the malfunctioning port, in addition to normal filling of the superior vena cava, there is filling of a pocket (*arrowheads*) around the catheter that is contained by a fibrin sheath. *B,* After the termination of contrast injection, contrast remains trapped between the catheter and the surrounding fibrin sheath (*arrowheads*).

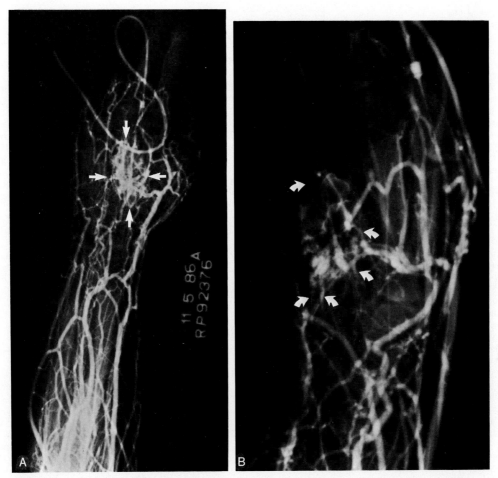

FIGURE 132–36. Venous malformation on closed-system venography. Anteroposterior (A) and enlarged oblique (B) views of the forearm and hand after compressive exsanguination and subsequent filling of the venous system with contrast medium. The venous malformation is delineated by *straight arrows*. The draining veins (*curved arrows*) are normal in caliber. Thrombi (filling defects) are present within the ectatic venous channels.

achieved with the complete forced filling obtainable with the closed-system venographic technique.[65] A peripheral vein in the vicinity of the suspected malformation is accessed with a plastic cannula. Exsanguination of the extremity being studied is accomplished with a 4- to 6-inch-wide Esmarch bandage (Cypress Medical Products, Buffalo Groves, IL), which is tightly wrapped from the digits centrally. The arterial inflow is temporarily occluded by a blood pressure cuff inflated to suprasystolic levels. The Esmarch bandage is removed. Contrast medium (30 to 45 per cent) is slowly injected by hand while venous filling is fluoroscopically monitored. Spot radiographs in multiple projections are obtained as the malformation and the feeding veins fill.

The malformation is characterized by a tangle of dilated, tortuous venous channels, which occasionally contain filling defects that represent thrombus caused by stasis of blood flow (Fig. 132–36). Capillary and venous malformations or angiodysplasias are characterized by feeding arteries that are smaller in caliber than the adjacent veins, whereas the arteries are larger in caliber in arteriovenous malformations. The dilated veins that connect the malformation to the normal venous system can often be fluoro-

scopically localized; marking the skin over the communicating veins may assist in the operative approach.

References

1. Berberich J, Hirsch S: Die röntgenologische Darstellung der Arterien und Venen im lebenden Menschen. Klin Wochenschr 49:2226, 1923.
2. Rabinov K, Paulin S: Roentgen diagnosis of venous thrombosis in the leg. Arch Surg 104:134, 1972.
3. Thomas ML: Phlebography. Arch Surg 1104:145, 1972.
4. Hull R, Hirsh J, Sackett DL, et al: Cost effectiveness of clinical diagnosis, venography, and noninvasive testing in patients with symptomatic deep vein thrombosis. N Engl J Med 304:1561, 1981.
5. Ramsay LE: Impact of venography on the diagnosis and management of deep vein thrombosis. Br Med J 286:698, 1983.
6. Lund F, Diener L, Ericsson JLE: Postmortem intraosseous phlebography as an aid in studies of venous thromboembolism with application on a geriatric clientele. Angiology 20:155, 1969.
7. Hull R, Hirsh J, Sackett DL, et al: Clinical validity of a negative venogram in patients with clinically suspected venous thrombosis. Circulation 64:622, 1981.
8. McLachlan MSF, Thompson JG, Taylor DW, et al: Observed variation in the interpretation of lower limb venograms. AJR 132:227, 1979.
9. Illescas FF, Leclerc J, Rosenthall L, et al: Interobserver variability in the interpretation of contrast venography, technetium-99m red blood

cell venography and impedance plethysmography for deep vein thrombosis. J Can Assoc Radiol 41:264, 1990.

10. Wille-Jorgensen P, Borris L, Jorgensen LN, et al: Phlebography as the gold standard in thromboprophylactic studies? A multicenter inter-observer variation study. Acta Radiol 33:24, 1992.

11. May R: Anatomy. In Surgery of the Veins of the Leg and Pelvis. Philadelphia, WB Saunders, 1979, pp 4–7.

12. Rose SC: Unpublished data.

13. Cotton LT, Clark C: Anatomical localization of venous thrombosis. Ann R Coll Surg Engl 36:214, 1965.

14. Nicolaides AN, Kakkar VV, Field ES, et al: The origin of deep vein thrombosis: A venographic study. Br J Radiol 44:653, 1971.

15. Stamatakis JD, Kakkar VV, Lawrence D, et al: The origin of thrombi in the deep veins of the lower limb: A venographic study. Br J Surg 65:449, 1978.

16. Browse NL, Thomas ML: Source of non-lethal pulmonary emboli. Lancet 1:258, 1974.

17. Coel MN: Adequacy of lower limb venous opacification: Comparison of supine and upright phlebography. AJR 134:163, 1980.

18. Mavor GE, Galloway JMD: Collaterals of the deep venous circulation of the lower limb. Surg Gynecol Obstet 125:561, 1967.

19. Ferris EJ, Lim WN, Smith PL, et al: May-Thurner Syndrome. Radiology 147:29, 1983.

20. Gothlin J: The comparative frequency of extravasal injection at phlebography with steel and plastic cannula. Clin Radiol 23:183, 1972.

21. Johns CM, Sumkin JH: US-guided venipuncture for venography in the edematous leg. Radiology 180:573, 1991.

22. Bhargava R, Millward SF: Contrast venography in patients with very edematous feet: Use of transdermal illumination to aid in vein puncture. Radiology 179:583, 1991.

23. Ansell G, Tweedie MCK, West CR, et al: The current status of reactions to intravenous contrast media. Invest Radiol 15:S32, 1980.

24. Cohan RH, Dunnick NR, Bashore TM: Treatment of reactions to radiographic contrast material. AJR 151:263, 1988.

25. Palmer FJ: The R.A.C.R. survey of intravenous contrast media reactions. A preliminary report. Australas Radiol 32:8, 1988.

26. Katayama H, Yamaguchi K, Kozuka T, et al: Adverse reactions to ionic and nonionic contrast media. A report from the Japanese Committee on the Safety of Contrast Media. Radiology 175:621, 1990.

27. Cochran ST, Wong WS, Roe DJ: Predicting angiography-induced acute renal function impairment: Clinical risk model. AJR 141:1027, 1983.

28. Taliercio CP, Vlietstra RE, Fisher LD, et al: Risks for renal dysfunction with cardiac angiography. Ann Intern Med 104:501, 1986.

29. Parfrey PS, Griffiths SM, Barrett BJ, et al: Contrast material-induced renal failure in patients with diabetes mellitus, renal insufficiency, or both. A prospective controlled study. N Engl J Med 320:143, 1989.

30. Schwab SJ, Hlatky MA, Pieper KS, et al: Contrast nephrotoxicity: A randomized controlled trial of a nonionic and an ionic radiographic contrast agent. N Engl J Med 320:149, 1989.

31. Ritchie WGM, Lynch PR, Stewart GJ: The effect of contrast media on normal and inflamed canine veins. Invest Radiol 9:444, 1974.

32. Albrechtsson V, Olsson C-G: Thrombotic side-effects of lower-limb phlebography. Lancet 1:723, 1976.

33. Walters HL, Clemenson J, Browse NL, et al: 125 I-fibrinogen uptake following phlebography of the leg. Comparison of ionic and nonionic contrast media. Radiology 135:619, 1980.

34. Laerum F, Holm HA: Postphlebographic thrombosis. A double-blind study with methylglucamine metrizoate and metrizamide. Radiology 140:657, 1981.

35. Bettman MA, Salzman EW, Rosenthal D, et al: Reduction of venous thrombosis complicating phlebography. AJR 134:1169, 1980.

36. Bettman MA, Robbins A, Braun SD, et al: Contrast venography of the legs: Diagnostic efficacy, tolerance, and complication rates with ionic and nonionic contrast media. Radiology 165:113, 1987.

37. Lensing AWA, Prandoni P, Buller HR, et al: Lower extremity venography with iohexol: Results and complications. Radiology 177:503, 1990.

38. Arndt RD, Grollman JH Jr, Gomes AS, et al: The heparin flush: An

aid in preventing post-venography thrombophlebitis. Radiology 130:249, 1979.

39. Brockman SK, Vasko JS: The pathologic physiology of phlegmasia cerulea dolens. Surgery 59:997, 1966.

40. Gothlin J, Hallbook T: Skin necrosis following extravasal injection of contrast medium at phlebography. Radiologe 11:161, 1971.

41. Spigos DG, Thane TT, Capek V: Skin necrosis following extravasation during peripheral phlebography. Radiology 123:605, 1977.

42. Gordon IJ: Evaluation of suspected deep venous thrombosis in the arteriosclerotic patient. AJR 131:531, 1978.

43. Montgomery S: Pulmonary embolism during venography: Report of a rare complication. Cardiovasc Intervent Radiol 12:196, 1989.

44. Thomas ML, McAllister V: The radiological progression of deep venous thrombus. Radiology 99:37, 1971.

45. Zachrisson BE, Jansen HJ: Phlebographic signs in fresh postoperative venous thrombosis of the lower extremity. Acta Radiol Diagn 14:82, 1973.

46. Martin EC, Cohen L, Sawyer PN, et al: Supine pedal venous pressure measurement in patients with venous disease. Radiology 131:75, 1979.

47. Thomas ML, Bowles JN: Incompetent perforating veins: Comparison of varicography and ascending phlebography. Radiology 154:619, 1985.

48. Herman RJ, Neiman HL, Yao JST, et al: Descending venography: A method of evaluating lower extremity venous valvular function. Radiology 137:63, 1980.

49. Morano JU, Raju S: Chronic venous insufficiency: Assessment with descending venography. Radiology 174:441, 1990.

50. Athanasoulis CA, Yucel EK: Venous reflux: Assessing the level of incompetence. Radiology 174:326, 1990.

51. Kistner RL: Transvenous repair of the incompetent femoral vein valve. In Bergan JJ, Yao TST (eds): Venous Problems. Chicago, Year Book Medical Publishers, 1978, pp 493–509.

52. Thomas ML, Bowles JN: Descending phlebography in the assessment of long saphenous vein incompetence. AJR 145:1255, 1985.

53. Gordon DH, Glanz S, Stillman R, et al: Descending varicose venography of the lower extremities: An alternate method to evaluate the deep venous system. Radiology 145:832, 1982.

54. Loveday EJ, Thomas ML: The distribution of recurrent varicose veins: A phlebographic study. Clin Radiol 43:47, 1991.

55. Thomas ML, Posniak HV: Saphenography. AJR 141:812, 1983.

56. Swinton NW Jr, Edgett JW, Hall RJ: Primary subclavian-axillary vein thrombosis. Circulation 38:737, 1968.

57. McCarthy WJ, Vogelzang RL, Bergan JJ: Changing concepts and present-day etiology of upper extremity venous thrombosis. In Bergan JJ, Yao JST (eds): Venous Disorders. Philadelphia, WB Saunders, 1991, pp 407–420.

58. Kinnison ML, Kaufman SL, Chang R, et al: Upper extremity venography using digital subtraction angiography. Cardiovasc Intervent Radiol 9:106, 1986.

59. Pang D, Wessel HB: Thoracic outlet syndrome. Neurosurgery 22:105, 1988.

60. Glanz S, Bashist B, Gordon DH, et al: Angiography of upper extremity access fistulas for dialysis. Radiology 143:45, 1982.

61. Gordon DH, Glanz S, Butt KM, et al: Treatment of stenotic lesions in dialysis access fistulas and shunts by transluminal angioplasty. Radiology 143:53, 1982.

62. Saeed M, Newman GE, McCann RL, et al: Stenoses in dialysis fistulas: Treatment with percutaneous angioplasty. Radiology 164:693, 1987.

63. Gmelin E, Winterhoff R, Rinast E: Insufficient hemodialysis access fistulas: Late results of treatment with percutaneous balloon angioplasty. Radiology 171:657, 1989.

64. Zajko AB, Reilly JJ Jr, Bron KM, et al: Low-dose streptokinase for occluded Hickman catheters. AJR 141:1311, 1983.

65. Braun SD, Moore AV Jr, Mills SR, et al: Closed-system venography in the evaluation of angiodysplastic lesions of the extremities. AJR 141:1307, 1983.

133

Laboratory Evaluation of the Patient With Chronic Venous Insufficiency

Enrique Criado, M.D.

· · ·

The fundamental pathophysiologic derangement found in patients with chronic venous insufficiency is persistent elevation of the venous pressure at rest and during exercise. This sustained increase in venous pressure is secondary to failure of the calf muscle pump mechanism to empty the lower extremity veins adequately. Failure of the calf muscle pump function may be caused by valvular incompetence, venous obstruction, calf muscle impairment, or a combination of these factors. Therefore, the diagnosis of chronic venous insufficiency should be directed toward elucidation of these problems and determination of how each contributes to the severity of chronic venous insufficiency.

The diagnostic evaluation of chronic venous insufficiency is both functional and anatomic. The investigation should determine whether the patient has valvular reflux, venous outflow obstruction, or both; should quantitate the severity of each; and should precisely localize which venous segments are involved in each problem. Valvular incompetence is the prevailing functional problem in patients presenting with chronic venous insufficiency. The majority of patients (more than 90 per cent) with advanced venous insufficiency who present with skin ulceration (class III chronic venous insufficiency, according to the Society for Vascular Surgery/International Society for Cardiovascular Surgery [SVS/ISCVS] reporting standards on venous disease[1]) have valvular incompetence as the prevailing problem, whereas only a minority have venous obstruction as an isolated underlying cause.[2–4] The old, widespread concept that chronic venous insufficiency leading to skin ulceration is always secondary to deep vein pathology and that superficial venous incompetence is rarely the cause is no longer sustainable. It has been shown that more than one third of patients with class III venous insufficiency have valvular incompetence confined to the superficial veins, the perforating veins, or both, without evidence of any deep vein involvement, and in one half of those patients, the valvular incompetence is isolated to the superficial system.[2] Patients with reflux confined to the superficial and communicating systems can be treated surgically, with predictably good results, whereas patients with deep venous valvular incompetence require complex venous reconstructions, which have lower success rates and worse long-term prognoses. Therefore, because of the significant therapeutic and prognostic implications, it is very important to determine whether the venous reflux involves the deep, superficial, or communicating veins.

Unfortunately, no single diagnostic tool is capable of delivering all of the information required to understand completely the pathophysiology of chronic venous insufficiency. To obtain this information, the author currently relies on several diagnostic tests that in combination are able to provide both anatomic and quantitative functional data. Some tests are purely qualitative (e.g., Doppler venous examination and photoplethysmography), some incorporate precise anatomic and functional information (e.g., duplex ultrasonography), and others assess venous function in a global quantitative fashion (e.g., ambulatory venous pressure measurement and air plethysmography). The physiologic approach to the treatment of the patient with chronic venous insufficiency requires knowledge of whether there is venous obstruction or valvular incompetence and to what extent the deep, superficial, and communicating systems are involved. The ability to conduct an appropriate work-up in a patient with chronic venous insufficiency and to reach a correct diagnosis that will enable optimal treatment depends on the clinician's understanding of the capabilities and limitations of all tests available.

The laboratory evaluation of chronic venous insufficiency is evolving rapidly. However, despite the enormous improvements made in the available technology, reliable and accurate quantitation of venous obstruction and reflux remains elusive.

AMBULATORY VENOUS PRESSURE

Venous hypertension, the main pathophysiologic consequence of chronic venous insufficiency, is the net result of venous outflow obstruction, valvular incompetence, calf muscle failure, or their combination. In 1949, Pollack and Wood observed that muscle contraction during exercise increases the blood return from the lower limbs, thus reducing lower extremity venous pressure.[5] They also noted that when walking stops, there is a gradual return to the resting venous pressure level. Arnoldi and associates demonstrated that variations in venous pressure are identical in the deep and superficial venous systems, which validated the use of superficial foot vein pressure monitoring for the investigation of deep venous disorders.[6] The ambulatory venous pressure (AVP) is defined as the venous pressure in the superficial foot veins after 10 tiptoe exercises performed by the patient in the standing position. Measurement of the AVP reflects the basic hemodynamic derangement present in patients with chronic venous insufficiency and is considered the hemodynamic gold standard for validating the results of noninvasive venous testing and for substantiating the results of venous surgery. The measurement of AVP quantitates the net effect of all hemodynamic factors involved in venous insufficiency, but it does not give any information about the individual components contributing to the problem. AVP measurement is an invasive procedure that cannot be used repeatedly or as a screening test.

The AVP is obtained by cannulating a superficial foot vein with a 21- or 23-gauge butterfly needle and connecting it to a pressure transducer and a pen recorder. The resting baseline venous pressure is measured with the patient standing and holding on to a frame to avoid calf muscle contraction. The patient performs 10 tiptoe exercises at a rate of 1 per second and returns to the original resting position, remaining steady as the venous refilling time is recorded. To determine the influence of the superficial and perforating veins on the refilling time, the procedure can be repeated with tourniquets or thin cuffs to occlude the superficial system above the knee, below the knee, or at the ankle. Correction of the refill time with a tourniquet implies the presence of an incompetent saphenous system, perforators above the level of the tourniquet, or both. Failure of the tourniquet application to improve refilling time is interpreted as incompetence of deep veins, communicating veins, or both. Deep venous obstruction may manifest as an increase, rather than a decrease, in venous pressure during exercise or when the resting baseline pressure is exceeded during the hyperemic phase after exercise.

AVP values in normal patients and in patients with venous disease are presented in Table 133–1. Nicolaides and Zukowski found that the highest venous pressure levels are associated with perforator and deep venous incompetence and that competence of the popliteal vein is an important factor in determining the severity of venous hypertension.[7] They also demonstrated the existence of a linear correlation between increasing levels of AVP and the incidence of leg ulceration (Table 133–2). AVP measurement is currently used for validation of new diagnostic techniques, for hemodynamic assessment of the results of deep venous surgery, and for clinical investigation.

Table 133–1.   Range of Ambulatory Venous Pressure Values in Normal Limbs and in Limbs With Venous Disease

Type of Limb	Ambulatory Venous Pressure (mmHg)
Normal	15–30
Varicose veins with competent perforators	25–40
Varicose veins with incompetent perforators	40–70
Deep valvular incompetence	55–85
Deep valvular incompetence with proximal obstruction	60–110
Proximal obstruction with a competent popliteal vein	25–60

Adapted from Nicolaides AN, Zukowski AJ: The value of dynamic venous pressure measurements. World J Surg 10:919, 1986.

Table 133–2.   Incidence of Skin Ulceration (Active or Healed) in Relation to the Ambulatory Venous Pressure Level in 251 Limbs

No. of Limbs	Ambulatory Venous Pressure (mmHg)	Incidence of Ulceration (%)
34	<30	0
44	31–40	12
51	41–50	22
45	51–60	38
34	61–70	57
28	71–80	68
15	>80	73

From Nicolaides AN, Sumner DS: Investigation of Patients with Deep Vein Thrombosis and Chronic Venous Insufficiency. Los Angeles, Med-Orion, 1991, p 30.

Despite the value of this test, AVP values are within normal limits in approximately 20 to 25 per cent of patients with stasis ulceration.[8] Furthermore, there is poor correlation between AVP measurements and the results of deep valvular reconstruction. These problems imply that other factors may be involved in the origin of stasis ulceration. To improve the predictive value of venous pressure measurement, Raju and Fredericks introduced the concept of a reflux index, which is defined as the product of multiplying the AVP by the venous pressure elevation that occurs in the supine position during a sustained Valsalva maneuver at 30 to 40 mmHg.[8] Using a reflux index of 150 as the discriminant point, these investigators found that 98 per cent of patients with ulcers fell beyond this level, implying that a reflux index below 150 has a 98 per cent predictive value in determining the absence of skin ulceration (Fig. 133–1). Furthermore, they showed that patients with successful valvular reconstructions experienced a significant decrease in the reflux index, whereas those who did not have clinical improvement had increased reflux indices.

The Valsalva-induced foot venous pressure elevation may represent the degree of transmission of venous pressure from the deep to the superficial system. If the communications between the deep and superficial systems are large and incompetent, the potential for pressure transmission is undamped, whereas with small and competent communications, the pressure transmission would be damped. In summary, although AVP measurement is the most accurate hemodynamic parameter currently available, it is not without limitations.

AIR PLETHYSMOGRAPHY

Air plethysmography is a noninvasive technique that allows detection of lower extremity volume changes in relation to gravity and exercise. Its application to the diagnosis of venous disease is based on the premise that acute changes in limb volume are almost entirely secondary to changes in venous blood content. Although this technique has been available for several decades, it was not until Christopoulos and Nicolaides introduced calibrated air plethysmography in the 1980s that it became useful for the quantitative evaluation of venous hemodynamics.

The air plethysmograph is a fairly simple device consisting of a 14-inch-long inflatable plastic sleeve with a 5-

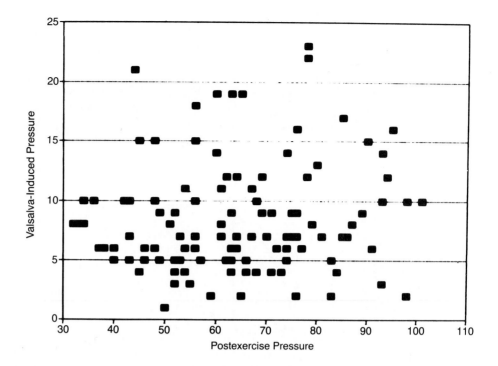

FIGURE 133-1. Valsalva-induced venous pressure elevation plotted against postexercise ambulatory venous pressure in 113 limbs with ulceration. Fifteen per cent of the limbs had normal Valsalva-induced venous pressure (4 mmHg or lower), whereas 22 per cent of the limbs had normal ambulatory venous pressure (50 mmHg or lower). However, only 2 per cent had a reflux index (Valsalva-induced venous pressure × ambulatory venous pressure) of less than 150. (From Raju S, Fredericks R: Hemodynamic basis of stasis ulceration—A hypothesis. J Vasc Surg 13:491, 1991.)

L capacity that is placed around the leg from below the knee to the ankle. The air chamber is connected with plastic tubing to a pressure transducer, an amplifier, and a pen recorder. With the patient supine, the heel resting on a support, and the leg externally rotated and slightly flexed to facilitate venous emptying, the chamber is inflated to a pressure of 6 mmHg to obtain good contact between the sleeve and the limb (Fig. 133–2). With the patient in this position, the plethysmograph is calibrated by injecting a standard volume of air (100 cc) into the chamber, measuring the change in pressure, and withdrawing the same volume again. Once the calibration is satisfactory, the volume changes are recorded during a sequence of exercises to elicit leg emptying with 45 degrees of elevation, leg refill

in the standing non–weight-bearing position, calf blood ejection during 1 bilateral tiptoe exercise and during 10 consecutive tiptoe exercises, and finally refill again in the standing non–weight-bearing position (Fig. 133–3). The performance of the test requires patient cooperation and fastidious technique to avoid artifacts derived from contact of the air chamber with any object or from muscle contraction in the standing position. A small number of patients cannot undergo testing with air plethysmography because of their extreme leg size or their inability to perform the exercise routine.

From the volume recording, measurements of venous hemodynamics are obtained directly or are calculated. The functional venous volume, venous filling time, calf ejection

FIGURE 133-2. Calibration of the air plethysmograph. With the patient supine, the heel resting on a support, and the leg slightly flexed and externally rotated, the air chamber is filled to a pressure of 6 mmHg. Calibration is performed by injecting and withdrawing a standard volume of air in the system (100 cc) and observing the variation in pressure on the recording.

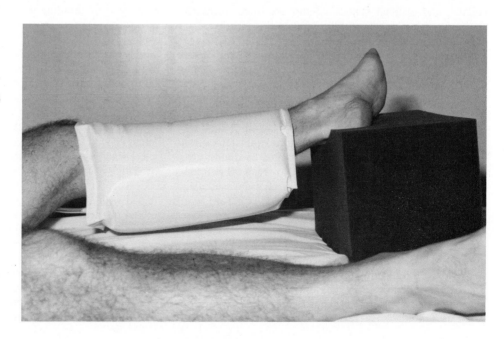

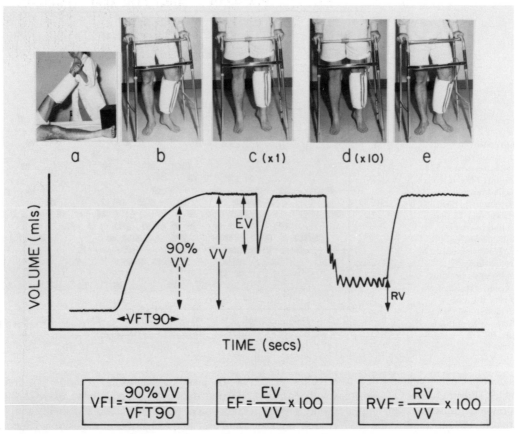

$$VFI = \frac{90\% VV}{VFT90}$$

$$EF = \frac{EV}{VV} \times 100$$

$$RVF = \frac{RV}{VV} \times 100$$

FIGURE 133–3.   Limb volume changes recorded during the standard sequence of postural changes and tiptoe exercises performed with calibrated air plethysmography. After calibration, the patient lies supine with 45-degree passive leg elevation with slight knee flexion and external rotation until maximal venous emptying occurs (*a*). The patient stands up without bearing weight on the leg under examination until maximal venous filling occurs (first plateau of the tracing) (*b*). The patient performs a single tiptoe exercise with both legs and returns to non–weight bearing (*c*). After reaching the second complete venous filling plateau, the patient performs 10 consecutive tiptoe exercises (*d*) and again returns to the non–weight-bearing position as in *b* (*e*). VV, functional venous volume; VFT, venous filling time; VFI, venous filling index; EF, ejection fraction; EV, ejected volume; RV, residual volume; RVF, residual volume fraction. (Courtesy of Cindy Burnham, R.N., R.V.T.)

volume, and residual venous volume are direct measurements, whereas the venous filling index, calf ejection fraction, and residual volume fraction are calculated values. The functional venous volume (VV) represents the increase in leg venous volume from supine leg elevation to the standing position and is given in milliliters. VV evaluates venous capacitance, which tends to be elevated in limbs with chronic venous insufficiency. The venous filling index (VFI) is a measure of the rate of venous refill of the limb expressed in milliliters per second, and it evaluates overall valvular competence. The VFI is calculated by dividing 90 per cent of the VV by the time taken to reach 90 per cent of the VV (VFT$_{90}$). The ejection volume (EV) measures the decrease in venous volume (in milliliters) achieved with one tiptoe exercise and represents the volume of blood expelled by the calf with a single calf muscle contraction. The ejection fraction (EF) is calculated by dividing the EV by the VV and multiplying the result by 100. This percentage represents the emptying power of one calf contraction. The residual volume (RV) measures the amount of blood left in the calf at the end of 10 consecutive tiptoe exercises, given in milliliters. The residual volume fraction (RVF) is

calculated by dividing the RV by the VV and multiplying by 100 to express the percentage of the total calf blood volume that remains in the calf after 10 tiptoe exercises, which evaluates overall calf muscle pump function. When the VFI is elevated, the test is repeated with an above-knee tourniquet to assess the influence of the superficial system on the degree of reflux. The coefficient of variability in the measurement on different days of VFI, EF, and RVF is lower than that for VV, VFT, EV, and RV because the latter depend on the daily fluctuations of venous compliance, whereas the former are normalized values not affected by daily variations.[9]

The reliability of the hemodynamic information obtained with air plethysmography is based on the direct correlation between the RVF and AVP (Fig. 133–4).[9, 10] Christopoulos and coworkers found that 80 per cent of limbs with venous disease had increased VV and that the VFI was less than 1.7 ml/sec in normal limbs, between 2 and 30 ml/sec in limbs with superficial incompetence, and 7 to 28 ml/sec in limbs with evidence of deep venous disease.[9] Furthermore, they demonstrated an increasing incidence of skin ulceration with increasing levels of RVF (Table

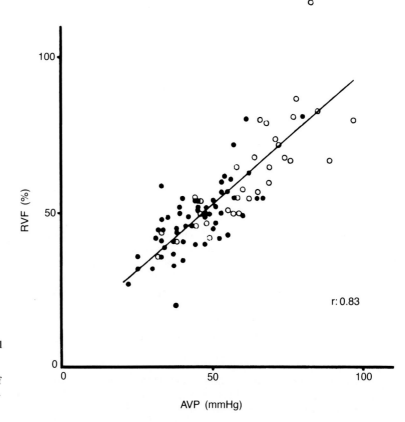

FIGURE 133–4. There is a linear correlation between the residual volume fraction (RVF) measured with air plethysmography and the ambulatory venous pressure (AVP) measured at the end of 10 tiptoe exercises. *Closed circles* represent limbs with superficial incompetence; *open circles*, limbs with deep venous disease. (From Christopoulos DG, Nicolaides AN, Szendro G, et al: Air-plethysmography and the effect of elastic compression on venous hemodynamics of the leg. J Vasc Surg 5:148, 1987.)

133–3). An increase in the incidence of ulceration was observed by Christopoulos and associates with increasing levels of reflux and decreasing values of calf EF.[11] In limbs with minimal reflux, a low EF is associated with a high incidence of ulceration, whereas limbs with severe reflux are protected from ulceration in the presence of a good EF (Table 133–4).[11] Accordingly, the incidence of leg ulceration escalates with increasing values of RVF.[11] More recently, Welch and colleagues reported that VFI values obtained with air plethysmography could differentiate normal limbs from those with reflux but could not differentiate between limbs with mild reflux and those with severe reflux as assessed with descending phlebography.[12] In summary, the combination of hemodynamic parameters obtained with air plethysmography offers quantitative information about the presence of reflux (VFI), the integrity of the calf muscle pump mechanism (EF), and the overall venous function (RVF).

The application of calibrated air plethysmography to the evaluation of chronic venous insufficiency appears scientifically and medically sound. The cumulative experience and available data with this test are limited, however. Although this technology is useful and promising, before it is embraced permanently, it would be optimal to see its reproducibility and clinical validity corroborated by a greater number of different laboratories.

EVALUATION OF VALVULAR INCOMPETENCE

Venous valvular incompetence, or venous reflux, is produced by the presence of pathologic reverse venous flow that occurs when vein valves are congenitally absent or, more commonly, when valves are damaged by acquired processes such as the recanalization of venous thrombosis or undue venous dilatation. Reflux can involve any of the valves of the superficial, deep, or communicating veins, and its severity is proportional to the number of valves and venous territories involved and to the amount of blood that refluxes in each vein.

To evaluate venous valvular function appropriately, it is essential to understand the physiology of valve closure. Because venous reflux is in great part the result of gravity, it should be measured in the standing position. It is impor-

Table 133–3. Incidence of Skin Ulceration (Active or Healed) in Relation to the Residual Volume Fraction Measured With Air-Plethysmography in 175 Limbs With Venous Disease

Residual Volume Fraction (%)	No. of Limbs	Limbs With Ulceration (%)
<30	20	0
31–40	24	8
41–50	48	18
51–60	43	42
61–80	32	72
>80	8	88

From Christopoulos D, Nicolaides AN, Cook A, et al: Pathogenesis of venous ulceration in relation to the calf muscle pump function. Surgery 106:829, 1989.

Table 133–4.   Incidence of Ulceration in 175 Limbs With Venous Disease in Relation to the Venous Filling Index and the Ejection Fraction of the Calf Muscle Pump

| | Ejection Fraction > 40 Per Cent | | | Ejection Fraction < 40 Per Cent | | | |
| | Total No. of Limbs | Limbs With Ulcers | | Total No. of Limbs | Limbs With Ulcers | | p Value* |
		No.	Per Cent		No.	Per Cent	
VFI < 5	41	1	2	19	6	32	< 0.01
5 < VFI < 10	37	11	30	19	12	63	< 0.02
VFI > 10	32	13	41	27	19	70	< 0.05

From Christopoulos D, Nicolaides AN, Cook A, et al: Pathogenesis of venous ulceration in relation to the calf muscle pump function. Surgery 106:829, 1989.
χ^2 test.
VFI, venous filling index.

tant to note that a certain degree of physiologic valvular reflux is found in normal subjects, and this reflux may become more pronounced during prolonged daily physical activity.[13] Valve closure does not occur with antegrade flow cessation alone: it requires reversal of flow to a minimum velocity of 30 cm/sec.[14] For this reason, venous valves remain open in patients in the supine position, and deep breathing will cause valve leaflet wobbling without closure. Reverse flow velocity above 30 cm/sec results in valve closure within 100 milliseconds.[14] With the patient in the supine position, manual compression of the thigh is unable to generate reverse flow velocities high enough to produce valve closure in many cases.[14] Likewise, the Valsalva maneuver generates sufficiently high reverse flow velocities to produce closure of the iliofemoral valves only, but in the limb this maneuver rarely produces enough reflux velocity to elicit valve closure unless the proximal valves are severely incompetent.[14] Therefore, proximal manual compression and Valsalva maneuvers in supine patients are not entirely reliable methods for the assessment of venous reflux.

Several tests are widely available to detect the presence of deep and superficial vein valvular incompetence and to quantitate its degree. These tests include venous refill time measured by photoplethysmography or direct venous pressure monitoring, continuous-wave Doppler ultrasound examination, VFI measured with air plethysmography, descending and ascending phlebography, and duplex scanning. The ideal test for the assessment of valvular reflux should be noninvasive, should precisely define the anatomic location of the incompetent venous segments, should measure the degree of reflux in each individual vein, should quantitate the global hemodynamic effect of venous reflux on the limb in question, and should be technically simple and inexpensive. Obviously, no single test that is currently available has all these features: several of these studies must be combined, depending on the questions to be answered in each individual patient.

Ideally, to confirm the validity of a noninvasive test for the evaluation of valvular incompetence, it should be compared with a known gold standard. Unfortunately, descending phlebography, considered as such, has limited value in the assessment of reflux for reasons explained later. Duplex scanning, and color flow imaging in particular, have become the most valuable tools for evaluating valvular incompetence and are becoming the new gold standards.

Photoplethysmography

Photoplethysmography (PPG) is an indirect, qualitative, noninvasive method of assessing the presence of venous reflux. It is very popular because of its simplicity, low cost, and ease of performance. Photoplethysmography is based on the emission of infrared light by a diode into the skin and the reception of the backscattered light by an adjacent photoreceptor. It allows continuous recording of instantaneous changes in cutaneous capillary network blood content, identifying reflux by measuring the time required for the skin capillaries to refill after they are emptied. The procedure involves the application of a phototransducer with double-sided tape to the anteromedial aspect of the lower leg above the medial malleolus. The test is performed as the patient sits with the legs hanging freely. Recording is performed with the patient at rest to obtain a baseline tracing, during five consecutive foot flexion-extensions, and finally until the tracing returns to baseline level again (Fig. 133–5). The venous refill time (RT) or venous recovery time obtained with PPG tracings measures the time taken to return to baseline capillary fullness at rest after capillary emptying with a standardized calf muscle exercise. The RT obtained with PPG tracings depends on the efficiency of dermal venous emptying with exercise, the arterial capillary inflow, and mainly, the degree of venous valvular competence. The RT obtained with PPG tracings correlates closely with the RT procured by direct venous pressure monitoring; however, it does not correlate with the AVP of the limb in question and therefore lacks quantitative value in terms of gauging the severity of venous reflux.[15, 16] Attempts to quantitate venous reflux with a calibrated PPG technique showed improved correlation of the RT with the AVP, but the technique was cumbersome and never gained widespread use.[17] More recent efforts to quantitate reflux using computer analysis of PPG RT with duplex scanning as the gold standard were unsuccessful in obtaining good separation between different clinical categories. Furthermore, the best criterion found to separate normal limbs from incompetent limbs was a 95 per cent RT of 15 seconds, which provided only a 50 per cent sensitivity and an 80 per cent specificity in identifying deep reflux.[18] Venous reflux as assessed by PPG is mainly determined by the presence of valvular incompetence in the saphenous system and distal deep calf veins, whereas proximal deep vein incompetence (i.e., incompetence of the common and su-

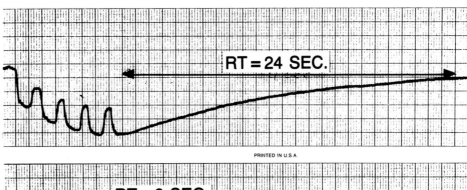

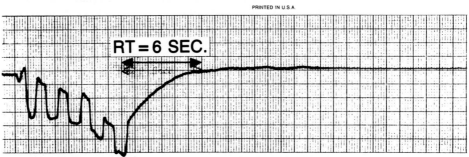

FIGURE 133–5.
Photoplethysmographic tracing. After a baseline tracing is obtained, the patient performs five tiptoe movements (*descending sawtooth tracing*). The recording continues until the initial baseline is reached again. The refill time (RT) is measured from the lowest point of the tracing to the point at which the baseline level is regained. *A*, The recovery time corrects after placement of an above-knee tourniquet to occlude the superficial system, implying reflux confined to the superficial system. *B*, Shortened refill time after five tiptoe exercises.

perficial femoral veins) has little influence on the PPG RT.[19, 20] The PPG RT is susceptible to variation, depending on the transducer position in the lower leg and on the type and amount of limb exercise performed during the recording.[21] Furthermore, there is substantial variability in repeated RTs in the same individual, and the RT is related more to the presence of superficial than of deep venous reflux.[21] Therefore, PPG RT appears to reflect local, rather than global, venous dysfunction. Despite its limitations, PPG RT has value as a screening test for venous valvular incompetence. A normal RT in an asymptomatic limb is a good predictor of venous competence in the superficial, calf communicating, and distal deep venous territories.[15, 20] A shortened RT that normalizes with a limb tourniquet occluding the superficial system implies incompetence of the superficial system alone or in combination with perforators located proximal to the tourniquet (see Fig. 133–5). If the RT does not correct with tourniquet application to the limb, it implies the presence of valvular incompetence in the deep system, in perforators located distal to the tourniquet, or in both. The normal value for PPG venous RT varies from 18 to 23 seconds among different laboratories and depends on the individual exercise protocol and instrumentation used.[15, 16] For this reason, every laboratory should develop its own data to obtain the value that separates normal patients from patients with venous reflux.

With the advent of duplex scanning, which allows direct assessment of valvular incompetence in combination with anatomic localization of the venous segments involved, the value of PPG for the diagnosis of venous reflux has been restricted. Its main role is in the evaluation of patients with varicose veins, in whom a shortened RT that corrects with an above-knee or a below-knee tourniquet predicts good results with superficial venous surgery.

Continuous-Wave Doppler Ultrasound Evaluation

Continuous-wave Doppler evaluation of venous reflux is based on the detection of the flow direction in the veins of the lower extremity.[22] Its main advantages are the speed of the technique and the low cost of the instrument. Doppler ultrasound evaluation offers merely a qualitative assessment of venous reflux; it cannot quantitate the severity of valvular incompetence and does not give any anatomic information. It is most suitable for the office evaluation of reflux at the saphenofemoral and saphenopopliteal junctions.

The examination is performed with the patient standing, holding on to a rail to ensure immobility, and bearing weight on the opposite leg to avoid muscle contraction. The saphenofemoral junction is examined with the physician facing the patient, whereas the saphenopopliteal junction is examined from behind, with the patient's leg slightly flexed. The Doppler probe is placed at a 45-degree angle to the skin, and the probe position is adjusted to obtain the optimal venous signal. The venous signal is confirmed by forward flow augmentation elicited with distal manual compression. Reverse flow is assessed during a Valsalva maneuver and coughing, and with the sudden release of distal manual compression. If no flow, or flow lasting less than 0.5 second, is detected during these maneuvers, it implies valvular competence in that venous segment; the detection of prolonged flow (more than 0.5 second) on release denotes the presence of reflux.[23] When reflux is documented with this maneuver, the examination can be repeated with finger or tourniquet compression of the greater or lesser saphenous vein a few centimeters distal to the examination site. If the reflux disappears, it means that the superficial vein is incompetent but the deep vein is competent, and if the reflux does not disappear, it is inferred that the deep system is incompetent. This method, in expert hands, has a very high sensitivity and specificity in detecting popliteal vein reflux. However, continuous-wave Doppler evaluation of venous valvular incompetence is a very limited test because the probe detects flow in all the vascular structures located in the path of the sound wave, making it impossible to determine in which vessel the reflux signal originated. For these reasons, the use of continuous-wave Doppler ultrasound should be restricted to the screening of valvular reflux at the level of the saphenofemoral and saphenopopliteal junctions, and therapeutic decisions regarding reflux should be based on further testing.

Duplex Scanning

The success and experience that have been accumulated with duplex scanning in the diagnosis of deep venous thrombosis since the early 1980s have prompted its application to the evaluation of valvular incompetence. Duplex scanning permits direct detection of valvular reflux in individual veins and allows visualization of valve leaflet motion (Fig. 133–6). Furthermore, it can quantitate the degree of incompetence by measuring vein cross-sectional area, reverse flow velocity, and duration of reflux, which allows the calculation of the amount of reflux in milliliters per second (flow = velocity × cross-sectional area) (Fig. 133–7). Reflux duration in the popliteal vein, measured in the standing position with the use of rapid-deflation cuffs in normal limbs, is usually less than 0.5 second.[14] The reflux volume at peak reflux velocity, average reflux flow, and mean peak reflux velocity have been shown to be significantly higher in patients with skin changes than in patients without them.[24]

The early experience with duplex scanning for the assessment of venous reflux was based on the identification of individual veins with B-mode ultrasonography and on the detection of pathologic reflux by placing the pulsed Doppler sample volume at multiple sites along the venous segment while performing limb compression and release maneuvers. The initial experience by pioneers in the field was encouraging and revealed an 84 per cent sensitivity and an 88 per cent specificity in the diagnosis of common femoral and popliteal vein incompetence.[25] However, the complete examination of all venous systems in both limbs with the use of this technique is time consuming and inadequate for screening purposes. The advent of color flow duplex scanning has dramatically reduced the time required for this evaluation by allowing real-time visualization of the flow direction without the need for repeated pulsed Doppler sampling (see Figs. 133–8 and 133–9 on Color Plate VII).

Duplex scanning–derived reflux velocity has been shown to correlate with the clinical severity of insufficiency as classified according to the Joint Council of the SVS/ISCVS reporting standards on venous disease.[24] More recently, Bergan and associates showed a promising correlation between reflux quantitation in individual veins and the clinical severity of venous insufficiency.[26] However, duplex scanning does not allow hemodynamic quantitation of overall limb reflux; this requires supplemental testing with air plethysmography and AVP measurement.

The maneuvers used to elicit valve closure during the evaluation of venous reflux are as important as the method employed to document the reversed flow. The standard physical methods of eliciting venous reflux are carried out with the patient in either the supine or the erect position. They include manual compression proximal to the insonation site, release of manual compression distal to the insonation site, and the sudden increase of intra-abdominal pressure with the Valsalva maneuver or coughing. However, it has been shown that these maneuvers are inadequate to elicit reflux.[27] Proximal manual compression of the horizontal limb does not result in valve closure but rather in prolonged reflux followed by flow cessation. Furthermore, manual proximal and distal limb compression produce such variability in reflux duration that they do not allow quantitative interpretation.[27] The Valsalva maneuver in the supine position allows physiologic reflux down to the knee level, but when the iliofemoral valves are competent, it does not produce flow reversal at more distal sites. In regard to the evaluation of reflux in the supine position, it has been shown that valves that clearly reflux with the patient standing may appear competent when the patient is supine and that the duration of reflux with the patient in the erect position is shorter than that with the patient supine.[27] It has also been suggested that the reflux assessed with the patient in the erect position correlates better with the clinical severity of chronic venous insufficiency than does that evaluated with the patient recumbent.[28]

The use of rapid-inflation and -deflation cuffs with the patient in the standing position provides standardization in the evaluation of reflux, avoiding the variability inherent in the use of manual compression or the Valsalva maneuver. Rapid distal cuff deflation simulates physiologic muscle relaxation and is the most reproducible method available for eliciting valve closure.[27] Pressures of 80 mmHg in the thigh, 100 mmHg in the calf, and 120 mmHg in the foot, with 3 seconds of inflation time and 0.3 second of deflation time, have been suggested as adequate for this examination.[27] The methodology for the investigation of venous reflux with duplex scanning is currently evolving; nevertheless, it appears essential that the evaluation be performed with the patient standing and with reproducible means used to elicit valve closure. More data are needed on the signifi-

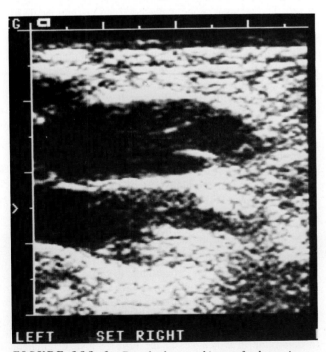

FIGURE 133–6. B-mode ultrasound image of a deep vein with an open valve. Real-time visualization of this segment would allow assessment of valve leaflet motion. (Courtesy of Patty Daniel, R.N., R.V.T.)

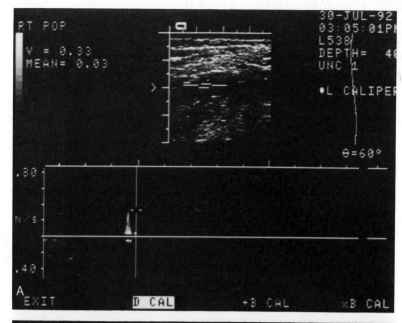

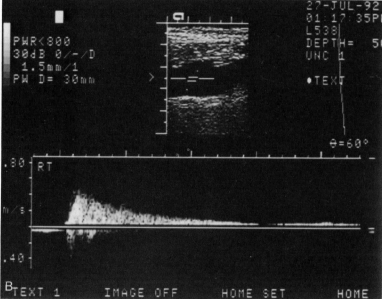

FIGURE 133–7. Popliteal vein reflux flow velocity spectra recorded in the standing position, with reflux elicited with a rapid-deflation cuff inflated to 100 mmHg at mid-calf (reflux flow above the zero line). *A*, Reflux spectrum in a normal popliteal vein in a subject without a history of venous disease. The peak reflux velocity is 33 cm/sec, and the reflux time is 72 milliseconds. *B*, Reflux spectrum of a severely incompetent popliteal vein in a subject with class III chronic venous insufficiency and venographically documented grade IV reflux. The reflux peak velocity is over 50 cm/sec, and the reflux time approaches 3 seconds.

cance of the duration and the velocity of reflux in individual veins in the evaluation and treatment of patients with chronic venous insufficiency. Despite this, duplex scanning and color flow imaging are currently the most valuable and promising tools for the assessment of venous incompetence.

Descending Phlebography

The reliability of noninvasive studies in the localization and quantitation of venous valvular incompetence has made phlebography rarely necessary in the evaluation of patients with chronic venous insufficiency. Descending phlebography offers morphologic information on the venous system, assesses valve function, and can identify residual post-thrombotic changes and the occasional cases of valvular aplasia. However, it allows visualization of the lumen of only those venous segments that contrast reaches in sufficient concentration and can reliably assess the competence of those valves only when contrast is injected in conjunction with maneuvers that produce enough retrograde flow velocity to elicit physiologic valve closure.

The technical aspects of descending phlebography are discussed in Chapter 132. It is important to recognize that because venous reflux is a dynamic phenomenon, static radiographs have limited diagnostic value. To avoid this problem, descending phlebographic images should be recorded on videotape to permit review of the reverse flow dynamics. The proximal valves located in the common femoral, superficial femoral, deep femoral, and greater saphenous veins are evaluated, and if any of them allows reflux, the distal extent is documented. Following Kistner and associates, the findings are categorized according to individual valve function (Table 133–5) and also according to the

Table 133–5.   Phlebographic Grading of Valve Reflux

Normal valve	Closes completely; no leakage regardless of Valsalva maneuver effort
Minimal leakage	Wisp of contrast goes through the valve with a forced Valsalva maneuver
Moderate leakage	Obvious retrograde flow during a Valsalva maneuver
Severe leakage	Contrast cascades distally without a Valsalva maneuver

Adapted from Kistner RL, Ferris EB, Randhawa G, et al: A method of performing descending venography. J Vasc Surg 4:464, 1986.

overall extent of reflux (Table 133–6).[29] Of note is that the presence of a competent valve in the distal superficial femoral or popliteal vein that prevents reflux into the calf minimizes the clinical significance of the degree of valvular incompetence.[29] The observation of intraluminal septations and valvular scarring suggests that the etiology of the valvular incompetence is post-thrombotic, whereas the absence of luminal abnormalities in a patient without a history of deep venous thrombosis is consistent with the diagnosis of primary valvular incompetence. The evaluation of reflux in the deep femoral vein may have important therapeutic implications because it has been suggested that valvular reconstruction of the superficial femoral and popliteal veins may fail to produce hemodynamic improvement in the presence of uncorrected reflux in the deep femoral vein.[30]

The quantitation of venous reflux based on descending phlebography has shown poor correlation with the clinical severity of chronic venous insufficiency in the limb. In this regard, Ackroyd and coworkers found that 67 per cent of limbs with chronic venous insufficiency that had skin changes, ulceration, or both had no evidence of pathologic reflux and that only 31 per cent of limbs with post-thrombotic changes documented by ascending phlebography had significant reflux on the descending venogram.[31] In contrast, studies done with duplex scanning showed that 87 to 93 per cent of limbs with skin changes, ulceration, or both had valvular reflux in at least one venous system.[2, 19] This discrepancy illustrates the inherent shortcoming of descending phlebography. Descending phlebography is limited by the presence of competent valves in a proximal venous segment because they prevent the passage of contrast, precluding evaluation of the distal segments. Furthermore, in patients without any evidence of deep venous disease, descending phlebography performed in the semi-erect and supine positions, with or without a Valsalva maneuver, demonstrates

Table 133–6.   Phlebographic Classification of Reflux

Grade 0	No evidence of reflux
Grade 1	Minimal reflux through one or more valves during a Valsalva maneuver
Grade 2	Considerable reflux in the thigh, but a competent valve is present in the distal femoral or popliteal vein
Grade 3	Considerable reflux in the thigh, with leakage through the popliteal vein into the proximal calf
Grade 4	Cascading reflux from the proximal femoral veins into the popliteal and calf veins

Adapted from Kistner RL, Ferris EB, Randhawa G, et al: A method of performing descending venography. J Vasc Surg 4:464, 1986.

physiologic reflux into the proximal or distal superficial femoral vein in most cases (grades I and II reflux).[31, 32] This is probably due to the inability of the Valsalva maneuver to elicit effective valve closure in many individuals and to the higher specific gravity of the contrast material (compared with blood) that trickles through relaxed valves by gravity.

Descending phlebography still remains an essential part of the evaluation of reflux for the planning of deep venous reconstruction, and for this purpose optimal anatomic information is obtained by combining both ascending and descending phlebography. Descending phlebography is also indicated in those rare instances when noninvasive studies fail to provide details of valvular competence.

EVALUATION OF PERFORATOR VEIN INCOMPETENCE

The clinical significance of the presence of incompetent calf perforating veins (ICPVs) was initially recognized by Linton.[33, 34] The hemodynamic relevance of ICPVs was documented by Zukowski and associates, who found that in an unselected population of patients with chronic venous insufficiency, 40 per cent of the patients presenting with varicose veins and no evidence of deep venous disease had ICPVs.[35] In 70 per cent of these patients, perforator incompetence had moderate to severe hemodynamic significance, whereas in one third, perforator incompetence appeared to be of no hemodynamic consequence. In this study, none of the patients with inconsequential ICPVs had skin changes or ulceration, whereas 68 per cent of those with moderate and 100 per cent of those with severe perforator incompetence had skin changes or ulceration. The normal direction of flow in perforating veins occurs during muscle relaxation and is from the superficial to the deep venous system. However, small perforating veins (less than 1 mm) that may not harbor valves may allow physiologic bidirectional flow.[36] Calf perforating veins follow a quite constant anatomic distribution and bear one to three valves, which are located deep to the muscle fascia.[37, 38]

The evaluation of calf perforator vein incompetence is based on the identification of reverse flow from the deep to the superficial system. However, it appears that outward flow in otherwise normal perforating veins can be elicited with proximal limb compression, and it has been suggested that a reliable demonstration of perforator vein incompetence is that of outward flow following the release of distal compression.[36] Therefore, any evaluation method should take these factors into consideration.

Continuous-wave Doppler detection of ICPVs was pioneered by Miller and Foote.[39] With the patient in the supine position, tourniquets are placed to occlude the superficial system proximal and distal to the area being examined. The medial aspect of the calf is scanned systematically while distal manual compression and relaxation are performed at each insonation site to elicit bidirectional flow. The presence of a Doppler flow signal during both compression and relaxation of the distal limb would correspond to the location of an ICPV. Using intraoperative assessment of perforator incompetence as the gold standard, O'Donnell and colleagues showed that Doppler examination is very sensitive in identifying limbs with ICPVs.[40] Unfortunately, this method has a very high false-positive rate in identifying individual incompetent perforators and is not more accurate than physical examination in predicting the presence or individual location of ICPVs.[40]

Ascending phlebography has been a popular method used for the diagnosis of ICPVs and was considered the gold standard. It is performed by injecting contrast material into a superficial vein of the foot and forcing the contrast into the deep system by applying a tourniquet as low as possible around the ankle.[41] With the patient supine or with the feet slightly down, contrast is injected under fluoroscopy and the study is recorded for later review. The presence of incompetent perforators is indicated by the passage of contrast from the deep to the superficial veins and by the presence of dilatation, irregularity, and tortuosity, which are common features of ICPVs. A tourniquet is placed just proximal to each ICPV that is identified to avoid further filling of the superficial system, which would obscure the evaluation of the more proximal segments. Despite the use of careful technique, as the ascending venogram progresses proximally, most of the superficial and deep systems is opacified by contrast material, making determination of the direction of flow difficult, if not impossible. Using this method, Thomas and coworkers were able to identify preoperatively 81 per cent of the incompetent perforators found at the time of surgery.[41] Ascending phlebography has a significant rate of false-negative findings in determining the overall presence or absence of ICPVs, an incidence that is even higher at the time of localization of the ICPV site.[40] Although phlebography has a significantly lower incidence of false-positive findings than does Doppler ultrasound evaluation, it has been shown that neither phlebography nor Doppler evaluation is superior to clinical examination in the diagnosis of the presence or localization of the site of an ICPV.[40]

Duplex imaging can identify both competent and incompetent perforating veins, whereas ascending phlebography cannot visualize most competent perforators. Hanrahan and associates found that duplex scanning identified all perforators seen on phlebography, but duplex scanning classified as incompetent a smaller number of veins than phlebography.[42] This discrepancy was probably produced by the use in this study of vessel size as the sole phlebographic criterion of incompetence. However, a good correlation between duplex identification of competent and incompetent perforators and operative findings was found. The diagnosis of ICPVs with conventional duplex scanning is time consuming because it requires placement of the pulsed Doppler sample volume in each vein identified by B-mode ultrasonography to ascertain the flow characteristics of the vessel. Perforating veins are sometimes small and tortuous, and the sample volume size of the pulsed Doppler may exceed the diameter of the vein in question, which could lead to mistakes in determining flow direction. The use of color flow duplex imaging overcomes this uncertainty to a great extent and expedites the procedure dramatically. The author is unaware of any data comparing color flow duplex imaging with other diagnostic modalities or with operative findings. However, in the author's experience, color flow duplex scanning is able to identify ICPVs with great certainty; unfortunately, the sensitivity of this

test has not yet been determined. The identification of bidirectional flow (red hue alternating with blue) during calf or foot compression maneuvers in a vein traveling fairly horizontally from the superficial to the deep system is diagnostic of an ICPV (see Fig. 133–10 on Color Plate VII). It is important to recognize that at the onset of calf muscle contraction, flow through ICPVs is from deep to superficial veins, but as muscle contraction progresses, flow is partially or completely interrupted. During passive muscle compression and release, outward flow is not interrupted in ICPVs, whereas it is in competent perforators. Color flow duplex scanning is superior to conventional duplex scanning for the evaluation of ICPVs and has the potential to become the new gold standard for this purpose.

EVALUATION OF VENOUS OUTFLOW OBSTRUCTION

The assessment of venous outflow obstruction is an essential part of the evaluation of chronic venous insufficiency. Screening for venous obstruction should be performed with noninvasive methods, with duplex scanning currently being the test of choice. The evaluation of venous obstruction with the use of duplex scanning is conducted in a fashion similar to that used for the evaluation of deep venous thrombosis and is not repeated here. Duplex scanning can directly visualize and locate intraluminal obstruction and can assess the characteristics of venous flow distal to the inguinal ligament. Duplex scanning can also identify the presence of collateral veins around the obstructed venous segments. However, duplex ultrasonography does not give any quantitative information about the degree of obstruction and cannot appraise obstruction in the iliac veins.

When duplex scanning is not available, an alternative method for the screening of venous obstruction is the use of the Doppler ultrasound venous survey. It is the simplest screening test for venous obstruction and requires minimal cost in instrumentation. Doppler ultrasonography is conducted with the patient erect or recumbent; the deep veins are located by their anatomic relation to major arteries, and the venous system is interrogated systematically from the groin to the ankle. The absence in the venous signal of flow spontaneity or phasicity with respiration and the lack of augmentation with distal limb compression are indirect signs of venous obstruction. Doppler evaluation is unable to identify double femoral or popliteal veins, cannot discern partial obstruction from no obstruction, may interpret well-developed collaterals as patent axial veins, and cannot evaluate pelvic, deep thigh, or calf veins. All these limitations are surmounted by duplex scanning. Doppler ultrasonography also does not give accurate information about the location and extent of venous obstruction and cannot quantitate the degree of obstruction present.

Ascending phlebography has long been considered the gold standard for the evaluation of venous obstruction. It offers accurate anatomic information regarding the extent and location of venous obstruction and the presence of collateral venous return; however, it does not quantitate the hemodynamic severity of venous outflow obstruction and is an invasive procedure that is inappropriate as a screening tool. With the advent of duplex scanning, the phlebographic evaluation of venous obstruction has been restricted to the preoperative assessment of patients undergoing venous reconstruction and to the diagnosis of pelvic vein obstruction in areas that duplex ultrasonography cannot access or in which its findings appear ambiguous. Pelvic vein patency is in many cases best evaluated with descending phlebography, mainly when there is more distal obstruction.

Quantitation of the degree of venous outflow obstruction is necessary to determine the impact of the obstructive component on the overall severity of chronic venous insufficiency. It is most important for assessing the results of different treatment modalities and for understanding hemodynamic changes in patients with chronic venous insufficiency. Venous pressure measurement and determination of the venous emptying rate are the currently used methods for appraising the degree of venous obstruction.

Quantitative Evaluation of Venous Outflow Obstruction

The severity of venous outflow obstruction is determined by the degree of blockage of the main axial veins and by the effectiveness of the development of collateral venous channels. The anatomic evaluation of venous outflow obstruction does not provide any assessment of the hemodynamic impact of the obstruction. In patients with severe chronic venous insufficiency thought to be secondary to venous outflow obstruction, quantitative evaluation is essential to correlate the degree of obstruction with the clinical status. Quantification of outflow obstruction is currently possible with the use of functional studies that measure volume changes after the release of proximal venous occlusion, the venous pressure differential between the foot and the arm, venous pressure changes following reactive hyperemia, and the combination of simultaneous pressure and volume change that permits the calculation of venous outflow resistance. The studies that measure pressure changes are invasive; they are not suitable for screening purposes and are more appropriate for the pre- and postoperative evaluation of patients undergoing venous reconstructive surgery and for clinical research.

Arm-Foot Venous Pressure Differential

Measurement of the arm-foot pressure differential was described by Raju.[43] It is performed by cannulating superficial veins of the foot and hand with butterfly needles in a patient in the supine position. Pressure transducers are placed at the level of the puncture sites, and the pressures are recorded simultaneously. Using ascending phlebography to assess the presence of venous obstruction, Raju found that the arm-foot pressure differential was 4 mmHg or less in patients without evidence of obstruction, whereas most patients with phlebographic evidence of obstruction had arm-foot pressure differentials greater than 4 mmHg. A normal arm-foot pressure differential found in several patients with deep venous obstruction was attributed to the presence of well-developed collaterals. To elucidate the contribution of collateral circulation to the venous outflow,

Raju measured the increase in foot venous pressure following reactive hyperemia and found better separation between normal patients and patients with phlebographically proven obstruction.[44] Normal patients were found to have an increase in venous pressure of less than 6 mmHg, whereas patients with proven obstruction had an increase of 8 mmHg or more. The combination of these two tests was 90 per cent sensitive and 93 per cent specific in diagnosing venous obstruction in the quoted study. The false-negative results found with this test were in patients who had phlebographic obstruction with good functional collateral channels, in whom the obstruction had few if any hemodynamic repercussions. On the basis of these two tests, Raju classifies the severity of outflow obstruction into four categories. Group 1 consists of patients with fully compensated obstruction from collateralization; these patients have a normal arm-foot pressure differential and a normal venous pressure response to hyperemia despite proven phlebographic obstruction. Patients in group 2 have partially compensated obstruction: they have collaterals that are adequate at rest (normal arm-foot pressure differential) but become insufficient during reactive hyperemia (elevated hyperemia-induced foot venous pressure). Group 3 consists of patients with minimal compensation of venous return with collateral flow; they have an abnormal arm-foot pressure differential and an abnormal hyperemic foot pressure elevation. Finally, patients in group 4 have the most severe form of outflow obstruction, with an elevated arm-foot pressure differential but no pressure elevation during reactive hyperemia because they have such a high degree of obstruction and fixed flow that reactive hyperemia cannot be induced. Although the described methods are fairly simple, their invasive nature makes them more suitable for the evaluation of patients with severe symptoms of obstruction, for the interpretation of results of deep venous reconstructions, and for investigational purposes.

Measurement of Venous Outflow Rate and Resistance

The rate of lower extremity venous emptying after the sudden release of venous occlusion reflects the net resistance of the limb venous outflow. The rate of venous outflow is directly proportional to the pressure gradient present between the calf veins and the inferior vena cava.[45] The venous emptying rate can be measured by the decrease in leg venous volume over a period of time after the release of venous occlusion, and it can be monitored with strain-gauge, impedance, air, or any other plethysmographic instrument. All tests that measure the venous outflow rate are performed with a similar technique. The patient lies in the supine position with the leg slightly elevated (10 to 15 degrees), externally rotated, and flexed to facilitate venous emptying. The volume monitoring device is placed on the calf, and a venous occlusion cuff is placed around the upper thigh and inflated to 50 to 70 mmHg. Maximal venous filling is allowed with the cuff inflated, then the cuff is suddenly deflated with the aid of a rapid-deflation valve. From the volume tracing recorded during the entire sequence, the maximal venous outflow and the 1-, 2-, or 3-second outflow fraction can be calculated. The rate of venous emptying is given by the maximal venous outflow,

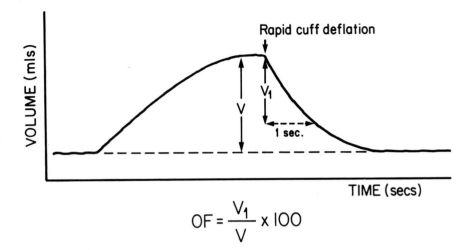

FIGURE 133–11. Typical outflow fraction tracing obtained with air plethysmography. After complete venous filling with a thigh tourniquet, rapid deflation (*arrow*) allows venous emptying. The outflow fraction (OF) obtained by dividing the amount of venous volume emptied in 1 second (V_1) by the venous volume (V) and multiplying by 100.

$$OF = \frac{V_1}{V} \times 100$$

which is calculated from the slope of the tangent to the initial downslope tracing. The outflow fraction is calculated by measuring the volume decrease during the first 1, 2, or 3 seconds from the onset of deflation (Fig. 133–11). Using mercury-in-Silastic strain-gauge plethysmography, Fernandes e Fernandes and coworkers found good separation of the maximal venous outflow between limbs with phlebographically proven deep venous obstruction and those without obstruction (Fig. 133–12).[46] In the same study, limbs with incompetent superficial or deep veins had maximal venous outflow values that overlapped with those of normal limbs but not with those of limbs that had obstruction.

The 1-second outflow fraction determined with air plethysmography is a rapid, noninvasive method of assessing outflow obstruction that can be obtained as part of the standard air plethysmography study. The test is performed with the patient supine, the leg slightly elevated, and the instrumentation set in the same manner as for standard air plethysmography. A venous occlusion cuff is inflated on the upper thigh to 70 mmHg, and the leg is allowed to fill until a volume plateau is reached on the tracing; the cuff is then suddenly deflated, and the outflow fraction is calcu-

lated from the volume drop observed during the 1st second of the outflow curve (see Fig. 133–11). The volume emptied in 1 second is divided by the total leg volume and multiplied by 100, which expresses the percentage of leg blood volume passively emptied in 1 second. Using this test, Nicolaides and Sumner found that limbs without evidence of obstruction have outflow fractions of greater than 38 per cent of the venous volume measured with the occlusion cuff inflated, limbs with moderate obstruction have fractions of 30 to 38 per cent, and limbs with severe obstruction have outflow fractions of less than 30 per cent.[47] The 1-second outflow fraction permitted good discrimination between extremities with a normal arm-foot pressure differential and those with an increased arm-foot pressure differential (greater than 5 mmHg).

Venous outflow resistance can be calculated by simultaneously monitoring foot venous pressure and leg volume changes. A standard AVP monitoring device is connected to a butterfly needle inserted into a superficial foot vein, while the venous outflow is recorded with air plethysmography. The outflow resistance can be calculated from the formula resistance = pressure/flow (mmHg/ml/min). At any given point of the outflow, the pressure is obtained

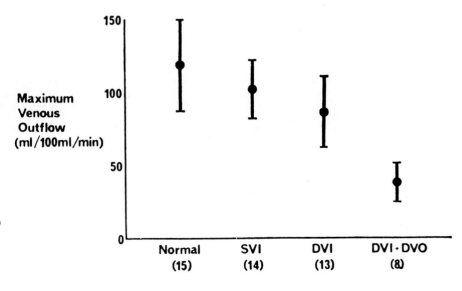

FIGURE 133–12. Maximal venous outflow measured with strain-gauge plethysmography in patients with chronic venous insufficiency. The maximal venous outflow in patients with deep venous incompetence and obstruction (DVI + DVO) is clearly lower than that in normal patients and in those with superficial venous incompetence (SVI) and deep venous incompetence (DVI). Note the overlapping between normal patients and patients with superficial and deep venous incompetence. (From Fernandes e Fernandes J, Horner J, Needham T, et al: Ambulatory calf volume plethysmography in the assessment of venous insufficiency. Br J Surg 66:327, 1979; by permission of the publishers Butterworth-Heineman Ltd.)

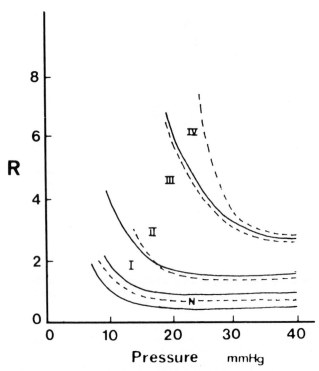

FIGURE 133–13. Relationship between outflow resistance curves and Raju's classification (grades I to IV) of outflow obstruction. With more severe forms of outflow obstruction, the resistance (R) is higher at any given venous pressure. The slope in the increase of outflow resistance with decreasing venous pressure levels is more pronounced in patients with severe outflow obstruction (grades III and IV). (From Nicolaides AN, Sumner DS: Investigation of patients with deep vein thrombosis and chronic venous insufficiency. Los Angeles, Med-Orion, 1991, p 59.)

from the pressure curve and the flow is calculated from the tangent of the corresponding point in the volume curve.[48] By plotting the resistance against the pressure obtained at multiple points of the outflow curve from a large number of patients with different degrees of venous obstruction, Nicolaides and Sumner found good separation between the pressure-resistance curves at various degrees of obstruction,[49] corresponding with the arm-foot pressure gradient classification established by Raju (Fig. 133–13).

References

1. Subcommittee on Reporting Standards in Venous Disease, Ad Hoc Committee on Reporting Standards, Society for Vascular Surgery/International Society for Cardiovascular Surgery–North American Chapter: Reporting standards in venous disease. J Vasc Surg 8:172, 1988.
2. Hanrahan LM, Araki CT, Rodriguez AA, et al: Distribution of valvular incompetence in patients with venous stasis ulceration. J Vasc Surg 13:805, 1991.
3. McEnroe CS, O'Donnell TF Jr, Mackey WC: Correlation of clinical findings with venous hemodynamics in 386 patients with chronic venous insufficiency. Am J Surg 156:148, 1988.
4. Killewich LA, Martin R, Cramer M, et al: An objective assessment of the physiologic changes in the postthrombotic syndrome. Arch Surg 120:424, 1985.
5. Pollack AA, Wood EH: Venous pressure in the saphenous vein at the ankle in man during exercise and changes in posture. J Appl Physiol 1:649, 1949.
6. Arnoldi CC, Greitz T, Linderholm H: Variations in the cross sectional area and pressure in the veins of the normal human leg during rhythmic muscular exercise. Acta Chir Scand 132:507, 1966.
7. Nicolaides AN, Zukowski AJ: The value of dynamic venous pressure measurements. World J Surg 10:919, 1986.
8. Raju S, Fredericks R: Hemodynamic basis of stasis ulceration—A hypothesis. J Vasc Surg 13:491, 1991.
9. Christopoulos DG, Nicolaides AN, Szendro G, et al: Air-plethysmography and the effect of elastic compression on venous hemodynamics of the leg. J Vasc Surg 5:148, 1987.
10. Welkie JF, Kerr RP, Katz ML, et al: Can noninvasive venous volume determinations accurately predict ambulatory venous pressure? J Vasc Technol 15:186, 1991.
11. Christopoulos D, Nicolaides AN, Cook A, et al: Pathogenesis of venous ulceration in relation to the calf muscle pump function. Surgery 106:829, 1989.
12. Welch HJ, Faliakou EC, McLaughlin RL, et al: Comparison of descending phlebography with quantitative photoplethysmography, air plethysmography, and duplex quantitative valve closure time in assessing deep venous reflux [Abstract]. J Vasc Surg 16:304, 1992.
13. Bishara RA, Sigel B, Rocco K, et al: Deterioration of venous function in normal lower extremities during daily activity. J Vasc Surg 3:700, 1986.
14. van Bemmelen PS, Beach K, Bedford G, et al: The mechanism of venous valve closure. Arch Surg 125:617, 1990.
15. Nicolaides AN, Miles C: Photoplethysmography in the assessment of venous insufficiency. J Vasc Surg 5:405, 1987.
16. Abramowitz HB, Queral LA, Flinn WR, et al: The use of photoplethysmography in the assessment of venous insufficiency: A comparison to venous pressure measurements. Surgery 86: 434, 1979.
17. Norris CS, Beyrau A, Barnes RW: Quantitative photoplethysmography in chronic venous insufficiency: A new method of noninvasive estimation of ambulatory venous pressure. Surgery 94:758, 1983.
18. Sarin S, Shields DA, Scurr JH, et al: Photoplethysmography: A valuable noninvasive tool in the assessment of venous dysfunction? J Vasc Surg 16:154, 1992.
19. Gooley NA, Sumner DS: Relationship of venous reflux to the site of venous valvular incompetence: Implications for venous reconstructive surgery. J Vasc Surg 7:50, 1988.
20. Pearce WH, Ricco J-B, Queral LA, et al: Hemodynamic assessment of venous problems. Surgery 93:715, 1983.
21. Rosfors S: Venous photoplethysmography: Relationship between transducer position and regional distribution of venous insufficiency. J Vasc Surg 11:436, 1990.
22. Folse R, Alexander RH: Directional flow detection for localizing venous valvular incompetency. Surgery 67:114, 1970.
23. Nicolaides AN, Sumner DS: Investigation of Patients With Deep Vein Thrombosis and Chronic Venous Insufficiency. Los Angeles, Med-Orion, 1991, p 31.
24. Vasdekis SN, Clarke GH, Nicolaides AN: Quantification of venous reflux by means of duplex scanning. J Vasc Surg 10:670, 1989.
25. Szendro G, Nicolaides AN, Zukowski AJ, et al: Duplex scanning in the assessment of deep venous incompetence. J Vasc Surg 4:237, 1986.
26. Bergan JJ, Moulton S, Beeman S, et al: Quantification of venous reflux in lower extremity venous stasis [Abstract]. J Vasc Surg 15:442, 1992.
27. van Bemmelen PS, Bedford G, Beach K, et al: Quantitative segmental evaluation of venous valvular reflux with duplex ultrasound scanning. J Vasc Surg 10:425, 1989.
28. Neglen P, Raju S: Should duplex Doppler scanning replace descending phlebography as the "gold standard" in evaluation of venous reflux? [Abstract]. J Vasc Surg 15:442, 1992.
29. Kistner RL, Ferris EB, Randhawa G, et al: A method of performing descending venography. J Vasc Surg 4:464, 1986.
30. Eriksson I, Almgren B: Influence of the profunda femoris vein on venous hemodynamics of the limb. J Vasc Surg 4:390, 1986.
31. Ackroyd JS, Lea Thomas M, Browse NL: Deep vein reflux: An assessment by descending phlebography. Br J Surg 73:31, 1986.
32. Thomas ML, Keeling FP, Ackroyd JS: Descending phlebography: A comparison of three methods and an assessment of the normal range of deep vein reflux. J Cardiovasc Surg 27:27, 1986.
33. Linton RR: The communicating veins of the lower leg and the operative technic for their ligation. Ann Surg 107:582, 1938.

34. Linton RR: The post-thrombotic ulceration of the lower extremity: Its etiology and surgical treatment. Ann Surg 138:415, 1953.
35. Zukowski AJ, Nicolaides AN, Szendro G, et al: Haemodynamic significance of incompetent calf perforating veins. Br J Surg 78:625, 1991.
36. Sarin S, Scurr JH, Coleridge Smith PD: Medial calf perforators in venous disease: The significance of outward flow. J Vasc Surg 16:40, 1992.
37. Criado E, Johnson G Jr: Venous disease. Curr Probl Surg 28:343, 1991.
38. Thomson H: The surgical anatomy of the superficial and perforating veins of the lower limb. Ann R Coll Surg Engl 61:198, 1979.
39. Miller SS, Foote AV: The ultrasonic detection of incompetent perforating veins. Br J Surg 61:653, 1974.
40. O'Donnell TF Jr, Burnand KG, Clemenson G, et al: Doppler examination vs clinical and phlebographic detection of the location of incompetent perforating veins. Arch Surg 112:31, 1977.
41. Thomas ML, McAllister V, Rose DH, et al: A simplified technique of phlebography for the localisation of incompetent perforating veins of the legs. Clin Radiol 23:486, 1972.
42. Hanrahan LM, Araki CT, Fisher JB, et al: Evaluation of the perforat-

43. Raju S: New approaches to the diagnosis and treatment of venous obstruction. J Vasc Surg 4:42, 1986.
44. Raju S: A pressure-based technique for the detection of acute and chronic venous obstruction. Phlebology 3:207, 1988.
45. Sumner D: Strain-gauge plethysmography. *In* Bernstein EF (ed): Noninvasive Diagnostic Techniques in Vascular Disease. 3rd ed. St. Louis, CV Mosby, 1985, p 746.
46. Fernandes e Fernandes J, Horner J, Needham T, et al: Ambulatory calf volume plethysmography in the assessment of venous insufficiency. Br J Surg 66:327, 1979.
47. Nicolaides AN, Sumner DS: Investigation of Patients With Deep Vein Thrombosis and Chronic Venous Insufficiency. Los Angeles, Med-Orion, 1991, p 61.
48. Barnes RW, Collicott PE, Mozersky DJ, et al: Noninvasive quantitation of maximum venous outflow in acute thrombophlebitis. Surgery 72:971, 1972.
49. Nicolaides AN, Sumner DS: Investigation of Patients With Deep Vein Thrombosis and Chronic Venous Insufficiency. Los Angeles, Med-Orion, 1991, p 59.

ing veins of the lower extremity using high resolution duplex imaging. J Cardiovasc Surg 32:87, 1991.

134

Venous Thromboembolism

Anthony J. Comerota, M.D., F.A.C.S.

• • •

PULMONARY EMBOLISM

Most current articles on venous thromboembolism begin with the statement that pulmonary embolism (PE) is a common problem and remains a significant cause of mortality in the United States today. In 1959, Coon and Willis estimated that PE caused 47,000 deaths each year in the United States.[1] In 1970, Hume and colleagues estimated that 142,000 patients died of pulmonary emboli and another 285,000 patients suffered nonfatal pulmonary emboli on an annual basis.[2] In 1975, the classic paper by Dalen and Alpert summarized the problem of venous thromboembolism and extrapolated available data.[3] These authors estimated that of approximately 200,000 patients who developed pulmonary emboli, 10 per cent died within 1 hour. Of the remaining 90 per cent, the majority (70 per cent) did not have the diagnosis correctly made, and in this group the mortality rate was 30 per cent. Among the 30 per cent who survived for longer than 1 hour and were correctly diagnosed and treated, the mortality rate dropped to 8 per cent. In a contemporary series, Carson and colleagues prospectively followed up 399 patients with PE and demonstrated a 9.5 per cent in-hospital mortality rate, although only 2.5 per cent died of PE.[4] There was a 23 per cent 1-year mortality rate. Clinically apparent recurrent PE was found infrequently (in 8.5 per cent of patients); however it was associated with a 45 per cent mortality rate.

In 1986, the National Institutes of Health (NIH) consensus conference reported that venous thromboembolism was responsible for approximately 300,000 hospitalizations and 50,000 deaths in the United States.[5] Unfortunately, since the mid-1980s, the rate of mortality from PE has not diminished.[6] Autopsy data from the Malmo General Hospitals provide an excellent look at the clinical problem.[7] During a 10-year period (the 1980s), autopsies were performed for 66 per cent of all in-hospital deaths and 76 per cent of all postoperative deaths. In 26 per cent of postoperative deaths, PE was the sole cause, and in another 35 per cent, PE was a major contributing cause of mortality. Thus, in more than 60 per cent of the patients who died, PE was either responsible for or a major contributor to mortality.

One likely reason that the incidence of venous thromboembolic disease has not decreased while the incidence of all other forms of cardiovascular disease has may be the failure of physicians to use adequate prophylaxis for deep venous thrombosis (DVT) in appropriate medical and surgical patients at risk. This was suggested by Anderson and coworkers when they studied more than 2000 patients with multiple risk factors for venous thromboembolism who were treated in 16 hospitals.[8] Appropriate DVT prophylaxis was given to only 32 per cent! Prophylaxis practices varied considerably between the different hospitals: prophylaxis was used in 9 to 56 per cent of patients, and the percentage was higher in teaching hospitals than in nonteaching hospitals (44 vs 19 per cent, $p<.001$). Despite the considerable body of evidence supporting DVT prophylaxis for pulmonary embolus and fatal PE, DVT prophylaxis continues to be underused.

Other factors that may be responsible for the continued high incidence of venous thromboembolic complications are (1) an aging population that puts more patients at risk, (2) operative procedures being performed on patients at higher risk, and (3) greater awareness, with the increased use of more sensitive diagnostic procedures.

Diagnosis

Clinical Diagnosis

The importance of making an accurate diagnosis is intuitively evident, because the mortality due to untreated PE is so high and the complications of unnecessary anticoagulation can be appreciable.

The clinical presentation of patients with PE is the consequence of the hemodynamic changes that occur as a result of the embolus, and it generally depends on the degree of pulmonary artery obstruction. The signs and symptoms of PE are nonspecific and can be part of any number of cardiopulmonary disturbances.[9] The clinical picture of patients with PE can generally be grouped into one of three clinical syndromes: (1) acute cor pulmonale, (2) pulmonary infarction, and (3) PE.[10] Patients presenting with *acute cor pulmonale* have massive PE. Their presentation is often sudden and dramatic, with rapid-onset dyspnea, cyanosis, right ventricular failure, and systemic hypotension. Patients presenting with *pulmonary infarction* had previous PE that was undiagnosed, either because it was asymptomatic or because the symptoms were mild or nonspecific enough that the diagnosis was not pursued. This patient usually complains of dyspnea, pleuritic pain, and hemoptysis and may have a pleural friction rub on physical examination. Patients suffering *acute PE* not causing severe cardiopulmonary disturbances often complain of sudden dyspnea, have vague complaints of not feeling well, and may have mild tachycardia and tachypnea as physical findings. Table 134–1 lists the signs and symptoms of PE that have been prospectively evaluated and proved with pulmonary angiography.

Dyspnea, chest pain, hemoptysis, and hypotension are classic signs and symptoms, but they are not specific to pulmonary emboli alone. Because dyspnea and tachypnea are the most frequent clinical findings, it is understandable that additional diagnostic studies are necessary. Interestingly, clinically evident DVT is noticeably infrequent in patients with PE, and fewer than 20 per cent of patients with fatal PE have DVT diagnosed at the time of the fatal event.

Diagnostic Testing

When a diagnosis of PE is considered, a chest x-ray, an electrocardiogram, and arterial blood gas measurements should be obtained immediately and can be thought of as part of the general "clinical" evaluation. In many patients with PE, the chest x-ray findings are normal. The x-ray study is used to exclude other pulmonary pathology and to assist in interpreting the ventilation-perfusion (V/Q) lung scan. Diminished pulmonary vascular markings in the distribution of the embolus, the classic Westermark sign,[11] may be evident; however, this is seldom identified prospectively. Electrocardiographic findings likewise are usually nonspecific. The classic findings of right-sided heart strain ($S_1Q_3T_3$) are observed in fewer than 10 per cent of patients. However, electrocardiography is useful in detecting myo-

Table 134–1.   Prevalence of Symptoms and Signs of Pulmonary Embolism Confirmed With Pulmonary Angiography

	Prevalence (%)		
	All Patients **(n = 327)**	**Massive** **(n = 197)**	**Submassive** **(n = 130)**
Symptoms			
Dyspnea	84	85	82
Pleural pain	74	64	85
Apprehension	59	65	50
Cough	53	53	52
Hemoptysis	30	23	40
Sweats	27	29	23
Syncope	13	20	4
Signs			
Respiration >16/min	92	95	87
Rales	58	57	60
Increased P$_2$	53	58	45
Pulse >100/min	44	48	38
Fever >37.8/min	43	43	42
Phlebitis	39	—	—
Sweating	36	42	27
S$_3$ or S$_4$	34	39	25
Cyanosis	19	25	9

From Bell WR, Simon TL, Demets DL: The clinical features of submassive and massive pulmonary emboli. Am J Med 62:355, 1977.

Table 134–2. Pioped Study: Pulmonary Embolism Status

Scan Category	No. of Patients With Embolism/No. of Patients (%)			
	CP of 80–100%	*CP of 20–79%*	*CP of 0–19%*	*All Probabilities*
High	28/29 (96)	70/80 (88)	5/9 (56)	103118 (87)
Intermediate	27/41 (66)	66/236 (28)	11/68 (16)	104/345 (30)
Low	6/15 (40)	30/191 (16)	4/90 (4)	40/296 (14)
Near-normal				
Normal	0/5 (0)	4/62 (6)	1/61 (2)	5/128 (4)
Total	61/90 (68)	170/569 (30)	21/228 (9)	252/887 (28)

From The PIOPED Investigators: Value of the ventilation/perfusion scan in acute pulmonary embolism: Results of the Prospective Investigation of Pulmonary Embolism Diagnosis (PIOPED). JAMA 263:2753–2759, 1990.
CP, clinical probability.

cardial ischemia or excluding myocardial infarction, as well as in identifying arrhythmias. Arterial blood gas measurements are obtained to evaluate the degree of hypoxia. Clinically, one would expect some degree of hypoxia associated with hypocarbia. Usually, patients have a widened alveolar-arterial gradient with a respiratory alkalosis; however, these are not invariable findings. Up to 8 per cent of patients have a normal PaO_2, and in 15 per cent the PaO_2 exceeds 80 mmHg. There was no difference in the PaO_2 on room air or in the alveolar-arterial oxygen gradient between patients with PE confirmed angiographically and those who had normal findings on pulmonary angiography but who were suspected of having PE.[12] Therefore, arterial blood gas results cannot be used to make the diagnosis; instead, they indicate the degree of oxygenation and serve as a guide to the patient's response to therapy.

V/Q lung scanning is the most widely used special diagnostic test for suspected PE. Scan results are used to distinguish between pulmonary vascular disease, in which perfusion is abnormal and ventilation is preserved (the classic V/Q mismatch), and pulmonary parenchymal disease, in which ventilation and perfusion defects occur in the same areas of the lung (matched defects). Because so much emphasis is placed on V/Q scans, the NIH supported the Prospective Investigation of Pulmonary Embolism Diagnosis (PIOPED) study, which evaluated V/Q lung scans in the diagnosis of acute PE.[12] The results of this large, modern prospective study should be familiar to all physicians taking care of patients with pulmonary emboli, and they are summarized in Table 134–2. The results of the lung scans were broken down into four categories: high probability, intermediate probability, low probability, and near normal or normal. Additionally, each patient was assigned by his or her physician to one of three categories, according to the patient's *clinical* probability of having PE (either 80 to 100 per cent, 20 to 79 per cent, or 0 to 19 per cent). On clinical assessment alone, when the physician thought the likelihood of PE was 80 to 100 per cent, patients had a PE documented 68 per cent of the time. A clinical assessment of a 0 to 19 per cent likelihood of PE was correct in excluding PE 91 per cent of the time. Therefore, clinical assessment was more often correct in excluding PE than in identifying patients with PE. In the majority of patients, however, the clinical assessment was noncommittal (20 to 79 per cent).

When clinical probability was combined with V/Q scan results, there was an improved overall chance of making a correct diagnosis. Among patients with a high clinical probability coupled with a high-probability V/Q scan finding, 96 per cent had PE. However, if a high-probability lung scan was obtained in a patient with an intermediate or a low clinical likelihood of PE, the probability of PE fell to 88 or 56 per cent, respectively. A low-probability clinical assessment coupled with a low-probability V/Q scan correctly excluded the diagnosis of PE in 96 per cent of patients. However, using the low-probability V/Q scan to exclude PE in patients with higher clinical risk categories would lead to error, whereas a near-normal or normal V/Q scan correctly excluded PE in 96 per cent of patients. In summary, the PIOPED study demonstrated that V/Q scan findings were not decisive unless a high-probability scan was associated with a high or an intermediate clinical probability of PE or, at the other extreme, unless the V/Q scan findings were normal. Unfortunately, fewer than 27 per cent of patients fell into one of these two categories. All other combinations were insufficiently diagnostic and required either the use of pulmonary angiography to confirm or exclude the presence of PE or the use of another diagnostic test to detect the presence of venous thrombosis.

In an earlier prospective study,[13] in which V/Q lung scan results were validated by pulmonary angiography in 305 consecutive patients with clinically suspected PE, findings were similar to those in the larger PIOPED study. Eighty-six per cent with a high-probability scan (mismatch of one or more segments) had PE demonstrated angiographically.

Although V/Q mismatch is the classic pattern, the finding of a good V/Q matched defect cannot be used to exclude PE. In the study by Hull and associates,[13] 25 to 36 per cent of patients with a V/Q matched defect were found to have PE, a finding that is consistent with the results of experimental studies indicating that V/Q matching may occur early in the course of PE.[14, 15]

Figure 134–1 is a suggested algorithm for the diagnosis of suspected PE. This is based on the PIOPED study and the McMaster angiogram series.[12, 13] It presumes that patients with venous thrombosis will be treated the same as those with PE.

Hull and associates demonstrated that impedance plethysmography could be used to evaluate the risk of recurrent PE in patients with suspected PE and a non–high-probability V/Q scan.[13] The premise was that if lower

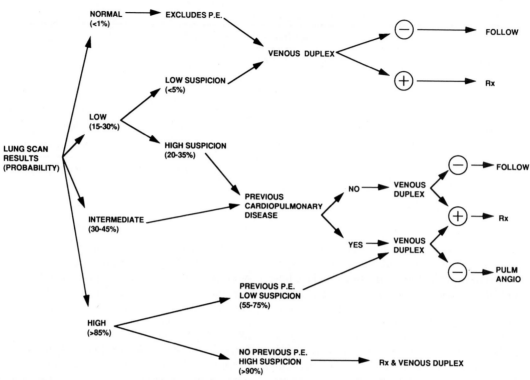

FIGURE 134–1. Diagnostic algorithm for pulmonary embolism (PE) based on lung scanning results. Numbers in parentheses indicate the likelihood of PE. (From Comerota AJ, Rao AK: Pulmonary thromboembolism. *In* Cameron JL [ed]: Current Surgical Therapy. 4th ed. Philadelphia, BC Decker, 1992.)

extremity DVT could be excluded, the risk of recurrent PE would be low. They found that patients with negative impedance plethysmographic findings who had non–high-probability V/Q scan findings had a low incidence of *clinically evident* recurrent venous thromboembolic disease. The current diagnostic algorithm uses venous duplex imaging, which is considerably more sensitive and specific than impedance plethysmography,[16–18] to assist in the evaluation of patients at risk for recurrent venous thromboembolism. In the author's institution, ascending phlebography was compared with venous duplex imaging in more than 225 consecutive patients within the same 24 hours. Duplex imaging had a sensitivity of 99 per cent and a specificity of 100 per cent for proximal DVT and a sensitivity for diagnosing isolated calf DVT of 70 per cent. If a patient suspected of having PE does not have lower extremity symptoms suggestive of DVT and then undergoes (hemodynamic) tests such as impedance plethysmography or phleborheography, approximately two thirds of proximal thrombi and essentially all calf thrombi will be missed.[17] Venous duplex imaging is considerably more sensitive than hemodynamic tests and is the diagnostic test of choice for DVT in most vascular laboratories. The cumulative reported sensitivity of venous duplex imaging for detecting proximal DVT is 96 per cent. If one considers those patients in the asymptomatic, high-risk surveillance group, the cumulative reported sensitivity of venous duplex imaging for proximal DVT falls to 75 per cent,[19] although in the author's experience, there is no difference in diagnostic sensitivity between these patient groups. A more complete review is presented in Chapter 131.

Treatment

To appreciate the impact of treatment on any disease, one must look at the natural history of the disease when it is not treated. The mortality of untreated PE is substantial. In a prospective, randomized trial of anticoagulation versus no active treatment, Barritt and Jordan found a 38 per cent mortality rate in the no-treatment group, compared with a rate of only 8 per cent in patients who were anticoagulated.[20] This prospective study was terminated early because it was considered unethical to withhold treatment from subsequent patients with PE. Other studies have demonstrated a similarly high mortality rate, ranging from 18 to 32 per cent. When treatment was instituted, however, the mortality rate fell significantly, to approximately 8 per cent.[21]

Patients who die of PE usually die within the first 2 hours of the acute embolic event, before any therapy is given. Those surviving longer have enough cardiorespiratory reserve to compensate for the large pulmonary embolus, or the pulmonary embolus is small enough that the patients' cardiopulmonary hemodynamics are not severely compromised.

Dalen and coworkers,[22] in a classic study, documented the natural history of anticoagulant therapy for PE. Fifteen patients diagnosed with pulmonary angiography were treated and had angiographically documented follow-up. Eighty-seven per cent of patients had more than 25 per cent obstruction of the pulmonary vasculature on their initial angiogram. Ninety-three per cent of patients had vena cava ligation, and 93 per cent were anticoagulated with heparin.

Therefore, the results of follow-up pulmonary angiography indicated the natural resolution of the initial pulmonary embolus, and subsequent findings were not due to recurrent pulmonary emboli during treatment. After a 2- to 3-week follow-up, 80 per cent of patients continued to have angiographically persistent PE, and 73 per cent had elevated pulmonary artery pressures.

In a larger study evaluating lung scan resolution with anticoagulation, 44 per cent of patients had persistent defects at 2 weeks, and 25 per cent had them at 3 months. The lung scan status at 3 months was predictive of the findings at 1 year.[23]

The Urokinase Pulmonary Embolism Trial[23] (Table 134–3) and the Urokinase-Streptokinase Pulmonary Embolism Trial[24] compared fibrinolytic therapy with standard anticoagulation in the treatment of PE. These were prospective, randomized, multi-center, angiographically confirmed clinical studies in which patients were randomly assigned to receive lytic therapy (streptokinase and urokinase) or anticoagulation. All patients had pulmonary angiogram and V/Q scan follow-up. The results demonstrated that thrombolytic therapy rapidly improved the angiographic and scan findings during the resolution of PE ($p<.05$). Thrombolytic therapy reduced pulmonary artery and right atrial pressure significantly. Although there was a 42 per cent bleeding complication rate with lytic therapy, this was mostly due to the multiple invasive procedures performed on patients in these studies. A high bleeding complication rate was also seen in patients receiving standard anticoagulation, who suffered a 27 per cent bleeding complication rate.

These NIH-sponsored trials demonstrated that thrombolytic therapy rapidly improved angiographic and scan resolution of pulmonary emboli. Perhaps more important, the hemodynamic status improved after lysis, with significantly reduced pulmonary artery pressures and right atrial pressures. There was no difference in mortality between the two treatment groups; however, death was not considered a primary end-point of the study during the protocol design. In addition, all patients with PE, not just those who were at risk of dying, were entered into these trials. Therefore, the absence of a documented survival benefit cannot be used in arguments addressing the merits of thrombolytic therapy for PE. If one were to propose a 50 per cent reduction in mortality in patients treated with lytic therapy versus anticoagulation, approximately 1000 patients would be required in each treatment arm of a study comparing these two methods of treatment.[25]

Table 134–3. Urokinase-Pulmonary Embolism Trial: Phase I

Parameter	Treatment	
	Urokinase	*Heparin*
Mortality (%)	7	9
Recurrent pulmonary embolism (%)	17	23
Angiographic improvement at 24 hr (%)	45	6
Scan improvement (%)		
24 hr	24	7
1 wk	45	42
Major bleeding complications (%)	27	14

From The Urokinase Pulmonary Embolism Trial. A national cooperative study. Circulation 47:1, 1973.

Long-term physiologic studies subsequently evaluated the functional unit of the lung by measuring pulmonary capillary blood volume and oxygen diffusing capacity.[26] At 1-year follow-up, significant benefit was observed in patients treated with lytic therapy, who demonstrated greater pulmonary capillary blood volume and oxygen diffusing capacity.

A 7-year follow-up study was reported in which the patients treated in the NIH trials were reevaluated with right-sided heart catheterization.[27] Pulmonary artery pressures and pulmonary vascular resistance were measured with the patient at rest and exercising. Patients treated with lytic therapy had significantly lower pulmonary artery pressures and pulmonary vascular resistance at rest and after exercise. Additionally, when patients' functional status was assessed, 73 per cent (8 of 11) of those treated with heparin were classified as New York Heart Association functional class III to IV, compared with 25 per cent (4 of 12) of those treated with a lytic agent.

More recently, echocardiography has been used to evaluate the short-term benefits of the dissolution of large pulmonary emboli on cardiac function.[28] In patients with pulmonary emboli causing hemodynamic compromise who were treated with recombinant tissue plasminogen activator (rt-PA), there was a significant reduction in pulmonary artery pressure, accompanied by a marked reduction in right ventricular diameter, an improvement in ventricular hypokinesis, and the resolution of tricuspid insufficiency. These early observations were evaluated at the completion of this study, which was the largest lytic therapy versus anticoagulation clinical study since the NIH-sponsored trials.[29] In a multi-center, prospective study, 101 patients with angiographically proven PE were randomized to receive either 100 mg of rt-PA over 2 hours followed by heparin (n=46) or heparin alone (n=55). Initial results have indicated that rt-PA provides marked improvement in right ventricular function and pulmonary perfusion compared with anticoagulation alone. On the basis of these data, it appears that eliminating thromboembolic occlusion in the pulmonary vasculature is functionally beneficial, both short-term and long-term.

Thrombolytic Therapy

Patients who have an objective diagnosis of PE and who have no contraindication to thrombolytic therapy, especially those who have a low risk of bleeding from the use of a lytic agent, appear to benefit substantially by dissolution of the PE. When thrombolysis for PE is being considered, an arbitrary upper age limit is no longer set. Data have suggested that older patients without risk factors associated with bleeding complications can be treated as safely as younger patients.[30] Additionally, cancer is no longer considered an exclusion criterion. Unlike patients with DVT, those with PE have a longer therapeutic opportunity for effective thrombolysis. Specifically, patients who receive thrombolysis up to 14 days after the appearance of new symptoms or signs seem to respond as effectively as those treated within the first 4 to 5 days after the onset of the PE.[31]

The next questions are which lytic agent to use and

which dose to administer. These two questions have not been resolved, although the results of prospective clinical trials will assist in answering them. The current clinical evaluations were based on experimental studies in venous thromboembolism indicating that rt-PA appeared more potent than urokinase or streptokinase and possibly was safer. Unlike streptokinase, rt-PA has not been reported to be antigenic[32] and has not been causally linked to allergic reactions. Additionally, urokinase has been shown to be safer and more rapidly effective than streptokinase in treating venous thromboembolic disease.[33]

In a plasminogen activator multi-center study,[34] patients randomized to rt-PA demonstrated significantly better post-treatment angiographic findings and a greater reduction in pulmonary artery pressures than those receiving heparin alone. Two patients in the rt-PA treatment group died (one of renal failure following cardiac tamponade and one of intracranial hemorrhage), and one patient who received heparin alone died (of recurrent PE).

European investigators compared 100 mg of rt-PA over 2 hours with standard-dose urokinase (a 4400-U/kg bolus followed by 4400 U/kg/hr for 12 hours).[35] They demonstrated a significantly better early hemodynamic response with rt-PA (2 hours), which disappeared by 6 hours.

Goldhaber and colleagues showed that rt-PA can be used effectively in patients with PE; however, if the duration of the infusion is extended, bleeding complications escalate during the 3rd and subsequent hours of rt-PA therapy, particularly at puncture sites used for invasive procedures.[36] In a subsequent study, they demonstrated that 100 mg of rt-PA over 2 hours was more effective than a standard-dose urokinase infusion for 24 hours in achieving rapid resolution and a rapid hemodynamic response.[37] When observed at 2 hours, patients who had received rt-PA had significantly greater resolution of their angiographic abnormalities and reduction in pulmonary artery pressures than those who had received urokinase. However, lung scanning performed 24 hours after the initiation of treatment demonstrated equivalent improvement in the two groups. This might not be surprising because at the 2-hour time point, patients randomized to rt-PA had received their entire dose, whereas those randomized to urokinase had received only 12 per cent of the suggested dose. Interestingly, bleeding complications were more common in the urokinase group, and in a surprisingly high number of patients, urokinase had to be discontinued because of a severe febrile response. This pyrogenic side effect of urokinase infusion has been observed more commonly with intravenous than with intra-arterial infusion and is thought to be mediated by interleukin 6.[38] The febrile response can be avoided by pretreating patients with meperidine or steroids and antihistamines.

A subsequent trial concentrated the 24-hour dose of urokinase to make it more comparable to the rt-PA infusion used.[39] This ''novel'' dose of urokinase was 3 million units given over 2 hours, with 1 million units given as a bolus over 10 minutes and a subsequent 2 million units infused over the remaining 110 minutes. These investigators did not have the problem with pyretic side effects of urokinase because all patients randomized to urokinase were pretreated with hydrocortisone, diphenhydramine, and acetaminophen. The rt-PA–treated patients received no premedi-

cation. The results indicated similar efficacy and safety for these two treatment regimens.

Anecdotally, the author has observed the rapid resolution of pulmonary emboli with select, catheter-directed intra–pulmonary artery (intraclot) infusion (Fig. 134–2). On the other hand, Verstraete and colleagues failed to demonstrate that selective intra–pulmonary artery infusion had better results than systemic thrombolysis.[40] However, in many of their patients treated with intra–pulmonary artery infusion, the catheter tip was not positioned in the thrombus. If the catheter tip were proximal to the thrombus, one would not expect noticeable benefit compared with systemic fibrinolysis (similar to observations of intra-arterial thrombolysis for arterial and graft occlusion).

Essop and colleagues evaluated the efficacy of intraclot infusion of streptokinase and aggressive catheter advancement in patients who had acute massive pulmonary emboli and were hemodynamically unstable.[41] Each patient was hypotensive and had markedly elevated right ventricular end-diastolic pressures, elevated pulmonary artery pressures, and a low cardiac output. After pulmonary angiography, mechanical clot agitation was performed with the catheter and the guidewire. Following catheter positioning, attempts were made to cross the occluding thrombus with the guidewire. A total of 600,000 units of streptokinase was infused over 30 minutes. Multiple hand injections of contrast were made to delineate the distal anatomy and guide the advancement of the guidewire. Streptokinase was infused at 100,000 U/hr for an additional 12 hours. Results demonstrated a significant resolution of pulmonary emboli, a return to normal blood pressure, and rapid improvement in cardiopulmonary hemodynamics with concurrent improvement in cardiac output. There was no hospital mortality; however, one patient died 2 weeks after discharge, presumably of recurrent PE. Similar observations were made by Brady and associates[42] and by Horstkotte and coworkers.[43]

Pulmonary Embolectomy

Massive pulmonary emboli frequently cause sudden death, but many patients, even those with massive embolism, survive several hours after the acute embolic event. Flemma and colleagues demonstrated that 55 per cent of patients who were in relatively good condition before their fatal PE lived longer than 2 hours, and 48 per cent survived 8 hours or more.[44] On the other hand, only 32 per cent of terminally ill patients lived for 2 or more hours after the embolic event.

The indications for emergency pulmonary embolectomy are persistent refractory hypotension despite maximal resuscitation in patients with documented massive PE. These patients must be transferred to the intensive care unit, and treatment must be initiated with a large bolus dose of heparin (10,000 to 20,000 units), followed by a continuous heparin infusion. The administration of vasopressors and inotropic agents and the use of ventilatory support should be routine. Ongoing evaluation of patients' cardiopulmonary status (in addition to continuous intra-arterial blood pressure recording), cerebral function, and renal function is necessary. The mortality rate for patients requiring pulmonary embolectomy is considerable.

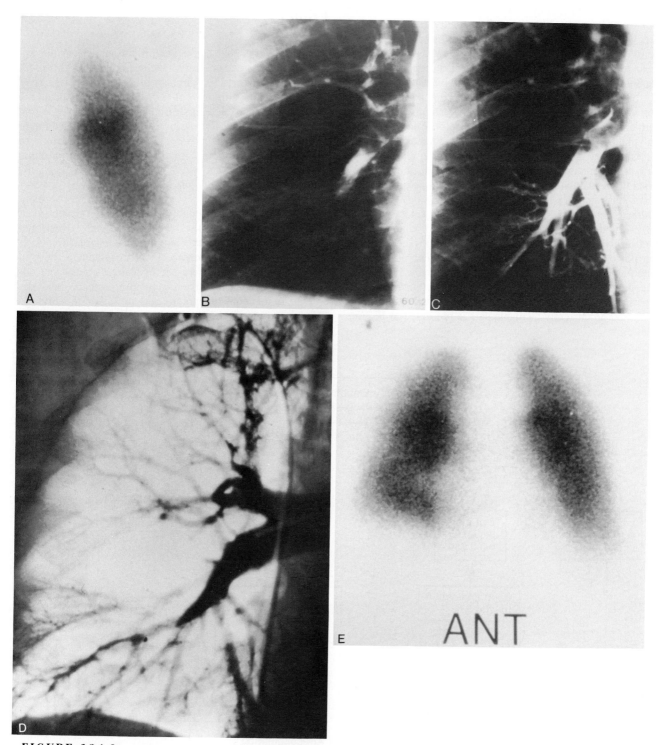

FIGURE 134-2. *A,* Pretreatment perfusion scan of a patient presenting with clinical signs and symptoms of PE. The scan showed no uptake of isotope in the right lung field. *B,* Initial pulmonary angiogram showing occlusion of the right main pulmonary artery. The patient had significant pulmonary hypertension at rest (60/20; mean, 34). *C,* Pulmonary angiogram after 1 hour of intrathrombus streptokinase infusion at a rate of 50,000 U/hr. Reperfusion of the right lower lung is observed, with a significant and rapid decrease in the patient's pulmonary artery pressures (42/15; mean, 20). *D,* Pulmonary angiogram after 24 hours of streptokinase infusion shows essentially complete reperfusion of the right lung, with normalization of the resting pulmonary artery pressures. *E,* Post-therapy perfusion scan shows reperfusion of the right lung field.

Numerous cases of pulmonary embolectomy have been reported since Trendelenburg's description of the first pulmonary embolectomy in 1908.[45] A collective review by Del Campo calculated an overall mortality rate of 40 per cent for pulmonary embolectomies performed when patients were placed on cardiopulmonary bypass.[46] Because these results include early experiences, contemporary series should demonstrate somewhat better survival rates, depending of course on patient selection. Clarke and Abrams reported a 74 per cent mortality rate in patients sustaining cardiac arrest before pulmonary embolectomy and a rate of only 11 per cent in patients operated on without prior cardiopulmonary arrest.[47] Similar results were reported by Gray and colleagues.[48] The importance of placing a vena caval filter, maintaining therapeutic anticoagulation, or both is demonstrated in Clarke and Abrams' series, in which the authors found that although 97 per cent of patients (35 of 36) without an episode of preoperative ventricular fibrillation survived the operation, 8 per cent (3 of 35) died during the postoperative period because of recurrent pulmonary emboli. Complications specific to revascularizing the ischemic lung include massive endobronchial hemorrhage and reperfusion pulmonary edema.[49] A treatment algorithm for PE based on currently available data is presented in Figure 134–3.

DEEP VENOUS THROMBOSIS

Etiology

The factors that cause venous thrombosis in the absence of direct venous injury have been of interest for more than a century. In 1856, Virchow proposed his classic triad elucidating the etiology of DVT.[50] He indicated that changes in blood elements, producing a *hypercoagulable state*; reduced blood flow velocity, causing *stasis*; and vein wall injury, resulting in *endothelial damage* combined to produce an environment that would naturally promote thrombus formation.

Although *procoagulant state* appears to be a better term, *hypercoagulability* is used because of convention. The effect of hypercoagulable states and the existence of stasis were extensively investigated by Stead.[51] Hirsh and associates demonstrated that an increased risk of thrombosis is associated with an increase in procoagulant activity in the plasma, including increases in platelet counts and adhesiveness, changes in the coagulation cascade, and decreased endogenous fibrinolytic activity.[52] Additionally, deficiencies of antithrombin III, protein C, protein S, and plasminogen, as well as the presence of a circulating lupus

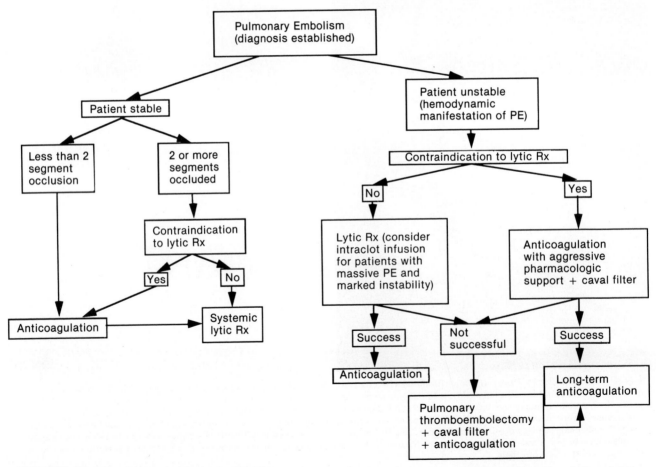

FIGURE 134–3.   Treatment algorithm for PE. When two or more pulmonary segments are occluded, as indicated by a high-probability ventilation-perfusion scan or pulmonary angiogram, the patient is considered a candidate for lytic therapy unless a contraindication exists.

anticoagulant, indicate either primary or secondary hypercoagulable states.

It is widely accepted by clinicians that *stasis* is a major factor causing DVT. It has been demonstrated radiographically as well as isotopically that venous stasis occurs,[53–55] especially in the lower leg. In his classic autopsy study of 1957, Gibbs demonstrated that the soleal sinuses are the principal site of origin of venous thrombosis.[56] A conclusion was naturally drawn that stasis was a causative factor for DVT. Although the evidence indicates that stasis occurs and although it is logical that reduced flow might prolong the contact time of activated platelets and clotting factors with the vein wall, thereby permitting thrombus formation, in no study to date has stasis alone been causally related to DVT.

The hypercoagulable state and stasis factors of Virchow's triad seem to have been well accepted in explaining postoperative DVT. However, the role of venous injury in the initiation of thrombosis has received relatively little attention. There is no argument that direct injury to the vein wall, either at the operative site or by penetrating or blunt trauma, leads to thrombus formation. Observing the overall problem of postoperative DVT, it is clear that the more distant veins are the most common sites of postoperative DVT, yet they are not directly damaged during the operative procedure.

To study the possibility that acute damage to the endothelium was caused by a distant operation, animal models were developed. The occurrence of endothelial damage in veins distant from the operative wound was investigated extensively in canine models of abdominal operations by Schaub and coworkers[57] and in a model of total hip replacement by Stewart and associates.[58] In canine models of three different types of abdominal surgery, Schaub and coworkers found that leukocytes adhered to and invaded the wall of jugular and femoral veins along their entire length.[57] They theorized that these lesions were induced by products of tissue injury that were released at the operative site and gained entry into the circulation. Stewart and associates created canine jugular and femoral vein endothelial damage with a continuous intravenous infusion of histamine and bradykinin, both of which are released from injured tissues.[59] It was subsequently demonstrated that mild venous endothelial damage occurred after abdominal operations and that much more severe endothelial damage was found after total hip replacement.[58] Scanning electron microscopic examinations showed endothelial tears located around the junctions of small side branches in the jugular and femoral veins (Figs. 134–4 and 134–5).[59] These tears extended through the endothelium and the basement membrane, exposing subendothelial collagen, which is highly thrombogenic. The lesions were infiltrated with leukocytes and platelets, trapping the blood cells and stimulating fibrin deposition. Interestingly, the constant location of this endothelial damage was explained anatomically by finding that the smooth muscle and connective tissue of the vein wall were markedly attenuated at the confluences of side branches[60] (the area of endothelial damage). This is also the area in which venous valves are found, and it fits with the common observation that venous thrombosis originates within a valve cusp.

Because the scanning electron microscopic images suggested that a tearing mechanism might create the observed injury, it was postulated that operative venodilatation might cause the initial intimal damage. Stewart and colleagues demonstrated that dilatation of the jugular vein

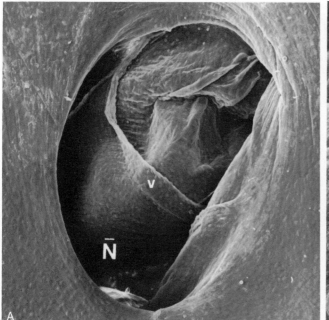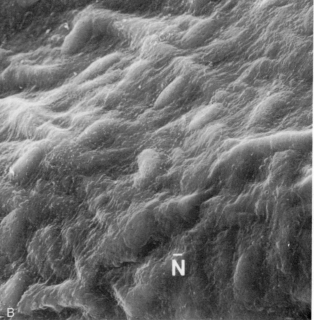

FIGURE 134–4. Scanning electron micrograph of the intimal surface of the jugular vein of a dog that was anesthetized but not operated on ($\bar{N}$). The ostium of a side branch is centered, with a valve (v) visualized. Both low-power (*A*) and high-power (*B*) magnification demonstrate an intact endothelial monolayer without evidence of damage. (*A* and *B*, Modified from Comerota AJ, Stewart GJ, White JV: Combined dihydroergotamine and heparin prophylaxis of postoperative deep vein thrombosis: Proposed mechanism of action. Am J Surg 150:41, 1985.)

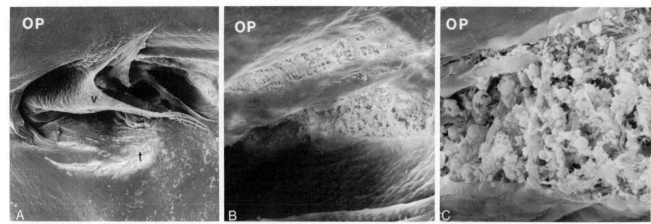

FIGURE 134–5.   Scanning electron micrograph of a jugular vein of a dog that underwent total hip replacement (OP) and had significant operative venodilatation. Note that under low-power magnification (A), an endothelial tear (t) is located in the area of a valve cusp (v). With progressively higher magnification, it appears that the endothelial damage occurred as a stretching (tearing) mechanism. The damage extends through the endothelium and basement membrane, exposing highly thrombogenic subendothelial collagen (B). One can appreciate the adherence of red blood cells, white blood cells, platelets, and fibrin strands to the area of damage (C). (A–C, Modified from Comerota AJ, Stewart GJ, White JV: Combined dihydroergotamine and heparin prophylaxis of postoperative deep vein thrombosis: Proposed mechanism of action. Am J Surg 150:41, 1985.)

beyond a certain critical point correlated with an increased frequency of venous endothelial lesions in the canine model.[61] Interestingly, the femoral veins appeared more susceptible to operative venodilatation than did the jugular veins in the frequency of endothelial lesions observed.[62]

Substantial clinical evidence supports operative venodilatation as a cause of postoperative DVT in humans, especially as one examines clinical studies of DVT prophylaxis. Observations made by Kakkar and associates,[63] the Multicenter Trial Committee,[64] and Beisaw and colleagues[65] demonstrated that the addition of a venotonic agent, dihydroergotamine, to low-dose heparin significantly reduced postoperative DVT. Therefore, there appeared to be a link between the clinical observations in humans and the experimental observations in laboratory animals. Clinical studies were then undertaken to evaluate the impact of operative venous dilatation in patients undergoing total hip and total knee replacement.

In the first study, patients undergoing total hip replacement were prospectively randomized to receive either dihydroergotamine plus heparin or placebo in a blinded fashion, and all patients had the diameter of their cephalic vein (contralateral to the operated hip) continuously recorded during the operation.[66] Ascending phlebography was performed in all patients postoperatively to assess for DVT. Results showed a significant difference in venodilatation between patients who had postoperative DVT and those who did not. Interestingly, patients with excessive operative dilatation were significantly older than patients with minimal or no dilatation. Patients who developed postoperative DVT had significantly greater dilatation and were significantly older than patients in whom DVT did not occur. All patients whose veins dilated more than 20 per cent of their baseline diameter developed postoperative DVT, whereas only 17 per cent of patients whose veins dilated less than 20 per cent developed postoperative DVT ($p<.002$). The addition of a venotonic agent prevented operative venodilatation and significantly reduced the incidence of postoperative DVT.

In a second study,[67] operative venodilatation was not observed in patients undergoing total knee replacement. There was a high incidence of ipsilateral postoperative DVT in patients undergoing total knee replacement, but they had no contralateral DVT, whereas a substantial number of patients undergoing total hip replacement are known to have contralateral postoperative DVT. Because total knee replacements are performed with the use of a thigh tourniquet (creating regional circulatory arrest), products of tissue injury do not gain entry to the circulation during the operation, and operative venodilatation should therefore not occur. On the other hand, high concentrations of these metabolic by-products in the wound and surrounding tissues are likely to lead to local venous injury, resulting in postoperative DVT. The observation that operative venodilatation occurs in humans has been confirmed by Coleridge-Smith and coworkers.[68]

Pathophysiology and Natural History

DVT represents a spectrum of disease patterns, ranging from asymptomatic calf vein thrombosis to venous gangrene (Fig. 134–6). Although venous thrombosis can affect every vein in the body, the present discussion is limited to DVT of the lower extremities.

The natural history of DVT has been of increasing interest since the mid-1960s. With today's technology, detailed information on patency, recanalization, and valvular function can be obtained quickly and easily and in a more objective fashion.

The signs and symptoms of venous thrombosis occur because of obstruction of the deep venous system, associated inflammation of the vessel wall or surrounding tissue, or fragmentation and embolization to the pulmonary arteries. It is well known that many patients with extensive DVT are asymptomatic. The physical examination findings are falsely negative in 50 per cent of patients with DVT, and they are falsely positive in patients with symptoms

Asymptomatic Calf Vein Thrombosis

↓

Symptomatic Calf Vein Thrombosis

↓

Femoral-Popliteal DVT
(below profunda)

↓

Femoral-Popliteal DVT
(above profunda)

↓

Phlegmasia Alba Dolens

↓

Phlegmasia Cerulea Dolens

↓

Venous Gangrene

FIGURE 134–6. Clinical spectrum of acute deep venous thrombosis (DVT).

and valvular incompetence. With recanalization of the thrombosed venous segment, patency is restored and maximal venous outflow study results may fall within the normal range. The fact that recanalization has occurred or that the venous outflow value at rest falls within the normal range does not mean that the vein is free of luminal obstruction. Figure 134–7 demonstrates this point. The ascending phlebogram (see Fig. 134–7A) of a patient with chronic venous insufficiency and venous ulceration demonstrates the classic appearance of a recanalized common and superficial femoral vein 15 years after acute DVT. The official interpretation described a patent superficial femoral vein without obstruction. Plethysmographic testing of the patient at rest failed to demonstrate any abnormality of venous outflow. Because this patient had had a classic Linton procedure, the superficial femoral vein was ligated and divided below the origin of the profunda femoris vein. A cross section of the superficial femoral vein high in the thigh is illustrated in Figure 134–7B. Although multiple channels due to recanalization can be observed, a large percentage of the normal luminal area remains obstructed. One can easily appreciate the extensive destruction of the venous valves and therefore the natural progression to the post-thrombotic syndrome. Shull and colleagues demonstrated additive effects of residual obstruction and valvular incompetence on ambulatory venous hypertension in post-thrombotic patients.[69] In general, patients with the highest ambulatory venous pressures have the most severe post-thrombotic syndrome, resulting from both residual venous obstruction and valvular insufficiency.

Studies have demonstrated that valvular reflux develops progressively from the time of acute venous thrombosis. Markel and colleagues followed up 268 patients who had acute DVT with venous duplex imaging.[70] At initial presentation, 14 per cent had valvular reflux. Patients were then restudied sequentially at 1 week, 1 month, 3 months, and 1 year. Reflux developed in 17 per cent of patients by the end of the 1st week. By the end of the 1st month, 40 per cent demonstrated reflux, and after 1 year, 66 per cent of patients showed reflux. In a cohort of more than 1000

related to conditions other than DVT. This is illustrated by the fact that 20 per cent or fewer of patients suffering fatal PE have the diagnosis of DVT at the time of the fatal event. This emphasizes the need for objective evaluation of patients suspected of having DVT and those at high risk.

The acute complication of DVT is PE, which was discussed earlier. The late complication of acute DVT is the post-thrombotic syndrome. The underlying pathophysiology of the post-thrombotic syndrome is ambulatory venous hypertension. The two components producing ambulatory venous hypertension are residual venous obstruction

FIGURE 134–7. *A,* Ascending phlebogram of a patient with a post-thrombotic syndrome. This patient had had acute DVT 15 years earlier. *B,* Cross-sectional view of the excised superficial femoral vein imaged by the ascending phlebogram in *A.* The specimen was obtained during a classic Linton procedure. One can appreciate significant residual luminal obstruction, multiple-channel recanalization, and destruction of the valves within this segment. This patient had normal impedance plethysmographic findings and phleborheography before operation.

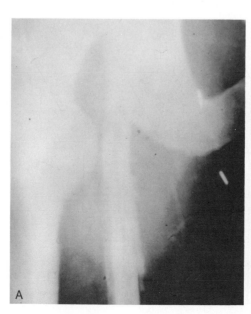
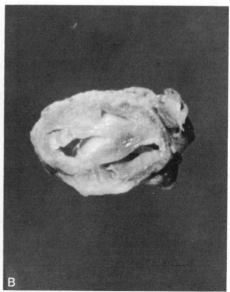

patients who had symptoms but did not have DVT, only 6 per cent demonstrated reflux at 1 year. Valvular reflux was more common in patients suffering occlusive thrombosis than in those with nonocclusive venous thrombosis. This important study demonstrates that increasing amounts of time are required for some valves to become incompetent. In an earlier analysis, it was shown that some patients developed incompetent valves in vein segments that were not involved in the thrombotic process.[71] This new observation leads to the conclusion that the mechanisms by which valvular incompetence occurs following DVT must involve more than a physical effect of the thrombus on the valve. Another important observation was that 38 per cent did not develop valvular incompetence during the study. The majority who maintained good valve function long term had complete recanalization of the original thrombi within 30 days. Therefore, these observations suggest that early lysis of the thrombus preserves valvular function.

Treatment

The appropriate treatment of patients with DVT is based on an awareness of the natural history of the disease and on the goals the physician wants to achieve with therapy. From the outset, the physician must clearly identify the therapeutic goal and then decide on a course of therapy that is most likely to ensure that end-point. Figure 134–8 lists potential therapeutic goals and the available treatment options that can be used to achieve these goals. The ideal treatment approach is to avoid embolization and to clear the venous system of thrombus, thereby restoring patency and maintaining valvular function. Preventing recurrent thrombosis is important and can be achieved in most cases with effective long-term anticoagulation.

Anticoagulation

Anticoagulants are the mainstay for treatment of patients with venous thromboembolic disease. Important advances made since the early 1980s have had a considerable impact on the efficacy and safety of anticoagulation, but many physicians have failed to appreciate these advances. Anticoagulant therapy is essentially prophylactic because these agents interrupt thrombus progression but do not actively resolve it. Of the antithrombotic agents currently available, only heparin and warfarin compounds have been approved for treating established venous thromboembolic disease. Preliminary results with the newer antithrombotic agents are promising; however, these drugs are not yet available for routine clinical use.

Heparin

Since it was discovered in 1916 by McLean,[72] heparin has been established as the most effective anticoagulant, and with the possible exception of aspirin, it is the drug most frequently used by vascular surgeons. To achieve its anticoagulant effect, heparin binds to antithrombin III, producing a conformational change that converts antithrombin III from a slow to a rapid inhibitor of fibrin.[73] Preparations of heparin in clinical use contain molecular weights ranging from 3000 to 30,000 daltons. Less than one half of the administered heparin is responsible for the anticoagulant effect by binding to the antithrombin III molecule.[74, 75] A secondary anticoagulant effect can be achieved through heparin cofactor II,[76] although higher doses of heparin must be administered than those usually given. Heparin has other effects independent of its anticoagulant activity that may play an important role in the patient's overall antithrombotic status. Heparin inhibits platelet function and prolongs bleeding time,[77, 78] and it inhibits vascular smooth muscle cells and binds to vascular endothelium.[79, 80] These secondary effects may become particularly important after invasive procedures such as angiography, cardiac catheterization, and angioplasty, both by improving results and by increasing complications.

The heparin–antithrombin III complex inactivates thrombin (factor IIa) and activated clotting factors IX, X, XI, and XII.[73] Evidence is increasing that heparin's inhibitory effect on coagulation is mediated through the inhibition of thrombin-induced activation of factor V and factor VIII.[81–83]

Goals of R$_x$	No R$_x$	Caval Filter	Anticoagulation	Thrombolytic Rx	Thrombectomy
Reduce P.E.	X	X	X	X	
Prevent Extension			X	X	±
Reduce Recurrence			X	X	±
Restore Patency				X	X
Preserve Valve Function				X	X
Reduce Chronic Venous Insufficiency			±	X	X

FIGURE 134–8. Goals of therapy for acute DVT and the treatment options available. ±, possibly.

Many physicians fail to appreciate that the biologic effect of heparin does not fit simple first-order kinetics. When higher doses of heparin are given, a longer disappearance time and decreased clearance are observed; therefore, the dose-response relationship is not linear. The anticoagulant response increases disproportionately as the dose increases.[84-87] Table 134-4 reviews the biologic activity of heparin in normal individuals, indicating a progressively longer half-life as the bolus dose of heparin increases.

Heparin's action may be prevented by platelets, fibrin, and circulating plasma proteins. Platelets secrete platelet factor 4,[88] which actively neutralizes the anticoagulant activity of heparin. Two other plasma proteins, histidine-rich glycoprotein[89] and vitronectin,[90] also neutralize the anticoagulant effect of heparin. Additionally, when factor Xa is bound to platelets, the anticoagulant effect of the heparin–antithrombin III complex is ineffective.[91, 92] The effect of heparin's interaction on the plasminogen-plasmin enzyme system has been studied, and heparin has been found to enhance the activation of circulating plasminogen to plasmin, but it paradoxically impairs the activation of the fibrin-bound plasminogen.[93, 94] The overall effect of heparin on endogenous fibrinolytic activity is small, and it most likely neither enhances nor inhibits endogenous fibrinolysis.[95, 96]

Heparin is poorly absorbed through the gastrointestinal tract or intrabronchially; therefore, it must be given parenterally for reliable therapy. Heparin is effective after subcutaneous injection and when given intravenously. The anticoagulant response to heparin in any individual is unpredictable, and close monitoring of the activated partial thromboplastin time (APTT) is therefore necessary to ensure the desired therapeutic response.

A number of studies have demonstrated that continuous intravenous infusion of heparin is safer and more effective than intermittent-bolus intravenous infusion.[97-99]

Clinical trials have demonstrated that failure to achieve an APTT ratio of 1.5 times control value is associated with an unacceptably high risk of recurrent venous thromboembolism. Hull and colleagues evaluated patients with proximal vein thrombosis who were treated either with continuous intravenous heparin or with intermittent subcutaneous heparin.[100] The respective routes of delivery produced markedly different intensities of anticoagulant response during the initial course of treatment. Sixty-three per cent of patients receiving subcutaneous delivery had an initial APTT response of less than 1.5 times control value and 19 per cent of these patients (11 of 57) developed recurrent venous thromboembolism. Twenty-nine per cent of those receiving continuous intravenous heparin had an inadequate APTT response, and 5 per cent of this group (3 of 58) developed recurrent thromboembolic events. Essen-

tially, the recurrent thromboembolic events in both groups were found in patients with a subtherapeutic anticoagulant response. When recurrent thromboembolic events were contrasted with efficacy of therapy, 24.5 per cent of patients (13 of 53) with an APTT response below 1.5 times control value for 24 hours or more had recurrent venous thromboembolism, compared with only 1.6 per cent (1 of 62) when an APTT ratio of 1.5 times control value or more was maintained ($p<.001$).

These findings were corroborated by Brandjes and associates.[101] These investigators compared intravenous heparin with oral anticoagulation alone for the initial treatment of patients with acute proximal DVT. Of course, patients receiving oral anticoagulants would always have an inadequate anticoagulant response during the first 48 to 72 hours because the onset of the anticoagulant effect is delayed by virtue of their mechanism of action (carboxylation of vitamin K–dependent clotting factors). In this randomized, double-blind study, recurrent venous thromboembolism was noted in 20 per cent of patients (12 of 60) treated with oral anticoagulants alone, compared with 6.7 per cent (4 of 60) who received intravenous heparin adjusted to maintain the APTT above 1.5 times control value plus oral anticoagulation. This study was terminated early by the data and safety monitoring committee because of the excessive number of symptomatic events in the group receiving oral anticoagulation alone. Additionally, asymptomatic extension of venous thrombosis was observed in 39.6 per cent of the oral anticoagulant group, compared with 8.2 per cent of patients in the heparin plus oral anticoagulant group ($p<.001$). Interestingly, major bleeding was infrequent, and its incidence was not different between the two treatment groups.

The optimal duration of intravenous heparin infusion has not been fully resolved for all patients with venous thromboembolic disease; however, efficient guidelines can be established based on objectively obtained data. Results of a prospective, randomized study suggest that heparin and oral anticoagulation can be started simultaneously, at the time of diagnosis.[103] The heparin can then be discontinued after 4 to 5 days, when the oral anticoagulants are therapeutic. Although this approach is applicable to most patients with venous thrombosis and PE, it remains to be established whether it is appropriate for patients with extensive disease.

It is commonly believed that the risk of bleeding with heparin increases as the dose increases and that patients with increased risk can be identified by in vitro coagulation tests used to monitor heparin therapy. There may be some merit to this observation in patients who have comorbid risk factors, which identify patients at high risk.[102] However, in patients without comorbid risk factors, the association between supratherapeutic APTT response and the risk of bleeding does not appear to be established.

Information about the upper limit of the therapeutic range for the APTT has been of interest, and data indicate that higher therapeutic ranges may be beneficial. Conti and colleagues evaluated two approaches to heparin therapy for acute DVT.[104] Patients were treated with either high-dose heparin without monitoring or conventional-dose heparin with monitoring. No thromboembolic complications occurred in the high-dose group, and symptom resolution was prompt. Significant bleeding occurred in 8 per cent. In the

Table 134–4. Heparin Kinetics: Biologic Activity of Heparin in Human Volunteers

Study	Intravenous Bolus (U/kg)	Plasma Biologic Half-Life (min)
Bjornsson et al, 1982[86]	25	30
Bjornsson et al[86]	75	60
Olsson et al, 1963[85]	100	56
Olsson et al[85]	400	152

conventional-dose group, thromboembolic complications occurred in 10 per cent, bleeding complications occurred in 12 per cent, and only 33 per cent of patients experienced prompt resolution of symptoms. In a more recent, randomized study, the clinical outcomes of patients with proximal DVT were evaluated after patients were randomized to receive initial treatment with either intravenous heparin alone or intravenous heparin plus simultaneous warfarin.[105] Both patient groups reflected adequate anticoagulation; however, the combined heparin and warfarin group received more intensive anticoagulation, and the majority exceeded an APTT ratio of 2.5 times control value. Sixty-nine per cent of patients (69 of 99) in the combined group had a supratherapeutic value for 24 hours or more, compared with 24 per cent (24 of 100) receiving heparin alone. Bleeding complications occurred with similar frequency in the two treatment groups, and the frequency of bleeding complications was no different in the supratherapeutic group than in those who did not have supratherapeutic values. Major bleeding occurred in 11 per cent of patients with comorbidities but in only 1 per cent of those at low risk for bleeding complications ($p = .007$). Therefore, available data demonstrate more effective anticoagulation in patients who have supratherapeutic APTT responses without an increased risk of clinically important bleeding complications (in the absence of comorbidities).

Hopefully, as physicians become more aware of these findings, improved practice patterns regarding anticoagulants will occur. Reviews of physician practices in the treatment of venous thromboembolism indicated that the majority of patients were inadequately treated during the first 24 hours[106] and that even after a subtherapeutic APTT was found, no alteration in heparin infusion was ordered in 33 per cent of patients. Landefeld and Anderson evaluated the effect of consultants and standard anticoagulation protocols on bleeding complications in patients receiving anticoagulants who were at increased risk for hemorrhagic complications.[107] They showed that guideline-based consultation reduced the number of anticoagulant-related bleeding complications, thereby making a strong case for the routine application of standard protocols to the treatment of most patients receiving anticoagulants.[108] Hull and coworkers confirmed that a prescriptive approach to heparin administration was more effective than the subjective, individual approach attempted by most clinicians.[105] These audits of heparin therapy indicate the need for ongoing quality assurance in patients receiving anticoagulants.

When patients are being followed up on a daily basis, it is advised that the APTT sample be drawn at relatively the same time, because a circadian variability in APTT response to the same heparin dose has been observed.[105]

Heparin is commercially available as a sodium or calcium salt and is derived from bovine (beef lung) or porcine (pig intestine) sources. There is no evidence that the pharmacokinetics or anticoagulant properties are different. Heparin-induced thrombocytopenia is a well-recognized and feared complication of heparin therapy that is usually observed 5 to 10 days after heparin use has begun.[109] This complication has been reported in 2 to 20 per cent of patients and is thought to occur more frequently in patients receiving bovine heparin than in those receiving porcine heparin.[110] Heparin-induced thrombocytopenia is an anti-

gen-antibody immunologic response that is not dose related. It is caused by heparin-induced antiplatelet antibodies leading to platelet aggregation, thrombocytopenia, and the subsequent thromboembolic complications. Cines and coworkers demonstrated that heparin-associated thrombocytopenia was a reaction requiring IgG and an intact classic complement pathway.[111] When studying patients with heparin-induced thrombocytopenia, they demonstrated that heparin administration was associated with complement-mediated platelet injury and that there was a dose-dependent relationship of complement activation in patients receiving heparin. The serologic studies of complement activation noted by Cines and coworkers differed from the clinical response to heparin-induced thrombocytopenia in terms of dose dependency. Interestingly, the thrombotic and embolic complications of platelet aggregation occur more frequently (both on the arterial and venous sides of the circulation) than the hemorrhagic complications of platelet depletion. Platelet counts must be monitored in all patients receiving heparin, regardless of the route of administration or the dose prescribed. A drop in the platelet count should indicate the likelihood of heparin-induced thrombocytopenia, and heparin should be discontinued and alternative antithrombotic therapy initiated.

Other complications infrequently associated with heparin administration are osteoporosis, alopecia, hypoadrenalism, and anaphylaxis.[112–114]

Oral Anticoagulation

Oral anticoagulants produce their anticoagulant effect by inhibiting the vitamin K–dependent coagulation factors II, VII, IX, and X.[115, 116] Oral anticoagulants also inhibit vitamin K–dependent carboxylation of proteins C and S. Because proteins C and S are naturally occurring anticoagulants that function by inhibiting activated factors V and VIII, any vitamin K antagonists can create a potential hypercoagulable state before they have their anticoagulant effect because the half-lives of proteins C and S are much shorter than the half-lives of the clotting factors. The warfarin compounds do not have an immediate effect on the coagulation system because the normal coagulation factors present must be cleared. Generally, the oral anticoagulants must be administered for 3 to 5 days to achieve therapeutic anticoagulation; therefore, patients should be treated during this time with intravenous heparin. As mentioned previously, primary therapy with oral anticoagulants without intravenous heparin is associated with unacceptably high recurrent thromboembolic complications.[101]

Guidelines for the appropriate intensity of oral anticoagulation have been clarified. Initial recommendations of prothrombin time levels of 2 to 2.5 times control value or an international normalized ratio (INR) of 4 to 7 have been revised. Evidence from prospective studies indicates that less intense warfarin therapy that achieves a prothrombin time ratio (PTR) of 1.3 to 1.5 (INR of 2.0 to 3.0) is equally effective in preventing recurrent venous thromboembolic events but results in significantly fewer bleeding complications.[117]

The duration of oral anticoagulation should be modified according to the needs of the individual patient. Patients with isolated calf vein thrombosis without ongoing risk factors can be treated differently than patients with more extensive disease with ongoing risk factors. Patients with documented hypercoagulable disease states and those with recurrent venous thromboembolic disease should remain on long-term and possibly lifelong anticoagulation.

Because guidelines for oral anticoagulation have been established, the importance of appropriate monitoring of patients receiving oral anticoagulants is evident. A little-recognized problem is that large differences exist in the sensitivity of thromboplastins used by hematology laboratories. The PTR, which is commonly used to guide oral anticoagulation, is based on the expectation that North American thromboplastin has an international sensitivity index (ISI) of 2.2 to 2.6. The INR is calculated by raising the PTR to the power of the ISI of the thromboplastin used in the assay (INR = PTR^{ISI}). Because the INR calculation adjusts for the sensitivity of the thromboplastin, the INR is therefore the PTR that would have been obtained if the World Health Organization reference thromboplastin had been used to perform the test. Therefore, one can appreciate the importance of using INR values in preference to PTRs. Unfortunately, few laboratories throughout the country report INR values, and the current guidelines for PTRs are no longer appropriate in the United States because many US thromboplastins have ISI values outside the range of 2.2 to 2.6. This was demonstrated by Bussey and colleagues when they evaluated 53 hospital laboratories and provided data on the sensitivity of the thromboplastin and whether the laboratory reported INR values.[118] They concluded that warfarin therapy in the United States is managed inappropriately, because most laboratories do not report INRs and the marked variability in thromboplastin sensitivity results in a misleading PTR. This means that the same blood sample could be processed in two laboratories using thromboplastins with different ISI values, and the results would appear markedly different. The sample might yield a PTR of 1.7 (20.5 seconds) in one laboratory and a PTR of 3.5 (42 seconds) in another laboratory. An understanding of this variability underscores the importance of standardized monitoring of oral anticoagulation, and the need for reporting the INR becomes evident.

The major side effect of oral anticoagulation is bleeding, which is usually related to the degree of anticoagulation as predicted by the prolongation of the prothrombin time.[119] Nonhemorrhagic complications include skin necrosis, which has been associated with a heterozygote protein C deficiency, and malignancy.[120–123] Warfarin compounds cross the placenta and have been associated with teratogenic effects when given during the first trimester of pregnancy.[124, 125] Because there are similar concerns during the second trimester, as well as the risk of fetal bleeding during and after delivery, warfarin compounds should be avoided during pregnancy. All women of childbearing potential who are taking warfarin must avoid becoming pregnant. Long-term adjusted-dose subcutaneous heparin is recommended in pregnant patients.[126]

Thrombolytic Therapy

Restoring patency by eliminating thrombus in the deep venous system is an ideal goal of therapy for acute DVT, although pharmacologic and mechanical methods designed to clear the deep venous system remain controversial. Reports demonstrate that lysis can be achieved and patency restored with thrombolytic therapy, and long-term post-thrombotic sequelae can be reduced when lytic therapy is successful in clearing the deep venous system. However, these results have not been uniform, and many physicians are unwilling to risk the potential complications or to encounter the additional expense associated with thrombolytic therapy. Although accumulated data have demonstrated that significantly more patients regain patency of the venous system when they are treated with thrombolytic therapy than when they receive standard anticoagulation,[127] in absolute terms there are a substantial number of failures. Therefore, a physician may not appreciate the advantages of lytic therapy because of his or her individual anecdotal experience.

The preservation of venous function is the long-term goal of thrombolysis for acute DVT; it includes restoring patency and maintaining valvular function. Those who argue against the use of lytic agents point to the risk involved, the cost of therapy, its limited application with respect to all patients with DVT, and the low success rate in selected studies. Proponents of lytic therapy, however, reiterate that treatment today is less risky than was quoted in earlier reports. They emphasize that the cost of the alternative outcome, the post-thrombotic syndrome, is exceptionally high, although it is spread over many years.[128] Although many patients with acute DVT are not candidates for lytic therapy (e.g., those in the early postoperative period and those with a history of intracranial disease), many patients who are eligible are young and are therefore likely to gain the most benefit from successful thrombolysis.

Some reports of the results of thrombolytic therapy are potentially biased because in many centers lytic therapy for acute DVT is reserved for patients with the most severe disease (i.e., those with massive iliofemoral DVT or phlegmasia cerulea dolens). In these patients, *systemic* thrombolysis is likely to fail because the iliofemoral venous system has extensive occlusion and is devoid of blood flow. Because flow is obliterated in the iliac veins, it is unlikely that the plasminogen activator will contact the clot, and lysis will therefore fail. In most medical centers, patients with less severe forms of acute DVT, who are likely to have a less severe post-thrombotic syndrome, are generally treated with anticoagulation alone.

In evaluating the use of thrombolytic agents for the treatment of acute DVT, several important questions should be answered: (1) What is the natural history of anticoagulant therapy? (2) Can venous thrombi be lysed? (3) Is lysis of venous clot important for long-term valvular function?

Thirteen studies reported in the literature compared anticoagulant therapy with thrombolytic therapy for acute DVT.[129–143] The diagnosis was established with ascending phlebography, and phlebography was repeated to assess the results of therapy. After the data were pooled (Table 134–5), it was found that only 4 per cent of patients treated with anticoagulants had significant or complete lysis, and an additional 14 per cent had partial lysis. The majority, 82 per cent, had either no objective phlebographic clearing or actual extension of their thrombi. Therefore, only a minority of patients had sufficient clearing of thrombus to expect the return of normal venous valvular function. In patients

Table 134–5. Phlebographic Outcome of Anticoagulation Versus Thrombolytic Therapy for Acute Deep Venous Thrombosis: Results of Pooled Data From 13 Reports

		Lysis (%)		
Treatment	**No. of Patients**	**None or Worse**	**Partial**	**Significant or Complete**
Heparin	254	82	14	4
Lytic therapy	337	37	37	45

Data from references 129 to 143 (references 134 to 136 report the result of the same patient group and are therefore considered as one report for tabulation purposes.)

treated with thrombolytic therapy, 45 per cent had significant or complete clearing of the clot, and 18 per cent had partial clearing. The conditions of 37 per cent failed to improve or worsened.

Four additional studies described the results of thrombolytic therapy for DVT but were considered unsuitable for inclusion in the collective data.[144–147] Two studies failed to include an anticoagulation cohort;[144, 145] therefore, comparative data were not available. Kakkar and Lawrence reported venous hemodynamic changes in patients followed up for 24 months after initial randomization to treatment with streptokinase or heparin for acute DVT.[146] Unfortunately, the patients reported on represent fewer than one third of those initially randomized. Because the initial response to therapy was not clarified in all patients, it would be incorrect to assume that the outcome of those followed up for the long term is representative of that of all patients initially randomized. Because symptomatic patients are more likely to seek continued care than are those who feel well, this report may have a pessimistic bias owing to patient self-selection. The fourth study that was excluded described the response of calf vein thrombosis to treatment with heparin or streptokinase.[147] Although these investigators reported the treatment group response with an average quantitative venographic score, they failed to report the individual patient responses to therapy. Two studies reported long-term symptomatic results of anticoagulation compared with thrombolytic therapy following randomized treatment of the acute episode (Table 134–6).[139, 148] Although the follow-up period was shorter for the study of Elliot and coworkers[139] than for that of Arnesen and associates[148] (1.6 vs 6.5 years, respectively), both treatment protocols were similar and the same drug (streptokinase) was used. Post-treatment evaluation indicated that the majority of patients who were free of post-thrombotic symptoms were treated with streptokinase, whereas the majority of patients who had the severe symptoms of the post-thrombotic syndrome were treated with anticoagulation alone.

The most important question to be answered is whether lysis of deep venous thrombi preserves venous valvular function. In a long-term follow-up of a prospective, randomized study, Jeffery and colleagues showed significant functional benefit 5 to 10 years after therapy for acute DVT in patients who had successful lysis. The acute response to streptokinase therapy was similar to that in the pooled data previously reviewed. Patients were then followed up long term for popliteal valve incompetence and regional venous insufficiency of the involved limb using photoplethysmography, foot volumetry, and direct Doppler

examination of the popliteal valve. Patients who had initially successful lysis were compared with patients who did not have lysis, regardless of the therapy they received. Patients who had lysis demonstrated normal findings on venous function tests compared with patients who did not have lysis. Nine per cent of patients who had successful lysis had an incompetent popliteal valve, whereas 77 per cent of those who did not have lysis had popliteal valve incompetence ($p = .001$). Therefore, it appears that in patients without a contraindication to thrombolytic therapy, systemic thrombolysis is preferred, especially when DVT is limited to the infrainguinal venous system. Another important issue currently being evaluated is whether lytic therapy for acute DVT reduces the incidence of recurrent DVT.

The causes of failure of thrombolytic therapy include poor patient selection, an inadequate fibrinolytic response, premature termination of therapy, and failure of the plasminogen activator to contact the venous thrombus.

Patients with acute DVT selected for lytic therapy are usually those with the most extensive venous thrombosis, namely patients with iliofemoral venous thrombosis or phlegmasia cerulea dolens. Because patients with extensive DVT are likely to have the most severe post-thrombotic sequelae,[149] the selection process represents an inherent bias when outcome evaluation is based on therapy. In such patients, the venous system is frequently occluded by the thrombus, and no blood flows through the involved veins. Therefore, plasminogen activators infused systemically do not reach the thrombus and cannot be expected to restore patency. Selecting patients with older thrombus also leads to failure, especially in patients receiving systemic infusion.

It has been demonstrated that the success of lysis is related to the amount of fibrin bound to plasminogen within the thrombus. Successful systemic therapy correlates with the age of the thrombus, and this therapy is unlikely to

Table 134–6. Long-Term Symptomatic Outcome of Patients Treated With Streptokinase or Heparin

	No. of Patients	Post-Thrombotic Symptoms		
Treatment		**Severe**	**Moderate**	**None**
Heparin	39	8 (21%)	23 (59%)	8 (21%)
Streptokinase	39	2 (5%)	12 (31%)	25 (64%)

Data from Elliot MS, Immelman EJ, Jeffery P, et al: A comparative randomized trial of heparin versus streptokinase in the treatment of acute proximal venous thrombosis: An interim report of a prospective trial. Br J Surg 66:838, 1979; and Arnesen H, Hoiseth A, Ly B: Streptokinase or heparin in the treatment of deep vein thrombosis: Follow-up results of a prospective study. Acta Med Scand 211:65, 1982.

dissolve a thrombus that is more than 1 week old. Unfortunately, clinicians cannot accurately predict the age of thrombi and must rely on the patient's symptoms. In many instances, symptoms and thrombus age may not be closely correlated.

All thrombolytic therapy depends on activation of plasminogen; therefore, systemic lytic therapy must be accompanied by a systemic fibrinolytic response. Failure to achieve adequate plasmin production is another reason for inadequate lysis.

Streptokinase has been the most frequently used plasminogen activator for the treatment of acute DVT. It is known that circulating antistreptococcal antibodies neutralize streptokinase and minimize its fibrinolytic activity. Likewise, urokinase inhibitors have also been demonstrated.[150] It is important that patients treated with systemic lytic therapy be followed up for appropriate fibrinolytic activation. Our practice is to obtain baseline coagulation study values, including the plasma fibrinogen. After a systemic infusion is begun, the partial thromboplastin time (PTT) and the fibrinogen are redetermined at 6 and 12 hours. A 25 per cent or greater drop in the fibrinogen and prolongation of the PTT are expected. This indicates that the drug is activating plasminogen and that a lytic effect is present. The infusion is continued, with the PTT and the fibrinogen monitored at 12-hour intervals. Although bleeding complications cannot be precisely correlated with laboratory studies of blood coagulation, we found that patients demonstrating the most severe induced coagulopathy (i.e., those with fibrinogen levels of less than 100 mg/dl) had the most frequent and severe bleeding complications. If profound hypofibrinogenemia occurs, the lytic infusion can be temporarily halted.

Although the goal of thrombolytic therapy is clot dissolution, it is surprising how few physicians appropriately monitor this end-point. In many patients, lytic infusions are discontinued before the desired end-point is reached, leaving patients with a residual thrombus burden and the continued risk of post-thrombotic sequelae. In a prospective evaluation of 28 patients receiving thrombolytic therapy for acute DVT at Temple University Hospital, 33 per cent had lytic therapy terminated while the clot was lysing.[151] In the group of patients who had partial lysis of their venous clot, 64 per cent had the lytic agent discontinued while the clot was lysing but before maximal resolution. These data indicated that a substantial number of patients had treatment discontinued before maximal lysis was achieved, which might be responsible for therapeutic "failure." Additionally, a predetermined duration of therapy may place the patient at higher risk for a bleeding complication if lysis occurs early and treatment is continued beyond the patient's maximal response. If the clot shows no lysis after 24 hours or if the clot completely resolves during this period, lytic therapy should be discontinued. On the other hand, if lysis occurs but is incomplete, lytic therapy should be continued until maximal lysis or resolution is documented. The author's group follows up patients with venous duplex imaging at 12- to 24-hour intervals to assess thrombus resolution. If no benefit is demonstrated after 24 hours, the lytic agent is discontinued. If the thrombus is completely lysed, the lytic agent is discontinued. If the thrombus continues to resolve, lytic infusion is continued until complete clearing occurs or until no change is apparent on two successive duplex examinations.

Catheter-Directed Thrombolysis

In the author's experience, patients with iliofemoral venous thrombosis frequently fail to have recanalization when they are treated with systemic infusions of fibrinolytic agents. This has also been reported by others.[152] Failure to respond to systemic lytic therapy is understandable because iliofemoral clot is "packed" into the iliofemoral segment, with little if any exposure to flowing blood. Because blood carries the plasminogen activator, very little of the activator reaches the thrombus. These patients therefore require different methods of delivery of the plasminogen activator than do patients with infrainguinal DVT. The author believes that thrombolytic therapy can be successful in these patients if the drug reaches the clot. Therefore, direct intraclot infusion for patients with iliofemoral venous thrombosis is recommended. Ipsilateral intra-arterial infusion with systemic doses of plasminogen activators has been given in the setting of severe phlegmasia cerulea dolens (early venous gangrene). Whether this is more advantageous than direct intraclot infusion remains to be established, although it is the author's impression that infrainguinal thrombus can be efficiently lysed with this technique but the iliofemoral thrombus will continue to require direct methods of therapy (intraclot infusion or thrombectomy).

Before treatment, patients are evaluated to delineate the extent of thrombosis. The infrainguinal leg veins can be accurately assessed with venous duplex imaging. The proximal extent of the thrombus is evaluated phlebographically, and the contralateral iliofemoral venous system and vena cava should also be studied. It is important to document if there is clot in the inferior vena cava because this will modify recommendations for therapy.

Direct intraclot infusion is achieved by placing a catheter from the contralateral femoral vein, the right jugular vein, or both (Fig. 134–9). Alternative access through an ipsilateral femoral vein catheter can be used at the discretion of the physician. Use of the contralateral femoral vein or the jugular vein allows placement of a vena caval filter, if indicated, before infusion. We have not routinely used caval filters for patients treated with catheter-directed thrombolysis for iliofemoral venous thrombosis unless they suffered acute pulmonary emboli during their current thrombotic episode or had irregular and nonocclusive caval thrombus. Current experience is limited; therefore, proper recommendations for caval filtration in this setting are in evolution. If a caval filter is placed, a subsequent venous thrombectomy, if necessary, becomes more difficult and requires fluoroscopic guidance, and the filter may be dislodged and malpositioned during the procedure. Temporary (removable) caval filters would be the answer in these patients.

Once a guidewire has been positioned appropriately in the thrombus, a multi–side-hole catheter is used to infuse systemic doses of the lytic agents. We have chosen to use urokinase, delivered as a 250,000- to 500,000-unit bolus followed by a continuous infusion of 250,000 U/hr. We have also used bolus doses of rt-PA (10 mg) followed by urokinase infusion to take advantage of synergistic lysis

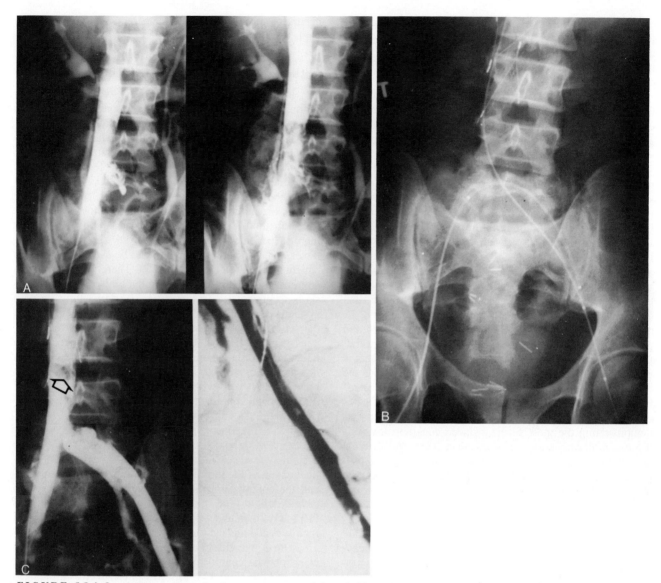

FIGURE 134–9. *A,* Iliocavagrams showing anteroposterior (*left*) and oblique (*right*) views of a patient with phlegmasia cerulea dolens. The entire left iliofemoral venous system is thrombosed, with thrombus partially occluding the distal vena cava. The patient had had total colectomy for ulcerative colitis 9 days earlier. *B,* A bird's nest filter was placed above the thrombus, and two multi–side-hole catheters were inserted into the clot, one from the right jugular vein and one from the contralateral femoral vein. A bolus dose of recombinant tissue plasminogen activator and a continuous infusion of urokinase were given through both catheters to regain patency of the iliofemoral venous system. *C,* After 72 hours, patency is restored, with an excellent clinical response. Note the embolus trapped by the caval filter (*arrow*).

with these agents.[153–155] We have observed an excellent response in a small number of difficult cases with this combination therapy. Repeated phlebography through the infusion catheter is performed at 8- to 12-hour intervals, and therapy is continued until maximal lysis is achieved. The iliac vein thrombi tend to lyse sooner than the more distal thrombi because of the direct activation of fibrin-bound plasminogen. Venous duplex imaging is used to follow lysis of the infrainguinal clot and as much of the iliac venous system as is accessible to ultrasound imaging. After completion of the lytic infusion, patients remain anticoagulated on heparin and are switched to oral anticoagulation.

If the infusion catheter cannot be appropriately positioned in the iliac vein thrombus, a venous thrombectomy is performed.

Venous Thrombectomy

The early experience with venous thrombectomy for iliofemoral venous thrombosis was enthusiastically received because of reports of excellent initial patency without severe post-thrombotic sequelae.[156, 157] Haller and Abrams reported an 85 per cent patency rate in patients operated on within 10 days of the onset of thrombosis, with 81 per cent of survivors having "normal legs" without post-thrombotic swelling.[157] Subsequent reports indicated higher rates of rethrombosis[158] and failure to prevent post-thrombotic sequelae despite patency, because valve competency had been destroyed. Perhaps the most important report was that of Lansing and Davis,[159] which was the 5-year follow-up of the patients originally described by Haller and Abrams. They reported that 94 per cent of those observed had sufficient edema and stasis changes to require elastic stockings and leg elevation. In addition, all patients who underwent long-term follow-up phlebography were found to have insufficient valves. Lansing and Davis also pointed out that two of the three postoperative deaths (in 34 patients) were from PE and that there was a 30 per cent wound complication rate, an average transfusion requirement of 1000 ml, and a mean hospital stay of 12 days. It is probably not reasonable to expect that similar complications of operative thrombectomy would be observed today, in light of the marked advances in all aspects of patient care and the substantial improvements in vascular surgical techniques. The report by Lansing and Davis suffered from a potential selection bias because it is likely that patients with the worst results were the most heavily represented. The patients followed up represented only 50 per cent of those initially operated on, and venographic documentation was achieved in even fewer. Nevertheless, this and other critical appraisals, plus the emergence of thrombolysis, soon relegated venous thrombectomy in most medical centers to the status of a procedure that was of historical interest only. Subsequent reports of successful thrombectomy from European centers (with success rates as high as 82 to 88 per cent without mortality) were for the most part ignored by surgeons in the United States.[160, 161] However, a number of vascular surgery centers persisted in using thrombectomy, and with ongoing experience and refinement in technique, the results improved.[161-167] Most notable among these technical improvements were intraoperative completion venography to ensure a complete thrombectomy, the creation of an arteriovenous fistula, and immediate and prolonged therapeutic anticoagulation to prevent rethrombosis. These improvements were tested in a Swedish prospective, randomized trial, in which much better results were obtained with thrombectomy and temporary arteriovenous fistula creation than with standard anticoagulation.[168] Equally important, the indications for iliofemoral venous thrombectomy have been refined. Therefore, a combination of more selective application and improved technique has reestablished a definite role for venous thrombectomy in the management of iliofemoral venous thrombosis.

Results of Iliofemoral Venous Thrombectomy

The three basic goals originally stated for iliofemoral venous thrombectomy were (1) to avoid PE (by removing the thrombus), (2) to eliminate early morbidity (by eliminating pain, swelling, and ischemic tissue loss), and (3) to minimize the post-thrombotic sequelae (by preserving patency and maintaining valve function). Whereas the mortal-

ity rate in Haller and Abrams' series was 9 per cent,[157] with two of three fatalities related to PE, by the mid-1980s a steady reduction was seen in operative mortality.[160, 167, 168] Ekloff and Juhan reported their experience in 230 patients undergoing thrombectomy for iliofemoral venous thrombosis: they had no fatal pulmonary emboli and only one operative death.[169] It is apparent that the application of venous thrombectomy now can be based not primarily on risk but on its effectiveness relative to competitive forms of therapy in reducing early morbidity or the late sequelae of iliofemoral venous thrombosis.

Successful iliofemoral venous thrombectomy will significantly reduce early morbidity in patients with phlegmasia cerulea dolens and phlegmasia alba dolens. The patient's pain and edema quickly subside, and the discoloration resolves. The definition of benefit, however, may be masked by the additional cost of the operation, transfusion requirements, incisional discomfort, and wound hematomas that may develop in anticoagulated patients. Interestingly, even if thrombectomy is not complete or is with some degree of rethrombosis, the limb rarely returns to its former threatened state if elevation and anticoagulation are continued. In our experience, thrombectomy has failed only when the guidelines were not observed, and although patients may not have benefited, no patient has been made clinically worse.

The long-term benefits of venous thrombectomy relate to its ability to achieve proximal patency and distal valve competence, which are influenced by initial technical success and avoidance of rethrombosis. Initial success in achieving patency is, in turn, influenced by treatment delay and attention to technical detail. Pooled data from a number of contemporary reports on iliofemoral venous thrombectomy (Table 134–7) have indicated that the early and long-term patency of the iliovenous segment is in the 80 to 85 per cent range, compared with 30 per cent patency in patients treated with anticoagulation alone.[176]

In the Scandinavian trial (results are summarized in Table 134–8), complete iliofemoral patency without significant filling defects was documented phlebographically in 76 per cent of thrombectomy patients at 6 months but in only 35 per cent of patients treated with anticoagulation alone. Distally, twice as many thrombectomy patients had patent femoropopliteal segments (52 vs 26 per cent), and valve reflux was demonstrated in four times as many anticoagulated patients (37 vs 9 per cent). Forty-two per cent of the operated patients were free of post-thrombotic symptoms at 6 months, compared with only 7 per cent in the anticoagulated group. Plate and coworkers reevaluated the randomized patients at 5 years.[173] Radionuclide phlebography showed patency in 76 per cent in the surgical group

Table 134–7. Contemporary Results of Venous Thrombectomy: Patency of Iliac Veins

	References	No. of Reports	No. of Patent Veins/ No. of Patients (%)	Follow-Up
Early results	165–168, 170–172	7	361/421 (86)	Not applicable
Late results	165, 166, 173–175	5	156/198 (79)	10–60 mo (mean, 28 mo)

Modified from Eklof B, Juhan C: Revival of thrombectomy in the management of acute iliofemoral venous thrombosis. Contemp Surg 40:21, 1992.

Table 134–8. Scandinavian Randomized Trial of Venous Thrombectomy and Temporary Arteriovenous Fistula (6-Month Results)

	Patients (%)	
Parameter	*Anticoagulant Group (n = 32)*	*Operative Group (n = 31)*
Proximal patency without defects	35	76
Competent distal valves	26	52
Valve reflux	37	9
Distal occlusion	39	37
Minimal or no symptoms	42	7
Dilated pelvic collaterals	65	24

From Plate G, Einarsson E, Ohlin P, et al: Thrombectomy with temporary arteriovenous fistula in acute iliofemoral venous thrombosis.

versus 20 per cent in the anticoagulation group. Long-term venous function was also evaluated. When the results of reflux, obstruction, and calf muscle pump function were considered together, 39 per cent of the operated patients had normal venous function, compared with 19 per cent of the anticoagulated patients. Fifty-five per cent of those operated on were free of post-thrombotic symptoms, compared with 27 per cent receiving anticoagulants alone.

Technique

The technical details important for successful venous thrombectomy are summarized in Table 134–9. It is always important to delineate the full extent of the thrombus. Venous duplex imaging is useful for evaluating the infrainguinal venous system. Ipsilateral iliofemoral phlebography may be required, and contralateral iliofemorocaval phlebography is important to evaluate the opposite iliac venous system and whether there is thrombus within the vena cava.

Although thrombectomy can be performed under local anesthesia, regional or general anesthesia is preferred. Because most patients will be receiving heparin and will remain anticoagulated postoperatively, regional (spinal or epidural) anesthesia is contraindicated. Our preference is general endotracheal anesthesia, with at least 10 cm of positive end-expiratory pressure applied. The patient will have 2 to 3 units of blood typed and cross-matched before the procedure. Autotransfusion devices are routinely used to salvage the patient's blood and minimize transfusion

requirements. A vertical inguinal incision is made over the femoral vessels, and the common femoral, superficial femoral, and saphenous veins are mobilized. The deep femoral vein is occasionally mobilized, although with experience it can be controlled with pressure. Patients are systemically anticoagulated with generous doses of heparin. A transverse or slightly oblique venotomy is made in the distal common femoral vein just proximal to the saphenofemoral junction (Fig. 134–10). The proximal thrombus is removed with passage of a No. 8 to 10 venous thrombectomy catheter. We do not place a balloon catheter up the contralateral iliofemoral system into the vena cava to occlude the cava before thrombectomy because the incidence of PE is low and positive end-expiratory pressure can be applied during the thrombectomy, further minimizing the likelihood of pulmonary emboli. In an awake patient, the Valsalva maneuver is performed. If the patient has a vena caval filter in place, fluoroscopy is used during the thrombectomy, with contrast liquid used to inflate the balloon of the thrombec-

Table 134–9. Technical Aspects of Successful Venous Thrombectomy

1. Completely visualize the thrombus; include contralateral iliofemoral phlebography and a cavagram.
2. Preferentially use general anesthesia with positive end-expiratory pressure.
3. Type and cross-match 2 to 3 units of blood.
4. Use an autotransfusion device during the procedure.
5. Use generous doses of heparin.
6. If a caval filter is in place, use fluoroscopy during thrombectomy, with contrast material used to inflate the venous thrombectomy balloon.
7. Consider intraoperative infusion of plasminogen activators after thrombectomy, with balloon occlusion of the iliac vein.
8. Use an extrusion technique to remove distal thrombus.
9. Perform completion iliofemoral phlebography to assess the adequacy of the thrombectomy (see Fig. 134–10E).
10. If the proximal thrombectomy is complete, an arteriovenous fistula is constructed with the saphenous vein or one of its large proximal branches to the proximal superficial femoral artery (see Fig. 134–10F).
11. If the iliac system remains occluded or if external compression exists, a cross-pubic venous bypass is performed with an 8- to 10-mm externally supported polytetrafluoroethylene graft with an associated arteriovenous fistula (see Fig. 134–11).
12. Apply external pneumatic compression devices in the recovery room.
13. Continue heparin throughout the postoperative period, switching the patient to oral anticoagulation.
14. Consider leaving the arteriovenous fistula functional if the anastomosis is small and problems do not exist.

FIGURE 134–10. Technique of venous thrombectomy and arteriovenous fistula creation. *A*, Preoperative ascending phlebogram of a 38-year-old woman who developed severe swelling of the left leg associated with constant pain and blue discoloration 6 days after spine reconstruction for scoliosis. All named veins of the left leg, below and above the inguinal ligament, are thrombosed. *B*, Through a longitudinal femoral incision, the common femoral, saphenous, and superficial femoral veins are exposed. A transverse venotomy is made in the common femoral vein (*arrow*), which is packed with thrombus. *C*, Within a short time, thrombus begins to extrude from the venotomy (*double arrow*) because of the high venous pressure. *D*, The leg is raised and a rubber bandage is tightly wrapped from the foot to the upper thigh in order to remove as much clot as possible from the infrainguinal venous system. *E*, After passage of a No. 8 to 10 venous thrombectomy catheter to remove the proximal thrombus, one can appreciate the extensive amount of thrombus retrieved. *F*, Completion venogram demonstrates a patent iliofemoral venous system without apparent residual thrombus. *G*, A small (4 mm) arteriovenous fistula (*arrow*) is created by sewing the end of the transected saphenous vein to the side of the superficial femoral artery. The proximal saphenous vein frequently requires thrombectomy before creation of the arteriovenous fistula. *H*, Photograph taken at the 2-year follow-up visit. The patient has only mild intermittent swelling, which is controlled with low-pressure compression stockings.

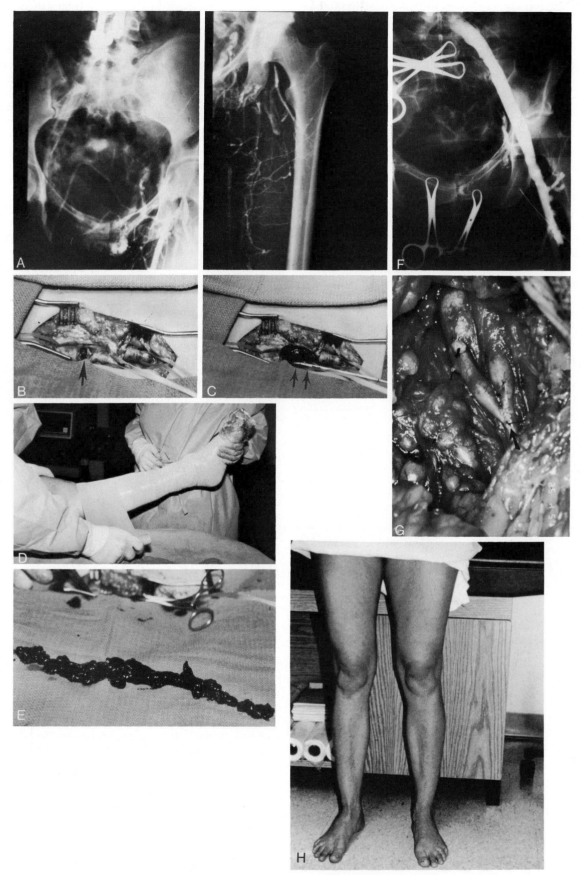

FIGURE 134–10.   *See legend on opposite page*

tomy catheter. At the completion of the proximal thrombectomy, the balloon can be reinserted and inflated, and intraoperative infusion of plasminogen activators may be of benefit in clearing residual adherent thrombus.

The proximal venous segment should be assessed with good completion venography, which can be performed with an injection of approximately 30 ml of contrast material. Because there is inflow occlusion, this technique generally gives good visualization of the entire iliac venous system (see Fig. 134–10). An alternative is to use direct venoscopy with a fiberbronchoscope, as reported by Loeprecht.[177] We have been unsuccessful with venous angioscopy owing to an inability to clear the lumen of blood draining from collateral veins.

If patency cannot be restored to the proximal venous segment or if it is found to be extrinsically compressed, a cross-pubic venous bypass is performed with an 8- to 10-mm externally supported polytetrafluoroethylene graft, with a 4-mm arteriovenous fistula created approximately 3 to 4 inches distal to the origin of the superficial femoral artery (Fig. 134–11).

After the proximal thrombectomy, attention is turned to removing the distal thrombus. As much clot as possible should be removed by the extrusion technique, either by stroking along the course of the distal veins or by using a tight Esmarch bandage wrapped from the foot proximally.

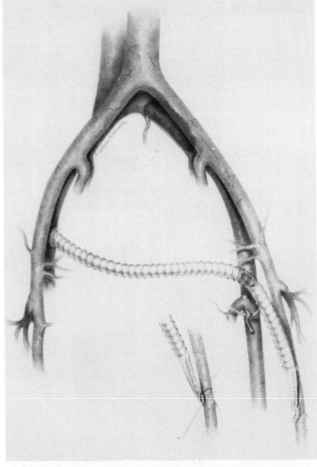

FIGURE 134–11. Preferred method of cross-pubic venous bypass with an 8- or 10-mm externally supported polytetrafluoroethylene graft. Note the small arteriovenous fistula (4 mm) to the superficial femoral artery.

A Fogarty venous thrombectomy catheter can be directed distally, although its passage is usually prohibited by venous valves. An alternative approach is to explore the posterior tibial vein, into which a catheter can be introduced up to the common femoral vein. A Fogarty catheter can then be attached and guided distally, at which time a thrombectomy of the entire leg can be performed.[169] Although we have no experience with this technique, this integrated approach may be an improvement over what can be achieved with the compression maneuvers. Additionally, venography can be performed through the same distal point of access.

An arteriovenous fistula is then constructed using the proximal saphenous vein, which usually is thrombosed and requires a thrombectomy to restore patency. A large proximal branch of the greater saphenous vein is used if available. The superficial femoral artery is mobilized 3 to 4 inches distal to its origin, and an end-to-side anastomosis no greater than 4 mm in diameter is performed. A double loop of Prolene suture material can be passed around this segment, with a silver or titanium clip holding its ends together, and left just under the incision. This can be readily accessed if the surgeon wishes to close the arteriovenous fistula. Since the late 1980s, we have chosen not to close the arteriovenous fistula routinely. Constructing a 4-mm or smaller arteriovenous fistula does not create a vascular steal or significant hemodynamic disturbances. If the iliofemoral venous segment is clear of obstruction, there will be no increase in venous pressure due to the arteriovenous fistula. Additionally, patients have suffered recurrent thrombosis as a result of routine ligation of arteriovenous fistulae.

Heparin is continued throughout the operative and postoperative period, with warfarin begun on the first postoperative day. External pneumatic compression devices are applied in the recovery room to further accelerate venous return and prevent recurrent thrombosis.

Clinical Treatment Strategies for Patients With Acute Deep Venous Thrombosis

On the basis of available information, patients with acute DVT can be stratified according to the magnitude of their disease, ongoing risk factors, and the likelihood of therapeutic success.

Because patients with the most extensive thrombosis have the poorest long-term prognosis and the highest risk of PE, it seems intuitive that measures designed to clear the deep venous system of thrombus would be the most attractive therapeutic option, assuming reasonable efficacy and safety. The location and extent of the acute thrombotic process should also be considered in the treatment of these patients. Unfortunately, in many medical centers, all patients with acute DVT, including those at the two ends of the thrombotic spectrum, are treated the same.

The treatment of *calf vein thrombosis* remains controversial. Because this represents the most minimal DVT, the acute complications of pulmonary emboli and the number of patients suffering post-thrombotic symptoms should be minimal. Moser and LeMoine supported the contention that the embolic risk was low with calf vein thrombosis.[178] They reported that 0 of 21 patients with venographically proven calf vein thrombosis suffered pulmonary emboli, whereas 8 of 15 (53 per cent) with proximal DVT had positive V/Q scan findings but only 1 was symptomatic. Their studies supported the contention that proximal DVT was associated with a high risk of pulmonary emboli and that embolic risk in patients with isolated calf vein thrombosis was negligible. On the other hand, Kakkar and colleagues, using radioisotopic techniques, demonstrated that 23 per cent of patients with calf vein thrombosis had extension of their thrombi into the popliteal or more proximal veins and that PE occurred in 10 per cent of patients with calf vein thrombosis.[179] Menzoian and colleagues also reported that 10 per cent of patients with calf vein thrombosis suffered PE.[180] Lohr and associates followed up 75 patients who had isolated calf thrombi with venous duplex imaging and demonstrated that 24 patients (32 per cent) had clot propagation and 11 patients (15 per cent) had clot extension into the popliteal or larger veins of the thigh.[181] Interestingly, none of the patients with proximal extension were adequately anticoagulated. No underlying risk factor was identified that was predictive of propagation.

Solis and colleagues followed up 42 patients with venographically documented asymptomatic calf vein thrombosis occurring after total joint replacement who were treated at the discretion of their attending physicians.[182] They found that anticoagulation did not alter the incidence of proximal extension, although the adequacy of anticoagulation in treated patients who had clot extension versus that in patients whose clot remained localized to the calf was not reported.

The importance of definitive therapy for calf vein thrombosis has been clarified by the prospective, randomized study of Lagerstedt and associates.[183] They treated 51 patients with venographically confirmed calf vein DVT, either with 3 months of oral anticoagulation or with minimal therapy. No patients treated for 3 months had recurrence during the 90 days of follow-up. In contrast, 8 (29 per cent) in the group not receiving long-term anticoagulation had objectively documented recurrence, with 5 patients having extension of clot into the proximal deep venous system and 1 patient suffering a pulmonary embolus.

In a study by Pellegrini and coworkers, 11 patients with isolated calf vein thrombosis following total hip arthroplasty were followed up, and none were treated after hospital discharge.[184] Thrombi were located either in the muscular veins (in 6 patients) or in the axial deep calf veins (in 5 patients). Three of 5 patients with axial deep vein calf thrombosis were readmitted for symptomatic PE, and 1 patient died.

On the basis of these overall data, it appears that treatment of patients with calf vein thrombosis is indicated, unless there is a high risk of a bleeding complication. Patients not treated should be placed in a follow-up surveillance program, with venous duplex imaging used to detect proximal extension if it occurs.

Schulman and associates reported using thrombolytic therapy for calf vein thrombosis.[147] Although lysis was demonstrated in patients receiving lytic therapy, it is difficult to determine how much these patients benefited compared with those treated with anticoagulation alone. The rationale for the use of lytic agents for calf DVT is that the majority of venous valves are located below the popliteal vein and that valvular function would therefore be preserved. We would consider lytic therapy for patients with calf DVT if it were extensive, involving the majority of the infrapopliteal veins. However, we have observed this condition only in patients who had total knee replacement and contraindications to lytic therapy. A definitive study has not been performed, and no data are available that suggest long-term benefit from thrombolytic therapy for acute calf vein thrombosis.

On the basis of available data, we suggest that all patients with calf DVT receive at least 3 months of anticoagulation, unless their risk for bleeding complications is high (Fig. 134–12). If not treated, patients should be monitored with venous duplex imaging until the high-risk period has passed and they return to full ambulation. If extension into the proximal venous system is demonstrated, patients must be reevaluated for definitive treatment.

Patients with femoropopliteal DVT have various symptoms, depending on the collateral drainage from the profunda venous system and the superficial veins. If thrombolytic therapy is not contraindicated and is successfully used, patients are likely to enjoy a better long-term outcome than those treated unsuccessfully or with anticoagulation alone.

If systemic thrombolytic therapy is selected as the treatment of choice, available data indicate that urokinase and streptokinase achieve equal efficacy; however, the duration of required therapy is shorter and the complications are fewer with urokinase.[33] If anticoagulation is chosen, immediate anticoagulation with intravenous heparin is preferred. If vascular access is a problem, subcutaneous administration can be effective;[185] however, one must ensure that enough heparin is injected subcutaneously to allow therapeutic anticoagulation. Oral anticoagulants are started immediately.

Hull and colleagues compared subcutaneous low-molecular-weight heparin with continuous intravenous heparin for the treatment of patients with proximal vein thrombosis.[186] In a prospective, double-blind clinical trial, a single daily dose of subcutaneous low-molecular-weight heparin was compared with a dose-adjusted continuous heparin infusion for the initial treatment of patients with proximal vein thrombosis, with objective documentation of clinical outcome. New episodes of venous thromboembolism occurred in 2.8 per cent of patients receiving low-molecular-weight heparin, versus in 6.9 per cent receiving intravenous heparin ($p = .07$). There were significantly fewer bleeding complications with low-molecular-weight heparin than with continuous intravenous heparin (a 91 per cent risk reduction). Interestingly, there was a more significant survival benefit from the long-term administration of low-molecular-weight heparin than in cancer patients receiving intravenous unfractionated heparin. Although low-molecular-weight heparin compounds are not yet approved for use in the United States, their approval by the Food and Drug Administration is certainly forthcoming, and they will offer an attractive alternative to continuous intravenous heparin for the acute treatment of patients with venous thromboembolic disease.

Part of the routine evaluation of patients with proximal DVT should include V/Q scanning. A substantial number

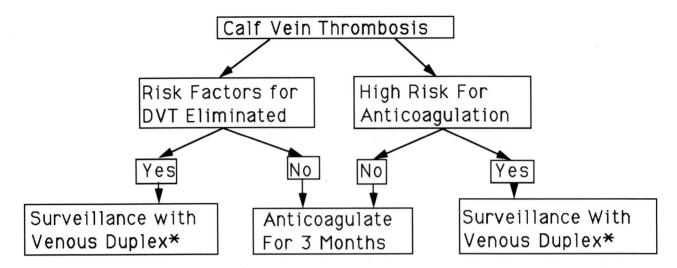

* Until high risk period is
over and patient is ambulatory.

FIGURE 134–12.   Algorithm for treating calf vein thrombosis. Because 20 per cent or more of calf vein thrombi will extend into the proximal veins, treatment is recommended unless the patient is at high risk for anticoagulation or unless all risk factors have been eliminated and the patient is ambulatory. Those not treated should be followed up in a surveillance program with venous duplex imaging.

of patients will have asymptomatic pulmonary emboli at the time their DVT is diagnosed. Monreal and colleagues obtained routine lung scans in patients presenting with DVT.[187] Six of 29 patients with V/Q scans suggesting a high probability of PE subsequently experienced acute signs or symptoms of PE while receiving heparin therapy. A repeated lung scan did not disclose new perfusion defects in any patient. In the absence of a baseline study, physicians would have assumed that PE occurred during therapy, and unnecessary caval interruption procedures might have been performed.

Patients with proximal vein thrombosis who have a contraindication to anticoagulation are treated with caval interruption procedures. Percutaneous placement of vena caval filters is both safe and effective. The current data on vena caval interruption are reviewed in Chapter 135.

Superficial femoral vein ligation has been abandoned as a method of treating DVT in patients with thrombus located distal to the profunda femoris vein. However, a series reported by Masuda and coworkers indicated that when the thrombus is limited to the infraprofunda venous system, superficial femoral vein ligation is effective in preventing PE and propagation to the more proximal venous system, without serious long-term sequelae.[188]

Iliofemoral venous thrombosis is the most extensive form of acute disease, and patients with it face the most severe post-thrombotic sequelae.[128] Clearing the iliofemoral system of thrombus will significantly improve short- and long-term venous function and reduce morbidity. If the femoropopliteal venous segments are open, patients will of course achieve the best short- and long-term results. However, if unobstructed venous drainage can be restored from the deep venous system, subsequent swelling and post-thrombotic symptoms can be reasonably controlled with

external compression, even if obstruction exists below the superficial femoral vein–profunda venous confluence.

Pharmacologic or mechanical thrombectomy is the treatment of choice for these patients. Because systemic lytic therapy frequently fails, direct delivery of thrombolytic agents into the thrombus via a multi–side-hole catheter should be considered. If patients have a contraindication to lytic therapy, venous thrombectomy with an arteriovenous fistula or venous bypass is considered (Fig. 134–13). Patients are then kept on long-term oral anticoagulation, maintaining an international normalized ratio of 2 to 3.

Venous Thromboembolism and Patients With Malignancy

Since the initial observation by Trousseau in 1868 relating thrombotic phenomena to cancer,[189] the relationship between malignant disease and venous thromboembolism has been well recognized. Prandoni and associates evaluated 105 patients with secondary venous thrombosis (DVT associated with a well-recognized risk factor other than cancer) and 145 patients with idiopathic venous thrombosis for the subsequent incidence of cancer.[190] During follow-up, only 2 of the 105 patients with secondary venous thrombosis (1.9 per cent) and 11 of the 145 patients with idiopathic venous thrombosis (7.6 per cent) developed cancer ($p = .043$). Overt cancers subsequently developed in 6 of 35 patients (17 per cent) with recurrent thromboembolism. The incidence of cancer in patients with recurrent idiopathic venous thrombosis was higher than that in patients with secondary venous thrombosis ($p = .008$) and that in patients with idiopathic venous thrombosis that did not

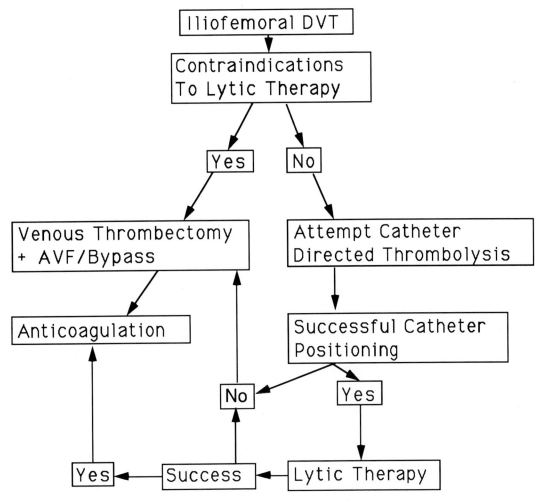

FIGURE 134–13. Algorithm for treating iliofemoral venous thrombosis. AVF, arteriovenous fistula.

recur ($p = .024$). Unfortunately, it is still not clear whether occult malignancy can be reliably detected at the time patients initially present with venous thromboembolism. These patients would undoubtedly require an extensive diagnostic evaluation, which is costly and has yet to be proven effective for the majority of patients with idiopathic DVT. Perhaps patients with recurrent idiopathic DVT represent a subset in which an intensive diagnostic work-up can be justified.

Once diagnosed, these patients represent therapeutic challenges. Moore and colleagues reported bleeding complications in 50 per cent of cancer patients treated with anticoagulants for venous thromboembolic disease.[191] Twenty-five per cent had major hemorrhages that led to cessation of therapy or death. Nineteen per cent of patients suffered a PE while receiving anticoagulants. These authors concluded that vena caval interruption or venous ligation would be a safer and more effective means of prophylaxis against PE in cancer patients. Altschuler and colleagues reported that anticoagulant therapy was safe and effective for patients with malignant glial tumors.[192] These particular tumors may be an exception. Most contemporary reports have confirmed Moore and colleagues' finding of high complication and failure rates when anticoagulants were used for venous thromboembolism associated with cancer.[193–195]

A new and interesting finding is the lower mortality rate in cancer patients treated with low-molecular-weight heparin for venous thromboembolic disease. In two prospective, randomized studies, patients with cancer who were treated with low-molecular-weight heparin had a significant survival advantage over those who were treated with standard anticoagulation.[186, 196] Interestingly, this difference could not be attributed to thrombotic or bleeding complications, which occurred with the same frequency in both groups. These findings suggest that low-molecular-weight heparin might exert an inhibitory effect on tumor growth that does not occur with standard heparin. The evidence from these two studies that low-molecular-weight heparin therapy is associated with lower mortality in cancer patients should renew interest in the use of these heparin fragments as adjuncts to other antineoplastic drugs and may provide valuable options for the long-term treatment of venous thromboembolism in patients with malignancy.

Because long-term anticoagulation with warfarin compounds has a high complication and failure rate, vena caval filtration is preferred as prophylaxis for PE. If patients are judged to have a low risk of a bleeding complication, adjusted-dose subcutaneous heparin is given to achieve prolongation of the mid-interval PTT to 1.5 times control.

Deep Venous Thrombosis of Pregnancy

In absolute numbers, DVT is a relatively uncommon complication of pregnancy. However, the pregnant woman faces a sixfold risk of venous thromboembolism compared with the nonpregnant woman,[197] and in the United States, PE is the most common medical cause of maternal mortality associated with live births.[198]

Two basic pathophysiologic processes account for the occurrence of venous thromboembolism during pregnancy. The first is the gravid uterus causing compression of the pelvic veins and the vena cava. The second is the hypercoagulability that occurs as a result of pregnancy. Pregnant patients have an increase in clotting factors, especially factors II, VII, VIII, and X, as well as an increase in fibrin split products and a decrease in clotting inhibitors. Plasma fibrinolytic activity and antithrombin III levels are also decreased.[199–201] There is evidence that platelet counts increase following labor.[202, 203]

Although the left leg is more frequently involved with DVT in general, the predilection for left-sided DVT is more pronounced in the pregnant patient. The diagnosis should be suspected when swelling occurs, especially when it is associated with atypical pelvic and lower abdominal complaints.[204]

Treatment of DVT in the pregnant patient warrants special consideration because coumarin derivatives must be avoided. Administration of coumarin derivatives to women during the first trimester causes a specific constellation of malformations in at least 25 per cent of the offspring. This is known as warfarin embryopathy or fetal warfarin syndrome,[205–210] the most consistent features of which are nasal hypoplasia and stippled epiphyses. The use of coumarin derivatives at any other time during pregnancy may increase the risk of central nervous system anomalies in the fetus.[211–215] Although the warfarin embryopathy syndrome is considered to be the most characteristic teratogenic consequence of oral anticoagulant use, the sequelae of central nervous system abnormalities are more significant and debilitating than the warfarin embryopathy itself.

Drugs with molecular weights of less than 1000 daltons pass through the placental membrane. Because the placenta acts as a selectively permeable barrier for substances with molecular weights of greater than 1000 daltons, coumarin anticoagulants cross the placenta. In addition to the teratogenic effects of warfarin, the coagulation system of the fetus can be affected. The fetus has low levels of vitamin K–dependent clotting factors throughout gestation, and the warfarin drugs will further deplete these already low levels. Hence, the coagulopathy present in the fetus is not necessarily related to that of the mother, and it may persist long after the mother's coagulation parameters have returned to normal following discontinuation of the drug. This therefore places the fetus at an increased risk of hemorrhage, especially during delivery.

Patients with DVT during pregnancy should be treated acutely with continuous intravenous heparin. Anticoagula-

tion for the duration of pregnancy should be maintained with intermittent subcutaneous heparin given every 12 hours, with the mid-interval PTT maintained at 1.5 times control. Subcutaneous heparin should be continued through childbirth and the immediate postpartum period. After delivery, the patient can be switched to warfarin and maintained on adequate anticoagulation for at least 6 months. During all subsequent pregnancies, the patient should be prophylactically treated with subcutaneous heparin, 5000 units every 12 hours. Any female of childbearing potential should be thoroughly counseled on the need for effective contraception during the time she is taking oral anticoagulants.

Venous thrombosis limited to the calf veins is usually treated with external elastic compression stockings with a 20 to 30 mmHg ankle gradient, continued ambulation, and ongoing surveillance with venous duplex imaging. Prolonged sitting or standing is discouraged.

Acute iliofemoral venous thrombosis during pregnancy is a particularly severe problem. These patients have a greater risk of post-thrombotic sequelae, which is especially morbid because these patients are so young.[216] A number of authors reported excellent results with thrombectomy and arteriovenous fistula creation for iliofemoral venous thrombosis during pregnancy.[216, 217] When followed by heparin anticoagulation, this appears to be safe and effective therapy. There is no need to interrupt pregnancy unless there is a specific obstetric reason. Because this is a particularly young group of patients and because the long-term results appear good, without having an adverse effect on the fetus, venous thrombectomy with an arteriovenous fistula should be seriously considered for severe iliofemoral DVT in these patients.

It remains to be seen whether low-molecular-weight heparin will be effective for treating DVT during pregnancy. The low-molecular-weight heparins do not cross the placenta barrier,[218–220] and reports have suggested that they might be safe and effective.[221]

All women who have a history of DVT and become pregnant should be treated prophylactically with subcutaneous heparin and good external support stockings throughout pregnancy in order to avoid recurrent venous thrombosis.

References

1. Coon WW, Willis PW: Deep venous thrombosis and pulmonary embolism: Prediction, prevention and treatment. Am J Cardiol 4:611, 1959.
2. Hume M, Sevitt S, Thomas DP: Venous Thrombosis and Pulmonary Embolism. Cambridge, MA, Harvard University Press, 1970.
3. Dalen JE, Alpert JS: Natural history of pulmonary embolism. Prog Cardiovasc Dis 17:259, 1975.
4. Carson JL, Kelley MA, Duff A, et al: The clinical course of pulmonary embolism. N Engl J Med 326:1240, 1992.
5. National Institutes of Health Consensus Development Conference. Prevention of venous thrombosis and pulmonary embolism. JAMA 256:744, 1986.
6. Lilienfeld DE, Godbold JH, Burke GL, et al: Hospitalization and case fatality for pulmonary embolism in the twin cities: 1979–1984. Am Heart J 120:392, 1990.
7. Lindblad B, Sternby NH, Bergqvist D: Incidence of venous thromboembolism verified by necropsy over 30 years. Br Med J 302:709, 1991.

8. Anderson FA, Wheeler HB, Goldberg RJ, Hosmer DW: Physician practices in the prevention of venous thromboembolism. Ann Intern Med 115:591, 1991.
9. Bell WR, Simon TL, Demets DL: The clinical features of submassive and massive pulmonary emboli. Am J Med 62:355, 1977.
10. Sasahara AA, McIntyre KM, Cella G, et al: Pulmonary thromboembolic disease. *In* Loscalzo J, Creager MA, Dzau UJ (eds): Vascular Medicine. Boston, Little, Brown and Company, 1993, pp 1049–1074.
11. Westermark N: On the roentgen diagnosis of lung embolism. Acta Radiol 19:357, 1938.
12. The PIOPED Investigators: Value of the ventilation/perfusion scan in acute pulmonary embolism: Results of the Prospective Investigation of Pulmonary Embolism Diagnosis (PIOPED). JAMA 268:2753, 1990.
13. Hull RD, Hirsh J, Carter CJ, et al: Diagnostic value of ventilation-perfusion lung scanning in patients with suspected pulmonary embolism. Chest 88:819, 1985.
14. Austin JHM, Sagel SS: Alterations of airway caliber after pulmonary embolization in the dog. Invest Radiol 7:135, 1972.
15. Robinson AE, Puckett CL, Green JD, Silver D: In vivo demonstration of small-airway bronchoconstriction following pulmonary embolism. Radiology 109:283, 1973.
16. Anderson DR, Lensing WA, Wells PS, et al: Limitations of impedance plethysmography in the diagnosis of clinically suspected deep vein thrombosis. Ann Intern Med 118:25, 1993.
17. Comerota AJ, Katz ML, Grossi RJ, et al: The comparative value of noninvasive testing for diagnosis and surveillance of deep vein thrombosis. J Vasc Surg 7(1):40, 1988.
18. Comerota AJ, Katz ML, Greenwald LL, et al: Venous duplex imaging: Should it replace hemodynamic tests for DVT? J Vasc Surg 11:53, 1990.
19. Comerota AJ, Katz ML, Hashemi HA: Venous duplex imaging for the diagnosis of acute deep venous thrombosis. Haemostasis 23:62, 1993.
20. Barritt DW, Jordan SC: Anticoagulant drugs in the treatment of pulmonary embolism: A controlled clinical trial. Lancet 1:1309, 1960.
21. Alpert JS, Smith R, Carlson CJ, et al: Mortality in patients treated for pulmonary embolism. JAMA 236:1477, 1976.
22. Dalen JE, Banas JS, Brooks HL, et al: Resolution rate of acute pulmonary embolism in man. N Engl J Med 280:1194, 1969.
23. The Urokinase Pulmonary Embolism Trial. A national cooperative study. Circulation 47:II-1, 1973.
24. Urokinase-Streptokinase Embolism Trial: Phase II results: A cooperative study. JAMA 229:1606, 1974.
25. Anderson DR, Levine MN: Thrombolytic therapy for the treatment of acute pulmonary embolism. Can Med Assoc J 146:1317, 1992.
26. Sharma GVRK, Burleson VA, Sasahara AA: Effect of thrombolytic therapy on pulmonary-capillary blood volume in patients with pulmonary embolism. N Engl J Med 303:842, 1980.
27. Sharma GVRK, Folland ED, McIntyre KM, Sasahara AA: Long-term hemodynamic benefit of thrombolytic therapy in pulmonary embolic disease [Abstract]. J Am Coll Cardiol 15:65A, 1990.
28. Come PC, Kim D, Parker JA, et al: Early reversal of right ventricular dysfunction in patients with acute pulmonary embolism after treatment with intravenous tissue plasminogen activator. J Am Coll Cardiol 10:971, 1987.
29. Goldhaber SZ, Feldstein ML, Haire WD, et al: T-PA versus heparin in acute pulmonary embolism: Effects on right ventricular function and pulmonary perfusion in a randomized multicenter trial [Abstract]. Circulation 86:I-409, 1992.
30. Schultz R, Meneveau N, Schele F, et al: Thrombolytic therapy in severe acute pulmonary embolism. Efficacy and safety in elderly patients [Abstract]. J Am Coll Cardiol 19:315A, 1992.
31. Goldhaber SZ: Thrombolytic therapy for pulmonary embolism. *In* Comerota AJ (ed): Thrombolytic Therapy for Peripheral Vascular Disease. Philadelphia, JB Lippincott, 1993.
32. Jang I-K, Vanhaecke J, De Geest H, et al: Coronary thrombolysis with recombinant tissue-type plasminogen activator: patency rate and regional wall motion after 3 months. J Am Coll Cardiol 8:1455, 1985.
33. Graor RA, Young JR, Risus B, et al: Comparison of cost effectiveness of streptokinase and urokinase in the treatment of deep venous thrombosis. Ann Vasc Surg 1:542, 1987.
34. Dalla-Volta S, Palla A, Santolicandro A, et al: PAIMS 2: Alteplase combined with heparin versus heparin in the treatment of acute pulmonary embolism. Plasminogen Activator Italian Multicenter Study 2. J Am Coll Cardiol 20:520, 1992.
35. Meyer G, Sors H, Charbonnier B, et al: Effects of intravenous urokinase versus alteplase on total pulmonary resistance in acute massive pulmonary embolism: A European multicenter double-blind trial. J Am Coll Cardiol 19:239, 1992.
36. Goldhaber SZ, Vaughan DE, Markis JE, et al: Acute pulmonary embolism treated with tissue plasminogen activator. Lancet 2:886, 1986.
37. Goldhaber SZ, Kessler CM, Heit J, et al: A randomized controlled trial of recombinant tissue plasminogen activator versus urokinase in the treatment of acute pulmonary embolism. Lancet 2:293, 1988.
38. Sasahara AA: Special considerations in the management of thrombolysis. *In* Update: New Developments in the Treatment of Thromboembolic Disease. Naples, Florida, November 6 and 7, 1992.
39. Goldhaber SZ, Kessler CM, Heit JA, et al: Recombinant tissue-type plasminogen activator versus a novel dosing regimen of urokinase in acute pulmonary embolism: A randomized controlled multicenter trial. J Am Coll Cardiol 20:24, 1992.
40. Verstraete M, Miller GAH, Bounazeaux H, et al: Intravenous and intrapulmonary recombinant tissue-type plasminogen activator in the treatment of acute massive pulmonary embolism. Circulation 77:353, 1988.
41. Essop MR, Middlemost S, Skoularigis J, Sareli P: Simultaneous mechanical clot fragmentation and pharmacologic thrombolysis in acute massive pulmonary embolism. Am J Cardiol 69:427, 1992.
42. Brady AJB, Crake T, Oakley CM: Simultaneous mechanical clot fragmentation and pharmacologic thrombolysis in acute massive pulmonary embolism. Am J Cardiol 70:836, 1992.
43. Horstkotte D, Heintzen MP, Stauer BE, Leschke M: Aggressive nonsurgical management of massive pulmonary embolism with cardiogenic shock [Abstract]. Eur Heart J 12(Suppl):52, 1991.
44. Flemma RJ, Young WG, Wallace A, et al: Feasibility of pulmonary embolectomy. Circulation 30:234, 1964.
45. Sabiston D: Trendelenburg's classic work on the operative treatment of pulmonary embolism. Ann Thorac Surg 35:570, 1983.
46. Del Campo C: Pulmonary embolectomy: A review. Can J Surg 28:111, 1985.
47. Clarke DB, Abrams LD: Pulmonary embolectomy: A 25 year experience. J Thorac Cardiovasc Surg 92:442, 1986.
48. Gray HH, Morgan JM, Paneth M, Miller GAH: Pulmonary embolectomy for acute massive pulmonary embolism: An analysis of 71 cases. Br Heart J 60:196, 1988.
49. Sabiston DC: Pulmonary embolism. *In* Textbook of Surgery: The Biological Basis of Modern Surgical Practice. 14th ed. Philadelphia, WB Saunders, 1991, pp 1502–1512.
50. Virchow R: Neuer Fall von todlicher Emboli der Lungenarterie. Arch Pathol Anat 10:225, 1856.
51. Stead RB: The hypercoagulable state. *In* Goldhaber SZ (ed): Pulmonary Embolism and Deep Venous Thrombosis. Philadelphia, WB Saunders, 1985, p 161.
52. Hirsh J, Barlow GH, Swann HC, Salzman EW: Diagnosis of prethrombotic state in surgical patients. Contemp Surg 16:65, 1980.
53. Almen T, Nylander G: Serial phlebography of the normal lower leg during muscular contraction and relaxation. Acta Radiol 57:264, 1961.
54. Clark C, Cotton LT: Blood flow in deep veins of the legs. Recording techniques and evaluation of methods to increase flow during operation. Br J Surg 55:211, 1968.
55. Nicolaides AN, Kakkar VV, Renney JTG: The soleal sinuses and stasis. Br J Surg 58:307, 1971.
56. Gibbs NM: Venous thrombosis of the lower limbs with particular reference to bed-rest. Br J Surg 45:209, 1957.
57. Schaub RG, Lynch RP, Stewart GJ: The response of canine veins to three types of abdominal surgery: A scanning and transmission electron microscopic study. Surgery 83:411, 1978.
58. Stewart GJ, Alburger PD, Stone AE, Soszka TW: Total hip replacement induces injury to remote veins in a canine model. J Bone Joint Surg 65A:97, 1983.
59. Stewart GJ, Schaub RG, Niewiarowski S: Products of tissue injury induce venous endothelial damage and blood cell adhesion in the dog. Arch Pathol Med 104:409, 1980.

60. Stone EA, Stewart GJ: Architecture and structure of canine veins with special reference to confluences. Anat Rec 222:154, 1988.

61. Stewart GJ: Personal Communication.

62. Comerota AJ, Stewart GJ: Operative venous dilation and its relation to post operative deep venous thrombosis. *In* Goldhaber SZ (ed): Prevention of Venous Thromboembolism. New York, Marcel Dekker, 1993, pp 25–50.

63. Kakkar VV, Stamatakis JD, Bently PG, et al: Prophylaxis for postoperative deep vein thrombosis. Synergistic effect of heparin and dihydroergotamine. JAMA 241:39, 1979.

64. The Multicenter Trial Committee: Dihydroergotamine/heparin prophylaxis of postoperative deep vein thrombosis. JAMA 251:2960, 1984.

65. Beisaw NE, Comerota AJ, Groth HE, et al: Dihydroergotamine/heparin in the prevention of deep vein thrombosis after total hip replacement. J Bone Joint Surg 70A(1):2, 1988.

66. Comerota AJ, Stewart GJ, Alburger PD, et al: Operative venodilation, a previously unsuspected factor in the cause of postoperative deep vein thrombosis. Surgery 106:301, 1989.

67. Stewart GJ, Lachman JW, Alburger PD, et al: Intraoperative venous dilation and subsequent development of deep vein thrombosis in patients undergoing total hip or knee replacement. Ultrasound Med Biol 16(2):133, 1990.

68. Coleridge-Smith PD, Hasty JH, Scurr JH: Venous stasis and lumen changes during surgery. Br J Surg 77:1055, 1990.

69. Shull KC, Nicolaides AN, Fernandes e Fernandes J, et al: Significance of popliteal reflux in relation to ambulatory venous pressure and ulceration. Arch Surg 114:1304, 1979.

70. Markel A, Manzo R, Bergelin R, Strandness DE: Valvular reflux after deep vein thrombosis: Incidence and time of occurrence. J Vasc Surg 15:377, 1992.

71. Killewich LA, Bedford GR, Beach KW, Strandness DE: Spontaneous lysis of deep venous thrombi: Rate and outcome. J Vasc Surg 9:89, 1989.

72. McLean J: The thromboplastic action of cephalin. Am J Physiol 41:250, 1916.

73. Rosenberg RD: The heparin-antithrombin system: A natural anticoagulation mechanism. *In* Colman RW, Hirsh J, Marder VJ, Salzman EW (eds): Hemostasis and Thrombosis: Basic Principles and Clinical Practice. 2nd ed. Philadelphia, JB Lippincott, 1987, pp 1373–1392.

74. Lam LH, Silbert JE, Rosenberg RD: The separation of active and inactive forms of heparin. Biochem Biophys Res Commun 69:570, 1976.

75. Andersson LO, Barrowcliffe TW, Holmer E, et al: Anticoagulant properties of heparin fractionated by affinity chromatography on matrix-bound antithrombin III and by gel filtration. Thromb Res 9:575, 1976.

76. Ofosu FA, Modi GJ, Hirsh J, et al: Mechanisms for inhibition of the generation of thrombin activity by sulfated polysaccharides. Ann NY Acad Sci 485:41, 1986.

77. Castellot JJ Jr, Favreau LV, Karnovsky MJ, Rosenberg RD: Inhibition of vascular smooth muscle cell growth by endothelial cell–derived heparin. Possible role of a platelet endoglycosidase. J Biol Chem 257:11256, 1982.

78. Heiden D, Mielke CH, Rodvien R: Impairment by heparin of primary haemostasis and platelet [14C]^5-hydroxytryptamine release. Br J Haematol 36:427, 1977.

79. Glimelius B, Busch C, Hook M: Binding of heparin on the surface of cultured human endothelial cells. Thromb Res 12:773, 1978.

80. Mahadoo J, Heibert L, Jaques LB: Vascular sequestration of heparin. Thromb Res 12:79, 1977.

81. Ofosu FA, Slie P, Modi GJ, et al: The inhibition of thrombin-dependent positive-feedback reactions is critical to the expression of the anticoagulant effect of heparin. Biochem J 243:579, 1987.

82. Ofosu FA, Hirsh J, Esmon CT, et al: Unfractionated heparin inhibits thrombin-catalyzed amplification reactions of coagulation more efficiently than those catalyzed by factor X_a. Biochem J 257:143, 1989.

83. Begiom S, Lindhout T, Hemker HC: The mode of action of heparin in plasma. Thromb Haemost 60:457, 1988.

84. de Swart CAM, Nijmeyer B, Roelofs JMM, Sixma JJ: Kinetics of intravenously administered heparin in normal humans. Blood 60:1251, 1982.

85. Olsson P, Lagergren H, EK S: The elimination from plasma of intravenous heparin: An experimental study on dogs and humans. Acta Med Scand 173:619, 1963.

86. Bjornsson TO, Wolfram BS, Kitchell BB: Heparin kinetics determined by three assay methods. Clin Pharmacol Ther 31:104, 1982.

87. Simon TL, Hyers TM, Gaston JP, Harker LA: Heparin pharmacokinetics: Increased requirements in pulmonary embolism. Br J Haematol 39:111, 1978.

88. Holt JC, Niewiarowski S: Biochemistry of alpha-granule proteins. Semin Hematol 22:151, 1985.

89. Lijnen HR, Hoylaerts M, Collen D: Heparin binding properties of human histidine–rich glycoprotein: Mechanism and role in the neutralization of heparin in plasma. J Biol Chem 258:3803, 1983.

90. Preissner KT, Müller-Berghaus G: Neutralization and binding of heparin by S protein/vitronectin in the inhibition of factor Xa by antithrombin III. J Biol Chem 262:12247, 1987.

91. Marciniak E: Factor X_a inactivation by antithrombin. 3. Evidence for biological stabilization of factor Xa by factor V–phospholipid complex. Br J Haematol 24:391, 1973.

92. Walker FJ, Esmon CT: The effects of phospholipid and factor Va on the inhibition of factor Xa by antithrombin III. Biochem Biophys Res Commun 90:641, 1979.

93. Andrade-Gordon P, Strickland S: Interaction of heparin with plasminogen activators in plasminogen: Effects on the activation of plasminogen. Biochemistry 25:4033, 1986.

94. Paques EP, Stohr HA, Heimbeurger N: Study on the mechanism of action of heparin and related substances on the fibrinolytic system: Relationship between plasminogen activators and heparin. Thromb Res 42:797, 1986.

95. Fry ETA, Sobel BE: Lack of interference by heparin with thrombolysis or binding of tissue-type plasminogen activator to thrombi. Blood 71:1347, 1988.

96. Agneli G, Pascucci C, Cosmi B, Neaci GG: Effects of therapeutic doses of heparin on thrombolysis with tissue-type plasminogen activator in rabbits. Blood 76:2030, 1990.

97. Glazier RL, Crowell EB: Randomized prospective trial of continuous versus intermittent heparin therapy. JAMA 236:1365, 1976.

98. Salzman EW, Deykin D, Shapiro RM, et al: Management of heparin therapy: Controlled prospective trial. N Engl J Med 292:1046, 1975.

99. Mant MJ, Thong KL, Birtwhistle RV, et al: Hemorrhagic complications of heparin therapy. Lancet 1:1133, 1977.

100. Hull RD, Raskob GE, Hirsh J, et al: Continuous intravenous heparin compared with intermittent subcutaneous heparin in the initial treatment of proximal-vein thrombosis. N Engl J Med 315:1109, 1986.

101. Brandjes DPM, Buller HR, Heijboer H, et al: Comparative trial of heparin and oral anticoagulants in the initial treatment of proximal deep vein thrombosis. N Engl J Med 327:1485, 1992.

102. Landefeld CS, Cook EF, Flately M, et al: Identification and preliminary validation of predictors of major bleeding in hospitalized patients starting anticoagulant therapy. Am J Med 82:703, 1987.

103. Gallus A, Jackaman J, Tillett J, et al: Safety and efficacy of warfarin started early after submassive venous thrombosis of pulmonary embolism. Lancet 2:1293, 1986.

104. Conti S, Daschbach M, Blaisdell FW: A comparison of high dose versus conventional dose heparin therapy for deep vein thrombosis. Surgery 92(6):972, 1982.

105. Hull RD, Raskob GE, Rosenbloom D, et al: Optimal therapeutic level of heparin therapy in patients with venous thrombosis. Arch Intern Med 152:1589, 1992.

106. Wheeler AP, Jaquiss RD, Newman JH: Physician practices in treatment of pulmonary embolism and deep-venous thrombosis. Arch Intern Med 148:1321, 1988.

107. Landefeld CS, Anderson PA: Guideline-based consultation to prevent anticoagulant-related bleeding: A randomized, controlled trial in a teaching hospital. Ann Intern Med 116:829, 1992.

108. Hirsh J, Poller L, Deykin D, et al: Optimal therapeutic range for oral anticoagulants: ACCP/NHLBI National Conference on Antithrombotic Therapy. Chest 2(Suppl):5S, 1989.

109. Silver D: Heparin-related complications. *In* Ernst CB, Stanley JC (eds): Current Therapy in Vascular Surgery. Philadelphia, BC Decker, 1992, pp 576–579.

110. King DJ, Kelton JG: Heparin-associated thrombocytopenia. Ann Intern Med 100:535, 1984.

111. Cines DB, Kaywin P, Bina M, et al: Heparin-associated thrombocytopenia. N Engl J Med 303:788, 1980.

112. Howell R, Fidler J, Letsky E, DeSwiet M: The risks of antenatal subcutaneous heparin prophylaxis: A controlled trial. Br J Obstet Gynaecol 90:1124, 1983.

113. Lechey D, Gantt C, Lim V: Heparin-induced hypoaldosteronism. JAMA 246:2189, 1981.
114. Wilson ID, Goetz FC: Selective hypoaldosteronism after prolonged heparin administration. Am J Med 36:635, 1964.
115. Vermeer C: Gamma-carboxyglutamate-containing proteins and the vitamin K-dependent carboxylase. Biochem J 266:625, 1990.
116. Furie B, Furie BC: Molecular basis of vitamin K-dependent gamma-carboxylation. Blood 75:1753, 1990.
117. Hull RD, Hirsh J, Jay R, et al: Different intensities of oral anticoagulant therapy in the treatment of proximal vein thrombosis. N Engl J Med 307:1676, 1982.
118. Bussey HI, Force RW, Bianco TM, Leonard AD: Reliance on prothrombin time ratios causes significant errors in anticoagulation therapy. Arch Intern Med 152:278, 1992.
119. Turpie GG, Gunstensen J, Hirsh J, et al: Randomized comparison of two intensities of oral anticoagulant therapy after tissue heart valve replacement. Lancet 1:1242, 1988.
120. McGehee WG, Klotz TA, Epstein DJ, Rapaport SI: Coumarin necrosis associated with hereditary protein C deficiency. Ann Intern Med 100:59, 1984.
121. Kamier FJ: Thromboembolism, coumarin necrosis, and protein C. Mayo Clin Proc 60:673, 1985.
122. Martin BF, Phillips JC: Gangrene of the female breast with anticoagulant therapy: Report of two cases. Am J Clin Pathol 53:622, 1970.
123. Everett RN, Jones FL: Warfarin-induced skin necrosis: A cutaneous sign of malignancy? Postgrad Med 79:97, 1986.
124. Hall JG, Pauli RM, Wilson KM: Maternal and fetal sequelae of anticoagulation during pregnancy. Am J Med 68:122, 1980.
125. Stevenson RE, Burton OM, Ferlanto GJ, et al: Hazards of oral anticoagulants during pregnancy. JAMA 243:1549, 1980.
126. Comerota AJ: Thrombophlebitis in obstetrics and gynecology. In Rakel RE (ed): Conn's Current Therapy. Philadelphia, WB Saunders, 1985, pp 903–907.
127. Comerota AJ: Thrombolytic therapy for acute deep vein thrombosis. Semin Vasc Surg 5(2):76, 1992.
128. O'Donnell TF, Browse NL, Burnand KG, Lea Thomas M: The socioeconomic effects of an ilio-femoral venous thrombosis. J Surg Res 22:483, 1977.
129. Browse NL, Thomas ML, Pim HP: Streptokinase and deep vein thrombosis. Br Med J 3:717, 1968.
130. Robertson BR, Nilsson IM, Nylander G: Value of streptokinase and heparin in therapy of acute deep vein thrombosis. Acta Chir Scand 134:203, 1968.
131. Kakkar VV, Franc C, Howe CT, et al: Treatment of deep vein thrombosis: A trial of heparin, streptokinase and Arvin. Br Med J 1:806, 1969.
132. Tsapogas MJ, Peabody RA, Wu KT, et al: Controlled study of thrombolytic therapy in deep vein thrombosis. Surgery 74:973, 1973.
133. Duckert F, Muller G, Hyman D, et al: Treatment of deep vein thrombosis with streptokinase. Br Med J 1:973, 1975.
134. Porter JM, Seaman AJ, Common HH, et al: Comparison of heparin and streptokinase in the treatment of venous thrombosis. Am Surg 41:511, 1975.
135. Seaman AJ, Common HH, Rosch J, et al: Deep vein thrombosis treated with streptokinase or heparin. Angiology 27:549, 1976.
136. Rosch JJ, Dotter CT, Seaman AJ, et al: Healing of deep vein thrombosis: Venographic findings in a randomized study comparing streptokinase and heparin. Am J Roentgenol 127:533, 1976.
137. Marder VJ, Soulen RL, Atichartakarn V: Quantitative venographic assessment of deep vein thrombosis in the evaluation of streptokinase and heparin therapy. J Lab Clin Med 89:1018, 1977.
138. Arnesen H, Heilo A, Jakobsen E, et al: A prospective study of streptokinase and heparin in the treatment of deep vein thrombosis. Acta Med Scand 203:457, 1978.
139. Elliot MS, Immelman EJ, Jeffery P, et al: A comparative randomized trial of heparin versus streptokinase in the treatment of acute proximal venous thrombosis: An interim report of a prospective trial. Br J Surg 66:838, 1979.
140. Watz R, Savidge GF: Rapid thrombolysis and preservation of venous valvular function in high deep vein thrombosis. Acta Med Scand 205:293, 1979.
141. Jeffery P, Immelman E, Amoore J: Treatment of deep vein thrombosis with heparin or streptokinase: Long-term venous function assessment. In Proceedings of the Second International Vascular Symposium. London, 1986, abstract no. S20.3.
142. Turpie AGG, Levine MN, Hirsh J, et al: Tissue plasminogen activator vs heparin in deep vein thrombosis. Chest 97:172s, 1990.
143. Goldhaber SZ, Meyerrovitz MF, Green D, et al: Randomized controlled trial of tissue plasminogen activator in proximal deep venous thrombosis. Am J Med 88:235, 1990.
144. Albrechtsson U, Anderson J, Einarsson E, et al: Streptokinase treatment of deep venous thrombosis and the post-thrombotic syndrome. Arch Surg 116:33, 1981.
145. van de Loo JCW, Kriessman A, Trubestein G, et al: Controlled multicenter pilot study of urokinase-heparin and streptokinase in deep vein thrombosis. Thromb Haemost 50:660, 1983.
146. Kakkar VV, Lawrence D: Hemodynamic and clinical assessment after therapy for acute deep vein thrombosis: A prospective study. Am J Surg 150:28, 1985.
147. Schulman S, Granqvist S, Juhlin-Danfelt A, et al: Long-term sequelae of calf vein thrombosis treated with heparin or low-dose streptokinase. Acta Med Scand 219:349, 1986.
148. Arnesen H, Hoiseth A, Ly B: Streptokinase or heparin in the treatment of deep vein thrombosis: Follow-up results of a prospective study. Acta Med Scand 211:65, 1982.
149. Lindner DJ, Edwards JM, Phinney ES, et al: Long-term hemodynamic and clinical sequelae of lower extremity deep vein thrombosis. J Vasc Surg 4:436, 1986.
150. Comerota AJ: Urokinase. In Messeril F (ed): Current Cardiovascular Drug Therapy. Philadelphia, WB Saunders, 1990, pp 1470–1478.
151. Comerota AJ, Katz ML, White JV: Thrombolytic therapy for acute DVT. How much is enough? Circulation (In press).
152. Hill SL, Martin D, Evans P: Massive vein thrombosis of the extremities. Am J Surg 158:131, 1989.
153. Collen D, Stump D, Van de Werf F: Coronary thrombolysis in patients with myocardial infarction by intravenous infusion of synergic thrombolytic agents. Am Heart J 11:1083, 1986.
154. Collen D, Stassen J, Stump D, Verstraete M: Synergism of thrombolytic agents in vivo. Circulation 14:838, 1986.
155. Gurewich V: Tissue plasminogen activator and pro-urokinase. In Comerota AJ (ed): Thrombolytic Therapy. Orlando, FL, Grune & Stratton, 1988, pp 209–223.
156. Mahorner H, Castleberry JW, Coleman WO: Attempts to restore function in major veins which are the site of massive thrombosis. Ann Surg 146:510, 1957.
157. Haller JA, Abrams BL: Use of thrombectomy in the treatment of acute iliofemoral venous thrombosis in forty-five patients. Ann Surg 158:561, 1963.
158. Karp RB, Wylie EJ: Recurrent thrombosis after iliofemoral venous thrombectomy. Surg Forum 17:147, 1966.
159. Lansing AM, Davis WM: Five-year follow-up study of iliofemoral venous thrombectomy. Am Surg 168:620, 1968.
160. Harris EJ, Brown WH: Patency after iliofemoral venous thrombosis. Ann Surg 167:91, 1968.
161. Lindhagen J, Haglund M, Haglund U, et al: Iliofemoral venous thrombectomy. J Cardiovasc Surg 6:411, 1962.
162. Goto H, Wada T, Matsumoto A, et al: Iliofemoral venous thrombectomy. J Cardiovasc Surg 21:341, 1980.
163. Provan JL, Rumble EF: Re-evaluation of thrombectomy in the management of iliofemoral venous thrombosis. Can J Surg 22:378, 1979.
164. Natali J, Tricot JF: Place de la chirurgie dans le traitement des phlébites aiguës des membres inférieurs. Phlébologie 35:187, 1982.
165. Piquet PH, Tournigand P, Josso B, Mercier C: Traitement chirurgical des thromboses ilio-caves: Exigences et résultats. In Keiffer E (ed): Chirurgie de la Vein Cave Inférieur et de Ses Branches. Paris, Expansion Scientifique Française, 1985, pp 210–216.
166. Juhan C, Cornillon B, Tobiana F, et al: Etude de la perméabilité des thrombectomies veineuse ilio-fémorales et ilio-caves. Ann Chir Vasc 1:529, 1987.
167. Einarsson E, Albrechtsson V, Eklof B: Thrombectomy and temporary arteriovenous fistula in iliofemoral vein thrombosis: Technical considerations and early results. Int Angiol 5:65, 1986.
168. Plate G, Einarsson E, Ohlin P, et al: Thrombectomy with temporary arteriovenous fistula in acute iliofemoral venous thrombosis. J Vasc Surg 1:867, 1984.
169. Eklof B, Juhan C: Revival of thrombectomy in the management of acute iliofemoral venous thrombosis. Contemp Surg 40:21, 1992.
170. Delin A, Swedenborg J, Hellgren M, et al: Thrombectomy and arte-

riovenous fistula for iliofemoral venous thrombosis in fertile women. Surg Gynecol Obstet 154:69, 1982.

171. Hutschenreiter S, Vollmar J, Loeprecht H, et al: Reconstructive Eingriffe am Venensystem: Spätergebnisse unter kritischer Bewertung funktioneller und gefassmorphologischer Kriterien. Chirurg 50:555, 1979.
172. Kniemeyer HW, Sandmann W, Waller S: Die embolisierende Venenthrombose: Therapiekoncept, Ergebnisse. Aktuel Chir 20:204, 1985.
173. Plate G, Akesson H, Einarsson E, et al: Long-term results of venous thrombectomy combined with a temporary arteriovenous fistula. Eur J Vasc Surg 4:483, 1990.
174. Einarsson E, Albrechtsson V, Eklof B, Norgren L: Follow-up evaluation of venous morphologic factors and function after thrombectomy and temporary arteriovenous fistula in thrombosis of iliofemoral vein. Surg Gynecol Obstet 163:111, 1986.
175. Torngren S, Swedenborg J: Thrombectomy and temporary arteriovenous fistula for iliofemoral venous thrombosis. Int Angiol 7:14, 1988.
176. Akesson H, Brudin L, Dahlstrom JA, et al: Venous function assessed during a 5 year period after acute iliofemoral venous thrombosis treated with anticoagulation. Eur J Vasc Surg 4:43, 1990.
177. Loeprecht H: Angioscopie veineuse. Phlébologie 41:165, 1988.
178. Moser KM, LeMoine JR: Is embolic risk conditioned by location of deep venous thrombosis? Ann Int Surg 94(Part 1):439, 1981.
179. Kakkar VV, Flanc C, Howe CT, Clarke MB: Natural history of postoperative deep-vein thrombosis. Lancet 2:230, 1969.
180. Menzoian JO, Sequeira JC, Doyle JE, et al: Therapeutic and clinical course of deep vein thrombosis. Am J Surg 146:581, 1983.
181. Lohr JM, Kerr TM, Lutter KS, et al: Lower extremity calf thrombosis: To treat or not to treat? J Vasc Surg 14:618, 1991.
182. Solis MM, Ranval TJ, Nix ML, et al: Is anticoagulation indicated for asymptomatic postoperative calf vein thrombosis? J Vasc Surg 16:414, 1992.
183. Lagerstedt CI, Olsson CG, Fagher BO, et al: Need for long-term anticoagulant treatment in symptomatic calf vein thrombosis. Lancet 7:515, 1985.
184. Pellegrini VD, Francis CW, Harris C, Totterman S: Embolic complications of calf thrombosis following total hip arthroplasty. Presented to the American Association of Orthopedic Surgeons, 1991.
185. Hommes DW, Bura A, Mazzolai L, et al: Subcutaneous heparin compared with continuous intravenous heparin administration in the initial treatment of deep vein thrombosis. Ann Intern Med 116:279, 1992.
186. Hull RD, Raskob GE, Pineo GF, et al: Subcutaneous low-molecular-weight heparin compared with continuous intravenous heparin in the treatment of proximal-vein thrombosis. N Engl J Med 326:975, 1992.
187. Monreal M, Barroso RJ, Manzano JR, et al: Asymptomatic pulmonary embolism in patients with deep vein thrombosis. Is it useful to take a lung scan to rule out this condition? J Cardiovasc Surg 30:104, 1989.
188. Masuda EM, Kistner RL, Ferris EB: Long-term effects of superficial femoral vein ligation: Thirteen-year follow-up. J Vasc Surg 16:741, 1992.
189. Trousseau A: Phlegmasia alba dolens. In Lectures on Clinical Medicine, Delivered at the Hôtel-Dieu, Paris. Translated by Cormack JR. London, New Sydenham Society, 1872, pp 281–295.
190. Prandoni P, Lensing AWA, Büller HR, et al: Deep vein thrombosis and the incidence of subsequent symptomatic cancer. N Engl J Med 327:1128, 1992.
191. Moore FD, Osteen RT, Karp DD, et al: Anticoagulants, venous thromboembolism, and the cancer patient. Arch Surg 405, 1981.
192. Altschuler E, Moosa H, Selker RG, Vertosick FT Jr: The risk and efficacy of anticoagulant therapy in the treatment of thromboembolic complications in patients with primary malignant brain tumors. Neurosurgery 27(1):74, 1990.
193. Calligaro KD, Bergen WS, Haut MJ, et al: Thromboembolic complications in patients with advanced cancer: Anticoagulation versus Greenfield filter placement. Ann Vasc Surg 5(2):186, 1991.

194. Cohen JR, Tenenbaum N, Citron M: Greenfield filter as primary therapy for deep venous thrombosis and/or pulmonary embolism in patients with cancer. Surgery 109(1):12, 1991.
195. Whitney BA, Kerstein MD: Thrombocytopenia and cancer: Use of the Kim-Ray Greenfield filter to prevent thromboembolism. South Med J 80(10):1246, 1987.
196. Prandoni P, Lensing AWA, Büller HR, et al: Comparison of subcutaneous low-molecular-weight heparin with intravenous standard heparin in proximal deep-vein thrombosis. Lancet 339:441, 1992.
197. Morris GK, Mitchell JRA: Clinical management of venous thromboembolism. Br Med Bull 34:169, 1978.
198. Centers for Disease Control: CDC surveillance summaries. MMWR 40:1, 1991.
199. Bonnar J: Blood coagulation fibrinolysis in obstetrics. Clin Haematol 12:213, 1973.
200. Daniel DG, Bloom AL, Giddings JC, et al: Increased factor IX levels in puerperium during administration of diethylstilboestrol. Br Med J 1:801, 1968.
201. Gallus AS: Venous thromboembolism: Incidence and clinical risk factors. In Maddan JL, Hume M (eds): Venous Thromboembolism. New York, Appleton-Century-Crofts, 1976, pp 1–32.
202. Bonnar J, McNicol GP, Douglas AS: Coagulation and fibrinolytic mechanisms during and after normal childbirth. Br J Med 2:200, 1970.
203. Ping WW, Lee TS: Thromboembolism in pregnancy. Med J Malaysia 30:169, 1976.
204. Bergqvist A, Bergqvist D, Hallbröök T: Deep vein thrombosis during pregnancy. Acta Obstet Gynecol Scand 62:443, 1983.
205. Becker MH, Genieser NB, Finegold M, et al: Chondrodysplasia punctata. Is maternal warfarin a factor? Am J Dis Child 129:356, 1975.
206. Pettifor JM, Benson R: Congenital malformations associated with the administration of oral anticoagulants during pregnancy. J Pediatr 86:459, 1975.
207. Shaul WL, Emery H, Hall JG: Chondrodysplasia punctata and maternal warfarin use during pregnancy. Am J Dis Child 129:360, 1975.
208. Hall JG: Embryopathy associated with oral anticoagulant therapy. Birth Defects 12:33, 1965.
209. Warkany J: A warfarin embryopathy? Am J Dis Child 129:287, 1975.
210. Shaul WL, Hall JG: Multiple congenital anomalies associated with oral anticoagulants. Am J Obstet Gynecol 127:191, 1977.
211. Warkany J, Bofinger M: Le rôle de la coumadine dans les malformations congénitales. Med Hyg 33:1454, 1975.
212. Warkany J: Warfarin embryopathy. Teratology 14:205, 1976.
213. Carson M, Reid M: Warfarin and fetal abnormality. Lancet 1:1127, 1976.
214. Holzgreve W, Carey JC, Hall BD: Warfarin-induced fetal abnormalities. Lancet 2:914, 1976.
215. Sherman S, Hall BD: Warfarin and fetal abnormality. Lancet 1:692, 1976.
216. Morgensen K, Skibsted L, Wadt J, Nissen F: Thrombectomy of acute iliofemoral venous thrombosis during pregnancy. Surg Gynecol Obstet 169:5054, 1989.
217. Delin A, Swedenborg J, Hellgren M, et al: Thrombectomy and arteriovenous fistula for iliofemoral venous thrombosis in fertile women. Surg Gynecol Obstet 154:69, 1982.
218. Forestier F, Daffos F, Capella-Pavlovsky M: Low molecular weight heparin (PK 10169) does not cross the placenta during the second trimester of pregnancy: Study by direct fetal blood sampling under ultrasound. Thromb Res 34:557, 1984.
219. Forestier F, Daffos F, Rainaut M, Toulemonde F: Low molecular weight heparin (CY 216) does not cross the placenta during the third trimester of pregnancy. Thromb Haemost 57:234, 1987.
220. Omri A, Delaloye JF, Andersen H, Bachmann F: Low molecular weight heparin NoVO (LHN-1) does not cross the placenta during the second trimester of pregnancy. Thromb Haemost 61:55, 1989.
221. Melissari E, Das S, Kanthou C, et al: The use of LMW heparin in treating thromboembolism during pregnancy and prevention of osteoporosis [Abstract]. Thromb Haemost 65:926, 1991.

135

Caval Interruption Procedures

Lazar J. Greenfield, M.D.

• • •

HISTORICAL PERSPECTIVE

It was John Hunter who performed the first femoral vein ligation for thrombophlebitis in 1784. However, it was not until 1893 that Bottini reported successful ligation of the inferior vena cava to prevent pulmonary embolism (PE). In the United States, venous ligation was also the earliest surgical technique used. Bilateral common femoral vein ligation was undertaken first as suggested by Homans, but an unacceptable incidence of recurrent PE and lower extremity venous stasis sequelae led to abandonment of the procedure. Ligation of the infrarenal inferior vena cava provided theoretical control of the final common path to the pulmonary circulation for most emboli and was performed commonly until the late 1960s. However, high postoperative mortality, recurrent PE, and adverse lower extremity sequelae were unacceptable outcomes. Nasbeth and associates[1] and Amador and coworkers[2] found mortality rates after inferior vena caval ligation of 19 and 39 per cent, respectively; rates were highest in patients with underlying cardiac disease (41 and 19 per cent). Among patients who had normal cardiac function and were classified as good preoperative risks, an operative mortality rate of 4 per cent was still observed; cited causes included recurrent PE arising at the site of caval ligation and phlegmasia cerulea dolens. In follow-up studies, Ferris and colleagues found recurrent PE in 3 of 20 patients within 2 months after vena caval ligation.[3] Although thrombus can form above the ligation, large ovarian and ascending lumbar venous collaterals were the probable conduits for emboli from lower extremity sources because acute thrombi were present below the ligation site in 40 to 50 per cent of cases. Lower extremity sequelae in the series of Nasbeth and associates included leg edema (40 per cent), development of new varicose veins (20 per cent), stasis pigmentation (18 per cent), leg discomfort (14 per cent), disabling venous claudication (14 per cent), and ulceration (6 per cent).[1] More recent data have also suggested an underappreciation of cardiac output limitation after vena caval ligation in patients without preexisting heart disease. Miller and Staats' exercise and gas exchange study of such patients found significant impairment of cardiac output secondary to inadequate venous return.[4]

Against this background, the first techniques to provide filtration of emboli without vena caval occlusion evolved. For more than a decade, vena caval suture, staple plication, and externally applied clip devices were used to provide a limited orifice flow through the inferior vena cava.[5–7] These techniques added the morbidity of general anesthesia and laparotomy. Although inferior vena caval clips are still being applied at the time of surgery in some instances, it is the author's opinion that there is considerably less morbidity if an intracaval filter is placed preoperatively. Despite promising early patency data, high rates of caval occlusion with external devices were noted after a relatively short follow-up.[8–10] The development of transvenous approaches under local anesthesia was the next logical step. The earliest transvenous approaches demonstrated the ease of access to the vena cava under local anesthesia and fluoroscopy. Although various devices were developed, the Mobin-Uddin umbrella became the most popular because it could be readily positioned below the renal veins. However, it was found to have a high rate of subsequent vena caval thrombosis and was associated with additional complications of proximal thrombus formation and occasional migration into the pulmonary artery.[11] It was withdrawn from the market and a new generation of devices was developed to facilitate placement, reliable capture of thromboemboli, and long-term caval patency.

INDICATIONS FOR VENA CAVAL FILTER PLACEMENT

Currently accepted indications for inferior vena caval filter insertion include (1) documented deep venous thrombosis (DVT) or PE with a recognized contraindication to anticoagulation, (2) recurrent PE despite adequate anticoagulation, (3) bleeding complications requiring that anticoagulation therapy for DVT or PE be discontinued, (4) after pulmonary embolectomy, and (5) failure of another form of caval interruption, demonstrated by recurrent thromboembolism (Table 135–1). Case-selective or relative indications include (1) the presence of iliofemoral thrombosis with a 5-cm or longer free-floating tail, (2) septic PE, (3) chronic PE in a patient with cor pulmonale, and (4) a high-risk patient (e.g., one who has significant cardiopulmonary disease, occlusion of more than 50 per cent of the pulmonary bed, or both) who would not tolerate any recurrent thromboembolism.

As long-term favorable experience with the Greenfield vena caval filter has accumulated, there have been suggestions to further liberalize the indications for filter insertion. Recommendations have included routine use of the filter for DVT in cancer patients and high-risk general surgical patients, general use in older or pregnant women with DVT

Table 135–1.   Indications for Insertion of a Vena Caval Filter

Absolute Indications

Deep venous thrombosis or documented thromboembolism in a patient
who has a contraindication to anticoagulation

Recurrent thromboembolism despite adequate anticoagulation

Complications of anticoagulation that have forced therapy to be
discontinued

Immediately after pulmonary embolectomy

Failure of another form of caval interruption, demonstrated by recurrent
thromboembolism

Relative Indications

A large free-floating iliofemoral thrombus demonstrated on venography
in a high-risk patient

A propagating iliofemoral thrombus despite adequate anticoagulation

Chronic pulmonary embolism in a patient with pulmonary hypertension
and cor pulmonale

A patient who has occlusion of more than 50 per cent of the pulmonary
vascular bed and would not tolerate any additional thrombus

Presence of recurrent septic embolism

or PE instead of anticoagulation, and general prophylactic use instead of anticoagulation.[12, 13] Additional studies are required to determine whether the risk of anticoagulation outweighs the risk of filter placement alone. At present, the author continues to recommend the use of appropriate anticoagulation to control the underlying thrombotic disorder in patients who are eligible for anticoagulant therapy.

STAINLESS STEEL GREENFIELD FILTER

The current benchmark for performance of transvenous vena caval filters is the stainless steel Greenfield filter, for which 20 years of long-term follow-up is available.[14] The Greenfield filter was developed to maintain caval patency after trapping emboli and to preserve prograde caval flow, avoiding stasis and facilitating lysis of the trapped emboli (Fig. 135–1). The cone-shaped filter is 4.6 cm long from apex to base. The base is formed by the filter's six legs, which provide for caval fixation by means of small recurved hooks at their distal ends. The spacing between the legs is 2 mm at the apex of the cone and a maximum of 5 to 6 mm at the base when the device is expanded, depending on inferior vena cava size. The spacing between limbs is such that the filter effectively traps most emboli 3 mm or greater in diameter.[15] The conical geometry allows progressive central filling while maintaining circumferential blood flow, thus avoiding progressive venous thrombosis, caval obstruction, and venous hypertension. When thrombus fills the filter to 70 per cent of its depth, only 49 per cent of the cross-sectional area is blocked. Experience has shown that no distal venous pressure increase occurs until 80 per cent of the filter is filled with clot, at which point more than 64 per cent of the cross-sectional area is blocked (Fig. 135–2). These design features result in superior patency rates and a minimal incidence of stasis sequelae. In addition, an unexpected result of flow preservation was the evidence of progressive lysis of the trapped thrombus over time.

The stainless steel Greenfield filter had a 4 per cent rate of recurrent embolism over a 12-year period of obser-

vation in 469 patients and a long-term filter patency rate of 98 per cent.[16] Similar results have been obtained in other follow-up series, with long-term patency rates in excess of 95 per cent.[11, 17] This high level of patency has allowed placement of the Greenfield filter above the level of the renal veins when needed because of thrombus at that level or in pregnant women to avoid contact between the gravid uterus and the filter. The results with suprarenal filter placement are quite comparable, with a 100 per cent patency rate in the 22 patients studied long term of the series of 69 filters placed at this level since 1976.[18]

The patency rate of the Greenfield filter is not dependent on prolonged anticoagulation, and the termination of anticoagulant therapy is dictated by the patient's underlying thrombotic disorder. The few associated complications include misplacement due to premature discharge or inaccurate fluoroscopic control of the carrier, rare limb penetration of the cava, and filter limb fracture. Although it is possible to retrieve a misplaced device, misplacements into the renal, hepatic, or iliac veins have not caused functional problems. The only functional consequence of venous misplacement may be inadequate filtration of vena caval flow.

Because of its reliable preservation of caval patency, the filter has adapted well to a variety of unusual clinical problems, such as the rare need for superior vena caval placement. The filter has also been a useful adjunct in the successful management of septic thrombophlebitis. This is possible because preserved prograde venous flow through

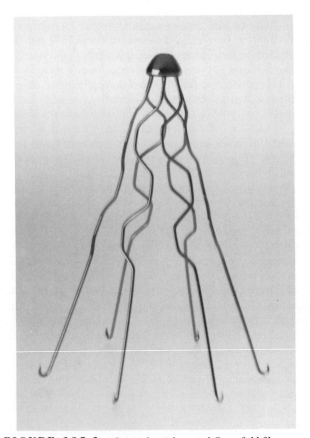

FIGURE 135–1.   Original stainless steel Greenfield filter introduced in 1972 for mechanical protection against pulmonary thromboembolism.

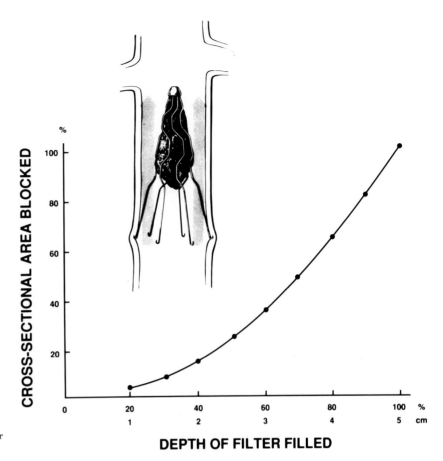

FIGURE 135–2. Relationship between the volume of thrombus trapped within the filter and the percentage of cross section occluded.

the filter permits in vivo sterilization of any infected thrombus within it by parenteral antibiotic treatment.[19]

Technical Considerations for Filter Insertion

The procedure should be performed under optimal fluoroscopy. This can be achieved in the operating room with a C-arm fluoroscope if the patient is not obese, or in the radiology suite, where better imaging can be obtained for the obese patient. A preoperative venacavogram should be obtained and available for review at the time of insertion. Operative insertion is usually undertaken via the jugular vein, which can be exposed under local anesthesia. The patient should be positioned with a small folded towel between the shoulder blades to extend the neck. With the head turned to the left, a short transverse incision is made over the base of the sternocleidomastoid muscle to allow separation of the sternal and clavicular heads of the muscle and expose the underlying jugular vein. Once a 4- to 5-cm length of jugular vein is exposed, it can be controlled by twill tape proximally and a vascular clamp distally, with care being taken not to injure the vagus nerve. The filter-carrier system, previously checked and filled with heparinized saline, is loaded with the filter and the plunger system locked securely. The guidewire should be removed from the carrier system to allow it to be positioned in the inferior vena cava before introduction of the carrier unit.[20] Although

a large-loop floppy J-wire is provided with the unit, it is often easier to use a straight 0.035-inch standard guidewire instead. The guidewire is introduced into the jugular vein through a No. 15 Jelco needle, and twill tape is used to secure the proximal vein. The guidewire is advanced under fluoroscopic guidance and is directed through the right atrium into the inferior vena cava as far as the bifurcation (Fig. 135–3).

The radiographic diameter of the vena cava should be measured, with correction for magnification, which can be as much as 25 to 30 per cent. Very large vena cavas (greater than 30 mm in diameter) may be found in patients with right-sided heart failure. In these patients, it is safer to introduce separate filters into each iliac vein. Fortunately, the vena cava is narrower in the anteroposterior diameter than it is in the transverse diameter, which provides an additional measure of security for fixation. Once the guidewire has been positioned in the inferior vena cava below the level of the renal veins, the external stiff end of the guidewire is passed retrograde through the carrier if the standard 24 Fr system is being used. The newer titanium Greenfield filter can also be used with this exposure, and its dilator-sheath system is described in the next section. The sheath provides a protected route for the filter-carrier system to the level of insertion, obviating the risk of premature discharge of the filter. With either system, the puncture hole in the jugular vein is enlarged by a short transverse incision, and then either the carrier or the dilator-sheath system is inserted into the vein and passed down to the level of L2 to L3. If the operator is using the dilator-

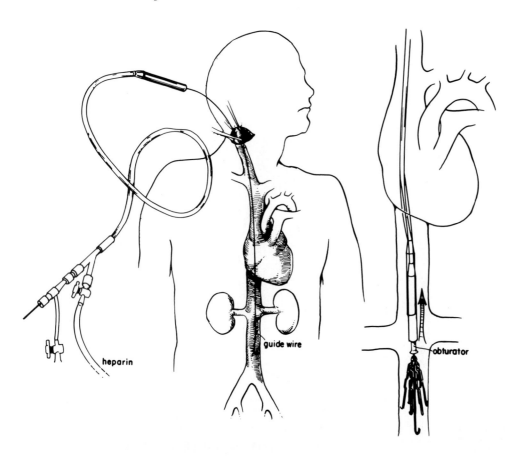

FIGURE 135–3. Technique of insertion of the stainless steel Greenfield filter using a guidewire for positioning of the carrier and for axial centering of the filter at discharge. (From Greenfield LJ, Stewart JR, Crute S: Improved technique for insertion of Greenfield vena caval filter. Surg Gynecol Obstet 156:218, 1983. By permission of Surgery, Gynecology & Obstetrics.)

sheath system, the dilator should be withdrawn once the sheath is in the infrarenal inferior vena cava, but not if the sheath is in the thorax, where negative pressure might allow air embolism to occur. The titanium Greenfield filter preloaded carrier is then inserted into the sheath until it is seen to exit the distal intravascular sheath completely at the desired level of filter introduction. Use of the standard stainless steel carrier follows a similar path over the guidewire to the level of L2 to L3. At this point, the stylet is unlocked and the stainless steel carrier is gradually retracted until the filter springs open at the appropriate level in the vena cava. The introducer system and the guidewire should then be withdrawn, with no further attempts being made to manipulate the filter. Any delay in positioning can be associated with thrombus formation inside the carrier; therefore, heparinized saline should be used to flush the system through the attached Luer-Lok connection either periodically or continuously. Contrast medium can also be injected, if necessary, to verify the filter's position as well as its proximity to any thrombus that might be in the inferior vena cava. Thrombus within the vena cava should not be allowed to contact the filter because this could lead to propagation of thrombus through the filter and above the level of mechanical protection. If thrombus does extend to the level of the renal veins or if the distal inferior vena cava is thrombosed, the filter should be inserted at the level of T12, above the level of the renal veins. After removal of the carrier system and the guidewire, the venotomy is closed with 5–0 monofilament suture, and the wound is closed without drainage after hemostasis has been ensured. A follow-up abdominal radiograph is obtained to confirm the position of the filter. Often, a discrepancy is noted between the fluoroscopic impression of the level of the filter and the filter level indicated by the abdominal radiograph; this difference is due to slight parallax of the fluoroscopic image.

PERCUTANEOUS FILTER DEVICES

Percutaneous insertion of devices designed to provide effective filtration of thromboemboli in the vena cava offers a number of potential advantages for the patient, including reduced discomfort, insertion time, and procedural cost because of the use of the radiology suite rather than the operating room.[21] Insertion is made possible by the use of the Seldinger technique, which allows the percutaneous insertion of progressively larger dilators and a sheath over a Teflon-coated guidewire. Enlarging the skin incision permits tract expansion either by a balloon or dilators to allow the insertion of a larger sheath. Percutaneously inserted caval devices are customarily placed through the right femoral vein, but they may also be inserted through the neck by way of the jugular vein. The latter route is less desirable because of the risk of air embolism.

Initial efforts at percutaneous introduction of the standard 24 Fr carrier system of the stainless steel Greenfield filter required a very large sheath (28 Fr) and prolonged compression of the insertion site; this resulted in a 30 to 40 per cent incidence of insertion site venous thrombosis.[22] This complication led to the enthusiastic proliferation of

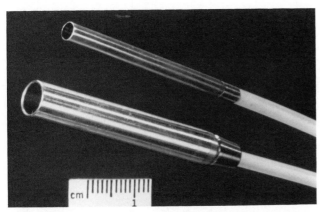

FIGURE 135–4. Comparison of the carriers used for the available models of the Greenfield filter: the 12 Fr carrier for the modified-hook titanium Greenfield filter (*top*) and the 24 Fr carrier for the stainless steel Greenfield filter (*bottom*).

many innovative devices that could be inserted percutaneously using smaller-diameter delivery systems (Fig. 135–4) in an effort to retain the advantage of percutaneous insertion while minimizing the incidence of insertion site venous thrombosis. Despite the insertion of large numbers of these alternative filter devices (Fig. 135–5), it has been difficult to obtain accurate follow-up information in order to compare their effectiveness (Table 135–2).

Bird's Nest Filter

In 1984, Roehm and coworkers reported the use of a percutaneously placed intracaval device that consisted of four stainless steel wires preshaped into a crisscrossing array of nonmatching bends.[23] Placement of such a complex array was intended to provide multiple barriers to thromboemboli. Each of these wires is 25 cm long, is 0.18 mm in diameter, and ends in a strut that is connected to a fixation hook. One strut is Z-shaped, so that a pusher wire can be attached. As initially described, the device was preloaded into an 8 Fr Teflon catheter. Problems with proximal migration of this model led to redesigning of the struts in 1986, with a stiffer, 0.46-mm wire used in an attempt to improve fixation. This modification required a concomitant increase in diameter of the catheter system to 12 Fr. During placement of this modified device, the pusher is used to set the first group of hooks into the caval wall; the wires are then extruded with the goal of closely packing the formed loops into a 7-cm-long segment of infrarenal vena cava (see Fig. 135–5). Finally, the second group of hooks is pushed into the caval wall. The pusher is then disengaged by being unscrewed from the filter, and the catheter is withdrawn. Purported but unproven advantages of this device include (1) the ability to trap smaller emboli by virtue of the tighter meshing of wires, (2) avoidance of the need for intraluminal centering with this configuration, (3) the ability to accommodate to vena cavas as large in diameter as 40 mm, (4)

FIGURE 135–5. Commercially available vena caval filter devices: the Vena Tech filter (*left*), the Simon Nitinol filter (*center*), and the bird's nest filter (*right*).

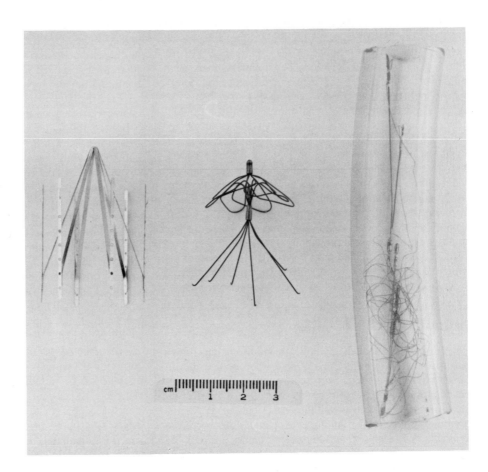

Table 135–2.   Comparison of Inferior Vena Caval Filters

Parameter	Greenfield Stainless Steel	Greenfield Titanium	Vena Tech	Bird's Nest	Simon Nitinol
Evaluation	Registry (1988)	Clinical trial (1991)	Clinical trial (1990)	Clinical trial (1988)	Clinical trial (1990)
Duration	12 yr	30 days	1 yr	6 mo	6 mo
Number	469	186 (123 at follow-up)	97 (77 at follow-up)	568 (440 at 6 mo)	224 (102 at follow-up)
Recurrent pulmonary embolism	4%	3%	2%	2.7% (33–67% in subset with objective follow-up)	4% based on those who had follow-up
Caval patency	98%	100%	92%	97%	81%
Filter patency	98%	Not reported	63% without thrombus	81%	Not reported
Insertion site deep venous thrombosis	41% (percutaneous)	8.7%	23%	Few reported clinically	11%
Migration	35% >3 mm	11% >9 mm	14% >10 mm	9% with original model	1.2% of those with follow-up
Penetration	Not reported	1%	Not reported	Not reported	0.6% of those with follow-up
Misplacement	4%	0.5%	Not reported	Not reported	Not reported
Incomplete opening	Not seen	2%	6%	Not reported	Not reported
Means of follow-up	Physical examination, inferior vena cava scan, x-ray study, noninvasive vascular examination	Physical examination, x-ray study, computed tomography, noninvasive vascular examination	Objective data vary by site (cavagram, computed tomography, duplex scanning, x-ray study)	Phone interview, objective data are random and only available for 40 of 440	Clinical, x-ray, laboratory tests

the possibility that wires may be able to occlude nearby collaterals, and (5) the lack of radially oriented struts, which limits the tendency toward caval wall penetration.

A series of 481 patients was reported on in 1988.[24] Only 37 patients with the filter in place 6 months or longer had been studied by venacavography or ultrasonography, so long-term data are limited. Of these patients, 7 (19 per cent) had an occluded vena cava. Three patients underwent pulmonary angiography for suspicion of recurrent embolism, which was confirmed in one case (3 per cent). As indicated previously, the original model showed a troublesome tendency to migrate proximally, despite what appeared to be adequate placement. This problem was encountered in 5 patients and resulted in the death of 1, who 10 days after placement was found to have the filter embedded within a massive pulmonary embolus. In a later series of 32 patients in whom the modified strut version was used, three instances of proximal migration were encountered. Two of these occurred within 24 hours of placement and could be corrected by angiographic manipulation. The third instance was not detected until 6 months after insertion, at which point the filter was not able to be repositioned from the right side of the heart, where it had become embedded.[25]

Nitinol Filter

Nitinol is a nickel-titanium alloy that can be drawn into a straight wire. Although pliable when cooled, it will rapidly transform into a previously imprinted rigid shape on warming to body temperature. Although a filter composed of this alloy was initially described in 1977, the preliminary results of a multi-center clinical trial were not available until 1989.[26] The filter design makes use of a 28-mm dome of eight overlapping loops, below which six diverging legs form a cone (see Fig. 135–5). Each leg has end-hooks designed to engage the caval wall. Insertion requires that iced normal saline be continuously infused through a 9 Fr delivery system. During placement, the cooled filter wire is rapidly advanced by the feeder pump and discharged from the storage catheter. Purportedly, the filter then instantly reshapes itself into its predetermined configuration and locks into place.

Of the 103 placements recorded in the initial multi-center trial, detailed information is available on 44. During a limited follow-up period, 2 patients sustained recurrent PE (5 per cent). In 1 individual, thrombus propagating above the filter was seen on venacavography. There were seven cases of confirmed vena caval occlusion, and in two cases occlusion was suspected on the basis of clinical findings, resulting in an overall caval occlusion rate of 18 per cent. Five patients (11 per cent) had stasis sequelae. Insertion site thrombosis was seen in 5 of 18 patients (28 per cent) studied with ultrasonography. Proximal migration was noted in one instance.

A subsequent report on the use of this device in 224 patients indicated that of the 102 individuals followed up and the 65 in whom 6-month follow-up evaluations had been completed, 4 patients experienced recurrent embolism (4 per cent) and 1 died (1 per cent). In addition, there were 20 documented caval occlusions (20 per cent).[27] A smaller series of 20 patients had follow-up in 16 patients for an average of 14 months. Caval penetration was seen in 5 patients (31 per cent), caval thrombosis was seen in 4 patients (25 per cent), filter migration into the pulmonary artery was found in 1 patient, and filter leg fracture was noted in 2 patients.[28]

Vena Tech Filter

The Vena Tech filter, introduced in 1986, is a stamped, cone-shaped filter made of Phynox, a material with properties similar to the alloy Elgiloy, which is used in temporary cardiac pacing wires. The filter cone consists of six angled radial prongs, each of which is connected to a hooked stabilizing strut; this array is designed to center and immobilize the device within the vena cava (see Fig. 135–5). It is generally inserted via a right internal jugular approach by means of a 12 Fr catheter system that is positioned over a guidewire. After the filter is pushed through the entire length of the insertion catheter, it is released by quick withdrawal of the catheter.

The initial reported experience was from France, where the design was introduced as the "LGM" filter.[29] In a series of 100 patients, the indication for filter placement was thromboembolism in 77 per cent, prophylaxis in iliocaval thrombosis in 13 per cent, and contraindication to anticoagulation in 9 per cent. As a result, most patients remained on anticoagulation after filter placement. In 100 attempted percutaneous insertions via the jugular route, 98 filters were discharged and 82 were positioned correctly. Eight filters had a 15 degree or greater tilt, 5 did not open completely, and 3 additional filters had both conditions, resulting in a 16 per cent incidence of malposition. The authors commented that many of these instances were early in their experience and may be operator dependent. Recurrent PE was seen in 2 patients (2 per cent), both of whom had incompletely opened filters. One-year follow-up demonstrated seven caval occlusions (8 per cent). Twenty-nine per cent of patients had lower extremity edema despite the use of support stockings. Migration of the device both proximally to the renal veins (4 per cent) and distally to the iliac veins (9 per cent) was observed. Another small series reported a 2.5 per cent incidence of recurrent embolism and an occlusion rate of 8 per cent.[30] There was a 13 per cent rate of either tilting or incomplete opening and a similar rate of distal migration. A more recent experience with this filter showed an occlusion rate of 22 per cent.[31] Breakage of stabilizer struts has also been reported in individual cases.[32]

Titanium Greenfield Filter

The most recent development in the Greenfield filter is the modified-hook titanium Greenfield filter, which is inserted using a 12 Fr introducer through a 14 Fr sheath. Its conical shape is similar to that of the stainless steel Greenfield filter, but it is 8 mm wider at the base and 0.5 cm taller (Fig. 135–6). The behavior of titanium in the tissues and its thrombogenicity in the circulation have been studied. It remains as inert as stainless steel in the tissues, and there is no evidence of any additional thrombogenicity. The mechanical properties of the titanium Greenfield filter have been tested extensively, and it shows remarkable resistance to flexion fatigue and induced corrosion.[33] Because this filter is sufficiently elastic to allow it to be folded into the 12 Fr carrier, modification of the original hook design was necessary to improve filter stabilization in the vena cava

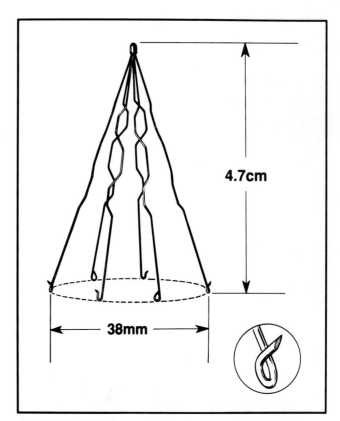

FIGURE 135–6. Modified-hook titanium Greenfield filter. The recurved hooks are set at an angle of 80 degrees for stabilization without full penetration of the vena cava.

against upward and downward vectors of force (see Fig. 135–6). This modified-hook design has reduced the incidence of filter migration and caval penetration found with the hook design of the original titanium filter.[34, 35] This filter can be inserted through either the jugular or the femoral vein, but usually the femoral vein is preferred for ease of entry. The titanium Greenfield filter can also be inserted at the time of laparotomy, either through a pursestring suture in the vena cava or through a small venous tributary. Under these circumstances, fluoroscopy is not required because the proper position of the carrier can be established by palpation and the filter can be discharged at the appropriate level.

Filter Insertion Technique

Under local anesthesia, a 4-mm stab incision is made over the right femoral vein, which is entered with a thin-walled needle that allows passage of a 0.035-inch guidewire (Fig. 135–7). The guidewire is passed into the upper reaches of the inferior vena cava, after which the dilator-sheath system is introduced and passed into the inferior vena cava (Fig. 135–8). The dilator is withdrawn, and the preloaded carrier is passed under fluoroscopic control through the sheath to the desired level of filter placement (Fig. 135–9). If resistance is encountered at the level of the common iliac vein as it angles out of the pelvis, the sheath and carrier should be advanced together, which will usually

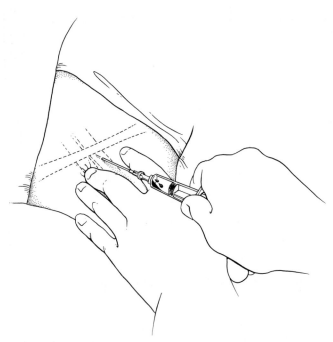

FIGURE 135–7. Percutaneous needle insertion into the common femoral vein is shown medial to the femoral artery, which is palpated with the middle finger. (Reprinted with permission from Greenfield LJ: Percutaneous placement of the Greenfield filter. *In* Vanoer Salm TJ, Cutler BS, Wheeler HB [eds]: Atlas of Bedside Procedures. 2nd ed. Boston, Little, Brown and Company, 1988, pp 107–110.)

facilitate passage. Once the carrier has been seen to exit the sheath, the base of the sheath should be secured to the carrier and the filter tip should be positioned at the desired level of introduction (Fig. 135–10). As a unit, the carrier catheter and sheath are retracted to release the filter. The carrier and sheath are then withdrawn, and gentle pressure is applied to the insertion site. An additional advantage to the use of the sheath-carrier is that premature discharge of the filter would be into the sheath rather than into the patient. The filter is preloaded into the carrier system, obviating concern about crossed limbs. The delivery system differs from that of the stainless steel version in that a guidewire is not used for axial stabilization of the filter during insertion. This may result in tilting of the filter and occasional asymmetry of the legs if the sheath-carrier is displaced against the wall of the vena cava; however, subsequent alignment of the legs of the filter has been seen on most follow-up radiographs.

Clinical Experience

Experience with the modified-hook titanium Greenfield filter is obviously limited because the device was approved by the Food and Drug Administration in 1991. The initial prospective, multi-center trial showed that filter insertion was successful in 181 of 186 patients (97 per cent); placement of the remainder was precluded only by unfavorable anatomy.[36] All but two of the insertions were per-

formed percutaneously. At the time of insertion, incomplete opening was seen in 2 per cent, but this was readily corrected by guidewire manipulation in each case. Leg asymmetry was seen in 5 per cent, but there was no association between this asymmetry and either recurrent embolism or penetration of the wall of the vena cava. Filter apex perforation of the vena cava at the time of insertion occurred in 1 patient after introduction from the left groin, and there was misplacement of one filter into a lumbar vein in another. No clinical sequelae were seen in either patient, although a second filter was inserted into each patient. The only symptomatic complication noted in the series was a hematoma at the insertion site in 1 patient. Initial follow-up data, obtained from all participating institutions at 30 days, showed minimal filter movement in 11 per cent; there was

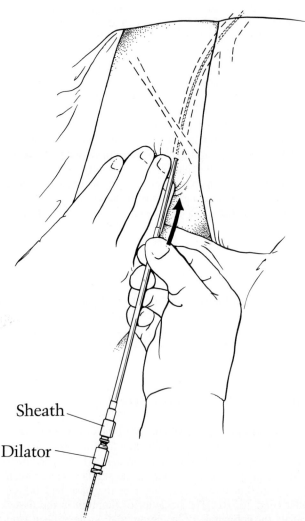

Sheath

Dilator

FIGURE 135–8. The dilator with attached sheath is passed under fluoroscopy over the guidewire to the desired level of discharge of the filter. The dilator and guidewire are then withdrawn, leaving the sheath in place. The sheath should then be flushed with heparinized saline. Digital control of the sheath orifice is necessary to minimize blood loss. (Reprinted with permission from Greenfield LJ: Percutaneous placement of the Greenfield filter. *In* Vanoer Salm TJ, Cutler BS, Wheeler HB [eds]: Atlas of Bedside Procedures. 2nd ed. Boston, Little, Brown and Company, 1988, pp 107–110.)

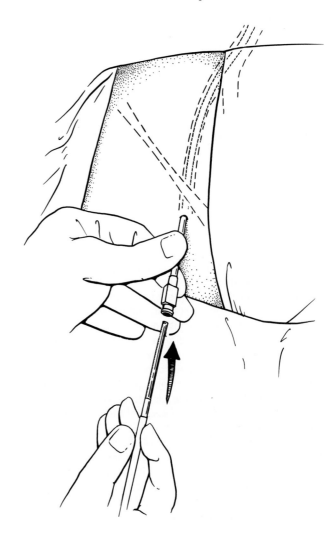

FIGURE 135-9.   The filter carrier is introduced into the sheath, and if difficulty is encountered in exiting the pelvis, both carrier and sheath should be advanced together. The carrier should be advanced through the sheath until the sheath hub contacts the control handle to prevent release of the filter into the sheath. (Reprinted with permission from Greenfield LJ: Percutaneous placement of the Greenfield filter. *In* Vanoer Salm TJ, Cutler BS, Wheeler HB [eds]: Atlas of Bedside Procedures. 2nd ed. Boston, Little, Brown and Company, 1988, pp 107–110.)

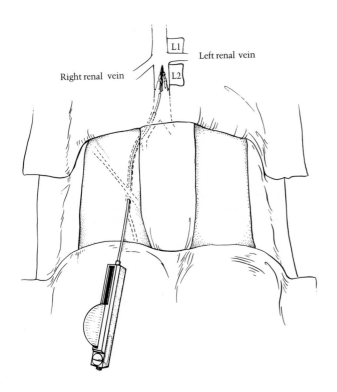

FIGURE 135-10.   The carrier tip should be positioned under fluoroscopy at the level of L2–L3. The locking mechanism on the control handle is released by moving the control tab with the thumb to the left. The control tab is then pulled backward to uncover the filter, which will be discharged within the vena cava. Once the filter has been discharged, no attempt should be made to alter its position. (Reprinted with permission from Greenfield LJ: Percutaneous placement of the Greenfield filter. *In* Vanoer Salm TJ, Cutler BS, Wheeler HB [eds]: Atlas of Bedside Procedures. 2nd ed. Boston, Little, Brown and Company, 1988, pp 107–110.)

no significant proximal migration. Computed tomographic scans were obtained when the diameter of the base of the filter was seen to have enlarged more than 5 mm. There was evidence of penetration of the wall of the vena cava in only one case (0.8 per cent), with no clinical sequelae. Long-term follow-up experience will be necessary to confirm that the performance of the modified-hook titanium Greenfield filter is equivalent to that of the stainless steel Greenfield filter, but it is obvious that this new device has made filter insertion easier, less expensive, and less invasive.

SUMMARY

There is considerable ingenuity in the numerous devices now available for clinical use as vena caval filters. The primary objective, to provide a safe and effective device for permanent implantation, should lead to continued evolution of materials and design. The standard for comparison, however, should remain the stainless steel Greenfield filter, on the basis of data available since its introduction in 1972. It seems clear that advances in percutaneous techniques will make percutaneous placement the obvious choice for the future, but the long-term safety and efficacy of the conical design of the Greenfield filter suggest that a new design may not be needed.

In the overall management of the patient with thrombotic disease, it is imperative to understand that any filtration device plays only a limited role and it is incumbent on the physician who treats the patient to assume the responsibility for the ongoing management and long-term follow-up of the underlying disorder.

References

1. Nasbeth DC, Moran JM: Reassessment of the role of inferior-vena-cava ligation in thromboembolism. N Engl J Med 273:1250, 1965.
2. Amador E, Ting KL, Crane C: Ligation of inferior vena cava for thromboembolism. JAMA 206:1758, 1968.
3. Ferris EJ, Vittimberga FJ, Byrne JJ, et al: The inferior vena cava after ligation and plication: A study of collateral routes. Radiology 89:1, 1967.
4. Miller TD, Staats BA: Impaired exercise tolerance after inferior vena caval interruption. Chest 93:776, 1988.
5. Spencer FC: Plication of the vena cava for pulmonary embolism. Surgery 62:388, 1967.
6. Adams JT, DeWeese JA: Partial interruption of the inferior vena cava with a new plastic clip. Surg Gynecol Obstet 123:1087, 1966.
7. Lindenauer SM: Prophylactic staple plication of the inferior vena cava. Arch Surg 107:669, 1973.
8. DeMeester TR, Rutherford RB, Blazek JV, Zuidema GD: Plication of the inferior vena cava for thromboembolism. Surgery 62:56, 1967.
9. Askew AR, Gardner AMN: Long-term follow-up of partial caval occlusion by clip. Am J Surg 140:441, 1980.
10. Couch NP, Baldwin SS, Crane C: Mortality and morbidity rates after inferior vena caval clipping. Surgery 77:106, 1975.
11. Cimochowski GE, Evans RH, Zarius CK, et al: Greenfield filter versus Mobin-Uddin umbrella: The continuing quest for the ideal method of vena caval interruption. J Thorac Cardiovasc Surg 79:358, 1980.
12. Cohen JR, Tenenbaum N, Citron M: Greenfield filter as primary therapy for deep venous thrombosis and/or pulmonary embolism in patients with cancer. Surgery 109:12, 1991.
13. Fink JA, Jones BT: The Greenfield filter as primary means of therapy in venous thromboembolic disease. Surg Gynecol Obstet 172:253, 1991.
14. Greenfield LJ, McCurdy JR, Brown PP, et al: A new intracaval filter permitting continued flow and resolution of emboli. Surgery 73:599, 1973.
15. Schroeder TM, Elkins RC, Greenfield LJ: Entrapment of sized emboli by the KMA-Greenfield intracaval filter. Surgery 83:435, 1979.
16. Greenfield LJ, Michna BA: Twelve year clinical experience with the Greenfield vena caval filter. Surgery 104:706, 1988.
17. Gomez GA, Cutler BS, Wheeler HB: Transvenous interruption of the inferior vena cava. Surgery 93:612, 1983.
18. Greenfield LJ, Cho K, Proctor M, et al: Late results of suprarenal Greenfield filter placement. Arch Surg 127:969, 1992.
19. Peyton JWR, Hylerman MB, Greenfield LJ, et al: Comparison of the Greenfield filter and vena caval ligation for experimental septic thromboembolism. Surgery 93:533, 1983.
20. Greenfield LJ: Technical considerations for insertion of vena caval filters. Surg Gynecol Obstet 148:422, 1979.
21. Hye RJ, Mitchell AT, Dory CE, et al: Analysis of the transition to percutaneous placement of Greenfield filters. Arch Surg 125:1550, 1990.
22. Glanz S, Gordon DH, Kantor A: Percutaneous femoral insertion of the Greenfield vena cava filter: Incidence of femoral vein thrombosis. Am J Roentgenol 149:1065, 1987.
23. Roehm JOF Jr, Gianturco C, Barth MH, et al: Percutaneous transcatheter filter for the inferior vena cava: A new device for treatment of patients with pulmonary embolism. Radiology 150:255, 1984.
24. Roehm JOF Jr, Johnsrude IS, Barth MH, et al: The bird's nest inferior vena cava filter: Progress report. Radiology 168:745, 1988.
25. McCowan TC, Ferris EJ, Keifsteck JE, et al: Retrieval of dislodged bird's nest inferior vena caval filters. J Intervent Radiol 3:179, 1983.
26. Simon M, Athanasoulis CA, Kim D, et al: Simon nitinol inferior vena cava filter: Initial clinical experience. Radiology 172:99, 1989.
27. Dorfman GS: Percutaneous inferior vena caval filters. Radiology 174:987, 1990.
28. McCowan TC, Ferris EJ, Carver DK, Molpum WM: Complications of the nitinol vena caval filter. J Vasc Interv Radiol 3:401, 1992.
29. Ricco JB, Crochet D, Sebilotte P, et al: Percutaneous transvenous caval interruption with the ''LGM'' filter: Early results of a multicenter trial. Ann Vasc Surg 3:242, 1988.
30. Maquin P, Fajadet P, Railhac N, et al: LGM and Gunther: Two complementary vena cava filters. Radiology 173:476, 1989.
31. Millward SF, Marsh JI, Peterson RA, et al: LGM (VenaTech) vena cava filters: Clinical experience in 64 patients. J Vasc Interv Radiol 2:429, 1991.
32. Awh MH, Taylor FC, Lu CT: Spontaneous fracture of a Vena-Tech inferior vena caval filter. Am J Roentgenol 157:177, 1991.
33. Greenfield LJ, Savin MA: Comparison of titanium and stainless steel Greenfield vena caval filters. Surgery 106:820, 1989.
34. Greenfield LJ, Cho KJ, Tauscher JR: Evolution of hook design for fixation of the titanium Greenfield filter. J Vasc Surg 9:345, 1990.
35. Greenfield LJ, Cho KJ, Pais SO, VanAman M: Preliminary clinical experience with the titanium Greenfield vena caval filter. Arch Surg 124:657, 1989.
36. Greenfield LJ, Cho KJ, Proctor M, et al: Results of a multicenter study of the modified hook titanium Greenfield filter. J Vasc Surg 14:253, 1991.

Varicose Veins: Patient Selection and Treatment

George Johnson, Jr., M.D., and Robert B. Rutherford, M.D.

• • •

Varicose veins have always bothered mankind; an early bas-relief shows a Greek sufferer, presumably asking for a cure, presenting the statue of a leg with a large varicosity to the god Aesculapius. As early as the 1st century A.D., Islamic physicians described the stab incision and avulsion method of surgery for varicose veins of the lower extremity. With continuing advances in methods of evaluating venous anatomy and hemodynamics, therapy for varicose veins is in a period of change.

ETIOLOGY AND DEVELOPMENT

Three factors dominate theories on the etiology of primary varicose veins: valvular incompetence,[1] weakness in the vein wall, and arteriovenous fistulae. It is likely that all three causes contribute to different degrees in different patients.

Valvular incompetence may be localized or segmental. Incompetence at key locations may lead to secondary incompetence and varicosities in tributary veins in one part of the superficial system. Thus, incompetent perforator vein valves may lead to localized varicosities. Varicosity of the entire saphenous vein is usually associated with valvular incompetence of the sentinel valve of the saphenofemoral or saphenopopliteal junction.[2, 3] On the other hand, valvular incompetence, and therefore varicosity, may be confined to discrete segments of the saphenous vein, most frequently the long saphenous vein below the knee. In contrast, valvular incompetence of the iliofemoral vein can be asymptomatic, with no apparent pathologic consequences.[4] The cause of the incompetence may be inherent in the valve, or it may result from physiologic abnormalities. The degree to which varicosities result may depend on hemodynamic stresses placed on the system (e.g., pregnancy).

It has been proposed that weakness of the vein wall is due to alterations in the biochemistry or to collagen defects, elastin defects, or both. European investigators have extensively researched this possibility.[5]

Arteriovenous fistulae may lead to varicose veins. Haimovici demonstrated microscopic arteriovenous fistulae,[6] and Baron and Cassaro found functional arteriovenous communication in patients with varicose veins.[7] Clarke and associates demonstrated a reduced vein wall elasticity and an increased arterial inflow in patients with superficial venous insufficiency and suggested this as an etiology for varicose veins.[2]

The degree to which these various "etiologic" factors play a primary versus a secondary role is difficult to discern from the study of patients with fully developed varicosities. Data on the relative importance and the sequence of development of each of these etiologies are difficult to obtain. Based on the authors' experience, valvular incompetence is the most important factor in the development of saphenous varicosities, and venous wall abnormality is most important in the development of nonsaphenous varicosities. It should be emphasized that except in the case of obvious congenital abnormalities, varicose veins develop because of some genetic or acquired predisposition. Superimposed physiologic or biochemical stresses, such as pregnancy, exercises that increase intra-abdominal pressure, or excessive standing, lead to the development of the varicosities. This is usually a progressive process, with sequential dilatation and incompetence of adjacent segments of the superficial venous system.

TYPES

Varicose veins of the lower extremity can be classified in several ways; this chapter concentrates on the therapeutic approach to *primary* varicose veins.

I. Spider angiomata: stellate clusters of small subcuticular veins, at times associated with a superficial "feeder" vein. These are described in greater detail in Chapter 137.

II. Varicose veins
   A. Segmental varicose veins: no evidence of association with incompetent saphenous or perforator vein valves.
   B. Varicose veins associated with incompetent perforator vein valves (i.e., no evidence of proximal saphenous incompetence).
   C. Incompetent saphenous system varicosities
      i. Long
         a. Competent saphenofemoral junction valve; incompetent saphenous valves below the knee.
         b. Incompetent saphenofemoral valve.

ii. Short
    a. Competent saphenopopliteal junction valve; incompetent valve below mid-calf.
    b. Incompetent saphenopopliteal valve.

According to Koyano and Sakaguchi's study from Japan, there can be several combinations of the pathology outlined.[3] The pathology most frequently seen by surgeons who operate on varicose veins is incompetence of the entire long saphenous vein (occurring in 66 per cent).[3] Patients with an incompetent long saphenous vein valve may also have varicose veins unassociated with the main saphenous trunk. Other patients present with isolated varicose veins, without incompetence of the saphenous system. Whether these are associated with local valve incompetence or weak vein walls may be determined with a Doppler probe by a skilled operator. Although this is not documented by Koyano and Sakaguchi's study, many surgeons encounter patients with isolated incompetence of the long saphenous vein below the knee. Giacomini's vein (the ascending branch of the short saphenous vein that communicates with the long saphenous vein) may transmit incompetence from the greater to the distal lesser saphenous veins below a competent saphenopopliteal junction. However, this is uncommon and occurred in only 1.4 per cent of Koyano and Sakaguchi's series. It is unusual to have a competent saphenopopliteal valve and to have incompetence in the short saphenous vein below the mid-calf.[3]

DIAGNOSIS AND EVALUATION

Varicose veins are usually quite apparent, although they can be missed in the morbidly obese patient. Therefore, the main diagnostic challenge is evaluation of the underlying valvular incompetence and the extent of segmental involvement.

Clinical Evaluation

Clinical evaluation is frequently the most important factor in deciding if therapy is indicated. Many patients are concerned about the appearance of their varicosities, which can be of major importance to the patient. However, the physician must separate patients suffering pain from those with primarily cosmetic concerns. Symptoms are usually worse at the end of the day and are alleviated by elevation. Tender varicosities, swelling of the ankle, and aching of the leg are common symptoms. However, bleeding, tender "knots" from phlebitis, and even stasis dermatitis and ulcers may also be present. Various clinical tests, such as Trendelenburg's and Perthes' tests,[8] have been replaced by more sophisticated technology (see Chapter 133).

Brawny edema, stasis dermatitis, subcutaneous fibrosis, cutaneous atrophy, pigmentation, and ulceration are signs of chronic venous insufficiency suggesting deep and perforator valve incompetence. However, these changes may be due entirely to superficial venous insufficiency in long-standing cases.[9]

Noninvasive Testing

A pencil *Doppler probe* can be helpful in evaluating the superficial venous system, but the results are highly dependent on the skill and experience of the operator. Incompetence of the valves of the deep venous system, incompetent perforators, and incompetence in the saphenous system can be identified by the skilled observer.

Although *photoplethysmography* has been discarded in many, if not most, laboratories because of inconsistent results, it may be useful when used in conjunction with a careful clinical examination. Its main weaknesses are the wide variations in normal venous refill time and the variable degrees to which reflux proximally in the superficial veins is transmitted to the subcutaneous plexus monitored at the ankle. Photoplethysmography will usually detect isolated saphenofemoral incompetence, on the basis of a rapid VRT which is corrected by a high thigh tourniquet, as opposed to more widespread incompetence, such as when perforator veins are also involved.

Duplex scanning is a useful, sensitive, specific, and less subjective test. The major drawbacks to its universal use are time and instrument cost. Except in the morbidly obese, it can more accurately appraise the same pathology as a Doppler probe. In addition, it is more accurate in identifying deep and superficial venous thrombosis and incompetent perforators. Incompetent valves may be identified by this method. The more complex the case, the greater the dividends from a careful duplex study.

Air plethysmography, as used by Belcaro and coworkers, appears to evaluate venous hemodynamics in a fashion that relates well to clinical findings (see Chapter 133).[10] This technique evaluates and quantitates reflux, the calf muscle pump, and the residual volume after exercise. With tourniquet occlusion of the saphenous vein in the thigh, its contribution to the pathologic hemodynamics can be assessed.

Summary

In summary, evaluation of varicose veins must be both anatomic and functional. Prior deep venous thrombosis must be excluded to ensure that varicose veins are not secondary to it. Clinical evaluation, including a history and a physical examination, is usually adequate before the initiation of therapy. However, because, currently, treatment is varied in order to deal with the underlying cause and not just the varicose veins, some objective evaluation of the underlying pathophysiology is required to identify the etiologic type of varicose veins and the extent of secondary changes. Central to this is an evaluation of the degree and extent of valvular incompetence.

INDICATIONS FOR THERAPY

After a thorough evaluation of the underlying pathophysiology, particularly the extent of valvular incompetence, therapy can be more logically directed toward the varicose veins and their cause.

Pain, aching, swelling, and recurrent thrombophlebitis are the unequivocal indications for therapy. Because this seems to be a progressive disease, the mere presence of varicosities can be an acceptable indication because early ablation can prevent the progression of valvular incompetence and simplify therapy.

In general, operative intervention is best used for the incompetent saphenous system and large varices, whereas sclerotherapy is best applied to the smaller varices and spider angiomas. Sclerotherapy is also being evaluated for ablation of larger varices and of the greater and lesser saphenous veins, but studies have indicated that sclerotherapy controls the underlying saphenous incompetence in only a minority of cases.[11] The results of this approach thus await more experience and longer follow-up.

SCLEROTHERAPY

Sclerotherapy has been used extensively throughout Europe and is gaining popularity in the United States. In the past, it was primarily used for cosmesis, but with increased skill in performance and knowledge of this technique, the indications for its use are being extended to larger varices. The technique of sclerotherapy and its indications are outlined in Chapter 137.

MULTIPLE LIGATION AND LOCAL EXCISION

Multiple ligation and local excision refers here to the popular practice of local excision of varicose veins through multiple small "stab" incisions. With this technique, it is important for the surgeon to identify the main sites of valvular reflux with a Doppler instrument beforehand and to mark these sites, and the course of the varicosities, with indelible ink before the operation. Vertical incisions give the best cosmetic result. With the leg elevated, the vein is identified by blunt dissection and delivered into the wound. This maneuver is aided by a small clamp, a crochet hook, or a specifically designed instrument. After as much vein as possible has been extracted by blunt dissection, the vein is avulsed without ligation. If bleeding persists, it indicates that an incompetent perforator has not been identified. This can be located by applying fingerpoint pressure in an exploratory fashion until the bleeding stops. Another stab wound over the source of the bleeding is made, and the vein is identified and ligated. The wounds are closed with subcuticular sutures, and the leg is firmly wrapped with elastic compression bandages while it is still elevated.

SAPHENOUS LIGATION AND STRIPPING

Long Saphenous Varicosities

If the entire long saphenous vein is pathologically involved, it is stripped after high ligation. It is exposed in the groin with an incision just below and parallel to the inguinal crease, over the fossa ovalis, and at the ankle with a vertical incision just anterior to the medial malleolus. At the ankle, the caudad portion of the saphenous vein is ligated with an absorbable suture and a disposable plastic stripper is inserted. Another incision may be needed along the course of the saphenous vein to facilitate further passage if the stripper "hangs up" on a tortuous segment of the vein.

In the groin, all tributaries entering the saphenous vein are identified by blunt dissection, tied, and divided. The saphenofemoral junction at the groin is never ligated until the stripper is felt in the saphenous vein as it is passed from below. This prevents inadvertent ligation of the superficial femoral vein. or even the femoral artery. A clamp is placed on the saphenous vein so as not to compromise the common femoral vein. When the ligature is applied, another two clamps are placed lower down cephalad and caudad to the anticipated venotomy for delivering the stripper passed up from below, and the vein is divided above them. The cephalad saphenous vein stump is tied, and then a transfixion suture is used. A head is placed on the end of the stripper in the groin, the handle is placed at the ankle end, and the stripper is removed by pulling down and removing the "telescoped" vein from the patient through the ankle incision. Compression is applied over the course of the saphenous vein for 5 minutes. At the end of this time, clotted blood is gently milked along the course of the saphenous vein and out through the two incisions. All incisions are closed with subcuticular sutures, and the leg is wrapped with a compression bandage. Some surgeons prefer to remove the stripper after the leg incisions have been closed and the leg has been wrapped with compression bandages.[12]

The patient's legs are kept elevated. After an initial period of complete bed rest (6 to 12 hours), walking is allowed whenever possible; sitting is discouraged. The patient is discharged the same day or the next day, is seen again in 1 or 2 weeks, and is advised to continue to wear support stockings.

Segmental or Distal Saphenous Varicosities

In the area of segmental or distal saphenous varicosities, the efficacy of sclerotherapy is being actively studied, but long-term results of this approach with good follow-up are still required. Meanwhile, with the new techniques of evaluating venous anatomy and function described previously, the operative approach can be nicely tailored to fit the pathology. Here, the long saphenous vein above the knee is often normal, whereas below the knee it is functionally incompetent. The short saphenous vein is much less involved than the long; thus, the operation required depends on the pathology found. The stripping of some main segments might be beneficial, but localized varices unassociated with major saphenous vein incompetence can be individually excised as described earlier.

Short Saphenous Varicosities

The short saphenous vein is removed through a small transverse incision placed posteriorly in the popliteal space at or just below the crease, with the exact site depending on the point of entrance of the lesser saphenous vein into the popliteal vein. The vein is removed by stripping with multiple stab incisions, with avulsion of tributary varicosities as indicated.

In the usual patient with extensive saphenous varicosities, the operation usually consists of a high ligation and stripping of the varicose saphenous vein, with multiple avulsions of tributary varices. It should be noted that more and more surgeons (and one of the authors) are recommending that the latter part of the procedure be accomplished with sclerotherapy at a later date.

Results and Complications

Major complications of this operation are infrequent and include damage to deeply placed arteries or veins, deep venous thrombosis, and saphenous nerve damage. Infection, bleeding, ecchymosis, and wound separation are complications of all operations and demand appropriate therapy. The incidence of saphenous nerve damage seems to vary considerably from series to series. It most frequently occurs with stripping of the saphenous vein below the knee. The use of a small stripper head decreases the incidence of this complication.

References

1. Anning ST: The historical aspects. *In* Dodd H, Cockett FB (eds): The Pathology and Surgery of the Veins of the Lower Limb. 2nd ed. New York, Churchill Livingstone, 1976, pp 3–17.
2. Clarke GH, Vasdekis SN, Hobbs JT, Nicolaides AN: Venous wall function in the pathogenesis of varicose veins. Surgery 111:402, 1992.
3. Koyano K, Sakaguchi S: Selective stripping operation based on Doppler ultrasonic findings for primary varicose veins of the lower extremities. Surgery 103:615, 1988.
4. Ludbrook J: Primary great saphenous varicose veins revisited. World J Surg 10:954, 1986.
5. Jurukova Z, Milenkov C: Ultrastructural evidence for collagen degradation in the walls of varicose veins. Exp Mol Pathol 37:37, 1982.
6. Haimovici H: Role of precapillary arteriovenous shunting in the pathogenesis of varicose veins and its therapeutic implications. Surgery 101:515, 1987.
7. Baron HC, Cassaro S: The role of arteriovenous shunts in the pathogenesis of varicose veins. J Vasc Surg 4:1248, 1986.
8. Dodd H, Cockett FB: Diagnosis of varicose veins. *In* The Pathology and Surgery of the Veins of the Lower Limb. 2nd ed. New York, Churchill Livingstone, 1976, pp 81–85.
9. Darke SG, Penfold C: Venous ulceration and saphenous ligation. Eur J Vasc Surg 6:4, 1992.
10. Belcaro G, Christopoulos D, Nicolaides A: Venous insufficiency: Noninvasive testing. *In* Bergan JJ, Kistner RL (eds): Atlas of Venous Surgery. Philadelphia, WB Saunders, 1992, pp 9–24.
11. Bishop CCR, Fronek HS, Fronek A, et al: Real-time color duplex scanning after sclerotherapy of the greater saphenous vein. J Vasc Surg 14:505, 1991.
12. Dale WA: Varicose veins: Modern management produces good results. *In* Management of Vascular Surgical Problems. New York, McGraw Hill, 1985, pp 441–460.

137

Sclerotherapy: Technique and Application

John J. Bergan, M.D.

• • •

The care of venous stasis in all of its manifestations is the responsibility of surgeons in general and of vascular surgeons in particular. With varicose veins, such care is directed toward ablation of pathologic vessels. This is achieved by removing them surgically or by obliterating them with sclerotherapy. Large varicose clusters, axial veins (e.g., the greater and lesser saphenous veins) that show gross reflux, and varicosities above the knee are best treated by removal.[1] Other vessels may be subjected to sclerotherapy.

Indications for the use of sclerotherapy are listed in Table 137–1. Sclerotherapy is the only modality effective in the ablation of telangiectatic blemishes. It can also erase reticular veins and varicosities, particularly when they are less than 4 mm in diameter. Below the knee, where effective compression is most efficient, sclerosants can ablate larger varicosities and small clusters of varices not associated with gross saphenous reflux. Furthermore, sclerotherapy is useful in obliterating residual varicosities after surgical treatment and those that appear at times remote from surgery after saphenous reflux has been totally corrected.

Many individuals, especially nonsurgeons, use sclerotherapy for nearly all varicosities.[2] Some even believe that axial reflux through saphenous veins can be halted effectively by sclerosants.[3] Furthermore, sclerotherapy is used by some for thigh varicosities of nonsaphenous origin and even for large varices associated with principal named perforating veins. As mentioned in Table 137–1, these are not ideal indications. It is the use of sclerotherapy in suboptimal situations that has contributed to its inferior reputation.

In general, sclerotherapy finds its greatest utility in the smallest incompetent vessels. These, then, may be telangi-

Table 137–1.   Indications for Sclerotherapy

Optimal Indications
Telangiectasias
Reticular varicosities and reticular veins
Isolated varicosities*
Below-knee varicosities*
Recurrent varicosities*

Less Than Optimal Indications
Symptomatic reflux
In the aged and infirm
In nonsurgical candidates

Questionable Indications
Greater saphenous reflux
Lesser saphenous reflux
Large varicosities

Contraindications
Allergy to the sclerosant

In the absence of gross saphenous reflux.

ectasias or small varices below the knee. Proximal venous reflux and venous hypertension must be corrected first. Under less than ideal circumstances, sclerotherapy also finds a distinct usefulness in palliation, such as in the aged and in the infirm. In addition, in situations that violate these guidelines, sclerotherapeutic ablation of symptomatic varicosities can temporarily prove to be gratifyingly beneficial.

HISTORICAL DEVELOPMENT

Although many attribute Pravaz with the invention of the syringe in 1851, it was actually Rynd who developed this radical advance in 1845.[4] Case reports of sclerotherapy appear throughout the latter half of the 19th century.[5] A variety of caustics were used, including carbolic acid. Profound inflammation and suppuration followed such treatments in the prelisterian era. All early agents were thrombogenic. After investigations showing that quinine obliterated small vessels by intimal damage, the focus of

sclerotherapy changed.[6] This led directly to the use of hypertonic saline in 1924 and sodium morrhuate in 1930.[7]

Credit should be given to Biegeleisen for the invention of microsclerotherapy after 1930.[8] The technique languished somewhat until after 1970, although in some centers treatment of varicosities of all sizes continued throughout this time.[9, 10]

RELEVANT ANATOMY

The gross anatomy of the venous system is well known to surgeons.[11] Valve-containing deep veins transport venous blood by means of muscular contraction. Less physiologically important superficial veins also contain valves that direct their flow upward, and these veins connect with the deep system by means of perforating veins that penetrate the deep fascia of the lower extremities. Check valves in these perforating veins protect the poorly supported venules superficial to the tela aponeurotica from compartmental exercise pressure. Less surgically appreciated is the reticular subdermic venous network, which also contains valves. Because it is the most superficially located vein network of the lower extremities, this plexus is the most poorly supported and is the source of the earliest subcutaneous varicosities.[12] Superficial to this network, in the dermis, postcapillary venules run horizontally, range in size from 12 to 35 μm, and empty into collecting venules twice as large in the mid-dermis.[11, 12] One-way valves are found in venules at the dermis-adipose junction and also in areas of anastomosis of small to large venules (Fig. 137–1). Larger venules also contain valves not necessarily associated with junctional points. Free edges of the valves are always directed away from the smaller vessels and toward the larger ones. These valves serve to direct blood flow toward the deeper venous system. The valve structure in these small venules is identical to that found in larger deep veins and includes valve sinuses, cusps, and aggeres in relation to vein walls.

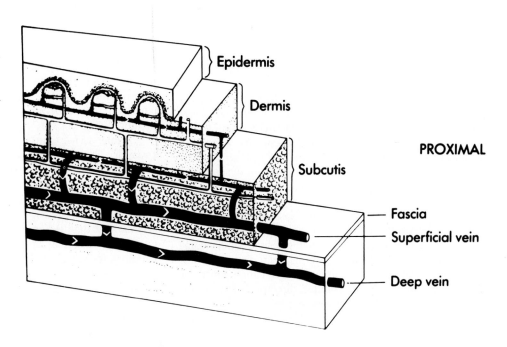

FIGURE 137–1. Dermal postcapillary venular network. Valves within these tiny vessels all direct blood flow deeper into large collecting veins. Failure of check valve function allows high-pressure venous blood to flow into unsupported dermal vessels, thus producing telangiectatic blemishes.

Epidermis

Dermis

PROXIMAL

Subcutis

Fascia
Superficial vein
Deep vein

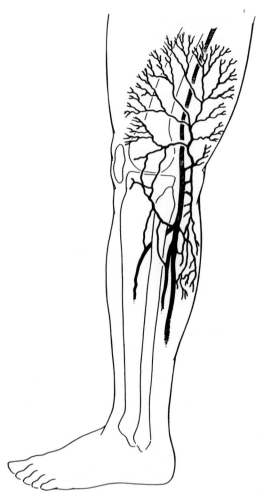

FIGURE 137–2. Medial side of the thigh and leg showing perforating vein connections with the deep circulation. Failure of check valve function allows intercompartmental exercise hydrodynamic pressure to be transmitted from the deep circulation directly to subcutaneous veins, reticular veins, and venules in the dermis. Thus, high-pressure effects can produce gross varicosities, reticular varicosities, and telangiectatic blemishes.

Postcapillary venules are composed of endothelial cells covered by a basement membrane, some collagen fibers, and rare smooth muscle cells. Collecting venules gradually receive more muscle cells, and larger veins have a continuous muscular coat.[13]

Simple telangiectasias are dilated channels in a normal dermal stroma. They usually have a single endothelial cell lining and a limited muscular cellular infiltration. "Sunburst" telangiectasias are widened cutaneous veins that demonstrate an intercellular collagenous dysplasia on electron microscopy.[14] This is similar to collagen dysplasia of varicose veins. Arteriovenous fistulae have been demonstrated as a component of dermal telangiectasias.[15] This can best be thought of as a venous hypertension–induced breakdown of the capillary barrier or opening of physiologic shunts rather than as the cause of the lesion. Direct communication of telangiectasias with the deep circulation has been demonstrated.[16] Such communications allow muscular exercise pressure to be transmitted directly to the unsupported subdermal and dermal venous network.[17, 18]

The practical value of knowledge of the relevant anat-

omy is understanding exactly where sclerotherapy should be performed to obtain a maximal effect. For example, telangiectatic blemishes may receive venous hypertension from a hydrostatic or gravitational effect from varicosities in subcutaneous tissue or reticular varices from the subdermal network. Elimination of the source of high pressure is critical to ablation of the telangiectatic blemish.

Furthermore, varicosities or telangiectasias may receive venous hypertension from a hydrodynamic source, muscular compartment pressure during exercise (Fig. 137–2). This is transmitted through incompetent perforating veins because of a check valve failure. Effective sclerotherapy in such instances depends on eliminating the source of hydrodynamic pressure.

SCLEROTHERAPEUTIC AGENTS

When telangiectasias are treated, the process is termed microsclerotherapy.[19] When sclerotherapy is used to obliterate larger veins, it is referred to as macrosclerotherapy. Drugs available for sclerotherapy may cause thrombosis, fibrosis, or both. Excessive thrombosis is undesirable and may lead to excessive perivascular inflammation and recanalization of the vessel. More desirable endothelial damage may be provoked by a number of mechanisms, including changing the surface tension of the plasma membrane, modifying the physical or chemical environment of the endothelial cell, and changing the intravascular pH or osmolality. For effective microsclerotherapy, the endothelial damage must produce vascular necrosis in a significant portion of the vascular wall.[10]

Agents that change the surface tension of the plasma membrane are detergents. They include sodium morrhuate, sodium tetradecyl sulfate, and polidocanol. Their action is to produce endothelial damage through interference with cell surface lipids.[20]

Hypertonic solutions, including hypertonic saline, hypertonic dextrose, and sodium salicylate, cause dehydration of endothelial cells through osmosis. Possibly fibrin deposition with thrombus formation occurs through modification of the electrostatic charge on the endothelial cells.[21]

Chemical irritants, such as chromated glycerin and polyiodinated iodine, act directly on the endothelial cells to produce endosclerosis. After endothelial damage occurs, there is fibrin deposition in the sclerosed vessels. Platelets adhere to the underlying elastin, collagen, or basement membrane.[22]

Table 137–2 ranks sclerosing agents according to strength. The strongest solutions are used in the largest veins, including the saphenopopliteal and saphenofemoral junctions, selective perforating veins, and larger varicose clusters. At the other end of the scale are the weakest solutions, which are used for telangiectasias and other vessels smaller than 0.4 mm in diameter. Weak solutions are useful for vessels of up to 2 mm in diameter, and strong solutions for vessels of 3 to 5 mm in diameter.

The only two sclerosing solutions approved by the US Food and Drug Administration (FDA) and listed in the *Physician's Desk Reference* are detergents. The oldest, sodium morrhuate, is a mixture of sodium salts of saturated

Table 137–2. Relative Strengths of Sclerosing Solutions

Category 1: Strongest
Sodium tetradecyl sulfate, 1.5–3.0%
Polidocanol, 3–5%
Polyiodinated iodine, 3–12%

Category 2: Strong
Sodium tetradecyl sulfate, 0.5–1.0%
Polidocanol, 1–2%
Polyiodinated iodine, 2%
Sodium morrhuate, 5%

Category 3: Moderate
Sodium tetradecyl sulfate, 0.25%
Polidocanol, 0.75%
Polyiodinated iodine, 1%
Hypertonic saline, 23.4%
Sodium morrhuate, 2.5%

Category 4: Weak
Sodium tetradecyl sulfate, 0.1%
Polidocanol, 0.25%–0.50%
Chromated glycerin, 50%
Polyiodinated iodine, 0.1%
Hypertonic saline, 11.7%
Sodium morrhuate, 1%

and unsaturated fatty acids present in cod liver oil. This agent experienced early popularity in the 1930s. This enthusiasm was dampened by reports of anaphylactic reactions. Sodium tetradecyl sulfate became widely used after 1950[23] and was advocated for use in dilute solution in the treatment of telangiectasias after 1978.[24] Although it is widely used, it does produce epidermal necrosis when infiltrated in concentrations of greater than 0.2 per cent. Allergic reactions have been reported, and postsclerotherapy hyperpigmentation is frequently seen. Curiously, the manufacturer recommends a test intravenous injection as a precaution against anaphylaxis.

Not approved by the FDA at present but undergoing phase II trials in anticipation of approval is the most widely used sclerotherapeutic agent, polidocanol. It was synthesized and introduced as a local and topical anesthetic that was clearly different from anesthetic agents that were "-caine" compounds. Polidocanol is a urethane whose optimum anesthetic effect is at a concentration of 3 per cent. Because its intravascular and intradermal instillation produced sclerosis of small-diameter blood vessels, polidocanol was withdrawn as an anesthetic agent and proposed as a sclerosing agent after 1967. An optimal concentration for treating telangiectasias is 0.5 per cent, whereas varicose veins may be treated with a 1 per cent or greater concentration.[25]

SCLEROTHERAPY OF VARICOSE VEINS (MACROSCLEROTHERAPY)

Indications for intervention in patients with varicose veins are for relief of symptomatology. Symptoms include aching pain, limb tiredness or heaviness after prolonged standing or sitting, and an exacerbation of symptoms at the termination of a menstrual cycle and on the 1st day of a menstrual period. Ugly appearance of varicose veins and telangiectasias is important to patients and is an indication

for treatment. Protuberant, saccular, bulging varicosities and the discoloration of dilated veins of telangiectasias or the purple stain of the corona phlebectatica at the ankle do bring patients to the physician.

If gross greater or lesser saphenous reflux is present, as determined by Doppler examination, it should be corrected surgically before sclerotherapy. However, palliation can be achieved for 2 to 4 years in the presence of axial reflux even though varix recurrence may be expected. For example, in an elderly patient who experiences external bleeding from varicose blebs, uncorrected axial reflux will not affect local sclerotherapy to obliterate the blebs and prevent further bleeding episodes. Similarly, if recurrent thrombophlebitis in varicosities has occurred, the varicosities themselves can be obliterated by sclerotherapy even without control of the proximal venous hypertension.

Contraindications to sclerotherapy include the presence of arterial occlusive disease, patient immobility, and the presence of uncontrolled malignant tumor. Other contraindications are hypersensitivity to the drug, acute thrombophlebitis, and huge varicosities with large communications to deep veins.

In addition to the clinical examination to determine the sites of varicosities and the origin of their venous hypertension, examination with a continuous-wave, hand-held Doppler instrument is essential (Fig. 137–3). This may be supplemented in particular cases with duplex scanning. Other tests of venous function, such as impedance plethysmography or photoplethysmography and venous pressure tests, are indirect and are not essential. Invasive phlebography is also not required. Classic tests, including the Perthes and Trendelenburg tests, have been replaced by the hand-held Doppler examination.

The objective of sclerotherapy is to produce endothelial damage and subsequent fibrosis of the entire vein wall without recanalization. Therefore, the ideal sclerosing solution would produce endothelial destruction with a minimum of thrombus formation. Unfortunately, FDA-approved agents are detergents, which are thrombogenic. Hypertonic saline is also used for sclerotherapy, although it is approved by the FDA for use only as an abortifacient. It does produce rapid endothelial damage. It is available in a concentration of 23.4 per cent and has been used extensively at this strength. Its single appeal is its total lack of allergenicity. However, it is common practice to add heparin, procaine, or lidocaine to hypertonic saline. Additives, of course, cancel the appeal of hypoallergenicity. Hypertonic saline at a concentration of 11.7 per cent is equal to that of 23.4 per cent in effect.[26]

Treatment of varicose veins 3 to 8 mm in diameter requires 0.5 to 1.0 per cent sodium tetradecyl sulfate or its equivalent. Such large varicosities require a stronger solution than telangiectasias.

Because of the commonplace nature of varicosities and the very large number of people who treat them, a variety of techniques have developed. In principle, small-caliber No. 25 butterfly needles are placed in varicosities while the patient is standing with the veins distended. The needles are attached to capped plastic extension tubing. A proximal tourniquet is neither necessary nor desirable. The multiple needles are placed either within a cluster of varicosities or in linear continuity in varices (Fig. 137–4). An attempt to

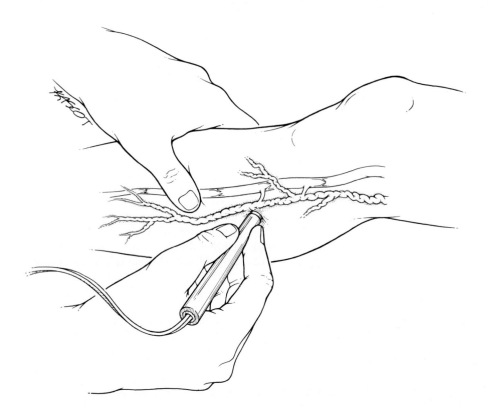

FIGURE 137–3.   Use of the Doppler instrument in identifying reflux in the region of Boyd's perforating vein. The continuous-wave, hand-held Doppler instrument confirms axial reflux as well as the general location of important refluxing perforators. These are intimately involved with the genesis of subcutaneous varicosities.

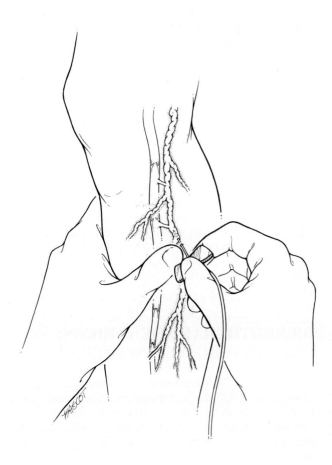

FIGURE 137–4.   Use of a No. 25 butterfly needle in macrosclerotherapy. The needle is securely placed in the offending varix near a perforating vein and is taped in place for use during injection using the empty vein technique.

identify and to inject into a source of reflux will aid in achieving long-term success. The needles are held in place with tape until all have been inserted, and then the patient is asked to assume a recumbent position and the leg is elevated so that the veins will be empty.

Duplex verification of superficial venous collapse with the leg elevated to 45 degrees has been confirmed.[27] While injection of 0.5 to 1.0 ml of solution proceeds, there should not be any pain, irritation, or burning sensation. The presence of any of these indicates extravasation rather than intravascular injection. Extravasation demands cessation of injection. At each injection site, after the needle has been withdrawn, a pressure pad of gauze, cotton, dental roll, or foam rubber is applied and taped in place with hypoallergenic tape. Elastic bandages may be used, wrapped from the toes proximally using gentle stretching. The wrap is carried to 3 inches above the most proximal injection site. An elastic stocking may be fitted over the elastic bandage for additional compression or used instead of the elastic bandage. The duration of compression will vary with the individual habits of the operator, but for varicosities of 3 to 8 mm in diameter, a constant compression for 3 to 7 days is advised. A large school of French phlebologists practice minimal or no compression, and the influential work of Fegan mandates 6 weeks of constant compression. The controversy over compression continues. Histologic studies suggest that 12 days of fibroplastic healing is required for obliteration of moderate-sized varicosities.[10, 28, 29]

Nearly all workers in this field advise that the patient should walk about the clinic for 30 minutes. This will allow symptoms and signs of an allergic reaction to appear and be treated. The comfort of the elastic compression can be evaluated, and the deep venous circulation will be stimulated to be flushed of any sclerosant that has entered from the superficial injection.

TREATMENT OF TELANGIECTATIC BLEMISHES (MICROSCLEROTHERAPY)

Telangiectatic blemishes may be thought of as extremely small varicose veins. Therefore, principles of treatment remain the same. The source of venous hypertension that has produced the elongation, tortuosity, and dilatation of the vessel must be controlled if treatment is to be effective. Telangiectasias may receive their pulse of venous hypertension directly through minute incompetent perforating veins.[16] This may be identifiable through careful Doppler examination, or more commonly, the offending perforating vein is not specifically identified. Treatment of the telangiectatic blemish in such a situation may fail simply because the sclerosant solution does not reach the feeding vein in a concentration sufficient to obliterate it.

On the other hand, telangiectasias may receive venous hypertension from the subdermal reticular network (Fig. 137–5). These are seen as thin-walled, blue, superficial dilated veins that are eventually tributaries to the main superficial venous system. Doppler studies have shown that free reflux occurs in such a network in association with telangiectasias. The reflux may proceed upward against the flow of gravity.[30] The reticular network may receive venous hypertension by gravitational effects or from incompetent perforators, hydrostatic, or hydrodynamic cause.

Knowledge of anatomy and the pathophysiology dictates that the treatment of telangiectasias begin with the source of venous hypertension. When it can be identified as a reticular dilated vein, the sclerosant solution may be seen to enter the telangiectasia directly from the feeding vein. The reverse may be true. Injecting telangiectasias may allow the observer to watch the sclerosing solution enter a

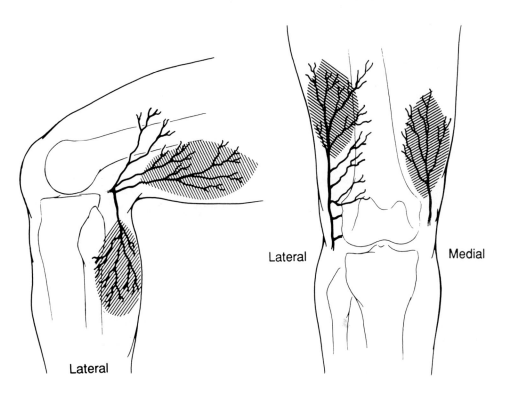

FIGURE 137–5. Common locations of telangiectatic blemishes on the medial distal thigh and the proximal leg both laterally and medially. Such telangiectatic blemishes may be connected to reticular feeding veins, which can be identified and sclerosed. Commonly, these feeding veins are connected to the deep venous circulation and transmit hydrodynamic forces to the dermal venules.

feeding vein from the site of injection. If it is impossible to identify the source of the venous hypertension, telangiectasias should be treated beginning at the point at which the branches converge. The actual injection method varies somewhat among authorities.[20, 31, 32]

The patient is in a horizontal position, either prone or supine. The skin is cleansed with alcohol to remove excess keratin and allow better visualization of the target vessel. Thirty-gauge needles are used, and they are bent to 10 to 20 degrees. The bevel of the needle may be placed either down or up, but the needle should be parallel to the skin surface. Small syringes, either 1 or 3 ml in volume, are most convenient. The skin adjacent to the blemish must be stretched, and the firmly supported needle and syringe are then moved so that the needle pierces the skin and vein while pressure on the plunger ejects the sclerosant solution (Fig. 137–6).

Magnification and good light may allow the operator to recognize the appearance of the needle within the lumen of the target vessel. Pressure on the plunger will allow the operator to see the development of a wheal if there is extravasation or a clearing of the telangiectatic web if intravascular injection is achieved. Some operators favor preceding injection of the sclerosant with a bolus (0.05 ml) of air. This allows the operator to check the position of the needle and may cause a greater spread of the sclerosant solution.[33]

Injections should be performed very slowly, and the amount of sclerosant should be limited to 0.1 or 0.2 ml. Injection over a 10- to 15-second period is optimal. If a precise intravascular injection with rapid clearing of the telangiectasias is achieved, the operator must control enthusiasm and sharply limit the amount of sclerosant given in any one particular site.

Minimizing the volume, pressure, and duration of the injection minimizes pain, risk of extravasation, and skin infarction. If persistent blanching of the skin to a waxy white color is seen or if a larger amount of sclerosant is inadvertently given in a single site, the area should be flushed thoroughly with hypodermic normal saline. This will dilute areas of extravasation and help to relieve vessel spasm. Vessels being treated that are larger than 0.5 mm and those that protrude above the skin surface should be compressed immediately, and compression should be maintained without interruption. Cotton balls, gauze, or foam rubber can be taped over the site with hypoallergenic tape in preparation for the eventual compression bandage or stocking.

After all telangiectatic blemishes and reticular varicosities have been injected and the injection session has been completed, elastic compression can be applied over the entire treated area. Again, practice varies, with some operators using compression elastic bandages and others elastic stockings. Furthermore, the duration of compression varies among authorities: some use no compression, some limit compression to 18 hours, and some advise compression for as long as 2 weeks. There is general agreement that protuberant telangiectasias or telangiectasias in association with large reticular veins should be treated with compression for 72 hours or more. Patients are encouraged to walk and not restrict their activities. The number of treatment sessions will depend on the degree of success of each session. However, it is common to treat telangiectasias for three or four sessions, and the interval between injection sessions is usually 2 to 4 weeks.

The treatment of reticular varicosities and feeding veins is slightly different from the treatment of telangiectasias. The patient is in a horizontal position. A No. 30 needle is optimal and can be inserted directly into the flat, blue-green reticular vein. A sensation of resistance will be felt at the skin level and also at the vein wall. After the vein has been pierced, the plunger may be pulled back and a flash of blood will be seen in the transparent syringe hub. This is possible even with a No. 30 needle. The volume injected

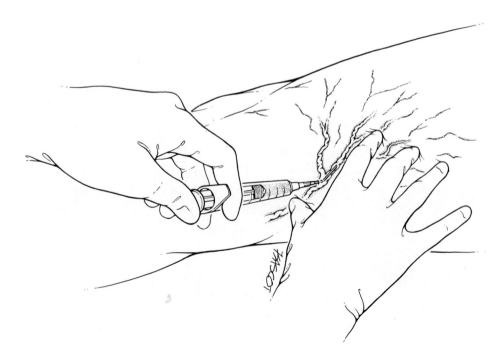

FIGURE 137–6. Placement of the needle in a feeding vein to treat the reticular varicosity found in association with a large telangiectatic blemish. Note the stretching of the skin, the penetration of the reticular varicosity with the needle, and the deft management of the plunger to clear blood from the entire blemish during injection.

should be maintained at less than 0.5 ml, and as in treating varicosities, multiple puncture sites aid in successful obliteration of the reticular varicosity.

Solutions used in treating reticular veins and telangiectatic blemishes must be dilute. The use of 0.1 or 0.2 per cent sodium tetradecyl sulfate or its equivalent is satisfactory. If 11.7 or 23.4 per cent hypertonic saline is used, and air block test of the injection site is advocated because this solution is caustic enough to cause cutaneous damage during extravasation. When polidocanol is approved by the FDA,[34] 0.5 per cent polidocanol solution may be used in treating reticular veins and telangiectatic blemishes.[35]

SIDE EFFECTS OF SCLEROTHERAPY

The fear of adverse sequelae of sclerotherapy keeps many physicians and surgeons from including this treatment modality in their therapeutic armamentarium. However, the incidence of complications is exceedingly low.[20, 32] Undesirable sequelae include anaphylaxis, allergic reactions, thrombophlebitis, cutaneous necrosis, pigmentation, and neoangiogenesis.[36, 37]

Anaphylaxis is an IgE-mediated mast cell–activated reaction that occurs within minutes of re-exposure to an antigen. Other classes of immunoglobulin may contribute to the reaction. Risk of anaphylaxis increases with repeated exposure to a given antigen, a fact that applies directly to repetitive episodes of sclerotherapy. Mast cell concentrations are high in the skin. Mediators derived from mast cells, including histamine, can produce clinical anaphylactic manifestations. These may range in severity from mild pruritus and urticaria to shock and death. Manifestations that should alert the physician to serious problems include itching, flushing, erythema, and developing angioedema. Mucous membranes of the eyes, nose, and mouth are frequently involved, and this involvement may precede upper airway obstruction caused by edema of the larynx. This, in turn, is heralded by respiratory stridor. Unrelated to respiratory obstruction can be hypotensive shock, which is thought to be due to peripheral vasodilatation and increased vascular permeability.

Rapid treatment is crucial. Therefore, the necessary equipment for resuscitation must be present and used aggressively. Epinephrine is the drug of choice for the treatment of systemic reactions. It will counteract vasodilatation and bronchoconstriction and will inhibit further release of mediators from mast cells. Antihistamines and corticosteroids are not the drugs of choice in initial treatment, but both may be administered after epinephrine. Endotracheal intubation, oxygen, and intravenous therapy may be necessary, and patients with serious reactions should be admitted directly to the hospital.

Sodium morrhuate has been implicated as the most frequent cause of anaphylaxis among the sclerosing agents. However, nearly all of the reactions reported occurred before 1950.

Goldman reviewed the medical literature regarding anaphylaxis and sodium tetradecyl sulfate and found only 47 cases of nonfatal allergic reactions in a review of 14,404 patients.[20] The product manufacturer has reported only two fatalities associated with the use of sodium tetradecyl sulfate, neither of which was from an anaphylactic reaction.

Polidocanol has the smallest incidence of allergic reactions, including anaphylaxis. Furthermore, patients allergic to sodium tetradecyl sulfate have been successfully treated with polidocanol. A single case of fatal anaphylactic shock has been reported with the use of polidocanol. Alone, hypertonic saline shows no evidence of inducing an allergic reaction or of having a toxic effect. However, additives such as lidocaine or heparin may, in and of themselves, induce allergic reactions.

Thrombophlebitis and its sequelae were commonly reported before the use of compression after sclerotherapy. The actual incidence of superficial thrombophlebitis is difficult to ascertain, but it ranges around 1 to 3 per cent. Duffy estimated that it occurred in 0.5 per cent of his patients.[31]

Deep venous thromboembolic events are obviated by postsclerotherapy exercise that flushes the deep veins. Scattered reports of pulmonary embolization following sclerotherapy have appeared.

Although serious reactions such as anaphylaxis, allergy, and thromboembolic events may be uncontrollable, the less severe complications of sclerotherapy can be diminished in frequency by attention to details of injection. Skin ulceration, cutaneous necrosis, may result from extravasation of solution. More commonly, it is due to arterial occlusion caused by sclerosant reaching a terminal arteriole. Other causes are reactive vasospasm from a too great volume of injection or excessive cutaneous pressure. Complications of extravasation are minimized by the use of extremely dilute solution, especially in the treatment of telangiectatic blemishes. Dilute 0.1 and even 0.2 per cent sodium tetradecyl sulfate may extravasate without complication. The same is true of 0.5 per cent polidocanol. However, extravasation of hypertonic saline in the skin may result in cutaneous necrosis if the solution remains undiluted. Intra-arterial infiltration of sclerosant is avoided by strict adherence to the practice of injecting small quantities into each individual site.

Postsclerotherapy hyperpigmentation is common after sclerotherapy for veins and telangiectatic blemishes. It may occur in up to 30 per cent of patients but is most common in patients treated with sodium tetradecyl sulfate and hypertonic saline. It is seen least in patients treated with polidocanol and is uncommon after the use of chromated glycerin. Neither of the latter two sclerosants had been approved by the FDA at the time of this writing.

The pigmentation is hemosiderin, and it is derived from extravasation of red blood cells, which may appear in the dermis either through diapedesis or the fracture of vessel walls. Postsclerotherapy pigmentation may be decreased in incidence by using weaker concentrations of solution, limiting the magnitude of intravascular pressure produced during injection, and removing the postsclerotherapy coagula that may appear in protuberant telangiectasias, reticular veins, or varicosities. Removal of such coagula can be achieved by incising the skin with a No. 21 or a No. 18 needle. This allows expulsion of the entrapped blood by pressure. During expression of the coagula, all must be evacuated in order to avoid tattooing the dermis with further extravasation of red blood cells. Postsclerotherapy hyperpigmentation will largely disappear over a prolonged period, and it has been estimated that 90 per cent will be gone after a 12-month period.

Treatment of hyperpigmentation is unsuccessful. Bleaching agents will affect only melanin, not hemosiderin. Exfoliants carry the risk of scarring and hypopigmentation. Topical retinoic acid has produced a varied response. Successful chelation of the iron with ethylenediaminetetraacetic acid ointment has been reported but is unconfirmed.

The new appearance of red telangiectasias in a site of prior sclerotherapy has been termed telangiectatic matting or neoangiogenesis. Although such matting may result from simple blockage of a crucial efferent vessel, it is usually thought to be a complex process in which new vessels actually grow in response to endothelial growth factors, mast cell products, or platelet-derived growth factors. Estrogen has been implicated as playing a role in the development of such neovascularization.

Prevention of neoangiogenesis is best achieved by using dilute concentrations of sclerosant solution, injecting under low pressure, and limiting the quantity of injectate to 0.1 to 0.2 ml per injection site. Treatment is relatively ineffective, but the process will usually resolve over a short period (3 to 6 months). Pulsed-dye laser therapy for neoangiogenesis has been successful but is expensive.

CONCLUSIONS

Like any surgical technique, sclerotherapy can be a part of every surgeon's armamentarium and should be made available by surgeons practicing the broadest forms of vascular surgery.

References

1. Bergan JJ: Surgery versus sclerotherapy in treatment of varicose veins. *In* Veith FJ (ed): Current Critical Problems in Vascular Surgery. St. Louis, Quality Medical Publishers, 1989.
2. Fronek A: Injection compression sclerotherapy of varicose veins. *In* Ernst E, Stanley J (eds): Current Therapy in Vascular Surgery. 2nd ed. Philadelphia, BC Decker, 1990, p 961.
3. Raymond-Martimbeau P: Two different techniques for sclerosing the incompetent saphenofemoral junction. J Dermatol Surg Oncol 16:626, 1991.
4. Garrison FH: Introduction to the History of Medicine. Philadelphia, WB Saunders, 1929.
5. Bergan JJ: History of surgery of the somatic veins. *In* Bergan JJ, Kistner RL (eds): Atlas of Venous Surgery. Philadelphia, WB Saunders, 1992.
6. Genevrier M: Du traitement des varices par les injections coagulantes concentrees de sels de quinine. Soc Med Mil Fr 15:169, 1921.
7. Rogers L, Winchester AH: Intravenous sclerosing injections. Br Med J 2:120, 1930.
8. Biegeleisen HI: Telangiectasia associated with varicose veins. JAMA 102:2092, 1934.
9. Foley WT: The eradication of venous blemishes. Cutis 15:665, 1975.
10. Fegan WG: Varicose Veins: Compression Sclerotherapy. Dublin, Wm. Heinemann Medical Books, 1967.
11. Bergan JJ: Common anatomic patterns of varicose veins. *In* Bergan JJ, Goldman MP (eds): Varicose Veins and Telangiectasias: Diagnosis and Management. St. Louis, Quality Medical Publishing, 1993.
12. Braverman IM: Ultrastructure and organization of the cutaneous microvasculature in normal and pathologic states. J Invest Dermatol 93:28, 1989.
13. Miani A, Rubertsi U: Collecting venules. Minerva Cardioangiol 41:541, 1958.
14. Wokalek H, Vanscheidt W, Martan K, Leder O: Morphology and localization of sunburst varicosities: An electron microscopic study. J Dermatol Surg Oncol 15:149, 1989.
15. deFaria JL, Moraes In: Histopathology of the telangiectasia associated with varicose veins. Dermatologica 127:321, 1963.
16. Bohler-Sommeregger K, Karnel F, Schuller-Petrovic SS, Sautler R: Do telangiectasias communicate with the deep venous system? J Dermatol Surg Oncol 18:403, 1992.
17. Wells HS, Youman JB, Miller DG: Tissue pressure (intracutaneous, subcutaneous, and intramuscular) as related to venous pressure, capillary filtration, and other factors. J Clin Invest 17:489, 1938.
18. Cockett HFB, Jones BE: The ankle blowout syndrome: A new approach to the varicose ulcer problem. Lancet 1:17, 1953.
19. Green D: Compression sclerotherapy: Techniques. Dermatol Clin 7:137, 1989.
20. Goldman MP: Sclerotherapy. St. Louis, Mosby–Year Book, 1991.
21. Imhoff E, Stemmer R: Classification and mechanism of action of sclerosing agents. Soc Fr Phlebol 22:143, 1969.
22. Lindemayer H, Santler R: The fibrinolytic activity of the vein wall. Phlebologie 30:151, 1977.
23. Reiner L: The activity of anionic surface active compounds on producing vascular obliteration. Proc Soc Exp Biol Med 62:49, 1946.
24. Tretbar LL: Spider angiomata: Treatment with sclerosant injections. J Kansas Med Soc 79:198, 1978.
25. Carlin MC, Ratz JL: Treatment of telangiectasia: Comparison of sclerosing agents. J Dermatol Surg Oncol 13:1181, 1987.
26. Sadick NS: Sclerotherapy of varicose and telangiectatic leg veins: Minimal sclerosant concentration of hypertonic saline and its relationship to vessel diameter. J Dermatol Surg Oncol 17:65, 1991.
27. Foley DP, Forrestal MD: A comparative evaluation of the empty vein utilizing duplex ultrasonography. *In* Raymond-Martimbeau P, Prescott R, Zummo M (eds): Phlebologie. Montrouge, France, John Libbey Eurotext, 1992, p 623.
28. Vin F: Principe, technique, et résultats du traitement rapide des saphènes internes incontinentes par sclérothérapie. *In* Raymond-Martimbeau P, Prescott R, Zummo M (eds): Phlébologie. Montrouge, France, John Libbey Eurotext, 1992, p 623.
29. Sigg K: The treatment of varicosities and accompanying complications. Angiology 3:355, 1952.
30. Tretbar LL: The origin of reflux in incompetent blue reticular/telangiectatic veins. *In* Davy A, Stemmer R (eds): Phlebologie 89. Montrouge, France, John Libbey Eurotext, 1989, p 95.
31. Duffy DM: Small vessel sclerotherapy: An overview. Adv Dermatol 3:221, 1988.
32. Goldman MP: Sclerotherapy of superficial venules and telangiectasias of the lower extremities. Dermatol Clin 5:369, 1987.
33. Bodian EL: Techniques of sclerotherapy for sunburst venous blemishes. J Dermatol Surg Oncol 11:696, 1985.
34. Goldman MP: Polidocanol (aethoxysclerol) for sclerotherapy of superficial venules and telangiectasias. J Dermatol Surg Oncol 15:204, 1989.
35. Sadick NS: Sclerotherapy of varicose and telangiectatic leg veins. J Dermatol Surg Oncol 17:65, 1991.
36. Bochner BS, Lichtenstein LM: Anaphylaxis. N Engl J Med 324:1785, 1991.
37. Bergan JJ, Goldman MP: Complications of sclerotherapy. *In* Bernhard VM, Towne JB (eds): Complications of Vascular Surgery. St. Louis, CV Mosby, 1991.

The Natural History, Pathophysiology, and Nonoperative Treatment of Chronic Venous Insufficiency

Gregory L. Moneta, M.D., Mark R. Nehler, M.D., Richard W. Chitwood, M.D., and John M. Porter, M.D.

• • •

EPIDEMIOLOGY

It is estimated that 27 per cent of the American adult population has some form of detectable lower extremity venous abnormality, primarily varicose veins or telangiectasias.[1] The incidence of chronic venous insufficiency (CVI) in the adult population based on American and European studies is between 0.5 and 3.0 per cent.[2–4] European data indicate that up to 1.5 per cent of European adults will suffer a venous stasis ulcer at some point in their lives.[5, 6]

Although the leg fatigue, discomfort, and edema associated with CVI alone are troublesome, the skin changes and their ulcerative sequelae are the most significant in terms of health care impact. Large epidemiologic studies have addressed this issue by examining patients with lower extremity ulcerations of all etiologies. Venous ulcers are identified wholly or in part on the basis of pulse status, skin changes, and the results of noninvasive vascular laboratory studies. An epidemiologic postal survey in Edinburgh, Scotland, identified 1477 patients within this community of 1 million people who were receiving treatment for lower extremity ulceration from the National Health Service.[7] From the 1477 identified patients, a representative sample of 600 patients, with a total of 827 ulcerated lower extremities, was examined in detail. Seventy-six per cent of the ulcerated limbs in this sample were classified as having a venous etiology, based in part on an ankle-brachial index (ABI) of greater than 0.9 in the ulcerated limb. Sixty-seven per cent of all the ulcerated limbs had a recurrent ulcer at the time of the survey. Thirty-five per cent of all ulcerated limbs had had four or more recurrences. Two hundred seventy patients (45 per cent) had had lower extremity ulceration for more than 10 years. Forty-two per cent of all venous ulcer patients noted moderate to severe limitation of their leisure activities, whereas 40 per cent of those employed at the time of the survey had their earning capacity limited by the presence of the presumed venous ulcer. Five per cent had lost their jobs secondary to lower extremity ulceration.[8]

Baker and associates studied 259 patients with chronic ulceration of 286 lower extremities.[9] On the basis of a shortened venous recovery time, 57 per cent of the ulcer-

ated limbs were diagnosed as having ulcerations secondary to CVI. The prevalence of venous disease increased progressively with age and was considered the primary etiology of lower extremity ulceration in 90 per cent of patients older than 60 years of age. At the time of the survey, 75 per cent of all patients had a history of recurrent ulceration, and 28 per cent had a history of 10 or more episodes of ulceration. Thirty-four per cent had had lower extremity ulceration for more than 10 years. These data clearly indicate the prevalence and the chronic nature of venous ulceration.

THE MACROCIRCULATION IN VENOUS INSUFFICIENCY

Diagnostic Advances

In the following discussion of CVI, the term *macrocirculation* is used to refer to the deep, superficial, and communicating veins of the lower extremity. Evaluation of the macrocirculation in CVI first used invasive measurements of ambulatory venous pressure (AVP) and venous recovery times as indicators of valvular dysfunction. Patients with an AVP of less than 40 mmHg were noted to have a minimal incidence of venous ulceration, compared with an 80 per cent incidence of venous ulceration in patients with an AVP of greater than 80 mmHg.[10] Unfortunately, AVPs clearly do not completely characterize the function of the lower extremity venous system. They have been found by some authors to correlate poorly with clinical outcome after deep venous reconstructive procedures and with symptoms of CVI.[11] A review of AVPs in 207 limbs found 25 of 52 limbs (48 per cent) classified as having severe ambulatory venous hypertension (a less than 25 per cent decrease in venous pressure with exercise) to be only mildly symptomatic or asymptomatic.[12]

As a result of the apparent limitations of AVPs, investigators have focused on developing additional measurements of valvular reflux. A reflux index has been proposed that incorporates AVP measurements and Valsalva-induced pressure elevations. While supine, the patient blows into a tube to obtain a 40-mmHg Valsalva pressure. Measurements are simultaneously made of changes in dorsal foot vein pressure. The reflux index is the product of the AVP and the Valsalva-induced change in venous pressure (normal value, less than 150 mmHg^2). Only 2 per cent of 113 ulcerated limbs have been found to have a normal reflux index.[13] Although the reflux index may prove to provide a more sensitive index of valvular insufficiency, it does not detail anatomic sites of reflux or examine the contribution of calf muscle function to CVI.

Air plethysmography has been reintroduced into the study of venous physiology.[14, 15] The air plethysmograph theoretically permits evaluation of individual components of calf muscle pump function. This device is a calibrated pneumatic plethysmograph. Through postural changes and a series of tiptoe exercises, the total venous volume (VV) of the leg and the rate of venous filling, the venous filling index (VFI), can be determined. In addition, by accepting geometric approximations, it is possible to measure the volume of blood expelled from the calf with a single calf muscle contraction (ejection volume [EV]). The expelled volume can be expressed as a percentage of the total venous volume (ejection fraction [EF] = [EV/VV] × 100%). It is also possible to determine the residual volume (RV) of venous blood after a series of calf muscle contractions as the percentage of blood remaining in the leg after exercise (residual venous fraction [RVF = [RV/VV] × 100%). (Fig. 138–1). This compares the venous volume after calf muscle contraction with the venous volume after leg elevation.

The RVF (normal value, less than 35 per cent) correlates well with AVP measurements and is an indicator of overall calf muscle pump function. The VFI (normal value, less than 5 ml/sec) measures the rate of venous filling as the patient moves from the supine to an upright, non–weight-bearing position. It is an indicator of the magnitude of valvular insufficiency. The ejection fraction (EF; normal value, greater than 60 per cent) serves as a measure of the

efficiency of calf muscle contraction, which could potentially be impaired by abnormalities within the gastrocnemius muscle or incompetence of venous valves distal to the calf muscle pump. Air plethysmography can therefore produce a measurement of the overall lower extremity venous function by calculation of RVF. Abnormalities in RVF are further delineated as inadequate calf muscle pump action (decreased EF), the presence of valvular reflux (increased VFI), or combinations of both. This type of information may allow more precise preoperative stratification of patients being considered for deep venous reconstructions or superficial vein ablative procedures. Patients with increased VFIs and normal EFs would theoretically appear to be appropriate candidates for antireflux procedures, whereas those with normal VFIs and diminished EFs would be unlikely to benefit from antireflux surgery.

Duplex scanning is now also employed for noninvasively detecting and quantitating venous reflux at specific anatomic sites. With the patient upright and non–weight bearing, pneumatic cuffs are deflated at different limb levels and reflux velocities are measured with the duplex scanner. Reproducible times to valve closure, venous diameters, peak reflux velocities, and calculated volume flow at peak reflux (VFPR) can be determined at specific locations in both the deep and the superficial venous systems. Ninety-five per cent of normal valves close within 0.5 seconds of cuff deflation (Fig. 138–2).[16] A high incidence of lipodermatosclerosis has been demonstrated in patients with a cumulative VFPR in the greater saphenous, lesser saphenous, and popliteal venous segments that is greater than 10 ml/sec.[17] This suggests that specific venous procedures may be tailored to the individual patient on the basis of the site and the severity of valvular reflux. For example, a patient with a venous ulcer and a combined VFPR of 12 ml/sec, 8 ml/sec of which is present in the superficial veins, may be adequately treated by obliteration of the superficial veins with either sclerotherapy or surgery. Likewise, a patient

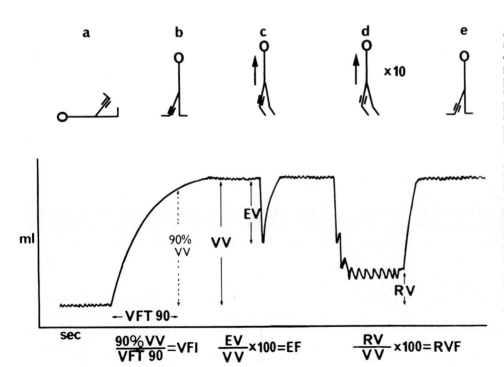

FIGURE 138–1. Typical recording of volume changes during a standard sequence of postural changes and exercise: patient in a supine position with the leg elevated 45 degrees (*a*); patient standing with weight on the nonexamined leg (*b*); patient performing a single tiptoe movement (*c*); patient performing 10 tiptoe movements (*d*); patient again standing with weight on the nonexamined leg (*e*). VV, functional venous volume; VFT, venous filling time; VFI, venous filling index; EV, ejected volume; RV, residual volume; EF, ejection fraction; RVF, residual volume fraction. (From Christopoulos DG, Nicolaides AN, Szendro G, et al: Air-plethysmography and the effect of elastic compression on venous hemodynamics of the leg. J Vasc Surg 5:148, 1987.)

$$\frac{90\% \, VV}{VFT \, 90} = VFI \qquad \frac{EV}{VV} \times 100 = EF \qquad \frac{RV}{VV} \times 100 = RVF$$

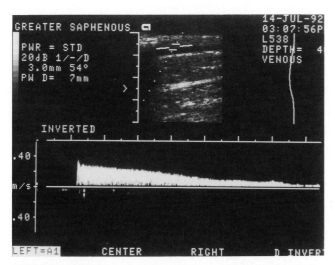

FIGURE 138–2. Reflux in the greater saphenous vein.

with a VFPR of 20 ml/sec in the popliteal vein would be unlikely to benefit from a superficial venous procedure alone and is perhaps better treated with deep venous reconstruction or nonoperative therapy.

Natural History

Venous insufficiency is usually described as primary or secondary. Primary valvular incompetence is diagnosed when no obvious underlying etiology of valvular dysfunction can be identified. Most cases of apparently isolated superficial venous insufficiency are considered examples of primary venous insufficiency. Such cases may develop from a loss of elasticity of the vein wall.[18] Patients with primary varicose veins have venous elasticity that is significantly lower than that of controls,[19] and loss of elasticity precedes valvular incompetence in patients identified as having primary venous insufficiency.[20] Valvular incompetence is described as secondary when there is an obvious antecedent event, most frequently a deep venous thrombosis (DVT), that may have led to destruction or dysfunction, or both, of the venous valves. Most information on the natural history of CVI derives from patients with presumed secondary CVI.

Several studies have followed up patients with documented DVT to determine the frequency of development of CVI symptoms, the location of valvular dysfunction, and the severity of disease in relationship to the extent and location of the initial thrombosis. In one study, 61 patients (65 limbs) with DVT documented by either contrast or isotope phlebography were followed up at 6-month intervals for 1 to 144 months (mean, 39 months).[21] Patients were evaluated for clinical symptoms or signs of CVI. Photoplethysmographic venous refill times were also determined. Continuous-wave venous Doppler examinations were used to demonstrate sites of venous obstruction, venous reflux, or both. No attempt was made to determine recanalization of the originally occluded segments by Doppler examination because of the difficulty in separating venous collaterals from a recanalized segment. Strain-gauge plethysmography was employed to evaluate venous outflow. Forty-one patients (66 per cent) had symptoms of pain, swelling, or both during follow-up. Nineteen limbs developed lipodermatosclerotic skin changes at or during follow-up, and 3 of these developed an ulcer. Doppler examination revealed that 39 limbs had deep veins distal to the most proximal site of the previously documented DVT that were either involved in the original occlusion or had developed reflux. Of these limbs with Doppler-determined distal deep venous abnormalities, 77 per cent were in patients with symptoms of pain, swelling, or both. Eighty-nine per cent of the limbs with lipodermatosclerotic skin changes and all of the limbs with venous ulceration had valvular incompetence or occlusion *distal* to the site of the previous DVT. Venous recovery times were shorter in patients with symptoms than in those who were asymptomatic. No differences were found in maximal venous outflow between symptomatic and asymptomatic patients.

Another series used photoplethysmographically determined venous recovery times and AVPs, in addition to Doppler examination of deep and superficial venous segments, to evaluate 47 patients (54 limbs) with phlebographically determined DVT at 5 and 10 years of follow-up.[22] Seventy-nine per cent of patients were symptomatic, but only 2 patients developed venous ulceration. Eighty-three per cent of patients had developed abnormal venous hemodynamics. Symptoms correlated with the extent of the initial thrombus, and 8 of 10 asymptomatic patients had DVT limited to the calf. However, only 3 of the 10 asymptomatic patients had normal venous hemodynamics.

A third study examined 21 heparin-treated patients with DVT who had duplex scanning at 7, 30, 90, 180, and 270 days after the diagnosis of their DVT.[23] Evidence of recanalization of the thrombosed venous segments was present in 44 per cent of patients at 7 days, in 94 per cent of patients at 30 days, and in all patients by 90 days after the diagnosis of DVT. The degree of venous segmental occlusion at each observation time was also determined as a percentage of the segments occluded at initial presentation. The percentage of segmental occlusion fell from 93 per cent at 7 days to 14 per cent at 90 to 270 days. Fifty-three per cent of patients had recanalization of all occluded segments by 90 days. Seven patients had thrombus propagation while they were receiving apparently therapeutic levels of anticoagulation. Thrombus propagation occurred in 3 patients within the first 7 days and in 4 patients between days 30 and 180. Valvular incompetence was determined as a percentage of all patent venous segments. At 30 days after the diagnosis of DVT, 8 per cent of patent venous segments were incompetent. This rose to 25 per cent by 180 days and then remained stable. There was great variability in the development of valvular incompetence, and 8 patients had no evidence of valvular incompetence at the end of the 270-day study period.

This important study demonstrates that venous recanalization following DVT generally occurs early, whereas valvular incompetence appears later. It suggests that incorporation of venous valves in the thrombotic process may not be the only etiology of venous reflux following DVT. In addition, the appearance and localization of valvular insufficiency following DVT in an individual patient appear unpredictable and may relate to the interval between thrombus formation and recanalization.

Several investigators have examined patients with CVI using either duplex scanning or phlebography in an attempt to correlate the anatomic location of reflux with clinical severity. Moore and associates used duplex scanning to examine the superficial and deep venous segments for sites of valvular reflux in 122 patients with CVI of various degrees of severity.[24] Ninety-three of the 174 symptomatic limbs (53 per cent) had a history of prior DVT. In addition, although 162 of the symptomatic limbs (93 per cent) had evidence of valvular incompetence by duplex examination, so did 41 of the asymptomatic limbs (59 per cent). Ten per cent of limbs with ulceration had isolated superficial venous insufficiency. Reflux in the distal (popliteal-tibial) deep venous system correlated most closely with clinical disease severity.

Hanrahan and coworkers used duplex scanning to examine the superficial and deep venous systems in 95 ulcerated limbs in 78 patients.[25] Twenty-six of the patients (33 per cent) had a history of DVT. Thirty-four limbs (36 per cent) had incompetence of the popliteal vein. The tibial veins were not evaluated, and 16 of the ulcerated limbs (17 per cent) had only isolated superficial venous incompetence.

An additional study of 98 consecutive patients (196 limbs) who had CVI of various degrees of clinical severity used phlebography and duplex scanning to evaluate the superficial and deep venous systems.[26] There was a history of DVT in only 13 limbs (7 per cent). Insufficiency of the posterior tibial veins was associated with more severe clinical disease. Valvular insufficiency was demonstrated in multiple asymptomatic limbs. There was no history of venous ulceration in any of the 38 limbs with isolated superficial venous insufficiency.

Depending on the series, 0 to 17 per cent of patients with venous ulceration appear to have reflux limited to the superficial system alone.[23–25, 27, 28] Incompetent communicating veins may also be present in patients with a competent deep system.[29] Communicating vein incompetence also appears to contribute to ulcer recurrence after vein-stripping procedures.[30]

In summary, a large percentage of patients with deep venous insufficiency do not have a known history of DVT. Deep venous insufficiency is not a prerequisite for developing venous ulceration. Many patients may have subclinical DVT as the etiology of their deep vein reflux because only an estimated 40 to 50 per cent of above-knee deep vein thrombi and 5 per cent of isolated calf vein thrombi are symptomatic.[31, 32] It is thus likely that asymptomatic DVT is important in the etiology of CVI, especially in view of the fact that distal valvular incompetence appears most important in the development of clinical symptoms[21, 23–25] and distal leg vein thrombi are much more likely to be clinically asymptomatic than proximal thrombi. The observation that the development of reflux in individual venous segments does not precisely correlate with the prior location of venous thrombus or the time course of recanalization after known DVT suggests that the mechanisms of the development of valvular incompetence are undoubtedly more complex than simple valvular destruction by organizing thrombi. Valvular incompetence may, in some instances, arise secondary to venous distention resulting from proximal obstruction. Prolonged distention of distal venous

segments may result in permanent valvular incompetence after several months of unrelenting distention.[33]

MICROCIRCULATORY CONSIDERATIONS

The end-organ in CVI is the skin and subcutaneous tissue. Several theories have been proposed to explain the abnormalities of the cutaneous microcirculation in patients with lipodermatosclerosis or venous stasis ulceration and to link these abnormalities with reflux in the deep venous system, the superficial venous system, or both. The end-result of microcirculatory abnormalities in CVI is a combination of the disruption of nutrient delivery to the skin and the release of toxic metabolites or enzymes that result in tissue destruction.

The oldest microcirculatory theory of venous ulceration comes from gross observations at the time of vein stripping. "Arterial" bleeding as well as pulsations within varicose veins at the time of operation led to the proposal that small arteriovenous fistulae were a cause of CVI.[34] It was postulated that microarteriovenous fistulae transmitted arterial pressure to the veins, leading to increased vascular permeability. This in turn induced abnormalities in the skin and subcutaneous capillaries that adversely affected tissue nutrition. The potential existence of such fistulae is supported by measurements of relatively high oxygen saturations in blood from varicose veins.[35] In addition, skin temperature has been found to be higher in limbs with varicose veins than in control limbs.[36] Finally, several radiologic studies have suggested an abnormally early venous phase during arteriography in patients with varicose veins.[37, 38]

Despite these historical studies, no recent data support the existence of microcirculatory arteriovenous fistulae in patients with CVI. Conversely, radiolabeled albumin has been used to measure the percentage of total shunt volume referable to the lower extremities. No difference has been found between patients with varicose veins and controls.[39] Arteriovenous fistula is no longer widely accepted as the primary mechanism for the cutaneous alterations associated with CVI.

Initial histologic studies of the perimalleolar skin and subcutaneous tissues in patients with CVI revealed an apparent increase in capillary number.[40] More recently, with the advent of video microscopy, these same capillary beds can be examined in vivo. Video microscopic studies reveal tortuous perimalleolar capillaries in patients with CVI. The absolute number is, however, similar to that in normal skin. The discrepancy between standard histologic studies and video microscopic examination may be a sectioning artifact in preparing the histologic specimens. In vivo microscopy studies also reveal areas of capillary microthrombosis in lipodermatosclerotic skin and reductions in capillary numbers in areas of prior ulceration (atrophie blanche). These data suggest that actual destruction of the cutaneous nutrient circulation may contribute to venous ulceration and recurrence.

Studies of the skin microcirculation in CVI indicate that diffusion abnormalities may be important in the development of lipodermatosclerosis. Burnand and associates[41] used implanted Guyton capsules[42] in the subcutaneous tissue to sample the interstitial fluid of canine hindlimbs in an animal model of venous hypertension. Radiolabeled sodium, albumin, and fibrinogen (selected for their increasing molecular weights) were injected intravenously. After circulation and diffusion times were allowed for, the contents of the Guyton capsules were aspirated and the radiolabeled substrates were assayed. Of the three molecules, fibrinogen was the only one found at higher concentrations within the interstitium of venous hypertensive limbs than within control limbs, suggesting a diffusion abnormality in CVI that increases large molecule capillary permeability.

Additional evidence of a diffusion abnormality in CVI is suggested by capillary video microscopy. Diffusion patterns of sodium fluorescein in patients with CVI and control subjects have been examined with appropriate filters, video techniques, and densometric analysis of light intensity.[43–45] Compared with those of controls, the cutaneous capillaries of patients with CVI developed much larger fluorescing pericapillary cuffs (''halos'') after intravenous injection of sodium fluorescein, suggesting increased transcapillary diffusion in these patients (Fig. 138–3).

The major theory of venous ulcer pathogenesis that depends in large part on capillary diffusion abnormalities is the so-called fibrin cuff theory.[46] It is postulated that semi-occlusive pericapillary fibrin cuffs result from leakage of fibrinogen into the interstitium. These cuffs then act as a barrier to oxygen and nutrient diffusion to interstitial tissues and cutaneous skin cells. Indeed, less fibrinolytic activity has been observed within vein walls of patients with varicose veins than within controls.[47] Lotti and associates demonstrated less plasma fibrinolytic activity in patients with CVI and lipodermatosclerosis than in controls.[48] In addition, studies in canine models of limb venous hypertension have documented increased pericapillary fibrin deposition and increased lymphatic concentration of fibrinogen.[49] Skin biopsy specimens from patients with CVI and lipoderma-

tosclerosis have demonstrated pericapillary fibrin deposition.[50] The presence of fibrin cuffs in CVI thus appears well documented. The importance of these cuffs in producing tissue hypoxia is more controversial. Investigators have been unable to demonstrate hypoxia of the perimalleolar tissues conclusively in patients with CVI.

Biochemical markers of ischemia have been reported in patients with CVI. Magnetic resonance spectroscopy of radiolabeled phosphate (phosphorus-31) from gastrocnemius muscle biopsy specimens has been used to evaluate levels of creatine phosphate, adenosine triphosphate, adenosine diphosphate, and inorganic phosphate as a measure of muscle energy stores in seven patients with symptomatic CVI.[51] All specimens demonstrated flattened spectral waveforms in the high-energy phosphate region, with increased spectral peaks in the low-energy phosphate region. Evidence of muscle atrophy was noted in each specimen on histologic sectioning. Despite the small sample size, these data are at least suggestive of a potential biochemical defect in cellular oxidative metabolism of the limb in patients with CVI.

Radioactively labeled oxygen (oxygen-15, a short-lived photon-emitting isotope) has been used during positron emission tomography to investigate oxygen levels in limbs of patients with CVI. Patterns of photon emission are mapped, permitting calculations of the original molecular distribution within the tissue. Eleven patients with venous stasis ulceration and five patients with lipodermatosclerosis underwent lower extremity positron emission tomography.[52] Regional blood flow was markedly *increased* in areas of venous ulceration, with reduced oxygen extraction at the same sites. This suggests an oxygen diffusion defect with resultant tissue hypoxia, although the study does not exclude the possibility of a defect in tissue oxygen delivery.

Multiple reports have described transcutaneous oxygen measurements of the lower extremity in various conditions. Transcutaneous partial pressure oxygen ($TcPo_2$) is meas-

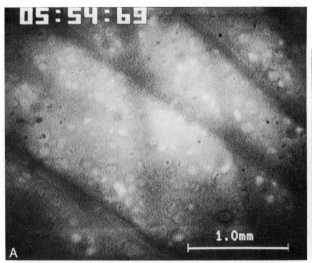
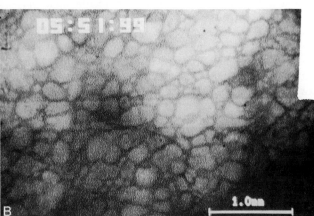

FIGURE 138–3. *A*, Normal capillary video microscopy findings after intravenous fluorescein injection. Note the uniform small pericapillary ''halos'' containing the fluorescein tracer. *B*, Abnormal capillary video microscopy findings after intravenous fluorescein injection in a patient with chronic venous insufficiency and lipodermatosclerosis. Note the irregularly sized large pericapillary halos containing the fluorescein tracer. (*A* and *B*, From Nehler MN, Moneta GM, Porter JM: The lower extremity venous system. II. The pathophysiology of chronic venous insufficiency. Perspect Vasc Surg 5[1]: 89, 1992.)

ured during heat-induced local hyperemia. Unfortunately, the techniques of obtaining perimalleolar TcPo$_2$ measurements in patients with CVI have not been consistent. By convention, TcPo$_2$ measurements are made with the probe heated to 43°C. Under these conditions, the TcPo$_2$ in the perimalleolar skin of CVI patients with venous ulcers is lower than normal.[53–55] However, when measurements of TcPo$_2$ are made with the unheated electrode, TcPo$_2$ is higher in limbs with CVI and venous ulcers than in controls.[56] There is no widely accepted explanation for these seemingly disparate findings. Perhaps low oxygen tensions detected with the heated sensor represent a deficiency in microvascular regulation that may act to prevent effective capillary recruitment and nutrient delivery in lipodermatosclerotic skin. There is some precedent for this reasoning because attenuated skin blood flow responses to hyperemia have also been demonstrated in patients with diabetes mellitus.[57]

A measure of local cutaneous blood flow can be obtained with laser Doppler flowmetry.[58] The scattering of laser light across skin capillary beds is measured using the Doppler principle. A baseline laser Doppler flux tracing is generated, and any deviations above or below baseline are considered a measure of increased or decreased net cutaneous blood flow in the area examined by the probe. Several reports have indicated higher resting skin blood flow in patients with CVI and venous ulcers than in controls.[59, 60] Cheatle and associates used laser Doppler flowmetry to examine skin blood flow in the limbs of 17 controls and 17 patients with CVI and lipodermatosclerosis.[61] With the use of inflatable cuffs of varying pressures, periods of arterial and venous occlusion were produced. Patients with CVI and lipodermatosclerosis showed no hyperemic response after 3 minutes of arterial occlusion, whereas areas of normal skin in the same patients demonstrated attenuated hyperemia. Control limbs also demonstrated attenuated hyperemia after 30 minutes of venous occlusion, possibly indicating that the changes in vascular regulation seen in patients with CVI can be reproduced in normals with periods of induced venous hypertension. These findings may partially explain the results of TcPo$_2$ measurements. Perhaps patients with CVI have resting hyperemia when compared with controls and are unable to recruit additional capillaries in response to stimuli that provoke a normal hyperemic response.

There is also evidence of abnormal activation of local neural control mechanisms within the subcutaneous microcirculation in CVI. A local sympathetic axonal reflex, the venoarteriolar reflex, results in microvascular vasoconstriction in response to venous pressures of greater than 25 mmHg.[62] Normally, this reflex is abolished by activation of the calf muscle pump and reduction in venous pressure.

In addition, axonal nociceptive C-fibers appear to be abnormal in CVI. These fibers are responsible both for transmitting pain sensation to the central nervous system, thereby preventing repetitive trauma to areas of injury, and for stimulating the release of vasodilator neuropeptides that act as growth factors for epidermal cells and fibroblasts.[63] Laser Doppler flowmetry has been used to study C-fibers in 15 elderly patients with venous ulcers.[64] Vasodilatation was measured by determining changes in skin blood flow in response to either electrical stimulation or chemical stim-

ulation with topical acetylcholine or nitroprusside and was compared in patients with CVI and controls. Patients with CVI demonstrated an attenuated electrically stimulated (neurogenic) vasodilatory response when compared with controls. There were no detectable differences in response to local stimulation by acetylcholine and nitroprusside between patients with CVI and controls. Because baseline foot skin blood flow was not significantly different between the two groups, it appears that the components of the cutaneous vasodilatory response mediated by nociceptive C-fiber input are dysfunctional in patients with severe CVI. This may contribute to venous ulceration by making the patient less sensitive to local trauma and diminishing vasodilator neuropeptides that could act as growth factors to stimulate healing after injury.

Thus far, the fibrin cuffs observed in lipodermatosclerosis have not been linked with any of the previously described abnormalities of the cutaneous microcirculation in patients with CVI. Although observable fibrin deposits do occur around skin capillaries in patients with CVI, at present these deposits appear to be primarily a histologic marker for lipodermatosclerosis. Data linking the anatomic finding of fibrin cuffs in CVI to the physiology of venous ulceration are inconclusive.

The most recent theory of venous ulceration to attract widespread interest suggests that white blood cell trapping within the skin microcirculation is important in venous ulceration. The proposed mechanism is that white blood cells become trapped in the microcirculation of patients with CVI, leading to microvascular congestion and thrombosis. The trapped white blood cells migrate into the interstitium and release lysosomal enzymes, resulting in tissue destruction. Originally, Moyses and colleagues incidentally discovered that venous blood from dependent limbs of normal subjects had proportionately lower white blood cell counts than did venous blood from the same limbs in the supine position.[65] The authors calculated an approximate 20 per cent loss of white blood cells, predominately monocytes, in lower extremity venous effluent after 40 minutes of dependency, suggesting that limb dependency resulted in microcirculatory white blood cell trapping or leakage into the interstitium.

Additional studies in patients with CVI have confirmed lower numbers of white blood cells in femoral venous samples after 30 minutes of dependency than in control limbs.[66, 67] Bollinger and associates, using capillary microscopy, also described capillary microthrombosis in the perimalleolar skin of patients with CVI.[68] Such thrombi may be secondary to sludging of white blood cells in the cutaneous microcirculation.

Additional work by Scott and associates is compatible with these data.[69] They used capillary microscopy to examine the perimalleolar skin in 10 patients with CVI, both with patients supine and after 30 minutes of limb dependency. In addition, femoral vein blood was obtained at the time of microscopy examination. After the dependent interval, there were fewer visible capillary loops on video microscopy in 9 of the 10 patients. Loss of visible capillary loops correlated with decreases in femoral vein white blood cell counts. Other investigators have also demonstrated that lipodermatosclerotic skin biopsy specimens taken from patients with CVI and a history of ulceration reveal significantly more white blood cells per cubic millimeter than do biopsy specimens from controls (217 vs 6.2 cells/mm^3),[69] presumably because of increased trapping of white blood cells within the microcirculation and the resultant migration into the interstitium.

Currently, no single proposed mechanism adequately explains all the observed changes within the microcirculation of patients with CVI. Venous hypertensive effects on the skin in patients with CVI are clearly much more complex than previously realized. Several suggested pharmacologic treatment strategies are based on these microcirculatory observations; they are discussed later.

NONOPERATIVE TREATMENT OF CHRONIC VENOUS INSUFFICIENCY AND VENOUS ULCERATION

Various forms of nonoperative therapy have been the basic treatment of CVI and venous ulceration for decades. Although bed rest with limb elevation is nearly universally accepted as effective treatment for venous ulceration, it is impractical for most patients as anything but a short-term solution to a refractory or enlarging ulcer. The goal of nonoperative therapy for venous ulceration is to promote healing of existing ulcers and prevent their recurrence while allowing the patient to maintain a normal ambulatory status.

Compression Therapy

Compression therapy remains the primary treatment for CVI despite progress in both ablative[70] and reconstructive[71, 72] venous surgery. The actual mechanism by which compression therapy obviates the adverse effects of venous hypertension on the skin and subcutaneous tissues remains unknown. Many studies, however, have focused on the possible venous hemodynamic effects of compression therapy. Some investigators have shown no change in AVP or venous recovery times with the use of both invasive and noninvasive techniques.[73–75] Whereas others have reported statistically significant improvements in AVP and venous recovery times with compression therapy.[76–81] However, even in the reports suggesting improved hemodynamics with compression, detected changes were often quite small and AVP measurements rarely normalized.

Another possible explanation for the benefits of compression therapy is a direct effect on subcutaneous interstitial pressures. An increase in interstitial pressure will counteract transcapillary Starling forces and promote fluid resorption and resolution of edema, leading to improved diffusion of nutrients to the skin and subcutaneous tissues. Several studies have examined the skin microcirculation in limbs with CVI after the resolution of edema following compression therapy. Skin capillary density, as determined by video microscopy, predictably increases after edema reduction.[82] Several authors have demonstrated an increase in skin TcPO$_2$ after edema reduction,[83, 84] although Nemeth and associates were unable to demonstrate a significant change in skin TcPO$_2$ after edema removal by pneumatic compression.[85]

Elastic Compression Stockings

Jobst invented gradient ambulatory compression therapy in the 1950s, after personally suffering for years from venous ulceration.[86] He observed that his leg symptoms were alleviated when he stood upright in a swimming pool. He therefore designed the first ambulatory gradient compression hosiery to mimic hydrostatic forces exerted by water in a swimming pool (Fig. 138–4). Forty years later, the use of ambulatory compression hosiery remains the primary treatment for CVI. At present, numerous manufacturers provide elastic compression stockings of various compositions, strengths, and lengths.

A number of clinical reports have demonstrated the benefits of compression stockings in the treatment of CVI and venous ulceration.[87–89] At the authors' institution venous ulceration was treated with local wound care and elastic compression therapy.[90] One hundred thirteen patients were treated over a 15-year period (from 1975 to 1990). Of these patients, 102 (90 per cent) were compliant with stocking use, and 105 (93 per cent) experienced complete ulcer healing, with a mean healing time of 5.3 months. Seventy-three patients had long-term follow-up (mean, 30 months). Fifty-eight (79 per cent) adhered to the recommendation of perpetual ambulatory compression therapy. The total ulcer recurrence in patients who were compliant with long-term therapy was 16 per cent. Recurrence was 100 per cent in patients who were noncompliant with long-term therapy. Recurrence was not related to previous ulceration, previous venous surgery, or arterial insufficiency.

In the authors' institution, patients with venous ulcers are first assessed for the presence of infection and the extent of lower extremity edema. When necessary, a period of bed rest of 5 to 7 days is prescribed to help to resolve the edema. Cellulitis is treated with short-term intravenous or oral antibiotics in conjunction with local wound care (dry gauze dressings changed every 12 hours). Topical agents are avoided. When the edema or cellulitis has resolved, patients are fitted with below-knee 30- to 40-mmHg elastic compression stockings. Two pairs are prescribed to permit laundering on alternate days. Patients are instructed to wear the stockings at all times while they are ambulatory and to remove them on going to bed. Wound care throughout the course of compression therapy consists of a simple daily soap-and-water washing of the ulcer. Topical corticosteroids may be applied to surrounding areas of significant stasis dermatitis, but they are not applied to the ulcer itself. The ulcer is covered with a dry gauze dressing held in place by the compression stocking. Once the ulcer has healed, the patient is instructed to continue ambulatory compression therapy.

Several problems have been recognized with compression therapy for venous ulcers. The most noteworthy is poor patient compliance.[91] Often patients have hypersensitive skin in the lipodermatosclerotic area adjacent to the ulcer or at the site of a previously healed ulcer. These patients are initially intolerant of the sensation of compression. Frequently, the stockings can be worn only for brief periods during the initial phase of therapy. The authors instruct patients to wear stockings for as long as tolerable (perhaps only 10 to 15 minutes at first) and to increase gradually the time they wear them. Occasionally, patients

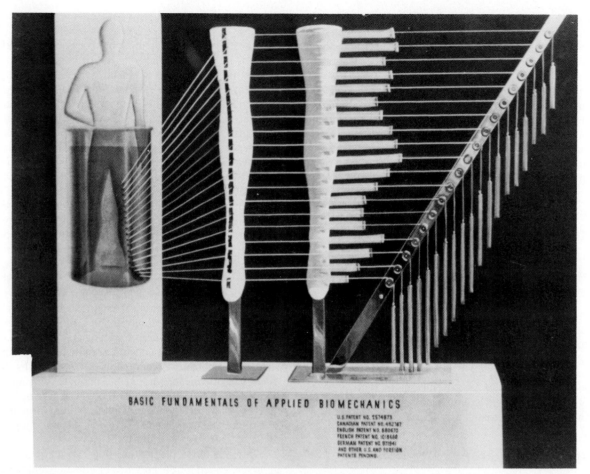

FIGURE 138–4. Model demonstrating the effect of hydrostatic pressure on the lower extremity in a water tank and its relationship to gradient compression hosiery. The pressure obtained by each is represented by the weights of various sizes, with the largest located at the ankle. (From Bergan JJ: Conrad Jobst and the development of pressure gradient therapy for venous disease. *In* Bergan JJ, Yao JS [eds]: Surgery of the Veins. Orlando, FL, Grune & Stratton, 1985, pp 529–540.)

initially have to be fitted with a lesser degree of compression (20 to 30 mmHg).

Many weaker, elderly, or arthritic patients have difficulty applying elastic stockings. The authors have found both silk "booties" and commercially available devices that assist in the application of the stockings to be useful for these patients. With open-toed stockings, an inner silk sleeve is placed over the patient's toes and forefoot to allow the stocking material to slide smoothly during application. The sleeve is removed through the toe opening after the stockings are on. Another device allows the patient to load the stocking onto a wire frame. The patient then simply steps into the stocking and pulls the device upward along the leg, applying the stocking (Fig. 138–5). These techniques, along with extensive counseling about the importance of compression therapy, are helpful in improving patient compliance.

An additional concern with elastic compression therapy is the possibility of exacerbating concomitant arterial insufficiency. One study noted that 49 of 154 general surgeons (32 per cent) had experience with a patient who had worsening of clinical leg ulceration after compression therapy.[92] Twelve cases resulted in amputation. Callam and associates analyzed 600 patients with 827 ulcerated limbs

and found an ABI of less than 0.9 in 176 limbs (21 per cent).[93] They concluded that arterial disease represented a serious risk for patients with leg ulcers and recommended against compression therapy in patients with evidence of arterial insufficiency. At present, the authors believe that the rare patients with a venous ulcer and significant arterial insufficiency should be considered for arterial reconstruction if the ulcer fails to make reasonable progress with elastic compression therapy. To date, this has been necessary in very few patients. Patients with critical leg ischemia (ABI of less than 0.4) are, however, offered arterial reconstruction as part of the initial management of their venous ulcer.

Paste Gauze Boots

The paste gauze compression dressing was developed by the German dermatologist Unna in 1896.[94] The current dressing (Dome paste) contains calamine, zinc oxide, glycerin, sorbitol, gelatin, and magnesium aluminum silicate and is popularly called the Unna boot. This dressing is designed to provide both compression and topical therapy. The Unna boot consists of a three-layer dressing. It is preferentially applied by trained medical personnel. The Dome

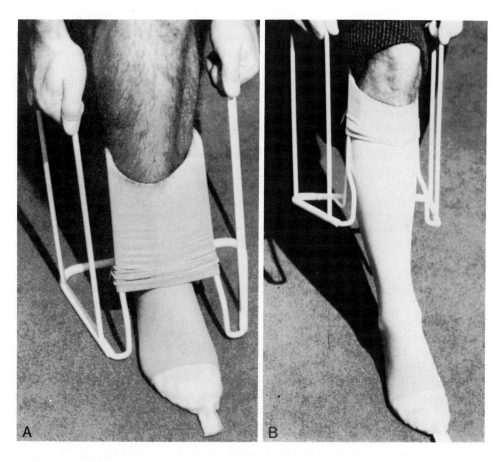

FIGURE 138–5. *A* and *B*, Compression stocking being sequentially fitted onto the leg with the Butler device. (*A* and *B*, From Mayberry JC, Moneta GL, Taylor LM, Porter JM: Nonoperative treatment of venous stasis ulcer. *In* Bergan JJ, Yao JS [eds]: Venous Disorders. Philadelphia, WB Saunders, 1991, pp 381–395.)

paste rolled gauze bandage is first applied with graded compression from the forefoot to just below the knee. The next layer consists of a 4-inch-wide continuous gauze dressing. An elastic wrap with graded compression comprises the outer layer. The bandage becomes stiff after drying, and the relatively unyielding nature of the Unna boot may aid in preventing edema formation. Bandages are changed weekly.

The Unna boot has the advantage that minimal patient compliance is required because the dressing is usually applied and removed by a health care professional. The disadvantages of its use include the inability to monitor the ulcer between dressing changes, the requirement for health care personnel to apply the bandage, the relative discomfort due to the bulky dressing, and the operator-dependent nature of the compression achieved after wrapping. In addition, contact dermatitis may occur secondary to the paraben preservative and may require boot removal.

Unna boots have been compared with other treatments. A randomized, prospective trial of 21 patients with venous ulcers that compared Unna boot therapy with mild compression stocking therapy (24 mmHg at the ankle) demonstrated that although both groups had healing of 70 per cent of the total number of ulcers, the average time for healing in the Unna boot group was 7.3 weeks, compared with 18.4 weeks in the compression stocking group.[95] The authors qualify this finding by noting that the average healing time for the compression stocking group was 11.8 weeks after the exclusion of a single patient in the stocking group who took 78 weeks to heal extensive calf ulcerations. Stronger compression therapy was not used in this study. An addi-

tional randomized study of 26 patients who had CVI and venous ulcers compared Unna boots with polyurethane foam dressings and elastic compression wraps.[96] After 12 months, patients in the Unna boot group had faster healing rates and greater overall wound healing. More than 50 per cent of the patients in the polyurethane dressing group withdrew before study completion. Unna boots were compared with hydrocolloid dressings (DuoDERM) in a 6-month trial treating 87 venous ulcers in 84 patients.[97] Seventy per cent of the ulcers treated with Unna boots healed, compared with only 38 per cent of those treated with the hydrocolloid dressings alone. A more recent study compared Unna boots with hydrocolloid dressings and elastic compression bandages and found no statistical difference in healing rates after 12 weeks.[98]

Other Forms of Elastic Compression

Additional forms of elastic compression include simple elastic wraps and multi-layered wrapped dressings. Although achieving and maintaining appropriate pressure gradients with elastic wraps of any sort is highly operator and technique dependent, satisfactory dressings can be applied. Ankle pressures achieved with a multi-layer wrap of orthopedic wool, crepe bandages, and elastic cohesive wraps (Coban) decrease only 10 per cent after 1 week.[99] A four-layer dressing used to treat 126 consecutive patients (148 ulcerated limbs) whose ulcers had previously been refractory to treatment with simple elastic wraps resulted in complete healing of 74 per cent of the ulcers at 12 weeks. In general, however, the results obtained with elastic wraps in the healing of venous ulceration have been inferior to those achieved with compression stockings or Unna boots.[100–103] This, in combination with the inconvenience and applicator dependency of elastic wraps makes them suboptimal for the treatment of most patients with venous ulcers.

A new legging orthosis (Circ-Aid) has become available.[104] It consists of multiple pliable rigid adjustable compression bands that wrap around the leg from the ankle to the knee and are held in place with Velcro tape. The device offers the rigid compression of the Unna boot with increased ease of application, and because of the adjustable nature of the bands, it can be tailored to the individual as limb edema resolves. Anecdotally, the orthosis appears to be efficient in promoting resolution of edema, especially in patients who for various reasons are unable or unwilling to wear compression hosiery. Clinical trials of this device are ongoing.

Adjunctive Compression Devices

External pneumatic compression devices serve as adjunctive measures in the treatment of lower extremity edema, venous ulceration, or both. Commercially available devices apply either intermittent compression of uniform strength or intermittent sequential gradient compression.

Those that provide sequential gradient intermittent pneumatic compression (IPC) have received the most attention. They have gained widespread use in the prevention of DVT in nonambulatory hospitalized patients. In addition, several reports have described the use of the device to treat venous ulcers. One group treated eight patients who had phlebographically documented CVI and stasis ulcers present from 1 month to 5 years with IPC for 45-minute sessions 5 days a week, for a total of 2 weeks.[105] IPC was then continued twice a week until the ulcer healed. Between treatments with IPC, the limbs were bandaged in elastic compression wraps and the ulcers were dressed with wet-to-dry dressings. All ulcers healed (mean time, 5 weeks). The authors compared this result with a mean healing time of 13 weeks in their previous patients who had had treatment with elastic compression bandages alone. They concluded that the addition of IPC therapy led to a superior rate of ulcer healing. A randomized study of 45 patients who had duplex-confirmed CVI and venous ulcers of at least 12 weeks' duration compared treatment consisting of IPC and 30- to 40-mmHg ambulatory compression stockings with the use of compression stockings alone.[106] The study continued until the ulcers had healed or 3 months had elapsed. Although only 1 of the 24 patients treated with stockings alone had ulcer healing, 10 of 21 patients in the IPC group had healing. The use of adjunctive intermittent compression has not, however, gained widespread acceptance despite the results of the few available studies indicating it may be useful in treatment of venous ulcers, especially those refractory to ambulatory compression therapy alone.

Pharmacologic Therapy

There are multiple pharmacologic strategies to treat lipodermatosclerosis and venous ulceration. These agents have primarily been studied in Europe and are relatively unknown in the United States. They can be separated into three groups: those based on a presumed nutritional defect in CVI, those based on the fibrin cuff theory, and those based on the white blood cell trapping theory.

Zinc

Several investigators have noted that patients with CVI and venous ulceration may have depressed levels of serum zinc.[107, 108] Greaves and Skillen subsequently reported complete ulcer healing after 4 months of oral zinc therapy and compression bandage use in 13 of 18 patients with low serum zinc levels and previously refractory venous ulceration of more than 2 years' duration.[109] A double-blind trial of 27 patients with venous ulceration and various serum zinc levels compared the combination of zinc therapy and compression bandage use with the use of compression bandages alone.[110] Additional zinc was found to be beneficial only if pretreatment zinc levels were low. A double-blind trial of 38 patients with venous ulceration and unknown zinc levels compared zinc therapy and compression bandage use with bandage use alone. Zinc did not result in an increase in ulcer healing.[111] Two additional studies of oral zinc therapy in patients with venous ulcers also showed no benefit of oral zinc in ulcer healing.[112, 113]

Fibrinolytic Agents

Treatments for venous ulcers derived from the fibrin cuff theory have been disappointing. Stanozolol, an androgenic steroid with significant fibrinolytic activity, has been used to treat patients with CVI and venous ulcers. Browse and associates originally reported encouraging results in 14 patients with CVI and lipodermatosclerosis who were treated for 3 months with stanozolol.[114] All patients had subjective and objective improvement (based on lipodermatosclerotic area). In addition, serum parameters of fibrinolytic activity improved. However, a placebo-controlled crossover study of 23 patients with CVI and long-standing lipodermatosclerosis refractory to stocking therapy demonstrated no difference between stanozolol and stockings versus stockings alone with respect to the area of lipodermatosclerosis.[115] Skin biopsies were unable to prove a reduction in tissue fibrin with the steroid treatment. Leg volumes demonstrated increased fluid retention with use of the drug. More recent studies have likewise been unable to demonstrate major benefits in patients with CVI, from anabolic steroid treatment.[116, 117]

Phlebotrophic Agents

Hydroxyrutosides are a class of flavanoid drug derived from plant glycosides. Initially, studies demonstrated a reduction in capillary permeability after thermal injury.[118] Studies of hydroxyrutosides in the treatment of patients with CVI without ulceration have suggested marginal subjective symptomatic improvement. The hydroxyrutosides also appear to be slightly more effective than placebo in controlling lower extremity edema as measured by ankle circumference.[119-121] They have not been demonstrated to promote healing of venous ulcers.[122]

Calcium 2,5-dihydroxybenzenesulfonate (calcium dobesilate) increases lymphatic flow and macrophage-mediated proteolysis. The net effect is a reduction in edema.[123-125] This drug has not been extensively evaluated in the treatment of CVI. Subjective improvements in the symptoms of CVI have been demonstrated in female patients with clinically "mild" CVI.[126] To date, no studies are available of calcium dobesilate in patients with venous ulceration.

Hemorrheologic Agents

Pentoxifylline is a well-known hemorrheologic agent also used in the treatment of venous ulceration. In addition to its hemorrheologic effects, it reduces white blood cell adhesiveness, inhibits cytokine-mediated neutrophil activation, and reduces the release of superoxide free radicals produced in neutrophil degranulation.[127] In one double-blind, placebo-controlled study of 59 patients with venous ulceration, 87 per cent of patients receiving the study drug had improvement in their venous ulcers, compared with 45 per cent of the placebo group.[128] In addition, a multi-center trial of 80 patients with venous ulceration treated with either pentoxifylline and compression stockings or compression stockings alone demonstrated a significant reduction in ulcer size after 6 months in the patients treated with pentoxifylline and compression stockings compared with those treated with compression therapy alone. Sixty per cent of the pentoxifylline-treated group had ulcer healing, compared with 29 per cent of the controls.

Free Radical Scavengers

Free radical scavengers have been evaluated in the treatment of CVI. One hundred thirty-three patients with CVI and venous ulcers were divided into three groups. Patients in the first two groups were treated with compression stocking therapy and either allopurinol or dimethyl sulfoxide as topical free radical scavenger agents.[129] Patients in the third group were treated with compression therapy alone and served as controls. At 12 weeks, patients treated with topical free radical scavengers had improved rates of ulcer healing. Average ulcer areas at 12 weeks were 0.2 to 0.3 cm^2 in the treatment groups compared with 1.3 cm^2 in controls.

Prostaglandins

Prostaglandin E_1 (PGE$_1$) has multiple microcirculatory effects. It reduces white blood cell activation, inhibits platelet aggregation, and decreases small vessel vasodilation.[130] This drug, which must be administered intravenously, has been used in the treatment of venous ulcers. In the largest trial of PGE$_1$ treatment of venous ulceration, 44 patients were treated with compression bandages and either placebo or PGE$_1$.[131] Patients receiving PGE$_1$ showed significant improvement in edema and ulcer healing. Forty per cent of the patients in the PGE$_1$-treated group had ulcer healing, compared with only 9 per cent in the control group.

Topical Therapies

Topical antibiotics have been advocated as a treatment of venous ulceration for years. However, without evidence of local infection, wound bacteriology appears to have little impact on healing.[132] The application of antiseptics is counterproductive to wound healing. Commercially available concentrations of povidone-iodine, acetic acid, hydrogen peroxide, and sodium hypochlorite are 100 per cent cytotoxic to cultured fibroblasts.[133]

Cadexomer iodine (Iodosorb) is an iodine-containing hydrophilic starch powder employed as a topical dressing for venous ulcers. It absorbs wound exudate and releases iodine as a bacteriocidal agent. Sixty-one patients with venous ulcers were treated with either Iodosorb or a standard topical antibiotic dressing.[101] Patients treated with the Iodosorb dressing demonstrated superior healing. A trial comparing Iodosorb with another hydrophilic powder containing propylene glycol (Scherisorb) in 95 patients with venous ulcers resulted in healing of 29 per cent of ulcers by 10 weeks.[100] There was no difference in healing rates between the two groups. Iodosorb was also compared with dextranomer powder (Debrisan) in the treatment of 27 patients with venous ulcers.[134] All limbs were also treated with elastic compression bandages. After 8 weeks, 64 per cent of the Iodosorb group and 50 per cent of the Debrisan group had had ulcer healing. Finally, a multi-center randomized trial compared Iodosorb treatment with saline dressing treatment in 93 patients whose venous ulcers had been present at least 3 months.[135] All limbs were also treated with elastic compression bandages. At 6 weeks, the mean ulcer size in the Iodosorb group had decreased 34 per cent, compared with 5 per cent in the saline group.

Several agents have been evaluated in attempts to promote ingrowth of granulation tissue in venous ulcer beds. Five days of treatment using human amnion as a topical occlusive dressing in combination with bed rest was reported in an uncontrolled trial of 15 patients.[136] The authors stated that amnion-treated ulcer beds had improved ingrowth of granulation tissue. The patients subjectively reported almost immediate pain relief with the application of the amnion dressings.

Ketanserin, a serotonin$_2$ antagonist, is reported to increase fibroblast collagen synthesis. A double-blind study of 23 patients with venous ulcers compared the use of topical 2 per cent ketanserin and compression bandages with bandage use alone.[137] Wound improvement was demonstrated in 91 per cent of the ketanserin-treated group, compared with 50 per cent of controls.

Hydrocolloid occlusive dressings (DuoDERM) maintain a moist wound environment, are often comfortable for the patient, and may promote more rapid epithelialization of granulating wounds.[138] A randomized trial of 55 patients with venous ulcers compared elastic compression bandages with either hydrocolloid occlusive dressings or gauze bandages for efficiency in ulcer healing. No difference in healing rate was found. In addition, it has been noted that occlusive hydrocolloid dressings may be associated with up to a 25 per cent infectious complication rate.[97] It therefore appears that although occlusive dressings may be more comfortable for the patient, they have not been conclusively demonstrated to produce more rapid healing and may lead to an increased number of local infectious complications.

SUMMARY

When all of the data on the nonoperative treatment of CVI are analyzed, elastic compression hosiery offers the best combination of simplicity and efficacy. Elastic compression therapy provides symptomatic relief, aids in ulcer healing, and prevents ulcer recurrence. The experience at the authors' institution over a 15-year period with a strict program of ambulatory compression hosiery use demonstrated excellent 93 per cent healing and 29 per cent 5-year recurrence rates. At present, elastic compression hosiery use continues to be the gold standard of nonoperative therapy for CVI against which all other adjunctive forms of therapy need to be measured.

References

1. Brand FN, Dannenberg AL, Abbott RD, Kannel WB: The epidemiology of varicose veins: The Framingham study. Am J Prev Med 4:96, 1988.
2. Coon WW, Willis PW, Keller JB: Venous thromboembolism and other venous disease in the Tecumseh community health study. Circulation 48:839, 1973.
3. Gjores JE: The incidence of venous thrombosis and its sequelae in certain districts of Sweden. Acta Chir Scand Suppl 2061:88, 1956.
4. Biland L, Widmer LK: Varicose veins (VV) and chronic venous insufficiency (CVI): Medical and socio-economic aspects, Basle study. Acta Chir Scand Suppl 544: 9, 1988.
5. Dale JJ, Callam MJ, Ruckley CV, et al: Chronic ulcers of the leg: A study of prevalence in a Scottish community. Health Bull (Edinb) 41:310, 1983.
6. Madar G, Widmer LK, Zemp E, Maggs M: Varicose veins and chronic venous insufficiency—A disorder or disease? A critical epidemiological review. Vasa 15:126, 1986.
7. Callam MJ, Harper DR, Dale JJ, Ruckley CV: Chronic ulcer of the leg: Clinical history. Br Med J 294:1389, 1987.
8. Callam MJ, Harper DR, Dale JJ, Ruckley CV: Chronic leg ulceration: Socioeconomic aspects. Scott Med J 33:358, 1988.
9. Baker SR, Stacey MC, Jopp-Mckay AG, et al: Epidemiology of chronic venous ulcers. Br J Surg 78:864, 1991.
10. Nicolaides AN, Zukowski AJ: The value of dynamic pressure measurements. World J Surg 10:919, 1986.
11. Raju S, Fredericks R: Valve reconstruction procedures for nonobstructive venous insufficiency: Rationale, techniques, and results in 107 procedures with two- to eight-year followup. J Vasc Surg 7:301, 1988.
12. Randhawa GK, Dhillon JS, Kistner RL, Ferries EB: Assessment of chronic venous insufficiency using dynamic venous pressure studies. Am J Surg 148:203, 1984.
13. Raju S, Fredericks R: Hemodynamic basis of stasis ulceration—A hypothesis. J Vasc Surg 13:491, 1991.
14. Christopoulos D, Nicolaides AN, Cook A, et al: Pathogenesis of venous ulceration in relation to the calf muscle pump function. Surgery 106:829, 1989.
15. Christopoulos DG, Nicolaides AN, Szendro G, et al: Air plethysmography and the effect of elastic compression on venous hemodynamics of the leg. J Vasc Surg 3:49, 1986.
16. van Bemmelen PS, Bedford G, Beach K, Strandness DE: Quantitative segmental evaluation of venous valvular reflux with duplex ultrasound scanning. J Vasc Surg 10:425, 1989.
17. Vasdekis SN, Clarke GH, Nicolaides AN: Quantification of venous reflux by means of duplex scanning. J Vasc Surg 10:670, 1989.
18. Clarke GH: Venous elasticity. Doctoral thesis, University of London, 1989.
19. Clarke H, Smith SR, Vasdekis SN, et al: Role of venous elasticity in the development of varicose veins. Br J Surg 76:577, 1989.
20. Clarke GH, Vasdekis SN, Hobbs JT, Nicolaides AN: Venous wall function in the pathogenesis of varicose veins. Surgery 111:402, 1992.
21. Strandness DE, Langlois Y, Cramer M, et al: Long-term sequelae of acute venous thrombosis. JAMA 250:1289, 1983.
22. Lindner DJ, Edwards JM, Phinney ES, et al: Long-term hemodynamic and clinical sequelae of lower extremity deep vein thrombosis. J Vasc Surg 4:436, 1986.
23. Killewich LA, Bedford GR, Beach KW, Strandness DE: Spontaneous lysis of deep venous thrombi: Rate and outcome. J Vasc Surg 9:89, 1989.
24. Moore DJ, Himmel PD, Sumner DS: Distribution of venous valvular incompetence in patients with the postphlebitic syndrome. J Vasc Surg 3:49, 1986.
25. Hanrahan LM, Araki CT, Rodriguez AA, et al: Distribution of valvular incompetence in patients with venous stasis ulceration. J Vasc Surg 13:805, 1991.
26. Rosfors S, Lamke LO, Nordstrom E, Bygdeman S: Severity and location of venous valvular insufficiency: The importance of distal valve function. Acta Chir Scand 156:689, 1990.
27. Sethia KK, Darke SG: Long saphenous incompetence as a cause of venous ulceration. Br J Surg 71:754, 1984.
28. Hoare MC, Nicolaides AN, Miles CR, et al: The role of primary varicose veins in venous ulceration. Surgery 92:450, 1982.
29. Burnand KG, O'Donnell TF, Thomas ML, Browse NL: The relative importance of incompetent communicating veins in the production of varicose veins and venous ulcers. Surgery 82:9, 1977.
30. Linton RR, Hardy IB: Postthrombotic syndrome of the lower extremity: Treatment by interruption of the superficial femoral vein and ligation and stripping of the long and short saphenous veins. Surgery 24:452, 1948.
31. Oster G, Tuden RL, Colditz GA: A cost-effective analysis of prophylaxis against deep-vein thrombosis in major orthopedic surgery. JAMA 257:203, 1987.
32. Lagerstedt CI, Fagher BO, Olsson CG, et al: Need for long-term anticoagulant treatment in symptomatic calf-vein thrombosis. Lancet 2:515, 1985.
33. van Bemmelen PS: Venous Valvular Incompetence: An Experimental Study in the Rat. Alblasserdam, Offsetdrukkerij Kaners BV, 1984.
34. Pigeaux AL: Traite Pratique des Maladies des Vaisseaux Conterent des Recherches Historiques Speciales. Paris, Labe et Ravier, 1843.
35. Blalock A: Oxygen content of blood in patients with varices. Arch Surg 19:898, 1929.
36. Haeger KH, Bergman L: Skin temperature of normal and varicose legs and some reflections on the aetiology of varicose veins. Angiology 14:473, 1963.
37. Piulachs P, Vidal-Barraquer E: Pathogenic study of varicose veins. Angiology 4:59, 1953.
38. Haimovich H: Abnormal arteriovenous shunts associated with chronic venous insufficiency. J Cardiovasc Surg 17:473, 1976.
39. Lindemayer W, Lofferer O, Mostbeck A, Partsch H: Arteriovenous shunts in primary varicosis? A critical essay. Vasc Surg 6:9, 1972.
40. Burnand KG, Whimster I, Clemenson G, et al: The relationship between the number of capillaries in the skin of the venous ulcer-bearing area of the lower leg and the fall in foot vein pressure during exercise. Br J Surg 68:297, 1981.
41. Burnand KG, Clemenson G, Whimster I, et al: The effect of sustained venous hypertension on the skin capillaries of the canine hind limb. Br J Surg 69:41, 1982.
42. Guyton AC: Interstitial fluid pressure. II. Pressure-volume curves of interstitial space. Circ Res 16:452, 1965.
43. Hasselbach P, Vollenweider U, Moneta G, Bollinger A: Microangiopathy in severe chronic venous insufficiency evaluated by fluorescence video-microscopy. Phlebology 1:159, 1986.
44. Bollinger A, Jager K, Geser A, et al: Transcapillary and interstitial diffusion of Na-fluorescein in chronic venous insufficiency with white atrophy. Int J Microcirc Clin Exp 1:5, 1982.
45. Fagrell B: Local microcirculation in chronic venous incompetence and leg ulcers. Vasc Surg 13:217, 1979.
46. Burnand KG, Whimster I, Naidoo A, Browse NL: Pericapillary fibrin in the ulcer-bearing skin of the leg: The cause of lipodermatosclerosis and venous ulceration. Br Med J 285:1071, 1982.
47. Wolf JH, Morland M, Browse NL: The fibrinolytic activity of varicose veins. Br J Surg 66:185, 1979.

48. Lotti T, Chimenti M, Bianchini G, et al: Cutaneous and plasmatic fibrinolytic activity in the subject of stasis dermatitis. Ital Gen Rev Dermatol 20:9, 1983.

49. Leach RD, Browse NL: Effect of venous hypertension on canine hind limb lymph. Br J Surg 72:275, 1985.

50. Vanscheidt W, Laaf H, Wokalck H, et al: Pericapillary fibrin cuff: A histologic sign of venous ulceration. J Cutan Pathol 17:266, 1990.

51. Taheri SA, Pollack L, Loomis R: P-31-NMR studies of muscle in patients with venous insufficiency. Int Angiol 6:95, 1987.

52. Hopkins NF, Spinks TJ, Rhodes CG, et al: Positron emission tomography in venous ulceration and liposclerosis: Study of regional tissue function. Br Med J 286:333, 1983.

53. Clyne CA, Ramsden WH, Chant AD, Webster JH: Oxygen tension on the skin of the gaiter area of limbs with venous disease. Br J Surg 72:644, 1985.

54. Mani R, White JE, Barrett DF, Weaver PW: Tissue oxygenation, venous ulcers and fibrin cuffs. J R Soc Med 82:345, 1989.

55. Franzeck UK, Bollinger A, Huch R, Huch A: Transcutaneous oxygen tension and capillary morphology characteristics and density in patients with chronic venous incompetence. Circulation 70:806, 1984.

56. Dodd HJ, Gaylarde PM, Sarkany I: Skin oxygen tension in venous insufficiency of the lower leg. J R Soc Med 78:373, 1985.

57. Rayman G, Williams SA, Spencer PD, et al: Impaired microvascular response to minor skin trauma in type 1 diabetes. Br Med J 292:1295, 1986.

58. Tenland T: On laser Doppler flowmetry: Methods and microvascular applications. Linkoping Studies in Science and Technology Dissertations. 1982, p 83.

59. Partsch H: Hyperaemic hypoxia in venous ulceration. Br J Dermatol 110:249, 1984.

60. Christopoulos DC, Nicolaides AN, Belcaro G, Kalodiki E: Venous hypertensive microangiopathy in relation to clinical severity and effect of elastic compression. J Dermatol Surg Oncol 17:809, 1991.

61. Cheatle TR, Coleridge Smith PD, Scurr JH: Skin microcirculatory responses in chronic venous insufficiency: The effect of short term venous hypertension. Vasa 20:63, 1991.

62. Henriksen O: Local sympathetic reflex mechanism in regulation of blood flow in human subcutaneous adipose tissue. Acta Physiol Scand Suppl 450:7, 1977.

63. Dalsgaard CJ, Haltgardh-Nilsson A, Haegerstrand A, Nilsson J: Neuropeptides as growth factors: Possible role in human diseases. Regul Pept 25:1, 1989.

64. Ardron ME, Helme RD, McKernan S: Microvascular skin responses in elderly people with varicose leg ulcers. Age Ageing 20:124, 1991.

65. Moyses C, Cederholm-Williams SA, Michel CC: Haemoconcentration and accumulation of white cells in the feet during venous stasis. Int J Microcirc Clin Exp 5:311, 1987.

66. Thomas PR, Nash GB, Dormandy JA: White cell accumulation in dependent legs of patients with venous hypertension: A possible mechanism for trophic changes in the skin. Br Med J 290:1693, 1988.

67. Thomas PR, Nash GB, Dormandy JA: Increased white cell trapping in the dependent legs of patients with chronic venous insufficiency. J Mal Vasc 15:35, 1990.

68. Bollinger A, Speiser D, Haselbach P, Jager K: Microangiopathy of mild and severe chronic venous incompetence (CVI) studied by fluorescence videomicroscopy. Schweiz Med Wochenschr (In press).

69. Scott HJ, Coleridge Smith PD, Scurr JH: Histologic study of white blood cells and their association with lipodermatosclerosis and venous ulceration. Br J Surg 78:210, 1991.

70. Cikrit DF, Nichols WK, Silver D: Surgical management of refractory venous stasis ulceration. J Vasc Surg 7:473, 1988.

71. Bergan JJ, Yao JST, Flinn WR, McCarthy WJ: Surgical treatment of venous obstruction and insufficiency. J Vasc Surg 3:174, 1986.

72. Raju S, Fredericks R: Valve reconstruction procedures for nonobstructive venous insufficiency: Rationale, techniques, and results in 107 procedures with two- to eight-year followup. J Vasc Surg 7:301, 1988.

73. Mayberry JC, Moneta GL, DeFrang RD, Porter JM: The influence of elastic compression stockings on deep venous hemodynamics. J Vasc Surg 13:91, 1991.

74. O'Donnell TF, Rosenthal DA, Callow AD, Ledig BL: The effect of elastic compression on venous hemodynamics in postphlebitic limbs. JAMA 242:2766, 1979.

75. Husni EA, Ximenes JOC, Goyette EM: Elastic support of the lower limbs in hospital patients: A critical study. JAMA 214:1456, 1970.

76. Noyes LD, Rice JC, Kerstein MD: Hemodynamic assessment of high-compression hosiery in chronic venous disease. Surgery 102:813, 1987.

77. Somerville JJF, Brow GO, Byrne PJ, et al: The effect of elastic stockings on superficial venous pressures in patients with venous insufficiency. Br J Surg 61:979, 1974.

78. Norris CS, Turley G, Barnes RW: Noninvasive quantification of ambulatory venous hemodynamics during elastic compressive therapy. Angiology 35:560, 1984.

79. Christopoulos DG, Nicolaides AN, Szendro G, et al: Air-plethysmography and the effect of elastic compression on venous hemodynamics of the leg. J Vasc Surg 5:148, 1987.

80. Jones NA, Webb PJ, Rees RI, Kakkar VV: A physiological study of elastic compression stockings in venous disorders of the leg. Br J Surg 67:569, 1980.

81. Horner J, Fernandes JF, Nicolaides AN: Value of graduated compression stockings in deep venous insufficiency. Br Med J 75:820, 1980.

82. Mahler F, Chen D: Intravital microscopy for evaluation of chronic venous incompetence. Int J Microcirc Clin Exp 106 (Suppl):1, 1990.

83. Neumann HA: Possibilities and limitations of transcutaneous oxygen tension. Measurements in chronic venous insufficiency. Int J Microcirc Clin Exp 105 (Suppl):1, 1990.

84. Kolari PJ, Pekanmaki K: Effects of intermittent compression treatment on skin perfusion and oxygenation in lower legs with venous ulcers. Vasa 16:312, 1987.

85. Nemeth AJ, Falanga V, Alstadt SA, Eaglstein WH: Ulcerated edematous limbs: Effect of edema removal on transcutaneous oxygen measurements. J Am Acad Dermatol 120:191, 1989.

86. Bergan JJ: Conrad Jobst and the development of pressure gradient therapy for venous disease. *In* Bergan JJ, Yao JS (eds): Surgery of the Veins. Orlando, FL, Grune & Stratton, 1985, pp 529–540.

87. Wright AD: The treatment of indolent ulcer of the leg. Lancet 1:457, 1931.

88. Anning ST: Leg ulcers—the results of treatment. Angiology 7:505, 1956.

89. Kitahama A, Elliot LF, Kerstein MD, Menendez CV: Leg ulcer: Conservative management or surgical treatment? JAMA 247:197, 1982.

90. Mayberry JC, Moneta GL, Taylor LM, Porter JM: Fifteen-year results of ambulatory compression therapy for chronic venous ulcers. Surgery 109:575, 1991.

91. Chant AD, Davies LJ, Pike JM, Sparks MJ: Support stockings in practical management of varicose veins. Phlebology 4:167, 1989.

92. Callam MJ, Ruckley CV, Dale JJ, Harper DR: Hazards of compression treatment of the leg: An estimate from Scottish surgeons. Br Med J 295:1382, 1987.

93. Callam MJ, Harper DR, Dale JJ, Ruckley CV: Arterial disease in chronic leg ulceration: An underestimated hazard? Lothian and Forth Valley leg ulcer study. Br Med J 294:929, 1987.

94. Unna PG: Ueber Paraplaste, eine neue Form medikamentoser Pflaster. Wien Med Wochenschr 43:1854, 1896.

95. Hendricks WM, Swallow RT: Management of stasis leg ulcers with Unna's boots versus elastic support stockings. J Am Acad Dermatol 12:90, 1985.

96. Rubin JR, Alexander J, Plecha EJ, Marman C: Unna's boots vs polyurethane foam dressings for the treatment of venous ulceration. Arch Surg 125:489, 1990.

97. Kitka MJ, Schuler JJ, Meyer JP, et al: A prospective, randomized trial of Unna's boots versus hydroactive dressing in the treatment of venous stasis ulcers. J Vasc Surg 7:478, 1988.

98. Cordts PR, Hanrahan LM, Rodriguez AA, et al: A prospective, randomized trial of Unna's boot versus DuoDERM CGF hydroactive dressing plus compression in the management of venous leg ulcers. J Vasc Surg 15:480, 1992.

99. Blair SD, Wright DD, Backhouse LM, et al: Sustained compression and healing of chronic venous ulcers. Br Med J 297:1159, 1988.

100. Stewart AJ, Leaper DJ: Treatment of chronic leg ulcers in the community: A comparative trial of Scherisorb and Iodosorb. Phlebology 2:115, 1987.

101. Ormiston MC, Seymour MT, Venn GE, et al: Controlled trial of Iodosorb in chronic venous ulcers. Br Med J 291:308, 1985.

102. Ryan TJ, Biven HF, Murphy JJ, et al: The use of a new occlusive

dressing in the management of venous stasis ulceration. *In* Ryan TJ (ed): An Environment for Healing: The Role of Occlusion. London, Royal Society of Medicine, 1984, pp 99–103.

103. Eriksson G: Comparative study of hydrocolloid dressing and double layer bandage in treatment of venous stasis ulceration. *In* Ryan TJ (ed): An Environment for Healing: The Role of Occlusion. London, Royal Society of Medicine, 1984, pp 111–113.

104. Vernick SH, Shapiro D, Shaw FD: Legging orthosis for venous and lymphatic insufficiency. Arch Phys Med Rehabil 68:459, 1987.

105. Pekanmaki K, Kolari PJ, Kiistala U: Intermittent pneumatic compression treatment for post-thrombotic leg ulcers. Clin Exp Dermatol 12:350, 1987.

106. Coleridge Smith P, Sarin S, Hasty J, Scurr JH: Sequential gradient pneumatic compression enhances venous ulcer healing: A randomized trial. Surgery 108:871, 1990.

107. Greaves MW, Boyde TR: Plasma zinc concentrations in patients with psoriasis, other dermatoses, and venous leg ulceration. Lancet 2:1019, 1967.

108. Withers AF, Baker H, Musa M, Dormandy TL: Plasma zinc in psoriasis. Lancet 2:278, 1968.

109. Greaves MW, Skillen AW: Effects of long-continued ingestion of zinc sulphate in patients with venous leg ulceration. Lancet 2:889, 1970.

110. Hallbook T, Lanner E: Serum-zinc and healing of venous leg ulcers. Lancet 2:780, 1972.

111. Greaves MW, Ive FA: Double blind trial of zinc sulphate in the treatment of chronic venous ulceration. Br J Dermatol 87:632, 1972.

112. Myers MB, Cherry G: Zinc and the healing of chronic ulcers. Am J Surg 120:77, 1970.

113. Phillips A, Davidson M, Greaves MW: Venous leg ulceration: Evaluation of zinc treatment, serum zinc and rate of healing. Clin Exp Dermatol 2:395, 1977.

114. Browse NL, Jarrett PE, Morland M, Burnand K: Treatment of lipodermatosclerosis of the leg by fibrinolytic enhancement: A preliminary report. Br Med J 2:434, 1977.

115. Burnand K, Lemenson G, Morland M, et al: Venous lipodermatosclerosis: Treatment by fibrinolytic enhancement and elastic compression. Br Med J 280:7, 1980.

116. McMullin GM, Watkin GT, Coleridge Smith PD, Scurr JH: The efficacy of fibrinolytic enhancement with stanozolol in the treatment of venous insufficiency. Aust NZ J Surg 61:306, 1991.

117. Layer GT, Stacey MC, Burnand KG: Stanozolol and the treatment of venous ulceration—an interim report. Phlebology 1:197, 1986.

118. Arturson G: Effects of 0-(B-hydroxyethyl)-rutosides (HR) on the increased microvascular permeability in experimental skin burns. Acta Chir Scand 138:111, 1972.

119. Balmer A, Limoni C: A double-blind placebo-controlled trial of venorutin on the symptoms and signs of chronic venous insufficiency. Vasa 9:76, 1980.

120. Pulvertaft TB: Paroven in the treatment of chronic venous insufficiency. Practitioner 223:838, 1979.

121. Pulvertaft TB: General practice treatment of symptoms of venous insufficiency with oxyrutins. Results of a 660 patient multicenter study in the UK. Vasa 12:373, 1983.

122. Mann RJ: A double-blind trial of oral 0. B-hydroxy-ethyl rutosides for stasis leg ulcers. Br J Clin Pract 35:79, 1981.

123. Casley-Smith JR, Casley-Smith JR: The effects of calcium dobesilate on acute lymphoedema (with and without macrophages) and on burn edema. Lymphology 18:37, 1985.

124. Casley-Smith JR: The effect of variations in tissue protein concentration and tissue hydrostatic pressure on fluid and protein uptake by the initial lymphatics, and the action of calcium dobesilate. Microcirc Endothelium Lymphatics 2:385, 1985.

125. Casley-Smith JR: A double-blind trial of calcium dobesilate in chronic venous insufficiency. Angiology 39:853, 1988.

126. Hachen HJ, Lorenz P: Double-blind clinical and plethysmographic study of calcium dobesilate in patients with peripheral microvascular disorders. Angiology 33:480, 1982.

126. Hachen HJ, Lorenz P: Double-blind clinical and plethysmographic study of calcium dobesilate in patients with peripheral microvascular disorders. Angiology 33:480, 1982.

127. Sullivan GW, Carper HT, Novick WJ, Mandell GL: Inhibition of the inflammatory action of interleukin-1 and tumor necrosis factor (alpha) on neutrophil function by pentoxifylline. Infect Immunol 56:1722, 1988.

128. Weitgasser H: The use of pentoxifylline (Trental 400) in the treatment of leg ulcers: The results of a double blind trial. Pharmatherapeutica 3(Suppl 1):143, 1983.

129. Salim AS: The role of oxygen-derived free radicals in the management of venous (varicose) ulceration: A new approach. World J Surg 15:264, 1991.

130. Sinzinger H, Virgolini I, Fitscha P: Pathomechanisms of atherosclerosis beneficially affected by prostaglandin E₁ (PGE₁)—An update. Vasa 28(Suppl):6, 1989.

131. Rudofsky G: Intravenous prostaglandin E1 in the treatment of venous ulcers—A double-blind, placebo controlled trial. Vasa 28(Suppl):39, 1989.

132. Gilchrist B, Reed C: The bacteriology of chronic venous ulcers treated with occlusive hydrocolloid dressings. Br J Dermatol 121:337, 1989.

133. Lineaweaver W, Howard R, Souey D, et al: Topical antimicrobial toxicity. Arch Surg 120:267, 1985.

134. Tarvainen K: Cadexomer iodine (Iodosorb) compared with dextranomer (Debrisan) in the treatment of chronic leg ulcers. Acta Chir Scand Suppl 544:57, 1988.

135. Hillstrom L: Iodosorb compared to standard treatment in chronic venous leg ulcers—A multicenter study. Acta Chir Scand Suppl 544:53, 1988.

136. Bennett JP, Matthews R, Faulk WP: Treatment of chronic ulceration of the legs with human amnion. Lancet 1:1153, 1980.

137. Roelens P: Double-blind placebo-controlled study with topical 2% ketanserin ointment in the treatment of venous ulcers. Dermatologica 178:98, 1989.

138. Alvarez OM, Mertz PM, Eaglstein WH: The effect of occlusive dressings on collagen synthesis and re-epithelialization in superficial wounds. J Surg Res 35:142, 1983.

139

Operative Management of Chronic Venous Insufficiency

Seshadri Raju, M.D.

• • •

Chronic venous insufficiency is a significant cause of disability in the workplace. Surveys have indicated that 4 per cent of the work force in the industrialized world may be affected.[1] The incidence in the overall population is estimated to be approximately 2 per cent.

ETIOLOGY AND CLASSIFICATION

Chronic venous insufficiency can result from congenital, cryptogenic ("primary"), or post-thrombotic causes of valvular reflux (Fig. 139–1). Congenital causes of reflux include valvular aplasia and dysplasias, such as avalvular duplication conduits that circumvent valve structures, and a wide variety of valvular malformations that predispose to poor valve function and reflux (Fig. 139–2). Klippel-Trenaunay syndrome is often associated with venous valve aplasia and dysplasias. Primary valve reflux, once thought to be a rare entity, is now recognized as a common cause of chronic venous insufficiency.[2] Currently, it accounts for about 30 per cent of valve reconstruction procedures in the author's center. In primary valve reflux, the valve leaflets appear normal in texture but are redundant, exhibiting lettuce-like folds with a tendency to evert. This results in poor coaptation of the leaflets, which leads to reflux (Fig. 139–3). Because thrombotic changes in and around the valve cusps are not usually evident, it is assumed that the defect arises from a developmental etiologic mechanism. The precise structural defect and its cause, however, have not been determined. Primary valve reflux may result in deep venous thrombosis from reflux stasis.[2] Such patients often present with primary reflux in the femoral area and with distal thrombosis in the calf veins. Recurrent bouts of deep venous thrombosis in these patients may be relieved by correcting the proximal valve reflux.

Deep venous thrombosis remains the most common cause of chronic venous insufficiency, accounting for about 70 per cent of such cases in the author's hospital practice. The precise incidence and evolution of chronic venous insufficiency following deep venous thrombosis are unknown because few longitudinal studies have been undertaken in the context of modern anticoagulant therapy. In a study that extended up to 4 years after the incidence of deep venous thrombosis, approximately one fourth of the patients studied were already severely symptomatic from postphlebitic syndrome.[3] Because the development of clinical manifestations of post-thrombotic venous insufficiency is a slow and insidious process, with a predilection for recurrent thrombosis, the full impact of the disease may not be apparent in many patients until 15 or 20 years after the initial onset. The valve structure may be completely destroyed by thrombosis and recanalization (see Fig. 139–3), or lesser degrees of damage, ranging from thickening of valve cusps, to shortening and fibrosis of the leaflets, perforations, or adhesion to each other or a sinus wall, may be evident. Reflux resulting from such deformities is often compounded by the presence of coexisting venous obstruction from the thrombotic process itself. Collaterals that develop are an important source of often massive reflux in the affected extremity. Collaterals that develop around an obstruction in the axial vein itself or those that develop between adjacent vessels, such as between the profunda and popliteal veins in the presence of femoral vein thrombosis, often persist even after the thrombus has become fully recanalized (Fig. 139–4). Post-thrombotic abnormalities of the calf venous pump mechanism, such as reduced venous capacitance and poor

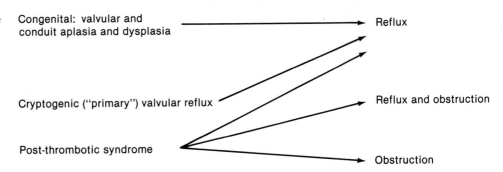

FIGURE 139–1. Etiologic mechanisms in chronic venous insufficiency.

Congenital: valvular and conduit aplasia and dysplasia ——————→ Reflux

Cryptogenic ("primary") valvular reflux ——→ Reflux and obstruction

Post-thrombotic syndrome ——→ Obstruction

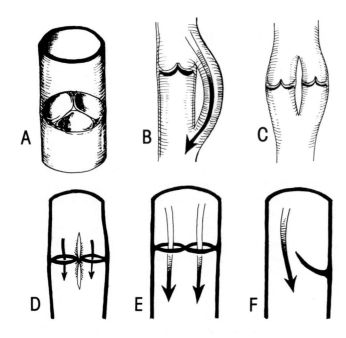

FIGURE 139–2. Congenital anomalies of the venous conduit and the valve structure. These are frequently associated with venous reflux. *A*, Tricuspid valve. *B*, Avalvular duplication conduit. *C*, Duplication conduit with refluxive valves. *D*, Duplication of the valve with an intervening septum. *E*, Duplication of the valve without a septum. *F*, Refluxive monocuspid valve.

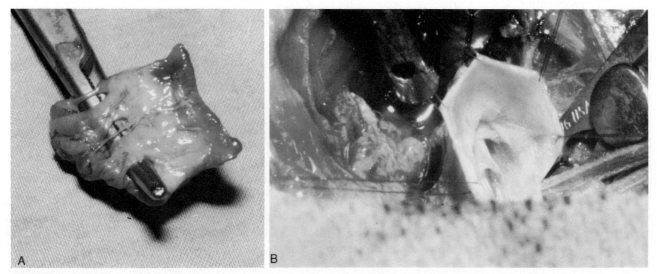

FIGURE 139–3. *A*, Postphlebitic valve with destruction of the valve structure. *B*, "Primary" valve reflux with everting valve cusps.

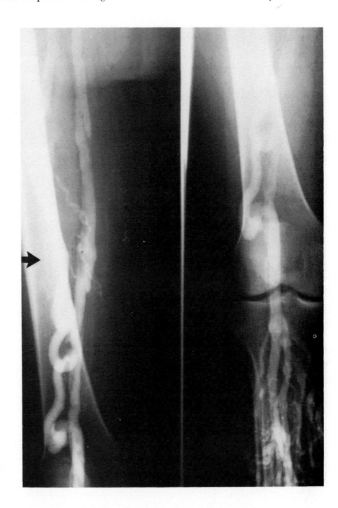

FIGURE 139–4. Profunda-popliteal collateral connection. Such collaterals *(arrow)* persist even after recanalization of the thrombosed superficial femoral vein. The rapid development of these collaterals suggests a putative collateral connection that may have an embryologic basis.

wall compliance (Fig. 139–5), compound the refluxive and obstructive pathologic mechanisms to produce the full-blown postphlebitic syndrome.

HEMODYNAMIC CHANGES

Reflux is clearly associated with stasis ulceration (Fig. 139–6). The resulting ambulatory venous hypertension can be shown to correlate with the incidence of stasis ulceration.[4] Approximately 25 per cent of patients who have reflux and develop stasis ulceration, however, record ambulatory venous pressures that are considered in the normal range (Fig. 139–7).[5] Thus, the precise interrelationship between venous reflux, ambulatory venous hypertension, and the genesis of stasis ulceration is not fully understood. There is increasing appreciation that the quantity of reflux is more important than its location (i.e., the superficial vs the deep system).[4] Thus, the traditional classification of chronic venous insufficiency into superficial and deep varieties appears obsolete. Patients who have massive reflux that is for the most part confined to the superficial system can develop stasis ulceration.[6] However, the proportion of patients with reflux confined entirely to the superficial system who develop stasis ulceration is small; the majority of patients with stasis skin changes demonstrate multi-valvular, multi-system reflux.[7] Deep system reflux, either alone or in association with superficial reflux, is commonly iden-

tified in this patient population (Table 139–1).[8] Symptom expression also correlates with increasing incidence of deep valvular and perforator reflux (Table 139–2).[9] The common association between deep venous reflux and stasis pathology is probably related to the large quantity of reflux required to overwhelm the compensatory mechanisms inherent in the calf venous pump.[10] Primary valve reflux is often global, affecting both the superficial and the deep systems. In postphlebitic syndrome, deep venous reflux is predominant following previous deep venous thrombosis. Thus, the high incidence of deep venous reflux in stasis ulceration should not be surprising, in view of the propensity of the major etiologic mechanisms to affect the deep system either alone or in combination with superficial venous insufficiency.

When both obstruction and reflux are present, the latter component is thought to be more important in the genesis of stasis skin changes.[11] Patients with deep venous obstruction primarily present with swelling and pain; stasis changes in the gaiter area develop with recanalization of the thrombosed vein and the onset of reflux.

CLINICAL PRESENTATION

The clinical presentation of chronic venous insufficiency can vary from mild to severe,[12] according to the extent of underlying pathology (Table 139–3). Patients who

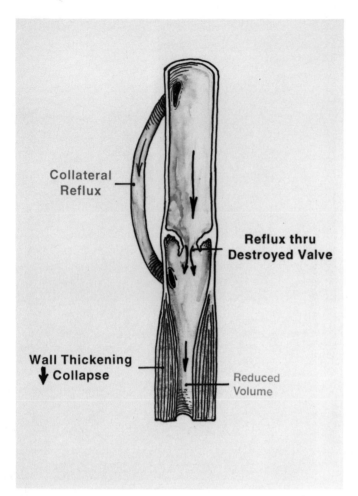

FIGURE 139–5.   Pathophysiology of postphlebitic syndrome: reflux through the postphlebitic valve and through collaterals is compounded by postphlebitic abnormalities of the calf venous pump. Reduced venous capacitance and post-thrombotic compliance changes decrease the efficiency of the calf venous pump and produce ambulatory venous hypertension.

FIGURE 139–6.   Incidence of leg ulceration in relation to the venous filling index (VFI) and the ejection fraction (EF) of the calf muscle pump as measured by air plethysmography in 175 limbs with venous problems. Normal range for these parameters is indicated by *inset* (N). (From Nicolaides AN, Sumner DS [eds]: Investigation of Patients With Deep Vein Thrombosis and Chronic Venous Insufficiency. Los Angeles, Med-Orion Publishing, 1991, p 49.)

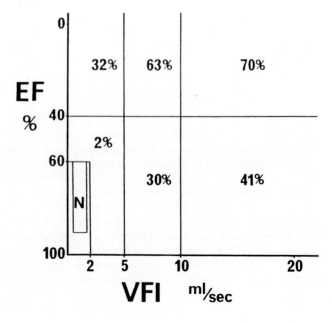

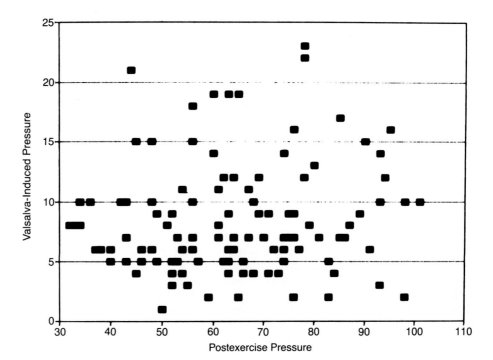

FIGURE 139–7. Plot of postexercise pressure and Valsalva-induced venous pressure in 113 limbs with stasis ulceration. Twenty-five limbs had ambulatory pressures of 50 mmHg or lower, which is considered normal. Most of these limbs, however, were found to have abnormal Valsalva-induced foot venous pressures (normal, 4 mmHg or lower). (From Raju S, Fredericks R: Hemodynamic basis of stasis ulceration—A hypothesis. J Vasc Surg 13:491, 1991.)

present with varicosities in the lower leg sometimes develop punctate skin necrosis over distended varices that can lead to impressive hemorrhage in the erect position. This should not be confused with the classic stasis ulcer with extensive areas of lipodermosclerosis and skin changes surrounding the "stasis" ulcer itself (Fig. 139–8).

PREOPERATIVE WORK-UP

The investigation of patients presenting with symptoms of chronic venous insufficiency focuses on providing the following information: (1) confirmation of the diagnosis of reflux and assessment of its degree and extent; (2) detection of the presence of associated obstruction and determination of its severity and location; (3) identification of a possible etiology (e.g., primary vs. post-thrombotic reflux), and (4) evaluation of the status of the lymphatics when swelling is a presenting symptom.

It is generally impossible to differentiate chronic venous obstruction from reflux on the basis of clinical pres-

entation alone. Similarly, primary valvular reflux cannot be differentiated with certainty from the post-thrombotic variety on the basis of history and physical findings. Patients who report previous episodes of "phlebitis" may have normal venographic findings. Conversely, extensive post-thrombotic changes may be evident on venography even when there is no history of deep venous thrombosis. All patients with evidence of prior thrombosis should undergo screening for clotting factor abnormalities. Older patients with thrombosis should be investigated for occult malignancies.

In most laboratories, duplex scanning has superseded other testing modalities in screening patients with suspected chronic venous insufficiency. The presence, extent, and location of reflux can be assessed noninvasively with this technique.[13] Modifications that provide for measurement of valve closure times[14] with the use of rapidly deflating cuffs have increased the sophistication of the duplex technique, allowing for quantification of reflux. The sensitivity of duplex scanning in detecting reflux is, however, in the range of only 75 per cent in most laboratories.[13] It is therefore recommended that additional independent techniques, such as air plethysmography or ambulatory venous pressure measurement, be incorporated in the investigative protocol.[13] Besides confirming the presence of reflux, the latter techniques provide important additional information about the efficiency of the calf venous pump mechanism. The presence and degree of hemodynamic obstruction cannot be reliably assessed with the duplex technique. Measurement of the arm-foot venous pressure differential[15] is used to provide this information.

Patients in whom valve reconstructive surgery is contemplated should undergo additional phlebographic examination including ascending and descending venography. These studies provide anatomic information essential for surgical exploration. Ascending venography provides infor-

Table 139–1. Incidence of Superficial and Deep Vein Reflux in 485 Descending Venograms

Reflux Location	Incidence (%)
Saphenous vein only	2
Superficial femoral vein only	19
Deep femoral vein only	12
Superficial and deep femoral veins	51
Saphenous vein with superficial femoral vein, deep femoral vein, or both	16

From Morano JU, Raju S: Chronic venous insufficiency: Assessment with descending venography. Radiology 174:441–444, 1990.

Table 139–2.   Frequency of Involvement of the Superficial Veins (on Ultrasonography), Perforator Incompetence (on Ascending Venography), Deep Vein Reflux (on Descending Venography), and Hemodynamic Tests in 56 Lower Limbs According to Clinical Severity Staging

Clinical Severity Class	No. of Limbs	Ambulatory Venous Pressure (% drop)*	Venous Filling Time (sec)	Superficial Incompetence (%)	Perforator Incompetence (%)	Reflux (%)
0	15	58 ± 7	39 ± 21	20	20	20
1	19	57 ± 5	33 ± 16	58	69	26
2	8	49 ± 12	16 ± 12	63	88	63
3	14	41 ± 11	9 ± 7	71	100	86

From Neglén P, Raju S: A comparison between descending phlebography and duplex Doppler investigation in the evaluation of reflux in chronic venous insufficiency: A challenge to phlebography as the "gold standard." J Vasc Surg 16:687, 1992.

Class 0 plus class 1 is significantly different from class 2 plus class 3 for ambulatory venous pressure (p<.001) and venous filling time (p<.001).

mation on the patency of axial channels, perforator incompetence, evidence of previous deep venous thrombosis, postphlebitic changes, sites of obstruction, and abnormal collaterals. Descending venography is performed to identify the presence and extent of reflux. It yields information on the location of refluxing valve stations and provides details of valve anatomy. Primary valve reflux can usually be differentiated from the postphlebitic variety on the basis of the descending venographic appearance. Although several grading systems have been devised to assess reflux on descending venography, correlation with hemodynamic parameters of reflux is inconsistent.[16] Findings on descending venography may be falsely negative for reflux in the presence of proximal venous obstruction.[9] Conversely, patients who are asymptomatic or only mildly symptomatic may demonstrate impressive reflux on descending venography.[9]

Therefore, a decision to operate should not be based on descending venographic findings alone; descending venography is most useful in aiding in surgical exploration once the decision to operate has been made on other grounds.

Nucleotide lymphoscintigraphy should be performed in patients who present with chronic leg swelling. The origin of the swelling may be purely venous, purely lymphatic, or a combination of the two. A surprisingly high percentage of patients with chronic venous insufficiency were found to have associated lymphatic abnormalities (25 per cent).[17, 18]

DIFFERENTIAL DIAGNOSIS

A wide variety of nonvenous conditions, such as periarteritis nodosa, acanthosis, restless leg syndrome, idio-

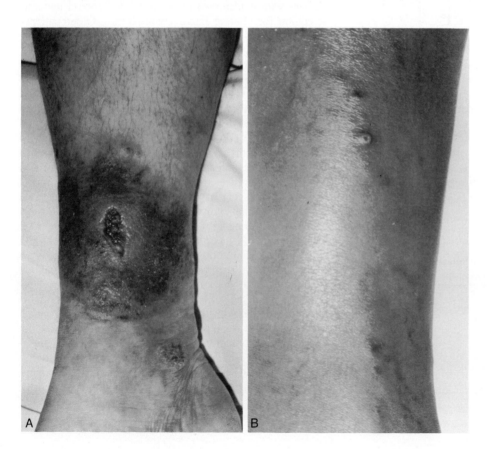

FIGURE 139–8.   *A,* Typical stasis ulcer with necrosis and surrounding areas of lipodermosclerosis. This should not be confused with the punctate pressure ulcers sometimes seen over prominent varicosities. *B,* Pinpoint ulcers can bleed profusely when the patient is in the erect position. Note the absence of skin changes around the punctate "varicose" ulcer.

Table 139–3.   Classification of Chronic Venous Insufficiency by Clinical Severity

Clinical Severity Class	Description
0	Asymptomatic
1	Mild signs and symptoms, including mild to moderate ankle swelling, mild discomfort, and local or generalized dilatation of subcutaneous veins
2	Moderate symptoms, including hyperpigmentation of the skin in the gaiter area, moderate brawny edema, and subcutaneous fibrosis, which may be either limited or extensive but is without ulceration
3	Severe symptoms, including chronic distal leg pain associated with ulcerative or preulcerative skin changes, eczematoid changes, and severe edema

From Subcommittee on Reporting Standards in Venous Disease, Ad Hoc Committee on Reporting Standards, Society for Vascular Surgery/North American Chapter, International Society for Cardiovascular Surgery: Reporting standards in venous disease. J Vasc Surg 8:172, 1988.

pathic calf cramps, lymphedema, Marjolin's ulcer, fungus infections, vasculitis of various types, and acrocyanosis, mimic some aspects of venous insufficiency. These conditions often coexist in some patients with demonstrable venous insufficiency because the latter is widely prevalent. Careful identification of the true basis of patient symptomatology is therefore essential. Atypical ulcers and skin lesions should always be biopsied.

INDICATIONS FOR SURGERY

Surgery may be considered when conservative therapy has failed to relieve severe stasis symptoms. Patients who develop complications such as recurrent cellulitis or recurrent deep venous thrombosis during conservative therapy may also be considered for surgery. Finally, certain ancillary factors such as relatively young age, desire for speedy rehabilitation to return to the work force or pursue an active lifestyle, or inability to pursue a strict regimen of conservative measures may be relative indications. Some patients find it difficult to wear stockings because of a warm climate or because of cosmetic or lifestyle considerations. Patients with arthritis or other disabling conditions of the extremities may not be able to maintain leg elevation or to apply tight-fitting stockings. For the most part, surgery should be confined to patients who present with class 3 symptoms (severe stasis skin changes or frank ulceration). Patients who present primarily with painful swelling or pain alone may be considered for surgery after the failure of conservative therapy if hemodynamically massive reflux can be demonstrated. Although considerable alleviation of leg swelling may be obtained with valve reconstruction surgery, complete resolution is rare. Painless swelling without skin changes is therefore a relative contraindication for surgery. Because of their chronic pain, personality alterations are common in patients with disabling venous insufficiency. Many of these patients have an exaggerated pain syndrome that is out of proportion to the existing venous disease. Other extraneous factors, such as a desire for disability or

workers' compensation payments, may also color the clinical presentation with exaggerated symptomatology. The treatment of this group of patients poses a difficult challenge because symptom relief may not follow successful surgical correction of reflux. Considerable clinical judgment is required in selecting patients from this group for surgery.

SURGICAL TECHNIQUE

Surgical correction is directed toward the valve stations that were identified to be refluxive on the preoperative work-up. The uppermost superficial femoral valve, which is nearly constant in location below the takeoff of the deep femoral vein, is the most frequently repaired. In post-thrombotic cases, the deep femoral vein may function as an important refluxive channel[11] and may be reconstructed. Less commonly, valve reconstruction procedures are undertaken at more distal locations, such as the distal superficial femoral vein in the adductor canal,[19] the popliteal vein, and the posterior tibial vein. When the etiology is cryptogenic reflux, it is unclear whether a single valve or multiple valves should be reconstructed, and the optimal site for single-valve reconstruction (i.e., femoral vs popliteal) has not been identified. Techniques of valve reconstruction in the post-thrombotic syndrome are currently evolving. Because of the presence of tributary and collateral reflux in this syndrome, reconstruction of multiple valves at various levels would appear to be logical.[20] Several reconstruction techniques are currently available to accommodate differences in valve pathology, valve location, and other factors, such as speed of execution.

Internal Valvuloplasty. The femoral and profunda valves are approached through a groin incision. Valve reflux is confirmed by performing the strip test (Fig. 139–9). The valve may be approached either through a longitudinal incision extending between valve cusp attachments (Kistner)[21] or through a supravalvular transverse (Raju)[18] or T (Sotturai)[22] incision. Fine sutures of 7–0 Prolene are used to gather up the redundant valve cusp edges at each commissure (see Fig. 139–9).

Kistner Segment Transfer. When the superficial femoral vein valve is refluxive but the profunda valve is competent, a segment transfer procedure[23] can abolish reflux in the femoral vein (Fig. 139–10).

External Valvuloplasty. An external technique for repairing the valve without a venotomy has been described.[24] When the valve is refluxive, the valve commissural angle is wide (Fig. 139–11).[20] The valve attachment lines, as seen through the vein wall, are brought together by externally placed sutures near each commissure. The technique is less precise than internal valvuloplasty but has the advantages of being more rapid and being applicable to small-caliber veins.

Placement of a Prosthetic Sleeve In Situ. A refluxive vein valve sometimes becomes competent with venoconstriction caused by surgical manipulation (Fig. 139–12).[18]

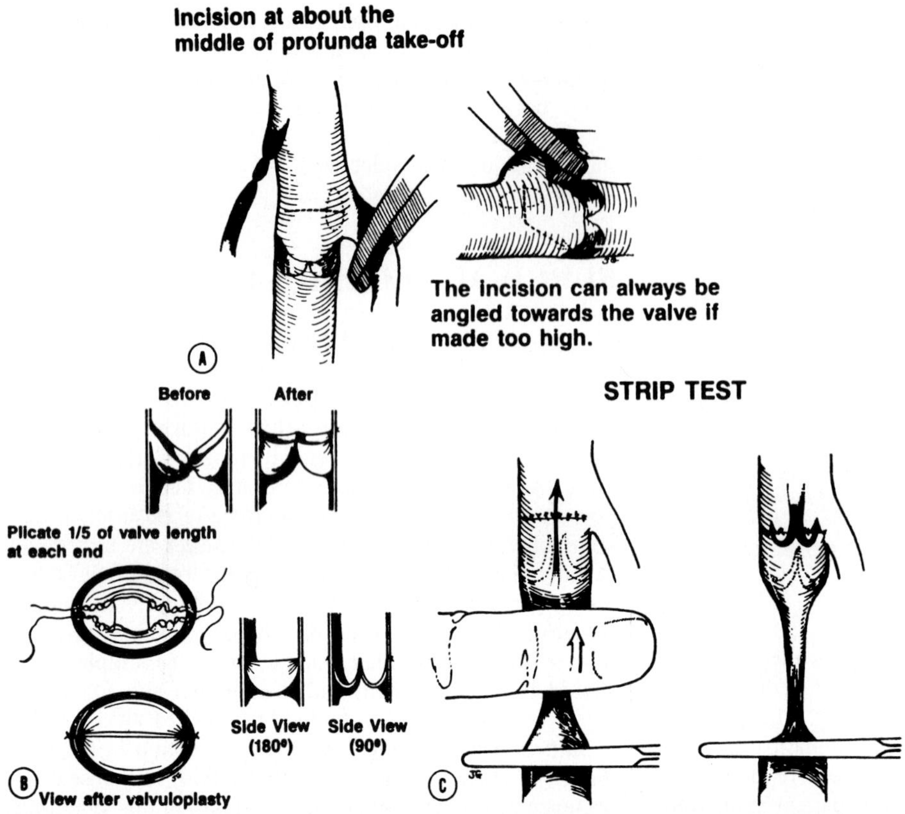

Incision at about the middle of profunda take-off

The incision can always be angled towards the valve if made too high.

STRIP TEST

Before   After

Plicate 1/5 of valve length at each end

Side View (180°)   Side View (90°)

B View after valvuloplasty

FIGURE 139–9. Strip test and technique of internal valvuloplasty. *A*, Transverse venotomy and placement of valvuloplasty sutures along the edge of redundant valve cusps near each commissure. *B*, View of tightened valve cusps. *C*, Strip test after valve repair demonstrates valve competency. (*A – C*, From Raju S, Fredericks R: Valve reconstruction procedures for non-obstructive venous insufficiency: Rationale, techniques, and results in 107 procedures with 2 – 8 year follow-up. J Vasc Surg 7:301, 1988).

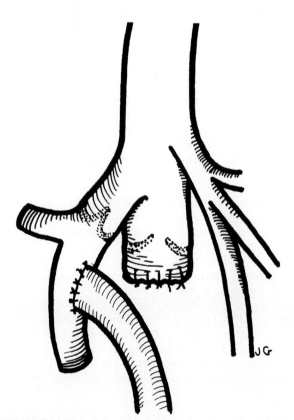

FIGURE 139–10. Kistner's segment transfer procedure. The superficial femoral vein is divided below an incompetent valve and anastomosed to the profunda vein below a competent valve.

An appropriately sized Dacron or polytetrafluoroethylene sleeve can be placed around the valve in the slightly contracted position to maintain competency. The technique is rapid, avoids a venotomy, and is applicable to small-caliber veins.

Axillary Vein Transfer. When the valve cannot be repaired by one of the previously mentioned techniques or has been completely destroyed by prior thrombosis, an axillary vein valve transfer may be considered.[25, 26] A competent valve-bearing segment of axillary vein is excised and transferred to the superficial femoral vein below the inguinal ligament at a more distal location, such as the superficial femoral vein in the adductor canal, the popliteal vein, or the posterior tibial vein below the knee. The axillary vein from which the valve segment was harvested is ligated without repair, because no obstructive malsequelae have been observed. The transferred axillary vein segment should be wrapped with a prosthetic sleeve to avoid late dilatation, which may occur from a compliance mismatch between the transferred venous segment and the native vein in the lower limb. This is especially important when the native vein is stiff from post-thrombotic changes. Axillary vein segments are prone to a higher incidence of failure[18] from both dilatation and stenosis (Fig. 139–13). Because the long-term results of axillary vein transfer are inferior to those of valvuloplasty, the former technique should not be used when valvuloplasty is feasible. In addition, 40 per cent of axillary vein valves are incompetent in situ.[18] A competent valve can usually be located, however, at a different

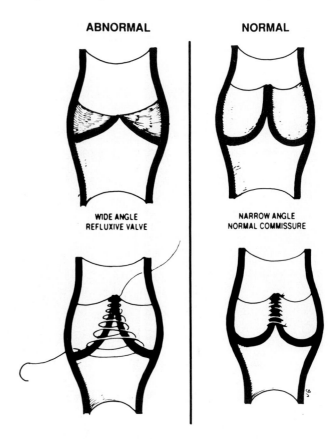

FIGURE 139–11. Technique of external valvuloplasty. Nonrefluxive normal valves have an acute commissural angle. This angle is found to be wide (greater than 12 degrees) when the valve is refluxive because of primary valvular insufficiency. The valve attachment lines near the commissure are clearly identified by adventitial dissection, and the obtuse valve angle is closed by sutures externally placed along valve attachment lines, as shown. (From Raju S: Multiple-valve reconstruction for venous insufficiency: Indications, optimal technique, and results. *In* Veith FJ [ed]: Current Critical Problems in Vascular Surgery—IV. St. Louis, Quality Medical Publishing, 1992, pp 122 – 125.)

location more proximal or distal on the same side or in the opposite axillary vein. Results of attempts to repair an incompetent axillary vein valve before transfer have been disappointing in the author's experience.

One or more of the previously described techniques can be combined to perform multiple-valve reconstruction (Fig. 139–14).

Other Antirefluxive Procedures. Saphenous vein stripping may be used alone or in combination with valve reconstruction when this vein has been identified as a major source of reflux. However, saphenous excision is commonly performed for cosmetic indications even when re-

fluxive symptoms are absent. A modified Linton procedure as described by DePalma may be a useful adjunct in the presence of marked perforator incompetence.[27] Even patients with combined obstruction and reflux tolerate this procedure well, without exacerbation of hemodynamic obstruction.[11] When it is used alone, however, a 50 per cent recurrence rate can be expected after perforator interruption. Reflux may be abolished by ligating persistent collateral connections, such as the profunda-popliteal connection shown in Figure 139–3. This should be performed only when the main venous axial channel has become satisfactorily recanalized because outflow obstruction may otherwise result.[20]

FIGURE 139–12.
Prosthetic sleeve in situ. A refluxive superficial femoral valve (*A*) becomes competent with surgical manipulation and venoconstriction (*B*). A prosthetic sleeve is fitted around the slightly contracted valve ring to maintain competency (*C*). The sleeve may be fashioned around the profunda-femoral junction as shown. SFV, superficial femoral vein.

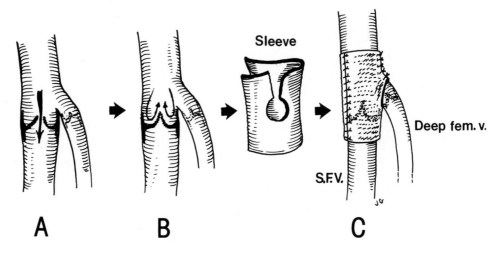

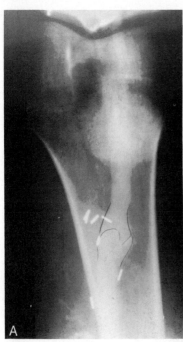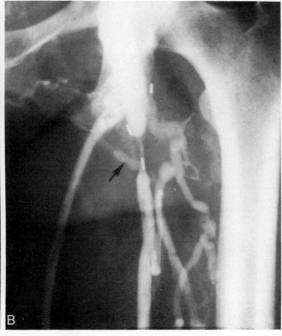

FIGURE 139–13.
A, Recurrent reflux through a transferred axillary vein valve that was not fitted with a prosthetic sleeve. *B*, Less commonly, the transferred valvular segment may become stenotic (*arrow*) after functioning satisfactorily for a number of years.

PERIOPERATIVE MANAGEMENT

Anticoagulation with heparin (2000 to 10,000 units) is used intraoperatively depending on the technique of valve repair chosen. When closed techniques of valve reconstruction, such as placement of a prosthetic sleeve in situ or external valvuloplasty, are used, the lower dose of heparin may suffice. Heparin is not reversed and is continued postoperatively for 48 to 72 hours as a continuous intravenous infusion at 400 to 800 U/h in adults of average weight. Oral warfarin sodium (2.5 to 5 mg/day) is started on the first postoperative day. In patients with clotting factor abnormalities, anticoagulation should be continued indefinitely. In others, it may be stopped after 4 months. The author has found low-dose warfarin (2.5 mg/day) to be associated with a low postoperative thrombotic complication rate without prolongation of the prothrombin time. This regimen may be used indefinitely. It has the advantage of negligible bleeding complications and avoids the need for frequent prothrombin time determinations necessary with higher dosages. A pneumatic or other compression device should be used in the postoperative period to reduce postoperative swelling. Prophylactic antibiotics are routinely used and are discontinued 48 to 72 hours after surgery.

POSTOPERATIVE COMPLICATIONS

Valve reconstruction carries a low morbidity (Table 139–4). Wound complications can be minimized by the routine use of closed drainage and meticulous surgical technique.

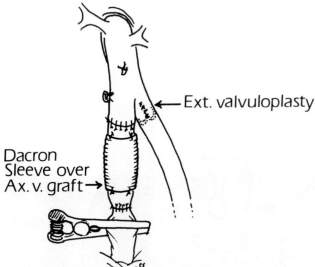

FIGURE 139 – 14. Different techniques can be combined to perform multiple venous valve reconstructions. An axillary vein (Ax. V.) transfer with a prosthetic sleeve to reconstruct the superficial femoral vein and an external (Ext) valvuloplasty of the profunda femoris venous valve are shown.

Table 139–4. Morbidity Following 107 Valve Reconstruction Procedures

Mortality	0%
Deep venous thrombosis	7%*
Infection	4%†
Wound seroma, hematoma only	5%

From Raju S, Fredericks R: Valve reconstruction procedures for non-obstructive venous insufficiency: Rationale, techniques, and results in 107 procedures with 2–8-year follow-up. J Vasc Surg 7:301, 1988.
*Reconstructed valve was involved in 2% of cases.
†Superficial vein, 2%; deep vein, 2%.

Table 139–5.   Results of Valve Reconstruction Procedures

		Postoperative Improvement*		
	Preoperative	0–12 Months	12–24 Months	>24 Months to Present
Valvuloplasty (n = 61)				
Pain	98% (60/61)	90% (54/60)	87% (52/60)	87% (52/60)
Swelling	98% (60/61)	83% (50/60)	83% (50/60)	83% (50/60)
Ulcer	66% (40/61)	85% (34/40)	75% (30/40)	63% (25/40)
Valvuloplasty/Dacron sleeve (n = 10)				
Pain	100% (10/10)	80% (8/10)	60% (6/10)	60% (6/10)
Swelling	100% (10/10)	80% (8/10)	60% (6/10)	60% (6/10)
Ulcer	60% (6/10)	83% (5/6)	50% (3/6)	50% (3/6)
Axillary vein transfer (n = 18)				
Pain	89% (16/18)	75% (12/16)	56% (9/16)	50% (8/16)
Swelling	100% (18/18)	66% (12/18)	50% (9/18)	39% (7/18)
Ulcer	72% (13/18)	69% (9/13)	46% (6/13)	46% (6/13)
Axillary vein transfer/Dacron sleeve (n = 6)				
Pain	100% (6/6)	83% (5/6)	50% (3/6)	50% (3/6)
Swelling	100% (6/6)	83% (6/6)	50% (3/6)	50% (3/6)
Ulcer	100% (6/6)	100% (6/6)	33% (2/6)	33% (2/6)
Dacron sleeve in situ (n = 12)				
Pain	100% (12/12)	100% (12/12)	83% (10/12)	83% (10/12)
Swelling	91% (11/12)	100% (11/11)	91% (10/11)	91% (10/11)
Ulcer	66% (8/12)	88% (7/8)	63% (5/8)	63% (5/8)

From Raju S, Fredericks R: Valve reconstruction procedures for non-obstructive venous insufficiency: Rationale, techniques, and results in 107 procedures with 2–8-year follow-up. J Vasc Surg 7:301, 1988.

*For stasis ulceration, improvement was defined as sustained and complete healing of the ulcer.

RESULTS

Valve reconstruction procedures carry a satisfactory long-term result (Table 139–5).[18] The results of internal valvuloplasty have been shown to be durable, with few recurrences after the first 3 or 4 years after surgery.[28] The results of axillary vein transfer are inferior,[18] for the reasons outlined previously. It may, however, be the only choice for patients in whom other reconstruction techniques are not possible because of extensive post-thrombotic valve destruction. Most patients in whom valve reconstruction is successful in healing stasis ulceration and relieving other stasis symptoms stop using support stockings.[18]

Hemodynamic Improvement

Significant improvement in postexercise pressure and recovery times has been documented after venous valve reconstruction.[18] Ambulatory venous pressure, however, does not normalize as a rule. This has been a source of skepticism about the value of valve reconstruction surgery. Determinants of ambulatory venous pressure are complex. Hitherto unappreciated is the role of the collapsible venous tube as a regulator of ambulatory venous pressure.[10] The nonlinear volume-pressure relationship in such collapsible tubes may explain the lack of improvement in ambulatory pressure despite a reduction in volumetric reflux by valve reconstruction.

References

1. Widmer LK: Peripheral Venous Disorders. Prevalence and Socio-medical Importance. Observations in 4529 Apparently Healthy Persons. Basle III Study. Bern, Hans Huber, 1978.
2. Raju S: Venous insufficiency of the lower limb and stasis ulceration: Changing concepts and management. Ann Surg 197:688, 1983.
3. Markel A, Manzo RA, Bergelin RO, Strandness DE Jr: Valvular reflux following deep vein thrombosis: Incidence and time of occurrence. J Vasc Surg 15:377, 1992.
4. Nicolaides AN, Sumner DS (eds): Investigation of Patients With Deep Vein Thrombosis and Chronic Venous Insufficiency. Los Angeles, Med-Orion Publishing Company, 1991.
5. Raju S, Fredericks R: Hemodynamic basis of stasis ulceration—A hypothesis. J Vasc Surg 13:491, 1991.
6. Bjordal RI: Pressure patterns in the saphenous system in patients with venous leg ulcers. Acta Chir Scand 137:495, 1971.
7. Raju S: Valve reconstruction procedures for chronic venous insufficiency. Semin Vasc Surg 1:101, 1988.
8. Morano JU, Raju S: Chronic venous insufficiency: Assessment with descending venography. Radiology 174:441, 1990.
9. Neglén P, Raju S: A comparison between descending phlebography and duplex Doppler investigation in the evaluation of reflux in chronic venous insufficiency: A challenge to phlebography as the "gold standard." J Vasc Surg 16:687, 1992.
10. Raju S, Fredericks R, Lishman P, et al: Observations on the calf venous pump mechanism: Determinants of post-exercise pressure. J Vasc Surg 17:459, 1993.
11. Raju S, Fredericks R: Venous obstruction: An analysis of 137 cases with hemodynamic, venographic and clinical correlations. J Vasc Surg 14:305, 1991.
12. Subcommittee on Reporting Standards in Venous Disease, Ad Hoc Committee on Reporting Standards, Society for Vascular Surgery/North American Chapter, International Society for Cardiovascular Surgery: Reporting standards in venous disease. J Vasc Surg 8:172, 1988.
13. Neglén P, Raju S: A rational approach to detect significant reflux using duplex Doppler scan and air plethysmography. J Vasc Surg 17:590, 1993.
14. van Bemmelen PS, Bedford G, Beach K, Strandness DE Jr: Quantitative segmental evaluation of venous valvular reflux with duplex scanning. J Vasc Surg 10:425, 1989.
15. Raju S: New approaches to the diagnosis and treatment of venous obstruction. J Vasc Surg 4:42, 1986.
16. Raju S, Fredericks R: Evaluation of methods for detecting venous

reflux: Perspectives in venous insufficiency with descending venography. Arch Surg 125:1463, 1990.

17. LePage PA, Villavicencio JL, Gomez ER, et al: The valvular anatomy of the iliac system and its clinical applications. J Vasc Surg 14:678, 1991.

18. Raju S, Fredericks R: Valve reconstruction procedures for non-obstructive venous insufficiency: Rationale, techniques, and results in 107 procedures with 2–8-year follow-up. J Vasc Surg 7:301, 1988.

19. Raju S: Axillary vein transfer for postphlebitic syndrome. *In* Bergan JJ, Kistner RL (eds): Atlas of Venous Surgery. Philadelphia, WB Saunders, 1992, pp 147–152.

20. Raju S: Multiple-valve reconstruction for venous insufficiency: Indications, optimal technique, and results. *In* Veith FJ (ed): Current Critical Problems in Vascular Surgery. 4th ed. St. Louis, Quality Medical Publishing, 1992, pp 122–125.

21. Kistner RL: Surgical repair of the incompetent femoral vein valve. Arch Surg 114:1304, 1979.

22. Sottturai VS: Supravalvular incision for valve repair in primary valvular insufficiency. *In* Bergan JJ, Kistner RL (eds): Atlas of Venous Surgery. Philadelphia, WB Saunders, 1992, pp 137–138.

23. Kistner RL: Transposition techniques. *In* Bergan JJ, Kistner RL (eds): Atlas of Venous Surgery. Philadelphia, WB Saunders, 1992, pp 153–155.

24. Kistner R: Surgical technique of external venous valve repair. Proc Straub Pacific Health Found 55:15, 1990.

25. Taheri SA, Lazar L, Elias S, et al: Surgical treatment of postphlebitic syndrome with vein valve transplant. Am J Surg 144:221, 1982.

26. Raju S: In discussion of Johnson ND, Queral LA, Flinn WR, et al: Late objective assessment of venous valve surgery. Arch Surg 116:1461, 1981.

27. DePalma RG: Surgical therapy for venous stasis: Results of a modified Linton operation. Am J Surg 137:810, 1979.

28. Kistner RL: Reflux disease: Valvuloplasty/transposition/valve transplant. Proc Straub Pacific Health Found 57:37, 1993.

140

Management of Chronic Obstructive Venous Disease of the Lower Extremity

Stephen G. Lalka, M.D.

• • •

With the realization that very significant chronic disability can be caused by obstructive venous disease, often in a relatively young vascular patient population, there has been a growing interest in venous reconstructive surgery to correct venous hypertension. In appropriately selected patients, estimated to be one third of those having deep venous insufficiency with a predominantly obstructive component, surgical management alone or in combination with more conservative methods may provide dramatic symptomatic relief.[1]

ETIOLOGY

It is usually estimated that 9 per cent of patients with deep venous insufficiency have predominantly chronic venous obstruction.[2–5] However, in a study of 29 limbs with phlebographically documented deep venous thrombosis evaluated hemodynamically 2 to 13 years later (mean, 7 years), Raju and Fredericks found that 31 per cent had insufficiency based on obstruction.[6] Of note is that the more severe symptoms were invariably associated with hemodynamic obstruction; in contrast, the patients with reflux had only mild to moderate symptoms. The overwhelming majority of cases of chronic venous obstruction result from absent or incomplete recanalization after deep venous thrombosis. This occlusive disease is commonly confined to an isolated segment of the iliac, common femoral, superficial femoral, or popliteal veins. Post-traumatic occlusion can also affect any segment of the venous system. Non-thrombotic proximal outflow obstruction at the iliofemoral level can be due to iatrogenic operative injury, pelvic tumor ingrowth or extrinsic compression, irradiation sequelae, retroperitoneal fibrosis, or left common iliac vein compression from the overlying right common iliac artery with or without associated intraluminal adhesions.[7, 8]

PATHOLOGIC ANATOMY AND PHYSIOLOGY

The natural history of a deep venous thrombosis, assuming it does not embolize, is determined by competition between fibrinolysis, organization, and recanalization.[9] These three major pathways of resolution of the thrombus may occur singly or, more frequently, in combination.[10] If clot lysis is the predominant mode of resolution, it may be complete in a matter of weeks. Indeed, findings on follow-up venography may appear essentially normal, with little or no evidence of prior clot.[10]

Recanalization of veins occluded by thrombus was demonstrated histologically by Edwards and Edwards.[11] Kwaan and Astrup found that recanalization originates in the open distal end of the venous segment.[12] Endothelial cells originate from the normal adjacent segment of vein and bring fibrinolytic activity to the thrombosed segment. This process results in phlebographically demonstrated vein wall irregularities, often with reduplicated lumina; and damage or destruction of the valves.[10] Recanalization occurs at different rates according to the anatomic site: the more cephalad the lower limb occlusion, the less likely it is to undergo recanalization. Regardless of the site, recanalization rarely occurs during the first 12 months following venous thrombosis.[13] Arenander[14] demonstrated a 95 per cent late patency rate after tibial and distal femoropopliteal thrombosis, whereas Thomas and McAllister[15] reported only a 50 per cent superficial femoral vein patency rate.

In iliofemoral thrombosis, persistent occlusion is the rule.[2, 16, 17] There are three possible explanations for this: (1) the iliac vein is commonly narrowed by a dense sheath of scar tissue, which is the end-result of an acute inflammatory periphlebitis stimulated by fresh thrombus in the iliac vein.[16, 18] (that such periphlebitis is not found to the same extent around infrainguinal deep veins may be related to the proximity of the thrombosed iliac vein to the pelvic lymph trunks); (2) iliac occlusion and absence of recanalization may be promoted by localized iliac vein stenosis occurring at the point where the left common iliac vein is crossed by the right common iliac artery at the lumbosacral junction, the so-called iliac compression syndrome (indeed, it has been observed that iliofemoral venous thrombosis is most frequently left sided, which is thought to be due to this chronic compression[16, 18]); and (3) finally, stenosis of the origin of the left common iliac vein may prevent proper recanalization by impairing the migration of endothelial cells, with their fibrinolytic capacity, from the adjacent vein wall at the open distal end of the vein segment.[12, 18, 19]

If chronic occlusion is the end-point of venous thrombosis, collateral veins develop around the area of occlusion (Fig. 140–1). The extent of collateral venous circulation decreases as the site of venous obstruction becomes more proximal.[20] Even if well-developed collaterals are present, these vessels have a higher resistance to flow than the native veins and rarely contain competent valves.[21, 22] Negus and Cockett demonstrated with femoral vein pressure measurements that phlebographically documented anatomic iliac obstruction does not correlate with functional obstruction to venous flow.[3] They found that resting venous hypertension,

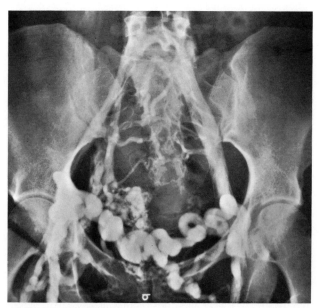

FIGURE 140–1. Chronic right iliofemoral vein occlusion with cross-pelvic venous collaterals.

exacerbated by increased venous flow with exercise, can exist with obstruction, whereas normal pressures may be obtained in other patients with similarly obstructed venous outflow. Negus and Cockett related the functional level of the post-thrombotic patient to the adequacy of collateral formation.[3]

Mavor and Galloway proposed three distinct patterns of anatomic abnormalities resulting from deep venous thrombosis (Table 140–1).[20, 23] Patients in the first group have marked skin changes and ulcerations in the lower calf but only minimal edema and minimal subjective aching and tiredness in the calf. Phlebography reveals the principal anatomic defect to be incompetent perforating veins in the calf and incompetent deep veins, with minimal residual occlusion and adequate collateral formation. Patients in the second group have significant calf and thigh swelling with marked aching and tiredness of the calf but no skin changes in the lower extremity. Their phlebograms reveal an occluded or stenotic iliofemoral segment with normal distal

Table 140–1. Clinical and Anatomic Patterns of Lower Extremity Venous Disease

	Pattern of Disease		
	Peripheral	*Central*	*Peripheral and Central*
Anatomic abnormality	Recanalized perforators and deep crural veins	Obstructed iliofemoral segment	Incompetent crural system Obstructed iliofemoral segment
Pathophysiology	Venous reflux	Venous outflow obstruction	Venous reflux and venous outflow obstruction
Major symptoms	Hyperpigmentation Ulceration	Edema Venous claudication	Stasis changes Edema Venous claudication
Therapy	Elastic support Ligation of incompetent perforators	Relief of proximal venous obstruction	Elastic support Ligation of incompetent perforators Relief of proximal venous obstruction

deep veins and perforators. Patients in the third group have the symptoms and signs of both preceding groups and, anatomically, have extensive proximal and distal deep venous disease. The actual incidence of each pattern of disease is poorly documented.

The significance of residual obstruction versus valve reflux and proximal versus distal deep venous disease in the development of the post-thrombotic syndrome remains unsettled. Pearce, Killewich, and Moore and their colleagues believe that valvular reflux involving the perforating and deep veins of the calf is the crucial factor in the development of postphlebitic signs and symptoms, as based on noninvasive vascular tests; residual proximal obstruction was not thought to play a significant role.[22, 24, 25] In contrast, Raju and Fredericks found that the more severe postphlebitic symptoms and signs (severe swelling, stasis dermatitis, or ulceration) were invariably associated with hemodynamic obstruction.[6] The anatomic site of obstruction was irrelevant; as long as the hemodynamic criteria (arm-foot venous pressure differential and venous pressure with reactive hyperemia) were met, obstruction at any level caused severe symptoms.

Nonthrombotic chronic obstructive venous disease occurs less frequently than post-thrombotic occlusion. Extrinsic compression can be caused by tumors, arterial aneurysms, or perivenous fibrosis secondary to irradiation, surgery, or retroperitoneal fibrosis. Trauma or iatrogenic surgical injury can cause short-segment venous occlusion. If there are sufficient collaterals around the obstruction, symptoms will be minimal. Irradiation, malignant disease, and retroperitoneal fibrosis often involve long segments and tend to obliterate potential collaterals. In these cases, obstructive symptoms may be severe.

Another mechanism of chronic lower extremity venous obstruction is the iliac compression syndrome, first described in 1965 by Cockett and Thomas.[26] The 3:1 predominance of left-sided iliofemoral thrombosis is explained by the peculiar anatomic relationship of the left iliac vein to the overlying right common iliac artery in its course along the pelvic rim. In addition to the extraluminal compression of the vein, fibrous adhesions or "webs" may develop within the lumen at the site of compression and produce intraluminal obstruction by binding the anterior and posterior walls of the vessel together.[7] In unselected autopsy series, the incidence of intraluminal iliac vein adhesions is 14 to 30 per cent.[7, 16, 27-30] Partial vein obstruction by this latter mechanism may be the cause of chronic mild left leg dependent edema.[7] The iliac compression syndrome may be unmasked by increased left iliac vein flow that occurs with angioaccess in the ipsilateral leg or after left pelvic renal transplantation.[31, 32]

Calnan and associates demonstrated that iliac vein compression in young girls at puberty was a consequence of the increased degree of lumbar lordosis caused by the backward tilting of the pelvis occurring at this age.[33] The L4 and L5 vertebrae are projected further forward, causing compression of the left common iliac vein between the vertebrae and the right common iliac artery. A similar mechanism may account for the bands of prevertebral fascia that were found by Connett to obstruct the left common iliac vein at its junction with the vena cava in three adolescent girls with unilateral leg edema.[34] Increased lumbar

lordosis may also be a cofactor along with compression or adhesion in other circumstances conducive to chronic venous stasis and subsequent thrombosis.[19] In the anesthetized surgical patient or the immobilized bedridden patient, the extended legs act as a powerful lever around the fulcrum formed by the patient's buttocks on the unyielding surface of the table or bed, causing a marked increase in lumbar lordosis. In the third trimester of pregnancy, the pregnant woman leans so far backward when erect in order to counter balance the forward weight of the pregnant uterus that a severe exaggeration of her lumbar lordosis is inevitable.

Three rare, nonthrombotic forms of chronic lower extremity venous obstructive symptoms caused by extravascular anatomic abnormalities are compression of the femoral vein (Gullmo's phenomenon),[35, 36] popliteal vascular entrapment,[37] and the soleal arch syndrome.[38] These may be of more phlebographic than physiologic significance. If they are found to be physiologically relevant, surgical therapy involves simple correction of the extravascular pathology.[39]

The underlying pathophysiology in all forms of chronic lower extremity venous obstruction is chronic venous hypertension. With significant deep venous obstruction as a component of chronic venous disease, the normal fall in ambulatory venous pressure is compromised. Indeed, with the most severe form of proximal venous obstruction associated with poorly developed collaterals, venous pressure may actually *increase* during exercise as outflow is impeded (Fig. 140–2). A detailed discussion of the pathophysiology of chronic venous disease is presented in Chapter 138.

DIAGNOSIS

The two most common signs and symptoms of segmental venous occlusive disease of the lower extremity are edema and pain on ambulation.[23] The edema resulting from proximal venous obstruction involves the entire lower extremity and is usually greater than that in patients with peripheral deep vein incompetence alone. Those who experience severe swelling within 2 to 4 hours of standing are distinguished as having a much more serious degree of venous insufficiency than those with lesser amounts of swelling noticed only at the end of the day. An occasional patient with only partial proximal obstruction may have episodic edema.

Comparison between patients with peripheral deep vein incompetence and those with outflow obstruction has shown that swelling of the affected limb in the latter group is usually less important to the patient than the exercise-induced calf pain.[18] The pain pattern of chronic obstructive venous disease is characteristic, described by the patient as a "bursting, stretching ache" with forceful exertion. Patients with peripheral deep vein incompetence alone often complain of "aching" or "heaviness" in the thigh or calf but not of pain sufficient to limit activity.[18] Because this bursting pain develops after exercise and requires the patient to be off his or her feet to obtain relief, it has been termed venous claudication by Cockett and Thomas.[26] They emphasized that it usually appears after walking at least a

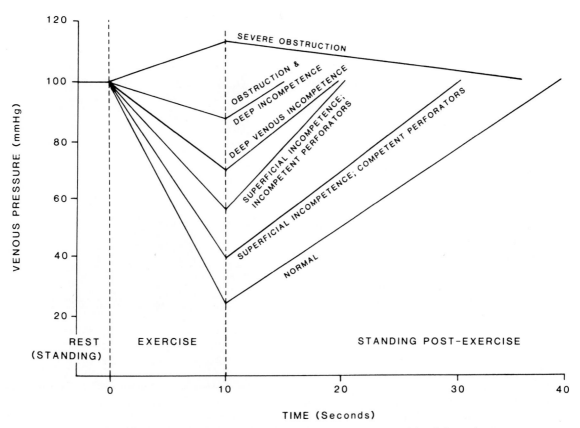

FIGURE 140–2. Ambulatory venous pressure measurements in normal and diseased states.

quarter of a mile but may occur sooner after climbing or running.[16] This was confirmed by Qvarfordt and associates, who found the claudication to be less severe than with arterial disease, with patients having a usual walking limit of 514 ± 255 m.[40] In addition, venous claudication may be accompanied by the appearance of cyanosis, a sensation of further swelling, and increased prominence of the superficial veins of the thigh. Cockett and Thomas established four criteria for the diagnosis of venous claudication: (1) leg pain with exertion, (2) iliac vein obstruction, (3) venous hypertension at rest, and (4) elevation of venous pressure with exercise.[26]

Qvarfordt and associates[40] and Christenson and colleagues[41] demonstrated that the pain in venous claudication is caused by increased intramuscular pressure, both at rest and with exercise.[40, 41] The increased pressure is apparently the consequence of increased transudation of fluid into muscle as a result of venous hypertension. The increased volume within a fasciae-enclosed compartment raises interstitial pressure and reduces capillary flow. It is postulated that the pain is mediated by Bassini's pain receptors associated with the fasciae.

The relative rarity of venous claudication despite the frequency of iliofemoral venous obstruction is thought to be due to two factors: (1) the presence of significant collaterals around an isolated iliac obstruction and (2) the fact that the symptoms occur only with vigorous exercise of the type not usually carried out by patients with chronic venous disease. In fact, these patients are usually able to carry out their normal daily activities without difficulty.[42, 43]

On physical examination, enlargement of the leg by more than 1 cm is considered a significant difference in size. A chronic difference of 2 cm or more suggests previous phlebitis in the larger leg unless another explanation is found.[44] Possible cardiac, renal, or hepatic causes should be ruled out by means of a thorough physical examination whenever bilateral edema is present. Chronic venous obstruction of the iliofemoral segment usually produces swelling of the entire lower extremity. If only the superficial femoral vein is occluded, the edema is primarily in the calf. Measurements of the circumference of both the normal leg and the abnormal leg should be taken at a constant marked position and should be done serially at a fixed time because edema may vary during the day.[23]

Stasis ulceration, hyperpigmentation, and severely swollen legs are thought by some to be uncommon with proximal venous obstruction alone, unless there is concomitant disease of the distal deep and perforating veins. Moore and associates found that obstruction played no discernible role in the severe postphlebitic syndrome.[24] Barnes and colleagues[45] and Killewich and Strandness[21] confirmed this by noninvasive testing. However, in the long-term follow-up of postphlebitic patients, Raju and Fredericks reported that severe swelling and ulceration can in fact be associated with a primarily obstructive pathology.[6, 46] The anatomic site of obstruction was irrelevant: obstruction at proximal or distal levels caused equally severe symptoms. In contrast, patients with reflux had only mild to moderate pain and swelling. Cockett and associates found in a series of 57 patients with chronic iliac vein obstruction that ulceration was rare before 5 years of symptoms but was almost always present after 15 years.[16] However, O'Donnell and associates demonstrated that these changes occurred much sooner after iliofemoral thrombosis.[47]

The various noninvasive diagnostic tests used to evaluate patients with symptomatic chronic venous disease are discussed in detail in Chapter 133. If the noninvasive tests indicate significant obstructive venous disease, venous pressure studies and phlebography are mandatory before surgical intervention. Ascending phlebography and foot venous pressure measurement can be performed at the same time, and descending phlebography and femoral venous pressure measurement can be done on a subsequent day, thus avoiding multiple percutaneous cannulations of the patient. Ascending phlebography for chronic venous insufficiency is designed to visualize the venous system distal to the inguinal ligament.[48] Descending venography is performed through the ipsilateral or contralateral femoral vein to assess the entire iliocaval system for patency and to identify extraluminal compression or intraluminal webs (Fig. 140–3). Under fluoroscopy in the 65-degree erect position, the valvular competence of the veins in the affected limb is also assessed.[49]

Cannulation of the common femoral vein allows measurement of iliac and femoral venous pressures. By the measurement of pressure gradients across intraluminal defects, partial obstruction of hemodynamic significance can be identified (Fig. 140–4). With simultaneous bilateral femoral pressure measurements, the hemodynamic significance of an iliofemoral obstruction is better delineated. According to Negus and Cockett, a significant obstruction exists if a vertical gradient of greater than 2 mmHg exists at rest or if the horizontal gradient (compared with contralateral femoral pressure) exceeds 2 mmHg (pressure measurement in the supine position) (Fig. 140–5).[3] Exercise pressures can

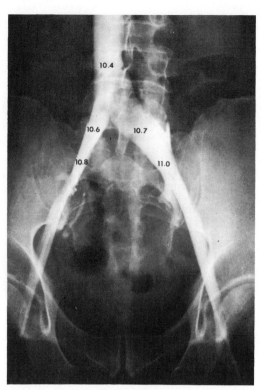

FIGURE 140–4.   Normal findings on bilateral iliac phlebography with saline manometric measurements. No horizontal or vertical venous pressure gradient (greater than 2 cm saline) is demonstrated in this patient. Note the indentation of the left common iliac vein by the overlying right common iliac artery.

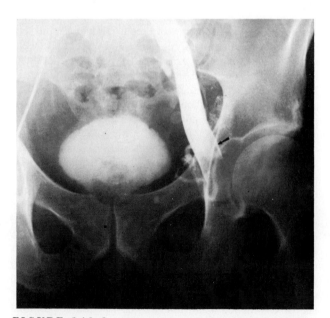

FIGURE 140–3.   Retrograde cannulation of the left common iliac vein from the right. Injection of contrast agent is coupled with a Valsalva maneuver to demonstrate intraluminal obstruction of the left common femoral vein. The *arrow* points to the rounded clot within the lumen.

be measured with a pedal ergometer while the patient is supine to detect subcritical partial obstruction that is magnified by the increase in venous flow with exercise. With this method, Negus and Cockett determined that an exercise venous pressure increase (from resting level) of greater than 3 mmHg indicated a significant proximal obstructive lesion.[3] They demonstrated that functional venous obstruction as indicated by direct pressure measurements is not present in all patients with phlebographic evidence of venous obstruction.

Raju has greatly refined the use of venous pressure measurements in the diagnosis of chronic obstructive venous disease.[46] Like Negus and Cockett, Raju found that patients with phlebographic obstruction may have normal hemodynamic function because of profuse collateral formation, whereas patients with patent but recanalized main venous channels as shown on phlebography may demonstrate significant hemodynamic abnormality. With the patient in the supine position, venous pressure is simultaneously measured in the dorsum of the foot and hand, and a resting arm-foot venous pressure differential is obtained. Next, a thigh cuff is inflated to 300 mmHg for 3 minutes and then released. This causes a foot venous pressure elevation due to the increased venous flow stimulated by reactive hyperemia. An arm-foot differential of greater than 4 mmHg and a foot venous pressure elevation of greater than 6 mmHg were found to be abnormal. Raju identified four grades of response to reactive hyperemia that were related to the arm-foot pressure differential and the extent of col-

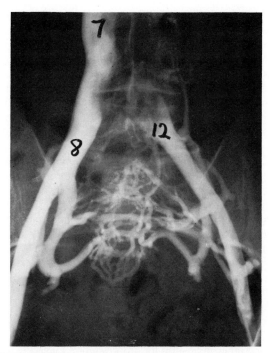

FIGURE 140–5. *Phlebogram of a young woman with long-standing edema of the left lower extremity. Near-total obstruction by the right iliac artery and the development of numerous collateral channels through the presacral plexus are evident. The superimposed numbers represent the manometric determinations at supine rest, indicating a horizontal gradient of 5 cmH₂O.*

lateralization seen on the venogram: (1) grade I (fully compensated)—normal arm-foot venous pressure differential and normal reactive hyperemia–induced venous pressure measurement (in this group, hemodynamic function was normal despite phlebographically documented obstruction due to hemodynamically adequate collaterals); (2) grade II (partially compensated)—normal arm-foot differential with abnormal response to reactive hyperemia, indicating that the collaterals were adequate at rest but insufficient during increased flow; (3) grade III (partially decompensated)—abnormal arm-foot differential and abnormal response to hyperemia; and (4) grade IV (totally decompensated)—abnormally elevated arm-foot differential and absent reactive hyperemia–induced venous pressure increase due to severely inadequate collaterals even at rest.[46] Raju concluded that large profuse collaterals on venograms can be hemodynamically inadequate owing to the presence of stenosis or other high-resistance areas not readily seen with phlebography. Such precise venous pressure studies are necessary to identify which patients will benefit from venous reconstructive surgery. Postoperatively, such pressure studies are required to assess the efficacy of various therapeutic modalities.

SURGICAL MANAGEMENT

Reconstructive surgery in the venous system has lagged far behind arterial repair despite the fact that there are 10 times as many sufferers of chronic venous disease as of symptomatic arterial disease.[50, 51] Vascular surgeons in general have had less enthusiasm for venous reconstruction and have opted for more conservative management, primarily consisting of elevation, elastic stocking compression, and ablative surgical techniques.[52] Depending on the patient's age, level of activity, and severity of deep venous insufficiency, these conservative measures may indeed be adequate. However, such a conservative approach has left a significant number of "venous cripples" who are young and active, relative to the patients with arterial disease.[53] Of patients with chronic deep venous insufficiency, it is estimated that 3 per cent have chronic obstructive disease amenable to surgical reconstruction.[1]

Experimental venous grafts in animals have revealed problems unique to venous surgery and have established technical principles for venous reconstruction. Autogenous vein grafts have been found to have uniformly greater patency than prosthetic grafts.[54–56] Increasing graft flow with an adjunctive arteriovenous fistula has been reported to improve graft patency.[57–59] Technical errors, which might be tolerated in the arterial system, will cause thrombosis of venous grafts.[23]

Experimental success with grafts in the venous system led to scattered clinical application. In 1953, Kunlin reported a brief success (3-week patency) with a saphenous vein bypass of an obstructed external iliac vein in a patient with postphlebitic syndrome.[60] Warren and Thayer (1954) described a saphenopopliteal bypass for the postphlebitic limb.[61] Hardin (1962) reported four cases of femorocaval bypass with saphenous vein for iliac occlusion and described venous angioplasty with lysis of intraluminal adhesions.[62] These early reports demonstrated the feasibility of direct venous reconstruction and laid the foundation for the various procedures employed presently for chronic obstructive lower extremity venous disease: cross-femoral venous bypass, in situ saphenopopliteal bypass, iliac vein decompression, femorocaval and iliocaval bypass, segmental venous replacement, and temporary arteriovenous fistula creation.

Indications

In the management of chronic venous disease, the goals are to treat the presenting symptoms and to prevent the adverse effects of continued venous hypertension on the skin and subcutaneous tissues by restoring the venous physiology of the limb to as normal a state as possible. Conservative treatment, which includes faithful (*every* day, *all* day) wearing of good-quality graded (30 to 50 mmHg at the ankle) knee-high elastic compression stockings, elevation of the legs whenever possible during the day, avoidance of any prolonged standing, nocturnal elevation by raising the foot of the bed 12 inches and propping the legs on pillows, and treatment of ulcers with medicated compression dressings, remains the first line of management and will be adequate for the overwhelming majority of patients with chronic venous disease. Conservative surgical therapy, including perforator ligation, stripping of saphenous and varicose veins, sclerotherapy, and grafting of ulcers, will provide adequate control for an additional large number of patients.[63–65] If these therapeutic modalities fail in a patient with class 3 (stage III)[66, 67] chronic venous disease, venous reconstructive surgery should be considered and the diagnostic plan as outlined previously should be instituted. Estimates of the number of patients with chronic venous insufficiency who are suitable candidates for deep venous reconstruction range from 1 to 5 per cent.[1, 63, 64] However, Kistner has found that in the subgroup of patients who have severe venous insufficiency (i.e., those with recurrent venous ulcers or disabling pain that has been resistant to conventional management), as many as two thirds of the patients can benefit from detailed diagnosis and aggressive surgical management.[64]

Cross-Femoral Venous Bypass

Segmental venous obstruction of the iliofemoral system can be bypassed by a crossover femoral vein–femoral vein graft. Palma and Esperon and their colleagues reported the first successful cross-femoral graft procedure in 1958.[68, 69] The technique was popularized in the United States by Dale.[70] This is the most frequently performed reconstructive procedure for chronic obstructive venous disease.

Patient Selection

The most suitable cases for a cross-femoral venous bypass involve persistent isolated unilateral iliac or common femoral vein occlusions in young and middle-aged patients with severe chronic deep venous insufficiency unresponsive to conservative measures. The venous outflow obstruction should be phlebographically and hemodynamically stable or worsening and of at least 1 year's duration, suggesting that no further resolution is likely to occur by recanalization.[61, 71] Venous claudication with appropriate anatomic and physiologic evidence of iliac obstruction is an indication for bypass surgery only in those patients with active enough lifestyles to elicit the pain on a regular basis. Consideration must be given to preceding or supplementing direct venous reconstructive surgery with conventional procedures such as perforator ligation and removal of superficial varicosities because the evidence shows that venous reconstruction alone is inadequate to cure a patient with severe deep venous insufficiency.[1, 63]

Vollmar has identified several prerequisites for an increased chance of success of cross-femoral grafts:[8] (1) patent contralateral iliofemoral and caval runoff; (2) the presence of a supine resting pressure gradient in excess of 4 to 5 mmHg between the femoral veins in the involved and contralateral limbs; (3) an adequate distal venous system: that is, a patent profunda femoris vein, preferably with an open or a partially recanalized superficial femoral vein; and (4) a patent, competent greater saphenous vein on the recipient (runoff) side with a minimal diameter of 4 to 5 mm and no varicosities. Gruss and associates found that a marked improvement in their results came with the introduction of venous pressure measurements to assess the functional efficacy of a reconstructive procedure, compared with their former sole reliance on phlebography, which provided evidence only of technical operability.[72, 73] They found that 10 per cent of patients with a post-thrombotic syndrome were operable according to phlebography,

whereas only one third of these patients should have reconstruction according to their venous function.[74] The main technical obstacle to reconstruction is the destroyed femoral vein with multiple septa resulting from recanalization in combination with poor outflow.[75]

A second, less frequent type of candidate for cross-femoral venous bypass is a patient with the subacute onset of progressive severe leg swelling secondary to extrinsic disease affecting one iliac vein. Diagnostic studies such as proctosigmoidoscopy and barium enema, computed tomography, cystoscopy, and intravenous pyelography should be performed. If the results of these studies are normal, lymphangiography should be considered in order to rule out a lymphoma. If the cause of vein compression is lymphoma, subsequent irradiation or chemotherapy may dramatically improve the extrinsic compression. If cervical, colonic, ovarian, prostatic, or bladder carcinoma is found, cross-femoral bypass should be performed, under the same anesthesia, for palliation if survival is estimated to be at least 6 months. The bypass should also be performed if the extrinsic compression is found to be due to periadventitial scarring from prior surgery, irradiation, or retroperitoneal fibrosis.[23]

One other indication for cross-femoral bypass is in the acute limb-threatening situation of phlegmasia cerulea dolens for which venous thrombectomy has failed to relieve the iliofemoral obstruction.[76] The rationale behind this approach is to perform reconstruction before the patency of the thrombectomized femoral vein and the competence of its delicate valves have been irreparably damaged by post-thrombotic changes.[75]

Operative Technique

The operative technique for cross-femoral vein bypass is demonstrated in Figure 140–6. If intra- or extraperitoneal exploration was initially undertaken for diagnosis of tumor, that incision should be closed, the instruments changed, and the patient and surgeons reprepared.[23]

General or spinal anesthesia can be used. Low-molecular-weight dextran (dextran 40 as a 1 ml/kg infusion over the first hour and then 20 ml/hr thereafter) is begun at the start of the case. The procedure may be performed with prosthetic graft (ringed polytetrafluoroethylene [PTFE]) or saphenous vein.

The first step with use of the saphenous vein is exposure of the donor greater saphenous vein in the leg contralateral to the iliofemoral obstruction. The saphenofemoral junction is first carefully exposed, and all branches are isolated and preserved. The vein is carefully exposed from the groin to the knee. The vein is left in situ, the adventitia is infiltrated with papaverine to relieve the spasm from dissection, and the vein is covered with an antibiotic-soaked sponge.

Next, a vertical groin incision is made in the affected limb, and the common femoral, proximal superficial femoral, and deep femoral veins; the saphenofemoral junction; and all other femoral branches in the field are exposed and encircled with vessel loops. To avoid such difficult dissection and to preserve every possible collateral, Dale dissects only the anterior 180 degrees of the common femoral vein in the affected limb and uses a U-shaped vascular clamp to

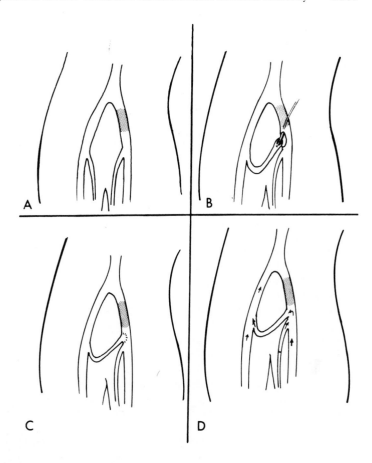

FIGURE 140–6. Technique of crossover saphenous vein grafting. *A*, The left ilofemoral segment is obstructed. *B*, The contralateral competent saphenous vein has been passed subcutaneously across the pubis to the left groin. *C*, An end-to-side anastomosis has been completed. *D*, Venous flow from the left leg crosses through the graft to the right iliac system. (*A–D*, Adapted from Dale WA: Chronic iliofemoral venous occlusion including 7 cases of cross-over vein grafting. Surgery 59:117, 1966.)

perform the anastomosis without complete dissection of the posterior aspect of the femoral vein.[77] In post-thrombotic proximal obstruction, the common femoral and superficial femoral veins should be dissected distally until a patent segment is found.[23] Palma and Esperon carried dissection caudally until a totally patent segment was reached, even if this necessitated anastomosis with the subsartorial femoral vein or the popliteal vein.[69]

If a prosthetic graft is to be used, the saphenous vein in the donor limb is left undisturbed and a vertical groin incision is used to expose the (outflow) common femoral vein.

A subcutaneous tunnel is dissected suprapubically between groin incisions. A moistened umbilical tape is used to measure the distance from the saphenofemoral junction of the outflow side, through the tunnel, and caudally to what appears to be a patent segment of vein on the inflow side; the length of outflow saphenous vein is then checked. After the dissections have been completed and inspected to ensure hemostasis, the patient is heparinized with a 100-U/kg bolus. (Heparin monitoring with activated clotting time is advisable.) The tributaries of the inflow femoral vein are controlled with vessel loops, the main femoral vein is controlled proximally and distally with soft-jaw vascular clamps, and an anteromedial longitudinal venotomy is made that is 1.5 to 3 times the diameter of the saphenous vein or prosthetic graft.[23, 78] A 2- to 5-mm ellipse of vein wall is removed. Sometimes the femoral vein at the site of anastomosis has intraluminal webs resulting from recanalization. The webs can be excised in the area of the anasto-

mosis as long as there is adequate inflow into this segment of vein.

The outflow saphenous vein is not dissected distally until after the femoral venotomy has been made on the involved side, in order to avoid having too short a vein graft. The vein graft length is again rechecked with the umbilical tape technique. The saphenous vein is then transected distally, and the caudal stump is suture ligated. The vein is then carefully filled with cold dilute heparin-saline-papaverine solution to locate any missed branches or areas of kinking due to adventitial bands. These bands are lysed under loupe magnification, and branches are ligated; missed branches with minimal stumps are carefully suture ligated with 6–0 polypropylene. The vein is rotated medially and passed through the subcutaneous tunnel, avoiding twisting or kinking. The saphenous vein is anastomosed to the affected common femoral vein either side-to-side (if an Edwards skip fistula is to be constructed[79]) or end-to-side with standard vascular surgery techniques. If prosthetic graft is used, the graft is anastomosed to both common femoral veins with the use of standard vascular surgery techniques. (The preferred graft is a 10-mm ringed PTFE, and the rings should be incorporated into the anastomoses.) Most authors recommend the creation of an adjunctive arteriovenous fistula with cross-femoral vein bypass (adjunctive arteriovenous fistulae are discussed in a later section).

An operative phlebogram, femoral venous pressure measurements, and duplex studies should be obtained. The heparin should not be reversed with protamine. All wounds should be closed in layers, with the placement of closed suction drains that remain for a maximum of 48 hours. Dextran 40 is continued for 36 hours. Heparin is restarted at 24 hours, and the dextran is stopped when the partial thromboplastin time exceeds 1.5 times control. Sodium warfarin (Coumadin) is begun when the patient is adequately anticoagulated with heparin and is continued as long as the graft is patent. Heparin is stopped after 5 days of concomitant heparin and warfarin therapy if the prothrombin time exceeds 1.3 times control. An intermittent pneumatic compression device is used to increase lower extremity venous flow while the patient is on bed rest for 72 hours. After this, the patient ambulates wearing elastic compression stockings.

In cases of venous reconstruction for acute iliofemoral venous thrombosis, Eklöf obtains a cannula phlebogram the day after iliofemoral thrombectomy (with arteriovenous fistula).[75] If this shows complete obstruction of the iliac vein with poor collateral capacity and the leg is severely swollen, the obstructed leg is revascularized with femorofemoral crossover bypass grafting using a 12-mm stented PTFE graft, with flow augmented by the previously constructed arteriovenous fistula. Anticoagulation is continued as long as the graft is patent. The adjunctive fistula is maintained for a much longer time than after thrombectomy (as long as 26 months in one case in which the graft remained patent at the 36-month follow-up visit).[75]

Results

Postoperatively, graft patency can be assessed with duplex scanning. Radionuclide venograms should be obtained at 1 month and then every 3 months for the 1st year, after which time conventional contrast venograms can be obtained with low risk of thrombosis.[80] Morano and Burkhalter described a useful method for evaluating venous graft patency while an adjunctive arteriovenous fistula remains open.[81] This technique involves simple foot venipuncture, temporary lower extremity venous occlusion with a thigh cuff during injection of contrast, and digital subtraction angiography during and after release of the cuff to opacify the graft with the rapid bolus of contrast. Halliday and associates found that serial venography is the only reliable method of postoperative follow-up of femorofemoral grafts because they could not distinguish between the patent graft and well-developed venous collaterals using Doppler ultrasonography or impedance plethysmography.[1] Eklöf has also found Doppler ultrasonography to be unreliable for assessing graft patency.[75]

In the most thorough study in the literature, involving 47 patients who underwent cross-femoral venous bypass, Halliday and associates found that 89 per cent of the grafts were clinically patent at 5 years, compared with a 75 per cent cumulative venographic patency.[1] The patients whose grafts were incorrectly thought to be patent clinically were shown to have either large venous collaterals or recanalized iliac veins on venography. The authors proposed that although recanalization of the iliac venous segment was uncommon, a slowly occluding cross-femoral graft may allow sufficient time for recanalization to occur silently or for collaterals to develop, so that the improvement gained with the bypass graft was not completely lost. Although early graft patency was found to be better in patients with normal

superficial femoral veins than in those with abnormal or occluded veins, there was no significant difference at 5 years.[1] Most patients with disabling venous claudication had relief of their symptoms, but return of their complaints suggested a stenosing graft, which was confirmed by venography. Those patients with minimal post-thrombotic changes in the calf but with disabling symptoms during exercise had the best clinical response to surgery. Resolution of venous ulceration was correlated with graft patency. Twenty-four patients with moderate to severe symptoms without ulceration did not require further surgical treatment to control their venous disease. There were no wound infections or hematomas, 6 per cent had recurrent venous thrombosis, and there was a 2 per cent incidence of postbypass pulmonary embolism. Although thrombosed venous grafts have been shown to recanalize in animal models and occasionally in clinical applications, Halliday and associates could not document recanalization of an occluded graft in their series.[1, 82] Using directional Doppler flow monitoring, they did document dilatation of the bypass over time, indicating that the valves in the transposed saphenous vein segment could become incompetent secondary to the dilatation.[1]

Dale reported a 75 per cent continuing patency in his cross-femoral bypass group, with excellent clinical results in 63 per cent and good results in 17 per cent, and a 20 per cent failure rate.[83] Husni reported a 180-month follow-up on 71 cross-femoral bypasses without, and 12 additional bypasses with, adjunctive arteriovenous fistulae, in which patency rates of 72 to 78 per cent, respectively, were achieved, with a 74 per cent clinical improvement.[84] Both Husni[84] and Dale[83] have observed that patients with extrinsic occlusion of iliac veins by tumor seemed to achieve greater symptomatic relief than patients who had major deep venous thrombosis as the indication for their surgery. Husni showed in properly selected patients that varicose vein stripping and perforator ligation enhance the clinical results.[84]

Danza and associates reported on 27 symptomatic patients with iliac vein thrombosis who underwent the standard Palma procedure (8 patients) or a modified Palma technique using a free femorofemoral saphenous vein graft (19 patients).[85] Their modified technique avoids the torsion that may occur when the proximal saphenous vein is left attached to the femoral vein. With this modified technique, 12 patients (63 per cent) had excellent results, 4 patients (21 per cent) had good results, and 3 patients (16 per cent) had no improvement. This is in contrast to the patients undergoing the standard Palma procedure, of whom only 3 (37.5 per cent) had excellent results, 3 (37.5 per cent) had good results, and 2 (25 per cent) had poor results.

Gruss reported on 23 crossover femoral venous grafts using PTFE conduits (8 or 10 mm) with adjunctive arteriovenous fistulae.[86] Twenty grafts maintained long-term patency; all patients with functioning grafts were free of subjective symptoms and did not require the use of elastic compression stockings.

O'Donnell and associates published one of the few long-term, detailed hemodynamic and anatomic follow-up studies of saphenous cross-femoral venous bypass grafts.[87] Their sequential study, which used impedance plethysmography to assess the degree of proximal venous resistance and light reflection rheography to determine the degrees of both venous reflux and venous emptying, confirmed the durability of a cross-femoral bypass procedure for relief of symptoms from iliac vein obstruction.

Additional reports in the literature on the clinical results with saphenous vein cross-femoral bypass grafts are presented in Table 140–2; the use of adjunctive arteriovenous fistulae varied in these series.

Saphenopopliteal Bypass

Venous reconstructive surgery to transpose the saphenous vein into the popliteal vein in order to bypass isolated occlusion of the femoropopliteal segment was first introduced by Warren and Thayer in 1954,[61] then revived by Husni, May, and Frileux and associates in the early 1970s.[88–90] This procedure is based on the principle that the calf muscle pump acts almost exclusively on the deep venous system to empty the leg. Thus, a new outflow connecting the deep system distally and proximally would provide relief from post-thrombotic venous hypertension.[72]

Patient Selection

Saphenopopliteal bypass is performed only if the following six conditions are met:[23, 91] (1) there is isolated occlusion of the superficial femoral vein, the popliteal vein, or both in the presence of patent tibial veins (inflow); (2) the common femoral and iliocaval systems (outflow) are patent; (3) the patient has a patent nonvaricosed saphenous vein unaffected by previous phlebitis (this is the most significant factor that limits this operation because the saphenous vein is so frequently affected either primarily or secondarily in deep venous insufficiency or else has been removed for cardiac or peripheral arterial surgery); (4) femoral phlebitis has been inactive for at least 1 year; (5) elevated ambulatory venous pressure exists: that is, after exercise (10 tiptoes or 10 knee bends), venous pressure on the occluded side should not drop by more than one third of the resting pressure on the contralateral side; and (6) compression and ablative surgery have failed to relieve

severe symptoms of deep venous insufficiency. The diagnostic evaluation should be the same as for a cross-femoral bypass, including noninvasive testing as well as phlebography and venous pressure studies.

Operative Technique

With the patient under either general or spinal anesthesia and with dextran 40 begun at the start of the case, a medial incision is made in the proximal calf immediately posterior to the medial border of the tibia, and the saphenous vein is carefully exposed without creation of a flap (Fig. 140–7). Intraoperative exposure of the saphenous vein is made easier by preoperative marking with indelible ink (using duplex imaging). The saphenous vein is mobilized over a distance of approximately 10 cm to provide enough length to allow it to lie in a gentle curve in its course to the popliteal anastomosis. The crural fascia is then incised, the gastrocnemius and soleus muscles are retracted posteriorly, and approximately 4 cm of popliteal vein is exposed. Occasionally, the posterior tibial veins are the most cephalad uninvolved vessels, and the dissection must expose them.[23] The popliteal vessels, the tibial vessels, or both are mobilized. When hemostasis in the dissection has been ensured, heparin (100 U/kg) is given systemically (intraoperative activated clotting time monitoring is helpful). After the tributaries to the inflow site have been controlled with vessel loops or micro-occlusion clips, a longitudinal venotomy 1.5 to 3 times the diameter of the saphenous vein is made in the anteromedial popliteal-tibial segment, and a 1-mm ellipse of vein is excised. The saphenous vein is transected only after the exact length required has been determined (with the knee in the extended position). The saphenous vein is carefully brought down to the recipient vein (without twisting or kinking) and anastomosed end-to-side to the popliteal-tibial vein using standard vascular surgical techniques. A generous window of gastrocnemius-soleus fascia is excised to avoid compression of the transposed vein graft. Both Bergan and coworkers[63] and Dale[71] described a side-to-side saphenopopliteal anastomosis; however, that technique is made possible only when the saphenous vein is elongated, as in the postphlebitic leg, allowing a side-to-

Table 140–2. Clinical Results With Saphenous Vein Crossover Grafting

Study	No. of Patients	Extrinsic Compression	Postphlebitic Syndrome	Results		
				Excellent	Good	Poor
Palma and Esperon, 1960[69]	7	0	7	4	2	1
Husni, 1981[150]	82	4	78	50	12	20
Frileux et al, 1972[88]	12	0	12	2	0	10
Riahi and Monafo, 1971[151]	5	2	3	3	1	1
Wagner et al, 1973[152]	14	0	14	9	4	1
Dale, 1979[71]	48	20	28	28	9	11
Aratzanov and Misev, 1976[153]	29	0	29	17	9	3
May, 1981[128]	66	0	66	48	0	18
Vollmar, 1977[8]	11	0	11	9	0	2
Raju, 1986[46]	8	0	8	2	1	5
O'Donnell et al, 1987[87]	6	0	6	5	1	0
Gruss, 1991[86]	15	0	15	10	0	5
Totals	303	26	277	187 (62%)	39 (13%)	77 (25%)

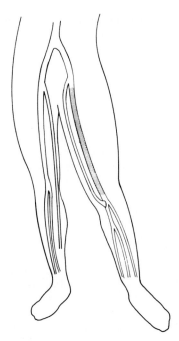

FIGURE 140–7. Completed in situ saphenopopliteal anastomosis for superficial femoral venous obstruction.

side anastomosis without tension. Annous and Queral reported 18-month patency in a case of mid-thigh superficial femoral vein occlusion for which a distal superficial femoral–greater saphenous bypass with an end-to-side anastomosis was performed.[92] The authors believed that such a configuration had an advantage over the typical saphenopopliteal bypass because the saphenous outflow collateral pathway was not interrupted and there was redirection of the total drainage of the popliteal vein into the saphenous vein.

If incompetent distal perforators have been diagnosed preoperatively, these should be ligated through a separate distal medial or posterior medial incision after the completion of the saphenopopliteal bypass.[23] An adjunctive arteriovenous fistula can also be performed, but the literature is less clear on its value in this procedure compared with cross-femoral bypass. Intraoperative and postoperative anticoagulation and serial graft surveillance techniques are the same as for cross-femoral bypass.

Results

Both Husni[84] and Dale[77] reported a 60 per cent patency rate in a combined total of 40 saphenopopliteal bypasses. Gruss reported on 14 operations (5 without and 9 with peripheral adjunctive arteriovenous fistulae).[91] Of the 14 patients with standard saphenopopliteal bypass, 3 developed postoperative thrombosis and continued to suffer severe venous hypertension symptoms. Four patients with patent bypasses exhibited worsening of their venous pressure and volumetric curves, which reverted to preoperative levels. Seven patients with patent grafts showed lasting improvement of function 10 to 15 years postoperatively despite varicose degeneration in two of these grafts. Gruss emphasized two important points: (1) the transposed saphenous vein can develop varicose degeneration without decreased function and (2) deterioration of function can occur despite having a phlebographically intact bypass graft.[91]

In rare cases of combined iliac and superficial femoral occlusion, a saphenopopliteal bypass can be combined with a cross-femoral bypass. Gruss reported long-term patency (11 and 16 years) in only two of five of such reconstructions.[91] Of the patients with graft thrombosis, all three had occlusion of the saphenopopliteal bypass but continued patency of the cross-femoral bypass.

A review of additional reports on the efficacy of saphenopopliteal bypass is presented in Table 140–3.

Obstruction of the popliteal vein and its tributaries more distally with inefficient perforator collaterals has been managed by Raju with direct saphenous vein–posterior tibial anastomosis.[46] Four of six patients had long-term graft patency with symptom resolution. In two cases, the "perforator bypass" thrombosed postoperatively but recanalized later to establish a useful outflow.

Iliac Vein Decompression

Cockett and Thomas first described the iliac compression syndrome in 1965 and then subsequently reported on

Table 140–3. Clinical Results With In Situ Saphenopopliteal Bypass

Study	No. of Patients	Results	
		Improved	*Unimproved*
Husni, 1979[89]	26	20	6
Frileux et al, 1972[88]	23*	15	2
May, 1972[148]	16	14	2
Totals	65	49 (75%)	10 (15%)

Six patients (10%) were lost to follow-up.

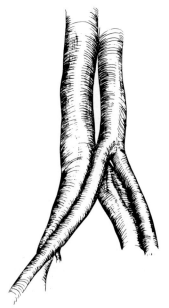

FIGURE 140–8. Anatomy of the iliocaval confluence, with the right iliac artery directly compressing the left iliocaval junction. This point directly overlies the most acutely lordotic portion of the sacral promontory.

its successful surgical management.[26] The problem is chronic compression of the left common iliac vein against the pelvic brim by the overlying right common iliac artery (Figs. 140–8 and 140–9). In approximately one fourth of the patients, intraluminal webs or adhesions form in the iliac vein, and surgical therapy requires not only relieving the compression but also excising the adhesions.

Patient Selection

The iliac compression syndrome is usually found in young women (2nd to 4th decade) who present with progressive leg edema.[23, 26] The edema may rarely involve both extremities, with the right side involvement related to (1) impingement on the right iliac vein by the crossing right iliac artery or (2) the development of collateral channels from the more severely compressed left side to the right, creating a relative flow overload and outflow obstruction on the right.[23]

Diagnostic tests include noninvasive, phlebographic, and venous pressure studies, as previously described (Fig. 140–10). In patients with the iliocaval compression syndrome, maximal venous outflow as determined by plethysmography may be within normal limits at rest or after exercise. Ambulatory venous pressure studies are required to identify those patients with inadequate venous collaterals. In the experience of Taheri and associates, ascending phlebography outlined the pelvic venous anatomic characteristics of the iliocaval compression syndrome in 90 per cent of patients; in the other 10 per cent, the syndrome was confirmed by transbrachial descending phlebography.[93]

Early operation is recommended in order to alleviate the primary problem of outflow obstruction before the

lower extremity sequelae of chronic venous hypertension ensue.[93] The basic approach is a direct repair of the involved segment. Contraindications are active thrombophlebitis or an occluded or severely stenotic iliac segment.[23] In the latter case, a cross-femoral bypass would be the most appropriate therapy.

Operative Technique

Through a transperitoneal abdominal incision, either mid-line or right transverse, the following vessels are exposed: the distal aorta, the distal half of the infrarenal vena cava, the entire common iliac artery and vein bilaterally, the hypogastric artery and vein bilaterally to below the superior gluteal branches, and the external iliac artery and vein bilaterally.[7, 94] The entire right common iliac artery is skeletonized, mobilized, and retracted to the left to expose the usual site of iliac vein compression (Fig. 140–11). After the pathology has been confirmed, the right internal iliac artery is dissected, and the superior gluteal branch is transected between suture ligatures. Next, the middle sacral and lowermost pair of lumbar arteries are likewise ligated and divided. This dissection mobilizes the distal aorta and left common iliac artery origin and exposes the left iliocaval confluence. Extreme care must be taken in handling the compressed iliac vein owing to the scarring and periphlebitis and the fragility of the vein itself.[7] If on excision of the constricting perivenous scar the previously compressed

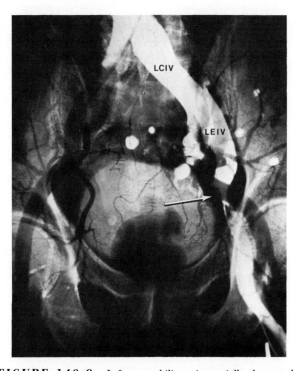

FIGURE 140–9. Left external iliac vein partially obstructed by a tortuous left external iliac artery in a man with marked swelling of the left leg. The x-ray picture was produced by superimposing the positive phlebogram on the subtracted arteriogram. The *arrow* points to the partially obstructed left external iliac vein (LEIV); the left common iliac vein (LCIV) is normal.

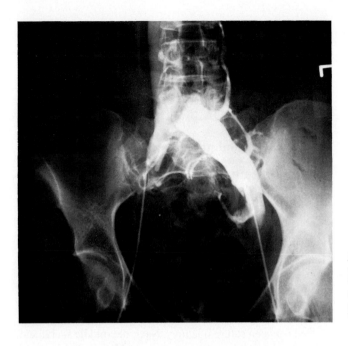

FIGURE 140–10. Iliac venous compression syndrome in a young woman, demonstrating widening of the proximal left common iliac vein, the notching created by the overlying right common iliac artery, an increased contrast density in the distal common and external iliac veins, and visualization of multiple collaterals without a Valsalva maneuver.

vein assumes a circular configuration and if no intraluminal webs were evident on preoperative phlebography, no further surgery is required. In the rare cases of presacral fibrous bands causing iliac vein compression, such perivenous excision should restore the normal luminal diameter.[34] If the normal vein diameter is not restored or if intraluminal webs are present, the vein must be entered.[23]

Skeletonization of the distal vena cava and both iliac veins is required before the left iliac vein is opened. All collateral veins are divided between ligatures so that one is able to pass a finger freely along the posterior wall of the

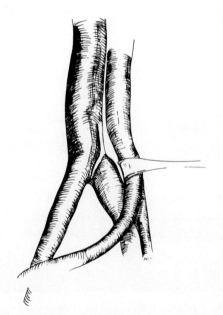

FIGURE 140–11. Leftward retraction of the artery reveals the dense fibrous band that surrounds the left iliocaval junction. This constrictive tissue presumably is a reaction to the continuous arterial pulsations, and its excision is required to allow the vein to assume a rheologically optimal circular configuration.

distal cava and down both iliac veins for a distance of at least 6 cm. After systemic heparinization, soft-jaw clamps are applied to the distal inferior vena cava and to the iliac veins just below the iliac bifurcation. The common iliac vein is opened through an anterior longitudinal incision from the iliocaval junction to the distal common iliac over the area of apparent scarring (Fig. 140–12). Several forms of intraluminal adhesions are typically encountered: (1) most commonly, there is a semi-circular septum oriented in the axis of the previously crossing right common iliac artery, and simple excision of the septum results in minimal intimal disruption and allows luminal expansion; (2) central adhesions that produce a double lumen may be present, and resection of the adhesions is required to restore luminal patency; and (3) there may be multiple intimal webs that form multiple channels, which can best be exposed and excised by retracting the vein walls with traction sutures.[23] Very careful attention must be directed to the posterior vein wall during web excision, in order to avoid inadvertent perforation. The venotomy is usually closed with a running 6–0 polypropylene suture (Fig. 140–13); however, if closure will significantly narrow the lumen, a patch angioplasty with cephalic vein (to preserve both saphenous veins) should be used to close the iliac vein. To resolve the compression problem, the right common iliac artery is isolated between proximal and distal soft-jaw clamps and is transected just proximal to the iliac bifurcation. The two ends of the artery are then transposed behind the left iliac vein and reanastomosed (Fig. 140–14).[95, 96] In the 10 per cent of cases in which the artery is too short to use this transposition technique, a Silastic Trimble bridge can be used to prevent recompression.[97] Taheri and associates described another technique, in which the right common iliac artery is transposed in a retrocaval position using an interposition autograft of the harvested right hypogastric artery to provide adequate artery length without tension on the anastomosis.[93] Intraoperative and postoperative anticoagulation and graft surveillance are as previously described.

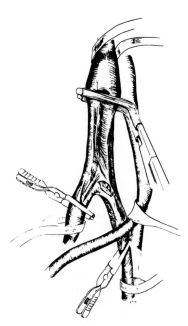

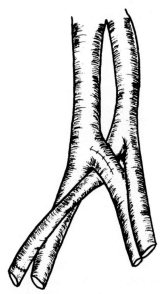

FIGURE 140–12. Total isolation of the iliocaval confluence, with a venotomy exposing intimal adhesions. Excision or lysis of these synechiae is then performed. On occasion, complete coaptation of the anterior and posterior walls may be encountered.

FIGURE 140–14. The right iliac artery has been divided just above the hypogastric artery, repositioned behind the left common iliac vein, and reanastomosed. This procedure prevents recompression of the left iliocaval confluence.

Results

A review of reported iliac decompression procedures indicates improvement in 75 to 85 per cent of cases without significant complications.[34, 93, 96, 98, 99] Selected reports of the clinical results of iliac vein decompression are presented in Table 140–4. If recompression occurs, a cross-femoral bypass should be performed.[100]

Several reports have introduced an efficacious new radiologic intervention for iliac compression syndromes.[101–103] This involves percutaneous transluminal balloon angio-

plasty with expandable intraluminal stent placement after thrombectomy or thrombolysis.

Inferior Vena Caval Reconstruction

Inferior vena caval (IVC) obstruction is an infrequent condition for which adequate surgical therapy is lacking. Although autogenous vein grafts yield the best patency rate in the venous system, they are of inadequate caliber to reconstruct the iliocaval system.[94] Large-caliber autogenous vein grafts have been created by paneling several segments of vein into a composite tube and also by constructing spiral grafts.[56, 94] However, these techniques are tedious and time consuming, and the created grafts may have a greater thrombogenic surface (because of the additional suture lines) than PTFE. The most promising solution for large vein reconstruction is a PTFE graft with external ring support and an adjunctive arteriovenous fistula (AVF).[46, 63, 104, 105] Bernstein and associates reported on IVC bypasses in animals using externally supported PTFE with a temporary (4 month) distal AVF. The overall patency was 75 per cent at 6 months (4 months after AVF closure).[104]

Patient Selection

Obstruction of the IVC can produce a severe, intractable, disabling form of chronic venous insufficiency that is not benefited by conservative compressive or ablative surgical management.[63] Patients presenting with this problem usually have a history of venous thrombosis, tumor invasion of the cava, or prior IVC interruption for pulmonary emboli. The caval obstruction is usually found to be caudal to the renal veins and frequently involves multiple skip areas.[104] The noninvasive work-up is as previously described. Venous pressure studies in addition to phlebogra-

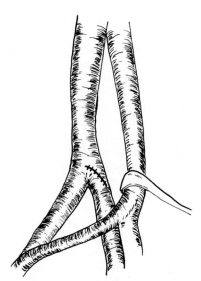

FIGURE 140–13. The iliac venotomy has been closed, the iliocaval confluence has assumed a normal circular configuration, and the lumen is uncompromised.

Table 140-4.   Clinical Results of Iliac Vein Decompression

Study	Procedure	No. of Patients	Improved	Unimproved
Cockett and Thomas, 1965[26]	Decompression only	17	13	4
	Venoplasty	9	8	1
	Venotomy and thrombectomy*	4	4	0
Connett, 1974,[34]	Decompression only	3	3	0
Dale, 1979[71]	Venotomy and patch	4	3	1
Jaszczak and Mathiesen, 1978[96]	Reposition artery behind vein	4	4	0
Rigas et al, 1970[99]	Fascia lata sling Venoplasty	8	8	0
Trimble et al, 1972[97]	Silastic bridge	14	11	3
Welter and Becker, 1981[149]	Venotomy and patch	2	2	0
Totals		65	56 (80%)	9 (14%)

Inguinal ligament obstruction of the external iliac vein in all four patients.

phy are required to document established venous hypertension amenable to iliocaval reconstruction.

Operative Technique

Through a mid-line abdominal exposure, the right colon, duodenum, and pancreas are mobilized to expose the vena cava from the suprarenal portion to the caval bifurcation. Retroperitoneal tunnels are made after exposure of the femoral veins through vertical groin incisions. Externally supported PTFE grafts 10 to 16 mm in diameter (appropriate to the diameter of the native vein) are employed.[46, 104, 105] A bifurcation can be created with a graft-graft anastomosis. Raju recommends separate femorocaval grafts for each side so that thrombosis of one graft would not jeopardize the contralateral lower extremity.[46] Bergan and coworkers believe that the suprarenal cava should be used for the proximal anastomosis because of its size and strength and because it is usually free of thrombus as long as no tumor is present.[63] Intra-, peri-, and postoperative anticoagulation are as previously described. The anastomoses are constructed using standard vascular surgery techniques. Raju incorporates the last reinforcing ring of the PTFE graft in the suture line at each end to stent the anastomoses.[46] Adjunctive femoral AVF should be employed to improve prosthetic graft patency.

Results

There are relatively few clinical reports in the literature on venous grafts for IVC occlusion. Eklöf and associates reported five iliocaval grafts (after thrombectomy), four of which were patent from 14 to 22 months.[106] Valentini and associates reported two IVC grafts that were patent at 12 and 14 months, respectively.[107] Dale reported patency of two grafts that replaced the IVC without use of an adjunctive AVF: a 14-mm ringed PTFE tube graft patent at 40 months and a 12-mm ringed PTFE bifurcated graft patent at 24 months.[105] Bernstein and associates reported 2-year patency for a right iliac vein–infrarenal IVC bypass with 10-mm ringed PTFE (with a 6-mm PTFE femoral artery–saphenous vein AV for a patient with an occluded IVC 7 years after interruption with a vena caval clip for pulmonary embolism.[104] Gloviczki and coworkers reconstructed the IVC and

its tributaries with PTFE in five patients, spiral saphenous vein grafts in two, and a Dacron conduit in one.[108] At follow-up, four of the five PTFE grafts remained patent (at 3 months and 3 years) with no symptoms. In the two patients with spiral vein grafts, the reconstruction was not successful: one graft occluded, and imaging to confirm patency of the other was inconclusive. Although the Dacron graft occluded by 3 years, the patient was only minimally symptomatic at 6 years. These investigators favor adding a temporary AVF at the femoral level to increase flow and improve graft patency.

Adjuncts to Venous Reconstruction: Prosthetic Grafts, Arteriovenous Fistulae, and Anticoagulants

Prosthetic Grafts

Grafts in the venous system, either autogenous or prosthetic, do not perform as well as their counterparts in the arterial system because of several unique characteristics of the venous environment: (1) a capacity for recanalization of native vessels with frequent formation of intraluminal adhesions, (2) low intraluminal pressure, (3) slow flow against a hydrostatic pressure gradient, (4) low oxygen tension, (5) irregular flow as a result of phasic nature and turbulence around valves, (6) thin, fragile vessel walls, and (7) a propensity for formation of large, profuse collateral pathways that can compete with and diminish flow in an implanted graft.[8, 54, 55, 109–111] The difficulty of venous surgery is emphasized in the cumulative literature review of Dale and Scott: only 60 per cent of 253 autogenous vein grafts inserted in the venous system of animals remained patent; this applied even to reimplantation of the same vein segment.[54]

Consistent problems unique to autogenous grafts in the venous system are marked anastomotic stricturing as a result of the organization of excessive fibrin and platelets at the suture lines and narrowing of the entire graft due to intense perigraft fibroblastic reaction in a low-pressure, low-flow, thin-walled, nonrigid conduit; synthetic grafts in the venous system also suffer the same fate.[8, 54, 112–114] Ijima and associates believe that cicatricial contraction occurring in the process of tissue healing after construction of the suprapubic subcutaneous tunnel for a cross-femoral bypass graft is an important factor in autologous vein graft occlusion.[115] Because of the thin, nonrigid, highly elastic vein walls, suture lines are under greater tension than in the arterial system; this adds to the tendency for anastomotic stricture.[111] To prevent excessive tension, it has been necessary to interpose a graft longer than the excised vein segment.[112]

There is unanimous agreement that the most nonthrombogenic conduit in the venous system is autogenous vein.[54, 55, 82, 105, 116] However, when autogenous vein is not available for distal vein reconstruction, or when large-diameter veins need to be replaced or bypassed, as in the common femoral iliocaval system, a prosthetic conduit (ringed PTFE) may be necessary. To prevent the anastomotic stricturing that invariably occurs in grafts in the venous system, attention initially centered on external rings to suspend the anastomotic sutures.[56, 117-120] The disadvantage of anastomotic rings was that they had a tendency to tilt and compress the vein, leading to thrombosis.[52, 56] However, experimental work by Fiore and associates with externally supported (ringed) PTFE thoracic caval grafts demonstrated the efficacy of this type of conduit in the venous position, with a patency rate equal to that of autologous vein.[121] External ring–supported PTFE has since become the venous prosthetic graft of choice.[104, 105] For caval bypass, the external ring support may also prevent graft narrowing as a result of extrinsic compression by the overlying abdominal viscera. In the subcutaneous position (cross-femoral bypass or saphenopopliteal bypass) or in the deep leg position (segmental vein replacement for trauma), the external ring support may prevent external compression.

It is generally agreed that iliocaval bypass grafts must be of PTFE because of the large-caliber vessels to be revascularized. However, controversy exists as to the preferential use of autogenous saphenous vein versus PTFE for cross-femoral venous bypass. Some investigators have noted that saphenous vein grafts often provide inadequate symptomatic relief of venous hypertension because of the high resistance of the small saphenous vein conduit.[46, 76, 122-125] One particularly tedious and time-consuming method of overcoming this problem was reported by Aschberg and colleagues, who created an AVF between the posterior tibial artery and the greater saphenous vein for 3 months until the diameter increased from 5 to 10 mm, after which the vein was used for a cross-femoral graft.[123]

The author and his associates have developed a clinically based mathematical model of unilateral iliac vein obstruction to establish a theoretical basis for selecting saphenous vein or a larger-diameter prosthetic conduit for cross-femoral bypass;[124] the validity of the mathematical model was previously confirmed by in vivo canine studies.[125] Common femoral vein resting and postexercise peak flows, and common femoral vein and saphenous vein diameters were measured in 18 healthy individuals. These measurements were used to estimate the pressure gradient across 20-cm-long cross-femoral venous bypass grafts of saphenous vein or 4-, 6-, 8-, 10-, and 12-mm prosthetic conduits, in the presence of a transpelvic venous collateral network of varied cross section. The upper limits of normal for the transfemoral pressure gradients in this model were set at 4 mmHg for resting flows and at 6 mmHg after exercise, based on clinical data.[3, 8, 126-128] The author and his associ-

ates found the mean saphenous vein diameter to be 4.3 ± 0.22 mm, which was 36.5 ± 1.73 per cent of common femoral vein diameter. When the saphenous veins of two thirds of the individuals in this study were used as theoretical cross-femoral venous bypass conduits, more than 80 per cent of postobstruction peak cross-femoral venous bypass graft flow had to be carried by collaterals to maintain a transfemoral pressure gradient within normal limits. This group demonstrated that saphenous cross-femoral venous bypass grafts 4.5 to 6.0 mm in diameter would be hemodynamically efficacious in relieving venous hypertension, but only when implanted in parallel with an existing venous collateral network that limited the preoperative transfemoral gradient to 4.5 to 7.5 mmHg at resting flows and 7.0 to 11.5 mmHg after exercise; only 44 per cent of saphenous veins were adequate for cross-femoral venous bypass grafts by these criteria. Prosthetic cross-femoral venous bypass conduits 8 mm or more in diameter eliminated venous hypertension even in the absence of collateral venous flow. After considering the cross-femoral venous pressure gradients generated by the physical dimensions of cross-femoral bypass conduits, diameter mismatch at the inflow anastomosis, wall shear stresses, and pseudointimal thickness, the author and his associates suggest that a 10-mm PTFE graft would be the most appropriate prosthetic conduit for cross-femoral venous revascularization of unilateral iliac vein occlusion.

Arteriovenous Fistulae

To avoid narrowing of venous grafts, early investigators emphasized the need to increase venous pressure. On the basis of experiments with AVFs distal to synthetic grafts, Bryant and associates in 1958 reported that elevation of intraluminal pressure to at least 37 mmHg was required for patency in the venous system.[112] Thereafter, increased pressure with an intraluminal "stenting" effect was thought necessary for improved patency in venous grafts. In 1968, Yamaguchi and associates demonstrated that remote distal AVFs minimally increased venous pressure but improved flow by 300 per cent and synthetic venous graft patency by more than 50 per cent.[59] The relatively greater importance of increased venous flow versus pressure has been confirmed by others.[58, 129, 130]

Multiple canine experiments using AVFs with short-segment venous reconstruction have been performed. Johnson and Eiseman in 1969 used a distal H-type fistula to improve venous graft patency.[131] Levin and associates reported that H-type distal fistulae were superior to side-to-side fistulae because of the more optimal direction of flow proximally through the vein graft and the smaller elevation in distal venous pressure.[132] Hobson and coworkers compared small-diameter (5 to 5.5 mm) with large-diameter (10 to 14 mm) H-type distal fistulae.[57] With the use of pressure and flow monitors, the hemodynamics of such fistulae were well delineated and confirmed the original work done by Holman and Taylor in 1952.[133] The only difference Hobson and coworkers found between small and large fistulae was the more significantly elevated distal venous pressures with the larger-diameter fistulae. Hobson and Wright later found that a peripheral distal side-to-side AVF (between muscular branches of the femoral artery and vein) augmented proximal venous flow only modestly but adequately enough for patency of the grafts; more important, the distal venous pressure was only minimally increased, hindlimb edema was avoided, and the AVF could be closed later without trauma to the venous graft.[134, 135]

The clinical application of adjunctive AVFs in venous reconstruction began with Dumanian and associates in 1968[136] and Frileux and colleagues in 1972;[88] they both reported improved patency with the addition of AVFs to cross-femoral venous bypasses. Gruss and associates in 1979,[73] Clowes in 1980,[137] and Ijima and coworkers in 1981[138] all reported success of cross-femoral venous bypasses in postphlebitic extremities using PTFE grafts with adjunctive AVFs. Adjunctive AVFs for venous reconstructive surgery, whether used with autogenous or prosthetic conduits, are now believed by many to be necessary for long-term graft patency. The minimal shunt flow required to keep both the adjunctive AVF and the bypass graft patent appears to be at least 100 ml/min if technical errors are excluded.[122, 139–141] Neglen and associates described eight patients in whom the mean fistula flow was 1.4 ± 0.2 L/min (range, 0.3 to 4.7 L/min) at the time of surgical obliteration.[140] However, even the patient with the high fistula flow had no adverse symptoms.

Various configurations of adjunctive AVFs have been used with venous reconstructions (Fig. 140–15). For IVC bypass, Bergan and coworkers anastomosed a 1- to 3-mm venous tributary of the superficial femoral vein (that crosses posterior to the superficial femoral artery and anterior to the origin of the profunda femoris artery) end-to-side to the superficial femoral artery with 7–0 monofilament suture (see Fig. 140–15A).[63] Bernstein and associates used a 6-mm PTFE graft to create a femoral artery–saphenous vein AVF; a 2–0 polypropylene suture was looped around the fistula, and the loosely knotted ends were left in the superficial subcutaneous tissue for later fistula ligation (see Fig. 140–15B).[104] For cross-femoral venous bypass, Vollmar,[8] Edwards,[79] and Halliday and associates[1] anastomosed the transposed contralateral saphenous vein side-to-side to the superficial femoral vein on the involved side and then joined the distal 3 to 4 cm of saphenous vein end-to-side to the femoral artery (see Fig. 140–15C). Gruss and associates, for both autogenous and prosthetic grafts, use a proximal branch of the ipsilateral saphenous vein for an end-to-side anastomosis to the femoral artery (see Fig. 140–15D).[72, 73] Raju described a side-to-side AVF for use with a prosthetic cross-femoral bypass (see Fig. 140–15E).[46] For saphenopopliteal bypass, Gruss creates an adjunctive AVF by an end-to-side anastomosis of the ipsilateral distal saphenous vein to the posterior tibial artery with 8–0 monofilament suture (see Fig. 140–15F).[91] The author and his associates,[142] from hemodynamic studies in their canine model of venous hypertension, have demonstrated that the peripheral caudal side-to-side AVF of Hobson and Wright[134] should be a particularly efficacious configuration; clinically, this would be represented by a side-to-side fistula between femoral artery and vein branches (Fig. 140–16).

Closure of an adjunctive AVF has been found to be technically difficult owing to the often severe desmoplastic reaction that occurs in the vicinity of venous reconstruction.

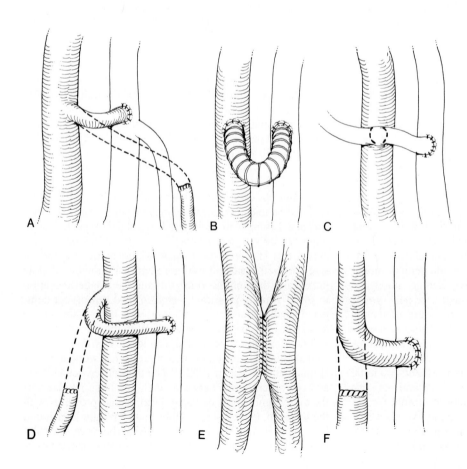

FIGURE 140–15. Configurations of adjunctive arteriovenous fistulae for venous reconstruction. *A,* Superficial femoral vein (SFV) tributary end-to-side to the superficial femoral artery (SFA). *B,* Polytetrafluoroethylene interposition graft between the SFA and SFV. *C,* Sequential or "skip" fistula: venous bypass graft side-to-side to the SFV and end-to-side to the SFA. *D,* Saphenous vein end-to-side to the SFA. *E,* Side-to-side SFA–SFV fistula. *F,* Distal saphenous end-to-side to the posterior tibial artery, which is used with saphenopopliteal bypass.

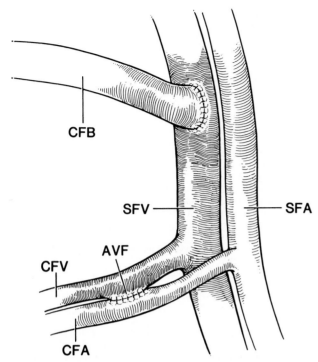

FIGURE 140–16. Peripheral caudal side-to-side arteriovenous fistula (AVF). Note that location of the fistula between femoral artery and vein branches allows closure with less risk of injury to the major vessels or the bypass anastomosis. CFB, cross-femoral bypass graft; SFV, superficial femoral vein; SFA, superficial femoral artery; CFA, circumflex femoral artery; CFV, circumflex femoral vein.

Edwards in 1982 described a simple technique to facilitate AVF ligation.[78] A heavy 0–0 nonabsorbable monofilament suture is doubly wrapped loosely around the body of the fistula. The two ends of suture are passed on a needle through the fascia to a subcutaneous position, where they are threaded through a button and loosely tied. The button is buried under the skin 2 to 3 cm medial to the vertical incision. At the time of fistula ligation, local anesthesia is used for a small skin incision over the button. The suture is untied, the button is removed, and the suture is then tied down snugly over the fascia to ligate the fistula.

Neglen and associates[140] and Endrys and colleagues[143] have introduced a percutaneous method for closure of temporary AVFs. Via entry of the contralateral femoral artery, a detachable balloon is placed in the fistula under direct radiographic control. Before inflation and detachment of the balloon, an arteriovenogram is obtained to evaluate the patency of the venous bypass graft. After release of the balloon, a repeated angiogram documents complete obliteration of the fistula.

The timing of closure of an adjunctive AVF remains unsettled. The AVF used by Bergan and coworkers for IVC reconstruction was of such small diameter that no fistula ligation was required.[63] Bernstein and associates' AVF for iliocaval bypass was closed after 3½ months.[104] Raju closes his adjunctive AVF for cross-femoral bypasses between the 1st and 3rd months.[46] Edwards[78] and Halliday and associates[1] ligate their adjunctive AVF for cross-femoral bypass at 6 weeks. Gruss and associates[72] and Vollmar[8] ligate their

AVF for cross-femoral bypass between the 2nd and 3rd months; the timing is the same for Gruss' saphenopopliteal bypasses.[91]

Bernstein and associates clearly define the controversy concerning adjunctive AVFs.[104] The benefits of the fistula are maintenance of an increased venous pressure to prevent collapse of the anastomotic suture line and higher flow velocity, which may wash away procoagulant substances and loosely adherent platelets. Because these two thrombogenic factors should not continue to be a problem after anastomotic healing is complete, AVF ligation at 3 to 6 months after venous reconstruction should be appropriate. Chronic effects of late AVF ligation include vein graft dilatation (with secondary valve incompetency) and stimulation of native venous collaterals.[78, 105] The latter effect argues for AVF ligation at an even later date. Arguments against prolonged maintenance of an AVF are that distal venous hypertension is created, causing peripheral edema and possibly caudad venous valvular incompetence. In addition, cardiac output is increased, there is a continuing threat of subacute bacterial endocarditis, and arterial ischemia may be exacerbated.[104] These facts argue for early closure of the AVF at 6 weeks.

Despite these numerous studies showing improved patency of venous reconstructions with adjunctive AVFs, their use has not become universally accepted because of the following: (1) they can be difficult to construct, (2) some types cause exacerbation of edema, (3) late ligation requires a second operation that can injure the venous reconstruction or the involved artery and vein, (4) reduction in arterial flow distal to the fistula can exacerbate arterial disease, (5) high venous pressure distal to the fistula may cause incompetency of residual valves and worsening of the venous hypertension for which the venous surgery was performed, and (6) there is a lack of consensus and sufficient experimental data on the proper time of fistula closure.[1, 57, 59, 114, 144]

The concept of ''adjunctive'' AVFs becomes even more confusing when one reviews Edwards' idea of a primary AVF between the femoral artery and vein in patients with occluded iliac veins who are not considered candidates for venous crossover grafts.[78] He had a patient whose cross-femoral bypass occluded in 10 days but whose AVF remained patent. The AVF was allowed to remain open for 2 months, after which time it was obliterated. Repeated phlebography showed enlarged pelvic collaterals, and repeated noninvasive testing showed a much less obstructive pattern. Edwards subsequently reported on two patients with primary femoral AVFs, one created with a segment of saphenous vein from the less affected leg and a second created with a 6-mm PTFE segment between the artery and the vein.[79] This work suggests that in selected patients, AVF creation without venous reconstruction is the surgical procedure of choice.

Raju performed seven posterior tibial–saphenous primary AVFs in patients with near-total obliteration of the deep venous system and outflow almost entirely by the superficial system.[46] All seven AVFs closed spontaneously a few days to several months after creation, with six of seven patients reverting to their preoperative levels of symptoms. Sawchuk and associates proposed one possible theoretical mechanism for the sustained effect of a temporary AVF: it may take more venous pressure and flow to open new or to dilate existing venous collaterals than to sustain them.[145]

Anticoagulation

The role of anticoagulant or antiplatelet therapy with venous reconstruction is also controversial. Eadie and DeTakats in 1966 reported that dextran 70 improved the patency of autogenous grafts in canine femoral vein from 8.3 per cent (controls) to 58 per cent (dextran 70); in that model, heparin was not beneficial.[113] In a similar model, Hobson and associates compared intra- and postoperative heparin with intra- and postoperative dextran 40.[146] Heparin did not improve patency, whereas there was a tendency for improved patency with dextran 40, although statistical significance was not achieved. In a study involving 3-mm PTFE segment interposition grafts in the jugular veins of rabbits, Friedman and Hamilton found that graft patency was maintained by pre- and postoperative administration of the anticoagulant warfarin or the antiplatelet agents aspirin and dipyridamole (either alone or in combination).[147] Their data suggested that without antiplatelet medication, platelet and fibrin thrombi build up on the nonendothelialized walls of the PTFE graft.

In the clinical situation, Raju presently leaves the intraoperative heparin bolus unneutralized and continues heparin at low levels (partial thromboplastin time of 1.5 times control) in the immediate postoperative period, with conversion to long-term warfarin anticoagulation on the 3rd to 5th postoperative day.[46] Gruss and associates also administer continuous heparin during the postoperative period with conversion to warfarin, which is maintained for 6 months.[72] Halliday and associates continue heparin in the postoperative period with conversion to warfarin, which is maintained for a minimum of 3 months.[1] For iliocaval decompression procedures, Taheri and associates, in addition to intraoperative systemic heparinization, use 5000 units of subcutaneous heparin 1 hour preoperatively and then every 8 hours thereafter until warfarin can be instituted and maintained for 3 months.[93] In contrast, Dale uses no adjunctive anticoagulation after the intraoperative heparinization for his venous reconstructions.[105] The anticoagulation protocol favored by the author has previously been discussed.

References

1. Halliday P, Harris J, May J: Femoro-femoral crossover grafts (Palma operation): A long-term follow-up study. *In* Bergan JJ, Yao JST (eds): Surgery of the Veins. Orlando, FL, Grune & Stratton, 1985, p 241.
2. Mavor GE, Galloway JMD: Iliofemoral venous thrombosis. Br J Surg 56:45, 1969.
3. Negus D, Cockett FB: Femoral vein pressures in post-phlebitic iliac vein obstruction. Br J Surg 54:522, 1967.
4. Raju S: Venous insufficiency of the lower limb and stasis ulceration. Ann Surg 197:688, 1983.
5. Sumner DS: Applied physiology in venous problems. *In* Bergan JJ, Yao JST (eds): Surgery of the Veins. Orlando, FL, Grune & Stratton, 1985, p 3.
6. Raju S, Fredericks RK: Late hemodynamic sequelae of deep venous thrombosis. J Vasc Surg 4:73, 1986.
7. Ellis PR, Delrosario VC: Left iliac vein "adhesions." Surgery 63:166, 1968.
8. Vollmar J: Reconstruction of the iliac veins and inferior vena cava.

In Hobbs JT (ed): The Treatment of Venous Disorders. London, MTP Press, 1977, p 320.
9. Ludbrook J: Post-thrombotic venous obstruction in the lower limb. Arch Surg 106:11, 1973.
10. Neiman HL: Venography in acute and chronic venous disease. *In* Bergan JJ, Yao JST (eds): Surgery of the Veins. Orlando, FL, Grune & Stratton, 1985, p 73.
11. Edwards EA, Edwards JE: The effect of thrombophlebitis on the venous valve. Surg Gynecol Obstet 65:310, 1937.
12. Kwaan HC, Astrup T: Fibrinolytic activity in thrombosed veins. Circ Res 17:477, 1965.
13. Bergvall U, Hjelmstedt A: Recanalization of deep venous thrombosis of the lower leg and thigh. Acta Chir Scand 134:219, 1968.
14. Arenander E: Varicosity and ulceration of the lower limb. Acta Chir Scand 112:135, 1957.
15. Thomas ML, McAllister V: The radiological progression of deep venous thrombus. Radiology 99:37, 1971.
16. Cockett FB, Thomas ML, Negus D: Iliac vein compression—Its relation to iliofemoral thrombosis and the post-thrombotic syndrome. Br Med J 2:14, 1967.
17. Luke JC: Venographic studies in the postphlebitic leg. J Cardiovasc Surg 6:411, 1965.
18. Negus D: The post-thrombotic syndrome. Ann R Coll Surg Engl 47:92, 1970.
19. DuPlessis JA: Iliac vein obstruction and the swollen leg of chronic venous stasis. S Afr Med J 42:174, 1968.
20. Mavor GE, Galloway JMD: Collaterals of the deep venous circulation of the lower limb. Surg Gynecol Obstet 125:561, 1967.
21. Killewich LA, Strandness DE Jr: The natural history of acute deep venous thrombosis. *In* Bergan JJ, Yao JST (eds): Surgery of the Veins. Orlando, FL, Grune & Stratton, 1985, p 123.
22. Killewich LA, Martin R, Cramer M, et al: An objective assessment of the physiologic changes in the post-thrombotic syndrome. Arch Surg 120:424, 1985.
23. Smith DE: Surgical management of chronic obstructive venous disease of the lower extremity. *In* Rutherford RB (ed): Vascular Surgery. Philadelphia, WB Saunders, 1984, p 1412.
24. Moore DJ, Himmel PD, Summer DS: Distribution of venous valvular incompetence in patients with the postphlebitic syndrome. J Vasc Surg 3:49, 1986.
25. Pearce WH, Ricco JB, Queral LA, et al: Hemodynamic assessment of venous problems. Surgery 93:715, 1983.
26. Cockett FB, Thomas ML: The iliac compression syndrome. Br J Surg 52:816, 1965.
27. Erich WE, Krumbhaar EB: A frequent obstructive anomaly of the mouth of left common iliac vein. Am Heart J 26:737, 1943.
28. May R, Thurner J: The cause of predominantly sinistral occurrence of thrombosis of the pelvic veins. Angiology 8:419, 1957.
29. McMurrick JP: The occurrence of congenital adhesions in the common iliac veins and their relations to thrombosis of the femoral and iliac veins. Am J Med Sci 135:342, 1908.
30. Reed DL, Gustavson RG: Anatomical factors in the etiology of "spontaneous" iliofemoral vein thrombosis. Am Surg 35:547, 1969.
31. Jacob ET, Bar-Nathan N, Heim M, et al: The "iliac vein compression syndrome" and lower limb vascular access for hemodialysis. J Cardiovasc Surg (Torino) 21:155, 1980.
32. Sorensen BL, Hald T, Nisson HM: Silent iliac vein compression syndrome as cause of renal vein thrombosis after transplantation. Scand J Urol Nephrol 6(Suppl 15):75, 1972.
33. Calnan JS, Kountz S, Pentecost BL, et al: Venous obstruction in the etiology of lymphoedema praecox. Br Med J 2:221, 1964.
34. Connett M: An anatomical basis for unilateral leg edema in adolescent girls. West J Med 121:324, 1974.
35. Gullmo A: The strain obstruction syndrome of the femoral vein. Acta Radiol 47:119, 1957.
36. Nylander G: Haemodynamics of the pelvic veins in incompetence of the femoral vein. Acta Radiol 56:369, 1961.
37. Rich NM, Hughes CW: Popliteal artery and vein entrapment. Am J Surg 113:696, 1967.
38. Servelle M, Babilliot J: Syndrome du soleaire. Phlebologie 21:399, 1968.
39. Eklöf B, Juhan C: Venous compression syndromes caused by anatomical anomalies. *In* Eklöf B, Gjores JE, Thulesius O, et al (eds): Controversies in the Management of Venous Disorders. London, Butterworths, 1989, p 291.

40. Qvarfordt P, Eklöf B, Ohlin P, et al: Intramuscular pressure, blood flow, and skeletal muscle metabolism in patients with venous claudication. Surgery 95:191, 1984.

41. Christenson JT, Al-Hassan HK, Shawa NJ: Subcutaneous and intramuscular pressures in the post-phlebitic limb. Scand J Clin Invest 46:137, 1986.

42. Killewich LA, Martin R, Cramer M, et al: Pathophysiology of venous claudication. J Vasc Surg 1:507, 1984.

43. Tripolitis AJ, Milligan EB, Bodily KC, Strandness DE Jr: The physiology of venous claudication. Am J Surg 139:447, 1980.

44. Kistner RL: Diagnosis of chronic venous insufficiency. J Vasc Surg 3:185, 1986.

45. Barnes RW, Collicott PE, Sumner DS, Strandness DE Jr: Noninvasive quantitation of venous hemodynamics in the post-phlebitic syndrome. Arch Surg 107:807, 1973.

46. Raju S: New approaches to the diagnosis and treatment of venous obstruction. J Vasc Surg 4:42, 1986.

47. O'Donnell TF, Browse NL, Bernand KG, Thomas ML: The socioeconomic effects of an iliofemoral venous thrombosis. J Surg Res 22:483, 1977.

48. Rabinov K, Paulin S: Roentgen diagnosis of venous thrombosis in the leg. Arch Surg 104:134, 1972.

49. Kistner RL: Venous valve surgery. In Bergan JJ, Yao JST (eds): Surgery of the Veins. Orlando, FL, Grune & Stratton, 1985, p 205.

50. Dale WA: Venous bypass surgery. Surg Clin North Am 62:391, 1982.

51. McLachlin AD, Carroll SE, Mead GE, Amacher AL: Valve replacement in the recanalized incompetent superficial femoral vein in dogs. Ann Surg 162:446, 1965.

52. Kunlin MJ, Kunlin A: Experimental venous surgery. In May R (ed): Surgery of the Veins of the Leg and Pelvis. Philadelphia, WB Saunders, 1979, p 37.

53. Bergan JJ, Flinn WR, Yao JST: Venous reconstructive surgery. Surg Clin North Am 62:399, 1982.

54. Dale WA, Scott HW: Grafts of the venous system. Surgery 53:52, 1963.

55. Haimovici H, Huffert PW, Zinicola N, Steinman C: An experimental and clinical evaluation of grafts in the venous system. Surg Gynecol Obstet 131:1173, 1970.

56. Shore JM, Greenstone SM, Massell TB, et al: A comparative study of canine venous autografts: The influence of graft diameter and external anastomotic support. J Cardiovasc Surg 6:67, 1964.

57. Hobson RW, Croom RD, Swan KG: Hemodynamics of the distal arteriovenous fistula in venous reconstruction. J Surg Res 14:483, 1973.

58. Stansel HC: Synthetic inferior vena cava grafts. Arch Surg 89:1096, 1964.

59. Yamaguchi A, Eguchi S, Iwasaki T, Asano K: The influence of arteriovenous fistulae on the patency of synthetic inferior vena caval grafts. J Cardiovasc Surg 9:99, 1968.

60. Kunlin MJ: The re-establishment of venous circulation with grafts in cases of obliteration from trauma or thrombophlebitis. Mem Acad Clin 79:109, 1953.

61. Warren R, Thayer TR: Transplantation of the saphenous vein for postphlebitic stasis. Surgery 35:867, 1954.

62. Hardin CA: Bypass saphenous grafts for the relief of venous obstruction of the extremity. Surg Gynecol Obstet 112:709, 1962.

63. Bergan JJ, Yao JST, Flinn WR, McCarthy WJ: Surgical treatment of venous obstruction and insufficiency. J Vasc Surg 3:174, 1986.

64. Kistner RL: Deep venous reconstruction (1968–1984). Int Angiol 4:429, 1985.

65. Browse NL, Burnand KG, Lea Thomas M: Primary (nonthrombotic) deep vein incompetence. In Diseases of the Veins. London, Edward Arnold, 1988, p 254.

66. O'Donnell TF Jr: Chronic venous insufficiency: An overview of epidemiology, classification, and anatomic considerations. Semin Vasc Surg 1:60, 1988.

67. Porter JM, Rutherford RB, Clagett GP, et al: Reporting standards in venous disease. J Vasc Surg 8:172, 1988.

68. Palma EC, Riss R, DelCampo F, Tobler H: Tratamiento de los trastornos post-flebiticos mediante anastomosis venosa safen-femoral controlateral. Sociedad de Cirugia de Uraguay, 25 Junio, 1958.

69. Palma EC, Esperon R: Vein transplants and grafts in the surgical treatment of the post-phlebitic syndrome. J Cardiovasc Surg 1:94, 1960.

70. Dale WA, Harris J: Cross-over vein grafts for iliac and femoral venous occlusion. Ann Surg 168:319, 1968.

71. Dale WA: Reconstructive venous surgery. Arch Surg 114:1312, 1979.

72. Gruss JD, Vargas-Montano H, Bartels D, et al: Direct reconstructive venous surgery. Int Angiol 4:441, 1985.

73. Gruss JD, Bartels D, Kawai S, et al: Application of plastic material in the Palma operation. Angiology 1:51, 1979.

74. Gruss JD, Bartels D, Tsafandakis E, Machedo JL: Blood vessel prosthesis in the Palma operation. In May R, Weber J (eds): Pelvic and Abdominal Veins: Progress in Diagnostics and Therapy. International Congress Series 550. Amsterdam, Excerpta Medica, 1981, p 550.

75. Eklöf B: Temporary arteriovenous fistula in reconstruction of iliac vein obstruction using PTFE grafts. In Eklöf B, Gjores JE, Thulesius O, et al (eds): Controversies in the Management of Venous Disorders. London, Butterworths, 1989, p 280.

76. McNeill AD, Sorour NN: Veno-venous internal saphenous crossover graft for phlegmasia caerulea dolens. Br J Surg 67:877, 1980.

77. Dale WA: Peripheral venous reconstruction. In Management of Vascular Surgical Problems. New York, McGraw-Hill Book Company, 1985, p 493.

78. Edwards WS: A-V fistula after venous reconstruction. A simplified method of producing and obliterating the shunt. Ann Surg 196:669, 1982.

79. Edwards WS: Femoral AV fistula as a complementary or primary procedure for iliac venous occlusion. In Bergan JJ, Yao JST (eds): Surgery of the Veins. Orlando, FL, Grune & Stratton, 1985, p 267.

80. Greenfield LJ, Alexander EL: Current status of surgical therapy for deep vein thrombosis. Am J Surg 150:64, 1985.

81. Morano JU, Burkhalter JL: Graft patency evaluations with DSA after reconstructive venous surgery. Radiology 160:267, 1986.

82. Hiratzka LF, Wright CB: Experimental and clinical results of grafts in the venous system: A current review. J Surg Res 25:542, 1978.

83. Dale WA: Crossover vein grafts for iliac and femoral venous occlusion. Res Staff Phys, March, p 58, 1983.

84. Husni EA: Reconstruction of veins: The need for objectivity. J Cardiovasc Surg 24:525, 1983.

85. Danza R, Navarro T, Baldizan J: Reconstructive surgery in chronic venous obstruction of the lower limbs. J Cardiovasc Surg 32:98, 1991.

86. Gruss JD: Venous bypass for chronic venous insufficiency. In Bergan JJ, Yao JST (eds): Venous Disorders. Philadelphia, WB Saunders, 1991, p 316.

87. O'Donnell TF Jr, Mackey WC, Shepard AD, Callow AD: Clinical, hemodynamic, and anatomic follow-up of direct venous reconstruction. Arch Surg 122:474, 1987.

88. Frileux C, Pillot-Bienayme P, Gillot C: Bypass of segmental obliterations of iliofemoral venous axis by transposition of saphenous vein. J Cardiovasc Surg 13:409, 1972.

89. Husni EA: In situ saphenopopliteal bypass graft for incompetence of the femoral and popliteal veins. Surg Gynecol Obstet 130:279, 1970.

90. May R: Der Femoralisbypass beim postthrombotischen Zustandshild. Vasa 1:267, 1972.

91. Gruss JD: The saphenopopliteal bypass for chronic venous insufficiency (May-Husni operation). In Bergan JJ, Yao JST (eds): Surgery of the Veins. Orlando, FL, Grune & Stratton, 1985, p 255.

92. Annous MO, Queral LA: Venous claudication successfully treated by distal superficial femoral-to-greater saphenous venous bypass. J Vasc Surg 2:870, 1985.

93. Taheri SA, Williams J, Powell S, et al: Iliocaval compression syndrome. Am J Surg 154:169, 1987.

94. Scherck JP, Kerstein MD, Stansel HC: The current status of vena caval replacement. Surgery 76:209, 1974.

95. Greenfield LJ, Alexander EL: Current status of surgical therapy for deep vein thrombosis. Am J Surg 150:64, 1985.

96. Jaszczak P, Mathiesen FR: The iliac compression syndrome. Acta Chir Scand 144:133, 1978.

97. Trimble C, Bernstein EF, Pomerantz M, Eiseman B: A prosthetic bridging device to relieve iliac venous compression. Surg Forum 23:249, 1972.

98. Cockett FB: Venous causes of swollen leg. Br J Surg 54:891, 1967.

99. Rigas A, Vomvoyannis A, Tsardakas E: Iliac compression syndrome. J Cardiovasc Surg 11:389, 1970.

100. Moller IW, Eickhoff JH, Hansen HJB, Lindewald H: The iliac vein compression syndrome. Acta Chir Scand 502:141, 1980.

101. Jakob H, Maass D, Schmiedt W, et al: Treatment of major venous obstruction with an expandable endoluminal spiral prosthesis. J Cardiovasc Surg 30:112, 1989.

102. Okrent D, Messersmith R, Buckman J: Transcatheter fibrinolytic therapy and angioplasty for left iliofemoral venous thrombosis. J Vasc Intervent Radiol 2:195, 1991.

103. Elson JD, Becker GJ, Wholey MH, et al: Vena caval and central venous stenoses: Management with Palmaz balloon-expandable intraluminal stents. J Vasc Intervent Radiol 2:215, 1991.

104. Bernstein EF, Chan EL, Bardin JA: Externally supported grafts for inferior vena cava bypass. In Bergan JJ, Yao JST (eds): Surgery of the Veins. Orlando, FL, Grune & Stratton, 1985, p 33.

105. Dale WA: Synthetic grafts for venous reconstruction. In Bergan JJ, Yao JST (eds): Surgery of the Veins. New York, Grune & Stratton, 1985, p 233.

106. Eklöf B, Broome A, Einarsson E: Venous reconstruction in acute iliac vein obstruction using PTFE grafts. In May R, Weber J (eds): Pelvic and Abdominal Veins: Progress in Diagnostics and Therapy. International Congress Series 550. Amsterdam, Excerpta Medica, 1981, p 259.

107. Valentini FB, Irace L, DiPietrantonio S, et al: Arterial reconstruction of the limbs in poor run-off conditions and surgical repair of vena cava with expanded PTFE (Impra-grafts). Int J Surg Sci 13:139, 1983.

108. Gloviczki P, Pairolero PC, Cherry KJ, Hallett JW Jr: Reconstruction of the vena cava and of its primary tributaries: A preliminary report. J Vasc Surg 11:373, 1990.

109. Krupski W, Fry WJ, Thal ER, et al: Endothelial response to venous injury. Arch Surg 114:1240, 1979.

110. Richardson JV, Wright CB, Hiratzka LF: The role of endothelium in the patency of small venous substitutes. J Surg Res 28:556, 1980.

111. Smith DE, Hammon J, Anane-Sefah J, et al: Segmental venous replacement. J Thorac Cardiovasc Surg 69:589, 1975.

112. Bryant MF, Lazenby WB, Howard JM: Experimental replacement of short segments of veins. Arch Surg 76:289, 1958.

113. Eadie DGA, DeTakats G: The early fate of autogenous grafts in the canine femoral vein. J Cardiovasc Surg 7:138, 1966.

114. Wilson SE, Jabour A, Stone RT, Stanley TM: Patency of biologic and prosthetic inferior vena cava grafts with distal limb fistula. Arch Surg 117:1174, 1978.

115. Ijima H, Hirabayashi K, Sakakibara Y, et al: Results of femoro-femoral vein bypass grafting with temporary arteriovenous fistula for femoro-iliac venous thrombosis: Differences between operations in the acute and chronic phases. Phlebology 5:237, 1990.

116. Herring M, Gardner A, Peigh P, et al: Patency in canine inferior vena cava grafting: Effects of graft material, size, and endothelial seeding. J Vasc Surg 1:877, 1984.

117. Egdahl RH, Hume DM: Nonsuture blood vessel anastomosis. An experimental study using polyethylene as the prosthetic material. Arch Surg 72:232, 1956.

118. Holt GP, Lewis FJ: A new technique for end to end anastomosis of small arteries. Surg Forum 11:242, 1960.

119. Kunlin MJ, Benitte AM, Richard S: The suspension of the venous suture. Experimental study. Bull Soc Int Chir 19:336, 1960.

120. Todd RS, Sive EB, Devore LR: Replacement of segments of the venous system. Arch Surg 87:998, 1963.

121. Fiore AC, Brown JW, Cromartie RS, et al: Prosthetic replacement for the thoracic vena cava. J Thorac Cardiovasc Surg 84:560, 1982.

122. Ijima H, Kodama M, Hori M: Temporary arteriovenous fistula for venous reconstruction using synthetic graft: A clinical and experimental investigation. J Cardiovasc Surg 26:131, 1985.

123. Aschberg S, Ankacrona H, Bergstrand O, Bjorkholm M: Temporary arteriovenous shunts to dilate saphenous crossover grafts and maintain patency. Acta Chir Scand 142:585, 1976.

124. Lalka SG, Lash JM, Unthank JL, et al: Inadequacy of saphenous vein grafts for cross-femoral venous bypass. J Vasc Surg 13:622, 1991.

125. Lalka SG, Unthank JL, Lash JM, et al: Hemodynamic effects of varied graft diameters in the venous system. Surgery 110:73, 1991.

126. Browse NL, Burnand KG, Lea Thomas M: Primary (nonthrombotic) deep vein obstruction. In Diseases of the Veins. London, Edward Arnold, 1988, p 271.

127. May R, DeWeese JA: Surgery of the pelvic veins. In May R (ed): Surgery of the Veins of the Leg and Pelvis. Philadelphia, WB Saunders, 1979, p 158.

128. May R: The Palma operation with Gottlob's endothelium preserving suture. In May R, Weber J (eds): Pelvic and Abdominal Veins: Progress in Diagnostics and Therapy. International Congress Series 550. Amsterdam, Excerpta Medica, 1981, p 192.

129. Kroener JM, Bernstein EF: Valve competence following experimental venous valve autotransplantation. Arch Surg 116:1467, 1981.

130. Scheinin TM, Jude JR: Experimental replacement of the superior vena cava: Effect of temporary increase in blood flow. J Thorac Cardiovasc Surg 48:781, 1964.

131. Johnson V, Eiseman B: Evaluation of arteriovenous shunt to maintain patency of venous autograft. Am J Surg 118:915, 1969.

132. Levin PM, Rich NM, Hutton JE: Role of arteriovenous shunts in venous reconstruction. Am J Surg 122:183, 1971.

133. Holman E, Taylor G: Problems in the dynamics of blood flow II: Pressure relations at site of an arteriovenous fistula. Angiology 3:415, 1952.

134. Hobson RW, Wright CB: Peripheral side to side arteriovenous fistula. Am J Surg 126:411, 1973.

135. Hobson RW, Wright CB: The peripheral arteriovenous fistula. In Swan KG (ed): Venous Surgery in the Lower Extremities. St. Louis, Warren H. Green, 1975, p 385.

136. Dumanian AV, Santschi DR, Park K, et al: Cross-over saphenous vein graft combined with a temporary femoral arteriovenous fistula. Vasc Surg 2:116, 1968.

137. Clowes AW: Extra-anatomical bypass of iliac vein obstruction. Arch Surg 115:767, 1980.

138. Ijima H, Sakurai J, Hori M, Kodama R: Temporary arteriovenous fistula for venous reconstruction using a synthetic graft. Clinical and experimental investigation. J Cardiovasc Surg 22:480, 1981.

139. Delin A, Swedenburg J, Hellgren M, et al: Thrombectomy and arteriovenous thrombosis in fertile women. Surg Gynecol Obstet 154:69, 1982.

140. Neglen P, Al-Hassan HK, Endrys J, et al: Iliofemoral venous thrombectomy followed by percutaneous closure of the temporary arteriovenous fistula. Surgery 110:493, 1991.

141. Okadome K, Muto Y, Eguchi H, et al: Venous reconstruction for iliofemoral venous occlusion facilitated by temporary arteriovenous shunt. Arch Surg 124:957, 1989.

142. Lalka SG, Unthank JL, McGue JG, et al: Arteriovenous fistulas as adjuncts to venous bypass grafts. J Invest Surg 4:125, 1991.

143. Endrys J, Eklöf B, Neglen P, et al: Percutaneous balloon occlusion of temporary femoral arteriovenous fistula after venous thrombectomy. Cardiovasc Intervent Radiol 12:226, 1989.

144. van Bemmelen SP, vanPapendrecht AAH, Hodde KC, Klopper PJ: A study of valve incompetence that developed in an experimental model of venous hypertension. Arch Surg 121:1048, 1986.

145. Sawchuk AP, Dalsing MC, Emerick SC, et al: A temporary distal arteriovenous fistula improves venous hemodynamics in a model of venous occlusion. Surgery 102:256, 1987.

146. Hobson RW II, Croom RD, Rich NM: Influence of heparin and low molecular weight dextran on the patency of autogenous vein grafts in the venous system. Ann Surg 178:773, 1973.

147. Friedman EW, Hamilton AJ: Polytetrafluoroethylene grafts in the peripheral venous circulation of rabbits. Am J Surg 146:355, 1983.

148. May R: Surgical treatment of the post-thrombotic state by a femoral bypass. Vasa 1:267, 1972.

149. Welter HF, Becker HM: Therapy of the pelvic venous spur and postoperative follow-up. In May R, Weber J (eds): Pelvic and Abdominal Veins: Progress in Diagnostics and Therapy. International Congress Series 550. Amsterdam, Excerpta Medica, 1981, p 172.

150. Husni EA: Issues in venous reconstruction. Vasc Diagn Ther 2:37, 1981.

151. Riahi GH, Monafo WW: Subcutaneous saphenofemoral venous crossover shunt: Simple palliation of iliac venous obstruction. Am J Surg 122:603, 1971.

152. Wagner O, Piza F, Lechner G: Indications and late results of Palma's venous bypass in chronic pelvic vein thrombosis. Vasa 2:347, 1973.

153. Aratzanov A, Misev B: Remote results of the treatment of postphlebitic syndrome. Folia Med (Plovdiv) 18:107, 1976.

The Management of Lymphatic Disorders

Edited by Peter Gloviczki, M.D.

141

Lymphedema: Introduction and General Considerations

Peter Gloviczki, M.D.

• • •

> I think I have proved, that the lymphatic vessels are the absorbing vessels . . . ; that they are the same as the lacteals; and that . . . with the thoracic duct, constitute one great and general system, dispersed through the whole body for absorption.
>
> *William Hunter, 1784*

If the transport capacity of the lymphatic system is reduced by obstruction or abnormal development of the lymph vessels or lymph nodes, protein-rich interstitial fluid accumulates, and lymphedema develops. Chronic limb swelling due to lymphedema is not only a marked cosmetic deformity, but in most patients it is also a disabling and distressing condition. Complications can be severe and include bacterial and fungal infections, chronic inflammation, wasting, immunodeficiency, and occasionally malignancy. Lymphedema, long a neglected field in medicine, has received considerable attention in recent years owing to progress in ultrastructural and physiologic investigations and to improvements in diagnosis and management of the disease. This new information and experience with lymphedema is based on a substantial knowledge of the lymphatic system that has been accumulating for centuries.

HISTORICAL BACKGROUND

Lymph vessels and nodes were mentioned in early times by Hippocrates (460–377 B.C.), who described "white blood" and "glands, that everyone has in the armpit,"[1] by

Aristotle (384–322 B.C.), who wrote about "nerves . . . which contain colorless liquids,"[2] and by Erasistratus (310–250 B.C.) from the Alexandrian School of Medicine, who recognized the lacteals as "arteries on the mesentery of sucking pigs full of milk."[3] It was not until the Renaissance, however, that further progress in this field was made. Eustachius in 1563 was the first to observe the thoracic duct during dissection in a horse, but he didn't recognize its significance and named it the "vena alba thoracis."[4]

The discovery of the lymphatic system is attributed to Gasparo Asellius, Professor of Anatomy and Surgery at Pavia, Italy. On July 23, 1622, during a vivisection he observed the mesenteric lymphatics in a well-fed dog.[5] Asellius named the lymphatics the vasa lactea and recognized their function of absorbing chyle from the intestines. He assumed, however, that the mesenteric lymphatics transported lymph to the liver. It was Jean Pecquet in 1651 who described the exact route of mesenteric lymphatic drainage to the "receptaculum chyli" and from there into the thoracic duct.[6] In subsequent years Bartholin and Rudbeck further clarified details of the lymphatic circulation and the anatomy of the thoracic duct (Fig. 141–1).[7, 8] The term lymphatic was first used by Bartholin. The valvular struc-

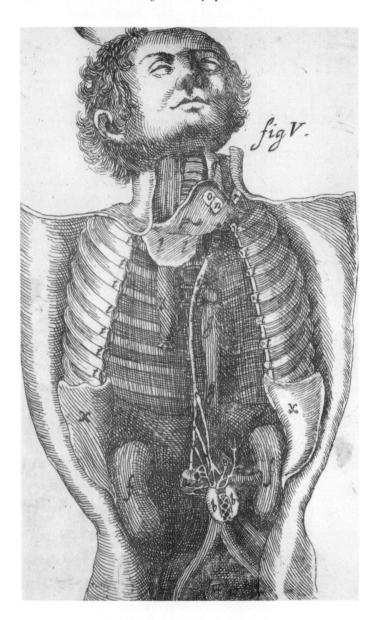

fig V.

FIGURE 141 – 1.   The receptaculum chyli and the thoracic duct in human. (From Bartholin T: Vasa Lymphatica. Hafniae, Petrus Hakius, 1653.)

ture in the lymph vessels was demonstrated by Ruysch[9] in 1665 and later in 1692 by Anton Nuck, who injected mercury into the lymph vessels for his anatomic studies.[10]

The gross anatomy of the lymphatic system was remarkably well documented by the great anatomists of the 18th century. Cruikshank, a student of William Hunter, published *The Anatomy of the Absorbing Vessels of the Human Body* in 1786.[11] His work, however, was surpassed by the atlas of Paolo Mascagni, who published exceptionally detailed and clear illustrations of the entire lymphatic system (Figs. 141–2 to 141–4).[12] It was not until one hundred years later that our knowledge of the anatomy of the lymphatic system was further broadened by the works of Sappey[13] and then by those of Ranvier.[14]

The lymphatics as an integrated system responsible for absorption were recognized at the end of the 18th century by William Hunter, his brother John, and two of his students, Hewson and Cruikshank.[15] However, their theory that the lymphatic system was the only absorbing system of the body was rightly criticized even by their peers.

Although Hunter thought that the lymphatics were closed tubes, Hewson suggested that they had physiologic orifices and acted as "capillary tubes" that are "capable of absorbing the chyle and the lymph."[16] The "open mouth" theory, that the lymphatics had completely open distal ends, was advocated by von Kölliker[17] and later by von Recklinghausen, who also discovered the endothelial lining of the lymphatics.[18]

As stated by Drinker,[19] however, "the modern history of lymph formation and lymph movement began with Starling." At the turn of the 20th century, Starling confirmed the relationship between the hydrostatic pressure in the blood capillaries and the oncotic pressure of the plasma proteins.[20] His work was a continuation of the theory of Ludwig, who suggested that lymph formed by filtration of the blood through the walls of the capillaries.[21] Drinker and his colleagues at Harvard University deserve the credit for explaining the absorption of proteins from the intercellular space via the lymphatic system.[22] Further details of lymphatic physiology were elaborated later by members of the

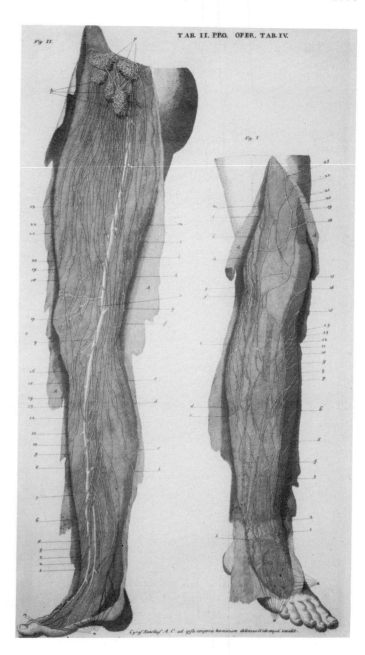

FIGURE 141–2. The lymphatic system of the lower extremity according to Mascagni. (From Mascagni P: Vasorum Lymphaticorum Corporis Humani Historia et Ichnographia, vol. 138. Senis, P. Carli, 1787.)

Hungarian school of lymphology, headed by Rusznyák, Földi, and Szabó.[23] With the introduction of a clinically usable technique of contrast lymphangiography in the early 1950s, Kinmonth gave a special impetus toward clinical research of the lymphatic system and focused much-needed attention on the diagnosis and management of chronic lymphedema.[24]

LYMPHEDEMA: AN ENIGMA?

Lymphedema, a disease known for centuries, has been considered by many clinicians to be one of the enigmas of medicine.[25] The reasons for this are legion. Lymphedema is caused by a fault in a system that is inconspicuous and hardly visible. It frequently occurs years after the initial insult to the lymph vessels and lymph nodes following a

long state of apparent well being and normal functioning. It is difficult and frequently frustrating to treat and almost impossible to cure.

Nonetheless, our understanding of lymphatic physiology has markedly improved in recent years. Chapter 142 provides new perspectives on the three-dimensional anatomy of the blood capillary–interstitial lymph interface and on the formation and propulsion of lymph. The spontaneous intrinsic contractility of the lymph vessels is recognized now as the pivotal mechanism by which lymph is propelled in normal conditions.

In discussing new theories of the pathophysiology of lymphedema, it is emphasized that the lymphatic system is not comparable to the venous system. They are not two identical unidirectional canalicular systems that are responsible for the return of excess interstitial fluid to the bloodstream and the heart. The major difference is that the ve-

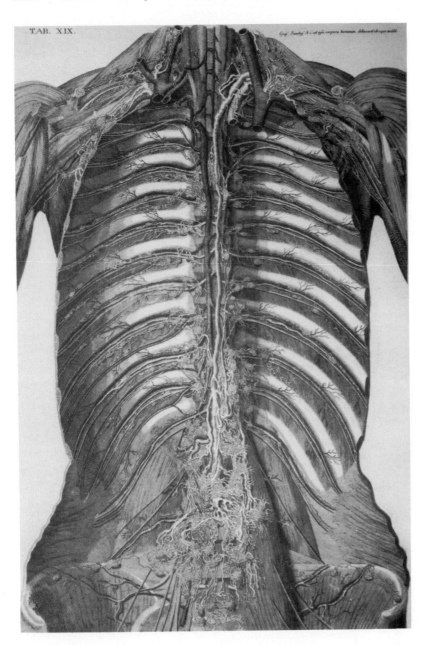

FIGURE 141–3.   The anatomy of the thoracic duct as illustrated by Mascagni. (From Mascagni P: Vasorum Lymphaticorum Corporis Humani Historia et Ichnographia, vol. 138. Senis, P. Carli, 1787.)

nous system is filled with a liquid column, which responds immediately to changes in pressure or resistance. The lymphatic system, however, is not fully primed, and only if there is longstanding stasis does the lymph column fill the lymphatic channels completely. Only in these conditions are factors other than intrinsic contractility, such as muscular contractions or external massage, important in the forward propulsion of lymphatic flow.

In most patients with limb swelling the diagnosis of lymphedema is based on the history and physical examination. Once a systemic cause of edema has been excluded, it should be remembered that chronic venous insufficiency is a more frequent local cause of limb swelling than lymphedema. Secondary lymphedema, on the other hand, is more common than primary lymphedema.[26] As detailed in Chapter 143, lymphoscintigraphy has become the test of choice in the 1990s to confirm that edema is lymphatic in origin.[27] It is still essential to perform computed tomography in most

adult patients with suspected lymphedema to exclude underlying malignancy. Magnetic resonance imaging is used with increasing frequency to image the anatomy of lymph nodes and has the potential to become the most useful test to complement the findings of lymphoscintigraphy. Although direct contrast lymphangiography still gives us the finest details of lymphatic anatomy,[24, 28] it is an invasive study with potential side effects, and its use has been markedly restricted in patients with lymphedema. In our practice contrast lymphangiography is reserved for the preoperative evaluation of patients with lymphangiectasia and for selected patients who are candidates for direct operations on the lymph vessels or the thoracic duct.

Prevention of primary lymphedema at present is not possible. The incidence of secondary lymphedema, however, can be reduced by preventive measures. Filariasis, which affects almost 100 million people in the world, was eradicated from Europe and North America by public health

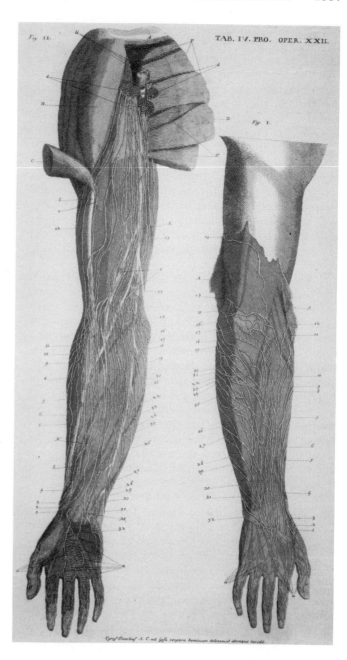

FIGURE 141 – 4. The anatomy of the lymphatic system of the upper extremity by Mascagni. (From Mascagni P: Vasorum Lymphaticorum Corporis Humani Historia et Ichnographia, vol. 138. Senis, P. Carli, 1787.)

measures and control of mosquito breeding.[29] The introduction of similar measures in Third World countries in addition to prophylactic antifilarial medications and immediate treatment of those infected could decrease a worldwide epidemic.

The most important form of secondary lymphedema in developed countries is postmastectomy lymphedema. The well-documented studies of Kissin and colleagues[30] noted that extensive axillary lymphadenectomy, axillary radiotherapy, and positive pathologic nodal status are the most important independent risk factors for lymphedema. Although treatment of malignancy should not be compromised, excision of any lymphatic tissue for either diagnostic or therapeutic reasons should be restricted to a minimum. The prevention of infectious complications is equally important in patients who have undergone lymph node dissection or have already developed lymphedema and is

achieved by adhering to meticulous personal hygienic measures, avoiding skin injury, and controlling fungal infections.

The mainstay of treatment of lymphedema continues to be conservative and includes leg elevation, elastic compression, manual physical decongestion, or intermittent pneumatic compression treatment. Leg elevation continues to be the simplest and most effective way of reducing lymphedema, although this form of treatment requires hospitalization, bed rest, and elevation of the extremity in an edema sling for several days. Manual physical decongestive therapy has been popularized in Europe by Földi and colleagues,[31] and this effective physical therapy regimen, as detailed in Chapter 144, is gaining acceptance in the United States. Intermittent pneumatic compression treatment is at present the most widely used conservative treatment for lymphedema. Data from a recent prospective study of Pappas and O'Donnell support the long-term effectiveness of this therapy.[32] Their protocol included a 2- to 3-day hospitalization with daily treatment with a sequential, high-pressure intermittent pneumatic compression pump. The edema status was then maintained with two-way stretch elastic compression stockings. Limb girth reduction was maintained in 90 per cent of patients, and excellent results were recorded in 53 per cent at a mean follow-up of 25 months.

Excisional debulking operations are recommended by Miller[33] to patients who have significant functional impairment due to excessive lymphedema (see Chapter 145). In the late stage of the disease when irreversible skin and subcutaneous changes have occurred, this may be the only way to decrease the volume of the extremity. Among the different excisional operations the staged subcutaneous excision beneath flaps has provided the most satisfying results.[33, 34]

Reconstruction of the obstructed lymphatic circulation has been attempted using direct operations on the lymph vessels (lymphovenous anastomoses, lymphatic grafting)[35–37] or operations designed to promote the formation of new lympholymphatic anastomoses (omental transposition,[38] mesenteric bridge operation,[39] lymph node transplantation[40]). Controversies on these procedures have been substantial. Although the long-term patency and function of lymphovenous anastomoses and lymphatic grafting are still not proved, recent well-documented studies from two centers have claimed long-term improvement in patients following microsurgical lymphatic reconstructions.[36, 37] As stated in a recent editorial, however, the lack of prospective clinical trials and the imperfect nature of current treatment modalities continue to generate disagreement about the optimal management of chronic lymphedema.[41]

The problems that we have to face in dealing with lymphatic diseases are still substantial. Lymphedema, however, should no longer be considered an enigma in medicine. The contributing authors on lymphedema in this new volume of Vascular Surgery sincerely hope that the information presented here will stimulate further basic and clinical research and much-needed prospective clinical trials in this difficult and long-neglected field. This section assigned to the management of lymphedema is a testimony to the indisputable progress that has been made in the past decades in the field of lymphatic diseases.

References

1. Kanter MA: The lymphatic system: An historical perspective. Plast Reconstr Surg 79:131, 1987.
2. Bartels P: Das Lymphgefässsystem. Jena, Germany, G Fischer, 1909, p 2.
3. Wolfe JHN: The pathophysiology of lymphedema. *In* Rutherford RB (ed): Vascular Surgery. 3rd ed. Philadelphia, WB Saunders, 1989, pp 1648–1656.
4. Eustachi B: Opuscula Anatomica. Venetiis, V Luchinus, 1564, p 301.
5. Asellius G: De Lactibus sive Lacteis Venis Quarto Vasorum Mesaraicorum Genere Novo Inuento. Mediolani, JB Biddellium, 1627.
6. Pecquet J: Experimenta Nova Anatomica, Quibus Incognitum Lactenus Chyli Receptaculum, et ab eo per Thoracem in Ramos Usque Subclavio Vasa Lactea Deteguntur. Paris, Cramoisy, 1651.
7. Bartholin T: Vasa Lymphatica. Hafniae, Petrus Hakius, 1653.
8. Rudbeck O: Novo Exercitatio Anatomica, Exhibens Ductus Hepaticos, Aquoso et Vasa Glandularum Serosa. Arosiae, kexud. e. Lauringerus 1653; English translation in Bull Hist Med 11:304, 1942.
9. Ruysch F: Dilucidatio Valvularium in Vasis Lymphaticis, et lacteis. Hagaecomitiae, Harmani Gael, 1665.
10. Nuck A: Adenographia Curiosa et Uteri Foeminei Anatome Nova. Lugduni Batavorum, Jordanum Luchtmans, 1692.
11. Cruikshank WC: The Anatomy of the Absorbing Vessels of the Human Body. London, G Nicol, 1786.
12. Mascagni P: Vasorum Lymphaticorum Corporis Humani Historia et Ichnographia. Senis, Pazzini Carli, 1787, vol. 138, p 27.
13. Sappey PC: Anatomie, Physiologie, Pathologie des Vaisseaux Lymphatiques, Considérés chez l'Homme et chez les Vertebrés. Paris, Delahaye et Lecrossier, 1874.
14. Ranvier L: Morphologie et developpment des vaisseaux lymphatiques chez mammiferes. Arch d'Anat Microscopique 1:69, 1897.
15. Hunter W: Hunter's Lectures of Anatomy. Amsterdam, Elsevier, 1972.
16. Hewson W: The Lymphatic System in the Human Subject, and in Other Animals. *In* Johnson J (ed): London, 1774.
17. von Kölliker A: Handbuch der Gewebelehre des Menschen. Leipzig, W. Engelmann, 1855.
18. von Recklinghausen F: Die Lymphgefässe und ihre Beziehungen zum Bindegewebe. Berlin, Hirschwald, 1862.
19. Drinker CK: The Lymphatic System: Its Part in Regulating Composition and Volume of Tissue Fluid. Stanford, CA, Stanford University Press, 1942.
20. Starling EH: On the absorption of fluids from the connective tissue spaces. J Physiol (Lond) 19:312, 1896.
21. Ludwig CFW: Lehrbuch der Physiologie des Menschen. 2nd ed. Leipzig, 1858–1861, p 562.
22. Yoffey JM, Courtice FC: Lymphatics, Lymph and the Lymphomyeloid Complex. New York, Academic Press, 1970.
23. Rusznyák I, Földi M, Szabó G: Lymphatics and Lymph Circulation. New York, Pergamon Press, 1960.
24. Kinmonth JB: The Lymphatics. Surgery, Lymphography and Diseases of the Chyle and Lymph Systems. London, Edward Arnold, 1982.
25. Olszewski W: The enigma of lymphedema—A search for answers [Editorial]. Lymphology 24:100, 1991.
26. Browse NL: The diagnosis and management of primary lymphedema. J Vasc Surg 3:181, 1986.
27. Gloviczki P, Calcagno D, Schirger A, et al: Non-invasive evaluation of the swollen extremity: Experiences with 190 lymphoscintigraphic examinations. J Vasc Surg 9:683, 1989.
28. Clouse ME, Wallace S: Lymphatic Imaging. Lymphography, Computed Tomography, and Scintigraphy. 2nd ed. Baltimore, Williams & Wilkins, 1985.
29. Reynolds WD, Sy FS: Eradication of filariasis in South Carolina: A historical perspective. J S C Med Assoc 85:331, 1989.
30. Kissin MW, della Rovere GQ, Easton D, Westbury G: Risk of lymphoedema following the treatment of breast cancer. Br J Surg 73:580, 1986.
31. Földi E, Földi M, Clodius L: The lymphedema chaos: A lancet. Ann Plast Surg 22:505, 1989.
32. Pappas CJ, ODonnell TF Jr: Long-term results of compression treatment for lymphedema. J Vasc Surg 16:555, 1992.
33. Miller AJ: The history of the lymphatics of the heart. *In* Miller AJ (ed): Lymphatics of the Heart. New York, Raven Press, 1982, pp 1–43.
34. Pflug JJ, Schirger A: Chronic peripheral lymphedema. *In* Clement DL, Shepherd JT (eds): Vascular Diseases in the Limbs: Mechanisms and Principles of Treatment. St. Louis, Mosby–Year Book, 1993, pp 221–238.
35. Gloviczki P, Fisher J, Hollier LH, et al: Microsurgical lymphovenous anastomosis for treatment of lymphedema: A critical review. J Vasc Surg 7:647, 1988.
36. O'Brien BMC, Mellow CG, Khazanchi RK, et al: Long-term results after microlymphatico-venous anastomoses for the treatment of obstructive lymphedema. Plast Reconstr Surg 85:562, 1990.
37. Baumeister RG, Siuda S: Treatment of lymphedemas by microsurgical lymphatic grafting: What is proved? Plast Reconstr Surg 85:64, 1990.
38. Goldsmith HS: Long-term evaluation of omental transposition for chronic lymphedema. Ann Surg 180:847, 1974.
39. Hurst PA, Stewart G, Kinmonth JB, Browse NL: Long-term results of the enteromesenteric bridge operation in the treatment of primary lymphoedema. Br J Surg 72:272, 1985.
40. Trevidic P, Cormier JM: Free axillary lymph node transfer. *In* Cluzan RV (ed): Progress in Lymphology XIII. Amsterdam, Elsevier Science Publishers B.V., 1992, pp 415–420.
41. Witte CL, Witte, MH: The enigma of lymphedema—A search for answers [Editorial comment]. Lymphology 24:100, 1991.

142

Lymphodynamics and Pathophysiology of Lymphedema

Charles L. Witte, M.D., and Marlys H. Witte, M.D.

• • •

Any proteid which leaves these vessels [blood capillaries] . . . is lost for the time to the vascular system. . . . it must be collected by lymphatics and restored to the [blood] vascular system by way of the thoracic or right lymphatic duct.

Starling, 1897

In a narrow sense, the lymph circulation is a unidirectional vascular system that merely transports surplus tissue fluid back to the bloodstream. In a wider sense, however, this network stabilizes the mobile intercellular liquid and extracellular matrix microenvironment to ensure parenchymal cellular integrity and function. In its entirety the lymphatic system is composed of vascular conduits, lymphoid organs including the lymph nodes, spleen, Peyer's patches, thymus, and nasopharyngeal tonsils, and circulating cellular elements such as lymphocytes and macrophages. These migrating cells cross the blood-capillary barrier, along with a multitude of immunoglobulins, polypeptides, plasma protein complexes, and cytokines to circulate in lymph back to the bloodstream. Whereas body water circulates very rapidly as a plasma suspension of red blood cells within the blood vascular compartment, it percolates slowly outside the bloodstream as a tissue fluid–lymph suspension of lymphocytes through lymph vessels and lymph nodes. As a specialized subcompartment of the extracellular space, therefore, the lymphatic system completes a closed loop for the circulation by returning liquid, macromolecules, and other blood elements that "escape" or "leak" from blood capillaries (Fig. 142–1). Disruption of this blood-lymph loop promotes tissue swelling and is also responsible for a variety of syndromes characterized by scarring, wasting, immunodeficiency, and dysangiogenesis.

TOPOGRAPHY

Macroscopic Anatomy

The discovery of chylous mesenteric lacteals in a well-fed dog by Gasparo Aselli early in the 17th century set off a flurry of anatomic dissections in England and continental Europe that established the nearly ubiquitous presence of lymphatics throughout the body and their important role in the absorption of nutrients.[1] These lymphatic "absorbents" accompany venous trunks everywhere except in the central nervous system and in the cortical bony skeleton. In general, lymph from the lower torso and viscera enters the bloodstream via the thoracic duct at the left subclavian-jugular venous junction. Lymphatics from the head and neck and the upper extremities enter the central veins either independently or by a common supraclavicular cistern. Numerous interconnections exist within this rich vascular network, and subvariant anatomic pathways are plentiful. For example, the bulk of cardiac and pulmonary lymph as well as the intraperitoneal fluid, which drains through fenestrae of the diaphragm into substernal mediastinal collectors, unites as a common trunk to empty into the great veins in the right neck. Intestinal lymph, on the other hand, which transports cholesterol and fat-soluble vitamins (vitamins A, K, and D) and long-chain triglycerides as chylomicra, unlike intestinal blood, which flows directly into the liver, courses retroperitoneally to the aortic hiatus to form with other visceral and retroperitoneal lymphatics the multi-channel cisterna chyli and the thoracic duct. The bulk of the lymph formed in the liver flows retrograde or countercurrent to the portal blood flow and joins intestinal lymph collectors just before the origin of the thoracic duct. Only a small amount of hepatic lymph drains antegrade along the major hepatic veins to the anterior mediastinum and right lymph duct. Although these topographic variants influence the development and progression of peripheral (lymph)edema only indirectly, they are nonetheless essential for a broad understanding of edema syndromes including those accompanied by visceral lymphatic abnormalities, celomic effusions, and chylous reflux. Although the brain and retina do not technically have a lymphatic apparatus, they possess analogous circulations such as the aqueous humor–canal of Schlemm (the anterior chamber of the eye) or the cerebrospinal fluid–subarachnoid villi (Pacchionian bodies) connections (the brain). Glial elements and nonendothelium-lined intracerebral perivascular (Virchow-Robin) spaces probably also serve to transport interstitial fluid to nearby intracranial

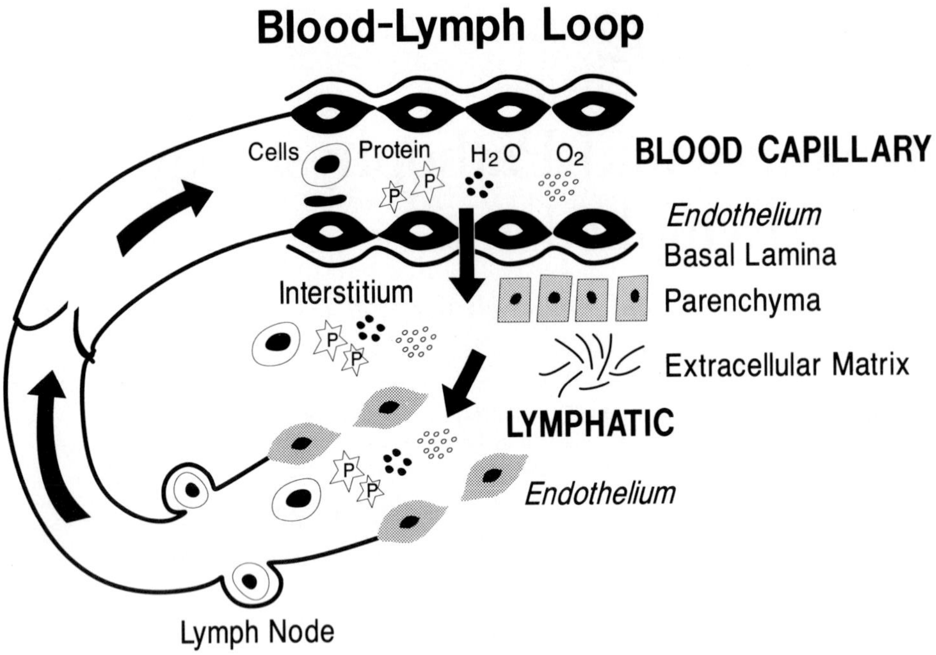

Blood-Lymph Loop

FIGURE 142–1. The closed liquid circulation of the body. Within the bloodstream, water flows rapidly as a plasma suspension of red blood cells; outside the bloodstream it flows slowly as a tissue fluid-lymph suspension of lymphocytes through lymphatics and lymph nodes. Small and large molecules including plasma proteins (P), cells, and respiratory gases cross the blood capillary–endothelial barrier to nourish the parenchyma and then return in the lymph stream.

venous sinuses. Extensive interruption of cervical lymphatic trunks (e.g., after bilateral radical neck dissection), therefore, causes prominent facial suffusion and a transient neurologic syndrome resembling pseudotumor cerebri,[2] whereas an infusion of crystalloid solution directly into the canine cisterna magna causing an elevation of intracranial pressure increases lymph flow from draining neck lymphatics.[3, 4] Although abundant lymphatic pathways thus exist for surplus tissue fluid to return to the bloodstream, homeostasis of the internal environment nonetheless still depends on an unimpeded, intact interstitial–lymph fluid circulatory system.

Microscopic Anatomy

As an afferent vascular system, the lymphatics originate within the interstitium as specialized capillaries, although in certain organs such as the liver, they seem to emanate from nonendothelialized precapillary channels (e.g., the spaces of Disse).[5] Lymphatic capillaries are remarkably porous and readily permit the entry of even large macromolecules (MW more than 1000 kd). In this respect, they resemble the uniquely "leaky" fenestrated sinusoidal blood capillaries of the liver but are in distinct contrast to most other blood capillaries, which are relatively impervious to macromolecules even the size of albumin (MW − 69 kd).[6]

Under light microscopy without preparaffin-embedded tracer or intravascular latex injection, it is difficult to distinguish between blood and lymph vessels, although the latter are usually thin-walled and tortuous, have a wider, more irregular lumen, and are largely devoid of red blood cells. Many staining features have been advocated to differentiate between blood and lymph microvasculature such as the endothelial marker, factor VIII:vWF (von Willebrand's factor). Although staining characteristics vary in both normal and pathologic states and at different sites (perhaps related

to endothelial cell dedifferentiation), in general, lymphatic staining resembles but is less intense than its blood vessel counterpart. In other words, the staining differences, if any, are more quantitative than qualitative.[7–9]

Ultrastructurally, lymph capillaries display both "open" and "closed" or so-called tight endothelial junctions, often with prominent convolutions.[8] Depending on the extent of tissue "activity," these capillaries can dramatically adjust their shape and lumen size. Unlike blood capillaries, a basal lamina (basement membrane) is tenuous or lacking altogether in lymph capillaries.[10, 11] Moreover, complex elastic fibrils, termed anchoring filaments, tether the outer portions of the endothelium to a fibrous gel matrix in the interstitium.[12, 13] These filaments allow the lymph microvessels to open wide with sudden increases in tissue fluid load and pressure in contrast to the simultaneous collapse of adjacent blood capillaries (Fig. 142–2). Just beyond the lymph capillaries are the terminal lymphatics. These, in contrast to more proximal and larger lymph collectors and trunks, are devoid of smooth muscle, although the endothelial lining is rich in the contractile protein actin.[7] Intraluminal bicuspid valves are also prominent features and serve to partition the lymphatic vessels into discrete contractile segments termed lymphangions.[14] These specialized microscopic features of the lymphatic network support the function of this delicate apparatus of absorbing and transporting lymph nodal elements and the large protein moieties, cells, and foreign agents of the bloodstream (e.g., viruses, bacteria) that have gained access to the interstitial space.

PHYSIOLOGY

General Principles

As a fine adjuster of the tissue microenvironment, the lymphatic system is often neglected in most treatises on vascular diseases. Yet this delicate system, so inconspicu-

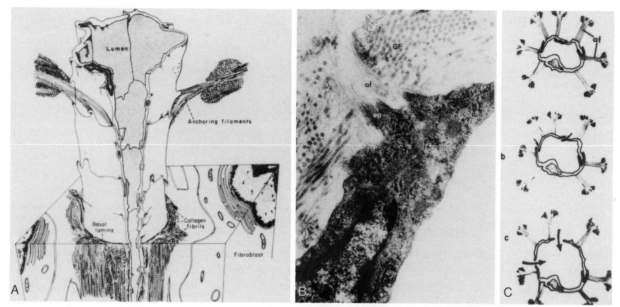

FIGURE 142–2. *A,* Three-dimensional diagram of a lymphatic capillary reconstructed from collated electron micrographs. The lymphatic anchoring filaments originate from the albuminal surface of the endothelial cells and extend into adjacent collagen bundles, thereby forming a firm connection between the lymphatic capillary wall and the surrounding interstitium. *B,* Transmission electron micrograph demonstrating anchoring filaments (af) that derive from the lymphatic endothelium (ep) and join nearby collagen bundles (CF).

C, Response of lymphatic capillaries to an increase in interstitial fluid volume. As the tissue matrix expands, the tension on the anchoring filaments (af) rises, and the lymph capillaries open widely to allow more rapid entry of liquid and solute (a–c). In contrast to the stretching of the lymph capillaries, a rise in matrix pressure collapses the blood capillaries, thereby restricting further plasma filtration. (*A–C,* From Leak LV, Burke JF: Ultrastructural studies on the lymphatic anchoring filaments. Reproduced from the *Journal of Cell Biology,* 1968, 30:129–149, by copyright permission of the Rockefeller University Press; and Leak LV: Electron microscopic observation on lymphatic capillaries and the structural components of the connective tissue–lymph interface. Microvasc Res 2:361, 1970.)

ous during life and collapsed after death, helps to maintain the liquid, protein, and osmotic equilibrium around cells and aids in absorption and distribution of nutrients, disposal of wastes, and exchange of oxygen and carbon dioxide in the local milieu interieur.

Two thirds of the body is composed of water, and most of this liquid volume is contained within cells. It is the remainder that exists outside cells, however, that continuously circulates. In a series of epochal experiments conducted nearly a century ago the English physiologist Ernest Starling outlined the pivotal factors that regulate the partition of extracellular fluid.[15, 16] In brief, the distribution of fluid between the blood vascular compartment and tissues and the net flux of plasma escaping from the bloodstream depends primarily on the transcapillary balance of hydrostatic and protein osmotic pressure gradients as modified by the character (i.e., the hydraulic conductance) of the filtering microvascular surface (Fig. 142–3). Normally, a small excess of tissue fluid forms continuously (net capillary filtration), and this surplus enters the lymphatics and returns to the venous system. In contrast to blood, which flows in a circular pattern at several liters per minute, lymph flows entirely in one direction and at rest amounts to only 2 to 2.5 L/24 hours. This limited volume derives from a slight hydrodynamic imbalance that favors fluid, salt, and macromolecular movement from plasma into tissue spaces. Although blood capillary beds vary in hydraulic conductance, in general, disturbances in the transcapillary hydrostatic and protein osmotic pressure gradients (Starling forces) tend to

promote edema that is low in protein content (less than 1.0 gm/dl), whereas impedance to lymph flow (lymph stasis) promotes (lymph)edema high in protein content (more than 1.5 gm/dl).

Unlike blood flow, which is propelled by a powerful and highly specialized muscular pump (the heart), lymph propulsion originates predominantly from spontaneous intrinsic segmental contractions of larger and probably also small lymph trunks[17–19] (Fig. 142–4), and to a lesser extent from extrinsic "haphazard forces" such as breathing, sighing, yawning, muscular squeezing (e.g., alimentary peristalsis), and transmitted arterial pulsations.[19, 20] As noted, the contractions of lymphatic segments between intraluminal valves (i.e., the lymphangions) are highly responsive to lymph volume. Thus, an increase in lymph formation is accompanied by more frequent and more powerful lymphangion contractions (Fig. 142–5), a lymphodynamic response that resembles Starling's other major physiologic principle, the Law of the Heart.[14, 21] Lymphatic truncal contraction, like venous and arterial vasomotion, is mediated by sympathomimetic agents (both alpha- and beta-adrenergic agonists),[22, 23] by-products of arachidonic acid metabolism (thromboxanes and prostaglandins),[24–27] and neurogenic stimuli[28, 29] (Fig. 142–6). Oddly, in different regions of the body, lymphatic trunks seem to exhibit varying sensitivity to different vasoactive and neurogenic stimulants.[23, 30, 31] Although the importance of truncal vasomotion as mediated by tunica smooth muscle is well established, it remains unclear whether terminal lymphatics or lymphatic

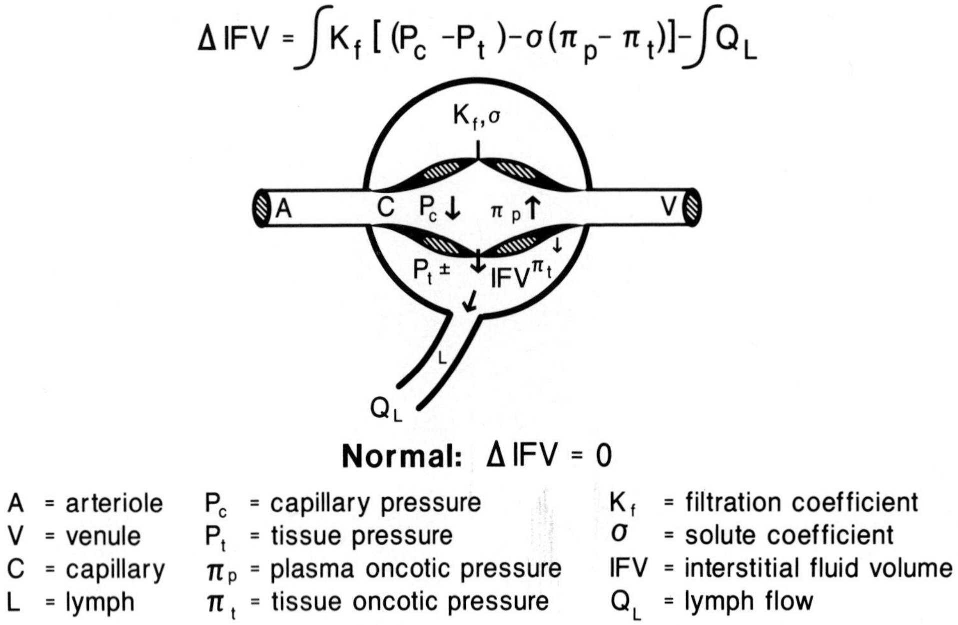

$$\Delta IFV = \int K_f \left[(P_c - P_t) - \sigma(\pi_p - \pi_t) \right] - \int Q_L$$

Normal: $\Delta IFV = 0$

A = arteriole
V = venule
C = capillary
L = lymph

P_c = capillary pressure
P_t = tissue pressure
π_p = plasma oncotic pressure
π_t = tissue oncotic pressure

K_f = filtration coefficient
σ = solute coefficient
IFV = interstitial fluid volume
Q_L = lymph flow

FIGURE 142–3.
Schematic diagram of the primary forces regulating fluid flux into the interstitium and the importance of lymph flow in maintaining a steady-state interstitial fluid volume and hence a stable partition of extracellular fluid between the bloodstream and the interstitium.

capillaries also are capable of vasomotion or are simply passive channels. In some ways, this controversy parallels the prolonged dispute about whether blood capillary endothelial cells are capable of vasoactivity, an issue now clearly resolved in the affirmative. Because lymphatic endothelium, like blood endothelium, is rich in actin[7] (a principal contractile protein), it is reasonable to assume that lymphatic microvessels also exhibit vasomotion.

In addition to their central immunologic role, lymph nodes are a potential site of impediment to the free flow of lymph. Unlike frogs, which lack lymph nodes but possess four or more strategically placed lymph hearts that propel large quantities of peripheral lymph back to the bloodstream,[32, 33] mammals possess immunoreactive lymph nodes, which, when swollen, fibrotic, or atrophic, may act to initiate or perpetuate lymph stasis.[34, 35] Perhaps the intrinsic contraction of mammalian lymphatic trunks represents a phylogenetic vestige of amphibian lymph hearts (see following section on flow-pressure dynamics for more details).

Flow-Pressure Dynamics

Although lymphatics, like veins, are thin-walled, flexible conduits that return liquid to the heart, the flow-pressure relationships in the two systems are quite different. The energy to drive blood in the venous system derives primarily from the thrust of the heart. The cardiac propulsive boost maintains a pressure head through the arteries and blood capillaries into the veins that is sufficient to overcome venous vascular resistance. Muscular contractions such as walking and running in the presence of competent venous valves supplements cardiac action in facilitating the return of blood to the heart.

Lymph vessels in tissues, on the other hand, are not directly contiguous with the blood vasculature, and the chief source of energy for lymph propulsion emanates from the intrinsic lymphatic truncal wall contractions (propulsor lymphaticum).[17–23] Like amphibian lymph hearts (cor lymphaticum), mammalian lymphatic smooth muscle beats

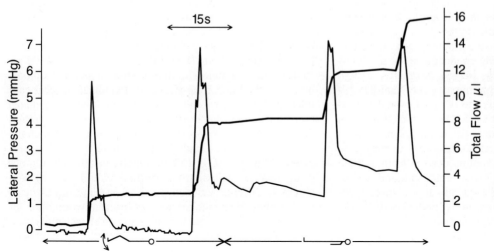

FIGURE 142–4. Lateral pressure *(curve with acute peaks)* and cumulative lymph flow *(stepwise rising curve)* in a subcutaneous leg lymphatic of a healthy man lying supine during movement of the foot and at rest. Note that lymph flow occurs only during rhythmic contraction of the lymphatic collector and specifically not by voluntary contraction of calf muscles (s, seconds). (From Olszewski WL, Engeset A: Intrinsic contractility of prenodal lymph vessels and lymph flow in the human leg. Am J Physiol 239:H775, 1980.)

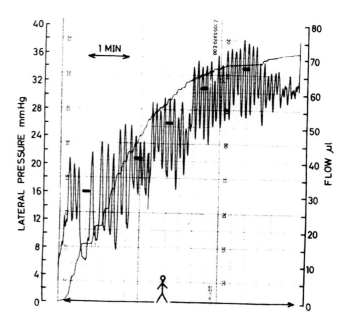

FIGURE 142–5. A human leg lymphatic has been cannulated retrograde, and the external tip of the cannula has been progressively raised, thereby gradually increasing hydrostatic pressure above the level of the cannulated lymphatic. While the man is upright *(upper tracing)*, sequential increases in outflow resistance cause an increase in lymphatic pulse frequency with subsequent decreases in pulse amplitude, lymph flow *(step-wise ascending curve)*, and stroke volume. When the intralymphatic pressure reaches 34 mmHg, lymph flow ceases despite a high pulsation rate. In the lower tracing the same man is now tiptoeing, and rising outflow pressure induces more frequent lymphatic pulsations. Note again that calf muscle contraction with up and down foot motion is not associated with greater lymph propulsion. Also note that at higher pressures each flow wave is followed by sporadic retrograde flow (reflux), which probably relates to intraluminal valve incompetence in the distending lymph vessel. (Reprinted with permission from Olszewski WL: Lymph pressure and flow in limbs. *In* Lymph Stasis: Pathophysiology, Diagnosis, and Treatment. Copyright CRC Press, Boca Raton, Florida, 1991, pp 136–137.)

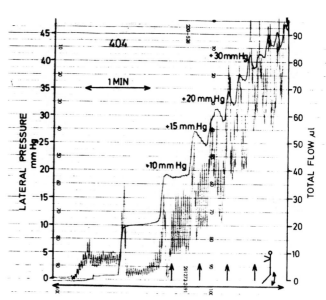

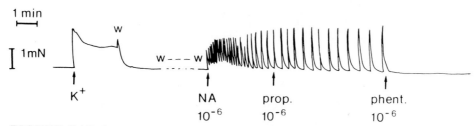

FIGURE 142–6. Tracing taken from a human lower leg lymphatic segment. Noradrenaline (NA) 10^{-6}M induces phasic lymphatic contractions that are unaffected by the beta-blocker propranolol (prop) 10^{-6}M but are abolished by phentolamine (phent) 10^{-6}M. K⁺ indicates previous potassium (124 mM)-induced contraction, and W indicates washout with fresh Krebs buffer solution. (From Sjöberg T; Steen S: Contractile properties of lymphatics from the human lower leg. Lymphology 24:16, 1991.)

rhythmically and in the presence of a well-developed intra-luminal valve system facilitates lymph transport (Fig. 142–7). In a sense, the lymphatics function as micropumps that respond to fluid challenges with increases in both rate and stroke volume.[14, 24] Ordinarily, resistance to flow in the lymphatic vessels is relatively high compared to the low resistance in the venous system,[37] but the pumping capacity of the lymphatics is able to overcome this impedance by generating intraluminal pressures of 30 to 50 mmHg (see Fig. 142–5) and sometimes even equals or exceeds arterial pressure.[17, 37, 38] This formidable lymphatic ejection force is modulated not only by filling pressure but also by temperature, sympathomimetics, neurogenic stimuli, circulating hormones, and locally released paracrine and autocrine cytokine secretions.[39]

It is often mistakenly thought that lymph return, like venous return, is directly enhanced by truncal compression from skeletal muscle and other adjacent structures. Whereas muscular contraction and external massage clearly accelerate lymph return in the presence of edema,[38] under normal conditions peripheral lymph flow is regulated primarily by spontaneous contraction of the lymphatics themselves.[38, 39] In peripheral lymphatics, unlike peripheral veins, the column of liquid is incomplete. Accordingly, with normal intralymphatic pressure, external compression is ineffective for propelling lymph onward (Fig. 142–8), although it may increase the frequency and amplitude of lymphatic contractions. In other words, lymphatics, in contrast to veins, are not sufficiently "primed."[40] During lymphatic obstruction and persistent lymph stasis, hydrostatic pressure in the draining tissue watersheds and lymphatics rises as intrinsic truncal contractions fail to expel lymph completely. In this circumstance, in contrast to the normal situation, the fluid column in the lymphatics becomes continuous, and skeletal muscle or forceful external compression then becomes an effective pumping mechanism that aids lymph transport.[38, 40]

Studies on the effects of gravity on peripheral lymphatic and venous pressure conform to these findings. Whereas assuming an erect position sharply raises distal venous pressure, peripheral intralymphatic pressure is unaffected, although lymphatic truncal pulsation increases both in frequency and amplitude.[40] This arrangement favors

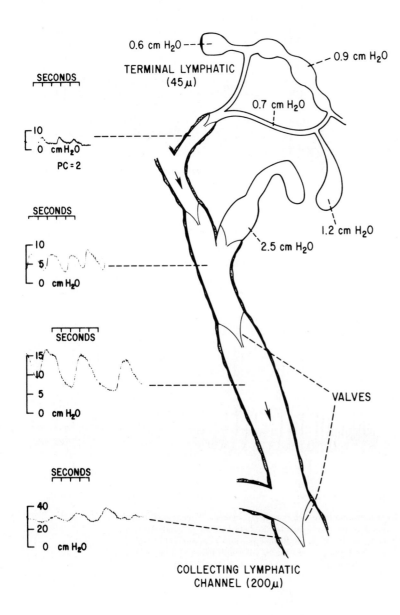

FIGURE 142–7. Composite drawing of terminal lymphatic network reconstructed from several mesenteric preparations in the rat demonstrating a gradual rise in intralymphatic pressure from 0.6 in the terminal lymphatics to 30 cmH₂O in the larger collecting duct. Note also the rhythmic pressure pulsations in the collecting trunks. (From Zweifach BW, Prather JW: Micromanipulation of pressure in terminal lymphatics in the mesentery. Am J Physiol 228:1326, 1975.)

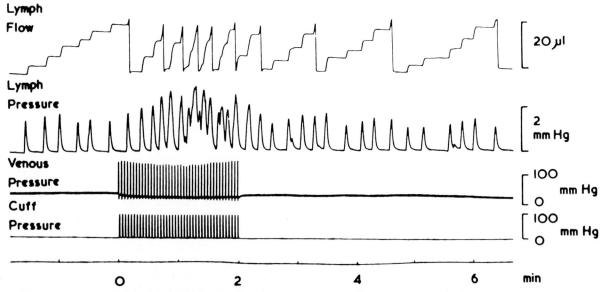

FIGURE 142–8. Effect of intermittent external pneumatic compression on the sheep foot on peripheral lymph flow, lymph outflow pressure, and venous pressure. Note that prior to external compression the lymphatic contracts spontaneously, and each contraction extrudes a small quantity of lymph, which appears as a step increment in the flow record. During the 2-minute time period when the foot cuff is inflated intermittently, each compression causes a synchronous pressure rise in peripheral venous pressure but not in lymph pressure. The frequency and amplitude of spontaneous lymphatic contractions increase, however, and this increase is associated with a concomitant rise in lymph flow. (From Pippard C, Roddie IC: Comparison of fluid transport systems in lymphatics and veins. Lymphology 20:224, 1987.)

the removal of tissue fluid by the lymphatics during dependency because, unlike the veins, the lymphatics operate at a much lower hydrostatic pressure. Once the lymphatics become obstructed, truncal contractions quicken at first, but then the intraluminal valves gradually give way, and as the lymph fluid column becomes continuous, this mechanical advantage is lost, and chronic lymphedema supervenes.

PATHOPHYSIOLOGY

Overview

Because congenital absence and radical excision of regional lymph nodes (and hence lymphatics) are both associated with edema, it seems straightforward that lymphedema is simply the end result of insufficient lymphatic drainage. Despite this reasonable conclusion, peripheral lymphedema has proved both hard to simulate in experimental animals and difficult to treat. Initial experimental attempts to simulate the clinical condition using lymphatic sclerosis and radical excision were notoriously unsuccessful and revealed a remarkable capacity of obstructed lymphatics to regenerate and "bridge the gap" or bypass the induced blockage with spontaneous opening of auxiliary lymphatic-venous shunts.[41, 42] Although transient swelling was common, these compensatory mechanisms were thought to preclude the development of chronic lymphedema solely on the basis of obstruction of lymphatic drainage. The general failure of early lymph stasis experiments to reproduce unremitting peripheral edema reinforced a long-held theory that overt or subclinical bacterial infection (lymphangitis) was indispensable to the evolution of chronic lymphedema.[43] By disrupting microvascular integrity and promot-

ing lymphatic obliteration, recurring infection was thought to exaggerate tissue scarring and eventually cause unremitting lymphedema. This widely held belief was consistent with the commonly observed delayed onset and unpredictability of arm and leg edema following radical mastectomy and groin dissection, respectively, and the grotesque deformities of tropical lymphedema (so-called elephantiasis) associated with filariasis (*Wuchereria bancrofti* and *Brugia malayi*).

Although understanding is still incomplete, it is nonetheless now clear that nonpitting, brawny extremity edema can arise from lymph stasis alone and the unremitting accumulation of protein-rich fluid in the extracellular matrix. By means of repeated intralymphatic injection of silica particles, Drinker and colleagues[44] first succeeded in simulating chronic lymphedema in dogs through extensive lymphatic sclerosis. Subsequently, Danese,[45] Olszewski,[35] Clodius and Altorfer,[46] and their associates established that refractory lymphedema could result solely from the mechanical interruption of peripheral lymphatics. Using an experimental model of circumferential lymphatic transection, tissue swelling was found to be prompt at first (acute lymphedema), disappeared by 4 to 6 weeks, and remained absent for months to years (latent lymphedema), but thereafter reappeared and persisted (chronic lymphedema). A similar sequence of events occurs in experimental filariasis (due to *B. malayi*).[47] During the latent phase, when edema is not visible, conventional oil lymphography corroborates ongoing lymphatic destruction.[35] Progressive truncal tortuosity and dilatation gives way to massive lymphangiectasis, valvular incompetence, and retrograde flow (dermal backflow). Serial microscopy discloses mononuclear cell infiltration, intramural destruction of lymphatic collectors, and collagen deposition throughout the soft tissues. Eventually the lymph trunks lose their distinctive smooth muscle and endothelial lining, and the boundary lines between lymph collectors and the surrounding matrix progressively blur.[35, 46] These studies definitively demonstrate that extensive impairment of lymph drainage is sufficient by itself to cause chronic lymphedema (Fig. 142–9). The key observation is the long interval between the disruption of the lymph trunks and the development of refractory edema, which helps to explain the inconstancy and unpredictability of limb swelling after radical operations for treatment of cancer and other disorders of defective lymphatic drainage. As with deep venous occlusive disease, which is associated with valve destruction, venous stasis, and eventually overt edema (post-thrombophlebitic syndrome) with characteristic trophic skin changes (hyperpigmentation and ulceration), the absence or obliteration of the lymphatics is associated with lymphatic valve incompetence, lymph stasis, and eventually intractable edema (postlymphangitic syndrome) with its characteristic trophic skin changes (thickened toe skin folds or Stemmer's sign, warty overgrowth, and brawny induration).[48]

Infection

Recurrent cellulitis is a devastating sequela of peripheral lymphedema. Erysipelas resulting from beta-hemolytic streptococcal infection is most common, but fulminant infection occurs with a variety of microorganisms.[49] To a certain extent, vulnerability to superimposed infection exists whenever tissue fluid stagnates. Thus, pyelonephritis

with urinary retention, cholangitis with common duct stones, and spontaneous bacterial peritonitis with "cirrhotic" ascites are vivid examples of this phenomenon. Yet lymphedema (in contrast to edema states arising from imbalances in transcapillary hydrodynamic forces) is so prone to recurring lymphangitis that at one time it was mistaken as the sine qua non of lymphedema (see earlier discussion).

The reasons for the extraordinary susceptibility of an extremity with lymphedema to secondary bacterial infection remain perplexing. Studies of canine-induced and human filarial lymphedema implicate defective complement activation and immunodysregulation.[35] Alternative hypotheses include the depopulation of regional lymph nodes with replacement by fat and scar[34] and deficient protease activity of extravascular macrophages.[50] It remains unclear, however, whether these immunologic perturbations are systemic, strictly regional, or even unique to lymphedema. Notwithstanding, the onset of overt lymphedema is often precipitated by sudden infection or injury in an extremity already exhibiting defective lymphatic function. Moreover, episodes of thrombophlebitis and trauma, including bony fractures and multiple insect bites, are associated with "lymphangitis" and worsening of peripheral lymphedema. Walking barefoot, particularly in Third World countries that lack proper hygiene, promotes overt and occult cellulitis and local foot infections that aggravate filaria-induced lymphedema and exaggerate exuberant skin verrucae and dermal scarring. In other words, in an extremity with marginal lymphatic drainage, even minor trauma and infection may initiate a protracted pernicious cycle that in extreme cases

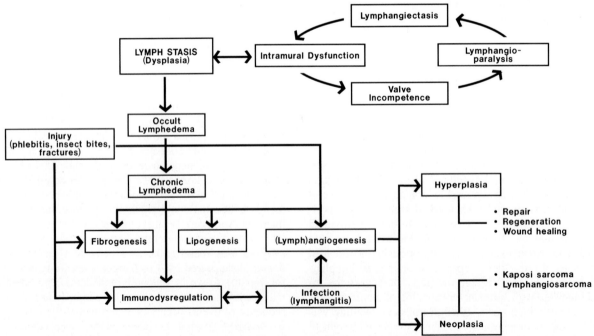

FIGURE 142–9. Flow chart illustrating the pathogenesis of peripheral lymphedema and some of its sequelae. According to this scheme, congenitally deficient or obstructed lymphatics promote lymph stasis, which is accompanied by deranged truncal contractility, progressive valve incompetence, destruction of contractile elements (lymphangioparalysis), and gradual ectasia of lymphatic collectors. After a variable period (occult lymphedema), sometimes aggravated by environmental trauma, a series of events is set into motion that culminates in chronic lymphedema. This clinical state is characterized not only by progressive swelling but also by fat and scar deposition, immunodysregulation, a propensity for cellulitis, and microvascular proliferation; these processes on the one hand are essential for repair and regeneration but on the other may result in bizarre and poorly understood vascular new growths.

culminates in a pachyderm-like deformity resembling an elephantine limb and on rare occasions leads to a highly aggressive vascular malignancy (see Fig. 142–9 and earlier discussion).

Fibrosis

Like the sequela of superimposed infection, the complications of progressive interstitial fibrosis also set lymphedema apart from other edematous states. Whereas the pathogenetic sequence linking scarring to lymphedema is still unclear, it has long been recognized that conditions associated with edema high in protein content (such as lymphedema) are characterized by fibrous proliferation. Altered cytokine production, perturbed immunoreactivity, accumulation of abnormal plasma protein moieties including growth factors in the extracellular matrix, proliferation of mast cells with release of vasomediators such as histamine,[51, 52] and activation of a complement cascade with ''fixation'' to immunocomplexes may exert, singly or in toto, both microvascular and chemotactic effects that facilitate tissue infiltration of chronic inflammatory cells (e.g., lymphocytes and macrophages).[53] As fibrin- and cell-binding circulating fibronectins accumulate in the stagnant edema fluid, they act as the scaffolding and support glue for the migration of fibroblasts and the laying down of collagen.[54] In addition, lymph stasis and the build-up of plasma proteins trapped in the interstitium overwhelm intrinsic neutrophil and macrophage proteases and provoke diffuse scarring.[55] Intensive neoangiogenesis associated with enhanced migration of endothelial cells further aggravates the pathologic picture. Ironically, these same processes are also critical for the repair of wounds, of which scar formation is also the final common pathway.

Neoplasia

A rare but nonetheless revealing sequela of long-standing peripheral lymphedema is the occurrence of (lymph)angiosarcoma. This aggressive vascular tumor was once thought to arise exclusively in the aftermath of radical mastectomy and irradiation for the local control of breast cancer (Stewart-Treves syndrome).[56, 57] Lymphangiosarcoma, however, has now been documented in other secondary lymphedemas and even in congenital or primary lymphedema.[58] Because the preexisting swelling has usually persisted for many years and may occur in either primary or secondary lymphedema or in the presence or absence of previous radiotherapy, the lymphedema process itself has been thought to be the prime causative factor. More recently, Kaposi's sarcoma, a vascular tumor akin to Stewart-Treves syndrome and allied closely with acquired immunodeficiency syndrome (AIDS), has been linked to an origin from lymphatic endothelium.[59–62] Perhaps immunodysregulation, particularly in the antigen-presenting afferent loop (i.e., dysregulated lymphangiogenesis and hemangiogenesis), underlies a wide range of bizarre vasoproliferative and lymphologic syndromes including hemolymphangioma, Kuppel-Trenaunay syndrome, angiofollicular hyperplasia (epithelioid hemangioma), lymphangioleiomy-

omatosis, and lymphangitic metastatic carcinomatosis (see Fig. 142–9).

Chylous Reflux

Abnormal retrograde transport of intestinal lymph is responsible for chylous disorders. Because cholesterol and long-chain triglycerides in the form of chylomicra are absorbed exclusively by the lymphatic system, dysfunction (in the form of disruption, compression, obstruction, or fistulization) of mesenteric lacteals, the cisterna chyli, and the thoracic duct is directly linked to chylothorax, chylous ascites, and chyluria. In some patients with high-grade blockage of intestinal lymph flow, the peripheral lymphatics gradually dilate and, with progressive valvular incompetence, lactescent lymph refluxes into the soft tissues of the pelvis, scrotum, and lower extremities (chylous vesicles and edema) (Fig. 142–10).

SUMMARY

Disturbances in microcirculatory perfusion and exchange of liquid, macromolecules, and cells across intact and abnormal microvessels and deranged lymph kinetics are, individually and together, associated with disorders of tissue swelling. Peripheral lymphedema manifesting as low-output failure of the lymph circulation is characteristically indolent for many years before lymphatic insufficiency and tissue swelling accelerate and become persistent. Nonetheless, impedance of lymph flow by itself is sufficient to explain at least mild to moderate forms of lymphedema. Chronic lymphedema is characterized by trapping in the skin and subcutaneous tissues of fluid, extravasated plasma proteins, and other macromolecules. It is typical to find impaired immune cell trafficking (lymphocytes, Langerhans' cells, monocytes), abnormal transport of autologous and foreign antigens, probably intact hydrodynamic (Starling) transcapillary forces,[63] and an increased propensity to superimposed infection. Additional characteristics include progressive obliteration of lymphatics (lymphangiopathy ''die-back'' or lymphangitis), defective lymphangion contractility, mononuclear cell infiltrate (chronic interstitial inflammation), epidermal cell–fibroblast proliferation, collagen deposition, altered immunoreactivity, and vasoactive mediator imbalance with increased production of local cytokines and growth factors including autocrine and paracrine hormones.

In contrast to the blood circulation, in which flow depends primarily on the propulsive force of the myocardium, lymph propulsion depends predominantly on intrinsic truncal contraction, a phylogenetic remnant of amphibian lymph hearts. Whereas venous plasma flows rapidly (2.5 to 3 L/min) against low vascular resistance, lymph ''plasma'' flows slowly (2.0 ml/min) against high vascular resistance. On occasion, impaired transport of intestinal lymph may be associated with reflux and accumulation or leakage of intestinal chyle into swollen legs. In extreme circumstances these factors operating together may be responsible for the hideous deformities known as elephantiasis.

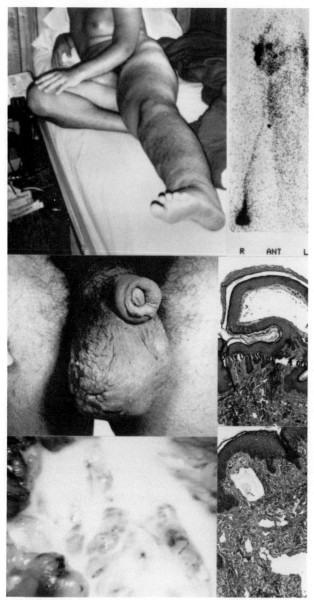

FIGURE 142-10. Sixteen-year-old boy with chylous reflux syndrome characterized by left leg, penile, and scrotal lymphedema with multiple small chyle-containing vesicles. Lymphoscintigraphy shows *(upper right)* that tracer (^{99m}Tc human serum albumin) injected intradermally into the right foot crosses to the left side and flows retrograde to outline dermal lymphatics in the contralateral leg. During a scrotal debulking operation, chylous lymph floods the operative field *(lower left)*, and light microscopy of the excised skin shows large endothelium-lined channels *(mid and lower right)* consistent with ectatic dermal lymphatics.

Transdifferentiation and transformation of endothelium and other vascular accessory cells associated with lymph stasis may also be pivotal to factors in a wide range of dysplastic and neoplastic vascular disorders including Stewart-Treves syndrome, AIDS-associated Kaposi's sarcoma, and lymphangitic metastatic carcinomatosis.

References

1. Rusznyák I, Földi M, Szabo G: History of the discovery of lymphatics and lymph circulation. *In* Lymphatics and Lymph Circulation. 2nd ed. Oxford, Pergamon Press, 1967, pp 15–24.

2. Földi M: Lymphogenous encephalopathy. *In* Diseases of Lymphatics and Lymph Circulation. Springfield, IL, Charles C Thomas, 1969, pp 91–117.

3. Bradbury MWB, Westrop RJ: Factors influencing exit of substances from cerebrospinal fluid into deep cervical lymph of the rabbit. J Physiol 339:519, 1983.

4. Leeds SE, Kong AK, Wise BL: Alternative pathways for drainage of cerebrospinal fluid in the canine brain. Lymphology 22:144, 1989.

5. Casley-Smith JR: Lymph and lymphatics. *In* Kaley G, Altura BM (eds): Microcirculation. Baltimore, University Park Press, 1977, vol. 1, pp 423–502.

6. Leak LV: Physiology of the lymphatic system. *In* Abramson DI, Dobrin PB (eds): Blood Vessels and Lymphatics in Organ Systems. Orlando, FL, Academic Press, 1984, pp 134–164.

7. Way D, Hendrix M, Witte MH, et al: Lymphatic endothelial cell line (CH3) from a recurrent retroperitoneal lymphangioma. In Vitro 23:647, 1987.

8. Gnepp DR, Chandler W: Tissue culture of human and canine thoracic duct endothelium. In Vitro 21:200, 1985.

9. Johnston MG, Walker MA: Lymphatic endothelial and smooth-muscle cells in tissue culture. In Vitro 20:566, 1984.

10. Casley-Smith JR: The lymphatic system. *In* Földi M, Casley-Smith JR (eds): Lymphangiology. Stuttgart, FK Schattauer-Verlag, 1983, pp 89–164.

11. Leak LV, Burke JF: Fine structure of the lymphatic capillary and the adjoining connective tissue area. Am J Anat 118:785, 1966.

12. Leak LV, Burke JF: Ultrastructural studies on the lymphatic anchoring filaments. J Cell Biol 36:129, 1968.

13. Leak LV: Electron microscopic observation on lymphatic capillaries and the structural components of the connective tissue-lymph interface. Microvascular Res 2:361, 1970.

14. Mislin H: The lymphangion. *In* Földi M, Casley-Smith JR (eds): Lymphangiology. Stuttgart, FK Schattauer-Verlag, 1983, pp 165–175.

15. Starling EH: Physiologic factors involved in the causation of dropsy. Lancet 1:1267, 1896.

16. Starling EH: The fluids of the body. The Herter Lectures. Chicago, WT Keener, 1909, p 81.

17. Hall JG, Morris B, Woolley G: Intrinsic rhythmic propulsion of lymph in the unanaesthetised sheep. J Physiol (Lond) 180:336, 1965.

18. Mawhinney HJD, Roddie IC: Spontaneous activity in isolated bovine mesenteric lymphatics. J Physiol 229:339, 1973.

19. Olszewski WL, Engeset A: Intrinsic contractility of prenodal lymph vessels and lymph flow in the human leg. Am J Physiol 239:H775, 1980.

20. Gnepp DR: Lymphatics. *In* Staub NC, Taylor AE (eds): Edema. New York, Raven Press, 1984, pp 263–298.

21. McHale NG, Roddie IC: The effect of transmural pressure on pumping activity in isolated bovine lymphatic vessels. J Physiol 261:255, 1976.

22. McHale NG, Roddie IC: The effect of intravenous adrenaline and noradrenaline infusion on peripheral lymph flow in the sheep. J Physiol 341:517, 1983.

23. Johnston MG: The intrinsic lymph pump: Progress and problems. Lymphology 22:116, 1989.

24. Sinzinger H, Kaliman J, Mannheimer E: Regulation of human lymph contractility by prostaglandins and thromboxane. Lymphology 17:43, 1984.

25. Johnston MG, Gordon JL: Regulation of lymphatic contractility by arachidonate metabolites. Nature 293:294, 1981.

26. Johnston MG, Feuer C: Suppression of lymphatic vessel contractility with inhibitors of arachidonic acid metabolism. J Pharmacol Exp Ther 226:603, 1983.

27. Ohhashi T, Kawai Y, Azuma T: The response of lymphatic smooth muscles to vasoactive substances. Pflügers Arch 375:183, 1978.

28. McHale NG, Roddie IC, Thornbury K: Nervous modulation of spontaneous contractions in bovine mesenteric lymphatics. J Physiol 309:461, 1980.

29. McGeown JG, McHale NG, Thornbury K: Popliteal efferent lymph flow response to stimulation of the sympathetic chain in the sheep. J Physiol 387:55P, 1987.

30. Sjöberg T, Alm P, Andersson KE, et al: Contractile response in isolated human groin lymphatics. Lymphology 20:152, 1987.

31. Sjöberg T, Steen S: Contractile properties of lymphatics from the human lower leg. Lymphology 24:16, 1991.

32. Swemer RL, Foglia VG: Fatal loss of plasma volume after lymph heart destruction in toads. Proc Soc Exp Biol Med 53:14, 1943.

33. Conklin R: The formation and circulation of lymph in the frog. I. The rate of lymph production. Am J Physiol 95:79, 1930.
34. Kinmonth JB, Wolfe JH: Fibrosis in the lymph nodes in primary lymphedema. Ann R Coll Surg 62:344, 1980.
35. Olszewski W: On the pathomechanism of development of post surgical lymphedema. Lymphology 6:35, 1973.
36. Zweifach BW, Prather JW: Micromanipulation of pressure in terminal lymphatics in the mesentery. Am J Physiol 228:1326, 1975.
37. Pippard C, Roddie IC: Resistance in the sheep's lymphatic system. Lymphology 20:230, 1987.
38. Olszewski WL: Lymph pressure and flow in limbs. In Lymph Stasis: Pathophysiology, Diagnosis and Treatment. Boca Raton, FL, CRC Press, 1991, pp 109–156.
39. McHale NG: Influence of autonomic nerves on lymph flow. In Olszewski WL (ed): Lymph Stasis: Pathophysiology, Diagnosis and Treatment, Boca Raton, FL, CRC Press, 1991, pp 85–107.
40. Pippard C, Roddie IC: Comparison of fluid transport systems in lymphatics and veins. Lymphology 20:224, 1987.
41. Reichert FL: The regeneration of the lymphatics. Arch Surg 13:871, 1926.
42. Blalock A, Robinson CS, Cunningham RS, Gray ME: Experimental studies on lymphatic blockade. Arch Surg 34:1049, 1937.
43. Halsted WS: The swelling of the arm after operations for cancer of the breast—Elephantiasis chirurgica—Its cause and prevention. Johns Hopkins Hosp Bull 32:309, 1921.
44. Drinker CK, Field MJ, Homans J: The experimental production of edema and elephantiasis as a result of lymphatic obstruction. Am J Physiol 108:509, 1934.
45. Danese CA, Georgalas-Bertakis M, Morales LE: A model of chronic postsurgical lymphedema in dogs' limbs. Surgery 64:814, 1968.
46. Clodius L, Altorfer J: Experimental chronic lymphostasis of extremities. Folia Angiol 25:137, 1977.
47. Case T, Leis B, Witte M, et al: Vascular abnormalities in experimental and human lymphatic filariasis. Lymphology 24:174, 1991.
48. Földi M: Lymphoedema. In Földi M, Casley-Smith JR (eds): Lymphangiology. Stuttgart, FK Schattauer-Verlag, 1983, pp 668–670.
49. Edwards EA: Recurrent febrile episodes and lymphedema. JAMA 184:102, 1963.
50. Casley-Smith JR, Casley-Smith JR: High-Protein Oedemas and the Benzo-pyrones. Sydney, Australia, JB Lippincott, 1986, pp 126–152.
51. Ehrich WE, Seifter J, Alburn HE, Begamy AJ: Heparin and heparinocytes in elephantiasis scroti. Proc Soc Exp Biol Med 70:183, 1949.
52. Dumont AE, Fazzini E, Jamal S: Metachromatic cells in filarial lymphoedema. Lancet 2:1021, 1983.
53. Gaffney RM, Casley-Smith JR: Lymphedema without lymphostasis: Excess proteins as the cause of chronic inflammation. Progress in Lymphology. Proceedings of the VII International Congress. Prague, Avicenum, 1981, pp 213–216.
54. Poslethwaite AE, Keski-Oja J, Balian G, Kang AH: Induction of fibroblast chemotaxis by fibronectin. J Exp Med 153:494, 1981.
55. Földi M: Insufficiency of lymph flow. In Földi M, Casley-Smith JR (eds): Lymphangiology. Stuttgart, FK Schattauer-Verlag, 1983, p 195.
56. Stewart FW, Treves N: Lymphangiosarcoma in post mastectomy lymphedema: A report of six cases in elephantiasis chirurgica. Cancer 1:64, 1948.
57. Unruh H, Robertson DI, Karasewich E: Post mastectomy lymphangiosarcoma. Can J Surg 22:586, 1979.
58. Woodward AH, Ivins JC, Sorle EH: Lymphangiosarcoma arising in chronic lymphedematous extremities. Cancer 30:562, 1972.
59. Dorfman RF: Kaposi's sarcoma: Evidence supporting its origin from the lymphatic system. Lymphology 21:45, 1988.
60. Witte MH, Stuntz M, Witte CL: Kaposi's sarcoma: A lymphologic perspective. Int J Dermatol 28:561, 1989.
61. Witte MH, Fiala M, McNeill GC, et al: Lymphangioscintigraphy in AIDS-associated Kaposi sarcoma. Am J Roentgenol 155:311, 1990.
62. Beckstead JH, Wood GS, Fletcher V: Evidence for the origin of Kaposi's sarcoma from lymphatic endothelium. Am J Pathol 119:294, 1985.
63. Kirk RM: Capillary filtration rates in normal and lymphedematous legs. Clin Sci 27:363, 1964.

143

Clinical Diagnosis and Evaluation of Lymphedema

Peter Gloviczki, M.D., and Heinz W. Wahner, M.D., F.A.C.P.

• • •

Chronic lymphedema is a progressive, usually painless swelling of the extremity that results from a decreased transport capacity of the lymphatic system. Lymphedema may be caused by developmental abnormalities of the lymph vessels, such as aplasia, hypoplasia, or hyperplasia with valvular incompetence,[1–2] or it may be the result of congenital or acquired obstruction of the lymph vessels and lymph nodes.[3–6] The diagnosis of lymphedema is suspected in most patients after obtaining the history and performing a physical examination. The goal of further evaluation is to confirm the cause and determine the type and site of lymphatic obstruction. It is equally important, however, to diagnose any underlying malignancy and to exclude other systemic or local causes of limb swelling such as venous disease or congenital vascular malformation.

In this chapter, the current classifications of lymphedema are presented and the clinical presentation of patients with this disease is reviewed. The methods of noninvasive evaluation are discussed, and the technique and interpretation of lymphoscintigraphy, which in the last decade has become the test of choice to confirm or exclude lymphatic disease, is presented in detail. The role of contrast lymphan-

Table 143–1.   Etiologic Classification of Lymphedema

I. Primary lymphedema
   A. Congenital (onset before 1 year of age)
      1. Nonfamilial
      2. Familial (Milroy's disease)
   B. Praecox (onset 1 to 35 years of age)
      1. Nonfamilial
      2. Familial (Meige's disease)
   C. Tarda (onset after 35 years of age)
II. Secondary lymphedema
   A. Filariasis
   B. Lymph node excision ± radiation
   C. Tumor invasion
   D. Infection
   E. Trauma
   F. Other

giography in the 1990s for the diagnosis of lymphatic disorders is reassessed. Finally, the differential diagnosis of lymphedema is discussed and a diagnostic protocol for the evaluation of patients with a swollen extremity is suggested.

CLINICAL CLASSIFICATIONS

Classic clinical classifications distinguish lymphedemas based on etiology (primary vs. secondary), genetics (familial vs. sporadic) and time of onset of the edema (congenital, praecox, tarda) (Table 143–1).[1, 2, 7] Although these systems are useful for categorizing all lymphedemas, they do not address the clinical severity of the disease and are usually not relevant to therapy. More recent classifications focus on the clinical stage of lymphedema[8] or emphasize the underlying anatomic abnormality of the lymphatic system in an attempt to plan therapy.[3, 4, 9]

Primary Lymphedema

The most accepted etiologic classification divides lymphedemas into two major groups, primary and secondary lymphedemas. These terms were suggested in 1934 by Allen from the Mayo Clinic, who evaluated 300 patients with lymphedema of the extremities.[7] He further divided the primary or idiopathic group into congenital and praecox types (Fig. 143–1). The former included patients who developed edema before 1 year of age. Kinmonth later added another group to the primary lymphedemas comprising those who develop the disease after 35 years of age (lymphedema tarda).[2]

Although it has been assumed that all primary or idiopathic lymphedemas have an underlying developmental abnormality in the lymphatic system, i.e., aplasia, hypoplasia, or hyperplasia of the lymph vessels, fibrotic occlusion of lymph vessels and lymph nodes has been described in primary lymphedema by Kinmonth and Wolfe.[10, 11] Studies by Browse suggest that the cause of primary lymphedema praecox in many patients is most likely acquired fibrotic obliteration of the lymph vessels and the lymph-conducting elements of the lymph nodes.[3, 4, 9]

Primary lymphedema is fortunately rare. Based on data

collected by the Rochester Group Study,[12] it affects 1.15/100,000 persons less than 20 years of age. It occurs more frequently in girls, and the incidence peaks between the ages of 12 and 16 years. In a group of 125 patients with primary lymphedema treated at the Mayo Clinic, 97 (78 per cent) were females and 28 (22 per cent) were males, yielding a female : male ratio of 3.5 : 1.0.[13] The ratio of unilateral to bilateral lymphedema was 3:1. Congenital lymphedema occurred more frequently in males than in females. In these patients, the edema was usually bilateral and involved the entire lower extremity. In contrast, the typical patient with lymphedema praecox was female and had unilateral involvement, with swelling usually extending up to the knee only.[13]

Familial Lymphedema

The familial form of primary lymphedema was described first in 1865 by Letessier,[14] and additional cases were published later by Nonne[15] and Milroy.[16, 17] The report of Milroy in 1892 described lower limb lymphedema that was observed in 22 members of the same family over six generations.[16] In all except two patients the edema was

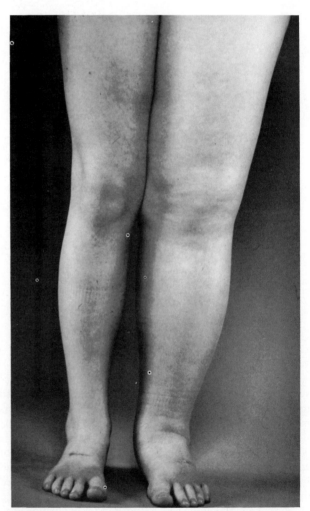

FIGURE 143–1.   Primary lymphedema praecox of both lower extremities, more significantly of the left. Leg swelling in this 9-year-old boy was first noted at age 4 years.

present at birth. The term Milroy's disease should be reserved for patients with familial lymphedema that is present at birth or is noticed soon thereafter. A familial form of lymphedema that becomes manifest only during puberty was described later by Meige.[18] The term Meige's disease, therefore, refers to the familial form of lymphedema praecox.

In a collected series of 291 patients with primary lymphedema 42 (14 per cent) had a family history of lymphedema. Fourteen patients (5 per cent) had congenital lymphedema, the onset of which was noted before 1 year of age, and 28 (9 per cent) had lymphedema praecox.[13] In the Mayo Clinic series, 10 of 125 (8 per cent) patients had a positive family history of lymphedema.

Functional Classification of Primary Lymphedemas

The functional classification of primary lymphedema by Browse is based on the underlying lymphatic anatomy as determined by lymphangiography.[3, 4] This classification describes three different anatomic abnormalities, which are associated with different clinical presentations. More important, however, the classification is treatment oriented and selects appropriate groups that may respond to medical or surgical treatment.

Based on the underlying anatomic abnormality of the lymphatic system, Browse subdivided primary lymphedemas into three groups: (1) distal obliteration, (2) proximal obliteration, and (3) congenital hyperplasia (Table 143–2).

Distal obliteration occurs in 80 per cent of patients and affects predominantly females. The swelling is frequently bilateral.[4, 9] Lymphangiography demonstrates absent or a diminished number of superficial leg lymphatics in these patients. This group was also described by Kinmonth and Wolfe as having aplasia or hypoplasia.[2, 10] The course of the disease is usually benign, progression is slow, and the edema is usually responsive to conservative compression treatment.

Ten per cent of patients with primary lymphedema have proximal occlusion in the aortoiliac or inguinal lymph nodes.[9] This disease is frequently unilateral and involves the entire lower extremity, affecting both males and females. This form of lymphedema frequently develops rapidly, and progression is usual. The edema responds poorly to conservative management. Distal dilatation with proximal occlusion, however, may be suitable for mesenteric bridge operation or for microvascular lymph vessel reconstruction (see Chapter 146).

Hyperplasia and incompetence of the lymph vessels are observed in the remaining 10 per cent of patients. Most of these patients have bilateral lymphedema, and males are more frequently affected than females.[11] One subgroup of these patients has megalymphatics, and because of concomitant involvement of the mesenteric lymphatics reflux of chyle frequently results. The leg edema is unilateral in most of these patients.[10, 11] Protein-losing enteropathy, chyluria, chylous drainage through the vagina, and chylorrhea from small vesicles in the labia majora, scrotum, or lower extremities may also develop (Fig. 143–2).[19–21] The leg edema responds well to elevation, but recurs rapidly with ambulation. These patients are candidates for surgical treatment consisting of ligation and excision of the incompetent retroperitoneal lymphatics (see Chapter 146).

Although this functional classification is helpful in selecting patients for further management, the overlap in the first two groups may be quite significant. In addition, without contrast lymphangiography, separation of the groups is not always possible.

Secondary Lymphedema

Secondary acquired lymphedema results from a well-defined disease process that causes obstruction or injury to the lymphatic system. The most frequent cause of secondary lymphedema in the world is parasitic infestation by filariasis.[22, 23] In North America and Europe the most frequent cause of secondary lymphedema is surgical excision and irradiation of the axillary or inguinal lymph nodes as part of the treatment of an underlying malignancy, most frequently cancer of the breast[24–29] (Fig. 143–3), cervical cancer,[30] soft tissue tumors (Fig. 143–4), or malignant melanoma of the leg.[31] Other causes of secondary lymphedema are tumors invading the lymph vessels and nodes,[32] bacterial or fungal infections, lymphoproliferative diseases, and trauma.[33] Less frequent causes of secondary lymphedema are contact dermatitis, tuberculosis, rheumatoid arthritis, and infection after a snake or insect bite. Factitious edema induced by application of a tourniquet on the arm or leg or by maintenance of the limb in an immobile or dependent state should also be considered in some patients.[34]

Table 143–2. Functional Classification of Primary Lymphedema

	Distal Obliteration (80%)	**Proximal Obliteration (10%)**	**Hyperplasia* (10%)**
Gender	Female	Male or female	Male or female
Onset			
Time	Puberty	Any age	Congenital
Location	Ankle; bilateral	Whole leg, thigh; unilateral	Whole leg; unilateral or bilateral
Progression	Slow	Rapid	Progressive
Family history	Frequently positive	None	Frequently positive

Adapted from Browse NL: The diagnosis and management of primary lymphedema. J Vasc Surg 3:181, 1986.
*With or without reflux of chyle.

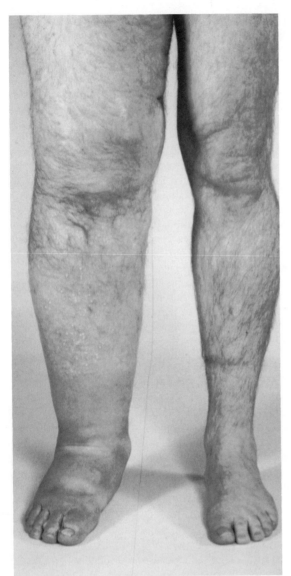

FIGURE 143–2. Primary lymphedema of the right leg caused by hyperplasia of the lymphatics and valvular incompetence. Note skin vesicles at mid-calf containing milky fluid because of reflux of chyle.

Filariasis

Lymphatic filariasis is caused by the developing and adult forms of three parasites: *Wuchereria bancrofti*, *Brugia malayi*, and *B. timori*. Of the estimated 90.2 million people in the world who are infected, more than 90 per cent have bancroftian filariasis.[23] The disease is most frequent in subtropical and tropical countries, such as China, India, and Indonesia. It is transmitted by different types of mosquitos, and transmission is closely related to poor urban sanitation.[35] Perilymphatic inflammation, fibrosis, and sclerosis of the lymph nodes are caused by the indwelling adult worms. Lymph node fibrosis, reactive hyperplasia, and dilation of the lymphatic collecting channels are caused by the worm products, by physical injury to the valves and vessel walls caused by the live worms, and by the immune response of the host.[36] Eosinophilia is found in the peripheral blood smear, and microfilaria can be demonstrated in peripheral

nocturnal blood, in the centrifuged urine sediment, or in the lymphatic fluid.[37] Filarial lymphedema rapidly develops into grossly incapacitating elephantiasis that is extremely difficult to treat.

Lymph Node Excision and Irradiation

Postmastectomy lymphedema is the most distressing and unpleasant complication following operation for breast cancer. During past decades, when radical mastectomy was routinely performed, clinically significant lymphedema was reported to occur in 6 to 60 per cent of patients.[24] Axillary vein obstruction and episodes of lymphangitis contributed significantly to the further development of edema (see Fig. 143–3). With the introduction of more conservative breast cancer operations, the incidence of postmastectomy lymphedema markedly decreased. The reported incidence of arm lymphedema following modified radical mastectomy is 15.4 per cent;[25] after local excision and total axillary lymphadenectomy it is 2.1 to 3.1 per cent,[26, 27] and after wide local excision and radiotherapy it is 2.3 per cent.[28] However, few studies have objectively documented the degree of limb swelling in these patients. Kissin and colleagues studied the development of lymphedema in 200 patients following different breast cancer operations.[29] Chronic lymphedema, with an increase of over 200 ml in the volume of the extremity, developed in 25.5 per cent of the patients. Independent risk factors contributing to lymphedema included extensive axillary lymphadenectomy ($p < .05$), axillary ra-

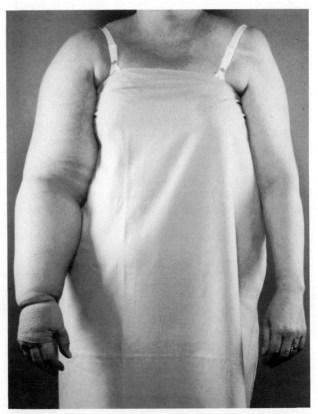

FIGURE 143–3. Right arm lymphedema following modified radical mastectomy and radiation treatment. The edema was aggravated by obstruction of the right axillary vein.

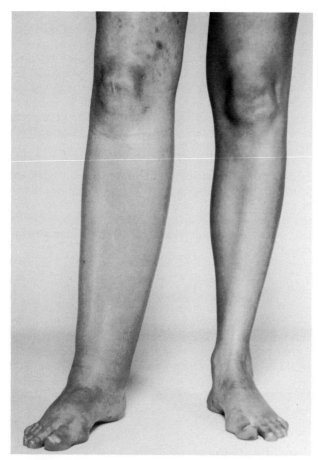

FIGURE 143–4. Twenty-nine-year-old woman with secondary lymphedema of the right leg following excision of Ewing's sarcoma of the thigh and irradiation.

diotherapy (*p* < .001), and pathologic nodal status (*p* < .10). Extensive axillary lymph node dissection followed by radiotherapy resulted in the highest incidence, with 38.3 per cent of the patients developing lymphedema.[29]

In a series of 91 patients who underwent regional lymphadenectomy for invasive primary melanoma, chronic lymphedema developed in 80 per cent of those followed for more than 5 years.[31] Most swelling occurred in the thigh. In a series of 402 patients from Norway who underwent radical hysterectomy and pelvic lymphadenectomy for cervical cancer, 5 per cent developed severe lymphedema, and 23.4 per cent developed mild to moderate lymphedema.[30] All patients with severe lymphedema had adjuvant preoperative and postoperative radiation treatment.

Tumor Invasion

Lymphedema may be the first manifestation of a malignant tumor infiltrating the regional lymph nodes. In a series of 650 patients with lymphedema, De Roo found 60 in whom limb swelling developed as the first clinical marker of a malignant process.[32] The most frequent tumor was metastatic ovarian carcinoma, followed by carcinoma of the uterus with inguinal metastases and lymphosarcoma. All these patients were 28 years old or older, and in two thirds of the patients, limb edema started in the *proximal*

region of the extremity. In our experience, the most frequent tumor causing secondary lymphedema is carcinoma of the prostate in men and malignant lymphoma in women.[33]

Infection

Obstructive lymphangitis, caused most frequently by beta-hemolytic streptococci or, rarely, staphylococci, is not only a severe complication of an already existing lymphedema but also is itself an important cause of secondary lymphedema. Swelling may develop following an episode of cellulitis caused by an insect bite, trauma, excoriation, or fungal infection. It is possible that many patients who present with inflammatory lymphedema already have an impairment of lymphatic transport due to lymphatic hypoplasia or primary fibrotic occlusion of the lymph vessels or lymph nodes.

Clinical Staging of Lymphedema

Because none of the classic classification schemes addresses the clinical stage of the disease, the Working Group of the 10th International Congress of Lymphology in 1985 suggested staging chronic lymphedemas regardless of etiology. A latent, subclinical stage and three clinical grades were established as suggested by Brunner.[8] Each grade was subclassified as mild, moderate, and severe.

In the latent phase excess fluid accumulates, and fibrosis occurs around the lymphatics, but no edema is apparent clinically. In *grade I*, edema pits on pressure and is reduced largely or completely by elevation; there is no clinical evidence of fibrosis. *Grade II* edema does not pit on pressure and is not reduced by elevation. Moderate to severe fibrosis is evident on clinical examination. *Grade III* edema is irreversible and develops from repeated inflammatory attacks, fibrosis, and sclerosis of the skin and subcutaneous tissue. This is the stage of lymphostatic elephantiasis.

The advantage of this classification is that it permits evaluation of the effectiveness of a treatment and comparison of different treatment modalities. A drawback, however, is that appropriate staging in some cases may be difficult without performing biopsy of the subcutaneous tissue.

CLINICAL PRESENTATION OF LYMPHEDEMA

History

A careful history of the disease frequently reveals the cause of swelling and suggests the diagnosis of lymphedema. A family history that is positive for leg swelling may indicate familial lymphedema. The development of painless leg swelling in a female in her teens without any identifiable cause strongly suggests *primary* (idiopathic) lymphedema. A history of diarrhea and weight loss is a clue to mesenteric lymphangiectasia, whereas intermittent drainage of milky fluid from skin vesicles in these patients indicates

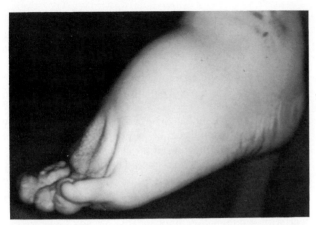

FIGURE 143–5. Lymphedema of the forefoot showing the typical "buffalo hump."

reflux of chyle. In patients with *secondary* lymphedema a cause of limb swelling is evident in the history, such as previous lymph node dissection, irradiation, tumor, trauma, or infection. In patients who have traveled in tropical countries filariasis is suspected. Although the etiology of primary lymphedema is different from that of secondary lymphedema, the clinical presentation and characteristic physical findings of the disease are frequently similar.

Signs and Symptoms

Edema

Patients with chronic lymphedema usually present with slowly progressive, painless swelling of the limb. The edema is partially pitting early in the course of the disease but is usually nonpitting in chronic lymphedema owing to the secondary fibrotic changes in the skin and subcutaneous tissue.

The distribution of swelling in lymphedema is characteristic. It starts distally in the extremity in most patients and involves the perimalleolar area, with disappearance of the contours of the ankle in advanced cases (tree trunk or elephantine configuration). The dorsum of the forefoot is usually involved, resulting in the typical appearance of a "buffalo hump" (Fig. 143–5). Squaring of the toes (Stemmer's sign) is also a characteristic feature and results from the high protein content of the excess tissue fluid (Fig. 143–6).

Skin Changes

In the early stage of lymphedema, the skin usually has a pinkish-red color and a mildly elevated temperature due to the increased vascularity. In longstanding lymphedema, however, the skin becomes thick and shows areas of hyperkeratosis, lichenification, and development of a "peau d'orange." The term pigskin reflects the reactive changes of the dermis and epidermis in response to the chronic inflammation caused by lymphatic stasis.[38] Recurrent chronic eczematous dermatitis or excoriation of the skin may occur, but frank ulcerations are rare. Unlike the situation in venous stasis, the skin maintains a higher degree of hydration and

elasticity for a long time in lymphedema, and ischemic changes due to high skin tension and disruption of the circulation to the skin and subcutaneous tissue are rare.[39]

Additional skin changes in chronic lymph stasis, primarily in patients with hyperplasia of the lymphatics and valvular incompetence, include verrucae or small vesicles, frequently draining clear lymph (lymphorrhea). In patients with lymphangiectasia and reflux of the chyle, drainage from the vesicles is milky in appearance (chylorrhea) (see Fig. 143–2).

Primary lymphedema may be associated with yellow discoloration of the nails.[40–42] In the yellow nail syndrome, pleural effusion is also present. The pale yellow color of the nails is most likely caused by impaired lymphatic drainage. Severe clubbing, transverse ridging, friability of the nail, and a decreased rate of nail growth are also observed.[41, 42]

Pain

Although some aching or heaviness of the limb is a frequent complaint, significant pain is rare. If the patient with lymphedema complains of marked pain, infection or neuritic pain in the area of scar tissue or radiation treatment should be suspected. Other possible causes of leg swelling, such as venous edema or reflex sympathetic dystrophy, should also be considered (see later section on differential diagnosis).

Complications

Infection

The lymphedematous limb is highly sensitive to fungal infections, such as dermatophytosis or onychomycosis (see

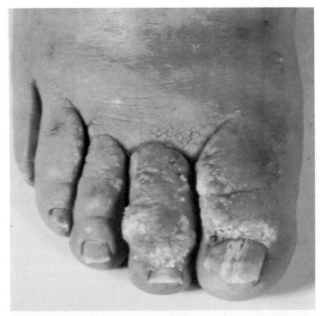

FIGURE 143–6. Squaring of the toes, small verrucae of the skin, and onychomycosis in a patient with primary lymphedema praecox. (From Gloviczki P, Schirger A: Lymphedema. *In* Spittell JA Jr [ed]: Clinical Medicine. Philadelphia, Harper & Row, 1985, pp 1–10.)

Fig. 143–6). Fungal infections in the interdigital spaces are also sites of entry for bacteria, most frequently beta-hemolytic streptococci, which may cause cellulitis or lymphangitis in the affected limb. Cellulitis may present with high fever and chills, and the skin of the affected extremity is red and tender. Repeated episodes of cellulitis aggravate lymphedema.

Malnutrition and Immunodeficiency

Lymphangiectasia with protein-losing enteropathy or chylous ascites or chylothorax may result in severe loss of proteins, long-chain triglycerides, cholesterol, and calcium.[19, 20] As discussed in Chapter 142, loss of lymphocytes, different immunoglobulins, polypeptides, and cytokines results in a state of immunodeficiency that decreases the ability of these patients to resist infections or malignancy.

Malignancy

Nonhealing ''bruises,'' the development of multiple rounded, purple-red nodules with persistent ulcerations should alert the physician to the possibility of malignancy.[43–45] Lymphangiosarcoma following longstanding secondary lymphedema, originally described by Stewart and Treves,[43] is a rare malignant disease that frequently results in loss of a limb or even the life of the patient.

NONINVASIVE EVALUATION

The most frequent noninvasive imaging modalities currently used to evaluate patients with lymphatic diseases include lymphoscintigraphy, computed tomography, and magnetic resonance imaging.

Lymphoscintigraphy

Interstitially injected colloids labeled with a radioactive tracer were used as long ago as 1953, when Sherman and Ter-Pergossian[46] injected radioactive gold (^{198}Au) into the parametrium to produce lymph node necrosis in an attempt to treat metastatic cancer. The first application of plasma protein labeled with radioactive iodine (^{131}I) for diagnostic evaluation of the lymphatic system in lymphedema was reported by Taylor and Kinmonth in 1957.[47] Because of advances in imaging techniques, the introduction of a better radioactive label (technetium-99), and selection of the optimal size of the labeled particles, the technique of diagnostic lymphoscintigraphy has improved continuously during the last two decades.[48–56]

At this time, lymphoscintigraphy with radiocolloids is used principally for evaluation of the swollen extremity. For detection of lymph node metastases, radiolabeled monoclonal antibodies are being used with increasing frequency.

Radiopharmaceuticals

The biokinetic behavior of interstitially applied colloid particles depends on their surface charge and particle size. Particles with small diameters are absorbed into capillaries, whereas those in the 10-nm range (antimony trisulfide [Sb_2S_3]) are absorbed into the lymphatic system. The time needed for activity to appear in the regional lymph nodes has been variably defined according to the physical characteristics of the imaging agent. For example, small particles such as ^{99m}Tc human serum albumin may appear in the pelvic nodes within 10 minutes,[55] whereas relatively large agents including rhenium and Sb_2S_3 colloid should arrive within 30 minutes[51] or 1 hour,[54] respectively. In our experience, which now includes studies in over 500 limbs, ^{99m}technetium-labeled Sb_2S_3 colloid (Cadema Medical Products Inc., PO Box 250, Middletown, NY 10940) has been used for lymphoscintigraphy with satisfactory results.[54, 57, 58] Others have reported similar success with the use of technetium-labeled human serum albumin.[52, 53, 55, 59]

Technique of Lymphoscintigraphy

Lymphoscintigraphy is performed with the patient comfortably positioned supine on the imaging table. The feet are attached to a foot ergometer, and the patient is instructed in the proper use of the device. For lymphoscintigraphy of the upper extremity, we employ a plastic squeezable ball the size of a tennis ball that is compressed on command.

After proper positioning and instruction, a subcutaneous injection of 11 MBq (350 to 450 μCi) of ^{99m}Tc-antimony trisulfide (Sb_2S_3) colloid is made into the web space between the second and the third toes (or fingers) bilaterally. The number of particles in the injected solution (0.1 to 0.2 ml) ranges from 10^9 to 10^{13}. The tracer dose is prepared previously in tuberculin syringes (one for each side), and the injection is made with a 27-gauge needle. The injection is associated with an often very intense stinging sensation lasting for 5 to 10 seconds. Absorption of Sb_2S_3 is rapid, and up to 30 per cent of the injected tracer is absorbed by 3 hours. In the United States this radiopharmaceutical is regulated as an investigational drug by the United States Food and Drug Administration.

Immediately after the injection, a gamma camera with a large field of view is positioned to include the groin region in the upper field of view. An all-purpose collimator is used, and a 20 per cent window is placed symmetrically around the 140-keV photopeak of the ^{99m}Tc isotope.

Dynamic anterior images (made every 5 minutes during the first hour, for a total of 12 frames in 1 hour) of the groin are obtained during the first hour (Fig. 143–7). The patient is requested to exercise with the foot ergometer for 5 minutes initially and then 1 minute out of every 5 minutes for the rest of the hour. The same exercise schedule is used for the upper extremity using the squeeze ball. Measured exercise is important to obtain reproducible appearance times in the groin.

At the end of the first hour the patient is scanned on a dual-headed gamma camera (Siemens) for a total body image. Imaging time is about 20 minutes. Similar total body images are obtained at 3 hours (Fig. 143–8) and, in selected patients, at 6 and 24 hours. The patient is encouraged to ambulate in the time span between the total body images. Like others, we have experimented with multiple injection sites (two or more sites on each side) or used an injection

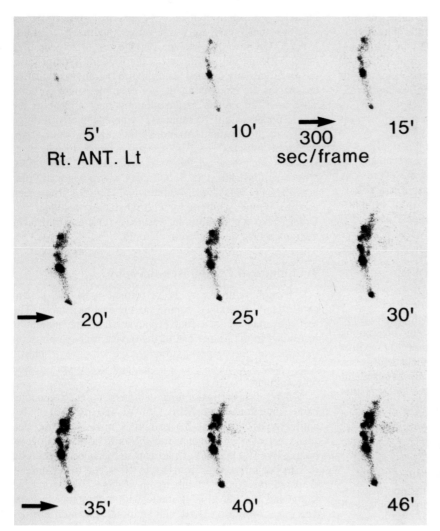

FIGURE 143–7. Lymphoscintigraphic images of the groin taken every 5 minutes after injection of the colloid into both feet. Normal lymphatic transport and image pattern of the inguinal nodes on the right, no visualization of the lymphatics of the left. This 30-year-old woman had primary lymphedema of the left leg.

site behind the lateral malleolus to obtain access to the deep lymphatic system. However, we have not been convinced that any advantage results from these modifications of the standard technique.

Reading a Lymphoscintigram

At the end of the study, the following information is available to the reviewer for diagnostic interpretation.

1. *Evidence of proper injection.* No uptake is seen in the liver initially, and only faint activity is present at 1 hour. Early liver uptake without activity in the abdominal nodes and channels suggests intravenous tracer injection.

2. *Appearance time of activity in regional lymph nodes (groin or axilla) after tracer injection.* Normal transit time is between 15 and 60 minutes. Less than 15 minutes indicates rapid transport, more than 60 minutes suggests delayed lymphatic transport (see Fig. 143–7).

3. *The absence or presence and the pattern of lymph channels in the leg; the number, size, and symmetry of tracer activity in the groin lymph nodes.* For the upper extremity, similar observations are made for the axilla and arms.

4. *The pattern of lymph nodes and channels in the*

pelvis and abdomen and activity in the liver. For the arm, the uptake pattern in axillary lymph nodes is observed.

The data are entered in a standardized report format, which helps to create reproducible reports when many physicians review these tracings. Such a report form is shown in Table 143–3 and is an adaptation of a form proposed by Kleinhans and colleagues for the estimation of a transport index.[60]

Uptake of the tracer by lymph nodes is not always predictable even in normal patients. Thus, when interpreting a lymphoscintigram, a detailed evaluation for the number of lymph nodes present in the groin is not possible. Nevertheless, abnormal patterns for nodes can be defined, such as (1) no lymph node uptake, (2) marked asymmetry, and (3) mild asymmetry.

The Normal Lymphoscintigram

Following the tracer injection, visible activity gradually ascends the anteromedial aspect of the leg. The injection site, because of the relatively large tracer dose given, does not show details, and no information about lymph distribution in the feet is obtainable. Several lymph channels may be identified in the calf. In the thigh, however,

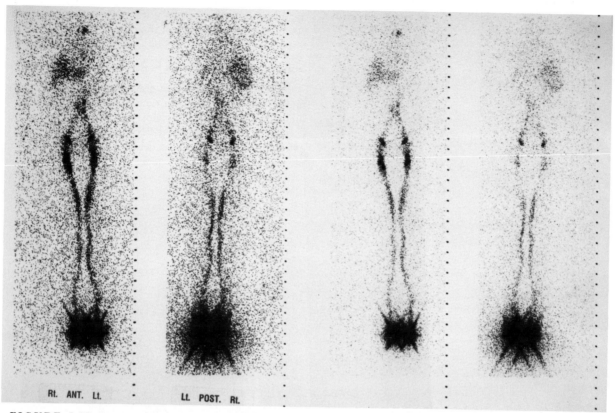

FIGURE 143–8. Image display from total body scan with dual-headed gamma camera. Anterior and posterior images are displayed in two intensity settings. *Left*, Anterior and posterior images of a normal lymphoscintigram. *Right*, Higher intensity settings in the same patient. Large area of high activity and scatter is seen at the feet where the injection was made. The single well-outlined band in each leg represents the main lymphatic channels. Lymph nodes in the groin, pelvic and para-aortic nodes, liver, and an area at the site of the upper thoracic duct are visualized.

Table 143–3. Evaluation Form for Calculation of Lymphatic Transport Index

Patient's Initials _____

Clinic Number_____ Date_____

LYMPHOSCINTIGRAPHY
DATA EVALUATION
☐ Arms ☐ Legs

Image	1 hr		3 hr		6 hr		24 hr	
	R	L	R	L	R	L	R	L
Lymph transport kinetics: 0 = no delay, 1 = rapid, 3 = low-grade delay, 5 = extreme delay, 9 = no transport								
Distribution pattern: 0 = normal, 2 = focal abnormal tracer, 3 = partial dermal, 5 = diffuse dermal, 9 = no transport								
Lymph node appearance time: Minutes								
Assessment of lymph nodes: 0 = clearly seen, 3 = faint, 5 = hardly seen, 9 = no visualization								
Assessment of lymph vessels: 0 = clearly seen, 3 = faint, 5 = hardly seen, 9 = no visualization								
Abnormal sites of tracer accumulation (describe)								

Adapted from Kleinhans E, Baumeister RGH, Hahn D, et al: Evaluation of transport kinetics in lymphoscintigraphy: Follow-up study in patients with transplanted lymphatic vessels. Eur J Nucl Med 10:349, 1985.

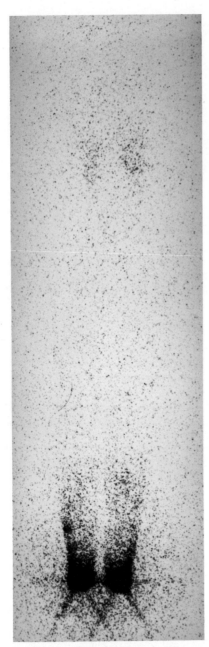

FIGURE 143-9. Lymphoscintigram of a 25-year-old woman with congenital familial lymphedema of both lower extremities. Note absence of lymph vessels and lymph nodes at 6 hours, with only minimal dermal backflow visible in the distal calves. This patient also had recurrent familial cholestasis due to absence of intrahepatic bile ducts (Aagenaes syndrome).

abdomen, and occasionally a tracer focus in the left supra-clavicular area at the site of the distal thoracic duct.

Scintigraphic Findings in Lymphedema

Abnormal lymphoscintigrams may show (1) an abnormally slow removal or no removal of the tracer from the injection site (Figs. 143–9 and 143–10), (2) the presence of collaterals or a cutaneous pattern (dermal backflow) in the extremities (Figs. 143–11 and 143–12A), (3) reduced, faint, or no uptake in the lymph nodes of the groin, the aortoiliac

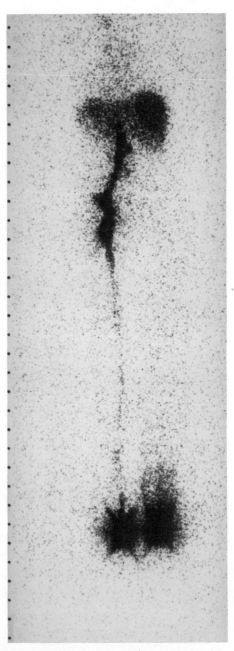

FIGURE 143-10. Lymphoscintigram of a 65-year-old woman with primary lymphedema tarda of the right lower extremity. There is minimal dermal backflow above the right ankle 3 hours after injection, and no lymph vessels or lymph nodes are visualized. Normal pattern in left leg.

the lymph vessels run close to each other; separate activity in each larger channel is seldom seen on lymphoscintigrams (see Fig. 143–8).

With standardized exercise, as mentioned before, tracer activity should be seen clearly in the inguinal lymph nodes by 60 minutes (range, 15 to 60 minutes). A faint hepatic uptake, activity in the bladder, and faint traces in the para-abdominal nodes are visible at 1 hour. Three-hour images show intense uptake in the liver, symmetric and good uptake in the lymph nodes of the groin, pelvis, and

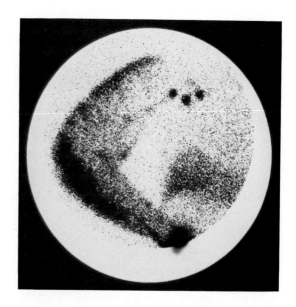

FIGURE 143–11. Lymphoscintigram of the right arm of a 51-year-old woman with postmastectomy lymphedema. Note extensive dermal backflow resulting from lymphatic obstruction. Three groups of axillary nodes are still visualized.

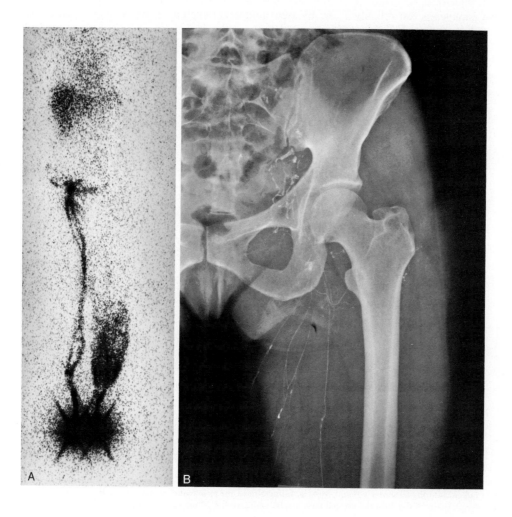

FIGURE 143–12. *A,* Lymphoscintigram of a 43-year-old woman with left lower extremity lymphedema following hysterectomy and bilateral iliac node dissection for cervical cancer. Dermal pattern is seen on left with no visualization of the inguinal nodes. Transport was mildly delayed in the clinically asymptomatic right limb. Note lack of visualization of iliac nodes bilaterally. *B,* Contrast lymphangiography in the same patient confirms the lymphoscintigraphic findings. Few small lymph vessels and two small nodes are seen only in the thigh.

nodes, and the axillary nodes, and (4) abnormal tracer accumulation suggestive of extravasation, lymphocele, or lymphangiectasia (Fig. 143–13A).

Primary and secondary lymphedema are associated with similar abnormalities on lymphoscintigraphy. These include a delay in transport from the injection site (Fig. 143–14), dermal backflow, the presence of large collaterals, occasionally extravasated activity, fewer visualized lymph nodes, and ''crossover'' filling of contralateral inguinal (or axillary) lymph nodes as a sign of collateral pathways.[54, 57, 58] In primary lymphedema it may be possible to distinguish aplasia from hypoplasia by imaging early in the evolution of the disease. In the former there is usually little or no (1) removal of tracer from the injection site, (2) tracer in regional lymph nodes on 1- and 3-hour images, (3) dermal backflow, and (4) visualized lymph channels. In hypoplasia these scintigraphic features may be variably present. Regardless of etiology, lymphatic vessels of normal caliber are not seen in patients with longstanding lymphedema.[55]

Qualitative interpretation of images has resulted in excellent sensitivity (92 per cent) and specificity (100 per cent) for the diagnosis of lymphedema.[57] Quantitative lymphoscintigraphy with measurement of lymphatic clearance may improve detection of early disease,[55] but the results obtained in our studies have been equivocal.[54, 57] Neither the image pattern nor quantitative parameters can reliably distinguish primary from secondary lymphedema.[54, 57, 58]

Scintigraphic Findings in Lymphangiectasia

Dilated lymph channels with only mild or no delay in lymph transport are frequently seen on lymphoscintigraphic images. Injection of the colloid into the unaffected lower extremity may reflux into the affected lymphedematous leg because of lymphatic valvular incompetence. Similar reflux of the colloid may be seen in the dilated mesenteric lymphatics (see Fig. 143–13A) or in the retroperitoneum, perineum, or scrotum (Fig. 143–15). Ruptured lymphatics cause extravasation of the colloid into the abdominal cavity or the chest of patients with chylous ascites or chylothorax. However, the images are generally not helpful in determining the exact site of the lymphatic leak.

Computed Tomography

The greatest value of computed tomography in the evaluation of patients with a swollen leg is to exclude any obstructing mass that may result in decrease of the transport capacity of the lymphatic system. In patients with lymphedema computed tomography confirms the presence of coarse, nonenhancing, tubular reticular structures in the subcutaneous tissue.[61–63] This honeycomb appearance in the subcutaneous tissue is caused either by lymphatic channels or by free fluid accumulating in tissue planes. However, computed tomography is not able to distinguish subcuta-

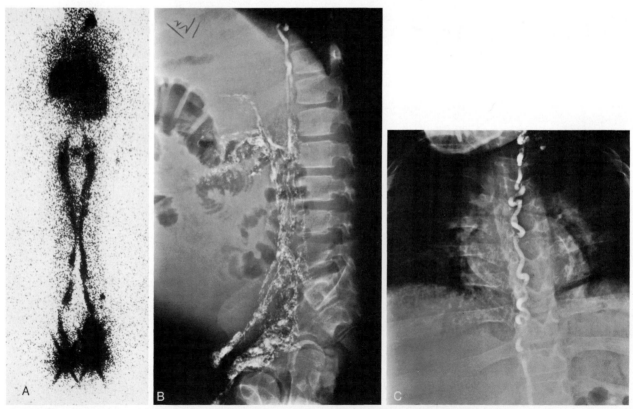

FIGURE 143–13.   *A*, Lymphoscintigram of an 18-year-old man with lymphangiectasia, protein-losing enteropathy, and chylous ascites. Note large leg lymphatics and reflux of colloid into the mesenteric lymph vessels, filling almost the entire abdominal cavity. *B*, Lymphangiogram of the same patient reveals reflux of dye into the dilated mesenteric lymphatics. *C*, Note extremely dilated and tortuous but patent thoracic duct.

FIGURE 143–14. Lymphoscintigram of a 47-year-old woman with primary lymphedema tarda of the right lower extremity. Note markedly delayed transport with dermal pattern in the right leg. The right inguinal or iliac nodes were not visualized.

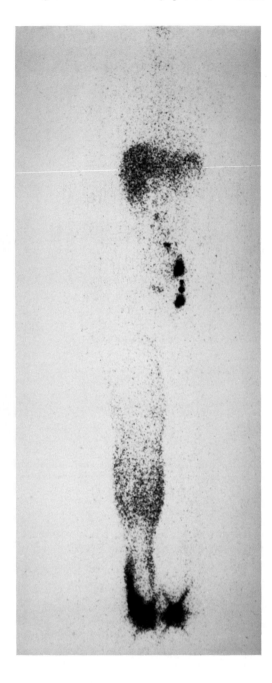

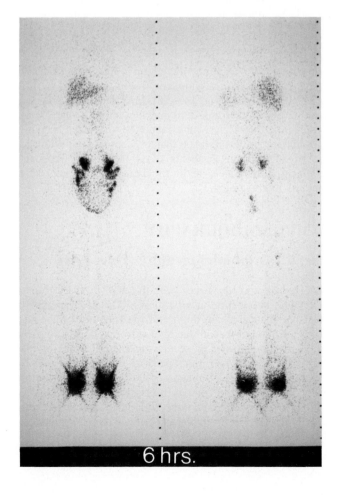

FIGURE 143–15. Bilateral leg scintigraphy with anterior *(left)* and posterior *(right)* views in a 24-year-old man outlines the swollen scrotum in the 6-hour image. Reflux of the colloid resulted from dilatation and valvular incompetence of the lymphatics.

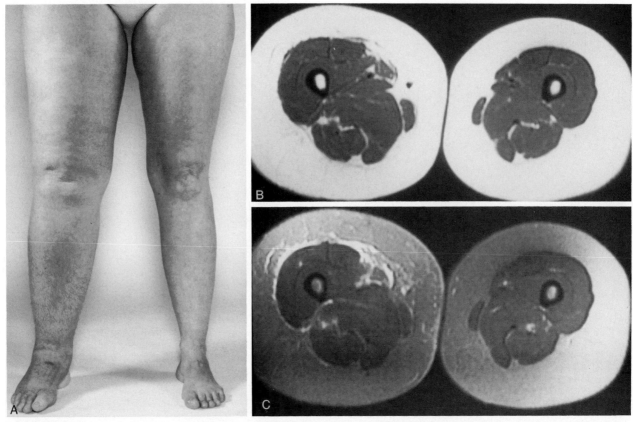

FIGURE 143–16. *A,* Thirty-six-year-old woman with secondary lymphedema of the right lower extremity. *B,* Magnetic resonance imaging of the legs reveals enlargement of the subcutaneous tissues and the deep compartment on the right with considerable stranding within the subcutaneous tissues, predominantly anteriorly and medially. *C,* T2-weighted image reveals the region of soft tissue stranding that is now of high signal intensity in the deep layers of the subcutaneous tissue.

neous fat from tissue fluid. In our experience, this test is not sensitive enough to define the cause of lower extremity swelling.

Magnetic Resonance Imaging

Because of continuous improvement in technology, magnetic resonance imaging (MRI) has become our most important noninvasive imaging test for the diagnosis of congenital vascular malformations and the identification of soft tissue tumors. The value of MRI in the diagnosis of the swollen leg, however, has not been evaluated until recently. Duewell and colleagues found MRI scanning useful in differentiating the three major forms of limb swelling: lipedema, chronic venous edema, and lymphedema.[64] Lipedema was characterized by an increased amount of subcutaneous fat without increased vascularity or signal changes suggesting excess fluid. The ratio of the superficial to the deep compartment was found to be increased. In lymphedema and venous edema, however, there was no change in the superficial-to-deep compartment ratio. Like findings observed on computed tomography, a honeycomb pattern was seen in the subcutaneous tissue of patients with lymphedema.[64]

MRI is particularly useful in complementing findings observed on lymphoscintigraphy.[65, 66] MRI is helpful for delineating nodal anatomy in addition to imaging soft tissue changes and the larger lymphatic trunks and nodes in different tissue planes (Fig. 143–16). MRI is also suitable for imaging lymphatic trunks and nodes proximal to the site of lymphatic obstruction, which cannot be visualized by lymphoscintigraphy. Experience that is accumulating with the use of supermagnetic agents (e.g., iron oxide) appears promising for delineation of the lymphatic truncal-nodal anatomy in greater detail.[67]

LYMPHANGIOGRAPHY

Visual Lymphangiography (Dye Test)

Hudack and McMaster were the first, in 1933, to use subcutaneous injection of vital dyes to visualize the superficial lymphatics of the thigh and the forearm.[68] Subcutaneous injection of patent blue V or isosulfan blue (Lymphazurin) dye in the first or second interdigital space of the foot results in fast, selective uptake of the large-molecular-weight dye into the lymphatic system. With normal lymphatic circulation the dye is transported to the inguinal lymph nodes 5 to 10 minutes after injection. In patients with lymphatic stasis in the superficial lymph collectors, dermal backflow is observed soon after injection (Fig. 143–17). If positive, the test is reliable to diagnose lymphatic

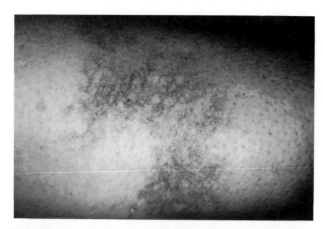

FIGURE 143-17. Visual lymphangiography in secondary lymphedema. Lymphazurine dye injected into the first interdigital space of the foot delineates the dermal lymphatics at the mid-calf owing to obstruction in the proximal main lymphatic vessels.

stasis but failure to demonstrate dermal backflow may also indicate extensive lymphatic obstruction, hypoplasia, or aplasia.

Direct Contrast Lymphangiography

Contrast lymphangiography was first performed by Servelle in 1943,[69] but the current technique using the subcutaneous injection of a vital dye to identify the foot lymphatics for cannulation and direct injection of the contrast material was developed by Kinmonth.[70] Lymphangiography using lipid-soluble contrast material provided a major stimulus to the investigation of the lymphatic system, in patients with both lymphedema and malignancy. With the availability of computed tomography and MRI, the utility of lymphangiography in the clinical staging of malignancies has significantly diminished. With the availability of isotope lymphoscintigraphy, the use of contrast lymphangiography in patients with lymphedema has also significantly decreased.

Technique of Pedal Lymphangiography

Contrast lymphangiography is performed under local anesthesia using a 1 per cent lidocaine (Xylocaine) solution. A small transverse incision is made in the mid-dorsum of the foot after 1 ml of isosulfan blue (Lymphazurin) dye has been injected subcutaneously into the first and second interdigital spaces. Since the dye injection itself is uncomfortable and painful, we mix the dye with equal amounts of 1 per cent lidocaine solution. The lymph vessels are dissected under loupe magnification, and a 30-gauge needle attached to a polyethylene tube is inserted into the lymph vessels. A constant infusion of lipid-soluble contrast material (ethiodized oil [Ethiodol]) is started at a rate of 1 ml in 8 minutes, as suggested by Wolfe.[71] A maximum of 7 ml is injected into each limb, making a total infusion that does not exceed 14 ml. If the injection is made too fast, the dye will extravasate through the wall of the lymph vessels, and interpretation of the images will be difficult (Fig. 143–18). If the amount of extravasation is significant, the rate of infusion

should be decreased. At the end of the procedure the needle is removed, and the incision is closed meticulously using interrupted 5–0 nylon vertical mattress sutures.

Serial films are taken of the lower extremities, groin, pelvis, lumbar area, and upper abdomen and chest during the injection. Additional films are taken several hours after injection and 24 hours later. The oily contrast material may remain in the lymph nodes for several months after injection.

Arm Lymphangiography

Lymphangiography of the upper extremity is now rarely performed. The technique is similar to that used for pedal lymphangiography, except that a small lymphatic on the dorsum of the hand is cannulated. The amount of contrast should be limited to 4 to 5 ml of ethiodized oil (Ethiodol).[71]

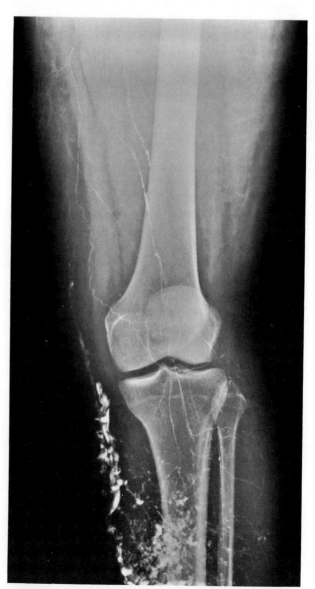

FIGURE 143-18. Extensive occlusion of most lymph vessels in the thigh with extravasation of the dye distal to the knee following contrast lymphangiography in patient with secondary lymphedema.

Interpretation of Lymphangiograms

Injection of a dorsal pedal lymph vessel will fill the superficial medial lymphatic vessels and most of the inguinal lymph nodes. Five to 15 lymph vessels are seen in normal patients at the medial aspect of the thigh (Fig. 143–19) with valves frequently visualized every 5 to 10 mm. Lateral lymphatics and deep lymphatics are not visible on normal lymphangiograms but may be seen in patients with lymphatic obstruction (Fig. 143–20). The deep lymph vessels are frequently paired and follow the main blood vessels of the extremity. The normal lymphatic nodes have a ground-glass appearance. Normally the iliac lymph vessels and lymph nodes fill within 30 to 45 minutes after the injection is started. The thoracic duct may only show up on images several hours after the injection (see Fig. 143–13C).

Most patients with primary lymphedema have an obstruction of some or most of the lymph vessels and lymph-conducting elements of the lymph nodes. As mentioned previously, distal obliteration of the lymph vessels in the leg is much more frequent than proximal, pelvic lymphatic obstruction. With pelvic obstruction the inguinal and iliac lymph nodes are few or absent, but the leg lymphatics are patent and are frequently distended and tortuous (Fig. 143–21). Backflow of the contrast into dilated dermal lymphatics is observed. The lymphangiographic findings in proximal obliteration are similar to those seen in secondary lymphedema. With time, however, fibrotic occlusion of the dilated distal lymph vessels frequently occurs. This retrograde occlusion of the lymph vessels (die-back) was observed in patients with both secondary and primary lymphedemas.[72]

Patients with lymphangiectasia frequently need larger amounts of contrast to image the dilated, incompetent lymphatics. The number of pelvic lymph nodes may be diminished. Contrast material may reflux into the mesenteric lymphatics (see Fig. 143–13B). The thoracic duct in some of the patients is occluded or absent, whereas in others it is dilated and tortuous (see Fig. 143–13C).

Complications of Lymphangiography

Contrast lymphangiography is an invasive and lengthy procedure that is frequently uncomfortable for the patient. Obstructive lymphangitis and progression of lymphedema following lymphangiography have also been noted.[73] Symptomatic pulmonary embolization due to the oily contrast material may complicate lymphangiography. This problem may be caused by using excessive amounts of contrast, or it may be the result of embolization through spontaneous lymphovenous anastomoses. In patients who have had previous pulmonary irradiation, cerebral embolization through pulmonary arteriovenous fistulae may also occur.[71] The use of ethiodized oil (Ethiodol) is contraindicated in patients who are allergic to iodine.

Current Indications for Direct Contrast Lymphangiography

Contrast lymphangiography remains a test that is now rarely and only selectively used for the diagnosis of lymphedema. It is indicated in some patients who are candidates for microvascular lymphatic reconstruction. It is also

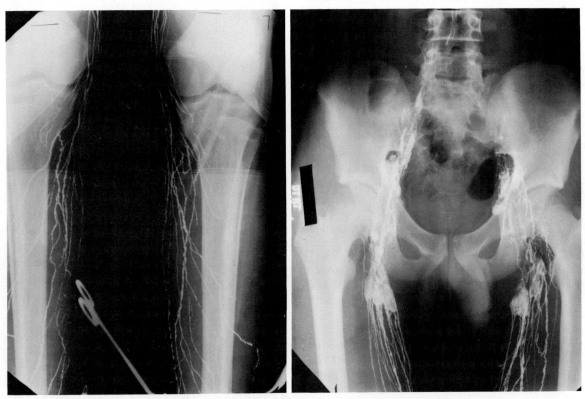

FIGURE 143–19. *A* and *B*, Normal bipedal lymphangiogram with only mild dilatation and tortuosity of the lymph vessels of the calf. Note the presence of 10 to 15 superficial lymphatic collectors in the thighs.

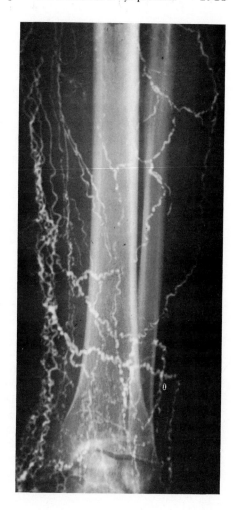

FIGURE 143–20.   Dilated tortuous lymph vessels with valvular insufficiency and filling of lateral lymph vessels in a patient with lymphedema praecox. (From Gloviczki P, Schirger A: Lymphedema. *In* Spittell JA Jr [ed]: Clinical Medicine. Philadelphia, Harper & Row, 1985, pp 1–10.)

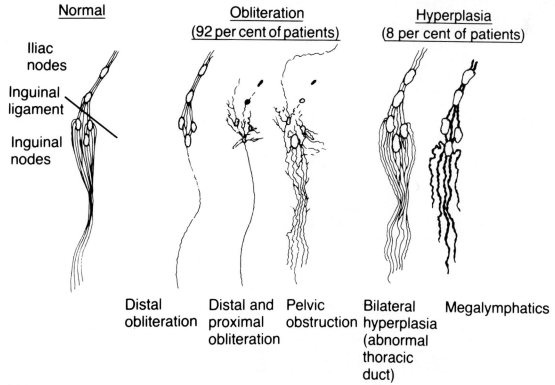

FIGURE 143–21.   Lymphangiographic pattern in normal patient and in patients with different types of primary lymphedema.

Table 143–4. Differential Diagnosis of Chronic Leg Swelling

Systemic Causes	Local or Regional Causes
Cardiac failure	Chronic venous insufficiency
Hepatic failure	Lymphedema
Renal failure	Lipedema
Hypoproteinemia	Congenital vascular malformation
Hyperthyroidism (myxedema)	Arteriovenous fistula
Allergic disorders	Trauma
Idiopathic cyclic edema	Snake or insect bite
Hereditary angioedema	Infection, inflammation
Drugs	Hematoma
Antihypertensives	Dependency
Methyldopa	Rheumatoid arthritis
Nifedipine	Postrevascularization edema
Hydralazine	Soft tissue tumor
Hormones	Hemihypertrophy
Estrogen	
Progesterone	
Anti-inflammatory drugs	
Phenylbutazone	
Monoamine oxidase inhibitors	

useful in the preoperative evaluation of patients with lymphangiectasia and reflux of chyle (see Chapter 146). Although the diagnosis of lymphangiectasia can be made with lymphoscintigraphy, the extent and location of the dilated lymphatics are best delineated by contrast lymphangiography. Lymphangiography remains the best test for imaging the thoracic duct and for identifying the exact location of some pelvic, abdominal, or thoracic lymphatic fistulae.

Indirect Contrast Lymphangiography

Because of the difficulties encountered with direct cannulation of the lymphatics and the use of oily contrast material, increasing research has focused in recent years on indirect lymphangiography. This is performed with subepidermal infusion of a water-soluble contrast material (iotasul, iopamidol [Isovist-300]).[74] The dermal lymphatics and in some patients the distal lymph collectors can be imaged with this technique. In primary lymphedema, absence, hypoplasia, or hyperplasia of the dermal lymphatics can be demonstrated using indirect lymphangiography. In secondary lymphedema, hyperplasia of the initial lymphatics is the most frequent finding. Although indirect lymphangiography is helpful for diagnosing lymphatic stasis and for imaging the fine initial lymph vessels, the limitations of the current technique are still important: larger lymphatic collectors or nodes distant to the site of the injection are not visualized.[75]

DIFFERENTIAL DIAGNOSIS OF LYMPHEDEMA

During the evaluation of patients with chronic limb swelling, a systemic cause of the disease should be excluded first. Underlying cardiac diseases such as congestive heart failure, chronic constrictive pericarditis, and severe tricuspid regurgitation are the most frequent systemic causes leading to pitting, bilateral leg swelling. Hepatic or

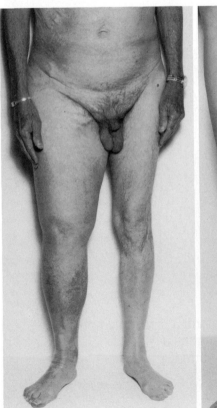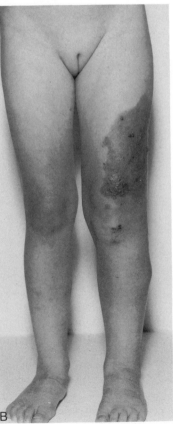

FIGURE 143–22. Venous disease in the differential diagnosis of limb edema. *A,* Right leg swelling due to venous insufficiency, caused by chronic iliofemoral venous thrombosis. *B,* Left leg edema associated with congenital vascular malformation (Klippel-Trenaunay syndrome).

renal failure, hypoproteinemia, malnutrition, and endocrine disorders (myxedema) are other possible causes of leg swelling. Allergic reactions, hereditary angioedema, and idiopathic cyclic edema are rare systemic causes that should be considered. Chronic use of diuretics may lead to generalized swelling, which most frequently affects the extremities and the face. Other drugs that may cause swelling include steroids, some of the antihypertensive, and antiinflammatory agents (Table 143–4).

It is important to remember that among the local or regional causes of limb swelling, chronic venous insufficiency is much more common than lymphedema. In some patients with chronic iliac or iliocaval obstruction, massive swelling of the entire extremity can develop (Fig. 143–22A). The usual causes of proximal venous occlusion are deep venous thrombosis or external compression of the vein by tumor or retroperitoneal fibrosis. Although lymphedema is usually painless, venous hypertension results in marked pain and cramps after prolonged standing or at the end of the day. Patients with proximal venous obstruction may complain of typical claudication, which presents with throbbing pain in the thigh or calf after walking. The pain resolves with rest, although elevation of the extremity provides the fastest relief. The presence of varicosity, pigmentation, induration, or venous ulcers makes the diagnosis of venous insufficiency easier. Chronic inflammation in the

subcutaneous tissue due to venous stasis may result in destruction of the collecting lymph channels, and a mixed venous-lymphatic edema develops in these patients.

Patients with congenital vascular malformations frequently have a larger extremity that may be difficult to distinguish from lymphedema (Fig. 143–22B). An increase in the length of the affected extremity, the presence of atypical lateral varicosity, and port-wine stain with underlying developmental abnormality of the deep venous system is characteristic of Klippel-Trenaunay syndrome.[76] Although hypertrophy of the soft tissues and bones is caused by an abnormality in mesenchymal development, congenital lymphedema may also be present in these patients. In patients with high-shunt, high-flow arteriovenous malformations the extremity is larger and is also frequently longer.[77] A bruit and thrill are present, the superficial veins are dilated and frequently pulsatile, and the distal arterial pulses may be diminished.

Lipedema is characterized by deposition of a large amount of fatty tissue in the subcutaneous layers. Most of these patients have morbid obesity, although some, mostly females, have fat deposition primarily localized to the lower half of the body. Evaluation of the lymphatic system with lymphoscintigraphy or lymphangiography shows essentially normal findings.

Trauma and subsequent reflex sympathetic dystrophy

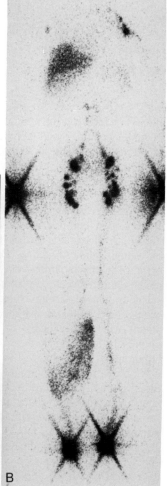

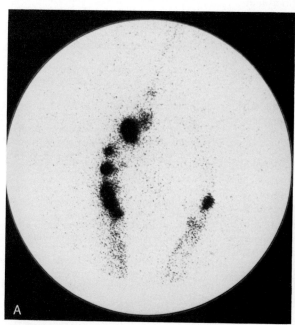

FIGURE 143–23. Lymphoscintigraphy in "high-output" lymphatic failure due to reflex sympathetic dystrophy of the right leg. *A,* Fast lymphatic transport in the affected right leg compared with the normal left leg on the image taken of the inguinal nodes 20 minutes after injection. *B,* Total body image taken at 3 hours shows dermal pattern on the right but no evidence of proximal lymphatic obstruction.

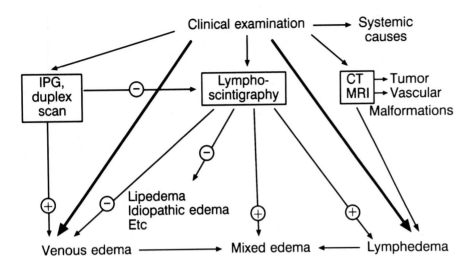

FIGURE 143-24. Diagnostic protocol in patients with chronic limb swelling.

may result in painful swelling of the extremity. Because of disuse, a varying degree of osteoporosis can be observed, and increased sympathetic activity occurs in the limb of these patients. The swelling is usually the result of a "high-output" lymphatic failure, and increased lymphatic transport on lymphoscintigraphy may be demonstrated (Fig. 143–23A and B). Baker's cyst, soft tissue tumor, hematoma, and inflammation such as tenosynovitis or arthritis are additional local causes of limb swelling that should be considered in the differential diagnosis of lymphedema.

DIAGNOSTIC PROTOCOL FOR EVALUATION OF CHRONIC EDEMA

Clinical examination of the patient frequently reveals the correct cause of limb swelling. Initial laboratory examinations should include routine blood tests to look for signs of renal or hepatic failure, eosinophilia, or hypoproteinemia. Urinalysis may indicate proteinuria. Once a systemic cause of edema is excluded, the local or regional cause should be confirmed (Fig. 143–24). Computed tomography has become a routine test in our practice in most adult patients with leg swelling to exclude underlying malignancy. Noninvasive venous studies, such as Doppler examination or strain gauge plethysmography, are frequently sufficient to diagnose venous disease. In some patients, however, duplex scanning is necessary to exclude obstruction of the deep veins. MRI provides the most accurate information in patients with clinical signs of congenital vascular malformation, soft tissue tumor, or retroperitoneal fibrosis. Lymphoscintigraphy is now the test of choice for the confirmation of lymphedema, and a normal lymphoscintigraphic examination essentially excludes the diagnosis of lymphedema. Patients with chronic venous insufficiency may have abnormal results on lymphoscintigraphic examination with delayed transport because of mixed, lymphatic, and venous edema. Direct contrast lymphangiography in the 1990s should be performed selectively and should not

be included routinely in the evaluation of patients with chronic limb swelling.

References

1. Kinmonth JB, Taylor GW, Tracy GD, et al: Primary lymphoedema: Clinical and lymphangiographic studies of a series of 107 patients in which the lower limbs were affected. Br J Surg 45:1, 1957.
2. Kinmonth JB: The lymphoedemas. General considerations. *In* Kinmonth JB (ed): The Lymphatics. Surgery, Lymphography and Diseases of the Chyle and Lymph Systems. London, Edward Arnold, 1982, pp 83–104.
3. Browse NL, Stewart G: Lymphoedema: Pathophysiology and classification. J Cardiovasc Surg 26:91, 1985.
4. Browse NL: The diagnosis and management of primary lymphedema. J Vasc Surg 3:181, 1986.
5. Gloviczki P, Schirger A: Lymphedema. *In* Spittell JA Jr (ed): Clinical Medicine. Philadelphia, Harper & Row, 1985, pp 1–10.
6. O'Donnell TF, Howrigan P: Diagnosis and management of lymphedema. *In* Bell PRF, Jamieson CW, Ruckley CV (eds): Surgical Management of Vascular Disease. Philadelphia, WB Saunders, 1992, pp 1305–1327.
7. Allen EV: Lymphedema of the extremities: Classification, etiology and differential diagnosis: A study of three hundred cases. Arch Intern Med 54:606, 1934.
8. Casley-Smith JR, Földi M, Ryan TJ, et al: Lymphedema: Summary of the 10th International Congress of Lymphology Working Group Discussions and Recommendations, Adelaide, Australia, August 10–17, 1985. Lymphology 18:175, 1985.
9. Browse NL: Primary lymphedema. *In* Ernst C, Stanley J (eds): Current Therapy in Vascular Surgery. Philadelphia, BC Decker, 1987, pp 454–457.
10. Kinmonth JB, Wolfe JH: Fibrosis in the lymph nodes in primary lymphoedema. Histological and clinical studies in 74 patients with lower-limb oedema. Ann R Coll Surg Engl 62:344, 1980.
11. Wolfe JHN: The prognosis and possible cause of severe primary lymphoedema. Ann R Coll Surg Engl 66:251, 1984.
12. Kurland LT, Molgaard CA: The patient record in epidemiology. Sci Am 245:54, 1981.
13. Smeltzer DM, Stickler GB, Schirger A: Primary lymphedema in children and adolescents: A follow-up study and review. Pediatrics 76:206, 1985.
14. Letessier EE: Cited by Schroeder E, Helweg-Larsen HF: Chronic hereditary lymphedemia (Nonne-Milroy-Meige disease). Acta Med Scand 137:198, 1950.
15. Nonne M: Vier Fälle von Elephantiasis congenita hereditaria. Arch Pathol Anat Physiol 125:189, 1891.
16. Milroy WF: An undescribed variety of hereditary edema. NY Med J 56:505, 1892.

17. Milroy WF: Chronic hereditary edema: Milroy's disease. JAMA 91:1172, 1928.
18. Meige H: Dystrophie oedemateuse hereditaire. Presse Med 2:341, 1898.
19. Servelle M: Congenital malformation of the lymphatics of the small intestine. J Cardiovasc Surg 32:159, 1991.
20. Kinmonth JB, Cox SJ: Protein-losing enteropathy in lymphoedema. Surgical investigation and treatment. J Cardiovasc Surg 16:111, 1975.
21. Gloviczki P, Soltesz L, Solti F, et al: The surgical treatment of lymphedema caused by chylous reflux. *In* Bartos V, Davidson JW (eds): Advances in Lymphology. Proceedings of the 8th International Congress of Lymphology, Montreal, 1981. Prague, Czechoslovak Medical Press, 1982, pp 502–507.
22. Lymphatic filariasis—Tropical medicine's origin will not go away [Editorial]. Lancet 1:1409, 1987.
23. Mak JW: Epidemiology of lymphatic filariasis. Ciba Found Symp 127:5, 1987.
24. Lobb AW, Harkins HN: Postmastectomy swelling of the arm with note on effect of segmental resection of axillary vein at time of radical mastectomy. West J Surg 57:550, 1949.
25. Leis HP: Selective moderate surgical approach for potentially curable breast cancer. *In* Gallagher HS, Leis HP, Snyderman RK, Urban JA (eds): The Breast. St. Louis, CV Mosby, 1978, pp 232–247.
26. Hayward JL, Winter PJ, Tong D, et al: A new approach to the conservative treatment of early breast cancer. Surgery 95:270, 1984.
27. Veronesi U, Saccozzi R, Del Vecchio M, et al: Comparing radical mastectomy with quadrantectomy, axillary dissection, and radiotherapy in patients with small cancers of the breast. N Engl J Med 305:6, 1981.
28. Osborne MP, Ormiston N, Harmer CL, et al: Breast conservation in the treatment of early breast cancer. A 20-year follow-up. Cancer 53:349, 1984.
29. Kissin MW, della Rovere GQ, Easton D, Westbury G: Risk of lymphoedema following the treatment of breast cancer. Br J Surg 73:580, 1986.
30. Martimbeau PW, Kjorstad KE, Kolstad P: Stage IB carcinoma of the cervix, the Norwegian Radium Hospital, 1968–1970: Results of treatment and major complications. I. Lymphedema. Am J Obstet Gynecol 133:389, 1978.
31. Papachristou D, Fortner JG: Comparison of lymphedema following incontinuity and discontinuity groin dissection. Ann Surg 185:13, 1977.
32. De Roo T: Analysis of lymphoedema as first symptom of a neoplasm in a series of 650 patients with limb involvement. Radiol Clin (Basel) 45:236, 1976.
33. Smith RD, Spittell JA Jr, Schirger A: Secondary lymphedema of the leg: Its characteristics and diagnostic implications. JAMA 185:80, 1963.
34. Földi M: Classification of lymphedema and elephantiasis. 12th International WHO/TDR/FIL Conference on Lymphatic Pathology and Immunopathology in Filariasis, Thanjavur, India, November 18–22, 1985. Lymphology 18:159, 1985.
35. Chernin E: The disappearance of bancroftian filariasis from Charleston, South Carolina. Am J Trop Med Hyg 37:111, 1987.
36. Case T, Leis B, Witte M, et al: Vascular abnormalities in experimental and human lymphatic filariasis. Lymphology 24:174, 1991.
37. Dandapat MC, Mohapatro SK, Dash DM: Management of chronic manifestations of filariasis. J Indian Med Assoc 84:210, 1986.
38. Schirger A: Lymphedema. *In* Spittell JA Jr (ed): Cardiovascular Clinics. Philadelphia, FA Davis, 1983, pp 293–305.
39. Chant ADB: Hypothesis: Why venous oedema causes ulcers and lymphoedema does not. Eur J Vasc Surg 6:427, 1992.
40. Samman PD, White WF: The "yellow nail" syndrome. Br J Dermatol 76:153, 1964.
41. Taylor JS, Young JR: The swollen limb: Cutaneous clues to diagnosis and treatment. Cutis 21:553, 1978.
42. Fields CL, Roy TM, Ossorio MA, Mercer PJ: Yellow nail syndrome: A perspective. J Ky Med Assoc 89:563, 1991.
43. Stewart FW, Treves N: Lymphangiosarcoma in postmastectomy lymphedema: A report of six cases in elephantiasis chirurgica. Cancer 1:64, 1948.
44. Alessi E, Sala F, Berti E: Angiosarcomas in lymphedematous limbs. Am J Dermatopathol 8:371, 1986.
45. Muller R, Hajdu SI, Brennan MF: Lymphangiosarcoma associated with chronic filarial lymphedema. Cancer 59:179, 1987.
46. Sherman AI, Ter-Pergossian M: Lymph node concentration of radioactive colloidal gold following interstitial injection. Cancer 6:1238, 1953.
47. Taylor GW, Kinmonth JB, Rollinson E, et al: Lymphatic circulation studied with radioactive plasma protein. Br Med J 1:133, 1957.
48. Ege GN: Internal mammary lymphoscintigraphy—The rationale, technique, interpretation, and clinical application. Radiology 118:101, 1976.
49. Jackson FI, Bowen P, Lentle BC: Scintilymphangiography with ^{99m}Tc-antimony sulfide colloid in hereditary lymphedema (Nonne-Milroy disease). Clin Nucl Med 3:296, 1978.
50. Sty JR, Starshak RJ: Atlas of pediatric radionuclide lymphography. Clin Nucl Med 7:428, 1982.
51. Stewart G, Gaunt JI, Croft DN, Browse NL: Isotope lymphography: A new method of investigating the role of the lymphatics in chronic limb oedema. Br J Surg 72:906, 1985.
52. Nawaz K, Hamad MM, Sadek S, et al: Dynamic lymph flow imaging in lymphedema. Normal and abnormal patterns. Clin Nucl Med 11:653, 1986.
53. Ohtake E, Matsui K: Lymphoscintigraphy in patients with lymphedema. A new approach using intradermal injections of technetium-99m human serum albumin. Clin Nucl Med 11:474, 1986.
54. Vaqueiro M, Gloviczki P, Fisher J, et al: Lymphoscintigraphy in lymphedema: An aid to microsurgery. J Nucl Med 27:1125, 1986.
55. Weissleder H, Weissleder R: Lymphedema: Evaluation of qualitative and quantitative lymphoscintigraphy in 238 patients. Radiology 167:729, 1988.
56. Collins PS, Villavicencio JL, Abreu SH, et al: Abnormalities of lymphatic drainage in lower extremities: A lymphoscintigraphic study. J Vasc Surg 9:145, 1989.
57. Gloviczki P, Calcagno D, Schirger A, et al: Noninvasive evaluation of the swollen extremity: Experiences with 190 lymphoscintigraphic examinations. J Vasc Surg 9:683, 1989.
58. Cambria RA, Gloviczki P, Naessens JM, Wahner HW: Noninvasive evaluation of the lymphatic system with lymphoscintigraphy: A prospective, semiquantitative analysis in 386 extremities. J Vasc Surg 18:773, 1993.
59. McNeill GC, Witte MH, Witte CL, et al: Whole-body lymphangioscintigraphy: Preferred method for initial assessment of the peripheral lymphatic system. Radiology 172:495, 1989.
60. Kleinhans E, Baumeister RGH, Hahn D, et al: Evaluation of transport kinetics in lymphoscintigraphy: Follow-up study in patients with transplanted lymphatic vessels. Eur J Nucl Med 10:349, 1985.
61. Gamba JL, Silverman PM, Ling D, et al: Primary lower extremity lymphedema: CT diagnosis. Radiology 149:218, 1983.
62. Hadjus NS, Carr DH, Banks L, Pflug JJ: The role of CT in the diagnosis of primary lymphedema of the lower limb. Am J Roentgenol 144:361, 1985.
63. Göltner E, Gass P, Haas JP, Schneider P: The importance of volumetry, lymphoscintigraphy and computer tomography in the diagnosis of brachial edema after mastectomy. Lymphology 21:134, 1988.
64. Duewell S, Hagspiel KD, Zuber J, et al: Swollen lower extremity: Role of MR imaging. Radiology 184:227, 1992.
65. Weissleder R, Thrall JH: The lymphatic system: Diagnostic imaging studies. Radiology 172:315, 1989.
66. Case TC, Witte CL, Witte MH, et al: Magnetic resonance imaging in human lymphedema: Comparison with lymphangioscintigraphy. J Magn Reson Imag 10:549, 1992.
67. Weissleder R, Elizondo G, Wittenburg J, et al: Ultrasmall superparamagnetic iron oxide: An intravenous contrast agent for assessing lymph nodes with MR imaging. Radiology 175:494, 1990.
68. Kanter MA: The lymphatic system: An historical perspective. Plast Reconstr Surg 79:131, 1987.
69. Servelle M: La lymphographie moyen d'étude de la physiopathologie des grosses jambes. Rev Chir 82:251, 1944.
70. Kinmonth JB: Lymphangiography in man: A method of outlining lymphatic trunks at operation. Clin Sci 11:13, 1952.
71. Wolfe JHN: Diagnosis and classification of lymphedema. *In* Rutherford RB (ed): Vascular Surgery. 3rd ed. Philadelphia, WB Saunders, 1989, pp 1656–1667.
72. Fyfe NCM, Wolfe JHN, Kinmonth JB: "Die-back" in primary lymphedema—Lymphographic and clinical correlations. Lymphology 15:66, 1982.
73. O'Brien BMcC, Mellow CG, Khazanchi RK, et al: Long-term results after microlymphatico-venous anastomoses for the treatment of obstructive lymphedema. Plast Reconstr Surg 85:562, 1990.

74. Partsch H, Urbanek A, Wenzel-Hora B: The dermal lymphatics in lymphoedema visualized by indirect lymphography. Br J Dermatol 110:431, 1984.

75. Gloviczki P: Invited commentary. In Gan JL, Chang TS, Fu DK, et al: Indirect lymphography with Isovist-300 in various forms of lymphedema. Eur J Plast Surg 14:109, 1991.

76. Gloviczki P, Stanson AW, Stickler GB, et al: Klippel-Trenaunay syndrome: The risks and benefits of vascular interventions. Surgery 110:469, 1991.

77. Gloviczki P, Hollier LH: Arteriovenous fistulas. In Haimovici H (ed): Vascular Surgery: Principles and Techniques. 3rd ed. Norwalk, CT, Appleton & Lange, 1989, pp 698–716.

144

Nonoperative Management of Chronic Lymphedema

Thom W. Rooke, M.D., and Peter Gloviczki, M.D.

• • •

Most patients with chronic lymphedema require conservative, nonoperative management. Nonoperative care of this distressing and frequently disabling condition should focus on several areas. These include measures to prevent the development or progression of the disease, drug therapy to decrease the edema and treat infectious complications, mechanical reduction of limb swelling, and maintenance of limb size. Because the psychological impact of this disease is significant, involving the deterioration of the quality of life and the patient's physical self-image,[1] these issues should also be addressed by the treating physician. A rare but severe late complication, lymphangiosarcoma, needs immediate attention and treatment.

PREVENTIVE MEASURES

It is generally easier to prevent lymphedema than to treat it. Although *primary* lymphedema occurs, by definition, in the absence of any known precipitating factors, many possible causes of *secondary* lymphedema can be avoided or minimized by taking appropriate measures.

Filarial Disease

In regions of the world where filarial disease is prevalent, the likelihood of infection can be reduced by taking simple precautions aimed at avoiding transmission of the parasites *(Wuchereria bancrofti, Brugia malayi)* by mosquito bites. These include public health measures to control mosquito breeding,[2, 3] use of protective clothing and mosquito netting, and, in some cases, prophylactic antifilarial medications. Prompt therapy with diethyl carbonate or ivermectin should be instituted when filarial infections are discovered.[4–6]

Malignancy

In North America and Europe secondary lymphedema is seen most commonly following surgical and radiation treatment for breast, pelvic, or prostate cancer. Although the extent of the surgical excision is ultimately dictated by the type and location of the malignant tumor, the incidence and severity of postoperative lymphedema may be minimized when less extensive axillary or inguinal lymph node dissections are performed.[7] Judicious use of adjuvant radiation therapy is equally important.[7, 8] In patients with suspected malignant disease who undergo lymph node biopsy, excision should be limited to the minimum lymphatic tissue needed for diagnosis.

Infection

Recurrent infection is a frequent cause of lymphatic destruction and may lead to the development of secondary lymphedema. The edematous limb is extremely susceptible to bacterial invasion. Therefore, there is a constant threat that infection may aggravate existing disease by causing further destruction of the already compromised lymphatics. Measures taken to prevent infection include rigorous protection of the limb from trauma, meticulous hygiene with eradication or control of chronic fungal infections, and prompt antibiotic therapy of lymphangitis when it occurs. Well-fitting clothing, shoes, stockings, and gloves can help to prevent trauma to the skin. The limb should be kept dry, washed gently with soap and water on a regular basis, and moistened as needed with an emollient to keep the skin soft and prevent the formation of cracks and fissures. Topical antifungal agents should be used to help control trichophytosis. Clotrimazole (1 per cent cream) or miconazole nitrate (2 per cent lotion or cream) is sufficient in most patients, although long-term systemic griseofulvin treatment (250 to 1000 mg daily) may be required in refractory cases. Prompt administration of appropriate antibiotic therapy in patients with lymphangitis is essential.[9] The causative agent is usually a penicillin-sensitive group A *Streptococcus; Staphylococcus* and other agents appear to be much less common causes of infection. Treatment should be started at the first sign of cellulitis using oral penicillin VK (250 or 500 mg four times daily). High-dose intravenous penicillin infusion, hospitalization, and bed rest with leg elevation may be needed in some patients with fulminant lymphangitis (erysipelas). Erythromycin or a first-generation cephalosporin is a reasonable alternative for patients who cannot take penicillin. Antibiotic therapy should be maintained for 5 to 7 days, or until all signs and symptoms of infection have clearly resolved. When spontaneous episodes occur frequently (more than four to six times a year), a regular prophylactic program consisting of penicillin VK (or its equivalent) 250 mg four times daily for 7 days of each month should be considered. An alternative regimen is penicillin G benzathine 1,200,000 units given intramuscularly once a month. In some patients, even this program may not be sufficient to prevent recurrent infections. In such patients, daily antibiotic prophylaxis may be necessary. If tolerated, two or even three different antibiotics can be taken on a monthly rotating basis.

Other Measures

Other conservative measures play a preventive role in the treatment of lymphedema. *Weight loss* should be encouraged in obese patients. *Periodic limb elevation* can help to reduce edema formation, especially early in the course of the disease. Prolonged periods of limb dependence must be avoided. *Exercise*, particularly walking, swimming, and certain forms of isometrics, should be encouraged as a means of promoting the circulation of lymphatic fluid.[10, 11] Some authors advocate a *nutritious low-sodium diet* with *avoidance of alcohol*.[11] Other considerations include avoidance of tight constricting clothing or a heavy breast prosthesis.

MEDICAL THERAPY

Pharmacologic agents have limited use in the direct treatment of lymphedema. Their role is best defined in the prophylaxis and treatment of bacterial infections by antibiotics as outlined earlier.

Diuretics are included in the treatment programs of some authors[12] but not others.[13] The authors of this chapter believe that regular treatment with diuretics is not appropriate for patients with chronic lymphedema. Their effect is temporary, and secondary hemoconcentration is a serious possible side effect.[14] In some circumstances, however, short-term use of diuretics may be helpful. In patients hospitalized for edema reduction (using strict bed rest, elevation of the extremity, and prolonged daily use of intermittent pneumatic compression treatment) the response to acute treatment can be maximized by administration of 40 to 80 mg of furosemide daily. In patients with a periodic increase in edema corresponding to the menstrual cycle, short-term use of diuretics may be helpful. Finally, in patients in the terminal phase of a malignant disease who have painful swelling of the extremity, diuretics may be needed to alleviate symptoms.

Benzopyrones (such as coumarin) are thought to decrease lymphedema by stimulating tissue macrophages and thus altering the macrophage-dependent relationship between protein deposition and lysis.[15–17] As a result of increased macrophage activity, the intercellular protein concentration is reduced, which promotes tissue softening and remodeling. In a recent randomized, double-blind study, 31 patients with postmastectomy lymphedema of the arm and 21 patients with leg lymphedema received 400 mg 5,6-benzo-(alpha)-pyrone or placebo, each for 6 months.[17] Limb volume measurements showed that the drug reduced the volume of the arms from 46 per cent to 26 per cent above normal ($p<.001$) and the volume of the legs from 25 per cent to 17 per cent above normal ($p<.001$). The softness of the limb tissue increased, the elevated skin temperatures decreased, and the episodes of infections also diminished. The authors concluded that 5,6-benzo-(alpha)-pyrone resulted in slow but safe reduction of lymphedema. This drug is used in Europe and Australia but has not yet been approved for use in the United States.

Intralymphatic steroid injections have been used to decrease fibrotic occlusion in lymph nodes and improve lymphatic transport. In a pilot study of 20 patients with primary lymphedema, 8 showed improvement up to 9 months after treatment.[18] The effectiveness of steroid treatment, however, remains unproved. Investigators in Japan have attempted to treat patients with secondary lymphedema by injecting autologous lymphocytes into the main artery of the affected limb.[19] Although five of seven patients showed short-term improvement, further evidence in support of this treatment is lacking. The beneficial effect of oral amitriptyline, reported to reduce postmastectomy lymphedema,[20] also awaits further confirmation.

MECHANICAL REDUCTION OF LIMB SWELLING

Reducing the size of the limb is usually the primary goal of therapy for lymphedema. Early in the course of the disease, when the tissues are still soft, it may be possible to return the limb to its original size. After fibrosis has developed, the brawny tissues typically do not become fully normal following reduction maneuvers, and residual swelling may have to be accepted. Changes in limb size can be followed subjectively or by objective measurements that include (1) circumferential determinations obtained at many levels or (2) volumetric assessments using water-displacement techniques. Reduction of limb swelling can be accomplished by a variety of techniques that may be employed individually or in conjunction with one another.

Elevation

Elevation is a simple and effective method for reducing lymphedema. The patient is positioned comfortably,

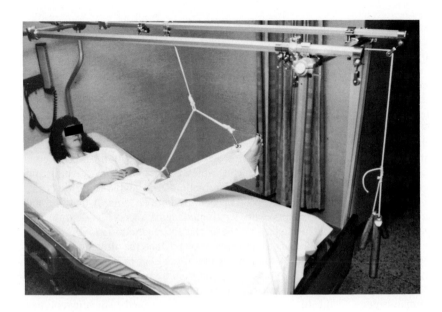

FIGURE 144–1. The lymphedema sling is used to elevate the patient's leg during bed rest, typically to 45 degrees or more.

and the limb is elevated as tolerated, usually to 45 degrees or more. A variety of arm boards and lymphedema slings[12] (Fig. 144–1) have been developed to facilitate this process. Gravity usually produces a maximal reduction in limb size within 2 to 5 days with continuous bed rest. This method of acute treatment of lymphedema has been used in the authors' institution for decades, with excellent early results (Fig. 144–2). Unfortunately, because the patient is confined to bed during the treatment period, therapy outside the hospital is difficult and not as effective. Still, the authors' outpatient limb reduction program incorporates overnight and regular daytime periods of limb elevation. O'Donnell and Howrigan[21] have suggested that 4- to 6-inch-high blocks be placed under the legs of the bed to provide adequate overnight elevation for patients with lower extremity lymphedema.

Massage or Manual Lymphatic Drainage

Simple massage of the affected limb, performed on a regular basis, can help to promote lymphatic drainage and keep the tissues soft and decompressed.[22] Manual lymphatic drainage (MLD) is a specific philosophical and technical approach to limb decompression that is based upon a unique application of massage popularized in Europe by Földi[13] and followed by others elsewhere.[23] An MLD treatment session is performed in sequential steps. The trunk is divided into four quadrants (upper and lower, right and left), and treatment is initiated by massaging the quadrant *contralateral* to the affected limb. In theory, massage stimulates lymphatic flow and helps to drain cutaneous lymph fluid from the "normal" skin located opposite the affected side, thus preparing it to receive lymph fluid from the adjacent involved area. Massage is performed next over the trunk quadrant adjacent to the affected limb. Fluid is pushed out, some of it draining directly into the veins or deep lymphatics and some of it crossing through the anastomotic lymph vessels into the freshly drained contralateral quad-

rant. The process is repeated in stages along the length of the limb, moving slowly in a proximal-to-distal direction, but massaging each segment in a distal-to-proximal fashion. Massage sessions are typically performed two times per week for up to a month to achieve the maximum reduction in limb swelling. At the end of the acute treatment program, the patient is fitted with an elastic stocking or sleeve.

Compression Pumping

An alternative method for achieving limb size reduction involves the use of intermittent pneumatic compression. The affected limb is placed in a pneumatic "cuff" or "sleeve," which is intermittently inflated and deflated; the subsequent pressure gradient thus created forces lymph fluid out of the affected limb and back into the trunk. These devices may utilize either a single uniform-pressure sleeve or a series of overlapping chambers within the sleeve that can be inflated sequentially.[24–31]

A theoretical disadvantage of the single-chamber device is that high pressure is exerted both proximally and distally and can potentially force fluid into the more distal extremity. Because of the longer duration of the pressure cycle, it may also be uncomfortable for the patient. In a controlled study, Richmand and associates[26] failed to achieve an acute response in 30 per cent of patients treated with a single-chamber pump. These authors also found that the proximal portion of the limb responded poorly to the unicell device. The data of Zanolla and colleagues,[27] however, support the effectiveness of the single-chamber device in the treatment of postmastectomy lymphedema. In this study, the acute treatment period of 1 week included 6-hour treatments daily, using a 90-mmHg cuff pressure with a ratio of 1:3 for compression and decompression. A 21 per cent reduction in limb circumference was achieved and maintained at 3 months in 20 patients.

With the sequential pneumatic compression device, developed by Zelikovski and colleagues,[25, 28] the chambers are inflated in a distal-to-proximal direction, thus producing a dynamic pressure gradient and a "milking" action on the

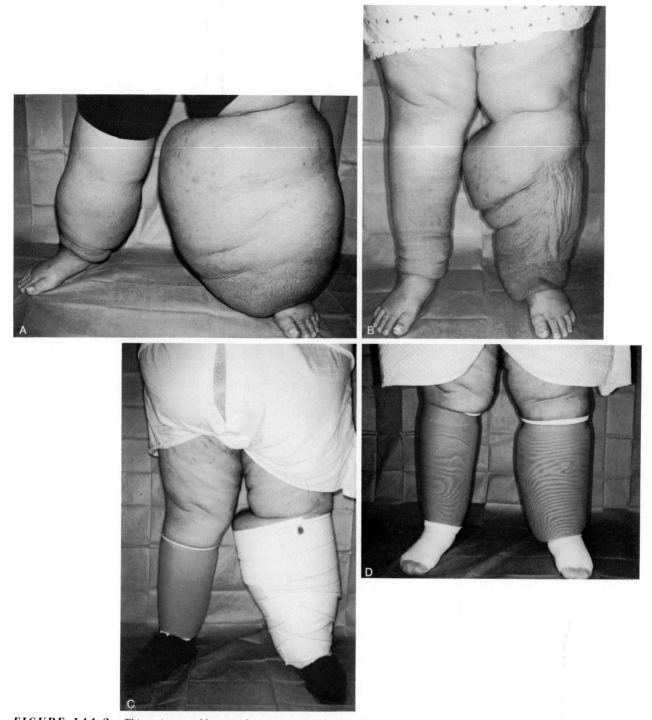

FIGURE 144–2.   Thirty-six-year-old man with severe primary lymphedema of the lower extremities. *A,* Limbs on presentation. *B,* The same patient after 2 weeks of continuous leg elevation, elastic wrapping, and pneumatic compression treatment. Much of the residual deformity distal to the knee is fatty deposition. *C,* The same patient after application of bilateral custom-made elastic stockings and a nonelastic wrapping to reinforce the stocking on the left. *D,* The same patient 1 month after initiation of therapy.

limb (Fig. 144–3). Pressures of 100 mmHg or more are typically tolerated with these devices owing to the short duration of each inflation cycle (typically ranging from 20 seconds to 1 or 2 minutes). Treatment sessions may last anywhere from 1 hour to as long as 8 to 10 hours or more, depending on the magnitude and refractoriness of the edema.

In a recent prospective nonrandomized clinical study,

Pappas and O'Donnell[29] confirmed the long-term effectiveness of compression treatment for lymphedema. Their protocol included a 2- to 3-day hospitalization and daily 6- to 8-hour treatment sessions with sequential high-pressure intermittent pneumatic compression using the Lymphapress device (Camp International, Inc., Jackson, MI). This was followed by maintenance of the limb volume by custom-made two-way stretch elastic compression stockings. Some

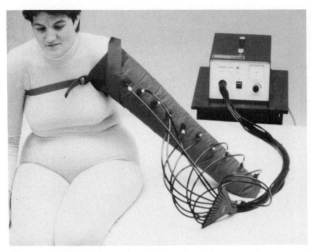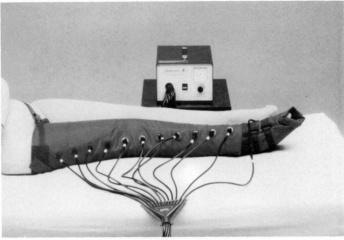

A   B

FIGURE 144–3.   Sequential pneumatic pump used for intermittent compression treatment of upper *(A)* or lower *(B)* extremity lymphedema. *(A* and *B,* Courtesy of Camp International, Inc., Jackson, MI.)

patients continued to use the Lymphapress at home. Limb girth measurements at nine levels were obtained serially during a follow-up period that averaged 25 months in 49 patients. This protocol resulted in long-term maintenance of limb girth reduction in 90 per cent of the patients, and the improvement remained excellent at late follow-up in 26 of 49 patients, with an absolute reduction in calf and ankle girths of 5.37 ± 1.01 and 4.63 ± 0.88 cm compared with pretreatment measurements. The most important factor affecting outcome was the degree of subcutaneous fibrosis involved. More than 80 per cent of patients with a poor response to the treatment had had lymphedema for more than 10 years. These data also confirm that conservative compression treatment should be started early, before a chronic inflammatory reaction has developed and irreversible fibrosis in the subcutaneous tissues has occurred.

Other multi cellular intermittent pneumatic compression devices include the three-celled Hemoflow II unit (Camp International, Inc., Jackson, MI) and the three-celled Wright linear pump (Wright-Linear Pump Inc., Imperial, PA). Klein and coworkers[30] used the Wright linear pump in 78 extremities in 73 patients with lymphedema. Acute treatment included 48 hours of hospitalization with bed rest and leg elevation, and pump treatment sessions lasting up to 8 hours. After therapy, 90 per cent of the patients showed a reduction in limb circumference at the ankle or at mid-calf ranging from 1.6 to 2.1 cm. The results of long-term maintenance of the reduced volume in this study were not reported. In comparing the three different multi-chamber devices in a small group of pediatric patients with congenital lymphedema, McLeod and colleagues[31] found that the Lymphapress was superior to the Hemoflow II and the Wright linear pump.

The use of intermittent, nonpneumatic high pressure using a mercury-filled chamber was introduced recently for the treatment of chronic lymphedema. The mercury-filled chamber generates a very high pressure gradient along the limb, with 500- to 800-mmHg pressures present at the ankle. These high pressures are applied in six cycles per treatment, each lasting for 6 minutes. In 12 patients, good early results were achieved without any apparent side effects, pain, or injury to the skin.[32] Larger experience with this technique is needed to evaluate the long-term results and the potential deleterious effects of the high pressures on the subcutaneous tissue. Temporary obstruction of arterial inflow in some patients carries an elevated risk of complications.

Heat

Heat therapy as a means of lymphedema reduction has been practiced in the Orient and elsewhere for centuries. Heating the limb presumably mobilizes fluid and softens the tissues; tight wrappings are applied between treatments to reduce and maintain limb size. In a study from China of 1045 patients with lymphedema, 68 per cent of the patients achieved an effective reduction in the volume of the extremity using heat therapy, with a subsequent decrease in the frequency of lymphangitis episodes.[33] Traditional methods have involved the use of ovens heated to 80 to 90° C, but newer methods involving microwave thermal stimulation are being explored.[34] However, no controlled trial is available to prove the effectiveness of this treatment. Theoretically, heat should *increase* lymph production.

MAINTENANCE OF LIMB SIZE

Although intermittent outpatient therapy with manual lymphatic drainage, pneumatic compression, elevation, or other methods can help to reduce the size of the swollen limb, elastic or nonelastic external support is necessary to maintain limb size.

Graduated Elastic Support

Strict daily use of properly fitting, appropriately graduated, elastic compression stockings remains the key to maintaining limb size for most patients.[35] Support stockings come in a variety of lengths, compression strengths, and materials, and the choice of each characteristic must be tailored to fit the needs and dimensions of the individual.[36] Although many patients with swollen limbs can be fitted with over-the-counter ready-made stockings, patients with significant swelling or an unusual leg shape may need custom-made stockings to obtain an optimal fit.

Compression. Stockings are classified according to the amount of compression they deliver at the ankle and may be graduated or nongraduated. Graduated stockings are made so that the highest amount of compression is obtained distally, with progressively less pressure in the proximal direction. Over-the-counter ''support'' stockings usually provide 7 to 15 mmHg of compression and are not graduated. ''Antiembolism'' stockings, such as TED hose, provide 15 to 20 mmHg of compression and tend to be graduated. ''Therapeutic'' elastic stockings, needed for patients with chronic venous insufficiency or lymphedema, come in a variety of compression categories (20 to 30, 30 to 40, 40 to 50, and 50 to 60 mmHg) and lengths depending on the patient's need. Limbs with lymphedema generally require 40 to 50 mmHg of compression pressure or more at the ankle to control the swelling. However, in patients with arthritis, arterial occlusive disease, or other problems that limit the use of high-compression stockings, stockings with pressures of 30 to 40 mmHg may be tried. Low-compression (less than 30 mmHg) or nongraduated stockings usually have little if any ability to control the swelling of even mild lymphedema.

Length. Stocking length is frequently an issue for patients with lymphedema (Fig. 144–4). As a rule, stockings should be long enough to cover the edematous portion of the limb. However, patient preference and physical limitations must be taken into account; if a stocking that is less than optimal from the physician's viewpoint provides more patient satisfaction and compliance than the alternatives, that stocking is probably the better long-term choice. This is especially true for male patients, in whom compliance tends to be better with below-knee stockings than it is with stockings that extend above the knee or are full length.

Materials and Brands. Stockings come in a variety of knits and materials; most are composed of a variable combination of latex, spandex, nylon, cotton, and silk.[36] Differences in construction, sizing, and materials can significantly

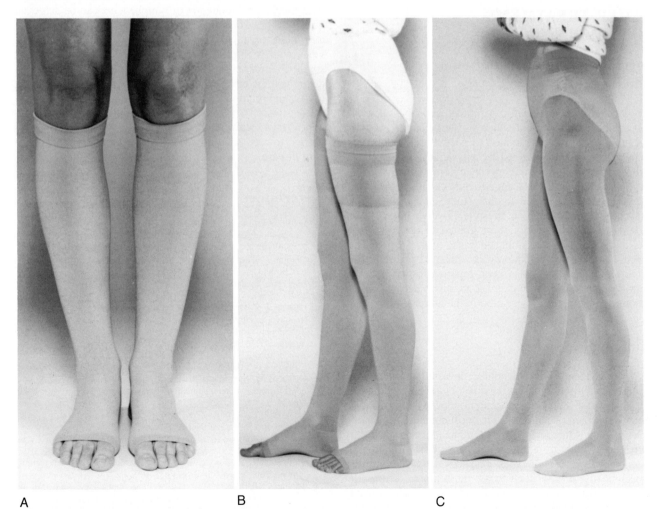

A   B   C

FIGURE 144–4. Different types of high-compression graduated elastic stockings for patients with lower extremity lymphedema (below-knee *[A]*, thigh-high *[B]*, and pantyhose *[C]* lengths).

affect the way a particular brand or style of stocking feels and functions in a given patient. Unfortunately, predicting which patient will do best with a particular stocking brand is almost impossible. For this reason, patients may need to try a variety of brands and styles before finding the one that works optimally for them. Like O'Donnell and Howrigan,[21] the authors prefer the two-way stretch elastic stockings, although no controlled study to prove the superiority of any of the available stockings (e.g., Sigvaris, Jobst, Camp, Medi Strumpf, Bell Horn, Juzo, Venosan) is available.

Nonelastic Support

Although nonelastic support was once widely used as a method for controlling limb swelling, it has been largely replaced by modern elastic stockings. Commercial devices employing the principle of nonelastic support have been reintroduced for the control of lymphedema. The Circ Aid (Shaw Therapeutics, Rumson, NJ) uses Velcro fastenings to readjust a series of nonelastic support bands around the leg and ankle. Whether this approach is superior or even comparable to conventional elastic support hose remains to be determined.

OTHER TREATMENT CONSIDERATIONS

Psychological and Functional Impairment

Smeltzer and associates[1] examined the psychological impact of lymphedema on patients. Their findings suggest that emotional problems related to edema are not uncommon and are often neglected by physicians. The need to address the psychological aspects of long-term disfigurement, especially in adolescent patients, cannot be overemphasized. Also discussed in this study is the functional impact of lymphedema on lifestyle. Twelve per cent of patients reported that they were limited to desk jobs (or jobs that allow frequent sitting) because of the edema. The impression that job promotion was withheld because of the employee's edema has also been reported. Some patients limit their participation in exercise or sports because of an uncomfortable or heavy sensation in the affected limb.

Malignancy

Malignancies are potentially devastating but fortunately uncommon complications of long-standing lymphedema. In most series, they occur in 1 per cent or less of patients with lymphedema.[1,37] The most common malignancies are angiosarcomas[38] and lymphangiosarcomas,[39, 40] which are thought to represent neoplastic transformation of blood vessels and lymphatics, respectively. Histologically and clinically, it is difficult to tell these tumors apart, and for most purposes they can be considered identical to each other. The association between angiosarcoma or lymphangiosarcoma and lymphedema is commonly called the Stewart-Treves syndrome.[38] Sarcomas can develop in patients with long-standing lymphedema of any cause, including primary lymphedema[41] or lymphedema secondary to filariasis,[42] hysterectomy,[43] trauma,[43] or mastectomy.[44] Other malignancies, including Hodgkin's and non-Hodgkin's lymphoma,[45] Kaposi's sarcoma,[46] squamous cell carcinoma,[47, 48] and malignant melanoma,[49] have been reported in association with chronic lymphedema. Limbs with edema must therefore be inspected frequently to permit early detection and appropriate treatment of tumors should they occur.

CONCLUSION

Conservative, nonsurgical management of lymphedema continues to be the mainstay of treatment for this debilitating condition. Preventive measures include immediate medical treatment for bacterial infections affecting the limbs or for parasitic infections known to cause filariasis. Effective pharmacologic treatment to decrease chronic lymphedema currently is not available in the United States, although a recent prospective randomized study from Australia confirmed the benefit of 5,6-benzo-(alpha)-pyrone in reducing lymphedema and decreasing the episodes of infections. Chronic use of diuretics is not recommended. Short-term mechanical reduction of lymphedema can be achieved with elevation, massage, manual lymphatic drainage, or intermittent pneumatic compression treatment. Pressure devices with multiple cells are generally preferred over the single-chamber compression pump. Maintenance of the reduced volume can be achieved in most patients with regular use of high-compression elastic stockings. The psychological aspects of the disease should be addressed to help patients cope with their disability. Regular follow-up is needed to recognize immediately and treat any late malignant disease.

References

1. Smeltzer D, Stickler GB, Schirger A: Primary lymphedema in children and adolescents: A follow-up study and review. Pediatrics 76:206, 1985.
2. Chernin E: The disappearance of bancroftian filariasis from Charleston, South Carolina. Am J Trop Med Hyg 37:111, 1987.
3. Mak JW: Epidemiology of lymphatic filariasis. Ciba Found Symp 127:5, 1987.
4. Ottesen EA: Description, mechanisms and control of reactions to treatment in the human filariases. Ciba Found Symp 127:265, 1987.
5. Subrahmanyam D: Antifilarials and their mode of action. Ciba Found Symp 127:246, 1987.
6. Dandapat MC, Mohapatro SK, Dash D: Management of chronic manifestations of filariasis. J Indian Med Assoc 84:210, 1986.
7. Kissin MW, Querci-della-Rovere G, Easton D, et al: Risk of lymphedema following the treatment of breast cancer. Br J Surg 73:580, 1986.
8. Markby R, Baldwin E, Kerr P: Incidence of lymphoedema in women with breast cancer. Prof Nurse 6:502, 1991.
9. Babb RR: Prophylaxis of recurrent lymphangitis complicating lymphedema. JAMA 195:871, 1966.
10. Stillwell GK, Redford JWB: Physical treatment of postmastectomy lymphedema. Mayo Clin Proc 33:1, 1958.
11. Thiadens SRJ, Rooke TW, Cooke JP: Lymphedema. *In* Cooke JP, Frohlich ED (eds): Current Management of Hypertensive and Vascular Diseases. St. Louis, Mosby-Year Book, 1992, pp 314–319.
12. Schirger A: Lymphedema. Cardiovasc Clin 13:293, 1983.

13. Földi E, Földi M, Weissleder H: Conservative treatment of lymphoedema of the limbs. Angiology 36:171, 1985.
14. Tiedjen KV, Kluken N: The lymphostatic edema? The therapeutic effect of diuretic treatment compared with physiological and physical methods in an isotope study. Presented at the 13th World Congress of the International Union of Angiology, Rochester, MN 1983.
15. Casley-Smith JR, Casley-Smith JR: The pathophysiology of lymphedema and the action of benzopyrones in reducing it. Lymphology 21:190, 1988.
16. Piller NB: Macrophage and tissue changes in the developmental phases of secondary lymphoedema and during conservative therapy with benzopyrone. Arch Histol Cytol Suppl 53:209, 1990.
17. Casley-Smith JR, Morgan RG, Piller NB: Treatment of lymphedema of the arms and legs with 5,6-benzo-(alpha)-pyrone. N Engl J Med 329:1158, 1993.
18. Fyfe NC, Rutt DL, Edwards JM, et al: Intralymphatic steroid therapy for lymphoedema: Preliminary studies. Lymphology 15:23, 1982.
19. Katoh I, Harada K, Tsuda Y, et al: Intraarterial lymphocytes injection for treatment of lymphedema. Jpn J Surg 14:331, 1984.
20. Winstone DJ: Amitriptyline and lymphoedema. Med J Aust 2:119, 1982.
21. O'Donnell TF, Howrigan P: Diagnosis and management of lymphoedema. *In* Bell PRF, Jamieson CW, Ruckley CV (eds): Surgical Management of Vascular Disease. Philadelphia, WB Saunders, 1992, pp 1305–1327.
22. Browse NL: The diagnosis and management of primary lymphedema. J Vasc Surg 3:181, 1986.
23. Casley-Smith JR, Casley-Smith JR, Mason MR: Complex physical therapy for lymphoedema in Australia. Phlebology 6:21, 1991.
24. Thiadens SRJ: Advances in the management of lymphedema. *In* Goldstone J (ed): Perspectives in Vascular Surgery. St. Louis, Quality Medical Publishing, 1990, pp 125–141.
25. Zelikovski A, Deutsch A, Reiss R: The sequential pneumatic compression device in surgery for lymphedema of the limbs. J Cardiovasc Surg 24:122, 1983.
26. Richmand DM, O'Donnell TF, Jr, Zelikovski A: Sequential pneumatic compression for lymphedema. A controlled trial. Arch Surg 120:1116, 1985.
27. Zanolla R, Monzeglio C, Balzarini A, et al: Evaluation of the results of three different methods of postmastectomy lymphedema treatment. J Surg Oncol 26:210, 1984.
28. Zelikovski A, Melamed I, Kott I, et al: The ''Lymphapress'': A new pneumatic device for the treatment of lymphedema: Clinical trials and results. Folia Angiol 28:165, 1980.
29. Pappas CJ, O'Donnell TF: Long-term results of compression treatment for lymphedema. J Vasc Surg 16:555, 1992.
30. Klein MJ, Alexander MA, Wright JM, et al: Treatment of adult lower extremity lymphedema with the Wright linear pump: Statistical analysis of a clinical trial. Arch Phys Med Rehabil 69:202, 1988.
31. McLeod A, Brooks D, Hale J, et al: A clinical report on the use of three external pneumatic compression devices in the management of lymphedema in a paediatric population. Physiother Can 43:28, 1991.
32. Palmar A, Macchiaverna J, Braun A, et al: Compression therapy of limb edema using hydrostatic pressure of mercury. Angiology 42:533, 1991.
33. Ti-sheng Z, Wen-yi H, Liang-yu H, et al: Heat and bandage treatment for chronic lymphedema of extremities. Report of 1,045 patients. Chin Med J 97:567, 1984.
34. Gloviczki P: Treatment of secondary lymphedema. *In* Ernst CB, Stanley JC (eds): Current Therapy in Vascular Surgery. 2nd ed. Philadelphia, BC Decker, 1991, pp 1030–1036.
35. Pierson S, Pierson D, Swallow R, et al: Efficacy of graded elastic compression in the lower leg. JAMA 249:242, 1983.
36. Johnson G Jr: Role of elastic support in treatment of the chronically swollen limb. *In* Bergan JJ, Yao JST (eds): Venous Disorders. Philadelphia, WB Saunders, 1991, pp 372–378.
37. Servelle M: Surgical treatment of lymphedema: A report of 652 cases. Surgery 101:485, 1987.
38. Schmitz-Rixen, Horsch S, Arnold G, Peters PE: Angiosarcoma in primary lymphedema of the lower extremity—Stewart-Treves syndrome. Lymphology 17:50, 1984.
39. Merli GJ: Lymphedema. Clin Podiatry 1:363, 1984.
40. Witte MH, Witte CL: Lymphangiogenesis and lymphologic syndromes. Lymphology 19:21, 1986.
41. Kobayashi MR, Miller TA: Lymphedema. Clin Plast Surg 14:303, 1987.
42. Muller R, Hajdu SI, Brennan MF: Lymphangiosarcoma associated with chronic filarial lymphedema. Cancer 1:179, 1987.
43. Alessi E, Sala F, Berti E: Angiosarcomas in lymphedematous limbs. Am J Dermatopathol 8:371, 1986.
44. Benda JA, Al-Jurf AS, Benson AB 3d: Angiosarcoma of the breast following segmental mastectomy complicated by lymphedema. Am J Clin Pathol 87:651, 1987.
45. Tatnall FM, Mann BS: Non-Hodgkin's lymphoma of the skin associated with chronic limb lymphoedema. Br J Dermatol 113:751, 1985.
46. Ruocco V, Astarita C, Guerrera V, et al: Kaposi's sarcoma on a lymphedematous immunocompromised limb. Int J Dermatol 23:56, 1984.
47. Shelly WB, Wood MG: Transformation of the common wart into squamous cell carcinoma in a patient with primary lymphedema. Cancer 1:820, 1981.
48. Epstein JI, Mendelsohn G: Squamous carcinoma of the foot arising in association with long-standing verrucous hyperplasia in a patient with congenital lymphedema. Cancer 1:943, 1984.
49. Bartal AH, Pinsky CM: Malignant melanoma appearing in a postmastectomy lymphedematous arm: A novel association of double primary tumors. J Surg Oncol 30:16, 1985.

145

Excisional Operations for Chronic Lymphedema

M. Samy Abdou, M.D., Eric R. Ashby, M.D., and Timothy A. Miller, M.D.

• • •

Nonsurgical therapy is the initial form of treatment for lymphedema, and most patients can be adequately managed without surgical intervention. For the 10 per cent of lymphedema patients who ultimately require surgical treatment,[1,2] the likelihood of benefit and satisfaction depends, in large part, on the indication for surgery. The patient with restricted movement due to gross enlargement of the extremity is most likely to benefit from surgical treatment. Functional impairment caused by inability to control the size of the extremity is the best indication for surgery. Those who experience frequent recurrent lymphangitis are also likely to benefit from surgical treatment. Patients with primary lymphedema of moderate severity who seek surgical correction for cosmetic reasons are less likely to be satisfied.

The aim of surgical therapy is to improve limb function and appearance by either improving lymphatic drainage or excising the lymphedematous skin and subcutaneous tissue. The operation should decrease the frequency of recurrent infections. The frustration encountered in the surgical management of lymphedema is reflected in the numerous techniques described during the past 80 years.

Operations for lymphedema can be divided into two major groups: physiologic procedures and excisional procedures. The physiologic procedures attempt to reconstruct lymphatic drainage either by bypassing a segmental lymphatic obstruction by constructing a lympholymphatic or lymphovenous shunt or by establishing communication between a lymphatic-rich flap and the edematous limb. The excisional procedures remove varying amounts of the involved skin and subcutaneous tissue. Thompson's buried dermis flap is intended to be both an excisional and a physiologic operation.[3]

In this chapter we discuss the three most frequently used excisional procedures. They are (1) total subcutaneous excision (Charles' procedure), (2) buried dermis flap (Thompson's procedure), and (3) subcutaneous excision underneath flaps (modified Homans' procedure). Excisional procedures continue to be the mainstay of surgical treatment for chronic whole-limb edema with poor distal lymphatic function. All patients must understand that surgery is palliative and that a cosmetically perfect result is unattainable. At present, no surgical procedure can be offered as a cure.

TOTAL SUBCUTANEOUS EXCISION (CHARLES' PROCEDURE)

Surgical Technique

Originally described by Charles in 1912, this operation is the most extensive of the excisional procedures.[4] In the lower extremity, all of the skin and subcutaneous tissue are excised from the tibial tuberosity to the malleoli (Fig. 145–1A). Tissues overlying the tibial tuberosity, malleoli, and tendons of the calcaneus are not removed. Although some surgeons resect the deep fascia in its entirety,[5] others remove only heavily fibrosed segments.[6] The excision of the tissue is tapered at the proximal and distal margins of the resection to prevent a step deformity (Fig. 145–1B). The defect is closed using a split-thickness or full-thickness skin graft from the resected specimen, or a split-thickness skin graft can be used from an uninvolved donor site (Fig. 145–1C). Some surgeons prefer to delay wound closure for 48 hours to achieve better hemostasis and reduce the likelihood of postoperative graft loss.[6] Coverage with a split-thickness skin graft is technically easier and gives a satisfactory initial appearance. However, these grafts are injured easily, ulcerate frequently, scar extensively, and may develop a severe hyperkeratotic weeping dermatitis. Hyperpigmentation of the grafted segment is also common. Coverage with a single full-thickness skin graft is technically more demanding but produces a better cosmetic result and a more durable graft site. Nevertheless, regions of graft breakdown and substantial scar formation can also occur with full-thickness grafts. A complete description of the operative procedure has been provided by Hoopes.[6]

Results

A few studies have assessed the long-term efficacy of the Charles' procedure. Preliminary results in patients who had the operation at the Johns Hopkins Hospital were reported in 1959,[7] and a long-term follow-up study of the same patients was published in 1977.[8] The later study contained 10 patients (12 extremities) who were reexamined an

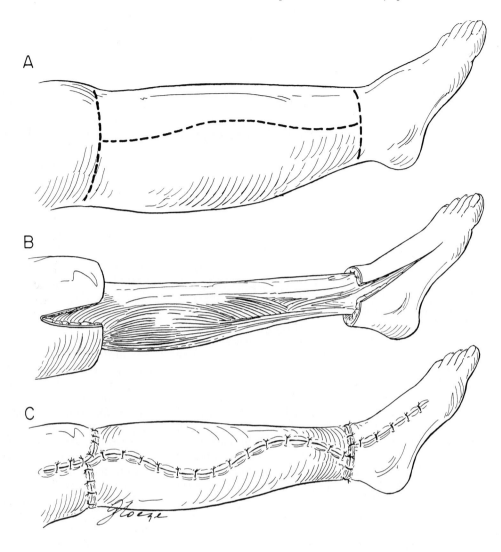

A

B

C

FIGURE 145–1. Total subcutaneous excision (Charles' procedure). *A,* The lines of incision are depicted. *B,* After removing the skin and subcutaneous tissue, the proximal and distal margins of the resection are tapered to prevent a step deformity. *C,* The defect is closed. A full-thickness graft is used for closure in this illustration.

average of 10½ years after the initial operation. Seven of the 10 patients were female, all had primary lymphedema, and 11 of the 12 limbs were lower extremities. All patients had a good functional result, and 9 of them were actively employed. Mild to moderate swelling of the grafted segment was reported by all after prolonged standing, but the swelling was well controlled by stockings. Two patients had notable swelling of the extremity distal to the graft site, and 2 required a subsequent procedure to revise scars or release contractures. None of the patients required a second operation for recurrent lymphedema. All had some degree of hyperpigmentation and hyperkeratosis of the grafted skin at the 12 graft sites. Both conditions were observed more frequently in segments covered with split-thickness skin grafts than in those covered with full-thickness grafts. Two of the 10 patients had recurrent cellulitis that required hospitalization, although the frequency of preoperative and postoperative cellulitis was not compared. Overall, all patients were said to be ''pleased'' with the improved appearance and function.

In 1965, Taylor reported a series of 34 patients who had undergone total subcutaneous excision followed by a split-thickness skin graft.[5] Thirty-six per cent of patients had a ''good'' result, 36 per cent had a ''satisfactory'' result, and 28 per cent had an ''unsatisfactory'' result. Despite its obvious limitations, this procedure is sometimes the only surgical option for patients with extensive swelling and extreme skin changes.

BURIED DERMIS FLAP (THOMPSON'S PROCEDURE)

In this operation, a portion of the lymphedematous subcutaneous tissue is resected beneath flaps, a flap edge is de-epithelialized, and the resulting ''dermis flap'' is buried in the underlying muscle compartment. Thompson's operation has three theoretical advantages: (1) The buried dermis permits the formation of lymphatic connections between the subdermal lymphatic plexus of the flap and the deep lymphatics of the muscle compartment, (2) muscle contractions increase the lymphatic flow rate through the subdermal plexus, and (3) the buried flap provides a physical barrier against deep fascia regeneration.[9] The operation is intended to be both excisional and physiologic in approach.[3]

Surgical Technique

In the lower limbs, the initial operation is usually performed on the lateral aspect of the involved extremity. If additional volume reduction is desired, the procedure is repeated on the medial aspect of the limb 3 months after the first operation. The surgical incision is placed at the junction of the anterior and middle thirds of the lateral thigh and leg but curves posteriorly at the knee to traverse its mid-lateral aspect (Fig. 145–2A). Anterior and posterior flaps 1 to 2 cm in thickness are elevated to the mid-sagittal line, thereby exposing 40 to 50 per cent of the entire limb circumference. The subcutaneous tissue and the underlying fascia are excised to expose the muscle compartments (Fig. 145–2B). Some subcutaneous tissue is retained over the proximal fibula, and the common peroneal nerve is carefully preserved. Overthinning of the flaps must be avoided to minimize the likelihood of postoperative flap loss. A 4- to 5-cm-wide split-thickness skin graft is harvested from the edge of the posterior flap. The entire epidermis must be removed; burial of the dermal flap with retained epidermal islands will lead to formation of draining sinus tracts at the suture line. The dermal flap is sutured to the lateral wall of the femoral canal in the thigh and to the intramuscular space between the tibialis anterior and the extensor hallucis longus muscles in the leg (Fig. 145–2C). A drain is placed beneath each flap, and the anterior flap is closed over the dermal flap in a "vest over pant" fashion using mattress sutures (Fig. 145–2D).

Depending on the extent of disease, this procedure may be limited to the leg and distal thigh or extended onto the proximal thigh and foot. A similar operation is available for the medial aspect of the lower limb and for both lateral and medial aspects of the upper extremity.[9–11] In planning the operation, the flaps are designed so that the direction of lymph flow in the superficial lymphatic plexus is toward the buried dermis. In most patients, the dermal flap is placed on the edge of a long posterior flap based on the mid-posterior line of the extremity (Fig. 145–3). In the small number of patients with primary hyperplastic lymphedema, Thompson stated that the "direction of lymph flow seems to be permanently reversed . . . in such cases the direction in which the shaved skin flap is buried should also be reversed; each skin flap is therefore based anteriorly and its shaved margin buried posteriorly . . . ."[11] He identified this small patient subgroup by the use of lymphangiography. However, there is growing evidence that lymphangiography can damage the remaining lymphatics, and the authors believe that it should not be routinely applied in the hope of identifying this patient subgroup.

Results

In 1980, Thompson and Wee published a study of the long-term results of this procedure.[3] One hundred fifty-one operations were performed on 140 patients, with bilateral procedures in 11 patients. Eighty-eight operations were performed for primary lymphedema of the leg, 14 for secondary lymphedema of the leg, and 49 for secondary lymphedema of the arm. One third of the patients were followed for up to 5 years, one third for 5 to 10 years, and the remainder for 10 to 20 years. Operative results were reported as "good," "satisfactory," or "unimproved." A "good" result indicated reduction of excess swelling by more than 75 per cent, a return to normal activity, and relief from the main complaints. A "satisfactory" outcome indicated significant reduction of swelling (but less than 70 per

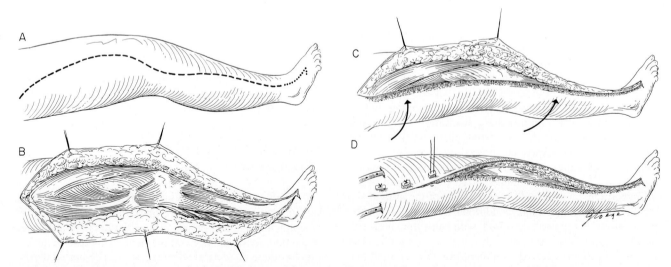

FIGURE 145–2. Buried dermis flap (Thompson's procedure). *A,* The line of the incision is demonstrated. If the foot is significantly involved, the incision is carried onto the dorsum *(dotted line). B,* The anterior and posterior flaps are elevated. The subcutaneous tissue and the underlying fascia are excised to expose the muscle compartment. *C,* The shaved margin of the posterior flap is buried into the intermuscular space between the tibialis anterior and the extensor hallucis longus muscles. Note that a portion of the shaved margin (dermal flap) remains visible after the flap has been buried *(stippled area). D,* The anterior flap is placed over the visible portion of the dermal flap in a "vest over pant" manner to close the wound.

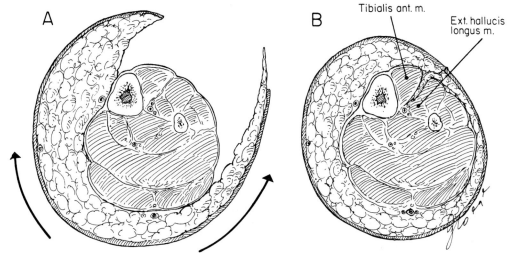

FIGURE 145–3. Buried dermis flap (Thompson's procedure). *A,* The leg is shown in cross section. The flaps have been elevated, and the subcutaneous tissue and fascia have been removed. The *arrows* represent the direction of lymph flow in the superficial lymphatic plexus. *B,* The shaved portion of the posterior flap is buried in the intermuscular cleft, and the anterior flap is reseated.

cent), a return to moderate activity, and alleviation of most complaints.

In patients with primary lymphedema, 51 per cent of the limbs had a good surgical result and another 32 per cent had a satisfactory outcome. Comparable results were reported for patients with secondary lymphedema of the lower extremity. In the upper extremity, 61 per cent had a good result, and 14 per cent were satisfactory. Flap necrosis, the most common complication, occurred in 47 per cent of the patients. Although most areas of tissue loss were small, 12 per cent of patients had significant tissue necrosis that exceeded 10 cm^2 and required excision and skin grafting under anesthesia. An additional 14 per cent of patients developed a draining sinus at the surgical incision. Two patients had inadvertent nerve injury during dissection.

Operative success is attributed to the formation of lymphatic connections between the flap and the muscle compartment, and radioactive iodine–tagged human serum albumin (RIHSA) clearance studies have demonstrated postoperative improvement in the rate of lymphatic isotope clearance.[11–13] However, postoperative lymphangiography has failed to demonstrate any lymphatic anastomosis.[3] Moreover, subcutaneous excision alone has been shown to increase the rate of RIHSA clearance.[14, 15] It may be the excisional component of the operation that actually produces most of the postoperative improvement.

STAGED SUBCUTANEOUS EXCISION UNDERNEATH FLAPS (MODIFIED HOMANS' PROCEDURE)

This operation was first described by Sistrunk in 1918[16] and was later modified and popularized by Homans.[17, 18] In our opinion, this approach provides the most reasonable surgical compromise among the excisional procedures. It offers reliable improvement while minimizing the likelihood of unfavorable postoperative complications. The operation is similar to the excisional component of Thompson's procedure and produces comparable results but with a lower complication rate. The third excisional operation, the Charles procedure, should be reserved for patients with severe skin changes.

Improvement is directly related to the amount of skin and subcutaneous tissue removed. The surgical procedure is offered to patients as a means of managing their lymphedema, not as a cure.[19] During the operation, as much subcutaneous tissue and skin are removed as possible while maintaining the ability to close the skin primarily.[19–21] The following section describes the surgical approach preferred by the authors.

Preoperative Care

All patients are placed on bed rest, and the extremity is elevated. Although this step can be started at home, the patient is usually admitted to the hospital 1 to 3 days preoperatively, and a modified Thomas orthopedic splint suspended from an overhead frame is used to elevate the lower extremity. The rate of edema resolution depends on the chronicity of the condition and the amount of subcutaneous fibrosis that exists. Diuretics are not employed. While the patient is in the hospital, the extremity is washed daily. Other than a single preoperative dose, antibiotics are not routinely used.

Operation on the Lower Extremity

Surgical Technique

A pneumatic tourniquet is placed as proximally as possible. A medial incision is made in the leg approxi-

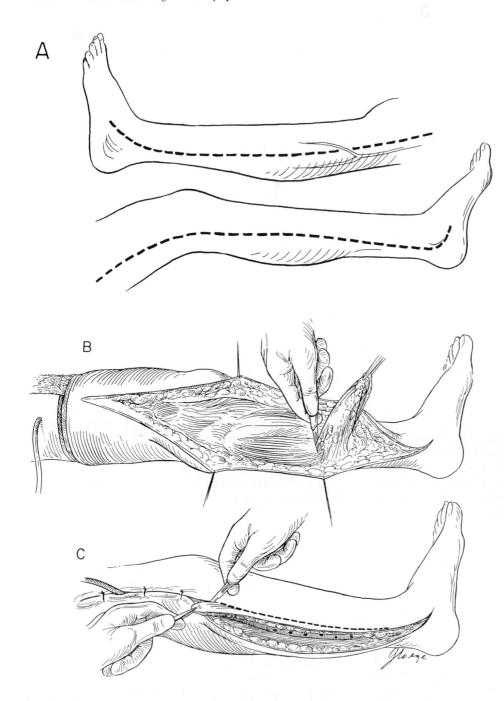

FIGURE 145–4.
Subcutaneous excision underneath flaps (modified Homans' procedure). *A*, The medial and lateral incisions are illustrated. *B*, Excision of the subcutaneous tissue on the medial aspect of the leg. *C*, Closure after excision of the redundant skin. (Reprinted with permission from Smith JW, Aston SJ [eds]: Grabb and Smith's Plastic Surgery. 4th ed. Boston, Little, Brown & Company, 1991.)

mately 1 cm posterior to the tibial border and extended proximally into the thigh (Fig. 145–4*A*). Flaps about 1.5-cm thick are elevated anteriorly and posteriorly to the midsagittal plane of the calf. The dissection is less extensive in the thigh and ankle. All subcutaneous tissue underneath the flap is removed. In both upper and lower extremities, more tissue is removed from the medial aspect than from the lateral. After the subcutaneous fat is excised from the periosteum of the tibia, the deep fascia is incised, permitting an easy plane of dissection to develop. The sural nerve is identified and preserved. All of the attached subcutaneous fat and deep fascia along the medial aspect of the calf are removed (Fig. 145–4*B*). The dissection is kept superficial to the deep fascia at the knee and ankle. Flaps in the ankle

are rarely longer than 6 cm. The redundant skin is excised after the subcutaneous fat has been removed. The tourniquet is deflated, and hemostasis is obtained. A suction catheter is placed in the dependent portion of the posterior flap and left in place for 5 days. Interrupted 4–0 nylon is employed for skin closure (Fig. 145–4*C*). No subcutaneous or dermal sutures are placed.

Postoperative Care

The extremity is immobilized with a posterior splint, gauze dressings are placed, and the leg is kept elevated. Sutures are usually removed on the 8th day. The patient is measured for an elastic compression stocking, and dependency of the leg is begun on the 9th day. Ambulation is started on the 11th postoperative day but only with the leg tightly wrapped. Postoperatively, elastic stockings must be used on a regular basis.

The second stage of the operation is performed on the lateral aspect of the limb 3 months later. The operation is essentially identical except that the deep fascia is not removed. Great care is taken to avoid damaging the common peroneal nerve.

Operation on the Arm

Surgical Technique

A medial incision is made from the distal ulna across the medial epicondyle of the humerus to the posterior medial upper arm. Flaps approximately 1-cm thick are elevated to the mid-sagittal aspect of the forearm, and the dissection is tapered distally and proximally (Fig. 145–5). The edematous subcutaneous tissue is removed, but the deep fascia is spared. The ulnar nerve is identified in the region of the medial epicondyle and preserved. The redundant skin is excised. The tourniquet is deflated, and hemostasis is obtained. (If necessary, the tourniquet can be removed, the area prepared, and the operation continued into the axilla.) A suction catheter is placed, and the skin is closed with 4–0 nylon suture. No subcutaneous or dermal sutures are placed.

Postoperative Care

The arm is immobilized and elevated for 5 days. The suction catheter can often be removed after the third day. Otherwise, postoperative management is similar to that described for the leg.

Results

Eighty-two lower extremity operations were performed by the authors' surgical team on 49 patients with chronic lymphedema. Sixty-five per cent of patients had a significant reduction in the size of the extremity. Of the remaining patients 10 per cent have experienced some improvement that has lasted through 2 years of follow-up. The remainder have returned to their postoperative levels of swelling or have continued to progress. Men have a worse prognosis than women, although the explanation for this is unclear. Only 3 postoperative complications related to ischemic necrosis of the flap have occurred. All have healed by secondary intention, and none has required further surgery. Although most patients experience some decreased sensation at the incision site, this has not been a source of complaint. None of these patients had inadvertent nerve injury, and no alteration in foot sensation has been observed. All patients have had some recurrence of swelling, and all must continue to wear support stockings. (The pre- and post-operative appearance of a patient who had the procedure is shown in Figure 145–6.)

The operative results for postmastectomy lymphedema have been more varied.[21] In patients with massive swelling, postoperative improvement is usually significant, and function is often restored (Fig. 145–7). In 10 of 14 patients, the postoperative arm volume was reduced by 250 to 1200 ml, and the reduced volume was maintained through the 6 years of the follow-up period. In the remaining 4 patients, arm swelling continued to progress despite the initial surgical reduction. One patient had a progressive increase in hand edema following surgery. Of the 4 patients with frequent recurrent cellulitis, 2 had a significant reduction in the frequency of infection. None of the patients experienced significant postoperative flap necrosis, and there was no inadvertent nerve injury.

CONCLUSIONS

The best indication for an excisional surgical procedure is functional impairment of the limb due to excessive lymphedema refractory to medical management. During the excisional procedures, a varying amount of skin and sub-

FIGURE 145–5.
Subcutaneous excision underneath flaps in the upper extremity. The flaps are elevated, and the subcutaneous tissue is excised. The ulnar nerve is identified and preserved.

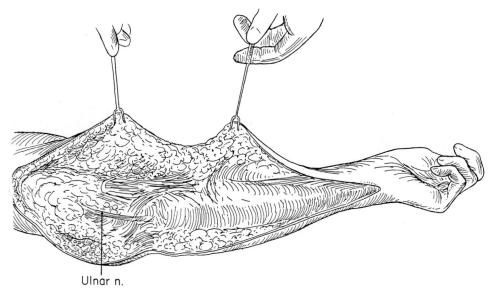

Ulnar n.

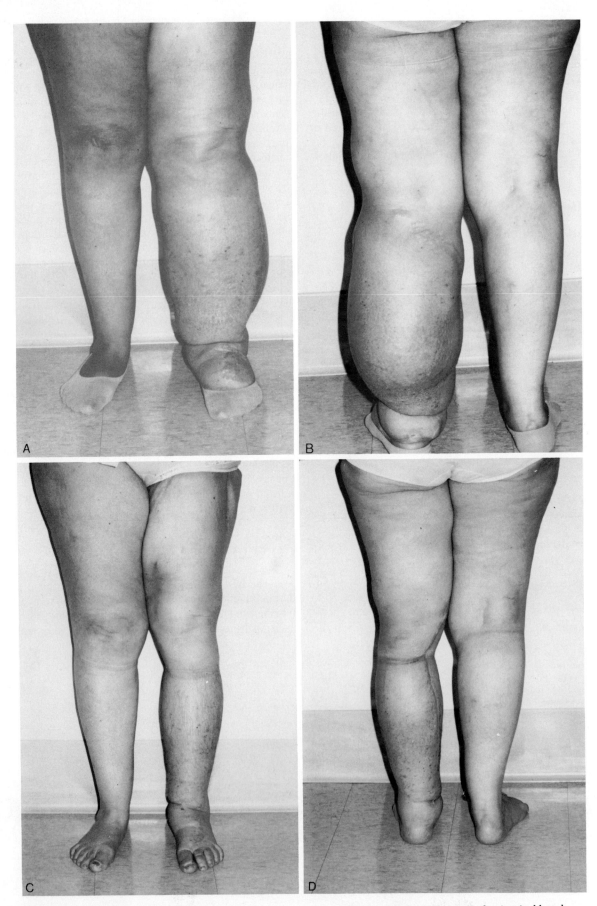

FIGURE 145–6. *A* and *B,* Legs of a 42-year-old woman with lymphedema of 18 years' duration after inguinal lymph node dissection. Two dermal flap procedures had been performed 5 years earlier. *C* and *D,* The patient's legs 1 year after lateral and medial subcutaneous excision underneath flaps. (Reprinted with permission from Smith JW, Aston SJ [eds]: Grabb and Smith's Plastic Surgery. 4th ed. Boston, Little, Brown & Company, 1991.)

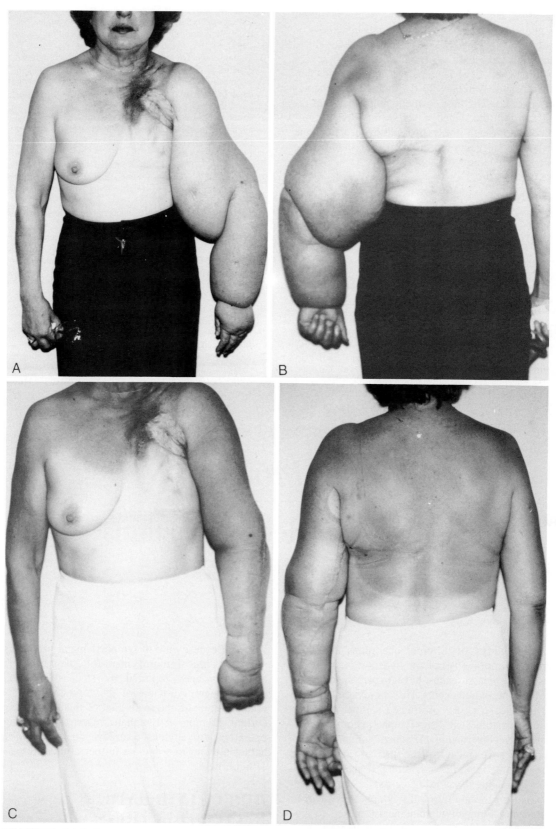

FIGURE 145–7. *A* and *B*, The arm of a 58-year-old woman 8 years after radical mastectomy. *C* and *D*, The patient's arm 1 year after medial and lateral subcutaneous excision underneath flaps. (Reprinted with permission from Smith JW, Aston SJ [eds]: Grabb and Smith's Plastic Surgery. 4th ed. Boston, Little, Brown & Company, 1991.)

cutaneous tissue is removed from the extremity. The Charles operation, which includes circumferential resection of all skin and subcutaneous tissue with split-thickness or full-thickness skin coverage, should be reserved for those few patients who have extreme lymphedema with severe skin changes. The benefit of Thompson's buried dermis flap operation is most likely related to the amount of subcutaneous tissue excised. The best cosmetic and functional result is achieved with the staged subcutaneous excision underneath flaps. Although these procedures decrease the volume of the extremity and improve function, they cannot cure chronic lymphedema.

References

1. Barsotti J, Gaisne E: Surgical treatment of lymphedema. J Mal Vasc 15:163, 1990.
2. Gloviczki P: Treatment of secondary lymphedema. *In* Ernst CB, Stanley JC (eds): Current Therapy in Vascular Surgery. 2nd ed. Philadelphia, BC Decker, 1991.
3. Thompson N, Wee JTK: Twenty years' experience of the buried dermis flap operation in the treatment of chronic lymphedema of the extremities. Chir Plast (Berl) 5:147, 1980.
4. Charles RH: Elephantiasis scroti. *In* Latham A (ed): A System of Treatment. Vol. 3. London, Churchill, 1912.
5. Taylor GW: Surgical management of primary lymphedema. Proc R Soc Med 58:1024, 1965.
6. Hoopes JE: Lymphedema of the extremity. *In* Cameron JL (ed): Current Surgical Therapy. Philadelphia, BC Decker, 1989, vol. 3, p 630.
7. McKee DM, Edgerton MT: The surgical treatment of lymphedema of the lower extremities. Plast Reconstr Surg 23:480, 1959.
8. Dellon AL, Hoopes JE: The Charles procedure for primary lymphedema. Plast Reconstr Surg 60:589, 1977.
9. Thompson N: Surgical treatment of chronic lymphedema of the lower limb. With preliminary report of new operation. Br Med J 2:1566, 1962.
10. Thompson N: The surgical treatment of chronic lymphoedema of the extremities. Surg Clin North Am 47:445, 1967.
11. Thompson N: Surgical treatment of primary and secondary lymphedema of the extremities by lymphatic transposition. Proc R Soc Med 58:1026, 1965.
12. Amar R, Rosello R, Meline F, Bureau H: L'utilisation de la serum albumine humaine marquee a l'iode-131 pour l'exploration des lymphoedemes chirurgicaux des membres. Etude preliminaire. Ann Chir Plast 21:49, 1976.
13. Harvey RF: The use of ^{131}I-labeled human serum albumin in the assessment of improved lymph flow following buried dermis flap operation in cases of post-mastectomy lymphedema of the arm. Br J Radiol 42:260, 1969.
14. Kinmonth JB: Primary lymphoedema of the lower limb: Response to discussion. Proc R Soc Med 58:1031, 1965.
15. Miller T, Harper J, Longmire WP: The management of lymphedema by staged subcutaneous excision. Surg Gynecol Obstet 136:586, 1973.
16. Sistrunk WE: Further experiences with the Kondoleon operation for elephantiasis. JAMA 71:800, 1918.
17. Homans J: The treatment of elephantiasis of the legs. N Engl J Med 215:1099, 1936.
18. Homans J: The treatment of elephantiasis of the legs: A preliminary report. N Engl J Med 215:1099, 1936.
19. Miller TA: Surgical management of lymphedema of the extremity. Plast Reconstr Surg 56:633, 1975.
20. Fonkalsrud EW, Coulson WF: Management of congenital lymphedema in infants and children. Ann Surg 177:280, 1973.
21. Miller TA: Surgical approach to lymphedema of the arm after mastectomy. Am J Surg 148:152, 1984.

146

Lymphatic Reconstructions

Peter Gloviczki, M.D.

• • •

The large number of different operations that have been proposed to improve lymphatic transport is testimony to the frustration that surgeons have experienced in the treatment of chronic lymphedema. Direct operations on the lymphatics to reconstruct the obstructed pathways include lymphovenous anastomoses[1-12] and lymphatic grafting.[13] Indirect lymphatic reconstructions designed to improve lymphatic drainage have included the use of an omental flap,[14, 15] the mesenteric bridge operation,[16, 17] and autotransplantation of lymphatic tissue as a free flap.[18] These procedures are based on the ability of the lymphatic system to form spontaneous lympholymphatic anastomoses to improve collateral lymphatic drainage to the mesentery or to regions of the body where lymphatic drainage is normal. Although some of these operations have been performed for several decades, the long-term effectiveness of none of them has been proved, and their use continues to be contro-

versial. Because cure of lymphedema at present is not possible and clinical improvement following each of the operations has been reported by at least one experienced surgical team, a review of these procedures is still warranted. Although the main goal of this chapter is to update current attempts at lymphatic reconstructions and discuss operations for chylous disorders, no less important is the author's intent to stimulate further clinical research in this difficult field.

DIRECT LYMPHATIC RECONSTRUCTIONS

Lymphovenous Anastomoses

Surgical lymphovenous anastomoses intended to bypass the obstructed lymphatic system in patients with

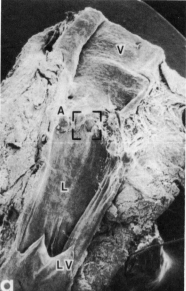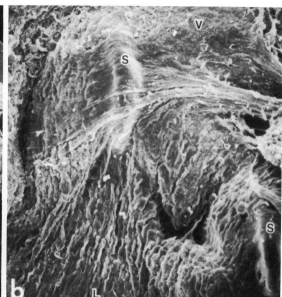

FIGURE 146–1. *a* and *b*, Scanning electron micrographs of patent lymphovenous anastomosis 4 weeks after operation in a dog. Endothelial cells cover suture line. A, anastomosis; L, lymph vessel; LV, lymphatic valve; S, suture; V, vein. (*a*, Original magnification, ×10; *b*, original magnification, ×200.) (*a* and *b*, From Gloviczki P, Hollier LH, Nora FE, Kaye MP: The natural history of microsurgical lymphovenous anastomoses: An experimental study. J Vasc Surg 4:148, 1986.)

chronic lymphedema have been performed in the last 3 decades.[1–12] The rationale for the operation is based on the observation that in patients with chronic lymphedema contrast lymphangiography occasionally demonstrates spontaneous lymphovenous anastomoses.[19] These are considered compensatory mechanisms of the body to decrease the lymphatic hypertension that occurs early in the course of the disease.

Nielubowicz and Olszewski suggested anastomosing the inguinal lymph nodes to the femoral or greater saphenous vein.[20] Although improvement in patients with lymph node–vein anastomoses has been reported,[3, 20, 21] enthusiasm for this operation faded because early occlusion due to thrombosis and fibrosis over the cut surface of the node is likely.[22]

The development of microvascular surgery and the availability of fine instruments and suture materials enabled microsurgeons to develop techniques to anastomose blood vessels less than 2 mm in diameter with excellent patency. Successful direct anastomoses between lymph vessels and veins were reported in experiments as early as 1962 by Jacobson,[23] and soon afterward by Laine and Howard.[24] Subsequent experiments from several groups documented a 50 to 70 per cent patency rate several months following surgery.[25–28] The author's group performed end-to-end anastomoses between normal femoral lymph vessels and a tributary of the femoral vein in dogs and noted a 50 per cent patency rate up to 8 months after the operation.[28] The anastomoses were done with 11–0 monofilament nonabsorbable interrupted sutures with the help of an operating microscope using high-power magnification. Cinelymphangiography and scanning electron microscopy were used to document patency (Figs. 146–1 and 146–2). Most anastomoses that occluded were performed at the beginning of the experiments, suggesting the importance of technical expertise in performing these operations. It should be noted, however, that Puckett and colleagues failed to confirm the patency of lymphovenous anastomoses 3 weeks after surgery in an experimental model of chronic lymphedema.[29]

Indication

Patients with secondary lymphedema of recent onset without previous episodes of cellulitis or lymphangitis are potential candidates for surgical treatment unless they can be managed easily with conservative measures. In the late stage of lymphedema, fibrosis and valvular incompetence of the main lymph vessels develop, the intrinsic contractil-

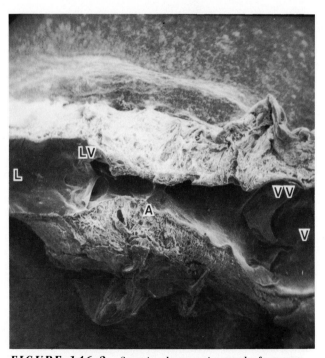

FIGURE 146–2. Scanning electron micrograph of a patent lymphovenous anastomosis 3 months after operation in a dog. A, anastomosis; L, lymph vessel; LV, lymphatic valve; V, vein; VV, venous valve. (Original magnification, ×10). (From Gloviczki P, Hollier LH, Nora FE, Kaye MP: The natural history of microsurgical lymphovenous anastomoses: An experimental study. J Vasc Surg 4:148, 1986.)

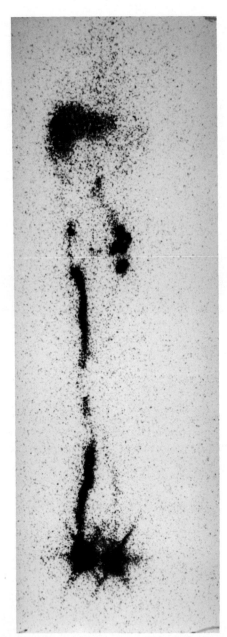

FIGURE 146–3. Bilateral lower extremity lymphoscintigraphy in a patient with right lower extremity lymphedema secondary to obstruction of the right iliac nodes. Note dilated lymph vessels in the right thigh distal to the obstruction suitable for direct lymphatic reconstruction.

ity of the vessel wall is lost, and interstitial pressure decreases owing to secondary changes in the subcutaneous tissue (see Chapter 142). The chances of success with lymphovenous anastomoses in such limbs are clearly diminished. Because venous hypertension impedes forward flow through the anastomoses, patients with chronic venous insufficiency are not candidates for this operation.

Preoperative Evaluation

Isotope lymphoscintigraphy is usually sufficient for preoperative imaging of the lymphatic system. In ideal candidates, it confirms the presence of dilated infrainguinal

lymph vessels with proximal pelvic lymphatic obstruction (Fig. 146–3). In selected patients, however, direct contrast lymphangiography can be performed to show the fine details of the lymphatics. Other preoperative tests include noninvasive venous studies and duplex scanning of the deep veins. Computed tomography is done in most patients to exclude any underlying mass or malignant tumor. Once surgery has been decided on, the patients are hospitalized for 28 to 48 hours to elevate the extremity in a lymphedema sling and to allow use of intermittent compression treatment with a pump to decrease the volume of the extremity.

Surgical Technique

Because the operation lasts many hours, general anesthesia is preferred. For lower extremity lymphedema, a transverse incision at the mid-thigh or a longitudinal incision close to the saphenofemoral junction is performed to allow dissection of the lymphatics of the superficial medial bundle (Fig. 146–4). The greater saphenous vein and any

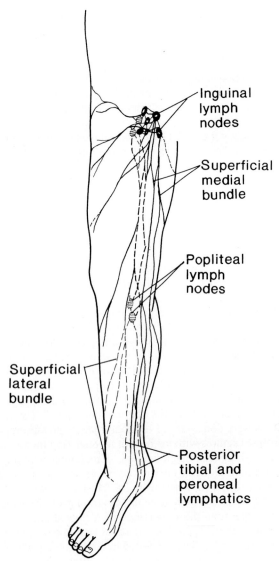

FIGURE 146–4. The lymphatic system of the lower extremity. (By permission of Mayo Foundation.)

tributary are also dissected. An attempt is made to visualize the lymph vessels with 5 ml of isosulfan blue (Lymphazurin) dye injected subcutaneously; half of this amount is directed toward the first interdigital space and half toward the area 10 to 15 cm distal to the site of incision. Because of lymphatic obstruction, however, lymph flow even in patent lymphatics may be minimal, and the dye is usually not visible during dissection. With experience, however, the whitish fluid-filled lymphatics, frequently with vascularized adventitia, can be distinguished from small subcutaneous nerves or fibrotic bands. If contrast lymphangiography is done within 24 hours of the operation, the contrast-filled lymphatics are easily identifiable and can be located during the operation using an image intensifier and a C-arm (Fig. 146–5*A*). Contrast lymphangiography in some patients helps to avoid many hours of unsuccessful searching for patent lymphatics at the groin. Once the lymphatic vessels

and the veins are isolated, a standard microsurgical technique is used to perform end-to-end anastomosis, using six to eight interrupted 11–0 monofilament sutures (Fig. 146–5*B–D*). The operation is performed using a Zeiss operating microscope with 4 to 40 times magnification.

For arm lymphedema, the lymphatics are dissected either through a transverse incision at the wrist or in the mid-cubital fossa or through a longitudinal incision at the medial aspect of the arm, a few centimeters proximal to the elbow. The lymphatics of the superficial medial lymphatic bundle are usually used for anastomoses (Fig. 146–6), which are performed with the mid-cubital, basilic, or brachial veins or their tributaries in an end-to-side or end-to-end fashion.

Postoperatively, the limb is wrapped with elastic bandage and elevated at 30 degrees using two pillows for the arm or elevating the foot of the bed for the lower extremity.

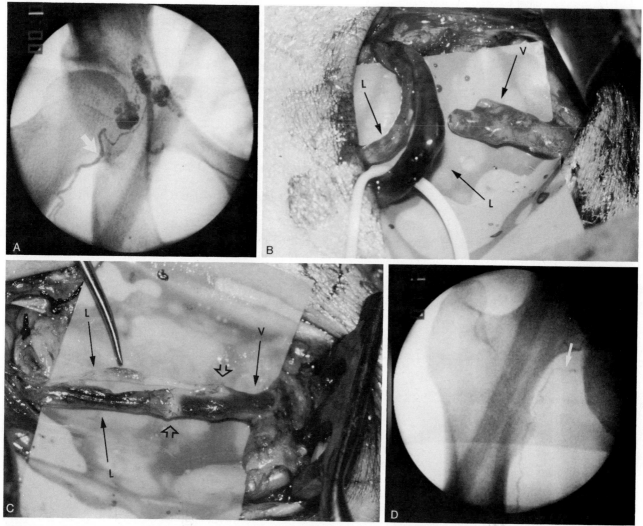

FIGURE 146–5. *A*, Localization of groin lymphatics before lymphovenous anastomosis operation. The patient underwent contrast lymphangiography 24 hours before operation. *Arrow* indicates the lymphatics selected for anastomosis. *B*, Two dilated lymphatics (L) and a tributary of the saphenous vein with a small side branch (V) were dissected for end-to-end lymphovenous anastomosis. *C*, End-to-end lymphovenous anastomosis completed between two lymph channels (L) and the bifurcated vein (V). *Open arrows* indicate the sites of the anastomoses. *D*, *Arrow* indicates patent lymphovenous anastomosis in the same patient. (*B* and *C*, From Gloviczki P: Treatment of secondary lymphedema—medical and surgical. *In* Ernst CB, Stanley JC [eds]: Current Therapy in Vascular Surgery. 2nd ed. Philadelphia, BC Decker, 1991, pp 1030–1036.)

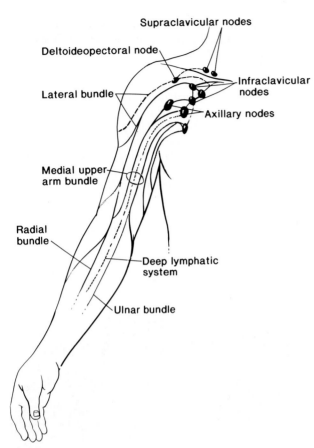

FIGURE 146–6. The lymphatic system of the upper extremity. (By permission of Mayo Foundation.)

Results

Objective evaluation of the long-term effectiveness of lymphovenous anastomoses in patients has been difficult (Table 146–1). Decrease in circumference or volume of the extremity, patient satisfaction, decrease in episodes of cellulitis, and improvement in lymphatic clearance as measured by lymphoscintigraphy have been used as the criteria

of success. In a review of 14 patients who underwent lymphovenous anastomosis in the author's institution, however, only 5 limbs were still improved at a mean follow-up time of 46 months after surgery.[10] Improvement was observed in 4 of 7 patients with secondary lymphedema but in only 1 of 8 patients with primary lymphedema. Improvement in lymphatic clearance from the injection site is the only indirect sign of patency of the shunts. Therefore, the author's group was not able to provide objective evidence of late patency of the lymphovenous anastomoses in these patients.

The largest experience with lymphovenous shunts has been reported in Australia. O'Brien and colleagues published a well-documented report with long-term follow-up on 90 patients who underwent lymphovenous anastomosis for chronic lymphedema.[12] Although a significant number of patients underwent additional excisional operation, improvement was documented even in patients who underwent only lymphovenous anastomoses: Of these patients, 73 per cent had subjective improvement, and 42 per cent had objective long-term improvement. Seventy-four per cent of all patients discontinued the use of elastic stockings. Because direct contrast lymphangiography occasionally has resulted in progression of lymphedema due to chemical lymphangitis or accumulation of the contrast material in the lymph nodes due to poor lymphatic transport, this test was not used to document late patency of the anastomoses. Therefore, objective evidence that the improvement in these patients was due to patent and functioning lymphovenous anastomoses is still lacking.

Lymphatic Grafting

Baumeister introduced lymphatic grafting for upper extremity and unilateral lower extremity secondary lymphedema.[13, 30–34] Because lymph is devoid of platelets and coagulates less than blood, the chances of patency in successful lympholymphatic anastomoses appear to be better than those in lymphovenous anastomoses. Also, an elevated venous pressure, which may at least intermittently interrupt flow through lymphovenous anastomoses, is not a factor in

Table 146–1. Clinical Results of Microsurgical Lymphatic Reconstruction

| Study | No. Patients | Extremity | | Type of Operation | Follow-up (mo) | Results: Excellent or Good (%) |
		Upper	Lower			
Krylov et al, 1982	50	+		LVA	?	30
Nieuborg, 1982	47	+		LVA	6–12	68
Gong-Kang et al, 1985	91		+	LVA	24*	79
Zhu et al, 1987	48		+	LVA	6–52	33
	185		+	LVA	6–52	73
Gloviczki et al, 1988	6	+		LVA	36.6*	50
	8		+	LVA		25
O'Brien et al, 1990	46	+		LVA		54
	30		+	LVA	51*	83
	6†	+		LVA		33
	8†		+	LVA		50
Baumeister et al, 1990	36	+		LG	>12	33
	12		+	LG	>24	8

*Mean.
†Lymphovenous anastomosis plus excisional procedure.
LVA, Lymphovenous anastomoses; LG, lymphatic grafting.

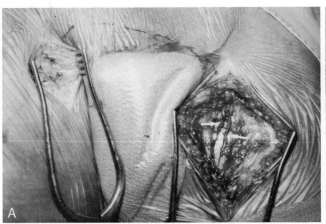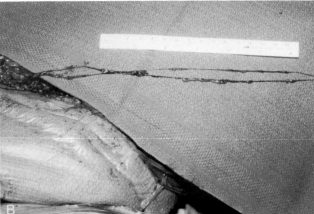

FIGURE 146–7.   *A*, Exposure of lymph vessels for suprapubic transposition. Note two major lymph vessels of the left thigh that will be used for grafting *(arrows)*. *B*, Two lymphatic grafts divided at the distal thigh are prepared for lymphatic grafting. (By permission of Mayo Foundation.)

this procedure. In his experiments, Baumeister achieved 100 per cent short- to medium-term patency of lymphatic interposition grafts.[30] Indisputably, this operation requires special microsurgical expertise.

Preoperative Evaluation

Preoperative evaluation is similar to that needed for patients who undergo lymphovenous anastomoses. It is important to image the donor leg lymphatics with lymphoscintigraphy because a normal lymphatic system is a prerequisite for the use of lymph vessels from the leg for grafting. In Baumeister's experience, which now amounts to 95 patients, postoperative leg swelling occurred in only one limb due to post-thrombotic venous disease.[34] Patients with bilateral leg edema are not candidates for this procedure.

Surgical Technique

The operation on the lower extremity is very similar to a suprapubic saphenous vein graft, as performed by Palma for unilateral iliac vein obstruction (see Chapter 140). As in lymphovenous anastomoses, the superficial thigh lymphatics in the edematous limb are dissected first through a longitudinal incision, made just distal to the saphenofemoral junction. Five ml of isosulfan blue (Lymphazurin) dye are injected subcutaneously into the first interdigital space of the normal foot, and the thigh lymphatics are exposed through a 25- to 30-cm incision along the greater saphenous vein using loupe magnification (Fig. 146–7). Two or three lymphatics are selected for grafting. They are transected distally after double ligation and tunneled subcutaneously above the pubis to the contralateral side, where end-to-end lympholymphatic anastomoses are performed under the operating microscope using 11–0 or 12–0 interrupted sutures (Fig. 146–8).

For postmastectomy lymphedema, the two or three lymphatics from the leg are harvested and used as free interposition grafts. They are placed in a subcutaneous tunnel from the upper medial arm to the neck and then sutured end-to-end first to the superficial medial bundle lymphatics in the arm, and then to the descending neck lymphatics in

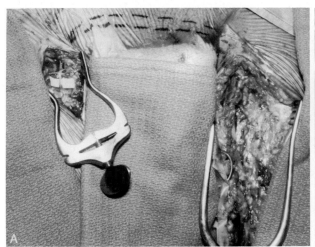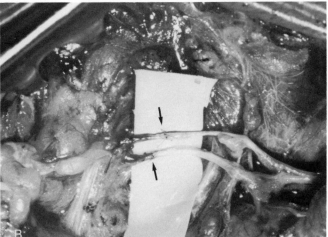

FIGURE 146–8.   *A*, Completed suprapubic lymph grafting with two lympholymphatic anastomoses at right groin. *Broken line* indicates position of suprapubic lymphatic grafts. *B*, Magnified photograph of two end-to-end lympholymphatic anastomoses *(arrows)* performed with 11–0 interrupted monofilament sutures. (By permission of Mayo Foundation.)

the supraclavicular fossa. Postoperative care for these patients is similar to that given to patients with lymphovenous anastomoses.

Results

In a report evaluating 55 patients undergoing this operation with a follow-up of more than 3 years, Baumeister and his associates documented a decrease in the volume of the extremity in 80 per cent of the patients.[13] Volume measurements showed significant improvement in 36 patients with arm lymphedema, and in 16 more than 2 years after surgery. Significant improvement was documented in 8 of 12 patients with lower extremity lymphedema more than 1 year after suprapubic grafting. Thirty patients were studied by lymphoscintigraphy. Using a semi-quantitative assessment with the help of a lymphatic transport index, some improvement in lymphatic clearance could be demonstrated in all patients. Although several grafts were imaged by lymphoscintigraphy, the patency rate of the implanted lymphatic grafts was not reported! Significant experience with this operation has not been gained by other surgical teams. In two of the patients operated on by the author's group using this technique, lymphoscintigraphy suggested graft patency (Fig. 146–9). This result, however, was associated with significant early reduction of the swelling in only one patient, in whom edema recurred at 2 years despite an apparently patent and functioning graft.

Conclusions

Meticulous microsurgical technique, fine instruments, and high-power magnification using the operating microscope now enable microsurgeons to perform anastomoses between lymph vessels or between a lymph vessel and a vein with good immediate success. Although long-term improvement in patients has been reported, these results remain to be confirmed by different surgical teams and then compared with results obtained in patients treated by conservative measures. Because lymph coagulates significantly less than blood, lympholymphatic anastomoses with lymphatic grafts have a potential advantage over lymphovenous anastomoses, in which thrombosis on the venous side may occur. However, the long-term patency and function of

these anastomoses in patients are still unknown. More important, the main questions remain unanswered: Does restoring the patency of two or three lymph channels result in restoration of normal lymphatic transport? Does lymphovenous anastomosis or lymphatic grafting reverse changes that have already occurred in the distal lymphatic circulation, the subcutaneous tissue, or the skin of patients with chronic lymphedema? Until these important questions are answered, patients should be made aware of the unproven benefit of this type of treatment.

INDIRECT LYMPHATIC RECONSTRUCTIONS

Mesenteric Bridge Operation

Patients with fibrotic occlusion or surgical excision of the iliac nodes may be candidates for the mesenteric bridge operation. Designed by Kinmonth and colleagues,[16] this procedure includes isolation of a segment of the ileum without division or ligation of its blood supply or lymphatic circulation (Fig. 146–10). The ileum is opened longitudinally, its mucosa is removed, and the bowel wall is sewn over the transected distal iliac or inguinal nodes. The continuity of the small bowel is reestablished by end-to-end ileostomy.

Hurst and colleagues reported the late results in eight patients who underwent enteromesenteric bridge operation for ilioinguinal lymph node obliteration.[17] Significant reduction in the volume of the swollen extremity and a decrease in discomfort was noted in five of the eight patients at a follow-up that extended more than 5 years. Lymphangiographic evidence of communications between the inguinal nodes and the mesenteric lymphatic circulation was obtained in five patients. Five of eight patients also had normal lymphatic clearance with lymphoscintigraphy 5 years after the operation, as reported later by Browse.[35] Unfortunately, patients with proximal lymphatic obstruction and intact inguinal or external iliac lymph nodes are rare. As Wolfe emphasized, the lymphatic obstruction for this procedure must be quite proximal for the pedicle to reach beyond it without tension.[36] In addition, patients who have obstruction proximal to the mesenteric vessels and those with hyperplasia are not candidates for this operation.

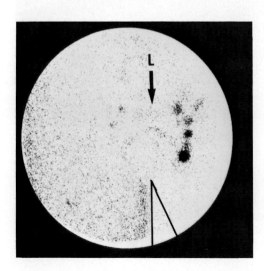

FIGURE 146–9. Lymphoscintigram 3 months after suprapubic lymphatic grafting for secondary lymphedema of the right lower extremity. Labeled colloid was injected into the right foot only. *Arrow* indicates suprapubic graft. Note intense filling of the left inguinal nodes. Preoperative lymphoscintigram in this patient showed no activity at the groin. L, lymphatic graft. (From Gloviczki P: Treatment of secondary lymphedema—medical and surgical. *In* Ernst CB, Stanley JC [eds]: Current Therapy in Vascular Surgery. 2nd ed. Philadelphia, BC Decker, 1991, pp 1030–1036.)

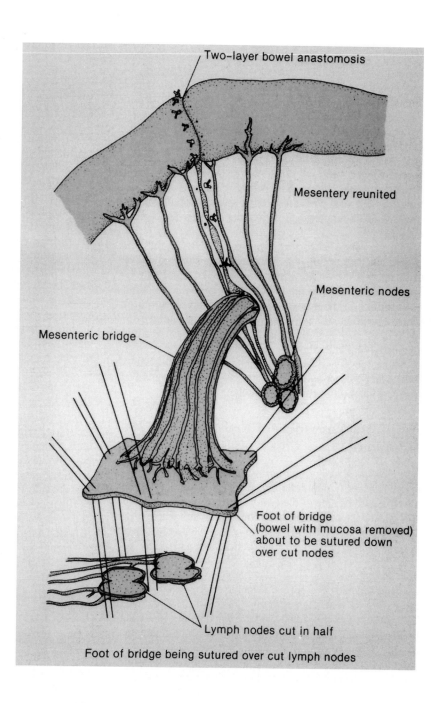

Two-layer bowel anastomosis

Mesentery reunited

Mesenteric nodes

Mesenteric bridge

Foot of bridge
(bowel with mucosa removed)
about to be sutured down
over cut nodes

Lymph nodes cut in half

Foot of bridge being sutured over cut lymph nodes

FIGURE 146–10.   Technique of mesenteric bridge operation.

Omental Flap

Goldsmith and associates suggested the use of an omental flap to improve lymphatic drainage of the swollen limb through spontaneous lympholymphatic anastomoses, which supposedly develop between patent lymphatics in the limb and the lymphatics of the greater omentum.[14] Using patent blue dye they documented passage of the dye, injected in the leg, to the omentum 1 month after surgery. In the experiments of Danese and associates, however, contrast lymphangiography failed to demonstrate similar communications 3 months after surgery.[37] At exploration the pedicles were found to have developed a fibrous capsule around them that prevented any communication between the leg lymphatics and the omentum.

In a follow-up study that extended up to 7 years and included 22 patients, Goldsmith admitted that poor results occurred in one third of his patients.[15] More important, he reported significant complications in 8 patients, including wound infection, bowel obstruction, pulmonary embolization, and hernia. For these reasons, this operation has largely been abandoned as a treatment option for lymphedema.

In the more recent experiments of O'Brian and associates, however, canine lymphedema was successfully decreased by the use of a vascularized free omental flap.[38, 39] Blue dye injected into the leg 6 months after surgery could be identified in the dilated lymphatics of the omentum implanted to bridge the lymphatic defect in the lower extremity in dogs. Although the ability of the omentum to provide adequate lymphatic drainage continues to be a controversial question, the easy availability of the omentum as a vascularized flap and at least some success in experiments warrant continuation of further research.

Autotransplantation of Free Lymphatic Flap

Trevidic and Cormier performed autotransplantation of a free axillary lymph node flap from the contralateral axillary fossa to the side of the lymphedematous arm in patients with postmastectomy lymphedema.[18] The inferior axillary nodes were removed with a vascularized flap, comprising a portion of the latissimus dorsi muscle with a segment of skin. The blood supply to the flap consisted of the subscapular artery and vein. This lymphatic tissue flap was then transplanted into the supraclavicular fossa, where anastomoses were created with the subclavian artery and vein. The authors reported results in 19 patients who underwent axillary lymph node transplantation. The graft failed in 1 patient. Improvement was documented in 75 per cent of patients, and direct contrast lymphography demonstrated the development of new lympholymphatic anastomoses in some patients. Lymphoscintigraphy showed improved lymphatic transport in 75 per cent of the patients. Further experience and longer follow-up with this operation are still needed to assess its efficacy.

Conclusions

Because of the paucity of lymphatics in the omentum and the reported complications, the author's group does not recommend omentoplasty for the treatment of lymphedema. The complexity of the mesenteric bridge operation, its possible complications, and the small number of suitable patients limit wide acceptance of this procedure as well. The most promising operation among indirect reconstructions of the lymphatic drainage is autotransplantation of a free vascularized lymphatic flap. The rich lymphatic tissue in the axillary flap provides the best opportunity for the spontaneous development of lympholymphatic anastomoses. Further research with this operation, therefore, is clearly warranted.

OPERATIONS FOR PRIMARY CHYLOUS DISORDERS

Chylous disorders are characterized by an accumulation of chyle in abnormal areas of the body. Chylous ascites, chylothorax, or chylocutaneous fistula may be caused by malignant tumors, most frequently lymphoma, or by trauma to the mesenteric lymphatics or the thoracic duct, which may also occur during vascular surgical procedures as discussed in detail in Chapter 40.

Primary chylous disorders are usually caused by congenital lymphangiectasia or megalymphatics, which in some patients are associated with obstruction of the thoracic duct. In patients with lymphangiectasia and lymphatic valvular incompetence, chyle may reflux into the lower extremities, the perineum, or the genitalia.[40–44] Depending on the site of the dilated lymphatics and the site of the chylous leak, these patients may also have protein-losing enteropathy, chylous ascites, chylothorax, chylopericardium, or reflux of chyle into the lungs and tracheobronchial tree.[40–46] Medical treatment is aimed at decreasing production of chyle by means of a medium-chain triglyceride diet or occasionally by parenteral nutrition (see Chapter 40). Repletion of proteins and calcium lost with chyle is as important as the need to strengthen the defense mechanism of the body because lymphocytes and important immunoglobulins are also wasted in these patients. Only surgical treatment can provide long-term improvement and occasionally cure by ligating the incompetent retroperitoneal lymph vessels and oversewing the site of the lymphatic leak. In some patients attempts to reconstruct the obstructed thoracic duct by creating thoracic duct–azygos vein anastomoses have also been reported.

Chylous Reflux Into the Lower Extremity or Genitalia

Although many patients with lymphangiectasia and reflux of chyle have lower extremity lymphedema that is unilateral in most cases, the main discomfort for the patients is intermittent or continuous discharge of chyle from cutaneous vesicles in the lower extremity or in the genitalia. The first five patients who suffered from this rare condition were described in 1949 by Servelle and Deysson.[47]

Preoperative evaluation of these patients should include lymphoscintigraphy (Fig. 146–11A).[48] Contrast lymphangiography, however, is the definitive test for confirming the diagnosis and localizing the dilated retroperitoneal lymphatics and frequently also the site of the lymphatic

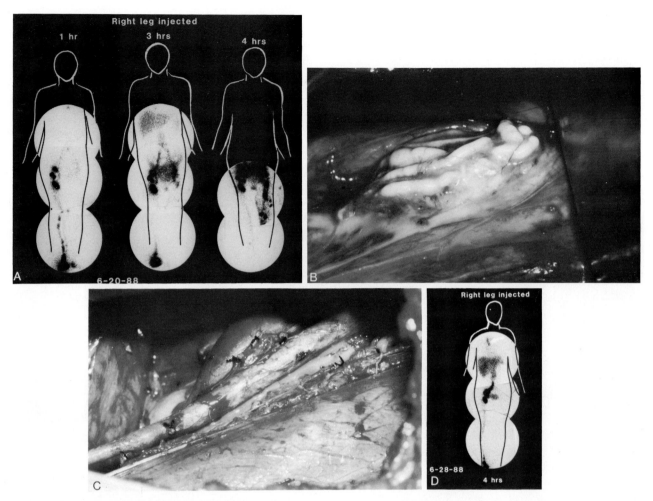

FIGURE 146–11. *A,* Right lower extremity lymphoscintigraphy in a 16-year-old female with lymphangiectasia and severe reflux into the genitalia and left lower extremity. Injection of the isotope into the right foot reveals reflux into the pelvis at 3 hours and into the left lower extremity at 4 hours. *B,* Intraoperative photograph reveals dilated incompetent retroperitoneal lymphatics in the left iliac fossa containing chyle. *C,* Radical excision and ligation of the lymph vessels were performed. In addition, two lymphovenous anastomoses were also performed between two dilated lymphatics and two lumbar veins. *D,* Postoperative lymphoscintigram performed in a similar fashion reveals no evidence of reflux at 4 hours. The patient has no significant reflux 4 years after surgery. (*A–D,* From Gloviczki P, et al: Noninvasive evaluation of the swollen extremity: Experiences with 190 lymphoscintigraphic examinations. J Vasc Surg 9:683, 1989.)

leak. Radical excision and ligation of the incompetent retroperitoneal lymph vessels is the only effective technique for controlling reflux of the chyle and its drainage through skin vesicles in the perineum, labia, scrotum, or lower extremity. The author's group uses the technique of Servelle[41] and performs the entire reflux operation in two stages through flank incisions using the retroperitoneal approach. The patient ingests 40 gm of butter melted in milk or cream 4 hours before the procedure. The fatty meal allows ready visualization of the retroperitoneal lymphatics during exploration (Fig. 146–11*B–D*). Ligation of the lymph vessels should be done with the utmost care to avoid tearing or avulsing the lymphatics, resulting in residual leaks or rupture. Lymphovenous anastomoses with the dilated lymphatics can also be performed.[45, 49]

Results

The largest experience has been reported by Servelle, who operated on 55 patients with this condition and reported durable benefit in most patients.[41] In a series of 19 patients who underwent ligation of the retroperitoneal lymphatics for chylous reflux to the limbs and genitalia by Kinmonth, permanent cure was achieved in 5 patients and alleviation of symptoms, frequently after several operations, in 12 patients.[40] No improvement or failure was noted in only 2 cases.

Chylous Ascites

Chylous ascites usually results from intraperitoneal rupture of the mesenteric or retroperitoneal lymphatics or from exudation of the chyle into the peritoneal cavity.[44] Evaluation of these patients should include computed tomography or magnetic resonance imaging to exclude abdominal malignancy. The diagnosis of lymphangiectasia is, however, confirmed by bipedal contrast lymphangiography. Paracentesis is both diagnostic and therapeutic. If conservative measures fail and ascites returns, abdominal exploration should be performed after a fatty meal as described previously. If chylous ascites is due to primary lymphan-

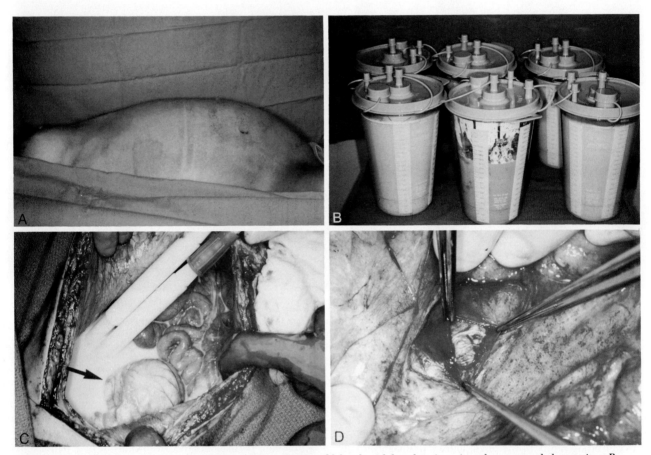

FIGURE 146–12.   *A*, Preoperative photograph of an 18-year-old female with lymphangiectasia and recurrent chylous ascites. *B*, During the operation, 12 liters of chyle were aspirated from the abdomen. *C*, The chylous ascites was caused by ruptured lymphatic and leaking large mesenteric lymphatic cysts *(arrow)*. *D*, The dilated retroperitoneal lymphatics containing chyle were ligated and excised. The patient has an excellent clinical result 8 months after the operation.

giectasia, abdominal exploration may reveal ruptured lymphatics, which can be oversewn. In some patients, large chylous cysts develop, which should be excised (Fig. 146–12). If the condition is associated with protein-losing enteropathy and the disease is localized to a segment of the small bowel, the bowel segment should be resected.

The outcome of the operation is usually good if a well-defined abdominal fistula is found. However, if the mesenteric lymphatic trunks are fibrosed, aplastic, or hypoplastic, and exudation of the chyle is the main source of the ascites, the prognosis is poor, and recurrence is frequent. In these patients, an attempt to control the ascites using a LeVeen peritoneal-venous shunt should be made. Results with peritoneal-venous shunts, however, have been mixed. It is noteworthy that in Browse's experience with nine peritoneal-venous shunts all became occluded within 3 to 6 months after insertion.[44]

Chylothorax

As with chylous ascites, the most frequent cause of chylothorax is trauma or malignant disease.[40] Primary lymphatic disorders causing chylothorax include lymphangiectasia with or without thoracic duct obstruction. However, chylothorax may also result from chylous ascites passing through the diaphragm. In these patients, the chylothorax is cured when the chylous ascites is controlled. Preoperative lymphangiography in these patients should be performed because it may localize the site of the chylous fistula or document occlusion of the thoracic duct (Fig. 146–13). Thoracentesis is usually not effective in curing the disease, and chyle that leaks from the thoracic duct or one of the large intercostal, mediastinal, or diaphragmatic collaterals reaccumulates. Injection of tetracycline is frequently ineffective because it is diluted by the leaking chyle. The best treatment for chylothorax is surgical pleurodesis with excision of the parietal pleura and prolonged pleural suction.[47] During thoracotomy, which is performed after a fatty meal, a careful search for the leaking lymphatics should be undertaken, and the site of the leak should be oversewn.

Thoracic Duct Reconstruction

If occlusion of the cervical or upper thoracic duct (Fig. 146–14) is the cause of lymphangiectasia and reflux of chyle into the pleural or peritoneal cavity, thoracic duct–azygos vein anastomosis can be attempted to reconstruct the duct and improve lymphatic transport. Preoperative imaging of the duct with contrast pedal lymphangiography is important because if occlusion of the entire duct is present it precludes anastomoses.

The operation is performed through a right posterolateral thoracotomy, and the anastomosis between the lower thoracic duct and the azygos vein is performed in an end-to-end fashion, with 8–0 or 10–0 nonabsorbable interrupted sutures and magnification using loupe or the operating mi-

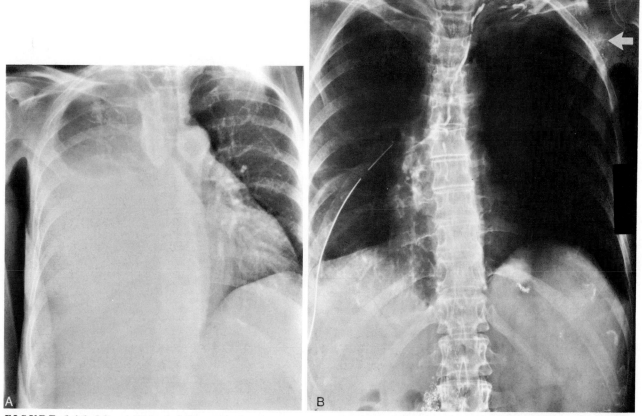

FIGURE 146–13. *A*, Right chylothorax in a 63-year-old woman. *B*, Bipedal lymphangiography confirmed thoracic duct obstruction at the base of the neck. Note contrast in the supraclavicular and left axillary lymphatics *(arrows)*.

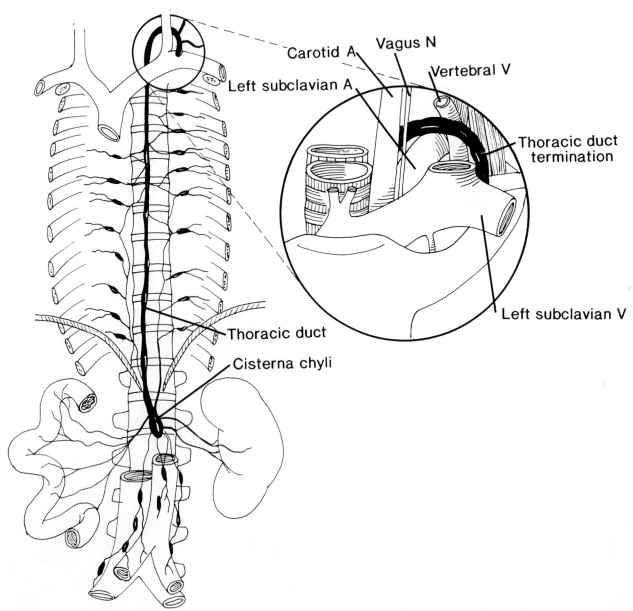

FIGURE 146–14. *A* and *B*, Cervical and thoracoabdominal anatomy of the thoracic duct.

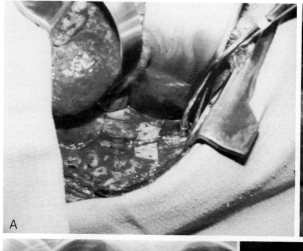

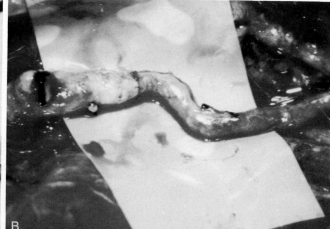

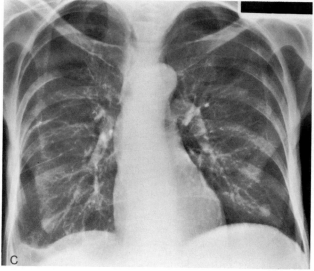

FIGURE 146–15. *A* and *B*, Thoracic duct–azygos vein anastomosis performed through a right posterolateral thoracotomy in an end-to-end fashion with interrupted 8–0 Prolene sutures. *C*, Chest roentgenogram 2 years later confirms absence of chylothorax.

croscope. Only a few patients with this operation have been reported.[40, 48] Both patients that the author's group operated on had good immediate patency, and excellent flow of chyle was observed through the anastomosis intraoperatively (Fig. 146–15). Although none had postoperative contrast lymphangiography, the recurrent chylothorax that was the main indication for the procedure ultimately resolved in both. Browse reported two successes in three patients who underwent thoracic duct reconstruction.[48] However, Kinmonth performed this procedure in two patients and concluded that the anastomosis alone is not effective for decompressing the thoracic duct; ligation of the abnormal mediastinal lymphatics and oversewing of the sites of the lymphatic leak are also necessary.[40]

Conclusions

Primary chylous disorders are fortunately rare. The underlying abnormality usually is congenital lymphangiectasia and fibrotic occlusion or atresia of the thoracic duct. Surgical treatment is frequently the only effective way to control chylous reflux or leak, and ligation of the incompetent retroperitoneal lymphatics and oversewing the ruptured lymphatics can produce long-term improvement or even

cure in many patients. In selected symptomatic patients with obstruction of the thoracic duct, a thoracic duct–azygos vein anastomosis may be considered as a surgical option.

References

1. O'Brien BMC, Shafiroff BB: Microlymphaticovenous and resectional surgery in obstructive lymphedema. World J Surg 3:3, 1979.
2. Huang GK, Ru-Qi H, Zong-Zhao L, et al: Microlymphaticovenous anastomosis for treating lymphedema of the extremities and external genitalia. J Microsurg 3:32, 1981.
3. Jamal S: Lymphovenous anastomosis in filarial lymphedema. Lymphology 14:64, 1981.
4. Krylov V, Milanov N, Abalmasov K: Microlymphatic surgery of secondary lymphoedema of the upper limb. Ann Chir Gynaecol 71:77, 1982.
5. Nieuborg, L: The Role of Lymphaticovenous Anastomoses in the Treatment of Postmastectomy Oedema. Alblasserdam, The Netherlands, Offsetdrukkerij Kanters BV, 1982.
6. Gong-Kang H, Ru-Qi H, Zong-Zhao L, et al: Microlymphaticovenous anastomosis in the treatment of lower limb obstructive lymphedema: Analysis of 91 cases. Plast Reconstr Surg 76:671, 1985.
7. Ingianni G, Holzmann T: Clinical experience with lymphovenous anastomosis for secondary lymphedema. Handchirurgie 17:43, 1985.
8. Campisi C, Tosatti E, Casaccia M, et al: Lymphatic microsurgery [in Italian]. Minerva Chir 41:469, 1986.
9. Zhu JK, Yu GZ, Liu JX, et al: Recent advances in microlymphatic surgery in China. Clin Orthop 215:32, 1987.

10. Gloviczki P, Fisher J, Hollier LH, et al: Microsurgical lymphovenous anastomosis for treatment of lymphedema: A critical review. J Vasc Surg 7:647, 1988.

11. Ipsen T, Pless J, Fredericksen PB: Experience with microlymphatico-venous anastomoses for congenital and acquired lymphoedema. Scand J Plast Reconstr Surg 22:233, 1988.

12. O'Brien BM, Mellow CG, Khazanchi RK, et al: Long-term results after microlymphatico-venous anastomoses for the treatment of obstructive lymphedema. Plast Reconstr Surg 85:562, 1990.

13. Baumeister RG, Siuda S: Treatment of lymphedemas by microsurgical lymphatic grafting: What is proved? Plast Reconstr Surg 85:64, 1990.

14. Goldsmith HS, De Los Santos R, Beattie EJ: Relief of chronic lymphoedema by omental transposition. JAMA 203:19, 1968.

15. Goldsmith HS: Long term evaluation of omental transposition for chronic lymphedema. Ann Surg 180:847, 1974.

16. Kinmonth JB, Hurst PAE, Edwards JM, Rutt DL: Relief of lymph obstruction by use of a bridge of mesentery and ileum. Br J Surg 65:829, 1978.

17. Hurst PA, Stewart G, Kinmonth JB, Browse NL: Long-term results of the enteromesenteric bridge operation in the treatment of primary lymphoedema. Br J Surg 72:272, 1985.

18. Trevidic P, Cormier JM: Free axillary lymph node transfer. In Cluzan RV (ed): Progress in Lymphology. Amsterdam, Elsevier Science Publishers, 1992, vol. 13, pp 415–420.

19. Edwards JM, Kinmonth JB: Lymphovenous shunts in man. Br Med J 4:579, 1969.

20. Nielubowicz J. Olszewski W: Surgical lymphaticovenous shunts in patients with secondary lymphoedema. Br J Surg 55:440, 1968.

21. Olszewski W, Clodius L, Földi M: The enigma of lymphedema—A search for answers [Editorial]. Lymphology 24:100, 1991.

22. Calderon G, Roberts B, Johnson LL: Experimental approach to the surgical creation of lymphatic-venous communications. Surgery 61:122, 1967.

23. Jacobson JH: Discussion. In Danese C, Bower R, Howard J: Experimental anastomoses of lymphatics. Arch Surg 84:9, 1962.

24. Laine JB, Howard JM: Experimental lymphatico-venous anastomosis. Surg Forum 14:111, 1963.

25. Yamada Y: The studies on lymphatic venous anastomosis in lymphedema. Nagoya J Med Sci 32:1, 1969.

26. Gilbert A, O'Brien BM, Vorrath JW, Sykes PJ: Lymphaticovenous anastomosis by microvascular technique. Br J Plast Surg 29:355, 1976.

27. Gloviczki P, LeFloch P, Hidden G: Anastomoses lymphaticoveineuses experimentales. J Chir (Paris) 116:437, 1979.

28. Gloviczki P, Hollier LH, Nora FE, Kaye MP: The natural history of microsurgical lymphovenous anastomoses: An experimental study. J Vasc Surg 4:148, 1986.

29. Puckett CL, Jacobs GR, Hurvitz JS, Silver D: Evaluation of lymphovenous anastomoses in obstructive lymphedema. Plast Reconstr Surg 66:116, 1980.

30. Baumeister RG, Seifert J, Wiebecke B: Homologous and autologous experimental lymph vessel transplantation—Initial experience. Int J Microsurg 3:19, 1981.

31. Baumeister RG, Seifert J: Microsurgical lymph vessel transplantation for the treatment of lymphedema: Experimental and first clinical experiences. Lymphology 14:90, 1981.

32. Baumeister RG, Siuda S, Bohmert H, Moser E: A microsurgical method for reconstruction of interrupted lymphatic pathways: Autologous lymph-vessel transplantation for treatment of lymphedemas. Scand J Plast Reconstr Surg 20:141, 1986.

33. Kleinhans E, Baumeister RGH, Hahn D, et al: Evaluation of transport kinetics in lymphoscintigraphy: Follow-up study in patients with transplanted lympatic vessels. Eur J Nucl Med 10:349, 1985.

34. Baumeister RGH, Frick A, Hofmann T: 10 years experience with autogenous microsurgical lymphvessel-transplantation. Eur J Lymphology 6:62, 1991.

35. Browse NL: The diagnosis and management of primary lymphedema. J Vasc Surg 3:181, 1986.

36. Wolfe JHN: Treatment of lymphedema. In Rutherford RB (ed): Vascular Surgery. 3rd ed. Philadelphia, WB Saunders, 1989, pp 1668–1678.

37. Danese CA, Papioannou AN, Morales LE, Mitsuda S: Surgical approaches to lymphatic blocks. Surgery 64:821, 1968.

38. O'Brien BM, Hickey MJ, Dvir E, et al: Microsurgical transfer of greater omentum in the treatment of canine lymphoedema. Br J Plast Surg 43:440, 1990.

39. Knight KR, Hurley JV, Hickey MJ, et al: Combined coumarin and omental transfer treatment for canine proximal obstructive lymphoedema. Int J Exp Pathol 72:533, 1991.

40. Kinmonth JB: Chylous diseases and syndromes, including references to tropical elephantiasis. In Kinmonth JB (ed): The Lymphatics: Surgery, Lymphography and Diseases of the Chyle and Lymph Systems. 2nd ed. London, Edward Arnold, 1982, pp 221–268.

41. Servelle M: Surgical treatment of lymphedema: A report on 652 cases. Surgery 101:485, 1987.

42. Servelle M: Congenital malformation of the lymphatics of the small intestine. J Cardiovasc Surg 32:159, 1991.

43. Kinmonth JB, Cox SJ: Protein losing enteropathy in lymphedema. Surgical investigation and treatment. J Cardiovasc Surg 16:111, 1975.

44. Browse NL, Wilson NM, Russo F, et al: Aetiology and treatment of chylous ascites. Br J Surg 79:1145, 1992.

45. Gloviczki P, Soltesz L, Solti F, et al: The surgical treatment of lymphedema caused by chylous reflux. In Bartos V, Davidson JW (eds): Advances in Lymphology. Proceedings of the 8th International Congress of Lymphology, Montreal, 1981. Prague, Czechoslovak Medical Press, 1982, pp 502–507.

46. Sanders JS, Rosenow EC III, Piehler JM, et al: Chyloptysis (chylous sputum) due to thoracic lymphangiectasia with successful surgical correction. Arch Intern Med 148:1465, 1988.

47. Servelle M, Deysson H: Reflux du chyle dans les lymphatiques jambiers. Arch Mal Coeur 12:1181, 1949.

48. Browse NL: The surgery of lymphedema. In Veith FJ (ed): Current Critical Problems in Vascular Surgery. St. Louis, Quality Medical Publishing, 1989, pp 408–409.

49. Gloviczki P, Calcagno D, Schirger A, et al: Noninvasive evaluation of the swollen extremity: Experiences with 190 lymphoscintigraphic examinations. J Vasc Surg 9:683, 1989.

Extremity Amputation for Vascular Disease

Edited by William C. Krupski, M.D.

147

Overview

William C. Krupski, M.D.

• • •

The principles discussed in previous chapters have substantially improved limb salvage rates in patients with peripheral vascular disease. Nevertheless, amputation may be the only practical treatment for a limb severely affected by trauma, infection, tumor, or the end stages of ischemia. Unfortunately, vascular surgeons often view amputations as manifestations of failure—failure to comprehend or control the disease process, failure of the referring physician or patient to seek help in a timely fashion, or failure of the vascular surgeon to perform adequate revascularization. This negative bias should be condemned because it may contribute to the poor results reported in many series of major limb amputations in contrast to the advances made in arterial reconstructions. Instead, amputation surgery should be considered an important *reconstructive* surgical technique in the total management of patients with limb-threatening disorders of the extremities.

Currently, most patients with peripheral vascular occlusive disease will have had a previous bypass graft, some other arterial reconstruction such as profundaplasty or thromboendarterectomy, or a percutaneous endovascular procedure such as transluminal angioplasty or atherectomy that was either unsuccessful or failed after a variable length of time. For these patients and for those who present with extensive tissue necrosis or infection, amputation may be preferable to increasingly complex reoperative vascular reconstructions, which carry attendant risks of morbidity and death. The decision to proceed to amputation rather than attempt revascularization must be individualized and is often complicated and difficult. Importantly, the patient must be a prominent participant in making this judgment.

The immediate aims of amputation are (1) removal of diseased tissue; (2) relief of pain; (3) primary healing at the amputation level chosen; and (4) construction of a stump and provision of a prosthesis that will permit useful func-

tion. The purpose of this introductory overview is to provide historical perspective and background for the detailed chapters that follow.

HISTORICAL PERSPECTIVE

The history of amputation surgery is long and colorful (Table 147–1). In neolithic times and in pre-Columbian America (as well as in some parts of the world even today) it was a religious ritual or a form of punishment.[1, 2] In the Babylonian era, the hands of the surgeon whose treatment caused blindness or death were amputated.[3] Hammurabi (King of Babylon in 1792–1750 B.C.) dictated that if a surgeon caused blindness, serious injury, or death in a free man, his hands were cut off, whereas the doctor was required only to replace a slave who died under his care.

Hippocrates (c. 460–370 B.C.) first reported extremity amputation as treatment for disease in patients with gangrene after vascular occlusion.[4] He advised amputation through devitalized tissue to avoid the greater risk of hemorrhage when cutting through living tissue. The Roman aristocrat and historian Aulus Cornelius Celsus (c. A.D. 25–50), often mistaken for a physician because of his meticulous treatises on medical subjects, elucidated important principles of amputation surgery. He proposed amputation through viable tissue, use of a rasp to smooth bone, and use of hemostatic ligatures.[5] In the latter part of the first century, Archigenes of Apamea, who lived under the rule of Emperor Trajan, advocated identification and ligation of blood vessels *before* completing an amputation.[6] Only if hemorrhage persisted did he resort to cautery with hot irons or boiling water.

The introduction of gunpowder in 1338 resulted in an unprecedented number of severe battle wounds requiring

Table 147–1.   Some Important Events in Amputation Surgery

Era	Notable Individuals	Dates	Events
Babylonian	Hammurabi	1792–1750 B.C.	Amputation as punishment
Greek	Hippocrates	c. 460–370 B.C.	First medical amputation
Roman	Celsus	c. A.D. 25–50	Amputation through viable tissue, hemostatic ligatures
Middle Ages	Hans von Gerssdorf	1485–1545	Opium for amputation, postoperative pressure dressings
Renaissance	Ambroise Paré	1510–1590	Abandoned scalding oil and reintroduced ligatures for hemostasis; designed prostheses; attention to rehabilitation
The "Enlightenment"	John Hunter	1728–1793	Surgeon-scientist, opposed primary amputation
Napoleonic wars	Dominique Jean Larrey	1766–1842	Expeditious evacuations of wounded; advocated primary amputation, débridement and healing by secondary intention
U.S. Civil War	Samuel D. Gross	1861–1865	Advised amputation of compound fractures, ignored asepsis
Franco-Prussian War	Joseph Lister	1827–1912	Successful treatment of compound fractures with carbolic acid dressings
World War I	Alexis Carrel	1914–1918	Abandonment of prophylactic amputation of compound fractures; developed Carrel-Dakin solution
World War II	Michael DeBakey	1939–1945	Blood banks, antibiotics; below-knee amputation more common than above-knee amputation
Korean conflict	"MASH" units	1950–1953	Sharp fall in amputation rate because of arterial injury repair
Vietnam War	Norman Rich	1965–1975	Improved vascular techniques; rapid evacuation
Post-Vietnam	Ernest Burgess	1975–present	Replantation, improved prostheses and rehabilitation

From Krupski WC, Bass A: Amputations for traumatic vascular injury. In *Bongard FS, Wilson SE, Perry MO (eds): Vascular Injuries in Surgical Practice. San Mateo, CA, Appleton & Lange, 1991.*

amputation.[3] Much of modern surgery was developed from lessons learned from war. Thus, it is not surprising that a German military surgeon, Hans von Gerssdorf, became a preeminent amputation surgeon, performing over 200 amputations for gangrene or erysipelas.[7] His two major contributions to amputation surgery were the administration of opium prior to the operation and the use of a pressure bandage fashioned from an ox bladder to reduce postoperative bleeding.

Ambroise Paré (1510–1590), the distinguished father of French surgery, ranks as one of the Renaissance's most acclaimed surgeons, whose contributions to amputation surgery are legendary. His accomplishments include (1) discontinuation of application of scalding oil for hemostasis; (2) reintroduction of hemostatic ligatures; (3) classification of amputation as a reconstructive procedure; (4) suggestion that amputation be performed through viable tissue; (5) description of phantom limb pain; (6) selection of amputa-

tion levels based on later prosthetic use; and (7) design of several upper and lower extremity prostheses.[8] Delivering advice that is equally befitting today, Paré wrote, "You say that tying up the blood vessels after amputation is a new method, and should therefore not be used. That is a bad argument for a doctor."[9]

Celsus had written about circular amputation incisions in the 11th century. This technique remained standard for 1600 years, until Verdusi (1696), Ravaton (1749), and Vermale (1765) advocated longitudinal incisions for the purpose of creating flaps for improved coverage of bone.[5, 6, 10] During this era, surgeons debated the proper timing of amputation for traumatic injuries. Some advocated primary amputation on the battlefield to prevent the fatal complications attendant on compound fractures and gangrene. Opponents argued that it was preferable to allow patients to recover from the initial trauma before imposing another injury.[3] Ironically, the brilliant London surgeon John

Hunter (1728–1793 [see Chapter 74]), esteemed for his contributions to the physiology of collateral circulation and repair of peripheral arterial aneurysms, was an ardent proponent of delayed amputation; his recommendations strongly influenced surgical practice in his day.[11]

At the age of 22, Pierre Joseph Desault (1744–1795) was already chief surgeon at the Hotel Dieu hospital in Paris. Although he became well known for private lectures, he later abandoned this teaching method in favor of bedside teaching. He spent much of his career observing wound healing and introduced the term débridement for treatment of traumatic wounds. Desault's most prominent student, Dominique Jean Larrey (1766–1842) became Napolean's surgeon. Larrey accompanied Napolean's troops in 400 skirmishes, 60 major battles, and 25 campaigns.[12] In Borodino on the road to Moscow, during the first great battle of the Russian campaign, Larrey performed 200 amputations in 24 hours—an amputation every 7 minutes![3] On the Russian front he learned to pack the amputation stump in ice and snow to decrease pain. Larrey contributed greatly to amputation and trauma surgery. He recognized the importance of prompt treatment after injury and developed the *ambulance volante* ("flying ambulance") corps of the French army to expedite evacuation of the wounded, who otherwise often remained unattended on the battlefield for days waiting for the fighting to end.[13] Larrey also was the first to perform amputation at the hip. He advocated extensive wound débridement, removal of all foreign bodies, delayed amputation only in severely infected wounds, closure of traumatic wounds by secondary intention, immobilization of extremities to promote healing, and therapeutic wound débridement with maggots.[3, 9] Remarkably, these achievements preceded the development of anesthesia or asepsis.

When ether and chloroform were introduced in 1846 and 1847, respectively, the need for excessive haste in performing amputations disappeared. On one occasion, the endeavor to complete the procedure with extraordinary speed resulted in amputation of not only the patient's extremity but also both his testicles and two fingers of an assistant![10] Robert Liston (1794–1847) routinely performed amputations in less than 30 seconds, holding the knife in his mouth.[3]

The catastrophic suffering in the American Civil War motivated interest in amputation surgery among American surgeons. Samuel D. Gross, the acclaimed Civil War surgeon and educator, published a treatise on amputations in 1862 that echoed the tenets proposed 50 years earlier by Larrey. Nevertheless, more limbs were lost by American soldiers in the Civil War than in any other military conflict, despite continuing development of more destructive weapons. Confederate soldiers suffered an estimated 25,000 major amputations, while in the Union army about 21,000 major amputations were performed.[3, 14] The mortality for major amputations approached 80 per cent because of the disastrous incidence of postoperative wound infection.[15]

Joseph Lister (1827–1912) reported successful treatment of 11 patients with compound fractures using occlusive dressings soaked in carbolic acid in 1867.[16] The surgical community was subsequently divided between those who advocated "laudable pus" and those in favor of aseptic technique. Surprisingly, Samuel D. Gross was a severe critic of Professor Lister. The Franco-Prussian war was instrumental in settling the issue when it became apparent that wounded Prussians, who were treated by the Listerian method, fared better than the French, who were not.[17]

Half a million men required amputations in World War I, including over 4000 Americans.[3, 18] Higher muzzle velocities and more powerful explosives produced more brutal injuries than in previous conflicts. Anaerobic bacteria from heavily fertilized European soil were responsible for the 28 per cent mortality from gas gangrene, which occurred in 5 per cent of wounds.[19] Nevertheless, several advances in amputation surgery arose from the lessons learned in World War I, including delayed primary closure of contaminated wounds after serial dressing changes with antiseptic solution, repudiation of prophylactic amputations in all compound fractures, and development of orthopedic external fixation splints.

The availability of antibiotics and blood transfusions transformed trauma surgery dramatically in World War II. Nonetheless, amputation rates after major extremity injury actually *increased* from 2 per cent in World War I to 5 per cent in World War II because of the violence caused by even more powerful weapons. Nearly 16,000 Americans underwent major amputations. There was improvement in treatment of compound fractures and preservation of the knee joint, thus resulting in better long-term rehabilitation. The ratio of above-knee to below-knee amputation in World War I was 2.5:1, falling to 1:1 in World War II.[14] Moreover, mortality from wound infections decreased from 8 per cent in World War I to 4.5 per cent in World War II.[20]

Mortality related to wounds continued to improve in the Korean conflict to 2.5 per cent.[14] Amputations were necessary in only 13 per cent of severely injured extremities because of improvements in rapid evacuation of the wounded and refinements in repair of vascular injuries. Similar rates were reported in the Vietnam war.[21, 22]

During the past three decades, the lessons learned from traumatic amputations were applied to amputations performed for nontraumatic causes. In the mid-1960s Burgess and associates introduced important advances in amputation techniques, increased acceptance of prostheses, and produced less psychological trauma postoperatively.[23, 24] The concept of immediate fitting of prostheses after amputation, proposed in 1958 by Berlemont in France,[25] was expanded by the group at the San Francisco Veterans Administration Medical Center in the 1970s.[26] During the last decade, most achievements in amputation surgery have involved lower limb vascular reconstruction, prosthetic materials and design, and better rehabilitation methods. Improvements in these areas have resulted in an increased number of useful extremities.

SCOPE OF THE PROBLEM

As the average age of the population has risen, the incidence of peripheral vascular disease and diabetes mellitus has increased. More than 90 per cent of the 60,000 amputations performed in the United States each year are for ischemic or infective gangrene.[27] Similar statistics have been reported in Great Britain.[28] Most lower extremity amputations are performed for vascular and infectious complications of diabetes mellitus, and 15 to 35 per cent of diabetic amputees will lose a second leg within 5 years.[29-31] Other indications for lower extremity amputation include nondiabetic infection with ischemia, ischemia without infection, chronic osteomyelitis, trauma, and miscellaneous causes. The evaluation and preparation of patients for amputation with respect to these different presentations are discussed in Chapter 148.

A recently published list of the 20 most commonly performed major procedures in general surgery based on the 1987 National Hospital Survey conspicuously omits extremity amputation, even though the number performed nationally would place it nearly in the top 10 operations.[32] This suggests that many amputations are performed by orthopedic surgeons and emphasizes the importance of exchanging information between disciplines. Moreover, few general surgery training programs offer extensive experience in the technical performance of amputation or, of equal importance, in postoperative rehabilitation or use of prostheses. It is therefore prudent for surgeons with experience in these areas to work closely with orthopedic colleagues and local prosthetists to develop a comprehensive program in amputation surgery.

Economic expenditures for amputations are substantial. In the United Kingdom, £33 million are spent per year on prostheses alone.[28] At the end of the 1970s, Malone and coworkers estimated that by applying a team approach to the treatment of potential amputees, the Veterans Administration could save $80 million over a 5-year period.[33] The actual expense of amputation varies widely depending on the locale, year, and success rate (i.e., primary healing). For example, in a comparison of the costs of revascularization versus amputation, Gupta and the group from New York City reported in a 1982 abstract that an uncomplicated amputation amounted to $27,225 ± 2896.[34] Mackey and colleagues in 1986 analyzed the extended costs of revascularization versus amputation, including the costs of secondary complications, and reported a value of $40,563 ± 4729.[35] Most recently, Cheshire found that the cost of primary amputation in the United Kingdom averaged £20,416.[36] The reasons for these discrepancies are discussed in Chapter 153.

LEVEL OF AMPUTATION

Amputation should be performed at the level at which healing is most likely to be complete but which will also permit the most efficient use of the limb after rehabilitation. In the upper extremity, circulatory impairment rarely constitutes an indication for amputation. In the lower extremities, in which vascular insufficiency is much more likely, the circulatory status at different levels may be determined by measurement of the peripheral pulses and the capillary refill time and by noting the presence of rubor, the condition of the skin, and the presence of ischemic atrophy. At present, no single measurement of blood flow can reliably predict the best level of healing. The best predictions are based on clinical assessment by an experienced surgeon, assisted by one of several techniques for determining amputation level. In patients with distinct lines of demarcation

and in those with tumors, the amount of tissue that must be removed is more obvious.

Maximum limb length should be preserved to maintain ambulation as near normal as possible with the least energy expenditure. For example, compared with normal walking, energy expenditure is increased 10 to 40 per cent for a unilateral below-knee amputation, 50 to 57 per cent for a unilateral above-knee amputation, and 60 per cent for crutch walking.[37] Consequently, whereas 70 per cent of below-knee amputees attain bipedal gait, only 10 to 30 per cent of above-knee amputees eventually walk again.[38-40]

Ancillary tests to assist in determination of optimal amputation level include segmental Doppler systolic pressure measurements, fluorescein dye measurements, laser-Doppler velocimetry, photoelectric skin perfusion pressure, isotope measurement of skin perfusion pressure, isotope measurement of skin blood flow, measurement of skin temperature, and measurement of transcutaneous oxygen tension. These techniques are elaborated in detail in Chapter 149. Specific lower extremity amputations are also discussed.

COMPLICATIONS OF AMPUTATION

Chapter 150 covers complications of amputation in depth. Adverse outcomes are unfortunately common despite refinements in *preoperative* assessment, *intraoperative* management, and *postoperative* care. The authors discuss complications in relation to these periods of time. In addition, late complications may affect the ability of amputees to use prostheses effectively. These unfavorable consequences include stump congestion, bulbous stump, excessive residual soft tissue, callosities and cysts, neuropathy and phantom limb, bone spurs, osteoporosis, bone overgrowth, adherent scar, loss of the contralateral limb, and requirement for revision of stumps.

THE TEAM APPROACH

Dramatic improvement in the rehabilitation of amputees has been achieved after institution of a team approach. In addition to the surgeon, the ideal group of individuals charged with caring for patients requiring amputation includes a physiatrist, rehabilitation nurse, physical therapist, occupational therapist, recreation or vocational therapist, prosthetist, medical social worker, and psychologist/counselor. Such a team enhances patient care immensely. Expectations for the amputee should be well defined and evaluated on a regular basis. The benefits of a team approach were established by Malone and colleagues, who compared the team approach with historical controls.[41] The results are summarized in Table 147-2. Chapter 151 presents the case for a comprehensive approach for the rehabilitation of amputees.

UPPER EXTREMITY AMPUTATIONS

Upper extremity amputations comprise 15 to 20 per cent of all amputations. Almost 8000 new upper extremity

Table 147-2. Team Versus Nonteam Approach to Rehabilitation

	Healing (%)	Hospital Days	Rehabilitation Days	Rehabilitation Rate (%)
Team approach	97	38	31	100
Nonteam approach	63	68	128	69

Adapted from Malone JM, Moore W, Leal JM, Childers SJ: Rehabilitation for lower extremity amputation. Arch Surg 116:93, 1981. Copyright 1981, American Medical Association.

amputations are performed each year in the United States.[42] Ten per cent of these amputees have involvement of the other upper extremity. In contrast to lower extremity amputees, most upper extremity amputations are performed for trauma. Other indications, in order of decreasing frequency, are tumor, congenital anomalies, vascular disease, infections, and iatrogenic causes (e.g., extravasation of caustic chemicals or vasopressor therapy). Reestablishment of a functional limb depends on preoperative counseling and explanation of realistic expectations, meticulous surgical technique, attention to the principles of prosthetic fitting and rehabilitation, and recognition and treatment of the psychological trauma imposed by loss of all or part of the upper limb. The features of upper extremity amputation are reviewed in Chapter 152.

AMPUTATION VERSUS REVASCULARIZATION

The final chapter in this section, Chapter 153, extensively reviews the arguments for and against amputation as opposed to revascularization for patients with end-stage peripheral vascular disease. Those in favor of primary amputation cite the large numbers of patients subjected to revascularization who ultimately require a major amputation, the level of which may be adversely affected by a failed bypass.[43, 44] Multiple reoperations increase morbidity and mortality rates. Furthermore, rehabilitation of amputees has become increasingly successful.

Proponents of revascularization note that limb salvage rates generally surpass bypass graft patency rates by 15 to 20 per cent.[45, 46] They point out that patients with severely ischemic extremities have a limited life expectancy, and a "palliative" revascularization is advantageous so that the patient can maintain as normal a lifestyle as possible for the remainder of life.

The reasons for this controversy arise from many factors, including differences in patient populations, different institutional philosophies, variable technical abilities of surgeons, different levels of expertise in support services (e.g., radiology versus rehabilitation medicine), and a lack of objective preoperative criteria on which to base the decision of when to attempt revascularization or primary amputation. Chapter 153 presents a comprehensive update of this problem. A analysis of fiscal considerations is also presented.

References

1. Brothwell D, Moller-Christensen V: Medico-historical aspects of a very early case of mutilation. Danish Med Bull 10:21, 1963.
2. Friedmann LW: Amputation in pre-Columbian America. Arch Phys Med Rehabil 54:323, 1973.
3. Aldea PA, Shaw WW: The evolution of the surgical management of severe lower extremity trauma. Clin Plast Surg 13:549, 1986.
4. Adams F: The Genuine Works of Hippocrates. Translated from Greek with preliminary discourse and annotations. New York, Williams, Wood, 1891.
5. Mettler CC: History of Medicine. Philadelphia, Blakiston, 1947.
6. Kirk NT: The development of amputation. Bull Med Lib Assoc 32:132, 1944.
7. Zimmerman LM, Veith I: Great Ideas in the History of Surgery. New York, Dover, 1967.
8. Garrison FH: An Introduction to the History of Medicine. 4th ed. Philadelphia, W.B. Saunders, 1929.
9. Haeger K: The Illustrated History of Surgery. New York, Bell Publishing, 1988.
10. Wagensteen OH, Smith J, Wagensteen SD, et al: Some highlights in the history of amputation reflecting lessons in wound healing. Bull Hist Med 41:97, 1967.
11. Hunter JA: Treatise on the Blood, Inflammation and Gunshot Wounds. Philadelphia, Thomas Bradford, 1796.
12. Dibble JH: DJ Larrey, a surgeon of the revolution, consulate and empire. Med Hist 3:100, 1959.
13. Larrey DJ: Memoires de Chirurgie Militaire et Campagnes. Paris, J Smith, 1812–1817.
14. Office of the Surgeon General, United States Army: Orthopedic Surgery in the Zone of the Interior: Surgery in World War II. Washington D.C., Medical Department, 1970.
15. Keen WW: The contrast between the surgery of the Civil War and that of the present war. NY Med J 101:817, 1915.
16. Lister J: On a method of treating compound fractures, abscesses, etc., with observations of the conditions of suppuration. Lancet 1:326, 1867.
17. Cartwright RR: The Development of Modern Surgery. New York, Thomas Crowell, 1968.
18. The Medical Department of the United States Army in the World War. Vol. 13, Part I—General Surgery, Orthopedic Surgery, Neurosurgery. Washington DC, U.S. Government Printing Office, 1927.
19. Hardaway RM: Vietnam wound analysis. J Trauma 18:635, 1978.
20. Simeone FA: Studies of trauma and shock in man: William S. Stone's role in the military effort. J Trauma 24:181, 1984.
21. Walter Reed Army Medical Center: Battle Casualties in Korea. Vol. 3. The Battle Wound: Clinical Experiences. Washington, DC, Army Medical Service Graduate School, 1955.
22. Rich NM, Braugh JH, Hughes CW, et al: Acute arterial injuries in Vietnam: 1000 cases. J Trauma 10:359, 1970.
23. Burgess EM, Romano RJ, Zettl JH, Schrock RD Jr: Amputation of the leg for peripheral vascular insufficiency. J Bone Joint Surg 53:874, 1971.
24. Burgess EM: Amputation surgery and postoperative care. *In* Banerjee SN (ed): Rehabilitation Management of Amputees. Baltimore, Williams & Wilkins, 1982.
25. Berlemont M: Notre expérience de l'appareillage précoce des amputées du membre inférieur aux établissements Helios Marius de Berck. Ann Med Phys 4:4, 1961.
26. Moore WS, Hall AP, Lim RC: Below-the-knee amputation for ischemic gangrene. Comparative results of conventional operation and immediate postoperative fitting. Am J Surg 124:127, 1972.
27. Krupski WC, Skinner HB, Effeney DJ: Amputation. *In* Way LW (ed): Current Surgical Diagnosis and Treatment, San Mateo, CA, Appleton and Lange, 1988, pp 704–714.
28. McColl I: Review of artificial limb and appliance centre services.

Department of Health and Human Services Report. London, Her Majesty's Stationery Office, 1986.

29. High RM, McDowell DE, Savin RA: A critical review of amputation in vascular patients. J Vasc Surg 1:653, 1984.

30. Whitehouse FW, Jurgensen C, Block MA: The later life of the diabetic amputee: Another look at fate of the second leg. Diabetes 17:520, 1968.

31. Powell TW, Burnham SJ, Johnson G Jr: Second leg ischemia: Lower extremity bypass versus amputation in patients with contralateral lower extremity amputation. Am Surg 11:577, 1984.

32. Wheeler HB: Myth and reality in general surgery. Bull Am Coll Surg 78:21, 1993.

33. Malone JM, Moore WS, Goldstone J, Malone SJ: Therapeutic and economic impact of a modern amputation program. Ann Surg 189:798, 1979.

34. Gupta SK, Veith FJ, Samson RH, et al: Cost analysis of operations for infrainguinal arteriosclerosis [Abstract]. Circulation 66(Suppl 2):II-9, 1982.

35. Mackey WC, McCollough JL, Conlon TP, et al: The costs of surgery for limb-threatening ischemia. Surgery 99:26, 1986.

36. Cheshire NJ, Wolfe JH, Noone MA, et al: The economics of femorocrural reconstruction for critical leg ischemia with and without saphenous vein. J Vasc Surg 15:167, 1992.

37. Waters RL, Perry J, Antonelli D, et al: Energy cost of walking amputees: The influence of level of amputation. J Bone Joint Surg 58:42, 1976.

38. Roon AJ, Moore WS, Goldstone J: Below-knee amputation: A modern approach. Am J Surg 134:153, 1977.

39. Couch NP, David JK, Tilney NL, Crane C: Natural history of the leg amputee. Am J Surg 133:469, 1977.

40. Steinberg FU, Sunwoo I, Roettger RF: Prosthetic rehabilitation of geriatric amputee patients: A follow-up study. Arch Phys Med Rehabil 66:742, 1985.

41. Malone JM, Moore W, Leal JM, Childers SJ: Rehabilitation for lower extremity amputation. Arch Surg 116:93, 1981.

42. Beasley RW: General considerations in managing upper limb amputations. Orthop Clin North Am 12:743, 1981.

43. Stoney RJ: Ultimate salvage for the patient with limb-threatening ischemia: Realistic goals and surgical considerations. Am J Surg 136:228, 1978.

44. Kazmers M, Satiani B, Evans WE: Amputation level following unsuccessful distal limb salvage operations. Surgery 87:683, 1980.

45. Veith FJ, Gupta SK, Samson RH, et al: Progress in limb salvage by reconstructive arterial surgery combined with new or improved adjunctive procedures. Ann Surg 194:386, 1981.

46. Bartlett ST, Olinde AJ, Flinn WR, et al: The reoperative potential of infrainguinal bypass: Long-term limb and patient survival. J Vasc Surg 5:170, 1987.

148

Patient Evaluation and Preparation for Amputation

Kenneth E. McIntyre, Jr., M.D., and Scott S. Berman, M.D.

• • •

Primary amputation of the lower extremity should rarely be performed before a complete evaluation of the feasibility of vascular reconstruction has been done. As techniques for vascular reconstruction of arteries below the knee have become increasingly successful, intuition dictates that amputation rates should decline. Unfortunately, the number of amputations has not decreased, largely because of the greater longevity of the population. Amputations are more prevalent in older patients.[1-3] In addition to circulatory impairment of the lower extremities, older patients may also have coexisting diseases that may affect the outcome after amputation.[4] Therefore, a thorough preoperative evaluation must be performed to minimize the high morbidity and mortality associated with lower extremity amputation.[5] Loss of a limb also engenders acute depression, which must be anticipated and treated to optimize postoperative rehabilitation.[6, 7] This chapter reviews the epidemiology of amputation and recapitulates the evaluation of concurrent diseases that influence the perioperative outcome and rehabilitation. A treatment algorithm is suggested to help identify and evaluate various preoperative conditions that contribute to postoperative morbidity in the patient who requires amputation.

EPIDEMIOLOGY OF LOWER EXTREMITY AMPUTATIONS

Nontraumatic amputations occur most commonly as a result of acute ischemia, chronic ischemia, or diabetes with infectious gangrene.[8, 9] The preoperative evaluation of patients with these conditions differs because the specific underlying condition that has resulted in the need for amputation may contribute to unique perioperative complications.[10] A discussion of the preoperative evaluation of amputations caused by each of these presentations follows.

Amputation for Acute Ischemia

Acute ischemia requiring lower extremity amputation results from either arterial thrombosis or arterial embolism.

More than 15 years ago, Blaisdell and associates documented the grim outcome of acute lower extremity ischemia following thromboembolism.[11] Today, acute lower extremity ischemia resulting from both thrombosis and embolism continues to challenge vascular surgeons.

It is often difficult to distinguish thrombosis from embolism as the cause of acute lower extremity ischemia. Classically, patients with embolism tend to be older and may or may not have an obvious embolic source. Arterial embolism may have a cardiac source such as arrhythmia (e.g., atrial fibrillation), valvular heart disease, acute myocardial infarction, or ventricular aneurysm. In addition, atheroembolism from a more proximal arterial source may occur.[12, 13] In contrast, thrombosis usually occurs in younger patients with a long history of vascular occlusive disease of the lower extremities including symptoms of claudication, ischemic rest pain, or prior vascular reconstructive procedures. It is incumbent on the surgeon to discern the cause of acute ischemia, although it is not always obvious.

A careful history suggests the cause of acute leg ischemia in most instances. The physical examination is also helpful. In patients with unilateral lower extremity ischemia secondary to embolism, pulses in the contralateral leg are usually normal. In addition, a murmur may indicate valvular heart disease. A chronic arrhythmia such as atrial fibrillation is readily diagnosed by the irregularly irregular pulse. In patients with thrombosis, diminished or absent pulses in the contralateral extremity may be present as well as other signs of chronic tissue ischemia. Findings on integumentary inspection such as absence of hair over the toes and dorsum of the foot, thickening of the toenails, atrophy of the subcutaneous tissue, pallor on elevation, and rubor on dependency in the contralateral extremity are important in this regard. Even with a thorough history and physical examination, however, the precise cause of tissue ischemia may be elusive. Additional tests are then required.

Two-dimensional echocardiography for evaluation of the heart for the presence of valvular heart disease or intracardiac thrombi is less accurate than transesophageal echocardiography (TEE) for this purpose. Although it is often difficult to identify thrombi by either method, ventricular wall motion abnormalities, which often lead to thrombus formation, can be readily identified.[14] Whether or not a cardiac embolic source is identified, anticoagulation with intravenous heparin should be instituted immediately. This therapy will prevent additional embolic episodes that may cause stroke, myocardial infarction, renal failure, or further lower extremity tissue ischemia[11, 15, 16] and is also useful for preventing propagation of thrombus in patients with acute thrombosis.

One of the most important contributors to the prognosis for both the patient and the extremity following an episode of acute thromboembolism is myocardial infarction. In addition, congestive heart failure greatly increases the risk.[13] A resting electrocardiogram and myocardial enzyme determination are obtained to exclude the presence of acute myocardial infarction, which may both precipitate limb ischemia and complicate its management. Myocardial infarction as a cause of acute thromboembolism is important to recognize not only during embolectomy but also prior to performance of the definitive amputation. Aggressive treatment of ventricular dysfunction and anticoagula-

tion therapy help to reduce the risk of operation to some degree. Chapters 2 and 22 discuss these issues in detail.

In patients who develop acute ischemia caused by thrombosis of preexisting disease, the diagnosis should generally be confirmed by arteriography. If adequate healing of a below-knee amputation is questionable, a more proximal arterial stenosis or occlusion that may be amenable to either surgical reconstruction or angioplasty may be identified by arteriography. Arteriography not only can identify the level of obstruction but also offers an opportunity for delivering intra-arterial thrombolytic agents.[17] Arteriography necessarily delays operative treatment, however, which some patients can ill afford. Even with optimal therapy for acutely ischemic limbs, postoperative mortality rates average 15 to 48 per cent.[11, 18, 19]

Chronic Ischemia

Even with modern arterial reconstructive techniques, chronic ischemia still accounts for nearly 20,000 amputations each year.[5] Usually patients are considered candidates for primary amputation only when a significant part of the weight-bearing surface of the foot is affected with gangrene or necrosis. However, in an elderly patient who does not ambulate, is mentally incompetent, has flexion contractures secondary to immobility or arthritis, has a concurrent terminal illness, or has no reconstructible vessels in the calf or foot, primary amputation is appropriate.[20]

As in patients with acute lower extremity ischemia, heart disease requires careful evaluation and treatment to prevent significant perioperative complications and obtain the best postoperative results.[21] In diabetic patients, silent (asymptomatic) myocardial infarction is particularly common, and therefore the absence of ischemic heart disease as documented by a negative history alone may be unreliable. In the presence of an abnormal electrocardiogram, a history of ventricular dysfunction (especially if manifested by congestive heart failure), or angina pectoris, further cardiac evaluation is advisable prior to proceeding with amputation (see Chapter 22).[22]

The standard test for the diagnosis of ischemic heart disease in the general population is the exercise treadmill stress test. This standardized examination has been validated as both specific and sensitive for identification of patients with ischemic heart disease.[23, 24] Unfortunately, the exercise stress test requires the ability to walk at a rate that elevates the heart rate to a target value.[25] In patients with claudication, ischemic rest pain, or a partially gangrenous extremity, the test is not applicable because these patients cannot walk at a rate of speed that will increase their heart rate sufficiently to ensure reliability of the examination.

An alternative to the exercise stress test is arm exercise ergometry,[25, 26] which monitors the electrocardiogram, heart rate, and blood pressure during a standard exercise protocol using an arm crank ergometer. This test has been shown to be a safe and effective alternative test for the detection of coronary artery disease in patients who cannot walk vigorously, although a direct concordance with coronary arteriographic findings has not been confirmed. Of note, ergometry has a role in determining safe exercise levels and may be predictive of successful prosthetic use in patients undergoing rehabilitation after amputations.[25, 26]

A currently popular test used to diagnose significant coronary artery disease in patients who cannot ambulate adequately is the dipyridamole-thallium myocardial perfusion scan. Although its sensitivity and specificity are controversial (see Chapter 22), the dipyridamole-thallium cardiac perfusion scan may be valuable in identifying patients who have an increased risk of myocardial ischemia during the operation.[27] If a reversible ischemic defect is identified on the dipyridamole-thallium scan, some practitioners recommend coronary arteriography in the hope of identifying a simple lesion that may be amenable to percutaneous transluminal angioplasty prior to amputation. If nonreconstructible coronary occlusive disease is identified, it is necessary to proceed with amputation using increased perioperative monitoring and pharmacologic cardiac support when indicated. In such a case, however, the patient is at greater risk for perioperative myocardial infarction.

Amputation in the patient with chronic ischemia generally is performed as an elective procedure. As such, time permits adequate preoperative evaluation and optimal treatment of comorbid conditions. The elective nature of amputation in these patients also allows for initiation of preoperative physical training and psychological counseling for better adaptation to amputation. Bradway and associates have described four stages of adaptation pertaining to amputation: preoperative, immediate postoperative, inhospital, and at-home rehabilitation periods.[6] All amputees must work through these adaptive stages. Ideally, the multi-disciplinary team of surgeon, prosthetist, physical therapist, occupational therapist, social worker, and psychologist or psychiatrist can begin working with the patient in the *preoperative* period to improve rehabilitation potential. Successful application of this team approach, paying attention to the psychological needs of the amputee, has been shown to enhance rehabilitation and prevent the need for long-term psychiatric care.[6]

Amputations for Infectious Gangrene

When infectious gangrene of the lower extremity is present, blood glucose and ketoacidosis may be difficult to control prior to amputation. Patients may be relatively "insulin resistant" and metabolically unstable. Dehydration caused by osmotic diuresis, ketoacidosis, and hyperosmolarity all contribute to worsening of peripheral vascular occlusive disease as well as coronary occlusive disease. Immediate and aggressive foot débridement with establishment of adequate drainage of abscesses is required to document the extent of infection and should be undertaken emergently.

If the foot is deemed unsalvageable by thorough inspection in the operating room, an ankle guillotine operation should be performed.[28] The authors have shown that preparatory guillotine amputation in patients with infectious gangrene substantially improves later outcome. Whereas stump infection occurred in 22 per cent of patients who underwent definitive amputation without preparatory guillotine amputation, infection supervened in only 3 per cent of those having staged procedures ($p < .005$).[28] Importantly, mortality from the two-stage amputation approach was not significantly greater than that with a one-stage operation.

Supramalleolar guillotine amputation provides an easy method of alleviating gangrenous foot infections that have destroyed the architecture of the foot. In addition, because the wound is left open to drain, lymphatics contaminated with bacteria are allowed to clear and rid the lower extremity of ascending infection. Immediately following a guillotine amputation, blood glucose is easily managed, and ketoacidosis resolves quickly, thereby facilitating metabolic and hemodynamic stabilization of the diabetic patient. After guillotine amputation, a more complete elective preoperative evaluation is undertaken before the definitive below-knee amputation is performed, generally 5 to 7 days later.

Infectious gangrene in the diabetic patient is generally polymicrobial and therefore requires administration of broad-spectrum antibiotics.[29, 31] Cultures obtained by either ulcer curettage or deep tissue biopsy are more accurate for defining the offending organisms than a superficial wound swab.[31] Even when the microbiology laboratory fails to culture anaerobic organisms, the characteristic putrid, foul-smelling odor emanating from the foot suggests their presence, including both obligate and facultative anaerobic bacteria.[30] In addition, a Gram stain of a wound specimen demonstrates a wide variety of different organisms.

Once the grossly infected and nonviable tissue has been removed by débridement or guillotine amputation, the wound must be closely observed before a definitive amputation is performed at a more proximal level. After infection is under control and sepsis has resolved, antibiotics may be discontinued. However, prior to performing the definitive below-knee amputation following resolution of sepsis, antibiotics should be given perioperatively to provide coverage for organisms cultured during the initial débridement or guillotine amputation. This helps to reduce the risk of subsequent infection in the definitive amputation stump.

SUMMARY

Lower extremity amputations are required as a consequence of acute and chronic leg ischemia as well as overwhelming infection, which occurs primarily in patients with diabetes mellitus. Although the indications for amputation differ, there are several common denominators that must be carefully considered by the surgeon prior to operation. First, the adequacy of tissue perfusion must be determined (see Chapter 149). There is no test currently available that will uniformly predict amputation healing at any given level.[32] However, before performing amputation, the surgeon must be reasonably confident that the blood supply is adequate to provide skin healing at the level of the amputation.

Second, the etiology of tissue ischemia must be determined. If acute tissue ischemia occurs as a consequence of embolism, further ischemia to the lower extremity or to other target organs may occur in the perioperative period. The surgeon must endeavor to salvage amputations at the below-knee level because rehabilitation potential is enhanced by preservation of the knee joint owing to the significantly lower energy expenditure required to ambulate with a below-knee prosthesis compared with an above-knee prosthesis.[33] Often a simple procedure such as iliac angioplasty may provide sufficient increase in blood flow to the ischemic extremity to ensure healing at the below-knee level.

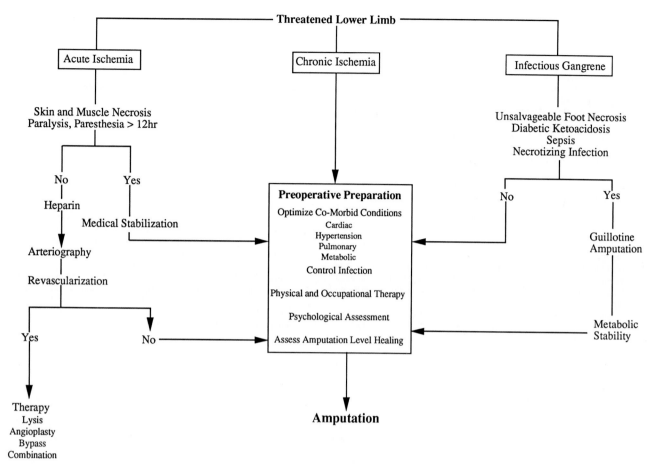

FIGURE 148–1. Algorithm for preoperative evaluation of amputation patients.

Third, infection must be eradicated prior to performing definitive amputation. This is most expeditiously accomplished by performing a guillotine supramalleolar amputation in patients with ascending infectious gangrene of the foot whose architecture has been destroyed. It is often necessary to perform this procedure emergently to achieve metabolic and hemodynamic stability in the unstable diabetic patient. However, before definitive amputation, an adequate evaluation of tissue perfusion at the proposed level of amputation should be performed.

Finally, myocardial ischemia is a major contributor to the high perioperative mortality rate associated with non-traumatic lower extremity amputations. Therefore, it is necessary to evaluate myocardial function in patients with a history of ischemic heart disease, ventricular dysfunction, or an abnormal electrocardiogram to identify those patients at greatest risk of an ischemic cardiac insult in the perioperative period. Figure 148–1 depicts an algorithm that can be applied in the setting of lower extremity amputation to direct appropriate timing of perioperative evaluation of co-morbid conditions to reduce periamputation morbidity and mortality and enhance rehabilitation and adjustment.

References

1. Veith FJ, Gupta SK, Wengerter KR, et al: Changing arteriosclerotic disease patterns and management strategies in lower-limb-threatening ischemia. Ann Surg 212:402, 1990.
2. Taylor LM Jr, Hamre D, Dalman RL, et al: Limb salvage vs amputation for critical ischemia. The role of vascular surgery. Arch Surg 126:1251, 1991.
3. Kald A, Carlsson R, Nilsson E: Major amputation in a defined population: Incidence, mortality and results of treatment. Br J Surg 76:308, 1989.
4. Roth EJ, Wiesner SL, Green D, et al: Dysvascular amputee rehabilitation. The role of continuous noninvasive cardiovascular monitoring during physical therapy. Am J Phys Med Rehabil 69:16, 1990.
5. Malone JM: Complications of lower extremity amputation. In Moore WS, Malone JM (eds): Lower Extremity Amputation. Philadelphia, WB Saunders, 1989, pp 208–214.
6. Bradway JK, Malone JM, Racy J, et al: Psychological adaptation to amputation: An overview. Orthot Prosthet 38:46, 1984.
7. Steinberg FU, Sunwoo IS, Roettger RF: Prosthetic rehabilitation of geriatric amputee patients: A follow-up study. Arch Phys Med Rehabil 66:742, 1985.
8. Bild DE, Selby JV, Sinnock P, et al: Lower-extremity amputation in people with diabetes. Epidemiology and prevention. Diabetes Care 12:24, 1989.
9. Gregory-Dean A: Amputations: Statistics and trends. Ann R Coll Surg Engl 73:137, 1991.
10. Thomas JH, Steers JL, Keushkerian SM, et al: A comparison of diabetics and nondiabetics with threatened limb loss. Am J Surg 156:481, 1988.
11. Blaisdell FW, Steele M, Allen RE: Management of acute lower extremity arterial ischemia due to embolism and thrombosis. Surgery 84:822, 1978.
12. Karmody AM, Powers SR, Monaco VJ, et al: "Blue toe" syndrome: An indication for limb salvage surgery. Arch Surg 111:1263, 1976.
13. Ljungman C, Adami HO, Bergqvist D, et al: Risk factors for early lower limb loss after embolectomy for acute arterial occlusion: A population-based case-control study. Br J Surg 78:1482, 1991.
14. Gottdiener JS, Gay JA, Van Voorhees L, et al: Frequency and embolic

potential of left ventricular thrombus in dilated cardiomyopathy: Assessment by 2-dimensional echocardiography. Am J Cardiol 52:1281, 1983.

15. Clagett GP, Graor RA, Salzman EW: Antithrombotic therapy in peripheral arterial occlusive disease. Chest 102:517S, 1992.

16. Elliott JP, Hageman JH, Szilagyi E, et al: Arterial embolization; problems of source, multiplicity, recurrence, and delayed treatments. Surgery 88:833, 1980.

17. Schilling JD, Pond GD, Mulcahy MM, et al: Catheter directed thrombolysis: An adjunct to PTA/surgery for management of peripheral vascular thromboembolic disease. Angiology (In press).

18. Tsang GMK, Crowson MC, Hickey NC, et al: Failed femorocrural reconstruction does not prejudice amputation level. Br J Surg 78:1479, 1991.

19. Ebskov LB: Lower limb amputations for vascular insufficiency. Int J Rehabil Res 14:59, 1991.

20. Harris KA, van Schie L, Carroll SE, et al: Rehabilitation potential of elderly patients with major amputations. J Cardiovasc Surg 32:463, 1991.

21. Moore TJ, Barron J, Hutchinson F III, et al: Prosthetic usage following major lower extremity amputation. Clin Orthop 238:219, 1989.

22. Brewster DC, Edwards JD: Cardiopulmonary complications related to vascular surgery. *In* Bernhard VM, Towne JB (eds): Complications in Vascular Surgery. St. Louis, Quality Medical Publishing, 1991, pp 23–41.

23. McCabe CJ, Reidy NC, Abbott WM, et al: The value of electrocardiogram monitoring during treadmill testing for peripheral vascular disease. Surgery 89:183, 1981.

24. Cutler B: Prevention of cardiac complications in peripheral vascular surgery. Surg Clin North Am 66:281, 1986.

25. Priebe M, Davidoff G, Lampman RM: Exercise testing and training in patients with peripheral vascular disease and lower extremity amputation. West J Med 154:598, 1991.

26. Finestone HM, Lampman RM, Davidoff GN, et al: Arm ergometry exercise testing in patients with dysvascular amputations. Arch Phys Med Rehabil 72:15, 1991.

27. Eagle KA, Singer DE, Brewster DC, et al: Dipyridamole-thallium scanning in patients undergoing vascular surgery. JAMA 257:2185, 1987.

28. McIntyre KE, Bailey SA, Malone JM, et al: Guillotine amputation in the treatment of nonsalvageable lower-extremity infections. Arch Surg 119:450, 1984.

29. McIntyre KE: Control of infection in the diabetic foot: The role of microbiology, immunopathology, antibiotics, and guillotine amputation. J Vasc Surg 5:787, 1987.

30. Fierer J, Daniel D, Davis C: The fetid foot: Lower extremity infections in patients with diabetes mellitus. Rev Infect Dis 1:210, 1979.

31. Sapico FL, Witte JL, Canawati HN, et al: The infected foot of the diabetic patient: Quantitative microbiology and analysis of clinical features. Rev Infect Dis 6(Suppl):S171, 1984.

32. Malone JM, Ballard JL: Complications of lower extremity amputation. *In* Bernhard VM, Towne JB (eds): Complications in Vascular Surgery. St. Louis, Quality Medical Publishing, 1991, pp 313–329.

33. Huang CT, Jackson JR, Moore NB, et al: Amputation: Energy cost of ambulation. Arch Phys Med Rehabil 60:18, 1979.

149

Lower Extremity Amputation Levels: Indications, Methods of Determining Appropriate Level, Technique, Prognosis

Joseph R. Durham, M.D.

• • •

Virtually every surgeon is presented with the unfortunate patient who has painful, dying, or infected tissue coupled with unreconstructable lower extremity arterial anatomy. Additionally, there are patients with established gangrene of an extremity such that even a patent vascular reconstruction could not revive the affected part. In such patients the surgeon must accept the multiple challenges of (1) providing the patient with an amputation that will remove the painful, infected, or dead part of the limb; (2) performing the amputation at a level that has an excellent potential for healing; (3) selecting a level of amputation that will provide the best chances for success in rehabilitation; (4) creating an amputation stump that will function in harmony with a prosthetic device; and (5) caring for the patient beyond the immediate postoperative period through

the arduous stages of rehabilitation. A thorough knowledge of the physiology of the underlying pathologic process coupled with experience with amputation and rehabilitation techniques is essential to achieve these goals.

In all instances, an experienced surgeon should be involved in the planning and execution of any amputation in a dysvascular patient. These operations should not be delegated to the novice surgeon, as so often happens. Any amputation for infection or ischemia should be regarded as a "rescue" from an egregious situation, with a potential new beginning for that patient. As Moore concluded, "A properly performed amputation cannot only be life-saving to the patient, but may often be a better therapeutic alternative than an ill-conceived, valiant, but often futile attempt at vascular reconstruction that is doomed to fail for lack of adequate recipient vessels to accommodate a distal extremity bypass."[83] The qualities essential to the successful amputation surgeon include objectivity, dedication, compassion, and technical excellence.

INDICATIONS

General indications for amputation of an ischemic lower extremity include (1) severe acute ischemia due to a truly unreconstructable arterial circulation, (2) irreversible tissue compromise by acute and prolonged ischemia, (3) unreconstructable chronic ischemia resulting in rest pain, gangrene, nonhealing skin lesions, osteomyelitis, or infection refractory to systemic antibiotics and aggressive local wound care measures, and (4) overwhelming foot sepsis in patients with diabetes mellitus (Table 149–1).

LEVEL SELECTION

Accurate selection of amputation level is of critical importance not only for morbidity and mortality results but also for rehabilitation potential. A proximal, mid-thigh amputation may deprive a patient of the opportunity for subsequent rehabilitation and ambulation, even though the amputation wound heals without difficulty. Conversely, if the amputation site is selected at too distal a level, inadequate blood supply may lead to wound dehiscence or infection, thereby requiring subsequent operative revisions to achieve healing. This latter approach is demoralizing to the patient, may result in increased morbidity and mortality, and may culminate in rehabilitation failure. Even so, more below-knee amputations should be performed than those at an above-knee level, resulting in an above-knee amputation (AKA) to below-knee amputation (BKA) ratio of less than 1.

The ultimate objective of preoperative amputation level selection is to determine the most distal site at which an amputation will heal reliably. The proposed level of amputation must accomplish removal of all infected, painful, or necrotic tissue and still yield a stump that may be readily fitted with an effective prosthesis. The objective determination of the adequacy of blood supply at the proposed amputation site is a challenging problem encountered by the amputation surgeon. Rehabilitation potential hinges on this determination because ambulation requires a *10 to 40 per cent* increase in energy expenditure for a unilateral below-knee prosthesis compared with a *50 to 70 per cent*

increase for a unilateral above-knee prosthesis.[135] Consequently, successful rehabilitation is achieved in about *70 per cent* of all below-knee amputees but in only *10 to 30 per cent* of all patients following above-knee amputation.[20, 29, 76, 109, 124]

Historically, amputations for ischemic disease were performed at above-knee level in virtually all patients; this level is still uniformly selected in some areas of the world. Although empiric above-knee amputation for ischemia does approach a 100 per cent healing rate, the overall rehabilitation potential of less than 30 per cent is unacceptable.

Many methods have been proposed to select optimum amputation levels objectively. Unfortunately, none of these methods is foolproof. The value of any objective test lies in its inherent *sensitivity*, which is its ability to predict accurately the actual presence of adequate local blood flow that would result in successful wound healing. The *specificity* of such a test is defined as its ability to detect a truly inadequate local blood flow that would lead to healing failure of the amputation stump at that level. No method of preoperative amputation level selection to assess local blood flow should be too specific, unless its sensitivity level is also high, because although it may produce 100 per cent healing rates, it may also result in unnecessarily high levels of amputation.

The following methods have been utilized for preoperative selection of amputation levels in the dysvascular patient: (1) clinical judgment, (2) Doppler systolic segmental blood pressure measurements, (3) fluorescein dye measurements, (4) laser Doppler velocimetry, (5) photoelectric skin perfusion pressures, (6) isotope measurement of skin perfusion pressures, (7) xenon-133 skin blood flow measurements, (8) skin temperature measurements, (9) transcutaneous oxygen measurements ($TcPO_2$), and (10) transcutaneous carbon dioxide measurements ($TcPCO_2$). The goal of each technique is to derive a numerical value above which all amputations will heal and below which none will heal. Suffice it to say that such an infallible technique does not presently exist. Many of these new techniques are useful guides, however.

Clinical Judgment/Empiric Amputation Level Selection

Empiric selection of the amputation site results in successful healing of roughly 80 per cent of below-knee amputations and 90 per cent of above-knee amputations.[16, 63, 70, 107] The results are even worse below the ankle, for empiric selection of this level results in a *failure* rate of 60 per cent.[119]

Most findings on physical examination are not helpful in improving the empiric healing rates just noted. Although the presence of pulses immediately above the proposed site of amputation is a good positive prognostic indicator, the absence of such a pulse does not necessarily lead to failure of healing.[51, 64, 147] Similarly, subjective assessment of skin temperature, correlation with arteriographic findings, and skin edge bleeding at the time of operation may lead to erroneous assumptions and suboptimal level selections. The only physical findings of consistent value are dependent

Table 149–1. Indications for Lower Extremity Amputation

	Percentage (Range)
Complications of diabetes mellitus	60–80
Nondiabetic infection with ischemia	15–25
Ischemia without infection	5–10
Chronic osteomyelitis	3–5
Trauma	2–5
Miscellaneous	5–10

From Malone JM: Lower extremity amputations. In Moore WS (ed): Vascular Surgery: A Comprehensive Review. 4th ed. Philadelphia: WB Saunders, 1993, p 810.

rubor and gangrene at the amputation level. Their presence indicates severe ischemia; amputation through ruborous or gangrenous skin will reliably fail and should not be performed. Unfortunately, the absence of dependent rubor does not ensure successful healing and cannot be used as a single indicator in selection of amputation level.

The value of an *experienced* clinical opinion cannot be overemphasized because objective tests are not infallible.[143] If clinical judgment contradicts laboratory values, the patient should not undergo a more proximal amputation based on vascular laboratory results alone. Amputation at a lower level should especially be attempted in a young, motivated patient, even if the findings of objective studies are marginal; in an older, sicker patient with limited rehabilitation potential, a higher level may be appropriate.[153]

Segmental Doppler Systolic Blood Pressure Measurements

Initial attempts at an objective determination of the potential for amputation wound healing employed measurement of segmental Doppler systolic blood pressures, as outlined in Chapters 4 and 5. Although this method can differentiate above-knee and below-knee amputation levels,[11, 97] its reliability and value diminish markedly for ankle, foot, and forefoot amputations.[34, 35, 82, 136, 137] Some of the problems with this technique stem from the falsely elevated pressure values that result from calcification of the arterial wall, especially in the tibial arteries of diabetics. The addition of adjunctive pulse volume recordings[34, 35, 101] and infrared photoplethysmographic determinations of toe blood pressures[4, 9, 51] helps to alleviate this shortcoming. Although these Doppler-derived segmental blood pressures are inexpensive, noninvasive, and easy to obtain, their major problem lies in their relative inability to predict which amputations will not heal. It is generally agreed that absence of *any* Doppler flow at the popliteal artery indicates that a distal amputation will not heal. Bone and Pomajzl[9] have shown that in diabetics toe blood pressures are of much greater utility than ankle-brachial ratios, with absolute pressures of less than 30 mmHg indicative of poor healing.

Fluorescein Dye Measurements

A technique utilizing ultraviolet Wood's light fluorescence in conjunction with new fiberoptic and microcomputer technology to quantitate skin blood flow based upon the measurement of local skin fluorescence was reported by Bongard and colleagues in 1984.[10] Following the intravenous injection of fluorescein dye, the skin at the proposed site of amputation is viewed with a fiberoptic fluorometer, which gives a digital numerical readout that is proportional to the amount of skin blood flow at that site. This technique appears to be applicable and reliable at all levels of amputation. When compared with segmental Doppler systolic pressures, skin fluorescence testing helps the surgeon to select a more distal level of amputation that has a high probability of healing.[79] Initial reports not only demon-

strated an optimum reference point between healing and nonhealing amputations but also led to the definition of a dye fluorescence *index* that could result in a 93 per cent accuracy for amputation level selection.[119] This test appears to be readily reproducible and is minimally invasive. For unclear reasons, however, this test has not gained widespread popularity.

Laser Doppler Velocimetry

The working principle of the laser Doppler velocimeter is derived from the fact that a laser light beam incident upon tissue is scattered by the static structures (skin) as well as by the moving components (red blood cells). According to the Doppler effect, light beams backscattered by the moving red cells undergo a frequency shift that is in proportion to the velocity of those cells. The beams scattered in the static tissue remain unshifted in frequency. These return signals are guided from the skin surface onto the probe's photodetector, extracted, and processed to produce a numerical value that is proportional to the flow in the microcirculation. This flow calculation is dependent not only upon the average velocity of the red cells but also upon the density of red cells per measured volume.

The advantage of using light as the tissue "probe" is the limited depth of penetration needed (approximately 1 mm), thus avoiding any interference from blood flow in the deeper major blood vessels, which would adversely influence accurate assay of the local microvascular flow in the skin (Fig. 149–1).

Resting measurements of cutaneous blood flow by the laser Doppler principle in dysvascular patients are in the same general range as similar measurements in patients *without* significant arterial disease. However, when the skin beneath the laser probe is heated to 44° C for 10 minutes, patients with significant arterial disease demonstrate mark-

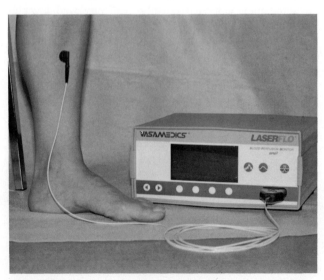

FIGURE 149–1. Laser Doppler velocimetry device with skin surface probe in place, connected to the monitor. This technique is noninvasive, reproducible, and portable. (Courtesy of Vasamedics, Inc., St. Paul, MN.)

edly diminished hyperemic responses compared with normovascular controls.[43, 46, 78] This use of local skin heating may make the laser Doppler technique more accurate as a potential preoperative assay for prediction of amputation healing. Enhanced reliability has been achieved by combining the results obtained by laser Doppler velocimetry with those derived from the transcutaneous assay of local skin oxygen tension (see the following section).[61] More recent work has suggested the utility of this technique in predicting accurately the successful healing of below-knee amputations.[139]

Photoelectric Skin Perfusion Pressure

The measurement of skin perfusion pressure may be obtained by isotope washout techniques, but these studies are time consuming and invasive and require expensive, sophisticated equipment. The photoelectric measurement of skin perfusion pressure is a less invasive and simpler means of determining skin blood flow.[47–53, 92, 125] The equipment consists of a photodetector that is placed upon the patient's skin and connected to a plethysmograph. External pressure is then applied over the photodetector with a blood pressure cuff to a suprasystolic level. As the pressure is gradually reduced at a constant rate, the plethysmographic tracing changes direction when capillary inflow begins. The skin perfusion pressure is defined as the minimum external pressure that prevents reddening of the skin after it has been blanched; this numerical value (mmHg) is the point at which the plethysmographic tracing changes direction and capillary inflow begins.[125]

In order to avoid the difficulties inherent in interpreting the tracings obtained in those patients with diminished lower extremity systolic blood pressures, a standardized reading technique has been developed such that the systolic pressure is measured directly by a strain gauge technique at the same level of the extremity at which the photoelectric tracing is being obtained.[125] Although the proponents of this technique conclude that it can replace isotope washout assays in many cases, if available, the isotope techniques should be the method of choice when technically satisfactory photoelectric tracings cannot be measured or when the systolic blood pressures cannot be accurately obtained.[92]

Isotope Measurement of Skin Perfusion Pressure

Estimation of local tissue perfusion pressure by isotope washout was originally described by Nilsen and Holstein and their associates[53, 91] using xenon-133 in muscle and skin. Holstein began with the radioisotope clearance method originally described for assay of muscle perfusion and modified it for use in skin perfusion pressure measurement, defining the skin perfusion pressure as the amount of external counterpressure necessary to stop the clearance of the intradermally injected isotope.[47]

Because xenon-133 can be trapped within the subcutaneous fat and because medical-grade xenon-133 is no longer commercially available, other isotopes have been proposed for this assay and now include sodium iodine-131, iodine-131 antipyrine, and technetium-99m pertechnetate. Several subsequent studies have verified the utility of Holstein's method.[47–50, 52, 86, 87] Although these reports do suggest that there is a correlation between isotopically derived skin perfusion pressure and successful amputation wound healing, until recently there was no discriminating skin perfusion pressure value above which all amputations would heal and below which none would heal. Data on skin perfusion pressure from the Netherlands (using a modified ^{123}I-iodoantipyrine technique) has demonstrated excellent amputation wound healing predictive values. The threshold value was 20 mmHg, with reliable healing occurring at values over 20 mmHg and poor healing occurring at values less than 20 mmHg skin perfusion pressure ($p < .001$; positive predictive value 89 per cent; negative predictive value 99 per cent).[147]

Isotope Measurement of Skin Blood Flow

Skin blood flow is determined by using an intradermal injection of xenon-133 gas that has been dissolved in saline[24, 76, 84] or an intracutaneous injection of iodine-125 iodoantipyrine;[136] the subsequent rate of isotope clearance from the point of injection is measured with a gamma camera interfaced to a minicomputer. Dual point testing with a separation of 1 cm is performed in order to eliminate injection error. As described by Malone and associates,[74, 75] the monoexponential washout rate of the intradermal xenon-133 during the first 6 minutes after injection is used to calculate the rate of skin blood flow in milliliters per minute per 100 gm of tissue.

One of the major drawbacks to the universal application of xenon-133 skin blood flow measurements for preoperative selection of amputation level has been the difficulty of reproducing results from one center to another. In addition, the technique is invasive and requires expensive, sophisticated nuclear scanning devices along with computing equipment and software. Nonetheless, in experienced hands, primary healing of amputation wounds has been accurately predicted from the toe (83 per cent success) to the below-knee level (93 per cent success), on up to the above-knee level (100 per cent success).[25, 75] These results were obtained by using the discriminate value of blood flow of 2.4 to 2.6 ml/min per 100 gm of tissue; blood flow above this level was associated with successful healing of amputations. However, Harris and associates[39] have suggested that these recommendations of the lowest flow consistent with healing have been set too high because they observed clinical success in 94 per cent of below-knee amputations with a local skin blood flow value of only 1.0 ml/min per 100 gm of tissue. A modification of this technique utilizes *epicutaneous* rather than intradermal injection of the xenon-133 with excellent results.[66] Again, the lack of availability of xenon-133 makes this test of largely historic interest.

Measurement of Skin Temperature

Although clinical assessment of the temperature of the skin by physical examination does not provide a sound basis for selection of amputation level,[51] studies have suggested that *objective* skin temperature measurement may yield valid data for preoperative selection of amputation level.[36, 122] This technique has been shown to be of particular value in discriminating between below-knee and above-knee levels with 90 per cent accuracy[36, 143] and has been correlated with isotopically derived measurements of skin blood flow.[122] Thus, thermographic mapping appears to hold considerable promise for objective preoperative amputation level selection, especially because the examinations are easily performed and may be tailored to provide a contoured isothermic map of the limb, which could be useful in the design of the amputation flaps.

Measurement of Transcutaneous Oxygen Tension ($TcPo_2$)

Use of a miniaturized, heated Clark electrode to measure the oxygen tension at the surface of the skin was reported simultaneously in 1972 by Huch and Eberhard and their associates.[26, 54] These reports led to widespread clinical application of this technique in the setting of neonatal critical care monitoring because the transcutaneous Po_2 values so derived were found to be highly correlated to more invasive arterial blood Po_2 values. Unfortunately, results were not reproducible in the adult populations.

At normal room temperature, the Po_2 on the surface of adult skin approaches zero.[28] Therefore, the clinically relevant measurements of transcutaneous oxygen rely on the maximal dilatation of the local vasculature in the upper dermis, an effect produced by local heating of the skin surface via heating the Clark electrode to 43 to 45° C. The theoretical basis of transcutaneous blood gas measurement has been presented in elegant detail by Lubbers.[72]

Several groups have reported encouraging work in the evaluation of the dysvascular patient using the modified Clark-type heated oxygen electrode.[14, 31, 41, 59, 62, 67, 77a, 78, 88, 102, 104, 123] All of these studies have suggested that the transcutaneous oxygen tension measurements can successfully predict the *healing* of a specific amputation level with a high degree of accuracy; however, the ability of $TcPo_2$ to predict accurately the *failure* to heal is not as reliable. Additionally, the failure of healing of an amputation wound may often be due to numerous perioperative factors, so that a preoperative test of any nature should not be expected to always predict the outcome with complete certainty.[102] Decreased $TcPo_2$ levels are correlated with an increased probability of failure to heal; however, even a $TcPo_2$ level of zero does not *invariably* lead to failure of amputation wound healing.

The discrepancy between $TcPo_2$ and actual skin blood flow measurements at low (less than 10 mmHg) $TcPo_2$ levels has been addressed in several studies that provide a partial explanation about why some amputations heal at low $TcPo_2$ levels that usually indicate failure.[78] Matsen and associates[78] reported that there is a nonlinear relationship between $TcPo_2$ and local cutaneous blood flow; they demonstrated that $TcPo_2$ readings of 0 mmHg were obtained in the presence of significant local cutaneous blood flow (arteriovenous gradients = 13 to 34 mmHg). $TcPo_2$ measurements are dependent on the ratio of arterial to venous gradients and vascular resistance. Heating the skin under the electrode minimizes local vascular resistance and tends to make the $TcPo_2$ measurements more parallel with the local cutaneous blood flow. Spence and associates[123] have suggested that the $TcPo_2$ values are not directly related to *actual* tissue Po_2 and thus may not represent the true local oxygen availability because oxygen extraction and utilization are significantly altered in ischemic tissue. However, they concluded that $TcPo_2$ may be closely related to the actual arterial perfusion pressure, especially in ischemic areas, since ischemic tissue is maximally vasodilated.

Other modifications to improve accuracy include $TcPo_2$ measurements while the patient is breathing supplemental oxygen[41, 85, 88, 149] and measurements following the intravenous infusion of naftidrofuryl, which increases oxydative cellular metabolism.[88] Ito and associates[59] have mapped out transcutaneous "isobars" on the lower limb based on circumferential $TcPo_2$ measurements; this technique should allow the objective preoperative modification of skin flap design to achieve maximal healing potential and to avoid any "islands of ischemia" described by Rhodes and Cogan.[103] Transcutaneous oxygen recovery half-time following temporarily induced limb ischemia has provided increased discrimination for objective evaluation of room air $TcPo_2$ values.[67] Harward[41] and Oishi[141] evaluated the accuracy of $TcPo_2$ measurements while patients were breathing room air and again while they were breathing supplemental oxygen; this technique increased the accuracy of amputation level selection at all levels. Finally, investigators at the Mayo Clinic defined successful healing of amputations as a $TcPo_2$ of more than 40 mmHg and failure of healing for $TcPo_2$ as less than 20 mmHg. In an attempt to enhance the predictability of the intervening "gray zone" of $TcPo_2$ between 20 and 40 mmHg, repeat $TcPo_2$ measurements were obtained during elevation of the lower limbs to 30 degrees for 3 minutes. *Decreases* in $TcPo_2$ of more than 15 mmHg were predictive of amputation wound healing failure, whereas *decreases* of less than 15 mmHg were usually associated with successful wound healing.[148]

Measurement of Transcutaneous Carbon Dioxide Tension ($TcPco_2$)

Most transcutaneous gas monitors now have available a combination sensor electrode that allows simultaneous monitoring of the transcutaneous carbon dioxide gas tension ($TcPco_2$) in addition to the $TcPo_2$. Less experience is available for assay of $TcPco_2$, and exact correlations among the $TcPco_2$, skin blood flow, and subsequent amputation healing have not yet been defined, thereby opening the door for future studies to determine whether the addition of $TcPco_2$ to the preoperative evaluation may assist in the selection of the optimal level of amputation.

Summary

In summary, the transcutaneous measurement of gases is a useful preoperative test to assist in the selection of the most distal amputation site that will successfully heal. Yet, the use of $TcPo_2$ and $TcPco_2$ values for such decisions requires a few caveats. First, different manufacturers of transcutaneous gas monitors often give different absolute numerical values for discriminatory purposes, making study comparisons very difficult from one institution to another. One possible solution to this problem is the use of an indexed value using the limb $TcPo_2$ or the limb $TcPco_2$ results as a numerator with a reference chest wall reading of $TcPo_2$ or $TcPco_2$ as the denominator, as described by Hauser and Shoemaker.[42] A second problem inherent in the interpretation of $TcPo_2/TcPco_2$ results is that excellent positive predictive values (approaching 100 per cent) are produced, whereas the negative predictive value is only 50 per cent.[25] This could lead to an increased number of amputations at a higher level (i.e., increased above-knee:below-knee ratio). Perhaps these problems may be resolved as more of the ongoing studies are completed. Malone and associates have reported a large experience with these tests.[77a]

AMPUTATION LEVELS: INDICATIONS, OBJECTIVE LEVEL SELECTION, TECHNIQUES, AND PROGNOSIS

General Principles

Precise surgical technique is essential to achieve optimal healing in amputations performed for complications of ischemia. As noted, one should strive to preserve the longest length stump that will reliably heal; at times, this requires a vascular reconstructive procedure prior to the planned amputation that will allow healing at a lower level, resulting in better potential for rehabilitation.

Because some amputations do follow revascularization operations,[105] atypical skin flaps are usually preferable to amputation at a more proximal site; these flaps may be mapped out preoperatively using the objective tests outlined in the previous section.

Transection of bones must be performed at a comfortable distance above the skin flaps. Appropriate beveling of angulated remnants and bony prominences should be performed exactly to create smooth contours. The periosteum should not be stripped away excessively because this may lead to bony overgrowth or sequestrum formation.

Division of small nerves should be performed sharply with firm but not excessive traction applied to the nerve trunk during transection. This allows retraction of the nerve remnant above the level of bone division, placing any subsequent neuroma well above any points of pressure. Excessive traction upon the nerve during division may lead to unnecessary neuralgia and stump pain. The blood supply to large nerves, such as the sciatic nerve, should be suture ligated proximally before transection because the vasa nervorum may cause substantial bleeding if not controlled.

Muscles may be divided sharply or with electrocautery. In either instance, hemostasis must be exact; mass ligature incorporating large clumps of tissue is unacceptable. The use of a proximal tourniquet is contraindicated during amputation of an ischemic limb. Myodesis procedures should not be performed in the amputation of an ischemic limb.

Hemostasis is essential to ensure optimal healing rates; a hematoma may elevate tenuous skin flaps or lead to subsequent infection of the hematoma. *Careful* use of electrocautery allows pinpoint control of bleeding sites. Indiscriminate use of electrocautery should be avoided to prevent damage to surrounding soft tissues. Likewise, the use of bone wax should be discouraged because it acts as a foreign body. If absolute hemostasis is not possible, the judicious use of closed system suction drains is indicated to prevent hematoma formation. Any such drains should be removed within 24 to 48 hours. Prior to closure of the wound, as hemostasis is being achieved, the wound should be thoroughly irrigated to remove clots and debris. Many surgeons use an antibiotic solution (e.g., bacitracin-kanamycin solution) for irrigation, although convincing data that "local" antibiotics are beneficial are lacking. Similarly, such an antibiotic solution should be used throughout the operation to prevent desiccation of the tissues and to keep bacterial counts down.

Closure of the skin of an amputation stump must be performed atraumatically using exact suture placement without the use of skin forceps. Perfect coaptation of the skin edges will be rewarded with enhanced rates of successful primary healing. In addition to monofilament sutures, metal staples or tape strips provide alternative, efficient, and effective means of closing the skin when atraumatic techniques with minimal use of tissue forceps are employed.

Lower limb amputation following a failed vascular reconstruction attempt may be complicated when the bypass conduit is a prosthetic material. Rubin and associates[111] documented that removal of the thrombosed graft in the presence of an infected wound or removal of an infected graft at the time of major limb amputation led to a decreased incidence of amputation wound complications and subsequent graft remnant infections. Rubin also provided evidence supporting removal of the *entire* failed prosthetic graft at the time of amputation, even if there is no evidence of wound or graft infection at that time.[112] Firm recommendation of this occasionally difficult addition to amputation awaits confirmation in other centers.

With the exception of digital or single ray level amputations, the immediate postoperative application of an exactly fitted rigid dressing leads to the most prompt and successful healing and rehabilitation of all amputations through or distal to the knee joint. The use of an immediately fitted rigid postoperative dressing does not always need to be combined with an immediate postoperative prosthesis. Of note, rigid postoperative amputation stump dressings are not panaceas and require an intimate knowledge of the technique; misuse can lead to serious wound problems. Some authors are quick to point out the disadvantages of such a rigid dressing protocol in the immediate postoperative period[19] and relate more successful postoperative courses when soft compression dressings are employed; however, such reports are old, reflect a lack of experience with rigid postoperative dressings, and are contrary to larger studies emphasizing the *team* approach that incorporates the surgeon, the prosthetist, and the physiatrist.[73]

Other important ancillary factors that may enhance the successful healing of amputations of the ischemic limb include optimal nutritional status,[24] preoperative hemodilution,[1, 32, 60] perioperative prophylactic antibiotic coverage,[55, 106, 121] and eradication of any existing septic focus. Control of the infected portion of the ischemic limb may be accomplished by using systemic intravenous antibiotics, local drainage, cryoamputation,[38, 56] or open guillotine amputation.[23, 80] Most often, a combination of these modalities is required. Surprisingly, the presence of diabetes mellitus has no significant impact on successful primary healing of major lower extremity amputations.[45, 57, 73–75] In fact, diabetics generally do better with management at an early stage. The worst patient profile is a white male nondiabetic smoker with coronary artery disease.[63, 144]

Toe Amputation

Indications

Amputation of a toe is the most commonly performed amputation of the lower limb. "Dry" gangrene is best treated by allowing autoamputation; epithelialization proceeds beneath the dead portion of the gangrenous but noninfected digit. This approach should be selected only for reliable, conscientious patients whose clinical course can be closely monitored. Also, the presence of dry gangrene permits preamputation vascular reconstruction, if warranted. However, when the gangrenous process is "wet," signifying an active infectious process that may be progressive, prompt surgical removal of all dead, infected tissue is mandatory. Antibiotics are a useful adjunct but are not to be used *alone* when the infection involves the entire toe or when osteomyelitis is present; rather, prompt digital amputation with concurrent antibiotic administration will enhance recovery and rehabilitation.[6]

Indications for toe amputation include gangrene, infection, osteomyelitis, or neuropathic ulceration that is confined to the mid or distal phalanx. Amputation of a painful but not infected ischemic toe may also be indicated.

Contraindications

Specific contraindications for the performance of an amputation at the toe level include (1) dependent rubor of the toes, (2) cellulitis proximal to the site of proposed toe amputation, (3) forefoot or plantar space infection, (4) infection or osteomyelitis involving the metatarsophalangeal joint or the metatarsal head, and (5) inadequate blood supply.

Prediction of Healing at This Level

The various methods of preoperative evaluation of the arterial circulation for amputation at the toe level are outlined in Table 149–2. Clinical findings still play a most important role in predicting the success of toe amputation.[140] Although empiric selection at this level yields a disappointing healing rate of 75 per cent in the absence of foot pulses, the presence of pedal pulses is associated with 98 per cent healing rates. If pedal pulses are not palpable,

Table 149–2.   Preoperative Level Selection: Toe Amputation

Selection Criterion	Successful Healing, Primary and Secondary/ Total (Per Cent)	Reference
Empiric	86/115 (75)	98
Presence of pedal pulses	357/365 (98)	120
Doppler toe pressure > 30 mmHg	47/60 (78)	53
Doppler ankle pressure > 35 mmHg	44/46 (96)	132
Photoplethysmographic digit or TMA pressure > 20 mmHg	20/20 (100)	116
Xenon-133 skin blood flow > 2.6 ml/100 gm tissue/ min	5/6 (83)	74

Key: *TMA, transmetatarsal.*

determination of the digit (or forefoot) systolic blood pressure via photoplethysmography is the best available predictor of healing. Further, more recent experience with photoplethysmographically derived toe, or transmetatarsal, pressures indicates that use of a systolic digital pressure of greater than 40 mmHg as the index for successful healing is the safest, most reliable prognostic parameter.[115]

Surgical Technique

Amputation of a single toe should never be performed by disarticulation through a phalangeal joint because this leads to exposure of the avascular cartilage of the proximal joint capsule; rather, the toe amputation is performed by transection of the proximal phalanx, thereby leaving a small button of bone to protect the metatarsal head. Skin flaps may be of any design (e.g., fish mouth, plantar-based, dorsally based, or side to side), but the most commonly used incision is circular (Fig. 149–2). Any flaps must be created to allow tension-free closure over the phalangeal stump.

A circular skin incision minimizes the length of the resultant wound and should help to reduce the possibility of skin edge devascularization that may occur with the construction of any type of skin flap. The incision is then

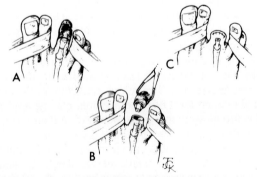

FIGURE 149–2. *A,* While the adjacent toes are retracted medially and laterally, a circular incision proximal to the proximal interphalangeal joint is made. *B,* Dissection exposes the proximal phalanx, which is divided. *C,* The circular incision is then closed in a transverse direction with interrupted, carefully placed, coapting sutures.

carried down to the phalanx, which is divided; the bony remnant may then be smoothed carefully with a rasp. Any tendinous structures must be sharply excised while they are placed on gentle traction. Electrocautery should be used sparingly, if at all. Irrigation fluid is used to cleanse the wound thoroughly. Exact hemostasis and careful, atraumatic, edge-to-edge skin closure will be rewarded with enhanced wound healing. Minimally reactive monofilament suture material is used because often these sutures must remain in place for extended time periods (3 to 4 weeks) to ensure complete wound healing. In the presence of an active infectious process, the amputation wound should be left open.

Advantages and Disadvantages of Toe Amputation

The primary advantages of simple toe amputation are the minimal amount of tissue removed and the minimal impact upon rehabilitation. Total resection of the great toe, or of *all* the toes of a given foot, however, may lead to minor imbalance during ambulation. The only disadvantage to a simple toe amputation is the risk of stump breakdown due to ischemia or intervening infection.

Prosthetic Requirements and Rehabilitation Potential

No prosthesis is required for the patient after toe amputation. The potential for rehabilitation should be 100 per cent. Amputation of all the toes of one foot causes minor disturbances in gait at a slow pace and becomes more troublesome at a fast pace because of the loss of "push-off"; also, squatting and tiptoeing are difficult or impossible. Consequently, a shoe filler is helpful for very active patients. Continued close follow-up care is essential because almost 75 per cent of these patients may require a more proximal amputation in the 3½-year period following the toe amputation.[71]

Ray Amputation

Indications

Localized gangrene or infection adjacent to the metatarsal-phalangeal crease or involving the metatarsal head precludes the performance of a simple toe amputation. In this instance, extension of the amputation to excise the metatarsal head accomplishes removal of all necrotic, infected, or compromised tissue and leaves adequate viable skin for successful wound closure without tension.

Contraindications

The presence of dependent rubor, cellulitis, infection, or gangrene proximal to the metatarsal-phalangeal crease are specific contraindications to performance of a ray amputation; osteomyelitis of a metatarsal shaft is also a contraindication to amputation at this level. Some instances of cellulitis that preclude immediate safe performance of a ray amputation may be initially treated with appropriate intra-

venous antibiotics as a first-line measure, followed by the ray amputation if the cellulitis subsides. Involvement of three or more toes presents a relative contraindication; a transmetatarsal amputation would be more suitable in this case. Ray amputation of the great toe may also be considered a relative contraindication *in the active patient* because removal of the first metatarsal head leads to unstable weight bearing, difficulties with ambulation, and late skin ulceration of the plantar surface. However, a ray amputation of the great toe is a worthwhile procedure in the patient with previously limited activity levels. Finally, caution has been advised in the performance of a ray amputation in the insensitive, dysvascular foot because these conditions may lead to a high failure rate owing to the subsequent development of a "transfer lesion." This is an ulceration resulting from abnormal weight bearing due to the transfer of pressure points following removal of a metatarsal head. When this type of ulceration develops in the ray amputee with an insensate foot, the amputation level must be revised, most often to the below-knee level.[33]

Prediction of Healing at This Level

The same preoperative objective parameters used for prediction of simple toe amputation are applicable to the evaluation of a patient for the potential success of a ray amputation (see Table 149–2).

Surgical Technique

A racquet-type incision is started with a vertical component (the "handle" of the racquet) on the dorsum of the foot to expose the metatarsal head (Fig. 149–3). This incision is then carried distally, bifurcating medially and laterally to encircle the toe; these two bifurcated limbs of the incision are then joined on the plantar aspect of the foot as a circular incision at the base of the toe (the "head" of the racquet). As the incision is taken down to the level of the

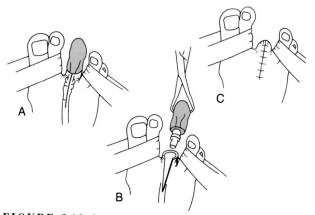

FIGURE 149–3. Artist's rendition of the steps involved in a single-ray amputation of the foot. *A*, The incision is designed to expose the distal metatarsal phalangeal region. *B*, The distal metatarsal is divided far enough proximally to permit closure without tension. *C*, Following excision of the specimen, including the intact metatarsal phalangeal joint, the dorsal portion of the incision is closed in its original direction, and the circular portion of the plantar incision is closed transversely.

bone, care must be exercised not to injure the digital arteries that course alongside the metatarsal shaft. Additional caution is employed to avoid entry into the deep tendon or joint spaces of the adjacent digits. The distal metatarsal shaft is divided at its neck, taking care to avoid damage to the adjacent tissues. Structures attached to the detached metatarsal head are divided sharply, and the intact specimen (consisting of the toe, the metatarsophalangeal joint, and the metatarsal head) may then be removed in continuity.

All tendon remnants are sharply excised as far proximally as possible. Hemostasis is achieved with careful, limited use of electrocautery. The space created by the removal of the metatarsal head is irrigated thoroughly with an antibiotic solution prior to closure of the skin. Monofilament sutures that incorporate the deep tissues are placed to coapt the skin edges exactly, or the wound may be closed in layers. A *closed* drain may be utilized only if hemostasis cannot be achieved and should be removed within 24 hours. If the metatarsal head is infected or if there is an extensive distal infection, the wound may be left open, packed, and allowed to heal by delayed primary closure or by secondary intention. A soft compression dressing will help to avoid tension on the suture line and to minimize the potential dead space in the bed of the metatarsal head.

Advantages and Disadvantages of Ray Amputation

The advantages of a ray amputation are minimal tissue loss and the absence of subsequent limitations upon activity. Disadvantages include the risks of nonhealing, chronic osteomyelitis of the metatarsal shaft remnant and hematoma or infection within the deep tissue space; certainly, these risks are minimized with proper patient selection and exacting surgical technique. Ray amputation of the great toe may lead to difficult ambulation and late plantar skin breakdown due to loss of the balance and pushoff provided by the first metatarsal head and the great toe.

Prosthetic Requirements and Rehabilitation Potential

Although no true prosthetic device is required for rehabilitation of the ray amputee, a specially constructed orthotic shoe will definitely improve the balance and minimize skin trauma for the very active patient following ray amputation of the great toe. Rehabilitation potential is 100 per cent.

Transmetatarsal and Forefoot Amputations

Indications

Gangrene or infection confined to several toes or encompassing the great toe represents the ideal indication for transmetatarsal amputation. This type of amputation may also be used if the disease process extends only a short distance past the metatarsal-phalangeal crease, provided that the plantar skin is healthy.

Contraindications

Specific contraindications to amputation at this level include (1) dependent rubor, cellulitis, lymphangitis, or osteomyelitis at the mid-foot; (2) deep forefoot (plantar space) infection; and (3) gangrene or ischemia of the plantar skin of the foot. Open transmetatarsal amputation may be successfully used in the presence of infection provided that the forefoot infectious process does not extend proximally beyond the level of the metatarsal heads and that no significant ischemia exists.[142]

Prediction of Healing at This Level

The most accurate objective techniques for preoperative determination of successful healing at the transmetatarsal level are fiberoptic fluorometry, xenon-133 (or iodine-125 iodoantipyrine) skin blood flow assay, and transcutaneous oxygen and carbon dioxide measurements (Table 149–3). Doppler ankle systolic blood pressure measurements are useful as a second-line technique if these tests are not available; however, these Doppler-derived pressures suffer from a lack of sensitivity, and the absolute ankle systolic pressure required to predict reliable healing success is at least 60 to 70 mmHg. If the objective tests listed earlier are not available, photoplethysmographic toe pressures of greater than 55 mmHg offer the most reliable guide to successful transmetatarsal amputation healing.

Surgical Technique

Excellent descriptions of the technique of transmetatarsal amputation have been presented by McKittrick and Effeney and their colleagues.[27, 81] The skin incision is designed to utilize a total plantar flap with virtually no dorsal skin flap component. A slightly curved dorsal incision is carried from one side of the foot to the other, just distal to the anticipated line of bone transection at the mid-portion of the metatarsal shafts. The incision extends to the base of the toes medially and laterally in the mid-plane axis of the foot and then extends across the plantar surface at the metatarsal-phalangeal crease (Fig. 149–4). Once the skin incision has been sharply defined, the dorsal component is carried down to the metatarsal shafts, which are transected 5 to 10 mm proximal to the line of the skin incision using a power oscillating saw with a small blade. The bony ends are carefully smoothed with a rasp if necessary.

The plantar tissues of the distal forefoot are sharply excised from the metatarsal shafts. Tendons are sharply transected under tension and are allowed to retract into the depths of the foot. The plantar skin flap is then tailored and thinned sharply to achieve a natural fit when it is rotated dorsally for closure. The avascular volar plates are sharply excised, as is any redundant muscle or fat. Meticulous hemostasis is essential; exacting use of electrocautery is preferable to the use of bone wax. Thorough irrigation with an antibiotic solution precedes closure of the deep tissues with a layer of absorbable interrupted sutures. Finally, a tension-free skin closure is performed using monofilament sutures in a vertical mattress technique. If there is tension present along the suture line at this point, the closure must be

Table 149–3. Preoperative Level Selection: Foot and Forefoot Amputation

Selection Criterion		Successful Healing, Primary and Secondary/ Total (Per Cent)	Reference
Empiric		11/24 (46)	98
		36/50 (72)	136
Doppler ankle pressure	< 40 mmHg	5/9 (56)	82, 136
	> 40 mmHg	20/60 (33)	8
	40–60 mmHg	4/5 (80)	136
	> 50 mmHg	14/21 (66)	53
	> 60 mmHg	68/91 (75)	82, 136
	> 70 mmHg	70/93 (75)	2, 90, 116
Doppler toe pressure	> 30 mmHg	4/5 (80)	53
Doppler ankle-brachial pressure index	> 0.45 (nondiabetic) > 0.50 (diabetic)	58/60 (97)	96
Photoplethysmographic toe pressure	> 55 mmHg	14/14 (100)	9
	> 45 < 55 mmHg	2/8 (25)	9
	< 45 mmHg	0/8 (0)	9
Fiberoptic fluorometry (Dye fluorescence index > 44)		18/20 (90)	119
Laser Doppler velocimetry		2/6 (33)	46
I-125 iodopyrine skin blood flow > 8 ml/100 gm tissue/min		18/18 (100)	136
Xenon-133 skin blood flow > 2.6 ml/100 gm tissue/min		23/25 (92)	25
Transcutaneous Po_2 > 10 mm (or a > 10 mm increase on $FIo_2 = 1.0$)		6/8 (75)	41
Transcutaneous Po_2 > 28 mmHg		3/3 (100)	25
Transcutaneous Pco_2 < 40 mmHg		3/3 (100)	25

revised by shortening the metatarsal shafts sufficiently to allow an absolutely tension-free wound closure.

The completed stump is then dressed with sterile bandages and protected by a well-padded short leg plaster cast. Such a rigid dressing helps to control edema and to prevent trauma to the vulnerable transmetatarsal stump. Ambulation on the amputated limb is not allowed for at least 7 to 10 days, at which time a cast change routine is initiated. Sutures are usually left intact for 3 to 4 weeks.

Once it has completely healed, the transmetatarsal amputation wound results in a very durable stump. Stumps thought to be at high risk for subsequent infection or wound breakdown may be left open (Fig. 149–5A). Rapid wound closure and rehabilitation may be accomplished by a partial-thickness skin graft placed on the open transmetatarsal stump when it is clean and covered by granulation tissue. Any ischemic or infectious process must be corrected for this approach to be successful. With time, wound contracture can lead to complete closure of the skin defect created by the open transmetatarsal amputation without the need for a potentially vulnerable partial-thickness skin graft (Fig. 149–5B).

Advantages and Disadvantages

The main advantage of a well-healed transmetatarsal amputation is its excellent function with minimal, if any, disability. It avoids the equinus and equinovalgus deformities inherent in the performance of the more proximal midfoot amputations:[130] (1) Lisfranc's amputation—forefoot disarticulation between the tarsal and metatarsal bones; (2) Chopart's amputation—forefoot disarticulation at the talonavicular and calcaneocuboid joints; and (3) Pirogoff's amputation—formal ankle disarticulation in which the talus is separated from the tibia and fibula, which are then tran-

sected immediately above the joint surface. These three mid-foot amputations are rarely indicated in the dysvascular patient.

The main disadvantage of a transmetatarsal amputation is the risk of nonhealing due to ischemia, infection, trauma, or hematoma, thereby requiring a subsequent revision to a higher level. When the appropriate objective preoperative

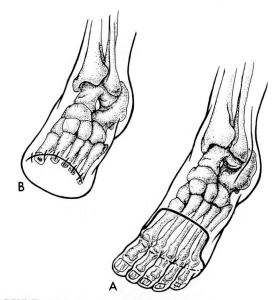

FIGURE 149–4. Illustration of the steps in a transmetatarsal amputation of the forefoot. *A*, The skin incision is placed to provide a total posterior flap while allowing excision of the forefoot with division through all five metatarsals in the mid-metatarsal region. *B*, Following excision of the forefoot, the plantar flap is thinned to remove capsule and tendinous material, and a meticulous closure of the plantar and anterior skin is performed.

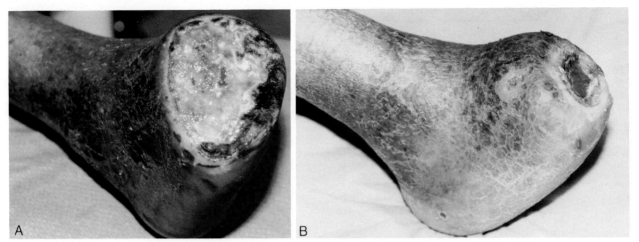

FIGURE 149–5. *A*, Open transmetatarsal amputation stump resulting from resection of all gangrenous and infected tissue in a patient with an advanced diabetic forefoot infection. *B*, The same patient 9 months later with almost complete wound closure owing to wound contraction. This patient was fully ambulatory.

tests to forecast healing potential are used, these risks are minimized. An open transmetatarsal amputation is a safe surgical option that is preferable to a mid-foot or below-knee amputation for the treatment of severe forefoot infection or gangrene, even if the distal plantar skin flap is nonviable. However, in some instances, the disease process precludes amputation at the transmetatarsal level. In these situations, a more proximal mid-foot procedure may be considered *if ischemia is absent or correctable* (Fig. 149–6).[150–152] Transmetatarsal amputation through neuropathic skin has a higher risk of developing a subsequent mal perforans ulceration than does one in the normally sensate

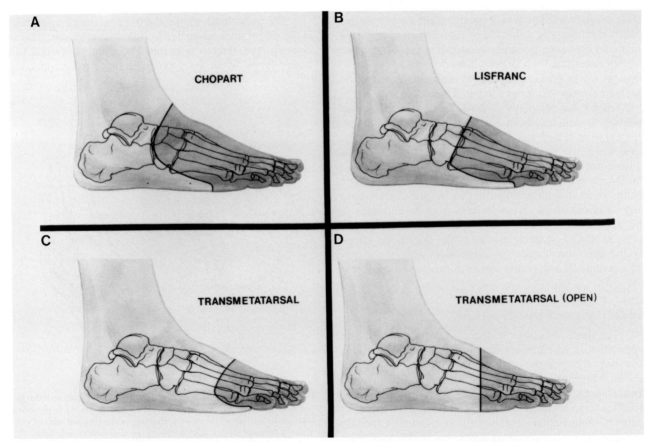

FIGURE 149–6. *A–D*, The various skin flaps required for closure of mid-foot and forefoot amputations. (*A–D*, From Durham JR, McCoy DM, Sawchuk AP, et al: Open transmetatarsal amputation in the treatment of severe foot infections. Am J Surg 158:128, 1989.)

foot.[81] Adjunctive revascularization enhances the rate of successful healing in the marginally ischemic limb.[145]

Prosthetic Requirements and Rehabilitation Potential

No specific prosthesis is required for adequate ambulation following transmetatarsal amputation, but a shoe modification incorporating a steel shank into the sole of the shoe will allow normal toe pushoff and will prevent excessive dorsiflexion. The steel spring shank reproduces the action of the longitudinal arch of the foot during ambulation. A custom-molded foam pad, lamb's wool, or a toe block is used to fill the toe portion of the shoe to prevent shoe buckling. A second shoe modification option is the creation of a custom-molded shoe that utilizes a roller-shaped sole to provide the toe pushoff motion during ambulation.[76] Forefoot amputations require only alterations in footwear in most instances. Aggressive physical therapy minimizes the chances of equinus or varus deformities that are sometimes associated with more proximal forefoot amputations.

There are no limitations on rehabilitation following transmetatarsal amputation, provided suitable footwear is furnished. Proper construction and fit will help to avoid subsequent problems with neuropathic ulceration and stump breakdown.

Syme's Amputation

Indications

The overall indications for a Syme amputation are generally the same as those for a transmetatarsal amputation, except that the Syme amputation does not require healthy plantar skin distally. The ideal indication for the performance of a Syme amputation is a distal forefoot or toe infection that involves the distal plantar skin, thereby precluding the performance of a transmetatarsal amputation. In this situation, an ankle-level amputation is indicated, as long as prognostic tests suggest a reasonable chance of successful healing. In the ischemic limb, the Syme amputation is preferable to the slightly more distal amputations of Lisfranc and Chopart and the above-ankle level amputation of Pirogoff. Two series report credible results using these techniques.[89, 96] However, healing of the Syme amputation is dependent on good blood supply to the skin flap via the posterior tibial artery, and thus this amputation is rarely indicated, or appropriate, in the truly ischemic limb.

Contraindications

Any abnormality of the heel or heel pad constitutes a contraindication to the performance of the Syme amputation: (1) gangrene or infection involving the heel, (2) an open lesion of the heel or ankle, or (3) dependent rubor, cellulitis, or lymphangitis of the heel. Pedal neuropathy in a diabetic patient that involves the heel is an absolute contraindication to amputation at this level because the absence of sensation invariably leads to eventual stump breakdown and failure. Moreover, the presence of diabetes mellitus should represent a relative contraindication to the Syme amputation because of the risk of subsequent development of distal neuropathy and ulceration of the stump, even after initial success. Malone reported[77] eventual long-term failure of the Syme amputation in 17 of 32 diabetic patients (53 per cent) who initially enjoyed successful postoperative healing and rehabilitation.

Prediction of Healing at This Level

The same objective parameters used preoperatively to predict the healing of foot and forefoot amputations are useful in the patient being considered for the Syme amputation (see Table 149–3).

Surgical Technique

The Syme amputation is indisputably one of the most demanding and least forgiving lower extremity amputations from a technical standpoint. Exacting attention to surgical details is crucial for its success because the skin flap is easily devascularized and the heel pad can migrate posteriorly if it is not properly affixed to the tibia and fibula. The two-stage Wagner's modification is superior to the classic one-stage Syme amputation[40] in the patient with ischemia of the lower extremity; the two-stage procedure also yields a less bulbous, more cosmetic, more easily fitted stump than does the one-stage technique. Wagner has described both techniques in elegant detail.[134]

The skin incision is planned to create a single long posterior flap incorporating the heel pad; the incision for the two-stage technique is begun 1 to 1.5 cm more distally than that for the classic Syme amputation to allow for the additional volume of the retained malleoli. The dorsal incision extends across the ankle from the tip of the medial malleolus to the tip of the lateral malleolus (Fig. 149–7). The plantar incision begins at a 90-degree angle from the dorsal incision and courses around the plantar aspect of the foot distal to the heel pad, cutting all layers to the bone. The dorsal incision is then carried through the subcutaneous tissues to the bone without dissection in the tissue planes. The tendons are sharply transected under tension and are allowed to retract. The anterior tibial artery is ligated. The capsule of the tibial-talar joint is entered across the dorsum of the talar neck. After dividing the posterior tibialis tendon, the foot is forced into plantar flexion, providing increased exposure of the tibial-talar joint. The mediolateral collateral ligaments are then divided, allowing the talus to be dislocated. Great caution must be exercised during dissection along the medial malleolus to avoid damage to the posterior tibial artery, which provides the only blood supply to the heel pad flap. The peroneus brevis and tertius tendons are transected. Beginning on its superolateral surface, the calcaneus is sharply dissected from the heel pad. At this point, direct inspection of the posterior tibial vascular bundle permits its transection *distal* to its branching into the medial and lateral plantar branches. Continued dissection distally allows medial retraction of the vascular bundle and medial dissection of the calcaneus. Transection of the

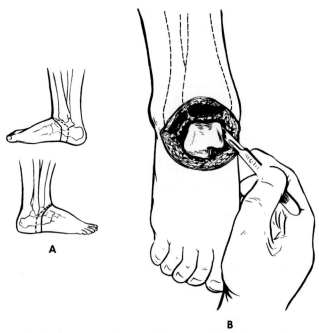

FIGURE 149–7. *A*, Incision for two-stage technique is 1–1.5 cm more distal than classic Syme's amputation to allow for volume of malleoli. *B*, Collateral ligaments are divided side to side to allow talus to dislocate distally. (*A* and *B*, Reproduced by permission from Wagner FW Jr: The Syme amputation. *In* Atlas of Limb Prosthetics: Surgical and Prosthetic Principles. American Academy of Orthopaedic Surgeons. St. Louis, 1981, The CV Mosby Co.)

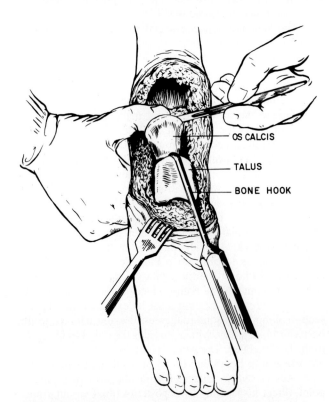

FIGURE 149–8. Care must be taken not to buttonhole skin when dividing the Achilles tendon, which is almost subcutaneous at this point. (Reproduced by permission from Wagner FW Jr: The Syme amputation. *In* Atlas of Limb Prosthetics: Surgical and Prosthetic Principles. American Academy of Orthopaedic Surgeons. St. Louis, 1981, The CV Mosby Co.)

Achilles tendon at its insertion to the calcaneus is performed with great care because at this point the tendon is virtually subcutaneous; penetration, or "buttonholing," of the skin at this step may lead to failure of wound healing (Fig. 149–8). Excision of the forefoot is completed by subperiosteal dissection of the calcaneus and division of the plantar aponeurosis.

Hemostasis is achieved and thorough irrigation of the wound is performed. A closed suction drainage tube is introduced through a separate small incision and is placed within the joint cavity. The heel pad is rotated anteriorly and placed against the malleoli and plafond; it is tailored to the exact length to enable a tension-free closure. The deep fascia over the anterior tibia and the remnants of the collateral ligaments are sutured to the deep fascia of the plantar flap. A single layer of monofilament interrupted vertical mattress sutures is used to complete the atraumatic skin closure. Either a soft compression dressing or a rigid plaster cast is used as the postoperative dressing; most authorities prefer a short leg plaster cast, which helps to maintain the correct alignment of the heel pad and helps to avoid trauma to the stump. Caution must be exercised with the use of a rigid dressing to avoid injury to the medial and lateral skin flaps, or "dog ears" (Fig. 149–9).

Most patients have adequate healing at about 6 weeks, and the second and definitive stage of the amputation may be performed at this time. Two elliptical incisions are made over the malleoli to remove the dog ears (Fig. 149–10). The amount of tissue removed must be equal to the volume of each malleolus. Sharp dissection is carried down to the bone, taking care not to damage the posterior tibial vascular bundle along the posteromedial aspect; close dissection around the medial malleolus will protect these vessels. Following periosteal resection, the malleoli are removed flush with the joint surface; the tibial articular cartilage is not disturbed (Fig. 149–11). The distal tibia and fibula are then exposed in a subperiosteal plane to a point 3 to 6 cm above the ankle joint; the tibial and fibular flares are removed with an osteotome and smoothed with a rongeur. This step results in a relatively square stump that subsequently simpli-

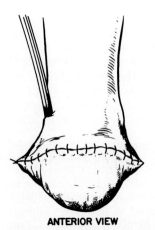
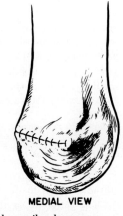

ANTERIOR VIEW   **MEDIAL VIEW**

FIGURE 149–9. No attempt is made to tailor dog ears at closure of first stage. Further posterior dissection narrows base of flap and jeopardizes its circulation. (Reproduced by permission from Wagner FW Jr: The Syme amputation. *In* Atlas of Limb Prosthetics: Surgical and Prosthetic Principles. American Academy of Orthopaedic Surgeons. St. Louis, 1981, The CV Mosby Co.)

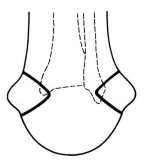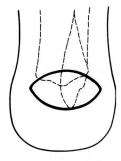

ANTERIOR   MEDIAL–LATERAL

FIGURE 149–10. Second-stage Syme's amputation. Elliptical incision removes tissue equal in volume to bone removed. (Reproduced by permission from Wagner FW Jr: The Syme amputation. *In* Atlas of Limb Prosthetics: Surgical and Prosthetic Principles. American Academy of Orthopaedic Surgeons. St. Louis, 1981, The CV Mosby Co.)

fies prosthetic fitting (Fig. 149–12). In closing the wounds, the heel pad must be anchored to bone; if the heel pad is loose following the removal of the malleoli, it must be secured to the tibia and fibula through drill holes. The skin is then closed with monofilament sutures, and a soft compression dressing, or rigid cast dressing, is applied to maintain the proper heel pad alignment.[76, 95, 134] Rehabilitation is initiated with a 3-week period of non–weight-bearing status followed by 3 to 4 weeks of a short leg walking cast.

Advantages and Disadvantages

The advantages of a well-healed Syme amputation are that rehabilitation is usually successful owing to minor increases in energy consumption over normal bipedal ambulation.[135] For daily use, a standard below-knee patellar-tendon–bearing (PTB) prosthesis is used; the stump is not sufficiently durable for long periods of end–weight-bearing. However, no prosthesis is required for short walks inside the home, such as a trip to the bathroom at night.

The disadvantages of amputation at the Syme level all stem from wound healing complications; hematoma formation and secondary infection are all too common. Failure of healing at this level leads invariably to reamputation at the below-knee level. As mentioned previously, a further problem with the Syme amputation in the diabetic patient is that progressive neuropathy at a later date may create problems in the Syme amputation stump.

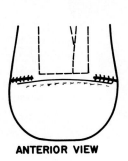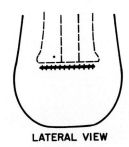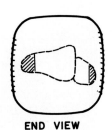

ANTERIOR VIEW   LATERAL VIEW   END VIEW

FIGURE 149–12. Second-stage Syme's amputation. Removal of malleoli and distal flare through lateral and medial incisions. (Reproduced by permission from Wagner FW Jr: The Syme amputation. *In* Atlas of Limb Prosthetics: Surgical and Prosthetic Principles. American Academy of Orthopaedic Surgeons. St. Louis, 1981, The CV Mosby Co.)

FIGURE 149–11. Second-stage Syme's amputation. Malleoli are removed flush with joint surface. Central cartilage is not disturbed. (Reproduced by permission from Wagner FW Jr: The Syme amputation. *In* Atlas of Limb Prosthetics: Surgical and Prosthetic Principles. American Academy of Orthopaedic Surgeons. St. Louis, 1981, The CV Mosby Co.)

Prosthetic Requirements and Rehabilitation Potential

As noted, the typical Syme amputee requires a PTB prosthesis consisting of a plastic foot and a lightweight plastic shell that incorporates the lower leg and stump. Ambulation around the home or for limited short distances may also be achieved using a simple strap-on cap slipper with a built-up heel. Since ambulatory energy consumption is, at most, 10 per cent above that of a nonamputee, no significant disability should be expected in the Syme amputee who has a well-healed stump and a well-fitted prosthesis. Most Syme-level amputees can resume normal daily and work activities.

Below-Knee Amputation

Indications

Amputation below the knee joint is indicated in patients who have gangrene, infection, unreconstructable rest pain, or nonhealing ulcerations of the foot that preclude a more distal amputation. A below-knee amputation should be considered as a first choice over a Syme amputation in the diabetic patient, as outlined earlier. Below-knee amputation is indicated as the definitive procedure following an initial staged open ankle guillotine amputation in the treatment of unsalvageable lower limb infections.[23, 80]

Contraindications

Any patient with a fixed flexion contracture of the knee of 15 degrees or more should not undergo below-knee amputation because prosthetic fit is impossible and the stump is subject to decubitus ulceration in the bedridden patient. Such knee flexion contractures are most common among stroke victims, demented patients, and in those with severe, chronic rest pain who have adopted the curled "fetal" position as a response to the chronic pain. Patients who are totally bedridden with no chance for ambulation should rarely undergo a below-knee amputation because the risk of nonhealing is not warranted in this population; rather, a through-knee disarticulation or a long above-knee amputation provides substantial limb leverage for mobility in bed but does not risk stump decubitus ulceration or breakdown should the patient develop a knee flexion contracture.

A gangrenous or infectious process that extends close to the tibial tuberosity or that encompasses the proposed skin flap consistently results in failure of a primarily closed amputation at the below-knee level, as does amputation through ruborous, cellulitic, or gangrenous skin. One technique that may allow salvage of the knee joint in infected cases is the performance of an open ankle guillotine amputation with concurrent administration of sensitivity-directed antibiotics; this may allow regression of the cellulitis to a point distal to the proposed skin flap margins, thus permitting safe performance of a below-knee amputation at a later date. Moreover, a patient who has been rid of systemic sepsis is more stable and is a much safer operative risk.[23, 80]

On occasion, especially in patients with trauma or gangrene due to hypotension and vasopressors, a sharp delineation between healthy skin and nonviable skin appears; this line of demarcation may prevent the creation of standard musculocutaneous flaps for primary closure of an amputation. With careful selection, an *open* below-knee amputation may be performed; retraction of the wound edges is minimized by gentle traction applied by skin hooks or even old-fashioned Buck's skin traction. Closure of the wound is subsequently accomplished by using partial-thickness skin grafts (Fig. 149–13). Because contemporary below-knee amputation prostheses place the weight burden on the patellar tendon and the femoral condyles, not the end of the stump, the skin graft covering the stump is not compromised.

A final contraindication to amputation at the below-knee level is the discovery by preoperative objective tests that the local blood flow is inadequate. These objective measurements are especially important when clinical ex-

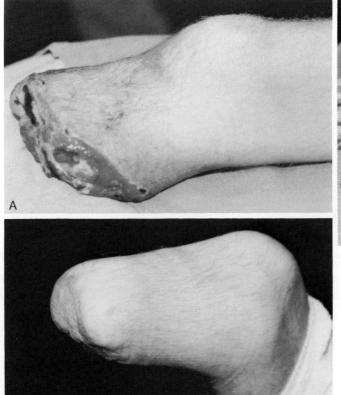
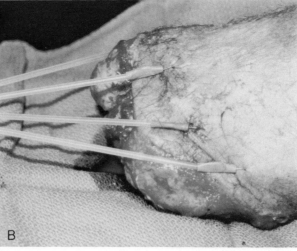

FIGURE 149–13. Series of photographs depicting the course of an open below-knee amputation performed for gangrene following disseminated intravascular coagulation due to systemic *Legionella* sepsis in a young carpenter. *A*, Proximal open below-knee amputation just proximal to eventual sharp line of demarcation between healthy skin and gangrenous tissue. *B*, Traction applied to skin wound edges by hooks placed under gentle traction (5 pounds). *C*, Result at 6 weeks following partial-thickness skin graft. Patient is now undergoing rehabilitation on bilateral below-knee prostheses.

amination of the patient indicates questionable healing potential.

It must be emphasized that *age* alone is not a contraindication to amputation at the below-knee level; impressive success may be achieved in the geriatric amputee who was ambulatory prior to the below-knee amputation.[15, 20, 64, 124]

Prediction of Healing at This Level

Because the below-knee amputation is the highest level of amputation at which rehabilitation potential is still good and above which rehabilitation attempts are poor, every patient in whom there is a *reasonable* chance of healing an amputation at the below-knee level should be offered this procedure. On the other hand, performance of a below-knee amputation in the patient with little chance of successful healing will result in the added morbidity and mortality that accompany wound breakdown, possible sepsis, and a setback in overall rehabilitation. The methods of planning below-knee versus above-knee amputation are listed in Table 149–4.

The tests available at this time for preoperative evaluation of the prospective below-knee amputee include fiberoptic fluorometry, laser Doppler velocimetry, photoelectric and radioisotope measurement of skin perfusion pressure, xenon-133 skin blood flow, and transcutaneous assay of oxygen and carbon dioxide. Table 149–4 shows that these methods are fairly comparable in accuracy. The particular test utilized will depend on the equipment and facilities available. Multi-sensor transcutaneous oximetric mapping of the anterior and posterior skin of the leg, particularly compared with skin $TcPO_2$ values at a reference site, is an accurate method of predicting successful wound healing after below-knee amputation.[146] If all these testing modalities are unavailable, careful interpretation of Doppler segmental systolic arterial blood pressures is a useful second-line technique.[11] When implemented properly, any of the objective tests will increase successful healing rates compared with the 80 per cent success that one may achieve by nothing more than *empiric* selection of the below-knee level for the site of amputation.

Surgical Technique

Design of the skin flaps for closure of the below-knee amputation depends on the distribution of gangrenous or infected tissues, the presence of surgical scars, and documented "islands of ischemia."[103] Three basic skin flap designs are utilized in the vast majority of below-knee amputations in the dysvascular patient: (1) equal length anterior and posterior flaps (fish mouth flaps), (2) the creation of a long posterior myocutaneous flap based on the underlying gastrocnemius and soleus muscles, and (3) the creation of equal length medial and lateral myocutaneous flaps via sagittal incisions. However, since open wounds or surgical incisions may exist at the time of amputation, ingenious atypical skin flap design is preferable to amputation at a more proximal level.

The long posterior flap technique is most commonly used owing to theoretical considerations related to the marginal blood supply to the ischemic leg. The theory is that the blood supply to the posterior gastrocnemius-soleus muscle group is usually better than that to the anterior compartment of the leg.[22, 131] Thus, according to this concept, the equal length anterior and posterior flap technique should exhibit higher failure rates. However, recent studies chal-

Table 149–4.   Preoperative Level Selection: Below-Knee Amputation

Selection Criterion		Successful Healing, Primary and Secondary/ Total (Per Cent)	Reference
Empiric		794/974 (82)	16, 63, 70, 98, 107
Doppler ankle pressure	< 30 mmHg	66/70 (94)	90, 101
Doppler calf pressure	> 50 mmHg	36/36 (100)	138
	> 68 mmHg	96/97 (99)	3, 6, 90
Doppler thigh pressure	> 100 mmHg	31/31 (100)	69
	> 80 mmHg	104/113 (92)	4, 35, 138
Fluorescein dye		24/30 (80)	79
Fiberoptic fluorometry (dye fluorescence index > 44)		12/12 (100)	119
Laser Doppler velocimetry		33/34 (97)	46, 139
Skin perfusion pressure			
Pertechnetate-99m		24/26 (92)	49
I-131 or I-125 antipyrine > 30 mm		60/62 (97)	51
Photoelectric skin perfusion pressure > 20 mm		60/71 (85)	92, 125
Xenon-133 skin blood flow			
Epicutaneous > 0.9 ml/100 gm tissue/min		14/15 (93)	17, 66
Intradermal > 2.4 ml/100 gm tissue/min		83/89 (93)	25, 44, 74, 118
Intradermal > 1.0 ml/100 gm tissue/min		11/12 (92)	39
Transcutaneous Po_2 = 0		0/3 (0)	14
> 10 mmHg (or > 10 mm Hg increase on FIo_2 = 1.0)		76/80 (95)	31, 41
> 10 but < 40 mmHg		5/7 (71)	25
> 20 mmHg		25/26 (96)	18
> 35 mmHg		51/51 (100)	14, 25, 62, 102
Transcutaneous Po_2 index > 0.59		17/17 (100)	62
Transcutaneous Pco_2 < 40 mmHg		7/8 (88)	25

lenge this contention and report excellent healing rates using the equal length anterior and posterior flap technique[30] and using sagittal incisions to create equal length medial and lateral myocutaneous flaps.[93, 127] Holloway and Burgess[44] reported a series of long posterior flap closures that were studied with the xenon-133 clearance skin blood flow method. They found that the postoperative blood flow of the posterior flap was actually lower than that of the undissected anterior skin flap.

Theoretical concerns notwithstanding, most surgeons report excellent results using the posterior myocutaneous flap method. The equally based sagittal incision flap method is useful in patients with infection, ischemia, or necrosis involving the boundaries of a proposed posterior flap. In both techniques, it is imperative that all vascular collaterals and vessels between the skin and the underlying muscle be preserved by avoiding any dissection along tissue planes; the creation of a myocutaneous flap preserves these essential blood vessels. One isolated study reported that plugging the medullary canal of the tibial stump with cortex of the removed bone led to a 67 per cent increase in blood flow to the amputation stump musculature.[94] These results have not been reproduced in other centers.

Because the long posterior myocutaneous flap technique is most commonly used and is the basis for comparison of other techniques, its construction is outlined in the following text. Details of the sagittal incision method for creating equal length medial and lateral myocutaneous flaps are described fully by Persson.[93]

For the routine below-knee amputation, the level of tibial transection is generally 10 to 12 cm below the tibial tuberosity (approximately one hand's breadth, including the thumb). When indicated by local disease processes, this may be shortened. The *absolute* minimum bone length for a functional below-knee amputation is just below the tibial tuberosity because the insertion of the patellar tendon *must* be preserved for knee extension. The skin incision should be placed about 1 cm distal to the planned level of tibial transection. Preincision measurement and outline of the skin flaps have been described by Sanders and Augspurger (Fig. 149–14).[114]

The skin incision is begun on the anterior surface of the leg and is carried down to the tibia; it then follows the marked outline laterally and medially before turning distally, initially penetrating only the skin and superficial fascia. The muscles of the anterior compartment are then divided, and the anterior tibial neurovascular bundle is identified, suture ligated proximally, and divided. Following circumferential scoring of the periosteum of the tibia, a periosteal elevator is used to mobilize the periosteum to a point just proximal to the site of planned bone division. The tibia is then divided in a steep bevel to avoid pressure on the overlying skin. The fibula is then transected at a point 1 to 2 cm proximal to the tibial stump.

Once the bony structures have been divided, the posterior tibial and common peroneal neurovascular bundles are identified; the arteries, veins, and nerves are suture ligated and divided. The posterior flap is then created, leav-

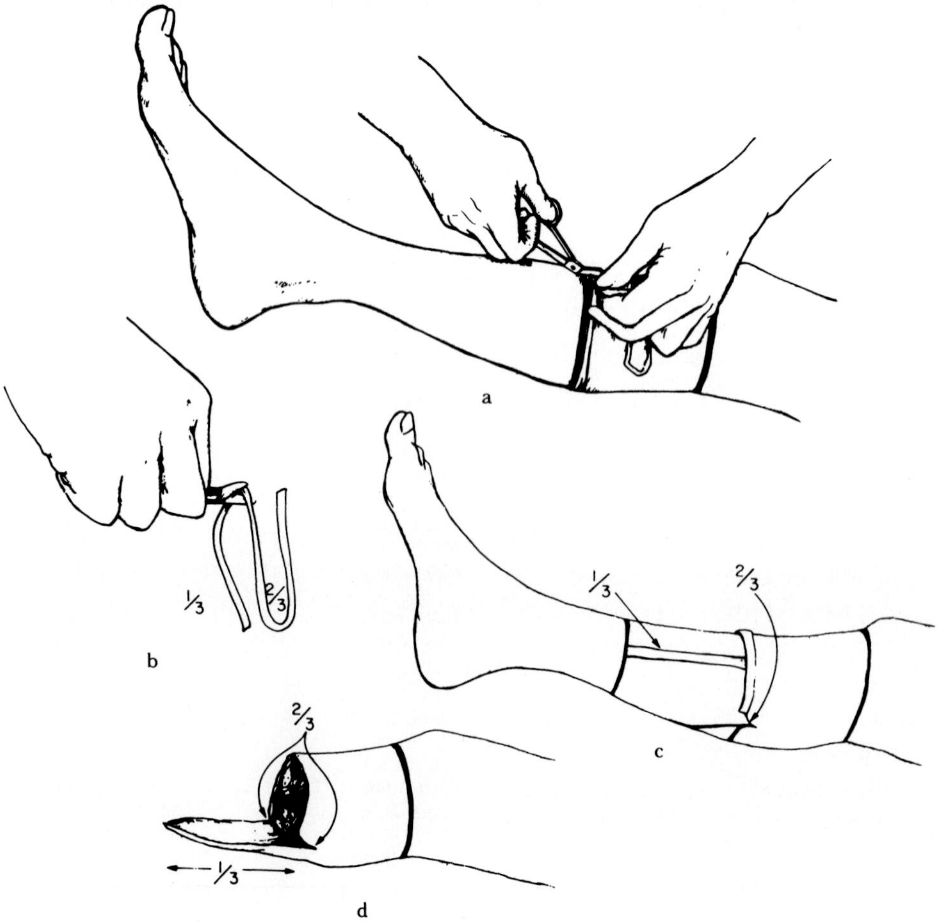

FIGURE 149–14.
Technique for measuring the length of skin flaps in below-knee amputations. *a*, Umbilical tape or string is used to measure the circumference of the leg at the point of bone transection. *b*, Tape is divided in one-third and two-third lengths. *c*, The one-third piece measures the length of the posterior flap. The two-thirds piece measures the length of the anterior incision. Dog ears at each corner are avoided by cutting a curved triangle of skin from the anterior flap. *d*, The completed amputation before closure. (*a–d*, From Sanders RJ, Augspurger R: Skin flap measurement for below-knee amputation. Surg Gynecol Obstet 145:740, 1977. By permission of Surgery, Gynecology & Obstetrics.)

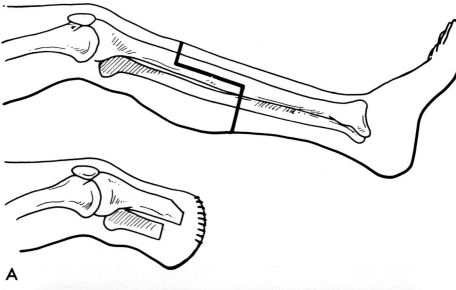

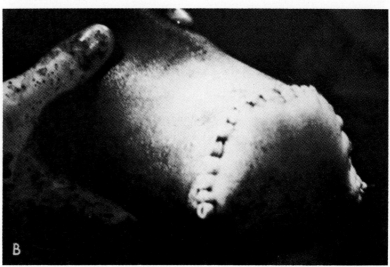

FIGURE 149–15. *A*, The standard posterior flap below-knee amputation. Notice the beveled tibia and the proximal shortening of the fibula compared with the tibia. *B*, An intraoperative photograph showing a below-knee amputation. Notice the skin coaptation with interrupted sutures and the minimal dog ears. (*A* and *B*, From Malone JM, Goldstone J: Lower extremity amputation. *In* Moore WS [ed]: Vascular Surgery: A Comprehensive Review. 2nd ed. Orlando, FL, Grune & Stratton, 1986, p 1165.)

ing the gastrocnemius and soleus muscles as the base of the myocutaneous flap. The posterior muscle mass may require additional tailoring to form a flap that may be readily rotated anteriorly to appose the anterior skin over the tibia. This beveling of the muscle flap must remove enough muscle so that the end of the stump is not bulbous, but caution must be exercised not to thin it so much that the tibia will have inadequate soft tissue coverage. The distal tibia is then beveled at a 45- to 60-degree angle, and all bony surfaces are smoothed with a rasp (Fig. 149–15).

Complete hemostasis is essential, followed by thorough irrigation with an antibiotic solution. A drain is usually not needed for amputations of an ischemic limb, but should one be required, it should be a closed suction drain because the use of Penrose-type drains may cause wound disruption.[60]

The posterior muscle flap is then rotated anteriorly, and the muscle fascia of the posterior flap is sewn to the anterior fascia using interrupted absorbable suture material. The skin edges are then atraumatically and exactly approximated using interrupted vertical mattress monofilament su-

tures, metal staples, or subcuticular sutures with sterile tapes for skin closure.

The use of a rigid postoperative dressing that incorporates the knee is ideal regardless of whether an immediate postoperative prosthesis is planned; a rigid dressing helps minimize edema, promote healing, protect the stump in the vulnerable immediate postoperative period, and prevent development of a flexion contracture. When used by a coordinated team of surgeons, prosthetists, and physiatrists, the use of immediate postoperative rigid dressings sets the standard for the optimal initiation of rehabilitation of the below-knee amputee.[73]

For those surgeons not thoroughly familiar with the application of the rigid dressings, the use of soft compression dressings is safer. An alternative method of managing the below-knee amputation stump in the immediate postoperative period is the use of an air splint; reports of the air splint claim that it helps to achieve primary goals of decreased wound edema, decreased pain, earlier mobilization, and improved primary healing.[117] An even more sophisticated device, the controlled environment unit, has been developed in Edinburgh; this particular unit not only offers an adjustable air pressure but also provides a flow of warmed, bacteriologically filtered air.[113] Although the limb and amputation stump are fully visible at all times with this technique, the theoretical advantages are offset, to some degree, by the practical disadvantages of immobility and noise.

Advantages and Disadvantages

The main advantages of the below-knee amputation are its durability following successful healing and its excellent potential for subsequent prosthetic ambulation. Disadvantages of the below-knee amputation include the need for a relatively expensive prosthesis and the increased energy expenditure required for prosthetic ambulation.

Prosthetic Requirements and Rehabilitation Potential

Some form of below-knee prosthesis is required to achieve energy-efficient ambulation following below-knee amputation. Advances have been achieved in lightweight, energy-storing prostheses, which are described in Chapter 151.

Crutch walking without a prosthesis is a very inefficient form of ambulation for the below-knee amputee, requiring considerably more energy expenditure than independent ambulation with a unilateral below-knee prosthesis.[135] Although ambulation using a well-fitted below-knee prosthesis requires a 10 to 40 per cent increase in relative energy cost compared with that of a normal non-amputee, the amputee modifies his walking speed to keep the heart rate, respiratory quotient, and relative energy costs within normal limits.[135] These results were compiled using conventional below-knee prostheses; newer lightweight prostheses should result in even less energy expenditure. It should be no surprise that successful independent prosthetic ambulation can be achieved in 70 to 100 per cent of all below-knee amputees, regardless of age, provided that they were ambulatory prior to amputation.[29, 76, 109, 124] Even the *bilateral* below-knee amputee has a surprisingly good rehabilitation potential, with successful ambulation in 33 to 71 per cent of such patients in good mental and physical condition.[20, 29, 124, 128, 133]

The amputation team must maintain a consistent follow-up protocol for below-knee amputees because there is substantial risk of arterial compromise of the *contralateral* limb as well as significant mortality during the ensuing years. Couch and associates[20] demonstrated 49 per cent survival at 3 years and 31 per cent survival at 5 years following unilateral amputation (below-knee or above-knee), which is similar to the 50 per cent 3-year survival rate reported by Bodily and Burgess.[7] Standard life table analysis also demonstrated that within 2 years of amputation, 50 per cent of the *surviving* amputees required a contralateral amputation.[7] Powell and colleagues have concluded that ". . . an independent, aggressive approach for evaluation and surgical revascularization should not be overlooked for the ischemic, remaining lower extremity in the dysvascular unilateral amputee."[99]

Knee Disarticulation

Indications

Disarticulation of the knee (or through-knee amputation) may be indicated in the occasional patient who has gangrene, infection, or cellulitis that precludes the creation of the flaps necessary for closure of a below-knee amputation. The patient with an uncorrectable flexion contracture of the knee and blood supply adequate to heal a below-knee amputation may also require a knee disarticulation. The bedridden, debilitated patient with no hope for ambulatory rehabilitation may avoid subsequent contracture of a below-knee amputation stump by undergoing a primary through-knee amputation; the resultant stump provides a long lever arm for mobility and balance in bed. Though it is most applicable in the young, healthy patient requiring lower limb amputation for trauma or tumor, the knee disarticulation has some limited utility in these particular dysvascular patients.

Contraindications

Preoperative objective findings of blood flow that is inadequate to heal a below-knee amputation should be considered a contraindication to knee disarticulation. Except for the patient with a specific contraindication to below-knee amputation as previously described, the knee disarticulation with loss of the knee joint should not be performed in preference to the below-knee amputation. Obvious ischemia, ulceration, gangrene, or infection involving the knee joint or its surrounding tissues contraindicates knee disarticulation. Finally, this amputation is contraindicated in the patient with a fixed hip flexion deformity of more than just a few degrees because the contracture would prohibit appropriate kinetic function of the intrinsic knee mechanism of the prosthesis. In this situation, a long above-knee amputation is preferable.

Prediction of Healing at This Level

Since disarticulation of the knee involves the creation of substantial skin flaps to enable a tension-free closure of the wound (especially if the femoral condyles are not remodeled), the same preoperative objective parameters for a below-knee amputation should be employed to determine the adequacy of blood supply at this level (see Table 149–4).

Surgical Technique

Two techniques have been described for disarticulation of the knee in the ischemic lower limb. The two main variations involve the management of the femoral condyles and the skin flap design. Transection of the femoral condyles requires more dissection but results in an easier and safer skin flap closure. Additionally, this remodeled stump accepts a prosthesis more readily. Alternatively, transection of the condyles is not indicated for the patient who is not expected to undergo any rehabilitation program aimed at prosthetic-assisted ambulation. When the condyles are left intact, the articular cartilage remains, and prolonged suction drainage of the amputation wound is essential to prevent the accumulation of joint fluid beneath the skin flaps.

Three basic skin flap designs are used for closure of the knee disarticulation: (1) the classic long anterior flap,[5] (2) equal length anterior and posterior flaps,[13] and (3) equal length medial and lateral flaps via sagittal incisions[65, 108] (Fig. 149–16). The sagittal incision technique (resulting in short medial and lateral flaps) and the equal length anterior and posterior flaps provide more reliable healing in the ischemic limb than the technique using the long anterior flap design.[130]

Operation may be performed with the patient in the prone or the supine position. The hip joint is hyperextended by placing a ''bump'' beneath the thigh, thereby providing ready access to the anterior or posterior aspect of the leg and thigh; the leg is flexed. A marking pen is used to outline exactly the desired skin flap design prior to incision; great care must be exercised to create flaps that will allow an absolutely tension-free skin closure.

The initial steps of the procedure involve dissection anteriorly down to the insertion of the patellar tendon on the tibia, at which point the tendon is divided. Deep medial dissection reveals the four inner hamstring muscle tendons, which are divided and allowed to retract. The deep fascia is then retracted along with the skin and tendon flap as a unit. Dissection along the lateral side of the knee reveals the biceps femoris muscle tendon and the iliotibial band, both of which are divided distally. The knee joint is then entered anteriorly and, as the knee is flexed, the cruciate ligaments are cut at their tibial insertions. The posterior structures are then transected following individual control and suture li-gation of the contents of the popliteal neurovascular bundle. The popliteal artery should be ligated distal to the origin of its superior geniculate branches. The tibial and peroneal nerves are transected sharply and allowed to retract. The patella is removed in a subperiosteal plane; the fascial defect thus created in the patellar tendon is closed with interrupted sutures.

The femoral condyles are transected transversely 1.5 cm above the knee joint (Fig. 149–17). Any sharp distal femoral margins are carefully remodeled into a smooth contour. Remaining articular cartilage on the femur, or any remaining synovium, need not be removed. Next, the patellar tendon is pulled well down into the intracondylar notch under moderate tension and is sewn to the stump of the cruciate ligaments. In similar fashion, the tendons of the semitendinous and biceps femoris muscles are pulled into the notch, tailored, and sewn to the stump of the patellar tendon and cruciate ligaments; this provides muscular stability. Following thorough irrigation and exacting hemostasis, the superficial fascia is closed with interrupted absorbable sutures. The skin is then closed atraumatically. Use of a closed suction drain is optional. An immediate rigid dressing is recommended, even if an immediate postoperative prosthesis is not employed.[13, 75, 76]

Advantages and Disadvantages

The advantages of the through-knee amputation include (1) excellent and durable end–weight-bearing capacity, (2) retention of a long and powerful muscle-stabilized femoral lever arm, (3) improved stump proprioception, and

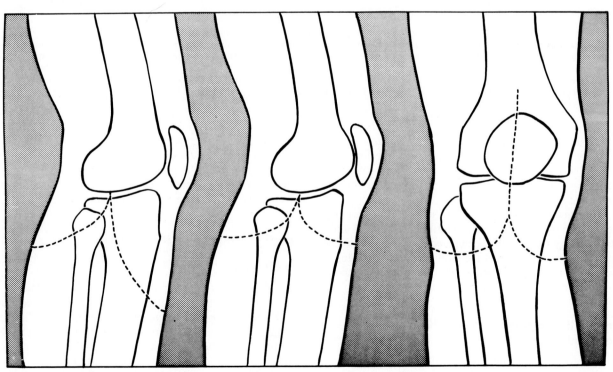

Classical long anterior   **Equal flaps**   **Sagittal flaps**

FIGURE 149–16. Skin incisions available for knee disarticulation. These may be modified further, depending on availability of suitable skin for development of flaps. (From Burgess EM: Disarticulation of the knee. A modified technique. Arch Surg 112:1250–1255, 1977. Copyright 1977, American Medical Association.)

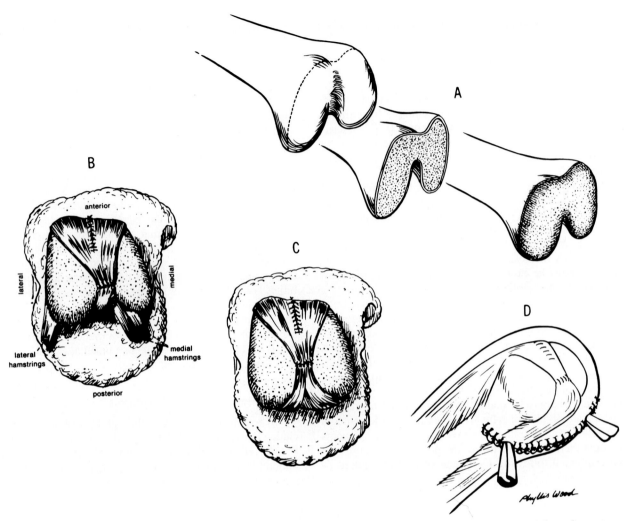

FIGURE 149–17. *A*, Weight-bearing surface of femoral condyles illustrating bone preparation: transverse cut 1.5 cm above condylar ends and femoral margins contoured. *B*, Muscle stabilization with patellar tendon sewn to cruciate ligaments. Biceps tendon and medial hamstrings are also sutured in intracondylar notch. One or more medial hamstrings may be stabilized. Site of patellar removal and repair is shown. *C*, Surgical closure of aponeurosis: hamstrings sutured through femoral notch to patellar tendon and cruciate ligaments. *D*, Closed wound over drainage using classic long anterior skin flap. (*A–D*, From Burgess EM: Disarticulation of the knee. A modified technique. Arch Surg 112:1250–1255, 1977. Copyright 1977, American Medical Association.)

(4) excellent potential for improved prosthesis control. Even for the bedridden, debilitated patient, the long lever arm allows easier mobility than an above-knee stump, and there is no risk of decubitus ulceration of a below-knee stump that becomes fixed in flexion.

The main disadvantages of this level of amputation are the absence of the knee joint, resulting in increased ambulatory energy expenditure (compared with the below-knee amputee), and the fact that the requisite long skin flaps are prone to result in wound healing problems in most ischemic limbs requiring amputation at this level.

Prosthetic Requirements and Rehabilitation Potential

Improved prosthetic design with lightweight polycentric hydraulic knee joints and endoskeletal systems has resulted in excellent rehabilitation results for the knee disarticulation patient, solving many of the former problems of nonsymmetrical knee axis alignment. In order to approach

the efficiency of a below-knee amputee's gait, the knee disarticulation prosthesis must have an effective knee joint mechanism. With the proper prosthetic design, the rehabilitation potential of the through-knee amputee should rival that of the below-knee amputee patient population.

Above-Knee Amputation

Indications

Indications for amputation of the lower limb at the above-knee level are usually a consequence of advanced ischemia that precludes reliable chances of healing at a more distal level. Rubor, infection, or open ischemic lesions at the level of the knee joint are contraindications to below-knee amputation and thus define instances in which an above-knee amputation is indicated. The disabled patient who is not expected to walk again constitutes another indication for above-knee amputation because disuse of a below-knee amputation may lead to a decubitus ulcer on the bottom of the stump in the bedridden patient. Similarly, a patient with a fixed flexion contracture of the knee presents another indication for an above-knee, rather than a below-knee, amputation.

Contraindications

The most common contraindication to amputation at the above-knee level is the presence of an infectious or gangrenous process that extends to the proposed level of amputation. A relative contraindication may be the preoperative objective documentation of inadequate local blood flow to ensure successful healing at this level. Bunt relates three specific situations that constitute relative contraindications to above-knee amputations *unless* there is definite *objective* evidence that the local blood flow is adequate to result in a viable stump: (1) acute thrombosis of a combined inflow and outflow revascularization attempt; (2) superficial femoral artery occlusion concomitant with an occluded, or highly stenotic, profunda femoris artery; and (3) the absence of a femoral pulse coupled with no detectable pulse volume recordings at the level of the high thigh.[12] Preamputation revascularization to correct any of these situations will result in more successful amputation wound healing.[12, 68]

Prediction of Healing at This Level

Many surgeons assume that virtually all amputations at the above-knee level will heal; unfortunately, this is not true; 2 to 10 per cent of amputation attempts at this level fail to heal.[76] Because this failure rate is relatively low, one may question the need for preoperative objective assay of blood flow in this patient group. However, the consequences of a failed above-knee amputation attempt may be disastrous, even fatal. Thus, appropriate selection of possible candidates for preamputation revascularization procedures may prevent such untoward sequelae in the severely ischemic thigh. Moreover, one may occasionally find that, following a revascularization procedure, an even more distal amputation will heal at the below-knee or through-knee level.

The most recent information reaffirms the notion that

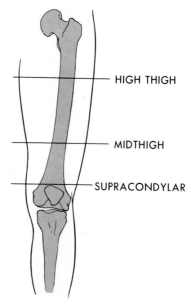

FIGURE 149–18. The potential levels of bone division of the femur. The three common levels are a supracondylar above-knee amputation, a mid-thigh amputation, and a high-thigh amputation.

empiric selection of amputation at the above-knee level will result in successful healing in 91 per cent of these patients.[63, 98] However, as outlined in Table 149–5, the proper use of preoperative testing methods should allow appropriate patient selection, resulting in successful healing of above-knee amputations at a rate approaching 100 per cent. The particular modality employed by each surgeon of course depends on the local availability of these various tests.

Surgical Technique

There are three general levels for amputation of the lower extremity above the knee (Fig. 149–18). Owing to the inherent loss of the knee joint, the length of the residual femur is crucial because of its function as the lever arm during prosthetic ambulation. In general, the longer the femoral shaft, the less energy required for prosthetic am-

Table 149–5. Preoperative Level Selection: Above-Knee Amputation

Selection Criterion	Successful Healing, Primary and Secondary/ Total (Per Cent)	Reference
Empiric	390/430 (91)	63, 88
Fiberoptic fluorometry (dye fluorescence index > 44)	6/7 (86)	119
Laser Doppler velocimetry	6/6 (100)	46
Photoelectric skin perfusion pressure > 21 mm	19/19 (100)	92
Skin perfusion pressure (I-131 or I-125 antipyrine)	44/48 (92)	50, 52
Xenon-133 skin blood flow intradermal > 2.6 ml/100 gm tissue/min	20/20 (100)	25, 74, 118
Transcutaneous P_{O_2}		
> 10 mmHg (or > 10 mmHg increase on FI_{O_2} = 1.0)	15/23 (65)	41
> 20 mmHg	12/12 (100)	18
> 23 mmHg	2/2 (100)	25
> 35 mmHg	21/24 (88)	25, 102
Transcutaneous P_{CO_2} < 38 mmHg	5/5 (100)	25

bulation and the more likely it is that the patient can successfully ambulate with a prosthesis. Amputation at a higher level, as dictated by infection, gangrene, or ischemia, lowers the chances of successful prosthetic ambulation because of the mechanical disadvantage of the shorter femoral shaft.

Two basic incision designs are applicable to above-knee amputation: the circular incision and the fish mouth incision. The circular incision is planned 2 to 3 cm below the level of proposed femur transection (Fig. 149–19). Fish mouth incisions define anterior and posterior skin flaps that are equal in length; the proximal extent of the incisions lies at the level of femur division, and the length of each flap is designed to be at least half the anteroposterior diameter of the thigh at the level of bone transection. With either type of flap design, the incision is carried through the skin, subcutaneous tissue, and fascia. Retraction of the skin and fascia superiorly allows division of the thigh muscles at a more proximal level. The femoral arteries and veins are identified in the subsartorial canal and are individually controlled and suture ligated. All remaining muscles of the anterior, medial, and lateral portions of the thigh are transected, allowing their proximal retraction to expose the femur. Many surgeons advise use of a long amputation knife to divide muscle groups in one swift incision, thereby avoiding creation of multiple tissue planes.

At the site of planned bone transection, the periosteum is scored circumferentially and is elevated superiorly, allowing transection of the femur well above the skin incision. The sciatic nerve is isolated; ligation and division are performed during gentle traction upon the nerve so that the proximal nerve remnant will retract well into the depths of the thigh muscle mass. Now the posterior musculature of the thigh may be divided.

The roughened edges of the femur stump are smoothed with a rasp, giving special attention to the anterolateral aspect, which must be flattened to prevent subsequent point pressure upon the overlying soft tissues. Thorough irrigation with an antibiotic solution will remove all bone frag-

ments and tissue debris. Hemostasis is achieved; no bone wax should be used. The skin edges are then manually coapted to ensure that the skin closure will be tension free. If there appears to be too much tension or if the soft tissue coverage appears inadequate, the femur may be shortened at this time to allow optimal closure of the soft tissues.

Once the adequacy of femoral coverage is ascertained, the wound is closed in layers. No myodesis procedures are utilized in the amputation of ischemic limbs. Perfect skin closure is achieved atraumatically with interrupted vertical mattress monofilament sutures. Only in instances of severe proximal gangrene or extensive infectious processes should the amputation wound be left open. As in any major amputation, any thrombosed prosthetic bypass graft should generally be removed at the time of amputation to decrease the incidence of wound healing complications and to prevent the subsequent infection of any retained graft material.[111, 112]

The use of a rigid dressing is not as advantageous for amputations above the knee and, in fact, is usually cumbersome. Consequently, application of a soft compression dressing is utilized; the dressing is suspended with a silesian-type elastic bandage or with a modified waist suspension belt to maintain its proper position.[100] Provision of a temporary prosthesis is often delayed until the wound has healed well, usually around 2 weeks postoperatively.

Advantages and Disadvantages

The main advantage of amputation at the above-knee level is the exceptionally high incidence of successful primary healing. The primary disadvantage is the lower rate of successful rehabilitation compared with more distal amputation.

Prosthetic Requirements and Rehabilitation Potential

The absolute minimum prosthetic requirements for the above-knee amputee are a wheelchair or a set of walking crutches; however, either of these options is a poor alternative to independent ambulation with a prosthetic limb. Newer designs of prosthetic devices for the above-knee amputee incorporate strong ultralightweight materials, endoskeletal design, sophisticated joints, and even energy storage capacity; all of these features combine to increase the rehabilitation rate of above-knee amputees, especially in the geriatric population.[58]

Rehabilitation potential following above-knee amputation of the ischemic limb is dependent on several factors, including the patient's nutritional and physical state, concurrent diseases, stump length, motivation, and rehabilitation training. Compared with normal bipedal ambulation, the relative energy cost for above-knee prosthetic ambulation is increased 50 to 70 per cent. Whereas *below-knee* amputees are able to modify their walking speed to maintain relatively normal energy costs, dysvascular *above-knee* amputees are less able to do this, resulting in increased oxygen consumption, increased heart rate, and a significantly increased respiratory quotient.[135] Crutch walking without a prosthesis imposes similar energy demands upon

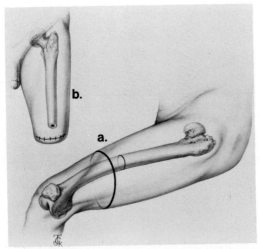

FIGURE 149–19. *a,* A circular incision is placed well distal to the point of proposed bone division. *b,* Each successive deeper tissue layer is circularly divided at a more proximal level to create a conical effect. The transverse closure of the fascia and skin following removal of the specimen is shown here.

the above-knee amputee, in contrast to all other amputee groups, who are able to walk with *less* energy using a prosthesis.[135]

Because of these dramatically increased energy requirements for ambulation following unilateral above-knee amputation, the rate of successful rehabilitation ranges from 36 to 76 per cent.[20, 76] Age alone need not be considered the major determinant of success or failure because rehabilitation failure is more often a result of concurrent medical disease or mental deterioration.[124]

As noted in the description of the patient course following below-knee amputation, the unilateral above-knee amputee who survives 2 years is at significant risk (up to 50 per cent) for development of problems requiring amputation of the contralateral limb.[7, 64] Ambulatory rehabilitation of the bilateral amputee with one above-knee amputation is successful in only 10 to 24 per cent of cases,[29, 76, 133] whereas that of the bilateral above-knee amputee approaches zero. The goal of the dysvascular bilateral amputee with at least one above-knee amputation is thus wheelchair mobility, which requires only a 9 per cent increase in relative energy costs over normal ambulation.[37]

Thus, long-term survivors of unilateral above-knee amputation must be closely followed postoperatively to detect quickly any imminent ischemic or infectious problems of the intact limb. This follow-up allows a possible aggressive approach to revascularization rather than the need for an amputation resulting in a bilateral amputee.

Hip Disarticulation

Indications

Typical indications for hip joint disarticulation are malignant bony tumors of the femur below the lesser trochanter and malignant soft tissue tumors of the middle or lower thigh.[126] Less frequent indications are extensive trauma, uncontrolled infections, extensive gangrene, or disruption of healing of a high above-knee amputation by infectious or ischemic complications.[110, 129] Objective preoperative evidence that local blood flow is inadequate to heal a high-level above-knee amputation may also constitute an indication for hip disarticulation if revascularization of the thigh is not feasible.

Contraindications

Contraindications include tumor, infection, or gangrene that involves the skin flaps or musculature at the proposed level of amputation. Performance of a hip disarticulation for ischemic complications of above-knee amputation may be hazardous unless proximal vascular reconstruction is considered prior to the disarticulation.[68]

Prediction of Healing at This Level

Owing to the fortunate fact that hip disarticulations are not often performed for ischemic complications, no data exist for objective preoperative determination of wound healing potential at this level. Consequently, observation of the contraindications outlined previously will ensure the

best results possible at this time. As an adjunct, transcutaneous mapping of the oxygen and carbon dioxide levels may help to guide the surgeon in the design of skin flaps, in much the same manner as is done for the more distal amputations.

Surgical Technique

An excellent detailed narrative with complete illustrations of the surgical technique for hip disarticulation has been published by Sugarbaker and Chretien.[126] An abstract of their technique follows (Figs. 149–20 and 149–21).*

> The operation is performed with the patient in a posterolateral position; in the first phase of the procedure the surgeon stands anterior to the patient. After incision of the skin and division of the femoral vessels and nerve, muscles of the anterior thigh are transected off the pelvic bone from lateral to medial starting with the sartorius and finishing with the adductor magnus. Muscles are divided at their origin except for the iliopsoas and obturator externus, which are divided at their insertion on the lesser trochanter of the femur. The quadratus femoris muscle is identified and preserved, then the flexor muscles are transected at their site of origin from the ischial tuberosity. During the next phase, the surgeon is posterior to the patient, and the pelvis is rotated from the posterolateral to the anterolateral position. After completion of the skin incision, the gluteal fascia, tensor fascia lata, and the gluteus maximus muscles are divided and dissected free of their posterior attachments to expose the muscles inserting by way of a common tendon onto the greater trochanter. These muscles are then transected at their insertion on the bone. The posterior aspect of the joint capsule is then exposed and transected. Finally, the sciatic nerve is divided and allowed to retract beneath the piriformis muscle. To close the wound the preserved muscles are approximated over the joint capsule and the gluteal fascia secured to the inguinal liga-

*From Sugarbaker PH, Chretien PB: A surgical technique for hip disarticulation. Surgery 90:546, 1981.

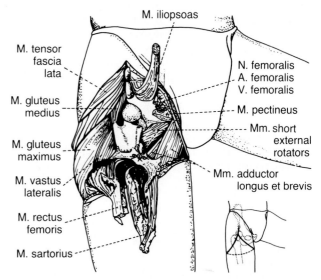

FIGURE 149–20. The stage of anatomic disarticulation following ligation of the femoral vessels and nerves and detachment of the sartorius, rectus femoris, pectineal, and iliopsoas muscles. *Insert* shows the line of the incision. (From Boyd HB: Anatomic dislocation of the hip. Surg Gynecol Obstet 84:346, 1947. By permission of Surgery, Gynecology & Obstetrics.)

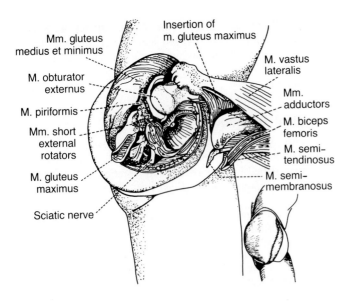

Mm. gluteus medius et minimus

M. obturator externus

M. piriformis

Mm. short external rotators

M. gluteus maximus

Sciatic nerve

Insertion of m. gluteus maximus

M. vastus lateralis

Mm. adductors

M. biceps femoris

M. semi-tendinosus

M. semi-membranosus

FIGURE 149–21. The stage of the anatomic disarticulation following separation of the gluteal muscles from their insertions, division of the sciatic nerve, severance of the short rotators, and detachment of the hamstring muscles from the ischial tuberosity. *Insert* shows the stump after closure of the wound. (From Boyd HB: Anatomic dislocation of the hip. Surg Gynecol Obstet 84:347, 1947. By permission of Surgery, Gynecology & Obstetrics.)

ment over suction drains. The skin is closed with interrupted sutures.

Advantages and Disadvantages

The only true advantage of hip disarticulation for ischemic problems is that it may result in a well-healed amputation wound that will allow prosthetic fit in situations in which an above-knee amputation has failed or is contraindicated. Also, disarticulation of the hip may be a life-saving procedure for the septic patient. The disadvantage of this amputation is its low incidence of successful ambulatory rehabilitation in the dysvascular patient population.

Prosthetic Requirement and Rehabilitation Potential

Although a number of prostheses exist for the hip disarticulation patient, most of them employ a Canadian-type pelvic bucket with an endoskeletal mode of construction to minimize weight; very few utilize sophisticated knee joints, ankle joints, or motion feet. Compared with normal bipedal ambulation, ambulation with the hip disarticulation prosthesis requires a 150 to 250 per cent increase in energy expenditure. Because of this massive energy requirement, successful ambulatory rehabilitation following hip disarticulation is distinctly uncommon, being less than 10 per cent in the dysvascular patient population;[76] thus, prescription of a prosthesis for this level of amputation is done very selectively.

References

1. Bailey MJ, Johnston CLW, Yates CJP, et al: Preoperative haemaglobin as predictor of outcome of diabetic amputations. Lancet 28:168, 1979.
2. Baker WH, Barnes RW: Minor forefoot amputation in patients with low ankle pressure. Am J Surg 133:331, 1977.
3. Barnes RW, Shanik GD, Slaymaker EE: An index of healing in below-knee amputation: Leg blood pressure by Doppler ultrasound. Surgery 79:13, 1976.
4. Barnes RW, Thornhill B, Nix L, et al: Prediction of amputation wound healing: Roles of Doppler ultrasound and digit photoplethysmography. Arch Surg 116:80, 1981.
5. Batch JW, Spittler AW, McFadden JG: Advantages of the knee disarticulation over amputations through the thigh. J Bone Joint Surg 36A:921, 1954.
6. Benton GS, Kerstein MD: Cost effectiveness of early digit amputation in the patient with diabetes. Surg Gynecol Obstet 161:523, 1985.
7. Bodily KC, Burgess EM: Contralateral limb and patient survival after leg amputation. Am J Surg 146:280, 1983.
8. Boeckstyns MEH, Jensen CM: Amputation of the forefoot: Predictive value of signs and clinical physiological tests. Acta Orthop Scand 55:224, 1984.
9. Bone GE, Pomajzl MJ: Toe blood pressure by photoplethysmography: An index of healing in forefoot amputations. Surgery 89:569, 1981.
10. Bongard FS, Upton RA, Elings VB, et al: Digital cutaneous fluorometry: Correlation between blood flow and fluorescence. J Vasc Surg 1:635, 1984.
11. Borozan PG, Schuler JJ, Flanigan DP: The accuracy of segmental Doppler pressures in predicting healing of below-knee amputation in diabetic patients. Unpublished data presented at the Association of VA Surgeons Meeting, Los Angeles, California, May 9–12, 1984.
12. Bunt TJ: Gangrene of the immediate postoperative above-knee amputation stump: Role of emergency revascularization in preventing death. J Vasc Surg 2:874, 1985.
13. Burgess EM: Disarticulation of the knee: A modified technique. Arch Surg 112:1250, 1977.
14. Burgess EM, Matsen FA, Wyss CR, et al: Segmental transcutaneous measurements of Po₂ in patients requiring below the knee amputation for peripheral vascular insufficiency. J Bone Joint Surg 64A:378, 1982.
15. Castronuovo JJ, Deane LM, Deterling RA, et al: Below-knee amputation: Is the effort to preserve the knee joint justified? Arch Surg 115:1184, 1980.
16. Cederberg PA, Pritchard DJ, Joyce JW: Doppler-determined segmental pressures and wound-healing in amputations for vascular disease. J Bone Joint Surg 65A:363, 1983.
17. Cheng EY: Lower extremity amputation level: Selection using non-invasive hemodynamic methods of evaluation. Arch Phys Med Rehabil 63:475, 1982.
18. Christensen KS, Klarke M: Transcutaneous oxygen measurement in peripheral occlusive disease: An indicator of wound healing in leg amputation. J Bone Joint Surg 68B:423, 1986.
19. Cohen SI, Goldman LD, Salzman EW, et al: The deleterious effect of immediate postoperative prosthesis in below-knee amputation for ischemic disease. Surgery 76:992, 1974.
20. Couch NP, David JK, Tilney NL, et al: Natural history of the leg amputee. Am J Surg 133:469, 1977.
21. Daly MJ, Henry RE: Quantitative measurement of skin perfusion with xenon-133. J Nucl Med 21:156, 1980.

22. Dellon AL, Morgan RF: Myodermal flap closure of below the knee amputation. Surg Gynecol Obstet 153:383, 1981.
23. Desai Y, Robbs JV, Keenan JP: Staged below knee amputations for septic peripheral lesions due to ischaemia. Br J Surg 73:392, 1986.
24. Dickhaut SC, Delee JC, Page CP: Nutritional status: Importance in predicting wound healing after amputation. J Bone Joint Surg 66A:71, 1984.
25. Durham JR, Anderson GG, Malone JM: Methods of preoperative selection of amputation level. *In* Flanigan DP (ed): Perioperative Assessment in Vascular Surgery. New York, Marcel Dekker, 1987, pp 61–82.
26. Eberhard P, Mindt W, Hammacher K: Percutane messung der sauer-statpartaldrukes. Methodick and Anwendungen. Stuttgart, Proc Medizin-Technik, May 16, 1972.
27. Effeney DJ, Lim RC, Schechter WP: Transmetatarsal amputation. Arch Surg 112:1366, 1977.
28. Evans NTS, Naylor PFD: The oxygen tension gradient across human epidermis. Respir Physiol 3:38, 1967.
29. Evans WE, Hayes JP, Vermilion BD: Rehabilitation of the bilateral amputee. J Vasc Surg 5:589, 1987.
30. Fearon J, Campbell DR, Hoar CS, et al: Improved results with diabetic below-knee amputations. Arch Surg 120:777, 1985.
31. Franzeck UK, Talke P, Bernstein EF, et al: Transcutaneous P_{O_2} measurement in health and peripheral arterial occlusive disease. Surgery 91:156, 1982.
32. Gatti JE, LaRossa D, Neff SR, et al: Altered skin flap survival and fluorescein kinetics with hemodilution. Surgery 92:200, 1982.
33. Gianfortune P, Pulla RJ, Sage R: Ray resections in the insensitive or dysvascular foot: A critical review. J Foot Surg 24:103, 1985.
34. Gibbons GW, Wheelock FC Jr, Hoar CS Jr, et al: Predicting success of forefoot amputations in diabetics by noninvasive testing. Arch Surg 114:1034, 1979.
35. Gibbons GW, Wheelock FC Jr, Siembrieda C, et al: Noninvasive prediction of amputation level in diabetic patients. Arch Surg 114:1253, 1979.
36. Golbranson F: Amputation level determination. Presented at the annual meeting of the American Academy of Orthotists and Prosthetists, San Diego, January 1983.
37. Gonzalez EG, Corcoran PJ, Reyes RL: Energy expenditure in below-knee amputees: Correlation with stump length. Arch Phys Med Rehab 55:111, 1974.
38. Harbrecht PJ, Netheny H, Ahmad W, Fry DE: A technic for freezing an extremity in preparation for amputation. Am J Surg 135:859, 1978.
39. Harris JP, McLaughlin AF, Quinn RJ, et al: Skin blood flow measurement with xenon-133 to predict healing of lower extremity amputations. Aust NZ J Surg 56:413, 1986.
40. Harris RI: Syme's amputation: The technical details essential for success. J Bone Joint Surg 38B:614, 1956.
41. Harward TRS, Volny J, Golbranson F, et al: Oxygen inhalation-induced transcutaneous P_{O_2} changes as a predictor of amputation level. J Vasc Surg 2:220, 1985.
42. Hauser CJ, Shoemaker WC: Use of a transcutaneous P_{O_2} regional perfusion index to quantify tissue perfusion in peripheral vascular disease. Ann Surg 197:337, 1983.
43. Holloway GA Jr, Watkins BW: Laser Doppler measurement of cutaneous blood flow. J Invest Dermatol 69:300, 1977.
44. Holloway GA Jr, Burgess EM: Cutaneous blood flow and its relation to healing of below-knee amputation. Surg Gynecol Obstet 146:750, 1978.
45. Holloway GA Jr: Cutaneous blood flow responses to injection trauma measured by laser Doppler velocimetry. J Invest Dermatol 74:1, 1980.
46. Holloway GA Jr, Burgess EM: Preliminary experiences with laser Doppler velocimetry for the determination of amputation levels. Prosthet Orthot Int 7:63, 1983.
47. Holstein P: Distal blood pressure as a guide in choice of amputation level. Scand J Clin Lab Invest 31(Suppl 128):245, 1973.
48. Holstein P, Lund P, Larsen B, Schomacker T: Skin perfusion pressure measured as the external pressure required to stop isotope washout. Methodological considerations and normal values on the legs. Scand J Clin Lab Invest 30:649, 1977.
49. Holstein P, Lassen NA: Assessment of safe level of amputation by measurement of skin blood pressure. *In* Rutherford RB (ed): Vascular Surgery. Philadelphia, WB Saunders Co, 1977, pp 105–111.
50. Holstein P, Sager P, Lassen NA: Wound healing in below knee amputations in relation to skin perfusion pressure. Acta Orthop Scand 40:49, 1979.
51. Holstein P: Level selection in leg amputation for arterial occlusive disease: A comparison of clinical evaluation and skin perfusion pressure. Acta Orthop Scand 53:821, 1982.
52. Holstein P, Trap-Jensen J, Bagger H, Larsen B: Skin perfusion pressure measured by isotope washout in legs with arterial occlusive disease. Clin Physiol 3:313, 1983.
53. Holstein P: The distal blood pressure predicts healing of amputations on the feet. Acta Orthop Scand 55:227, 1984.
54. Huch A, Huch R, Mentzer K, et al: Eine schnelle, behitze problachenelektrode zur Kontinuier lichen uberwach ung des P_{O_2} bemenschen. Elektrodenaut bau und-eigen schaften. Stuttgart, Proc Medizin-Technik, May 16, 1972.
55. Huizinga WFJ, Robbs JV, Kritzinger NA: Prevention of wound sepsis in amputations by peri-operative antibiotic cover with an amoxycillin-clavulanic acid combination. South Afr Med J 63(15):71, 1983.
56. Hunsaker RH, Schwartz JA, Keagy BA, et al: Dry ice cryoamputation: A twelve year experience. J Vasc Surg 2(6):812, 1985.
57. Huston CC, Bivins BA, Ernst CB, Griffen WO Jr: Morbid implications of above-knee amputations. Report of a series and review of the literature. Arch Surg 115:165, 1980.
58. Isakov E, Susak Z, Becker E: Energy expenditure and cardiac response in above-knee amputees while using prostheses with open and locked knee mechanisms. Scand J Rehab Med Suppl 12:108, 1985.
59. Ito K, Ohgi S, Mori T, et al: Determination of amputation level in ischemic legs by means of transcutaneous oxygen pressure measurement. Int Surg 69:59, 1984.
60. Kacy SS, Wolma FJ, Flye MW: Factors affecting the results of below-knee amputation in patients with and without diabetes. Surg Gynecol Obstet 155:513, 1982.
61. Karanfilian RG, Lynch TG, Zirul VT, et al: The value of laser Doppler velocimetry and transcutaneous oxygen tension determination in predicting healing of ischemic forefoot ulcerations and amputations in diabetic and nondiabetic patients. J Vasc Surg 4:511, 1986.
62. Katsamouris A, Brewster DC, Megerman J, et al: Transcutaneous oxygen tension in selection of amputation level. Am J Surg 147:510, 1984.
63. Keagy BA, Schwartz JA, Kotb M, et al: Lower extremity amputations: The control series. J Vasc Surg 4:321, 1986.
64. Kihn RB, Warren R, Beebe GW: The "geriatric" amputee. Ann Surg 176:305, 1972.
65. Kjolbye J: The surgery of through-knee amputation. *In* Murdock G (ed): Prosthetic and Orthotic Practice. London, Edward Arnold, 1970, pp 255–257.
66. Kostuik JP, Wood D, Hornby R, et al: Measurement of skin blood flow in peripheral vascular disease by the epicutaneous application of xenon-133. J Bone Joint Surg 58A:833, 1976.
67. Kram HB, Appel PL, White RA, et al: Assessment of peripheral vascular disease by postocclusive transcutaneous oxygen recovery time. J Vasc Surg 1:628, 1984.
68. Kwaan JHM, Connolly JE: Fatal sequelae of the ischemic amputation stump: A surgical challenge. Am J Surg 138:49, 1979.
69. Lepantalo MJA, Haajanen J, Linfors O, et al: Predictive value of preoperative segmental blood pressure measurements in below-knee amputations. Acta Chir Scand 148:581, 1982.
70. Lim RC Sr, Blaisdell FW, Hall AD, et al: Below-knee amputation for ischemic gangrene. Surg Gynecol Obstet 125:493, 1967.
71. Little JM, Stephen MS, Zylstra PL: Amputation of the toes for vascular disease: Fate of the affected leg. Lancet 2:1318, 1976.
72. Lubbers DW: Theoretical basis of the transcutaneous blood gas measurements. Crit Care Med 9:721, 1981.
73. Malone JM, Moore WS, Goldstone J, Malone SJ: Therapeutic and economic impact of a modern amputation program. Ann Surg 189:798, 1979.
74. Malone JM, Leal JM, Moore WS, et al: The "gold standard" for amputation level selection: Xenon-133 clearance. J Surg Res 30:449, 1981.
75. Malone JM, Goldstone J: Lower extremity amputation. *In* Moore WS (ed): Vascular Surgery: A Comprehensive Review, 1st ed. New York, Grune & Stratton, 1984, pp 909–974.

76. Malone JM, Goldstone J: Lower extremity amputation. *In* Moore WS (ed): Vascular Surgery: A Comprehensive Review. 2nd ed. Orlando, FL, Grune & Stratton, 1986, pp 1139–1209.

77. Malone JM: Unpublished data, personal communication, 1987.

77a. Malone JM, Anderson GG, Lalka SG, et al: Prospective comparison of noninvasive techniques for amputation level selection. Am J Surg 154:179, 1987.

78. Matsen FA, Wyss CR, Robertson CL, et al: The relationship of transcutaneous Po_2 and laser Doppler measurements in a human model of local arterial insufficiency. Surg Gynecol Obstet 159:418, 1984.

79. McFarland DC, Lawrence PF: Skin fluorescence. A method to predict amputation site healing. J Surg Res 32:410, 1982.

80. McIntyre KE Jr, Bailey SA, Malone JM, et al: Guillotine amputation in the treatment of nonsalvageable lower-extremity infections. Arch Surg 119:450, 1984.

81. McKittrick LS, McKittrick JB, Risby TS: Transmetatarsal amputation for infection or gangrene in patients with diabetes mellitus. Ann Surg 130:826, 1949.

82. Mehta K, Hobson RW II, Jamil Z, et al: Fallibility of Doppler ankle pressure in predicting healing of transmetatarsal amputation. J Surg Res 28:466, 1980.

83. Moore WS: Introduction to amputation symposium. Arch Surg 116:79, 1981.

84. Moore WS, Henry RE, Malone JM, et al: Prospective use of xenon Xe-133 clearance for amputation level selection. Arch Surg 116:86, 1981.

85. Moosa HH, Makaroun MS, Peitzman AB, et al: TcPo₂ values in limb ischemia: Effects of blood flow and arterial oxygen tension. J Surg Res 40:482, 1986.

86. Munck O, Anderson AM: Decomposition of iodine labelled antipyrine. Scand J Lab Invest 19:256, 1967.

87. Munck O, Anderson AM, Binder C: Clearance of 4-iodo-antipyrine-125-I after subcutaneous injection in various regions. Scand J Lab Invest Suppl 99, p 39, 1967.

88. Mustapha NM, Jain SK, Dudley P, Redhead RG: The effect of oxygen inhalation and intravenous naftidrofuryl on the transcutaneous partial oxygen pressure in ischemic lower limbs. Prosthet Orthot Int 8:135, 1984.

89. Nakhgevary KB, Rhoads JE Jr: Ankle-level amputation. Surgery 95:549, 1984.

90. Nicholas GG, Myers JL, Demuth WE: The role of vascular laboratory criteria in the selection of patients for lower extremity amputation. Ann Surg 195:469, 1982.

91. Nilsen R, Dahn I, Lassen NA, Wastling GA: On the estimation of local effective perfusion pressure in patients with obliterative arterial disease by means of external compression over a xenon-133 depot. Scand J Clin Lab Invest 99(Suppl):29, 1967.

92. Ovesen J, Stockel M: Measurement of skin perfusion pressure by photoelectric technique—An aid to amputation level selection in arteriosclerotic disease. Prosthet Orthot Int 8:39, 1984.

93. Persson BM: Sagittal incision for below-knee amputation in ischaemic gangrene. J Bone Joint Surg 56B:110, 1974.

94. Pilegard HK, Madsen MR, Hansen-Leth C, et al: Muscle blood flow after amputation: Increased flow with medullary plugging. Acta Orthop Scand 56:500, 1985.

95. Pinzur MS, Jordan C, Rana NA: Syme's two stage amputation in diabetic dysvascular disease. Ill Med J 160:23, 1981.

96. Pinzur M, Kaminsky M, Sage R, et al: Amputations at the middle level of the foot. J Bone Joint Surg 68A:1061, 1986.

97. Pollack SB, Ernst CB: Use of Doppler pressure measurements in predicting success in amputation of the leg. Am J Surg 139:303, 1980.

98. Porter JM, Baur GM, Taylor LM Jr: Lower extremity amputations for ischemia. Arch Surg 116:89, 1981.

99. Powell TW, Burnham SJ, Johnson G Jr: Second leg ischemia: Lower extremity bypass versus amputation in patients with contralateral lower extremity amputation. Am Surg 50:577, 1984.

100. Puddifoot PC, Weaver PC, Marshall SA: A method of supportive bandaging for amputation stumps. Br J Surg 60:729, 1973.

101. Raines JK, Darling RC, Buth J, et al: Vascular laboratory criteria for the management of peripheral vascular disease of the lower extremities. Surgery 79:21, 1976.

102. Ratliff DA, Clyne CAC, Chant ADB, et al: Prediction of amputation wound healing: The role of transcutaneous Po_2 assessment. Br J Surg 71:219, 1984.

103. Rhodes GR, Cogan F: "Islands of ischemia": Transcutaneous Ptco₂ documentation of pedal malperfusion following lower limb revascularization. Am Surg 51:407, 1985.

104. Rhodes GR: Uses of transcutaneous oxygen monitoring in the management of below-knee amputations and skin envelope injuries (SKI). Am Surg 51:701, 1985.

105. Rhodes GR, King TA: Delayed skin oxygenation following distal tibial revascularization (DTR): Implications for wound healing in late amputations. Am Surg 52:519, 1986.

106. Robbs JV, Kritzinger NA, Mogotlane KA, et al: Antibiotic prophylaxis in amputations (débridement) with or without arterial reconstructions for septic ischaemic lower limb lesions. South Afr J Surg 19(3):181, 1981.

107. Robbs JV, Ray R: Clinical predictors of below-knee stump healing following amputation for ischaemia. South Afr J Surg 20(4):305, 1982.

108. Robinson K: Amputation in vascular disease. Ann R Coll Surg Engl 62:87, 1980.

109. Roon AJ, Moore WS, Goldstone J: Below-knee amputation: A modern approach. Am J Surg 134:153, 1977.

110. Rosental JJ: Discussion in Kwaan JHM, Connolly JE: Fatal sequelae of ischemic amputation stump: A surgical challenge. Am J Surg 138:52, 1979.

111. Rubin JR, Yao JST, Thompson RG, et al: Management of infection of major amputation stumps after failed femorodistal grafts. Surgery 98(4):810, 1985.

112. Rubin JR, Marmen C, Rhodes RS: Management of failed prosthetic grafts at the time of major lower extremity amputation. J Vasc Surg 7:673, 1988.

113. Ruckley CV, Rae A, Prescott RJ: Controlled environment unit in the care of the below-knee amputation stump. Br J Surg 73:11, 1986.

114. Sanders RJ, Augspurger R: Skin flap measurement for below-knee amputation. Surg Gynecol Obstet 145:740, 1977.

115. Schuler JJ: Unpublished data, personal communication, 1987.

116. Schwartz JA, Schuler JJ, O'Connor RJA, et al: Predictive value of distal perfusion pressure in the healing of amputation of the digits and the forefoot. Surg Gynecol Obstet 154:865, 1982.

117. Sher MH, Liebman P: The air splint: A method of managing below-knee amputations. J Cardiovasc Surg 23:407, 1982.

118. Silberstein EB, Thomas S, Cline J, et al: Predictive value of intracutaneous xenon clearance for healing of amputation and cutaneous ulcer sites. Radiology 147:227, 1983.

119. Silverman DG, Rubin SM, Reilly CA, et al: Fluorometric prediction of successful amputation level in the ischemic limb. J Rehab Res Dev 22:29, 1985.

120. Sizer JS, Wheelock FC: Digital amputations in diabetic patients. Surgery 72:980, 1972.

121. Sonne-Holm S, Boeckstyns M, Menck H, et al: Prophylactic antibiotics in amputation of the lower extremity for ischemia. J Bone Joint Surg 67A(5):800, 1985.

122. Spence VA, Walker WF: The relationship between temperature isotherms and skin blood flow in the ischemic limb. J Surg Res 36:278, 1984.

123. Spence VA, McCollum PT, Walker WF, et al: Assessment of tissue viability in relation to the selection of amputation level. Prosthet Orthot Int 8:67, 1984.

124. Steinberg FU, Sunwoo I, Roettger RF: Prosthetic rehabilitation of geriatric amputee patients: A follow-up study. Arch Phys Med Rehabil 66:742, 1985.

125. Stockel M, Ovesen J, Brochner-Mortensen J, et al: Standardized photoelectric technique as routine method for selection of amputation level. Acta Orthop Scand 53:875, 1982.

126. Sugarbaker PH, Chretien PB: A surgical technique for hip disarticulation. Surgery 90:546, 1981.

127. Termansen NB: Below-knee amputation for ischaemic gangrene. Prospective, randomized comparison of a transverse and a sagittal operative technique. Acta Orthop Scand 48:311, 1977.

128. Thornhill HL, Jones GD, Brodzka W, et al: Bilateral below-knee amputations: Experience with 80 patients. Arch Phys Med Rehabil 67:159, 1986.

129. Tooms RE, Hampton FL: Hip disarticulation and hemipelvectomy amputation. *In* Atlas of Limb Prosthetics, Surgical and Prosthetic

Principles. American Academy of Orthopoedic Surgeons, St. Louis, CV Mosby, 1981, p 403.

130. Tooms RE: Amputation of the lower extremity. *In* Crenshaw AH (ed): Campbell's Operative Orthopaedics. 7th ed. St. Louis, CV Mosby, 1987, vol. 1, pp 607–627.

131. Towne JD, Condon RE: Lower extremity amputations for ischemic disease. Adv Surg 13:199, 1979.

132. Verta MJ, Gross WS, Van Bellan B, et al: Forefoot perfusion pressure and minor amputation surgery. Surgery 80:729, 1976.

133. Volpicelli LJ, Chambers RB, Wagner FW: Ambulation levels of bilateral lower extremity amputees. J Bone Joint Surg 65A:599, 1983.

134. Wagner FW: The Syme amputation. *In* American Academy of Orthopoedic Surgeons: Atlas of Limb Prosthetics: Surgical and Prosthetic Principles. St. Louis, CV Mosby, 1981, pp 326–340.

135. Waters RL, Perry J, Antonelli D, et al: Energy cost of walking amputees: The influence of level of amputation. J Bone Joint Surg 58A:42, 1976.

136. Welch GH, Leiberman DP, Pollock JG, et al: Failure of Doppler ankle pressure to predict healing of conservative forefoot amputations. Br J Surg 72:888, 1985.

137. Wyss CR, Robertson C, Love SJ, et al: Relationship between transcutaneous oxygen tension, ankle blood pressure, and clinical outcome of vascular surgery in diabetic and non-diabetic patients. Surgery 101:56, 1987.

138. Yao JST, Bergan JJ: Application of ultrasound to arterial and venous diagnosis. Surg Clin North Am 54(1):23, 1974.

139. Kram HB, Appel PL, Shoemaker WC: Prediction of below-knee amputation wound healing using noninvasive laser Doppler velocimetry. Am J Surg 158:29, 1989.

140. Light JT Jr, Rice JC, Kerstein MD: Sequelae of limited amputation. Surgery 103:294, 1988.

141. Oishi CS, Fronek A, Golbranson FL: The role of non-invasive vascular studies in determining levels of amputation. J Bone Joint Surg [Am] 70A:1520, 1988.

142. Durham JR, McCoy DM, Sawchuk AP, et al: Open transmetatarsal amputation in the treatment of severe foot infections. Am J Surg 158:127, 1989.

143. Wagner WH, Keagy BA, Kotb MM, et al: Noninvasive determination of healing of major lower extremity amputation: The continued role of clinical judgment. J Vasc Surg 8:703, 1988.

144. Stewart CPU: The influence of smoking on the level of lower limb amputation. Prosthet Orthot Int 11:113, 1987.

145. Miller N, Dardik H, Wolodinger F, et al: Transmetatarsal amputation: The role of adjunctive revascularization. J Vasc Surg 13:705, 1991.

146. Kram HB, Appel PL, Shoemaker WC: Multisensor transcutaneous oximetric mapping to predict below-knee amputation wound healing: Use of critical P_{O_2}. J Vasc Surg 9:796, 1989.

147. Dwars BJ, van den Broek TAA, Rauwerda JA, Bakker FC: Criteria for reliable selection of the lowest level of amputation in peripheral vascular disease. J Vasc Surg 15:536, 1992.

148. Bacharach JM, Rooke TW, Osmundson PJ, Gloviczki P: Predictive value of transcutaneous oxygen pressure and amputation success by use of supine and elevation measurements. J Vasc Surg 15:558, 1992.

149. Scheffler A, Rieger H: A comparative analysis of transcutaneous oximetry (TcPo$_2$) during oxygen inhalation and leg dependency in severe peripheral arterial occlusive disease. J Vasc Surg 16:218, 1992.

150. Roach JJ, Deutsch A, McFarlane DS: Resurrection of the amputations of Lisfranc and Chopart for diabetic gangrene. Arch Surg 122:931, 1987.

151. Christie J, Clowes CB, Lamb DW: Amputations through the middle part of the foot. J Bone Joint Surg 62B:473, 1980.

152. Hamit HF: The Boyd-Syme forefoot amputation technique. Contemp Orthop 23:321, 1991.

153. Yao JST: Choice of amputation level. J Vasc Surg 8:544, 1988.

150

Complications of Amputation

Frank A. Gottschalk, M.D., F.R.C.S.(Ed.), F.C.S.(S.A.) Orth.,
and Daniel F. Fisher, Jr., M.D.

• • •

Despite improved techniques in amputation surgery, patients frequently develop one of the various complications related to the procedure itself or to the postoperative rehabilitation. The patient's ability to deal with these complications is often affected by his or her overall premorbid condition and ultimate desire to walk again. Multiple smaller complications can be just as devastating as a single major complication.

The authors of this chapter have arbitrarily divided the list of complications into *preoperative, intraoperative,* and *postoperative* problems in an attempt to identify individually the multitude of complications that can occur. In reality, this division oversimplifies the total situation because many of these problems are integrally interrelated and fre-

quently coexist. Any treatment directed at a specific complication should take into account the overall status of the patient, the potential for recovery, and the desire for ultimate ambulation.

PREOPERATIVE CONSIDERATIONS TO AVOID COMPLICATIONS

Patients about to undergo amputation may have several preexisting medical conditions that can markedly affect the approach to surgery.

Cardiovascular Status. Many elderly patients undergoing amputation for vascular insufficiency have compromised cardiac function (see Chapters 2, 22, and 148). Detailed attention by a team of physicians including an internist or cardiologist should be directed at improving the patient's cardiac status to minimize anesthetic complications. In extreme cases of congestive heart failure, Swan-Ganz catheterization may help to monitor the patient's cardiac output and manage inotropic support. Occasionally, in severely ill patients with septic extremities, a "medical" (i.e., packing the extremity in ice) or guillotine amputation may afford time to improve the patient's hemodynamics.[10, 21, 25, 31, 35] A definitive amputation can later be performed under more optimal conditions.

Respiratory Status. In general, most lower extremity amputations can be performed adequately under spinal or epidural anesthesia, which avoids having to extubate a patient who may have severely compromised pulmonary reserve. However, spinal anesthesia may be associated with severe hypotension unless the patient's preoperative volume status is satisfactory. Central venous pressure or Swan-Ganz catheter monitoring in conjunction with the judicious administration of fluids and systemic vasodilators or vasopressors may help to correct volume deficits and to avoid hypotensive complications at the onset of spinal or general anesthesia.

Preoperative Activity Level. Before any amputation is performed, the surgeon should critically evaluate the patient's rehabilitation potential. This may require consultation with physicians specializing in rehabilitation medicine.[26, 56, 61, 81] Inactive and bedridden patients, such as those with preexisting stroke or dementia who are not candidates for prosthetic fitting, may develop flexion contractures and stump breakdown if below-knee amputations are performed, ultimately requiring revision to the above-knee level (see Chapter 149). The authors generally perform above-knee amputations in patients with no rehabilitation potential, to avoid the development of knee flexion contractures and subsequent stump complications.[57]

Joint Deformities. Preexisting joint problems, such as severe knee or hip flexion contractures, may compromise the potential for walking. In these circumstances, the authors usually perform above-knee amputations to ensure healing, with less emphasis on femur length. Severe arthritis in the knee joint would be a relative contraindication to a below-knee amputation. Failed total knee replacement associated with an ischemic limb would necessitate an above-knee amputation.

Previous Orthopedic Surgery. Before any patient is taken to the operating room for amputation surgery, the surgeon should question the patient about any previous orthopedic operations and examine the extremity for scars indicative of an orthopedic procedure. Prior hip or femur surgery may involve the placement of an implant, *which cannot be cut with standard saws.* If there is a question about the type of orthopedic implant at the site of the proposed bone transection, standard bone radiographs, which should include the joint above and below, may be

helpful in planning the amputation. It may be advisable to plan to remove an intramedullary nail through a separate hip incision before performing bone transection for an above-knee amputation. Long-stemmed hip implants may have to be transected with special saws. Stemmed total knee replacements may present similar problems.[72]

Osteomyelitis. Bone infections unresponsive to intensive antibiotic and surgical therapy require amputation at a level *above* the infection itself. If circulation in the leg is adequate, osteomyelitis in the digit generally requires a ray amputation. Osteomyelitis in the tibia or fibula requires a knee disarticulation, and osteomyelitis of the knee or femur requires an above-knee amputation. If an amputation is performed in close proximity to a site of osteomyelitis, a specimen of bone at the amputation margin should be sent to the bacteriology laboratory for culture and sensitivity determination.

Soft Tissue Infections. Diabetic patients with insensitive feet are particularly prone to severe forefoot ulceration and infection. Medical management of such patients should include antibiotics (which cover aerobic and anaerobic organisms) and an assessment of local arterial circulation.[46, 70, 85] If septicemia ensues, an open guillotine ankle amputation can be easily performed for quick relief of sepsis and any associated lymphangitis that may accompany the foot infection.[16, 21, 53] Revision to a formal below-knee amputation is accomplished after resolution of any cellulitis or lymphangitis in the residual extremity.

Neurotrophic Ulcers. Patients with peripheral neuropathies from any cause are extremely prone to develop plantar ulcers, which may not be secondary to arterial ischemia per se.[14, 37] If treated early, these ulcers can be healed with a combination of shoe modification and patient education. If a toe or forefoot amputation becomes necessary, recurrent ulceration at a later date frequently occurs unless the amputation is performed above the level of insensitivity. Likewise, a transmetatarsal or Syme amputation in these patients with diminished sensation may also be unsuccessful on a long-term basis.[19, 54, 83]

Diabetes or Renal Failure. The combination of these two metabolic problems leads to poor wound healing, especially of the skin. Some authors have suggested that a primary amputation is the operation of choice in all dialysis-dependent diabetics with gangrene of the foot because the healing potential of these patients is so poor, regardless of the success of a bypass graft. Because of the risk of wound edge necrosis in these patients, the surgeon should pay the utmost attention to gentle handling of tissues and precise skin closure.[18, 41, 80]

Traumatic or Crush Injuries. A combination of bone, nerve, muscle, and skin trauma occasionally dictates that an emergency amputation must be performed, and this is one setting in which a tourniquet can be used. If the lower leg is involved, a knee disarticulation may lead to a very functional amputation level.[12] If the knee is involved, an above-knee amputation may be the only reasonable choice. Usually, the level of amputation is dictated by the injury.

Absent Femoral Pulse. Approximately 10 per cent of all patients undergoing an above-knee amputation do not have a palpable femoral pulse. These patients are at high risk for necrosis of the stump, even if the amputation is performed at the mid-thigh level. If wound edge gangrene occurs or if persistent, excruciating stump pain develops, the authors recommend hip disarticulation to the patient in whom revascularization of the profunda femoris artery cannot be accomplished. If the disarticulation is performed before infection develops in the above-knee amputation incision, the patient has an 80 per cent chance of healing the hip disarticulation.[43, 82]

Deep Venous Thrombosis. A severe case of deep venous thrombosis may result in secondary arterial compromise of the leg (phlegmasia cerulea dolens).[7] If anticoagulation, lower leg fasciotomy, and possibly venous thrombectomy do not help the patient, the lower leg may develop gangrene. Most of these very unusual patients require an above-knee amputation. Necrosis of skin flaps may occur because of venous hypertension in the residual limb. Distal compression with an elastic bandage may help to reduce the residual edema.

Postphlebitic Syndrome. Rarely, patients require amputation for refractory venous stasis ulcers alone, and others need amputation for a combination of arterial and venous insufficiency. Patients with hyperpigmentation of the lower leg are particularly prone to develop posterior skin flap ulceration after a below-knee amputation that otherwise has enough arterial circulation to heal. If a below-knee amputation is chosen in this setting, immediate stump compression with some type of rigid plaster dressing or elastic bandage is mandatory until well after the stump has healed (up to 6 weeks). Thereafter, a support stocking is recommended whenever the patient is ambulatory.

Smoking. Most studies confirm that cigarette smoking contributes to atherosclerosis. A Danish study found that the risk of infection and reamputation was twice as high in smokers as in nonsmokers. By measuring digital blood flow, platelet aggregation, hematocrit, and fibrinogen levels of patients who smoke, it was concluded that patients should stop smoking for at least a week to reduce the nicotine effects of cutaneous and subcutaneous vasoconstriction.[47]

Blue Toe Syndrome. Distal microembolization can occur from any embolizing lesion located more proximally in the arterial tree. If the patient is an operative candidate, the embolizing lesion should be corrected to prevent recurrent embolization to the remaining limb regardless of whether a distal amputation is necessary.[22] Progressive embolization can lead to necrosis of a healed stump, or, depending on the location of the embolic source, it can threaten the contralateral extremity. In the classic case of blue toe syndrome associated with normal pedal pulses, a distal toe disarticulation or a formal ray amputation usually cures gangrene in the forefoot. In more severe cases in which pedal pulses may not be present (such as those associated with embolization of large amounts of debris from aortic, femoral, or

popliteal aneurysms), a below-knee or higher amputation may be necessary.

Impending Gangrene, Unreconstructable Vessels. Patients in this category usually have ischemic rest pain with or without open foot lesions. Arteriography demonstrates vessels that may be too diseased to bypass. Nevertheless, in 80 to 85 per cent of these patients a carefully performed below-knee amputation will heal unless a more compelling reason to perform an above-knee amputation exists.[13, 34] Overall, amputation healing can be raised to over 90 per cent if an above-knee amputation is offered to those patients who do not have an audible popliteal Doppler signal.[3]

Previous Incisions. If possible, old scars should be excised or used to create amputation flaps to prevent the chance of skin necrosis between old and new incisions. This becomes an issue more often in patients who have failed vascular procedures in the lower leg and who are thought to be candidates for a below-knee amputation. Although most authorities believe that below-knee amputations are best performed using long posterior and shorter anterior flaps, other flaps can be used in selected circumstances to prevent "skin island" necrosis. A skew flap provides good closure and has healing rates similar to those of long posterior flaps. Equal sagittal flaps may also provide satisfactory healing.[20, 32, 67]

Failed Bypass. In an effort to prevent amputation, it is always reasonable to consider distal reconstruction initially unless the extremity is unsalvageable. However, there is an unresolved controversy in the literature about whether a failed distal bypass will compromise healing at the below-knee amputation level (see Chapter 153).[15, 20, 30, 39] If the bypass fails and amputation becomes necessary, it still may be feasible and desirable to attempt a below-knee amputation. Amputation success will most likely depend on whether the graft thrombosis extends into the host vessels beyond the insertion of the graft in patients in whom bypasses end *above* the proposed level of amputation. In general, the longer the time interval between the presumed graft thrombosis and amputation, the greater the chance of below-knee amputation healing. In such cases, the surgeon should plan the operation to start initially with a below-knee amputation, and if bleeding is totally inadequate, he or she can proceed with an above-knee amputation. The experience of the authors has demonstrated that below-knee amputation healing frequently occurs after bypass surgery (Fig. 150–1).

Unsalvageable Foot, Patent Bypass. Since the advent of in situ bypass grafting, the authors have seen patients with distal foot lesions that have not healed despite a patent bypass.[52] The surgeon reluctantly may have to perform an amputation in this situation but may have concern that a below-knee amputation will result in acute graft thrombosis that might severely jeopardize stump healing.[80] In an effort to try to preserve the knee joint, the authors have had reasonable success in performing below-knee amputations in this circumstance. If possible, the posterior flap should

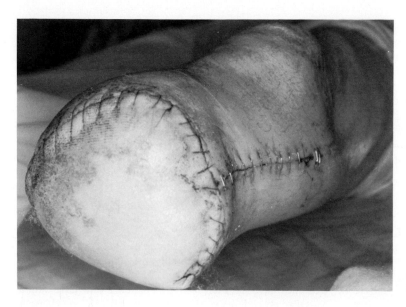

FIGURE 150–1.   Healing of below-knee amputation and incision for bypass surgery.

be created as long as possible to avoid graft ligation. Another alternative to below-knee amputation is to use the patent bypass as a source of arterial inflow for a microvascular free myocutaneous flap.

INTRAOPERATIVE PROBLEMS

Cardiovascular Collapse With Induction of Anesthesia. This complication usually occurs in patients who have deficient intravascular volume to compensate for the vasodilatory effects of spinal or general anesthetics. If this occurs, it is generally better to postpone the amputation until the patient's specific problem can be elucidated and treated appropriately. If the patient's hypotension is thought to be secondary to sepsis from a foot infection, an expeditious open guillotine amputation can be performed in less than 5 minutes.[16, 21, 53] This can significantly improve the patient's hemodynamic status in a matter of hours.

Stump Failure Secondary to Technical Problems. There are a variety of problems that may severely affect prosthetic utilization but may not cause pain or threaten stump viability. Frequent problems include an excessively long fibula or inadequate beveling of the tibia in below-knee amputations; an excessively long femur in above-knee amputations; an excessive muscle or soft tissue mass in the end of the stump, which may cause pistoning in a prosthesis; and skin separation after suture removal. In most stumps with an adequate blood supply, these problems can be improved or cured by local remedial surgery without having to shorten the residual limb and jeopardize the overall amputation level.[29] If the bone has to be resected, the residual bone should be kept as long as feasible. Bulky soft tissue or muscle masses always interfere with optimal prosthetic fitting, which is facilitated by revision to a tapered, cylindrical stump. In many instances, the stump remodels itself with wrapping, as do the dog ears of a posterior flap.

Inadequate Bleeding in Skin and Muscle. Patients with ruborous lower extremities at the mid-calf level, pre-

viously failed distal bypasses, or no Doppler popliteal or femoral pulse are likely to be poor candidates for healing at the below-knee amputation level. These patients should have the entire lower leg prepared for surgery. If the skin incision does not bleed or if the muscle does not react when stimulated with electrocautery, the surgeon should abort plans for a below-knee amputation.[4, 6] The next best level for predictable healing is the above-knee level because knee disarticulations have unpredictable healing in very ischemic extremities.[36, 40, 57, 63]

Inadequate Posterior Skin Flap. In optimal circumstances, the authors transect the tibia at least 9 cm distal to the tibial tubercle in below-knee amputations to allow maximal below-knee stump length.[33, 69] In amputations with equal flaps the length of the posterior skin flap should always be at least as long as the anterior skin flap, and in patients who have an excessively large lower leg, the posterior flap should be longer (12 to 14 cm). Redundant posterior skin can always be trimmed and discarded. If the posterior flap is cut too short, the tibia should be cut shorter to determine whether the posterior flap can then be closed. This may require removal of more muscle in the posterior flap. If the flap still cannot be closed, the tibia can be shortened more, but the residual stump function will be compromised severely. Nevertheless, a short below-knee stump is better than an above-knee stump.

Excessive Muscle in Posterior Flap. The posterior flap should be carefully fashioned to prevent a bulky, noncylindrical stump. If this flap contains too much gastrocnemius and soleus muscle, preventing a snug fit of the flap over the end of the tibia, prosthetic fitting may be a serious problem. Ideally, the soft tissue in the posterior flap should be a direct extension of the tibia.[2, 50] Soft tissue redundancy at the end of the stump serves no useful purpose and complicates prosthetic fitting and wearing. Excessive muscle and soft tissue should be excised during the amputation procedure to prevent the need for later revisional surgery.

Inadequate Beveling of the Tibia. The tibia must be beveled (45 to 60 degrees) so that there is no residual sharp point on this bone. Beveling can be done with a variety of saws, but the authors have found that pneumatic saws are especially useful for this purpose. A file can also be useful to smooth sharp edges.

Use of Foreign Material. Any material that can cause a foreign body reaction should be avoided. This includes the use of bone wax to stop bone marrow bleeding and the use of multi-filament sutures such as silk. The authors routinely use Dexon, Vicryl, or PDS sutures for fascial closure.

Avoiding Excessive Tissue Destruction. Electrocautery should not be used to transect muscle when performing an amputation for ischemia because it may make residual muscle tissue more ischemic than it was originally. Excessive bleeding in these patients is rarely a major problem. All skin and muscle transection should be accomplished with sharp instruments such as a scalpel. Electrocautery may be used to obtain hemostasis for smaller vessels.

Stump Hematoma. Often there is a slow ooze of blood after the posterior flap is fashioned despite an inability to find a focal bleeding point. The use of drains is controversial. The authors routinely drain all amputation stumps with subfascial closed suction (Hemovac) drains for this reason. These can be removed in 24 to 48 hours in almost all circumstances except knee disarticulations, which may require prolonged drainage for up to 7 days to evacuate synovial fluid. Postoperative stump hematomas, which can become secondarily infected, should be totally avoidable with routine drainage. Others have reported good results without using wound drains.[53, 66]

Redundant Edges (Dog Ears). Ideally, the extent of the anterior skin incision in below-knee amputations should be equal to that of the posterior skin (see earlier section, Inadequate Posterior Skin Flap). This is rarely the case because the posterior skin flap is usually longer. This can be partially avoided by extending the anterior skin incision farther posteriorly on the medial and lateral aspects of the flap. Most small dog ears remodel spontaneously. Unless the dog ears are extremely large, they should not be excised

because injudicious excision can jeopardize the blood supply to the remaining flap (Fig. 150–2). With the use of long posterior flaps, dog ears can be minimized by rounding the corners of the flap.

Wound Edge Necrosis. The surgeon should always try to avoid wound edge necrosis because it may cause the demise of an otherwise perfect amputation (Fig. 150–3). It is best to avoid picking up the skin with instruments. Delicate skin forceps should only be used, if needed, to pick up the subcutaneous tissue, not the skin. Plastic surgery skin hooks may be useful. Sutures should gently approximate the skin and should not be pulled too tight. Because fascial sutures are placed so close to the wound edge, subcutaneous sutures are generally not necessary. Usually, good skin approximation can be achieved with simple sutures placed close to the wound edge. Occasionally, vertical mattress sutures may be required to achieve good skin coaptation.

Residual Stump Problems. The immediate postoperative dressing for below-knee amputees should prevent swelling and external trauma, avoid knee flexion contracture, and be comfortable. All of these objectives can easily be accomplished with a rigid plaster dressing that is correctly applied.[58] If the surgeon has no experience in applying this device, the stump should be wrapped snugly in an elastic bandage, and the knee can be held in full extension with a knee immobilizer or a posterior plaster splint. If the latter is used, care should be exercised to avoid a skin plaster burn by placing an adequate amount of cotton wrapping between the skin and the plaster. In addition, tape applied directly to ischemic skin can result in a severe "tape burn" when it is removed. This should be avoided.

POSTOPERATIVE COMPLICATIONS
General Considerations

Death. Because of improvements in preoperative and intraoperative management, mortality should be 6 per cent

FIGURE 150–2. Redundant edges as a result of inadequate fashioning of flaps.

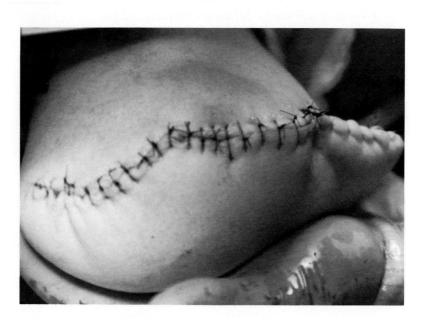

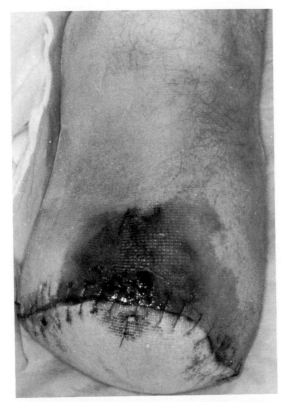

FIGURE 150–3. Wound edge necrosis with incipient gangrene of anterior flap.

or less for below-knee amputations and about 11 to 12 per cent for above-knee amputations.[8, 68] The higher mortality for above-knee amputations reflects the fact that these patients, in general, are older and have more extensive atherosclerosis. Death is typically secondary to ischemic heart disease and stroke. Despite a successful operation, the elderly amputee is still at significant risk for death. By using life table survival curves, Burgess showed that 50 per cent of all elderly lower extremity amputees died within 36 months of the initial amputation.

Prevention of Stump Infection. Amputations performed for noninfected indications should have prophylactic perioperative antibiotic coverage that covers staphylococcal organisms primarily.[42, 55] Most surgeons today use cephalosporins for this purpose. Amputations performed for wet gangrene or other infectious indications should have coverage with culture-specific antibiotics if this information is available. If not, broad-spectrum coverage should include antibiotics active against gram-positive, gram-negative, and anaerobic organisms.

Stump Trauma. This potentially avoidable complication occurs with alarming frequency. Some patients forget that their leg has been amputated and may even try to ''walk'' on their stump. Rigid plaster dressings or knee immobilizers can help to prevent the complications of stump trauma.[5, 58] If a hematoma develops and the stump remains viable, expectant therapy is adequate. If the stump is forced open by the trauma itself or opens up sponta-

neously to decompress the hematoma, it will almost certainly need reamputation to a higher level (Fig. 150–4).

Swelling. All stumps tend to swell, especially below-knee amputation stumps. Excessive swelling may significantly prolong the interval between amputation and prosthetic fitting. Rigid plaster dressings should be rapidly reapplied to below-knee stumps to prevent swelling between changes. If swelling continues to be a problem, careful compressive wrapping with an elastic bandage will usually result in an eventual loss of edema.

Deep Vein Thrombosis. This complication occurs in 5 to 40 per cent of amputation operations.[38] The diagnosis should be considered whenever the surgeon observes that a stump has suddenly become more swollen. In addition, the *contralateral* leg is also at risk; hence, prophylaxis against deep venous thrombosis (e.g., a sequential compression stocking or low-dose subcutaneous heparin) should be considered. Deep vein thrombosis usually occurs about 3 to 7 days after amputation. Documentation by the standard venogram may be impossible, but a Doppler examination of the femoral venous system is usually diagnostic. If deep venous thrombosis is strongly suspected or diagnosed, therapeutic doses of heparin can be instituted with little fear of bleeding into the amputation site, especially if the stump is immobilized in a plaster cast or knee immobilizer. Stump swelling may be a significant problem and may mandate removal of a plaster dressing. Excessive swelling may tend to pull skin edges apart, jeopardizing stump viability. If anticoagulation is contraindicated, a Greenfield inferior

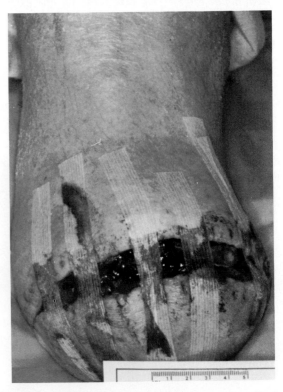

FIGURE 150–4. Stump gaping after minor trauma. Taping of wound is not correct, and additional surgery is required.

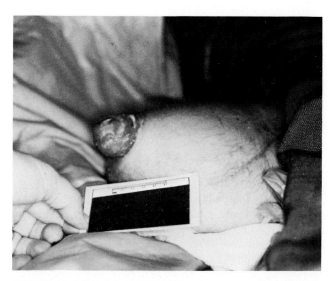

FIGURE 150–5.   Erosion of distal femur through anterior aspect of skin.

vena cava filter can be placed to prevent the development of pulmonary embolism.

Decubitus Heel Ulcers. Bedridden patients are extremely prone to develop heel ulcers on the contralateral foot. The ulcer can quickly cause necrosis of all the thin subcutaneous tissue covering the calcaneus, leading to an amputation of this limb.[8] All patients should have foam heel protectors applied to the contralateral limb to avoid this preventable complication. Frequent changes in position are mandatory. Occasionally, the authors apply a total contact cast to this contralateral leg to distribute the weight of the leg over the entire surface area of the cast.

Decubitus Sacral Ulcers. Nonambulatory patients frequently develop this type of ulcer. Special mattresses and frequent turning are invaluable in preventing this calamity. Occasionally, more radical amputation surgery is necessary to cure these pressure problems by removing the underlying bone.[44, 60, 78, 79, 82]

Overall Nutrition. Optimal wound healing and ambulation training require good nutrition. In patients who have inadequate caloric intake, temporary tube feedings may be indicated. However, if tube feeding is necessary for longer than 2 to 3 weeks, it is extremely unlikely that the patient will be a candidate for rehabilitation. Because of the expense and complications involved with intravenous hyperalimentation, it has little applicability to most amputees.

Upper Body Strength. It should be remembered that ambulation training for lower limb amputations requires upper body strength, especially in the arms. While patients are recuperating from the amputation itself, it is important to start early upper body rehabilitation to maintain the patient's upper body strength.

Bone Erosion. Below-knee amputation bone erosion typically occurs because the tibia was inadequately beveled. If this complication occurs, and revision becomes neces-

sary, an elliptical incision should be used that encompasses the old incision and the area of bone erosion through the skin. The tibia should be shortened 1 to 2 cm and beveled correctly. If the stump is also bulbous, the posterior flap can be modified appropriately.

Above-knee amputation bone erosion typically occurs because the femur was left too long. Because the hip flexors are stronger than the hip extensors, the femur tends to erode through the anterior aspect of the skin incision (Fig. 150–5). The authors have generally reamputated the entire above-knee stump, making sure that the femur is adequately short. If the patient is expected to ambulate, the femur should be left as long as is consistent with adequate wound closure.

Early or Late Ischemic Stump Ulceration. When this problem occurs, revision to a higher level of amputation may be the only feasible option.[43] Occasionally, lower extremity vascular reconstruction to save an ischemic amputation stump is technically possible. Most below-knee amputation failures will heal at the above-knee level, and most above-knee failures will heal at a very high above-knee level. Occasionally, hip disarticulation is necessary in very ischemic limbs that have totally occluded the common femoral and profunda femoris arteries.[9, 79, 82] The authors have a small experience with dismal results at trying to salvage failing stumps with a variety of revascularization procedures, although others have reported limited success with these procedures.[11]

Early Postoperative Complications

Local

The most common complications seen in the early postoperative period (first 3 to 4 weeks) are infection, gangrene, and poor wound healing (Fig. 150–6). Frequently, these are directly related to an inappropriately low level of amputation and are further compounded by the patient's poor medical and nutritional condition. Despite the current

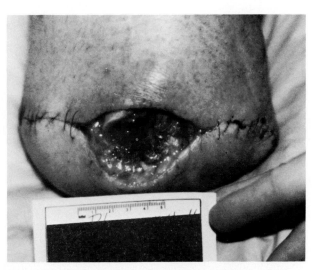

FIGURE 150–6.   Wound breakdown and infection of soft tissue. Note sharp end of tibia as a result of inadequate beveling.

trend to amputate at as low a level as possible, in some instances this may result in unnecessary complications that delay patient rehabilitation. Once a local problem is identified, the surgeon must decide whether revision surgery or local débridement is required. This should be done expeditiously to encourage early rehabilitation.

Early Excessive Pain. Most amputations, regardless of level, cause a tolerable amount of pain in 4 to 7 days. Stumps that seem to be causing excessive amounts of pain after this time may have underlying ischemic muscle or frank muscle necrosis. Such extremities almost always require reamputation at a higher level for pain relief.[43]

Infection

The incidence of stump infection is directly related to the indication for the amputation and ranges from 12 to 28 per cent.[46, 48, 49, 53] In patients with a preexisting infection, antibiotic therapy together with a guillotine amputation or wide drainage of the infection prior to the definitive amputation is usually effective in reducing the incidence of this complication.[16, 53] It has been shown that an ankle guillotine amputation prior to definitive below-knee amputation for a septic foot significantly decreased the rate of stump infection from 22 per cent for a one-stage procedure to 3 per cent for a two-stage operation.[16, 21, 53]

The authors recommend treating patients who have preoperative infections with broad-spectrum antibiotics that provide aerobic and anaerobic coverage. The combination of gentamicin and clindamycin has proved to be very effective in reducing postoperative infections in diabetic patients, in whom the incidence of mixed anaerobic infections may be as high as 60 per cent. However, there are many nonnephrotoxic broad-spectrum antibiotics that provide good coverage without the high risks of renal inefficiency.

An established infection in an amputation stump must be adequately drained with a widely opened incision. The result of this is almost always a revision to a higher level amputation. The seriousness of the complication is emphasized by the fact that in the elderly patient, conversion from a below-knee to an above-knee amputation is often the difference between successful ambulation and not walking.

Prevention of stump hematoma is very important because there is a high correlation between hematoma formation and the development of infection. Hemostasis in flaps must be meticulous. The authors recommend placing closed suction drains for all amputations in which there is any significant oozing from the tissues.

Wound Healing

Failure of a wound to heal may be due to (1) inadequate blood supply at the level selected for amputation, (2) rough or traumatic intraoperative handling of marginally vascularized tissue, (3) a stump hematoma with or without secondary infection (Fig. 150–7), or (4) metabolic factors (e.g., malnutrition, immunosuppression). The incidence of nonhealing after major lower extremity amputation varies from 3 to 28 per cent.[4, 6, 48, 49, 66] An overall healing rate of 80 to 85 per cent for below-knee amputations and 85 to 90 per cent for above-knee amputations can be expected.[13]

The authors' experience with forefoot and Syme's amputations in the dysvascular patient is not as good as that quoted in the literature.[24, 62] It has been disappointing to notice how few patients show healing in a transmetatarsal or Syme amputation, especially those patients with diabetes mellitus who do not have a palpable ankle pulse prior to amputation.[24] Appropriate vascular reconstruction may help lower the level of amputation by improving the local blood supply.

Failure of an amputation stump to heal may be related to any of the four categories previously listed. With respect to nutrition, several investigators have shown that if the lymphocyte count is less than $1500/mm^3$ or the serum albumin is less than 3.5 gm/dl, wound healing may be severely compromised.[17] This may occur in both diabetic and nondiabetic patients. Although the nutritional status cannot be immediately corrected, awareness of the patient's debilitated state allows provision for prolonged wound healing and delayed fitting of a prosthesis.

Poor surgical technique resulting in inadequate skin

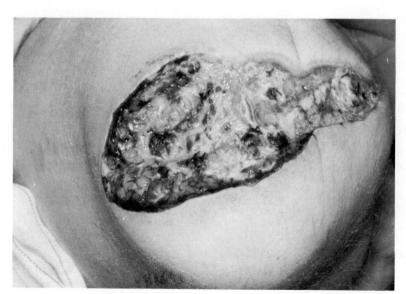

FIGURE 150–7. Failure of wound to heal, with necrotic tissue in base. Revision to higher level is necessary.

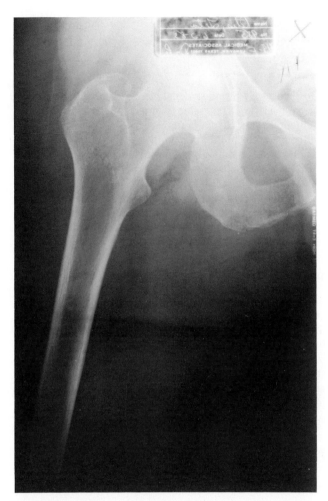

FIGURE 150–8. Residual femur in fixed abduction. (From Gottschalk F, Kourosh S, Stills M, et al: Does socket configuration influence the position of the femur in above knee amputation? J Prosthetics Orthotics 2[1]:97, 1989.)

flaps that have an excessive amount of tension often contributes to wound breakdown in the early postoperative period. Excessive postoperative swelling may further aggravate an already compromised skin flap. Prevention and reduction of the swelling can best be controlled by either a rigid dressing or a pneumatic sleeve applied to the stump. Previous venous congestion in a limb, which may involve part of the skin flap, has also been noted to be a contributing factor to postoperative stump congestion and wound breakdown.

Flexion Contractures

Flexion contractures of the hip or knee joint are not uncommon following major lower limb amputation. The contractures are prone to occur early in the postoperative phase in ambulatory and nonambulatory patients if the patient is not adequately monitored.[48, 49, 58] Pillows placed under the thigh or the knee should be avoided, and patients should be encouraged to avoid positions that keep the joints flexed. The rigid dressing for below-knee amputations will prevent flexion contractures at the knee by keeping the knee

straight. The role of the therapist in the early postoperative phase is extremely important in helping to prevent these deformities. The presence of joint contractures compromises the fitting of a prosthesis and thus the patient's ability to walk. It is generally accepted that a flexion contracture of *10 degrees* or more at the hip and *15 degrees* or more at the knee cannot be satisfactorily fitted with a prosthesis and limits the patient's ability to walk.

Muscle Stabilization

Inadequate and insufficient muscle stabilization at the time of surgery may result in a stump that is too flabby or contains too much bony prominence. Another effect of the poor stabilization is poor stump control and unopposed muscle action of the opposing muscle group. This is frequently seen in above-knee amputations when the femur may be pulled into abduction because of inadequate anchoring of the adductor group of muscles (Fig. 150–8). The eventual outcome is tenting of the skin on the lateral side of the thigh with callus formation. Although the frequency of this problem has not been rigorously studied, it does affect the fitting of a prosthesis.[27]

Preservation of the adductor magnus and use of muscle myodesis to hold the residual femur adducted prevent some of the fitting problems and gait abnormalities associated with above-knee amputation[28] (Fig. 150–9). In below-knee amputations, anchoring the gastrocnemius tendon to the periosteum of the anterior tibia helps to reduce the posterior muscle sag and popliteal fossa discomfort associated with wearing a prosthesis.

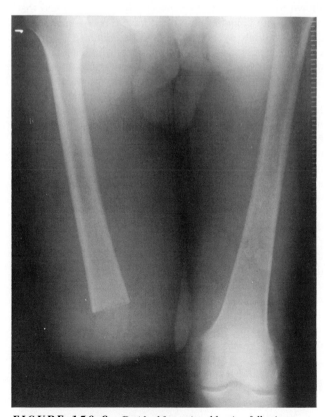

FIGURE 150–9. Residual femur in adduction following muscle-preserving adductor myodesis.

Pain

Phantom limb sensation is a painless limb image that is experienced by most amputees. It is a feeling that the limb is still present and varies in intensity. Phantom limb pain, however, is poorly localized and may be burning, cramping, aching, or stabbing.[1] Melzack noted that phantom limb pain had four major properties: (1) pain lasted long after healing of the injured tissue; (2) the pain had trigger zones that could spread to healthy areas; (3) pain developed in patients who had experienced pain for some time before amputation, and resembled in quality and location the pain present before amputation; (4) the pain could be abolished by temporary increases or decreases in somatic input.[51]

A study of 59 patients who had hemipelvectomy or hip disarticulation showed that phantom limb sensation occurred in all patients and that 14 of 16 patients who had preamputation pain developed postoperative phantom limb pain. Eight of nine patients with no preamputation pain subsequently developed postoperative phantom limb pain.[84]

Various reports in the literature cite the incidence of disabling stump pain and phantom limb pain following major lower extremity amputation as between 5 and 30 per cent.[1, 59, 73–76] Sherman and associates noted that 85 per cent of patients responding to a survey had significant stump pain.[73–76] The explanation for the high incidence of postoperative pain was in part based on the fact that most reports have not closely assessed its presence. Phantom limb pain is very difficult to treat. Common treatment modalities for phantom limb pain include drug therapy, local injections, and surgery. No single or combined treatment has been shown to have any type of success. It has been noted that patients with phantom pain often have a personality disorder and exhibit psychologic aberrations. This seems to occur more frequently in younger patients who have had amputations for trauma. Severe pain is less common in older patients undergoing amputation for vascular disease.

Amputations occurring as a result of trauma may be followed by a local agonizing burning pain associated with trophic changes in the remaining part of the limb. This burning pain, originally called causalgia, is now considered to be part of the syndrome of reflex sympathetic dystrophy.[71] The skin of the involved limb becomes mottled, cool, and shiny, and the bones become osteopenic. Early sympathetic anesthetic blocks or surgical sympathectomy may abort the process, but there is no one individual modality that is invariably successful.

The experience of Malone and others showed that in an aggressive amputation rehabilitation program, the incidence of disabling pain problems following major lower extremity amputations was less than 5 per cent, especially when the amputation was done for vascular rest pain or gangrene.[48, 49, 65, 66] This was attributed to the rapidity and success of rehabilitation as well as postoperative rigid dressings.

Late Complications

Various types of long-term complications may occur in the stump, with many related to loss of adequate fitting of the prosthesis and some due to the patient's general condition.

Stump Congestion

Incorrectly fitting sockets may predispose the stump to edema because of pressure distribution that disturbs the circulation. This edema is unrelated to the surgical trauma and is due more to mechanical factors of poor prosthetic fit and obesity. A commonly seen problem is *verrucous hyperplasia*, which results in a wart-like appearance of the entire distal stump (Fig. 150–10).[45] The cause is thought to be a result of lymphatic and venous congestion due to a poor-fitting prosthesis. The treatment of the condition is not surgery but rather a better-fitting prosthesis with total contact distally to support the stump.

Bulbous Stump

The persistence of a bulbous end to the stump after the early maturation phase may complicate the fitting of prosthesis and lead to uneven pressure distribution and skin breakdown. Excessive residual soft tissue may have to be surgically revised to produce a more cylindrically shaped stump. This applies equally to below-knee and above-knee amputations. The commonest cause of bulbous stumps is insufficient excision of muscle bulk to allow for flap closure.

Excessive Residual Soft Tissue

An excessively flabby stump owing to redundant soft tissue severely compromises an adequate prosthetic fit so

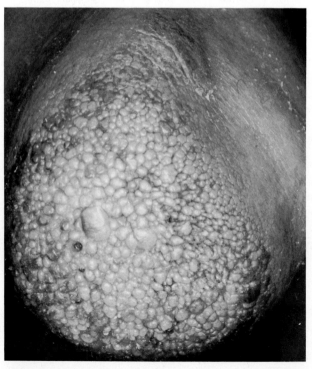

FIGURE 150–10.   Verrucous hyperplasia of distal stump due to poor-fitting prosthesis.

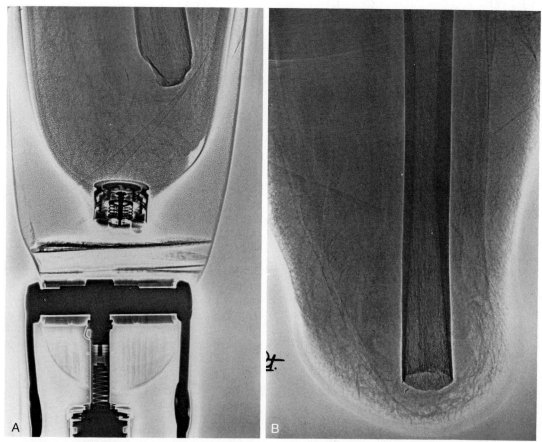

FIGURE 150–11. *A,* Xerogram of excessive residual soft tissue squeezed into prosthetic socket. *B,* Postoperative xerogram showing excision of redundant soft tissue.

that the prosthesis cannot be adequately suspended. Pressure areas may develop where the soft tissue is compressed in the prosthesis (Fig. 150–11).

Calluses and Cysts

The development of calluses around the knee or the groin area may occur with long-term prosthetic users and is associated with areas of increased weight bearing in a prosthesis, particularly over bony prominences. Occasionally, these areas may break down or become painful. Calluses are commonly seen at the end of the stump when insufficient soft tissue has been left over the tibial tuberosity and the ischium.

Other frequently seen problems related to long-term prosthetic wear are inspissated hair follicles and epidermoid cysts. Both are caused by mechanical pressure and are seen in hairy limbs, especially in the popliteal area and the inguinal-groin area.[45] If realignment of the prosthesis or adjustment of the socket does not help to relieve the problem, surgical drainage or excision is recommended. However, recurrence of the cysts at the same site or in close proximity is not uncommon.

Neuroma and Phantom Limb

Neuroma formation cannot be uniformly prevented and is a manifestation of a natural repair phenomenon. If the neuroma forms in an area that is subjected to pressure or is not well buried in the deep muscle tissue, the patient experiences a deep aching pain that may be unresponsive to treatment.[23] The best way to ensure that the neuroma is least likely to cause a problem is to cut the nerve deep in muscle tissue. *Gentle* traction on the nerve and division with a sharp scalpel are recommended. If central vessels in the nerve bleed, they should be cauterized or *individually* ligated. A heavy ligature will not prevent neuroma formation and may irritate that portion of the nerve to which it is applied.

It is generally agreed that a neuroma buried in scar or situated in a vulnerable position may be symptomatic enough to impair the amputee severely. It has also been noted that rigid dressings in the early postoperative phase have reduced the symptoms from the neuroma and also phantom pain.[48, 49, 58]

Phantom limb pain appears to be difficult to control and is more common in patients who have had chronic pain prior to their amputation (see discussion under Early Postoperative Complications). Most patients seem to be resistant to therapy and do not respond to injections, therapy, or medication. Repeat surgery does not resolve the pain either.

Bone Spurs

Although bone callus does not form around the cut end of an amputated bone, it is not unusual for bone spurs to form at some point on the circumference, probably related to periosteal stripping. If the spur is in a location near the subcutaneous border, it may lead to a pressure problem.

Osteoporosis

Long-standing amputees develop osteoporosis of the residual bone in the stump as a result of disuse (Fig. 150–12). The bone is not stressed during activities because it is shielded by the prosthesis. In itself, osteoporosis is asymptomatic, but it may cause the bone to be prone to fracture.

Bone Overgrowth

Amputations through the long bones in children are uncommon and are usually a result of major trauma. Bone overgrowth has been noted in the femur, tibia, and humerus. This does not occur in congenital amputations of these bones. The cause of the overgrowth relative to the soft tissues is not known, but it is proposed that because of the periosteum's contribution to bone growth in children and the lack of stimulation for growth of the soft tissues, bone overgrowth occurs.[77] Overgrowth does not occur in disarticulations. Surgical attempts at preventing the overgrowth include capping the cut end of the bone with cartilage.

Adherent Scar

Adherent skin and scar tissue, which is subjected to weight-bearing stresses, may break down and become in-

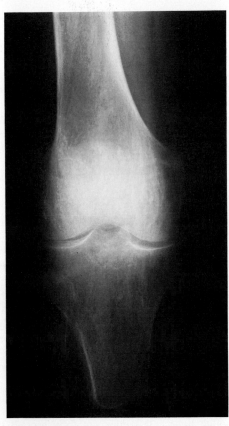

FIGURE 150–12. Osteoporosis of remaining tibia. Note loss of cortical thickness and trabeculae.

fected. Placement of surgical incisions is important to prevent the soft tissues prone to injury from becoming adherent to the underlying bone as the wounds heal.

Opposite Limb

The patient's other limb may be prone to vascular complications (see Chapter 149). In addition, contractures and skin problems may develop if care is not appropriate and if the patient is bedridden. The risk of contralateral amputation is very high in the diabetic or dysvascular patient, and all precautions should be taken to prevent further complications. It is reported that contralateral limb amputation may be as high as 40 per cent within a mean time interval of 17.2 months.[8]

Revision Surgery

Because of increasing longevity, more stump problems requiring surgical treatment are becoming evident. However, the need for revision is related to the level of amputation, adequate prosthetic fitting, and well-supervised postoperative follow-up and care. In long-term prosthetic users with chronic stump problems, revision surgery may be the only means of resolving the problem stump.

References

1. Abramson AS, Feibel A: The Phantom phenomenon: Its use and disuse. Bull NY Acad Med 57:99, 1981.
2. Abrahamson MA, Skinner HD, Effeney DJ, et al: Prescription options for the below knee amputee. Orthopedics 8:210, 1985.
3. Barnes RW, Thornbill B, Nix L, et al: Prediction of amputation wound healing. Roles of Doppler ultrasound and digit photoplethysmography. Arch Surg 116:80, 1981.
4. Baur GM, Porter JM, Axthelm S, et al: Lower extremity amputation for ischemia. Am Surg 44:472, 1978.
5. Behar TA, Burnham SJ, Johnson G: Major stump trauma following below-knee amputation: Outcome and recommendations for therapy. J Cardiovasc Surg 32:753, 1991.
6. Berardi RS, Keonin Y: Amputations in peripheral vascular occlusive disease. Am J Surg 135:231, 1978.
7. Bernstein EF: Operative management of acute venous thromboembolism. *In* Rutherford RB (ed): Vascular Surgery. 2nd ed. Philadelphia, WB Saunders Co, 1984, pp 1367–1384.
8. Bodily RC, Burgess EM: Contralateral limb and patient survival after leg amputations. Am J Surg 146:280, 1983.
9. Boyd HB: Anatomic disarticulation of the hip. Surg Gynecol Obstet 84:346, 1947.
10. Bunt TJ: Physiologic amputation for acute pedal sepsis. The Am Surg 56(9):530, 1990.
11. Bunt TJ: Gangrene of the immediate postoperative above-knee amputation stump: Role of emergency revascularization in preventing death. J Vasc Surg 2:874, 1985.
12. Burgess EM: Disarticulation of the knee. Arch Surg 112:1250, 1977.
13. Burgess EM, Matsen FA, Wyss CR, et al: Segmental transcutaneous measurements of PO_2 in patients requiring below the knee amputation for peripheral vascular insufficiency. J Bone Joint Surg 64A:378, 1982.
14. Ctercteko GC, Dhanendran M, Hutton WC, et al: Vertical forces acting on the feet of diabetic patients with neuropathic ulceration. Br J Surg 68:608, 1981.
15. Dardik H, Kahn M, Dardik I, et al: Influence of failed vascular bypass procedures on conversion of below-knee to above-knee amputation levels. Surgery 91:64, 1982.
16. Desai Y, Robbs JV, Keenan JP: Staged below-knee amputations for septic peripheral lesions due to ischemia. Br J Surg 73:392, 1986.
17. Dickhaut SC, DeLee JC, Page CP: Nutritional status: Importance in predicting wound-healing after amputation. J Bone Joint Surg 66A:71, 1984.

18. Edwards JM, Taylor LM, Porter JM: Limb salvage in end-stage renal disease (ESRD): Comparison of modern results in patients with and without ESRD. Arch Surg 123:1164, 1988.

19. Effeney DJ, Lim RC, Schecter WP: Transmetatarsal amputation. Arch Surg 112:1366, 1977.

20. Evans WE, Hayes JP, Vermillion BD: Effect of a failed distal reconstruction on the level of amputation. Am J Surg 160:217, 1990.

21. Fisher DF, Clagett GP, Fry RE, et al: One-stage vs. two-stage amputation for wet gangrene of the lower extremity: A randomized study. J Vasc Surg 8:428, 1988.

22. Fisher DF Jr, Clagett GP, Brigham RA, et al: Dilemmas in dealing with the blue toe syndrome: Aortic versus peripheral source. Am J Surg 148:836, 1984.

23. Fisher GT, Boswick JA: Neuroma formation following digital amputations. J Trauma 23:136, 1983.

24. Francis H, Roberts JR, Clagett GP, et al: The Syme amputation: Success in elderly diabetic patients with palpable ankle pulses. J Vasc Surg 12(3):237, 1990.

25. Garrison AF, Jelenko C III, Brahn G, et al: The MCG boot: A device which facilitates physiologic amputation. Am Surg 39:637, 1973.

26. Gonzales EG, Corcoran PJ, Reyes RL: Energy expenditure in below-knee amputees: Correlation with stump length. Arch Phys Med Rehabil 55:111, 1974.

27. Gottschalk F, Kourosh S, Stills M, et al: Does socket configuration influence the position of the femur in above-knee amputation? J Prosthet Orthot 2:97, 1989.

28. Gottschalk F: Transfemoral amputation. *In* Bowker J, Michael J (eds): Atlas of Limb Prosthetics. 2nd ed. St. Louis, CV Mosby, 1992.

29. Hadden W, Marks R, Murdock G, Stewart C: Wedge resection of amputation stumps: A valuable salvage procedure. J Bone Joint Surg 69B:306, 1987.

30. Haimovici H: Failed grafts and level of amputation. J Vasc Surg 2:271, 1985.

31. Harbrecht PJ, Nethery H, Ahmad W, et al: A technique for freezing an extremity in preparation for amputation. Am J Surg 135:859, 1978.

32. Harrison JD, Southworth S, Callum KG: Experience with the ''skew flap'' below-knee amputation. Br J Surg 74:930, 1987.

33. Hicks L, McClelland RN: Below-knee amputations for vascular insufficiency. Am Surg 46:239, 1980.

34. Holloway GA Jr, Burgess EM: Cutaneous blood flow and its relation to healing of below-knee amputation. Surg Gynecol Obstet 146:750, 1978.

35. Hunsaker RH, Schwartz JA, Keagy BA, et al: Dry ice cryoamputation: A twelve-year experience. J Vasc Surg 2:812, 1985.

36. Huston CC, Bivins BA, Ernst CB, et al: Morbid implications of above-knee amputations. Report of a series and review of the literature. Arch Surg 115:165, 1980.

37. American Academy of Orthopaedic Surgeons. Instructional Course Lectures. XXVIII. St. Louis, CV Mosby, 1979, pp 118–165.

38. Johnson G Jr: Superficial venous thrombosis. *In* Rutherford RB (ed): Vascular Surgery. 4th ed. Philadelphia, WB Saunders, 1995.

39. Kazmers M, Satiani B, Evans WE: Amputation level following unsuccessful distal limb salvage operations. Surgery 87:683, 1980.

40. Kihn RB, Warren R, Beebe GW: The ''geriatric'' amputee. Ann Surg 176:305, 1972.

41. Knighton DR, Fylling CP, Fiegel VD, Cerra F: Amputation prevention in an independently reviewed at-risk diabetic population using a comprehensive wound care protocol. Am J Surg 160:466, 1990.

42. Krebs B: The use of antibiotic prophylaxis in amputations of the lower extremity. Acta Orthop Scand 56:179, 1985.

43. Kwaan JHM, Connolly JE: Fatal sequelae of the ischemic amputation stump: A surgical challenge. Am J Surg 138:49, 1979.

44. Lawton RL, DePinto V: Bilateral hip disarticulation in paraplegics with decubitus ulcers. Arch Surg 122:1040, 1987.

45. Levy SW: Skin Problems of the Amputee. St. Louis, Warren H Green, 1983, p 153.

46. LeFrock JL, Joseph WS: Lower extremity infections in diabetics. Infect Surg 5:135, 1986.

47. Lind J, Kramhoft M, Bodtker S: The influence of smoking on complications after primary amputation of the lower extremity. Clin Ortho 267:211, 1991.

48. Malone JM, Moore WS, Leal JM, Childers SJ: Rehabilitation for lower extremity amputation. Arch Surg 116:93, 1981.

49. Malone JM, Moore WS, Goldstone J, et al: Therapeutic and economic impact of a modern amputation program. Ann Surg 189:798, 1979.

50. Medhat MA: Rehabilitation of vascular amputee. Orthopaed Rev 12:51, 1983.

51. Melzack R: Phantom limb implications for treatment of pathological pain. Anesthesiology 35:401, 1971.

52. Memsic L, Busuttil RW, Machleder H, et al: Interval gangrene occurring after successful lower extremity revascularization. Arch Surg 122:1060, 1987.

53. McIntyre KE Jr, Bailey SA, Malone JM, et al: Guillotine amputation in the treatment of nonsalvageable lower-extremity infections. Arch Surg 119:450, 1984.

54. McKittrick LS, McKittrick JB, Risley TS: Transmetatarsal amputation for infection or gangrene in patients with diabetes mellitus. Ann Surg 130:826, 1949.

55. Moller BN, Krebs B: Antibiotic prophylaxis in lower limb amputation. Acta Orthop Scand 56:327, 1985.

56. Mooney V: Innovations in care of the amputee. Tex Med 75:43, 1979.

57. Mooney V: Above-knee amputations. *In* American Academy of Orthopaedic Surgeons: Atlas of Limb Prosthetics: Surgical and Prosthetic Principles. St. Louis, CV Mosby, 1981, pp 378–382.

58. Mooney V, Harvey JP Jr, McBride E, et al: Comparison of postoperative stump management: Plaster vs. soft dressings. J Bone Joint Surg 53A:241, 1971.

59. Parkes CM: Factors determining persistence of phantom pain in the amputee. J Psychosomat Res 17:97, 1973.

60. Pearlman NW, McShane RH, Jochimsen PR, Shirazi SS: Hemicorpectomy for intractable decubitus ulcers. Arch Surg 111:1139, 1976.

61. Perry J, Waters RL: Physiological variances in lower limb amputees. *In* American Academy of Orthopaedic Surgeons: Atlas of Limb Prosthetics: Surgical and Prosthetic Principles. St. Louis, CV Mosby Co, 1981, pp 410–416.

62. Pinzur M, Kaminsky M, Sage R, et al: Amputations at the middle level of the foot. A retrospective and prospective review. J Bone Joint Surg 68A:1061, 1986.

63. Pinzur MS, Smith DG, Daluga DJ, Osterman H: Selection of patients for through-the-knee amputation. J Bone Joint Surg 79A:746, 1988.

64. Porter JM, Baur GM, Taylor LM Jr: Lower extremity amputation for ischemia. Arch Surg 116:89, 1981.

65. Potts JR, Wendelken JR, Elkins RC, et al: Lower extremity amputations. Review of 110 cases. Am J Surg 138:924, 1979.

66. Roon AJ, Moore WS, Goldstone J: Below-knee amputation: A modern approach. Am J Surg 134:153, 1977.

67. Ruckley CV, Stonebridge PA, Prescott RJ: Skewflap vs. long posterior flap in below-knee amputations: Multicenter trial. J Vasc Surg 13:423, 1991.

68. Rush DS, Huston CC, Bivins BA, et al: Operative and late mortality rates of above-knee and below-knee amputations. Am Surg 47:36, 1981.

69. Sanders RJ, Augspurger R: Skin flap measurement for below-knee amputation. Surg Gynecol Obstet 145:741, 1977.

70. Sapico FL, Whitte JL, Canawati HN, et al: The infected foot of the diabetic patient: Quantitative microbiology and analysis of clinical features. Rev Infect Dis 6:S171, 1984.

71. Schnell MD, Bunch WM: Management of pain in the amputee. *In* American Academy of Orthopaedic Surgeons: Atlas of Limb Prosthesis: Surgical and Prosthetic Principles. St. Louis, CV Mosby Co, 1981, pp 464–472.

72. Schwartz ME, Harrington EB, Harrington M, et al: Above-knee amputation in patients with prior hip surgery: A caveat. J Vasc Surg 11:480, 1990.

73. Sherman RA: Published treatment of phantom pain. Am J Phys Med 59:232, 1980.

74. Sherman RA, Sherman CJ, Gall NG: A survey of current phantom limb pain treatment in the United States. Pain 8:85, 1980.

75. Sherman RA, Sherman CJ, Parker L: Chronic phantom and stump pain among American veterans: Results of a survey. Pain 18:83, 1984.

76. Sherman RA, Tippens JK: Suggested guidelines for treatment of phantom limb pain. Orthopaedics 5:1595, 1982.

77. Speer DP: The pathogenesis of amputation stump overgrowth. Clin Orthop 159:294, 1981.

78. Strinden WD, Mixter RC, Dibbell DG: Internal hemipelvectomy as a treatment for end-stage pressure sores. Ann Plast Surg 22:529, 1989.

79. Sugarbaker PH, Cretien PB: A surgical technique for hip disarticulation. Surgery 90:546, 1981.

80. Taylor LM, Hamre D, Dalman RL, Porter JM: Limb salvage vs.

amputation for critical ischemia: The role of vascular surgery. Arch Surg 126:1251, 1991.

81. Traugh GH, Corcoran PJ, Reyes RL: Energy expenditure of ambulation in patients with above-knee amputations. Arch Phys Med Rehabil 56:67, 1975.

82. Unruh T, Fisher DF, Unruh TA, et al: Hip disarticulation: An 11-year experience. Arch Surg 125:791, 1990.

83. Wagner FW Jr: The Syme amputation. *In* American Academy of Orthopaedic Surgeons: Atlas of Limb Prosthetics: Surgical and Prosthetic Principles. St. Louis, CV Mosby Co, 1981, pp 326–340.

84. Wall R, Novotny JP, MacNamara T: Does preamputation pain influence phantom limb pain in cancer patients. South Med J 78:34, 1985.

85. Wheat IJ, Allen SD, Henry M, et al: Diabetic foot infections. Arch Int Med 146:1935, 1986.

151

Rehabilitation of the Person With an Amputation

Robert H. Meier III, M.D.

• • •

PHILOSOPHY OF THE AMPUTATING SURGEON

Amputation surgery must be viewed as a means of providing patients with improved function, which requires the removal of nonviable tissue, alleviation of pain, extirpation of dysfunctional tissue, and construction of a limb that can be fitted with a prosthesis if the patient is a prosthetic candidate. Neither the surgeon nor the patient should view the amputation as a failure of therapy but instead should approach the operation as the prelude to more comfort and improved function—with or without a prosthesis.

The level of amputation largely determines the prognosis for the functional outcome. In most cases, the longer the residual limb, the better the function. Three levels may not follow this rule: a hindfoot amputation, a long transtibial amputation (distal to the taper of the gastrocnemius–soleus belly), and a long transfemoral amputation (distal to the junction of the middle and distal thirds of the femur).

PHASES OF REHABILITATION

The rehabilitative phases of amputee management are divided into nine phases (Table 151–1):

1. Preoperative.
2. Amputation surgery reconstruction.

Table 151–1. Phases of Amputee Rehabilitation

Phase	Hallmarks
1. Preoperative	Assess body condition, patient education; discuss surgical level, postoperative prosthetic plans
2. Amputation surgery reconstruction	Length, myoplastic closure, soft tissue coverage, nerve handling, rigid dressing
3. Acute postoperative	Wound healing, pain control, proximal body motion, emotional support
4. Preprosthetic	Shaping and shrinking amputation stump, increasing muscle strength, restoring patient locus of control
5. Prosthetic fabrication	Team consensus on prosthetic prescription, experienced limb prosthetic fabrication
6. Prosthetic training	Increase wearing of prosthesis and mobility skills
7. Community reintegration	Resume roles in family and community activities; regain emotional equilibrium and healthy coping strategies; pursue recreational activities
8. Vocational rehabilitation	Assess and plan vocational activities for future. May need further education, training, or job modification
9. Follow-up	Provide lifelong prosthetic, functional, medical, and emotional support; provide regular assessment of functional level and prosthetic problem solving

3. Acute postoperative.
4. Preprosthetic.
5. Prosthetic fabrication.
6. Prosthetic training.
7. Community reintegration.
8. Vocational rehabilitation.
9. Follow-up.

Preoperative Phase

Optimal functional outcome results when the patient is in the most favorable cardiovascular condition and has been mobile prior to the amputation. At minimum, the potential amputee should avoid being wheelchair-bound and should ambulate with a walker or crutches, at least for short distances. Strengthening the hip extensor and abductor muscles as well as the knee extensors hastens postamputation rehabilitation. Additionally, this is an appropriate time to discuss phantom limb sensation, phantom pain, and residual limb pain with the patient. The postoperative rehabilitation plan, the stages of prosthetic use, and the approximate timetable for the rehabilitation program should be presented. Discussion of the emotional adaptive process is also helpful during the preoperative phase. It is essential to prevent flexion contractures of the hip or knee joints of the affected limb and the opposite leg. Any hip or knee contracture of more than 5 to 10 degrees from full extension substantially increases the difficulty of using the prosthesis and augments the energy expenditure required.

Amputation Surgery Reconstruction

This topic has been extensively covered elsewhere in this text, but it cannot be stated strongly enough that careful reconstruction of the amputated limb at the time of surgery is the sine qua non for optimal rehabilitation results. The techniques that seem to determine successful prosthetic fit and comfort are related to (1) identification of a level of tissue viability that will heal primarily, (2) formation of a cylindrical residual limb (Fig. 151–1), (3) myoplastic closure for prevention of movement of the residual limb in the soft tissues, (4) beveling of the ends of the residual bones, (5) control of postoperative edema with immediate postoperative rigid dressings, and (6) burying the ends of major peripheral nerves.

Acute Postoperative Phase

At the conclusion of the amputation, the residual limb is best placed in an immediate postoperative rigid dressing to diminish postoperative edema, enhance wound healing, and decrease pain. Various postoperative rigid dressing protocols have been proposed and are part of a comprehensive coordinated amputee management system.[1,2] If a soft dressing is applied at the conclusion of the surgery, no attempt should be made to use elastic compression to shrink the stump or to decrease the edema until the wound shows evidence of primary wound healing (at least 3 weeks on average). An alternative to the soft dressing that can pro-

vide important protection to the fresh incision is the removable rigid dressing.[3] It can be applied shortly after the patient has had the amputation. This cap protects the stump from trauma and can be changed as edema decreases. If a rigid dressing is not employed postoperatively, a long posterior splint should be affixed behind the knee to hold it in extension. In addition, an elevating leg rest for wheelchair mobility will assist in keeping the knee in full extension. Prolonged periods of lying prone should be mandated to assist in maintaining full extension of the hip. Limiting the time spent in the sitting position will diminish the development of hip flexion tightness.

After skin sutures or staples have been removed, a more aggressive program of residual limb shaping and shrinking can begin. Suture removal marks the beginning of the preprosthetic phase if the patient has the potential for using a prosthesis. The important components of rehabilitation during this phase consist of controlling pain, promoting wound healing, and increasing upper limb, trunk, and remaining limb muscle strength. These activities enhance mobility before use of a prosthesis is desirable or practical. This is an ideal time for the patient to adjust to the new appearance of the body and to teach functional skills without using a prosthesis.

The debate over rigid, semi-rigid, or soft dressings after amputation continues in the United States. A consen-

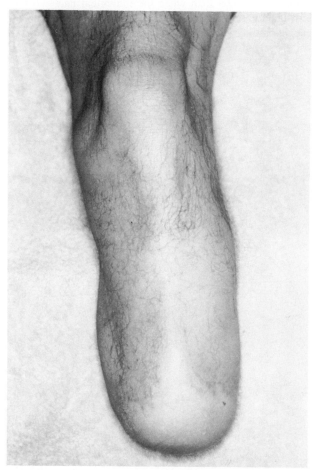

FIGURE 151–1. Transtibial amputation residual limb demonstrating the preferred cylindrical shape of the soft tissues below the knee.

sus conference on amputation surgical techniques was held at Strathclyde, Scotland, in 1990.[4] Whether rigid dressings or some other dressings are employed, a center-specific protocol for amputee care should be developed. Members of the team caring for amputees should understand their roles in effecting the goals of rehabilitation.[5]

In addition to the surgeon, an ideal amputee team includes a physiatrist, rehabilitation nurse, physical therapist, occupational therapist, psychologist, medical social worker, recreational therapist, vocational rehabilitationist, prosthetist, and pastoral counselor. These team members can evaluate the individual amputee and design a plan with functional goals that can be measured objectively at regular intervals. This team should be able to predict accurately the patient's expected function at 1 month, 3 months, 6 months, and 1 year from the time of the amputation. It should provide a complete array of services to facilitate the patient's return to optimal function in the most timely and cost-effective manner. Amputation rehabilitation has progressed beyond the point at which the patient with a healed amputation was sent to the prosthetist with a generic prosthetic prescription in hand. If the patient's quality of life is to reach its zenith, he or she should be carefully guided through each phase of amputee rehabilitation with input from this team of health professionals.

Nail and preventive foot care for the remaining limb should be established early because this limb must always sustain more force than when the individual had two feet on which to bear weight during ambulation. The health care team should inspect the shoes customarily worn and ensure that properly fitted shoes are acquired.

Preprosthetic Phase

Once the wound has developed adequate tensile strength, the stump must be shaped and shrunk. A rigid dressing, changed weekly, can be applied, or an Unna paste dressing can be employed. Elastic compression with a shrinker garment or elastic rolled bandages can be utilized.[6] If elastic rolled bandages are used, they must be applied in a figure-of-eight fashion (Figs. 151–2 and 151–3). The elastic bandages are anchored by incorporating the next proximal joint, and bandages should be rewrapped every 4 hours. When they are removed, they should not remain off for more than 15 minutes so that extracellular fluid does not reaccumulate. Usually, 2 weeks of shaping and shrinking should produce enough residual limb change to permit creating a cast for the initial prosthetic socket.

During this phase, increasing the strength of the residual and opposite limb muscles is of paramount importance. These remaining muscles must compensate for those lost in the amputation. Knee stability is enhanced not just by the quadriceps muscle but, more importantly, by the hip extensors, including the gluteus maximus and the hamstrings (Fig. 151–4).[7] These muscles are essential for knee stability in the amputee. The hip abductor mechanism, generated by the gluteus medius, minimus, and tensor fascia lata, is of prime importance for pelvic stability during the stance phase of prosthetic gait (Fig. 151–5). In addition, trunk and upper limb strengthening is essential during this phase. This is also a time to improve cardiovascular fitness and endurance.

Psychosocial issues are of great importance during the

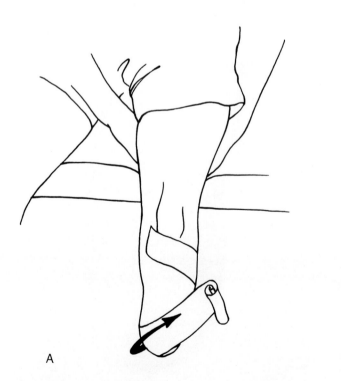
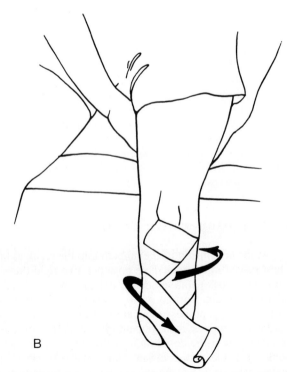

A   B

FIGURE 151–2. *A,* All turns should be on the diagonal. Never use horizontal turns because they tend to constrict circulation. *B,* Do not encircle the end of the residual limb with one turn because this tends to cause skin creases in the scar. Alternatively, cover the inside and outside of the end in successive turns.

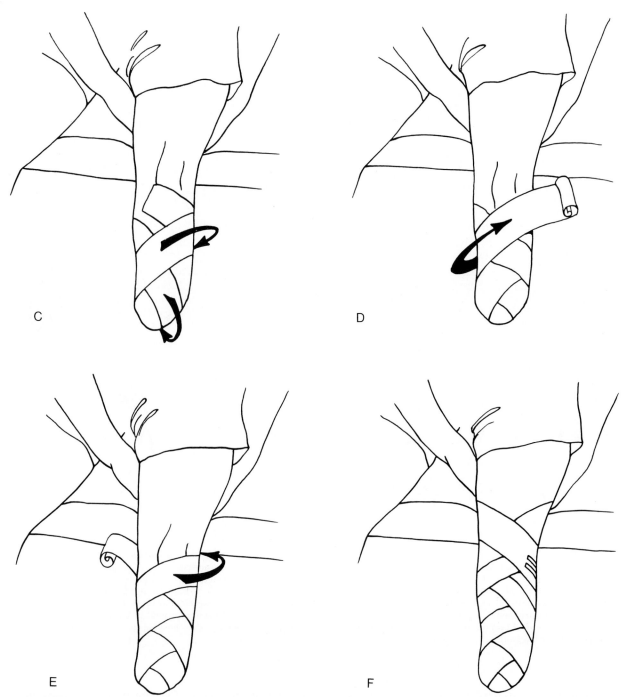

FIGURE 151–2 *Continued C*, Continue making diagonal turns, exerting firm pressure over the distal end of the residual limb.
D, Bandage pressure should become lighter as you continue to wrap proximally. *E*, Extend the wrap above the knee. There should be at least one turn above the kneecap. *F*, Return to below the knee. If there is bandage remaining, finish the bandage with diagonal turns *over the end* of the residual limb. Anchor the bandage with tape. Do not use safety pins. Rewrap the residual limb every 3–4 hours, or more often if necessary. (Reprinted from *Lower Extremity Amputation*, 2nd ed, by LA Karacoloff, CS Hammersley, and FJ Schneider, pp 16–17, with permission of Aspen Publishers, Inc., © 1992.)

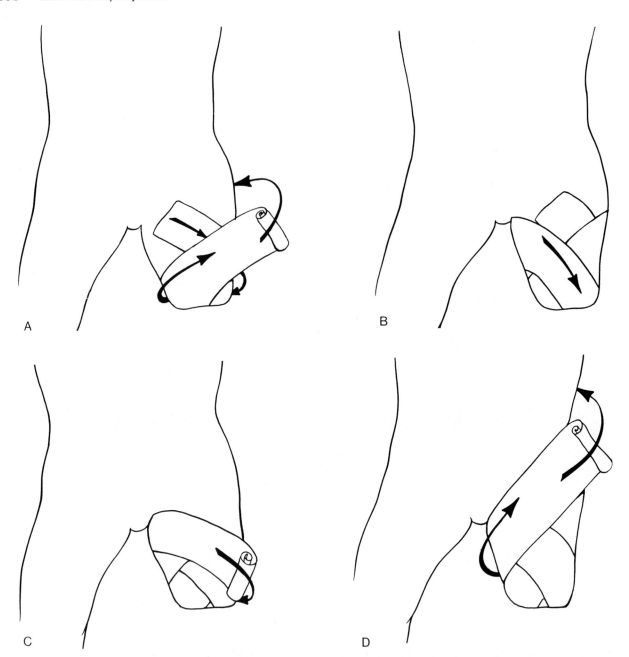

FIGURE 151–3. *A*, Start with the bandage in the groin area. Roll toward the outside, then behind and around the residual limb, covering the medial thigh. Be certain to keep the bandage smooth. Avoid wrinkles because they may cause skin irritations. *B*, Roll around the posterior residual limb. Continue down and around the lateral half of the distal end. *C*, Continue making diagonal turns around the residual limb until all skin is covered with at least two layers of bandage and firm pressure is obtained over the end. Avoid encircling the end with one turn because this tends to cause skin creases in the scar. Never use circular turns, because this constricts circulation. Pressure should be greatest at the end, becoming lighter as you wrap toward the hip. Include all soft tissue on the medial thigh at the groin. *D*, Begin the hip spica as shown here. The bandage should be placed as high as possible on the medial thigh and then crossed over the hip joint.

preprosthetic period.[8] All rehabilitation team members play important roles in the patient's psychosocial adaptation to limb loss. A psychologist or social worker experienced in the process of adapting to limb loss and change in body image is essential for optimal rehabilitation. Often these aspects of rehabilitation, not simply the provision of the prosthesis, are the basis of a successful outcome. Psychological counseling enhances the coping mechanisms of the amputee adapting to altered body image and function, with

or without a prosthesis. Team members responsible for psychosocial issues should actively interact with the amputee throughout all phases of the rehabilitation program.

This phase of rehabilitation is concluded when the patient is ready for prosthetic fitting, a prosthetic prescription is generated, and the prosthesis is fabricated. In general, if the amputee can stand independently and walk for short distances on one leg using a walker or crutches, he or she is a potential prosthetic candidate. Even if the prosthesis

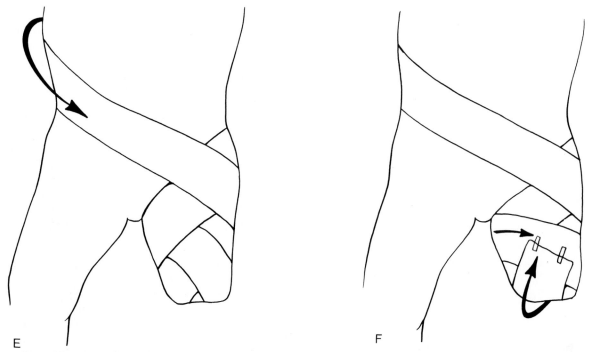

E

F

FIGURE 151–3 *Continued E,* Carry the bandage behind and around the pelvis, crossing just below the waist on the sound side. Returning to the amputated side, cross over the hip joint again. *F,* Finish the bandage by making diagonal turns around the end of the residual limb. Anchor the bandage with tape. Do not use safety pins. The bandage should not cause pain. If it does, remove it and rewrap. Rewarp the residual limb every 3–4 hours, or more often if necessary. (Reprinted from *Lower Extremity Amputation*, 2nd ed, by LA Karacoloff, CS Hammersley, and FJ Schneider, pp 17–18, with permission of Aspen Publishers, Inc., © 1992.)

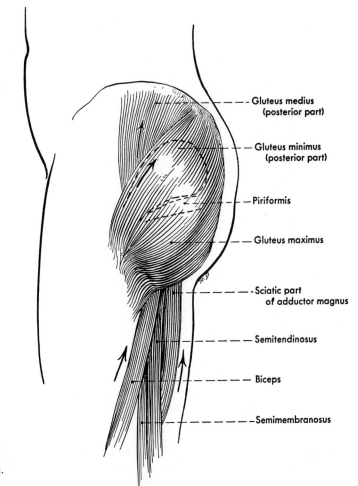

FIGURE 151–4. Extensors of the thigh. According to electromyographic evidence, the posterior part of the gluteus minimus, usually regarded as an extensor, may not participate in extension. (From Jenkins DB: Movements of the thigh and leg. *In* Hollinshead's Functional Anatomy of the Limbs and Back. 6th ed. Philadelphia, WB Saunders, 1991, p 272.)

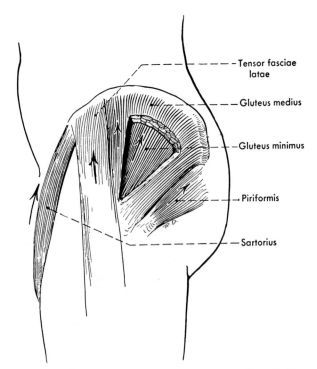

FIGURE 151–5. The abductors of the thigh. (From Jenkins DB: Movements of the thigh and leg. *In* Hollinshead's Functional Anatomy of the Limbs and Back. 6th ed. Philadelphia, WB Saunders, 1991, p 273.)

is to be used only for transferring from a wheelchair to another surface, provision of a prosthesis may be warranted. Only rarely should a leg prosthesis be prescribed for purely cosmetic reasons.

The preprosthetic period usually lasts from 6 to 10 weeks from the date of surgery in the dysvascular amputee and often is shorter for the primarily healed traumatic leg amputee. In general, the patient should first be fitted with a preparatory (temporary) prosthesis, which should last from several weeks to months. These preparatory prostheses are best made by an experienced prosthetist from thermoplastic materials rather than from plaster. A definitive prosthesis of plastic laminate should be fabricated when the soft tissues have responded to the pressure of weight bearing using the preparatory prosthesis. The process of stump shaping occurs over several months to several years. However, in most cases, the residual limb tissues stabilize within the first 12 months. Less frequent prosthetic adjustments are required after this initial period.

Prosthetic Training

The phase of prosthetic training begins with the delivery of the prosthesis from the prosthetic laboratory and should start within 6 to 10 weeks of the amputation surgery. Training should occur under the guidance of an experienced physician, therapist, and prosthetist, all of whom understand the biomechanics and principles of prosthetic use.[9–11] The decision of whether to use an inpatient or outpatient setting for teaching prosthetic use depends on many factors. In most instances, a patient with unilateral transtibial or trans-

femoral amputation can be rehabilitated as an outpatient. The transfemoral amputee with significant cardiopulmonary compromise or multiple medical problems, however, probably will need an initial inpatient training period.

Short periods of wearing the prosthesis and instruction in donning and doffing it should be the initial focus. Walking while wearing the prosthesis, although a very exciting prospect for the amputee, is often inappropriate early in training because the proximal leg muscles have not yet been properly strengthened to provide adequate knee, hip, or pelvic stability. Periods of standing supported by parallel bars with weight shifting should be attempted initially. Good hip and knee stability must be attained prior to advancing to the next stage—walking with a gait aid. Whenever possible, the amputee should be discouraged from using a wheelchair and encouraged to walk with a walker and then to walk using crutches or a cane. Use of a walker never permits a normal gait pattern and frequently limits the environment in which the prosthesis can be used. Use of the prosthesis in the home should be observed by the training therapist, and training on curbs, ramps, and stairs should be offered to maximize mobility. Most older persons have a dreadful fear of falling. Training in falling techniques and arising from a fall help to minimize the dangers and fear associated with falling. Exploration of the use of the prosthesis for driving, recreation, and vocational needs should also be part of this phase.

Assessment should be made of the amputee's perception of the prosthesis, its meaning to the quality of life, the effort needed to use it, and how closely it simulates the lost leg. Often the artificial limb does not meet the fantasized expectations of the amputee in regard to what a prosthesis should look like, what function it provides, and how it feels to walk with it compared to normal walking before the amputation.

This training phase is completed when the amputee achieves full use of the prosthesis. A proficient team experienced in amputee rehabilitation and knowledgeable about prosthetic function is required to make this assessment.

Community Reintegration

Reentering society with an altered body image and function is often an emotionally stressful time for an amputee. Identification of a meaningful support structure in the community is one of the most important roles of the rehabilitation team. Often this is a time in an elderly amputee's life when changes in support systems are overwhelming. Spouse and friends are dying, living settings are changing, vocational lives are winding down or have stopped, and there may be fewer things to enjoy and to which the amputee can look forward. Whenever possible, previous community supports need to be enlisted. However, on occasion, an extended care facility may provide the best environment for the leg amputee in which to enhance his or her prosthetic skills and proficiency in activities of daily living before returning to previous living conditions. All aspects of an individual's life should be addressed during this phase. The individual's function in society, although changed, should be made as meaningful and satisfying as possible. This integrative model really draws on all persons and resources in the community: spouse, family, merchants, employer, senior citizens' center, clergy, social workers, health professionals, municipal government, and the federal government working in concert to assist in restoring the individual to his or her rightful place in society. This phase of rehabilitation continues to influence the amputee for the remainder of his or her life.

Vocational Rehabilitation

Unfortunately, for the geriatric amputee the phase of vocational rehabilitation is often overlooked. More and more today, individuals over the age of 65 years find that continuing to work is an important part of their senior years. Despite the loss of a limb, their dreams and plans should not be discouraged. They may still retain significant potential for full-time or part-time employment. A careful discussion of vocational plans should occur. Knowledgeable vocational services should be provided for the older amputee who has questions about her or his future vocational options. In such cases, an understanding of the amputee's maximal prosthetic functional skills should help in proper vocational rehabilitation planning. For the younger person with a traumatic amputation, this is an essential part of amputee care.

Follow-Up

Careful patient follow-up remains the single most important phase of amputee rehabilitation following inpatient discharge. It is during this lifelong phase that attention to functional outcome, with or without a prosthesis, follows the quality of life achieved by the amputee.[12] Emphasis should not be placed on the prosthesis but instead on the ultimate functional capability achieved by the amputee. The emotional well-being and role in the family and community are continually assessed and enhanced whenever possible by the rehabilitation team. Follow-up visits to the physiatrist should be as frequent as visits to the internist or vascular surgeon. Any prosthetic fitting problem should receive prompt attention, and any decrease in the level of function should be investigated. Often, correction of the problem requires more than just a visit to the prosthetist, and the problem should be discussed with the rehabilitation team. Only with this comprehensive array of services can the wide variety of amputee issues be dealt with thoroughly and in a coordinated fashion. This highly structured system provides health care to the amputee in the least frustrating and most cost-effective manner. Such a system results in the best functional outcome and quality of life following an amputation.

PROSTHETIC PRESCRIPTION AND COMPONENTRY

During the past decade, the variety of prosthetic components for lower limb prostheses has increased tremendously. However, few data exist to support the superiority of this new technology over that developed in the 1950s. Certainly the cost-effectiveness of these more expensive designs has not been established. Subjective patient feedback, however, does affirm that these newer designs provide improved comfort and function.

Partial Foot

Usually the portion of the foot missing is replaced with a molded toe filler approximately the size of the opposite foot. The toe filler is usually attached to an insole that slips into a blucher shoe or sneaker that laces to hold the residual foot and insole with minimal shear at the skin-insole interface.[13] To achieve improved rollover and simulation of toeoff, a rocker bar built into the shoe sole and a long steel or carbon graphite shank approximate a more anatomic gait. In hindfoot amputations, the prosthetic foot restoration can be attached to a molded plastic shell that crosses the ankle and extends up the lower leg (Fig. 151–6). This design helps to provide better ankle and hindfoot control and a larger surface over which to distribute the pressures.

Syme's Amputation

Two basic prosthetic designs are generally used: (1) a windowed plastic shell or (2) an expandable inner lining. Both of these systems have outer walls of plastic laminated material that extend up to the knee region and may provide some patellar tendon weight bearing rather than allow loading of all the weight directly on to the end of the Syme heel pad. The windowed plastic shell permits the bulbous end of the residual limb to pass through the window into the end of the socket. The window is closed and held in place, providing a means of self-suspension. The alternate suspension design provides an inner distensible lining through which the residual limb is placed. The lining closes over the bulbous end, and the prosthesis is self-suspended. Although fewer prosthetic feet are available for this level of amputation, some do provide dynamically responsive features.

Transtibial Amputation

The traditional design developed for this amputation level became popular in the 1950s and has proved to be very durable. This design, the patellar-tendon-bearing (PTB) prosthesis, places weight-bearing pressures in pressure-tolerant areas while relieving pressure in pressure-intolerant areas.[14] In the past, this prosthesis was held in place with a supracondylar cuff and had a solid-ankle-cushion-heel (SACH) foot attached. This remains a durable option, but newer systems have been designed. Most frequently, an inner lining of cushioning material is placed on the residual limb and then inserted into the plastic laminate socket. Today, an increasingly more popular way of suspending the socket makes use of an elasticized sleeve that fits around the outside of the prosthesis and is unrolled up onto the knee and thigh (Fig. 151–7). This sleeve does not appear to have any adverse effect on circulation to the skin or distal

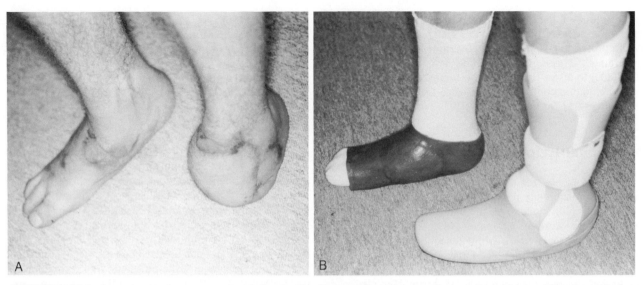

FIGURE 151–6. *A*, Left Lisfranc amputation. *B*, Bivalved hindfoot prosthesis that extends above the ankle to stabilize the residual hindfoot in the prosthesis while wearing a shoe.

leg. Another popular new system is referred to as the "triple S" (silicone suction suspension) system; it uses a silicone sleeve placed against the below-knee skin and then unrolled over the knee and locked inside the prosthesis (Fig. 151–8). This is a self-suspending design that works much like the Chinese finger trap.[15]

There are many prosthetic foot and ankle design options. Michael[16] and Esquenazi and Torres[17] have nicely categorized them in a systematic way (Table 151–2). The dynamically responsive designs include the Seattle Lightfoot, the Flex-Foot, the Carbon Copy Foot, and several others (Fig. 151–9). These designs presumably restore more

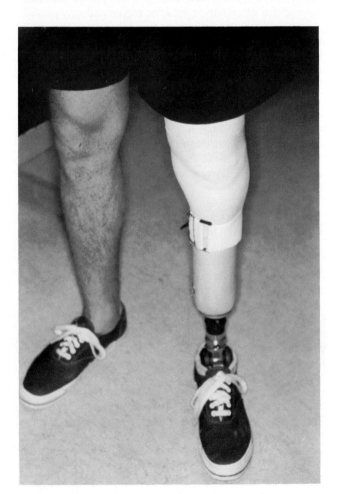

FIGURE 151–7. Transtibial below-knee (BK) amputee with patellar-tendon-bearing (PTB) prosthesis utilizing elastic sleeve suspension.

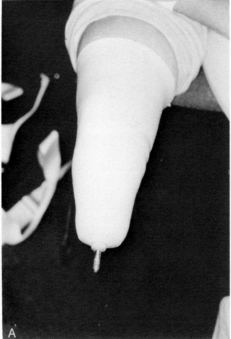
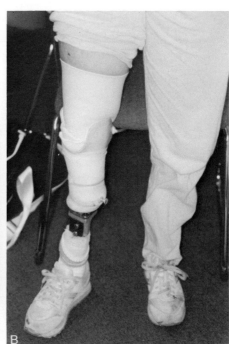

FIGURE 151–8. *A*, Triple S (Silicone Suction Socket, ICEROSS) suspension system for a PTB prosthesis. Silicone sleeve is placed against the skin of the residual limb, and distal pin locks into the inside of the prosthetic socket. *B*, Prosthetic socket locked in place over the silicone sleeve.

normal foot and ankle dynamics and permit a greater amount of physical activity. Some of these designs also significantly decrease the weight of the total prosthesis and therefore change the location of the center of mass of the prosthesis. This change may cause less skin friction and decrease stump-socket interface forces, permitting greater tolerance for the below-knee prosthesis.

Socket design has been modified to place windows or cutouts in the pressure-sensitive areas, permitting tissue expansion into these windowed areas. Such a design is seen in the Icelandic–Swedish–New York University (ISNY) socket (Fig. 151–10).[18] In this device, a thermoplastic, vacuum-molded inner socket is formed from polypropylene or polyethylene.

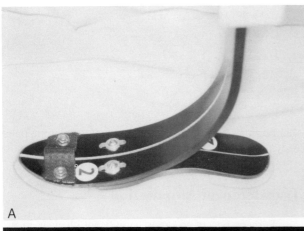
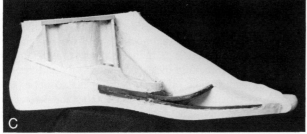
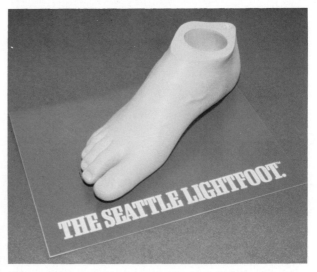

FIGURE 151–9. Dynamically responsive (energy-storing) feet. *A*, Modular III Flex-Foot. (Courtesy of Flex-Foot, Inc., Laguna Hills, CA.) *B*, Seattle Lightfoot. (Courtesy of Model and Instrument Development Corp., Seattle, WA.) *C*, Carbon Copy II. (Courtesy of The Ohio Willow Wood Co., Mt. Sterling, OH.)

Table 151–2.   Recommended Foot-Ankle Systems According to Level of Amputation and Level of Activity

	Weight (gm)	Below-Knee Sedentary	Above-Knee Sedentary	Syme's Sedentary	Bilateral Sedentary	Below-Knee Active	Above-Knee Active	Syme's Active	Bilateral Active
Carbon Copy II	495	2	1	2	1	3	3	2	2
Carbon Copy III	900	2	NA	NA	0	3	NA	NA	3
Dynamic	550	1	1	NA	1	1	2	NA	1
Flex-Foot	900	0	0	NA	1	3	3	NA	2
Flex-Walk	550	1	1	NA	1	3	1	NA	3
Flex Syme's	900	NA	NA	1	NA	NA	NA	3	NA
Graph-Lite	600	1	2	NA	1	2	2	NA	2
Greissinger	850	1	1	NA	1	1	2	NA	1
Endolite with ankle	800	0	0	NA	1	1	2	NA	1
Multiflex	540	3	3	NA	3	2	2	NA	2
Quantum	540	2	2	2	2	1	1	1	1
RAX	425	2	1	NA	2	1	1	NA	1
Sabolich	500	0	0	NA	0	3	3	NA	2
S.A.F.E. I & II	750	1	1	2	1	2	1	3	2
Seattle Lightfoot with ankle	715	1	1	NA	1	2	1	NA	2
Seattle Lightfoot	470	3	3	2*	2	2	1	1*	2
Spring-Lite	900	0	0	NA	0	3	3	NA	2
STEN	685	1	0	NA	0	1	0	NA	1

From Esquenazi A, Torres MM: Prosthetic feet and ankle mechanisms. Phys Med Rehabil Clin North Am 2:299, 1991.
Key:
    0, Not recommended
    1, Good
    2, Very good
    3, Excellent
    NA, Not available
    *To be used without ankle

Knee Disarticulation

This level of amputation has become more popular because it provides a weight-bearing surface for prosthetic use. The minor disadvantage of this amputation level is the wide appearance of the distal end of the thigh socket when a prosthesis is worn. This cosmetic appearance may not be acceptable to persons with slim thighs. The prosthetic prescription for this amputation level may provide a socket window that closes over the femoral condyle protrusions and is therefore self-suspending. Another form of suspension uses suction with an ischium-containing narrow mediolateral socket. A few knee units that can be fitted close to the end of the thigh socket are now available and have improved the cosmetic appearance of the prosthetic knee axis, matching the axis of the remaining limb. The distal shin portion should usually be of endoskeletal components. A dynamically responsive foot completes this prescription.

Transfemoral Amputation

Perhaps one of the most significant changes in prosthetic design in the past few years has been the move away from quadrilateral above-knee sockets to the ischium-containing narrow mediolateral socket.[19, 20] This design, with its variety of fabrication methods, is meant to lock onto the pelvis by encompassing the ischial tuberosity and the inferior pubic ramus. The proximal brim of the socket extends higher on the residual limb and contains the lateral and posterior gluteal muscle masses (Fig. 151–11). This permits better stabilization of the superincumbent body over the

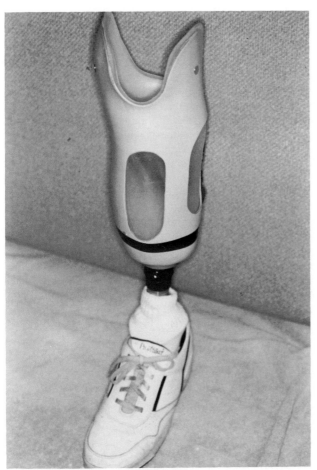

FIGURE 151-10. PTB prosthesis of endoskeletal design showing the cut-out windows in the plastic laminate socket that are present in an Icelandic–Swedish–New York University (ISNY) design.

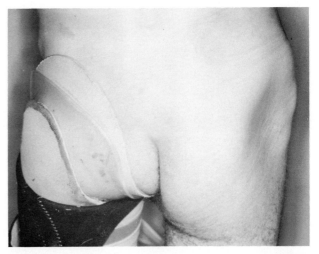

FIGURE 151-11. Posterior aspect of transfemoral amputee with ischial containment socket. The socket includes portions of the gluteus medius and maximus muscles.

in geriatric patients to provide a friction brake for added knee stability in the extended position. Hydraulic knee mechanisms can also be used in prostheses for more active dysvascular patients. A rotator unit that permits rotation of the prosthetic socket on the distal components should also be considered for those who play golf or participate in other outdoor activities requiring rotational movement.

prosthesis. This socket design is also frequently fabricated with an ISNY design utilizing suction suspension (Fig. 151–12). This socket can be applied without the traditional pull sock; instead, a skin lotion or gel is applied to the skin, and the residual limb is slipped into the suction socket with minimal effort. A total elastic suspension (TES) belt, which is flexible and encircles the waist, can be used for supplemental suspension (Fig. 151–13).

The positioning of the femur in the socket has become a point of controversy, but it is generally agreed that the femur should be kept in as normal anatomic adduction as possible.[21] This femoral alignment permits better hip abductor muscle mechanics, which enhance better pelvic stability and more normal gait. Gottschalk[22] has discussed the surgical handling of the adductor muscles when performing a transfemoral amputation (see Chapter 150).

Most geriatric amputees prefer a lighter-weight prosthesis. The weight of the finished prosthesis can be decreased with use of an endoskeletal design. The supporting skeletal structure is fabricated from aluminum, titanium, or carbon-graphite pylons and couplings (Fig. 151–14). In addition, some of the dynamically responsive feet and newer knee units can help to decrease the total prosthetic weight so that currently an above-knee prosthesis should weigh between 6 and 8 pounds. Safety knee units are often used

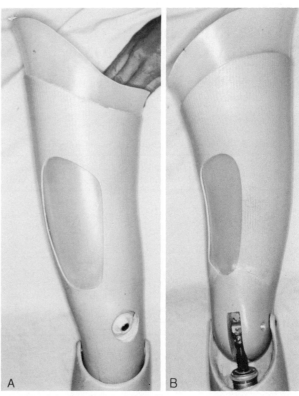

FIGURE 151-12. *A,* Anterior view of transfemoral prosthesis with ISNY socket design and suction suspension. *B,* Posterior view of the same prosthetic socket.

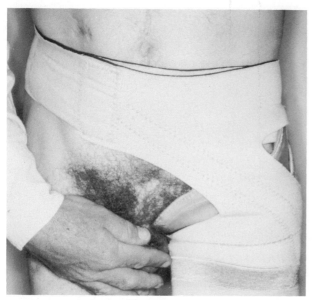

FIGURE 151–13.   Total elastic suspension (TES) system for suspension of a transfemoral prosthesis.

Hip Disarticulation

Geriatric dysvascular amputees can rarely tolerate the energy expenditure required to use this level of prosthesis. Certainly, if a prosthesis is considered, an endoskeletal design is preferred. The lightest components must be employed to minimize the total weight of the final design.

ENERGY EXPENDITURE OF PROSTHETIC AMBULATION

A number of authors have discussed the energy costs of prosthetic use and have compared these costs in younger traumatically injured amputees with those in the older dysvascular amputee population (Table 151–3).[23, 24] From these studies it is apparent that all efforts should be made to salvage the knee joint because it may make the difference between a successful prosthetic ambulator and an amputee who is wheelchair-bound. The below-knee amputee walking with a prosthesis requires 25 to 40 per cent more energy expenditure than normal. In contrast, the above-knee amputee walking with a prosthesis requires 65 to 100 per cent more energy expenditure than normal. Wheelchair use on level surfaces requires an energy expenditure that is 8 per cent greater than normal. It is apparent why some dysvascular amputees with cardiopulmonary disease are not able to sustain the increased energy demands of ambulating with a prosthesis. Instead, they choose to be sedentary and to get around with a wheelchair. A slower speed of ambulation with a prosthesis puts less demand on cardiopulmonary reserves. Nonetheless, even amputees with limited cardiopulmonary function will benefit from prosthetic restoration for transfers and short distance ambulation, especially for toilet and hygiene activities.

Table 151–3.   Energy Expenditure: Unilateral Amputees

Amputees*	Speed (m/min)	O₂ Rate (ml/kg • min)	O₂ Cost (ml/kg • m)	Pulse (beats/min)
Vascular				
TF	36	10.8	0.28	126
TT	45	9.4	0.20	105
AD	54	9.2	0.17	108
Surgical				
TP	40	11.5	0.29	97
HD	47	11.1	0.24	99
Traumatic				
TF	52	10.3	0.20	111
KD	61	13.4	0.23	109
TT	71	12.4	0.16	106

From Waters RL: The energy expenditure of amputee gait. In Bowker JH, Michael JW (eds): Atlas of Limb Prosthetics: Surgical, Prosthetic, & Rehabilitation Principles. 2nd ed. St. Louis, Mosby–Year Book, 1992, p 385; data from Nowroozi F, Salvanelli ML, Gerber LH: Energy expenditure in hip disarticulation and hemipelvectomy amputees. Arch Phys Med Rehabil 64:300–303, 1983; and Waters RL, Perry J, Antonelli D, et al: The energy cost of walking of amputees—influence of level of amputation. J Bone Joint Surg (Am) 58:42–46, 1976.

*TF, transfemoral; TT, transtibial; AD, ankle disarticulation; TP, transpelvic; HD, hip disarticulation; KD, knee disarticulation.

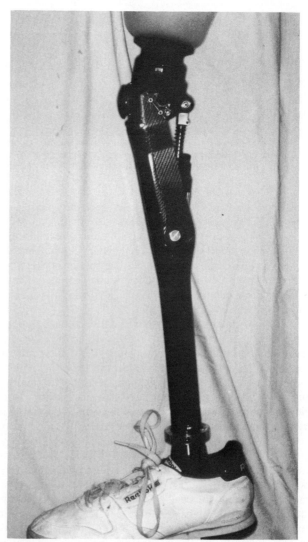

FIGURE 151–14.   Endoskeletal (Endolite) device is made of carbon graphite material to decrease the final weight of the prosthesis.

FUNCTIONAL EXPECTATIONS FOR LOWER LIMB AMPUTEES

Partial Foot Amputation

With a prosthetic toe filler, most amputees should be able to ambulate around the house, including level surfaces and stairs. They can also negotiate uneven terrain, curbs, and ramps. They may have a shortened stride from the affected foot onto the normal foot and will have difficulty with jogging and some sports-related activities.

Syme's Amputation

With good prosthetic restoration, these amputees should be quite functional in most if not all activities in which they would have participated prior to the amputation. They may be able to do even more than they could before the amputation if the dysvascular leg prevented them from actively walking and functioning on two legs.

Transtibial Amputation

With 10 to 18 cm of leg remaining below the medial tibial plateau, adequate soft tissue, and a well-placed scar, these amputees should be very functional in almost any desired activity that is tolerated by their heart, lungs, other leg, and muscles. These amputees should be encouraged to lead a very active and "normal" life.

Knee Disarticulation

The long femoral lever arm permits excellent powering of the prosthesis but does require more energy than amputation at the transtibial level or below. If there is good cardiopulmonary reserve and the other leg is strong, these amputees should be very functional on all surfaces and can enjoy many recreational opportunities.

Transfemoral Amputation

Functional expectations at this level vary with residual limb length and the cardiopulmonary condition of the amputee. With a mid-thigh to long residual femoral lever arm and a well-fitted prosthesis, such amputees should be able to perform all ambulatory activities including negotiation of stairs, ramps, curbs, and uneven terrain. Athletic endeavors of all types may be possible including running, golf, baseball, hunting, and fishing. With a shorter residual limb or significant cardiopulmonary compromise, even level ambulation may be compromised. In these individuals, transfer activities and short distance ambulation may be all that is possible. The use of a walker, crutches, or cane may also be important for safe ambulation. The combination of a prosthesis and a wheelchair may provide the most functional combination for household and community activities.

Hip Disarticulation

Prosthetic restoration for this level is best accomplished in the younger, previously active person who has no significant cardiopulmonary problems. Even the most physically fit person may find the energy expenditure and discomfort of wearing this prosthesis excessive. These amputees find that walking with crutches or using a wheelchair may be preferable to the slow gait achieved with a hip disarticulation prosthesis.

Bilateral Amputations

Various combinations of bilateral leg amputations permit different functional abilities. Loss of portions of both feet shortens the stride length but generally does not limit activities other than running. Bilateral Syme's amputations present minimal functional limitation. Walking with bilateral transtibial prostheses increases the energy expenditure needed to 40 per cent above normal but yields good functional results. However, a combination of transtibial and transfemoral amputations is severely limiting for the elderly amputee (Table 151–4). Bilateral transfemoral amputations

Table 151–4. Bilateral Amputees

Amputees*	Speed (m/min)	O₂ Rate (ml/kg · min)	O₂ Cost (ml/kg · m)	Pulse (beats/min)
Traumatic				
TT/TT†	67	13.6	0.20	112
TF/TF†	54	17.6	0.33	104
Vascular				
AD/AD†	62	12.8	0.21	99
TT/TT†	40	11.6	0.31	113
Stubbies‡	46	9.9	0.22	86

From Waters RL: The energy expenditure of amputee gait. In Bowker JH, Michael JW (eds): Atlas of Limb Prosthetics: Surgical, Prosthetic, & Rehabilitation Principles. 2nd ed. St. Louis, Mosby–Year Book, 1992, p 386.

*TT, transtibial; TF, transfemoral; AD, ankle disarticulation.

†Data from Waters RL, Perry J, Chambers R: Energy expenditure of amputee gait. In Moore WS, Malone JM (eds): Lower Extremity Amputation. Philadelphia, WB Saunders Co, 1989, pp 250–260.

‡Data from Wainapel SF, March H, Steve L: Stubby prostheses: An alternative to conventional prosthetic devices. Arch Phys Med Rehabil 66:264–266, 1985.

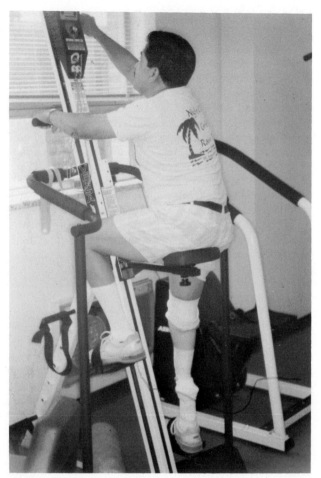

FIGURE 151–15. Versaclimber equipment can be used for cardiopulmonary conditioning for the transtibial or transfemoral amputee.

are catastrophic for successful function. Even a healthy young amputee finds this combination excessively difficult to utilize for walking. For most bilateral transfemoral amputees, the wheelchair becomes the most practical method of achieving mobility.

Activities

Recreational activities should be explored for all individuals who have an amputation.[25] With satisfactory prosthetic restoration, many preamputation leisure activities can be resumed. These activities include swimming, golf, tennis, dancing, hunting, fishing, running, and many others.

Another area of functional concern is the amputee's ability to drive an automobile. Driving should be possible for below-knee and above-knee amputees without major alteration of their cars, although it is always advisable for the vehicles to have automatic transmissions. Driver evaluation and, when indicated, driver training may be necessary. When the remaining foot is the left one, a left-footed accelerator can be useful.

A total body conditioning program should be initiated to enhance cardiopulmonary function and endurance. A variety of exercise equipment can be utilized, but we have found the Versaclimber to be especially adaptable to the lower limb amputee (Fig. 151–15).

GAIT TRAINING WITH A LEG PROSTHESIS

The requirements for fulfilling functional prosthetic expectations include a rigorous preprosthetic training program to prepare the entire body for the increased energy expenditure imposed by use of the prosthesis.[8, 26] These preprosthetic elements include:

1. Strengthening of the upper body and trunk.
2. Strengthening of the remaining lower extremity.
3. Stretching of any lower extremity joint that does not have full range of motion.
4. Specific programs aimed at increasing the strength and endurance of the hip extensors and abductors bilaterally.
5. Increasing the strength of the remaining knee extensors.
6. Cardiovascular conditioning (usually requiring upper arm ergometry).

Once these preprosthetic goals have been achieved, the prosthesis is fabricated, and early prosthetic gait training is initiated. Certain therapeutic guidelines must be followed, including careful attention to the details of gait to decrease energy requirements and provide enhanced function. Gait training should emphasize:

1. Equal stride length.
2. Active hip extension to provide knee stability, especially at heel strike.
3. Encouraging a heel strike to footflat pattern rather than initiating stance with a footflat position.
4. Stance phase training to load the prosthetic toe during pushoff.
5. Discouraging significant lateral trunk bending (Fig. 151–16).
6. Withdrawal of the wheelchair and gait aids at the appropriate time to enhance reliance on and use of the prosthesis.

VOCATIONAL FUNCTION

Loss of a limb does not necessarily signal the end of a productive vocational life. Most below-knee amputees can return to their previous employment. A transfemoral amputee who has a job requiring prolonged standing, walking on uneven surfaces, or climbing ladders may need to consider alternative employment. Such a person may also benefit from vocational rehabilitation if the preamputation job is not feasible.

PREVENTIVE CARE OF THE REMAINING LIMB

Every effort must be made to protect the remaining foot and leg from the need for amputation. Perhaps the

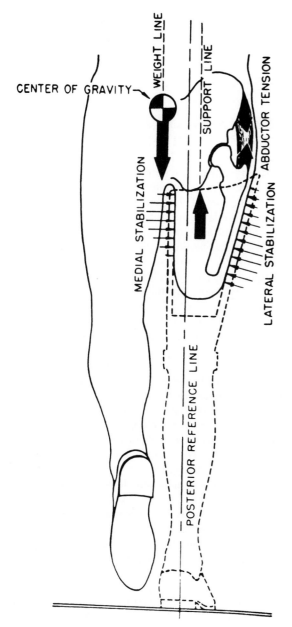

FIGURE 151–16. Use of hip abductors for lateral stabilization of the pelvis can be achieved only by providing adequate lateral support to the femur. (Reprinted with permission from CW Radcliff, Artificial Limbs 2:38, 1955. Courtesy of the National Academy of Sciences, Washington, DC.)

single most important preventive measure is the use of proper footwear. The author normally recommends careful fitting of appropriately sized shoes, which provide even pressure distribution over the plantar aspect of the foot. Shock-absorbing systems should be used through the addition of insoles that conform to the plantar contours. An alternative is the use of sneakers that have an air or gel cushion built into the forefoot and the heel. When significant edema is present, the use of compressive stockings providing 30 to 40 mmHg of pressure is helpful. The patient should be instructed in the proper care of calluses and toenails.

EMOTIONAL ADAPTATION TO LIMB LOSS

The process of emotional adaptation to an amputation is an individual one that follows a variable course.[27] In many persons there is a period of grieving as though a close family member has died. This emotional process can be supported through open discussion of the amputee's feelings of body loss, the presence of pain, anxiety, concern about the loss of control, uncertainty about the future, and frustration with the condition that caused the change in body image. Any team member may lend an ear and support, but it is desirable to have an experienced psychosocial team available to counsel the patient and the family. Ideally, this team includes a psychologist, a social worker, and a pastoral counselor. Emotional adaptation to amputation may proceed at varying rates. This is a time for amputees to be open about their feelings and concerns with their immediate support system and the health team members. Acknowledgment of feelings of loss, anxiety, and depression is often helpful in dealing with this difficult event. The adaptive process and the way in which the emotional needs of the amputee are met are among the most important aspects of amputee rehabilitation.

COMPLICATIONS OF WEARING A PROSTHESIS

Many prosthetic complications are related to the presence of excessive pressure at the stump-socket interface, which produces redness, blistering, and ulceration. Shear forces resulting from pistoning of the residual limb against the wall of the socket cause these skin problems. Common areas of skin trauma occur near the fibular head, the anterior distal tibia (kick point), the proximal medial and lateral tibial flares, and at points of scar that meet normal soft tissue. In addition, hair follicles become plugged and, as they build up bacteria, form a folliculitis.[28] This process may progress to involve the pilosebaceous apparatus, forming an infected sebaceous cyst. The skin of the residual limb may become sensitive to the materials used in the prosthesis or the substances used to clean the socket. Superficial infections usually respond to broad-spectrum antibiotics, whereas an infected sebaceous cyst may need to be incised, drained, and excised. An allergic response should be handled by discontinuing use of the prosthesis and applying topical steroids. The development of painful redness, blisters, or ulcerations requires discontinuation of wearing the prosthesis until the proper adjustments can be made by the prosthetist. On occasion, the addition or removal of stump socks can help to alleviate the excessive pressure. Changes in size and shape of the residual limb also cause frequent fitting problems. These changes require the addition or deletion of stump socks or modifications in the prosthetic socket.

PHANTOM LIMB PAIN

Phantom limb pain, phantom limb sensation, and residual limb pain must be differentiated to be understood by the amputee and to determine the best modalities for treatment. Phantom limb sensation occurs in almost everyone with an acquired amputation and does not usually require treatment. It is usually no more than a minor annoyance and on occasion may be useful during the phase of prosthetic training. It is felt most strongly in the immediate postoperative period and normally decreases in intensity but may continue throughout life. Phantom limb pain begins in the acute postamputation period, generally subsides, and is seldom a long-term problem. However, in a few amputees, this pain becomes problematic and results in a chronic pain syndrome that may be refractory to treatment. Such pain may alter lifestyle and may become the focus of the patient's existence.

Treatment methods are numerous and have produced inconsistent success.[29, 30] During the immediate postoperative period, narcotic medications are necessary. The use of narcotics, synthetic narcotics, or other addictive substances is contraindicated past the immediate postoperative phase. Other modalities commonly used to diminish this pain are (1) transcutaneous electrical nerve stimulation (TENS), (2) percussion, (3) vibration, (4) massage, (5) acupuncture, (6) biofeedback, (7) hypnosis, and (8) relaxation techniques. Regional neurologic blockade has had some success, especially if sympathetic nervous tone appears to be a significant part of the pain. Injection near or into a neuroma is useful. More invasive procedures for pain control include sympathectomy, neuroma excision, dorsal root entry zone rhizotomy, epidural spinal cord stimulation, and sensory thalamic stimulation.

Medications that are currently available to diminish phantom limb pain are (1) analgesics, (2) neuroleptics, (3) anticonvulsants, (4) tricyclic antidepressants, (5) beta-blockers, and (6) sodium channel blockers. These medications should be tried in an orderly fashion and for problematic pain should be used in the maximally tolerated doses. They may also need to be administered in combination for optimal pain relief.

Residual limb pain is defined as pain in the residual limb that does not descend into the phantom. This pain may be related to neuroma formation or be caused by physical changes in the residual limb. A common cause is the pressure caused by an ill-fitting prosthesis. Prosthetic modification often improves this type of pain. If the pain seems to be related to a neuroma, local infiltration with an anesthetic with or without steroids may improve the pain. Local resection of the neuroma or relocation of the terminal end of the nerve deeper into the residual limb may improve the situation.

BONE LENGTHENING AND SOFT TISSUE COVERAGE TECHNIQUES

Very short transtibial and transfemoral residual limbs should now be considered for lengthening techniques using a free bone graft or an Ilizarov procedure. These reconstructive operations can add significant length, providing a longer lever arm to power the prosthesis. Inadequate soft tissue coverage or significant scarring can be removed and replaced with a full-thickness skin graft or a myocutaneous

flap.[31] The provision of scar-free skin and full-thickness subcutaneous tissues can result in much improved prosthetic function and can enhance the outcome. Occasionally, these procedures should be considered before prosthetic fitting is attempted.

UPPER LIMB AMPUTATION AND PROSTHETIC REHABILITATION

The tragedy of arm amputation occurs most frequently in the formative and productive years of a young man's life.[32, 33] The loss of this particular body part often results from a work-related injury and often robs the victim of his dominant hand and arm. Postoperatively, this type of patient should also be fitted with an immediate postoperative rigid dressing to control edema and pain. Within 30 days of the amputation, the individual should be fitted and trained to use a preparatory prosthesis that will help him incorporate the prosthesis as a functional assist to the remaining limb. This golden window of opportunity for successful wear and function of a prosthesis has been studied by Malone and colleagues.[34] It appears that the upper limb amputee becomes "one-handed" after this time and has increasing difficulty in incorporating the prosthesis successfully into his daily activities.

There are three types of prosthetic systems used in the United States to replace the upper limb. The first system is primarily a cosmetic system that is passive in nature and has no moving parts. A few laboratories in this country specialize in this type of design. The materials from which such prostheses are made are fairly life-like but are not particularly durable. They do provide some assistive function but cannot actively grasp and release, nor do they provide any sensory feedback. They are the lightest in weight of all the upper limb prostheses and provide the most acceptable facsimile of the usual body appearance.

The most frequently prescribed upper limb system is a body-powered prosthesis that is controlled through straps, harnesses, and cables that capture residual body movement to actively power the moving parts of the artificial arm. These moving parts are most frequently the terminal device and the elbow for use with the transhumeral or more proximal amputation levels. The body-powered terminal devices used are most commonly voluntary opening hooks or hands, and a few voluntary closing devices are also currently available. The voluntary opening devices are limited in their pinch force by the number of rubber bands or the spring mechanism built into the hand. These terminal devices are opened by pulling on a cable using the force provided by residual scapular abduction and humeral flexion. Voluntary closing devices also operate through a cable control and can generate more closing pinch force but are heavier. The voluntary opening hand is heavier than the voluntary opening hook but does appear more natural. However, because of its bulk, it covers more of the visual sight lines than the hook does. It is thought by proficient body-powered wearers that the harnessing and cable control systems actually provide the user with some sensory feedback, which is useful in sensing where the terminal device is located and how much pinch force has been applied to an object that has been grasped.

The third system is an externally powered prosthesis that is available in two types: myoelectric and switch control. Except in some unusual, patient-specific circumstances, the myoelectric design is most widely applied. Myoelectric prostheses take advantage of human-generated electrical signals normally transmitted to the residual limb muscles from the nervous system. These signals are picked up from the surface of the skin through contact electrodes placed inside the prosthetic socket. They are amplified and fed into motors that drive the movable prosthetic fingers and may also move a rotating wrist unit or an electric elbow. These designs diminish the amount of harnessing and cable strapping necessary to operate the body-powered design. This decrease in strapping often makes the prosthesis more comfortable, but the motors and electrical components add weight. Another advantage of this prosthesis is provided by the electric motors, which supply greater grip force than body-powered methods. A disadvantage of these designs is that they are significantly more expensive than their body-powered counterparts.

Despite the advantages and disadvantages of these design options, less than half of unilateral amputees wear and use an arm prosthesis for most of the day. If the patients are fitted within 30 days of the amputation or if they are rehabilitated in an experienced, comprehensive medical center treating upper limb amputees, these results appear to be improved. Successful upper limb prosthetic use may be related to how the amputee perceives his future and how he interprets the role of the prosthesis in that future.

The emotional well-being of the amputee should always be the primary focus of the amputee rehabilitation team's effort because the amputee's future may or may not include a prosthesis. Even if the arm amputee becomes a successful prosthetic user, will society permit him to return to a productive and fulfilling vocation? Our vocational systems have a poor understanding of the functional abilities of a one-handed person or of someone who uses an artificial arm. There certainly is a societal "Captain Hook" stigma for anyone who wears a terminal device that looks different from a human hand. American society has difficulty in recognizing individuals who have significant contributions to make when they appear different. However, with the advent of the Americans with Disabilities Act,[35] hopefully the public will begin to see the fallacy of these beliefs and behaviors.

For the best prosthetic functional outcomes and the most cost-effective care, upper limb amputees should be treated in a comprehensive rehabilitative center experienced in upper limb amputee care. These centers provide multidisciplinary rehabilitation for many arm amputees each year.

References

1. Burgess EM, Romano RL, Zettl JH: The Management of Lower Extremity Amputations. Bulletin TR 10–6. Washington, DC, US Government Printing Office, 1969.

2. Malone JM, Moore WS, Goldstone J, Malone SJ: Therapeutic and economic impact of a modern amputation program. Ann Surg 189:789, 1979.

3. Wu Y, Krick H: Removable rigid dressing for below-knee amputees. Clin Prosthet Orthot 11:33, 1987.

4. Murdoch G, Jacobs NA, Wilson AB (eds): Papers presented at the ISPO Consensus Conference on Amputation Surgery. University of Strathclyde, Scotland, October 1990.

5. King JC, Titus MD: Prescriptions, referrals, and the rehabilitation team. *In* DeLisa JA (ed): Rehabilitation Medicine: Principles and Practice. Philadelphia, JB Lippincott, 1993.

6. Banerjee SN (ed): Rehabilitation Management of Amputees. Baltimore, Williams & Wilkins, 1982.

7. Anderson MH, Bray JJ, Hennessy CA: Prosthetic Principles—Above-Knee Amputations. Springfield, IL, Charles C Thomas, 1960.

8. Dise-Lewis J: *In* Atkins DJ, Meier RH (eds): Comprehensive Management of the Upper Limb Amputee. New York, Springer-Verlag, 1989, Chapter 15.

9. Gailey RS, McKenzie A: Prosthetic Gait Training Program for Lower Extremity Amputees. University of Miami School of Medicine, Department of Orthopaedics and Rehabilitation, Division of Physical Therapy, 1989.

10. Karacoloff L, Hammersley CS, Schneider FJ: Lower Extremity Amputation: A Guide to Functional Outcomes in Physical Therapy Management. 2nd ed. Gaithersburg, MD, Aspen Publishing, 1992.

11. Mensch G, Ellis P: Physical Therapy Management of Lower Extremity Amputation. Rockville, MD, Aspen Publishing, 1986.

12. Fuhrer MJ (ed): Rehabilitation Outcomes: Analysis & Measurement. Baltimore, Paul Brookes, 1987.

13. Wu KK: Foot Orthoses. Baltimore, Williams & Wilkins, 1990.

14. Radcliffe CW, Foort J: The Patellar-Tendon-Bearing Below-Knee Prosthesis. Biomechanics Laboratory, University of California Berkeley, 1961.

15. Kapp S, Cummings D: Transtibial amputation—Prosthetic management. *In* Bowker JH, Michael JW (eds): Atlas of Limb Prosthetics: Surgical, Prosthetic, & Rehabilitation Principles. 2nd ed. St. Louis, Mosby–Year Book, 1992.

16. Michael J: Energy-storing feet: Clinical comparison. Clin Prosthet Orthot 11:154, 1987.

17. Esquenazi A, Torres MM: Prosthetic feet and ankle mechanisms. Phys Med Rehabil Clin North Am 2:299, 1991.

18. Fishman S, Berger N, Krebs D: The ISNY (Icelanic–Swedish–New York University) flexible above-knee socket. Phys Ther 65:742, 1985.

19. Michael JW: Current concepts in above-knee socket design. Instr Course Lect 39:373, 1990.

20. Staros A, Rubin G: Prescription considerations in modern above-knee prosthetics. Phys Med Rehabil Clin North Am 2:311, 1991.

21. Long I: Normal shape-normal alignment (NSNA) above-knee prosthesis. Clin Prosthet Orthot 9:9, 1985.

22. Gottschalk F: Transfemoral amputation—Surgical procedures. *In* Bowker JH, Michael JW (eds): Atlas of Limb Prosthetics: Surgical, Prosthetic, & Rehabilitation Principles. 2nd ed. St. Louis, Mosby–Year Book, 1992.

23. Gonzalez EG, Corcoran PJ, Reyes RL: Energy expenditure in below-knee amputees: Correlation with stump length. Arch Phys Med Rehabil 55:111, 1974.

24. Waters RL, Perry J, Antonelli D, et al: The energy cost of walking of amputees—Influence of level of amputation. J Bone Joint Surg (Am) 58:42, 1976.

25. Kegel B: Adaptations for sports and recreation. *In* Bowker JH, Michael JW (eds): Atlas of Limb Prosthetics: Surgical, Prosthetic, & Rehabilitation Principles. 2nd ed. St. Louis, Mosby–Year Book, 1992.

26. Slocumb DB: Atlas of Amputations. St. Louis, CV Mosby, 1949.

27. Kohl SJ: The process of psychological adaptation to traumatic limb loss. *In* Krueger DW (ed): Emotional Rehabilitation of Physical Trauma and Disability. New York, SP Medical and Scientific Books, 1984.

28. Levy SW: Skin Problems of the Amputee. St. Louis, Warren H Green, 1983.

29. Sherman R: Stump and phantom limb pain. Neurol Clin 7:249, 1989.

30. Davis R: Phantom sensation, phantom pain and stump pain. Arch Phys Med Rehabil 74:79, 1993.

31. Shenaq SM, Krouskop T, Stal S, Spira M: Salvage of amputation

stumps by secondary reconstruction utilizing microsurgical free-tissue transfer. Plast Reconstr Surg 79:861, 1987.

32. Atkins DJ, Meier RH (eds): Comprehensive Management of the Upper-Limb Amputee. New York, Springer-Verlag, 1989.

33. Leonard JA, Meier RH: Upper and lower extremity prosthetics. *In* DeLisa JA (ed): Rehabilitation Medicine: Principles and Practices. Philadelphia, JB Lippincott, 1993.

34. Malone JM, Fleming LL, Leal JM, et al: Immediate, early and late postsurgical management of the upper extremity amputation. J Rehabil Res Dev 21:33, 1984.

35. Anmuth CJ, Kamen L: Small business concerns regarding compliance with the Americans with Disabilities Act. Arch Phys Med Rehabil 73:978, 1992.

152

Upper Extremity Amputation

Michael J. V. Gordon, M.D., and Lawrence L. Ketch, M.D., F.A.C.S., F.A.A.P.

• • •

Upper extremity amputations comprise 15 to 20 per cent of all amputations. In contrast to lower extremity amputees, those requiring amputations of the upper extremity are younger, with a mean peak age ranging from 20 to 40 years. Psychological, emotional, and financial considerations play an even greater role in upper than in lower extremity amputations. The great majority of upper extremities are lost to trauma (90 per cent), with tumors, congenital anomalies, vascular insufficiency, infections, and iatrogenic causes (e.g., cardiac catheterization mishaps, extravasation of vasopressors) accounting for the remainder. It has been estimated that there currently are 75,000 upper extremity amputees in the United States with 7800 new amputations each year.

GENERAL CONSIDERATIONS

There are three primary issues to be considered when evaluating a patient requiring an upper extremity amputation. First, a thorough evaluation of the injury, tumor, or ischemia is required to determine the best surgical procedure for the patient. Only through extensive experience can one estimate the degree of functional recovery possible at the time of an injury. Nevertheless, such information is important in determining the best surgical procedure for the patient. Second, evaluation of "extrinsic" factors including the patient's age, sex, handedness, general medical condition, other associated injuries, occupation, and hobbies is necessary. These elements help determine the suitability of the patient for initial repair, secondary operations, and extended rehabilitation, and thus guide the surgeon in recommending either replantation, definitive amputation, or alternative complex reconstructive options. Finally, the most difficult assessment involves evaluation of the patient's "intrinsic" factors. These include the patient's own self-image and desires for the final functional and cosmetic result. Consideration must be given to the patient's social and cultural background. In some cultural settings, even a minor cosmetic deformity is more debilitating than *any* functional impairment.

Following this overall evaluation of the patient, a decision must be made about the immediate care. Often this involves a determination about whether replantation is either surgically possible or functionally desirable. If replantation has been eliminated as a possibility, closure of the wound must be considered. The timing of wound closure is critical and depends on several factors. In cases of traumatic injury, the nature of the wound (the contamination of the offending agent) and the amount of time elapsed since the injury dictate whether immediate closure is possible. It is best to adhere to general surgical principles of wound management. Although it is technically possible to close upper extremity traumatic amputation sites immediately most of the time, one cannot be faulted for deciding to perform a delayed closure if conditions warrant.

A much more difficult problem is deciding what type of closure to perform. This decision is dependent on the level of amputation and is discussed in detail in subsequent sections with reference to each amputation level. General considerations in this regard are determined by the principles of the reconstructive ladder. This approach dictates that one begin with the simplest closure and progress to more complex closure patterns as required by lack of simpler methods or by functional (or aesthetic) considerations. In practical terms, one considers direct closure first, and then skin grafting, local flaps, distant flaps, and finally free flap coverage. Before dealing with these issues in detail, attention must be paid to how the different anatomic structures are handled. In general, one usually considers bone, cartilage, tendons, muscles, nerves, vessels, and cutaneous coverage.

Length

Although preservation of length is a fundamental principle of amputation surgery, length does not always determine improved function, depending on what type of prosthetic application is contemplated. In certain cases, it may be wise to sacrifice length in favor of better prosthetic fit. Such decisions are almost never possible in acute situations, and ideally it is desirable to consult with an experienced prosthetist or rehabilitation specialist in these matters.

Bone

Whatever length is ultimately chosen for the amputation, the bony prominences must be optimally contoured. Lack of attention to the bony prominences or irregularities in contour leads to aesthetic abnormalities and difficulties with prosthetic fit. This results from inadequate débridement of traumatized and displaced bony fragments, improper initial contouring of the bone, or failure to identify or address bone-producing periosteum, which must also be contoured. Visual identification of the periosteum is easiest at the time of the initial injury, and achievement of a natural contour of the bone is greatly assisted by palpating the end of the bone through the skin prior to closure. This is even more important in amputations through joints, where natural anatomic flairs of the bone produce aesthetically unnatural contours and interfere with prosthetic fitting.

Vessels

After proper débridement of the bony structures, the vessels are identified and ligated or coagulated depending on their size and location.

Tendons

The hand represents a very delicate balance between extensor and flexor forces. It is extremely difficult to duplicate the balance of these forces through *myodesic* methods (suturing of tendons or muscles to bones) or *myoplastic* techniques (suturing of tendons or muscles to tendons or muscles of the opposite functional group; e.g., suturing an extensor tendon directly to a flexor tendon over a bony amputation site). In general, then, such techniques are not used distally in the fingers and hand because they often *add* to the functional deficit. However, they do have value more proximally, where the balance is not as critical and reeducation and adaptation are not as difficult.

Nerves

Prevention of neuroma is the major and most difficult problem with upper extremity amputation. As in all of medicine, the existence of many methods of treatment usually indicates that none of them is exceptionally good. Such is the case with neuromas. Distal ligation, proximal ligation, coagulation, chemical ablation of the end, simple division, traction and division, nerve repair to other divided nerves, and immediate burial of the transected nerve end have all been attempted with varying degrees of success. The desire to eliminate painful focal sensation must be

balanced against the secondary loss of sensibility induced by many of these techniques. One must accept the fact that a divided nerve always attempts to regenerate and in so doing produces a neuroma of variable clinical significance. Thus, in reality the goal is not to prevent the formation of a neuroma altogether but to prevent the patient from experiencing pain or dysesthesias from the neuroma that will predictably form. In general, locating the divided, free nerve end as far from external stimuli as possible and placing it in a healthy, nonscarred bed of tissue are the best preventive measures. In addition, early postoperative therapy (desensitization or sensory reeducation) is an extremely important determinant of the patient's ability to tolerate the dysesthesias that result from an amputation.

Soft Tissue Coverage

Historically, the issue of soft tissue coverage has been indistinguishable from the issue of length. Previously, if soft tissue coverage was not adequate, one merely shortened the extremity until closure could be achieved. The concept of grafts and flaps has dramatically changed this approach. Skin grafts are applicable when the underlying bed is acceptable; but one must be sensitive to the ultimate functional needs of the amputation site, and in some cases skin grafts may not be durable enough. Local flaps (as discussed later under fingertip amputations) abound, but their applicability, owing to the anatomy at more proximal amputation sites, is limited. Pedicled flaps (regional or distal) have a long, productive history in hand surgery; however, these have been increasingly replaced by free tissue transfers. This change is based on (1) better matching of the tissue transferred (in terms of thickness and ultimate functional performance), (2) lack of need for secondary surgery (whether for division or thinning of the flap), and (3) lack of the joint limitations that result from the immobility that is necessary until the pedicled flap is divided.

SPECIFIC AMPUTATIONS

Fingertip Amputation

Distal digital amputations are extremely common. The most frequent mechanism causing such injuries is a crushing blow such as from a closing door. Although many people arrive in the emergency room with the tips of the finger available for reattachment, this injury is usually too distal for microsurgical reattachment. Many surgeons have attempted composite reattachment (that is, reattachment without specific revascularization) with generally poor results. At present, such composite grafts are not indicated except in younger children (less than 2 years of age), in whom there is an increased chance of graft survival. The reason for failure of these composite grafts is twofold: (1) the amount of tissue that is expected to survive is generally too great, and (2) the zone of injury is greater than the area of amputation (i.e., the tip is usually damaged and thus is not capable of surviving as a composite graft).

Closure of the amputation site is then the problem. If the proximal portion of the distal phalanx is not severely injured so that the insertions of the flexor digitorum profundus and extensor tendons are intact, preservation of that portion of bone is indicated for functional length. If these areas are involved beyond repair, disarticulation through the distal interphalangeal joint is indicated. The overriding issues are the status of the nail and what type of coverage can be provided. Generally, the amputation occurs through a portion of the nailbed. If enough proximal nailbed (approximately 50 per cent) is present to provide a functional nail, the bed should be repaired under optical magnification with absorbable 6–0 or 7–0 sutures.

The distal phalanx is usually rongeured back so that the end of the bone is not exposed. If the final cutaneous defect is then less than 1 cm,[2] simply allowing the wound to close by secondary intention is acceptable. Other wound closures have been attempted, including every conceivable type of local or regional flap. However, given the fact that the flap closures are frequently insensate, the ultimate functional recovery appears to be better after secondary healing because the resulting scar contracture diminishes the size of the sensory defect.

If the cutaneous defect is greater than 1 cm,[2] the amount of time needed for closure and the ultimate functional result no longer warrant healing by secondary intention. If there is no exposed bone, a skin graft is possible. The temptation is to use the amputated part as a donor source for the skin graft. This should be avoided because the amputated portion has been traumatized, and therefore the overall success of these skin grafts is less than might be expected. Nevertheless, one advantage of such grafts is that they may serve as temporary biologic dressings even if they do not survive. Nontraumatized skin graft donor sites that may be considered are (1) the ulnar border of the palm (within the operative field and a good color match), (2) the forearm (the medial portion of the forearm or the elbow crease, although hypertrophic scarring can lead to some cosmetic deformity), and (3) the groin (a well-hidden donor area, although the color match is not good and some unwanted hair may also be transferred).

As previously mentioned, there are many alternative flaps that are variably useful for cutaneous defects of the fingertip. Some of the more common local flaps are the Kutler flap[1] (a lateral V-Y flap for closure of a central tip defect), Atasoy flap[2] (a palmar V-Y flap), palmar flap[3] (based on both digital neurovascular bundles in which the entire soft tissue coverage of the digit above the tendon sheath is elevated and advanced to cover the tip of the finger), and radially or ulnarly based local flaps that preserve the cutaneous innervation on the appropriate digital nerve[4] and use skin grafting of the donor area if necessary. In addition to these local flaps there are also numerous regional flaps that can be used. These include dorsal skin cross-finger flaps, palmar skin cross-finger flaps, and thenar flaps. Although it is sometimes necessary to use these regional pedicled flaps, they carry significant additional morbidity by creating joint stiffness because of the obligatory period of immobility needed for attachment of the flap. Even in fairly young people with good physical therapy, this can cause a long-term problem. In addition, rarely, a patient may require distant pedicled flaps for coverage. Many such flaps have been described: abdominal flaps, infraclavicular flaps, supraclavicular flaps, cross-arm and cross-hand flaps, and others. Again, secondary morbidity resulting from immobility is usually higher than warranted, and other simpler techniques are preferable. Free tissue transfer is almost never indicated for these injuries except in the case of thumb tip amputations (discussed later).

Digital Amputations

Digital amputations are classified by level. Amputations that leave more than half of the proximal phalanx may be functional for the patient. These amputations, then, represent variations of fingertip amputations. First, the bone is rongeured back a short distance to allow soft tissue coverage. Tendons that have been separated from their bony insertions by the amputation are placed on traction, divided, and allowed to retract into the palm. Digital nerves are a potentially more difficult problem. It is preferable to divide them under mild traction and allow them to retract under healthy vascularized tissue. Too much traction may denervate the new tip of the digit. No traction leaves the cut nerve adjacent to the amputation site, allowing postinjury trauma and producing significant pain. The associated soft tissue defect is managed in the same manner as a fingertip amputation.

Amputation proximal to the mid-portion of the proximal phalanx typically is not a functional amputation. If enough digit remains it may be possible for the patient to wear a cosmetic prosthesis that may allow some functional restoration. However, most patients find the remaining digit a nuisance (Fig. 152–1). Each time they reach into their pocket or a purse for a small object, it falls through the opening left in the hand by the remaining short digit, which cannot flex to close the space. As a result, these patients frequently choose to undergo a secondary ray amputation. Regardless of the certainty of this denouement, *ray amputation should not be offered to the patient at the time of the initial wound closure.* Elective deletion of the remaining portion of the digit is a decision each patient should come to by experience. Ray amputation often provides a far more cosmetically acceptable hand; in most cases, the appearance of a three-fingered hand with normal border contours is so natural that it goes unnoticed. Nevertheless, the operation is not without its own set of risks. First, the procedure narrows the palm by approximately 20 to 25 per cent. This reduces the hand's ability to stabilize objects. Second, the operation is a more extensive procedure, producing more proximal postoperative pain, edema, and stiffness than were produced by the injury to the digit. However, in the final analysis, ray amputation is very beneficial functionally and cosmetically, and there are few dissatisfied patients.

Thumb Amputations

Comprising 40 per cent of the function of the hand, the thumb deserves special attention in any amputation involving the hand. Clearly, the major emphasis is on reattachment of the thumb. However, the desire for reattachment has led some surgeons to attempt replantation in circumstances that would otherwise be considered contraindications (e.g., severe avulsion injuries). Although not uni-

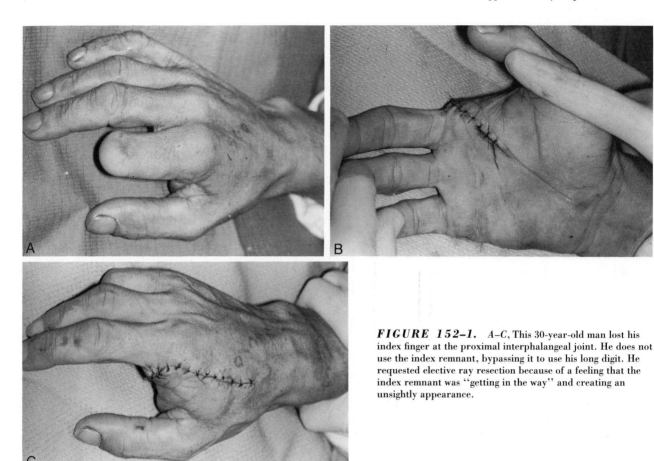

A
B
C

FIGURE 152–1. *A–C,* This 30-year-old man lost his index finger at the proximal interphalangeal joint. He does not use the index remnant, bypassing it to use his long digit. He requested elective ray resection because of a feeling that the index remnant was "getting in the way" and creating an unsightly appearance.

versally accepted, thumb replantation even after avulsion injuries has produced encouraging results.[5] Nonreplantable amputations at the level of the interphalangeal joint are quite functional, and most patients will not request or require additional reconstruction. More proximal thumb amputations may be reconstructed by pollicization, osteoplasty, bone-lengthening techniques, or toe-to-thumb transfer (great toe, second toe, or toe wrap-around). The issues of closure of the amputation site are basically the same as those already discussed with respect to digital amputations except that there must be greater emphasis on retention of length. Local flaps such as the neurovascular island flap from the dorsum of the index finger may be quite useful in these injuries.[6]

Hand-Wrist Amputations

Whatever can be salvaged from a hand amputation should be salvaged. A short palm hand may seem dysfunctional, but as an assist hand it may be preferable to a prosthesis in some individuals. Each patient should be allowed to function with such a partial hand to determine whether she or he would prefer to have a more proximal amputation with subsequent fitting of a standard prosthesis. The advantage of the short palm to the patient is that it retains some valuable wrist flexion-extension (particularly if the remaining portion has good sensibility). If, however, the injured extremity is the dominant one and the patient

wants to rehabilitate the extremity to an independently functional unit, she or he will probably benefit from wrist disarticulation and fitting with a hook prosthesis (Fig. 152–2).

After removal of the proximal carpal row, the radial and ulnar styloid processes are trimmed but not completely resected. This allows secure fitting of the prosthesis and good transmission of pronation and supination capability without causing wear by the bony prominences. The radial,

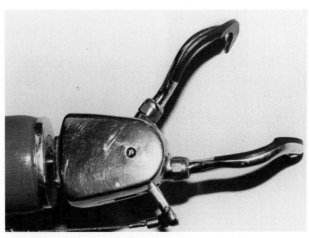

FIGURE 152–2. This is an example of a voluntary-closing terminal device. Internal springs provide opening power.

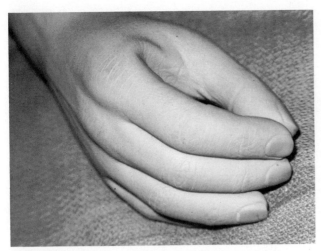

FIGURE 152–3. An Otto Bock myoelectric hand with standard rubber glove.

ulnar, and median nerves can present difficulties. The ulnar and median nerves are frequently avulsed at a more proximal level with these traumatic amputations; if they are apparent in the wound, they can be severed with mild traction. Retraction of the ends usually positions the nerves away from contact with a prosthesis. The sensory branch of the radial nerve, however, is quite superficial throughout its course in the forearm (covered only by the brachioradialis muscle). Neuromas from this nerve are not uncommon, and division of the nerve in the proximal forearm may be considered at the time of the initial amputation.

The wrist is the most distal level of amputation at which tenodesis may be safely considered. Suturing of the flexor and extensor tendons over the amputation stump may provide some extra soft tissue padding at the amputation site as well as maintaining some forearm muscle mass.

A difficult problem that is sometimes encountered is whether the patient is best rehabilitated with a hood prosthesis or a myoelectric hand. The myoelectric prosthesis adds a certain length to the amputation site and is more cosmetically positioned with removal of several additional centimeters of distal forearm (Fig. 152–3). The amputee is usually unable to make such decisions near the time of the initial injury. Proximal revision of these amputations may be done at any time in the future, and no bridges should be burned until the patient has had ample time to evaluate the consequences of her or his decision.

Forearm Amputations

There are two considerations in forearm amputation. First, as much length as possible should be preserved to maintain maximal pronation and supination. The more proximal the amputation, the less moment arm remains for rotation, and if far enough proximal, the muscles that create pronation and supination are lost. This principle is illustrated graphically in Figure 152–4. The other issue in forearm amputation is the patient's ability to wear a prosthesis. Preservation of the elbow joint is critical, and a prosthesis must fit well without interfering with the motion of the joint. With the exception of very short below-elbow amputations, heroic efforts at preserving length are not indicated. Heeding these caveats, the bony tissues can be trimmed adequately to permit soft tissue closure. Flexor and extensor tendons (or muscles more proximally) should be sutured to each other over the ends of the amputation site. Nerves (radial, median, ulnar, and superficial cutaneous nerves) are either transposed to the deeper structures or placed on traction and divided (allowing them to retract to deeper, more protected, and healthier tissue).

Reconstruction of the amputation is generally accomplished by means of a fitted prosthesis. As outlined by

FIGURE 152–4. Residual forearm rotation after amputation.

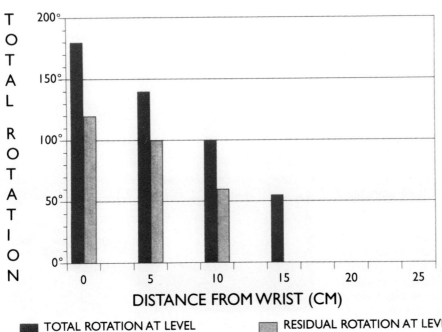

DISTANCE FROM WRIST (CM)

■ TOTAL ROTATION AT LEVEL WITHOUT AMPUTATION

■ RESIDUAL ROTATION AT LEVEL WITH AMPUTATION

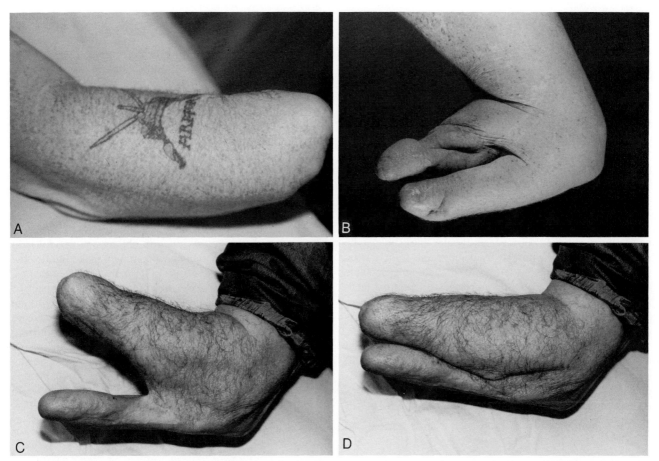

FIGURE 152–5. A–D, In the bilateral blind amputee, use of any standard prosthesis is impossible because of the absence of visual feedback or proprioception in the prosthesis. Under such circumstances, separation of the radius and ulna with Krukenberg's procedure will provide a proprioceptive "feeling" extremity capable of simple grasp-release action.

Tubiana,[7] however, bilateral upper extremity amputations can be functionally improved by using the Krukenberg procedure, in which a sensate pincer is created between the radius and the ulna (Fig. 152–5). Although the cosmetic result is far from desirable, the functional improvement is great, and the procedure should be given serious consideration in those rare instances of bilateral injuries in blind individuals.

Elbow Disarticulation and Upper Arm Amputations

Surgical recommendations for specific amputations are still dependent on the type of prosthetic fitting that can be expected. Although improvements in upper extremity prostheses continue, the rate of improvement and the funds available for research are limited. Many systems that have been proposed are very expensive, and funding through insurance coverage is a substantial financial issue (e.g., the Utah elbow with terminal device can run from $35,000 to $45,000).

Compared with the forearm, which has two bones with a functional noncircular cross section and thin soft tissue

coverage that allows transmission of rotational forces (pronation and supination), the upper arm has a single bone with a relatively circular cross section and less transmission of rotational forces to the skin because of its thicker soft tissue. Thus, there has been considerable emphasis on retention of the full length of the humerus to take advantage of the flare of the condyles as a method of achieving a better prosthetic fit (prevention of rotation of the prosthesis) and preserving some rotational movements of the upper arm. However, in so doing, the upper arm will appear longer than the normal arm in order to accommodate an internal elbow joint. It is possible to fit the patient with an external elbow joint, but these joints are substantially less durable. Another approach to this problem involves the construction of an artificial asymmetry by means of angulation osteotomy. Although this method has gained popularity in Europe, it is not routinely practiced in the United States because of the obvious cosmetic deformity induced in the proximal remaining stump.

Surgical considerations with above-elbow amputations are essentially the same as those in forearm amputations with respect to the treatment of bone, muscles, tendons, nerves, and skin. Wood and Cooney have reported that replantation should be considered even in these high amputations. Although functional recovery of the hand may not be expected, it may be possible to convert an above-elbow amputation to a below-elbow amputation, which is much more functional.[8]

The shorter the remaining stump, the more difficult the prosthetic fit and the less functional the prosthesis will be. As a result, several new techniques have been developed to facilitate this type of reconstruction. The use of free flaps can provide additional soft tissue and bone length for a short upper arm amputation. Functional restoration of the glenohumeral joint may be accomplished using a free fibular transfer. The proximal humerus can be completely replaced with the fibula and its proximal joint with reattachment of the muscular insertions. Particularly in patients with malignant tumors, limbs that would otherwise have to be sacrificed can now be salvaged. Fibular flaps can also be used in conjunction with soft tissue coverage from a latissimus dorsi flap (pedicled or free) to provide an acceptable length of upper arm for fitting a prosthesis. One final technique being explored for short amputations (upper arm or forearm) is that of distraction osteogenesis. Initial reports of this method of treatment have been encouraging.

As indicated previously, every effort should be made to avoid high amputations. Even when the amputation will be a functional shoulder disarticulation (amputation proximal to the insertions of the deltoid and pectoralis major), the maximal proximal length of humerus should be salvaged for either prosthetic fitting or reconstruction.

Shoulder Disarticulation and Forequarter Amputations

These are the most complex and difficult amputations from a prosthetic and functional standpoint. Considerations are (1) loss of potential motor units as drivers of the prosthetic device and (2) difficult of fitting the prosthesis to contour. The shoulder disarticulation (after rounding off the bony prominences that may cause wear) will leave a contour adequate to provide a snug fit for the prosthesis. In addition, scapular function is retained and can be used (with some difficulty) as a motor unit for the prosthetic device. The forequarter amputation (which is done almost exclusively for malignant processes), however, offers little hope for functional restoration of the limb.

The surgical techniques for these amputations are well described in the literature. The anterior approach, described by Berger,[9] and the posterior approach, described by Littlewood,[10] differ only in the exposure of the vascular structures hidden behind the clavicle. Both approaches are well accepted. The same principles described previously apply in terms of removing the bony prominences, treating the nerves and muscles, and providing adequate soft tissue coverage.

Postoperative Management

Aside from routine postoperative care, several other issues deserve mention. Application of postoperative prostheses immediately has been advocated by many. The advantages of this approach are decreased edema and earlier rehabilitation. The poor vascularity and problems in wound healing found inherently in lower extremity amputees are rarely encountered in the upper extremity.

A major issue frequently overlooked in the amputee is the psychological disturbance created first by the amputation itself and then by the subsequent impact on the patient's life. The hand and upper extremity are so intricately involved in daily existence that the complete or partial loss of either demands psychological readjustment in *all* cases. This principle applies as much to children as to adults. In many cases, a young man or woman may make light of the psychological issues and insist that there are no problems. Although as surgeons we welcome quick adjustment to disability and anticipate the patient moving ahead with the rest of his or her life, it is necessary for the amputee to experience a grieving process similar to that encountered with the death of a close relative. In detailing some of the principles learned in the treatment of hand injuries during World War II, Cleveland pointed out that ''. . . the hand is more important than the eye, and is next in importance to the brain itself . . . .''[11] Grunert and colleagues investigated some of the psychological issues involved and reported their treatment results.[12]

References

1. Kutler W: New method for fingertip amputation. JAMA, 133:29, 1947.
2. Atasoy E, Ioakimidis E, Kasdan M, et al: Reconstruction of the amputated fingertip with a triangular volar flap. J Bone Joint Surg, 52(A):921, 1970.
3. Snow JW: The use of a volar flap for repair of fingertip amputations: A preliminary report. Plast Reconstr Surg 40:163, 1967.
4. Venkataswami R, Subramanian N: Oblique triangular flap: A new method of repair for oblique amputations of the finger tip and thumb. Plast Reconstr Surg 66:296, 1980.
5. Bowen CVA, Beveridge J, Milliken RG, et al: Rotating shaft avulsion amputations of the thumb. Hand Surg, 16A:117, 1991.
6. Foucher G, Braun J: A new island flap transfer from the dorsum of the index to the thumb. Plast Reconstr Surg 63:344, 1979.
7. Tubiana R: Krukenberg's operation. Orthop Clin North Am 12:819, 1981.
8. Wood MB, Cooney WP: Above-elbow limb replantation: Functional results. J Hand Surg 11A:682, 1986.
9. Berger P: L'amputation du Membre Supérieur dans la Contiguité du Tronc (Amputation Interscapulo-Thoracic). Paris, G Masson, 1887.
10. Littlewood H: Amputations at the shoulder and at the hip. Br Med J 1:381, 1922.
11. Cleveland M: Hand injuries in the European theater of operations. *In* Surgery in World War II: Hand Surgery. Washington, DC, Office of the Surgeon General, Department of the Army, 1955.
12. Grunert BK, Matloub HS, Sanger JR, et al: Treatment of post-traumatic stress disorder after work-related trauma. J Hand Surg 15A:511, 1990.

153

Revascularization Versus Amputation

T. J. Bunt, M.D., F.A.C.S., and Jerry D. Mohr, M.D.

•   •   •

A thoughtful surgeon will conduct a well thought out operation, and thereby finds himself well thought of.

From *The Epistle According to T.J.*

The selection of revascularization versus amputation for a given patient presenting with advanced ischemia is a decision faced frequently by all vascular surgeons; such decisions are integral to vascular surgery and embody the melding of art and science that is intrinsic to this discipline. The development of ever more sophisticated and innovative distal arterial reconstructive procedures to salvage ischemic extremities raises the question of when to capitulate. Even when it is technically possible to perform revascularization, is the overriding probability of early failure ever so high that a primary amputation is more appropriate? How many *re*operations should be performed for revascularization of the same extremity? In other words, "when is enough, enough" relevant to the limits of revascularization?

Historically, many variables have been considered in choosing between amputation and arterial reconstruction, including patient age and predicted longevity, operative risk (including cardiac dysfunction, pulmonary disease, and renal failure), variables once associated with poor outcome (diabetes, foot sepsis), functional status of the patient and the involved limb, risk of graft failure (previous graft failure, graft sepsis, poor runoff, lack of suitable autogenous vein), and cost-effectiveness. Although we all wish to provide optimal care for every patient, opinions vary about what procedure should be performed in any given patient.

Part of this disparity in approaches can be attributed to the variables and the conflicting data associated with revascularization versus amputation. In fact, the variables themselves are a continuum with different degrees of severity (e.g., cardiac dysfunction, diabetes, renal failure, foot sepsis, or atherosclerosis itself). Although we try to assess the variables independently, the spectrum of disease *within* each variable may not be comparable, giving rise to further conflicting results. This chapter examines the variables or factors that make up the framework for designing a therapeutic plan. The discussion is limited strictly to patients with limb-threatening ischemia.

The answer to the question posed in this chapter is as much philosophic as it is scientific. The complexity of the issue hinges on the absence of objective criteria with which to identify which patients would benefit from revascularization and which would be best served by early amputation

and rehabilitation. Surgeons and institutions are addressing the issue of limb salvage, which has become an increasingly large part of the practice of vascular surgery. Their analyses must consider the quality of life and cost-effectiveness as well as the details of graft patency rates, complication rates, rehabilitation rates, and long-term outcomes.

Proponents of revascularization, even to the level of the ankle and foot, base their position on the uncontestable value of limb preservation, pointing out that limb salvage rates are usually 15 to 20 per cent higher than graft patency rates; the percentage of patients who die of other causes but are still ambulatory on a salvaged limb is high; and the mortality rates of revascularization in more aged and medically compromised patients becomes progressively lower. They challenge the concept that a failed revascularization may cause a higher level of amputation and cite low morbidity and mortality rates. They argue that increased familiarity with complex distal bypasses as well as experience with such special clinical situations as peripheral graft infection, contralateral amputation, end-stage renal disease, and so on favor revascularization over primary amputation.

Those favoring primary amputation base their arguments on the shortened patient hospitalization and lower *overall* morbidity. They call attention to the increased morbidity and mortality associated with amputations done after failed revascularizations with eventual levels of amputation higher than expected in 20 to 40 per cent of patients. Proponents of primary amputation have been able to demonstrate a decreased (or even equivalent) initial operative mortality, particularly in the elderly or medically compromised patients usually selected for this procedure. Finally, they cite exceptional series of amputations that demonstrate high rates of postoperative prosthesis use or ambulation, and they suggest that early rehabilitation is a frequently obtained goal with primary amputation. (In fact, many such studies have emanated from highly specialized units, and the results are not necessarily applicable to health care in the community.)

The natural history of the limb-salvage patient must be taken into account when deciding on revascularization or amputation. Consideration must be given to the facts that limb salvage is decreased with increasingly distal or repeated revascularizations, and expected survival is decreased in such patients, particularly in diabetic or elderly amputees in nursing homes. Thus, the decision for limb salvage or ablation is made within the confines of often limited survival and may be most appropriately directed at *palliation of the quality of remaining life.*

The reality of this controversy is that the issue is really not a matter of opposing alternatives but rather a continuum of possible choices. No treatise on this subject can provide a definitive answer because there is none, or at least there is no single answer to all the questions. As is so often the case in vascular surgery, the surgeon is faced with a judgment that must be made individually according to the patient and the clinical situation. The purpose of this chapter is to present the data that the surgeon may employ to present the options, alternatives, and relative risks intelligently to the patient, who must then ultimately make the choice.

Table 153–1 details the basic considerations that must go into formulation of an algorithm for primary amputation. One must consider the *changing* clinical situation. In the past, valid indications for amputation, which no longer have the same predictive value, would have included absence of the pedal arch, the presence of diabetes, distal infection, graft infection, and so on. The most important factors for selecting primary amputation are psychosocial (nonambulatory status, nontransfer, significant cognitive disorders) and an expected survival of less than 1 year. In nearly every other situation, the decision can be reasonably based on comparison of relative risk and cost. The bias of the author, and that of most other vascular surgeons, is that the basic mission of vascular surgery is to salvage tissues, whether cerebral, visceral, or of the lower extremity. The decision in favor of revascularization or amputation then becomes a matter of comparing the risks to the patient (comparative morbidity and mortality) and, to a lesser extent, the real costs to the system or patient (comparative costs.)[1]

Table 153–1.   Indications for Primary Amputation

Absolute	
Psychosocial situations	Patient is nonambulatory, has no transfer capability, or has limited cognitive capability
	Patient has ipsilateral paralysis or ipsilateral insensate leg
Anatomic considerations	There are no reconstructible vessels
	There is uncontrolled diabetic pedal sepsis despite patent bypass
Relative	
Situational considerations	Patient has expected survival of less than 1 year
	There is life-threatening sepsis or hemorrhage from graft infection
	Only a synthetic conduit is available for a distal bypass site
	The surgeon is not skilled in distal bypass techniques
Anatomic consideration	There is a hindfoot ulcer requiring free flap, and no donor vessel is available

COMPARATIVE MORBIDITY AND MORTALITY

Although it might seem straightforward to compare the operative mortality and morbidity of revascularization with those of amputation and to utilize these data to decide who would best benefit from either procedure, such a comparison is severely handicapped by the limitations of the studies available. Conclusions deduced from four major recent series are listed in Table 153–2.

Gregg in 1985 reviewed a community experience of 18 surgeons at several hospitals over four years; 275 patients underwent 289 procedures, including 62 aortic reconstructions (AR), 69 extra-anatomic bypasses (EAB), and 158 infrainguinal bypasses.[2] The *overall* mortality was 15

Table 153–2.   Comparative Morbidity and Mortality for Revascularization Versus Amputation

Author (Year)	Procedure	No. Patients	Mortality (%)	Long-Term Survival
Hobson (1985)[3]	Revascularization	375	3	58% at 5 years
	Amputation	172	13	57% at 5 years
			(*p* < .01)	
Ouriel (1988)[4]	Revascularization	204	2.9	
	Amputation	158	7.6	
			(*p* < .05)	
Bunt (1991)[5]	Age < 70			
	Revascularization	183	2.2	
	Amputation	212	1.5	
			(NSS)	
	Age > 70			
	Revascularization	119	8.0	84 per cent at 1 year
	Amputation	253	1.5	50 per cent at 1 year
			(*p* < .01)	
Schina (1992)[6]	Revascularization	211	2	
	Amputation	122	4	
			(NSS)	

NSS, not significant.

per cent for 101 patients over 70 years versus 3 per cent (6/188) for those under 70 years; with respect to limb operations, the mortality for amputations (16 per cent) and revascularization (17 per cent) was comparable in the over-70 age group. The mortality for 80 primary amputations (17 per cent) was not significantly different from that for 49 amputations done after failed revascularizations (12 per cent). The proportion of above-knee amputations rose from 16 per cent (2/16) for those under age 55 to 50 per cent for those over 55; however, 40 per cent of patients 75 years old or older were ambulatory with a prosthesis.[2]

Gregg estimated the influence of specified risk factors on comparative mortality; for revascularization these were angina, prior infarction, atrial fibrillation, significant hypertension, cardiac decompensation perioperatively, pacemaker, chronic obstructive pulmonary disease, and stroke with residua. Ten of thirty-two (18 per cent) high-risk patients died, and 18 per cent (6/32) required subsequent amputation; only seven were ambulatory 1 year later. In contrast, 110 low-risk patients sustained a 4 per cent (4/110) mortality, and 13 per cent (14/110) eventually required amputation. A 100 per cent mortality was noted if four risk factors were present.[2]

In 1985 Hobson and colleagues reviewed a 5-year period during which the institutional policy was one of preferential revascularization.[3] Three hundred and seventy-five patients underwent revascularization, 64 per cent femoropopliteal and 37 per cent femorotibial; there was a 3 per cent operative mortality and a 58 per cent long-term survival. One hundred and seventy-two patients underwent primary below-knee amputation with 13 per cent mortality and 57 per cent long-term survival; 64 per cent of patients were successfully rehabilitated and 23 per cent of these procedures were revised to above-knee amputations. The requirement for a higher level amputation revision was 19 per cent in those with primary revascularization and 23 per cent in those with failure of prior revascularization.[3]

Hobson and colleagues' series presents acceptable mortality and patency rates for revascularization while contrasting a higher mortality rate for amputation but does not state the indications for primary amputation and includes 92 secondary amputations in that series. In addition, the mortality for the amputation series is excessive; reasons for this are not delineated.[3]

In 1988 Ouriel and colleagues analyzed 362 patients over a 25-year interval at an institution that favored primary amputation for patients with substantial medical compromise.[4] Two hundred and four patients underwent revascularization (56 per cent femoropopliteal, 44 per cent femorodistal) for distinct limb salvage indications; 158 underwent primary below-knee amputation for equivalent limb salvage indications, specifically excluding secondary failures, trauma, infection, and nonreconstructable limbs, so that the populations receiving the two approaches were fairly equivalent.[4]

Patient risk was assessed by both Dripps anesthesia and Goldman cardiopulmonary risk protocols, and the patients were divided into low-risk (A), moderate-risk (B), and high-risk (C) categories. Ouriel and colleagues found significantly lower mortality rates, shorter hospital stays, and higher rates of ambulation for the revascularization group. Mortality for revascularization was 2.9 per cent versus 7.6 per cent for primary amputation ($p < .05$), with nearly all deaths occurring in class C patients. Hospital stays for revascularization patients were 10 ± 1.1 days for class A and 14 ± 2.1 days for class C patients, respectively, significantly less than the 19 ± 2.1 and 31 ± 3 days for similar categories of patients in the amputation cohort ($p < .05$). Eighty-seven per cent (177/204) of revascularization patients attained ambulatory status versus 63 per cent (100/158) of amputees ($p < .01$). These authors concluded that their conservative approach, in which amputation was offered preferentially to patients deemed medically compromised by a poor Dripps or Goldman class, was not supported by the data because revascularization was performed with lower mortality than amputation, particularly in class C patients. One can, however, criticize both the Dripps and Goldman classifications as being insensitive to real perioperative risk (see Chapter 22); furthermore, the amputation group had significantly more class C ($p < .01$) and fewer class A ($p < .05$) patients.[4]

In 1991 the authors' group looked at the effect of an aggressive policy of limb salvage in most patients, with amputation reserved for psychosocial considerations or *operatively determined* inability to perform revascularization. The amputation cohort was divided into operations performed urgently for pedal sepsis and those done electively (which more closely approximated the clinical profile of the revascularization group). The independent effect of age on mortality and morbidity was also analyzed.[5]

Three hundred and two primary revascularizations and 465 primary amputations were performed, 62 per cent of these in patients over age 70. Mortality for revascularization and amputation in the under-70 group was equivalent—2.2 per cent versus 1.5 per cent, respectively; in the over-70 group mortality for revascularization (8 per cent) was significantly higher ($p < .01$) than that for *elective* amputation (1.5 per cent). However, the overall mortality of urgent amputations was 22 per cent, ranging from 66 per cent (12/18) for emergency definitive amputation to 25 per cent (3/12) for guillotine amputation to 8 per cent (6/69) for "medical" amputation ($p < .01$). The 1-year survival for the over-70-year-old cohort was 84 per cent for revascularization and 50 per cent for amputation.[5]

Schina and coworkers in 1992 presented a review of 266 patients treated over a 7-year period; 211 patients underwent 295 infrainguinal limb salvage operations, and 122 patients underwent 23 transmetatarsal, 70 below-knee, and 29 above-knee amputations.[6] Amputations were performed for nonreconstructible situations, including 39 patients with failed revascularizations. Mortality for revascularization was 2 per cent (6/295), and for amputation it was 4 per cent (6/122—not significant). They further looked at comprehensive morbidity, defined as *all* perioperative complications, and found that this was 48 per cent for primary revascularization procedures, 35 per cent for secondary revascularization ($p < .05$), and 37 per cent for amputation ($p < .05$). The most common complications were cardiac-, wound-, or graft-related, and there was a significantly greater ($p < .05$) incidence of cardiac complications after primary revascularization.[6]

First, the four series described in this section examine the comparative morbidity and mortality of revascularization and amputation from different viewpoints, using different indications for amputation; in particular, there is a wide variation in the clinical indications for amputation. Most series include but do not specifically identify patients presenting with *acute* foot sepsis requiring *urgent* amputation—a situation clearly recognized as carrying a higher operative mortality. This essentially precludes any meaningful comparison of mortality rates because elective revascularization is being compared with *both* elective and emergency amputation. Mortality rates for the truly comparative situation of emergency lower extremity revascularization (thromboembolectomy, for example) carry just as high a mortality as emergency amputation!

Second, the factor of age is poorly controlled in most studies. The authors' series specifically addressed this problem and noted the effect of increasing age on mortality for both revascularization and amputation; such data are consistent with large community studies, although they are also disputed by smaller single institution studies. Thus, Plecha's Cleveland Metropolitan Registry data demonstrated the linear effect of increasing age on operative mortality in vascular surgery, noting that mortality for distal revascularization increased from 2.2 per cent for patients 75 years old or less (55/2377) to 6.7 per cent for patients 75 or older (38/571) ($p < .01$), and for amputation it increased from 9.8 per cent (77/783) to 14.7 per cent (62/421) ($p < .01$), respectively. Gregg presented similar data from a community experience, describing an operative mortality in the 275-patient study of 3.5 per cent for those under 70 years to 15 per cent for those over 70.[2] Conversely, Scher and colleagues presented a single-institution study of 168 patients over 80 years old who had limb salvage procedures with a 6 per cent overall mortality.[8] Friedman and associates reported a series of 50 patients over 80 years old with 3.1 per cent mortality,[9] and Edwards and coworkers analyzed 65 patients over 80 years old who underwent infrainguinal operations with a 3.5 per cent mortality. The smaller series notwithstanding, it seems reasonable to expect greater difficulty in treating elderly patients; therefore, if the amputation series is heavily weighted with elderly nursing home patients who were never psychosocial candidates for revascularization, the mortality comparisons may be invalid.[7–10]

Third, data on "medical" amputations clearly show that it is precisely the combination of the elderly patient with sepsis or urgent indications that predisposes a series to excessive mortality when such individuals are subjected to emergency amputation. The authors reported 106 patients undergoing physiologic ("medical") amputation with a 5.1 per cent mortality; use of this modality for all urgent situations involving medically compromised or elderly patients was an integral factor in the authors' overall 2.7 per cent mortality for 262 above-knee and 0.5 per cent mortality for 213 below-knee amputations. The rationale for physiologic amputation is that it defers the anesthesia or operative risk to an elective time frame while allowing immediate control of sepsis and time for metabolic and hemodynamic stabilization.[11–12]

The authors' comparison of revascularization versus amputation isolated the effects of *both* age and urgent indications; the comparative mortality for nonurgent revascularization and amputation was the same (2.2 per cent vs. 1.5 per cent) for patients less than 70 years of age, and was higher for revascularization than for amputation in the over-70 years age group (8 per cent vs. 1.5 per cent) owing to the increased cardiac morbidity encountered with that group.[5]

The authors draw the following conclusions from these studies:

1. Comparative morbidity and mortality of revascularization and primary amputation are roughly equivalent for *elective* operations.

2. Morbidity and mortality increase for *both* operations with increasing age and for more urgent operations.

3. Amputation in the elderly is best performed *early*, before tissue loss leads to frank sepsis.

4. If amputation is required for urgent indications in the elderly, physiologic ("medical") amputation is preferable to definitive procedures.

COST-BENEFIT RATIO COMPARISON

The increasing importance of economic costs in health care planning must be recognized, but it should also be realized that the choice of procedures cannot ethically be based on economic factors alone. For the question of revascularization versus amputation, economic comparisons are not obliging because the two procedures carry equivalent costs (Table 153–3).

Initially, information was provided by Gupta and colleagues in a 1982 analysis of their institutional policy of aggressive limb salvage evaluated over 3 years in 313 patients.[13] Two hundred and eighty-nine patients underwent either femoropopliteal (166) or femorodistal (123) reconstruction, whereas 24 underwent primary amputation based on inability to achieve revascularization, advanced gangrene, or psychosocial reasons. The patient groups were comparable except for a higher incidence of foot necrosis in the amputation group (88 per cent vs. 72 per cent); analyzed costs included all hospital, physician, and rehabilitation charges. The cost of revascularization averaged $26,194 ± 876 and required an average of 50 ± 2.3 days of hospitalization, and the cost of amputation averaged $27,225 ± 2896 with an average hospitalization of 60 ± 4.3 days. Amputations following unsuccessful revascularization cost considerably more at $42,107 ± 486 with an average hospital stay of 78 days.[13] Unfortunately, these widely quoted data appeared only in abstract form; a complete manuscript was not published.

Mackey and colleagues in 1986 analyzed the *extended* costs of revascularization versus amputation, looking at the long-term secondary complications as well as the initial hospital costs. Seventy-eight patients underwent revascularizations, and 28 had primary amputations; there was a mean patient age of 62 versus 66.6 years, respectively. Costs were limited to direct hospital and rehabilitation charges but did not include physician fees. The cost for revascularizations was $40,769 ± 3726 with an average of 2.4 ± 0.2 hospitalizations and an average total hospital stay of 67 ± 6 days. Amputation costs averaged $40,563 ± 4729 with 2.2 ± 0.3 hospitalizations and 85 ± 10 days total hospital stay. A successful initial revascularization procedure cost

Table 153–3. Comparative Costs of Revascularization Versus Amputation

Author (Year)	No. Patients	Surgery	Costs	Hospital Stay (Days)
Gupta (1982)[13]	289	Revascularization	$26,194 ± 876	50 ± 2.3
	24	Amputation	$27,225 ± 2896	60 ± 4.3
		Failure to amputate	$42,107 ± 486	78
Mackey (1986)[14]	78	Revascularization	$40,769 ± 3726	67 ± 6
		Average	$28,374	
		Simple	$56,809	
		Complex		
	28	Amputation (average)	$40,563 ± 4729	85 ± 10
Raviola (1989)[15]	94	Revascularization		
		Simple	$20,300	15.4
		Complex	$42,200	
	53	Amputation		
		Simple	$20,400	18.4
		Complex	$40,600	
Cheshire (1992)[16]	130	Revascularization		
		Simple		
		Complex (PTFE)		
		Complex (autologous)		
		Amputation		

$28,374, whereas a failed revascularization led to costs of $56,809. On analysis of the indications for limb salvage, it was evident that patients presenting with tissue loss cost more than those with rest pain alone; an amputation done for tissue loss cost more, but one done for rest pain cost less than revascularization for the same indication.[14] Because most surgeons charge more for revascularization than for amputation, it is reasonable to assume that inclusion of these costs would add to the costs of revascularization.

In 1988 Raviola and associates reported the costs of 147 patients undergoing procedures from 1975 to 1979 (presumably during her much earlier tenure at UCLA).[15] Hospital costs and professional fees were included; rehabilitation costs were averaged at $6400 per patient because all services were performed on an outpatient basis. The average cost for 53 primary below-knee amputations was $20,400 (18.4 hospital days), which increased to $40,600 if there were complications; the average cost for 94 femoropopliteal grafts was $20,300 (15.4 hospital days), which increased to $28,700 if the grafts were successfully revised and to $42,200 if failure led to amputation.[15]

In 1992 Cheshire and colleagues looked at total primary and secondary expenses for revascularization versus amputation and specifically analyzed the variable of more extended (i.e., femorodistal) bypass in cost analysis.[16] One hundred and thirty patients who presented with limb salvage indications over a 5-year period underwent femorodistal reconstruction (41 with a polytetrafluoroethylene [PTFE] graft and 89 with autologous grafts), and their costs were compared with the cost of primary amputation at the same tertiary care institution. Operative mortality was less than 1 per cent for revascularization procedures but was 10 per cent for amputations; survival was 80 per cent at a mean follow-up of 20 months for both groups. The mean cost of a revascularization procedure was $6898 for both PTFE and autologous grafts, which increased by an additional $7074 per operation for revisional surgery; however, the probability of a revision being necessary was 0.375 for

autologous grafts but 0.61 for PTFE grafts, leading to total costs of $15,024 for autologous and $20,416 for PTFE grafts. The cost of an amputation was $21,726. (Of note, these figures seem quite low for 1992 dollars.) The authors summarized their data with the statement that revascularization was 44 per cent less expensive than amputation for autologous and 6 per cent less expensive for synthetic grafts; furthermore, only one third of amputees achieved ambulatory status, as opposed to 80 per cent of revascularization patients.[16]

Analysis of these series leads us to the following conclusions:

1. An amputation done without furnishing a subsequent prosthesis is less costly than one that involves rehabilitation costs; this might be a factor in decisions made for a more elderly patient whose rehabilitation prospects are small.

2. Amputation done for relief of rest pain is less costly than that done for tissue loss; this echoes the mortality findings and should be used to justify decisions to perform amputation earlier in the course of events rather than waiting for a more acute clinical situation to develop.

3. Complications of *either* revascularization or amputation operations markedly increase the costs.

Put more succinctly—the surgeon's judgment and skill greatly influence the comparative costs. For early limb salvage situations, a well-done revascularization procedure costs the least; untimely delay leading to frank tissue loss ensures that any procedure costs more. This fact indicates that the decision to perform one or the other should be made early and not late in the course of the illness.

RISK OF HIGHER AMPUTATION

Proponents of primary amputation suggest that failure of a primary revascularization can lead to a higher than expected level of eventual amputation and perhaps an increased overall morbidity from the combined procedures. Proponents of primary revascularization point out that both the rate and level of amputation would be higher without arterial reconstructions, and that revascularization resulting in limb salvage is worth the effort. Both groups admit that there are situations in which poorly planned or poorly executed operations of either type can result in amputations of a higher level than expected.

There is an abundance of studies supporting one view or the other; however, it is difficult to assess the merits of each position because of the number of uncontrolled variables. As discussed earlier, primary amputation in some reports was performed for both urgent and elective indications, and age was not factored into the analyses; equivalent degrees of peripheral vascular disease were not present in both groups and higher-risk patients were often over-represented in the amputee group.

Stoney summarized his primary amputation philosophy succinctly in 1979, noting that in four series of revascularizations half of all failures led to higher level amputations.[17] He suggested that the surgeon recognize his or her obligation to provide the operation most likely to benefit the patient, *not* the surgeon. Dardik and colleagues in 1982 suggested that femoropopliteal grafts failed more often than femorotibial grafts and resulted in an unanticipated higher amputation level.[18] Other authors, however, have reported little difference in the healing rates of below-knee amputations between those done as primary amputations and those done after failure of primary revascularization, with 75 to 85 per cent healing rates in both cohorts.[17–22]

In 1981 Kazmers and coworkers examined the outcome of 40 limbs amputated after failed bypass and compared the eventual level of amputation obtained with that predicted by Doppler pressure measurements performed prior to bypass. An arbitrarily determined value of 60 mmHg Doppler popliteal arterial pressure was used as a control, basing this on an observed 87 per cent rate of healing of below-knee amputation (BKA) stumps in a published series. Thirty-three limbs after failed bypasses had had a pregnative pressure of 60 mmHg or more; the healing rate of BKA stumps with this pressure was 52 per cent. Four of seven patients with pregnative pressure of 60 mmHg or less also healed. The authors suggested that this observed decrease in healing rate (87 per cent [theoretical] to 52 per cent) was related to the failed bypass. However, the study group included seven patients who had had tibial explorations *without* revascularizations, and seven patients who underwent above-knee (AKA) procedures without attempt at BKA based on ''clinical judgment.'' Only 14 patients underwent determination of the popliteal artery pressure after bypass failure and before amputation, and in these, only six had a *decreased* pressure of more than 20 mmHg.[23]

Evans and colleagues in 1990 updated the same institutional data, looking at 210 amputations following failed revascularization procedures and comparing these with 551 primary amputations.[24] Three hundred and nineteen primary amputations were performed with a 6.6 per cent (21/39) mortality and a 92 per cent (274/298) healing rate; 92 per cent (108/118) of patients with a popliteal pressure of 60 mmHg or more healed, and 56 per cent (8/14) of those with

pressures of less than 60 mmHg also healed. One hundred and forty-seven BKAs following failed bypass had only a 3 per cent (4/147) mortality but also had only a 77 per cent rate of primary healing ($p < .01$); of these 147 patients, 61 per cent (31/51) with pressures of 60 mmHg or more and 64 per cent (39/61) of those with pressures of less than 60 mmHg healed primarily ($p < .05$).[24]

Although at face value a 77 per cent healing rate for BKA is quite acceptable, it pales in comparison with the very high 92 per cent rate reported for primary amputations at the same institution. One has to question whether comparable clinical situations are being compared. Why was such an unusually high rate of BKA healing obtained in the control series? Why were equivalent rates of BKA healing obtained for those with popliteal pressures above or below the threshold value of 60 mmHg? Perhaps the failures were *not* a matter of inadequate vascular supply. It also does not make sense that the mortality rate for amputations following failed revascularizations was very low (3 per cent), half of that usually observed for primary amputations.

In 1986 Sethia and colleagues noted in a review of 193 amputations performed over 3 years that 37 per cent of patients had undergone prior revascularization procedures, and this proportion increased to 58 per cent of patients requiring revision to a higher level. Half of these had undergone revascularization within 2 weeks of amputation ($p < .02$). Although they concluded that injudicious attempts at bypass increased the level of amputation, the procedures performed or their appropriateness were not given and healing problems were almost as frequent (23/150) with AKA as with BKA (29/63).[25]

Other recent papers have added to the confusion over this issue. Bloom and Stevick in 1988 followed 59 patients with femorodistal grafts for a median 24 months and noted that only 3 of 12 subsequent amputations were at the (presumably unexpected) above-knee level.[26] However, Epstein and colleagues in 1989 noted a significantly higher ($p < .05$) proportion of AKA in 32 failed revascularizations compared with 43 primary amputations, and they reported that primary BKA healing occurred in 84.4 per cent of primary amputations but in only 64.3 per cent of secondary amputations.[27]

The findings discussed in the preceding section can be used to support either hypothesis. One should note that the data are flawed by lack of control of variables. It is reasonable to conclude that attempts at revascularization, if successful, will result in prolonged limb salvage but, if unsuccessful, may result in a higher level of amputation, particularly if thrombosis occurs early, if synthetic rather than autologous grafts are used, and if secondary complications supervene.

SPECIAL CLINICAL SITUATIONS

Technical Considerations

Calcific Vessels

Diabetics commonly demonstrate medial calcinosis; in some, rigid pipe-like casts of the trifurcation vessels form and are visible on plain roentgenograms. The success of tibial or distal revascularization is highly dependent on technical perfection in performing the distal anastomosis, which is complicated by this calcific arterial wall. Arteriotomy is difficult and tends to fragment the wall; suturing is equally difficult, and application of excessive force results in frank arterial lacerations. Consequently, some surgeons consider heavily calcified vessels a contraindication to revascularization. However, the vessels can be bypassed if the surgeon uses perseverance and patience. Use of a special tempered steel needle designed for calcific vessels or application of the fracture-crush technique described in 1986 by Ascer and colleagues may facilitate difficult anastomoses.[28] Ascer and his colleagues presented experience with 36 patients who had heavily calcified tibial vessels that were fractured with hemostats applied circumferentially over a 3- to 4-cm segment, followed by repair of intimal injuries and subsequent vein-graft anastomoses. The patency of grafts to severely calcified vessels at 30 days was 75 per cent and at 3 years it was 47 per cent—not significantly different from patencies reported for anastomoses to less severely calcified vessels.[28]

Poor Outflow

Intuitively, one would think that a long graft into a compromised outflow system would have a high rate of failure. This might apply to isolated popliteal arteries (defined as segments of 7 cm or more in length and with no named branch outflow vessels), to isolated segments of tibial vessels, or to the terminal vessels of the foot such as the tarsal or calcaneal arteries. However, there are reports of reasonable success with bypasses in these situations. Thus, there is little reason to prohibit revascularization based on outflow alone; if there is a vessel, it may be used with reasonable expectations of patency provided that a satisfactory venous conduit exists.[29, 30]

Synthetic Versus Autologous Grafts

It is well recognized that synthetic grafts require a higher flow to maintain patency and are more likely to incite neointimal hyperplasia of the distal anastomosis. Virtually all series note a pronounced decline in patency rate for below-knee procedures and especially for femorodistal synthetic reconstructions compared with autologous grafts.

Should a distal reconstruction be attempted if an autologous conduit is inadequate or unavailable? It should be noted that the lesser saphenous, basilic, and cephalic arm veins and the basilic complex of arm veins may all be used as conduits. Dardik and associates have described an advantage of adding an arteriovenous fistula distally to increase total graft flow, but few others have reproduced their results.[31] Again, the surgeon intent on limb salvage can nearly always find an autologous conduit; if no autologous conduit is truly available, a synthetic conduit with a distal fistula may be constructed. Absence of an autologous vein should seldom represent an indication for primary amputation.

Situational Considerations

Contralateral Amputation

A small number of patients present with a prior contralateral amputation and a new ipsilateral limb salvage situation. The decision to revascularize the second leg should be made using the same clinical and psychosocial indications used for other patients; the ability to ambulate with or without a prosthesis and the ability to transfer on the good leg are important considerations for continued self-care. Powell and colleagues in 1984 specifically addressed the problem, looking at 12 cases from a larger series of 108 distal bypasses. The incidence of diabetes was higher in the study group (42 per cent vs. 31 per cent), but pedal arch visualization was similar (85 per cent vs. 83 per cent). Operative mortality was not significantly higher (8 per cent vs. 3 per cent—not significant), and 25-month survival was 68 per cent versus 82 per cent with graft patencies of 59 per cent versus 38 per cent (not significant). Thus, in this small series, there were no significant differences between those with and those without contralateral amputation.[32]

Large Forefoot or Hindfoot Ulcer

Ulcers larger than 4 cm in size, particularly those involving the calcaneus, in the past have been thought to represent a contraindication to successful revascularization. Some extensive forefoot or hindfoot wounds *do* pose daunting problems of wound healing and reconstruction that cannot be minimized; however, per se they do not represent a convincing deterrent to revascularization. Dedicated local wound care and repeated débridement, even into the tarsal or calcaneal marrow, can be successful. Occasionally, primary closure of the defect may be obtained with free flaps based on the revascularization conduit. In 1990 Greenwald and coworkers reported successful free flap transfer in 10 patients, 8 of whom were revascularized first. Six flaps were based on the pedal vessels. Eight of the 10 patients achieved ambulatory limb salvage.[33]

End-Stage Renal Disease

The presence of end-stage renal disease (ESRD) requiring dialysis, particularly when it occurs in the presence of diabetes, has been uniformly associated with lessened chances of successful limb salvage after revascularization. In 1988 Edwards and colleagues at the University of Oregon analyzed 19 such patients undergoing autologous distal reconstruction and compared them with 226 patients without renal failure who had distal revascularizations. The 18-month patency was similar in the two groups (85 per cent vs. 89 per cent), but limb salvage was significantly worse in the ESRD patients (76 per cent vs. 95 per cent, $p < .005$), with 5 of the 19 undergoing amputation, all of whom had *patent* grafts but persistent foot sepsis.[34]

Based on these data, these authors suggested that primary amputation should be performed in patients presenting with profound limb ischemia and ESRD. An alternative interpretation of these findings is that a salvage rate of 76 per cent at 18 months is quite acceptable and is not significantly different from other reported limb-life salvage rates for medically compromised patients. The reported 20 per cent annual mortality for dialysis patients must also be considered in the decision to attempt limb salvage procedures or perform primary amputation.

In 1990 Harrington and colleagues described 39 patients with ESRD undergoing limb salvage procedures for

59 limbs. Primary patency was 77 per cent at 1 year and 68 per cent at 2 years; operative mortality was 7.7 per cent. Long-term survival was only 39 per cent at 3 years, but 84 per cent of those alive had a salvaged limb.[35] Thus, ESRD confers a dismal prognosis for survival, and a small number of patients are available for late outcome analysis.

Revision Surgery

When do further attempts at limb salvage pose excessive additional risk to the patient or are of such unlikely long-term success that they warrant primary amputation? The answer involves both philosophy and judgment. Suffice it to say that *failing* grafts *can* be successfully revised to result in long-term patencies not dissimilar to those of primary grafts. Revision of a *failed* graft presents the same problems as those of primary grafts, and the surgeon must weigh successful revascularization rates against patient risk. If a suitable distal site for anastomosis and a suitable conduit can be found in a patient with an acceptable medical risk, limb salvage is justifiable; if the remaining sites are marginal or the conduit can only be synthetic, a primary amputation is more reasonable.

Graft Infection

The generally pessimistic attitude toward lower extremity peripheral graft infection prompted Kitka's group in 1987 to suggest that primary amputation was the preferable solution to such infections.[36] However, increasing experience with distal and complicated revascularizations has led to lower mortality and amputation rates associated with infrainguinal graft infections. Flinn in 1992 reported successful extra-anatomic reconstruction of perigeniculate infection in six of eight patients,[37] and Bunt in 1992 also noted uniform success in 33 patients with peripheral graft infections. Ten of these, for psychosocial reasons, underwent graft resection only, with four amputations. However, another 15 patients underwent graft resection and ''extra-anatomic'' distal reconstruction, and an additional 8 underwent successful local therapy of mid-shaft infection; no mortality or major amputation was reported in all 23 patients undergoing reconstruction or graft salvage.[38]

SUMMARY

As is so often the case, the data presented in the literature can be interpreted in different ways. The issue of revascularization versus primary amputation has been isolated as an important individual issue when in reality it is a microcosm of the continuum of vascular disease. None of the variables discussed in this chapter is in itself an absolute factor in resolving this question. Furthermore, multiple variables often coexist and are difficult to separate from each other, explaining some of the conflicting conclusions of different studies.

It is clear that the basic approach should be one of limb salvage, not at all costs, but with reasonable appreciation of the relative risks and benefits of attempts at limb salvage. For the majority of vascular surgeons and patients, limb salvage is a highly desirable goal that can usually be obtained at morbidity-mortality and monetary costs that are equivalent to those of primary amputation.

References

1. Mohr JD, Rutherford RB: The role of primary amputation in critical limb ischemia. Semin Vasc Surg 4:4:227, 1991.
2. Gregg RO: Bypass or amputation? Concomitant review of bypass arterial grafting and major amputations. Am J Surg 149(3):397, 1985.
3. Hobson RW, Lynch TG, Zafor J, et al: Results of revascularization and amputation in severe lower extremity ischemia: A five year experience. J Vasc Surg 2(1):174, 1985.
4. Ouriel K, Fiore WM, Geary JE: Limb threatening ischemia in the medically compromised patient: Amputation or revascularization? Surgery 104(4):667, 1988.
5. Bunt TJ, Malone JM: Revascularization or amputation in the > 70 year old. Am J Surg (In press).
6. Schina MJ, Atnip RG, Healy DA, Thiele BL: The relative risk of limb revascularization and amputation in the modern era. J Vasc Surg (In press).
7. Plecha FR, Bertin VS, Plecha EJ, et al: The early results of vascular surgery in patients 75 years of age and older: Analysis of 3,259 cases. J Vasc Surg 2:769, 1985.
8. Scher LA, Veith FJ, Ascer E, et al: Limb salvage in octogenarians and nonogenarians. Surgery 99(2):160, 1986.
9. Friedman SG, Kerner BA, Friedman MS, Moccio CG: Limb salvage in elderly patients—Is aggressive surgical therapy warranted? J Cardiovasc Surg 30(5):848, 1989.
10. Edwards WH, Mueherin JL Jr, Rogers DM: Vascular reconstruction in the octogenarian. South Med J 75:648, 1982.
11. Bunt TJ: Physiologic amputation for acute pedal sepsis. Am Surg 56(9):520, 1990.
12. Bunt TJ, Manship LR, Bynol RP, Haynes JL: Lower extremity amputation: A low mortality operation. Am Surg 50(11):581, 1984.
13. Gupta SK, Veith FJ, Samson RH, et al: Cost analysis of operations for infrainguinal arteriosclerosis [Abstract]. Circulation 66(Suppl 2):II-9, 1982.
14. Mackey WC, McCullough JL, Conlon TP, et al: The costs of surgery for limb-threatening ischemia. Surgery 99(1):26, 1986.
15. Raviola CA, Nichter LA, Baker JD: Cost of treating advanced leg ischemia: Bypass graft vs. primary amputation. Arch Surg 123(8):495, 1988.
16. Cheshire NJW, Wolfe SHN, Noone MA, et al: The economics of femorocrural reconstruction for critical leg ischemia with and without autologous vein. J Vasc Surg 15(1):170, 1992.
17. Stoney RJ: Ultimate salvage for the patient with limb-threatening ischemia. Am J Surg 136(8):228, 1978.
18. Dardik H, Kahn M, Dardik I, et al: Influence of failed vascular bypass procedures on conversion of below knee to above knee amputation levels. Surgery 91:64, 1982.
19. Samson RH, Gupta SK, Scher LA, Veith FJ: Level of amputation after failure of limb salvage procedures. Surg Gynecol Obstet 154(1):56, 1982.
20. Burgess EM, Marsden FW: Major lower extremity amputations following arterial reconstruction. Arch Surg 108:655, 1976.
21. Schlenker JD, Wolkoff JS: Major amputations after femoropopliteal bypass procedures. Am J Surg 129:495, 1975.
22. Kihn RB, Warren R, Beebe GW: The geriatric amputee. Ann Surg 176:305, 1972.
23. Kazmers M, Satiani B, Evans WE: Amputation level following unsuccessful distal limb salvage operations. Surgery 87(6):683, 1980.
24. Evans WE, Hayes JP, Vermilian BD: Effect of a failed distal reconstruction on the level of amputation. Am J Surg 160(8):217, 1990.
25. Sethia KK, Berry AR, Morrison JD, et al: Changing pattern of lower limb amputation for vascular disease. Br J Surg 73(9):701, 1986.
26. Bloom RJ, Steviek CA: Amputation level and distal bypass salvage of the limb. Surg Gynecol Obstet 166(1):1, 1988.
27. Epstein SB, Worth MH, El Ferzli G: Level of amputation following failed vascular reconstruction for lower limb ischemia. Curr Surg May–June, p 185, 1989.
28. Ascer E, Veith FJ, Flores SAW: Infrapopliteal bypasses to heavily

calcified rock like arteries: Management and results. Am J Surg 152(8):220, 1986.

29. Ascer E, Veith FJ, Gupta SK: Bypass to plantar arteries and other plantar arteries: An extended approach to limb salvage. J Vasc Surg 8(4):434, 1988.

30. Rubin JR, Pitluk HC, Graham LM: Do operative results justify tibial artery reconstruction in the presence of pedal sepsis? Am J Surg 156:144, 1988.

31. Dardik H, Berry SM, Dardik A, et al: Infrapopliteal prosthetic graft patency by use of distal adjunctive arteriovenous fistula. J Vasc Surg 3(5):685, 1991.

32. Powell TW, Burnham SJ, Johnson G Jr: Second leg ischemia: Lower extremity bypass vs. amputation in patients with contralateral lower extremity amputation. Am Surg 50(11):577, 1984.

33. Greenwald LL, Comefota AJ, Mitra A, et al: Free vascularized tissue transfer for limb salvage in peripheral vascular disease. Ann Vasc Surg 4(3):244, 1990.

34. Edwards JM, Taylor LM, Porter JM: Limb salvage in endstage renal disease (ESRD): Comparison of modern results in patients with and without ESRD. Arch Surg 123(9):1164, 1988.

35. Harrington EB, Harrington ME, Schnazer H, et al: Endstage renal disease—is infrainguinal limb revascularization justified? J Vasc Surg 12(6):691, 1990.

36. Kitka MJ, Goodson SF, Bishara RA, et al: Mortality and limb loss with infected infrainguinal bypass grafts. J Vasc Surg 5:566, 1987.

37. Baytes BT, Mesh CL, McGee GS, et al: Lung-threatening ischemia complicated by perigeniculate infection. J Surg Res 54:163, 1993.

38. Bunt TJ: Vascular graft infections: a personal experience. J Cardiovasc Surg 1:489, 1993.

Note: Page numbers in *italics* refer to illustrations; page numbers followed by t refer to tables.

ISBN 0-7216-3838-4

90038

9 780721 638386